THE TRAIL OF THE INVISIBLE LIGHT

Publication Number 579
AMERICAN LECTURE SERIES®

A Monograph in
The BANNERSTONE DIVISION *of*
AMERICAN LECTURE IN ROENTGEN DIAGNOSIS

Edited by

LEWIS E. ETTER, B.S., M.D., F.A.C.R.
Professor of Radiology, Western Psychiatric Institute
and the Falk Clinic
School of Medicine, University of Pittsburgh
Pittsburgh, Pennsylvania

THE TRAIL
OF THE
INVISIBLE LIGHT

From X-Strahlen to Radio(bio)logy

By

E. R. N. GRIGG, M.D.

Attending Radiologist, Cook County Hospital, Chicago
Consulting Radiologist to the Illinois Department of
Public Welfare and to the hospitals in Charleston,
Harvard, Paris, and Paxton (Illinois)

With a Foreword by

BENJAMIN H. ORNDOFF, M.D.

Chairman, Department of Radiology
Loyola University, Chicago

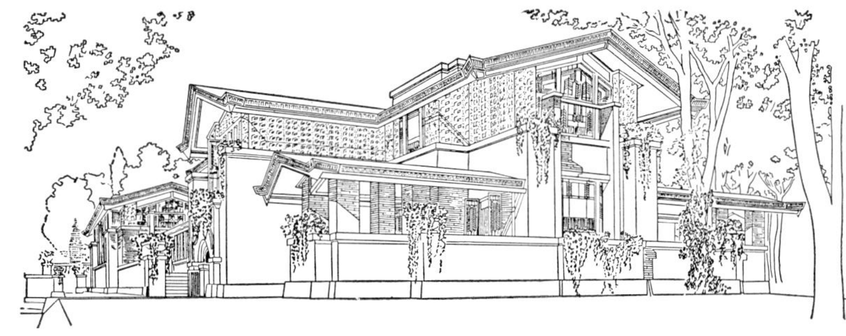

CHARLES C THOMAS • PUBLISHER

Springfield • Illinois • U.S.A.

Published and Distributed Throughout the World by

CHARLES C THOMAS • PUBLISHER

BANNERSTONE HOUSE

301-327 East Lawrence Avenue, Springfield, Illinois, U.S.A.

NATCHEZ PLANTATION HOUSE

735 North Atlantic Boulevard, Fort Lauderdale, Florida, U.S.A.

Library of Congress Catalog Card Number: 64-11653

With THOMAS BOOKS careful attention is given to all details of manufacturing and design. It is the Publisher's desire to present books that are satisfactory as to their physical qualities and artistic possibilities and appropriate for their particular use. THOMAS BOOKS will be true to those laws of quality that assure a good name and good will.

Printed in the United States of America

I-2

Qui va plus tost que la fumée,
Si ce n'est la flamme allumée ?
Plus tost que la flamme ? le vent;
Plus tost que le vent ? c'est ma femme:
Monique !
Quoi plus ? rien, elle va devant
Le vent, la fumée et la flamme !

A la manière d'Agrippa d'Aubigné (1551-1630)

FOREWORD

In order to chronicle early steps in the birth of a branch of science, legendary records must be considered. Legends have the propensity to expand and often fancy is added to a point where historical values are sacrificed. Facts and fancy cannot always be separated by the most conscientious historian. However, careful research will usually document the facts and the legendary phases become apparent.

Where personalities, accomplishments, and historical facts are to be assembled and recorded in an interesting and reliable manner, there must be a proper blending of the facts with the legendary phases.

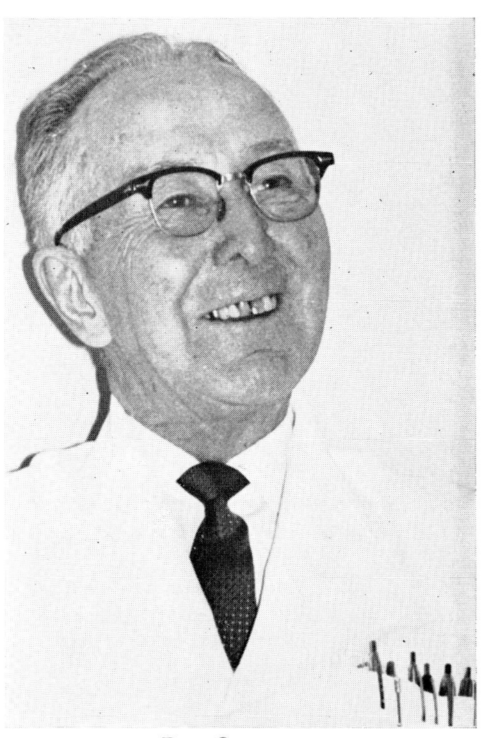

Ben Orndoff

The story of the discovery and the development of Radiology with its integration into the medical science is fascinating and educational. No division of science has exerted so great an influence on medicine, as we know it today, as has radiology. Its contributions to a better knowledge of living anatomy and physiology to structural changes from disease, as well as its profound influence on the discipline and art of the practice of all phases of medicine, has indeed been revolutionary.

The author has extended his research into fields that have not been fully recorded. His manner of presentation is unique and entertaining. I believe it is accurate and basically educational.

Before Roentgen or Radiological Societies were organized by physicians in America, electrotherapeutic groups moved to include in their membership all who concerned themselves with x rays. The early Roentgen Societies created interesting history in their formative days. The author has presented such data in this book in a very commendable way.

Readers will find detailed facts linked with personalities and individuals who became engaged with the current events of a rapidly changing world, toward an era of great scientific expansion and achievement. This book will do much to clarify the step-by-step history that has placed radiology in the position of not only being an important section of medicine, but a high ranking division of the physical sciences.

Benjamin H. Orndoff, M.D.

Park Ridge, Illinois

MOTTO PAGES

Οὐδὲν χρῆμα μάτην γίνεται, ἀλλὰ πάντα ἐκ λόγου τε καὶ ὑπ' ἀνάγκης. (Nothing happens capriciously; there is a necessary reason for everything.) LEUCIPPUS, *On Mind* (5th Century B. C.).

Ἱστορία φυλοσοφία ἐστὶν ἐκ παραδειγμάτων. (History is philosophy teaching by examples.) THUCYDIDES, interpreted by DIONYSIUS OF HALLICARNASSUS, *De Arte Rhetorica* xi, 2 (1st Century B. C.).

Iamque opus exegi, quod nec Iovis ira, ne cignis, Nec poterit ferrum, nec edax abolere vetustas. (And now I have finished the work which (I hope) neither the wrath of Jove, nor fire, nor the sword, nor devouring age shall be able to destroy.) PUBLIUS OVIDIUS NASO, *Metamorphoses* xv, 871 (7 A.D.).

Mais où sont les neiges d'antan? (But where are the snows of yesteryear?) François Villon, *Ballade des Dames du Temps Jadis* (about 1470).

It is as easy to count atomies as to resolve the propositions of a lover. WILLIAM SHAKESPEARE, *As You Like It,* iii, ii, 246 (1599).

Poco vale lo que poco cuesta. (Of little worth is that which little costs.) BALTAZAR GRACIAN, *Oráculo Manual,* 18 (1647).

Discreto amigo es un libro: Qué á propósito que habla Siempre en lo que quiero yo! (A book is a thoughtful friend who always speaks when and what I would like to hear!) PEDRO CALDERÓN DE LA BARCA, *Cual es Mayor Perfeccion?* ii, 2 (1668).

Tous les genres sont bons, hors le genre ennuyeux. (All styles are good, except the boring style.) FRANÇOIS MARIE AROUET (Voltaire), Preface to *Enfant Prodigue* (1738).

All history, so far as it is not supported by contemporary evidence, is romance. SAMUEL JOHNSON, *Boswell's Tour to the Hebrides* (November 20, 1773).

Ein Märchen aus alten Zeiten, Das kommt mir nicht aus dem Sinn! (An old time tale stays on my mind!) HEINRICH HEINE, *Die Lorelei* (1825).

Even when we are quite alone, how often do we think with pleasure or pain of what others think of us — of their imagined approbation or disapprobation. CHARLES ROBERT DARWIN, *The Descent of Man,* chap. 4 (1871).

There was things which he stretched, but mainly he told the truth. MARK TWAIN, *The Adventures of Huckleberry Finn,* chap. 1 (1885).

Le mal de prendre une hyppalage pour une découverte, une métaphore pour une démonstration, un vomissement de mots pour un torrent de connaissances capitales, et soi-même pour un oracle, ce mal naît avec nous. (The folly of mistaking a syntactic exchange for a discovery, a metaphor for a demonstration, a regurgitation of words for a torrent of capital knowledge, and oneself for an oracle, that folly is born with us.) PAUL VALÉRY, *Note et Digressions* (written in 1919 as a preface to a reprint of *Introduction à la Méthode de Leonarde de Vinci* of 1894).

Vittorio Maragliano per questo si è battuto fin dall'inizio; per una Radiologia integrale, comprendente tutta la gamma delle radiazioni. (For this Vittorio Maragliano fought from the very beginning, for an integral Radiology, comprising the entire gamut of radiations.) GIAN GIUSEPPE PALMIERI, Preface to *La Scuola Elettroradiologica Genovese* (July, 1938).

Der Techniker will und der Röntgenarzt soll den Weg von einfachen Anfängen zur jetzigen vervollkommneten Form kennenlernen. Dann wird er auch nachsichtiger in der Beurteilung der noch heute fühlbaren technischen Mängel. (The technician wishes to, and the roentgen physician should, find out about the transition from simple beginnings to the current, perfected forms. He would then become more tolerant in the evaluation of the technical shortcomings discernible even today.) RUDOLF GRASHEY, Preface to ALBERS-SCHÖNBERG'S *Die Röntgentechnik,* Ed. 6 (1941).

En el momento que vivimos, y seguramente todavía por muchos anos, se ha de seguir empleando el bisturi . . .; pero . . . el progreso . . . poco a poco hasta encuadrarlo en los limites de utilización reparadora y no mutilante. (For the time being, and certainly for many years to come, the scalpel will be utilized; but progress will gradually restrict its utilization to repair and not to mutilation.) ALFONSO C. FRANGELLA, Initial Words to *La Radioterapía en Clínica* (1942).

I do not believe that civilization will be wiped out in a war fought with the atomic bomb. Perhaps two thirds of the people of the earth might be killed, but enough men capable of thinking, and enough books, would be left to start again, and civilization could be restored. ALBERT EINSTEIN, *On the Atomic Bomb* in *Atlantic Monthly* (November, 1945).

After adequate consultation . . . the radiotherapist treating a case (should be) in charge of, and responsible for, that case. . . Division of responsibility is not in the patient's best interests. RALSTON PATERSON, Introduction to *The Treatment of Malignant Disease by Radium and X-Rays* (1947).

Он заметил, что эти лучи распространяются прямолинейно и поэтому дают совершенно четкие тени. И тот факт, что они распространяются прямолинейно, заставил его назвать их лучами. Но, так как неизвестно было, какие это лучи, он назвал их Х-лучами. (He noted that those rays travelled in a straight line, thus giving perfectly circumscribed shadows. That very fact, the straightforward propagation, made him call them rays. But since those rays, whatever their nature, were unknown, he called them X rays.) ABRAM F. YOFFÉ, *Reminiscences about Wilhelm Konrad Röntgen,* in *Ocherka Razvitiy Medizinskoe Rentgenologiy* (1948).

Man muss sich schon bescheiden in dem Bewusstsein der Unvollkommenheit alles . . . menschlichen Strebens. (One must resign himself in the realization of the incompleteness of all human endeavor.) HERMANN HOLTHUSEN, *Letter* (1953).

A ciência pode falhar no mundo incoerente em que se vive . . . Não importa, resta a esperança, resta acima de tudo a ilusão de estar no caminho certo. (Science may fail in the incoherent world in which we live. . . It does not matter, there remains the hope, there remains above all the illusion of being on the right path.) MANOEL DE ABREU, *Speech* (1958), cf. *Rev. Brasil. de radiol.,* 2:96 (1959).

Honor is so frequently bestowed upon the wrong, the false, and the scheming that it has become a prize rather than a virtue. DAGOBERT D. RUNES, *Dictionary of Thought* (1959).

Radiation is dangerous because fear of it attacks people's ability to think rationally. Radiation presents two medical hazards. It will give some people ulcers from worrying about it, and it will give other people ulcers from worrying about the people who worry about radiation. EDWARD TELLER, *Talk* before AMA's Conference on Disaster Medical Care (November, 1960).

Shortly after the peak of the radiation hysteria in 1958, federal laws were passed in the USA to prevent scientists from mistreating dogs at first, then all vertebrates — this being intended as an obvious indication that scientists must be an immoral lot, as they seemed to mistreat their experimental animals. It was the same federal mentality which has shifted the US Constitution from a document that prohibited the government from oppressing the people, to a document that prohibited the people from oppressing the government. MARSHALL BRUCER, *Letter* (1961).

(In the very beginning) anyone, simply by the purchase of an x-ray set . . . became *ipso facto* a radiologist. FREDERICK GORDON SPEAR, *Questioning the Answers* (1961).

(One of) the essentials of the (historic) "relativism" — of Carl Lotus Becker and Charles Austin Beard — (is) that what is accepted as truth (fact) by historians and the public will shift markedly from time to time due to emotional factors. . . James Harvey Robinson went (far) in arguing the utilitarian and pragmatic view of historical facts. He proclaimed that the "objective historian" is an historian without any object and, hence, a rather useless person unless somebody comes along to utilize the facts he has collected. HARRY ELMER BARNES, *The New History* in *A History of Historical Writing* (1962).

Not until each of the great powers had produced a full atomic arsenal would the threat of one-sided atomic war pass. Once this state was finally achieved, and I feel that it has been, with sane national leadership, major was is impossible. . . While it is tragic that the forces for destruction that we unleashed are stronger than man's present ability to control them, it is fortunate indeed for humanity that the initiative in this field was gained and kept by the United States. GENERAL LESLIE R. GROVES, *Now It Can Be Told* (1962).

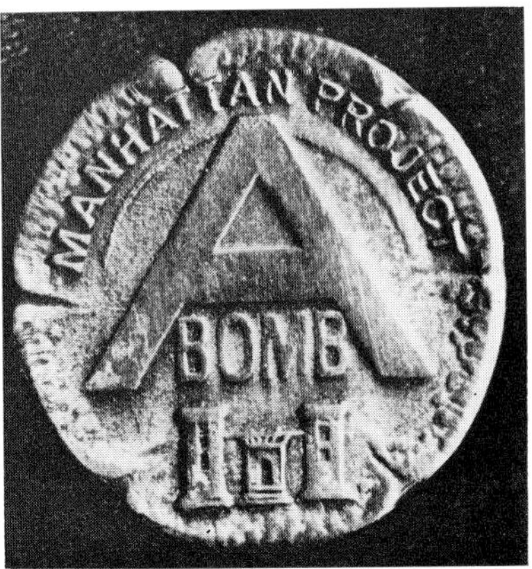

The Era of the Roentgen Pioneers

HEMISPHERE OF NON-ACTIVITY

HEMISPHERE OF X RAY ACTIVITY

The Trail of the Invisible Light

The Golden Age of Radiology

MPLS

X-Ray

The Atomic Phase

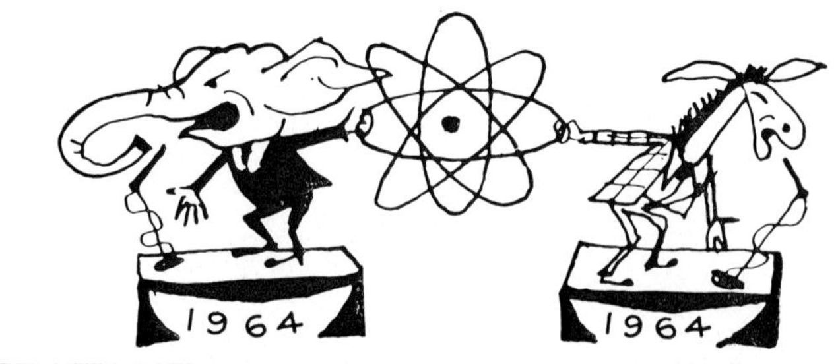

FROM X-Strahlen TO RADIO (BIO) LOGY

THE AUTHOR TO THE READER

I wish thee as much pleasure in the reading as I had in the writing
FRANCIS QUARLES (1592-1644)

AMONG THE PROSPECTIVE readers there is always at least one who would like to know how, why, and when a given book has been written. In the preface to his beautiful *Anatomy of Bibliomania* (1930-1931), the bookman *par excellence* Holbrook Jackson (1874-1948) stated: ". . . the questions (are) clear and reasonable in themselves, but I owe thee no answer, for if the contents please thee 'tis well; if they be useful, 'tis an added value; if neither, pass on. . .!" Since Jackson relented and answered the questions, so will I.

Most people have no single reason for writing, nor for reading. In general, writers are extroverts and readers are introverts, albeit I cannot conceive of a serious author who is not a voracious reader, *i.e.,* a proper companion to Jackson's whimsical "book-eaters" and "book-drinkers."

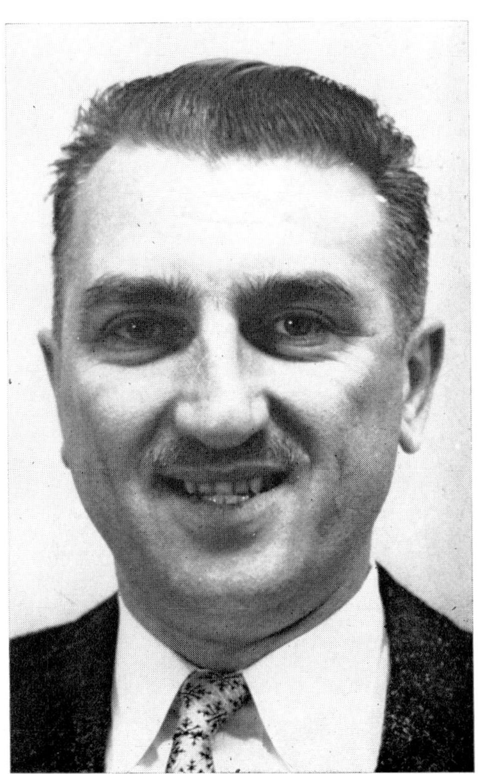

E. R. N. GRIGG

I am a confessed bibliophagist, display as a rule extrovert tendencies, and have always liked to indulge both in historic and in bibliographic endeavors. Still, I never planned to write this book. It all started in 1957 when I decided to investigate the manner in which radiologic findings are reported to the referring clinicians. First I requested samples of modern reports from leading radiologists in active practice, then copies of old reports from retired colleagues. The chore proved to be more frustrating than anticipated because so many of those queried never bothered to answer my letters.

Halfway through writing that piece I became aware of the varied terminology employed by American radiologists. Some speak of x-ray reports, others call them roentgen reports. In digging further, I discovered a double morality of sorts. Most people in the profession say "take an x-ray" or "to x-ray a patient," but many will *write* "expose a roentgenogram," or "to roentgenograph a patient." They act as if that other set of terms were too fancy for verbal usage (which, indeed, they are). Moreover, I often found that those who subscribe to the eponymic form, *i.e.,* to vocables formed with the root roentgeno- (such as roentgenologist, roentgen diagnosis, and

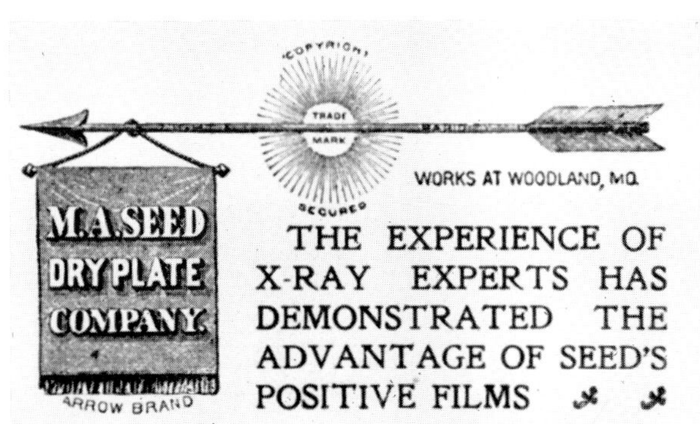

roentgen therapy), formally frowned not only on hearing the verb to x-ray, but also upon words derived from the etymon radio- (such as radiography, radio-diagnosis, and radio-therapy).

Throughout the year 1958 I searched for the origins of this terminologic controversy between roentgenology and radiology. The analyses of, and the explanations for, these antagonistic etymologies were put on paper during the last half of the year 1959. That was the first draft of the *Radio-Semantic Treatise*. It was submitted in January, 1960 to *Radiology* in 70 manuscript pages under the title *From X-Strahlen to Radio(bio)logy.*

A few months earlier, in September of 1959, I had flown to the meeting of the American Roentgen Ray Society (ARRS) in Cincinnati. Application for membership in the ARRS requires submission of an original thesis. Back home, from my bulging bibliographic boxes I selected the material for the initial version of the *First Clinical Roentgen Plate*. Rejected, relegated to the shelves, then revised as well as refurbished, it became the first chapter in the book, but that did not come about until later.

In April, 1960 the editor of *Radiology* returned the manuscript of the *Semantic Treatise*. The "committee" had decided it was too long for their journal. With the rejection came the suggestion to submit the manuscript for publication as a monograph in the *American Lecture Series*. Thereupon the (untouched) manuscript of the *Semantic Treatise* was sent to Prof. Lewis Elmer Etter, who teaches radiology in the University of Pittsburgh, and also edits the *American Lectures in Roentgen Diagnosis* for its publishers, the firm of Charles C Thomas, Publisher in Springfield (Illinois): Prof. Etter's reply was very encouraging.

A copy of the original *Semantic Treatise* had also been sent to Prof. Benjamin Harry Orndoff, who has been for over half a century in active general practice of radiology, while serving at the same time as chairman of the Department of Radiology of Stritch School of Medicine in Loyola University (Chicago). He liked the manuscript, but told me of his long-held belief that the contributions of the x-ray industry to the growth of radiology have yet to be properly recognized. Thereupon Prof. Orndoff strongly suggested that information on manufacturers of x-ray equipment be inserted into the text of the semantic monograph.

I was quite willing to agree on this count. Antique oriental rulers were often buried together with an adequate retinue, including several wives, many slaves and soldiers, perhaps here and there a lone court medicus. *Mutatis mutandis,* radiologists might as well enter history together with the technologic members of the profession, meaning both x-ray technicians and manufacturers of radiologic equipment.

I agree with Frank Berry (*JAMA* of September 22, 1962) that it is difficult to be both a chronicler (accurate recorder) and historiographer (interpreter of events), but I have always tried to combine these two aspects of the historic trade. To compensate for the inherent difficulty related to such a task, I tend to write my pieces in a contrapuntal manner, in some ways similar to Bach's polyphonics, wherein two or more melodies are simultaneously carried on different musical planes. This causes at times a degree of unintentional "obscurity," when a certain meaning is partially hidden in between the lines. But at least I always try to show "malice toward none," except for "ignoring" a few obviously unimportant personages.

By sheer luck I happened to find an x-ray report written in May, 1896 by William James Morton of New York City. This is how I first became interested in one of the most intriguing figures among American radiologic pioneers. The historic past resembles a string of railroad stations which recede further and further as the departing train (time) advances. If one were able to temporarily reverse the flow of time, and return to the point or departure, all the old familiar faces would still be waiting in their original stations. Any historian worth his salt must be able to

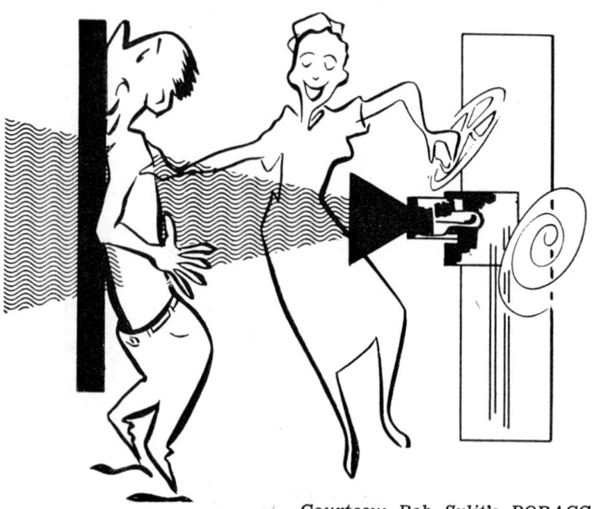

Courtesy: Bob Sulit's PORACC

"take such a train back" to the era under consideration. But even in day-dreams the shadows of bygone days eventually go up in smoke. A sensible way of honoring those shades is to go on record with a description of their station in life, and this I attempted to do in Morton's biography.

The first draft of Morton's life story was submitted to Prof. Etter, and then to Messrs. Thomas, whereupon we signed the contract in September, 1960. This is also when the present title — *The Trail of the Invisible Light* — was adopted. As first planned, the book contained five chapters, beginning with the *Semantic Treatise,* followed by Morton's biography, after which came the *First Clinical Roentgen Plate,* and the *Plea for Palliation,* the last chapter being the

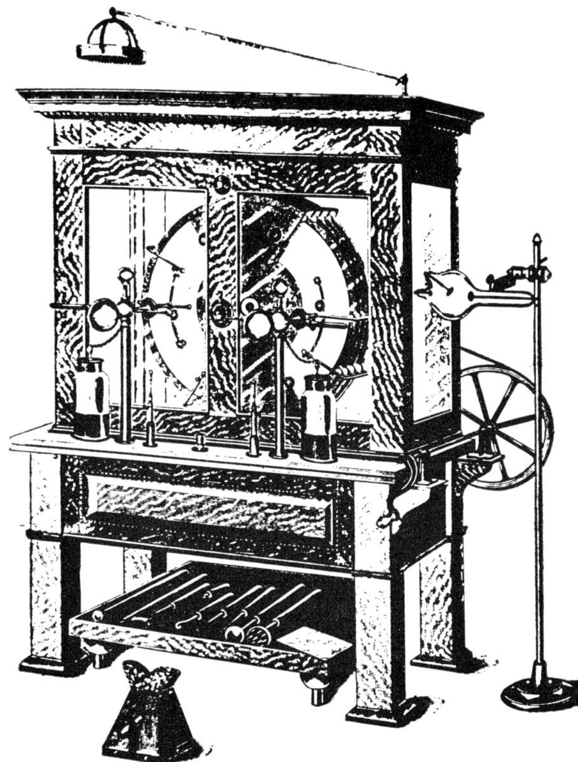

STATIC MACHINE with gas tube and cryptoscope, sold by Friedländer (1905).

monograph on x-ray reporting. The latter was initially sailing under the peculiar title, *A (Fairly) Sober Entreaty to Strengthen Virtuousness in the Labeling of Shades.* Work on the chapter on reporting progressed very slowly (because of the time spent in research on early x-ray manufacturers). It was finally finished in September, 1961. In the process, its title had been modified to *The Power of Wishful Thinking.*

In the summer of 1961, in the Wheaton (Illinois) country home of Dr. Irvin Franklin Hummon, Jr.,

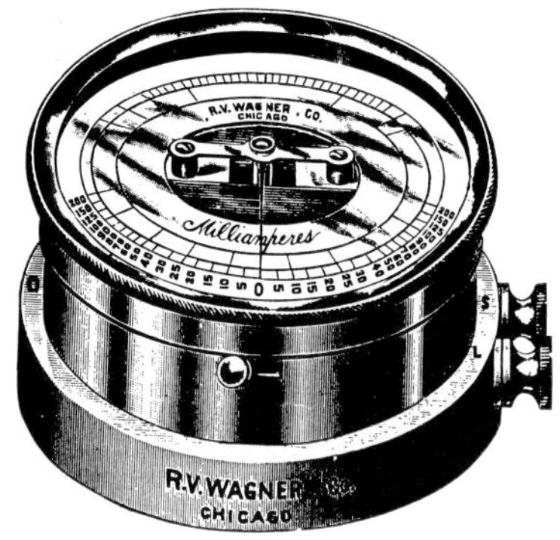

director of the Department of Radiology in Cook County Hospital (Chicago), about one thousand slides of advertisements of American x-ray products were shown to a select audience. Their response was gratifying. The material had been collected for inclusion in the *Radio-Semantic Treatise,* to illustrate the "x-ray names" given to commercial products. But there was so much material that it had to be made into a separate chapter, even though it covers only *American X-ray Makes and Makers* until World War II. "X-ray names" of later, and of foreign, extraction had to be sandwiched into the *Radio-Semantic Treatise.* Those foreign listings provided a good pretext to attempt a survey of the x-ray industry around the globe.

The names of the various radiological organizations had to be listed for a similarly semantic scope. Whenever possible, the date of organization and the names of the founding or important members are also given. As in the case of x-ray manufacturers, here as well as abroad, no wilful discrimination was made, political or otherwise. In most instances in which significant information along these lines was not included in the text, it is only because such information had not been received, and could not be otherwise elicited. Whatever data will arrive after publication deadline shall be preserved just in case another edition may some day be issued.

A mandala is a mystic symbol — often a geometric combination of one or more squares and circles — used in oriental religions as a stare-on aid to meditation. The idea of mandala is as old as man: rounded (sun?) symbols have been found in prehistoric cave drawings. Society seals (crests), and commercial trade-marks are all cousins to the mandala. Occasionally the very square-in-a-circle pattern will emerge, as in the beautiful sign of the Portuguese Society of

Radiology and Nuclear Medicine.* The Swiss psycho-mystic Carl Gustav Jung thought that modern man's addiction to mandalas stems from mankind's insecurity. Orderly geometric patterns are seemingly suggestive of security. Jung's mind was unquestionably pure. When one of his patients dreamed of being "attacked" by a circling snake — somewhat in the manner in which RB (meaning Radium Belge), in their exquisite seal, is circled by a "medical" snake — Jung interpreted her dream as a representation of a mandala. Jung's former magister, Sigmund Freud, would undoubtedly have offered a more candid interpretation of the snake.

I am willing to agree that it seems puerile to de-

*As explained in the *Radio-Semantic Treatise,* in languages of Latin origin the terms derived from the root *radio-* often do not cover nuclear medicine.

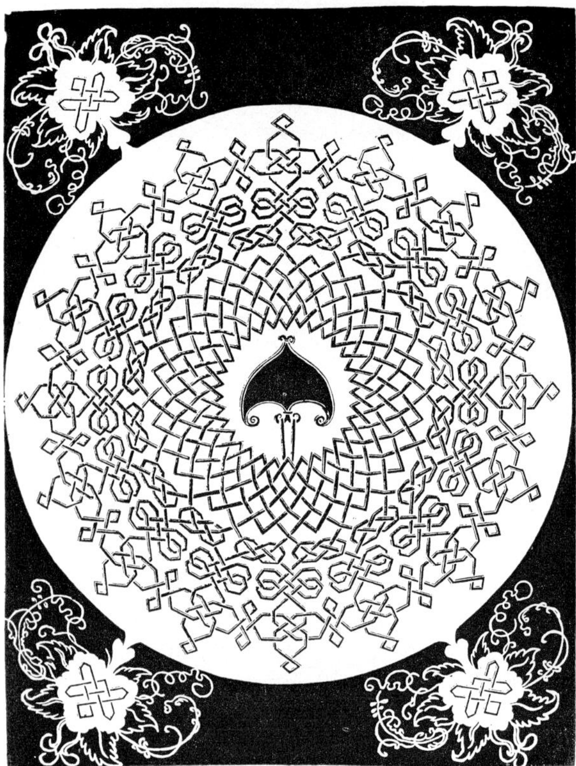

ALBRECHT VON DÜRER'S "Knotty" Mandala

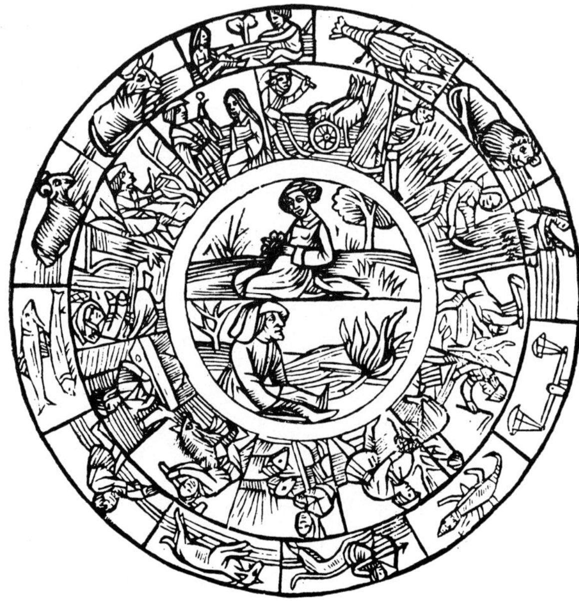

HOROSCOPIC MANDALA OF LIFE

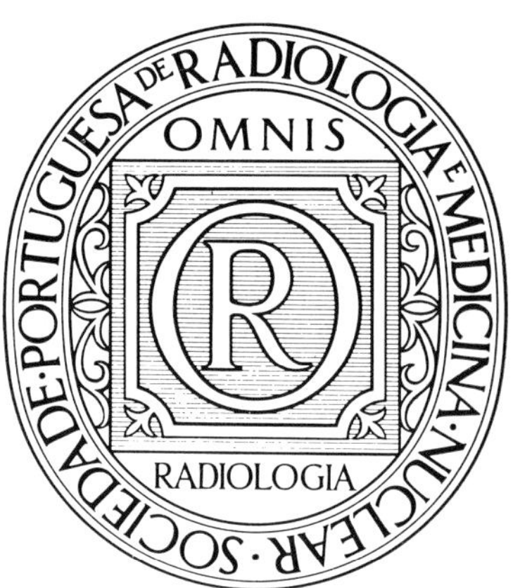

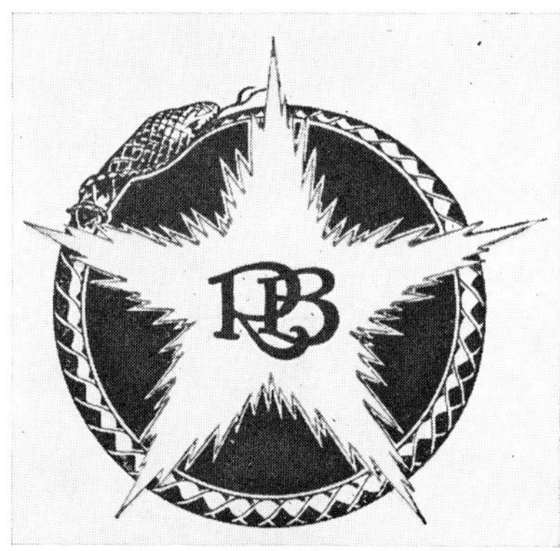

RADIUM BELGE

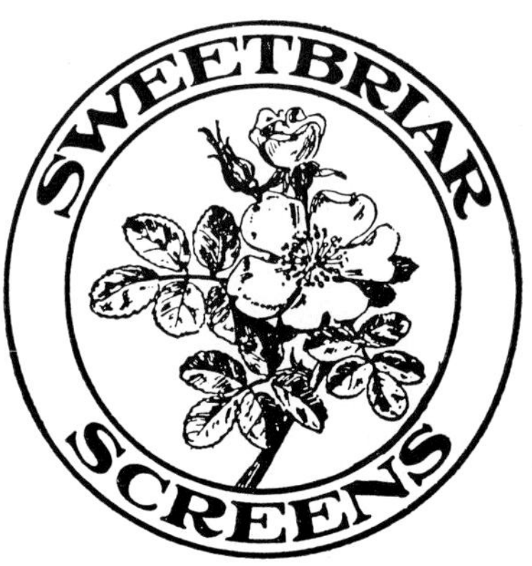

vote much time to mandalas, regardless of their origin. And yet the multitude of mandalas and of other symbols found along the radiologic trail prove that very many people — including radiologists — are obviously preoccupied with these signs.

As a belated atomism permeated the world, the mandalas adopted a new shape, derived from a (now known to be erroneous, but very popular) concept of the orbiting electrons. The spread of this new symbol has been marked in the book by including the reproductions of several of these ultra-modern mandalas. The historian feels that these images must be saved for posterity, even if he were to believe that such preoccupation with mandalas is at best a fancy. Every so often, though, a radio-mandala comes along that is really well done, or at least unusual (I, too, am at times human).

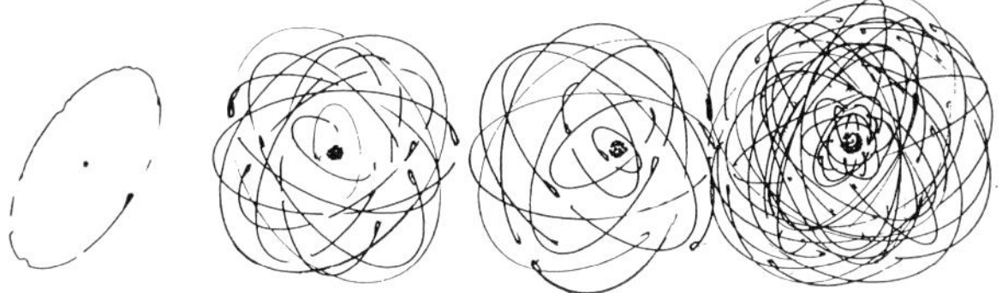

Courtesy: Bulletin of the Atomic Scientists

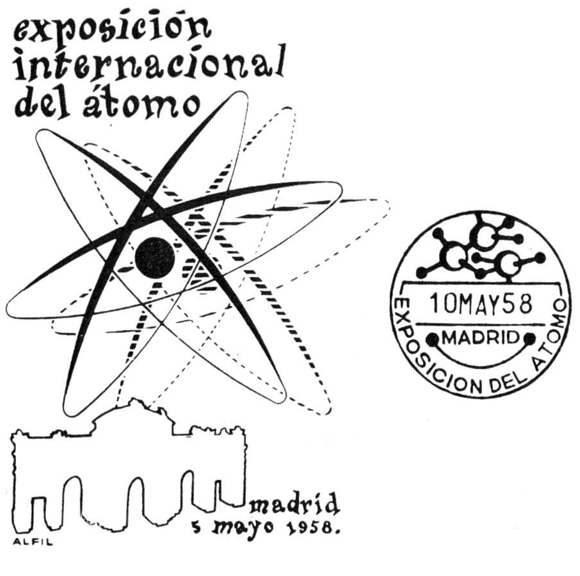

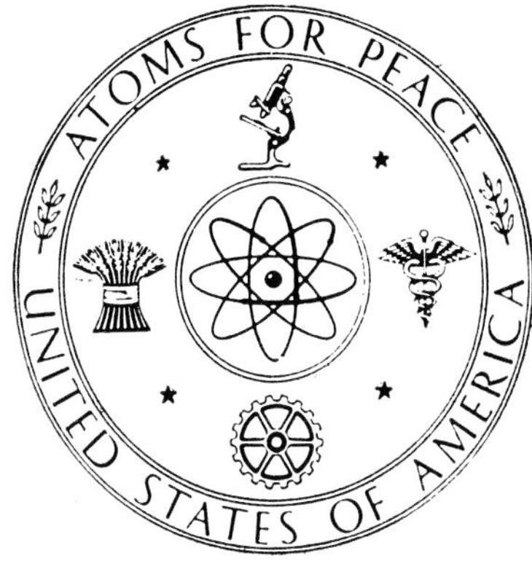

In November, 1956, I wrote an editorial for the *American Journal of Roentgenology,* entitled *Etymologic and Other Aspects of Palliation.* My original text, submitted on that occasion, had been "palliated" in the Journal's editorial office, to comply with their selectively serene style. An amplified version of my original text is included in this book under the title *A Plea for Palliation.* As I had said before, I am (also) an extrovert.

With the passing of time, the *Semantic Treatise* became overcrowded with an assortment of titles of periodicals from the radiologic literature, utilized simply for their names. An effort was then made to complete this *List of Radiologic Periodicals* by consulting the Index Catalogue, the Union Catalogue, the World List of Periodicals, and other possible sources. The list soon exceeded all sensible proportions and was therefore relegated to a separate section, which comes in the book after Morton's biography. The radiologic periodicals are also indexed by country of publication, just in case someone remembers *where* a given journal had appeared but cannot recall its title.

Throughout the book there is an emphasis on word lore, which needs no special justification. There is today a growing concern for etymologic and related problems. Electronic translating machines have to be fed very accurate corresponding terms in the respective languages. Besides, intra-professional communication is in dire need of improvement. These are some of the reasons for which the National Science Foundation is sponsoring investigations into the semantic content of terms used in various scientific disciplines.

Three "orthographic" items deserve a special mention. *One* is my exalted hypheno-philia (the "correct" spelling is hyphenomania), used in this text mainly as a means of emphasizing the root radio- in its many derivations. *Next* are the "wrong" ways of indicating the elements, for instance radioiodine — which can be found as I-131, Iodine^{131}, or iodine^{131} (the two "approved" ways are I^{131} and iodine-131), depending on the year in which the respective section had been written. The *third* concerns alliteration, something which is regarded as denoting an elegant use of the language: for this purpose I have included an "alliterated" paragraph (to end all alliterations) in the sixth chapter, Morton's biography.

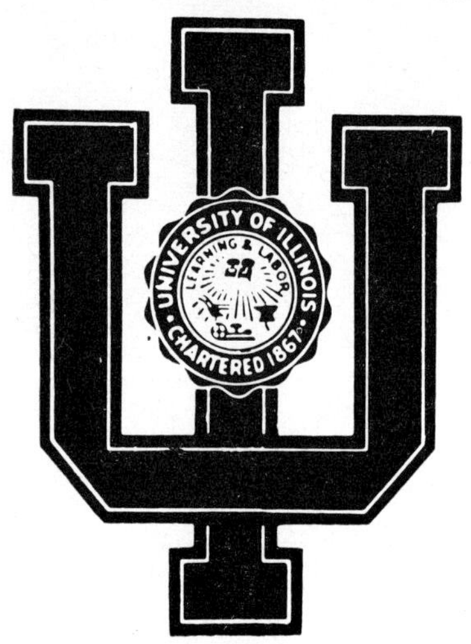

The desire to "quote" from previous authors is undoubtedly older than writing itself. It was commonly and quite successfully used by the ancient Greeks, it bloomed in religious texts, and then it became the mainstay of medieval scholasticism. The "father of (universal) bibliography" was Conrad Gesner (1516-1565) of Zürich. The first systematic attempt at medical bibliography was made by James Douglas (1675-1742) of London. Largely forgotten is the real initiator of modern medical bibliography, the German with the French name, Wilhelm Gottfried von Ploucquet (1744-1813), author of 17 volumes of *Literatura Medica Digesta.* The 33 tomes of the *Medicinisches Schriftsteller-Lexicon* by the Danish surgeon Adolph Carl Peter Callisen (1787-1866) became the forerunner of the *Index Medicus,* started in New York City in 1879 by John Shaw Billings (1838-1913), a native of Indiana and former Civil War surgeon, and by Robert Fletcher (1823-1912), a physician born and bred in Bristol (England).

In 1927, the *Index Medicus* merged with the *Quarterly Cumulative Index to Current Medical Literature* (which existed since 1916 and for a while was published in France) and was continued by the American Medical Association. Billings (who also organized the New York Public Library) began the famous *Index Catalogue* of the Surgeon's General (Army Medical) Library in 1880. The last of Billings' successors in that job, Dr. Claudius Francis* Mayer, resigned in 1954 as the *Index Catalogue* was discontinued at the volume M_2 of its fourth series (that last volume contained entries printed up to 1951, and monographic literature printed mostly before 1952).

In the meantime, the *Current List of Medical Literature* (started in 1941)) was turned over from the Army Medical Library to the National Library of Medicine (NLM) as the latter acquired the former's holdings, which were recently moved to a new building in Bethesda (Maryland). The NLM issues now the *Current List* under the name *Index Medicus,* using IBM cards, film reproduction of cards, and mechanical transfer of these data directly to the printing presses. The AMA provides since 1958 a *Quarterly Cumulative Index* of the monthly issues of NLM's *List.* In addition, there is a *Cumulated Index,* which comes out once a year.

Connoisseurs insist that these indices, from the old *Index Catalogue* to the new *Index Medicus,* with its *Cumulated Index,* are the greatest American contribution to universal medical science. Much of the early bibliography, on which my book is based, can easily be identified by collating my text with the respective items in these American indices.

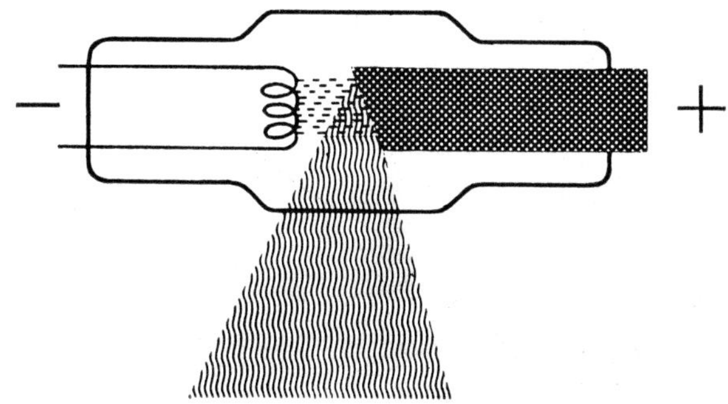

Courtesy: Deutsches Röntgen-Museum

In his scholarly *Natural History of Love* (1959) Morton M. Hunt mentions (also) the Greek hetaera

*Francis was the name given to Dr. Mayer at the time of his baptism, in 1899. In 1914, as he entered the novitiate of the Cistercian Order, he received the name Claudius, and kept it even after returning to secular life in 1918. He is now a physician in the Pentagon's Civilian Employee's Health Service, and contributor of historic items to the periodical *Military Medicine.*

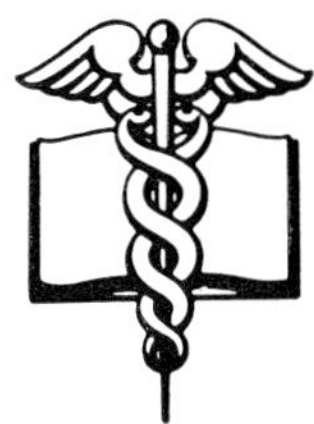

Phryne (4th Century, B.C.), reputed to have been the most beautiful woman of her time. Hunt emphasizes that Phryne had a different "face" for each of her many lovers. Likewise bibliography — which can be many things to different people — is simply a reflection of the image of its creator. A bibliography can be brief or boundless, bashful or bombastic, brazen or boring. A "dead" bibliography is an amas of roughly related references, collected after completion of the text, and appended only because it is demanded by current custom. By contrast, an adequate bibliography is a "living" part of the text, and often reaches beyond the indices (which, in the way of all human strive, can never achieve completeness). To accommodate the excessive number of references available for my text, instead of burdening it with a "general" bibliography, or with bibliographic footnotes, throughout most of the book quotations include (and can easily be identified from) the name of the periodical, the month (also the day, when necessary), and the year of publication. In the case of cited books, the author's name alone would often suffice, but the quotations (usually) contain also the title of the book and the year of publication.

There are three exceptions to the above rules. The chapter on *Wishful Thinking* has its own *Roentgen Reporting References.* Morton's biography carries the quoted titles in footnotes, while Morton's own publications are posted in chronologic order at the end of the chapter; the numbering of Morton's works corresponds to similar numbers used *only in that chapter* as references in parentheses. There is, in addition, a completely separate chapter entitled *Annotated "Radio-Historical" Bibliography,* which contains a listing of and comments on articles and books devoted (mainly) to the history of radiology. As expected, the selection of those titles reflects my personal preferences for the respective author, for his text, or for both.

Just before the *Author to the Reader* was written (in February, 1962), I decided to re-arrange the order of the chapters. It was again altered during the manuscript's proof-reading, in the summer of 1962, when the chapters were placed in the order in which they are now included in the book. That is also when it was decided to append three indices, one of manufacturers, another by subjects, and finally an index of names.

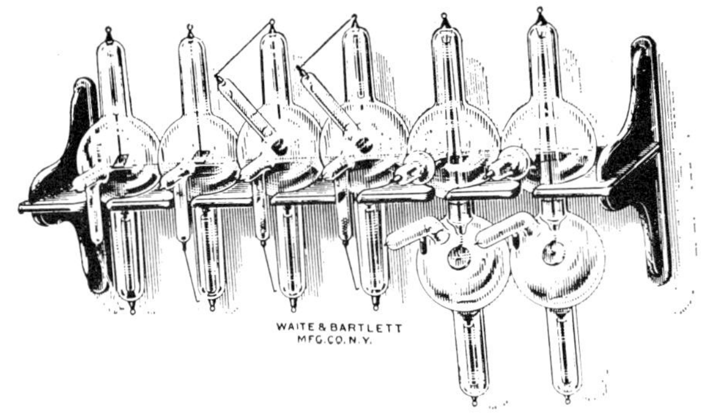

"To dear-bought wisdom give the credit due . . ." is an often quoted quip of the master-versifier Alexander Pope (1688-1744). In this instance his advice will be taken seriously.

Prof. Ben Orndoff spent many hours in discussing with me various passages from the book. In so doing, he often gave color and depth to shadows from the radiologic past. Many of these conversations took place at the Orndoff summer residence on Fox Lake (in Northern Illinois); there, in a converted barn, are preserved many of his radiologic memorabilia. Orndoff was president of the Radiological Society of North American (1918), and of the American College of Radiology (1936); and secretary-general of the American Congress of Radiology (1933), and of the Fifth International Congress of Radiology (1937). He kindly gave permission to use in this book the half-tone cuts from the portrait-catalogs of these two congresses. Prof. Orndoff has received many honors, such as the ACR Gold Medal and more recently the Stritch Gold Medal. He is very actively engaged in private medical practice, and his 80th birthday was celebrated on February 5, 1961 with an open house at his office in Park Ridge (a Northern suburb of Chicago). To all this must be added his activity as an educator: he has been on the faculty of the Medical School of Loyola University ever since its creation, and in his quiet manner, he has contributed considerably to the overall growth of that institution. In

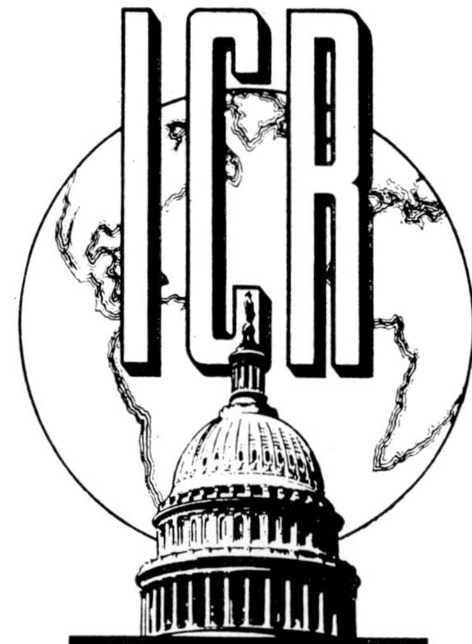

Official Seal of the fifth International Congress of Radiology, held in Chicago in 1937.

many ways, this book may be regarded as a homage to Prof. Orndoff.

Prof. Lewis Etter, the well known skull specialist and "glossarist" from Pittsburgh, recommended my book for publication: that recommendation was given after a brief (but animated) interview, and subsequent reading of excerpts from two chapters (the *Semantic Treatise* and Morton's biography). Prof. Etter also offered constructive criticism, and friendly advice on many aspects of the preparation of this manuscript.

Dr. Irvin Hummon furthered the collection of material in several ways. He did not hesitate to fly with me to "far-away places" such as Oak Ridge, Colorado Springs, and Cleveland, to mention only the longer trips. Being always available, and having a good memory, he had to answer many technical questions, especially on teletherapy and isotopic equipment.

The basic philosophy expounded in *A Plea For Palliation* comes from the teachings of (and from my conversations with) Dr. Marion Frank Magalotti, director of the Radiation Center in Cook County Hospital, who provided also several cases to illustrate some of the points made in that chapter.

Dr. Marshall Brucer, the former director of the Medical Division of the Oak Ridge Institute for Nuclear studies (ORINS), kindly permitted lengthy quotations from his writings. He contributed much historic information on several of the "atomic" developments considered in the book. His co-worker, Mrs. Betty Anderson, a technical editor in the Medical Division of the ORINS, offered many interesting details on Oak Ridge operations, details which were transmitted in an extended exchange of correspondence.

Mr. Ed. Goldfield, former managing director of the Waite-Picker Manufacturing Division (Cleveland), placed at my disposal his collection of old catalogs and advertisements, many of them collector's items, some from "competitors" long since gone out

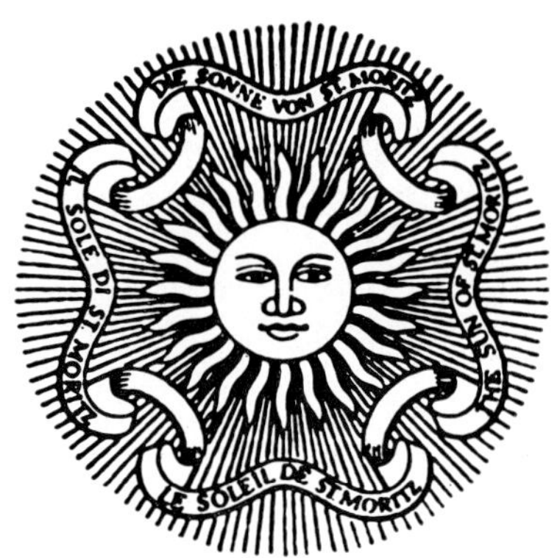

Unofficial Seal of the fourth International Congress of Radiology, held in Switzerland in 1934.

of business. We also corresponded intensely for over one year, then Mr. Goldfield read the chapter on *American X-ray Makes and Makers,* and offered valuable criticism. That chapter was then reviewed by Dr. Bob Laudauer, Sr., physicist in Cook County Hospital (Chicago), who contributed advice also on other phases of the manuscript.

Mr. Byron Hess, a vice-president of the Standard X-ray Company (Chicago), permitted utilization of material from his historic files.

Mr. David Shields of Cleveland, a former president of the American Society of X-Ray Technicians, graciously sent me a set of glossy photographic prints, depicting technical achievements of the American x-ray industry. At the time of this writing, Dave is fighting a valiant battle with skin grafts, placed after the amputation of an arm because of radiogenic osteosarcoma.

Aside from Prof. Orndoff, half-tone cuts of portraits have been contributed by the following: Prof. Boris Rajevsky, president of the 9th ICR in München (Germany); the Girardet Verlag in Wuppersthal-Elderfeld (Germany); and the American Society of X-Ray Technicians.

Mr. Charles W. Smith, of the Pennsylvania X-ray Corporation in Philadelphia, allowed me to inspect

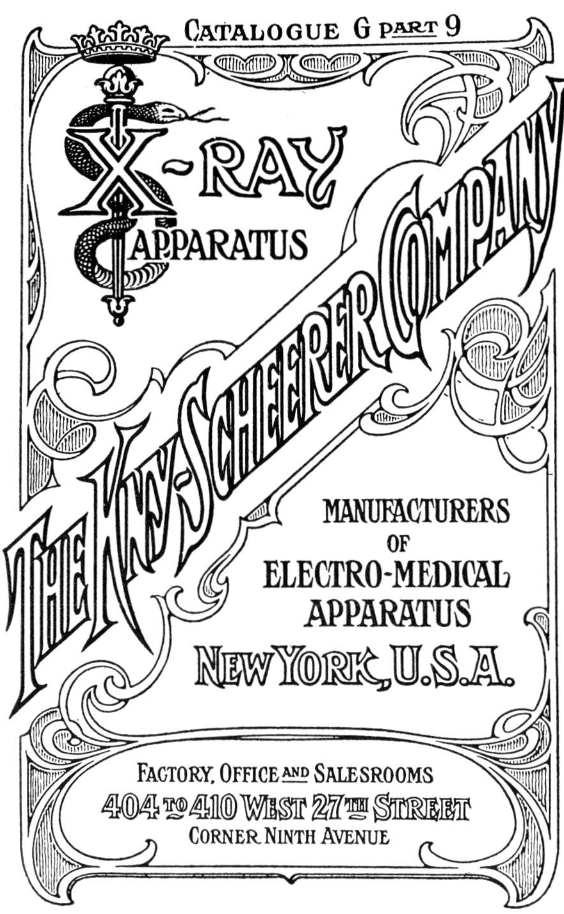

his valuable holdings of primeval x-ray catalogs; the covers of several of them have been used as illustrations.

Dr. Stanley Paul Bohrer, a budding radiologist, has assembled a large collection of philatelic material re-

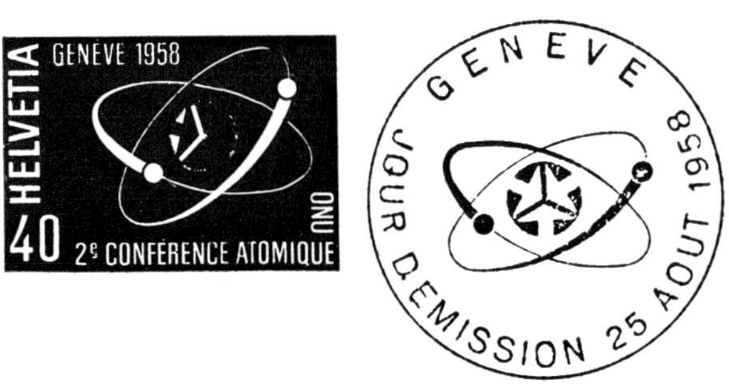

lated to radiology. Many (but not all) of the stamps inserted in these pages have been reproduced from his albums.

Mr. Byron Montelle Smith, R.T., the accomplished chief x-ray technician in the Hospital and Clinic in Paris (Illinois), personally executed the photographic work for the reproduction of x-ray films used in the chapter on reporting.*

Steve Andrew Grigg, the oldest of my nine children — who is now in college — developed the negatives and the prints for the book, and made most of the several thousand slides on the history of radiology, which I have accumulated in the interim. My three next-oldest children (Madelyn, Richard, and Sandra) did the ferrotyping.

Mrs. Mary Tweedy of Paris (Illinois) typed most portions of the manuscript — several times. Then — after it was seen by the publisher — the manuscript was re-typed by Mrs. Mary Ann Little of Paris (Illinois), and Mrs. Betty Moore of Champaign (Illinois).

The largest part of the bibliographic research was done at the friendly John Crerar Library in Chicago, with the invaluable help of Miss Ella Salmonson, Mrs. Frances Johnson, and Miss Millie Booker. Many items were found in the Library of the University of Illinois in Urbana, and in the Medical Li-

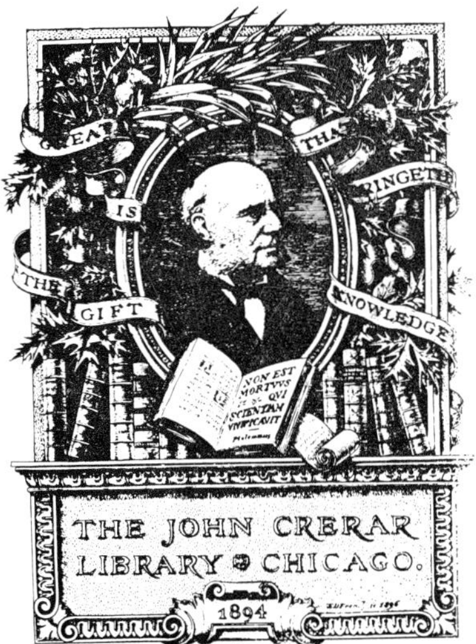

brary of the University of Illinois in Chicago. Further help was obtained from Miss Louise Annan, the chief-librarian of the New York Academy of Medicine. And when nobody else had a given title, it was (usually) available in the National Library of Medicine in Washington (D.C.).

Very important material was collected for my book by and from overseas friends. In this respect first

*After this was written, my friend Byron suddenly passed away, regretted by all those who knew him. A brief eulogy has been inserted into the fifth chapter (on reporting).

place credit goes to Mademoiselle Antoinette Béclère, the secretary and founder of the Centre Antoine Béclère (named after her father) in Paris. Aside from portraits and other documentary material, I was permitted to use historic information printed in their *Bulletin d'Information.*

Both valuable and invaluable data were also obtained from the following countries: in Argentina from Dr. Lidio Gianfranco Mosca of Córdoba; in Austria from Prof. Ernst Ruckensteiner of Innsbruck; in Brazil from Prof. Walter Bonfim Pontes of Sao Paulo; in Ecuador from Dr. Mario Hinojosa Cardona of Guayaquil; in England from the erudite bi(bli)ographer Mr. Leslie Thomas Morton, lately with the (British) National Research Council, and from Dr. Thomas Henry Hills, chief-radiologist of Guy's Hospital in London; in Germany from Dr. Heinrich Chantraine of Neuss-am-Rhein, and from

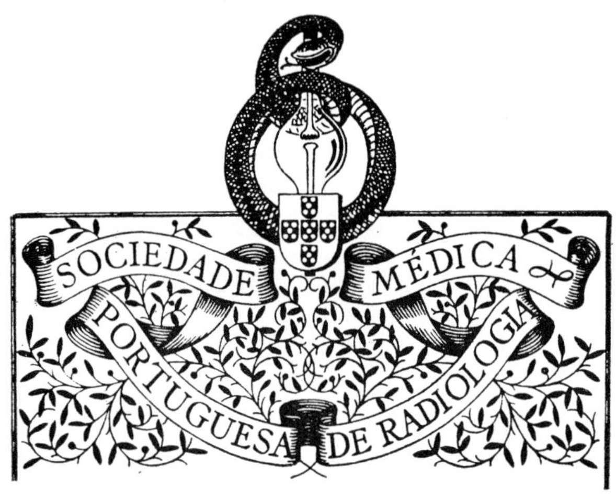

Dr. Kurt Walther of Leer (Ostfriesland); in India from Dr. Ved Prakash of New Delhi; in Italy from Prof. Alessandra Vallebona of Genova, Prof. Arduino Ratti of Milano, and Prof. Ettore de Bernardi of Salerno; in Portugal from Prof. Ayres de Sousa of Lisbon; in Sweden from Prof. Elis Berven and Prof. Åke Lindbom of Stockholm; in Uruguay from Prof. Helmut Kasdorf of Montevideo; and in the USSR from Prof. Georg Zedgenidze of Moscow, and Prof. Boris Shtern of Leningrad.

Credit for the overall appearance of the book goes to my publishers, Messrs, Charles C Thomas and Payne Thomas. With remarkable faith they accepted for publication, sight unseen, an historical manuscript which (at the time the contract was being signed) existed only in my imaginative intention. In charge of the actual production of the book have been Mr.

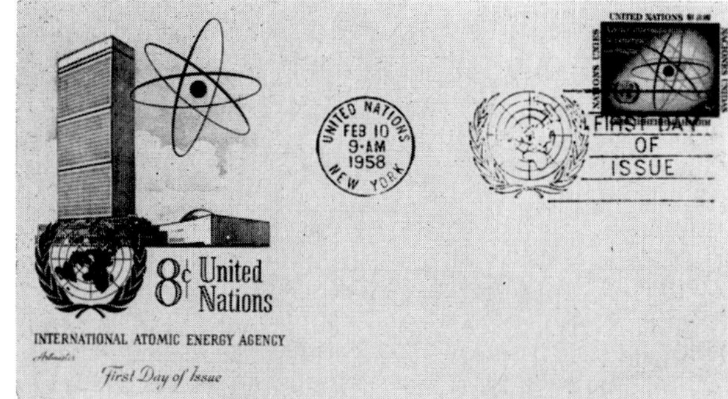

Courtesy: Artmaster, Louisville (Kentucky)

W. H. Green in Fort Lauderdale (Fla.), and Mr. R. S. Schinneer and Mr. W. N. Lyon in Springfield (Ill.).

Credit for the quality of the illustrations goes to the G. R. Grubb Engraving Company of Champaign (Illinois). In charge of the actual production of the zinc cuts and halftones has been Mr. George McKinley Floyd ("Kinkey"): together we went at least twice over all the illustrations. I suspect Kinkey of having subsequently "doctored" some of those photographs, because a few of the engravings turned out better than the respective originals. Actually, as with all historic material, a number of photographs were simply not good enough for faultless reproduction, and had to be included "as is." The size of halftones used for portraits was determined, not by the importance of the subject portrayed, but by the source of the halftone cuts (those made by Kinkey are in the 9 pica width, those from the 5th ICR are 7 picas wide, those from the 9th ICR are 6 picas wide, and those from Girardet are 19 picas wide).

To the many others who contributed smaller parts, appropriate credit was given — whenever possible — in footnotes, or otherwise. A few may have been omitted or forgotten, and to those I humbly apologize.*

No radiologic organization had any part in the making of this book. The *Trail* was all along one man's effort, printed by a private publisher, with no public monies or any other institutional subsidies. In its own way, this book (which the publisher insisted on producing in a lavish format) is a vivid exemplification of what individual initiative can achieve in a climate of private enterprise.

*For instance, several cartoons — including the one with the obviously (educationally!) imprudent, x-ray technician — have been reproduced from Dr. Robert Sulit's exquisitely illustrated three volumes of (Naval) Principles of Radiation and Contamination Control (PORACC), published in 1960-1961 by the Government Printing Office in Washington (D.C.).

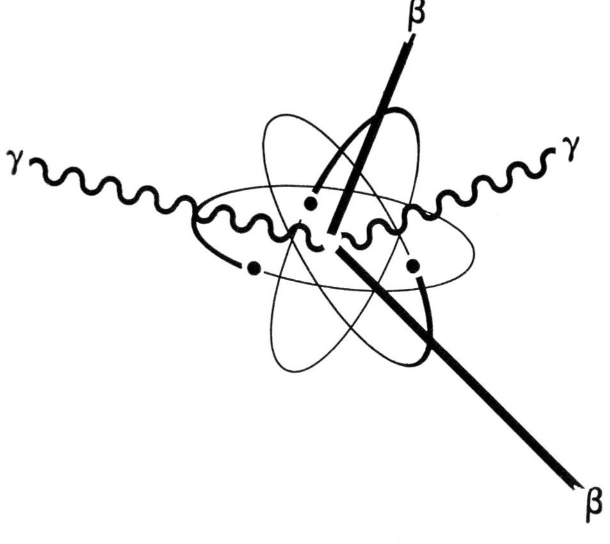

There is one item which I had to include in this lengthy preface, but there seemed to be no place for it in any other paragraph. Amateur historians are delighted when they can show that there is nothing new under the sun. (Incidentally, the very first mandalas were representations of the sun's circle, with "radiating" rays of light — and a few stylized sun rays have been inserted into the square radio-mandala of the British Institute of Radiology.) But Joseph Agassi, who teaches philosophy in the University of Hong Kong, has warned amateurish historians of science not to confuse physics with metaphysics. He specifically objected to the currently common "ludicrous identification" of the (metaphysical) atomism of Democritus with the (physical) atomism of Dalton. I, for one, am not willing to subscribe to Agassi's anti-meta-atomistic animadversions. Today the electron enjoys the same *conditions* of indivisibility, identity, and stability, postulated by Sir Joseph John Thomson in 1897 when he "recognized" that cathode rays were streams of electrons. But those same *conditions* had been for millenia the very essence of metaphysical atomism.

As a final introductory remark, I wish to mention that many passages in the book have first been dictated on a portable tape recorder installed in my plane (I use a plane in commuting between the hospitals I serve — see *The Flying Physician* magazine, November, 1964). This is why some of my phrases may

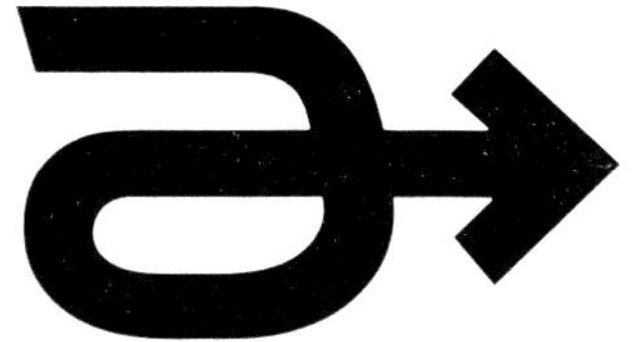

not be as polished as I had wanted them to be. Even otherwise I could hardly have hoped to achieve the perfection, clarity, and forcefulness of the style of the flyer-reporter-warrior-statesman-writer Sir Winston Leonard Spencer Churchill. To prove the point I have only to quote from a speech which he delivered on November 10, 1942 at the Mansion House in London: "This is not the end. It is not even the beginning of the end. But it is, perhaps, the end of the beginning."

E. R. N. Grigg, M.D.

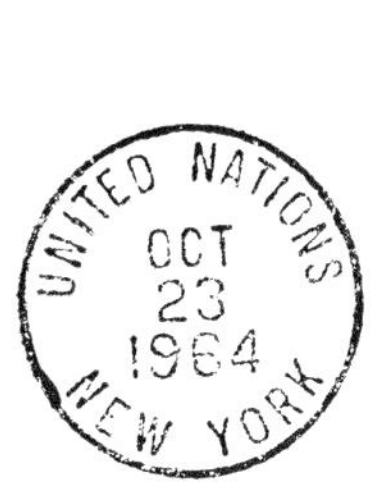

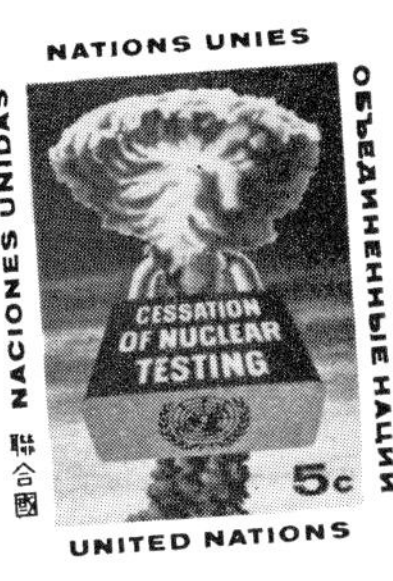

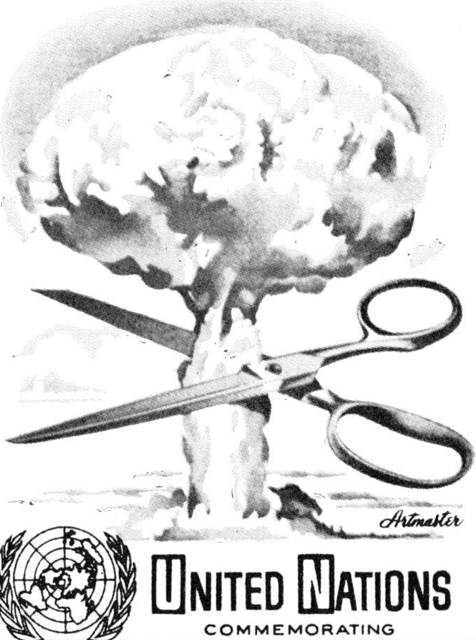

CONTENTS

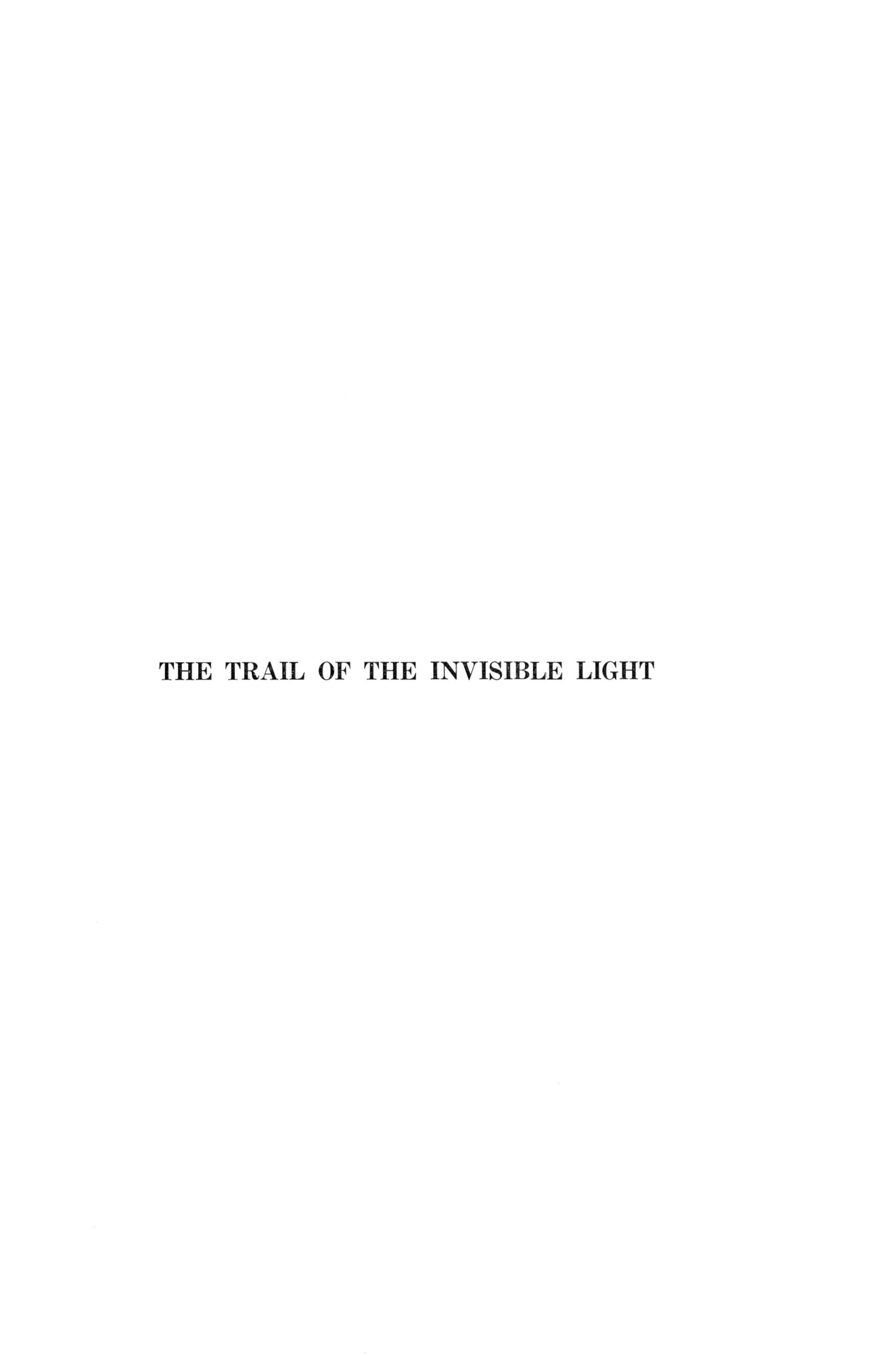

THE TRAIL OF THE INVISIBLE LIGHT

Chapter 1

THE FIRST CLINICAL ROENTGEN PLATE AND RELATED "FIRSTS" FROM THE YEAR 1896

Progress . . . is not an accident,
but a necessity
HERBERT SPENCER

A NEW SCIENTIFIC discipline may be based on a single, ground breaking advance, but has to be built with (*i.e.*, it cannot be built until after the development of) practical applications. And since relatively few people comprehend abstract notions, the importance given to the new discipline will depend on its "actual usefulness."

The author of the initial scientific breakthrough is usually well known, and so are most of his scientific forefathers. As the new discipline develops, diverging priority claims are attached to its practical contributions, because the latter tend to emerge at about the same time in different geographic locations (multicentric pattern). The authors of these "secondary" achievements deserve proper credit, and it is only fair to try to identify them. Besides, historic research in the sciences has its own rewards. It is always fascinating to go over the devious trails, unexpected twists, and odd time schedules which seem to prevail in the advancement of almost any discipline.

INTRODUCTION

In roentgen chronologies it is customary to encounter as a first authenticated entry the date of Sat-

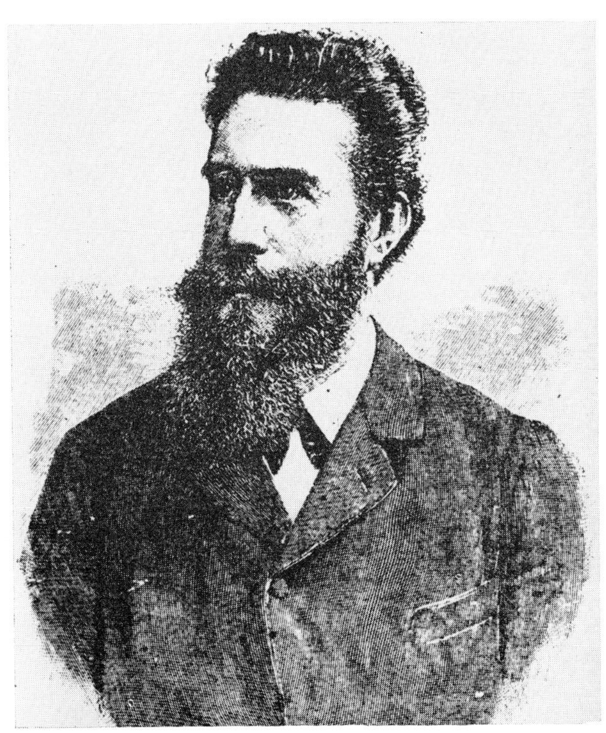

WILHELM CONRAD RÖNTGEN (1845-1923). A melted medal, a papered prize, and the *Diener* as discoverer — what price glory!

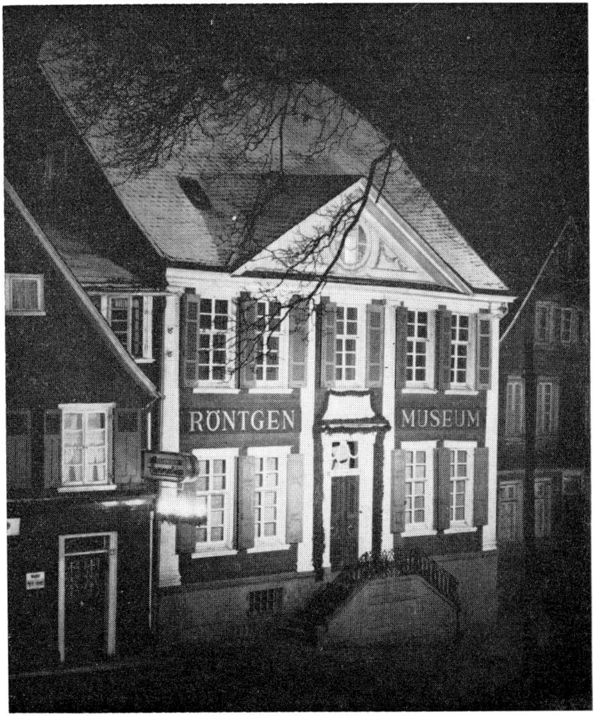

Coutesy: Ernst Streller.

RÖNTGEN-MUSEUM. It is located in Remscheid-Lennep (Germany), the birthplace of Wilhelm Conrad Röntgen.

urday, December 28, 1895. On that day Wilhelm Conrad Röntgen (1845-1923) submitted his now famous first "provisorial" communication, *Ueber eine neue Art von Strahlen* (On a New Kind of Rays): it was printed in the Proceedings of (as if it had been read before) the Würzburg Physico-Medical Society.

On Thursday, January 23, 1896 — before the same Würzburg society — Röntgen made his first oral presentation of the discovery. It was a slightly revised version of his initial text. To honor the occasion, as reported by Hoffa in the *Münchener Medicinische Wochenschrift* of January 29, the chair was held by the famous anatomist Albert Rudolf von Kölliker (1817-1905). After the lecture, Röntgen produced an x-ray picture of Kölliker's hand: among the preserved relics (seen by Etter in 1945), this is the glass plate of the hand with two rings. Thereupon Kölliker proposed the eponymization of the new agent, to be known henceforth as Roentgen's rays. On that same day (January 23) Arthur Stanton published in *Nature* the first British translation of the *New Kind of Rays.*

Röntgen was born in Lennep (Germany) on March

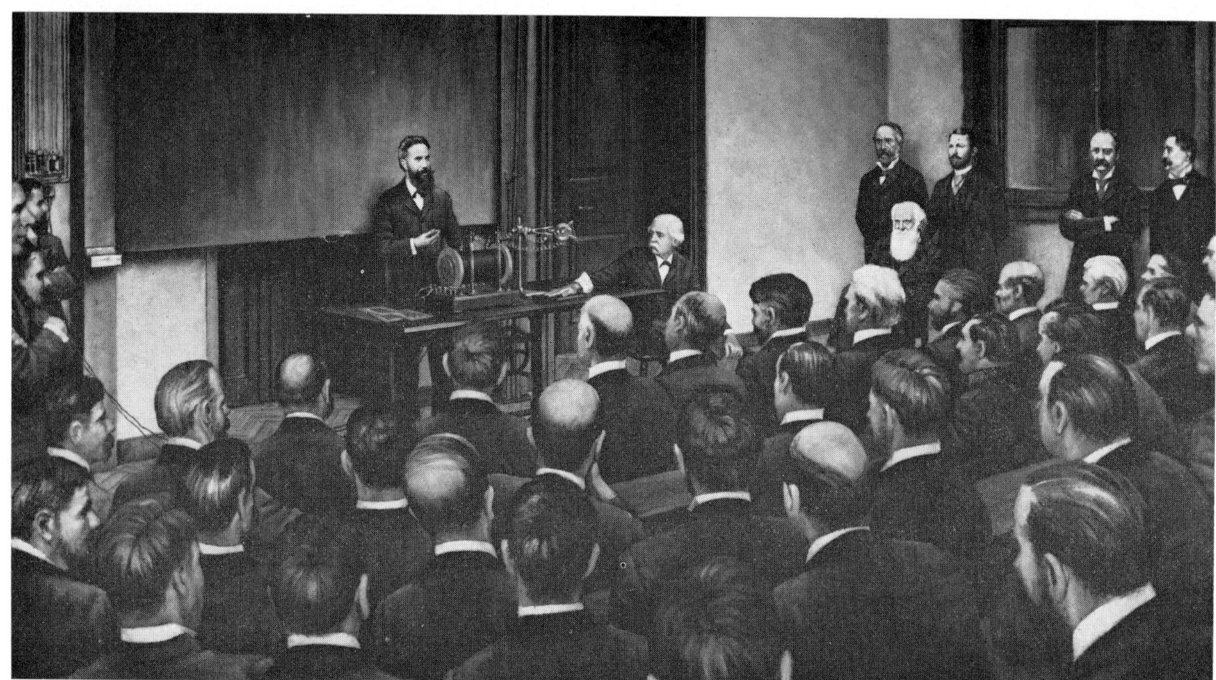

Courtesy: Parke, Davis & Co.

Röntgen's first public demonstration of x rays. This painting (copyright 1962, Parke, Davis & Co.) is one of a continuing series, the beautiful *History of Medicine in Pictures.* The first thirty pictures were published in book form (1961), after appearing in *Therapeutic Notes,* a promotional publication of Parke, Davis & Co., a Detroit drug manufacturer. The project is written and directed by a pharmacist-historian, George Almon Bender, while the paintings are executed by Robert Alan Thom. The paintings reveal a painstaking quest for historic accuracy. The research for this painting was conducted in Würzburg. The lecture hall of the Physics Institute (where this demonstration actually took place) had been destroyed. The lecture room of the Physiological Institute (constructed by the same architect, at the same time as the Physics Institute) provided the background for Thom's painting. This was fortunate because today also the Physiologic lecture room has been torn down. Of help in the collection of details and local color were two professors in the University of Würzburg, Robert Herrlinger (medical history) and Heinrich Schröer (physiology). In the painting Röntgen speaks, while Kölliker's hand is exposed to the rays. In the right-hand corner can be recognized several of those who had been present at that demonstration, for instance the sitting, white-bearded Von Leydig (anatomy), and standing, in front of the window, at the far right of the picture, the bow-tied Rindfleisch (pathology), seen in profile.

27, 1845. His eyes were kind (he was color blind, and had serious retinal damage in one eye, due to a childhood illness). His disposition was usually happy, but he was very shy. For the discovery, Röntgen received many distinctions, an honorary MD degree from the University of Würzburg, the (very first) Nobel Prize, the Rumford Gold Medal of the (British) Royal Society, the Iron Cross from Hindenburg, and others. During World War I, as a good patriot, Röntgen gave his Rumford medal to be melted down for its gold – he is said to have regretted the loss of the medal, but only after the armistice.

Röntgen refused to patent any part of his discovery, and rejected indignantly all "commercial" offers connected therewith. His professorial income provided him with financial security until the end of the war. During the postwar inflation he lost all his savings. Even the Nobel Prize money, which he had donated to the University of Würzburg for scientific purposes, turned into worthless paper.

In the last years of his life, Röntgen suffered deprivations, both financial and of other nature. He was also exasperated by humiliating remarks. One of the crucial moments of his discovery had occurred when a screen began to fluoresce, even though the energized Hittorf tube was covered with dark paper. That fluorescence was first noticed by Röntgen's laboratory servant (*Diener*, in German). This trivial fact was so distorted in some accounts as to have Röntgen complain he was being accused of stealing his *Diener's* discovery.

Röntgen's wife, born Anna Bertha Ludwig (they were married on June 19, 1872: no children, one adopted daughter) passed away in 1919. Röntgen himself died on February 10, 1923 with a carcinoma of the rectum, which had remained unsuspected to the very last. He is buried at his wife's side in the family grave in Giessen.

The actual date of Röntgen's discovery (*i.e.*, the day when he first grasped the significance of the penetrating quality of the new agent) has been a matter of debate. He was a man of few words, and of fewer friendships. Unwarranted personal attacks embittered the last two decades of his life, whence he became for all private purposes a recluse. Finally, in accordance with Röntgen's will, all his notes were destroyed after his death (Etter, 1946).

In December, 1908 Elmer Ellsworth Burns published in the *Popular Scientific Monthly* an interview with a practising physician from Chicago, Thomas Smith Middleton (1868-1934), who had allegedly been a "research student in physics" under Röntgen in the early 1890's. Middleton offered an involved fairy tale, regarding a photographic plate, and a book with a metallic key as a page marker. The book was lying on top of the plate and, when Mrs. Röntgen called for lunch, Mr. Röntgen laid an energized Hittorf tube on top of the book (and took off for the coffee break). The same "underlying" plate was subsequently used in outdoor photography and, when developed, revealed *also* the shadow of the key. Röntgen showed this puzzling photograph to the undergraduates, but nobody could offer any sensible explanation for the silhouette of the key. The master himself did not have an answer, but he kept on searching, and finally found one. As the Italians say, *se non è vero, è ben trovato* (if it is not true, it is well concocted). When asked about the date of the key incident, Middleton placed it before October of 1893, perhaps as early as 1892 (*sic*).

This little fable was widely quoted in the English literature, especially in this country. In 1931, Trostler communicated with Middleton himself, and obtained from him yet another date for that quaint affair with the key, the plate, and the luncheon, namely April 30, 1895.

As a matter of fact, it would have been out of character for the methodical Röntgen to leave an energized tube unattended. Middleton's narrative (which harbors also other technical flaws) is hardly more than barely plausible fiction, but it is intriguing, and has inspired a few bookplates, for instance that of the Canadian radiologist Gordon Richards.

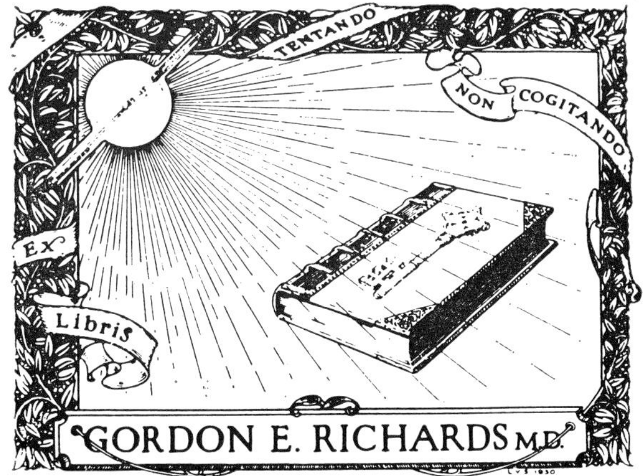

RICHARDS' PLAUSIBLY FICTITIOUS BOOKPLATE. "Professor Röntgen, what were you thinking when you made the discovery?" "I didn't think, I tried." *(tentando, non cogitando)!*

Röntgen's biographer, Otto Glasser (the physicist from the Cleveland Clinic), saw a letter written in March, 1896 by Röntgen's wife Bertha. The letter was for one of Röntgen's cousins, Mrs. L. R. Grauel of Indianapolis. In that letter Bertha recalled that one evening in November of 1895 she became angry with her husband who had failed to compliment her on the quality of the food. In the guise of explanation, he took her downstairs to his laboratory (which was in the same building), and introduced her to the wonders of the new rays.

The plate with the hand of Röntgen's wife—among the relics seen by Etter in 1945 it is the one with a single ring — was probably exposed on Friday, November 8, 1895. The latter date was mentioned by the reputable Scottish scholar, Edgar Ashworth Underwood (1946), director of the Wellcome Historical Museum. More recently, the same date was acknowledged by Konrad Weiss, the historiographer of the Austrian Röntgen Society. That date of November 8, 1895 is also accepted by Otto Glasser, and by most of the currently knowledgeable roentgenophiles.

LITERARY PRECURSORS

It is possible to locate roentgen-like descriptions in passages of poetic provenience, printed before 1895. One such example appeared in 1884 in the introduction to excerpts from the *Runes of Kalevala,* translated by Patricio Lafcadio Hearn (1850-1904) who, at that time, was still in New Orleans (*i.e.,* before his Japanese adventure). The passage reads:

"So fair was the virgin (daughter of the witch Louhi) that her beauty gave light like the moon; so white were her bones that their whiteness glimmered through the transparency of her flesh; so clear was the ivory of her bones that the marrow could be seen within them . . ."*

Roger Bacon (1214?-1294), the Franciscan monk better known as *Doctor Mirabilis,* offered a very definite premonition: ". . . there are many dense bodies which altogether interfere with the visual and other senses of man, so that rays cannot pass with such energy as to produce an effect on the human sense and yet nevertheless rays do really pass through without our being aware of it."

The name of John William Draper (1811-1882) is associated with that of the melancholic (and ultimately suicidal) Russo-German physicist Christian Johann Dietrich Theodor von Grothuss (1785-1822) in the eponym of a fundamental truism in radiology: only that amount of radiant energy which is absorbed can produce physical or chemical changes in matter or tissue. Draper, who became in 1850 the president of the Medical School of the University of the City of New York, had developed in 1841 the concept of "dark (invisible) tithonic rays" (a sort of light rays). This tithonistic theory (for which its author coined a long list of vocables, from tithonography to detithonescence) was first expounded in several articles in the *Philosophic Magazine,* and later incorporated in a book, the *Treatise on the Organisation of Plants . . . with a Memoir on the Chemical Action of Light* (1844), which contains many surprising sentences, such as:

"A large number of bodies obstruct the radiation of the tithonic rays, so that apparently shadows will remain on a sensitive plate. . ." Other passages are tantalizingly close to predicting the existence of what is known today as gamma radiation in sunshine. The latter quotations appear in his book on page 161 which – to complete the forebode – carries as the binder's signature the Roman numeral ten, *i.e., X.*

The German industrialist and natural philosopher Baron Karl von Reichenbach (1788-1869) published in 1846 his odd volume on the *od.* In his opinion, the *od* was a natural power which among other things was supposed to produce the phenomena of hypnotism. It could be incorporated in, or rather was emanating from, all matter. When it resulted from electrolytic action, it was called *electrodyle* or *electrod,* when it came from a magnet it was called *magnetod,* from the sun, *solod,* from the moon, *lunod.* By further developing his theory, Reichenbach came to believe that his *odic* rays passed through solids. Moreover, after experimenting with a magnet and a vacuum tube, he described odylic rays, to which he ascribed feats very similar to those later found with x rays.

In this context, another precursor was a Boston inventor and professor of physics at Tufts, Amos Emerson Dolbear (1837-1910), who wrote in April, 1894 in the *Cosmopolitan*:

"It is actually possible to take a photograph of an object in absolute darkness, with the ether waves set up by working an electric machine."

During the first days of February, 1896 Dolbear referred to his previous statement and claimed then to have photographed a five-point iron star by means of electric sparks from a static machine "through an ordinary table top, about one inch in thickness." This remarkable exploit — called "brush discharge effect" in contemporary jargon (Morton, Pupin) — is unfortunate in that it removes most of the significance from Dolbear's otherwise disturbing forecast of 1894.

ACTUAL PRECURSORS

Practically every historian of Röntgen's discovery begins his account by referring to the good, old names of those who contributed to the knowledge of electricity. Some go as far back as Gilbert's *De Magnete, Magneticisque Corporibus* (1600), a few recall even

*The *Kalevala* is a collection of heroic poetry, preserved in the folklore of Finland. It was first printed by two Finnish physicians, Zakarias Topelius in 1822, and then Elias Lönnrot in 1835 and 1849. The standard English translations of the *Kalevala,* by J. M. Crawford (1889) and W. F. Kirby (1907), contain nothing similar to Hearn's description of the "radiolucent" virgin.

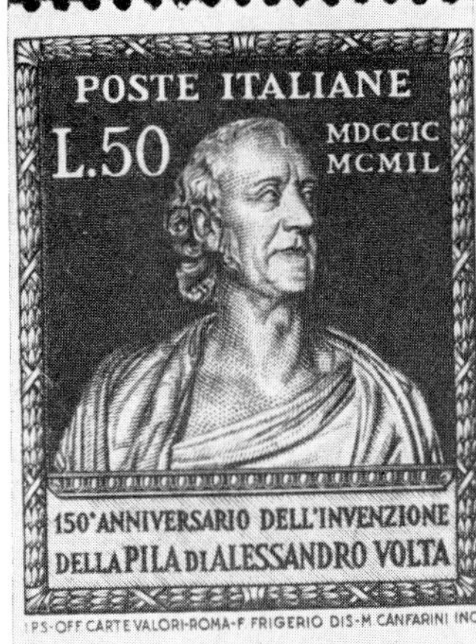

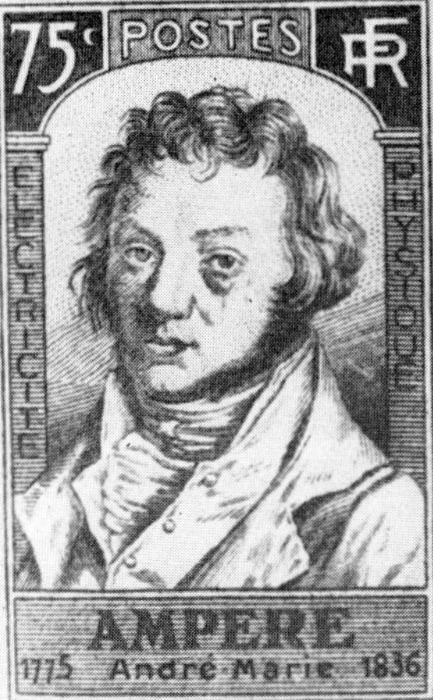

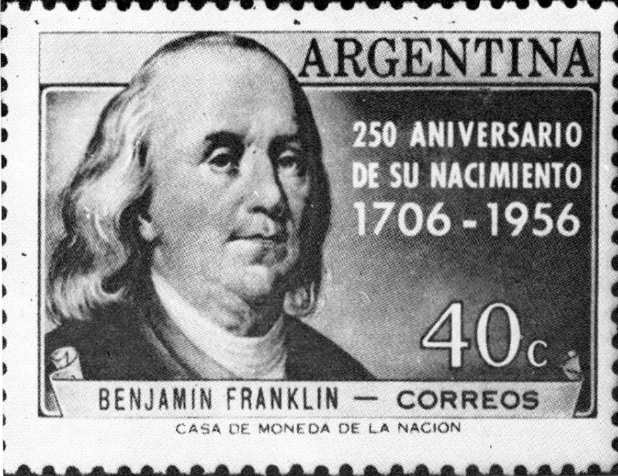

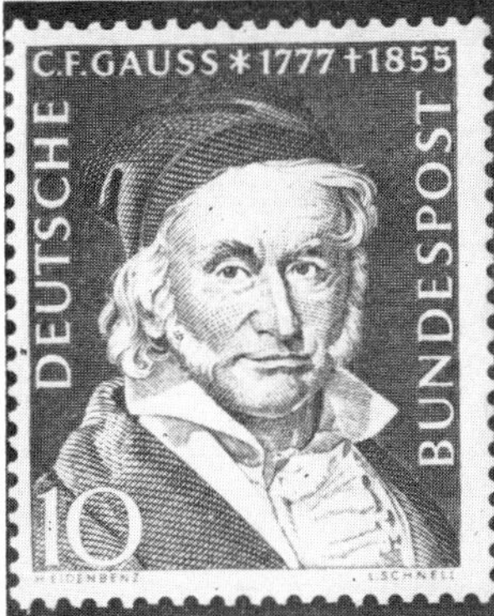

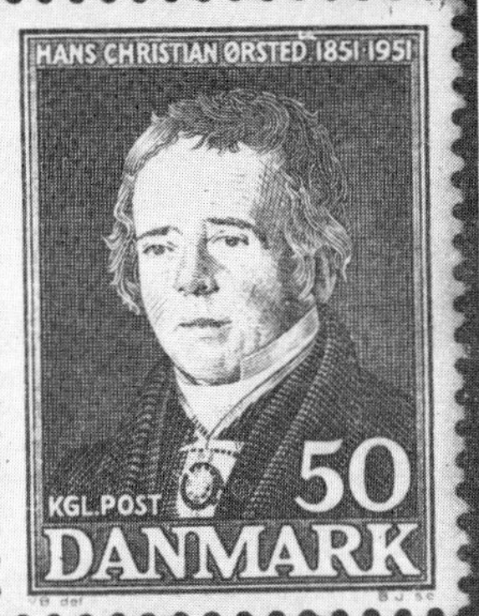

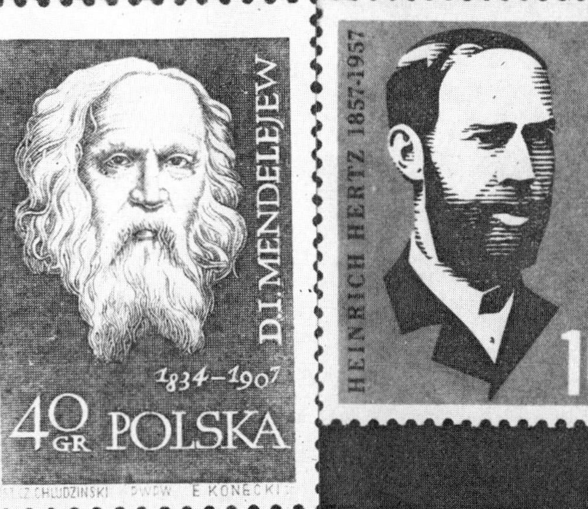

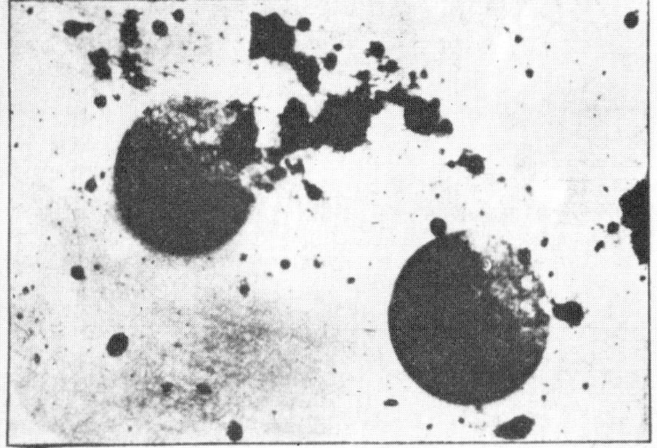

Courtesy: Bob Morrison

GOODSPEED'S FIRST SHADOW PICTURE. Produced in the University of Pennsylvania on February 20, 1890. The rounded shadows are coins representing Bill Jennings' carfare on the Woodland Avenue trolley. Goodspeed told Charlie Smith that Jennings was a plan-everything-beforehand type. Jennings was leaving and had just counted his coins. At that point Goodspeed asked Jennings' help in photographing the spark gap of a Ruhmkorff coil, so Jennings placed his coins on top of a plate while assisting in the positioning of the electrodes. They paid little or no attention to those circular shadows, but —after Röntgen's announcement—they repeated the experiment and understood the relationship.

the ancient times when the Phenicians (and the Egyptians before them) learned to carress the amber. It is less well known that x rays had been produced experimentally before Röntgen's date of 1895.

In the information given to *Who's Who,* Morris Wilbur Stine (1863-1934), a New York physicist and *bona fide* roentgen pioneer, noted that his first "sciagraph" had been exposed on February 14, 1892. In a letter to Glasser, the Philadelphia experimenter Arthur Willis Goodspeed (1860-1943) specified that he had obtained actual images of metallic objects in the winter of 1890, but he expressly and repeatedly denied any claims to priority, because at that time he had failed to interpret these unexpected shadows. The German physicist Philipp Lenard (1862-1947) — who had described (before 1895) the penetration of "cathode rays" through aluminum — was not so gracious and (as narrated by Etter), during the Nazi reign, Lenard used his political influence to revendicate at least part of Röntgen's glory.

Actually, all those who worked with electric discharges in rarefied gasses – as they were produced in the tubes of Heinrich Geissler (1814-1879), Johann

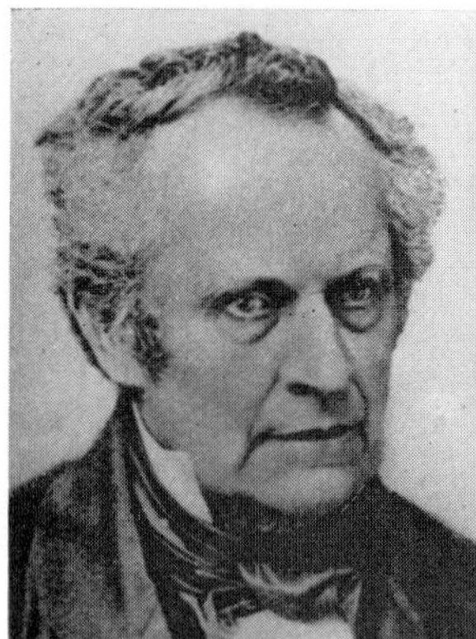

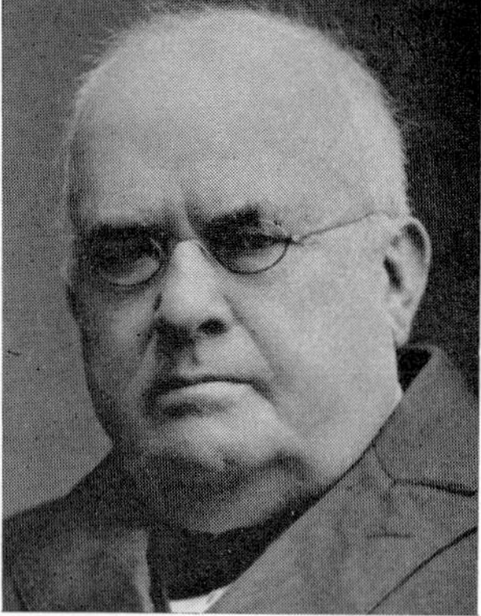

Courtesy: Deutsches Röntgenmuseum

JULIUS PLUCKER WILHELM HITTORF

Wilhelm Hittorf (1824-1914), and Sir William Crookes (1832-1919) – had obtained roentgen rays, at one time or another. The very first in this category was Julius Plücker (1801-1868), professor of mathematics in Bonn (Germany), who investigated–among other things–the effect of a magnetic field on electrical discharges in rarefied gasses.

In 1879, Crookes produced x rays when the vacuum of his tubes was high enough to give a pale green flourescence. He often found that photographic plates stored near his work table were fogged, in fact he complained to the manufacturer, and returned the "defective" plates. Crookes was obviously unaware of the real cause of this fogging (Russell Reynolds). Lenard had noticed that "cathode rays" penetrated through aluminum, and had established that these "cathode rays" were absorbed to a different degree by various materials: he was indeed on the threshold of the big discovery. But Röntgen was undoubtedly the first who realized the true significance of such a penetration – that was when he stepped – figuratively – through the magic door, as well as into the history of science.

The English "electrician" Francis Hauksbee, Sr. (?-1713) found that shaking mercury in a glass vessel produces light – which he called "mercurial phosphorus" – and noticed that this light was very vivid when the glass globe was exhausted of air, even changed color upon slight "attrition" (apposition) of the hands on the globe. In the 18th Century, experiments with electricity were quite fashionable, for instance the ecclesiastic French electrotherapist Jean Antoine Nollet (1700-1770) – who developed the "electrical egg" – actually repeated the experiments of

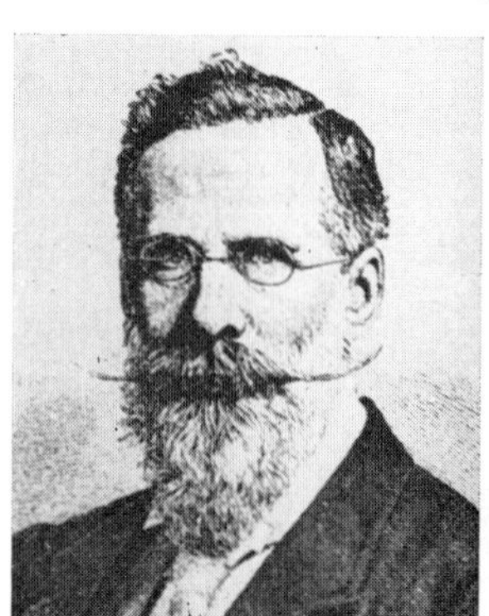

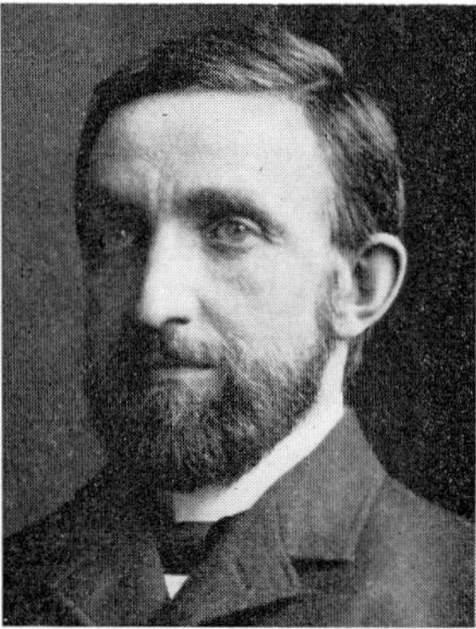

SIR WILLIAM CROOKES (1832-1919). Basically a chemist (discoverer of thallium in 1861), Crookes was knighted in 1897, one year after the vacuum tube (which he had improved sufficiently in 1873 to "spoil" his photographic plates in 1879) became in 1896 a household word because of its association with the Invisible Light. Crookes had come very close to discovering the x rays, because in 1896 he produced a satisfactory roentgen plate with one of the (Crookes) tubes made in 1876. Another contender came almost as close. PHILIPP LENARD (1862-1947)–on the viewer's right–was no more than a few months away from the discovery of the rays at the time Röntgen made his announcement.

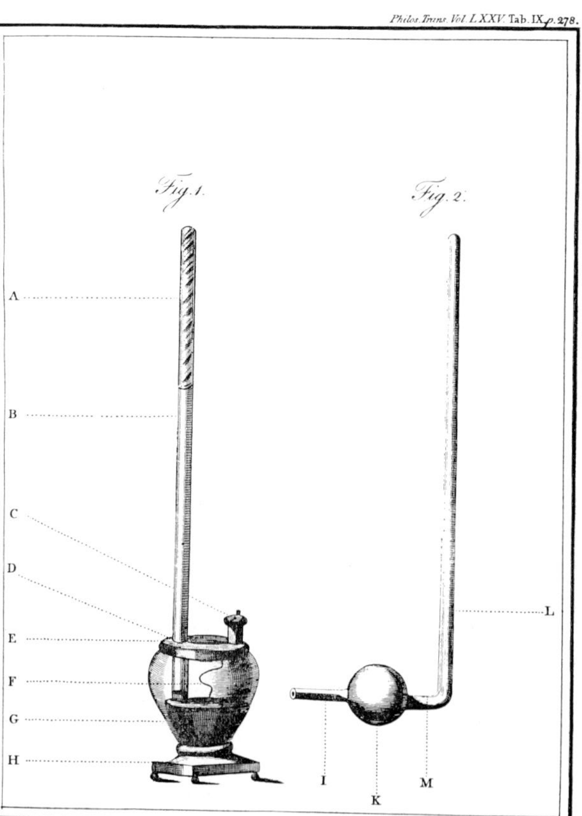

WILLIAM MORGAN'S "PERFECT VACUUM" MACHINE. He reported in the *Philosophical Transactions* of February, 1785 that – according to the length of time during which the mercury was boiled – the "electric" light turned violet, then purple, then a beautiful green . . . and then the light became invisible!

a certain (now no longer definitely identifiable) Boze.*

The first to produce (extremely soft) roentgen rays was probably the Welsh mathematician and chief-actuary of the (British) Equitable Assurance Society, William Morgan (1750-1833); his success was based on the use of a better vacuum, made possible by "boiling the mercury" which was a method originated by a certain (now no longer identifiable) Walsh. Morgan's unique communication was presented to the Royal Society on February 24, 1785 by an eye-witness, his uncle, the Rev. Richard Price (1723-1791). Morgan's experiments, made in 1784, were also witnessed by one of Price's good friends, an American "electrician" named Benjamin Franklin (1706-1790)!

JOURNALISTIC "FIRSTS"

In Glasser's chronology, it is noted that on January 2, 1896 Röntgen mailed reprints of the December 28, 1895 paper to his physicistic colleagues, for instance to Franz Serafin Exner (1849-1926) in Vienna, to Friedrich Wilhelm Georg Kohlrausch (1840-1910) in Göttingen, to Henri Poincaré (1854-1912) in Paris, and to Sir Arthur Schuster (1851-1934) in Manchester. Exner is said to have communicated the information thus received to a group of friends, one of whom was the physician Ernst Lecher* (1856-1926), son of the publisher of the *Freie Presse* (Vienna): this is how and why the news of Röntgen's discovery was first printed on Sunday, January 5, 1896 in the *Freie Presse.* From there it reached several European newspapers on Monday, and on the same day (January 6, 1896) a world cable was sent from the London *Standard.* It was received in the United States on January 7, and was reprinted on January 8 in several American newspapers (for instance in the New York *Sun*). Russell Reynolds has obtained from the British Museum a photostatic copy of the first account published in the morning paper Standard (London) on Tuesday, January 7, 1896:

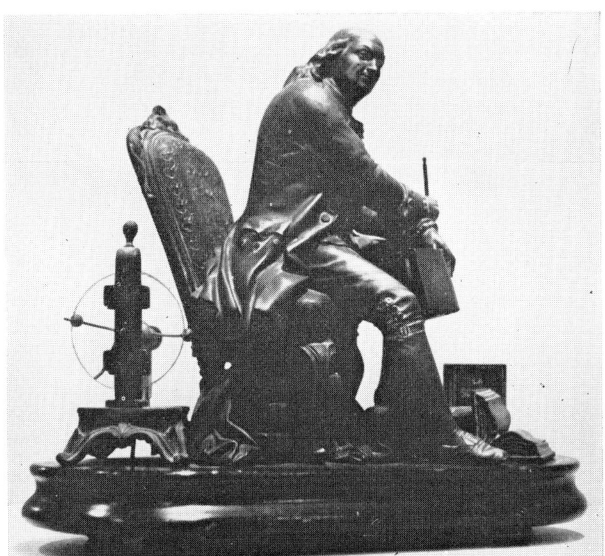

HE SAW THE LIGHT TURNING INVISIBLE. Statuette of Ben Franklin with the "electrical wheel", by unknown artist (courtesy of the American Philosophical Society: the statuette stands on a bookcase in the Auditorium of their Library in Philadelphia).

Vienna, Monday night

A very important scientific discovery has recently been made by Professor Röntgen, of Wurtzburg (*sic*) University, the details of which have already reached Vienna, and are now being carefully examined by several scientific authorities here. Professor Röntgen uses the light emitted from one of Crookes' vacuum tubes, through which an electric current is passed, to act upon an ordinary photographic plate. The invisible light rays, of whose existence there is already ample evidence, then show this peculiarity, that to them wood and various other organic substances are transparent, whilst metals and bones, human and animal alike, are opaque to those rays. That is to say, they will, for instance, absorb the rays which have passed through a wooden case in which bones or metals are enclosed. Thus it is possible to photograph in the manner described any bone or metals which may be contained in wood or woolen coverings. Moreover, as human flesh being organic matter acts in the same way as such coverings towards the invisible rays from the Crookes' vaccum tube, it has become possible to photograph the bones, say, of the human hand, without the flesh surrounding the bones appearing on the plate. There are photographs of this description already in Vienna. They show the bones of a hand together with the rings that were worn on the fingers — metals, as I remarked above, being opaque to these rays — but they show nothing else. They are ghastly enough in appearance, but from a scientific point of view, they open up a wild field for speculation. Among the practical uses of the new discovery, it is stated that it will henceforth be possible for surgeons to determine by help of this new branch of photography the exact position of any bullet that

*It was probably Bose, who taught natural philosophy at Wittemberg. He is quoted in the *Universal Magazine* (London) of July 1761 as having observed that the kisses of a lady, standing or sitting on pitch, and electrified by a glass globe, are as bad as wounds, in regard to the smarting pain felt by them.

* Incidentally, Lecher was the author of the first medical article on roentgen rays published (geographically speaking) in Czechoslovakia. It appeared in the *Prager Medicinische Wochenschrift* of February 6, 1896.

may be imbedded in the human body, or, again, to render visible any fractures there may be in the bones prior to performing any operation on the respective part of the body. And there are various other uses to which the new method may be put as for example, in connection with caries and other bone diseases. The *Presse* assures their readers that there is no joke or humbug in the matter. It is a serious discovery by a serious German Professor.

In the same Viennese newspaper, *Neue Freie Presse,* in date of January 23, 1896, was to appear

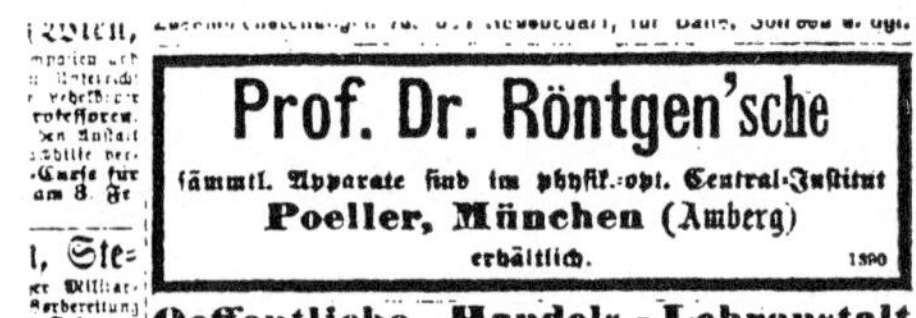

Courtesy: C. H. F. Müller Co.

World's first roentgen advertisement. This classified ad appeared on page 14 of the *Neue Freie Presse* (Vienna) of January 23, 1896, the same newspaper which had printed the very first news of Röntgen's discovery.

the world's first advertisement of x-ray equipment. It was printed in the classified section, indeed one wonders how did anybody ever pick it out, let alone preserve it for posterity.

The first notice of Röntgen's discovery in a scientific periodical was published under the title *Electric Photography Through Solids* in the *Electrical Engineer* (New York), dated January 8: it contained the text of the world cable. The first notice in the medical press came out on January 11,* both in the New York *Medical Record* and in the London *Lancet.* The former maintained a non-committal attitude (justified in the face of not otherwise confirmed newspaper reports), while the latter indulged in Dickensian jokes (Underwood). These, though, were by far not as painful (in retrospect) as the "famous last word" printed on January 10, 1896 by the London *Electrician:* their editorial writer belittled this "revolution in photography" mainly because "very few persons . . . would care to sit for a portrait which would show only the bones and the rings on the fingers."**

On January 24, the same *Electrician* (London) published a full translation of Röntgen's original communication together with a brief abstract of a lengthy and seemingly important paper by Jaumann, which had appeared in *Wiedemann's Annalen* under the striking title *Longitudinal Light.* Now the editorial writer remarked that "Röntgen, Lenard and others would appear to have discovered what Professor Silvanus Thompson has, with characteristic preference for the picturesque, termed "ultra-violet sound."

*In his reminiscences (1931), Trostler regarded Howard Van Rensselaer's article in the *Albany Medical Annals* of February, 1896 as the first medical notice.

**In his autobiography (1930), Swinton recalled that the x-ray plate of his own hand was shown in 1896 to the then Prince of Wales (later King Edward VII), who remarked, "how disgusting!"

Soon, physicists were asked to give written opinions on the subject, for the benefit of medical audiences. Their impressions were obviously favorable, like Schuster's article in the January 18 issue of the *British Medical Journal;* or a similar note in the February 3 issue of the *Berliner Klinische Wochenschrift,* signed by Eugen Goldstein (1850-1930), the astronomer who had discovered the canal rays. Medical editorials — which at that stage were better informed and thus more realistic than the very first one in the *Lancet* of January 11 — were published on February 1 in the *Medical Journal* and in the *Medical Record* of New York, and in the *British Medical Journal,* and on February 8 in the *Wiener Medicinische Wochenschrift.* Subsequent leading articles became more and more enthused, for instance in the retrodated February 15 issue of the *Maryland Medical Journal,* in the *Boston Medical and Surgical Journal,* finally even in the *Journal of the American Medical Association (JAMA)* in date of February 15, 1896.* It was an editorial, which *Radiology* reprinted in its (commemorative) issue of November, 1945. That editorial contained the following sentences:

"The further fact that in a general way only the density of the medium penetrated seems to affect them is suggestive of practical medical and surgical possibilities; it hints at future valuable physiological revelations as well as diagnostic aids. It is only a hint, however, and whether it is to be ever realized to any extent is perhaps open to serious question."**

The London *Standard's* correspondent in Vienna, when first learning of the new discovery, exhibited more medical insight as well as practical foresight

*The appealing title, *A New Formula for Craniographers,* in the *JAMA* of January 18, was a disappointment, in that it had no connection with roentgen rays. In fact, satisfactory views of the skull did not become available until much later.

**L. H. Friedburg, who taught chemistry and toxicology in the New York Homeopathic College, wrote in the *North-American Journal of Homeopathy* of April, 1896: "As far as the application of this new-born babe (the x radiance) for the purpose of medical diagnosis is concerned, very little can be said as yet."

than — five weeks later! — the *JAMA* editorialist. But then, the AMA is by definition and mandate obliged to be ultra-conservative in matters scientifical, which makes a both significant and inevitable difference in the manner of approach.

FIRST "INTENTIONAL" ROENTGENOGRAMS

Since (perhaps even before) Crookes' date of 1879, photographic plates had been exposed to roentgen rays — unintentionally, of course. Who was the first (after Röntgen) to produce an "intentional" roentgenogram?

In this regard, one of the most legitimate claims is that of the Scottish engineer Alan Archibald Campbell Swinton (1863-1930) who subsequently reconstructed the following timetable of his early endeavors: first (poor) roentgenogram on Tuesday, January 7; first satisfactory "metallic" roentgenogram (a razor in its paperboard casing) on January 8; first roentgenogram of a hand on January 13 (this is the one shown to the Prince of Wales); and first exhibit of these two plates on January 16, 1896.

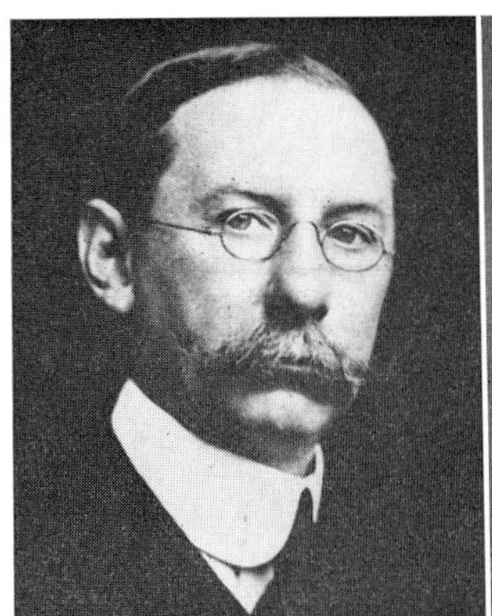
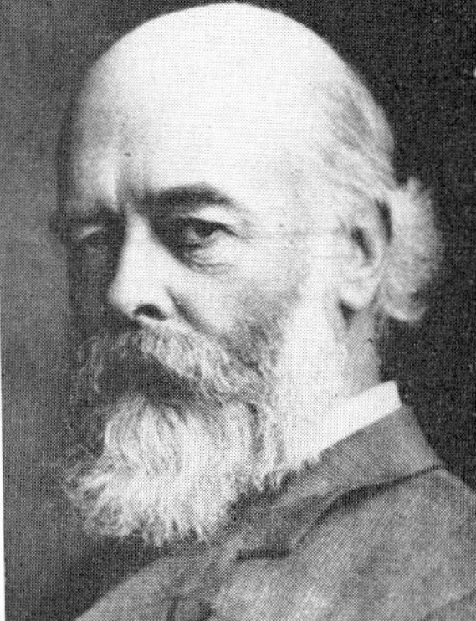

Campbell Swinton and Bearded Oliver Lodge

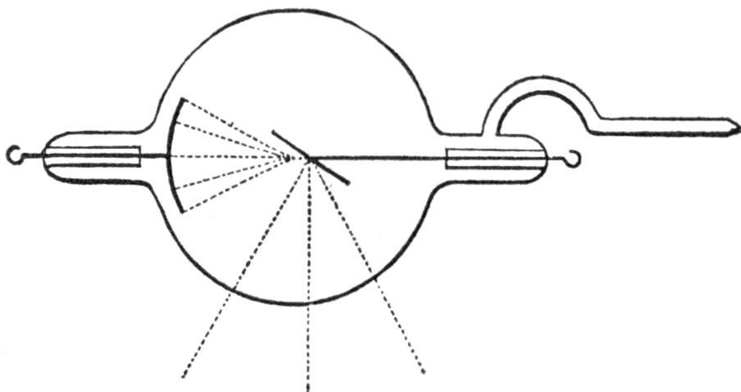

Focus tube. Claimed by, and ascribed to, many – it was originally designed by Sir Herbert Jackson (1863-1936).

It is interesting to note that the homemade tube Swinton used was operated, not by the usual induction coil, but by a Tesla high-frequency generator (Stead). His plates were first reproduced in *Nature* on January 23, and the following day in *Industries and Iron,* and in the *Electrical Review,* of London. These first English plates are now in the custody of the British Institute of Radiology.

Sir Oliver Joseph Lodge (1851-1940), who taught Physics in the University of Liverpool, wrote on Lenard's and Roentgen's rays in the London *Electrician* of January 31, 1896. A few days later, at the Royal Southern Hospital, Lodge – using a coil with a two-inch spark, energized by five storage cells – produced an "X-Ray Photograph" of a bullet embedded in a wrist: it was shown before the Liverpool Medical Institution on February 13, and published in both *Lancet* and *British Medical Journal* of February 22, 1896. That, however, was about one month after similar feats had been done in Germany and Austria.

Evidently, Sir Herbert Jackson (1863-1936) – who perfected the focusing cathode-ray tube, used extensively in the early years for the production of x rays – produced early plates in England. So did Schuster, and others, but they left no definite (or only late) dates.

In the *Moseley Society Journal* (Birmingham) of February, 1896 appeared the reproduction of the roentgen print of the hand of a local physician, J. R. Ratcliffe. The print had been made by the famous physician-photographer who was to become the famous radiologist John Hall-Edwards – but the date on that roentgen plate was February 12, 1896.

In this country a very bold claim was made by a former Serbian immigrant, the learned Michael Idvorsky Pupin (1858-1935), who had become professor of Mechanics and Electricity at Columbia University. In 1924, he wrote: "I obtained the first x-ray photograph in America on January 2, 1896, two weeks after the discovery was announced in Germany . . ." Surprisingly enough, this claim was widely ac-

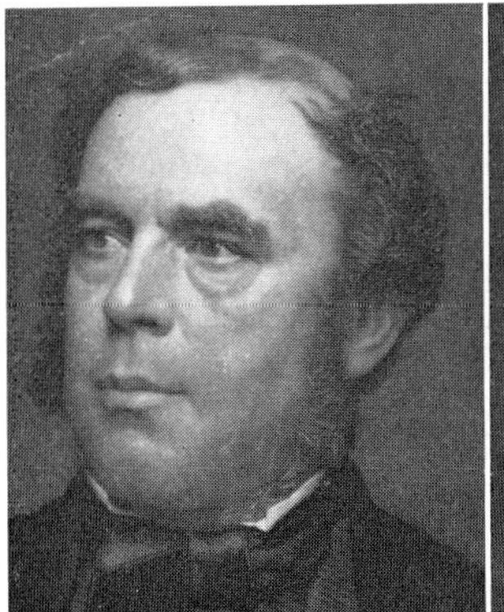
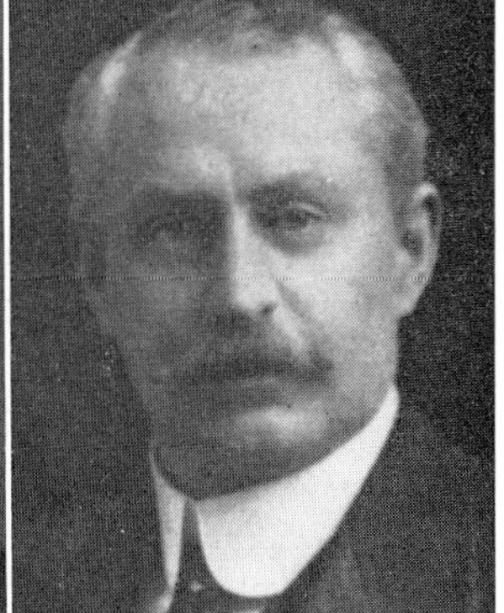

Courtesy: National Library of Medicine

John William Draper and mustachioed Sir Herbert Jackson

cepted in the American literature, as if it had been incontrovertibly substantiated.

Pupin's claim was acknowledged and believed by Robert Harvey Lafferty (1878-1950) of Charlotte (North Carolina), by the otherwise circumspect William Albert Evans, Sr. (1878-1940) of Detroit (in *Science of Radiology*), even by one of the most longevous pioneers of 1896, Leon Theodore LeWald (1874-1962) of New York City. Glasser, for one, did not accept Pupin's claim, and intimated that Pupin could have taken Röntgen's oral communication of January 23, 1896 as a baseline for his "two weeks," which would then bring his date closer to reality. I believe Pupin meant February 2, 1896.

ROENTGEN RAYS

AND

PHENOMENA

OF THE

ANODE AND CATHODE.

PRINCIPLES, APPLICATIONS AND THEORIES

BY

EDWARD P. THOMPSON, M.E., E.E.

Mem. Amer. Inst. Elec. Eng.
Mem. Amer. Soc. Mech. Eng.
Author of "Inventing as a Science and an Art."

CONCLUDING CHAPTER

BY

PROF. WILLIAM A. ANTHONY,

Formerly of Cornell University.
Past President Amer. Inst. Elec. Eng.
Author, with Prof. Brackett of Princeton, of "Text-Book of Physics."

60 Diagrams. 45 Half-Tones.

NEW YORK:
D. VAN NOSTRAND COMPANY,
23 MURRAY AND 27 WARREN STREET.

A PHYSICO-MEDICO-HISTORICAL CLASSIC. Edward Pruden Thompson was also the author of the *Inventor's Guide*. The reviewer of the *Electrical Engineer* called him a mechanical engineer, electrical engineer, chemist, professor, editor, expert, and patent attorney; this text proves that he must have been quite good at all of these.

The question deserved a bit of "literary" search. It turned out that on January 18, 1896, Pupin addressed the Henry Electrical Club (New York), and gave a very conventional talk on transformers. His first paper on roentgen rays (dated Saturday, February 1, and published on Wednesday, February 5, in *Electricity* of New York) was a summary of data from European sources.

Pupin's first roentgen plate is mentioned in his article written for *Science*, dated February 8, and printed on or about February 14. The reproduction of a roentgen print of metallic objects made visible (albeit "hidden") inside an aluminum box appeared in *Electricity* of February 12 (his date on that paper was February 11).

There is in addition an eye-witness account: on Friday, February 7, 1896 Pupin was seen exposing a photographic plate to roentgen rays "reinforced" by a fluorescent screen. The eye-witness was Edward Pruden Thompson.*

And since Pupin took his first "intentional" roentgenogram sometime between February 1 and February 7, it is quite possible that he worked on Sunday, February 2. During the first few days in a "new" month, it is not unusual to see the "old" month creeping up in some of the dates. This is how Pupin may have found in his notes the date of January 2, 1896 (which should have read February 2, 1896) as the day on which he first succeeded in producing a roentgen plate. He certainly deserves credit for having been the first who used a ("reinforcing") screen to shorten the time of roentgen exposure, and for this he was given credit in the editorial which appeared in *Electricity* of February 12, 1896. In such use of the fluorescent screen, Pupin edged ahead of Nikola Tesla (1856-

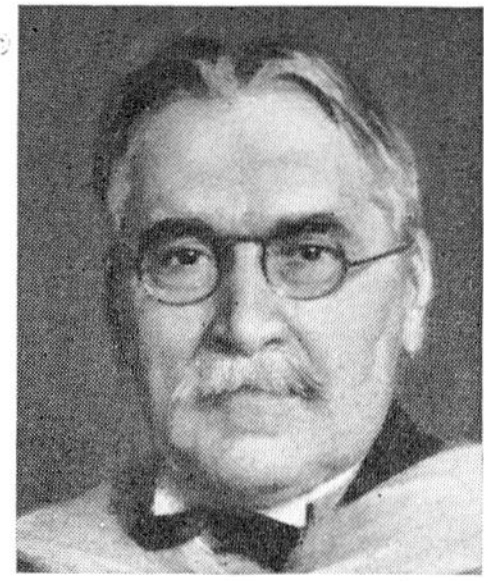

MICHAEL IDVORSKY PUPIN (1858-1935). Was it two weeks after the first or two weeks after the second beginning? Or was it simply misdated?

*Not much is known about Thompson, except that he was a patent attorney, and very knowledgeable in matters of electro-physics. He was also a stickler for dates, as he specified in one of his papers that on February 1, 1896 he conceived the idea (recently corroborated by roentgencinematography) that motion makes visible on the fluoroscent screen certain objects which were invisible while stationary.

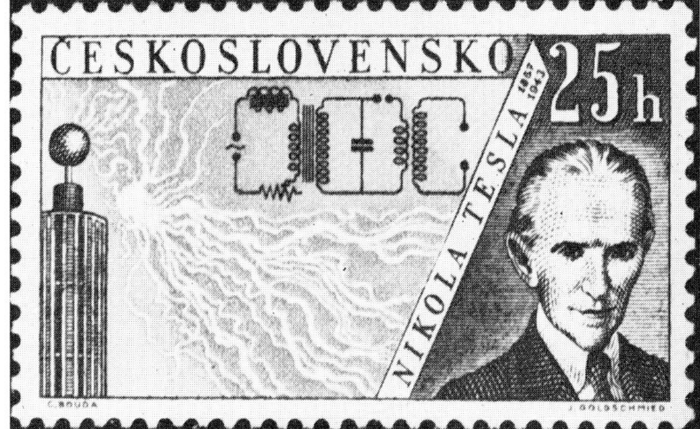

NIKOLA TESLA (1856-1943). A Yugoslavian immigrant (like Pupin), former associate and friend of Edison (like Pupin), electrician (like Pupin), with more laurels (Tesla motor, Tesla arc lighting, principle of rotating magnetic field) than Pupin: And yet, Pupin "invented" intensifying screens ahead of Tesla.

1943), and of Swinton, by a slim margin of weeks, perhaps only days.

It may be mentioned that in May, 1896 the British firm B. J. Edwards & Co. marketed the short-lived *cathodal plates,* which were photographic plates with fluorescent salts incorporated in the emulsion (the idea had been offered by Oliver Lodge).

In 1928, Preston Manasseh Hickey (1865-1930) contended that the first "intentional" roentgenogram in America was obtained by Thomas Alva Edison (1847-1931), the master mechanic who excelled in planned research for industrial purposes. Edison disdained "intellectuals" (not officially) and boasted that he could hire as many college graduates in mathematics (at $15.00 per week) as he wished, while no mathematician could hire him.

In 1927, Hickey asked Edison for details about his early work with roentgen rays. The answer, signed by Edison's secretary, William Henry Meadowcroft (1853-1937), stated: "Mr. Edison was the first to recognize the importance of the cable announcement of Dr. Röntgen's discovery. The same day he started to make the apparatus and had it finished and working the next day. Three of the metropolitan dailies heard of it, and for three weeks more than twenty newspaper reporters were stationed at the Laboratory." This sounded like a statement which one should be able to substantiate with reference to contemporary newspaper accounts. The earliest months of the collection of the New York *Times* of 1896 were perused, and this is what they yielded.

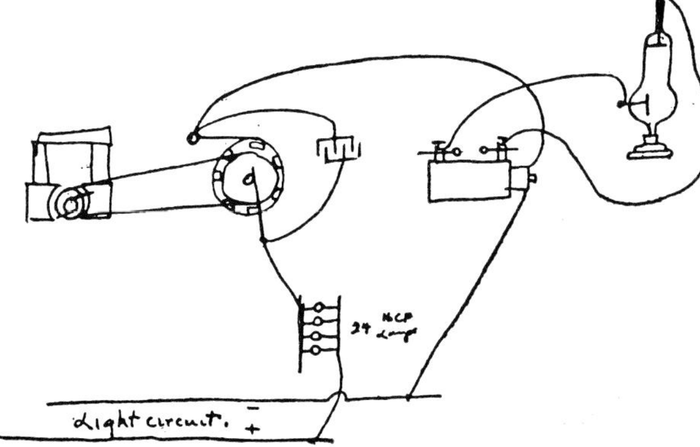

EDISON X-RAY WIRING DIAGRAM. One of his earliest experiments, with Hittorf tube, similar to one used by Röntgen.

Most of the attention was then focused on the Anglo-German crisis, caused by the Kaiser's telegram of January 3, 1896 in which he congratulated the (South-African Boer) Kruger for having successfully repressed a (British-inspired) raid, led by the Scottish-born physician Sir Leander Starr Jameson (1853-1919)). This is the "War" referred to in the world cable announcing Röntgen's discovery in the *Electrical Engineer* of January 8. The New York *Times* was obviously Anglophile, and its hostility toward the Kaiser permeated even some of the comments so sparingly bestowed upon Röntgen's discovery. In mid-January, the Anglo-German tension had abated somewhat, and an interview with Ogden Nicholas Rood (1831-1902), professor of physics at Columbia, published on January 16 (9-5) was labeled *Hidden Solids Revealed.* The big change-over came with the glowing account of the achievements of William Francis Magie (1858-1943), professor of physics at Princeton, printed on February 7 (9-3). The next day, on February 8 (9-7), *Times* brought its first interview with Edison – which had taken place on Friday, February 7, and which was followed by many write-ups during the remainder of February (these were the three weeks mentioned by Meadowcroft!). In his interviews, Edison stated repeatedly that his staff was trying to find the most favorable conditions for taking roentgen photographs, in the hope that some practical (*i.e.,* marketable) application would emerge from Röntgen's "purely scientific" discovery. During those three weeks, public interest was maintained by various publicity stunts, thus Edison mentioned that preparations were being made for a roentgen picture of his brain. These, though, were only intended as a stopgap. Edison's attempts to achieve something practical in this field were already centered on fluoroscopy.

In this respect, many claims and counter claims have been launched. People forgot that in the 1880's and 1890's cathode ray researchers knew of, and experimented with, fluorescence. Röntgen's use of a screen painted with barium platinocyanide was simply a continuation of these earlier experiments. Enrico Salvioni (1863-?) first showed his *criptoscopio* in Perugia (Italy) on February 5, 1896. Magie's *skiascope* came a few days later, while the screening device of Edison (it was called *vitascope* for a while, and then *fluoroscope*) was first mentioned on March 25, in Edison's first paper on roentgen rays, published in the *Electrical Engineer*. Salvioni and Magie had provided only more or less suitable enclosures for their screens, but Edison's staff tested a large number of substances (between 1200 and 8000, the actual number remained a secret), and came up with calcium tungstate, which was an obvious improvement over barium platinocyanide.

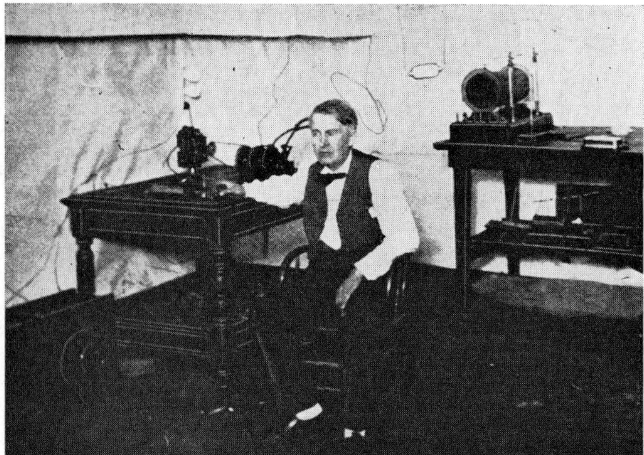

X-RAY BUTTON-PUSHING EDISON I. This promotional photograph was to have been an illustration of attempts at getting an "x-ray photograph" of the brain.

For that, Edison received much editorial praise, for instance in the *American Journal of Photography*, dated April 8, 1896.

From then on, Edison advocated fluoroscopy to the exclusion of plates, hoping that wide acceptance of this procedure would lead to the sale of so many more fluoroscopes. In the meantime, Edison also tried to develop a tube in which the energy was said to be transformed into light, and only very little, if any, into roentgen rays. This turned out to be mainly wishful thinking, because one of Edison's assistants, the glassblower Clarence Madison Dally (1865-1904) suffered visible radiation damage (alopecia), at which point Edison, always safety-minded, dropped all research on fluoroscopy.

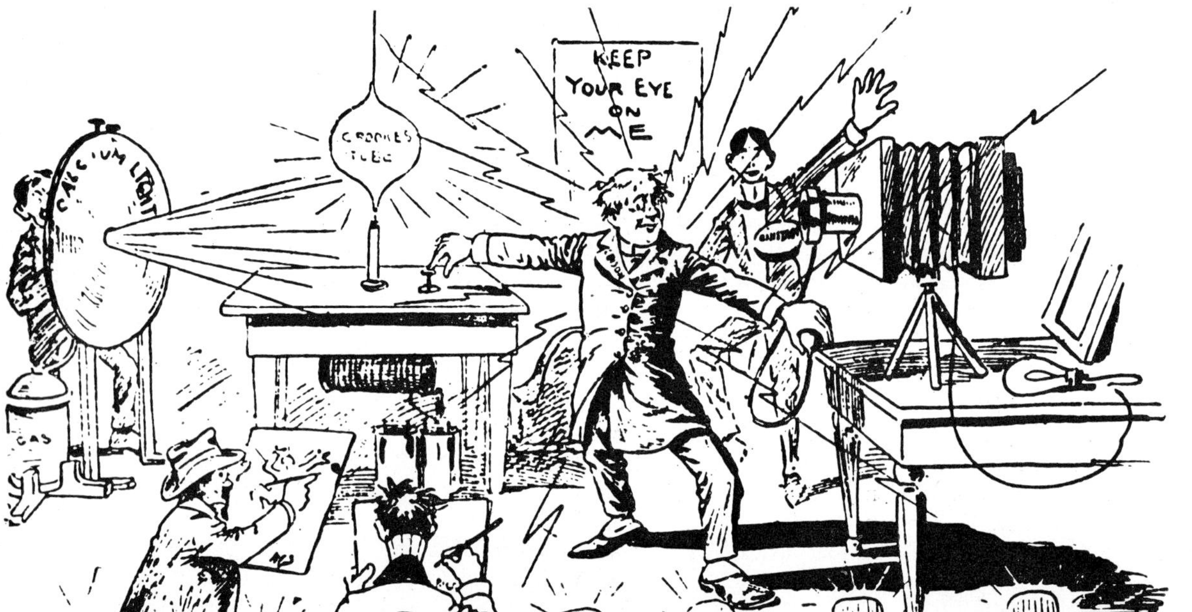

X-RAY BUTTON-PUSHING EDISON II. This shows much the same scene viewed by an irreverent, nay sacrilegious cartoonist.

Dally became the first radiation fatality in this country, but the first "x-ray burn" was inflicted in December, 1895 to the left hand of the Chicago roentgen pioneer Emil Herman Grubbé, a former chemist and subsequent homeopathic physician, who was then producing (and experimenting with) Crookes tubes: the ensuing "dermatitis" became visible in mid-January, 1896. A physician who saw that "dermatitis" referred to Grubbé a Mrs. Rose Lee, who received — on Wednesday, January 29, 1896 — from Grubbé the first therapeutic application of x rays. She had an advanced carcinoma of the left breast (years later, Grubbé would contend that the treatment improved her condition noticeably). Grubbé died in 1960, after almost one hundred mutilating operations for radiogenic neoplasia.

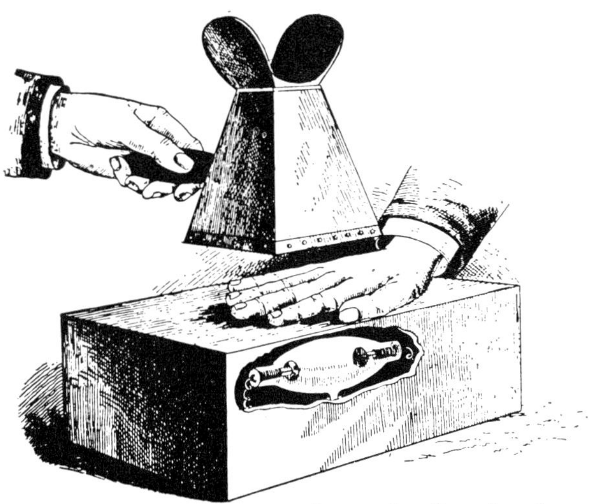

EDISON'S FIRST VITASCOPE. This is the first drawing of what was to be called forever after the fluoroscope. The term is regarded as an Americanism, and its coinage credited to Edison.

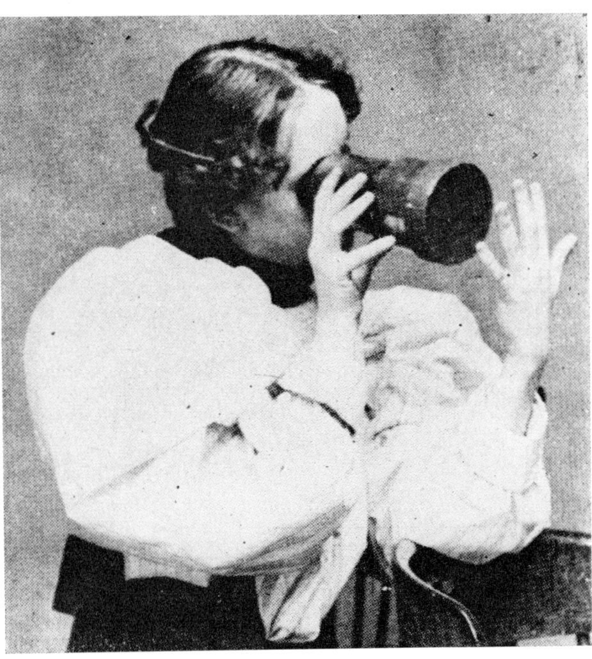

FEMALE FLUOROSCOPIC FAN. Photographs of female x-ray gazers are not common; this is a particularly becoming example.

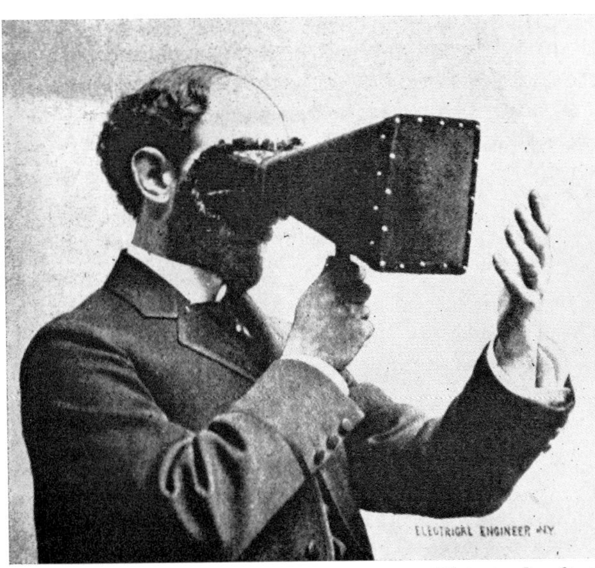

AFTER THE STOPGAP, A SELLING POINT. This is the first photograph of an Edison fluoroscope in actual use. This classic stance of 1896 cost many people the skin of their hands.

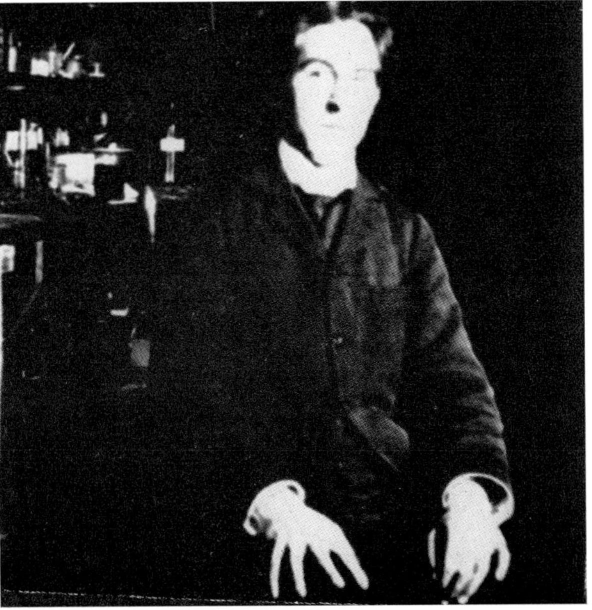

EMILE HERMAN GRUBBÉ (1875-1960). Photograph taken in 1895 shows the young assayer-chemist's impeccable hands shortly before their radio-scorching started.

There is another definite priority claim for the first "intentional" roentgen plate in America. The educator Henry Louis Smith (1859-?) had built a set-up to demonstrate cathode-ray experiments to his junior class. The set-up was located in the physics laboratory at Davidson College in North Carolina. On Sunday night, January 12, 1896, three of the students – Osmond Barringer, Eben Hardie, and Pender Porter (the latter became subsequently a practicing physician in New York) – returned surreptitiously to the laboratory, and with three hours of exposure obtained the roentgen image of several objects (egg, keys, etc.) on a Kodak plate. Its print was recently reproduced in the *Du Pont X-Ray News* (nr. 22, no date).

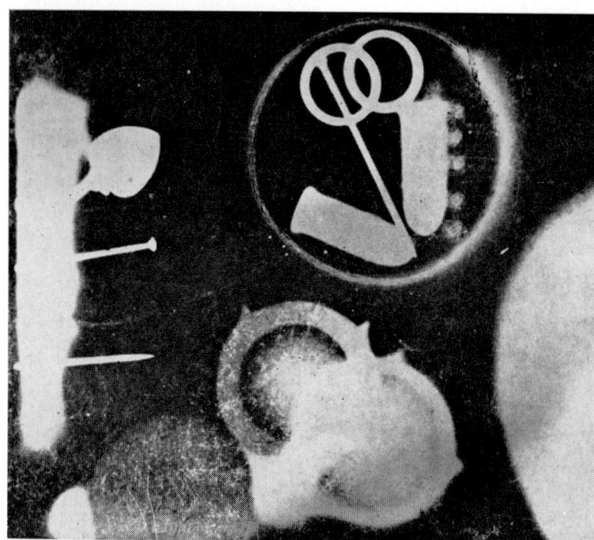

Courtesy: DuPont X-Ray News.

Varsity victory voided. Both early and authentic metallogram, initially embellished with the apocryphal date January 12, 1896.

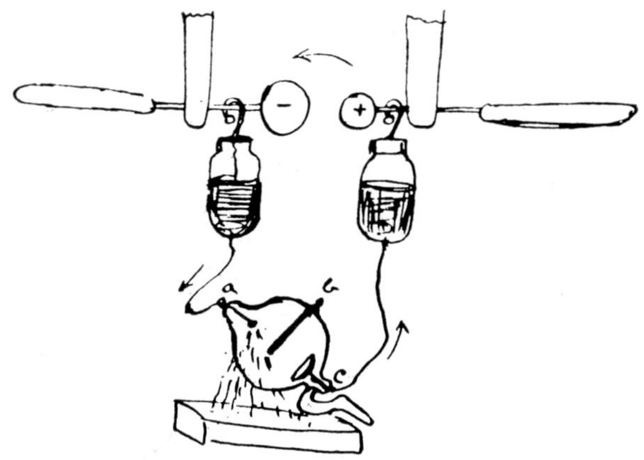

Meanwhile at Lynn (Massachusetts). Autographed wiring arrangement of first roentgen experiment of Elihu Thomson (1853-1937), founder and director of General Electric's first Research Laboratory.

The students were at first afraid to confess their deed, and when they finally gave the news to Smith, he had to verify their statement experimentally. All these delays taken into account, it still seems odd that the first newspaper story of this event did not appear earlier than on Thursday, February 27, 1896 in the Charlotte (North Carolina) *Observer*.

One can hardly assume an inadvertent alteration of the month, which would transfer the event from the almost mythical January 12 to a very reasonable February 12. In 1896, Lincoln's birthday (February 12) fell on Wednesday – which may not have been too religiously observed in a Southern college – or else the "Sunday night" detail was added by consulting a calendar.

The technical flaw in the story seems to be the excessive exposure. It would indicate that previous experiments, with shorter exposures, had been attempted. Otherwise, why did they decide on three hours of exposure when the usual was one to one and one-half hours? Furthermore, at that time, not too many tubes (if any at all) withstood continuous operation for three hours. Nevertheless, the first "intentional" roentgenogram in America was probably produced in the physics laboratory of an educational institution, if not in the first, certainly in the second half of January, 1896. This is why the story of the junior student trio seemed so credible to many previous writers (Evans, Sr., Glasser, Trostler, Lafferty), including the respectable Charles Goldie Sutherland (1877-1951) from the Mayo Clinic.

Others have tried to determine who obtained the first roentgenogram in America, for instance Otto Glasser listed twenty-three names of possible contenders among the pioneers: Albert Algernon Atkinson (1867-?), professor of physics in Ohio University at Athens; Florian Cajori (1859-1930), a mathematician from Colorado College; William Hermann Dieffenbach (1865-?), a New York physician who specialized in hydrotherapy and short wave applications; Daniel

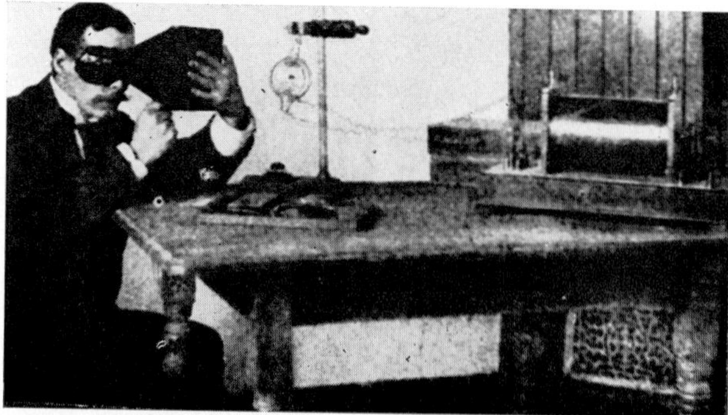

Daniel Webster Hering (1850-1938). Photograph taken in March, 1896, shows the noted science writer and columnist in the classical stance of the pioneer testing the hardness of the tube during the exposure of the objects placed on top of the plateholder.

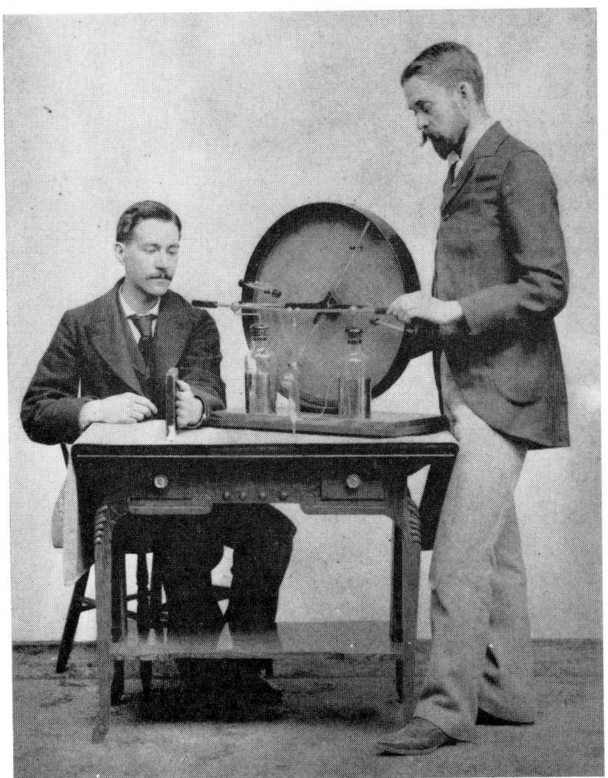

Courtesy: General Electric

ED JERMAN IN 1896, turning the static machine while unidentified friend has his hand in the beam.

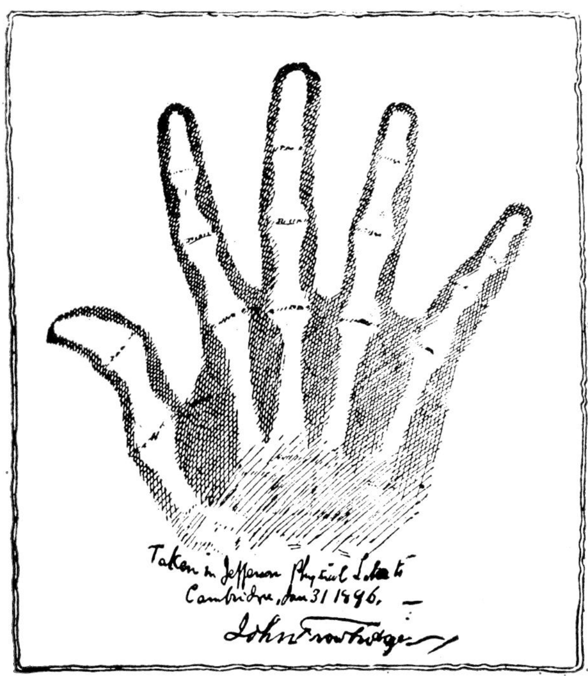

ALMOST BUT NOT QUITE THE FIRST. Autographed drawing of roentgen plate executed at Harvard University by John Trowbridge (1843-1923) on January 31, 1896. He came in second-best, one day after Wright at Yale.

Webster Hering (1950-1938), a New York physicist who wrote the well known *Foibles and Fallacies of Science;* the electrical engineer Edwin James Houston (1847-1914) of General Electric; the expert in gaseous radiation Charles Clifford Hutchins (1859-?) from Brunswick, Maine; Edward Clifford Jerman (1865-1936), who at the time was building Patee static machines, and later joined General Electric X-Ray Company; Arthur Edwin Kennelly (1861-1939), who

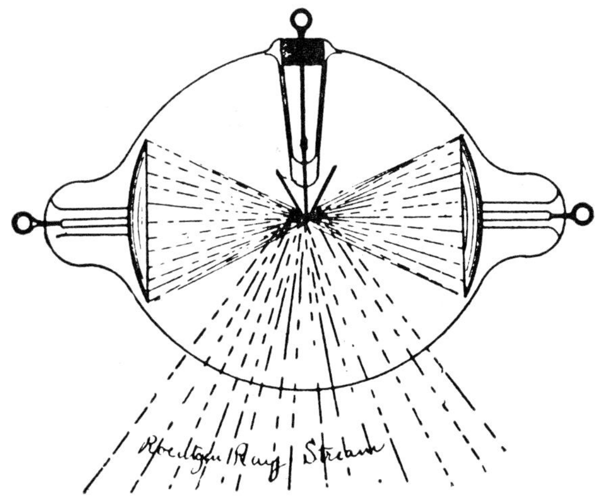

THOMSON'S STANDARD ROENTGEN TUBE. Diagram of a twin-focus arrangement usable for either direct or alternate current: the vertical electrode with twin deflectors is the anode, while the other two are cathodes, connected to a single pole when direct current is employed.

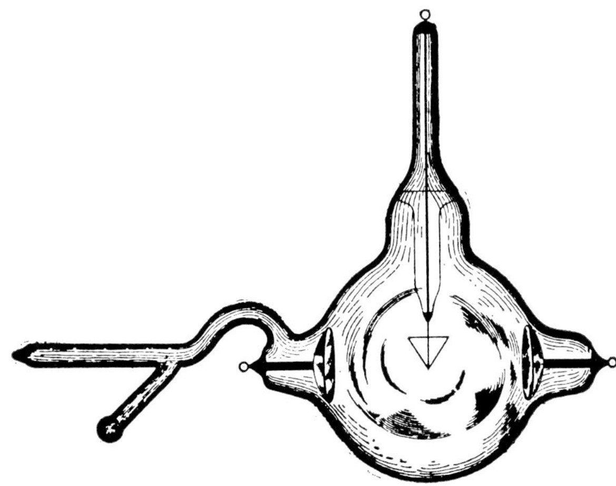

THOMSON'S TWIN-FOCUS TUBE. Drawing of actual design, with platinum wedge-shaped anode and two concave aluminum cathode cups; usable on either the low or the high-frequency coils, including Thomson's roentgen-ray transformer of 1896; the additional outpouch was filled with a chemical mixture which, when heated, would give off "steam" to reduce vacuum and thus correct over-hardening.

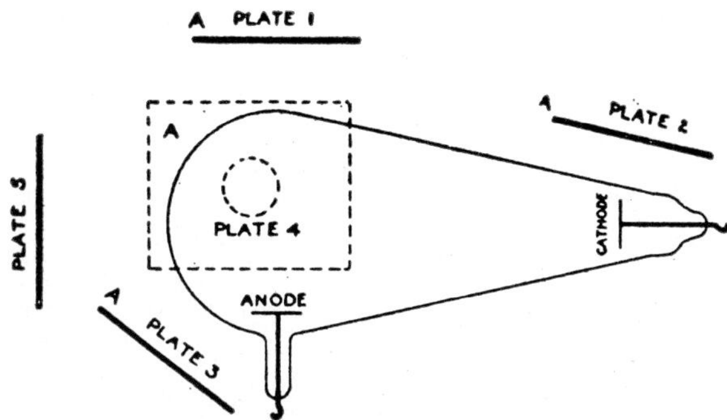

Early endeavors. With this excellent experimental arrangement of photographic plates around an energized tube (*Electrical World* of April 11, 1896), Morris Wilbur Stine proved that the "invisible rays" were produced in the glass of the tube (he also hypothesized: on the inside part of the glass!).

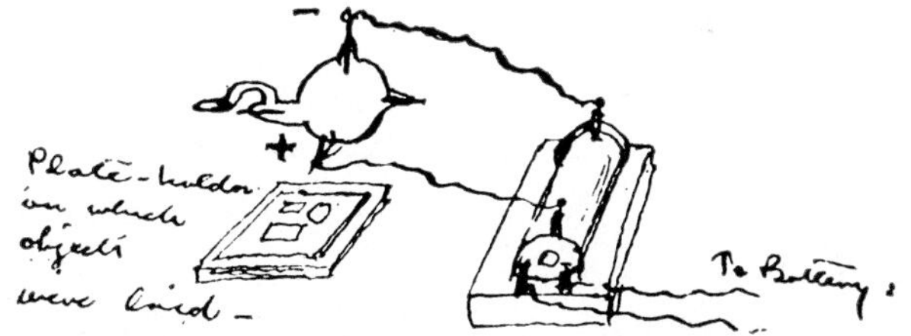

Wright's wiring diagram. Autographed sketch of arrangement for producing first metallogram in the U.S.A. by Arthur Williams Wright (1836-1915) at Yale University on January 30, 1896.

first worked with Houston, then gave his name to the ionized (Kennelly-Heaviside) atmospheric layer; Ernest George Merritt (1865-1948), a physicist from Cornell; George Sylvanus Moler (1851-?), also at Cornell; James Powell Cocke Southall (1871-?) of the Miller Training School in Albermarle, Piedmont; and the famous John Trowbridge (1843-1923), who reformed the teaching of physics at Harvard. Glasser mentioned also Cattell, Cox, Edison, Frost, Goodspeed, Meadowcroft, Miller, Norton, Pupin, Stine, and Wright, whose full names are given elsewhere in this paper. As with any listing, other "contending" names could be added, for instance the physicist Benjamin Franklin Thomas (1850-1911) of Ohio State University, who became a (questionable) radiation casualty; the historian of American homeopathy, William Harvey King (1861-

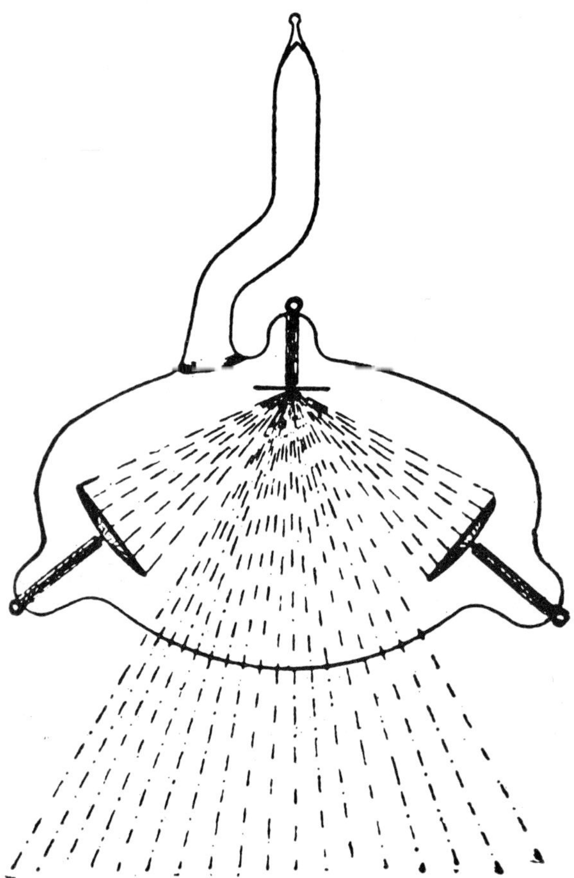

Swinton's Alternate Current X-ray Tube. British model of twin-focus tube, for use on Tesla high-frequency transformer; tube made by Alan Archibald Campbell Swinton (1863-1930), who was also the first (after Röntgen) to produce a roentgen plate – on January 7, 1896.

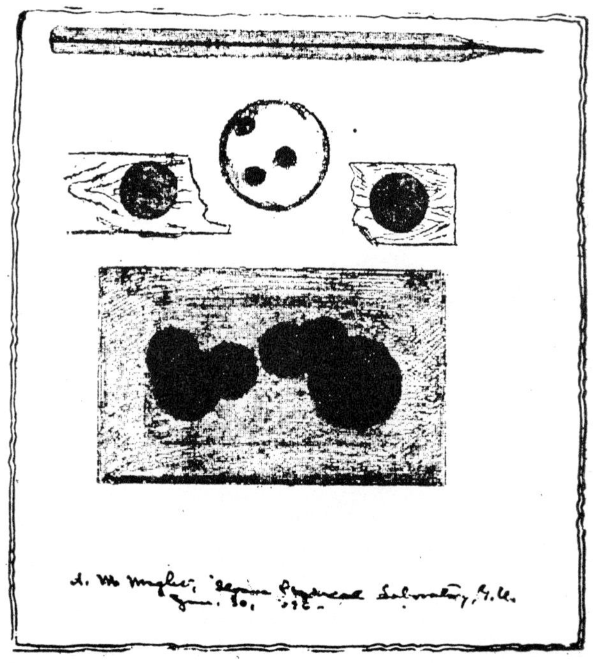

First metallogram at Yale. Autographed and dated drawing of Wright's first "metallic" roentgen plate (January 31, 1896). This remains to date the first authenticated roentgen plate produced in America.

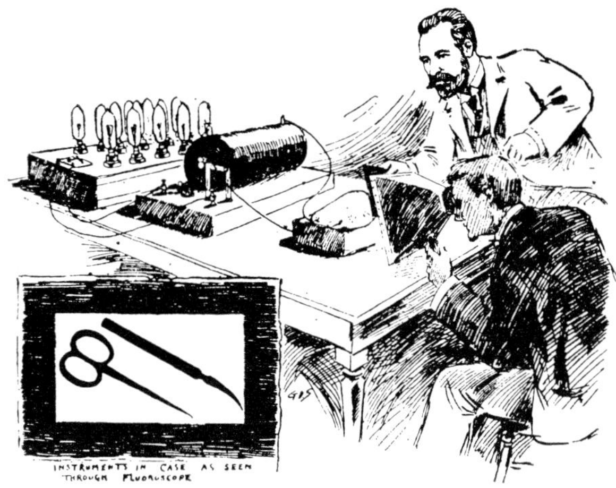

John Townsend Pitkin (1858-1935). He is the bearded figure watching as his friend, Edgar H. Stevens (a physicist and chemist) gazes into the home-made cryptoscope – the insert shows what he saw.

Pitkin, a physician, became a roentgen martyr.

1942) of New York Medical College; and Elihu Thomson (1853-1937) who originated stereo-roentgenography.

As far as records go, in America the earliest "intentional" roentgen plate was a *cathodograph* produced on January 27, 1896 by the Yale physicist Arthur Williams Wright (1836-1915) in his laboratory at New Haven (Connecticut). It was reported in the *Electrical Engineer* of February 5, in *Science* of February 14, and in the *American Journal of Science* of March, 1896.

There was some controversy over who initiated metallography. Röntgen himself produced a plate showing a double barreled shotgun with "thin spots." An editorial in the *Electrical Engineer* (New York) reported that x-ray plates, investigating the solidity of a weld, had been made at Carnegie Steel in Pittsburgh, with little or no success. Another American editorial, printed in the *Electrical World* of February 8, 1896, credited Swinton of London with the first successful roentgen examination of a weld. In 1927, however, in *X-Rays, Past and Present,* the British authors Pullin and Wiltshire bestowed upon Wright of Yale the priority for the first adequate roentgen examination of a weld.

In Russia, the first intentional roentgen plate was produced on January 16, 1896 in the Physical Institute in Petrograd, by N. G. Egorov. Another important Russian roentgen pioneer was the physicist Prince Boris Borisovich Golitsyn (1862-1916). Alexander Stepanovich Popov (1859-1906) — the renowned radio engineer who first used a wire high in the air as an antenna — was the first to install a "floating" roentgen department on the Russian cruiser "Aurora" in Kronstadt harbor.*

60-ЛЕТИЕ ИЗОБРЕТЕНИЯ РАДИОТЕЛЕГРАФА
1895–1955
А.С.ПОПОВ
1 РУБ.
ПОЧТА СССР
1 РУБ.

ПОЧТА СССР
А.С.ПОПОВ ДЕМОНСТРИРУЕТ АДМИРАЛУ МАКАРОВУ ПЕРВУЮ В МИРЕ РАДИОУСТАНОВКУ
50 коп

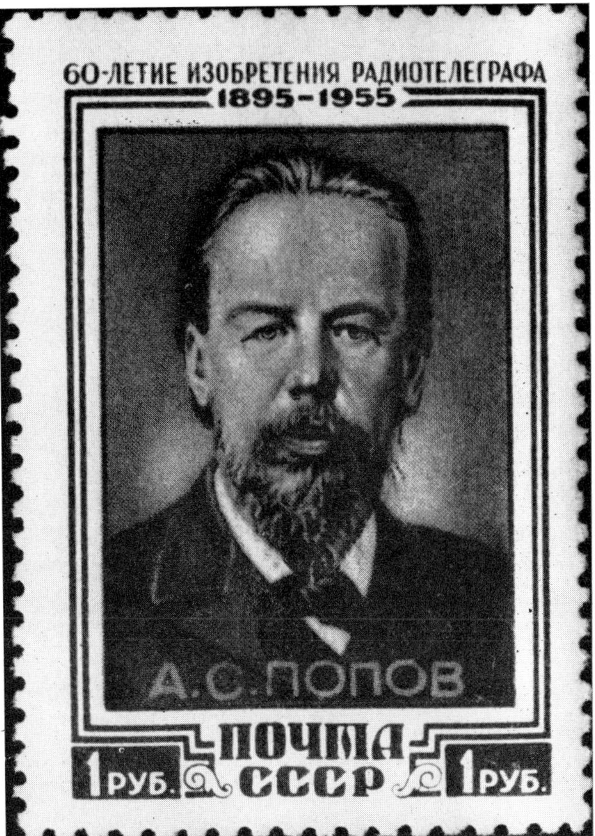

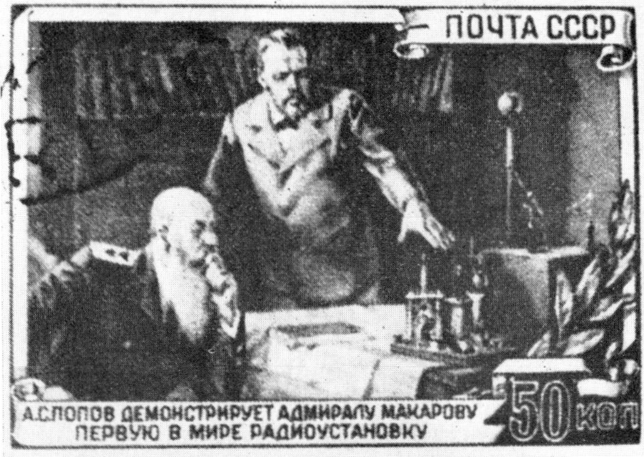

Alexander Stepanovich Popov (1859-1906). Russian roentgen pioneer – better known for his inventions in "wireless telegraphy," especially the antenna. This and other (but not all of the) topical stamps herein reproduced are from Stanley Paul Bohrer's collection.

*It soon became fashionable to use the same apparatus (and the same energy sources) for both wireless telegraphy and for the production of x rays on board of warships. A thesis on this subject, by H. J. Voille, was printed in 1896 at Bordeaux (France).

In Australia, the first announcement of Röntgen's discovery appeared in the form of two small paragraphs in the Sydney *Daily Telegraph* of January 31, 1896. The following day, a reporter from that paper made an inquiry with all sorts of people, from photographers to university professors, but nobody seemed to have heard of Röntgen or his rays.

The first intentional roentgen plate on Australian soil was produced on March 3, 1896 in the Physics Laboratory of Melbourne University by Sir Thomas Rankin Lyle. It was the representation of the right foot of the professor of chemistry Orme Masson, as mentioned in the Melbourne *Argus* of March 4. The print was reproduced in the *Australasian* of March 14, 1896.

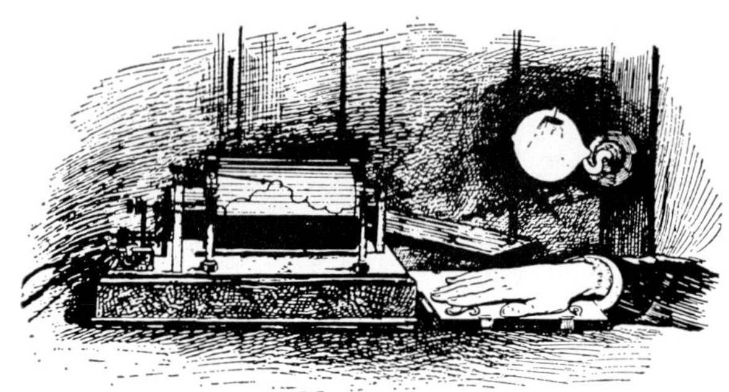

AUSTRALIAN ARRANGEMENT. The engraving is reproduced from the *Australasian* of March 14, 1896, but it could not be the drawing of the very first roentgen plate produced at Melbourne University on March 3, 1896 – because that was the plate of a foot.

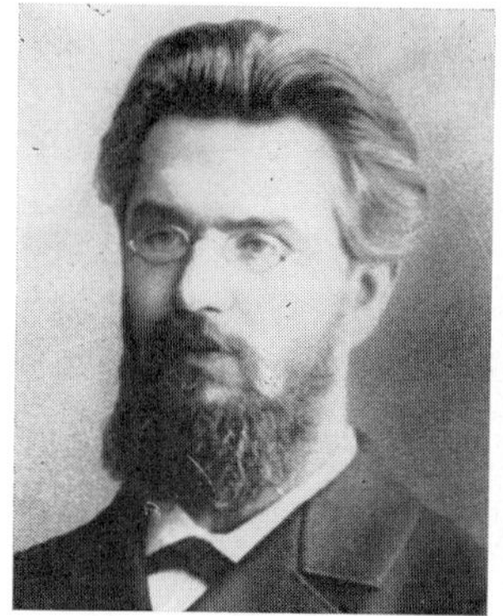

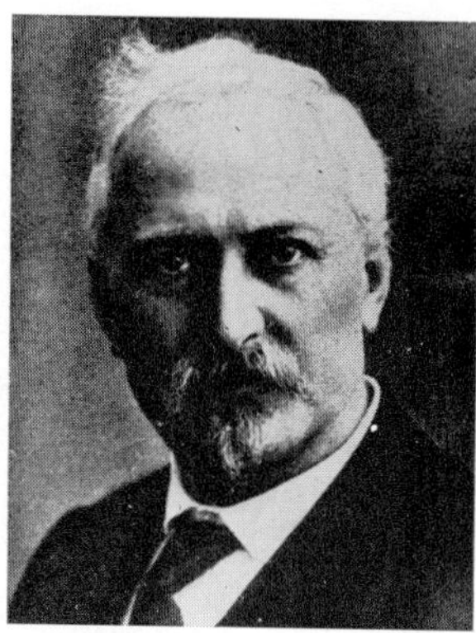

Courtesy: André Bruwer

NIKOLAI GRIGORIEVICH EGOROV (1849-1918). A mathematical physicist, director of the Physical Institute in Petrograd, who produced the first roentgen plate in Russia. On the right, in black tie, is white haired ANGELO BATTELLI (1863-1916). During his tenure as chairman of the Department of Physics in the University of Pisa, Battelli produced the first roentgen plate in Italy, and showed it on January 25, 1896.

In Italy, Angelo Battelli (1863-1916), director of the Istituto di Fisica in the University of Pisa, showed his first "metallic" roentgen plate on January 25, 1896. His first publication, jointly with the professor of mathematical physics Giorgio Antonio Garbasso (1871-?), appeared in the *Nuovo Cimento* of February, 1896: it contained a mention of the possibility of photofluorography, which chronologically preceded that of Bleyer. The first "scientific" article on roentgen rays printed in Italy was a review of foreign achievements, presented by Monsignor Francisco Regnani before the *Accademia dei Nuovi Lincei* on January 19, 1896. Augusto Righi (1850-1920), the experimental physicist in the University of Bologna, published in 1896 a dozen papers on x-ray technology.

The only possible contender to Swinton's priority remains Jenö Klupathy (1861-1931), a Hungarian cathode ray expert who was professor of physics in the University of Budapest. A newspaper release, based on a world cable, originated in London on Saturday, January 11, 1896 and reproduced in the *Electrical Engineer* (New York) of January 15, stated that Klupathy had repeated Röntgen's experiments and had tested the penetrability of several substances.

At this point Jozsef Végh of Budapest – who is the publisher of *Magyar Radiologia* – was asked to clarify the question. He referred it to his associate Balazs Bugyi (a radiologist from Budapest who is currently compiling the history of early Hungarian radiology): he informed me that, as far as could be determined, Röntgen's original communication was published in translation in the *Pester Lloyd* on January 16, 1896. On that same afternoon, in the auditorium of the Mathematical-Physical Association of Budapest, Klupathy demonstrated the production of x rays, then exposed and developed the plate of the hand of their famous physicist, Baron Lorand von Eötvös (1848-1919). On January 21, E. Hogyes published in the *Orvosi Hetilap* the first medical paper on (bone) radiology, then V. Wartha summarized current knowledge for the *Termeszettudomanyi Közlöny*. The latter article contained a print of von Eötvös' hand, but the text of Klupathy's first communication was never published. Klupathy's early date (at least January 10, 1896) is substantiated by the original cable, but otherwise Swinton's priority of January 7, 1896 is still valid.

IN BERLIN

The hagiographer of American radiation martyrs, Percy Brown (1875-1950) of Boston, stressed the fact that there occurred everywhere a distinct "premedical" stage, during which (medical) radiology was in lay (meaning non-medical) hands. This is true if only by reference to Röntgen, who was a physicist. For various reasons, the "premedical" roentgen stage was shorter in Germany and Austria than it was in England and America.

Early radiologists were recruited among all medical specialties, but two groups prevailed numerically: former surgeons, because of their interest in fractures and foreign bodies, and former neuro-psychiatrists, because of their knowledge of electricity (they were the ones to apply most of the electrotherapy then in current use.) The first physician ever to address a medical audience (actually the first individual to address any audience) on the subject of roentgen rays was the psychiatrist Moritz Jastrowitz (1839-1912): on Monday, January 6, 1896, he presented before the Verein für Innere Medicin (Berlin) a summary of Röntgen's preliminary communication, and showed the "single ring" plate (as reported in the *Berliner Klinische Wochenschrift* of January, 13). One week later, on January 13, before the same audience, Jastrowitz exhibited a "metallic" roentgenogram, made by Paul Spiess, chief-physicist of a manufacturing plant (Urania-Werke) in Berlin.

On Wednesday, January 15, Richard Neuhauss (1851-?), a general practitioner from Posen – it is today's Poznan (Poland) – brought before another society, the Berliner Medicinische Gesellschaft, a few roentgen plates, but still only of metallic objects. That was reported in the same *Berliner Klinische Wochenschrift* of January 27.

Finally, on January 20, Jastrowitz demonstrated before the same Verein several "clinical" roentgen plates, one of which was reproduced in the text of his paper in the *Berliner Klinische Wochenschrift* of January 30: it reveals a glass splinter retained in the middle finger of the left hand (of a glassblower from the Urania-Werke). Jastrowitz noted that this plate had been exposed eight days before – counted back from the day of presentation (January 20) – which would mean January 12, and that day was Sunday. If he had the plate on Sunday, why did he not show it on Monday, January 13, together with the "metallographs"? Such retroactive dating (of which we shall see several other instances) was facilitated by the date of publication of his text (January 30). It indicates that priority claims were already being handed out. Incidentally, in the paper dated January 30, Jastrowitz mentioned that during the session of January 20 he showed several other "clinical" plates (not reproduced as illustrations in the text), including the stump of an amputated phalanx, and a fractured limb in plaster cast, both from children. All these had been produced by Spiess.

The *Electrical Engineer* (New York) of March 4, 1896 related that on Thursday, January 30, Baron von Büol-Berenberg, president of the German Reichstag, invited ministers and members of the legislature to the Session Hall, where "Professor Spiess" demonstrated the production of x rays. In his explanatory remarks, Spiess predicted that science would soon develop a method to photograph the contents of secret documents through letter boxes. The only solution to such inconvenience would be to use lead in the construction of mailboxes.

IN PARIS

There was no true "premedical" roentgen stage in France. At the time, the Académie des Sciences turned out to be the clearing house for the earliest communications on roentgen rays. The champion in this field became the physicist Jean Baptiste Perrin (1870-1942). And yet in France the very first "intentional" roentgen plate (that of a healthy hand) was produced, on or before Friday, January 20, 1896, by two physicians, Paul Oudin (1851-1923) and Toussaint Barthélemy (1852-1906).

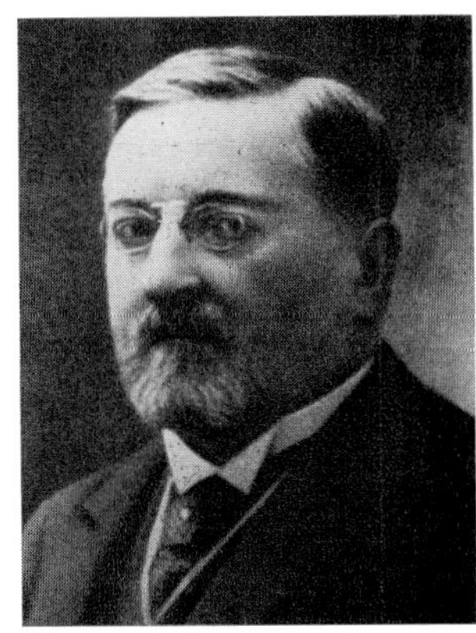
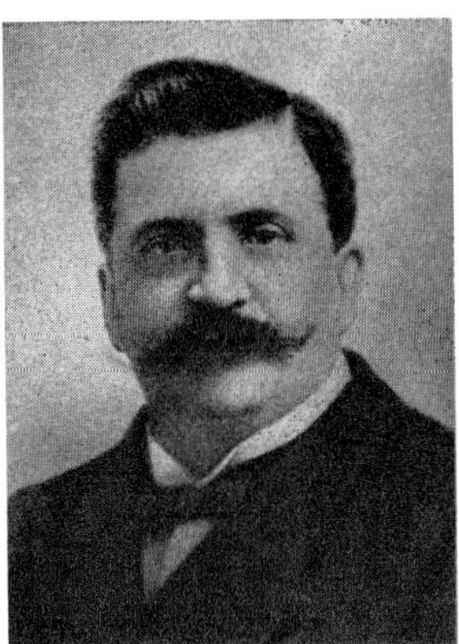

Courtesy: Oudin's photo from Mlle Elizabeth Baudry, French Ministry of Public Health; Barthélemy's photo from Mlle Antoinette Béclère.

First roentgen flash in France. Paul Oudin (1851-1923) and Toussaint Barthélemy (1852-1906) produced the first roentgen plate in France. It was a hand, and the plate was shown by Henri Poincaré to the Académie des Sciences on January 21, 1896, and by Fournier to the Académie de Médecine on January 28. Oudin (left) became a well known radiumologist and therapist, Barthélemy was trained syphiligrapher.

As was the custom in Romanic countries, the chief of their department – in this case the famous surgeon from *Hôpital Trousseau,* Odilon Marc Lannelongue (1840-1911) – appeared as the senior author of their first communications. On January 27, 1896 they showed to the Académie des Sciences their first clinical roentgen plate: it was a case of tuberculosis of the distal interphalangeal joint of the third finger on the left hand, which they also presented to the French Académie de Médecine on January 28, this time without Lannelongue.

On January 27, before the Académie des Sciences,

the physician and sociologist Gustave Le Bon* (1841-1931) delivered what was probably the first (honest) roentgen hoax: he assumed the existence in visible light of a "dark component" (including roentgen rays), and exhibited photographic plates "darkened" by the "black light" of a kerosene lamp, "filtered" through a steel plate (*sic*). Believe it or not, this method was "improved upon" by Murat (of Havre): he replaced the kerosene lamp with a Bunsen burner, hoping to thus adapt it to clinical problems. Murat's first "results" were reported in the *Bulletin Médical* (Paris) of February 19, and were abstracted in the *JAMA* of March 21, 1896. In line with AMA policy, this article, having been published in a legitimate periodical, was classified as a legitimate clinical study and as such deserved proper recognition.

IN PRAGUE

A letter from Wenzl Karl Friedrich Zenger (1830-1908) — a specialist in sunspots, residing in Prague — was read, on February 10, before the Académie des Sciences in Paris. He first referred to his extra-large induction coil, custom-built in 1865 by Heinrich Daniel Ruhmkorff (1803-1877) himself: it delivered a kingsize spark of 45 cm (about 17 inches).** A Crookes tube, energized by this coil, could be placed at 60 cm from the photographic plate.

With Zenger's letter came three prints, one of a thumb with a retained glass splinter, one of a healthy hand, and one of a hand with bone destruction (allegedly) caused by syringomyelia. On February 24, before the same Paris Academy, was read a second letter from Zenger — dated February 17 — in which he explained that the plates shown on February 10 had been made at the Bohemian Technical Institute in Prague by the professor of physics Karl Domalip (1846-1909), and by his assistant Brozet. And Zenger specified that these plates had been produced between January 11 and January 20, 1896.

At the time, professor of physics in the Prague Electrotechnical Institute was Johann Puluj (1845-1918), who in 1882 had perfected a "phosphorescent" version of the Crookes tube. Puluj soon adapted his tube to the "new" procedure. On January 31, 1896, the laryngologist Friedl Johann Pick (1867-1926) showed to the German Medical Society of Prague a clinical roentgen plate (made by Puluj) of a hand with bone tuberculosis: this was reported in the *Prager Medicinische Wochenschrift* of February 13. And Puluj made a report to the Wiener Königliche und Kaiserliche Akademie on February 20, 1896.

Had local competition forced Zenger and associates to select faraway Paris for the exhibition of their products? Zenger's revendicatory (second) letter of February 17 was just two days older than the publication date of the minutes of the session during which Pick showed his first case in Prague. And Zenger's retroactive date of January 11 seems to provide a trim margin even over the (alleged) date of January 12, given by Jastrowitz. In fact, it appears quite likely that Jastrowitz's printed text reached Prague after the mailing date of Zenger's first letter to the Paris Academy of Sciences, but before the mailing date of his second letter.

IN VIENNA

There is an even more intriguing Austrian anecdote.* The main figure in this case was Gustav Kaiser (1871-1954) who lived the last years of his life in Solbad Hall (Austria).

Because of extensive radiation damage to both hands, Kaiser came under the care of Ruckensteiner, who teaches radiology in near-by Innsbruck. After they became good friends, Kaiser gave to Ruckensteiner three original glass plates, and Ruckensteiner turned them over to the Austrian Roentgen Society.

One of these plates (the famous double-toe) was thereafter reproduced in the February, 1956 issue of *Radiologia Austriaca* in a commemorative article, signed by Weiss. A print of that plate will be included in the last volume of *Codex Austriacus* with a caption saying in effect, that Röntgen — before making his epochal provisional communication dated December 28, 1895—had given all the details of his discovery to Franz Exner

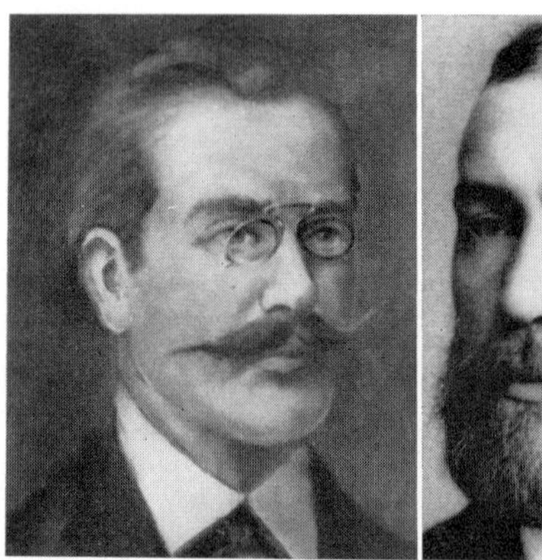

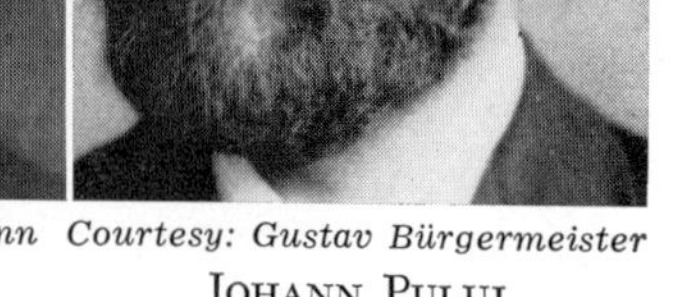

Courtesy: Vladimir Teichmann *Courtesy: Gustav Bürgermeister*

KARL ZENGER JOHANN PULUJ

*Le Bon was identified with the help of Mr. Pierre Gauja, secretary-archivist of the Paris Academy of Sciences. Data on Barthélemy were furnished by Mlle Antoinette Béclère.

**The largest coil on record was constructed by the English physicist William Spottiswoode (1825-1885): its giant sparks would span across 42 inches of air (about 107 cm).

*Most of this information was obtained from Prof. Ernst Ruckensteiner of Innsbruck (Austria), some details from Prof. Konrad Weiss of Vienna, and the remainder from contemporary sources.

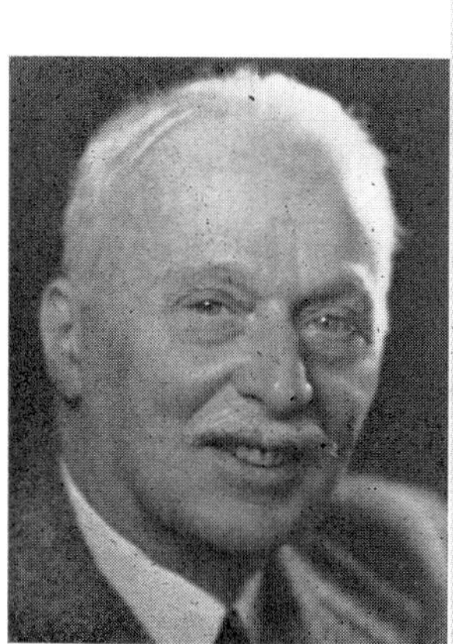

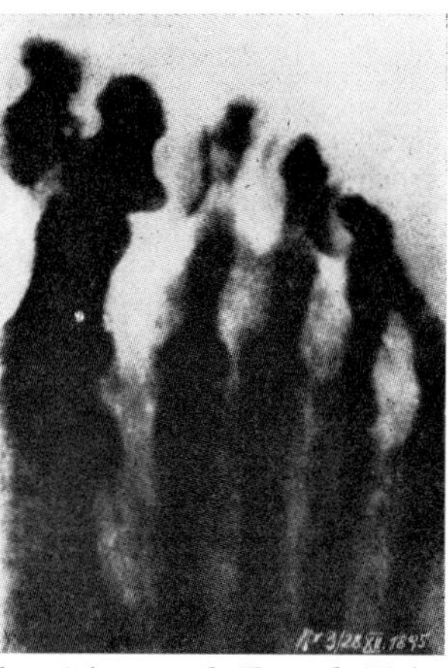

Courtesy: Ernst Ruckensteiner and Konrad Weiss.

THE PRE-HISTORIC DOUBLE-TOE. A tale from the Vienna (roentgen) woods purports that Röntgen gave advance notice of his coming initial communication to Franz Exner, in whose laboratories roentgen plates were thereupon produced during December of 1895. Gustav Kaiser (1871-1954), who was the first radiologist in the position later graced by Holzknecht, left three glass plates, all of which he contended were exposed in the last week of 1895. One of them is this famous double-toe, which was originally reproduced during January and February, 1896 by major medical and non-medical periodicals around the globe. In the absence of corroborative documentary evidence (that legendary "preview" letter from Röntgen to Exner), it is hard to believe in this *Röntgen-Märchen.*

(they were close friends since college days in Switzerland), asking him to confirm the findings obtained in Würzburg.

The intimation is that "intentional" roentgen plates had been produced in Vienna in December of 1895. Kaiser had graduated from medical school in the summer of 1895, was interested in physics, and was well acquainted with Eduard Haschek (1875-1947), the first assistant of the physicist Franz Exner. This is how and why Kaiser was allowed to assist at, and later to participate in, Exner's first experiments with roentgen rays. Kaiser, at the time a simple cohort in the second Medical Clinic of the famous internist Edmund von Neusser (1852-1912) at the Allgemeines Krankenhaus, told his chief about the potential value of the new tool – and was promptly assigned to evaluate its diagnostic possibilities. In the course of the association with Haschek, Kaiser exposed (also) the roentgen plate of a forester's left hand, which revealed a retained gunshot.

Kaiser became the first director of the Central Roentgen Institute in the Allgemeines Krankenhaus (that is the job subsequently held by Holzknecht). Kaiser never published anything, nor is there any record of his having talked before a medical audience.

Kaiser told Ruckensteiner that he (Kaiser) remembered perfectly having produced the plate of the forester's hand on December 28, 1895. Thereupon, all three plates given by Kaiser (via Ruckensteiner) to the Austrian Roentgen Society were marked in white ink with the date of *28. XII. 1895* (which, in Ruckensteiner's words, may not have been the correct date, certainly not for all three plates).

What can be substantiated in contemporary references? After the Christmas vacation, in the first session held by the Vienna Medical Society on Friday, January 10, 1896, the famous neuro-physiologist Siegmund Exner (1846-1926) – older brother to Franz Exner, the physicist – presented (just like Jastrowitz had done in Berlin, a few days earlier) a summary of Röntgen's provisorial communication, and showed the print of the "single ring" plate. We know from the *Standard* press release that that print had arrived in Vienna. The session of the Vienna Medical Society of January 17 was of historic importance. That is when Siegmund Exner exhibited all sorts or roentgen plates made in Vienna*, including the inevitable weights "hidden" in a wooden box, a "healthy hand and foot," a phalanx with callus formation after trauma due to pistol shot, and finally the very first angiogram (vessels of the hand, injected during autopsy).** The angiogram — the hand came from the Anatomical Institute directed by Julius Tandler (1869-1936) – was used as an illustration in a paper by Haschek (the physicist) and Otto Theodor Lindenthal (a physician on Neusser's staff), published on January 23, 1896 in the *Klinische.*

In the January 24 session of the Viennese Medical Society, the surgeon Albert von Mosetig-Moorhof (1838-1907) demonstrated two instances in which the roentgen examination had been of obvious surgical value: the first was a gunshot in the left hand of a forester (removal of the foreign body was facilitated by knowing its location), while the second was a supernumerary left great toe in a twenty-year old female servant (it was important to know which of the two toes articulated with the metatarsal, and this the plate revealed at a glance). In both cases, an appropriate surgical procedure had been successfully performed, and in each case Exner's installation had been used to produce the roentgen plates. As a curiosity, it may be mentioned that a newspaper account of the successful pre-operative evaluation of the double-toe had

*All these plates had been produced in Franz Exner's laboratory, except for the "healthy hand and foot" which came from the office of the famous photochemist Joseph Maria Eder (1855-1944).

**The minutes of the sessions of the Vienna Medical Society appeared both in the then up-and-coming *Wiener Klinische Wochenschrift,* and in the venerable *Wiener Medicinische Wochenschrift.* The currently "accepted" German spelling is *Medizin* and *medizinische,* but before the turn of the century it was *Medicin* and *medicinische.*

appeared in the *Freie Presse* (Vienna) of January 22, *i.e.*, two days before the presentation to the above cited Viennese Medical Society.

The January 31 session was somewhat anticlimactic as only plates of gallstones (from specimens, not *in-situ*) were introduced, while Neusser is said to have shown "calcareous deposits in liver and kidney" two days before, on January 29, as reported in the *Electrical Engineer* (New York) on February 12.

Kaiser (just like Pupin) recalled the facts correctly, but may have mixed up the dates, albeit there exists the remote possibility that Exner instructed his assistants to wait until the last moment before taking "literary" advantage of Röntgen's friendly gesture. It meant to postpone the showing of the first plates made in Vienna until after Röntgen's first oral communication. When it became clear — after the January 13 session in Berlin — that Jastrowitz was on the verge of coming up with the first clinical roentgen plate, the *pièces de resistance* were suddenly exhibited in the January 17 session in Vienna. This would explain Jastrowitz's subsequent ante-dating to January 12, and Zenger's to January 11. As far as authenticated records go, the first "clinical" roentgen plate was the bone callus on the phalanx, shown by Siegmund Exner on January 17 in Vienna. Kaiser's earlier date may have been true, but it could hardly be substantiated, short of retrieving a copy of that legendary mid-December, 1895 letter from Röntgen to Franz Exner.

In *Fortschritte auf dem Gebiete der Röntgenstrahlen* of January, 1962 Hellmut Hubert Ellegast and Bruno Thurnher summarized the beginnings of roentgenology in Vienna. There is no mention of Kaiser's date of 1895, but emphasis is placed on the fact that Kaiser should be remembered as one of the most respected Viennese roentgen pioneers, and that Kaiser was Holzknecht's teacher. It seems that Kaiser had been a forgotten man until Konrad Weiss published his obituary in 1955 in the *Radiologia Austriaca.* Another interesting detail in the paper by Ellegast and Thurnher is the supposition of the rivalry which, at that early date, existed between the two primeval Viennese roentgen locations, Neusser's II. Medicinische Universitätsklinik and Eder's Königliche und Kaiserliche Versuchstanstalt für Photographie und Reproductionsverfahren. Indeed, Leopold Freund – who may rightfully be regarded as the first radiation therapist (of consequence) – was refused by Neusser, and had to go to (and was gladly accepted by) Eder: that is where Freund treated, beginning in November, 1896, his first case of hypertrichosis.

Be all that as it may, by the end of January, 1896 — with regard to advances in the field of clinical roentgen rays — both Austria and Germany were almost one month ahead of England and America. In the *Münchener Medicinische Wochenschrift* of February 4, 1896 Franz Mink published his first series of results of tests on the vitality of roentgen-irradiated bacteria (there seemed to be no detectable bactericidal effect). On the same day, in Heidelberg, Walther Petersen presented before the Naturhistorisch-Medicinischer Verein a number of "surgical" roentgen cases. Before the Berliner Medicinische Gesellschaft, on February 7 — and not on January 5, as Gocht erroneously recollected — the surgeon Franz König (1832-1910) was the first ever to correlate roentgen appearance, surgical findings, and pathologic examination (in the case of a patient in whom the leg had been amputated because of sarcoma of the tibia).* König's "technician" had been (canal-ray) Goldstein. The article appeared in the *Berliner Klinische Wochenschrift* of February 17, 1896.

On that very day Antoine Henri Becquerel (1852-1908) presented to the French Academy of Sciences

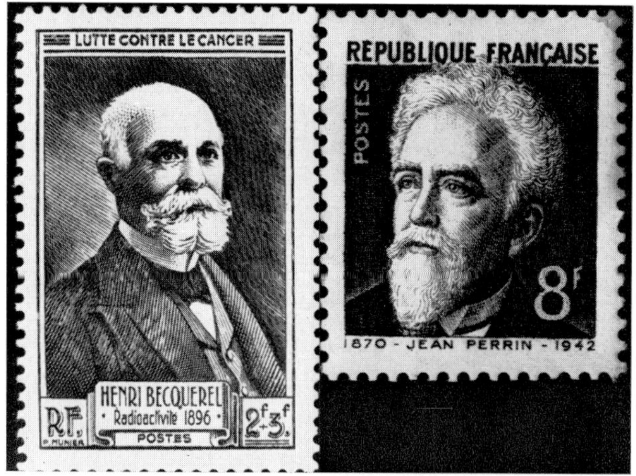

his first communication on the rays emitted by uranium. His investigation had been prompted by a suggestion offered by the French physicist Lucien Poincaré (1862-1920), who thought it might be of interest to investigate the radiation caused by phosphorescence. Radium, of course, was not to appear until 1898.

CLINICAL PLATES IN AMERICA

The first roentgen illustration in American medical literature appeared on February 15 in the *Medical*

*The *Western Electrician* (Chicago) of March 7, 1896 related that Burry and Scribner had made a sciagraph of a woman's right thigh. It showed "absence of bone," meaning metastases from a "sarcoma" of the kidney.

Record: it was the reproduction of a German original (a healthy hand, taken on January 17 in Hamburg). The second roentgen illustration(s) appeared in the same journal on February 29, and reproduced Viennase originals (the double-toe and Haschek's angiogram).

Obviously, the editors of the New York *Medical Record* were unaware of the fact that the first clinical roentgen plate in America had been produced on Monday, February 3, 1896 by the astronomer Edwin Brant Frost (1866-1935) in the Physics Laboratory (Reed Hall) of Dartmouth College in Hanover (New Hampshire): the date is authenticated by an appropriate post-script in Frost's original paper, published in *Science* of February 14.

The proceedings had also been photographed, and a print of the photograph was reproduced in the November 1945 issue of *Radiology* by a Dartmouth alumnus, the New York dermatologist Anthony Cipollaro. The photograph reveals (in addition to the various spectators) the Puluj tube energized by an induction coil and batteries. The patient's name was Eddie McCarthy, his physician was the astronomer's brother Gilman Dubois Frost (1864-1947), and the lesion was a Colles fracture of the left wrist.* The apparatus used at that time, as well as this and other original roentgen plates, can be seen in the museum of the Wilder Laboratory of Physical Sciences at Dartmouth.

The second ascertainable clinical roentgen plate in

*Prints from the original plate and from the original photograph were made available for inspection — in a very gracious manner — by the radiologist of Mary Hitchcock Memorial Hospital in Hanover, Leslie Kenneth Sycamore, who has assembled a recent historic exhibit on early roentgen procedures at their hospital.

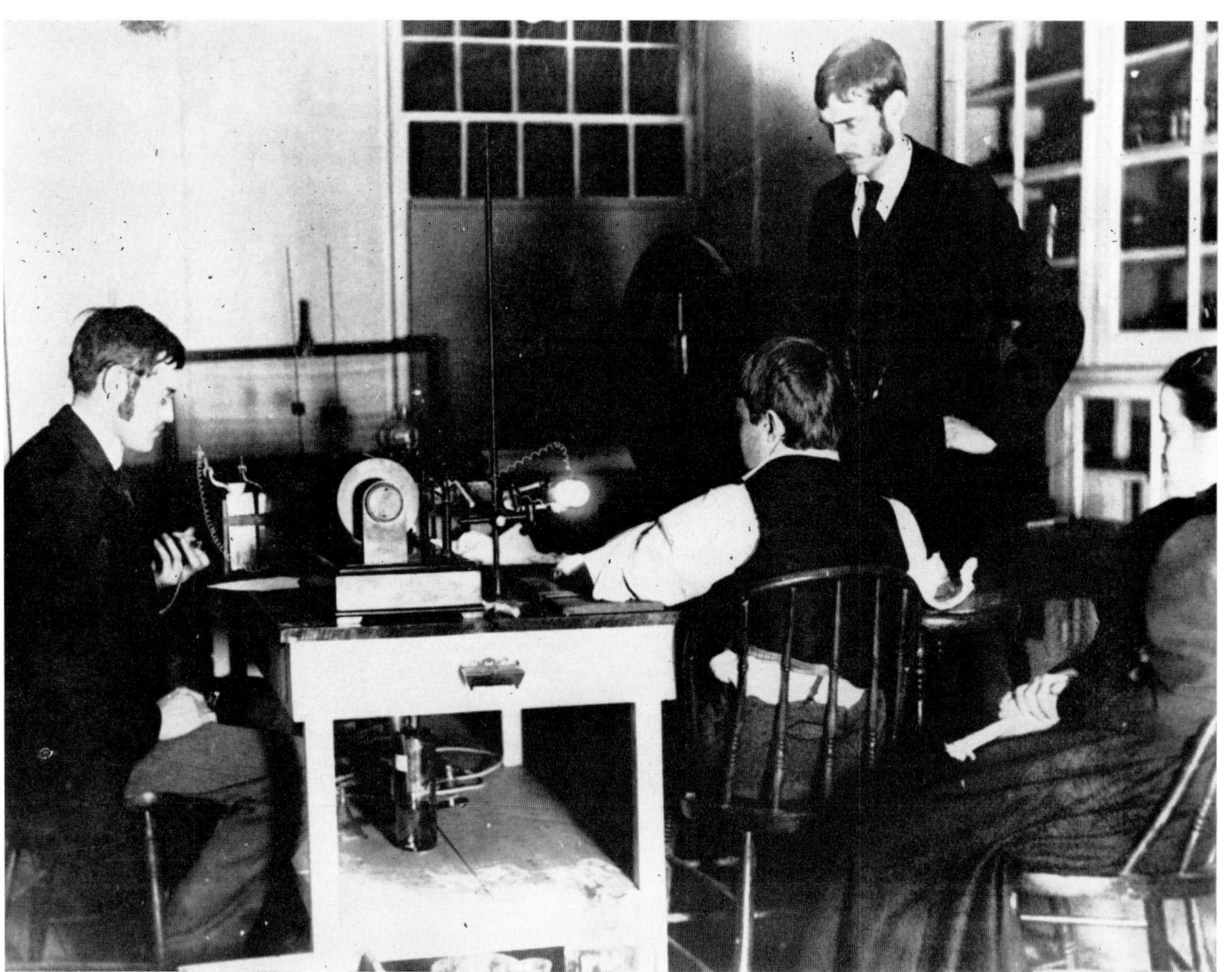

FIRST "CLINICAL" ROENTGEN PLATE IN AMERICA. On the evening of February 3, 1896 – in the Physics Lab of Dartmouth College – Edwin Frost (left) produced a plate of the Colles fracture of Ed McCarthy. The referring physician, Gilman Dubois Frost (1864-1947) and his wife watch the incandescent Puluj tube.

America was produced on Friday, February 7, 1896, by John Cox (1851-1923), professor of physics in McGill University, and published in the March issue of the *Montreal Medical Journal.*

The patient's name was Tolson Cunning, his physician was Robert Charles Kirkpatrick (surgeon to Montreal General Hospital), and the diagnosis was bullet lodged between tibia and fibula. This information appeared in part in a news item carried on February 8 (9-7) in the New York *Times* with a slight typographical error: Fox instead of Cox. On Saturday, February 8, 1896, Cox addressed the Montreal Medico-Chirurgical Society, and showed them both the patient and the plate. This was the first presentation of a roentgen subject before an American medical audience: among those present was Gilbert Prout Girdwood (1832-1917) who subsequently became the first radiologist of Montreal General Hospital.

Bob Kirkpatrick, who was instructor in surgery at McGill, died of tuberculosis in 1897.

In the Université Laval, the beginnings of radiology are associated with the name of Joseph-Clovis Kemner-Laflamme (1849-1910), who is also hailed as the first French-Canadian geologist.* Actually, he taught all sorts of Natural Sciences, from Physics to Astronomy, and from Botany to Patriotism. Laflamme was three times Rector at Laval.

In the historical review of French-Canadian radiology, Louis-Philippe Bélisle states that in Canada the

*These details were courteously obtained from Laflamme's biographer, René Bureau, professor of Geology at Laval in Quebec. The family name of Laflamme used to be Quémeneur, later changed to Kemner. Laflamme had been a nickname, adopted as the family name. Thus, the correct spelling was J.-C. K -Laflamme.

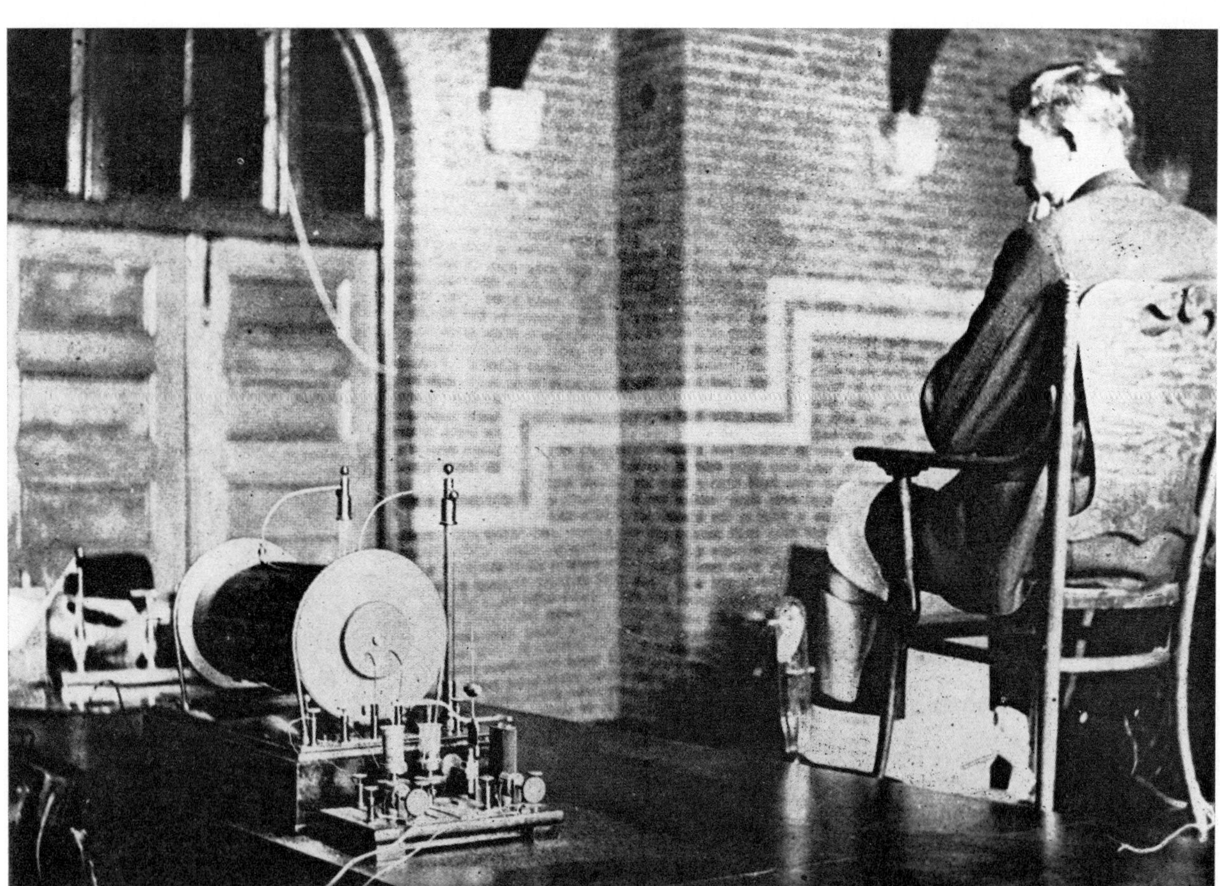

Courtesy: Charles Roland.

FIRST "CLINICAL" ROENTGEN PLATE IN CANADA. Arrangement used in the Physics Lecture Theatre of McGill University by John Cox in exposing the plate of Tolson Cunning's leg; this photograph first appeared in the *Montreal M. J.* of March, 1896, and was reproduced by Charles Roland in the *Canadian Journal of Surgery* of July, 1962. In Cox's article it is not made clear whether the subject shown was the patient whose case is reported, or whether the photograph was made at a later date.

first notice of Röntgen's discovery appeared in *La Presse* of February 6, 1896. Laflamme's first (unsuccessful) attempts to produce a roentgen plate (with 20-25 minutes of exposure) were made on February 12. On February 17, he received a catalog with x-ray apparatus made by the firm Ducretet of Paris. At that time, firms from France were preferred among French-

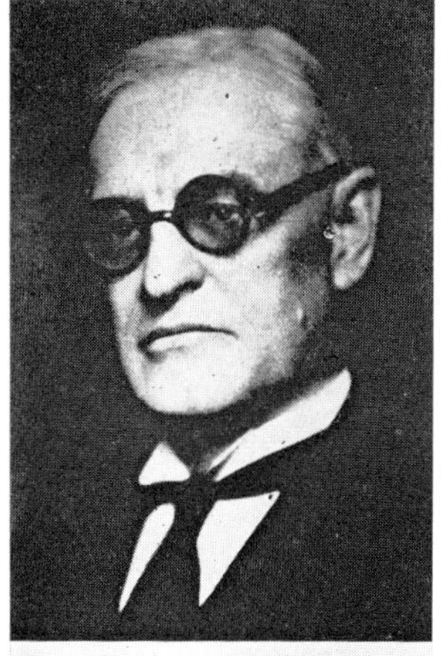

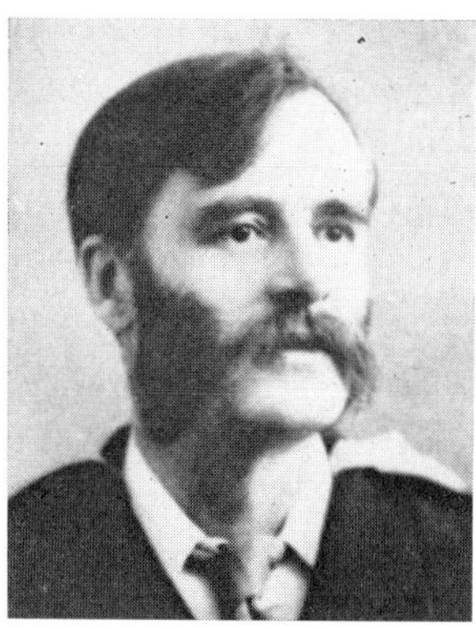

Edwin B. Frost

Courtesy: John Crerar Library.

Edwin Brant Frost (1866-1935). A well-known astronomer, shown here a few years before his death, had produced the first "clinical" roentgen plate on the American continent. On the right, with burnsides, is John Cox (1851-1923). He was the professor of physics in McGill University who produced the first roentgen plate in Canada, on February 7, 1896.

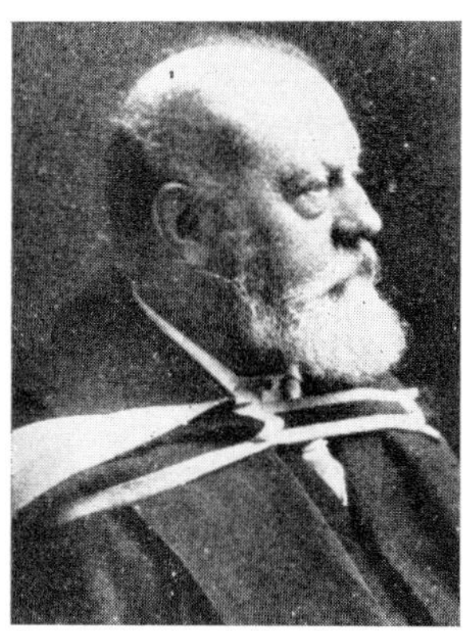

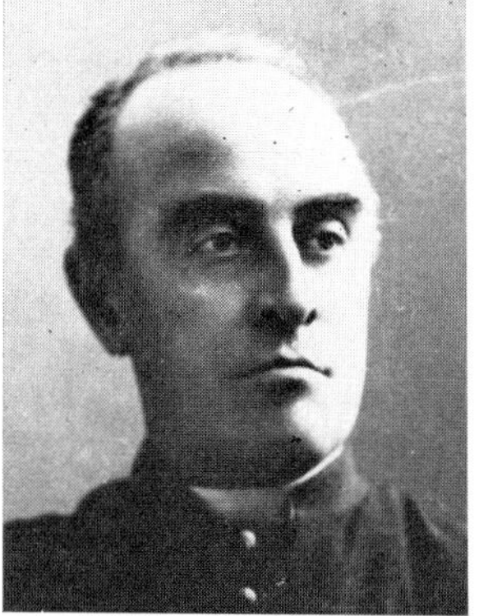

Courtesy: Prof. René Bureau of Laval University in Québec.

Gilbert Prout Girdwood (1832-1917). A physician who was in the audience on February 8, 1896, when John Cox showed the first roentgen plate obtained in Canada. Girdwood later became the first radiologist of Montreal General Hospital, and held the office of president of the ARRS. The smooth-chinned priest is Joseph-Clovis Kemner-Laflamme (1849-1910). The first French-Canadian geologist (three times Recteur of Université Laval), Monsignor Laflamme, produced the first French-Canadian roentgen plate on April 5, 1896.

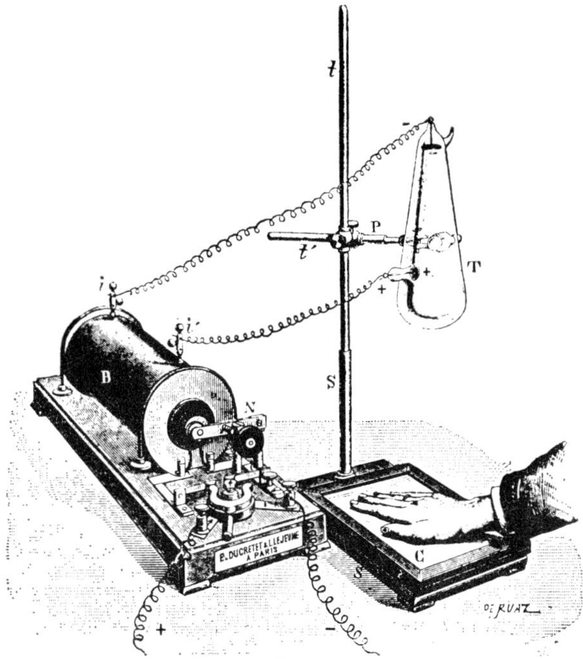

Early French roentgen apparatus. This is from an advertisement by E. Ducretet and L. Le Jeune (of Paris), which appeared also in the *Electrical Review* (London) of March 27. They recommend the use of a mercury or mechanical interruptor, and suggest to operate the tube for four minutes, then let it cool one minute, again energize it for another four minutes, again shut if off for one minute, and so on. "Longer" Crookes tubes are of advantage because they will hold the vacuum better than "shorter" ones.

MAX KOHL'S ROENTGEN RAY OUTFITS.

Having made a specialty of the manufacture of ROENTGEN RAY OUTFITS from the beginning, I can now offer at the following prices:—

INDUCTION COILS OF THE HIGHEST EFFICIENCY.

8 inch ... £15 10	16 inch ... £41 10	24 inch ... £86 5	30 inch ... £122 10	35-36 inch ... £1[illegible] 0
10 „ ... £19 0	18 „ ... £51 10	26 „ ... £97 10	31-32 inch ... £135 0	37-38 „ ... £175 0
12 „ ... £26 10	20 „ ... £64 0	28 „ ... £110 0	33-34 „ ... £147 10	40 „ ... £192 10
14 „ ... £34 0	22 „ ... £75 0			

My Induction Coils are of acknowledged superior efficiency.

The adoption of a new and improved method of winding has enabled me to add to their efficiency without a corresponding increase in prices.

All the Coils are tested to considerably more than their guaranteed length of spark, which they maintain even when the interruption works with great rapidity.

The insulating materials are chosen with the greatest care, so that it becomes impossible for the Coils to break down, or to get damaged during transit.

The Coils can be used on 110 volt as well as on battery circuits.

ROTATING INTERRUPTOR, greatly improved model, producing unsurpassed results for Photography and Screenwork, £7 15s.

First-class Vacuum Tubes, Practical Stands for Tubes, Accumulator Batteries, Fluoroscopes, Intensifying Screens for reducing time of exposure, Dry Plates for the same purpose, as well as all other appliances.

References from Leading Experts.

Catalogues containing numerous Testimonials.
Estimates for complete outfits, explicit directions for use, &c., will be promptly forwarded upon request.

MAX KOHL, Chemnitz, Germany,
ELECTRICAL AND PHYSICAL INSTRUMENT MAKER.
Special Manufacturer of Roentgen Ray Outfits.

Courtesy: John Crerar Library.

Early German roentgen outfit. The "chemical" firm of Max Kohl in Chemnitz entered the roentgen business in the first months after the discovery, and was quite active; by the turn of the century it had again restricted itself to "chemistry." This ad is from a late 1896 issue of the *Archives of Skiagraphy*.

Canadians – while in English-speaking laboratories in Canada, most of the equipment was furnished by the firm Max Kohl of Chemnitz (Germany). On April 2, Laflamme obtained new photographic plates, and on April 5 he succeeded in producing his first roentgen plate with one half hour of exposure: the hands and feet of an infant. That plate was mentioned in the *Electrical World* (New York) of May 16, 1896.

IN PHILADELPHIA

On Thursday, February 13, the pathologist Henry Ware Cattell (1862-1936) addressed the Pathological Society of Philadelphia on the subject of roentgen rays, as mentioned in the February 29 issue of the *Medical Record.* This was the first presentation of such a topic to a medical audience in the United States (second only

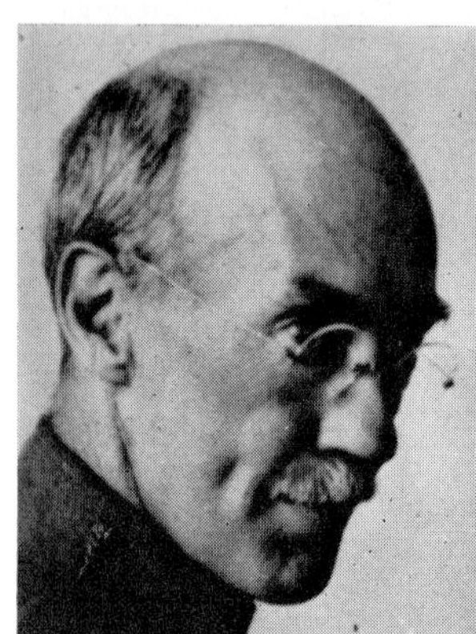

HENRY CATTELL

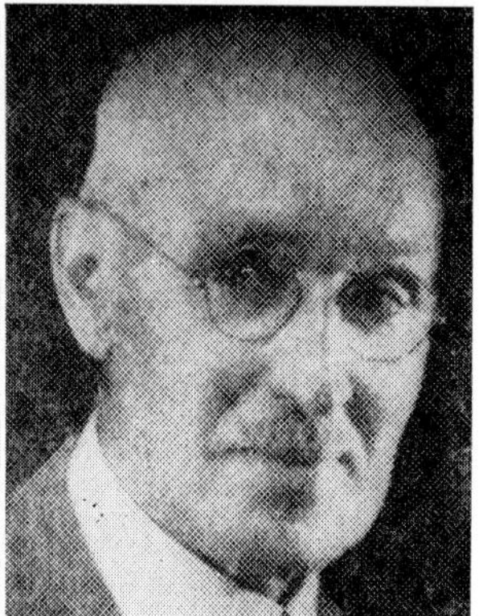

BILL JENNINGS

to that of Cox for all of America). It was described in *Medical News* of February 15. Cattell's plates were produced by Arthur Goodspeed, of whom William Williams Keen (1837-1932) – who was both the author of a well-introduced *System of Surgery,* and a clinical roentgen pioneer (for his paper in the March, 1896 issue of the *American Journal of Medical Sciences*)– would later say that he (Goodspeed) accumulated a pathologic roentgen file of unequalled priority and superiority in both quality and variety.

Actually Cattell's presentation was to some extent

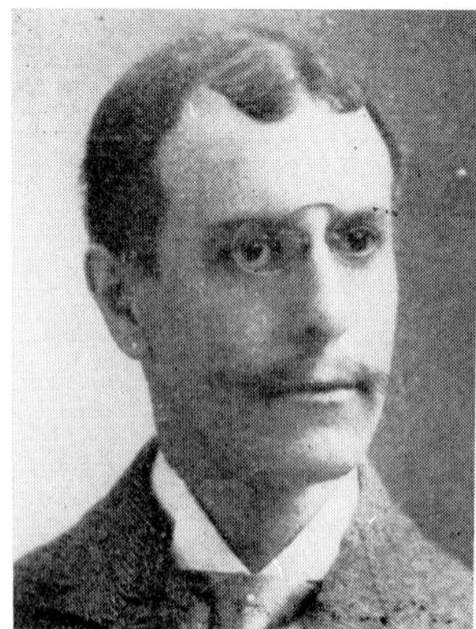

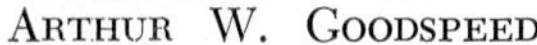

ARTHUR W. GOODSPEED

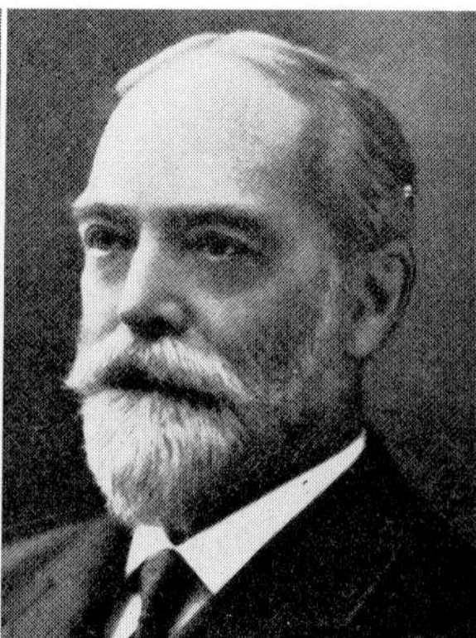

ARTHUR W. WRIGHT

anticlimactic because the night before, on February 12, at the Philadelphia Photographic Society – as mentioned in the *Electrical World* of February 22 – various plates were exhibited by John Carbutt (a plate manufacturer), by a certain now unidentifiable Jennings,* and by Goodspeed himself. They showed "lines of flesh, bone, diamond, gold, and so on" and Carbutt an-

*Charlie Smith identified him as English-born William N. Jennings (1860-1945), who came to this country in 1879, produced in 1882 the first known photograph of a lightning (he called it "Jove's autograph"), and in 1893 the first aerial picture of Philadelphia (from a balloon).

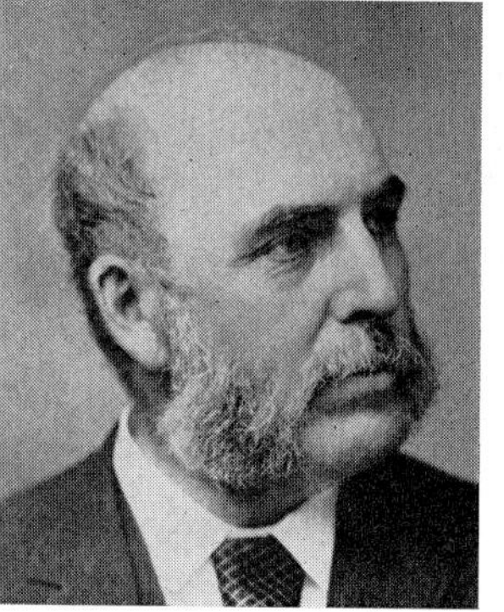

JOHN CARBUTT

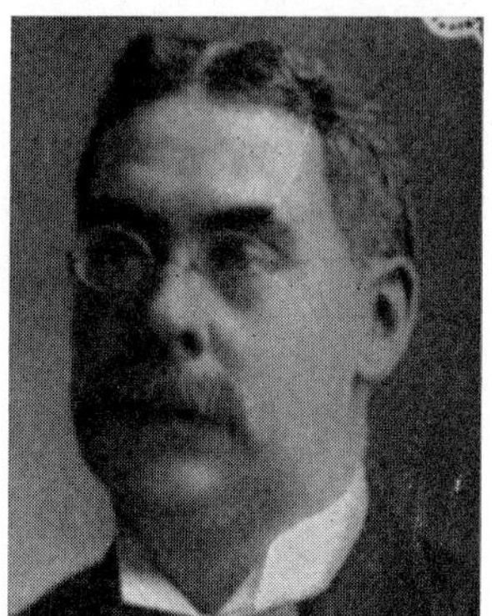

EDWARD DAVIS

Amateurs and Professionals

SHOULD USE

THE OLDEST AND BEST

THE Carbutt Plates, Films AND Specialties

USE • • • UNDOUBTEDLY HAVE THIS DISTINCTION

"Eclipse" for Portraiture and Hand Camera exposures, and you have a Plate that has **Rapidity with Quality.**

Orthochromatic **Sen. 27,** about equal in speed to the Eclipse gives correct color values.

X Ray Plates for making **Radiograph Negatives.** These plates have the special quality of absorbing the X Rays of a Crookes Tube, allowing of short exposures. They are used by Prof A. W. Goodspeed of the University of Pa., who has produced fine results with exposures as short as 4½ seconds, Nikola Tesla and Dr. William J. Morton, of New York, and many other Scientists also use them.

For View Photography use

Ortho **Sen. 23,** also for photographing Flowers, Architecture, etc Can be used with or without a Color Screen as circumstances necessitate.

B **Sen. 16,** for Landscape and Architecture. Unparalleled latitude of exposure makes it the "**Standard**" for beginners.

Lantern Plates have no equals for Brilliancy and Uniformity

J. C. Developing Tabloids. Put up in boxes containing 96 Tabloids, enough to develope 8 to dozen 4x5 Plates. **Price, 75 cents.** Mailed postpaid, on receipt of price. Sample box 10 cents.

FOR SALE BY ALL DEALERS.

Send to Factory for full list of PLATES, FILMS and SPECIALTIES.

MANUFACTURED BY

JOHN CARBUTT,

KEYSTONE DRY PLATE AND FILM WORKS.

Wayne Junction, PHILADELPHIA

Courtesy: Library of the University of Illinois.

EARLY CARBUTT AD. This advertisement appeared in October, 1896 in the *American Journal of Photography.*

nounced his plate, especially sensitive to x rays, with which twenty minutes of exposure sufficed instead of the usual hour. The reporter noted that "all the Crookes tubes in Philadelphia for sale, have been purchased, which certainly illustrates the universal interest in these new and important phenomena."

Carbutt's special plate was immediately adopted by several researchers in Philadelphia, for instance by Edward Parker Davis (1856-1937) professor of midwifery in Jefferson Medical College. In his article, printed in the *American Journal of Medical Science* of March, 1896, Davis provided a vivid word-picture of his procedure. "The child was bandaged upon a sensitized plate . . . very much as the Indian papoose is fastened to its board. The bandage was the ordinary surgical roller and entirely covered the front of the child's body. It was then exposed to the direct action of the rays, the tube being 10″ from the body, for forty-five minutes. The child remained quiet, did not seem annoyed by the crackling of the tube, and experienced no apparent discomfort . . . the accompanying illustration shows a faint outline of the ribs . . ."

IN CHICAGO

The first roentgen ray experiments in Chicago were performed on February 6, 1896 in the laboratory of the Western Electric by their chief electrical engineer Charles Ezra Scribner (1858-1926). The physician in the picture was James Burry (1853-1919), chief-surgeon of the Illinois Steel Company. At first they had some "tube trouble," but by Saturday, February 8 they had obtained a satisfactory plate of Scribner's own hand.

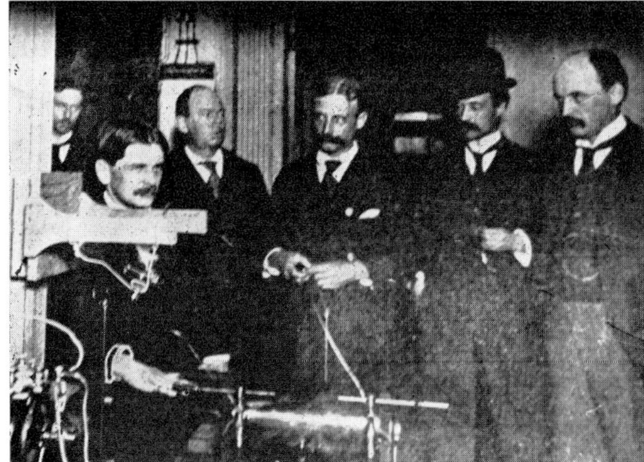

Courtesy: Library of the University of Illinois.

FIRST ROENTGEN PLATE IN CHICAGO. Charles Ezra Scribner (1858-1926) submits his right hand to the roentgen rays, while his medical adviser, James Burry (1853-1919) is the mustachioed, balding watcher on the extreme right. Place: laboratories of the Western Electric Company; date: February 8, 1896.

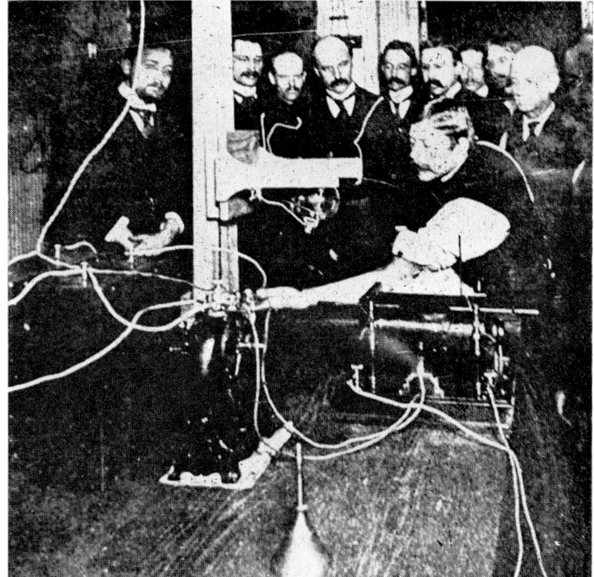

Courtesy: Library of the University of Illinois.

ORTHOPEDIC CHECK-UP IN CHICAGO. Patient was an employee of Western Electric. The plate (dated February 15, 1896) showed a Colles fracture with fragments healing in good position. Burry is among the spectators, with goateed F. R. McBerty on the far left.

Photographs of the induction apparatus, lay-out, and spectators appeared in the *Western Electrician* (Chicago) of February 15.

Word got around and on Monday, February 10, a certain Louis Burkhart (who resided at 725 West Madison Street) came to the plant of Western Electric and wanted to have his hand examined. A plate was exposed and demonstrated the presence of a bullet, which had been lodged there for several years, ever since an "encounter" in Strassbourg (then part of Germany). On Tuesday, February 11 Burry (assisted by J. S. Rankin and J. L. Miller) removed the bullet in the operating room at Mercy Hospital. This is described in Burry's article in the *JAMA* of February 29; that paper contains also an account of experimental irradia-

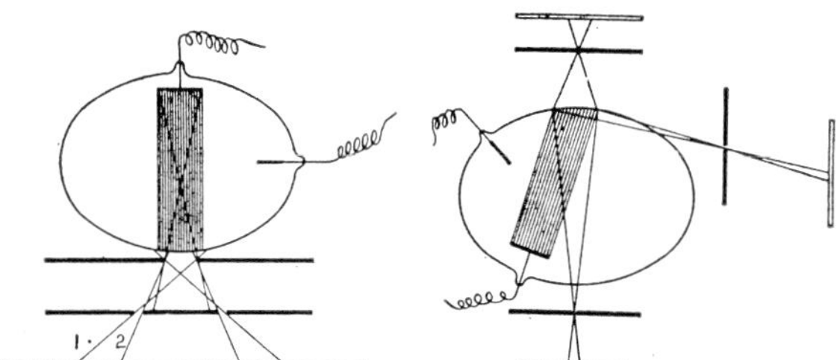

Courtesy: Mid-West Inter-Library Center.

WHERE ARE THESE RAYS COMING FROM? Scribner and McBerty answered the question by placing lead screens with various openings at strategic locations in relation to the anode. Photographic plates did the rest.

tions of tubercle bacilli, but it reproduces the plate of a healthy hand, not the hand with the bullet. Scribner, and his assistant F. R. McBerty, investigated the part of the tube (glass!) where the x rays are coming from and their contribution, first published in the *Electrical Engineer* (New York) on April 8, was widely quoted and reprinted.

OTHER PIONEERS

Pupin claimed also a priority with regard to a clinical roentgen plate. Two years before his death, Pupin sent a positive print (showing a hand with multiple

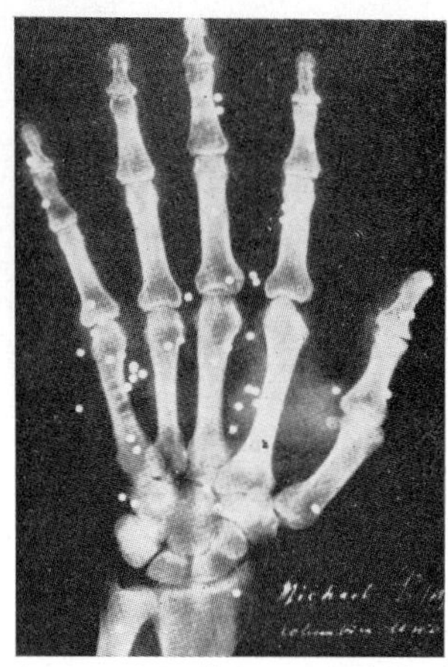

Courtesy: Department of Radiology of Cook County Hospital.

PUPIN'S PRIORITY PROCLAMATION. This is the famous gunshot-ridden hand of Prescott Hall Butler, which Pupin examined on February 14, 1896. The print is so much better than anything available at that time, one would be inclined to regard it as a forgery – but it is authentic, and had been reproduced in the *Scientific American* of March 21, 1896.

retained gunshots) to Maximilian John Hubeny (1880-1942), who was at that time chief-radiologist of Cook County Hospital and chairman of the Historical Roentgen Committee for the American Congress of Radiology. Together with the print came a letter* with the following text:

Michael I. Pupin
One West Seventy-Second Street
New York City

Norfolk, Conn.
August 5, 1933

Dr. M. J. Hubeny, M.D.,
Chairman,
25 East Washington Street,
Chicago, Ill.

My dear Dr. Hubeny:

I send you the X-ray picture taken by myself in February, 1896. It was the first X-ray picture to guide a surgical operation in the United States. I also enclose a brief account of this picture and of the discovery of the method of shortening the time of exposure in X-ray photography. This description was copied from pages 307-308 of my autobiography "From Immigrant to Inventor."

Yours sincerely,
(ss) M. I. Pupin

Encl.

The patient's name was Prescott Hall Butler (a New York attorney), the surgeon was William Tillinghast Bull (1849-1909), the injury was due to the (accidental) discharge of a shotgun at short distance, and the final outcome was successful surgical removal of the gunshots. This print had been reproduced in contemporary publications, for instance in the March 21, 1896, issue of the *Scientific American*. It had been exposed, in all probability, on Friday, February 14, 1896.* As such, it was at the most the first roentgen plate to guide a surgical operation in New York. Still, it is the best of all early roentgen prints as far as technical quality (and bone detail) is concerned which is quite unusual when one considers the fact that the x rays were produced in the glass of the tube, and were in no way focused.

IN CALIFORNIA

The San Francisco *Examiner,* stimulated by civic pride, sponsored a Committee, under the direction of Philip Mills Jones (1870-1916). Their laboratory was established first in the Thurlow Building at Kearny and Sutter Streets. After three days of experimentation with the largest coil available in San Francisco, they produced roentgen rays on Wednesday, February 19, 1896.**

Leo Henry Garland, the current professor of radiology at Stanford, in his article on the *History of Radiology in California,* mentions that when the little x-ray plant in the Thurlow Building broke down, the researchers moved to the State University, and continued the work with Professor Cory. The latter made the first surgical roentgen diagnosis in California on February 25, 1896, when he located a bullet in a boy's hand with a ninety-minute exposure.

Philip Jones, who shortly before that had migrated from Brooklyn to 'Frisco, opened his own private roent-

*Both the letter and the print have been preserved, and can be seen in the Department of Radiology of Cook County Hospital.

*This date was established by Mr. Arthur Wolfram Fuchs, from the Eastman Kodak Company (personal communication).

**This information was obligingly contributed by Dr. Robert Reid Newell, the ever-so-active (although allegedly retired) professor of radiology emeritus at Stanford.

gen office at the Walbeck Hospital. He reported his observations to the San Francisco Medical Society on March 10, 1896. When mentioning those very early days (in the *JAMA* of November 6, 1897), Jones said: "In the beginning, the desire of experiencing the creeping sensation of seeing one's own bones resulted in a great deal of kindergarten research."

Meanwhile, in Los Angeles, a physician, F. E. Yoakum was reported as having demonstrated a functioning x-ray apparatus to the County Medical Association on March 6, 1896.*

CONTINUING PROGRESS

On February 22, 1896, the *Western Electrician* reported that "from all over Europe photographs of hands and feet, the discovery of bits of copper wire, needles, and the like are taken almost daily. A needle was seen in a woman's hand in Birmingham last week. In London an effort is being made to form a society for making serious experiments in the new photography. Harold Frederick, the London correspondent relates (that) the Vienna Museum possessed an Egyptian mummy, swathed to resemble a human being, but with an inscription which suggested it to be an ibis instead. The thing was too rare and precious to run the risk of unwinding its bandages to solve this paradox, but the shadow photograph now plainly reveals the skeleton of a large bird.† A Toronto dispatch dated February 14, says: "Today in Grace Hospital the value of Röntgen's discovery was again demonstrated. A woman whose foot had caused her intense pain was submitted to the cathode rays and the photograph revealed the presence of a needle. Professor Wright of University College, who conducted the experiment, pointed out to the surgeon the exact location of the foreign body and an operation at this point, proved the photograph to be a true one."

In Portugal, the first news of Roentgen's discovery appeared in the daily newspapers; for instance, in January in *Novidades,* while on March 1, 1896, *O Seculo* gave its first page to the first roentgen plates produced: in Coimbra on February 3, by the physicist Alvaro Teixera Bastos, in Oporto by Araujo e Castro and Emilio Biel, and in March, in Lisbon by Vergilio Machado.

*This information comes from Mrs. Viola Warren, and reached me *via* Prof. Garland.

†Similarly, but for promotional purposes, the previously mentioned John Carbutt of Wayne Junction, Pennsylvania, made the radiograph of a mummy hand, encased in gold leaf, and proved with 2 minutes exposure that his x-ray dry plates were quite sensitive, and that the form contained, indeed, the skeleton of a hand (*cf.,* the report in the September 26, 1896, issue of *Western Electrician*).

The first medical reference to roentgen rays appeared on February 1, 1896, in *Coimbra Medica,* while in the same year a photographer, A. Bobone set up the first "X-Ray Laboratory" in Lisbon. In February, 1896, after learning of Oudin's exploit, Daniel de Matos, who was teaching surgery in Coimbra, had a roentgen plate exposed of a metacarpal bone tuberculosis, for use in his clinical demonstration. This is regarded as the beginning of radiologic teaching in Portugal.

In Latin America the very first x-ray plate (of a hand) was made in Chile by Arturo Salazar-Valencia (1855-1943), who reported it on March 27, 1896 before the Sociedad Cientifica de Chile. The second such plate (on record) was shown on May 16, 1896 in the

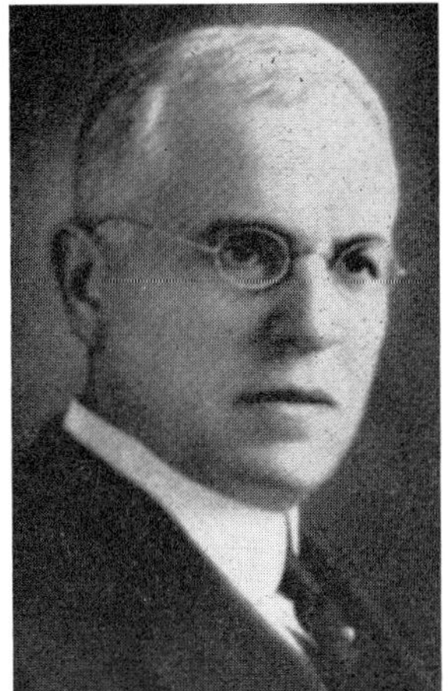

A. Salazar Valencia.

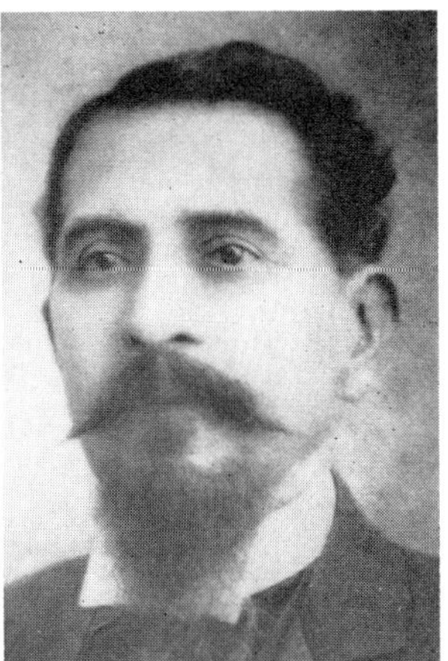

Dario Gonzalez

meeting of the Escuela de Medicina y Farmacia of Guatemala City by Dario Gonzalez, their professor of Medical Physics (who became their first radiologist); at that meeting Gonzalez, Sr. lectured on Röntgen's discovery, and his lecture was printed in the *Diario de Centro-America* of May 19, 1896.*

In Brazil, the first roentgen plate was obtained by Ferreira Ramos from the Polytechnic School in Sao Paulo. He used a Ruhmkorff coil and a small Crookes tube: this occurred sometime in 1896. Clinical roentgen pioneers in Sao Paulo were Edmundo Xavier (professor of medical physics), A. Alvin (who became a radiation fatality – *cf.,* stamp on page 45), and Jorge Dodsworth.

The news of Röntgen's discovery reached Japan – by boat – around the middle of February, 1896. In Tokyo the first x-ray plate was produced at the Imperial University, in March, 1896 by a physicist, Kenjiro Yamakawa (1854-1951). At about the same time, independently, Binnojo Mizuno (1864-1944), a high-school physics teacher, succeeded in reproducing Rönt-

*This information, and the photograph of Gonzalez, have been graciously provided by Prof. Armando Gonzalez, third generation radiologist in Guatemala (Dario's grandson). The photograph of Salazar-Valencia is from the collection of Agfa's "x-ray director," Georg Grössel.

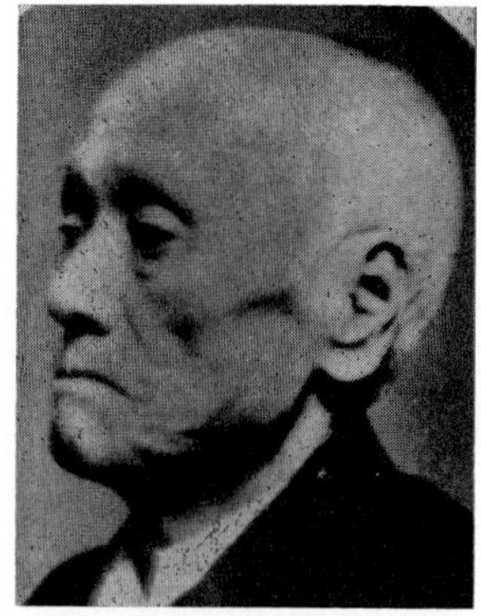

YAMAKAWA

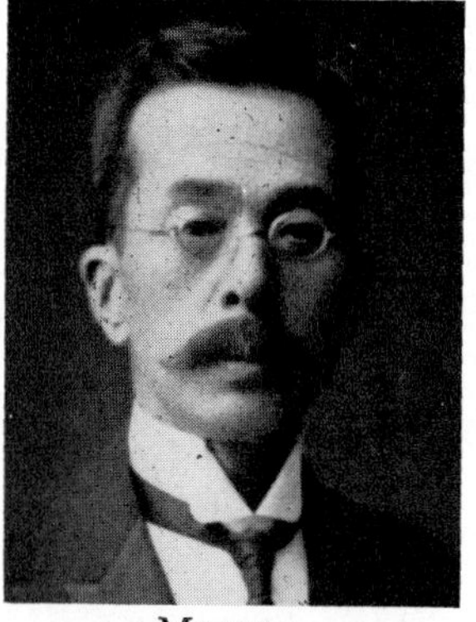

MIZUNO

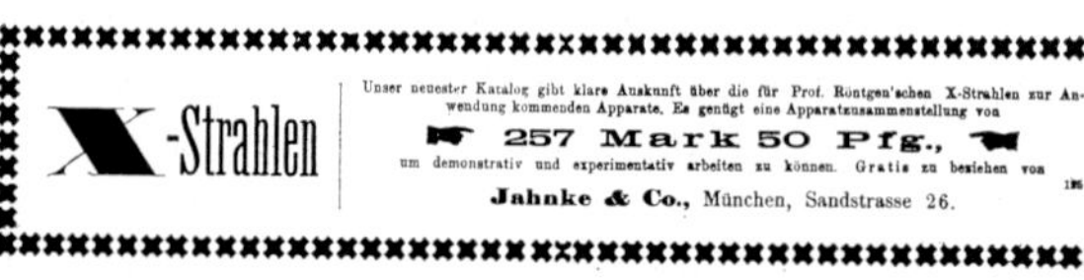

X-Strahlen

Unser neuester Katalog gibt klare Auskunft über die für Prof. Röntgen'schen X-Strahlen zur Anwendung kommenden Apparate. Es genügt eine Apparatzusammenstellung von

257 Mark 50 Pfg.,

um demonstrativ und experimentativ arbeiten zu können. Gratis zu beziehen von

Jahnke & Co., München, Sandstrasse 26.

Röhren für Röntgen-Strahlen.

Die **Glühlampenfabrik Hard** in Zürich III 177

ist die **alleinige** Herstellerin bester, genau geprüfter Vacuum-Röhren für X-Strahlen

System Prof. Dr. Zehnder*).

Diese Röhren zeichnen sich durch intensive Wirksamkeit und durch Dauerhaftigkeit aus und liefern scharfe Bilder bei sehr kurzer Expositionszeit. Preis in Etui: 40 Fr. = 32 Mark.

*) Prof. Zehnder in Freiburg i/B., ein ehemaliger Schüler von Prof. v. Röntgen, ist Constructeur der bekannten „Zehnder-Röhren" für Hertz'sche Versuche.

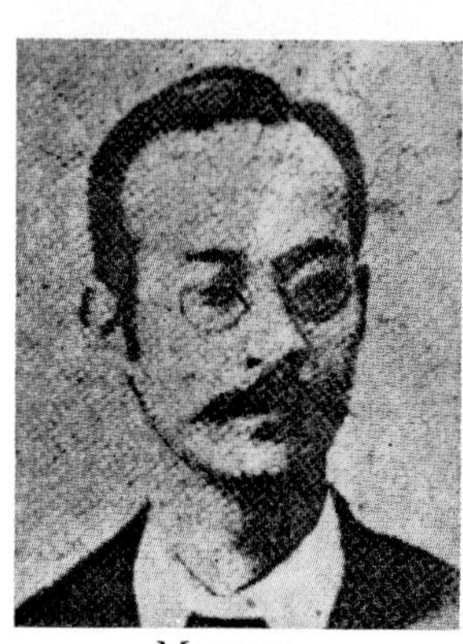

MARUMO

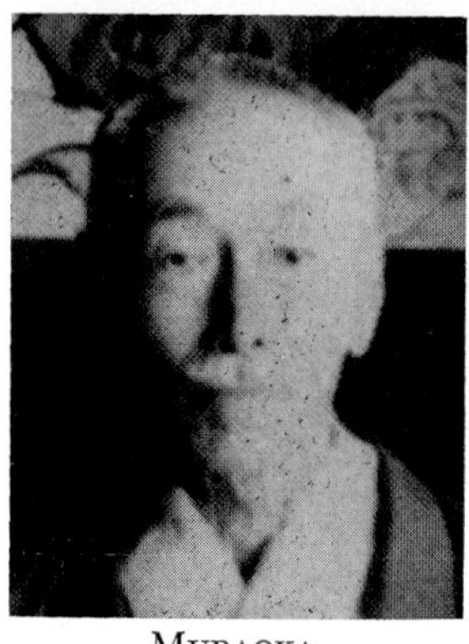

MURAOKA

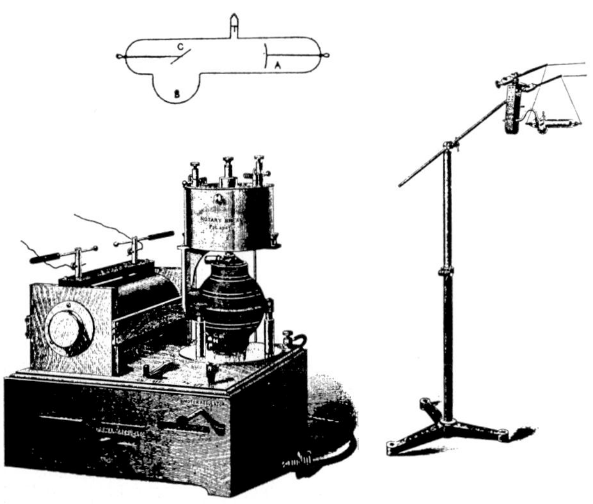

WILLYOUNG EQUIPMENT OF 1896. The roentgen ray machine consisted of the Willyoung Coil (with the wiring set into molten insulation to exclude air), topped by a motor-driven interrupter. Above it is the original drawing of the Bowdoin tube, as it appeared in the *Electrical Engineer* of June 10, 1896. The tubestand was illustrated (with the roentgen ray machine) in the *Electrical World* of December 26, 1896, but its Bowdoin tube is more stylized than the schematic version.

gen's experiments. A surgeon, Bunryo Marumo (1852-1906), made the first medical applications of the procedure in Japan. The physicist Hanichi Muraoka (1853-1929) was interested in the technologic aspects.*

TRANSIENT COMMERCIAL VENTURES

It would be near impossible to collect, let alone to tell the story of the many short-lived attempts to make fast money out of the fact that Röntgen had refused to claim legal rights over any part of his discovery.

Beginning in April, 1896, Jahnke & Co. (of München) offered complete installations "from 257.50 mark up." Moreover, their copywriter "misplaced" the word *gratis* so that it promised something free (the catalog, of course).

A few weeks after Jahnke's first publicity campaign, one finds that in Switzerland a lightbulb factory (Hard of Zürich) has expanded its production to include Zehnder tubes. Particular emphasis was placed in their ads on the former relationship between Röntgen and Zehnder (they were friends), Zehnder being called Röntgen's disciple.

The American firm which is going to be mentioned in this context came into the roentgen business a bit later (around the middle of the year 1896), but was very serious and stayed in it longer than the previous two. Elmer Willyoung started out in Philadelphia, and his first product was a coil. By the end of 1896, he had on the market a roentgen machine, consisting of a coil with motor-operated rotary interrupter. His tubestand looked fairly good, and — as shown in a sizable spread in the *Electrical World* (New York) of December 26, 1896 — Willyoung had decided upon using the Bowdoin focusing x-ray tube, so named because it was constructed by Hutchins and Collins, two physics teachers at Bowdoin College. In 1899 Willyoung sold his Philadelphia business to a friend, Morris Leeds, and this is how today's well-known instrument manufacturer Leeds & Northrup started.

*Above data were courteously offered by Prof. Goro Goto, the unofficial historian of Japanese radiology.

POPULAR MISCONCEPTIONS

The penetration of opaque materials by the roentgen rays resulted in certain misapprehensions. These may have been well expressed in the versified complaint *X-Craze,* signed Wilhelmina: it appeared *X-actly So* in *Photography* (London) in February, 1896,

The Röntgen rays, the Röntgen rays,
What is this craze?
The town's ablaze
With this new phase
Of X rays ways.
I'm full of daze,
Shock and amaze,
For nowadays
I hear they'll gaze
Thro' cloak and gown — and even stays!
These naughty, naughty Röntgen rays!

It has often been pointed out that advertisements of that time extolled "x-ray proof" garments. Buckskin impervious to rain, wind and x rays was publicized on February 16, 1896, in the Canadian *La Presse* (Bélisle).

The "convincing powers" of a publicity campaign must not be underestimated. And yet, extensive advertising by health faddists does not necessarily mean that a large or even significant segment of the population believes in food fads.

There is the famous "bill of the opera-glasses" — mentioned by Alan Ralph Bleich (and by Glasser before him). That trivial incident was reported in a totally different manner to the contemporaries. In the *Electrical Engineer* (New York) of February 26, 1896, appeared the notice: ". . . a loud laugh went over the State of New Jersey on February 15, when Assemblyman Reed of Somerset County introduced a bill in the House, at Trenton, prohibiting the use of x rays in opera glasses in theaters." This removes most of the zest from all comments on the so-called "delightful" ignorance of Röntgen's contemporaries.

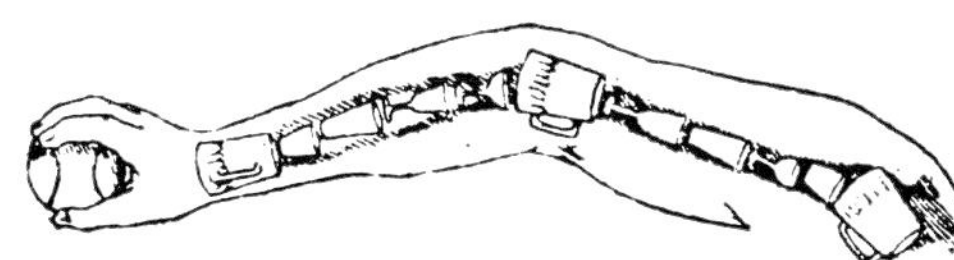

BASEBALL PLAYER'S GLASS ARM. The caption to this obvious take-off was "Another application of Röntgen's discovery." It allegedly deplored the fact that dipsomaniac pitchers will no longer be able to hide their vice because the "rays" will reveal the (effects of the) beer, gin, or whiskey glasses in their arms.

There are people, though, who want to believe in amusing things. For their benefit are reproduced the following less well known sentences from an editorial which appeared in the (British) *Pall Mall Gazette* in March of 1896:

"We are sick of the Röntgen rays. It is now said, we hope untruly, that Mr. Edison has discovered a substance — tungstate of calcium is its repulsive name— which is potential, whatever that means, to the said rays. The consequence of which appears to be that you can see other people's bones with the naked eye and also through eight inches of solid wood. On the revolting indecency of this there is no need to dwell. But what we seriously put before the attention of the Government is that the moment tungstate of calcium comes into anything like general use, it will call for legislative restriction of the severest kind."

The "transparent clothes" idea was obviously quite repulsive to the puritanic Victorian mind. This reminds one of Macaulay's quip about the Puritan who hates bear-baiting, not because it gives pain to the bear but because it might please the spectators.

FIRST MEDICAL RADIOLOGIST

When a successful revolution has turned into an organized authority, few of the original revolutionists are permitted to retain commanding positions. Some of the early radiologists experienced similar difficulties. In London, Sidney Donville Rowland (1872-1917) was catapulted into fame after the first few (of a total of sixteen) installments on the *New Photography,* published in the *British Medical Journal* in 1896. Rowland had a private office with a roentgen apparatus as early as February, 1896: in the *British Medical Journal* of February 22, Bertram Leonard Abrahams (1870-1908) described the surgical removal of a post-traumatic spur on the right little

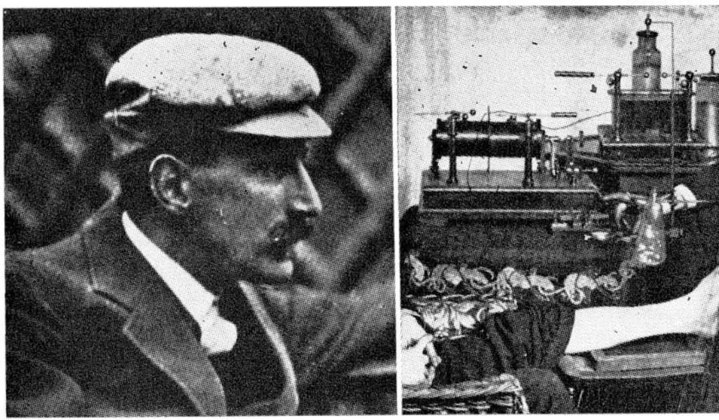

Courtesy: John Crerar Library.

FIRST BRITISH MEDICAL RADIOLOGIST. Sidney Donville Rowland (1872-1917) is shown in one of the two extant reproductions of his face (the other is that of a *bas relief*). The photograph on the right (from the *Archives of Skiagraphy,* of which Rowland was the founder and first editor) shows his hand, and a patient's foot. Rowland did not like clinical medicine, and soon left the roentgen business; otherwise he would have probably turned into a radiation casualty.

finger of one of his patients — the respective roentgen plate had been made by Rowland.

In 1897, Rowland faded out of radiology, went back to finish medical school, changed his avocation, and became an excellent bacteriologist. He died of meningitis in France, while on military duty, during World War I. There are some who regard James Mackenzie Davidson (1856-1919) as the first British radiologist, others bestow this honor on the Scottish ear, nose and throat specialist John Macintyre (1857-1928). The latter was

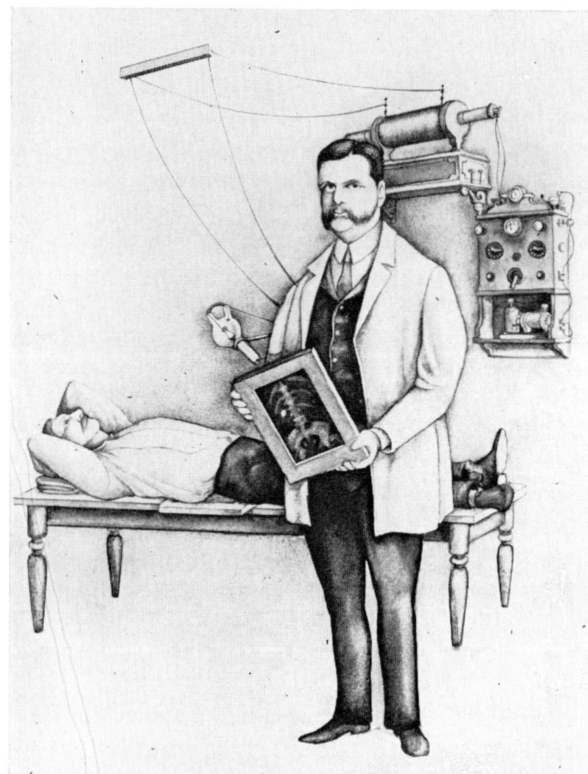

JOHN MACINTYRE (1857-1928). This illustration was done by Blake Hampton for a Gantrisin advertisement in the June, 1962 issue of *Image* (a promotional periodical of the Hoffman-La Roche Laboratories through the courtesy of which it is herein reproduced). The drawing refers to Macintyre as having been the first to identify a kidney stone on a roentgen plate.

the first (in the very year 1896) to splice single roentgen frames into what appeared to be a crude, but moving picture of living human articulations. His earliest roentgen plates – according to his own recollections (published in June, 1907) – were exposed only in the Spring of 1896. I checked the records and found that Macintyre's first "x-ray paper" appeared in *Nature* of February 20, but it was similar to William Morton's first production (brush discharge effect); his first roentgen plate was reported in *Nature* of March 19, 1896. Mackenzie Davidson's first (the picture of a broken needle in the foot) was published in the *British Medical Journal* of February 29, 1896. Undoubtedly, Rowland was the first British radiologist.

Rowland founded, and was the first editor of, the first periodical devoted exclusively to roentgen rays, the *Archives of Clinical Skiagraphy*. Its first installment (dated April 2) was issued in May, 1896. In America, the first specialty journal in this field was started in 1897, but during the year 1896, several periodicals devoted entire numbers to the "new discovery." Such were the March issue of the *Journal of Electricity* (San Francisco), or the July issue of the *Bulletin* of the Electrotherapeutic Laboratory at the University of Michigan (Ann Arbor).

In Trostler's opinion (which I share), the first radiologist in this country was William James Morton (1845-1920), a neurologist from New York City. Morton's "x-ray beginnings" had been somewhat quaint: he claimed he could obtain "plates" without using Crookes tubes. A spelling gremlin caught his tail in that provocative title in the *Electrical Engineer* of February 5, and changed it to "Brookes" tube. That method of obtaining plates was the so-called

Archives

— of —

Clinical Skiagraphy.

BY

SYDNEY ROWLAND, B.A., CAMB.,

LATE SCHOLAR OF DOWNING COLLEGE, CAMBRIDGE, AND SHUTER SCHOLAR OF ST. BARTHOLOMEW'S HOSPITAL.
SPECIAL COMMISSIONER TO "BRITISH MEDICAL JOURNAL" FOR INVESTIGATION OF THE APPLICATIONS OF THE NEW PHOTOGRAPHY TO MEDICINE AND SURGERY.

A SERIES OF COLLOTYPE ILLUSTRATIONS WITH DESCRIPTIVE TEXT, ILLUSTRATING APPLICATIONS OF THE NEW PHOTOGRAPHY TO MEDICINE AND SURGERY.

London:
THE REBMAN PUBLISHING COMPANY, LIMITED,
11, ADAM STREET, STRAND.

1896.

"brush discharge," advocated before and after Morton by several inventors, Dolbear, Bell, and Crumbie in this country, Moreau in France, or Thompson in

PHOTOGRAPHY OF THE INVISIBLE WITHOUT THE AID OF A BROOKES TUBE.

BY

William James Morton, M.D.

MISSPELLED TITLE. This is the way it was printed in the *Electrical Engineer* (New York) of February 5, 1896. How can anyone make such mistakes, when it should have read "Krookes."

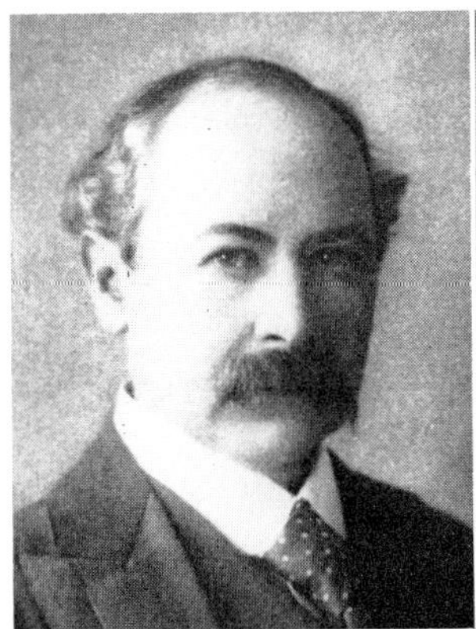

SYLVANUS THOMPSON

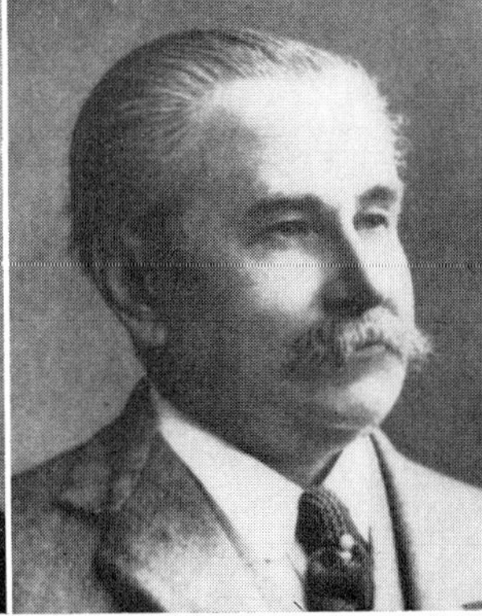

MACKENZIE DAVIDSON

England. The latter was the well known Sylvanus Phillips Thompson who also coined the term anticathode, and came very close to discovering natural radioactivity.

Morton had a facile pen, but it was a mistake to tackle Pupin at that early stage. In *Electricity* of February 19, Morton accused Pupin of having copied a design for producing x rays with a static machine, a design which Morton had published in the New York *World* of February 10. Pupin dipped his pen in poison and prepared a sardonic reply, which was printed in the same *Electricity* of February 10 together with Morton's comparatively mild *Letter to the Editor*. In his rebuttal, Pupin referred to Morton as the "learned electrotherapeutist" who " talked wildly about cathode rays" but who – at the time of Pupin's visit to Morton's office on Sunday evening, February 9, 1896 – had no roentgen plates to show. Moreover, wrote Pupin, Morton tried repeatedly to return to the question of "brush discharges," a subject which Pupin rejected as outrageously obsolete. Pupin was probably correct in assuming that Morton talked so much about "sparks" simply because as of February 9 Morton had not yet produced a roentgen plate. But he was soon to make the grade, indeed Morton added a very lucrative private radiologic practice to his already thriving electro-

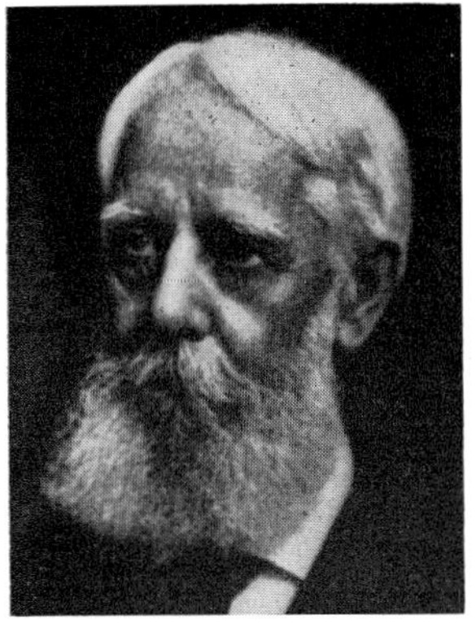

FRANCIS WILLIAMS

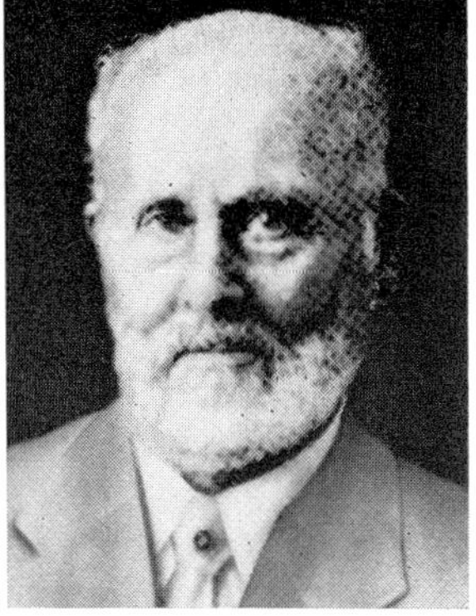

HERBERT ROLLINS

therapeutic clientele. Morton proposed (*Dental Cosmos* of June, 1896) the use of intraoral films for dental purposes. The first to actually produce a dental x-ray plate in this country was C. Edmund Kells, Jr., of New Orleans. Kells suffered severe radiation damage, had over one hundred operations for radiogenic neoplasia, and – in desperation – committed suicide.

IN BOSTON

In Boston, the first clinical fluoroscopies were performed at the Massachusetts Institute of Technology on Wednesday, April 22, 1896.

As reported in the *Electrical World* of May 23, the technical side was the domain of Charles Ladd Norton (1870-1939), who invited a respected physician, Francis Henry Williams (1852-1936). The latter brought patients from Boston City Hospital, and this is how and where the first "diagnostic" fluorescopies (sic) were done in the Hub. They soon decided it would be easier to install an apparatus on the hospital premises, as described in Williams' reminiscences. Williams gives credit to another MIT physicist, Ralph Restieaux Lawrence, and especially to the Boston dentist William Rollins (1852-1929), who was a mechanical genius.

Information on the beginnings of radiology in Massachusetts General Hospital comes from the pages by George Winslow Holmes, included in the 1921 Memorial and Historical Volume of the MGH. While no specific date is given, corroboration with other sources makes it reasonable to assume that Walter James Dodd, their pharmacist and photographer, did not obtain good results until after June or perhaps July, 1896. He also availed himself of a portentous x-ray coil, built by Hermann Lemp of the General Electric Company. That coil was placed in the old Kingsley Studio where Dodd and his assistant Joseph Godsoe (who later became the chief-pharmacist at the hospital) used it steadily. The amount of current needed by that coil was excessive and blew the fuses on the mains; the machine was pronounced unsafe, and remained in the hospital at least until the 50th anniversary of "ether day" when it was purchased as a souvenir and moved to the old West Room under the Bulfinch steps.*

Also in 1896, at a medical convention in Washington (D.C.), Reginald Heber Fitz (1843-1913) – remembered for his description of pancreatitis – showed a radiograph of the entire human body, produced by Dodd, the subject being Godsoe.

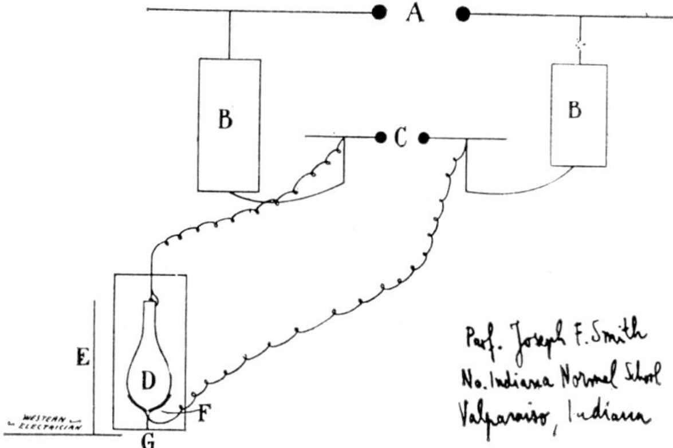

INCANDESCENCE IN INDIANA. On March 21, 1896 in the *Western Electrician* (Chicago) was reproduced this scheme showing the arrangement whereby roentgen rays had been produced with a modified incandescent bulb. The author was Joseph F. Smith, who taught physics in the Normal School in Valparaiso (Indiana).

ELSEWHERE IN THE U. S.

Actually, the first total body radiograph was the work of Dayton Clarence Miller (1866-1941), who was then dean of the Physics Department at the old Case School of Applied Sciences in Cleveland. Miller was his own subject for the total body radiograph. He had himself strapped in a frame so he would not move during the one and one-half hour exposure. His wife operated the controls.† Prior to that momentous exploit Miller lectured before the Cleveland Medical Society on April 3, 1896, together with the biophilosophical surgeon George Washington Crile, Sr. (1864-1943), who later founded the Cleveland Clinic. In the same year and city, a distraught woman rushed her gasping husband to a hospital and announced that he had swallowed his false teeth. The man was radiographed and the foggy prints indicated that the teeth were lodged in his gullet. After two inconclusive operations on the victim's neck, the missing teeth were found under a bed post. Then the man expired from a cardiac condition, and the Cleveland papers came out with the headline, "Patient who didn't swallow teeth is dead."‡ By that time, x rays were being produced in most of the forty-five states (after renouncing polygamy, Utah had been admitted into the Union in 1896 as the 45th).

At Grinnell College in Iowa, Frank Fayette Almy (1866-1932), their professor of physics, had made "cathodic ray photographs" reproduced on February 29 in *Scholars in Black*, the school's house organ.§ In this respect, Minnesota trailed Iowa because the first notice or roentgen rays at the University of Minnesota appeared in the March 21 issue of the *Western Electrician*. On February 29, in the same magazine, had appeared the news that on February 15, the "electrician" Thomas E. Duncan and A. B. Crowe (from the local schools) had produced their first roentgen plates (of coins) in the Laboratory of the Fort Wayne Electric Corporation.

The beginning of medical radiology in Chicago would fill a very colorful chapter. It had everything from quacks to apostles. In February 1896, Harry Preston Pratt located a foreign body in the hand of a patient, which brought him local fame. Friedrich Curt Harnisch, an opthalmologist by trade, began work with a 6″ spark coil (from the McIntosh Battery Co.) installed in his own home. By April 1896, he had moved with another physician, Otto Schmidt, into the Schiller (later called the Garrick Theatre) Building. They hired an electrician from the Cicero and Proviso Railroad, a German immigrant called Wolfram Konrad Fuchs (1856-1908). The office got a big write-up in the *Western Electrician* of August 29, and soon became known as the Fuchs X-Ray Laboratory. It was very successful and before the end of 1896, Fuchs had performed over 1400 examinations in that office.

Lay X-Ray Laboratories had appeared in many cities. In the *Electrical Engineer* of June 3, 1896, was inserted the following notice: "Mr. M. F. Martin has opened an x-ray studio at 110 E. 26th St. in New York City, where pictures of interior human structure will be taken. The consultation hours are from 1:00 to 2:00 and from 5:00 to 6:00. A lady assistant is in attendance."

Still, by and large, there were more physicians than lay people among practicing radiologists. In February 1896, Heber Robarts (who subsequently founded the American Roentgen Ray Society) installed x-ray equipment in his office on Grand Avenue, near Locust Street in St. Louis. His assistant at that time was Fred Summa

*The current director of radiology at Massachusetts General Hospital, Dr. Laurence Robbins, could not locate the Lemp coil, nor any information on it, except what Percy Brown had taken from the same source (Holmes).

†This total body radiograph was not in one piece, nor was Dodd's. The first single piece total body radiograph was obtained in 1897 by Morton using Eastman-Kodak film. Dayton Miller's total body radiograph was exhibited at the 1949 RSNA meeting in Cleveland.

‡This information comes from an article by Jack Warfel in the *Cleveland Press* of November 2, 1949. It was called to my attention by Mr. Ed Goldfield from Picker.

§This information was courteously supplied by Mrs. Elizabeth Anderson, the technical editor of the Medical Division of the Oak Ridge Institute of Nuclear Studies.

WONDERFUL NEW RAY SEES THROUGH HAND!

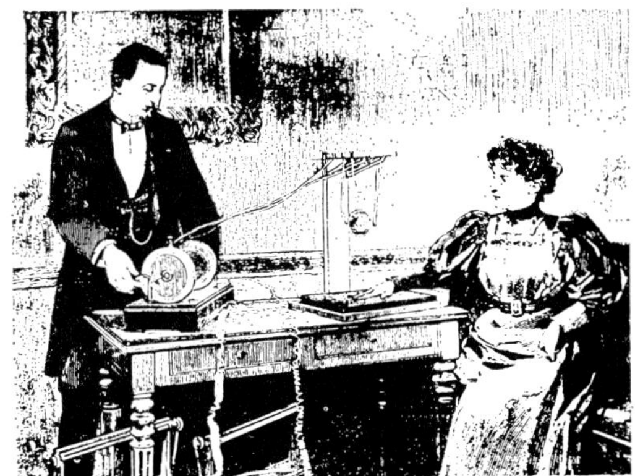

X-Ray Studio . . .

110 East Twenty-Sixty Street,

. . . . New York City.

O'Hara (who subsequently founded the Radiological Society of North America).

On March 9, 1896, the Denver *News* reported the x-ray examination performed by a doctor W. F. Hassenplug.*

FIRST "FOREIGN" RADIOLOGISTS

An attempt was also made to identify "first" radiologists in foreign lands. In such matters the personal impression of the "judge" (or of his sources) may not agree with everybody else's opinion. It has already been stated that Kaiser was the first radiologist in Austria, Oudin the first in France, and Rowland the first in Great Britain. In Hungary, Karoly Kiss opened his x-ray office on February 7, 1896. In Czechoslovakia, the first radiologist was Rudolf Jedlicka (1869-1926), in Denmark the first was L. J. Mygge (1850-1935), in Sweden the first was Thor Stenbeck. In Roumania the first was G. T. Michaescu. In Canada, the previously mentioned Girdwood qualifies in this category. In Australia, F. J. Clendinnen (1860-1913), of Melbourne, was the first medical radiologist, and also their first radiation casualty. In Argentina, Carlos Heuser was the first medical radiologist; in the Netherlands, this priority goes to J. K. A. Wertheim-Salomonson (1864-1922). In Russia, N. N. Cherkassov of Moscow may be regarded as the first. In Germany the choice is very difficult: this epithet of first medical radiologist is not a purely chronologic qualification, the "candidate" must also have created something (at least a trend): the German selectee is Herman Gocht (1869-1938), who began to operate on March 20, 1896 the Roentgen Department installed by the surgeon Hermann Kuemmell (1852-1937) – remembered for his description of pancreatitis – in the Eppendorf Hospital in Hamburg.*

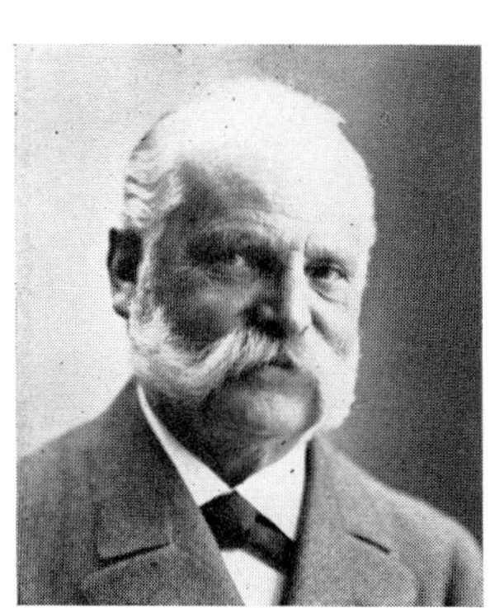

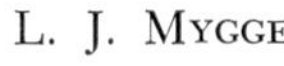

L. J. MYGGE

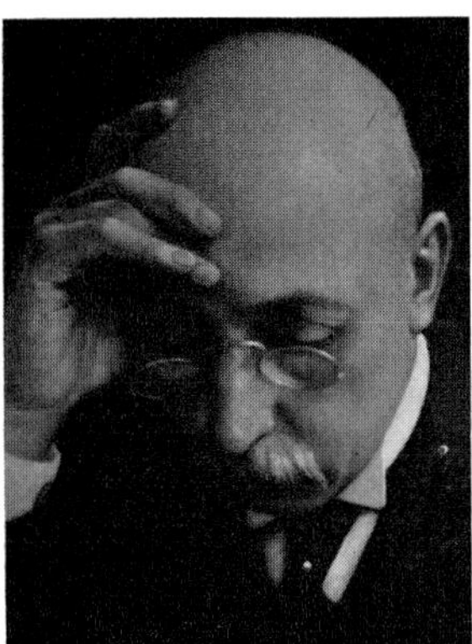

WERTHEIM-SALOMONSON

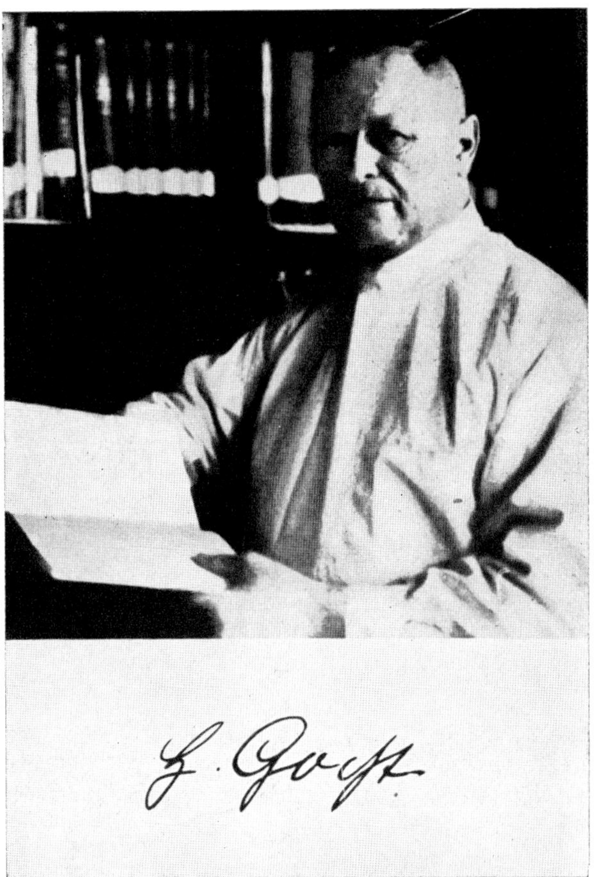

Courtsey: Röntgen-Blätter & Girardet-Verlag

HERMANN GOCHT

*This information comes from Dr. William Walter Wasson, who has compiled a *History of Radiology in Colorado.* So far it has been circulated as a manuscript.

*Heinrich Ernst Albers-Schoenberg (1865-1921) did not open his office (together with Gustav Deycke) until 1897.

LEGAL X-RAY "FIRSTS"

In the *Electrical Engineer* of June 10, 1896, appeared the information that in May, Miss Gladys Ffolliett, a burlesque actress, had sued the Nottingham Theater Company (England) for damages incurred during a fall (in the line of duty). A roentgen plate of her left foot was recommended by Dr. Frankish and made at the University College Hospital. It demonstrated a displacement of the cuboid bone, was accepted by the jury and compensation was awarded for "contributory carelessness."

The Denver case, reported by Sanford Martin Withers (1891-1938), was initiated in April, 1896, but decided only on December 2 (Judge Owen Lefevre's decision to accept x-ray plates in evidence was then published in the Denver *Republican*). The case was brought to court by one James Smith who had a fracture of the femur, overlooked by Dr. W. W. Grant. Patient was then seen by another physician, Dr. Tennant, and the latter asked a photographer, H. Buckwalter, to expose plates of the thigh. These were then presented in court by the plaintiff's attorneys, Benjamin B. Lindsey (afterwards founder of the Denver Juvenile Court), and Fred W. Parks (later U. S. Senator).*

Carleton Barnhart Peirce, the current professor of radiology in McGill University, called my attention to the fact that there is some question regarding whether or not Cox or one of his assistants took that first Canadian roentgen plate. On Peirce's advice I wrote to Hugh Ernest MacDermot, medical historian of the Montreal General Hospital, and this is what he answered:

"It is not easy to say whether Cox himself exposed the plate in question. I should have thought it likely that he did, as the case was the first of its kind to be sent to him, but he may have left it to one of his assistants, of whom Nevil Norton Evans was one. On the other hand I have recently come across a statement from one of the early radiologists in Montreal (Walter Wilkins, who was radiologist at Montreal General Hospital from 1900 for several years) to the effect that it was one Charles O. Jost who exposed the plate in question. I don't know what his authority for saying that was, as he died lately and I never had a chance to question him about it. However, it is a small point. I got hold of the newspaper report of the incident today; it appeared in the *Montreal Star* of March 11, 1896, and was a description of the case in court. The name of the gunman was George Holder, and the article stated that this was the first time that x-rays had been used as evidence in court, *in the world!* I don't know who was the authority for that large statement, except the *Star* itself, but I shouldn't be surprised if it was accurate."

*In 1954, the forensic radiologist *par excellence* Samuel Wright Donaldson remarked that early "timorous acceptance" of x-ray evidence by the court has since changed to "implicit trust."

Yes, indeed, it came ahead of Miss Ffolliett, and will have to be accepted as the very first. As to the question whether Cox himself made the first exposure it may be said that Charles Roland, a physician from Winona (Ontario), made no mention whatsoever of the existence of such a doubt in his note on Cox and Kirkpatrick's first report (*cf., Canadian Journal of Surgery* of July, 1962).

OTHER MEDICAL USES

The first utilization of roentgen rays on wounded soldiers is credited to Giuseppe Alvaro, who in February, 1896, employed this method in the Military Hospital in Naples. The *Electrical Engineer* (New York) of July 15, 1896, reported that the British War Office had sent two sets of roentgen ray apparatus up the Nile to be used by Army surgeons in locating

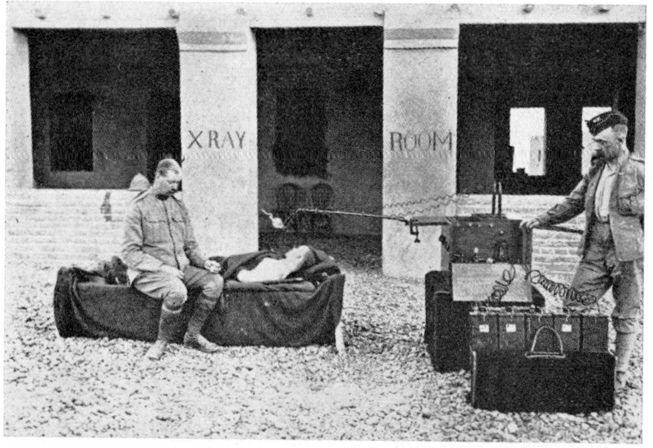

Courtesy: David Shields.

ROENTGEN WARPATH ON THE NILE. The original caption was: "Major Battersby and his orderly taking a radiograph".

bullets and determining the extent of fractures. Those units, operated with pedal-pushing "power supply," gave good service on actual battle casualties.

Similar interest was manifested by the German War Department. They assigned Otto von Schjerning (1853-1921), the "father" of their Medical Military Corps, and Fritz Kranzfelder (1858-1907), a ballistic expert, to evaluate the surgical usefulness of the roentgen method. Their carefully worded, but other-

H. PRESTON PRATT, M. D., President. R. S. GREGG, M. D., Secretary.

Dr. Pratt's X-Ray

...AND...

Electro-Therapeutical Laboratory,

MASONIC TEMPLE, CHICAGO.

Long Distance Phone, Central 1910.

The Oldest X-Ray Laboratory, established February 7, 1896, is well equipped for

General Electro-Therapeutical Work of all kinds. Dr. Pratt's long experience enables him to guarantee

No Injurious Effects from the X-RAY or other treatments in his laboratory.

X-Ray Pictures, both snap shots and time exposures.

Cancer, Lupus, and other forms of tuberculosis, inflamed joints, and numerous other ailments, are successfully treated.

Interests of Physicians and Surgeons protected.

Expert Evidence rendered in medico-legal cases.

Professional Correspondence receives prompt attention.

Published Articles on X-Rays and Electro-Therapeutics will be sent on application.

wise promising report was published in April, 1896 in the *Deutsche Medicinische Wochenschrift.*

In the July 22 number of the *Electrical Engineer* appeared the information that "Professor H. P. Pratt (with Prof. Hugo Wightman) had treated an almost hopeless case of consumption with results 'so far but little short of marvelous.' " The patient had his chest bared, the

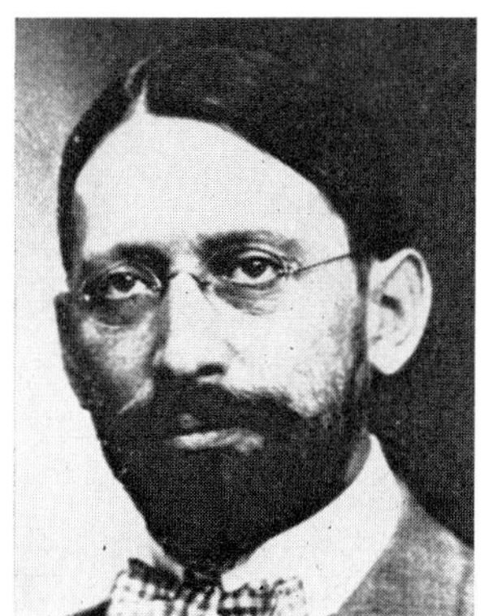

Harry Preston Pratt. A well-known Chicago roentgen pioneer who came closer to the margin of the profession than his New York City counterpart (Monell).

tube placed in direct contact with the flesh, for an exposure of three hours, after which they noticed a decrease of 2° in temperature . . . and with subsequent treatment a continual improvement occurred during five weeks. Signed statements of the doctors who attended the treatment of the young man appeared in the Chicago *Times-Herald.*

Also in the *Electrical Engineer,* on December 9, appeared a notice that the Rochester *Democrat & Chronicle* gave credit to Dr. G. Waverly Clark, of San Francisco for having discovered that blind persons could see with the help of cathode rays. The Rochester *Herald* chided the *Democrat* & *Chronicle* for bestowing such honor on Clark, when Edison had discovered it. Thereupon, Edison wrote a letter to the *Democrat* & *Chronicle,* saying that Clark's reported experiment is incomprehensible as the blind person was supposed to have seen motion on the fluoroscopic screen which is ordinary light, while Edison's experiments were made with blindfolded viewing of so-called cathode rays directly by the eye. We know today that x rays cause faint luminosity on the retina.

ROENTGEN DAMAGE

As previously stated, Grubbé was the first person to incur deleterious effects from roentgen irradiation. It began to happen to other people as well and word got around. The *bona-fide* pioneers were fluoroscopists and they resented the implication that their "hobby" was in any way dangerous. On April 30, 1896, during the meeting of the *Association of American Physicians,* Francis Williams was asked whether he was in danger of losing his hair. "I have had my head in the rays for some time," he replied, "and I do not think I have any less hair than I had a few weeks ago."

On December 12, 1896, in the *Western Electrician,* Wolfram Fuchs admitted having had "but four instances of the slow healing burns which have lately attracted considerable attention through the columns of the press . . . the injury may be regarded as slight in comparison with the benefits resulting from this wonderful discovery. However, it is desirable to prevent the inconvenience and pain of these sun burns and as a result of a number of experiments, the last four months, I offer the following suggestions: 1. Shorten exposure to a minimum. 2. Place tube not nearer than 12″ from body, and 3. Rub vaseline well into the skin and leave coating over part to be exposed." After a few whimsical explanations concerning "vasomotoric nerves," Fuchs added, "the x-ray burns are not more dangerous than ordinary burns," and finally, "when the x rays are applied to the head very long, the hair drops out, but it grows in again with no attendant bad effects."

Elihu Thomson exposed his left little finger over one of those crackling gas tubes for half an hour, and one week later he noticed erythema, tenderness, and finally blistering (*Western Electrician,* November 21). By contrast, E. A. Frey (*Electrical Engineer,* December 23) claimed to have seen no ill effects from exposing his left foot to the rays emitted by a tube energized with a static machine. He "treated" his foot from one-half hour to one hour every four days but allegedly noticed neither discoloration nor anything else. Frey was not a physician: he was the owner of the Frey & Co. of Boston, which had just placed on the market a Toepler-Holtz Machine with 2000 revolutions per minute. His claim was that x rays produced by a static machine were not dangerous as opposed to the x rays produced by coil.

EARLY X-RAY MANUFACTURERS

At this point several of the more colorful electromedical firms will be listed among those which were in operation in 1896, and have survived to this day. Some have retained their original name, although ownership has changed through mergers or purchase.

In the *USA,* General Electric (GE) is the oldest firm in the "x-ray business," even though they have discontinued production of certain equipment at one time or another. The text of their initial announcement of entering the field was printed in the *Electrical World* of August 22, 1896 (it is reproduced in the chapter on American X-Ray Makers).

GE x-ray equipment was then produced mainly but not exclusively at Edison's plant in Harrison (New Jersey). Elihu Thomson, with his associate Hermann Lemp (who developed, patented, and used in 1896 the world's first rotary switch as well as a transformer), were active at GE's Research Laboratories in Lynn (Massachusetts): that was the birthplace of Thomson's Inductorium (an oil-immersed coil with

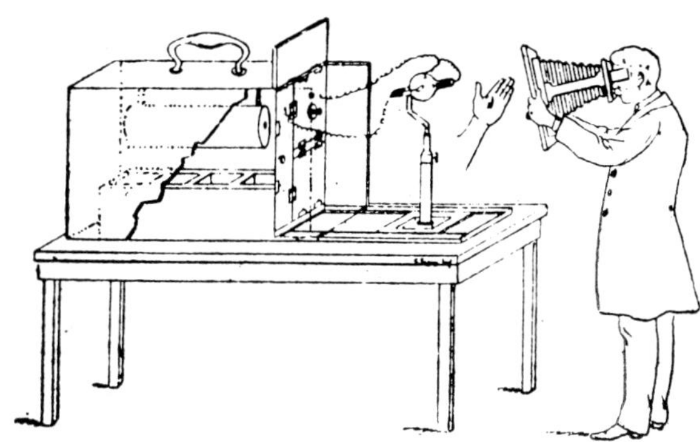

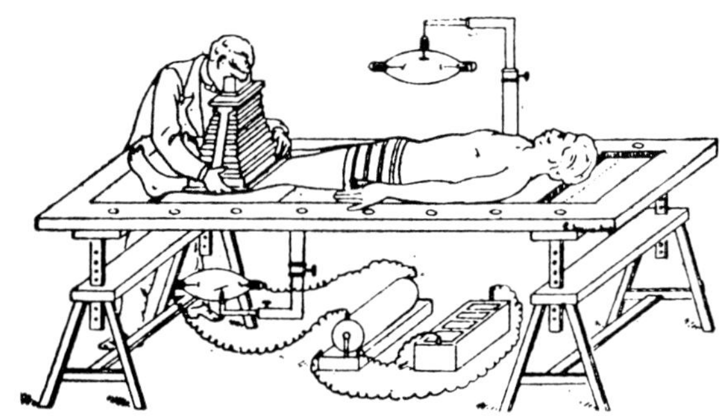

FLUOROSCOPIC WORKBENCH. Much improvisation was done in the very beginning, but by the end of 1896, manufacturing had set in. The twin-tube arrangement is by George Séguy of Paris.

LE ROY'S IMPROVED ALUMINUM **X-RAY** FLUOROSCOPE

FOUR TIMES AS POWERFUL AS ANY YET MADE.

TUNGSTATE OF CALCIUM mounted on an Aluminum Window.

Weight, 6 Ounces.

Complete Portable X-Ray Outfits for Physicians

LOW PRICE.
HIGH QUALITY.
WRITE FOR PRICES.

AND OTHERS DESIRING AN OUTFIT FOR EXPERIMENTAL USE.

TOTAL WEIGHT ONLY 55 TO 60 LBS. TRADE SUPPLIED WITH FLUOROSCOPES.

J. A. LE ROY, 143 E. 13th ST., NEW YORK.

ROENTGEN ADVERTISEMENT FROM BYGONE DAYS. It appeared in the *Electrical Engineer* (New York) of June 24, 1896. The true roentgen pioneers, from Williams to Holzknecht, and from Albers-Schönberg to Macintyre, were fluoroscopists: in the very beginning plates were often regarded as self-evident, *i.e.,* needing no interpretation.

X-RAY OUTFITS.

The Edison Manufacturing Company

ARE PREPARED TO SUPPLY

MR. THOMAS A. EDISON'S ORIGINAL APPARATUS

As exhibited at the recent Electrical Exhibition in New York.

OUTFITS FOR TRAVELLING EXHIBITORS.
OUTFITS FOR SCIENTIFIC INSTITUTIONS.
OUTFITS FOR PHYSICIANS.
EDISON X-RAY TUBES.
EDISON-LALANDE BATTERIES FOR X-RAY APPARATUS.

WRITE FOR PARTICULARS.

EDISON MANUFACTURING COMPANY,

110 East 23d St., New York City.

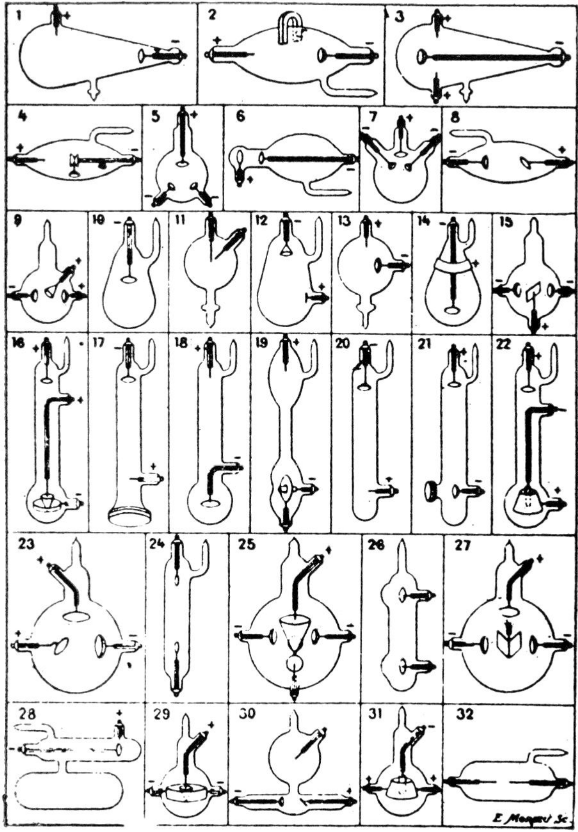

GAS TUBES OF 1896. This often reproduced (and most of the time wrongly attributed) representation of early gas tubes appeared in *La Nature* (Paris) in November of 1896. It was Séguy's personal collection, and contained tubes both with and without reflector. Some of the shapes are identifiable: 1, 2, 20 Crookes; 3, 5, 7, 9, 11, 13, 21, 22, 23, 29 Séguy; 4 Wood; 8 Thomson; 10 D'Arsonval; 12 Puluj; 24 Röntgen; 28, 30 Colardeau.

motor-driven interrupter, giving a continuous shower of 6″ or 12″ sparks), and of the Standard Double Focus Tube. Thomson built also a special roentgen ray "transformer," which consisted mainly of a combination of a conventional and a high frequency coil, coupled with a condenser, so that it could be operated from either direct or alternate current. Thomson's machines were described in detail in the *Electrical Engineer* of October 21, 1896. Another GE team was that of Houston and Kennelly who had produced a workable hospital x-ray installation (based on a Tesla type coil), described in the *American Electrician* of August, 1896.

In Chicago, William Scheidel, who had worked for Kaiser & Schmidt in Berlin, began to construct x-ray coils soon after the announcement of Röntgen's discovery. After a few unsuccessful attempts, he produced the first x-ray coil in Illinois (and perhaps in the United States) to be sold to a physician, Benjamin Hamilton of Shawnee (Oklahoma). Soon thereafter, Scheidel & Co. went into business and its first three coils were delivered to H. P. Pratt, James Burry, and F. H. Blackmarr, all in Chicago. Eventually, though, after three mergers Scheidel & Co. became part of General Electric.

In that first year (1896) x rays were produced not only with low-frequency (Ruhmkorff) or high-frequency (Tesla) coils. A third modality was the static machine, so dear to the electrotherapists.

One of the most famous makers of static machines was the Waite & Bartlett of New York, founded in 1889 by Henry E. Waite, a physician, Civil War vet-

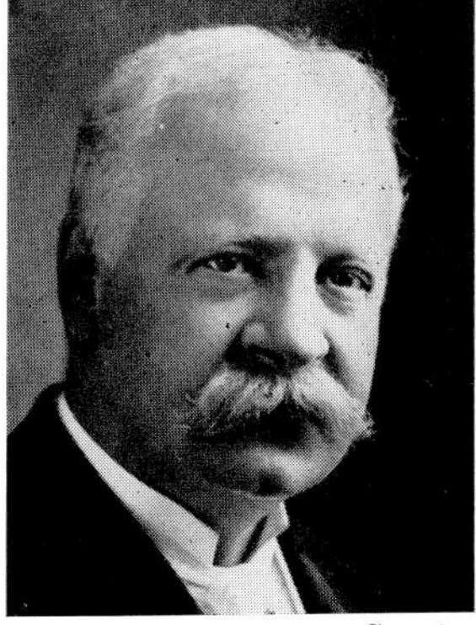

Courtesy: Ed Goldfield.

HENRI E. WAITE (1848-1916). A physician, electrotherapist, and inventor (of the "molecular," long-distance telephone), Waite, Sr. founded, with a certain Bartlett, the Waite & Bartlett Co. in 1889. Bartlett died, but his name persisted until Picker purchased the W & B in 1929.

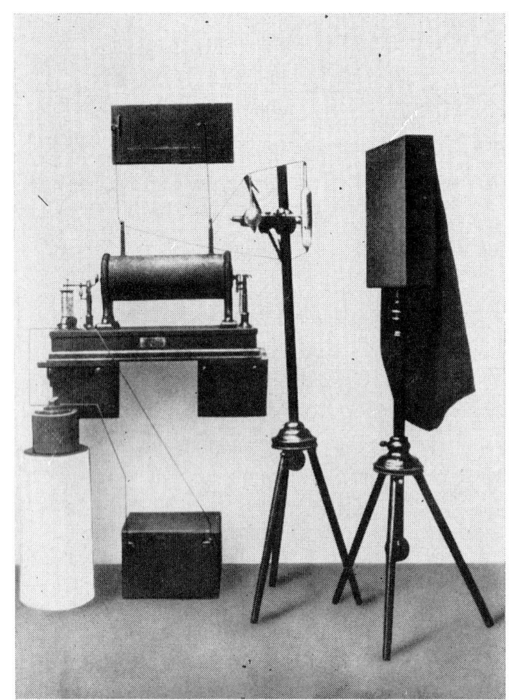

Courtesy: Archives of Siemens-Reiniger-Werkes.

SIEMENS & HALSKE EQUIPMENT OF 1896. It consisted of a battery-operated coil with their own, peculiarly-shaped, vacuum-regulated x-ray tube. The height of the screen was adjustable. The black drape retarded deterioration of the screen, and provided a dark space for the fluoroscopist's head.

eran, and instructor in electrotherapy in the New York Postgraduate Medical School. He was an inventor in his own rights (he patented the molecular telephone, for some time the only available device for long distance communications). During the Big Depression, Waite & Bartlett was purchased by Picker.

In *Germany,* electromedical equipment was being produced since 1847 by Werner von Siemens (1816-1892). In 1896, Siemens & Halske made and sold x-ray equipment: their coils were conventional, but they manufactured special x-ray tubes with a device for the regulation of vacuum, patented in Germany (DRP 91028) on March 24, 1896.

The firm of Reiniger, Gebbert & Schall was founded in 1886 in Erlangen (Germany) by Erwin Reiniger (1854-1909), Max Gebbert (1856-1907), and Karl Schall (?-1925). Shortly after the announcement of the discovery, Gebbert contacted Röntgen himself: there are letters to prove it. Röntgen was very polite, replied courteously to all his correspondents, and always thanked for the tubes, coils, and other items which people sent him, but he never endorsed anybody's products. Actually RGS managed quite well without special endorsements. Their original name was "Vereinigte physikalisch-medizinische Werkstätten Reiniger, Gebbert und Schall, Erlangen-

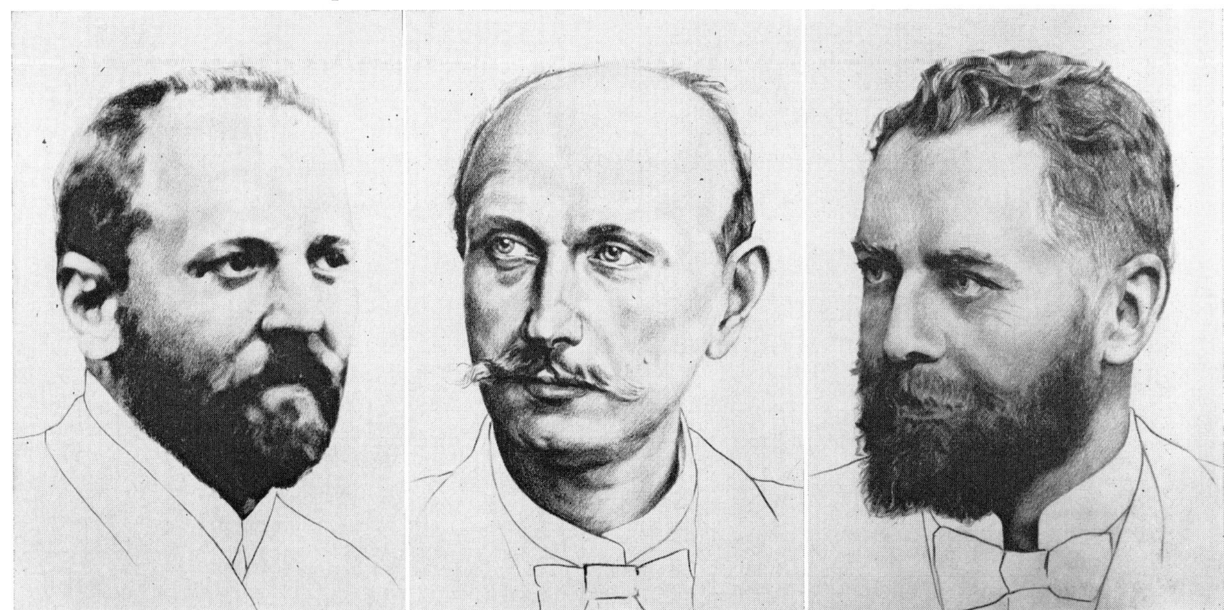

Courtesy: Archives of Siemens-Reiniger-Werke

REINIGER, GEBBERT & SCHALL. The real soul of their company was the center figure, Max Gebbert (1856-1907), but in the current appelation of the firm, only the name of Erwin Reiniger (1854-1909) has been preserved, although he had left the firm in 1895. Karl Schall (right) had gone to London in 1887, and was successful in establishing his own business.

New York-Stuttgart," Gebbert had lived in New York and Philadelphia from 1883 to 1885, and was considering to expand and return to the States to start a manufacturing plant. In 1887 Schall left the firm, emigrated to London, and created there his own organization, which is still in part directed by his son. Reiniger left the firm in 1895, so that it was actually Max Gebbert who decided in 1896 to devote much

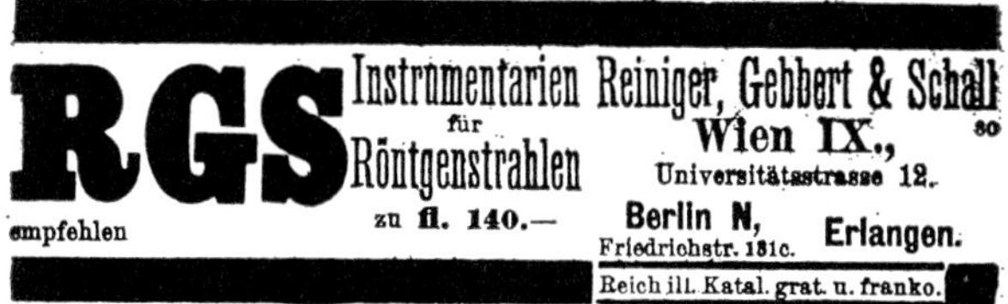

Courtesy: Library of the University of Illinois.

RGS AD OF 1896. This insert was printed for most of the second half of 1896 in every other issue of the *Wiener Medicinische Wochenschrift.*

of the company's time and money to the production of x-ray equipment. Eventually RGS and Siemens & Halske merged into what is today the Siemens-Reiniger-Werke A. G. (SRW).

In Hamburg existed since 1865 the glassblowing shop of Carl Heinrich Florenz Müller (1845-1912) who made and sold Crookes and Geissler tubes since 1874. Also in Hamburg existed since 1892 the Richard Seifert & Co. — its owner being Friedrich Wilhelm Richard Seifert (1862-1929). Röntgen had communicated with Voller (director of the Physikalischen Staatslaboratorium) and with Voller's associate Walter, who wanted immediately to produce roentgen rays. They called on Seifert to furnish the coil, and on Müller to make the tube, and this is how around January 15, 1896, they came up with the roentgen plate of a hand, which was duly circulated in the periodicals of the time. For a long time Seifert and Müller maintained this business relationship wherein the first would produce the machines, the other the tubes. Today Müller's firm is owned by the Dutch company Philips. Seifert, however, is the only firm in the x-ray business which is still privately owned by the same family: its director is Heinrich Wilhelm Richard Seifert, son of the founder.

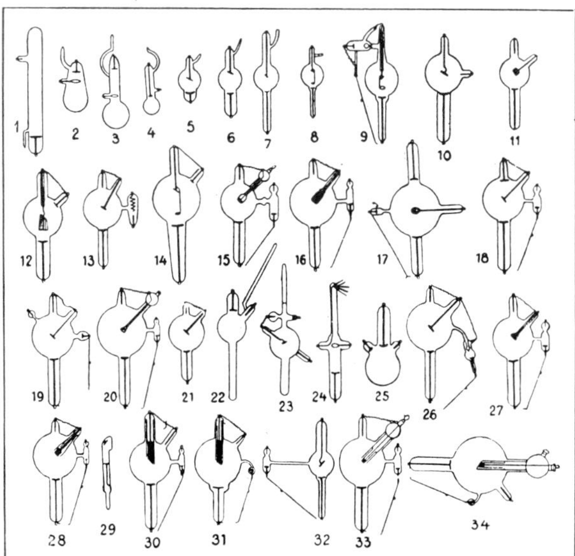

Courtesy: David Shields.

EARLY MÜLLER ROENTGEN TUBES.

In *Great Britain* the microscope makers Watson & Sons were manufacturing also electro-medical equipment since 1837 — they are apparently the world's oldest electro-medical manufacturer, and are said to have made and sold some x-ray equipment in 1896, but so far I have been unable to substantiate this by printed (dated) ads. Subsequently, Watson & Son (Electro-Medical) separated from the mother firm,

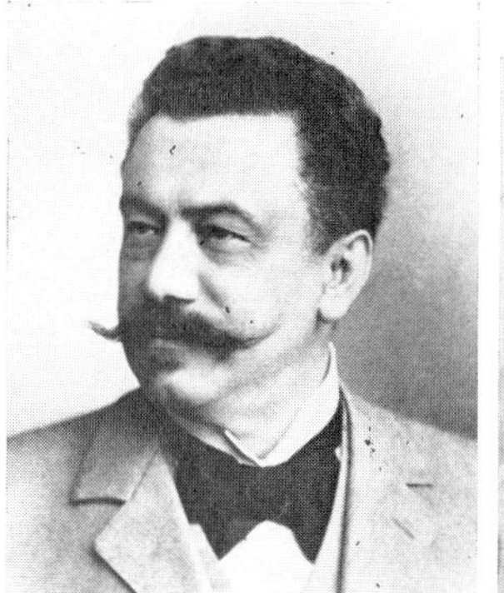

Courtesy: Archives of the C. H. F. Müller Co.

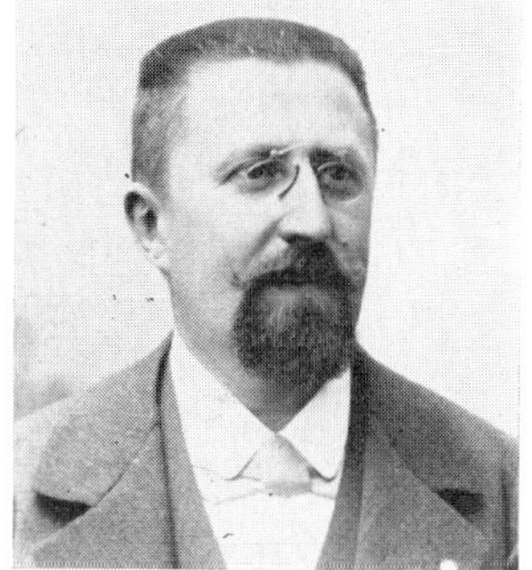

Courtesy: Archives of the Massiot-Philips Company.

CARL HEINRICH FLORENZ MÜLLER (1845-1912). The corporate name and image of this former glassblower from Hamburg is now owned by a Dutch company (Philips). Müller was a true roentgen pioneer, and is remembered as a radiation casualty. Man with goatee is ARTHUR RADIGUET (1850-1905). Manufacturing roentgen pioneer, and one of the earliest recognized radiation casualties in France; his firm changed its name to that of his son-in-law (Massiot), and is now owned by a Dutch company.

later yet they were bought out by the (British) General Electric Company, but continued to operate under the good old name of Watson's. In the last months of 1896, Alfred Ernest Dean (1866-1927) founded a company which is still in the manufacture of x-ray equipment; it is no longer family-owned, but Dean's son was until recently its director. Harry William Cox (1870-1937) started making x-ray machines in that same year 1896, but after World War I he had to merge with the Cavendish Electrical Company; they are currently in business, but no longer manufacture x-ray equipment proper.

In *France,* there existed a family of opticians, who had been in business since the 18th Century. The head of the firm in 1896, Arthur Radiguet (1850-1905) began to produce x-ray equipment, and made several communications to the French Academy of Sciences (in February and March of 1896) on his improvements of the fluoroscope. Among Radiguet's customers were many of the French pioneers, Oudin, Bouchard, Guilleminot, Bergonié and others. Radiguet became a radiation casualty, but the firm was continued by his son-in-law, Georges Massiot (today it has become the Massiot-Philips).

While Radiguet produced conventional low-frequency coils, Georges Gaiffe (1857-1943), who in 1896 had a going manufacture of electromedical equipment, adapted for x-ray apparatus the high-frequency coils he was producing for d'Arsonval. Through several mergers Gaiffe's company became part of today's Compagnie Générale de Radiologie, France's largest x-ray manufacturer.

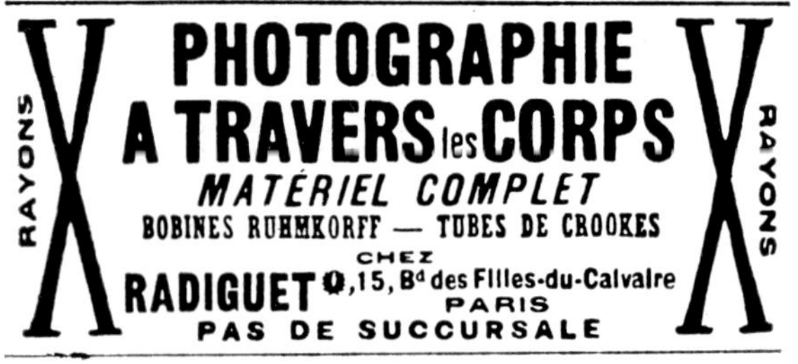

In *Italy,* Luigi Gorla had an electro-medical company which in 1896 began making x-ray apparatus; today, his successor is the Gorla-Siama, a subsidiary of the SRW.

LUIGI GORLA

MILANO -- Corso S. Celso, 17 — MILANO

Premiato alle Esposizioni di Medicina ed Igiene

MILANO 1892 -- ROMA 1894

Apparecchi completi per esperienze di RADIOGRAFIA ROENTGEN.

Rocchetti RUHMKORFF da L. 600 - 520 - 350 - 230.

Tubi di CROOKES modello *B* **L. 30** - modello *C* **L. 25** - modello *D* **L. 20.**

L'Agenzia del Giornale **Il Policlinico,** Roma, Via Convertite, 8, assume commissioni per questa Ditta.

Courtesy: National Library of Medicine.

GORLA AD OF 1896. This appeared for several months in the *Policlinico.*

In *Japan,* roentgen plates were produced in 1896 in the laboratories of the firm founded in 1875 by

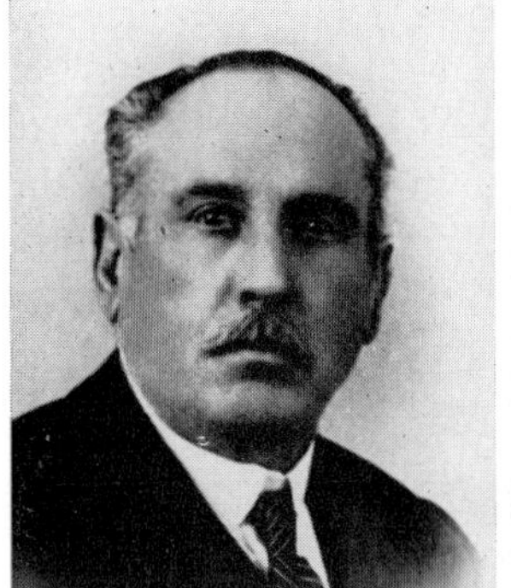

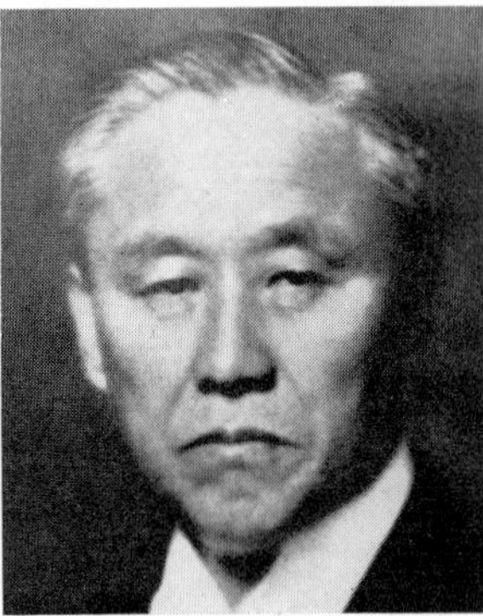

Courtesy: Gorla-Siama and Shimadzu.

LUIGI GORLA. His electro-medical manufacturing shop was in operation since 1889, and in 1896 he began to connect Crookes tubes to Ruhmkorff coils, and sell them as x-ray equipment. Today his old firm is owned by Siemens-Reiniger-Werke. The other portrait is that of GENZO SHIMADZU (1869-1951), the electrical engineer who built the first commercial x-ray unit in Japan in October, 1896.

Genzo Shimadzu — it is today the respected Shimadzu Seisakusho Ltd.

In *Australia,* there existed in 1896 the Watson & Son, founded by a descendant of, but not otherwise connected with, the British Watson. In 1896 Watson & Son, then in Melbourne, purchased an 8″ coil from the Australian experimenter G. W. Selby (a former accountant, who had found himself as a genial electrical experimenter). Incidentally, Selby also sold the first x-ray equipment on May 21, 1896, to the previ-

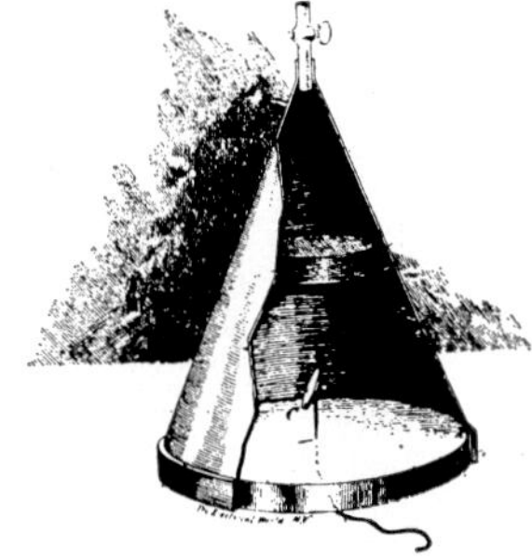

METALLIC X-RAY TUBE. In the *Electrical World* of February, 1896 appeared this drawing of a "novel form of ray lamp," the sides being made of aluminum sheet, the base of solid glass, with a metal ring holding the glass and the aluminum together. A circular wooden disc, fastened on the inside of the metallic cone, prevented collapse of the walls as the tube was being evacuated. Air tightness was achieved with plaster-of-Paris. It proved that glass was not necessary for the production of x rays. This metal tube, built by E. A. Woodward, preceded by almost three decades Albert Bouwers' Metallix.

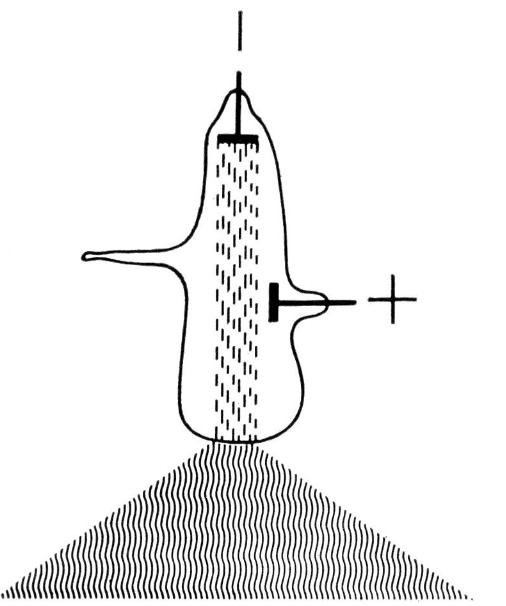

Courtesy: Deutsches Röntgen-Museum.

Stylized Hittorf tube. This is the type Röntgen was using at the time he discovered the Invisible Light.

ously mentioned first Australian medical radiologist, F. J. Clendinnen. The (Australian) Watson & Son is today the largest x-ray manufacturer in that part of the world.

X-RAY ODDS AND ENDS

A certain H. G. Davis from Parkersburg (Virginia) had in the *Electrical Engineer* a "fascinating" report of his discovery which made opaque objects transparent to ordinary light rays. This was allegedly done by passing the light through chemical solutions, the nature of which he refused to disclose. The explanation is in its' "foolish" date: April 1, 1896.

On May 27, the *Electrical Engineer* printed a letter from one H. A. Falk, president of the X-Ray Shadowgraph Company of New Orleans. It was a bitter protest against the "diabolical falsehood" of a regular correspondent of said periodical who, in its May 13 issue, had asserted that, all claims to the contrary notwithstanding, Falk was unable to make roentgen plates of the brain.

Under the title *X-Ray Foolery,* the *American Electrician* of June, 1896, reported that at Vanderbilt University, an operating roentgen tube was held for one hour at one-half inch distance from a patient's head, in an attempt to obtain an *x-radiograph* of his brain: a few weeks later, the spot on the head opposite the site of the tube became bald.

On July 4, the *Western Electrician* noticed the existence — on Madison Street in Chicago — of an *X-Ray Saloon and Restaurant.*

The *Western Electrician* of September 26 described the *X-Ray Illusion,* provided on street corners by fakers. For a small consideration, the naive spectator was allowed to view his hand "through" a brick or steel plate. The secret was an ingenious arrangement of mirrors.

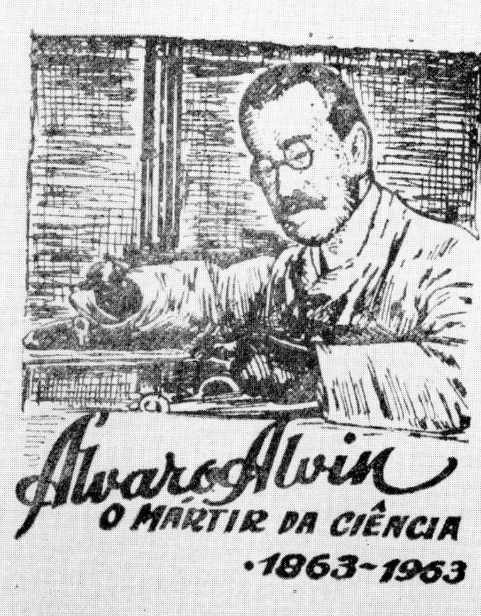

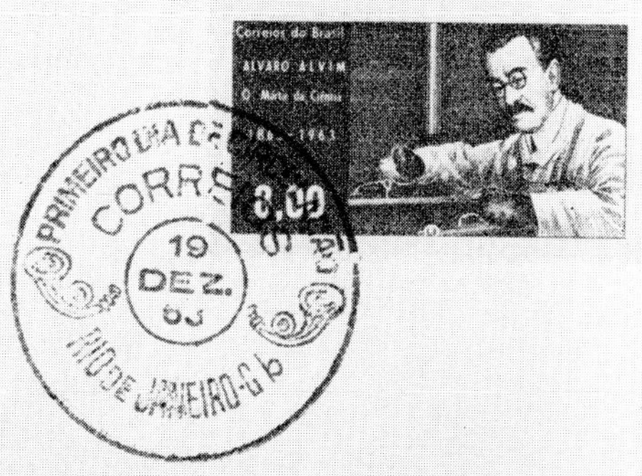

E. R. N. GRIGG, M.D.
BOX 293
CHAMPAIGN, ILLINOIS 61823

By way of contrast, it may be recalled that Otto Glasser appended to his biography of Röntgen more than one thousand very serious (among them many ground-breaking) bibliographic titles devoted to some phase of radiology: all those titles had in common the fact that they had been printed in that first momentous year of the x-ray era, 1896.

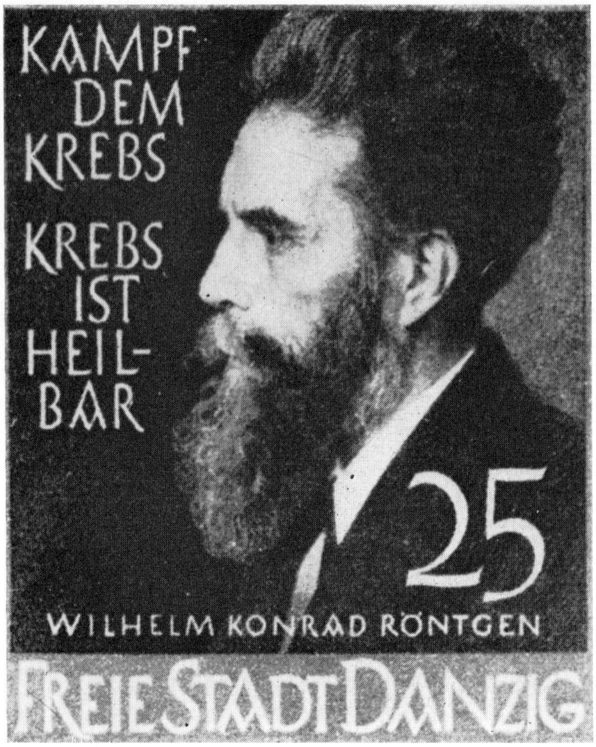

CLOSING PARAGRAPHS

At any given time in recorded history, there are among the younger generation a number of individuals who profess to be self-reliant (to the point of over-confidence), sophisticated (meaning bored), and disdainful of earlier achievements (in this regard they are often close to crass ignorance).

Some of these strong young men who enter scientific careers would reject as absurd the idea that they could ever indulge in a priority fight over "literary" contributions. Maturity must exert a certain uncanny influence on their strong characters because so many periodicals now print on the face of the article the date on which the respective manuscript was received for publication, which is obviously done to "insure" it against future priority claims.

In fact, with advancing age most people become more appreciative of the value of accurate records for the History of Science. True intellectual maturity demands in addition a dash of humility. One must be able to comprehend the truth in the sentence of Jonathan Swift (1667-1745), "It is a maxim that those to whom everybody allows the second place, have an undoubted title to the first!"

Chapter 2

AMERICAN X-RAY MAKES AND MAKERS

Agriculture, manufactures, commerce, and navigation, the four pillars of our prosperity, are the most thriving when left most free to individual enterprise.
THOMAS JEFFERSON, *Message to Congress* (1801).

WILHELM CONRAD RÖNTGEN was the first who purposely produced the *Invisible Light* on or before November 8, 1895. By January, 1896 that particular type of light was being purposely produced in most scientific centers around the globe. Such purposeful production required certain equipment.

Röntgen had used an induction coil, a Hittorf tube, and a photographic plate to record the shadow of his wife's hand (the two-ring picture).

Photographic (dry) plates were readily available, and were stocked in quantities. Coils were also available, but not in stocks. Tubes – whether of the Hittorf, Crookes, Geissler, Puluj, or of any other type – were in short supply: soon thereafter they could be had only on order, and competent glassblowers were few and far apart. Every dignified electric laboratory had several coils, and everything else could be purchased or improvised, except the tubes which were the big problem in the very beginning. In the first two weeks of February, 1896 James Burry complained that he could not purchase these tubes in Chicago, and had to order them from Philadelphia.

Soon several lightbulb plants began to include x-ray tubes in their production, as did the Beacon Lamp Co., located at Harcourt Street in Boston until October 1, 1896 when they moved to New Brunswick

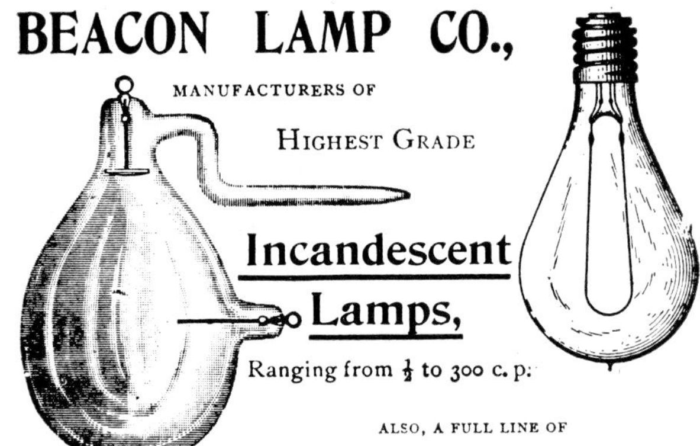

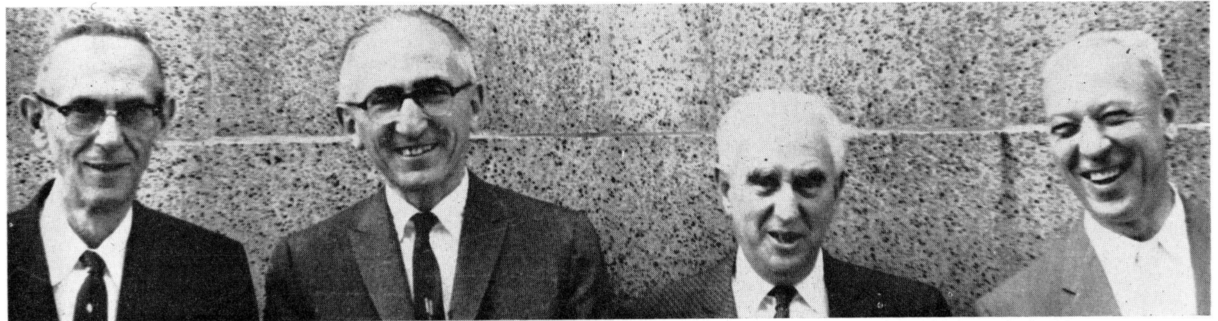

MY SENIOR X-RAY ADVISERS. From the left (the two with glasses) are Ed Goldfield (Picker) and Byron Hess* (Standard), then Bob Landauer (physicist at Cook County Hospital), and Walt Petrie (General Electric). These four gentlemen have between them over 150 years of activity in the x-ray business. Much of what is good in this chapter can be credited to them, the mistakes are my responsibility.

*Hess started at Standard at the bottom of the ladder, and advanced to vice-president. Petrie, now retired, was at the time advertising manager.

August 22, 1896

ICAL WORLD. Vol. XXVIII. No. 8.

Röntgen-Ray Apparatus.

Investigators and others practically interested in Röntgen-ray work will without doubt be greatly interested in noting the appearance of the General Electric Company as manufacturer of all kinds of Röntgen-ray apparatus. As will be seen in our advertising columns, the Edison Decorative and Miniature Lamp Department (General Electric Co.), Harrison, N. J., is in the field with an entire line of Röntgen-ray apparatus of all kinds. The name of this concern is a guarantee of the completeness and efficiency of any apparatus that it may put out.

We hope to be able to present to our readers shortly some further description of the apparatus which is now being made and extensively sold by the above concern.

(New Jersey). Small glassblowing shops appeared here and there in response to local demand. One such enterprise was started by Emile Herman Grubbé at 12 Pacific Avenue in Chicago. His glassblower was a German immigrant named Albert Schmidt. They made and sold incandescent lightbulbs, Geissler and Crookes tubes, and other glassy appurtenances.

OLDEST AMERICAN X-RAY MAKER

In the *Electrical World* of August 22, 1896 appeared the first ad in which the Edison Decorative and Miniature Lamp Dept. of the General Electric Company, located in Harrison (New Jersey) announced that it was producing a complete line of x-ray apparatus.

Elihu Thomson (1853-1937) was an electrician and inventor, born in Manchester (England), who came to the United States as a boy. Edwin James Houston (1847-1914) was an American electrical engineer, who became well known for having invented the system of arc lighting (1881). Together, they formed in 1883 the

ROENTGEN RAY

APPARATUS

EDISON DECORATIVE AND MINIATURE

LAMP DEPARTMENT

GENERAL ELECTRIC COMPANY

HARRISON, N. J.

No. 9050 June 28, 1897

Thomson-Houston Electric Co., which in 1892 merged with the Thomas Edison Co., to form the General Electric Co. (GE).

Edison christened and manufactured the fluoroscope. During February, 1896 his crew tested numerous compounds, of which about 1800 gave some results: the crystals of calcium tungstate appeared to be many times "stronger" than barium platinocya-

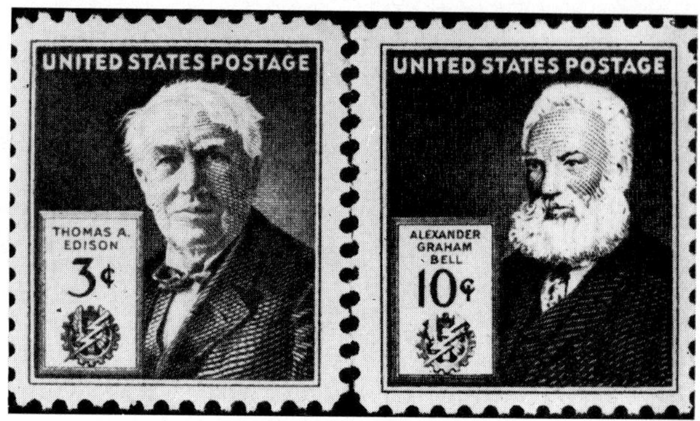

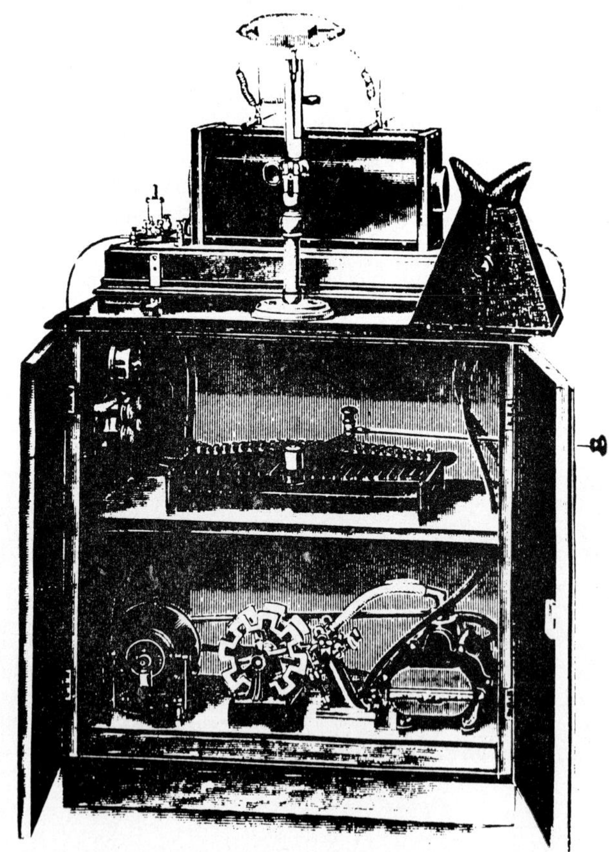

Edison Portable X-ray Outfit. First x-ray installation in the U. S. Navy, on the Hospital ship "Solace." The unit was immediately placed in operation in Santiago de Cuba during the Spanish War.

nide. A piece of cardboard was coated with a matrix of collodion, and on it were pasted crystals of calcium tungstate. This was Edison's first fluoroscope, a noticeable improvement despite its great fluoroscent lag and fairly rapid deterioration.

Edison advertised on a large scale. His "Beneficent X-Ray Exhibit" was shown at Grand Central Palace (New York City) on May 5-7, 1896 during the Electrical Exposition. A special room was fitted out by Edison's Luther Stieringer with somber black drapings and dull red lights. An 18x22″ fluorescent screen was mounted on a platform so that two persons could come together and see their anatomy. During the exhibit, the staff was supervised by Max Osterberg. The exhibit was visited – among others – by George Westinghouse, Jr., Cornelius Vanderbilt, Chauncey M. Depew, and Charles Delmonico. And a pompous meeting was arranged between Edison and Alexander Graham Bell – they were to meet again, this time in effigy, on commemorative stamps of the US Post Office.

For several years thereafter, GE built and sold Thomson's "inductorium," his electrolytic interrupters, and his "standard double focus tube" (intended for use with alternating current, so as to produce x rays during both phases of the cycle). But Edison's machines, especially the so-called Portables, were more popular.

The *Electrical World* of September 10, 1898 recorded the fact that when the US Navy needed an x-ray outfit in a hurry, an Edison Portable was installed in less than 48 hours from the time the order was received. On that Portable the induction coil had no vibrator. It had instead the instantaneous air-brake wheel device (set on the bottom of the cabinet). The device consisted of two touch-wheels mounted on the same shaft: their projections or teeth made and broke contact with two flat brushes. A rheostat controlled the current in the primary coil. The tube holder was sufficiently versatile for use also on reclining patients. The Portable was installed on the Hospital Ship "Solace," placed immediately in service, and used in Santiago de Cuba during the Spanish War. It was the very first floating x-ray equipment in the US Navy.

Another GE subsidiary was the Edison Manufacturing Co. at 110 East 23rd Street, in New York City. They offered for sale Edison x-ray tubes, Edison-Lalande batteries for x-ray apparatus, and complete x-ray outfits for both physicians and traveling exhibitors.

In 1899, GE advertisements claimed that "powerful x rays, abundant and penetrating" were being obtained with their "well known" x-ray tubes with Iridium targets. Their coils had a 4-40″ spark capacity.

Most of these tubes were blown and tested by Clarence Madison Dally (1865-1904), for whom Edison had a personal friendship. When Dally made history as the first American radiation fatality, Edison decided against further exposing his co-workers to such deadly hazards, and the entire x-ray line was silently dropped. Based on these documented antecedents, GE is the oldest American firm in the x-ray industry, but in this field it is not the oldest firm in continuous business.

EARLY COMPETITION

The initially heavy demand coupled with a minimal supply attracted many firms into the x-ray business, but most such ventures were ephemeral, with a casualty rate comparable to that of the automobile industry.

Powerful X-Rays,

Abundant and Penetrating,

Are obtained from our well-known X-Ray Tubes.

We have recently made some very excellent special tubes with Iridium targets.

Our Barium Fluoroscopes

Have hosts of good friends.

We Have Coils From 4 to 14 inch spark capacity.

Candelabra, Miniature, Decorative and Battery Lamps.

EDISON DECORATIVE AND MINIATURE LAMP DEP'T

(GENERAL ELECTRIC CO.) HARRISON, N. J.

ROENTGEN OUTFIT.

Photographing Invisible Objects.

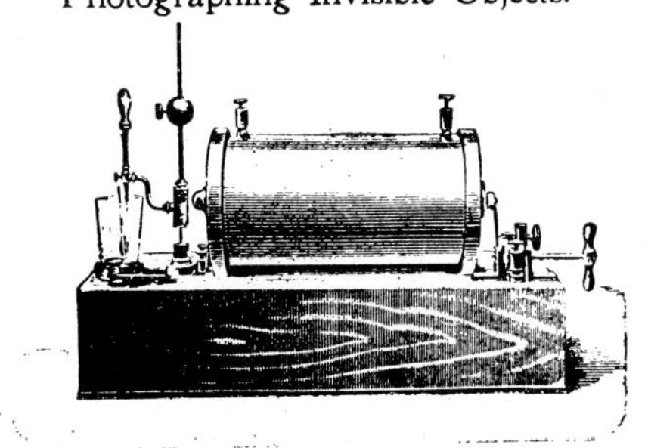

NEWTON'S FOCUS TUBES, PROF. E. THOMSON'S FOCUS TUBES,

COVERING LARGER FIELD THAN ANY OTHER.

Low Ampère Coils. Secondary Batteries. Fluoroscopes and Fluorescent Salts.

Glass-blowing done to Order.

EIMER & AMEND, DEALERS IN CHEMICAL APPARATUS AND CHEMICALS,

205, 207, 209, 211 Third Avenue, New York.

A relatively large number of early x-ray firms were located in New York City. Eimer & Amend, suppliers of chemical apparatus offered also induction coils and gas tubes, the latter glass-blown (apparently not by their own glassblower who at the time was Machlett but) by Emil Greiner at 146 William Street.

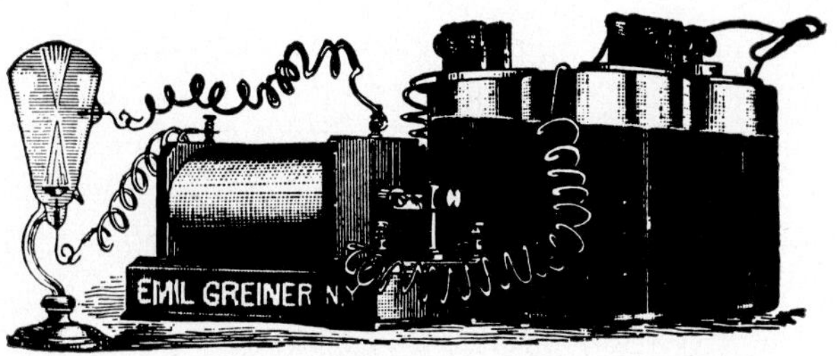

Foote, Pierson & Co. at 82-84 Fulton St. (New York) built their own coils, but purchased barium platinocyanide fluoroscopes from Aylsworth & Jackson in East Orange (New Jersey), who had built the very first fluoroscopes in this country – certainly ahead of Edison, whose merit was to have changed to calcium tungstate as a better base.

In the *Electrical Engineer* of June 24, 1896 appeared the advertisement of the improved Aluminum X-Ray Fluoroscope ("four times as powerful as any yet made: calcium tungstate mounted on an aluminum window, weighing only 6 oz."), sold by J. A. LeRoy, 173 East 13th Street in New York City.

The Standard Electric Lamp & Novelty Co., 248 West 23rd St., advertised Crookes tubes but they were also willing to furnish induction coils as well as complete x-rays outfits. In that company Charles R. Fowler was the president; J. L. Somoff, the electrician; and William R. Powell the treasurer and secretary.

KNOTT

In the *Electrical World,* of July 25, 1896 was published the notice that L. E. Knott Apparatus Co., at 14 Ashburton Place in Boston, had "perfected a new coil for Roentgen-Ray work." It was a high frequency coil of the Tesla-Thomson type, called for the purpose the "new influence machine." Its secondary coil was insulated, and also the condensor was immersed in oil. It could be used either with a 52 or 104 volt current and another improvement was the mechanical spark-gap, claimed to render the discharge of the condensor absolutely uniform. This high frequency coil was more expensive than the conventional model (Foote & Pierson sold complete outfits with the regular coil for $175.00).

In the *Electrical World* of December 12, 1896 Knott announced the introduction of flexible photographic paper to be used instead of photographic glass negatives in x-ray work. They stressed the obvious advantage of unbreakability, and claimed that any number of copies could be obtained at once. George Eastman embarked on a similar venture, but

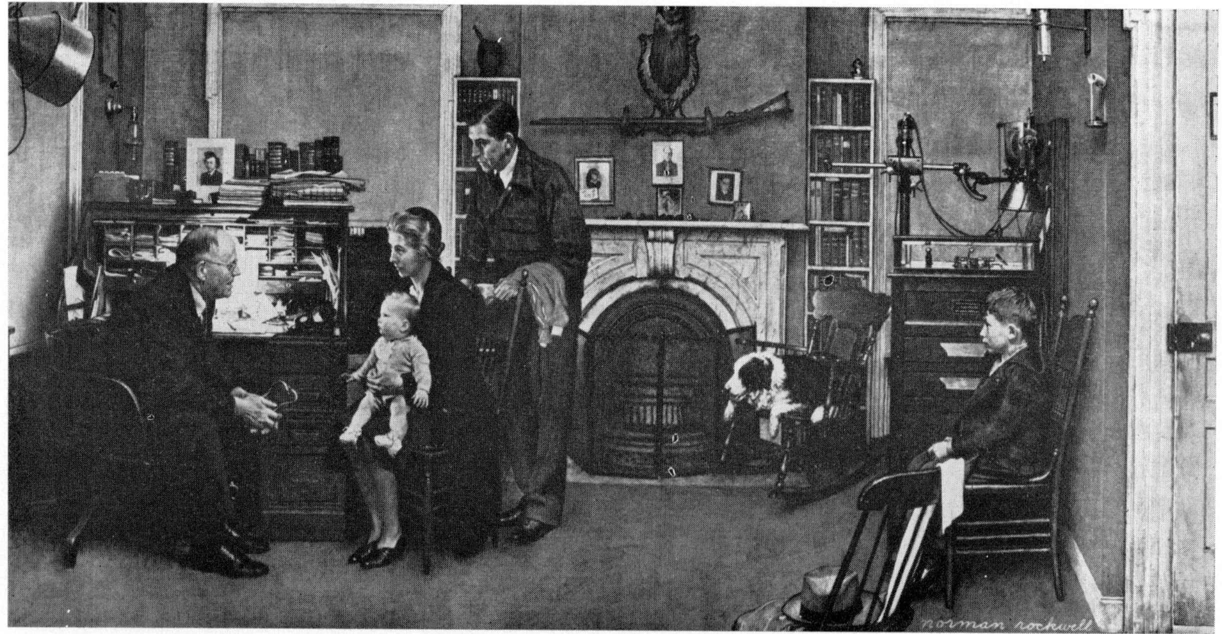

Courtesy: Charles W. Smith

THE FAMILY DOCTOR, a painting by the well-known illustrator Norman Rockwell features a Thompson & Plaster "Electrical Cabinet" (in the corner on viewer's right) with x-ray tube in a glass bowl.

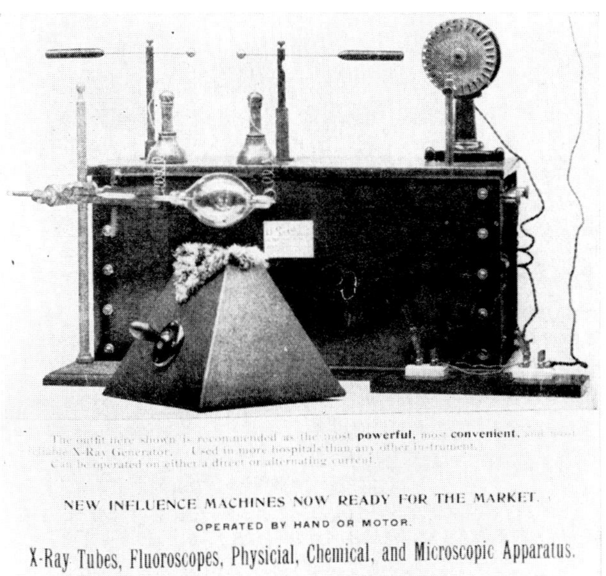

neither product could then be manufactured at a satisfactory quality level.

Popular among country physicians in the first quarter of the century was the "Electrical Cabinet" of the Thompson & Plaster Co. of Leesburg (Virginia). These cabinets were quite versatile, and furnished not only x rays, but also high-frequency sinusoidal, cautery, and other currents, ozone, tankless compressed air, hyperemia by vacuum, and several other conveniences. A Thompson & Plaster catalog from the turn of the century is in the Charles W. Smith Collection. The Thompson & Plaster Co. went out of business during the depression. Charles Smith made a special trip to Leesburg, and saw the deserted plant still standing.

ENTER THE STATIC MACHINE

On February 5, 1896 Wm. James Morton published an article in the *Electrical Engineer* in which he claimed that roentgen rays were produced in the open air between the discharge rods of a static machine. Later on, he became more amenable and agreed to interpose a gas tube between those discharge rods. Very satisfactory roentgen plates were then obtained.

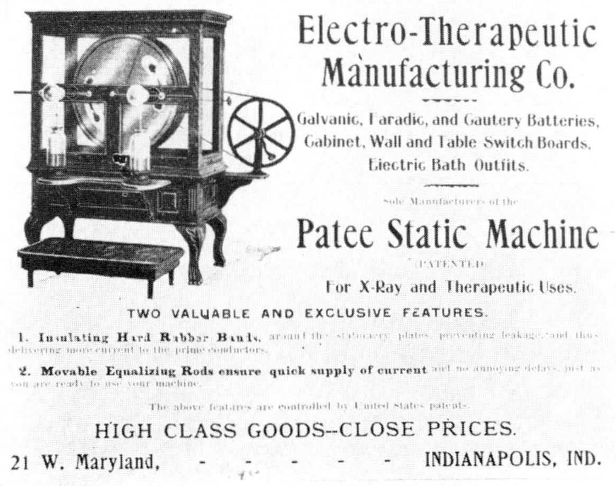

The electrostatic induction machine, with its familiar discs and brushes, had been invented in 1865 by the German physicist, Wilhelm Holtz (1836-1913). It was subsequently improved by many others, for instance the English engineer James Wimshurst (1832-1903) gave it the duplex generator. In 1896, the static machine was in current use among electro-therapists all over the world. Within certain limitations it turned out to be a fairly satisfactory generator for the production of roentgen rays.

By the stroke of a pen all manufacturers of static machines had joined the budding x-ray industry.

There was, for instance, the Electro-Therapeutic Manufacturing Co. at 21 W. Maryland in Indianapolis, which offered the Patee Static Machine, built by Ed. Jerman.

The Western Static Machine Co., located at 116-18 Main Str., in Kansas City (Missouri), manufactured until about 1900 a static unit which delivered not only x rays, but also had an attachment for ozone therapy. It was called the Static X-Ray Ozone Machine.

In Chicago, the McIntosh Electrical Co. at 39-41 W. Randolph St. had its own McIntosh Static Machine.* Competition from the Western Surgical Instrument House, 647-653 W. 59th St., in the same city of Chi-

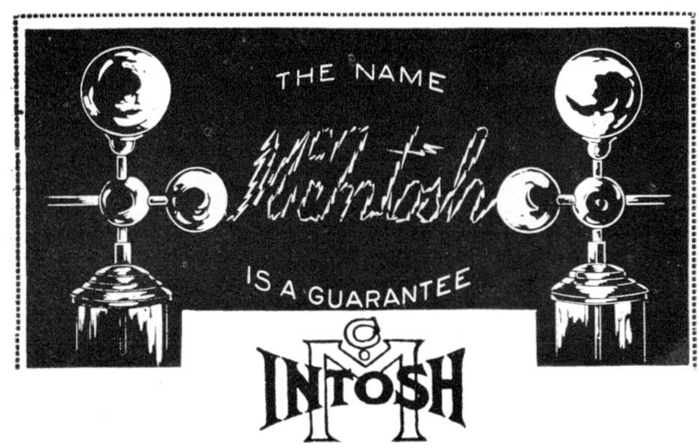

*Years later, when the firm had moved to 322 W. Washington Street, and had modified its name to McIntosh Battery & Optical Company, they manufactured the Hogan Silent X-Ray Transformer, advertised as being interrupterless, motorless, commutatorless, and noiseless on alternating current. The tube acted as its own valve.

cago, with the offer of a 16 plate static (and x-ray) machine for $125.00 in cash.

The bottom was probably reached by the Snyder Electric Co., 1626 S. Broadway, in St. Louis, in selling a complete outfit for $100.00 in cash.

Reducing prices at the expense of quality is not the mark of a reputable manufacturer.

The N. O. Nelson & Co. at 171 E. Randolph St., in Chicago, insisted that $99.00 could not possibly be the price of one of their static machines. They declared that any Nelson Machine is "built in honor and will last a lifetime. It is built more especially for heavy x-ray work, using the thick, fast, and rapid spark required for trunk illumination. Highly recommended by those who saw it at the Roentgen Society Meeting held in Chicago, December 10-11, 1902."

Two resalers were located in St. Louis, one of them the long since defunct X-Ray Outfitting Company at 2902 Morgan St. the other is still very much around, the A. F. Aloe Co., at 517 Olive St.* The latter sold at that time x-ray apparatus built by Fessenden Mfg. Co., of Pittsburgh – with a conventional coil "patented" by Reginald Aubrey Fessenden (1866-1932), who was teaching physics in the University of Pittsburgh.

The Jerome Kidder Mfg. Co., at 820 Broadway in

*Aloe is a well known hospital and surgical supply house, and will seldom venture out of their field, but occasionally they have, as in 1959 with the short-lived Cineray.

$99.99 is not the price of this machine. The erroneous notion exists that a good Static Machine can be built for some such price. Skilled labor comes high. The Glass Trust we *must* patronize. Other materials never were so high as at present.

NELSON NELSON

THE NELSON MACHINE is built on honor and will last a lifetime. It is built more especially for heavy x-ray work, giving the thick, fat and rapid spark required for trunk illumination.

Highly recommended by those who saw it at the Roentgen Society meeting held at Chicago, December 10-11, 1902.

Write for new colortype catalogue.

N. O. NELSON & CO.

171 E. Randolph Street CHICAGO

Have You Got It?

Not $300, not $200, not $150 for an 8-plate, but

$125.00 CASH,

for a High Grade Perfection

16-PLATE Static and X-Ray MACHINE.

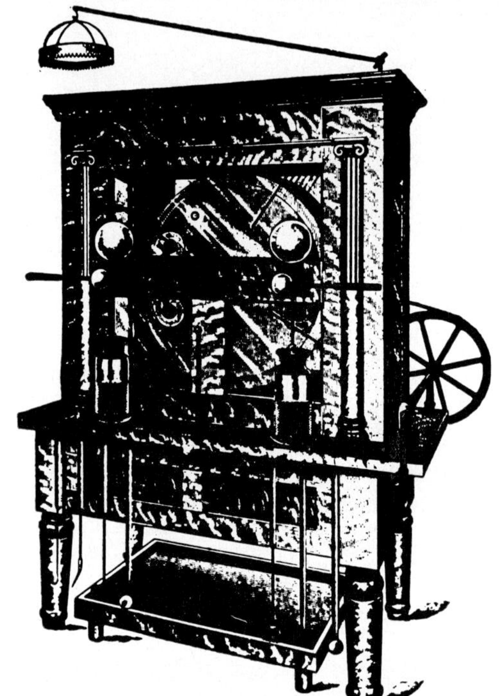

Elegant Oak Case. Platform, Crown Breeze, Electrodes, Etc., Etc. All Complete.
For a limited time only. Send for our bargain bulletin.

Western Surgical Instrument House,
647-653 W. 59th St., Chicago, Ill.

"Roentgen"

Induction Coils

and other

X-Ray Apparatus.

JAMES G. BIDDLE

General Sales Agent

1112-1114 Chestnut Street,

PHILADELPHIA, U. S. A.

New York City, made several sorts of electro-medical apparatus, some of which could produce x rays.

The Morris E. Leeds & Co. in Philadelphia marketed all their equipment through James G. Biddle at 1020 Stephen Girard Bldg., in the same city. They introduced the Leeds 1901 Type Portable Induction Coil mounted in two cases, one with the coil itself, the other containing the accessory working parts, independent variable speed vibrator, adjustable condenser, interlocking reversing switch, and fuse block. This coil was said to give "a very heavy discharge, sufficient in the hands of an expert for the most difficult x-ray work that has been undertaken heretofore with coils of 12 to 15″ spark. To secure maximum current output from the Leeds Portable Coil, it should be connected to a storage battery of six cells, with normal discharge of five to sixteen amperes." This type of portable coil was purchased by the St. Louis X-ray Laboratory, by Charles Leonard in Philadelphia, by the Montreal General Hospital, and by the St. Joseph's Hospital in Reading, Pennsylvania.

QUEEN'S TUBE

Operation of gas tubes presented many problems not the least of which was preservation of adequate vacuum. The tubes contained a certain amount of gas, necessary to permit passage of the current. As this gas was gradually "used up" the tube would get harder, that is higher voltage would be required to "get through" (occasionally, some also became the opposite, too "gassy"). The solution to this problem was the adjustable tube, which meant adding an "appendix" with a metal cap. Unscrewing the metal cap, and immediately tightening it up again, a minute air passage was opened thus giving the tube a reserve of "gas." A better method was the application of heat to a suitable chemical placed in that "appendix." The heating was done at first with a flame, later by electrical means. Soon, self-regulating devices were introduced, among which one of the most successful was known as "Queen's Self-Regulating Tube," created by Sayen.

The Queen & Co., J. G. Gray, President, had its headquarters at 1010 Chestnut St. in Philadelphia (with branches at 59 5th Ave. in New York and 480 Monroe Bldg. in Chicago). They were also manufacturing other items, such as an early table, Sweet's

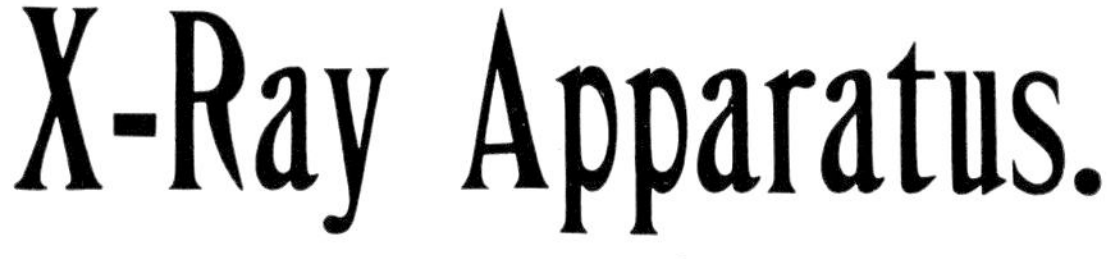

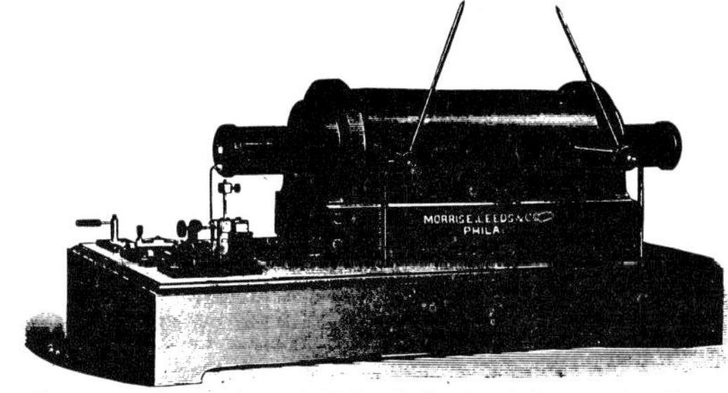

B5475. 15-in. Spark Leeds X-Ray Induction Coil—Hospital Type.

Leeds Induction Coils.
Self-Regulating Tubes.
B. P. C. Fluoroscopes.
Storage Batteries.
Motor Generators.

Complete X-Ray Equipments for Hospitals, Medical Colleges and Private Offices.

Write for Illustrated Pamphlets 350 and 365.

JAMES G. BIDDLE.
1020 Stephen Girard Building, Philadelphia.

We consider it a demonstrated fact that radiographs can be made with an **Induction Coil** which show **superior definition** for a given time of exposure, when compared with those obtained with a **static machine.**

1901

The LEEDS 1901 Type
PORTABLE INDUCTION COIL.

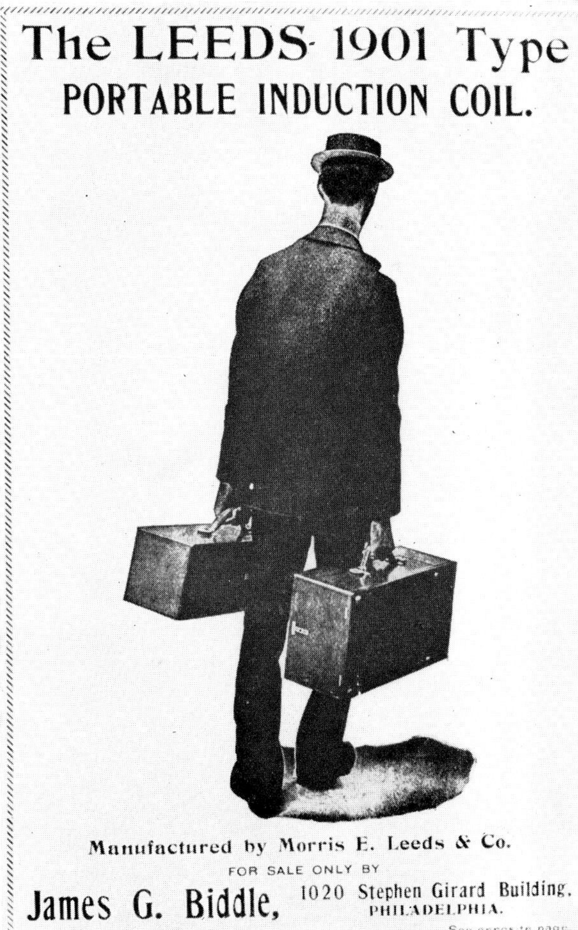

Manufactured by Morris E. Leeds & Co.
FOR SALE ONLY BY
James G. Biddle, 1020 Stephen Girard Building, PHILADELPHIA.

See opposite page.

Localizer for foreign bodies in the eye, and they were the sole licensees of Johnston's Mercury Interrupter. Nevertheless, they were best known for their tube.

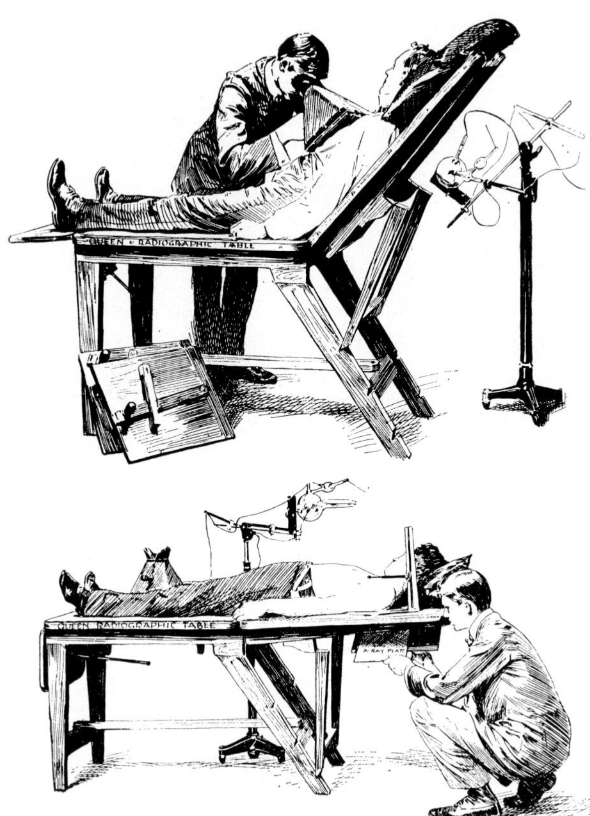

Courtesy: Charles W. Smith.

QUEEN'S RADIOGRAPHIC TABLE (1903). It is shown in position for fluoroscopy with under-the-table tube, as well as with the special localization device, and under-the-table arrangement for changing plates. In 1906, the Queen Co. became C. H. F. Mueller's USA representative, and began to import German x-ray tubes, but things did not work out so well. In some ways Snook's firm was a successor to Queen's.

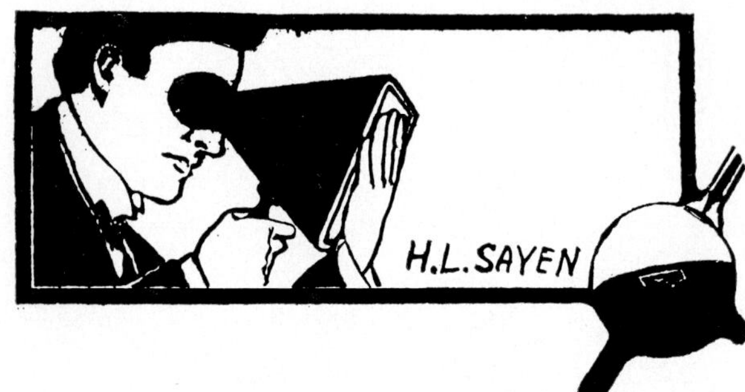

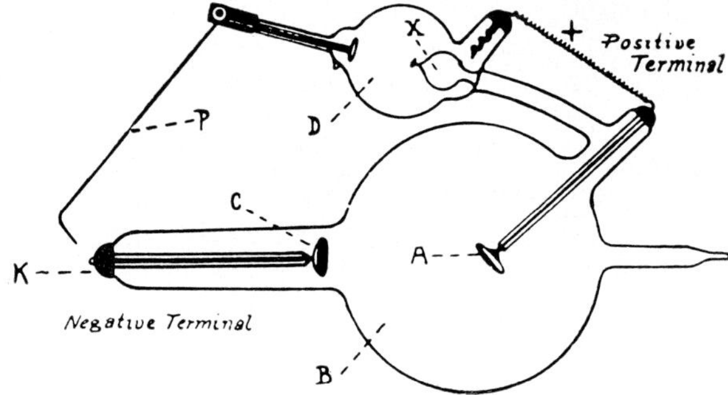

QUEEN'S SELF-REGULATING TUBE. Their best-seller, developed by Sayen.

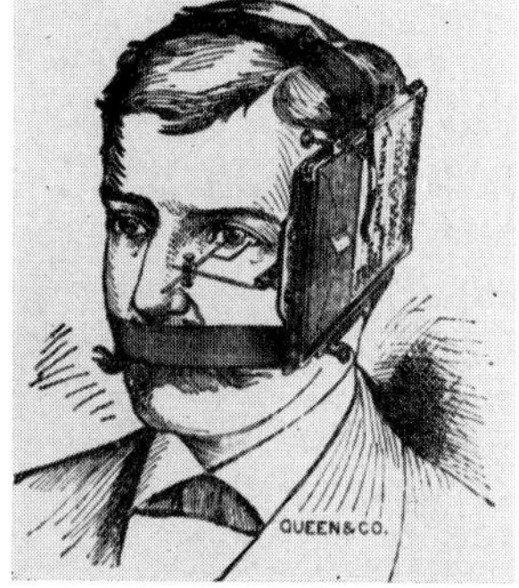

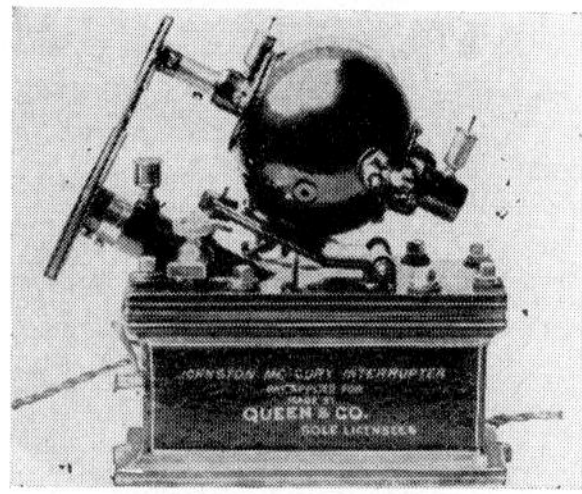

QUEEN'S SECOND BEST-SELLERS. Sweet's appliance for localizing foreign bodies in the orbit is still being sold today (by Keleket). Johnston's Mercury Interrupter must have made more money for Queen than Sweet's localizer.

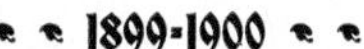

* * 1899-1900 * *

Queen Standard
X-Ray
Apparatus

Made and Sold by

Queen & Co., Philadelphia and New York

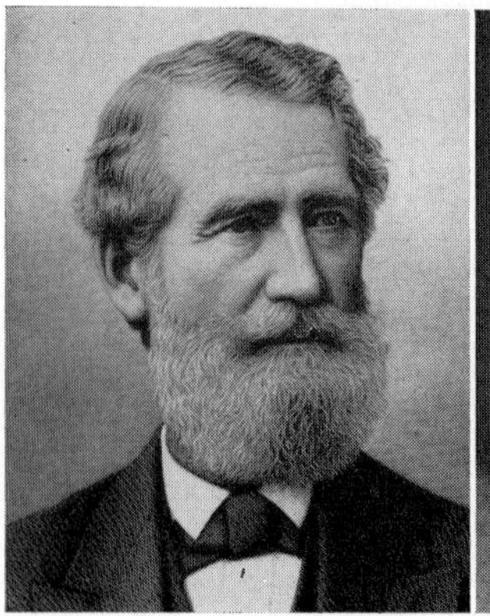

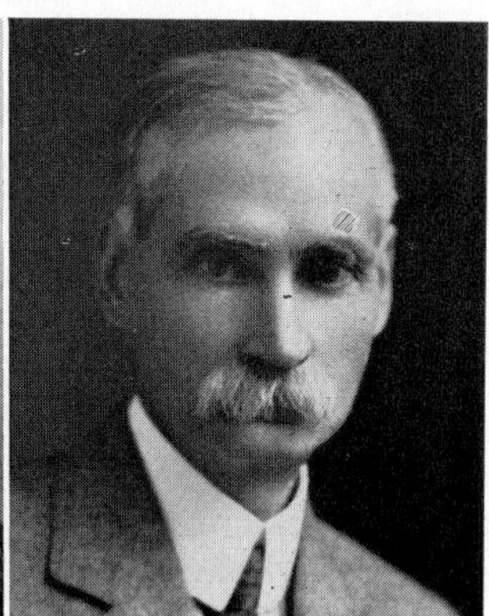

Courtesy: Charles W. Smith

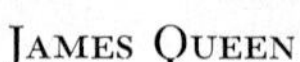

JAMES QUEEN JOHN GRAY

On December 29, 1902 appeared in the *Western Electrician* an editorial which mentioned that the Queen Co. had built an x-ray machine for the Mikado Mints. "With an x-ray machine to face, the bland, coin-laden Jap, with perhaps a rouleau of gold snugly concealed in the intestinal tract, will doubtless be less imperturbable as he approaches the exit with his unmasticated gains. And thus, with oriental ingenuity, is another laurel added to the brow of Roentgen."*

*Joseph Arthur Burns, Sr. told me that he was once approached by a radiologist in the name of a gambling establishment near Washington (D.C.). They had suffered several hold-ups. If a concealed fluoroscope were installed at the entrance of the gambling spot, suspicious incomers could be discreetly "examined," knowing that the invisible light would detect guns, knives, and other "hidden tools." Westinghouse, represented by Burns, turned down the offer — it is not known whether the competition went along with the gambler's request. "Frisking fluoroscopes" were in use in Defense plants during World War II. The Illinois Radiation Law of 1960 forbids the use of ionizing radiation on humans for any but medical diagnostic and therapeutic purposes. This is when the fluoroscope used at Joliet State Prison for the examination of visiting relatives, and all the shoefitting fluoroscopes in the state of Illinois were dismantled.

The Queen Self Regulating X-Ray Tube

Has advantages possessed by no other Tube. Ask for special circular.

"Especially Ingenious."—Prof. Dr. W. C. Roentgen.
"Most Satisfactory."—Lord Kelvin.
"The best I have yet seen."—Dr. A. W. Goodspeed, Univ. Pa.
"Operator can make it do exactly as he desires."—Dr. C. L. Leonard, Univ. Pa.
"Perfectly satisfied in every respect."—Elliott Woods, Washington, D. C.
"It can take care of itself."—Dr. H. P. Bowditch, Harvard College.
"Self regulating feature a success."—Prof. D. C. Miller, Case School.

We make the LARGEST and BEST INDUCTIONS COILS, Localization Apparatus, Sweet's Indicator, Radiographic Table.

(All described in our new Catalogue of X-Ray Apparatus.)

QUEEN & CO., Inc.,
J. G. GRAY, Pres.

89 Fifth Aveuue, New York, 480 Monroe Bldg., Chicago. 1898 *1010 Chestnut St., Philadelphia, Pa.*

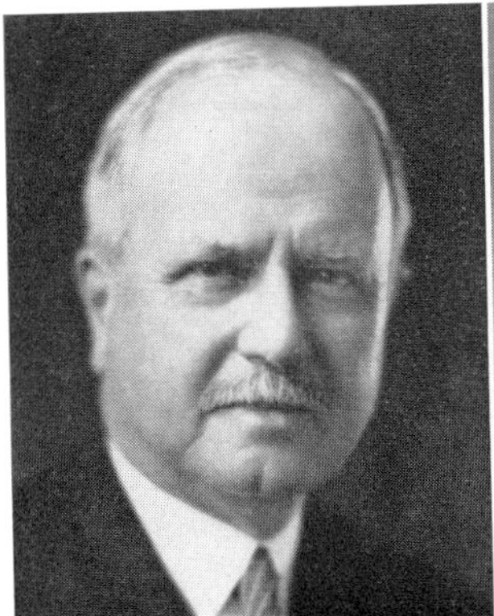

James Biddle

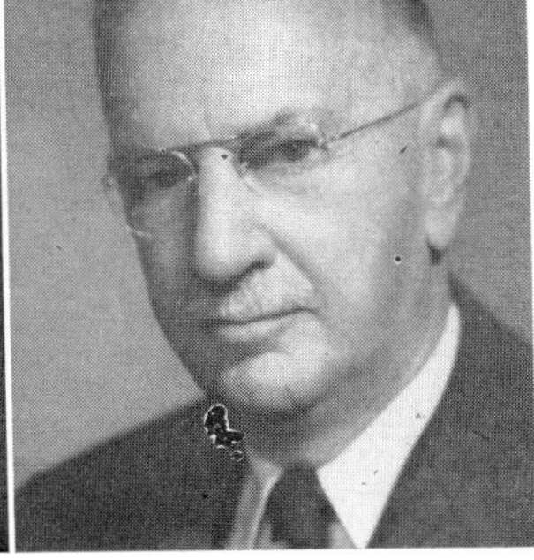

Courtesy: Charles W. Smith

Morris Leeds

If care was taken not to permit a tube to become too evacuated, and if its vacuum was reduced as soon as it showed a four to six inch spark resistance, the tube would rarely puncture. The vacuum could be lowered by "baking" the tube. When heated, the glass would become sufficiently porous to permit the passage of air into the tube. This, at least, was the opinion accepted at the time (Wm. Benham Snow, 1905). It is more likely that the heating liberated gas trapped between the glass molecules themselves. Snow recommended placing the tube on a piece of asbestos for 5-10 minutes in the lower oven of a "perfect" gas range, *i.e.*, one burning with a cool blue flame. The baking could lower the vacuum of some tubes to where they would no longer fluoresce, except with a ball interrupter. Such soft (gassy) tubes could then be used in treating acne or lupus until their vacuum was again raised (hardened) to where they could be returned to diagnostic tasks.

Charles Warner Smith, after reading the galley for this chapter, decided to find more information on the Queen Company. At the Pennsylvania Historical Society he discovered a sixteen-page brochure, entitled *Fifty Years, 1853-1903.* It was the history of the Queen & Co. In Philadelphia, in 1783, John McAllister, Sr. started in business as an optician, and became a well-known maker of "glasses for philosophical experiments." James W. Queen was an optician who started in business with W. Y. McAllister, dealer in "philosophical apparatus" at 48 Chestnut Street, the very same firm which dated back to 1783. Queen founded his own business in 1853, and began to import scientific materials from Europe, especially instruments. Queen retired in 1870 and his interests were purchased by S. L. Fox. In 1893 the business was turned into a corporation, with Fox as president and principal stockholder. The depression of 1893-1894 resulted in temporary financial embarrassment, and John G. Gray was appointed assignee. Fifteen months later, the entire indebtedness of the firm ($200 thousand) had been repaid, Gray bought out Fox's interests, and remained president. By 1903 Queen & Co., at 1010 Chestnut Street in Philadelphia, consisted of four floors—eight sales departments, each with its own manager. They had four factories, and a New York City branch.

The accumulation of talents at the Queen & Co. was unusual. Between 1894 and 1900 numerous people left the company and started their own businesses, which have turned out to be extremely successful.* Among there were the founders of the well known Arthur H. Thomas Co., Williams, Brown and Earle, James Biddle,

*Some of this information was also included in a letter written by Arthur H. Thomas in 1938 to H. N. Ott of Spencer Lens Company, for a book which covered the history of microscopy in the USA. Additional information appears in Ernest Child's *The Tools of the Chemist* (Reinhold, 1940).

Leeds, Willyoung, Snook, to name only some of those connected with roentgenology. In his historical tract on roentgenology, Homer Snook recalled that the Queen Co., using an old French coil and a Maltese cross tube obtained x rays very early in 1896, ahead of many other manufacturers. Soon thereafter, Queen x ray apparatus became the "standard" for America. In the Queen laboratories, H. Lyman Sayen developed the automatic vacuum regulator for x ray tubes—his patent was filed on April 29, 1897—for which the Franklin Institute awarded the Queen Co. the John Scott Medal.

Returning now to the anniversary brochure, it contained the mention of two Queen coils, built for the Japanese government. These coils had a 45 inch spark —the Queen Co. was willing to build coils with 60 inch spark.

At this point Charlie Smith continued his search, and to his surprise discovered that the Queen Co. was still in business. They stayed at 1010 Chestnut until 1912 when the name was changed to Queen-Gray Co., and the locale moved to 64½ W. Johnson St. in Germantown (Pennsylvania). John Gray died in 1925, the name of the firm was then changed to Gray Instrument Co., and they moved to 448 Mill Road in Andalusia (Pennsylvania), where they remained until they merged with the James G. Biddle Co. in 1963. It is difficult to pinpoint the time when the Queen Co. gave up the x-ray business, but it must have been around 1912, when they moved away from 1010 Chestnut Street, where such notables as Goodspeed, Pancoast, Pfahler, Newcomet, Manges and Bowen were familiar figures.

Some data can be gleaned from the history of Leeds & Northrup*, the precision instrument maker. Morris Evans Leeds, James G. Biddle, and Elmer Willyoung were boyhood friends and (just like James Queen), of old Quaker stock. When Leeds went into business for himself in 1899, he left behind an investment of $10,-000 in the Queen Co. To start out, he bought the Philadelphia instrument shop of Willyoung; later took in a partner, Edwin F. Northrup, a brilliant researcher who did not stay very long, and became professor at Princeton (Northrup was also a former Queen employee). James G. Biddle had gone into business in 1895. Again it would be difficult to determine when they discontinued their x-ray line, but it was some time before the end of the Era of the Roentgen Pioneers.

COOLING THE TARGET

The Boston dentist and x-ray inventor, Wm. Rollins, made many groundbreaking advances in x-ray technology. One of his most interesting was an x-ray tube with cooled target, called the A-W-L X-Light

*The name of the book is *Precision, People and Progress* by Wm. P. Vogel, Jr. (Philadelphia, 1949). A copy was courteously forwarded to me by Mr. Kenneth Wray Conners from Leeds & Northrup.

THE A-W-L X-LIGHT TUBE.

DESIGNED BY WILLIAM ROLLINS.

Power—Definition—Long Life.

The Only Tube With a Cooled Target.

All other targets are destroyed by powerful currents. This target will bear any current.

The only tube in which the vacuum is lowered from the exterior. All other regulators fail.

THIS NEVER FAILS.

OELLING & HEINZE,

70 Washington St., BOSTON, MASS., U. S. A.

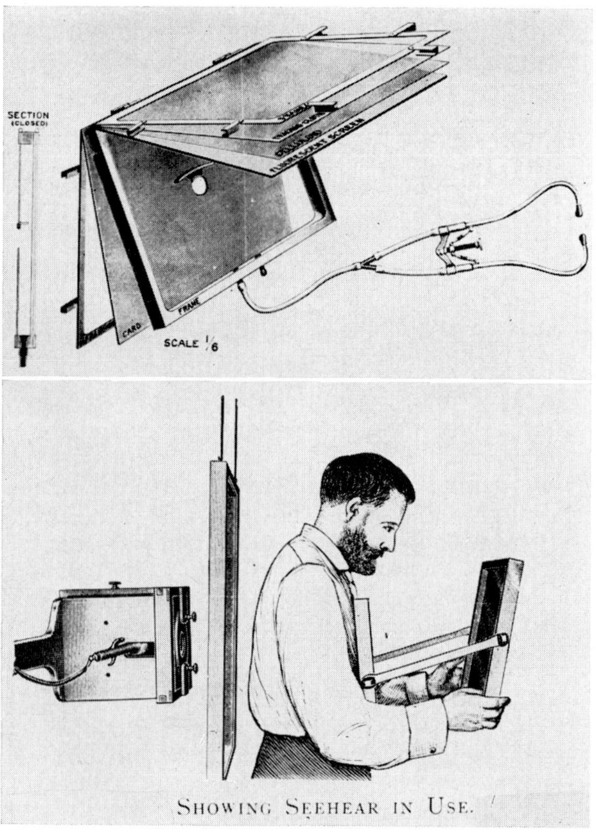

Showing Seehear in Use.

Tube, manufactured at 70 Washington St. in Boston by Oelling & Heinze.

Oelling & Heinze contended that when conventional tubes were used with powerful currents, their targets were sooner or later destroyed. By the same token they claimed that the A-W-L "cooled target" would bear with impunity even the strongest tube currents then available. In that particular tube the vacuum could be lowered from the exterior, with a regulator which was never supposed to fail. Oelling & Heinze built also the A-W-L Universal Coil.

Rollins described several of his early inventions in the *American X-Ray Journal,* later assembled them into *Notes on X-Light.* He constructed in 1898 a tube with rotatable target and the See-Hear (a fluoroscope with built-in stethoscope) usable even for autoscreening, as illustrated by Rollins himself.

A well-publicized automatic resistance regulator was then manufactured by the Bario-Vacuum Co., located at 106 East 23rd St. in New York City.

All these companies were also producing induction coils. One of the best such coils was made by Elmer G. Willyoung, first in Philadelphia, then at 11 Frankfort St., in New York City.

TUBE IMPORTERS

In the early 1900s, Ottomar Carliczek at 908 Schiller Bldg. in Chicago imported German tubes, for instance the famous Gundelach or the Mueller. Of course, Carliczek was willing to repair gas tubes.

Also in Chicago, at 42 Wabash Ave., Truax, Green &

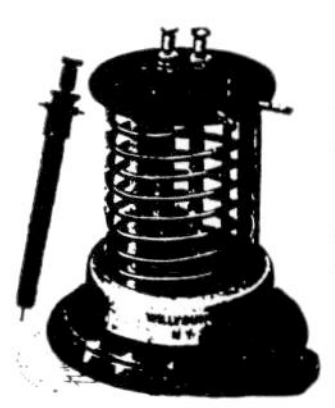

W. C. Electrolytic Interruptor.

The continuously adjustable electrode gives Interruptions from 200 to 5,000 per second and enormous discharges with any Coil.

(Circular No. 510, 4 pages, describes it.)

The Cunningham Mercury Jet Interruptor.
(Patent applied for.)
Will Soon Be Ready.

Interruptions variable at will from 10 to 10,000 per minute at any current up to 30 amperes.

Absolutely Instantaneous Breaks. Needs no attention and can be placed in another room if desired. No sticking and short circuiting possible. Current simply stops if break stops.

Write for particulars.

The Caldwell Tube and Radiographic Stand.

(As devised by Mr. E. W. Caldwell, inventor of the Caldwell Interruptor and Radiographer in Chief of the Riggs X-Ray Laboratory of Bellevue Hospital, New York City.)

A necessity to the up-to-date Radiographer. Tube clamp has no screws, the jaws opening by mere pressure and holding any size tube firmly but gently. Entire stand is practically free from metal except for the heavy base. For the radiography of fractures and other troubles in the limbs, a small table, about 11" x 18", on ball and socket joint, attaches to the stand and adjusts vertically upon it; spring clips drop into holes drilled into the board and carry straps by which the limb is firmly held against the plate.

Write for Circular No. 519.

Elmer G. Willyoung, 11 Frankfort Street, New York, N. Y.

CATALOGUE OF HIGH-GRADE

X-Ray and High Frequency Apparatus

INCLUDING

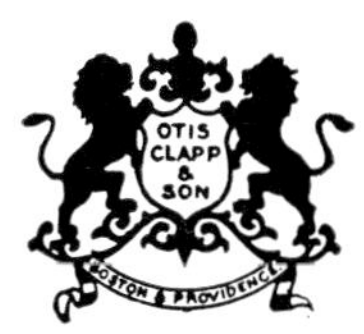

Standard X-Ray Coils
Mercury Interrupters
Wehnelt Electrolytic Interrupters
Finest Imported X-Ray Tubes,
Fluoroscopes, Tube Holders, High Frequency Apparatus, Etc., Etc.

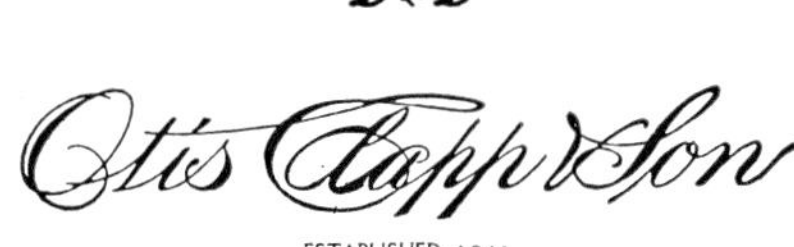

ESTABLISHED 1840.
INCORPORATED 1901.

Eastern Agents for the SCHEIDEL COIL.

New England Agents for R. F. GERMAN TUBES.

HEADQUARTERS:

10 PARK SQUARE, - BOSTON, MASS.

Branches at

48 Beacon Street, Boston, Mass. 417 Westminster St., Providence, R. I.

—THE—

DENNIS FLUOROMETER.

Necessary Surgical Adjunct of X-Ray Work.

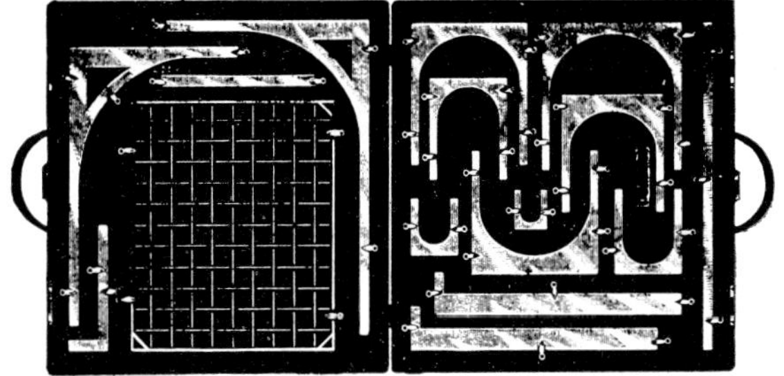

Patented April 27, 1897. Velvet Lined Case.

THE DENNIS FLUOROMETER is the only instrument that furnishes accurate cross-sections and measurements, rectifies distortion of position and distortions caused by the divergence of the rays.

It forms a perfect shadow of any por ion of the anatomy, making it indispensable in cases of dislocations and fractures. It gives protection to the surgeon or physician in courts, and equips him for expert testimony. Precise instruments and accurate methods produce precise results. It accurately locates bullets, needles, and metal of every description, including gall stones, and the operation for their removal can be undertaken at once, eliminating any danger from delay.

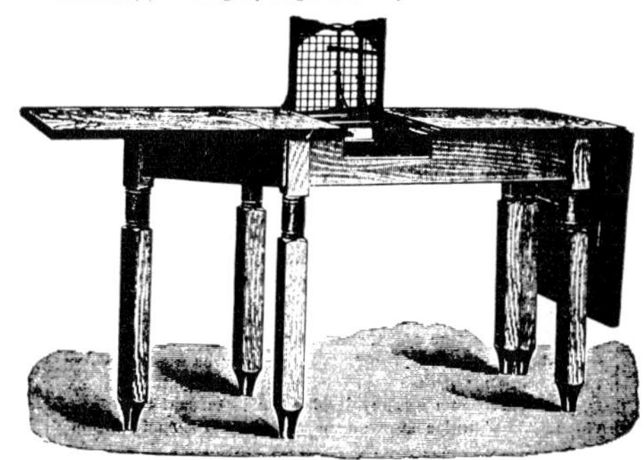

Observation and Operating Table. Quarter Oak, highly finished.

Write for illustrated catalogue, giving full description, prices and terms.

The Rochester Fluorometer Co.

225 Cutler Building, Rochester, N. Y.

Co. offered improved x-ray tubes in regular size ($12.00) or extra large ($20.00), and their improved x-ray stand ($10.00). These, too, were imported from Germany.

One of the larger importers on the East Coast, with headquarters at 10 Park Square in Boston, and a branch in Providence (Rhode Island), was Otis Clapp & Son, a firm which dated since 1840, but was not incorporated until 1901.

X-RAY MOTORS

The Holtzer-Cabot Electric Co., at 395 Dearborn St. in Chicago, had its home office and factory in Brookline (Massachusetts), with another branch at 143 Liberty St. in New York.

X-ray batteries were sold by the Northwestern Storage Battery Co. at 465 West 22nd St. in Chicago. This information comes from an advertisement dated 1903.

X-RAY PICTURES

At the turn of the century it was common practice to sell significant (and in many cases insignificant) positives made from roentgen plates. William J. Morton put on the market one of the earliest collections of such prints.

The American X-Ray Publishing Co. (which also issued the *American X-Ray Journal*) advertised its ability to supply "skiagraphs of any portion of the anatomy at cost, ranging from 40¢ for the wrist and hand to $1.50 for the shoulders and pelvis. Pathological and anatomical skiagraphs of injected vessels are furnished at a cost of 50¢ to $2.00. These are all actual reproductions of the original and are most artistically finished. None better in the world. State in letter just what you want and we will give you prices."

FOREIGN BODY LOCALIZER

Various methods for localization of foreign bodies were developed with the help of roentgen rays. Many of the earlier workers devised their own apparatus for this purpose.*

The Dennis Fluorometer, patented April 27, 1897, was manufactured by the Rochester Fluorometer Co.,

*Sir James Mackenzie Davidson described his method (in which use of stereoscopy was optional) in a monograph first published in 1916. In Germany, Grashey advocated placement of an x-ray transformer and tube under the operating table; he used the term *röntgenoskopische Operation.* A surgical stereoscopist, L. Druener of Hamburg, strapped a small tubular fluoroscopic screen over his left eye, leaving the right eye uncovered; during the operation, whenever he needed fluoroscopy, he simply closed the right eye and looked with the left. Carlos Heuser (Buenos Aires) improvised a similar, and just as hazardous, gadget.

225 Cutler Bldg., in Rochester (New York). It was a fluoroscopic localizing method and required examination in two successive planes, against a square pattern of wires strung on a glass.

PLATES

It is not generally known that celluloid (cellulose nitrate) coated with sensitive photographic emulsion (film) was available since 1889. Roentgen himself had used film in some of his experiments, but the single coated films of that time were not very satisfactory for radiographic purposes.

The stock item was called "dry plates." At the turn of the century, very well known were the plates manufactured by John Carbutt of Philadelphia. He is the one, previously mentioned, who "sciagraphed" the severed hand of the Egyptian mummy. Carbutt's factory, called the Keystone Dry Plate and Film Works was at Wayne Junction in Pennsylvania.

Carbutt produced (with the help of Goodspeed) a special emulsion for what they called the Roentgen X-Ray Plate. It was first tested on February 11, 1896 at the Maternity Hospital in Philadelphia. It permitted exposure of twenty minutes where previously one or more hours was required.* In June, 1897 Carbutt

*By 1906, with further improvements, the exposure came down to a few seconds for a hand; thirty to sixty seconds were needed for heavier parts of the body.

KEYSTONE
ELECTRIC
INCORPORATED COMPANY

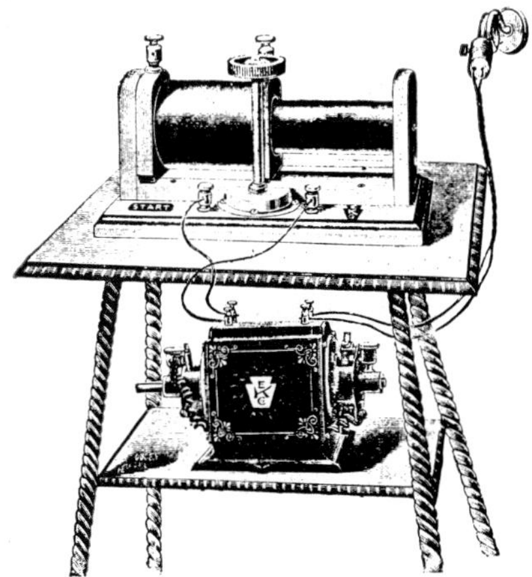

Manufacturers of

Electro-Therapeutic Instruments
Cabinets
Storage Batteries
Static Machines
X-Ray Outfits
Physiological Laboratories Equipped

OFFICE, SALESROOM AND FACTORY
135 SOUTH TENTH STREET
PHILADELPHIA, PA.

DO NOT DEPEND
UPON YOUR FLUOROSCOPE
FOR X-RAY DIAGNOSIS
Get a Permanent Record
BY USING THE
Gramer X-Ray Plate
Specially made for this work. It gives fullest detail and contrast, rendering diagnosis of even difficult cases easy and certain.
Sold by all dealers in Photo Supplies.
Write us for X-Ray Manual and Pyro-acetone X-Ray Eormula.
G. Cramer Dry Plate Co.
ST. LOUIS NEW YORK CHICAGO

CRAMER MISSPELLED GRAMER. This "gremlinized" ad appeared in the very first issue of the *American Quarterly of Roentgenology* (1907).

All Dry Plates Work Best When Fresh.
CRAMER PLATES WILL HEREAFTER BE
PROTECTED WITH A LABEL
On the bottom of each box of plates, limiting the time within which the plates should be used for best results.
We consider this protection necessary to guard our patrons against plates which have deteriorated by age.
We feel that this long delayed action is in the right direction, and will be appreciated by our friends and the trade generally.
G. CRAMER DRY PLATE CO.,
ST. LOUIS, MO.
NEW YORK DEPOT: 32 East 10th Street

Compact, Authoritative, Practical
Our NEW Manual of
X-Ray Practice and Technique
FREE ON REQUEST
G. Cramer Dry Plate Co.
St. Louis 1913 Missouri

summarized the proper characteristics of a roentgen ray emulsion: "It should be of medium sensitiveness, have a good body of emulsion, be capable of absorbing the x rays, thereby giving more detail and perspective to the bones. . ." (Fuchs).

In another of his advertisements, Carbutt stated that "x-ray plates for making radiograph negatives have the special quality of absorbing the x rays of a Crookes tube, allowing a short exposure. They are used by Professor A. W. Goodspeed of the University of Pennsylvania who has produced fine results with exposures as short as 4½ seconds. Nicola Tesla and Dr. Wm. J. Morton of New York and many other scientists also use them."

OTHER PLATE MANUFACTURERS

The M. A. Seed Dry Plate Co., located at 2005 Locust St. in St. Louis, had another outlet at 57 E. 9th St. in New York City.

Another company from St. Louis, the G. Cramer Dry Plate Co., had also offices in New York (32 E. 10th St.), in Chicago (1211 Masonic Temple), and in San Francisco (Room 38, 819 Market St.) The Cramer Co. introduced in 1901 a label, placed on the bottom of each box of plates, limiting the time in which the plates should be used for the best results.

GREEN & BAUER

The first company which produced x-ray tubes in fairly large quantities was headed by two roentgen "saints." One of them, John Bauer, died in 1908. Henry Green (1860-1914) succumbed also to radiation exposure: this was the lot of many early manufacturers who received unwittingly large doses of lethal radiation while testing tubes.

C & B

TRADE MARK.

The Celebrated

Clover Leaf Tungsten Transformer Tube

NEW MODEL

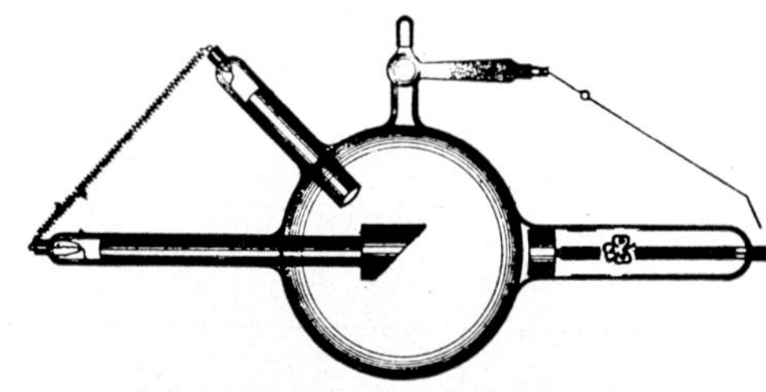

WE GUARANTEE

No more cracked cathode necks
Absolute unshifting focus
That these tubes will not go cranky in use

THE MOST DURABLE TUBE EVER PRODUCED

DOUBLE THE LIFE OF THE OLD-TYPE TUBE

None are genuine unless bearing the Clover Leaf Trade-Mark

Manufactured only by us under U. S. Patent, July 29, 1913
Demand them of your dealer or order direct

GREEN & BAUER, INC.
HARTFORD, CONN.

1913

Improved Transformer Tube

A tube for transformer use embodying an improvement to eliminate the possibility of the tube's cracking at the cathode neck.

The tube can be operated until the anode becomes white hot.

The danger point in operating our new tube is the melting of the copper in the tungsten target. From a large number of tests we find that the tungsten disc will stand heavy impacts without being apparently damaged.

GREEN & BAUER INC.
CHICAGO ILL. HARTFORD CONN.

1916

The Kinraide High-Frequency Coil.

The best apparatus for use with the direct or alternating current.

SEND FOR DESCRIPTIVE CIRCULAR.

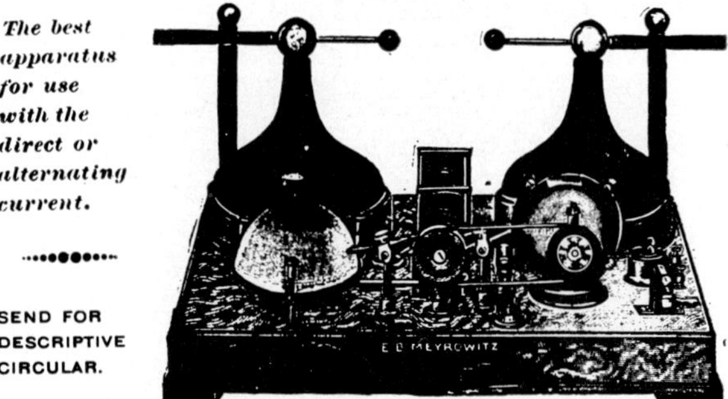

E. B. Meyrowitz,

Maker of Ophthalmological Apparatus, Complete Standard Electro-Therapeutic Equipments, X-Ray Apparatus and High Grade Eye, Ear, Nose and Throat Instruments.

104 East Twenty-third Street, 125 West Forty-second Street, 650 Madison Avenue, NEW YORK.

604 Nicollet Avenue, Minneapolis. 360 St. Peter Street, St. Paul. 3 rue Scribe, Paris, France.

1899

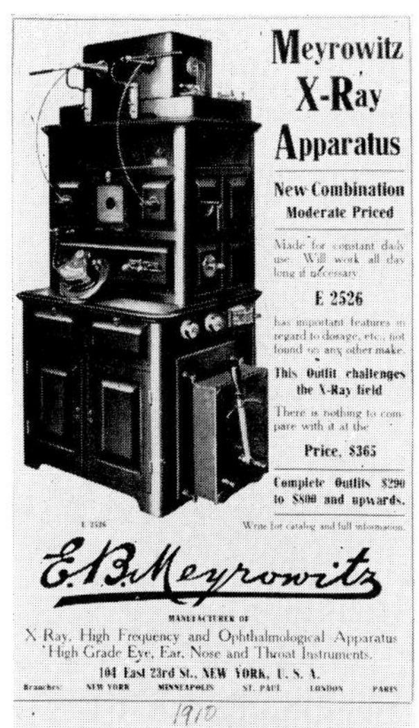

American Electro-Therapeutic

AND X-RAY ERA August 1903

OFFICE OF PUBLICATION:

504 Masonic Temple, Chicago, Illinois

F. W. BUTTERMANN, M.D. . . . . EDITOR
Radiographer and Radiotherapeutist St. Joseph Hospital, Chicago.

C. H. TREADWELL, B.S. . MANAGING EDITOR

EDITORIAL STAFF OF PHYSICIANS:

J. RUDIS JICINSKY, M.D. . . . Cedar Rapids, Ia.
E. H. GRUBBE, M.D. . . . . Chicago, Ill.
RUSSELL H. BOGGS, M.D. . . . . Pittsburg, Pa.
Radiographer at the Allegheny General Hospital.
G. G. BURDICK, M. D. . . . . Chicago, Ill.
WILLIAM H. DIEFFENBACH, M.D. . New York City
NOBLE M. EBERHART, M.S., M.D., F.S.S.c. Chicago, Ill.
A. DECKER, M.D. . . . . Chicago, Ill.

Publisher: R. FRIEDLANDER.

SUBSCRIPTION, PER ANNUM, ... $2.00
SINGLE COPIES, ... 20c

Make all checks payable to R. Friedlander, Publisher.

THIS JOURNAL IS DEVOTED ENTIRELY TO ALL BRANCHES OF ELECTRO-THERAPEUTICS

Contributions of actual experience by physicians using the X-Ray as a therapeutic agent are highly valued by this journal, and the editor is always willing to reserve space for such communications.

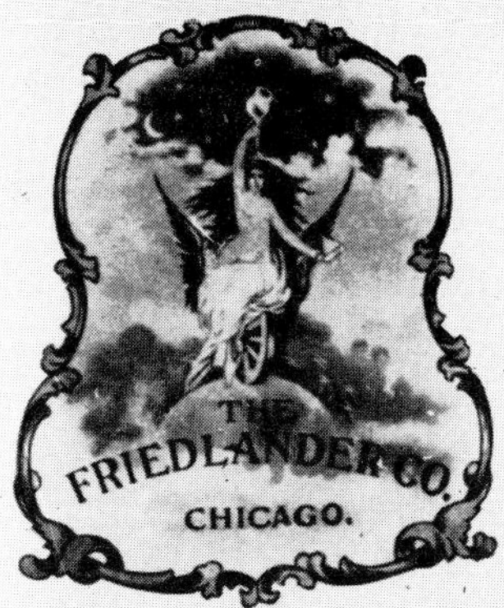

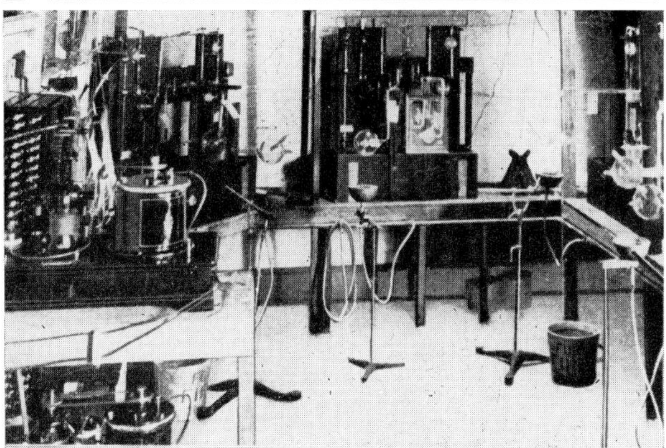
Courtesy: Herbert Pollack.

EXHAUST ROOM AT FRIEDLÄNDER'S. This is the place where the tube manufacturers got their deadly dose of x radiation — while testing the tubes after they were exhausted. A catastrophic device, the cryptoscope (seen on the table in right background), permitted a check of the tube's vacuum without darkening the room.

The Green & Bauer Co. was very well introduced. It had a clover leaf as its trade-mark. Their tubes were quite dependable, and many of them lasted well into the early 1930s. The firm was best known for the Tungsten Transformer Tube, patented as of July 29, 1913. The last advertisements of this firm appeared around 1920.

MEYROWITZ

In New York City existed the E. B. Meyrowitz Co., at 104 East 23rd St. They boasted of branches in Minneapolis, St. Paul, London, and Paris. In 1910, they were willing to sell for $365.00 a very impressive coil placed on top of a wooden cabinet, which contained all necessary accessories for x-ray diagnosis and for electro-therapy. Meyrowitz was Ilford's representative in the U.S.A.

CHICAGO

The Friedlander Co., with the main office at 41-45 State St. in Chicago, had a branch at 1411 Flat Iron Building in New York City. Their catalog* contained a full line of roentgen equipment, from tubes to tube-stands, and from coils to fluoroscopes. Friedlander sold many protective devices, including their patented protective x-ray tube shield (prices of this tube shield varied by size from $10.00 to $14.00), but died as a radiation casualty.

Information on Friedländer is scarce. In a biographical dictionary I found that he was born in Baltimore in 1868, his profession being listed as scientific electrician.

*This information was taken from a Friedländer catalog, which is in the possession of Dr. Herbert Pollack, chairman of the Section of Radiology in the International College of Surgeons. The catalog is preserved in the Hall of Fame (their museum of surgical history) in Chicago.

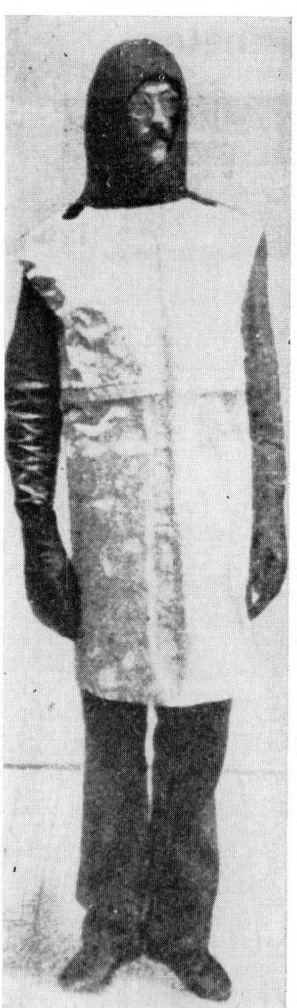

FRIEDLÄNDER X-RAY PROTECTIVE SUIT. The complete outfit (apron, hood, gloves and spectacles) was $30; the apron alone $16.50, the hood $8.50; the year: 1907.

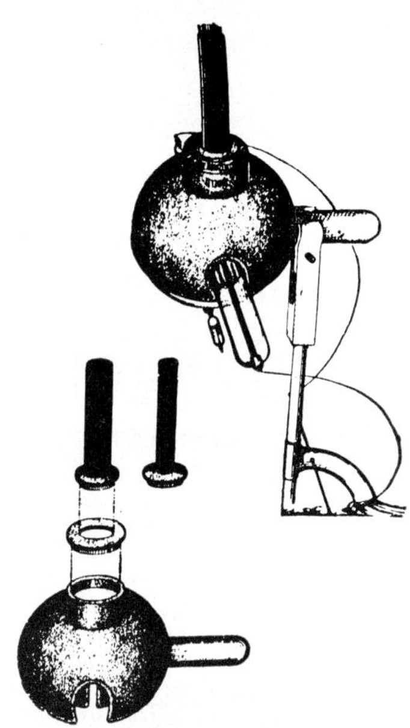

FRIEDLÄNDER PROTECTIVE X-RAY TUBE SHIELDS. All shields fitted with the various diaphragms and hard rubber extensions.

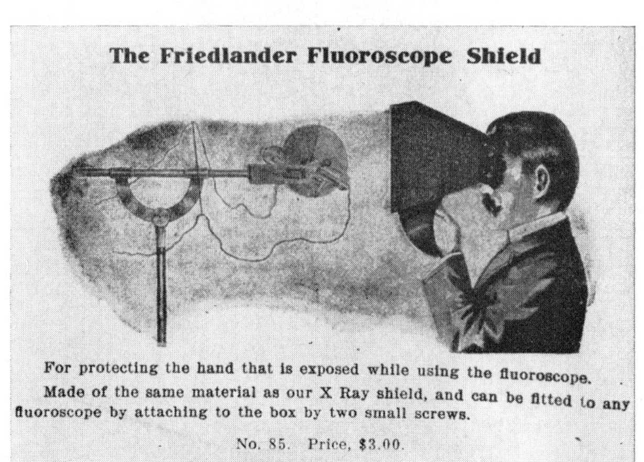

Complete X-Ray Outfits for Office, Hospital and Portable Work.

THE HUTTON SYSTEM

..FOR...

X-RAY WORKERS.

Anyone can make a coil. But to build a **good coil** that will **work well, work always** and **work economically,** takes years of experience and a thoro knowledge of electricity.

Mr. Hutton's eight years of experience in different laboratories of this country is a **guarantee** of his ability to do the best work.

Each coil may be used effectually for Therapeutic, Diagnostic, or Radiographic work.

We build coils ranging in prices from $25.00 to $1,000.00.

Special coils built according to the specifications of those wishing their own designs.

Send for circulars and prices.

Louis F. Nafis & Co.,

...MANUFACTURERS OF...

SCIENTIFIC INSTRUMENTS.

120-122 Randolph St., CHICAGO, ILL.

Complete X-Ray Outfits for Office, Hospital and Portable Work.

THE HUTTON SYSTEM

..FOR...

X-RAY WORKERS.

Anyone can make a coil. But to build a **good coil** that will **work well, work always** and **work economically,** takes years of experience and a thoro knowledge of electricity.

Mr. Hutton's eight years of experience in different laboratories of this country is a **guarantee** of his ability to do the best work.

Each coil may be used effectually for Therapeutic, Diagnostic, or Radiographic work.

We build coils ranging in prices from $25.00 to $1,000.00.

Special coils built according to the specifications of those wishing their own designs.

Send for circulars and prices.

Hutton & Co.,

1902

...MANUFACTURERS OF...

SCIENTIFIC INSTRUMENTS.

55 State St., CHICAGO, ILL.

At the last meeting of the American Roentgen Ray Society the latest thing in Fluoroscopes was exhibited and described. The

Fluoroscope

was designed by Dr. H. Preston Pratt. It is superior in every respect to anything on the market. Will last four times as long as the old style. It cuts out all reflected rays, protects the eyes against particles thrown off from the screen and gives an absolutely perfect image, **something heretofore unknown.**

ALL FORMS OF

X-Ray Coils and Hyperstatic Induction Coils at Greatly Reduced Rates for the Next 90 Days.

The latest forms of special X-Ray tubes, and every variety of electro-therapeutical and X-Ray apparatus supplied at lowest rates.

STANDARD X-RAY SCREEN.

In treating patients for malignant growths in which frequent and prolonged exposure is required, some efficient means of protecting the healthy tissues is absolutely necessary.

The operator himself if exposed repeatedly to even a mild amount of the x-radiance may suffer considerable injury, as many experimenters have found to their cost.

The screen is made of sheet steel and can be folded into small compass when not in use.

Since using this protection Dr. Pratt has had no trouble on account of x-ray burns, even in cases in which exposure has been pushed to an extreme degree in order to destroy malignant growths.

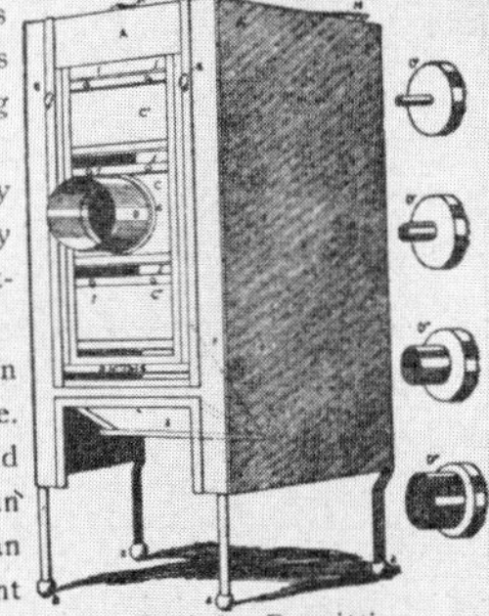

Send for Description.

S. T. Hutton & Co.

120-122 Randolph St. CHICAGO, ILL.

PRATT'S
Improved Fluoroscopes

will fill a long felt want.

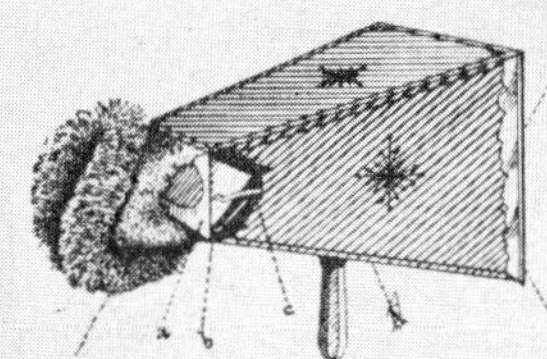

The screen is protected from dust by a glass plate, which also protects the eyes, preventing the decomposed particles from the screen striking the eyes and setting up a conjunctivitis.

The hood is of metal, thus cutting out the reflected rays, which in other fluoroscopes blurs the shadows.

A shutter closes the upper portion when not in use, keeping the compartment free from dust; and when placed on a metal plate it acts as a shield, preventing the further decomposition of the screen by the x-rays which are thrown off from the tube.

The screen is mounted on a metal frame, and warping is impossible. A new screen may be substituted for the old one at a moment's notice.

This Fluoroscope will last several times longer than any other on the market.

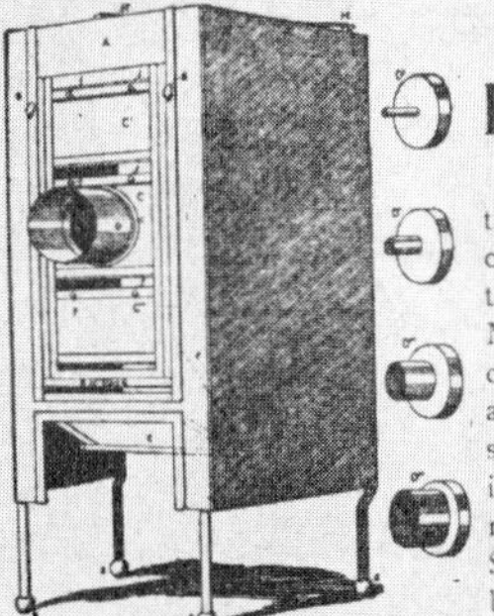

Pratt's Standard Protection X-Ray Screen

The x-ray operator who has suffered from the effects of continued exposures will appreciate the value of an appliance as here illustrated. It will afford him perfect protection. Many who have suffered from the effects of constant exposures are now using the apparatus and indorse it. The screen is made of sheet steel, can be folded into small space when not in use. A series of attachments enables treatment of various parts to be given with safety. Screens made in different sizes and shapes embodying the same principle for reasonable price. Will save operator a damage suit.

Write for further information.

AMERICAN X-RAY CO.,

35-37 Randolph St. CHICAGO, ILL.

He organized and incorporated the Friedländer Co. in 1896, and by 1905 owned 23 patents on x-ray and electrical items. He established in 1901 the *Archives of Electrology and Radiology*, of which he was the first editor. He died around 1915.

Recessions, re-adjustments, and re-possessions were not infrequent among early x-ray manufacturers. Some of their "tragedies" have been "immortalized" in contemporary ads in the *American X-Ray Journal.* In August, 1902 the Louis F. Nafis & Co. (at 120-122 Randolph Street, in Chicago) advertised the "Hutton System for X-Ray Workers." The same text was used in September, 1903 as an offering of the Hutton & Co. (at 55 State Str., in Chicago). Through April, 1903 Hutton & Co. had a nice spread on Harry Preston Pratt's eponymized fluoroscope and steel screen. The first ad of the American X-Ray Company (35-37 Randolph Str., in Chicago) appeared in March, 1903. Hutton's last ad came out in April, 1903 – in June, 1903 Pratt's fluoroscope and screen were being offered by the American X-Ray Company.

The American X-Ray Company started out as a tube (glass) shop, retailing Queen's self-regulating tubes ($15 to $35); Gundelach tubes ($6 to $16); and special Wehnelt tubes ($15.75 to $40) for use with coils that had electrolytic interrupters. They expanded slowly, the first item other than tubes being the McIntosh Reduction Oven for "baking" tubes. Then they bought out Hutton's business.

On October 19, 1901 the *Western Electrician* editorialized that "the x-ray and the slot machine are modern utilities that have finally combined their energies to make a sidewalk show for the curious possessor of the nickel indispensable to operation." On March 22, 1902 in the same *Western Electrician* appeared the information that Jacob M. Hunter had a patent of a Coin-

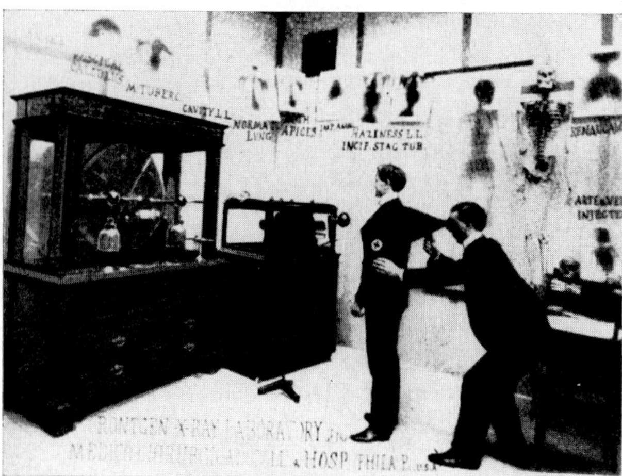

Kassabian's roentgen x-ray lab. Is the resemblance fortuitous?

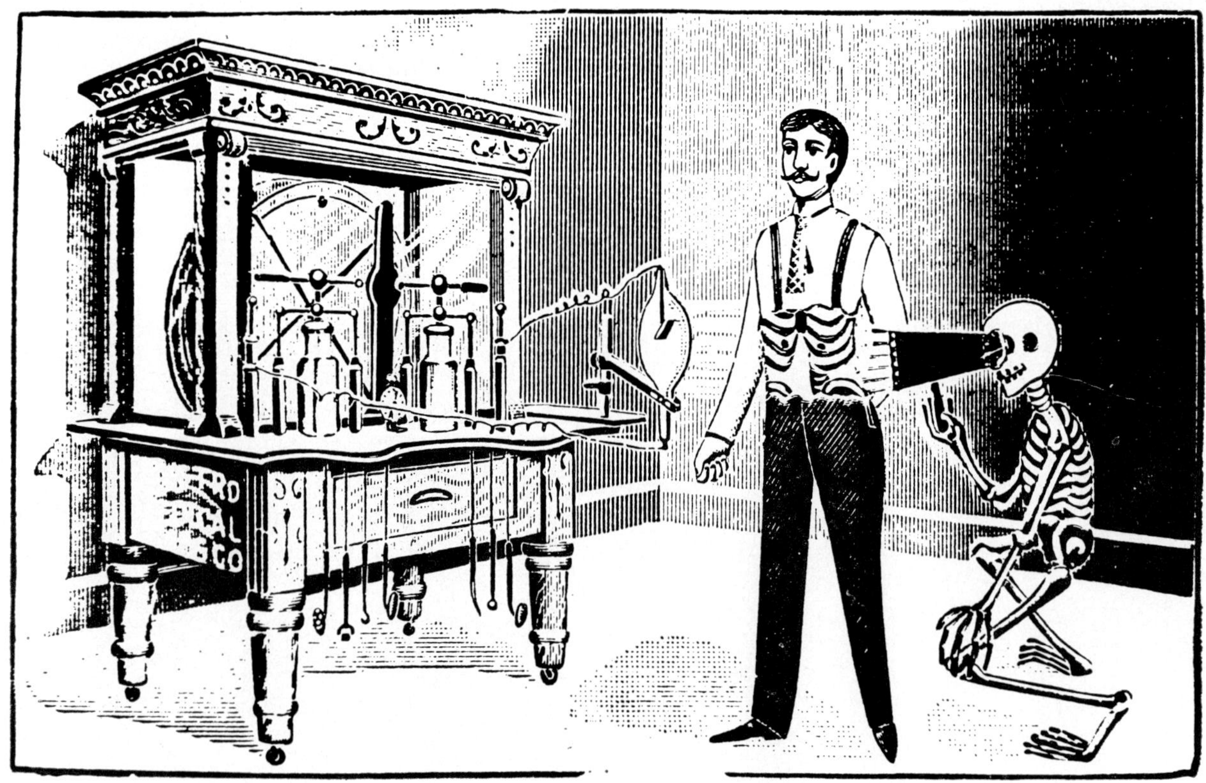

Promotional roentgen-pioneering parody. Part of an advertisement of the Electro-Medical Manufacturing Co. of Chicago.

Controlled X-Ray Machine issued on March 11, which he had assigned to William T. Blaine: the machine was being manufactured by the American X-Ray Company. It was a simple, battery-energized coil, with a coin-controlled contact wheel. At the end of the brief cycle, a spring-operated handle would break the contact. The editorial writer mentioned that about forty such machines were in operation in and around Chicago, and appeared to be quite popular.

At almost the same address, 37, 39, and 41 on Randolph St., was located the Frank S. Betz & Co., which offered 4000 "electric" and other articles, sold directly to physicians at wholesale prices. It was a successful mail-order business. As they brought out the famous Betz 1903 Static Machine and X-Ray Outfit, their catalog listed 5000 items.*

The Electro-Medical Mfg. Co., at 350 Dearborn St. in Chicago, carried in their advertisements a very in-

*Mr. Ed Goldfield (from Picker) has a Betz catalog from the year 1920, published from Hammond (Indiana), with branch offices at 634 S. Wabash in Chicago, and at 6-8 W. 48th St. in New York. That catalog no longer contained x-ray apparatus, only electrotherapeutic equipment. It may be of interest to mention that from 1905 to 1907 Betz printed and promoted a pseudomedical periodical, the *Journal of Physical Therapy,* edited by G. M. Blech.

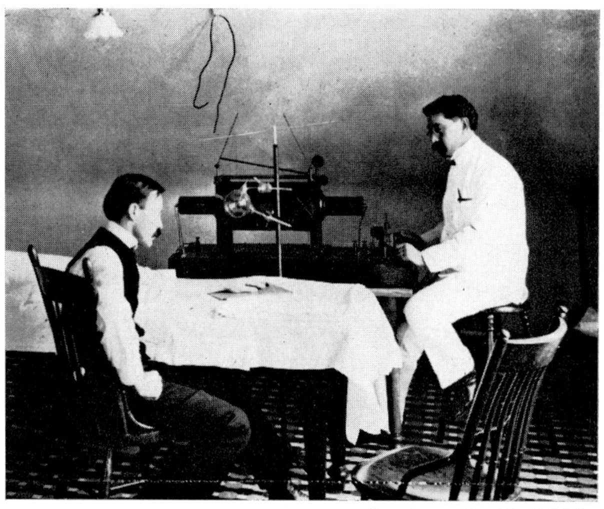

Courtesy: David Shields.

Dr. X-ray Smith with patient and coil. This view of the x-ray room at Presbyterian Hospital (Chicago) around 1900 was once part of the collection of Julius Wantz.

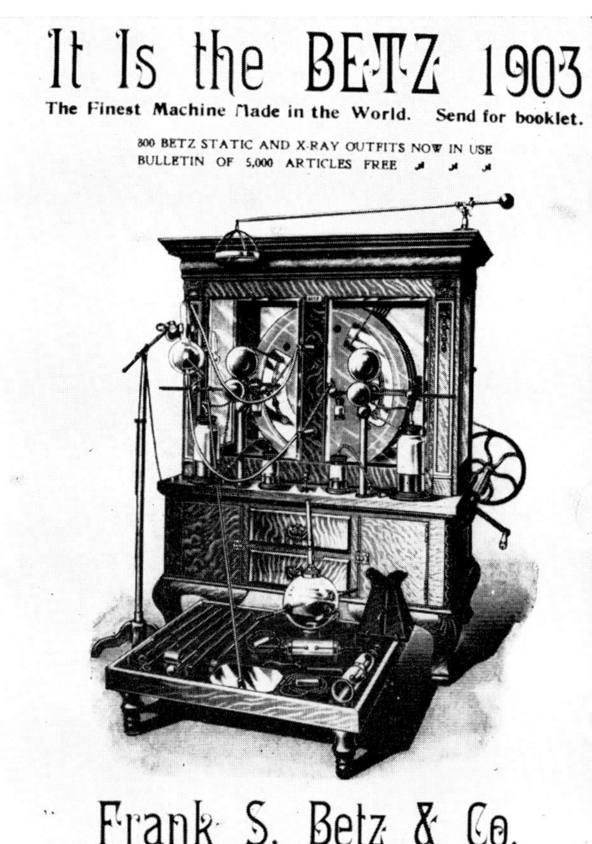

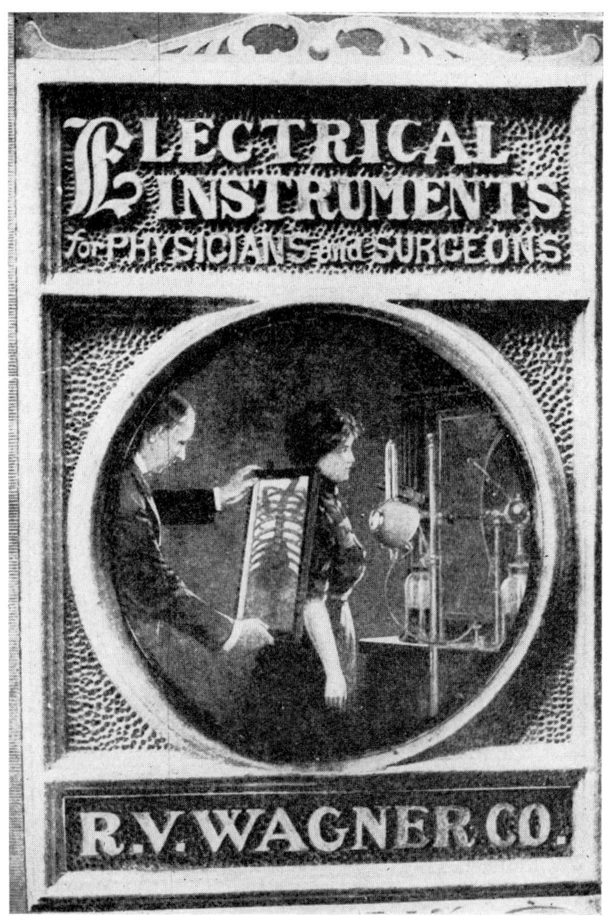

Courtesy: Mrs. Emma (Geo. W.) Brady.

Wagner catalogue of 1907.

teresting cartoon, modeled after the central figures in a famous photograph showing Kassabian at work in his hospital department in Philadelphia.

Around 1898, at the Presbyterian Hospital in Chicago, the orthopedist Joseph F. Smith became the first designated radiologist of that institution. He was nicknamed X-Ray Smith. An early photograph shows him with a patient and a coil, in the city which was to become, so to speak, the hometown of the static machine.

ROME WAGNER FLUOROSCOPING. Note the motor-driven static machine, the hard rubber shield around the tube, and the unconcerned model.

MICA PLATES

Since the beginning of Electrotherapy, there had existed a running competition between static machines and induction coils.

For x-ray work, the coils were less bulky, and when of sufficiently high voltage (12-14″ spark) in conjunction with low vacuum tubes, were preferable for heavy work, as when looking for gallstones. But the coils needed interrupters and those were quite noisy, and otherwise unpleasant.

Static machines required less adjustment and fewer repairs. Tubes would puncture less often with static machines than with induction coils. An electric motor could be used to turn the static machine but this was

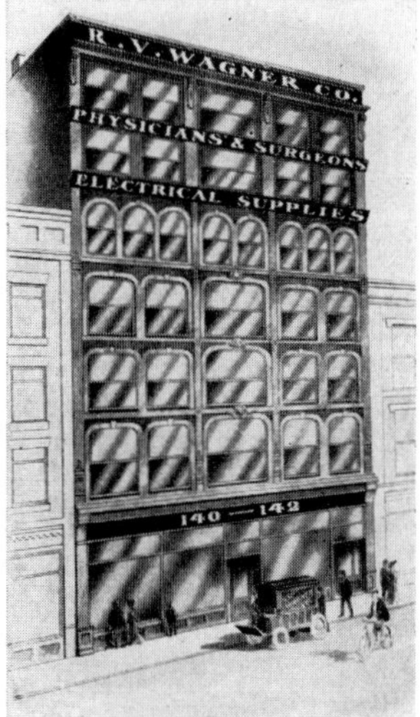

WAGNER'S SHOWROOMS IN 1907. Location: 140-142 Wabash Avenue, near Madison Street in Chicago. The vintage "horseless delivery-carriage" is inscribed with the firm's name.

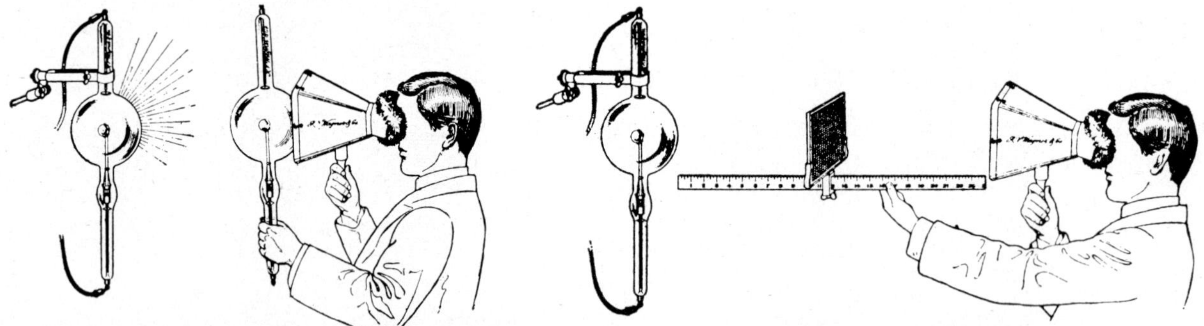

TREACHEROUS TUBE TESTING. Drawings of Rome Wagner shown fluoroscoping a tube, to determine degree of radiotransparency of its glass, and checking adequacy of focus. Writes he: "The nearer it is necessary to bring the screen to the surface of the fluoroscope, the more the tube is out of focus . . . with a perfectly focused tube the holes in a 20-mesh screen will stand out perfectly clear at least 12 inches away from the fluoroscope, having the fluoroscope 24 inches away from the tube."

not strictly necessary, it could also be turned by hand, by water, or by any other power source. Of all things, humidity was a serious handicap to the static machine because it would interfere directly with its operation.

Obviously, there were as many pros as there were cons on each side. The opponents could extoll the virtues of their own product, denigrate the rival's ware, and still be safe from "exposure." One such "battle" took place between two proponents of the static machine, the argument being over mica plates.

Just before the turn of the century, a revolutionary improvement in static machines was made in Chicago by Rome Wagner. Instead of using the glass plates introduced by Wimshurst, he adapted mica plates, imported from India, split to the thinnest lamina, put into dies with cement and turned out under hydraulic pressure with molds at a temperature of 700° F. With these plates he ran the machines at 2000 revolutions per minute (RPM). Glass plates of the same size would break at a speed higher than 300 RPM. Since the current depended on the speed with which the machine was run, machines with four mica plates were supposed to produce more current (and thus do better x-ray work) than larger glass plate machines.

WAGNER
IDEAL EQUIPMENT FOR RADIOGRAPHY

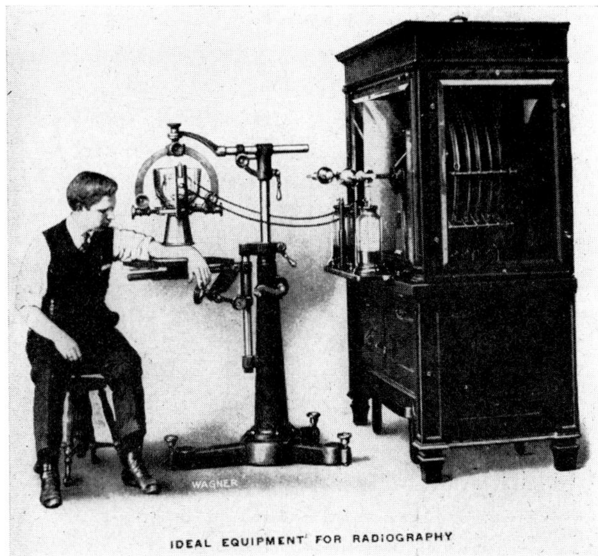

WAGNER'S "IDEAL EQUIPMENT." This extremely sturdy piece resembles a modern Bucky stand. A very well preserved specimen (albeit without that table attachment) stands in the Hall of Fame of the International College of Surgeons in Chicago.

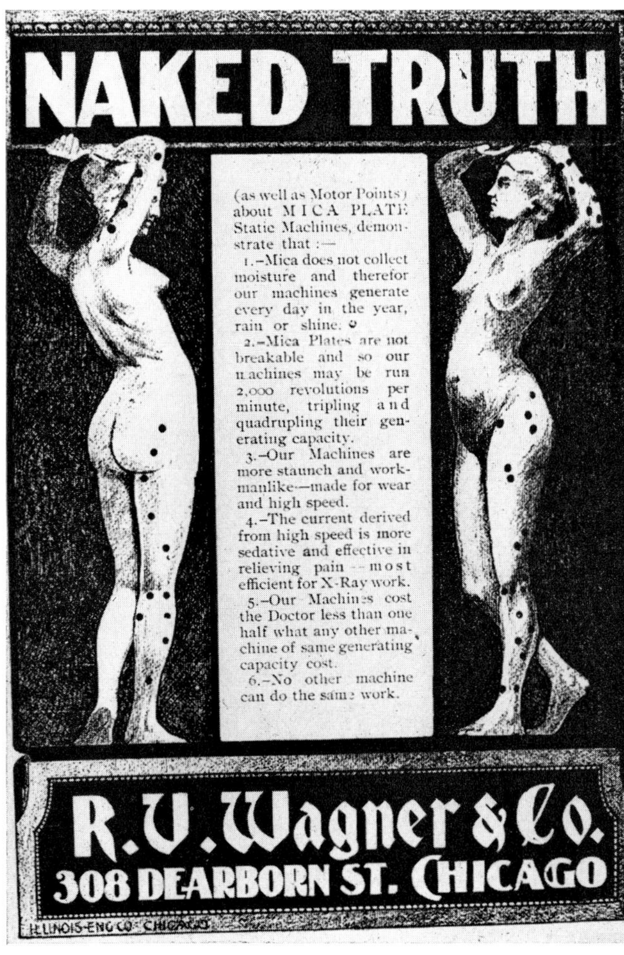

FACTS NOT FANCIES
A BEAUTY
Comes from good stock and is well put together.
As to shape, the form compared with others, is that of a Venus de Milo. Sparks every day Rain or Shine. Is absolutely independent of the case which prevents getting out of adjustment and loss by leakage. Does not change polarity while in operation. MICA PLATES for high speed developing highest mode of molecular motion in the current. Will do all you ask in Therapeutic and X-Ray work.
New Catalog gives much information.
R. V. WAGNER & CO., 308 Dearborn Street, Chicago.
1899

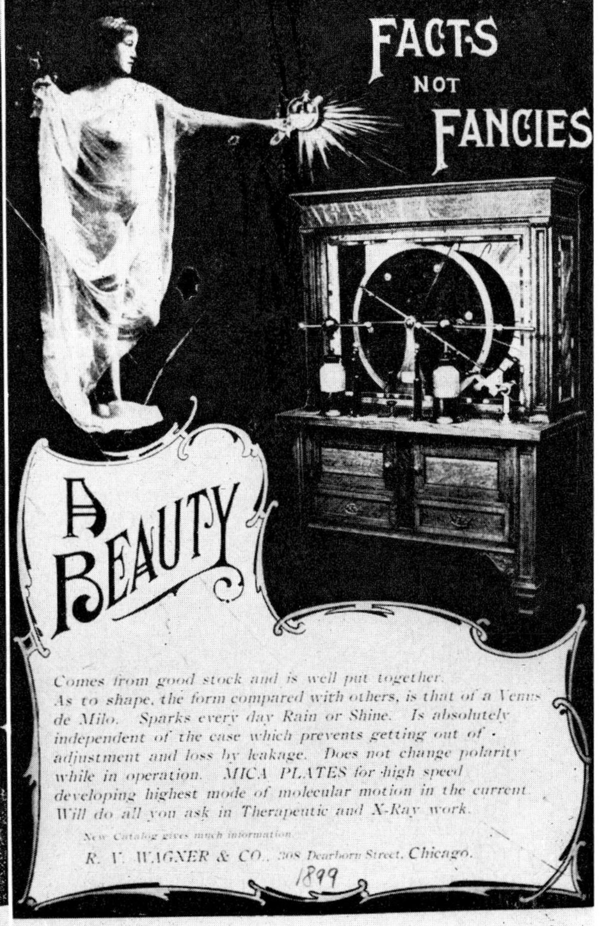

WAGNER & CO.

Rome Vernon Wagner (1869-1908) was a physician (he had served as an apprentice to an established practitioner) but his main interest concerned the construction of electrical appliances for medical use. He developed the process by which melted shellac was used to cement the mica plates under hydraulic pressure. The toughness of the resulting plate was comparable to that of sheet metal.

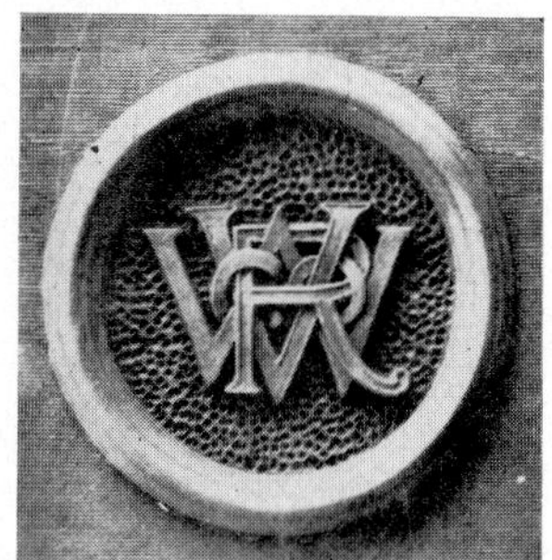

WAGNER'S TRADE-MARK. Monogram made from the initials of Rome Vernon Wagner – the "Patron Saint of the Static Machine".

Their first location was at 52 State St. because Wagner had bought out and become successor to the Electro-Medical Supply Co. By 1900, a larger shop was acquired at 308 Dearborn St. and this is also the address given on the frontispiece of a catalogue of that time. His brother, Truman Lester Wagner (1876-1912) was likewise a physician (a graduate of the College of Physicians and Surgeons in Chicago). They both died from prolonged and repeated exposure to radiation incurred while testing x-ray tubes.

Some of their ads, while a bit risqué, have a classic quality. In one of them, the copy refers both to the veil-clad lady and to the static machine (shown side by side on the poster) as coming from good stock and being well put together. Wagner equipment was indeed very sturdy and certainly well put together. A Wagner tubestand is on exhibit in the Hall of Fame of the International College of Surgeons in Chicago. It is rumored that a few of those Wagner tubestands, provided with modern tubes, are still in operation. As a fitting tribute to the industry of the older Wagner, the *American X-ray Journal* called him appropriately, "the Patron Saint of the Static Machine."

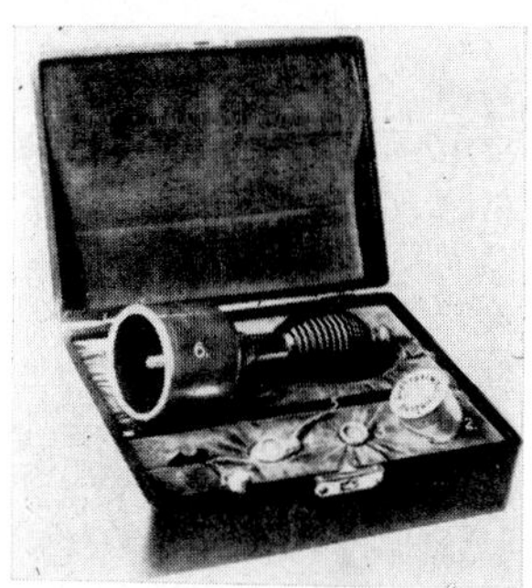

FANCY RADIUM EQUIPMENT. This box, made and sold by Swett & Lewis (Boston) around 1910, contained a brass receptacle (1) for radium; a small round box (2) for containing the receptacle "when carried in pocket"; and applicators of solid silver, and lead.

Static Machines
For all Purposes. . . . .
Crookes
. . . Tubes..
X-Ray . .
Apparatus . . .
Send for Catalogue No. 25.
SWEET & LEWIS CO.
11 BROOMFIELD STREET.
BOSTON, : : MASS.
1900

SPELLING GREMLINS AT WORK. Swett's reaction to the misspelling of his name was hardly akin to honey.

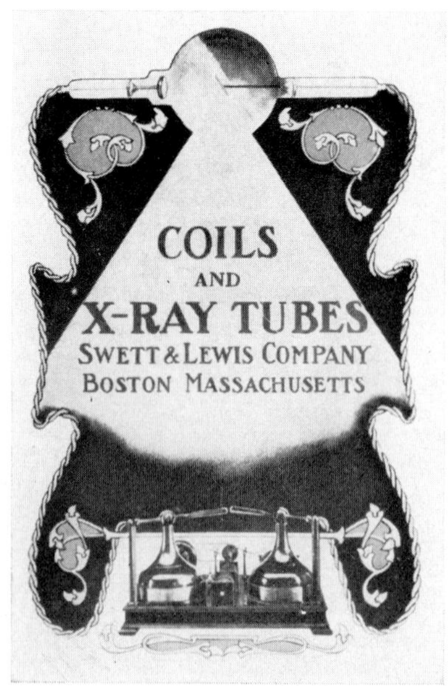

MEANWHILE IN THE EAST

In Connecticut, Burton Eugene Baker (1871-1913), was a counter-part of Wagner. He used mica plates in his static machines, and he got himself "burned" (with "fatal" consequences) while testing gas tubes. He had established in 1905 the Baker Electric Co., which was supported, according to Percy Brown (1936), by two physicians, W. E. Clark and the well known J. C. DaCosta, both of Philadelphia. In 1910, Baker formed also the Baker X-ray Tube Co., but after his death from metastatic carcinoma, the companies distintegrated.

In Boston, at 11 Broomfield St. the Swett & Lewis Co. (successors to the E. A. Frey & Co.) manufactured tubes as well as static machines with conventional glass plates. The main figurehead was Frank Howard Swett (1868-1929) whose name will be mentioned again in connection with the Victor Co. Swett & Lewis were also producing very fancy brass receptacles for radium.

South of Connecticut, in New York City, at 304 - 4th Ave. there existed since 1870 the Van Houten & Ten Broeck Co.: their advertised advice was to "look before you leap." They were offering the Morton-Wimshurst-Holtz influence machine* which was just a conventional static apparatus. It is of interest to mention that this was the first x-ray equipment purchased by the Osteopathic College in Kirksville (Missouri).

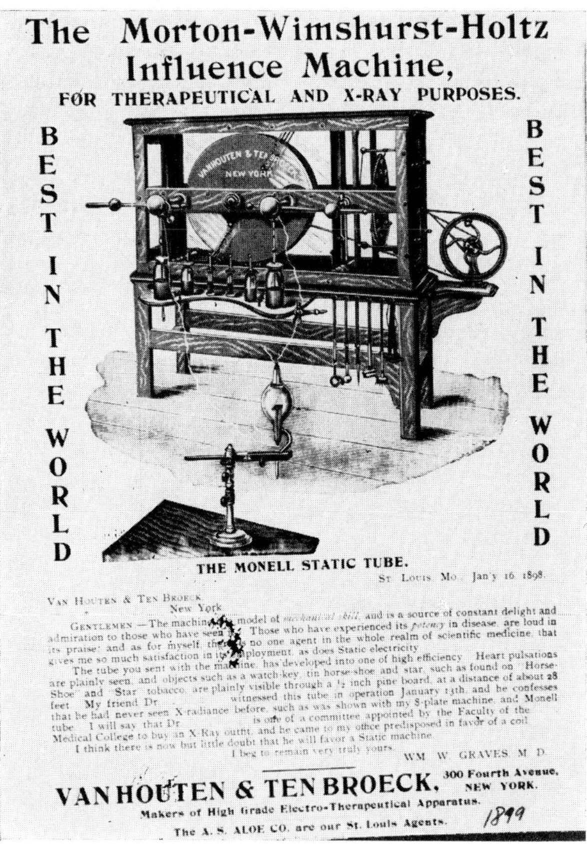

WAITE & BARTLETT

At 108 East 23rd Street, in New York City, existed the Waite & Bartlett Co., founded in 1879. In June, 1902 its president, Henry Waite, Sr. (1848-1916) printed in the *American X-Ray Journal* a challenge to the Wagners, offering

". . . to make the test to prove that two mica plates will not give the same amount of current that ten glass plates of equal size will give. Furthermore (I will) prove that a machine with two glass plates, same size as two mica plates, will equal and do more and better work (x-ray or otherwise) under same conditions, than

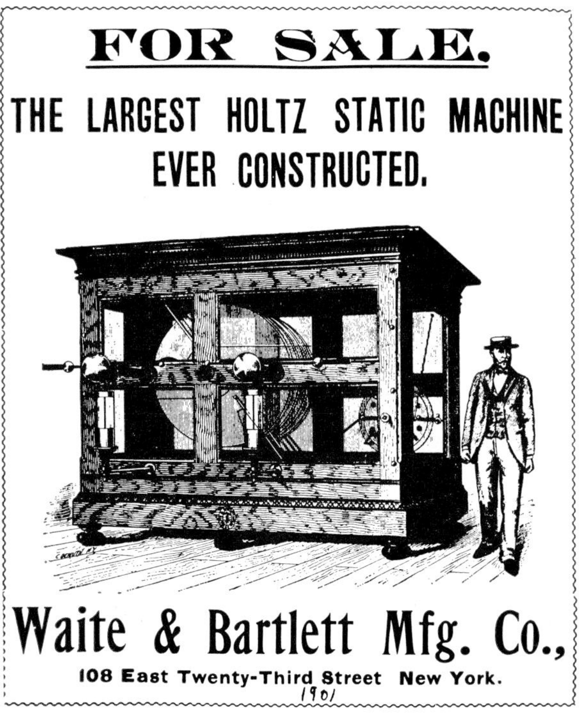

*Edmund A. Crain (1853-1909) was one of the first physicians who used an x-ray machine in Montana, while he practised at Missoula. In 1899 Crain moved to Great Falls (Montana), and purchased a Morton-Winshurst-Holtz "influence machine," with x-ray attachment. He advertised that this machine would photograph organs and bones of the body, and was effective in treating muscular and nervous diseases. Such advertising won him the ill will of the colleagues who did not have x-ray equipment, *cf.* p. 285 in Paul C. Phillips and Lewellyn L. Callaway, *Medicine in the Making of Montana* (Missoula, 1962). Other physicians who used x rays in Montana before the turn of the century were James F. Spelman (1868-1917) of Anaconda, regarded as one of their early experts in this field (p. 430); and Daniel McHeffey McKay (1842-1914) at White Sulphur Springs (Montana), a criminal lawyer who later graduated as a physician (p. 326).

the mica plate machine can do. This advertised statement gives them (the manufacturers of the mica plate) the opportunity to prove the same and have it settled, which is the most efficient in actual practice."

In the *American X-Ray Journal* of July of 1902, under the caption *A Bluff Called,* Wagner retorted:

". . . We accept the challenge and name the following conditions, the fairness of which is obvious!! 1. The test to be made at Chicago. 2. The Medical and Scientific Electricians who shall decide the contest are to be chosen, one by our opponent, one by ourselves, and the two to appoint a third. 3. The machine selected for the test shall have been sold in the open market by the respective contestants, within two years, and shall be selected from the offices of parties now using the same or trying to do so. We, to furnish the machine manufactured and sold by our opponent, he to furnish any four-plate Mica Static Machine which has been sold by us. It is understood that these machines shall not be broken or otherwise injured, and that each party shall have six hours prior to the test to produce necessary adjustments for making the machine work at its best, but not to replace or add parts."

In August, 1902 the editor of the *American X-Ray Journal,* T. Proctor Hall (he had just started after the one month interregnum of Charles P. Renner), suggested that the meeting of the ARRS slated for December 10th in Chicago, could provide an adequate background for the contest between Wagner and W & B. Moreover, the editor thought that new machines could also be tested in addition to used models.

To this, Rome Wagner replied in a letter published in the *American X-Ray Journal* of October, 1902. He explained that a manufacturer could select carefully from a large number of glass plates those well grounded and well balanced which would permit higher speed in a test machine. He could also have those plates heavier bushed with soft rubber which would decrease the amount of vibration. His tougher mica plates were superior simply because they could be run at higher speeds. This is why he insisted on used rather than on new models. As far as could be determined, the contest between Wagner and Waite never took place.

The advertising genius of Waite & Bartlett (W & B) was in many ways comparable to that of the Wagner Co. W & B built the largest static machine* then in existence, with eight revolving glass plates, five feet in diameter, and place to put in two more. This machine was made for a physician in Washington (D.C.), F. A. Gardner. It would give a spark of 30-36″. Later Gardner wanted to sell the machine, and it was purchased by another physician, Kellogg, owner and operator of the Sanitarium in Battle Creek (Michigan).

W & B had a very fancy trade-mark, with a lightning-sparked caduceus, of which there were several

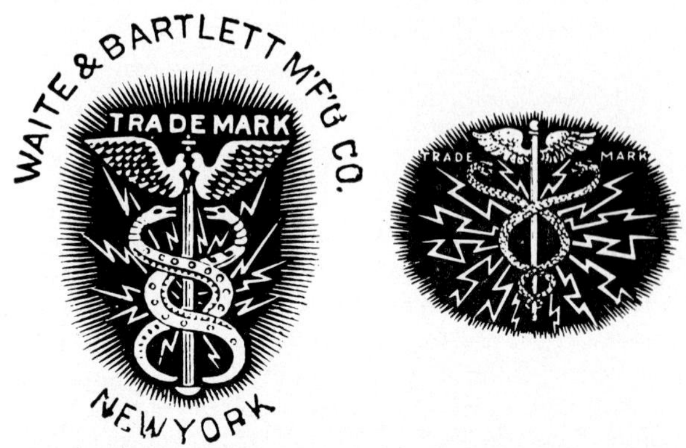

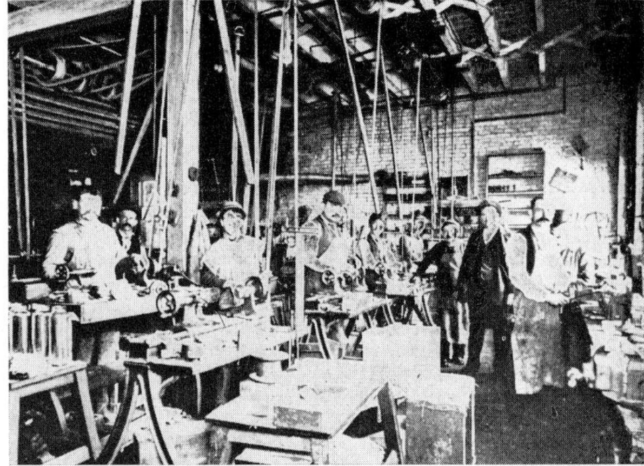

Courtesy: Ivor Bennett

WAITE & BARTLETT CONSTRUCTION ROOM (about 1912).

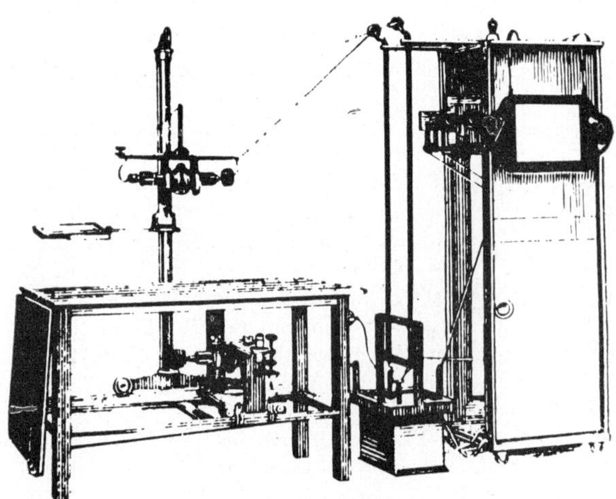

W & B UNIT ADVERTISED IN 1920. At that time the unit was outdated, but in 1910 when it had first been issued, it represented the last word.

*Later, Henry Hulst built one with 36 plates.

variants. They never had a nationwide sales organization, but they were well known because a potential customer who came to New York received friendly attention and other courtesies.

W & B sold all sorts of accessories. Around 1915, fluoroscopic screens cost from $35.00 for the 8x10″ to $99.00 for the 14x17″ A 5x7″ hand-held cryptoscope was $10.00. $18.50 would buy an Eagle Electric Ruby Lamp, and for $10.35 you could get a 14x17″ plate washer. A negative illuminator (viewbox) with rheostat sold for $30.00.

By 1920, many were still using two separate units for fluoroscopy, one in recumbency, the other for upright position. Actually, some of the equipment herein illustrated is more or less transitional between the Pioneering Era and the Golden Age of Radiology.

A personal friendship existed between Waite, Jr. (son of the founder of W & B) and the famous radiologist Lewis Gregory Cole of New York City. The latter "fathered" the Cole Golden Flame X-Ray Coil. In a photograph, dated 1905, we see the young but already bald Cole adjusting the gas tube. In the background is his famous Golden Flame Coil on the face of which is a huge ma-meter. In the W & B catalogues, Cole's Coil is much fancier and encased. Incidentally, in 1918 the cost of that huge ma-meter had reached $25.00.

Cole designed for the W & B also a radiographic and fluoroscopic "surface" which shows why this contrivance was originally called a table. Today's epigones

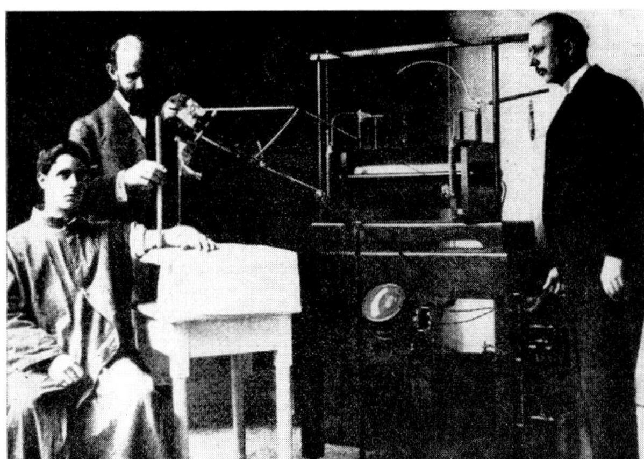

Cole's Golden Flame Coil. Young Lewis Gregory Cole shows his "modern" technic – while technician throws the switch.

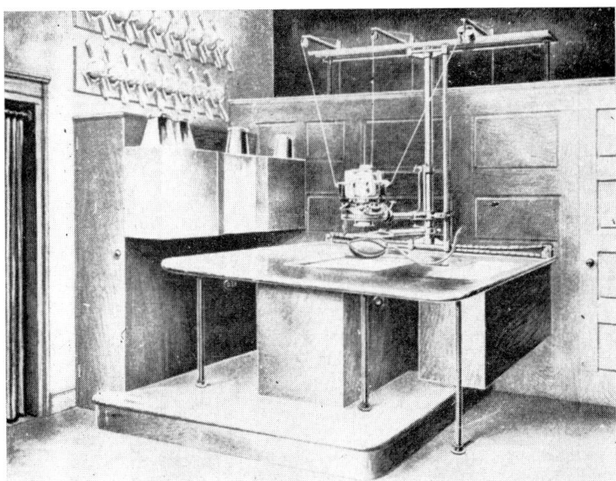

Cole's Table. It was called radiographic and fluoroscopic table.

The Cole Floor Push

No. 17

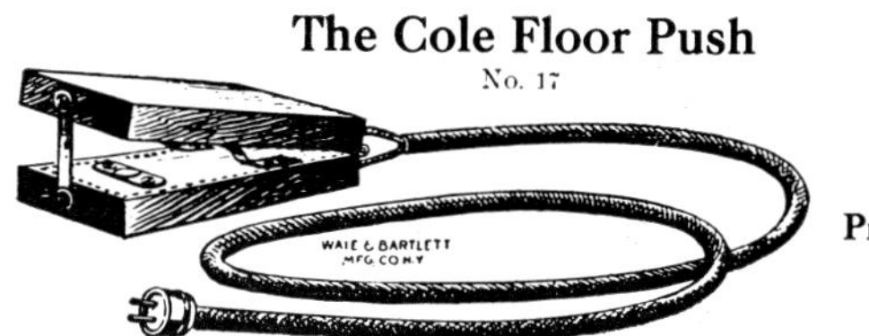

Price, $7.50

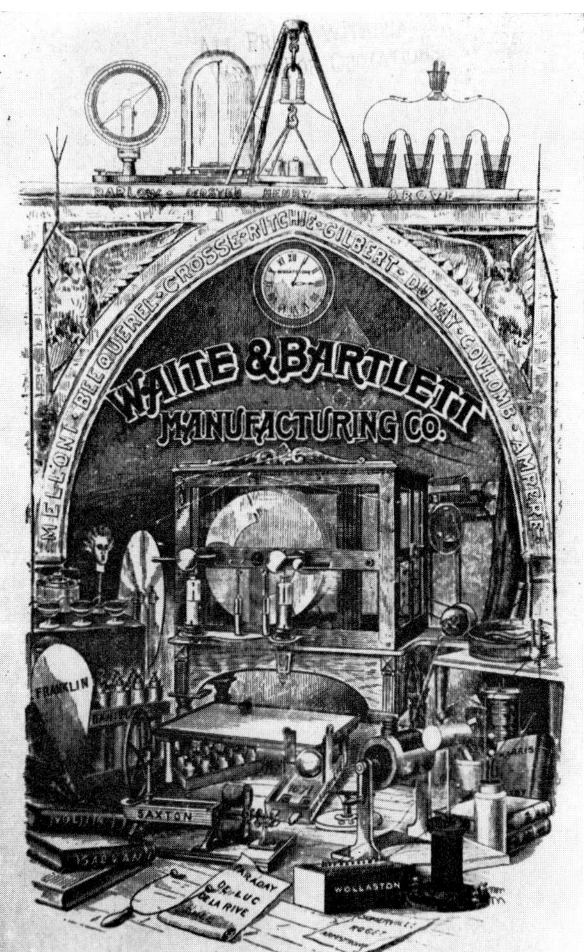

Courtesy: Dave Bennett from the Picker Co.

W & B Catalog of 1918.

are still called tables but their resemblance to tables is only perfunctory. In Great Britian, they are called couches and this term is sometimes encountered also in the American x-ray literature in the 1920s, but only with regard to treatment tables. Cole's eponym was also used by W & B for their Cole Floor Push, marked $7.50; it was simply a foot-switch.

At the time, just before 1920, W & B sold reflecting stereoscopes, made by both Wappler and Keleket; they were priced at $150.00.

W & B's most famous machine was the Army Bedside Unit. After the end of World War I, they renamed it (for civilian users) the Moderate Power Machine. I have seen a photograph of Frank Borzell using an Army Bedside Unit (at bedside) in the Base Hospital in Grand Blottereaux (France) in 1918. An original Army Bedside Unit, restored and in perfect functioning order, is one of the showpieces in the exhibit room of the Waite Mfg. Division (Cleveland) of the Picker Company. The Army Bedside Unit was the first stock x-ray equipment provided with a Coolidge hot cathode tube.

The W & B issued many revolutionary designs, for instance a new type of transformer for deep therapy apparatus. They had also a Solace Duplex Tubestand, named after the U. S. Hospital Ship Solace, which in 1912 was re-equipped with W & B x-ray apparatus. This particular tubestand was used for simultaneous therapeutic application from one tube to two patients.

After the war was over, the Army Bedside Unit was also adapted as a civilian mobile unit which sold for $800.00. It was the last "open" unit before introduction of the revolutionary oil-immersed model, the brainchild of Henry (Harry) Fuller Waite, Jr., (1874-1946), son of and successor to Waite, Sr.

After graduating in 1897 from New York University as a full-fledged physician, the young Waite returned to work in the factory in which he had practically grown up. The collection of patents issued to Waite is preserved in the archives of the (above mentioned) Waite Mfg. Division in Cleveland. The first of Waite, Jr.'s patents is no. 514,524 dated February 13, 1894 which concerns an influence machine. The collection contains also no. 876,166 dated June 11, 1901, which is a method for regulating roentgen ray tubes. Another one, no. 1,471,081 dated October 16, 1923, is a vibrating Bucky diaphragm, a feature which was not introduced (re-discovered) until three decades later.

An interesting gadget is a day-light fluoroscope, no. 1,936,342, dated June 22, 1932, which contains even a fan to provide air conditioning of sorts within the enclosure draped about the radiologist's bust. Fifty-one patents are preserved in above mentioned book. The last of them, no. 2,025,139 dated December 24, 1938 concerns a casing for x-ray apparatus.

Additional personal information was obtained from Ted Koch, who had been since 1925 with W & B,

BORZELL AT BLOTTEREAUX. The stern sergeant is in control of the controls, while Frank Borzell stands on a wooden chair to look into the cryptoscope. I asked him a few years ago if he remembers how long he had to accommodate, and he said they wore red goggles, only with two layers of glass, one for adaptation (which could be raised on hinges), the other made of transparent lead glass.

H. F. WAITE.
X-RAY APPARATUS.
APPLICATION FILED JAN. 31, 1919.

1,334,936. Patented Mar. 23, 1920

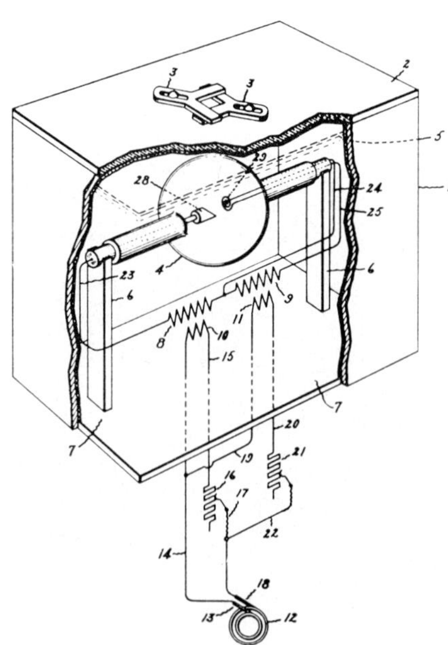

WAITE'S OIL-IMMERSION PRINCIPLE. One of the basic patents in modern x-ray technology.

then worked for Picker, and finally "retired" to form the Koch X-Ray, Inc. in Miami. Following are some excerpts from his letters:

"Henry Waite was an officer in the Civil War, and since then an avid gun, sword, and sabre collector. The W & B factory basement was full of crated guns. Bartlett died in New York City about two years after W & B was formed: Waite retained his name on the masthead because of their close friendship.

"It is interesting to note the various addresses of Waite & Bartlett; first at 108 East 23rd Street, then at 217 East 23rd Street, next at 252 West 29th Street, following at 113 West 31st Street, and finally at 53 Jackson Avenue in Long Island City.

"There were two brothers Garretson, born in Scotland. They were electrical engineers, had a transformer business in New York City, and were making the transformers for W & B. One of the brothers was killed in a train wreck in 1910, then W & B bought out their business – that was just before W & B moved to Long Island City – and H. D. Garretson came to work for W & B as electrical engineer and designer. There was close and very fruitful co-operation between Waite and Garretson. But the Garretson Dental X-Ray Chair was not named after this Garretson: it was eponymized for John L. Garretson, professor in the College of Dentistry of the University of Buffalo (New York).

"Among the people at W & B, I would like to mention Herbert H. Watjen, who was the accountant. He became an executive of the Lepel High Frequency Company in New York City. Henry Hollmann, Sr. had been for many years W & B's general manager; he went out on his own, sometime in the 1930s, and formed the XRM Co., which manufactures dental x-ray equipment. Henry Hollmann, Jr. succeeded his father, and

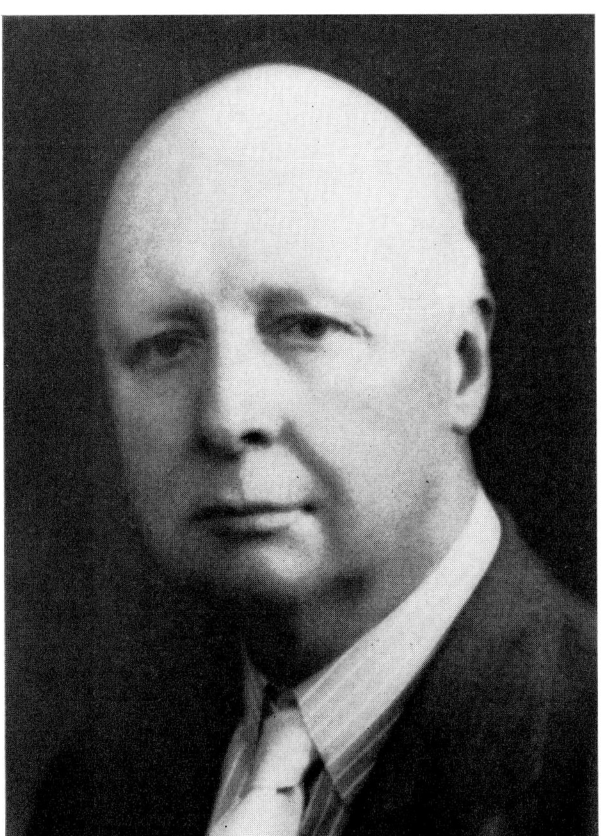

HARRY FULLER WAITE, JR. (1874-1946). One of the most imaginative among American X-Ray Makers.

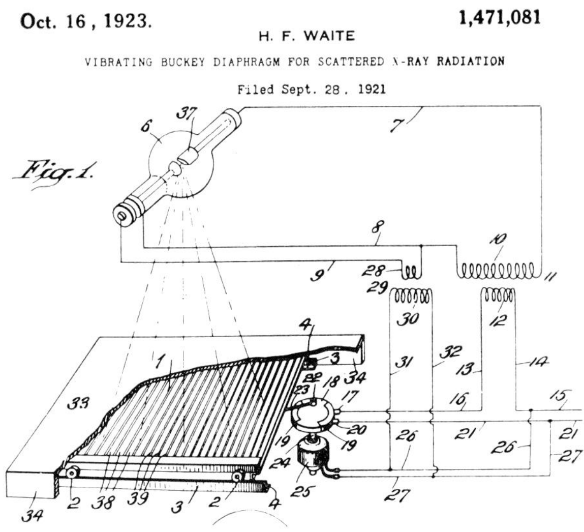

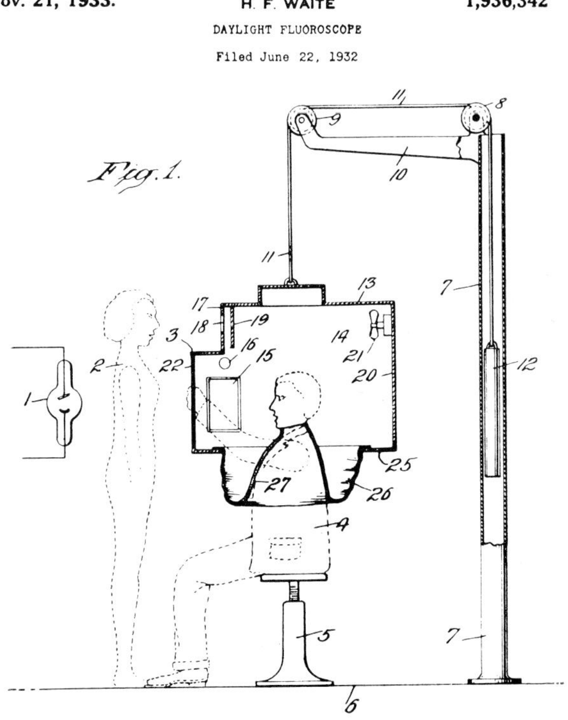

continued with the S. S. White Mfg. Co., of which the XRM is now a subsidiary.

"Tom White worked for many years for the City of New York as an x-ray electrician: he had assembled most of W & B's custom-built units. Tom Ford retired after fifty years of service with W & B. Brustlein & Brustlein were also located at 53 Jackson Ave.: they did all the machine shop work for W & B.

"Incidentally, between 1926 and 1928 W & B were manufacturing a shockproof cable unit and special tubestand under license, but I cannot recall the name of the man they were working with. Approximately ten units of that type were made, then they gave up the idea."

There were many devices which carried Waite's name, for instance a Wave Selector. The one which made him famous had patent no. 1,334,936, issued on March 23, 1920. It was a very simple design: the x-

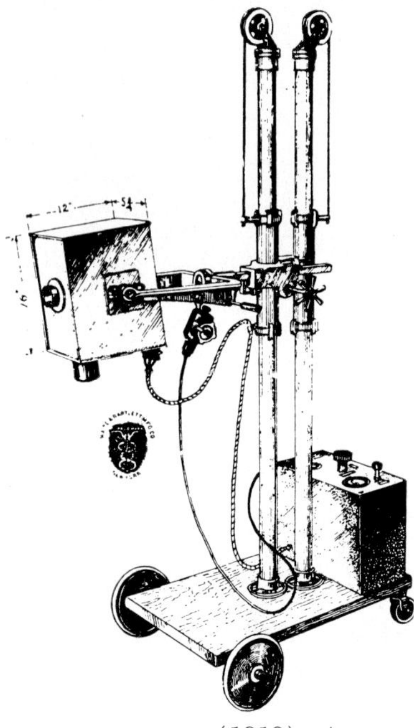

FIRST OIL-IMMERSED UNIT (1919). A most important first created by Waite was this shock-proof, radiation-proof mobile unit. It had a Coolidge hot cathode tube. Its basic design – transformer encased together with the tube in an oil-filled container – is still utilized in all portable, mobile, and in a few stationary combinations.

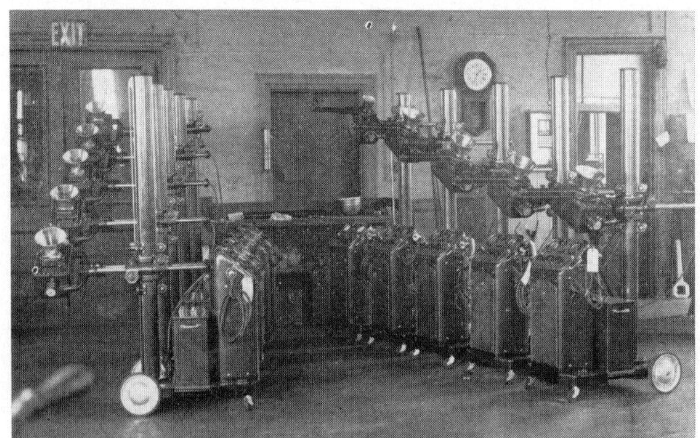

Courtesy: Ted Koch.

W & B's THIRD FLOOR (1928). Ten mobile (oil-immersed) units in the Long Island City plant were quite a production for that time.

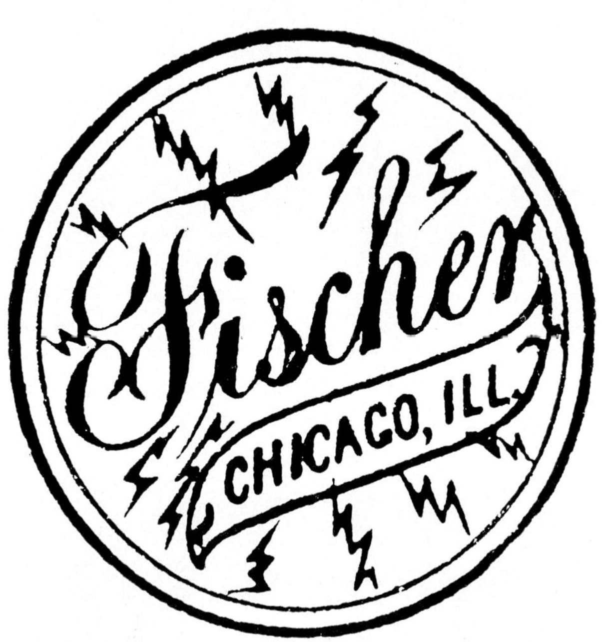

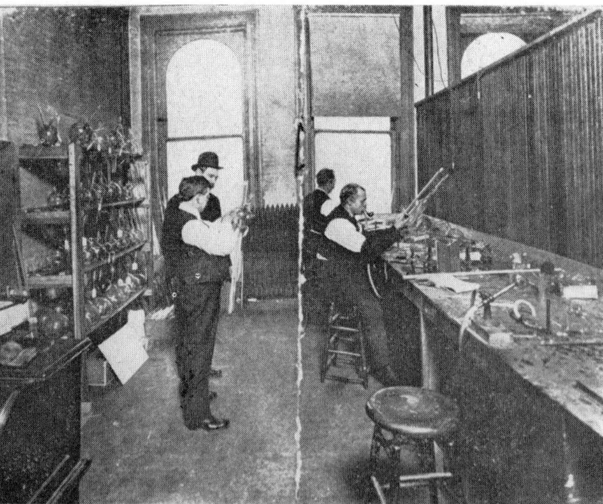

X-RAY TUBE "FACTORY" (ABOUT 1900). Location: 100 East Lake Street in Chicago. Owner: Heinz Wandner, the bespectacled gentleman in shirt sleeves, "selling" a glassy contraption to the customer wearing a derby bowler. A crease is seen running down the middle of the picture. The company was later called Wandner & Son. It disappeared before World War I.

ray tube was encased together with the transformer in a box filled with oil. This was the first oil-immersed, shock-proof and later (when the box was lined with lead) also the first "radiation-proof" apparatus. The then available models of Coolidge's hot cathode tube were too large for a reasonably sized casing. Around that time Coolidge came forth with a similar idea, and wanted to build a dental unit based on the oil-immersion principle. By the force of circumstances — unavailability of tubes which would fit into the casing — Waite entered into an agreement with General Electric whereby he received $1,000 and the assurance that GE would sell him every year 300 Coolidge tubes in exchange for the rights to the oil-immersion patent. I have in my possession a copy of that agreement (courtesy of Ted Koch), together with a letter from Hollmann, mentioning the fact that the Australian Watson wanted to purchase some of the W & B dental units, but wondered what could be done about the tubes, and W & B offered to sell the units, and let Watson purchase his tubes directly from GE, because the agreement between Waite and GE contained a limiting clause with regard to x-ray tubes.

As the Big Depression kept on deepening, an aging Waite, Jr. was looking for a buyer, and this is how and when Picker bought out the W & B Company.

W & B is now a name from the radiologic past, but in that past it holds a place of honor, achieved through the genius and industry of Waite, Sr. and Waite, Jr., together with their associates. The page occupied by W & B is as bright as any in the history of the American x-ray industry.

SMALL MANUFACTURERS OF TUBES

Toward the end of the era of gas tubes there were in the large cities a number of shops which specialized in the repair and rebuilding of such tubes.

There was for instance the Kesselring X-Ray Tube Company at 136 W. Lake Street in Chicago, where Matz got his first contact with the trade. This is also the way in which the H. G. Fischer & Company, 2235-2341 Wabansia Avenue in Chicago, had its beginning.

The Heinz Wandner X-Ray Tube Company was at 100 East Lake Street in Chicago. A few years later, the Wandner & Son X-Ray Tube Company (as seen from

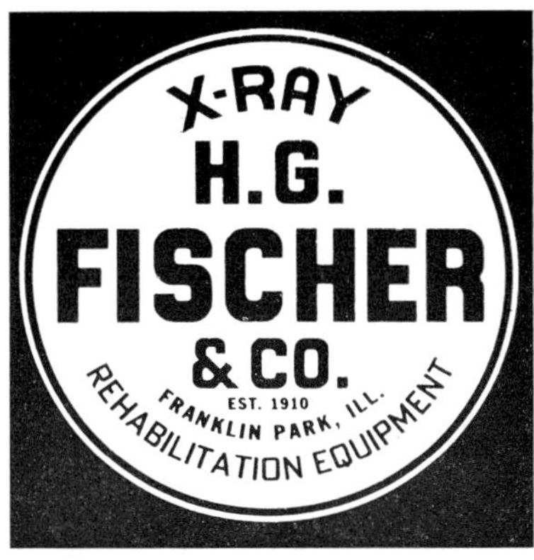

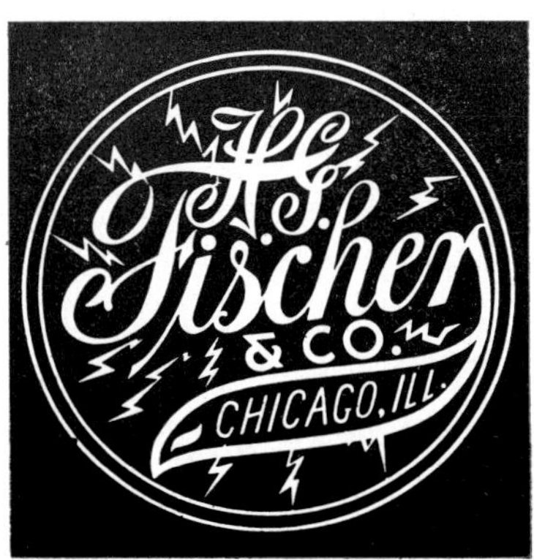

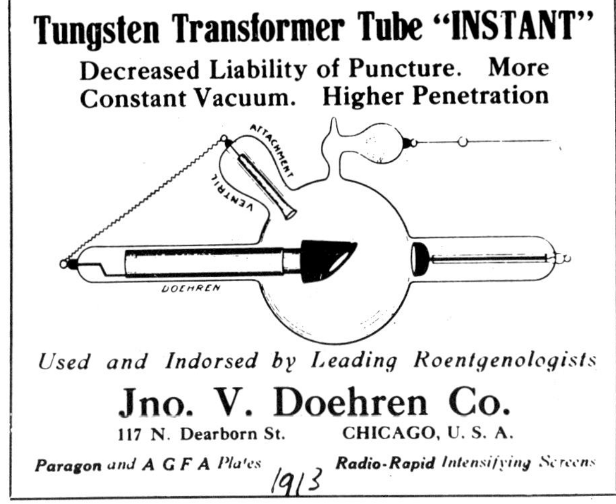

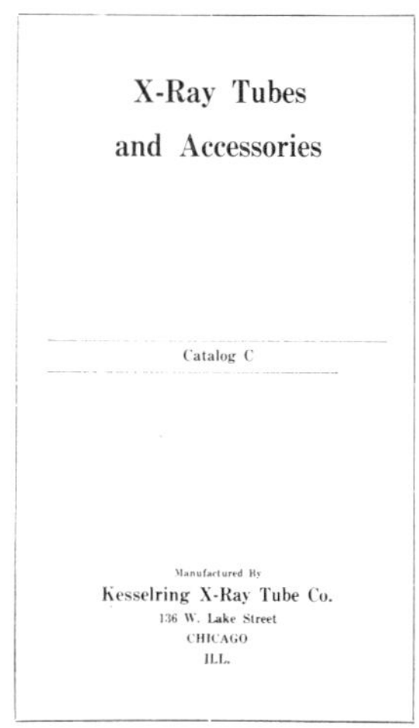

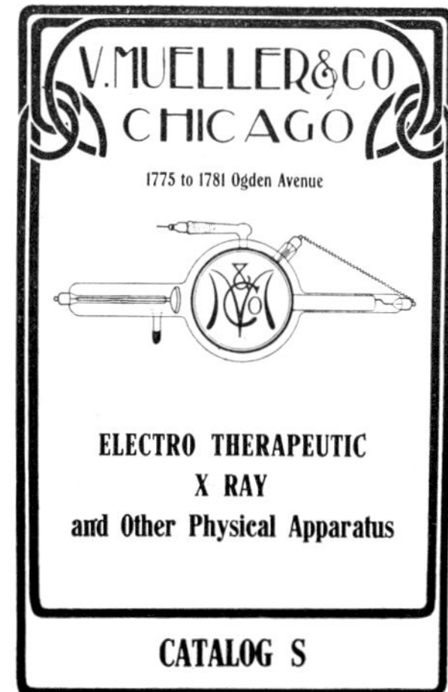

a catalog which is in the possession of Charles W. Smith) gave its address at 160 N. Fifth Ave., also in Chicago. They were making also screens and other accessories, for instance "the most complete portable High Frequency Apparatus at the lowest price of $15."

The Jno. V. Doehren Company, at 117 North Dearborn Street, in Chicago, marketed the Tungsten Transformer Tube called *Instant,* said to decrease the liability of punctures; its vacuum was supposedly more constant, and therefore it produced higher penetration. Doehren sold also plates, as well as screens and other accessories.

V. Mueller & Company, 1775-1779 Ogden Avenue, in Chicago advertised in 1912 a full line of x-ray apparatus and accessories, including foreign makes, for instance Gehler, Prima, and Rotax intensifying screens. They sold, for $7.50 a pair, improved goggles, made of smoked glasses hinged to heavy lead glass spectacles. In a darkened room, the smoked glasses could be raised while the lead glass would still provide the necessary shielding for the eye during fluoroscopy. This improved model had been designed by Trostler himself.

Some of the tube shops developed into small manufacturers, as the (comparatively short lived) Vacuum Glass Company of Lynn (Massachusetts).

Other glass shops turned to the sale of accessories, foı instance Cooper & Cooper, Inc., 23 Cliff Street, in New York City. They advertised "x-ray immunizing protecto-gloves" — just a resounding name for the usual leather-covered lead-rubber. The term opaque gloves was used in the Keleket catalogue no. 25, dated October, 1920.

RADIUM

A few of the pioneers attempted to obtain diagnostic information by exposing photographic plates on the surface of the body, after placing a radium source into the esophagus, stomach, or rectum. Needless to say that the procedure never gained much acceptance. Nevertheless, the necessary receptacles were available commercially for instance one of the manufacturers was Geo. Tiemann & Company in New York City. Needles for radium treatment were manufactured by many others and including Williams, Brown and Earle in Philadelphia.

Perhaps the most ambitious operation was that of the Radium Co. of Colorado, located in the Radium Building in Denver. They advertised themselves on the trade-mark as being like Colorado's greatest peak, pre-eminent and everlasting. They published a journal, the *Radium Therapist.* They maintained branch offices at 582 Market St., in San Francisco, at 815 Peoples Gas Building in Chicago, at 244 Madison Ave. in New York, and best of all at 118 Avenue des Champs Elysées in Paris (France). Fortunately for Colorado, Pike's Peak is still standing, as pre-eminent as ever. Unfortunately for the Radium Company of Colorado, the radium extracted from the Belgian Congo brought the prices down: the Radium Company then tried to sell Belgian radium, struggled valiantly for a few years, and just before the depression it joined the other glorious bygones of the radiologic past.

In the Era of the Pioneers, the most famous American radium firm was the Radium Chemical Co. in Pittsburgh. The Radium Emanation Corporation and the

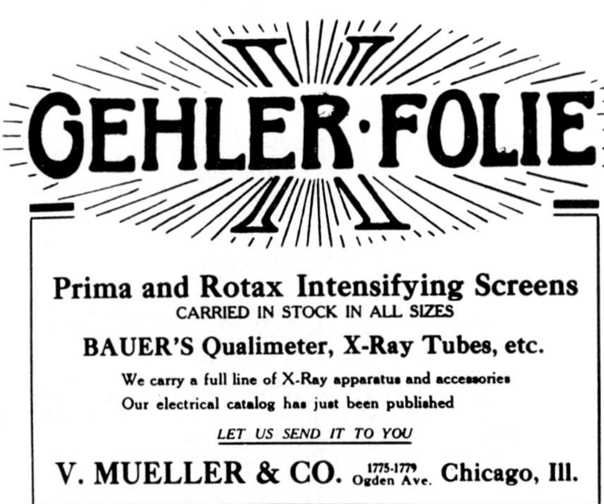

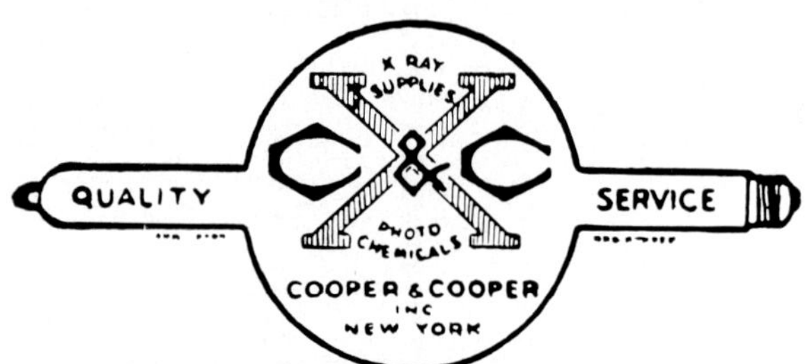

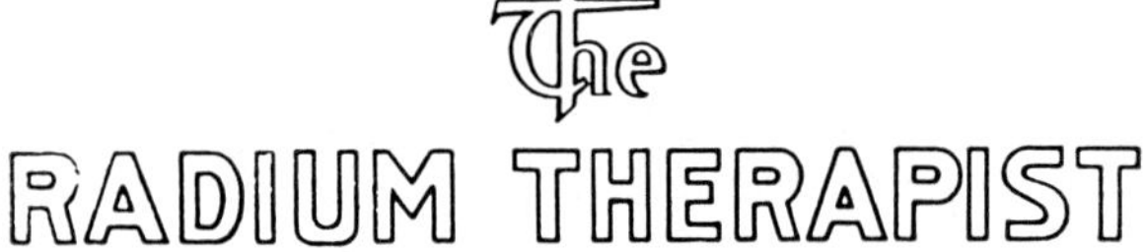

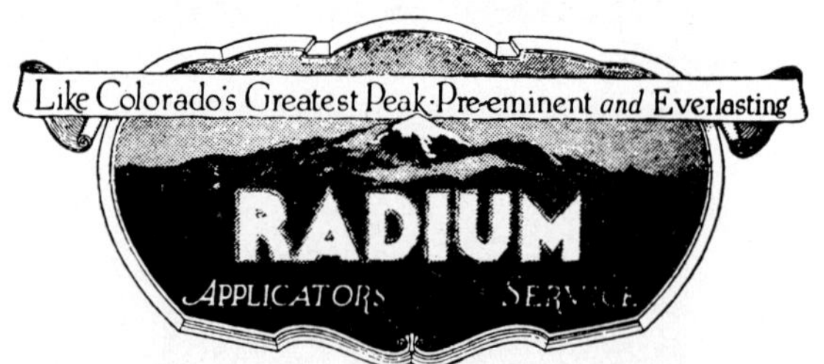

The Mark of a Complete and Careful Radium Therapeutic Service

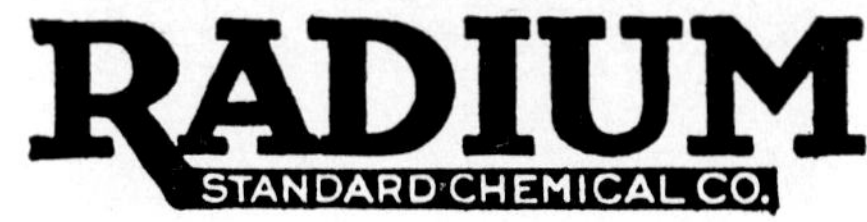

US Radium Corporation (both in New York City), and the Radium Service Corporation of America (in Chicago) came up after World War I.

THE GOLDEN AGE OF RADIOLOGY

The typical roentgen machine of the pioneers was the induction coil with interrupter and gas tube. The transition to the Golden Age of Radiology did not come as a sudden change. Like all things in life, it was prepared gradually. Several contributions were outstanding and the most important of these was the Hot Cathode Tube. This is usually credited to William David Coolidge (born in 1873), who at that time was director of GE's Research Department in Schenectady (New York).

In the early 1920s Orndoff went to Schenectady to purchase several (otherwise hard to get) Coolidge tubes. He happened to talk to the wife of a man by the name of Fink who had worked for GE's Research Laboratory at the time of Coolidge's discovery. She told Orndoff that her husband had actually invented the Hot Cathode Tube, and that it was supposed to have been patented in her husband's name. After the (surprising) move to make out the patent in Coolidge's name, her husband was called in and assured of adequate financial reward, including permanency in his job. He realized how difficult it was to prove that he had been the real inventor. On the other hand there was assured security in his current employment. All this made him decide against interfering with the course of events.

Orndoff, while telling me this anecdote, insisted that in his opinion it was, if not a complete fabrication, certainly not more than wishful thinking related to a minor

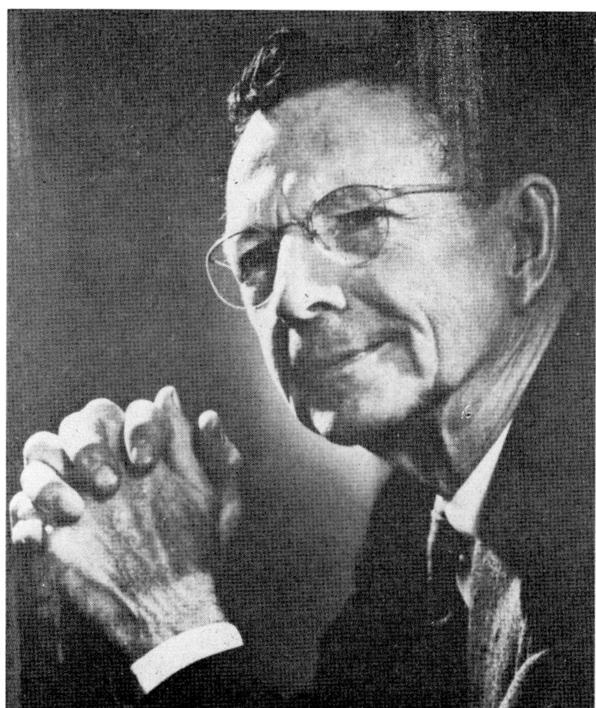

Courtesy: GE

William David Coolidge

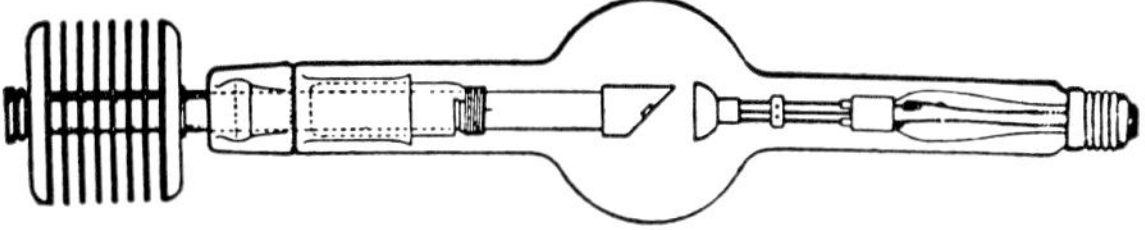

Courtesy: GE Archives.

Coolidge's Hot Cathode Tube. With a heated tungsten filament as a source of electrons, and the highest attainable vacuum, one can control both the intensity (ma) and the penetrating power (kvp) of the x rays produced, thereby making possible standardized technics. Coolidge brought out the first hot cathode tube in 1913. This diagram is of a 1916 model with radiator, and with a sufficient margin so as to rectify its own current, obviating—within certain limitations—the need for a mechanical rectifier.

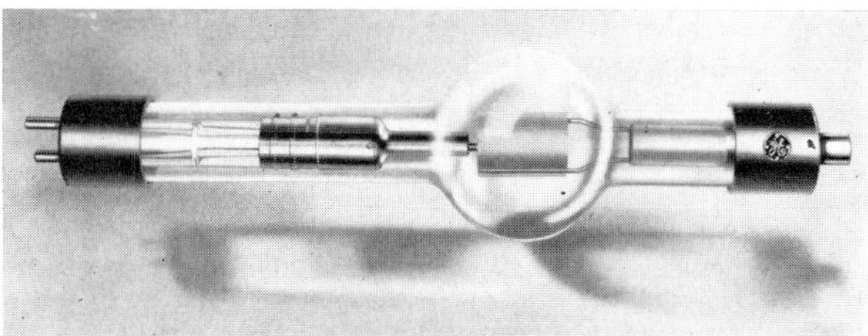

Courtesy: GE Archives.

Saul Dushman's Kenotron. In 1914, at GE's Research Lab in Schenectady, Dushman developed the hot cathode valve tube. This is the first commercial model (KR-3). Its long life stemmed, in part, from the fact that the anode surrounded the cathode, thus precluding erratic voltage drops from charges developed on the inner surface of the glass.

contribution to the actual discovery. In larger institutions, when the chief is working on a project, it is only natural that various tasks of lesser importance be assigned to subordinates.

In this particular instance, the situation was altogether different. In his reminiscences of 1933, and again in 1945, Coolidge started by recalling that in the 1880's Edison had shown that in the vacuum of the incandescent light bulb, current would flow from the hot filament to another electrode. The relationship between the temperature of the heated filament (actually between the temperature of any hot body) and the emission of electrons was elucidated in 1903 by the British physicist Owen Willans Richardson (1879-1959). In 1913, the American chemist, and Nobel Prize winner, Irving D. Langmuir (1881-1957) demonstrated that electron emission from tungsten filament continued in vacuum. In the same year Langmuir was issued patent no. 1251388 regarding the controllability of the electron emission by varying the current which heated the filament (Langmuir also built the mercury vapor vacuum pump).

To all this, Coolidge added only one thing which in itself is so much more important for technology in general (than for the relatively restricted x-ray territory): he succeeded in making ductile tungsten from what was previously regarded to be a brittle, non-workable metal. Walter Petrie recalled that his first job in the Schenectady plant was "graining tungsten contacts" at $9.00 per week.

As a matter of fact, Coolidge produced ductile tungsten in 1910. He filed for patent on the hot cathode, high vacuum tube in 1913 and was granted that patent in 1916.

Zed Jarvis Atlee, after reading the galley proofs for the chapter, urged me to tone down this anecdote. He had worked from 1929 to 1932 with Coolidge, and there was no doubt in his mind that Coolidge was the inventor. In a big company, no such inadvertencies are permitted, if only because the patent might be invalidated. There was no doubt in my mind about the integrity of Coolidge, whose paternity of the tungsten process was documented beyond any question. I inserted this story simply as an illustration of what is so often rumored about great men.*

The first Hot Cathode Tube was installed in the private office of Lewis Gregory Cole. On this occasion, Cole gave a dinner in the honor of Coolidge, on December 27, 1913, at the Hotel St. Dennis in New York City. A select group of radiologic notables was invited, and Harry Waite put up the high voltage generator necessary to demonstrate how the tube functioned. Obviously, the importance of this new development was recognized from the very beginning.

*There has appeared a biography of Coolidge, entitled *Yankee Scientist* by John Anderson Miller (Schenectady, 1963), where all dates and circumstances of the tungsten story are detailed.

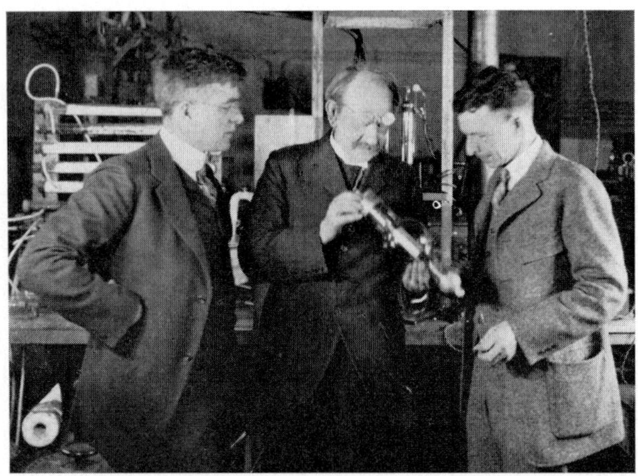

Courtesy: GE Archives.

Hot Cathode Kenotron. Irving Langmuir watches intently as old Sir Joseph John Thomson (1856-1940) inspects a contraption, which was to prove extremely useful over the years, the kenotron (valve tube); explanations are given by William Coolidge, director of the GE Laboratory in Schenectady, where this photograph was taken at an unknown date.

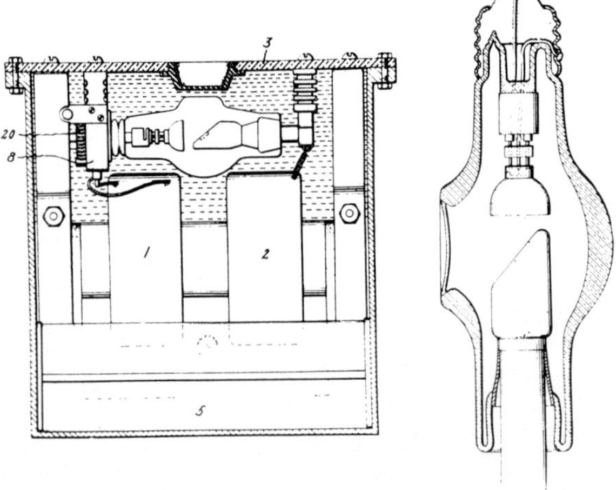

Courtesy: American Journal of Roentgenology.

Coolidge's Dental Unit. The description of this oil-immersion, fully shock-proof unit appeared in the *American Journal of Roentgenology* of April, 1920. It was based on the principle for which Waite, Jr. had filed a patent in January, 1919, granted one month before the publication date of this paper. Subsequently, a barter deal was made between GE and W & B, whereby for the use of Waite's patent, GE sold to W & B 300 hot cathode tubes per year. Thereafter both companies built self-contained dental units.

In 1914 Saul Dushman, at the same General Electric Research Laboratory, developed the hot cathode, high voltage valve tube (kenotron). In 1915 Coolidge introduced the hooded-anode x-ray tube, and in 1917 the self-rectifying x-ray tube. The latter had those famous radiating fins, a very recognizable feature, preserved for two decades, until all tubes were encased in protective lead shields.

In 1918 Coolidge introduced a portable x-ray unit with protection built right in (lead glass with lime glass window). In 1919 Coolidge published the announcement of the CDX shock-proof dental x-ray unit, built on the oil-immersion principle developed by Waite, Jr. The days at Schenectady represent the second period in GE's contributions to the development of x-ray apparatus.

Vacuum tubes had been constructed in Germany in 1905 by Wehnelt, but the radiation emitted was too soft. In 1911, in Austria, Lilienfeld produced a gas-free tube based on the field-current principles, whereby electrons were extracted from cold metals by high potential gradients. This tube was used in 1912 and 1913 by Rosenthal and Holzknecht. None of these approached the major advantage of the Coolidge tube which was the possibility of duplicating results with an accuracy never hoped for in the time of the gas tubes.

Coolidge's high vacuum, hot cathode x-ray tube,* more than any other single development, ushered in the Golden Age of Radiology. Several important advances — wave rectification, use of transformers and of the auto-transformer, grid diaphragms, tilting tables, the oil-immersion principle — were either of American origin, or had been changed into workable tools in this country. All these developments were available in 1920. Thereafter, throughout the Golden Age of Radiology, the x-ray industry searched for shapes, rather than for solutions.

MACHLETT

In the beginning, Ernst Machlett (I) and his son Robert (II) worked as glassblowers for Eimer &

*In a W & B catalog of the 1920s, a 30 ma Coolidge tube, advertised for the Moderate Power Machine, was listed at $125.00 with $15.00 for the optional protective lead glass cover. A 10 ma tube, with finer focus, for bone detail, was also offered.

ANNOUNCEMENT

Those who purchase and re-sell or use in the United States of America Coolidge X-Ray tubes or complete outfits involving Coolidge X-Ray tubes manufactured by the General Electric Company are hereby assured that the General Electric Company is prepared to, and will, defend any suit brought against them, in so far as it is based on such purchase and re-sale or use, provided that it is promptly notified of any suit or threat of suit involving such tubes or outfits and is given full power to defend the same.

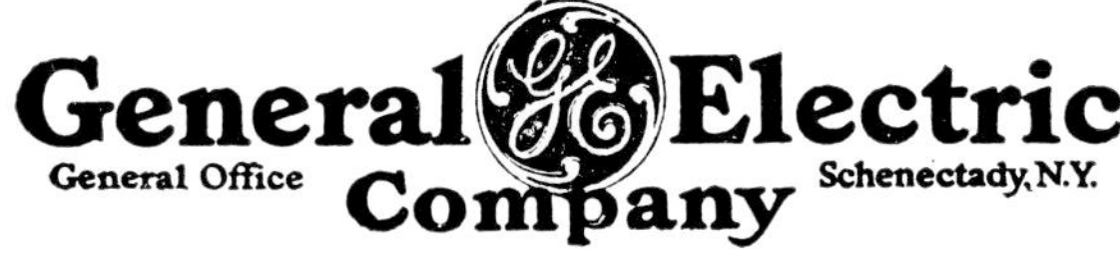

35B-17

CURIOUS AD, dated 1917, reprinted in the *Journal of Roentgenology* of 1920. Neither GE in Milwaukee, nor GE in Schenectady could explain it to me. Eddy Ernst said it had nothing to do with the RSNA lawsuit, which did not begin until years later. Who could possibly have challenged the Coolidge priority?

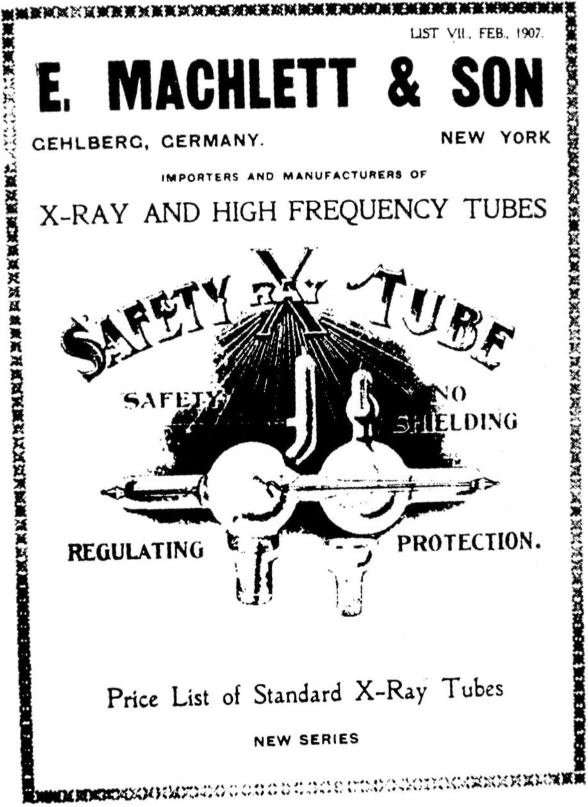

Amend in New York City. In 1897, the Machletts set up their own shop, which was incorporated in 1899 as E. Machlett & Son, with the son as president. The claim has been made that in the Summer of 1897 Robert Machlett (II) produced the first x-ray tube commercially manufactured in the USA.

That claim appears on page 13 in the Memorial Issue of *Cathode Press,* authored by Robert Keith Leavitt (an "outsider" as far as the Machlett Company is concerned), commissioned to write the History of Machlett's. The History is excellent, and well illustrated with both dated and more recent photographs. A few minor and obviously unintentional inadvertencies have slipped into its text, such as the contention that Grubbé was in 1896 a medical student in the University of Chicago: that medical school did not come into existence until four decades later. Altogether, though, Leavitt's History of Machlett is very pleasant, highly readable, and generally accurate. While it may have been issued for promotional purposes, it has unquestionable historic value, and will be a priceless account one century hence. Other manufacturers have issued similar histories of their organizations, for instance the drug firm Abbott Laboratories of North Chicago published *The Long White Line* (1963). Another pharmaceutic organization. Eli Lilly and Company (Indianapolis) printed its *Threescore Years and Ten, 1876-1946.* All significant companies should seriously consider the preparation and publication of their corporate histories.

With reference to the first x-ray tube commercially manufactured in the USA, it may be of interest to quote from a paper by Harry Miles Imboden, published in the *American Journal of Roentgenology* of October, 1931:

"It seems that the earliest roentgen tubes in this country were made by a glass-blower named Greiner for Eimer & Amend but very shortly after this, Robert Machlett of New York started making tubes, to be followed very shortly by Green & Bauer of Hartford, who were the first ones to make the tubes in any quantity. They were manufacturers of incandescent lamps at the time that Roentgen made his announcement. Other manufacturers of this period are Friedländer, Baker, and Macalaster & Wiggins."

As a matter of fact, Imboden misspelled several names in his last cited sentence (they were corrected in this text). He is also otherwise quite in error. It cannot be said that one year means "shortly," and Emil Greiner (a chemical firm) made tubes in 1896, while Machlett claimed to have started making some in 1897. I have seen a Machlett advertisement of 1936 in which their beginning is given as 1898, but

MACHLETT

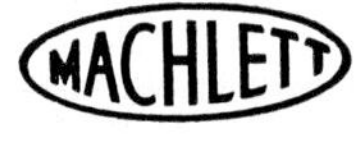

"Quality Since 1898"

X-RAY AND VALVE TUBES

Technical Information on Products of

MACHLETT LABORATORIES, Incorporated

Springdale, Connecticut

Manufacturers of X-Ray and Valve Tubes Exclusively

Fig. 2-69. Advertisement printed in 1936. The year 1898 is a printing error, because the original Machlett shop was started in 1897. Since World War II they have expanded, and the largest part of Machlett's production is now in "power" tubes.

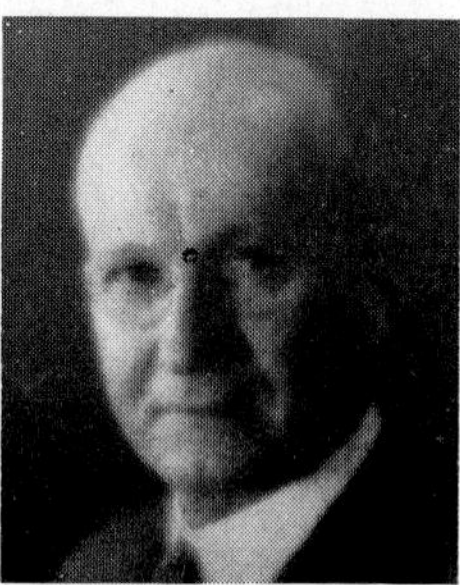

Harry Imboden, Sr.

Skill—
Born of
1904
A Machlett glass blower displays one of Dr. Piffard's lead-glass x-ray tubes—the earliest self protected type.
1936
The same glass blower seals the elements in a Machlett CYR tube — the latest self protected type.

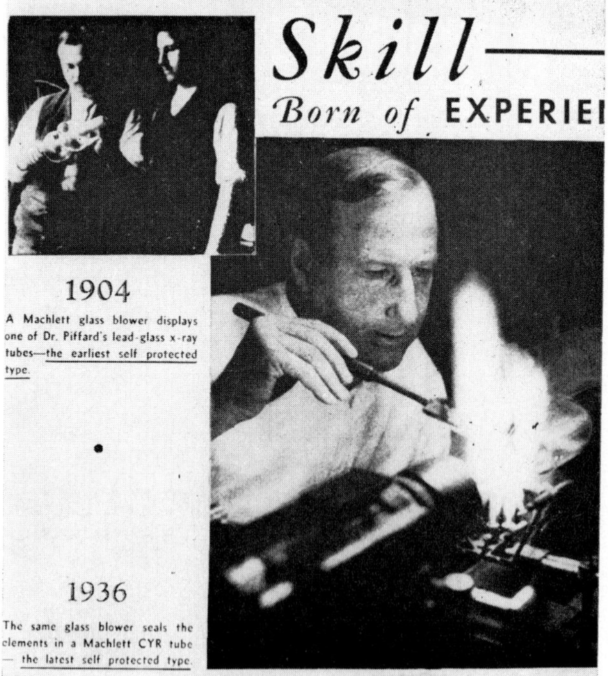

Then and "now." Ernst Zitzmann, mastercraftsman in glass-blowing, at two periods in his long life, a life-long Machlett employee.

that may have been a printing error. There are dated advertisements proving that in 1896 x-ray tubes were made and sold by the Edison Company, and by the now defunct Beacon Lamp Company. Others, for instance Grubbé, hired their own glassblower(s), and went into the x-ray tube business. More important is the fact that the Machlett Company is now making all sorts of tubes, both for x-ray equipment and for power purposes. But so does Edison's General Electric Company. And if GE did not make and sell x-ray tubes continuously from 1896 to this day, neither did Machlett. Indeed, GE was the very motive for which Machlett's went — temporarily — out of the x-ray business.

During the gas tube era Machlett's shop was on the second floor of a battered building at 143-147 East 23rd Street, near Manhattan's (then fashionable) business center. Their staff was composed of a young apprentice, Ernst Zitzmann, Machlett I and II, and a bookkeeper. The reputation of Machlett's skill attracted many customers. One of them was Peter Cooper Hewitt (1861-1921), remembered for a mercury-vapor electric lamp and for having discovered the principle of vacuum-tube amplification. Hewitt gave Machlett the idea to manufacture x-ray tubes.

At that time, Machlett produced not only simple Crookes tubes, but also the Jackson concave cathode tube, Monell's truncated cone, Morton's safety tube for cavity treatment, Caldwell's water packet cavity treatment tube, and so on.

Frank Farrelly, the Machlett employee who later became president of the Green & Bauer X-Ray Tube Company, recalled that Robert Machlett built in 1904 the pilot sample of Piffard's "safety" tube, made from lead glass with a small window of ground glass through which the rays could emerge. To that, Machlett added an innovation, an interchangeable cup. Piffard initially objected to the change, but Waite, Jr., who by coincidence was there at the time, pointed out its advantages (interchangeability) and the innovation was permanently adopted. Piffard's tube is seen on the cover of Machlett's catalog of 1907 (*cf.* page 79).

In October, 1912 Robert Machlett bought a building at 153 East 84th St. the Yorktown district, heart of the German neighborhood.

There he developed the Bellevue Interrupterless Transformer Tube – with a small spear-point projecting from the face of the anode – a design which was later improved to where it would withstand a current as high as 25 amperes passing through the primary of its induction coil without affecting the internal part of the tube or destroying its efficiency.

In 1913, Machlett brought out the "Hydrex" tube, which is usually represented in a heavy lead glass bowl. It was quite an improvement over the previous models, but it happened to arrive at a time when the hot cathode principle was just introduced. Indeed, for as long as Coolidge's patent was valid, the Machlett Company withered slowly on the vine.

In the meantime Robert's son, Raymond Robert Machlett (1900-1955), who had just come of age, founded the Rainbow Light Company, which was the name of a new, brilliantly luminous tube — the neon light. The enterprise, located first on 84th St., and later on 44th Road (Long Island City), flourished in the business boom of the 1920s.

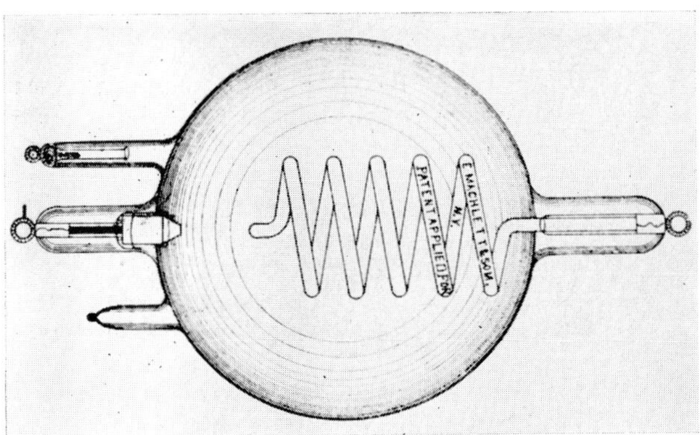

Gas valve tube. Date about 1912; note the vacuum regulator, and the spring-shaped anode, reminiscent of the DeForest audion tube.

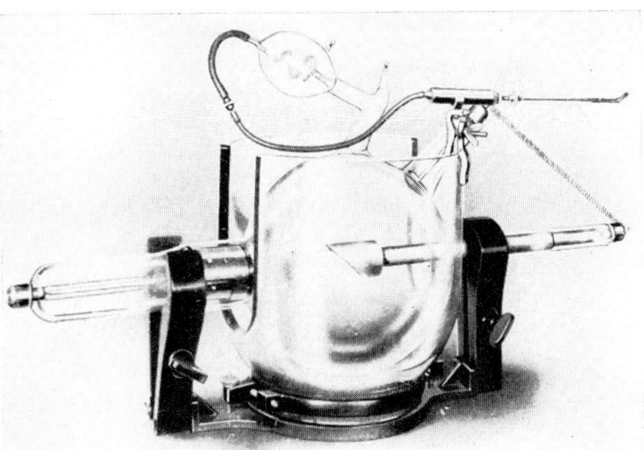

Hydrex in lead glass bowl. In 1912, Machlett brought out a tube which contained hydrogen instead of the usual residues of gas. It was a significant improvement over the conventional ionic tube, but it happened to "collide" with Coolidge's hot cathode, for which it was no match. This was the last "x-ray" effort of the old E. Machlett & Son. That company is still in business, but in chemical glass and other wares, in combination with Fisher Scientific in New York City.

In 1926 Robert Herman Machlett died of radiation malignancy. The old E. Machlett & Son was continued by Robert's son-in-law, Richard Schnier, who turned to the manufacture and distribution of scientific laboratory glass equipment (it is still in that business). Rainbow became involved in patent suits, then its financial backbone, Charles V. Bob, turned out to be a fraud and was sent to jail. The Rainbow Light Company was taken over by creditors.

During the years of hot cathode monopoly, in this country most of the x-ray industry was under a sort of servitude because of the Coolidge patent. General Electric would deliver tubes, even allow others to produce them under franchise, but in the absence of competition, tube models were designed to fit into GE's own production at Victor. One year or two before expiration of the patent, several companies decided to cut the Gordian knot by putting on the market hot cathode tubes. Their assumption that GE would not prosecute, proved to be correct. There was also a patent suit in which the RSNA became involved.

Waite, Jr. (W & B), Wilbur Werner (Keleket), and Edwin Goldfield (Engeln), among others, urged Ray Machlett to re-enter the x-ray tube business. Thereupon he created a *new* firm, called the Machlett Laboratories, which he incorporated in 1931 under the laws of the State of New York.

He started out in small quarters, provided by the old E. Machlett & Sons, and purchased from Schnier whatever had been left from their old machines and parts used in manufacturing gas tubes. Ray Machlett reorganized the business, even went on a study trip to see the European production of x-ray tubes, and slowly succeeded to place his enterprise on a solid footing.

In 1932, they brought out the MR50 and the MR100: these tubes embodied both the line focus principle and a new method of massive copper casting of the heavy copper backed anode. In 1933, they came out with the "Conex," a shock-proof as well as ray-proof tube housed in a combination lead-impregnated bakelite and metallic lead shield. Sales-wise, the Conex was only moderately successful, but it created much good-will because it proved that Machlett intended to keep up with progress (European makers had then introduced similar metallic containers for their x-ray tubes).

Steady growth forced Machlett to move to a new location. In 1934 they purchased a building in Springdale (Connecticut), and incorporated also in that state.

In the same year they introduced the CYR tube, which embodied what they called "geometry of design."

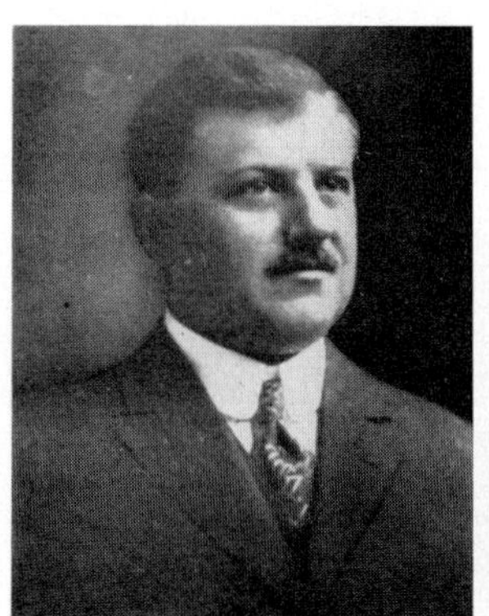

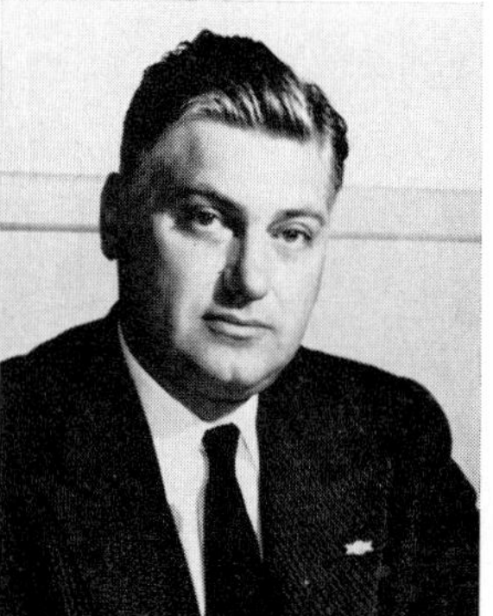

Courtesy: Wilbert Stevenson.

ROBERT HERMAN MACHLETT (1872-1926). Gas-tube Machlett (II), with mustache, who founded the first firm, became a roentgen martyr as his firm was fading away during the hot cathode monopoly. He had a son, RAYMOND ROBERT MACHLETT (1900-1955). The third and most successful direct descendent from Ernst Machlett, was the actual founder of what is known today as Machlett Laboratories.

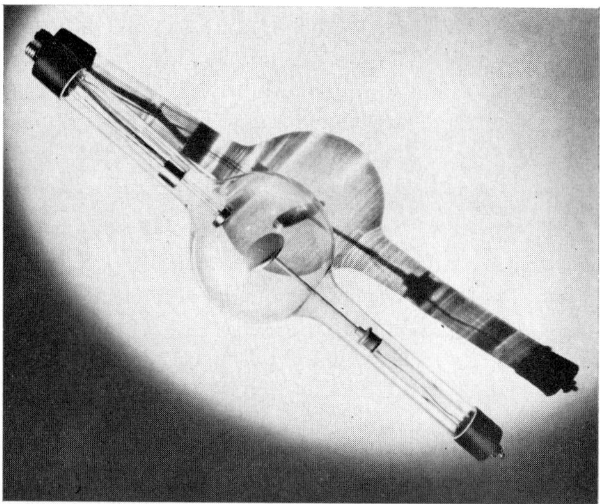

Courtesy: Machlett Archives.

MACHLETT'S XT. First hot cathode therapy tube made in early 1930's. Note the light target, supported on a slender stem. Heavy copper anodes were yet to come.

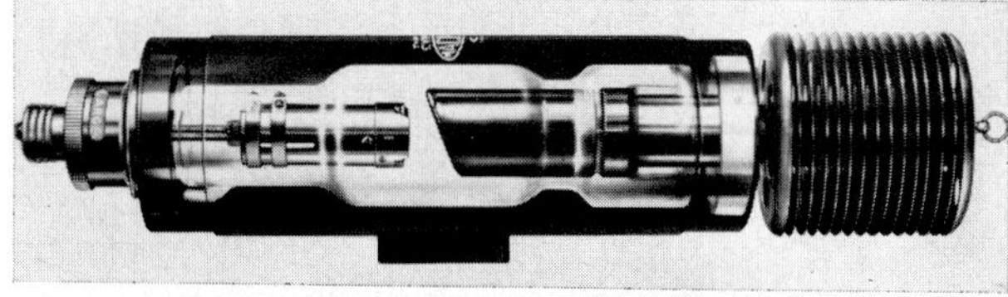

Courtesy: Machlett Archives.

MACHLETT'S CYR. Schematic view of Machlett's first satisfactorily protected x-ray tube, put on the market in 1934. Its precursor was the somewhat similar, but bulkier Conex of 1933.

On the outside of the housing it had fins, similar to those made famous by GE.

In 1937, they began work on a rotating anode. In their early models, the target was backed with the usual heavy copper. It was not satisfactory, so they turned to a rotor of solid tungsten which could stand considerable thermal overload. Heat dissipation was achieved by radiation, using a tungsten disc on a thin stem. Their main problem was the "lubrication" of ball-bearings, and this they solved by coating with silver the steel balls after degassing in vacuum. Machlett placed its first rotating anode on the market in 1939: its name was (and still is) Dynamax.

During World War II, Machlett added a plant at Norwalk (about 10 miles from Springdale). This was done mainly to take care of large sub-contracts for radio and radar triodes, obtained from Westinghouse's Henry J. Hoffman.* From that moment on — as far as volume of production was concerned — x-ray tubes would never (?!) again become Machlett's main line of business.

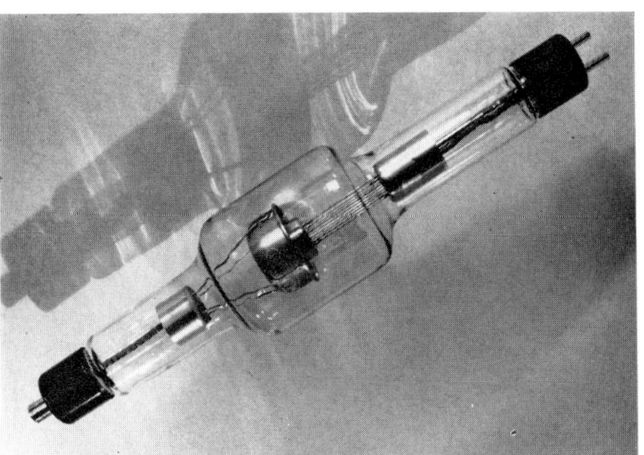

Courtesy: Machlett Archives.

MACHLETT'S ML-80. A rectifier tube, issued about 1940.

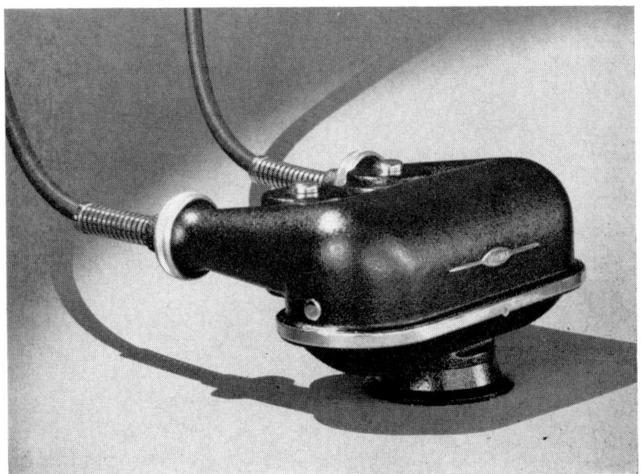

Courtesy: Machlett Archives.

MACHLETT'S DYNAMAX D. Machlett put its first rotating anode on the market in 1939 – it had silver-coated steel ball bearings.

EUREKA

The Eureka X-Ray Tube Company was started in Chicago in 1919 by Emil F. Matz, joined later by Arthur Klinckmann. In the beginning they manufactured gas tubes and electrodes for electrotherapy. Then they moved to a building near Chicago Ave. and Franklin Str.

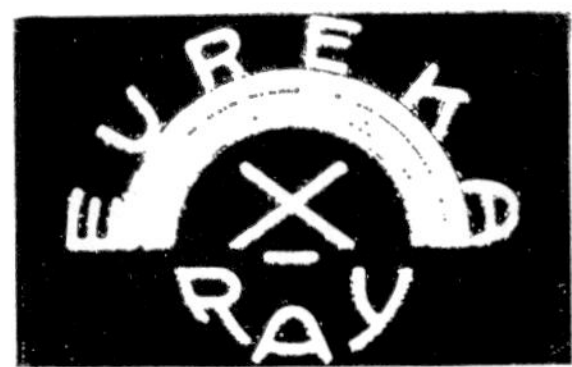

Their production followed the trends of the industry. Like everybody else, they "jumped the gun" on Coolidge's patent one or two years before its actual expiration. Next came the round focus tube, the slender anode shank, and the loose fitting radiator. These were replaced by the line focus (made under the Goetze patent), massive anodes with uniformly tapered shanks, and tight fitting copper radiators. A hard glass (Pyrex) displaced lead and lime glass in all tubes.

The private partnership prospered, and in 1933 Eureka was incorporated. Ownership has since changed, but the old name was preserved to this day.

MEYER

In the early 1900s the William Meyer & Co. had its location at 56 Fifth Avenue in Chicago. At that time their trade-mark was a super-imposition of the owner's initials M and W, which became more stylized as time went on.** In 1920 they were at 1644 North Girard Str., and advertised a combination stereo-radiographic table and Klinoscope.

The very first advertisements of the Klinoscope had appeared in 1916, and showed the possibility of changing that table from horizontal to vertical with the patient in position. This may have been theoretically pos-

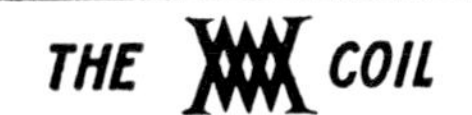

*In most industries, the leading concerns follow such practices. Today, Machlett supplies certain tubes to friendly competitors, and buys other types from them. It is not unusual to see big firms "farming out" entire tables, transformers, or control stands.

**A similar trade-mark is used today by the Midwestern Coil Company, which produces automobile accessories in Chicago.

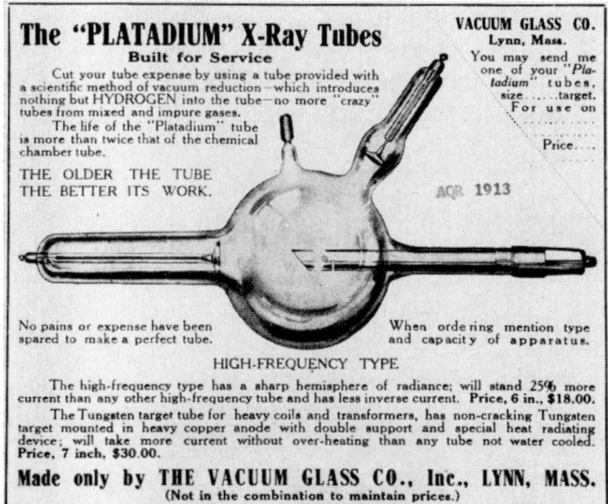

sible, but it required Herculean strength as the original Klinoscope was not counterbalanced.

CAMPBELL

At that time only Campbell's Tube Tilt Table could be reclined with the patient on the table. Before that, one needed a separate stand for upright fluoroscopy, in addition to the horizontal table (a makeshift upright fluoroscopy could be performed at the end of horizontal tables, by using an over-the-table tube). The world's first tilting table was devised by Caldwell* at Bellevue Hospital in New York City. The first commercial model was built (on a request from the Mayo Clinic) by the Campbell Electric Company (successors to the Platadium "tube shop," the Vacuum Glass Co.) in Lynn (Massachusetts).

Campbell produced also a high frequency coil, which required a special tube because the oscillatory character of its current would soon destroy the efficiency of the ordinary tube of the uni-directional type. Campbell had a combination called "Seven outfits in one." It came in a portable, or in a table model and permitted the production of x rays as well as electro-therapeutic applications. For bedside applications they had the Clinette, a conventional mobile unit.

In the Campbell catalogue of 1920 appeared the Surex transformer, advertised as reducing "roentgenology to a mathematical science." It proved that their copywriter was very efficient.

Campbell's most ambitious and glorious venture was the Clinix table, an improved and beautified version of the tilting model of 1916. Its classic lines have often been copied — or, shall we say, the Clinix of-

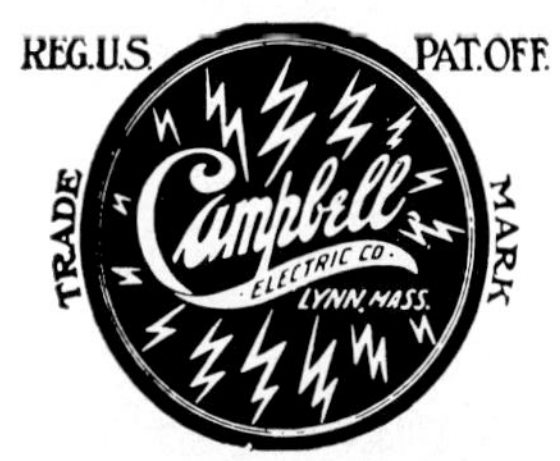

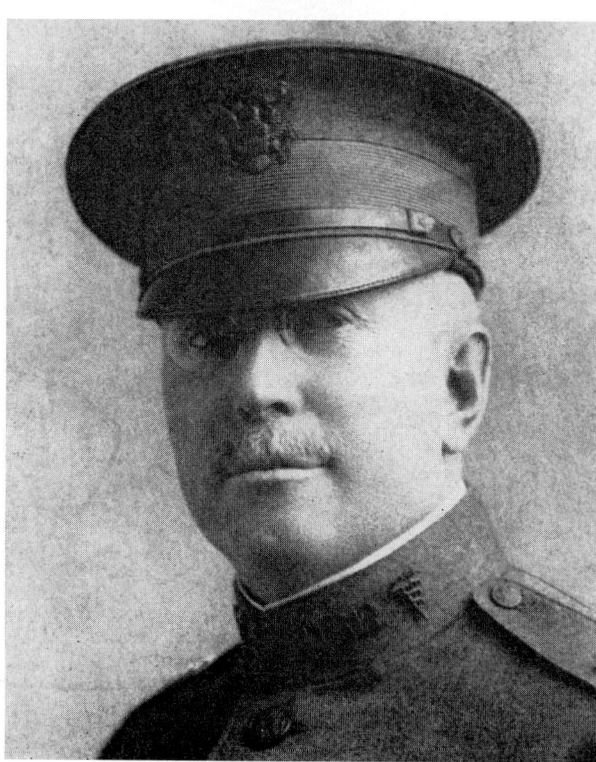

EUGENE WILSON CALDWELL

*In the *American Journal of Roentgenology* of October, 1931 Imboden wrote: "Upon returning from a European trip in the fall of 1912, Caldwell was very much impressed with the necessity for fluoroscopy and the advantages of a tilting table. He accordingly set to work to develop such a table and it was actually placed in operation that winter." It was the world's first truly tiltable, motor-operated table, *cf.* George Hanchett in the *American Journal of Roentgenology* of December, 1918 and Rudolf Grashey in Albers-Schönberg's *Die Röntgentechnik,* ed. 6, 1941, p. 250.

Patented 1,173,409

Campbell-Tube-Tilt-Table

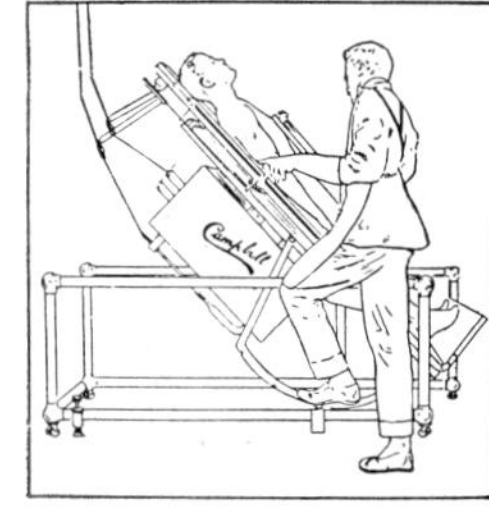

ANGULAR FLUOROSCOPY
One of the many positions. Note that tube tilts with table

Horizontal / Angular / Vertical } STEREOSCOPIC RADIOGRAPHY AND FLUOROSCOPY

TUBE TILTS WITH TABLE

Pronounced by Leading Roentgenologists as one of the Greatest Strides in Years in the Development of X-Ray Apparatus

Easily movable, with patient, to any position

Patient once on table remains there until complete X-Ray examination has been made, including the radiographs

SAVES SPACE RENT TIME INVESTMENT

Send for description and prices

TUBE TILT TABLE

CAMPBELL ELECTRIC CO., LYNN, MASS. 1916

fered inspiration for much of the equipment manufactured during the first half of the Golden Age of Radiology.

The price of a Campbell Clinix Tilt Tube Table, with automatic plate changer, 11x14 fluoroscopic screen and holder, two 17x17 cassettes, and a foot board, cord reel, etc., boxed ready for shipment, f.o.b., was $1,550.00. The high tension transformer attached under the table (with control case) cost $550.00. In addition, a no. 6 tubestand was $300.00, the extra high tension transformer for the tubestand was $450.00, and two Coolidge radiator x-ray tubes were $250.00. The complete Clinix x-ray plant sold for $3,200.00. Dark room equipment, illuminators, and other accessories had to be purchased (and paid) separately. For those who did not have alternating current (100-120 volts, 50-60 cycles) one needed a rotatory converter and transformer giving four kw (for the 30 ma tube). It could be operated on either 110 or 220 volts, and sold for $525.00.

7 Outfits in 1
X-RAY
TESLA
D'ARSONVAL
THERMO-FARADIC
SINUSOIDAL
CAUTERY
DIAGNOSTIC LIGHT
Model "E" Coil
(See page 13)
PORTABLE POWERFUL PRACTICAL
OPERATES FROM ANY ELECTRIC LIGHT SOCKET
1916

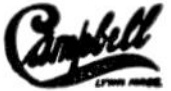

VARIABLE VOLTAGE and VOLUME for VARYING — DENSITY DETAIL

CAMPBELL NUMBER 12 SureX TRANSFORMER

Reduces Roentgenology to a Mathematical Science
For all kinds of Radiography, Fluoroscopy, and Radio-Therapy. Secondary Voltmeter.
Unit Rectifier. Polarity Indicator.
Auto Transformer.

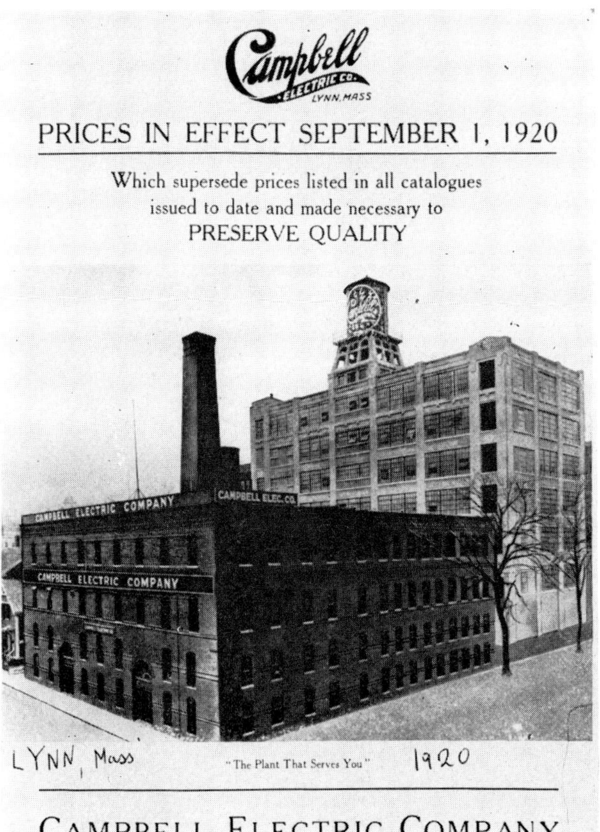

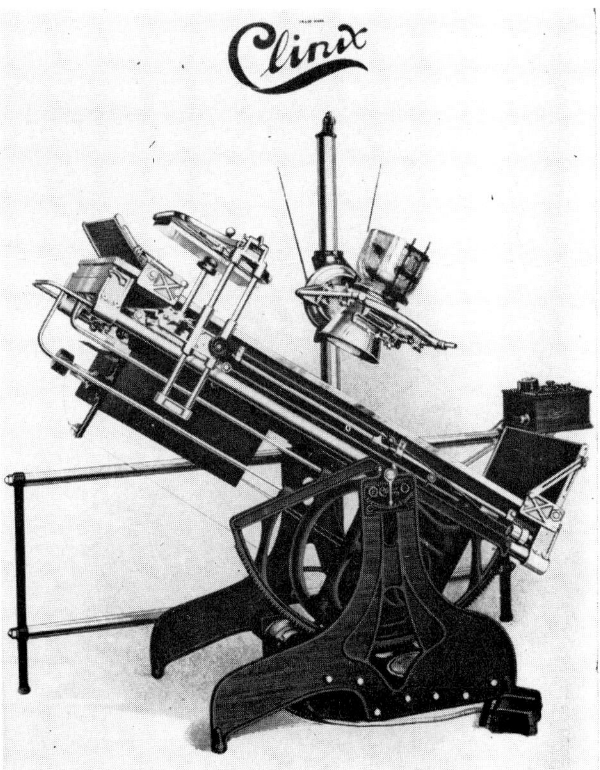

CAMPBELL'S FAMOUS TABLE. This classic design marked a turning point in the styling of x-ray equipment.

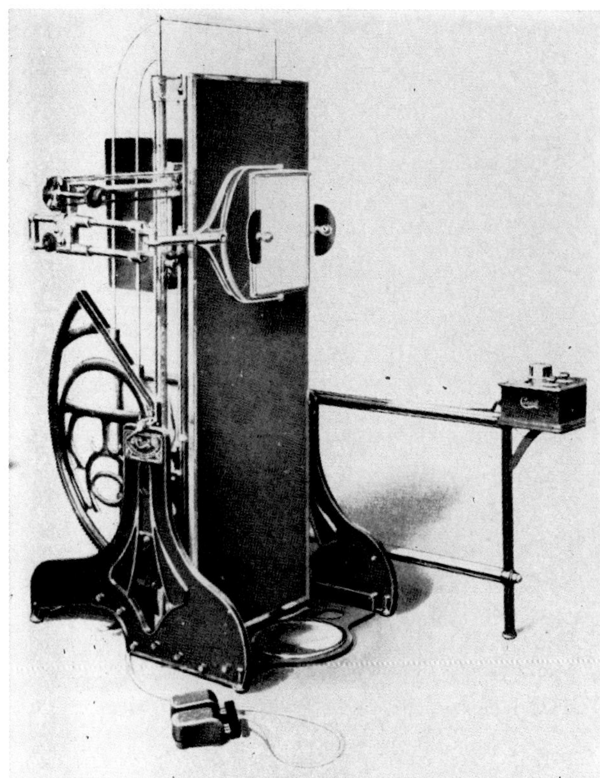

Campbell ClinıX. In upright position access of the patient was not yet very simple, but otherwise it looks quite modern.

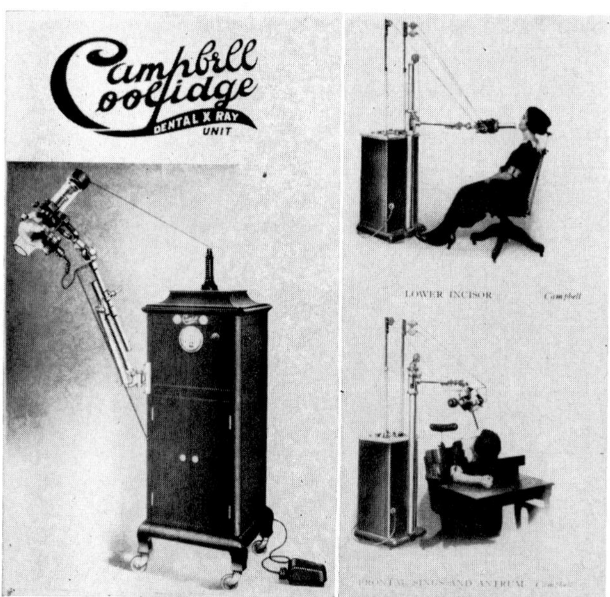

Campbell Dental Unit. This came out before (and was displaced by) Coolidge's oil-immersed combination. The two samples on the right are from a total of six positions illustrated in that catalog. The label for the one on top reads "lower incisor," the other is "frontal sinus and antrum."

Another important item to remember was the Campbell Coolidge Dental X-ray Unit. By using a tube with radiator type cooling, one could approach the oral cavity from most sides.

RAPER

At this point, a digression will attempt to bring a few details on the beginnings of Dental Radiology.

The first dental x-ray plate was exposed in April or May of 1896 by Charles Edmund Kells, Jr. (1856-1928), a dentist from New Orleans. As mentioned by Raper in his *Notes on the Early History of Radiodontia* in *Oral Surgery* of January, 1953, for fourteen years after the first dental plate made by Kells, nothing much happened. Fewer than a dozen American dentists were using x rays in their work. Indeed, no such device as a dental x-ray unit existed in 1909 when Howard Riley Raper, then a full-time instructor in the Indiana University School of Dentistry in Indianapolis (Indiana) became interested in this field.

In 1909, Raper convinced the School's dean, Edwin Hunt, to purchase an x-ray machine, and in 1910 they

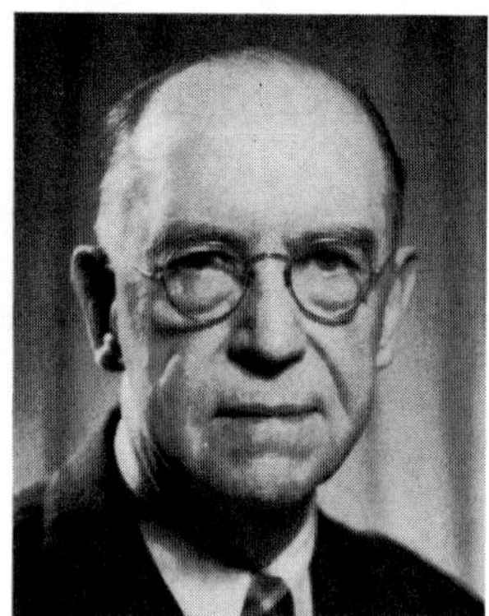

Howard Riley Raper. Had first scientific dental radiologic office in the U. S. A., and coined the word *radiodontia.*

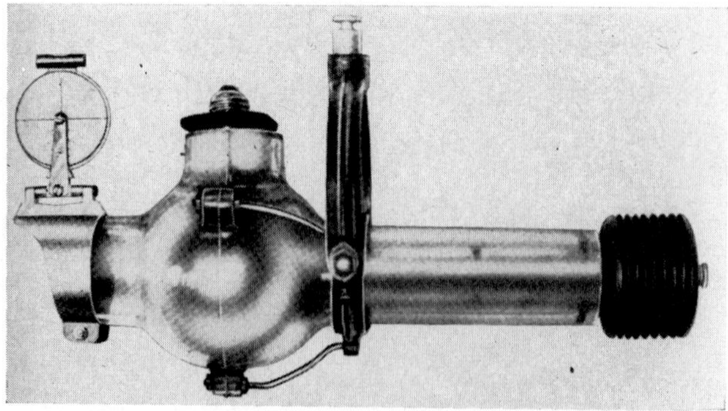

Courtesy: Buck Xograph Co.

Raper's Angle Meter. It is that dial-shaped contraption mounted on the x-ray tube's lead glass shield by use of an adjustable collar.

acquired an 18-inch Scheidel coil, which was then one of the largest in the state of Indiana. As a result of work performed with that coil, Raper became in 1911 professor of roentgenology in said Indiana Dental College. Between February, 1911 and March, 1913 Raper published a series of articles on *Elementary and Dental Radiography* in Ottolengui's *Items of Interest* (New York City). That series of articles was made into a textbook, using the same title (the first edition had about 200 dental radiographic illustrations). It was the first and only text on the subject until the professor of physics (not a dentist)* of the New York College of Dentistry published *Dental Radiology* (with about 30 illustrations). Raper was also the author of a paper on the *Teaching of Dental Radiography,* which was read at the Twentieth Annual Meeting of the National Institute of Dental Pedagogics in January of 1913. This is also when they changed the name from Pedagogics to Teachers.

Raper's work attracted the attention of local dentists who, by 1913, were referring patients to him for examination. In 1915 he opened, at 506 in the Hume-Mansur Building in Indianapolis, the first office devoted exclusively to dental x-ray diagnosis. He had created a new discipline, and had to find a name for it: this is why he coined the word *radiodontia,* patterned after the two then outstanding dental specialties, orthodontia and exodontia. The term radiodontia was immediately accepted in *Items of Interest* whose editor, Ottolengui, was himself a "radiocoiner," who fathered the terms radioparent, radiolucent, and radiopaque.

But Raper's most significant achievement was the development of a radiographic dental angle meter. Early in the game, Raper had agreed with C. O. Simpson (of St. Louis) that for either the upper or the lower teeth, the occlusal plane must be horizontal during x-ray procedures, meaning that when the mouth was open, the head had to be tipped backward (chin-lifted), to bring about this horizontality. A Polish dentist, Cieszynski, first suggested that facial landmarks could be used to locate the occlusal planes of teeth.

Raper, who had acquired considerable experience in x-ray examination of teeth, realized that different teeth required different angles of beam incidence so as to minimize distortion. He was working on a device intended to facilitate measurement of the proper angle when – in the Fall of 1916 – he came down with an acute phase of pulmonary tuberculosis. He gave up the office, and moved in 1917 to Albuquerque where he still resides (in 1956 the University of New Mexico conferred upon him an honorary LL.D).

In 1917, from Albuquerque, Raper sent drawings to Otto Krueg, owner of the Dental X-Ray Supplies Company of Terre Haute (Indiana): that is where the first experimental models of Raper's Angle Meter were produced in 1918. Raper used the meter for the first time in 1919. The first public announcement of the instrument appeared in *Oral Hygiene* of June, 1921. That meter was so important because it supplied not a single specific angle for the various teeth, but a range of angles, and that range embraced most if not all possible anatomic variations. The significance of Raper's Angle Meter is still discernible after 40 years, because all "charts of angles" are taken, directly or indirectly, from his meter's measurements. Raper's Angle Meter was manufactured in quantity by Buck in St. Louis. Raper also designed a dental film holder, which is still very popular in a slightly improved version (Buck All-Rubber Holder).

BUCK

Arthur Wells Buck (who celebrated in 1962 his 83rd birthday by having his picture taken) founded the Buck X-Ograph Company in 1918 — it was not incorporated until 1930. Buck's first of many patents was the impressionable metal backed dental film. The first products he manufactured were intended for the dental profession, such as special films, mounts, safes, holders, illuminators, charted envelopes, and the Raper Angle Meter.

By 1924 — as shown in Buck's brown-cover catalog no. 3 — many items had been added to that list, for instance developing and fixing powders, intensify-

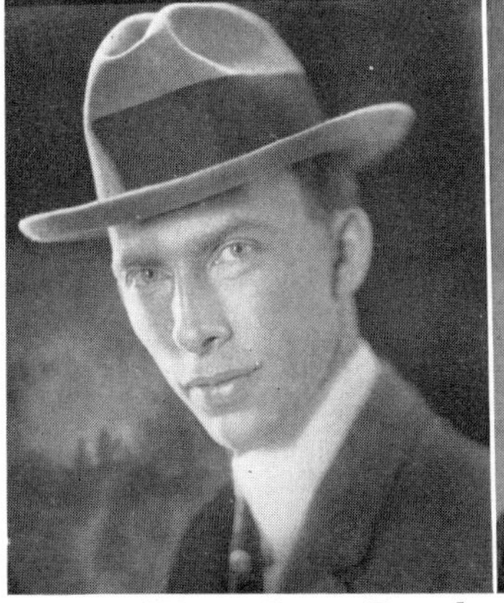

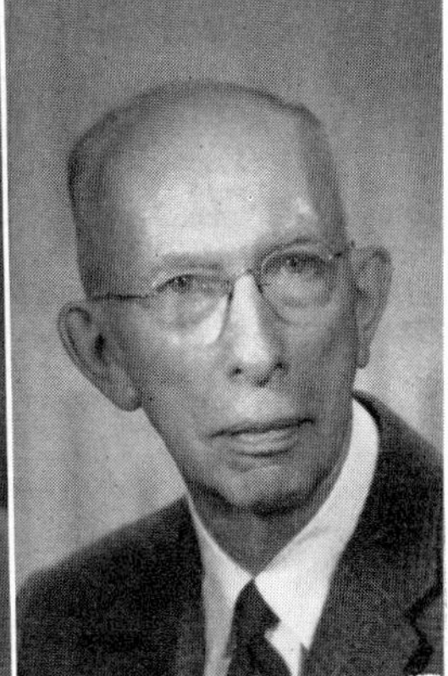

ARTHUR WELLS BUCK. Founder and President of Buck Xograph Company in St. Louis. One picture of the x-ray industry's elder statesman was taken on his 83rd birthday, the other dates from the time when he was employed by Eastman Kodak.

*His name was Francis Le Roy Satterlee (1881-1935). *Webster's Biographical Dictionary* (Merriam Co., 1943) summarized his data as follows: "American roentgenologist, born New York City. At age of fifteen, took first x-ray photograph in America; invented protective shield for x-ray operators; first to x-ray mouth and teeth." The source of information for these credits (*nay,* claims) is not stated.

ing screens and cassettes. Between 1924 and 1927 came out the (large-sized) Buck X-Ray Film, the Buck Kidney Films, and the Buck Thermonel Developing Tank.*

Buck x-ray film, introduced in 1926, was very well received. Their representative in Chicago, A. Frederick Knies (who is now working for Eastman Kodak in Oklahoma), had always been a very personable salesman. He made an excellent introduction of Buck wares in Chicago. With the depression and the consequent losses, instead of continuing to sell the merchandise through independent dealers, Buck decided to open a branch office in Chicago. This brought about the wrath of many Chicago x-ray dealers, who then refused to handle Buck film altogether. Still, many of the customers remained faithful to Buck film (including the special kidney shaped 3¼″ x 4¾″, for use on the operating table). But the demand decreased, and in 1959 Buck discontinued the sale of x-ray films. To the very last moment, though, some of their fans, for instance Augustana Hospital (Chicago), used exclusively Buck film.

Buck's first intensifier screen was introduced in 1924, their first fluoroscopic screen in 1925. Buck's first film

*Byron Hess remembers the McPhedries X-Ray Company, located in a Chicago suburb. It had been founded to manufacture the Buckeye Tank (a molded developing tank) — the rights to that patent were held by George McFedries, Buck, and George W. Brady.

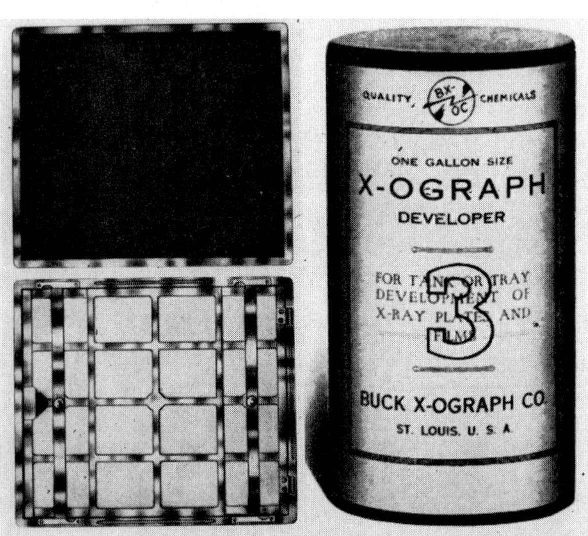

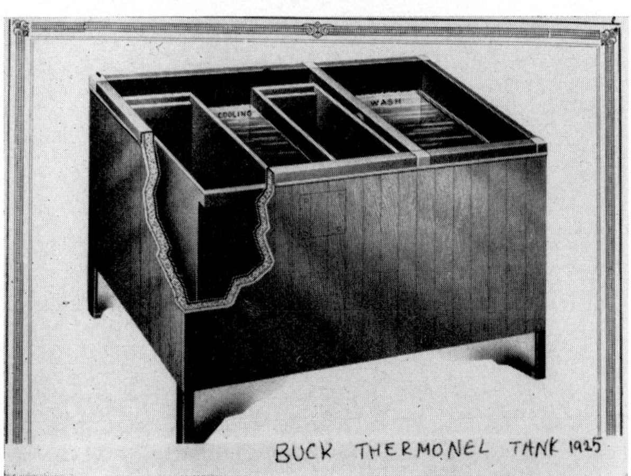

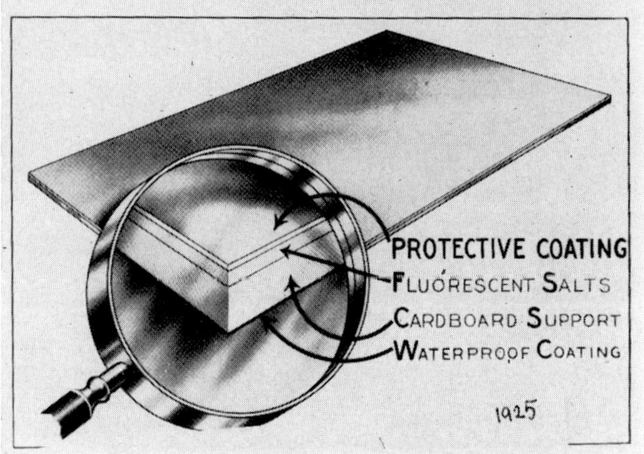

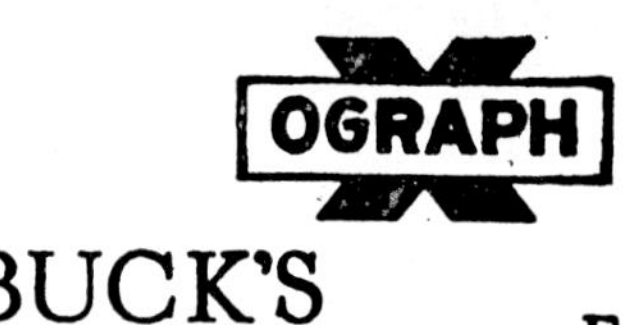

BUCK'S X-OGRAPH PACKETS

For Dental X-Ray Work

An extremely thin, metal-backed dental film packet, with smoothly rounded corners. Readily conforms to the curves of the mouth.
¶ Easy to hold in position.
¶ Two speeds, suitable for any kind of equipment.
¶ Produces roentgenograms of wonderful detail and brilliancy.

IT'S THE PERFECT PACKET—TRY IT

MANUFACTURED AND PATENTED BY

A.W. BUCK, St. Louis, Mo.

DEALERS IN ALL PRINCIPAL CITIES

Buck's first ad. It appeared in 1919, in the *American Journal of Roentgenology* (through courtesy of which it is herein reproduced).

dryer was sold to Ernest Charles Samuel, a radiologist from New Orleans.

Today, the Buck X-Ograph Company is a respected manufacturer of darkroom equipment. Their decades of tradition are exteriorized also in the fact that their street address is called after the company — Xograph Ave. — because at the time the plant was built, there were only fields around; then the expanding town caught up with the plant. Buck's first trade-mark, a stylized version of X and OGRAPH, was introduced in the summer of 1918, but had to be discontinued after two years because it produced objections (some regarded it as an infringement, albeit not legally so). The next trade-mark contained the name Buck and the eternal sign of electricity, the lightning. Finally a globe was adopted (in both white-on-black and black-on-white versions), to show the company's intent to achieve world-wide distribution.

At the time of this writing, Arthur Wells Buck (after recovering from a partial colectomy for neoplasm) continues as an active head of the company, and as one of the cherished elder statesmen of the x-ray industry.*

INTENSIFYING SCREENS

In 1896, Pupin had employed one screen of calcium tungstate to reinforce the x-ray image on his dry plate. Other early users of such reinforcing action of the screen were Tesla in this country, and Campbell-Swinton in England. During the Era of the Roentgen Pioneers, intensifying screens made of natural calcium tungstate were imported from Germany under the name of Gehler Folie, or from France – there existed the France Screen Co., located at 406 McKerchey Bldg., 2631 Woodward Ave. in Detroit (their screens were made by Caplain St. André Fils & Co. of Paris). The reason why screens were not used more often was that they possessed extreme fluorescent lag and excessive graininess: the large sized crystals obscured, rather than brought out, details.

Herbert Threlkeld-Edwards (1870-1922) manufactured the T-E Intensifying Screens. They were advertised as the first American-made intensifying screens, "made by a roentgenologist for roentgenologists."

*Some of this information was contributed by another executive of the Buck Company, Mr. I. J. Matlock.

X-OGRAPH PACKETS

FOR DENTAL X-RAY WORK

THE PERFECT DENTAL FILM PACKET

SEVEN ADVANTAGES

No. 1—Extremely Thin With Smoothly Rounded Corners
No. 2—Permits a Record on the Back of Each Packet
No. 3—Special Metal Back Increases Detail and Contrast
No. 4—No Secondary Rays Means Clearer Definition
No. 5—Less Tendency to Nauseate the Patient
No. 6—Readily Conforms to the Curvatures of Mouth
No. 7—Easily Placed and Held in Position

X-OGRAPH PACKETS WILL IMPROVE YOUR DENTAL X-RAY WORK

BUCK X-OGRAPH CO.

Dealers in all Principal Cities ST. LOUIS, MO.

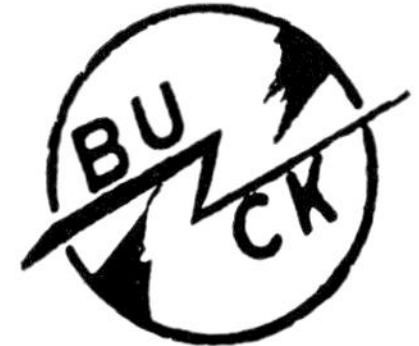

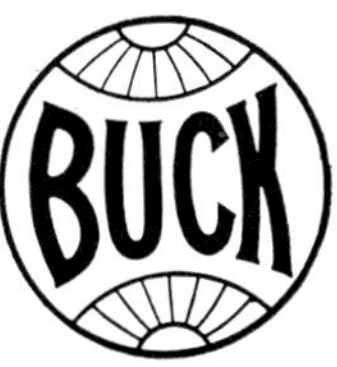

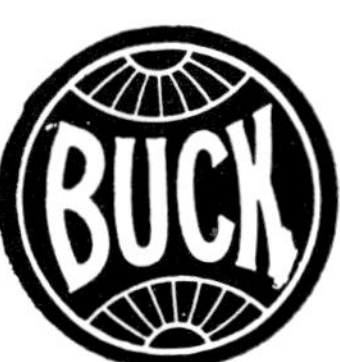

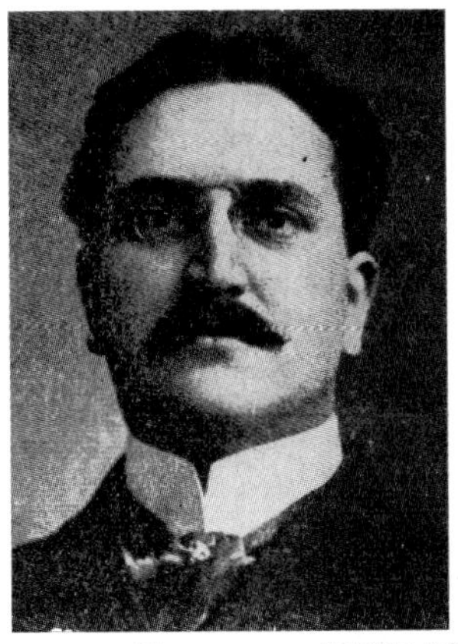

HERBERT THRELKELD-EDWARDS (1870-1922). Owner of the "X-ray Laboratory" in Bethlehem (Pennsylvania), who perfected and then successfully marketed the first (and for its time quite satisfactory) intensifying screens in the U. S. A.

The Premier American Screen

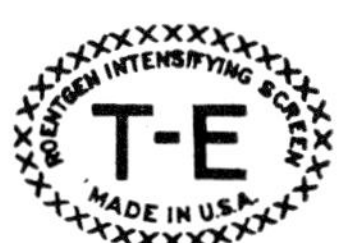

Dr. H. Threlkeld-Edwards
South Bethlehem, Pa.

"Made by a Roentgenologist for Roentgenologists"

+ SPEED – GRAIN

THIS IS THE FORMULA BY WHICH YOU ARE ASKED TO JUDGE ALL "T-E" SCREENS.

The "T-E" is GUARANTEED to be faster and have less grain than others and is SOLD WITH THIS UNDERSTANDING.

NEW "THIN" MODEL FOR DOUBLE SCREEN TECHNIQUE.

Threlkeld-Edwards first showed his screen at the 1912 meeting of the ARRS in Niagara Falls. While its base was the same calcium tungstate, it appeared to be of good quality and high speed, though still quite grainy. It had a very hard, smooth surface, which could be washed with soap and water. As advertised, the inventor's "X-Ray Laboratory" was at 314 W. 4th St., in South Bethlehem (Pennsylvania).

After the death of Threlkeld-Edwards, his business was purchased by Carl V. S. Patterson. The latter had been employed by Snook in Philadelphia and had introduced in 1913 the Snook Lagless Intensifying Screen, very similar to the T-E Screen. Later, Patterson went out on his own, founded the Patterson Screen Co. in Towanda, Pa., and in 1916 introduced another screen, not quite as fast as the T-E but with much finer grain. This, however, was actually the second step. The first had been in 1914 when he introduced the Patterson Fluoroscopic Screen, based on the use of a new chemical, Cadmium Tungstate. Very soon, Patterson fluoroscopic screens became the recognized standard in the US.

In 1918, after the introduction of "duplitized" (double coated) film by Eastman Kodak, Patterson developed the double screen technique with "thin" front screen and "thick" back screen.

As a matter of interest, it may be stated that these double screens were only slightly more expensive than the competitive T-E screen. For instance, in 1919, the Patterson special double intensifying screen (sold only in pairs, the price being that of one pair) ranged from \$15.00 for the 5x7″ to \$20.00 for the 14x17″ size. The respective cassette cost from \$7.00 for the 5x7″ to \$15.00 for the 14x17″.

By comparison the T-E screens ranged from \$8.00 for the 5x7″ to \$57.20 for the 14x17″ size. His cassettes were from \$8.80 for the 5x7″ to \$16.50 for the 14x17″ size.

The price of the Solace Intensifying Screen, offered at that time by the Waite & Bartlett Co. ranged from \$12.00 for the 6½x8½″ screen to \$45.00 for the 14x17″ screen. Their cassettes sold from \$8.00 for the smallest to \$15.00 for the largest.

None of them offered any discount when cassettes were purchased with screens. Incidentally, Patterson manufactured also the screens which W & B sold as their own brand.

Carl Patterson, who was born near, and lives in, Towanda (Pennsylvania), offered the following data. He graduated as a chemical engineer from the University of Pennsylvania in 1911, and in the same year and from the same school Fred Reuter graduated as a mechanical engineer. Patterson joined Snook in June of 1912. In march of 1914, Patterson returned to Towanda, and opened his own business, into which he

Important Announceme

AMERICAN INTENSIFYING SCREEN

THE perfected "T-E" Screen is now ready for distribution. It is far superior to the foreign screens and is more than 25 per cent faster than its prototypes.

"After-glow" or phosphorescence has been eliminated and so the pictures are full of detail, and without fog or grain.

The emulsion surface is smooth and hard and may be washed with soap and water. Cassetts of original design can also be supplied.

For further particulars and for prices and samples write to

Dr. H. Threlkeld-Edwards

314 W. Fourth St. 1912 **South Bethlehem, Pa.**

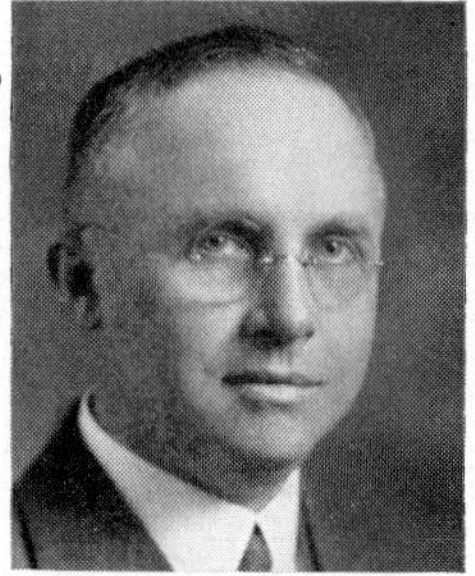

C. V. S. Patterson

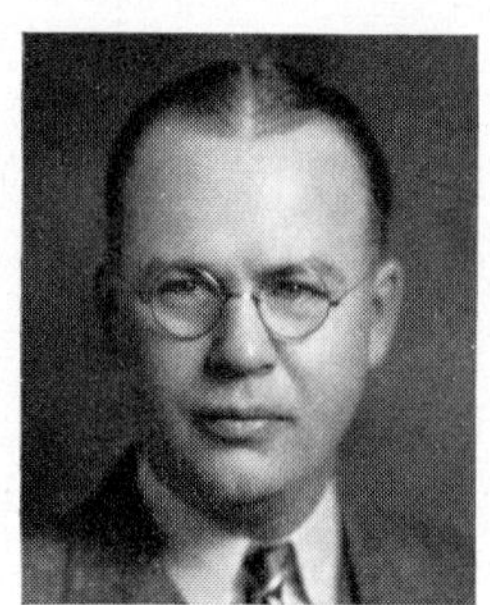

F. W. Reuter

Patterson Cleanable Intensifying Screens are accepted as standard in the roentgenological laboratories of America, Europe, and Asia for these reasons:

1. *They are grainless*
2. *They are free from afterglow*
3. *They are absolutely uniform*
4. *They are completely cleanable with soap and water*
5. *They do not deteriorate with age*
6. *They are pliable and flat*
7. *They are the fastest of their type*

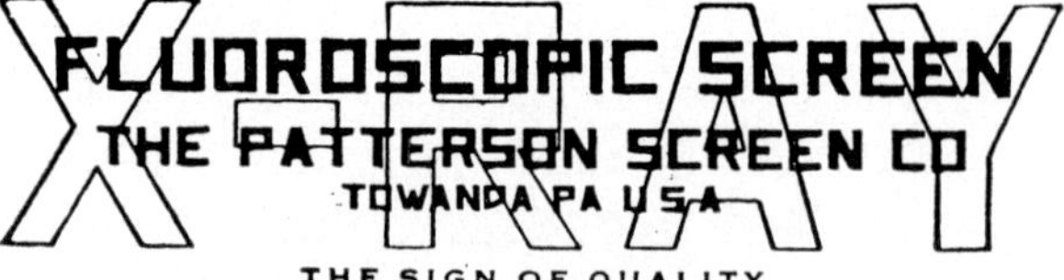

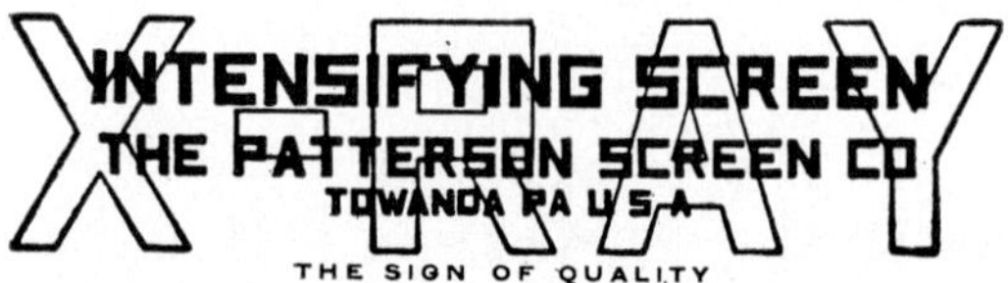

THE PATTERSON SCREEN COMPANY

TOWANDA, PENNSYLVANIA, U. S. A.

soon took a partner, the above named classmate Fred Reuter. For several years the two worked alone, performing all the required operations for manufacturing screens, from sweeping the quarters and typing to mixing the chemicals and shipping the finished products. In 1925 they incorporated their firm, in the same year in which they purchased the business of Threlkeld-Edwards, which was being operated after Threlkeld-Edwards' death by the estate. The Patterson Company developed a procedure for coating fluorescent lights, and that part of their business was sold to Sylvania Electric Products in 1941. The x-ray screen part of the business was sold to Du Pont in 1943. Carl Patterson remained as manager of the Patterson Science Division of Du Pont, and Reuter as assistant manager, until their retirement in 1950.

In the early 1920s several short-lived firms entered the manufacture of screens, such as the Sweetbriar Laboratories, at 1120-1228 Hotchkiss St. in Pittsburgh or, in Chicago, the National X-Ray Screen Co. at 24 North Wabash Ave., and the F. Blume X-Ray Screen Co. at 6423 Irving Park Blvd.

BARIUM

Barium is being produced from ore in Nebraska. The Basor Co., at 314 S. 12th St. in Omaha, specified in their advertisements that its laboratories were devoted exclusively to refining, testing, and packing this article.

Barium Sulfate is completely inert and therefore non-toxic but Barium Sulfide is very poisonous. A few instances, in which confusion resulted in catastrophy, made it worthwhile to sell packaged "x-ray" barium, absolutely safe for consumption. Some call it simply pure Barium Sulfate, USP, as does the chemical firm Mallinckrodt in St. Louis. Others market the substance under their own brand name, for instance GE's Bari-o-Meal was introduced in 1928.

Barium sulphate cannot be dissolved in water, it can only be suspended, and suspensions are not very stable. Many attempts have been made in the hope of stabilizing a barium suspension. The fact that "new" and "improved" formulas are still being advertised indicates that the problem has not been solved. This is true, today, but perhaps to-morrow . . . the ideal formula will be found. One of the first such preparations was I-X Barium Meal, prepared by the Industrial X-Ray Research Laboratories in St. Louis, and sold especially by the Dick Company, also of St. Louis.

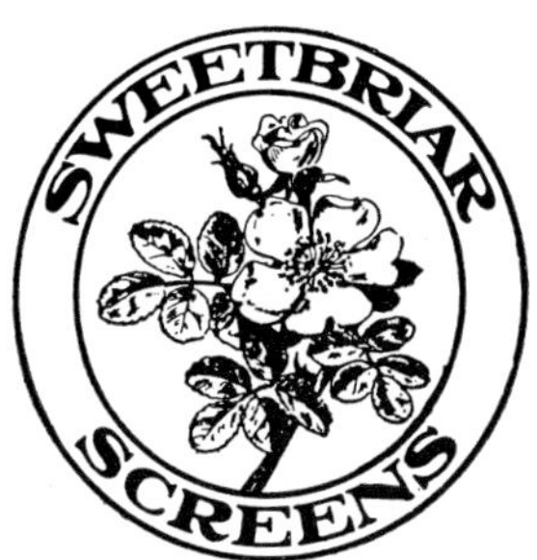

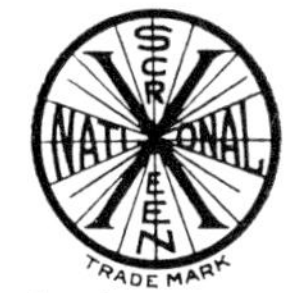

National X-Ray Screen Co.
INC.

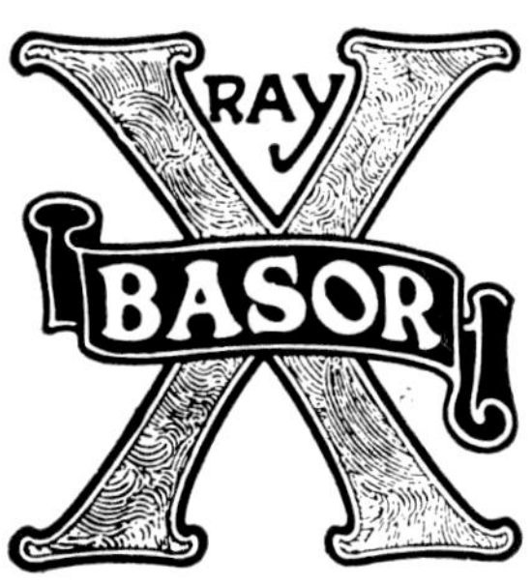

FORBES DRY PLATES

To Insure Getting the Best Results, Use

FORBES X-RAY PLATES

THERE is no Plate on the market that has caught on more readily and created a more steady demand. Easy to work, full of detail and intensity, and very rapid. TRY THEM.

FORBES DRY PLATE CO., 26 Armour St., ROCHESTER, N.Y.

GENERAL AGENTS:

MACALASTER-WIGGIN CO., Boston, Mass.

THE APPENGOLD CO., 193 Third Avenue, New York, N.Y. 1913

"Paragon"

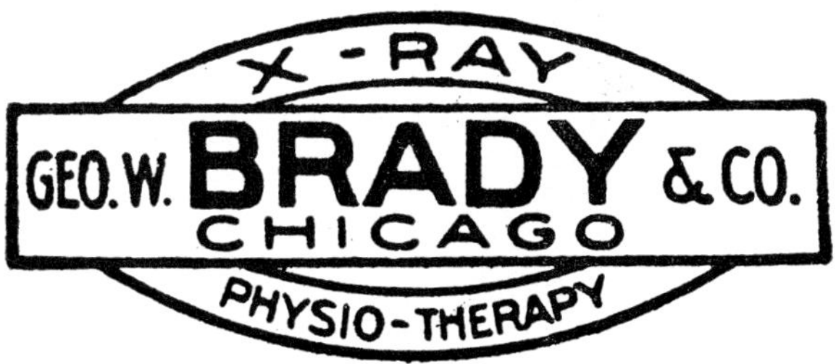

Most companies "packed" barium, either themselves or with the help of others, for instance, Picker had the Basolac, prepared by the Kerasol Company of New York City; Keleket sold Sta-Barium; Victor had the Bari-Meal, whereupon Acme "continued" with the Bariumeal.

DRY PLATES

A few of the companies which made this product lasted for quite some time, for instance the Forbes Dry Plate Co. (in business since 1883) at 26 Armour St. in Rochester (New York). Among their agents was the Macalaster & Wiggins in Boston, and the Appengold Co. at 193 Third Ave. in New York City.

The American Photochemical Co. was then located in the "Photographic City" Rochester (New York). In an advertisement dated 1916, they claimed that their Diagnostic X-Ray Plates were 25 percent faster than anything available at that time.

The Paragon X-Ray Plates "made especially for fine radiographic work" were sold only by the Geo. W. Brady & Co., 761 South Western Ave. in Chicago. They also retailed miscellaneous supplies, including screens, cassettes, Coolidge tubes, developers, x-ray gloves, aprons, and so on. George Brady was a well known figure among mid-western radiologists, indeed, he was involved personally in the founding of the original Western Roentgen Society, forerunner of the RSNA. Brady had for some time a financial interest in the Standard X-Ray Co. Byron Hess told me nostalgically of the day when Bill Hettich accompanied Brady to a tailor for the fitting of a new suit: Brady asked the tailor to line his pockets with very strong material, as he always carried tools with him. To this day, a good x-ray salesman must be willing (and often able) to make on-the-spot, small repairs on x-ray equipment and accessories, even on those manufactured by a competitor. The inherent good will thus created among "customers" always pays off in increased sales.

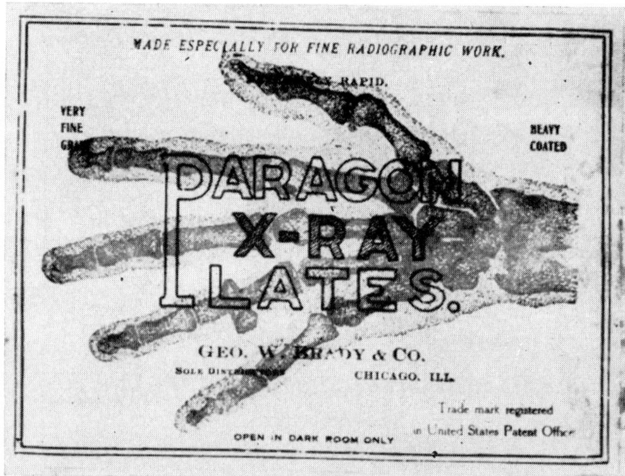

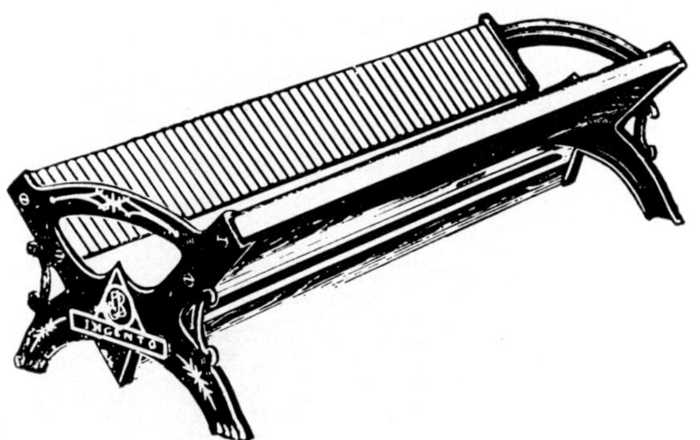

Ingento Negative Rack. This was a professional type, with a trough to catch the drippings, while the vertically placed glass plates were drip-drying. Price: $1.25.

EASTMAN-KODAK

This firm was founded by George Eastman (1845-1932), whose phenomenal, self-made success based on hard work and ingenuity can hardly be duplicated. His memorabilia are preserved in the George Eastman House of Photography in Rochester (New York), his former home converted into a museum.

The history of the development of x-ray films has been written by Arthur Wolfram Fuchs, a longtime technical executive of the Eastman-Kodak Company. It appeared in several places: a summary can be found in the *American Journal of Roentgenology* of January, 1956.

Eastman Transparent Film — New Formula was still being manufactured in 1896, and was used on a very limited scale also in radiography. Neither gelatin, nor celluloid films were then desirable because of their

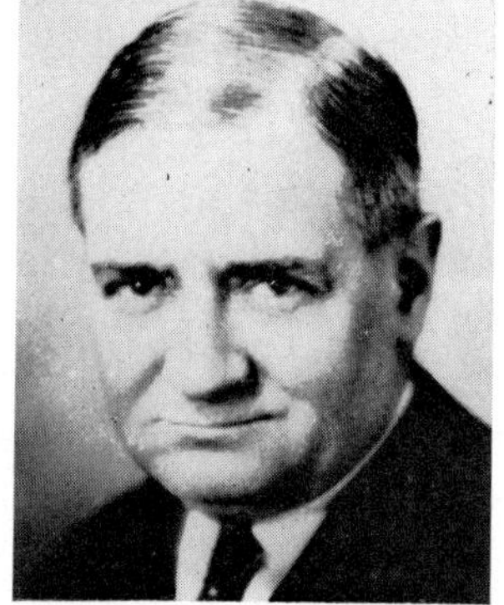

George William Brady (1881-1932). A manufacturer of x-ray accessories, who started in the Era of the Roentgen Pioneers, but was typical of the Golden Age of Radiology. Well remembered are his Paragon X-ray Plates, his financial support of the beginnings of the RSNA, and his having brought out the first commercial model of Bucky-Potter's moving grid diaphragm. Brady died in the Big Depression.

tendency to curl and crack, but they had the advantage of being thin, which permitted the usage of one or even two intensifying screens.*

Before World War I, the glass for making glass plates in America was brought in from Belgium. This source of supply was curtailed after the war started. But even while glass was easily available, its bulk and fragility were serious drawbacks. It is of interest to note that film was being used all along in dental radiography.

Otto Walkhoff, the physician from Braunschweig (Germany) who produced the first roentgen plate of teeth (his own) only weeks after Röntgen's discovery, used for this purpose an ordinary photographic plate cut to a small size and wrapped in black paper. Frank Harrison was the first to describe the method of employing film in dental radiography: his paper appeared in the *Journal of British Dental Association* of September, 1896. William James Morton, of New York City, used Eastman NC roll film when he examined teeth in April, 1896. About 1900, Weston Price, a Cleveland dentist, designed a celluloid-base dental film; it was said to be thick enough to prevent curling, but flexible enough to be introduced into the mouth; the product was made by the Seed Dry Plate Company, it came in large sheets, which the user himself cut to size, and wrapped in black, unvulcanized dental rubber. Charles Edmund Kells, Jr., of New Orleans, first suggested to use two dental films in one "packet" to have a duplicate in case one was lost, or sent to the referring dentist. In 1913 a red, waxed, moisture-proof, hand-wrapped paper packet was introduced (containing two single-coated dental films). In 1921, came out the machine-wrapped packets, since 1925 double-coated with fine-grain, high-contrast ("radia-tized") emulsion. In 1926 Howard Riley Raper designed and introduced the first "bite-wing" film packet.

Eastman-Kodak's contribution to the coming of the Golden Age of Radiology was the double-coated film. Before that, in 1914, they manufactured a single-coated 14x17″ film, on a cellulose nitrate base, with an emulsion of greater sensitivity than any glass plates offered at that time. The urgency of World War I speeded up the development. The then current practice of tray development was a deterrent to the adoption of Eastman-Kodak's "duplitized" (double-coated) films, introduced in 1916. The first satisfactory film hanger did not become available until about 1920.

Cellulose nitrate was quite satisfactory as a base, but its incendiary potentialities made storage hazardous, and resulted occasionally in disasters. Its replacement with cellulose acetate was first suggested in 1906, but many practical problems had to be solved prior to actual production. Basic inventions and patents in the matter were offered by several foreign manufacturers (Agfa, Schleussner), but George Eastman and his company made outstanding contributions in the three main areas of difficulty: reduction in brittleness, improved

*In England, prior to 1901, the Austin-Edwards snapshot film, and the Cristoid, made by the Sandell Plate Company, were also used in radiography. The emulsions were first coated on glass, then stripped off, thus some "films" were made of gelatin. The emulsions consisted of a mixture of a very rapid and a regular speed emulsion. In Germany — in the very year 1896 — Schleussner made such an x-ray film with a double emulsion on each side, four coats in all. The results were very good, but the manufacturing difficulties considerable and the cost high. Even so, it is hard to understand why production of x-ray film ever declined, but so it did until after coming of the Golden Age of Radiology.

AN IMPORTANT RADIOGRAPHIC DISCOVERY.

EASTMAN'S

...X-RAY PAPER

ENTIRELY SUPERSEDES DRY PLATES WITH THEIR ATTENDANT DRAWBACKS.

Of Unparalleled Advantage in Surgical Diagnosis by means of the Röntgen Rays.

Courtesy: Arthur Wolfram Fuchs.

ADVERTISEMENT FROM THE YEAR 1897. Wishful thinking.

EASTMAN

X-Ray Films

EASTMAN X-Ray Films mean— convenience in *handling, developing, mailing* and *filing*. They are flexible, light and unbreakable and in quality are *at least* the equal of the best X-Ray plates make.

The present extensive use of cut films for professional portraiture is proof that the film's advantage over glass plates is appreciated by the photographer—the advantages to the Roentgenologist are even more marked.

For sale by all Supply Houses. Illustrated booklet, "X-Ray Efficiency" by mail on request.

EASTMAN KODAK CO.,

ROCHESTER, N. Y.

Courtesy: Arthur Wolfram Fuchs.

ADVERTISEMENT FROM THE YEAR 1914. Prophetic peroration.

clarity, and greater strength. Eastman-Kodak's first roentgen film on a safety base of cellulose acetate was produced and placed on the market in 1924.

Meanwhile, Eastman-Kodak had been growing all along, and developed into an industrial giant. Its main plant at Rochester (New York) became a city in itself. Eastman-Kodak's X-Ray Division expanded proportionately, and came to manufacture (almost) every item needed in the darkroom. They developed an educational program for x-ray technicians, and issued numerous editions of a booklet, which was first printed in 1918 under the title *X-Rays.* They also published since 1932, under varied names, the excellent *Medical Radiography and Photography.* A similar periodical appeared for dentists, both with Spanish editions.

ANSCO

In 1842 Edward Anthony established a daguerreotype supply company at 308 Broadway, in New York City. In 1852 Edward took his older brother Henry into the business, and the partnership flourished under the name E. and H. T. Anthony & Company.

The Anthonys conducted the world's first photographic prize contest in 1853; the prize ($500) went to Jeremiah Gurney, a famous "daguerreotype artist." In 1855 an Anthony print was the world's first ever to appear as an illustration in a magazine. In 1859 Henry Anthony was the first ever to take a photographic snapshot. In 1860 a wet plate made by Anthony was used for the first American aerial photograph (from a captive balloon hovering over Boston).

In London, Frederick Scott Archer had discovered the use of collodion as a vehicle for coating glass plate negatives in 1851. The English "wet plate" method was introduced in America in 1857. When used as an "ambulatory" procedure, it required carrying around a darkroom and facilities for coating as well as for on-the-spot processing. But it was a major advance for its time, and was soon adopted by the trade. In 1861, when the famous New York, Philadelphia, and Washington high society daguerreotype artist Mathew B. Brady (1822-1896) went to photograph the Civil War his equipment came along in a "prairie schooner," a modified Conestoga wagon. James D. Horan (who wrote Brady's biography, *Historian with a Camera,* New York, 1955) tells us that the materials used for making those war pictures were advanced on credit by the Anthonys, but were never repaid, because Brady lost all his money in the process, and he never quite recuperated from that episode. But his collection of Civil War photographs remains as an invaluable record, both human and historic, of those troubled times.

In the late 1870s appeared the so-called dry plates. At first the Anthonys imported such plates from England. Later they contracted to sell the spare-time output of a bank clerk from Rochester (New York), whose hobby was photography. That clerk's name was George

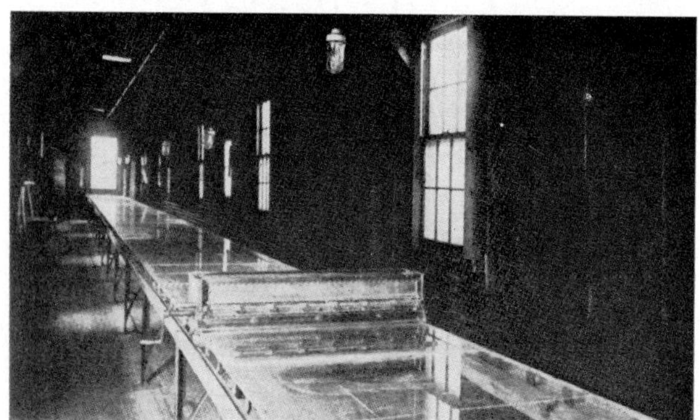

EARLY FILM-COATING. In the very beginning, Eastman film was coated on glass-topped tables 200 feet long.

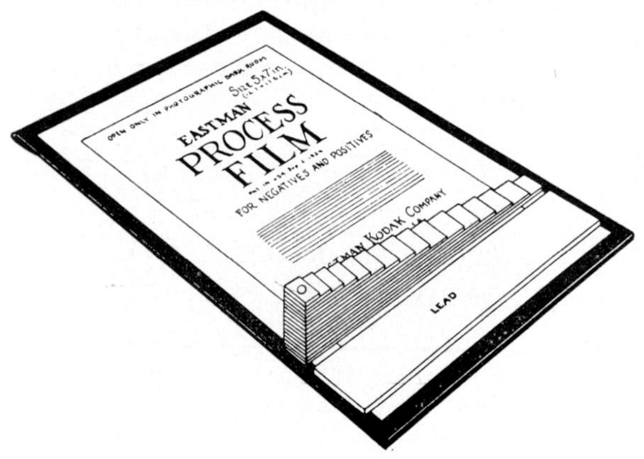

X-RAYS

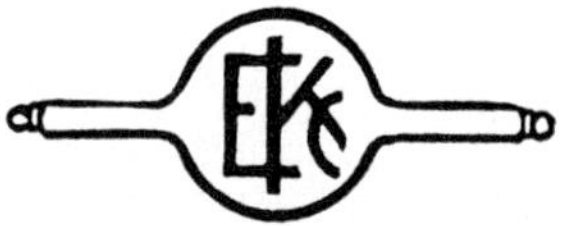

EASTMAN KODAK CO.
ROCHESTER, N. Y.
1918

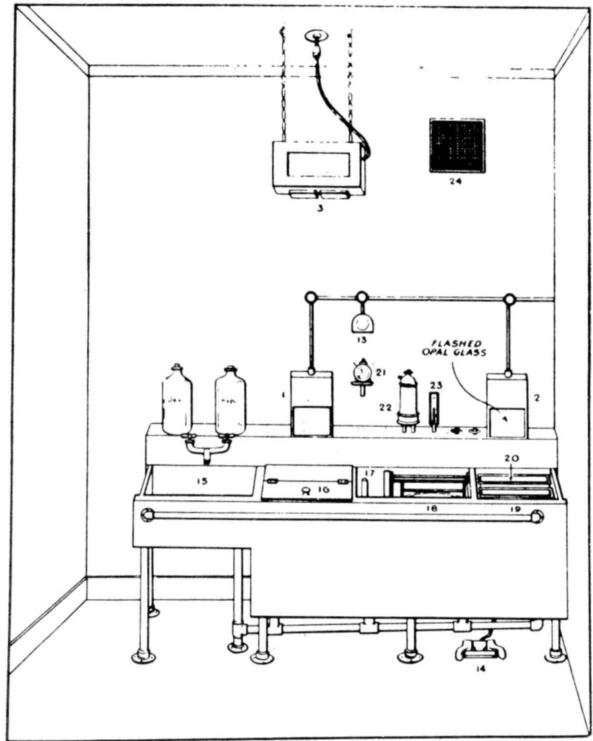

EASTMAN DARKROOM OF 1918. Tray-processing was satisfactory for plates, but not for films. Therefore Eastman, if he wanted to make a go of the films, had to push for tank-processing. Good film-hangers did not become available before 1920, but otherwise the darkroom underwent no significant changes until the advent of automatic film-processors.

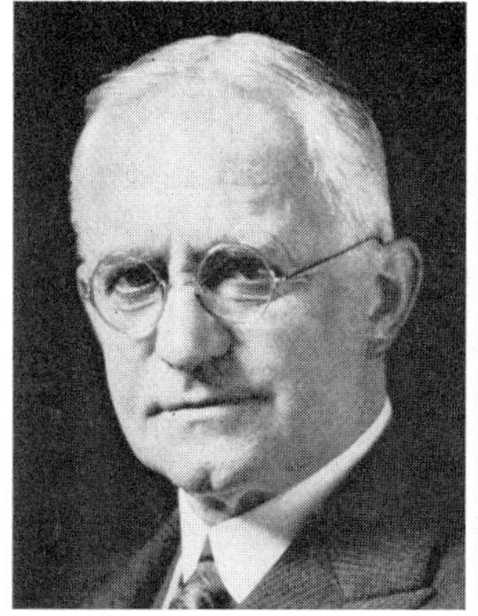

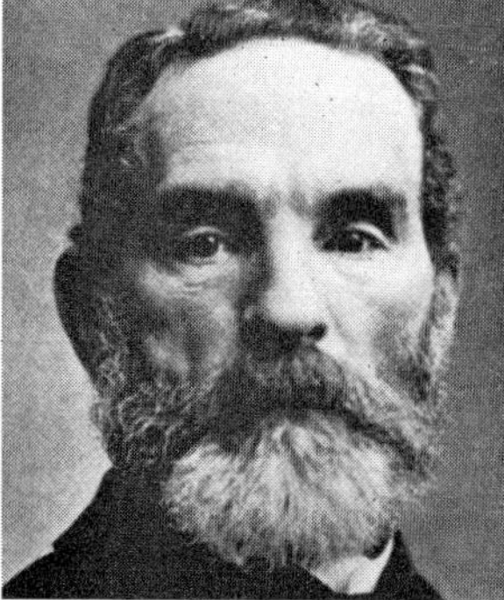

EDWARD ANTHONY, bearded founder of Ansco. No portrait has been preserved of the other eponymic half, Scovill. In a famous patent litigation over rollfilm, Anthony obtained a favorable settlement. "Defeated" winner was GEORGE EASTMAN (1854-1932). Eastman's most important invention was the snapshot (Kodak) camera of 1888. His most significant achievement remains the Eastman-Kodak Company. His most cherished creation is the Eastman School of Music in Rochester, New York.

Eastman, and the Anthonys sold Eastman's dry plates until 1885.

On May 2, 1887, the American Episcopal clergyman Hannibal Williston Goodwin (1822-1900) applied for a patent on the first flexible photographic rollfilm, and the Anthonys purchased his rights. At about that time George Eastman had developed his own rollfilm. In 1888, Eastman put on the market the world's first portable box camera: it was called the Kodak, and this is where the current appellation Eastman-Kodak originated. In 1889 Eastman started to sell rollfilm for his Kodak. This tremendous departure from the cumbersome paraphernalia needed until that time made amateur photography possible, but it also produced a bitter patent fight between the Anthonys and Eastman. Goodwin's patent was finally issued on September 13, 1898 following a settlement between Eastman and the Anthonys.

The Scovill Manufacturing Company was the earliest manufacturer of copper daguerreoplates in America. In 1889, they set up a special division, the Scovill and Adams Company, which specialized in the manufacture of cameras, lenses, and shutters. In 1900 the Anthonys moved their manufacturing operations to Binghamton (New York). In 1901 they merged with Scovill & Adams, whereupon the Scovill Camera Works were also moved to Binghamton. Finally in 1907 the name of the new firm was abbreviated to ANSCO from Anthony and Scovill.

George Eastman combined "his" rollfilm with an apparatus built simultaneously by Thomas Edison, and this fortunate combination made motion pictures successful. Eastman was forever striving to achieve a mass market, thus in 1923 the Eastman-Kodak introduced the 16 mm film which brought amateur cinematography with it. Eastman's first Kodak camera, introduced in June of 1888, was sold loaded (including shoulder strap) for $25; anybody could "press the button," after which that "amateur" would send the whole camera to Eastman's at Rochester, where the exposed strip was removed, processed, and printed, and a new one inserted at a charge of $10.

While Eastman-Kodak was getting bigger and bigger, Ansco underwent a process of attrition: in 1928 it was purchased by the German firm Agfa, with the resulting change of name to Agfa-Ansco. About that time they went into the x-ray field, and in 1936 Agfa-Ansco placed on the American market the first commercially available non-screen x-ray film. Then came World War II, and Agfa-Ansco came under government control as an Enemy Alien property. About the time of that forcible scission from Agfa, Ansco had started to publish a series of ads devoted to the history of radiology, with emphasis on American pioneers (that series is now being reprinted in the Ansco X-Ray News).

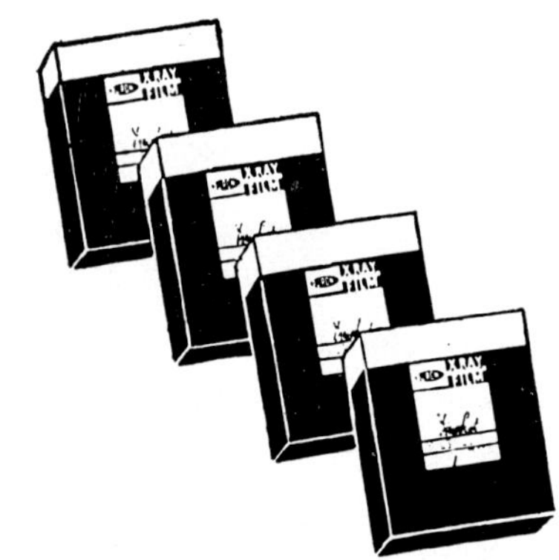

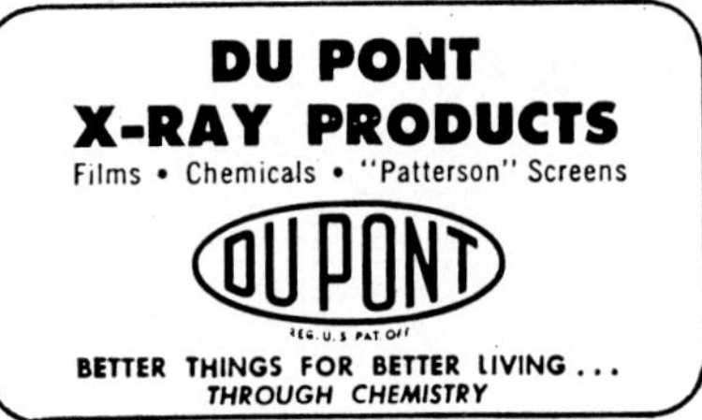

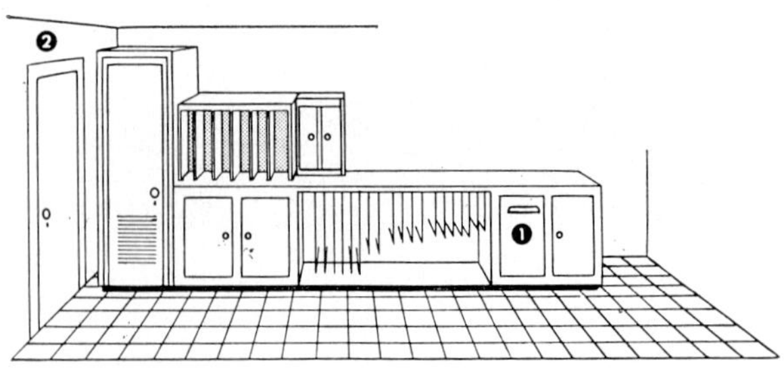

DU PONT

The E. I. Du Pont de Nemours & Co. of Wilmington (Delaware) — established initially as a gunpowder factory in 1802 — is older as a firm than most (if not all) those herein mentioned, but it did not come into the x-ray business until 1932.

Du Pont's early production of x-ray film was on both cellulose acetate (safety) and cellulose nitrate (flammable) bases. Soon, though, everybody discontinued the manufacture of the incendiary base, especially after the Cleveland hospital fire. In 1933 Du Pont added a blue tint to their base, which enhanced the diagnostic quality of the film. This procedure, which was original with Du Pont, has since been adopted universally by all manufacturers of x-ray film. Packaged x-ray chemicals were made part of the Du Pont Photo Products line in 1934, at which time they also introduced industrial x-ray film.

Du Pont Photo Products disposes of three plants. Radiographic screens are produced in the Towanda (Pennsylvania) plant — Du Pont purchased in 1943 the Patterson Screen Company, until then the principal manufacturer of intensifying and fluoroscopic screens. In 1945 Du Pont bought out the Defender Photo Supply Company, whose Rochester (New York) factory became the second plant. Du Pont x-ray films are produced in the largest (third) manufacturing facility of their Photo Products Section, a plant located in Parlin (New Jersey), a southwestern New York City exurbia.

Their promotional leaflets are printed under the

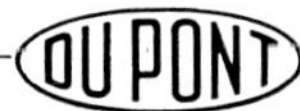

Patterson Screens

Light the paths of X-Ray

BETTER THINGS FOR BETTER LIVING . . . *THROUGH CHEMISTRY*

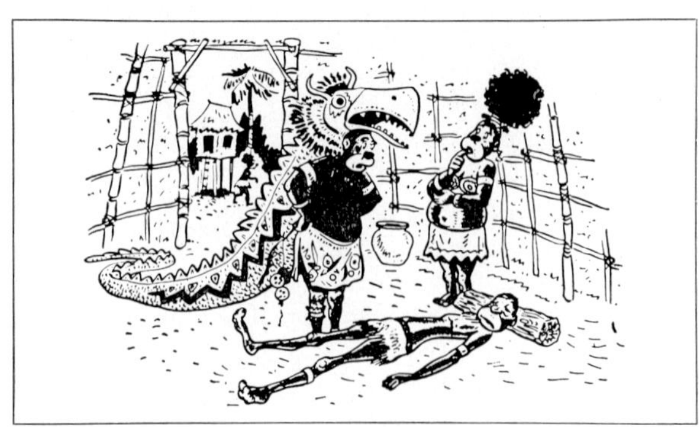

"I'll dance around him a few times. But, if that doesn't help, you'll have to get him down to my office for some x-rays."

name *DuPont X-Ray News,* and are best known for their "x-ray cartoons." One of these holds the unofficial record of having been pinned on more x-ray bulletin boards for a longer time than anything else on record: it purports the x-ray indications of a witch doctor as a sly parallel to the habits of certain (more orthodox?) practitioners.*

CONVERTERS

The Electric Conversion Co., at 114 Cypress St., in Brookline (Massachusetts) was selling in 1913 the Cabot High Potential Direct Current Converter.

In 1916 the Rieber Laboratories, 121 Second St. San Francisco, promoted the Rieber Converter Unit, emphasizing its greater standardization of control, silence, ease of operation, and higher potentials for use in therapy. This company changed soon into the Roentgen Manufacturing Co., 209-211 Tihuana St. in San Francisco, and then into the Roentgen Appliance Company. Later they marketed the Rieber Stabilizer, advertised as the modern means for achieving exact control of Coolidge tubes.

*In the *AMA News* of May 27, 1963 appeared the information that the medicine men of Central Africa—they call themselves *chirembas*—have formed an association (annual dues: $3) to build a school to train new chirembas.

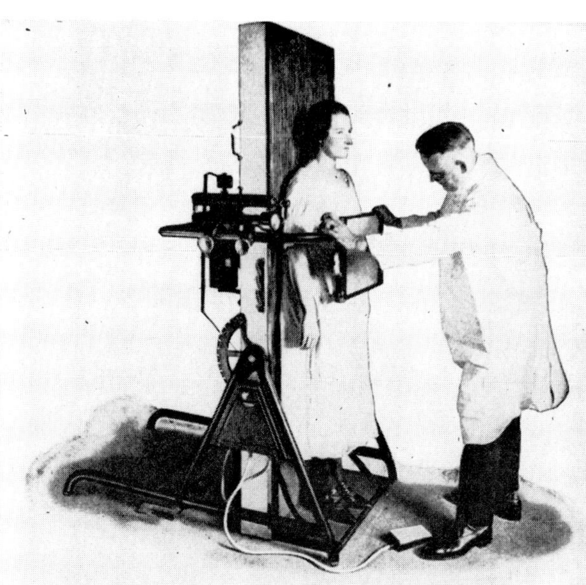

SNOOK

Under the same name of Roentgen Manufacturing Co. there existed a firm in Philadelphia, located in the Mariner & Merchant Building. It became famous in 1907 with Snook's cross-arm rectifier.

In 1897, in GE's Lynn Laboratories, Herman Lemp developed the "automatic wave selector" which may be regarded as the first mechanical high voltage rectifier (switch). His patent, for which GE applied on December 1, 1897, was granted on November 1, 1904. In January, 1904 the German physicist Franz J. Koch was given an English patent for a high tension mechanical rectifying system. Together with K. A. Sterzel, he had described it in 1903 in the *Annalen der Physik* and the following year in the *Fortschritte.*

Beginning in 1903 Homer Clyde Snook (1878-1942), while a graduate student in the Randal Morgan Laboratory of Physics at the University of Pennsylvania, undertook a series of studies with the intention to improve the discharge from a spark coil. He made an oscillographic study of the spark and was impressed by the amount of inverse discharge. He developed a synchronous series spark gap which led to the building of a synchronous reversing high tension switch to put both the direct and inverse discharges through the tube. The discharges came from a coil with a mercury inter-

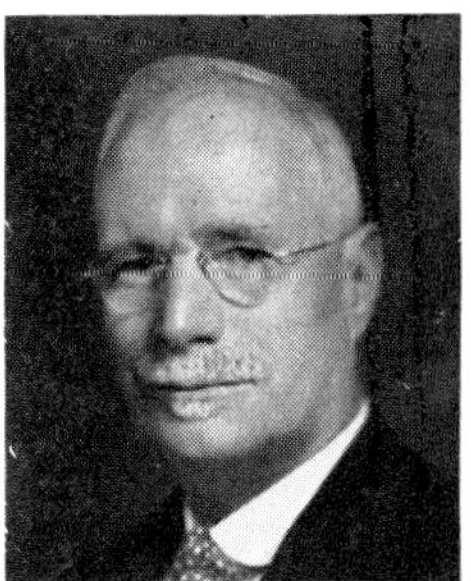

HERMANN M. LEMP

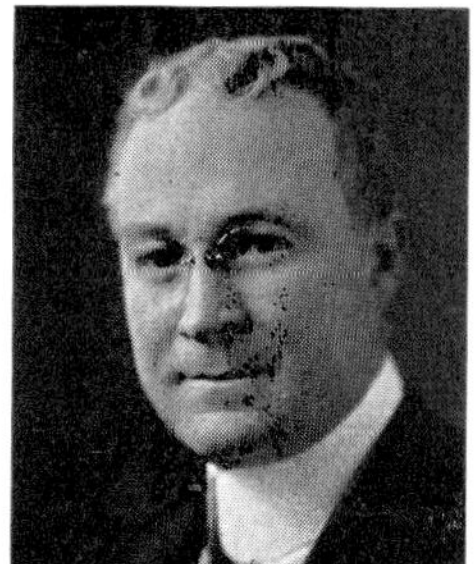

HOMER SNOOK

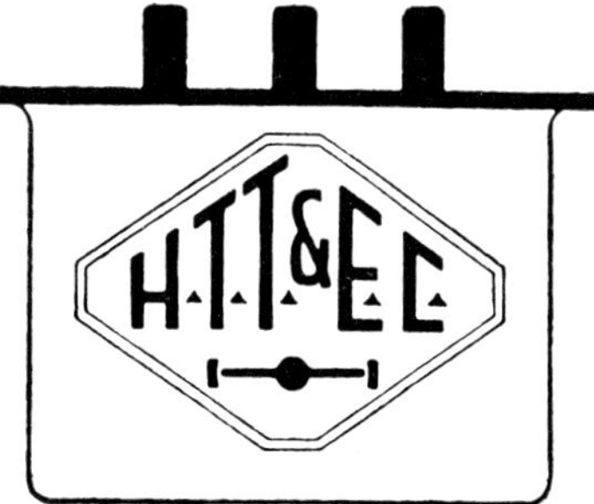

Trade Mark Registered
HIGH TENSION TRANSFORMER AND ELECTRICAL CO.

rupter. Additional oscillographic studies showed much time waste between the waves, and poor wave form. Thereupon, Snook built a closed core transformer (for alternating current), to which he added that high tension rotary switch: this was his "interrupterless" apparatus. By the testimony of Imboden (1931), Snook had been unaware of the work of either Lemp, or Koch and Sterzel.

In 1916, Snook published an (anonymous) *Brief History of Roentgenology,* which contains important details on the American x-ray industry in the Era of the Pioneers. Snook's first contact with the new rays occurred while he was still an undergraduate student at Ohio Wesleyan University: he helped W. G. Hormell to put together a coil and a Crookes tube and their experiment "terminated successfully." Then Snook went to work for the Queen & Co. in Philadelphia. In 1903 Snook with two other Queen employees (G. Herbert White and Edwin W. Kelly) went out on their own, and formed the Radioelectric Company. Their first office and workshop was a second story room at 226 Ionic Street in Philadelphia. A few months later they changed the name to Roentgen Manufacturing Company.

The experimental design and early production of the interrupterless transformer was done there on Ionic Street. The first unit for hospital use was installed in the service of Willis Manges at the Jefferson Hospital in Philadelphia in June of 1907. If not the second, perhaps the third or fourth of those very early models was sold to Baetjer at Johns Hopkins in the same year of 1907: the equipment was still in operation, carrying a heavy clinical load, as late as 1946. In 1908, at the International Congress in Amsterdam, Snook described his interrupterless transformer. Time has proved that their 1907 advertisement was correct in stating "the day of the Induction Coil is passing." His patent was granted in 1910. By then, the Roentgen Manufacturing Company had moved to fancier quarters in the Mariner & Merchants Building, also in Philadelphia.

A

Brief History

of

ROENTGENOLOGY

and the part played

by the

SNOOK-ROENTGEN

MANUFACTURING CO.

in its development and

perfection

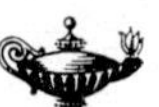

Phila., 1916

In 1906, a gas type valve tube had been used in the so called Hutton Atrema Transformer. The frailty of early gas valves made the whole project too expensive for practical purposes. GE's Dushman introduced the hot cathode valve in 1915, but it did not become commercially available before 1926. Until that time Snook's interrupterless transformer (or some of its competitive variants) remained unquestionably the best available generator.

In 1945, Paul Hodges explained the "interrupterless" name in the following manner. Only those fortunate few whose hospitals and offices were provided with alternating current power were spared the inequities of the electrolytic interrupter (Wehnelt's rectifier). The latter was noisy, not entirely reliable, it needed quite a bit of maintenance, and produced dangerous acid fumes. When Snook introduced the closed-core A.C. transformer with motor-driven rotary switch, instead of being called mechanical rectifier, it was hailed by radiologists as the *Interrupterless Transformer* meaning

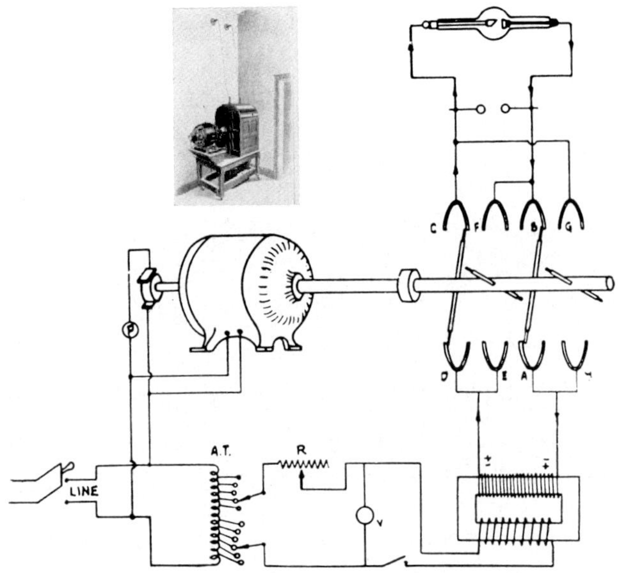

SNOOK'S RECTIFYING SWITCH. The insert shows the first Snook (at Jefferson Hospital in Philadelphia).

something, however noisy, which spared you from having to put up with those undesirable interrupters.

Snook was very successful, so much so as to change the name of the firm to the Snook-Roentgen Manufacturing Company. In 1913, it was located at 1206 Race Street in Philadelphia. By then, Snook had acquired a dramatic trade-mark with his name superimposed upon a gas tube.

Snook employed a rotating cross-arm rectifying switch in combination with a closed core, high tension transformer, a synchronous motor for operating the switch, a ma-meter and a rheostat control for use with alternating current supply (with the addition of a rotary converter for direct current). Even the earliest models gave 100 kvp at over 100 ma, which was more than existing tubes could carry. In 1915 he redesigned the transformer and in 1916 a thirty button autotransformer was included in the mainline circuit. Actually, the first autotransformer had been introduced about 1909. With its stable characteristics, it came into general use soon after the introduction of the Coolidge tube.

The mechanical rectifying principle was employed by many others. In 1910, the Kny-Sheerer Company, 404-410 West 27th St., New York City, advertised an Interrupterless X-Ray Current Generator which could be operated with equal results from the direct or from the alternating current "365 days in the year."

It may be of interest to evaluate the significance of Snook's switch. It had been developed on Ionic Street (so named by a classicist not by an electrician), but it achieved its big-time popularity only when ionic tubes were replaced by Coolidge's hot cathode. These two developments, together with Bucky-Potter's Diaphragm and Caldwell's (Campbell's) Tilting Table brought about the Golden Age of Radiology. It seems, though, as if Coolidge's tube was the most important of the four, because in the beginning, even without rectification (but with an autotransformer) the hot

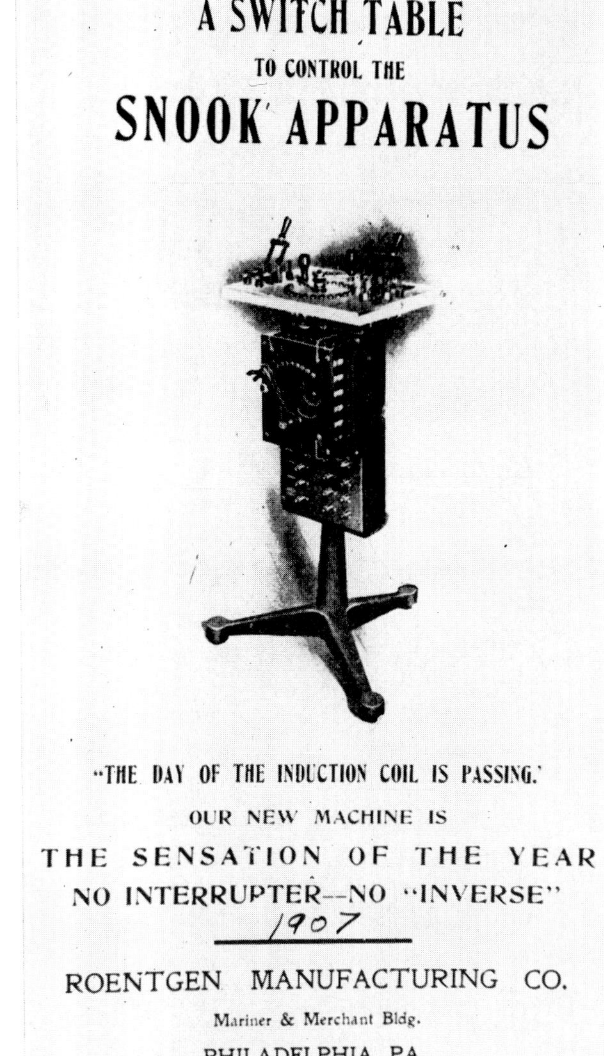

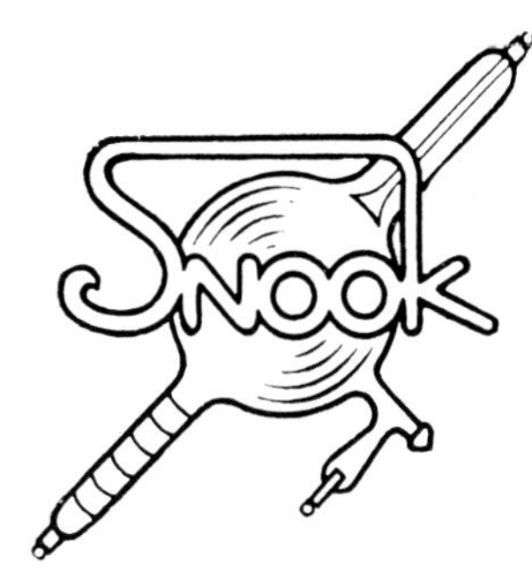

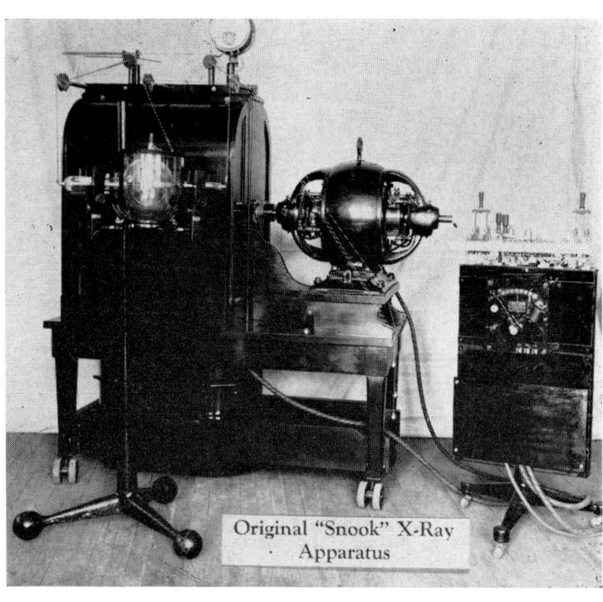
Original "Snook" X-Ray Apparatus

THE VICTOR
SEMI-MONTHLY X-OGRAM
A Newspaper for Boosters. Latest News, Prices and Information
No. 1 IMPORTANT—READ AND SAVE Aug. 1, 1916

cathode permitted fair duplication of factors, which was the most important thing.

VICTOR

In the first issue of the *Victor Semi-Monthly X-ogram,* "a newspaper for boosters, latest use, prices and information" printed on August 1, 1916, appeared a phrase from H. Clyde Snook, Vice-President, To our Salesmen:

"You men out on the sales firing line may find it hard to realize that 'Scheidel,' 'M&W.,' 'Victor,' and 'Snook,' are actually pulling together in the same harness – but it's true."

To understand this quotation, one would have to go back in history. The first name meant the Scheidel-Western X-Ray Coil Co., 411 S. Jefferson St. in Chicago. This company had resulted from the merger in 1907 of the Scheidel Coil Co. and of C. W. Howe's Western Coil Company, located at 171-172 East Randolph Street — they called themselves manufacturers, originators, and patentees. The former had been organized in 1898 as the W. Scheidel & Company, which was incorporated in 1905. After the merger with Western, they advertised themselves as the largest manufacturers of x-ray apparatus in the world. This statement may have been correct if one qualified it to exclusive manufacturer of x-ray equipment.

Wilhelm Scheidel was born in Frankfurt-am-Main (Germany) in 1863. He came to Chicago around 1890, entered the x-ray business in 1896, and in 1900 incorporated W. Scheidel & Co., at 171-173 East Randolph Street. At the time of the sale to Victor, he was already marked as a radiation casualty. He sur-

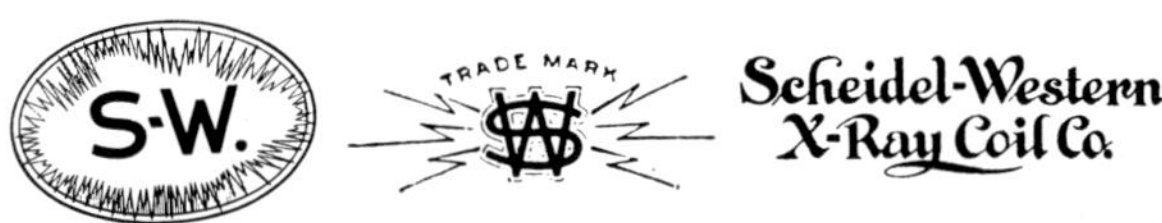

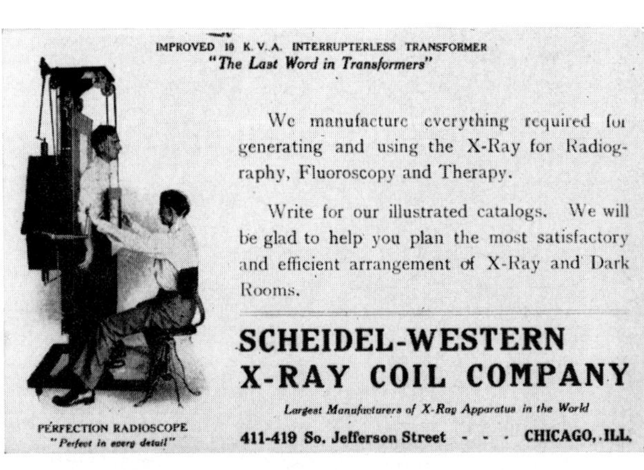

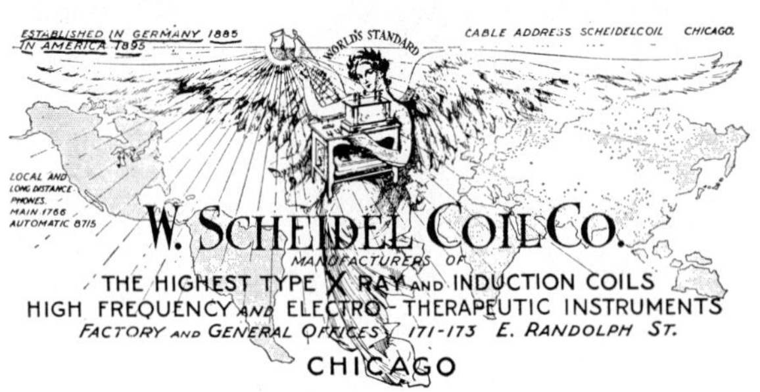

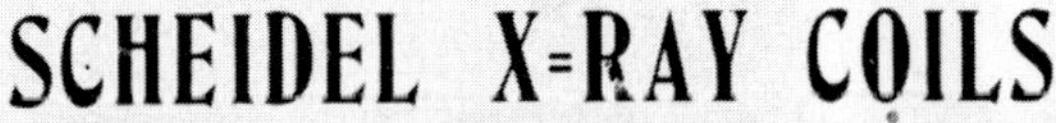

Do you want perfect work with trouble eliminated? Then purchase the **Scheidel**

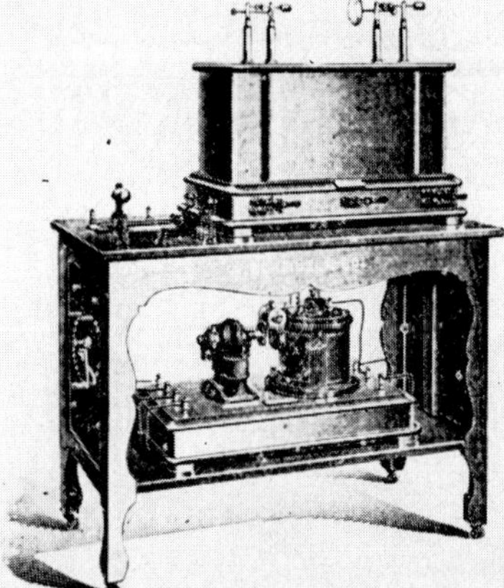

We furnish everything electrical for the physician.

N. B.—You Should write and ask us about our "Scheidel" Special," constructed to do **instantaneous radiographic work.**

"SCHEIDEL"
(The Name is a Guarantee)

OUR REFERENCES:
U. S. Government,
Every large Hospital in Chicago,
Thousands of **satisfied** users throughout the world.

W. SCHEIDEL COIL CO., Inc.
Manufacturers, Originators and Patentees
171-172 East Randolph St., Chicago, Ill.

vived, however, beyond the date on which he would have made Percy Brown's book. In his last years, Scheidel was given a desk in the Standard X-Ray Company in Chicago, which at the time was owned and operated by one of his nephews, Bill Hettich. Scheidel's widow was still alive in the late 1950s, but she could not be located, and none of the other living relatives had a portrait of the "first Chicago x-ray manufacturer."

The M & W was the Macalaster-Wiggin Company, with two addresses, 600 Sudbury Bldg. in Boston, and 154 West Lake Street in Chicago. This firm was successor to the glass-blowing segment of the Frey X-Ray Company founded in 1896. In 1897 Frey's business had been purchased by Swett & Lewis, and they in turn in 1902 sold the "glass" portion to M&W. The latter firm was known for their tungsten target tubes, used with heavy generators. Frank Swett became a vice-president of Victor. For some time during the year 1916 Victor Electric Corporation advertised themselves as the successors to Macalaster-Wiggin Co., and gave their addresses as 66 Broadway in Cambridge, Mass., and 737-739 West Van Buren St. in Chicago.

The Victor Co. was founded in 1893 by Charles Frances Samms (1868-1934) and Julius Benjamin Wantz (1873-1952), and their first achievement was to "electrify" a dental "engine" in Wantz's basement in Chicago.

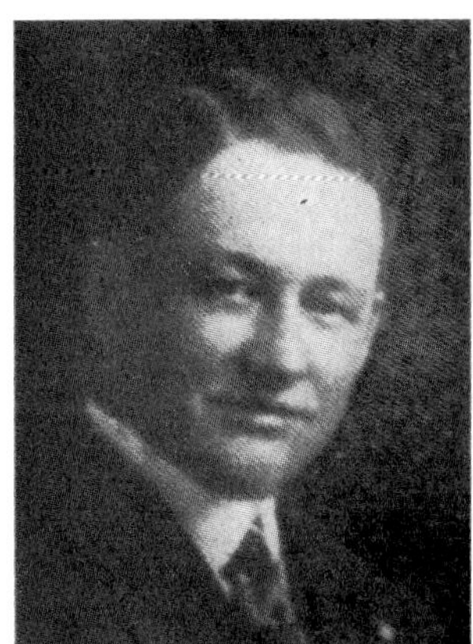
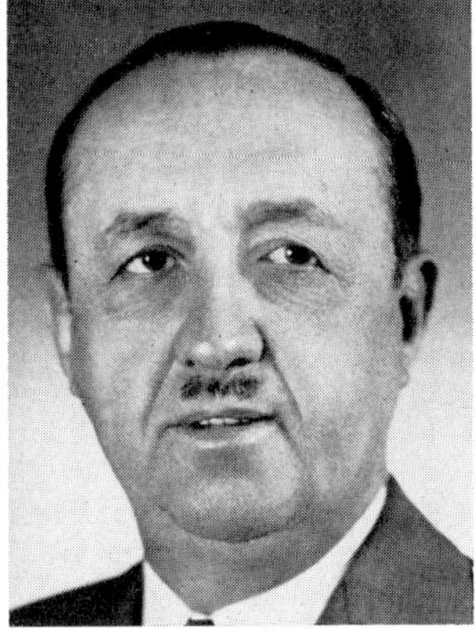

C. W. Howe. Founder of the Western Electric Company — at the time of the merger Howe was made vice-president of Victor, but later turned out to be one of the leaders of the Acme "defection". When GE took over Victor, W. S. Kendrick (with mustache, on the viewer's right) came from Schenectady to Chicago, and became one of GEX-RAY's best salesmen.

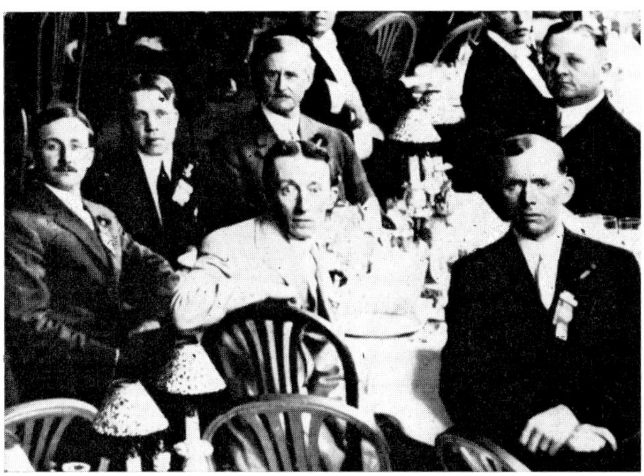

Coutesy: Mrs. Emma (George) Brady.

Convivial X-Ray Table. This photograph was taken on June 16, 1914, at the Sherman Hotel (Chicago) during the fourteenth annual banquet of the American Surgical Trade Association. The surprised lad in the light suit is McFedries (of the McFedries X-Ray Co. at 245 North Wolcott); McFedries' head projects over the chest of the serious-faced William Scheidel; the round head of George Brady can be recognized in the right upper hand corner.

"Western" Mercury Turbine Interrupter and Condenser

For Use on 110 or 220 Volt Direct Circuits

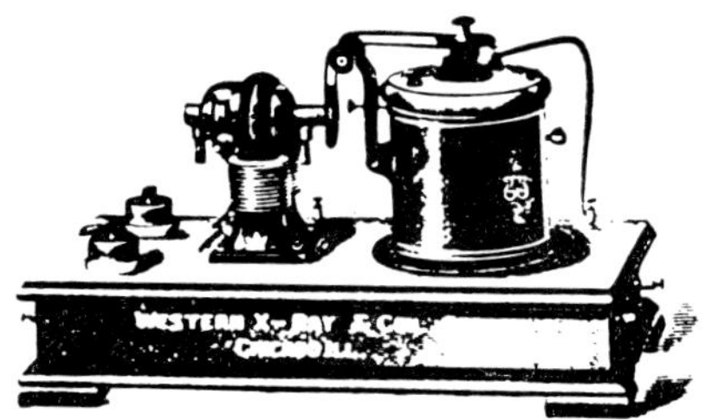

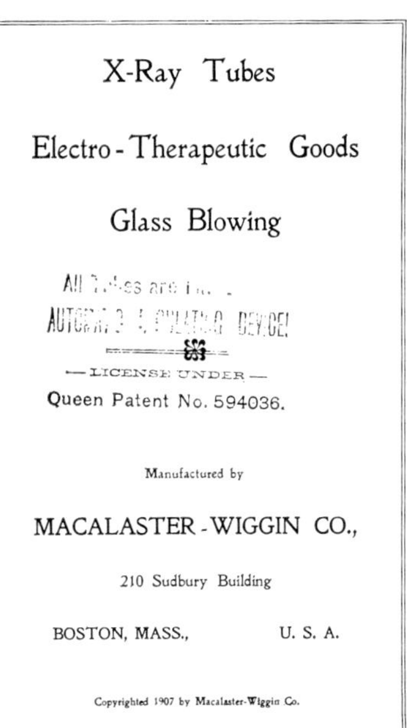

They were incorporated as the Victor Electric Co. in 1895, being then located at 87 on Washington St. In 1896 they started producing static machines for x-ray and electrotherapy. The shop was located at 218 Washington St. Two years later they moved to larger quarters at 418 Dearborn St., and in 1903 they acquired two floors at 55 Market St.

In October, 1910 there appeared an advertisement of Victor, in which they offered for sale a high frequency coil. In 1911, in the *Journal of the AMA,* they offered the Wantz Radiographic Apparatus which was simply a coil, with about 10″ spark. For a short time between 1910 and 1915, they used not only the Victor trade-mark (which was to become so famous), but also a Wantz seal.

In its days of glory — since 1911 — Victor had its factory on the corner of Jackson and Robey (now Damen) in Chicago. After 1916, and until the move to Milwaukee, it was the largest x-ray plant in the United States, and could boast of an impressive accumulation of talents on its staff.

In 1917, Ed Jerman inaugurated the Victor Educational Department, and later founded the American Society of X-Ray Technicians. Elihu Thomson came to Victor in 1920 when GE acquired interest in the company (GE had it re-incorporated as Victor X-Ray Corporation). Victor took over the manufacture of Coolidge tubes and the whole "glass and tungsten" operation was moved from Schenectady to the plant at Jackson and Robey. At one time or another, many other famous names had been connected with GE, for instance Lemp, Langmuir, and W. S. Kearsley, Jr.

Snook did not stay very long with Victor: from 1918 to 1925 he was with the Western Electric Company in Chicago, in 1925 he joined the Bell Telephone Laboratories, and in 1927 he became an independent consulting engineer. Another name which must be recalled is that of Winfield Smith Kendrick (1885-1960): he had been a Coolidge tube salesman in Schenectady, and after coming to Chicago, he grew in stature, and became vice-president in charge of sales. Kendrick is still very well remembered for his efficiency, friendliness, and witty repartees.

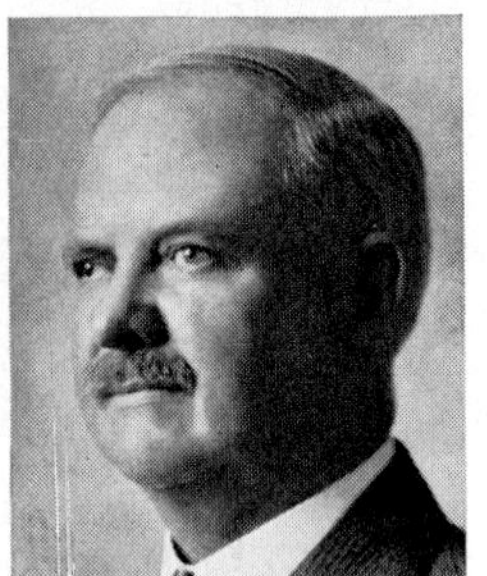

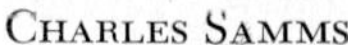
CHARLES SAMMS

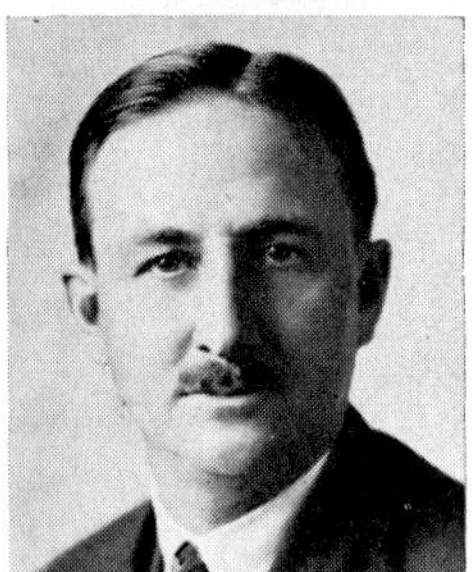
JULIUS B. WANTZ

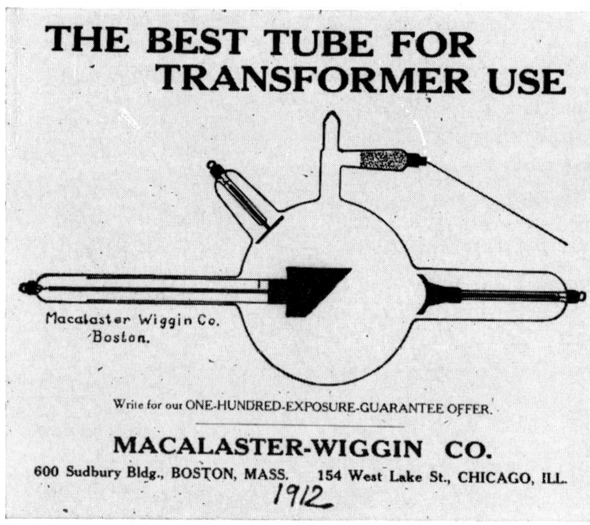

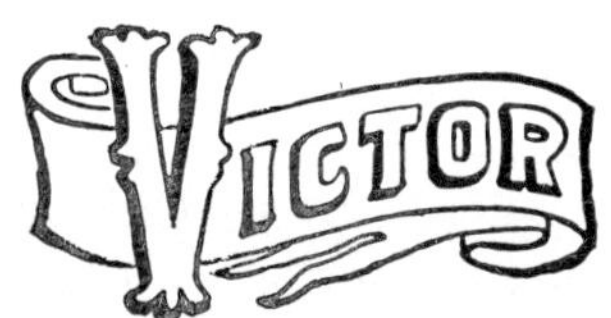

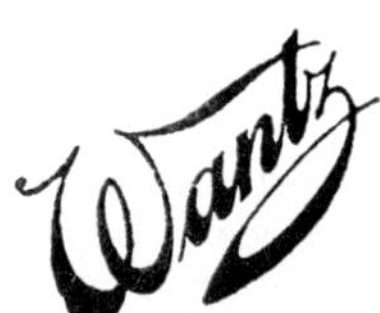

CONFIRMING a DIAGNOSIS by RADIOGRAPHY

—IN BOTH—

Tissue and Bone Structure

generally means that the radiographer must have available two separate X-Ray equipments—one suitable for soft tissue work and one for deep seated bone work.

THE OPERATOR WHO USES THE

Wantz Radiographic Apparatus

owing to the great range and flexibility of the outfit, is enabled at his discretion to show the finest detail of either tissue or bone, as the case may be—tissue radiography requiring a relatively low potential and high milliamperage—these conditions being reversed in deep seated bone radiography.

This is a unique feature in the construction of an induction coil.

AS A COMPANION APPARATUS, WE OFFER THE

Victor Compression Diaphragm Protective Shield and Tube Stand

—a very necessary adjunct to the coil for those who are anxious to secure the best results in radiography.

Means are provided by which the tube can be adjusted to any conceivable position for fluoroscopy and radiography, facilities being such that the tube can be arranged either over or underneath the patient.

SEND FOR DESCRIPTIVE LITERATURE

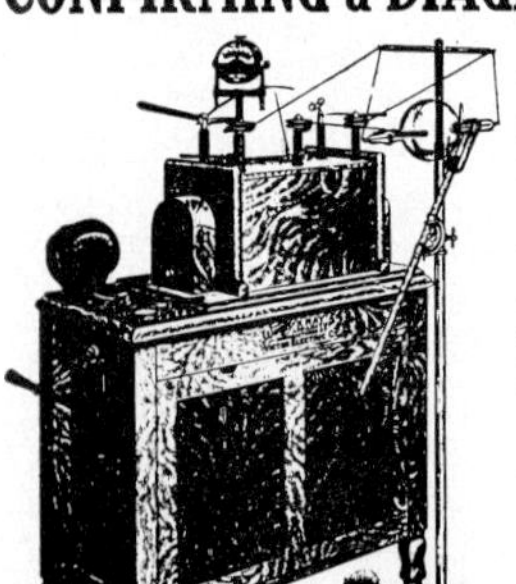

VICTOR ELECTRIC COMPANY BRANCHES AND AGENCIES IN ALL PRINCIPAL CITIES **55 to 61 Market Street, CHICAGO**

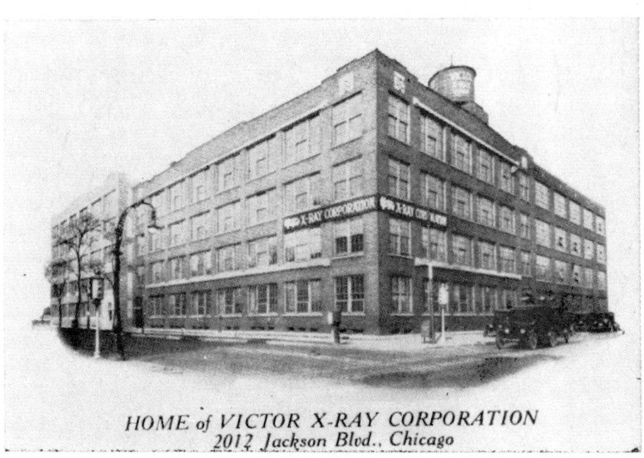
HOME of VICTOR X-RAY CORPORATION
2012 Jackson Blvd., Chicago

Victor created a classical line of x-ray equipment. Most of those who had used it were willing to praise its remarkable solidity (if not its "overweight").

Improved versions of Snook's transformer were sold well into the 1930s. In 1929 appeared the ("100 percent electrically safe") shock-proof* models of Victor apparatus. Its Snook rectifier could be mounted either on a special supporting frame, or in a separate booth. There were two basic control stands, one with black marble; the other had that famous stabilized timer, which was a large circular contraption bolted on top of the controls. Another stock item was the Victor Sphere Gap. More impressive yet was the unforgettable, suspended, king-size ma-meter, and the Kearsley stabilizer with its shaft bringing the switch down to within the reach of the operator's hand.

Around 1923 was introduced the Victor Water-Cooling System. It consisted of a radiator, behind which was located a high pressure pump and ventilating fan, the latter two connected to the motor by an insulating shaft. In 1929 they were mounted "high and dry" to preserve the shock-proof principle.

*The first truly shock-proof x-ray appartus was the dental all-in-one (tube and transformer under oil) machine based on Harry Waite, Jr.'s patent. Equipment with separate units could not be made adequately shock-proof until after the development of high-tension cables by the General Cable Company of Boston.

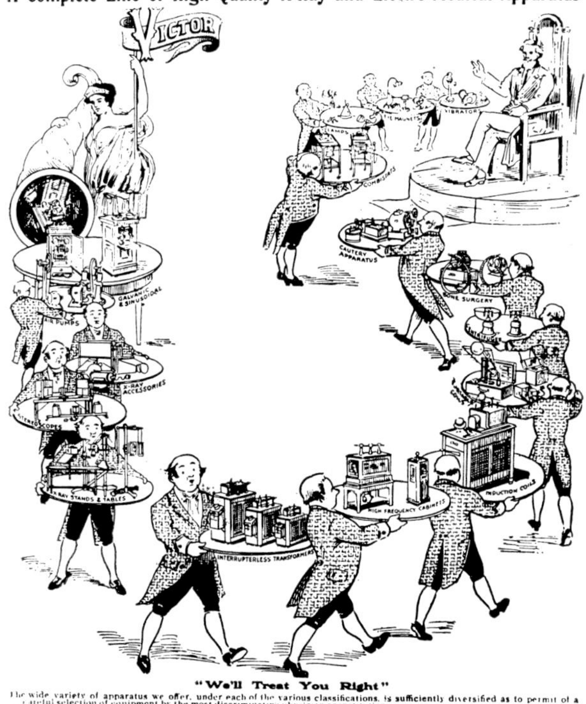

Victor maintained a constant advertising campaign, reaching not only those directly interested in x rays, but also the general public. On April 15, 1925 Victor's New York Branch placed in the hands of the American Telephone & Telegraph Co. in New York an "x-ray picture" of the hand, and had it transmitted by teletype to Chicago. Seven minutes later, a duplicate had been recorded on film at the receiving end in Chicago. After delivery, Victor's experts were amazed at the diagnostic quality of the duplicate, which was immediately passed on to the newspapers.

There was much concern regarding the technical updating of Victor employees. Regular sales classes were held. There were sales competitions between districts: in 1919, with but three months of the year gone, the Minneapolis district turned in their full year's quota of business. The chief at Minneapolis was then F. L. Pengelly. The most successful salesman was Waller, dubbed the wizard from Minneapolis; the *X-ogram* asked sheepishly "when you stick two 110 volt lamps in series with a ground wire, what horsepower do you develop?" The cartoon showed a "wiry" Waller.

At Victor they used both the carrot and the stick. A sample of the latter comes from the same *X-ogram;* "A man's mind is like a pool of water. It must be fed by fresh streams from outside, or it will become stagnant. Just as a machine is a finished product so is the employee who does not look beyond his present work."

Since its inception, Victor worked with independent dealers, who acted as field representatives and gave service on existing apparatus. Victor actively cultivated togetherness among its dealers, but it backfired. One day a group of dealers put their heads together, and decided to compete with Victor. This is how the Acme defection came about. Along that time, GE — deciding to reap more benefits from

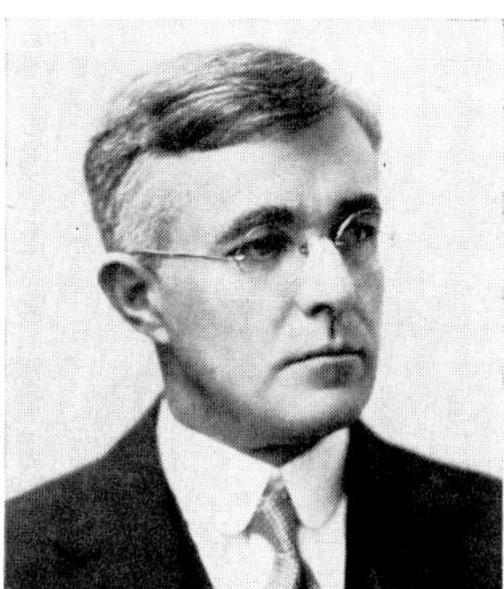

IRVING LANGMUIR. Developed gas-filled tungsten electric lamp, an electron-discharge apparatus, a process of welding using atomic hydrogen, and was awarded 1932 Nobel prize in chemistry for his work in surface chemistry.

Coolidge's hot cathode tube — was investigating several firms in the x-ray business for possible "affiliation." One of those investigated was the Engeln Company in Cleveland, but Victor was more diversified in its "electro-medical" coverage. GE began buying Victor stock, and as soon as they gained control — in 1920 — they had it re-incorporated as the Victor X-Ray Corporation.

Its first main decision was to change the methods of operation, to discontinue all dealerships, and to rely on a factory operated field sales and service organization. Among their personnel, one name was quite outstanding, W. C. Dee, their sales manager in Chicago until 1935.

Victor had many significant "brainchildren." in 1921 Kearsley developed the first x-ray tube current stabilizer. In 1922 a 200 kv machine was installed at Waterstown Arsenal for industrial work. In 1924, Coolidge tube manufacture (which was also done at Nela Park, near Cleveland, since about 1919) was discontinued in Schenectady and transferred to Victor in Chicago. The relationship became closer yet, and in 1926 GE bought all remaining Victor stock: Victor became its wholly owned affiliate, but both Samms and Wantz were maintained as president and vice-president. In 1926, J. Grobe patented for Victor the over-under-table tube mounting. In 1929, Wantz developed an oil-immersed x-ray unit for medical diagnosis, on the principle established by Waite, Jr. a decade before. In 1930, the name Victor was altogether discontinued in the title of the firm which became the General Electric X-ray Corporation (GEXCO).

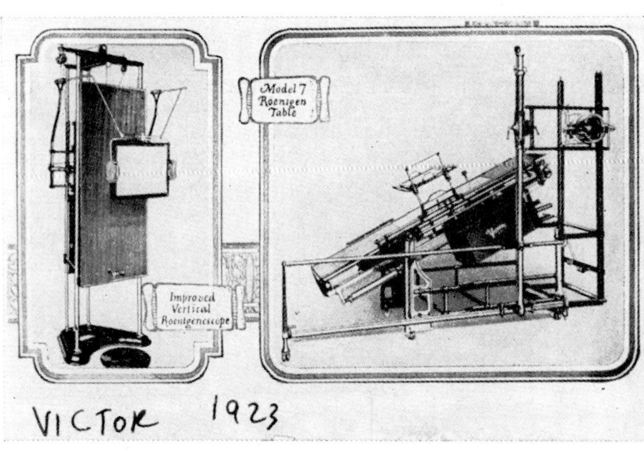

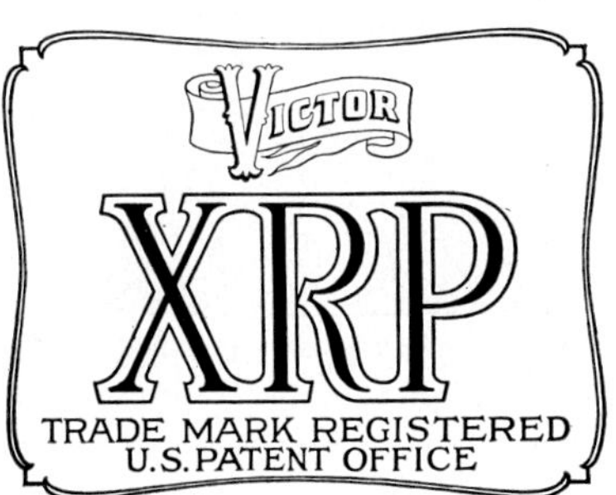

Victor's Brand of Radiopaques

Aside from Coolidge and Gross (who were actually involved in research), the Vacuum Tube Engineering Department of General Electric, first at Schenectady, then at Chicago, had a number of other talents. One of them was Zed J. Atlee. Since that Department was at the time the most important American manufacturer of x-ray tubes, I requested Zed Atlee to provide us with a brief history of the time when he was their chief-engineer. He sent instead (on May 15, 1963) a list of patents, and added:

"It is not a complete list by any means, but I feel it is representative of the range of patent activity of GEX-Ray during the 14 years I was there (1932-1946). Obviously the dates are not those of conception of the ideas or reduction to practice which may have been considerable time, up to several years, earlier than the filing date."

1. U. S. Patent No. 2,090,582: H. Mesick, Rotating x-ray tube; filed February 9, 1934; issued August 17, 1937.
2. U. S. Patent No. 2,118,434: M. J. Gross, Z. J. Atlee, Shockproof cable type therapy tube 220 kilovolt (the original XPT workhorse tube), filed March 16, 1934; issued May 24, 1938.
3. U. S. Patent No. 2,121,630: M. J. Gross, Z. J. Atlee, Oil immersed rotating anode x-ray tube solid tungsten disk type; filed May 11, 1936; issued June 21, 1938.

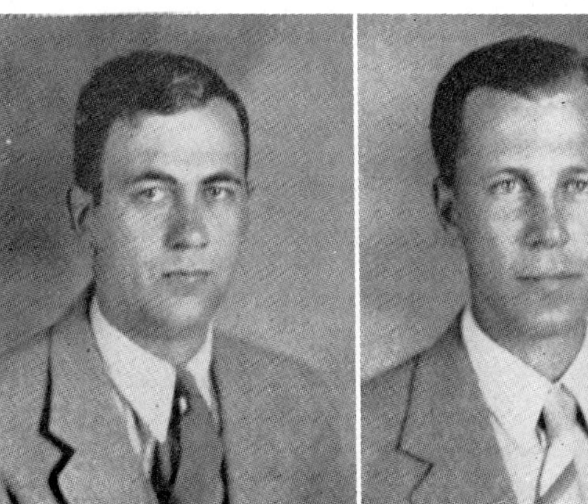
Malvern Gross Zed Atlee

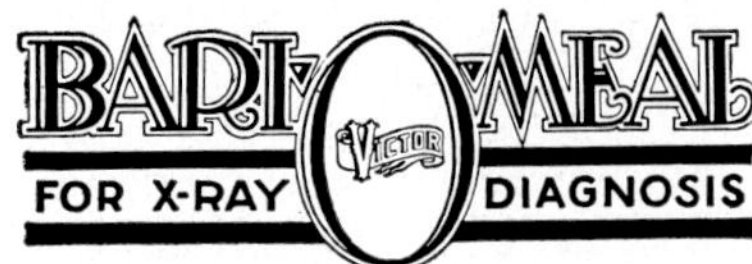

4. U. S. Patent No. 2,121,631: M. J. Gross, Z. J. Atlee, Rotating anode x-ray tube cathode cup structure with angled slots to provide parallel and superimposed focal spots; filed May 11, 1936; issued June 21, 1938.
5. U. S. Patent No. 2,121,632: M. J. Gross, Z. J. Atlee, Rotating anode x-ray rotor construction with squirrel cage vacuum cast copper and ball bearings G.E. tungsten cobalt steel; filed May 11, 1936; issued June 21, 1938.
6. U. S. Patent No. 2,141,860: M. J. Gross, Z. J. Atlee, Oil immersed shockproof cable type radiographic tube unit with double focus and expansion chamber design for easy tube replacement; filed March 22, 1935; issued December 27, 1938.
7. U. S. Patent No. 2,167,275: M. J. Gross, Z. J. Atlee, 400 kilovolt x-ray tube for operation on all circuits including self rectification; filed October 7, 1935; issued July 25, 1939.
8. U. S. Patent No. 2,185,826: Z. J. Atlee, Protective circuit for rotation check of rotating anode x-ray tube; filed June 7, 1938; issued January 2, 1940.
9. U. S. Patent No. 2,230,858: Z. J. Atlee, Magnetic pickup in vacuum to hold bearing wear particles of rotating anode x-ray tube; filed July 13, 1939; issued February 4, 1941.
10. U. S. Patent No. 2,242,100: Z. J. Atlee, Getter in self rectified therapy tube (SRT and SRT-2 types) filed May 26, 1939; issued May 13, 1941.
11. U. S. Patent No. 2,242,101: Z. J. Atlee, Lubrication of bearings by vaporized metallic films of elements such as barium etc., also serving as getter; filed November 25, 1940; issued May 13, 1941.
12. U. S. Patent No. 2,242,182: J. C. Brown, D. C. Braking, For rotating anode x-ray tube; filed November 24, 1939; issued May 20, 1941.
13. U. S. Patent No. 2,256,229: Z. J. Atlee & J. T. Wilson, Four post Lindemann glass shielded x-ray diffraction tube; filed February 12, 1940; issued September 16, 1941.
14. U. S. Patent No. 2,298,335: Z. J. Atlee, Multiple target x-ray diffraction tube; filed September 10,

Mid-West Sales Class Held at Chicago

Week of May 19-24, 1919

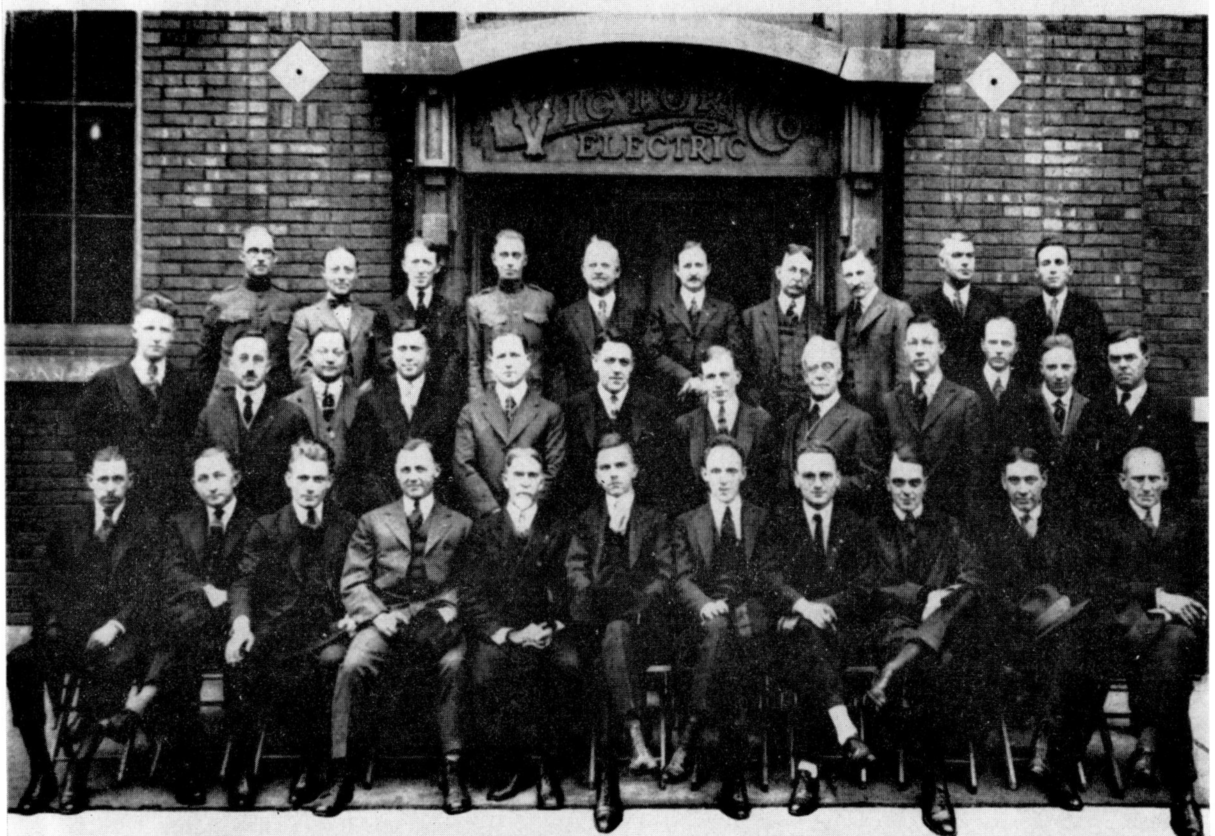

Top Row (Left to right)—Myers, Stiner, McFedries, Robbins, C. F. Samms, J. B. Wantz, F. H. Sweet, White, Jones, Keys.
Center Row—Running, Manuel, Miller, Rosenthal, H. E. Pengelly, Waller, Martin, Wainwright, Reed, Bloomquist, McCorquadale, Kahl.
Bottom Row—BeGole, Taylor, Ovens, Tourville, Ed. C. Jermans, Bolin, Jewel, Ardit, Pennington, Tatman, Schuman

1940; issued October 13, 1942.

15. U. S. Patent No. 2,310,567: Z. J. Atlee & H. W. Brackney, Vacuum tight brazed beryllium window x-ray tube; filed January 8, 1941; issued February 9, 1943.
16. U. S. Patent No. 2,311,724: Z. J. Atlee, Self propelled rotating anode by use of magnetic material cyclically heated through the curie point; filed April 25, 1941; issued February 23, 1943.
17. U. S. Patent No. 2,329,318: Z. J. Atlee & H. W. Brackney, Transmission target gold plated beryllium window x-ray tube; filed September 8, 1941; issued September 14, 1943.
18. U. S. Patent No. 2,329,318: Z. J. Atlee, Multiple element rectifier to provide full wave rectification in one vacuum unit; filed November 12, 1941; issued September 14, 1943.
19. U. S. Patent No. 2,329,320: Z. J. Atlee, X-Ray target for diffraction tube prepared by evaporation in final vacuum; filed April 25, 1942; issued September 14, 1943.
20. U. S. Patent No. 2,332,428: Z. J. Atlee & R. F. Wilson, Thoriated tungsten filament rectifier tube; filed March 26, 1942; issued October 19, 1943.
21. U. S. Patent No. 2,332,422: M. J. Zunick, Electroplated target for x-ray diffraction tubes; filed March 28, 1942; issued October 19, 1943.
22. U. S. Patent No. 2,336,769: Z. J. Atlee, Metal envelope rotating anode tube; filed March 26, 1942; issued December 14, 1943.
23. U. S. Patent No. 2,336,774: H. W. Brackney & J. B. Gosling, Multisection high voltage x-ray tube with interchangeable intermediate electrodes; filed August 18, 1941; issued December 14, 1943.
24. U. S. Patent No. 2,340,361: Z. J. Atlee & H. W. Brackney, Four beryllium window appendages glass envelope x-ray diffraction tube; filed October 2, 1941; issued February 1, 1944.
25. U. S. Patent No. 2,340,362: Z. J. Atlee & H. W. Brackney, Glass envelope high voltage x-ray tube with beryllium window; filed February 27, 1942; issued February 1944.
26. U. S. Patent No. 2,340,363: Z. J. Atlee & F. R. Abbott, Variable focus 400 kilovolt x-ray tube; filed March 3, 1942; issued February 1, 1944.
27. U. S. Patent No. 2,343,729: Z. J. Atlee, Delay loading generator circuit to avoid cracking of tungsten target; filed July 10, 1942; issued March 7, 1944.
28. U. S. Patent No. 2,343,730: Z. J. Atlee, Convex target superficial therapy tube; filed November 30, 1942; issued March 7, 1944.
29. U. S. Patent No. 2,345,723: Z. J. Atlee & J. C. Filmer, Rotating anode diffraction tube of a permanently evacuated type; filed August 17, 1942; issued April 4, 1944.
30. U. S. Patent No. 2,348,184: Z. J. Atlee & R. F. Wilson, Thoriated tungsten filament x-ray tube incorporating method to measure vacuum; filed December 11, 1941; issued May 9, 1944.
31. U. S. Patent No. 2,365,855: Z. J. Atlee, X-Ray tube and high voltage radio frequency generator in same

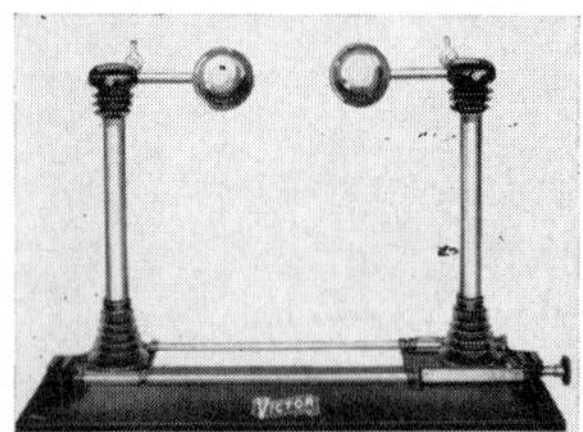

VICTOR SPHERE GAP

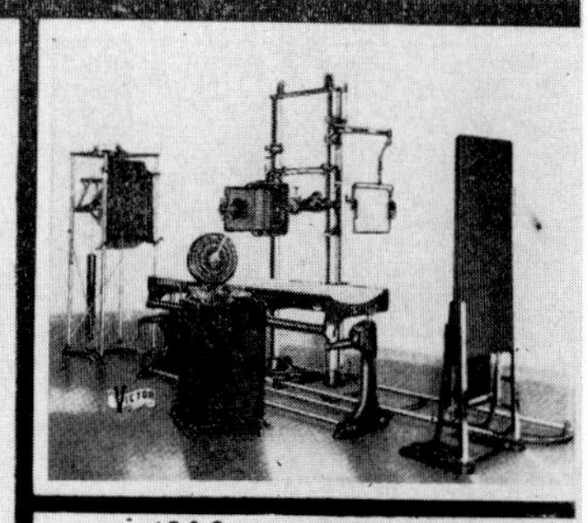

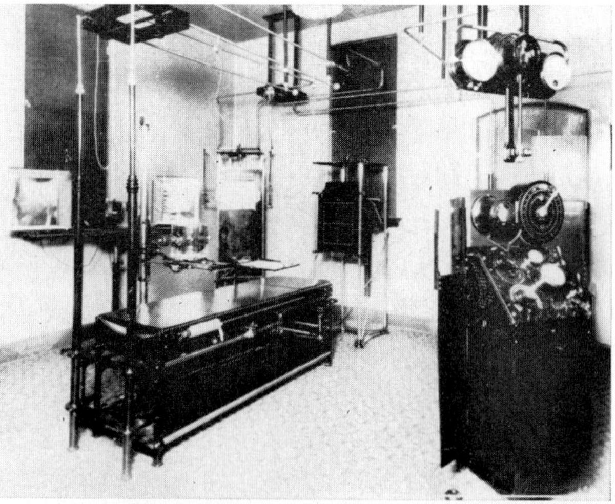

VICTOR INSTALLATION OF 1929. The overhead tubing, the upright stereoscopic chest stand, the large milliamperemeter with the Kearsley stabilizer, and the round face of the timer on top of the control stand are well seen. The Snook mechanical rectifier is in part hidden by the control stand.

vacuum tube envelope; filed December 7, 1942; issued December 26, 1944.

32. U. S. Patent No. 2,387,427: Z. J. Atlee & J. C. Filmer, Gas filled shockproof rotating anode tube housing; filed October 22, 1942; issued October 23, 1945.
33. U. S. Patent No. 2,471,298: Z. J. Atlee, Focussing cathode to obtain multiple emitting filament area; filed October 2, 1943; issued May 24, 1949.
34. U. S. Patent No. 2,477,110: Z. J. Atlee & W. W. Lange, Thoriated tungsten filament high voltage power rectifier tube; filed March 11, 1946; issued July 26, 1949.
35. U. S. Patent No. 2,640,167: Z. J. Atlee & J. B. Gosling, Semi-conducting glass for x-ray tube envelope; filed May 29, 1947; issued May 26, 1953.

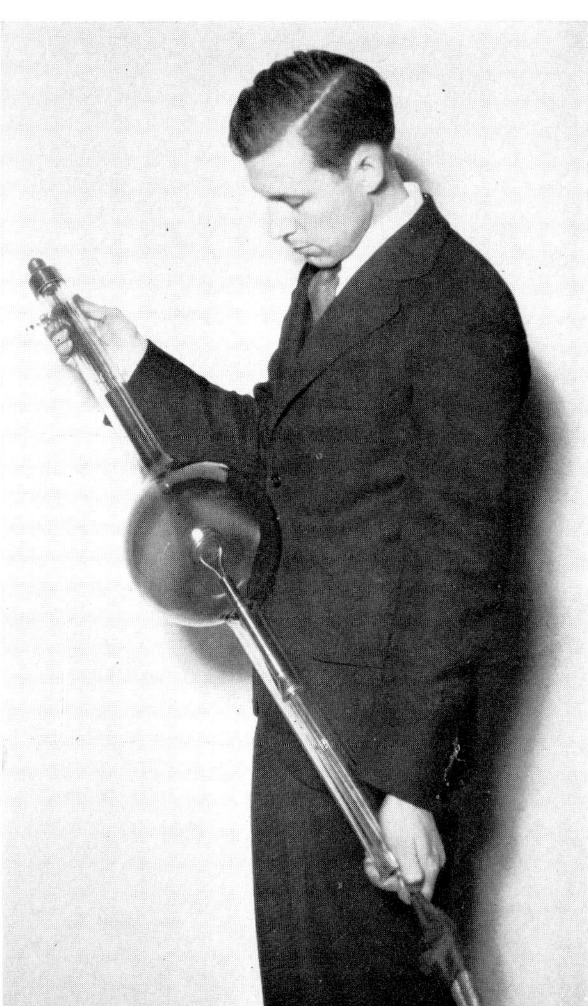

Courtesy: Zed Atlee

GE 440 KVP Tube (1931). This cut, which appeared in the *GE Monogram* of March, 1932, announced the commercial availability of thick-walled tubes suitable for water-cooled operation at 340 kvp and 10 ma; or 440 kvp and 5 ma. This development permitted radiography of four-inch steel forgings in 15 minutes. Incidentally, since 1928 Lauritsen (at the California Institute of Technology in Pasadena) had built 1000 kvp x-ray tubes, and by 1930 Mudd gave 1 mev x-ray therapy to patients.

The flow of innovations continued unabated. 1000 ma diagnostic and 300 kvp therapy tubes were first made in 1931, in the same year in which experimental work with yet higher tension therapy tubes was started at Memorial Hospital in New York City, 800 kvp x-ray therapy units were first installed in 1933, both at Mercy Hospital in Chicago, and at the Swedish Hospital in Seattle. A 400 kvp constant potential x-ray unit was marketed beginning in 1935. The one-million-volt x-ray unit was created in 1939: it incorporated the basic principles of multi-section tube, resonant transformer, and gas insulation, developed through the joint efforts

GENERAL ELECTRIC
X-RAY CORPORATION
Formerly Victor X-Ray Corporation
Manufacturers of the Coolidge Tube and complete line of X-Ray Apparatus
Physical Therapy Apparatus, Electrocardiographs, and other Specialties
2012 Jackson Boulevard *Branches in all Principal Cities* Chicago, Ill., U.S.A.

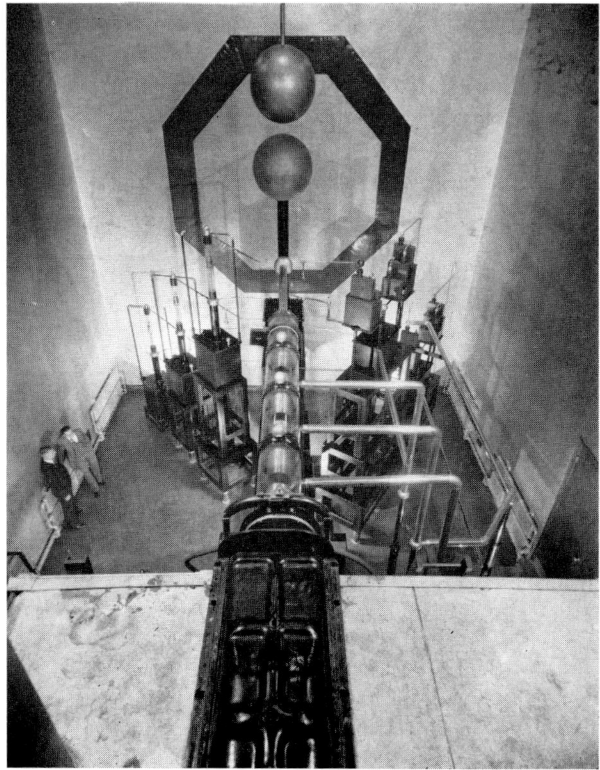

Courtesy: GE Archives.

Multi-section therapy tube. This is the 800 kvp therapy unit installed in 1933 by GE at Mercy Hospital (Chicago).

of T. E. Charleston, W. F. Westenthorp, L. E. Dempster, and G. Hotaling. On the same principles was then built in 1943 the two-million-volt x-ray unit. In 1944 Glenn W. Files introduced the high-ratio Bucky-Potter grid, patented in 1946.

Following is the text of a letter by James Thomas Case, requested for, and used by Harry Miles Imboden, Sr. in the historical paper of 1931. The text is herein reproduced through courtesy of (the estate of) Harry Miles Imboden, Jr.

August 11, 1931
Dr. H. M. Imboden
30 West 59th Street
New York, New York

My dear Dr. Imboden:

Thanks for your inquiry. I am sure my machine for deep therapy was the first one manufactured in the United States. Before I went to France, during the war, I had foreseen the coming of high voltage therapy and we had secured from the Scheidel Western Company a transformer which would deliver 196,000 volts. I was unable to use it at anything like its full capacity because I had no tube.

One day, in 1920, I was seated in my office, when a woman was brought in by her husband for a breast treatment. I asked him why he had come to me to Battle Creek from their home (in Fort Wayne), for they had already given her x-ray therapy such as we gave in those days, 125,000 volt stuff. He told me he understood I could give deeper x-ray therapy than ordinarily available. I explained to him that I had a transformer to permit me to give 196,000 volts, but I had no tube.

"I will get you a tube and have it here in two days," he said.

I explained to him that Dr. Coolidge was experimenting with a tube for deep x-ray therapy and had completed one, but that it was not yet on the market. True, Dr. Coolidge had given me one half dozen of his original tubes for experimental purposes at the same time he gave some to Dr. Cole, of New York, back in 1913, I think; but I could not ask Dr. Coolidge for a treatment tube.

My visitor said: "All right, I will telephone him tonight."

I continued to explain that Dr. Coolidge was a scientist; that when he got ready to put the tube on the market, he would do so; and that I could not *ask* him for a tube, although I would be very glad to accept one if he offered one to me.

My visitor then said: "All right, I will have a tube here in 48 hours."

"Who are you, anyhow?" I asked.

"I am the General Manager of the Fort Wayne Branch of the General Electric Company," answered my visitor.

I immediately warmed up to the fact and asked not only that he try to get me a tube but also a heavier transformer. The tube arrived in 48 hours and we promptly burned out the 196,000 vole transformer on

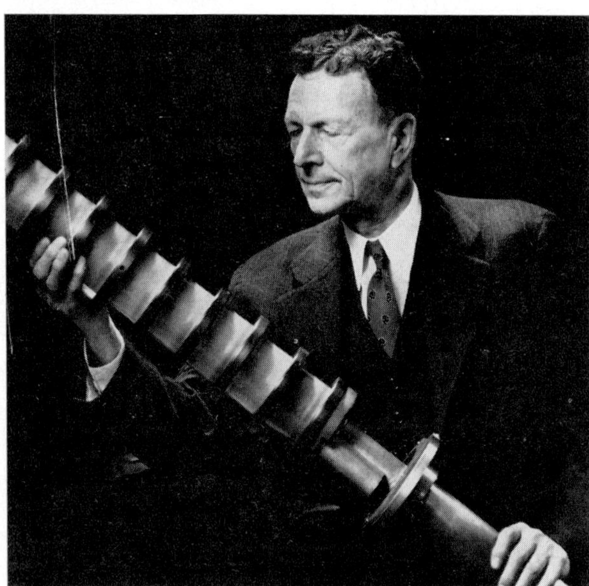

WILLIAM DAVID COOLIDGE recently celebrated his 80th anniversary, on which occasion he received another gold medal. His hot cathode x-ray tube, more than any other single advance, brought about the Golden Age of Radiology.

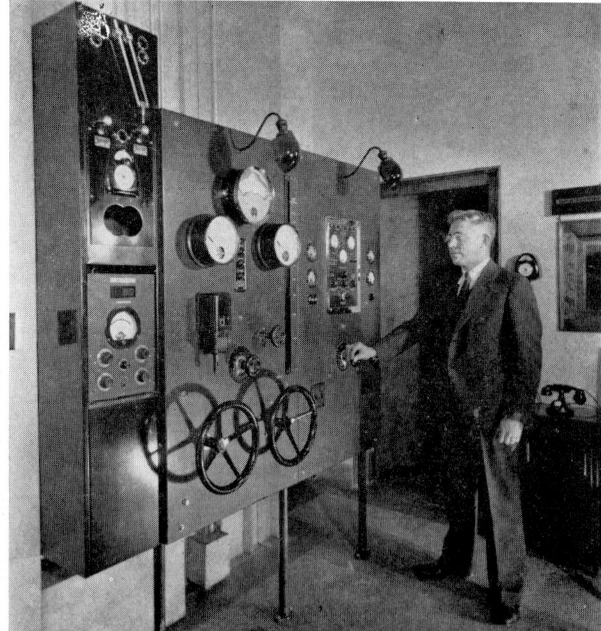

Courtesy: GE Archives

W. C. DEE at the controls of the 800 kvp at Mercy Hospital (Chicago) in 1933.

the first treatment. Dr. Coolidge immediately shipped me a 300,000 volt transformer, and we continued working with this until we received from the factory the 280,000 volt outfit, which was installed at Battle Creek and was the first one manufactured and installed in the United States. Several had been shipped from Germany, one anyhow, but I understand that they were never actively used because they did not have the necessary tube.

This patient, by the way, who had been operated for carcinoma of the breast and had had recurrence, proven by biopsy of a cervical gland, lived nine years before she finally died of the carcinoma. Eight years of that time she was in ordinarily fair health.

It might interest you to know that during the war, back in 1916, when I was attempting to use higher than the ordinary voltage, I was perplexed by the filter. I was able to get up to something like 155,000 or 160,000 volts, judging by the old point to plate spark gap, but I wanted to increase my filter above the four millimeters of aluminum I was then using. There appeared in the Muenchener med. Wochenschrift the first installment of an article by Prof. Kroenig of Freiburg, who recommended copper but the details were not quite complete. The number of the Muenchener containing the second installment of this article apparently did not arrive in the United States, probably for some war reason. So I wrote to Prof. Kroenig asking

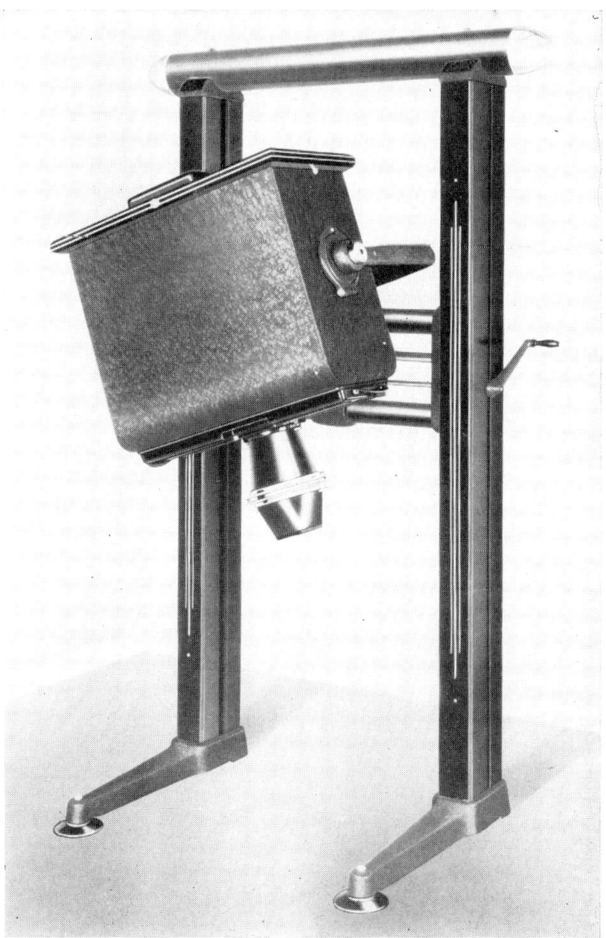

Courtesy: GE Archives

GE MAXIMAR 200. Transformer and tube with all high-tension parts oil-immersed within the (fairly) movable head. This was introduced in 1936, and was followed a few years later by the Maximar 220, more flexible and with higher output; 200 and 220 meant kvp, giving up to 15 or 25 ma.

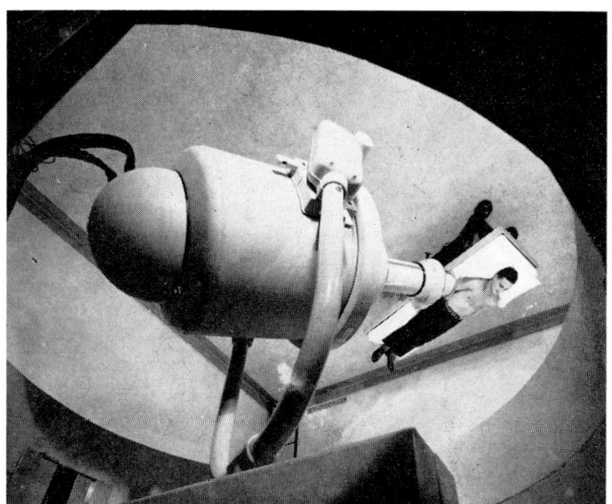

Courtesy: GE Archives.

GE's FIRST MAXITRON 1000. GE's first million volt (supervoltage) therapy unit – resonant transformer with multi-section tube – was placed on the market in 1941.

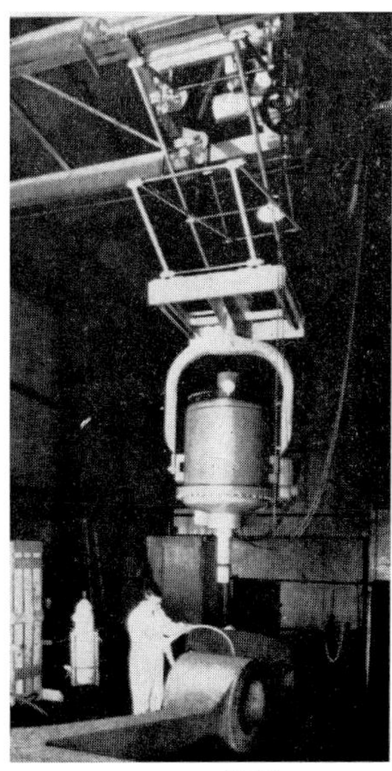

MAXITRON INDUSTRIALIZED. GE's one megavolt unit adopted for radiography of castings during World War II.

whether I should use pure copper or an alloy, and what about dimensions? He replied in a brief letter stating that the filters should be copper and that he hoped I would use pure copper of as large dimensions and thickness possible "so that your munitions manufacturers would have less copper to make explosives for our enemies!"

I really was interested in deep therapy back in 1915 and 1916 and prepared for it, using as high as 150,000 and 160,000 volts before I went to the war in 1917.

Sincerely yours.
(ss) James T. Case
jtc/erm

The passing of the Victor era was concluded belatedly — in 1946 — by closing GE's x-ray plant at 2012 West Jackson Blvd. (a few blocks from Cook County Hospital) in Chicago. They moved into Wisconsin and renamed their "new" street, so that the new address became 4855 Electric Avenue in Milwaukee.

STORY OF THE STANDARD

William Hettich, son of a well-known Chicago jeweler, had learned the x-ray trade from his uncle William Scheidel. Bill Hettich worked later for Wagner's. After the Wagner brothers' death, he took over the remains of the firm, and founded the Wm. Hettich X-Ray Co.: the latter went broke in a few years, only to re-appear as the Static X-Ray Machine Co., located at the same address, 19 Lake Street. Soon another re-adjustment became necessary, and the Standard X-Ray Company — with Bill Hettich as president — was created in 1916 (rumors have it that gambling money furnished a large portion of the initial investment). Standard's location was then established at Throop, Harrison, and Congress in Chicago.

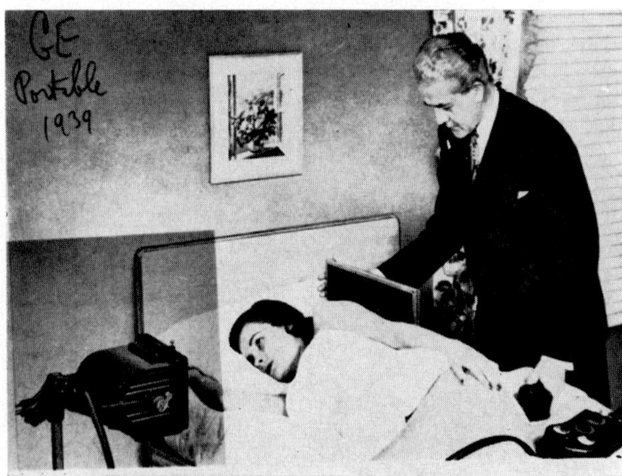

UNADULTERATED ANATHEMA. This photograph from a GE ad on its pre-World War II portable unit is typical of the carefree Golden Age of Radiology.

Standard manufactured very solid equipment, as was customary at the time. In 1917, they introduced the Standard Interrupterless Transformer, guaranteed against breakdown for five years. By then, Standard had already changed its address to 19-21 West Lake Street. In 1920, they had a somewhat primitive fluoroscopic, radiographic, and stereoscopic combination tilt table. But their motor-driven table, dated 1928, exhibited a beautiful, classic line with cast-iron ornamental legs, and other luxuries.

In 1922, Standard had the DM X-Ray Machine, listed at 100 pKv, which meant about seven inches of spark. It was a mobile, mechanically rectified unit, quite noisy, but with the MA-meter right there on the cart.

They manufactured a treatment couch which permitted simultaneous therapeutic irradiation from twin tubes, one overhead, the other hidden in the "couch" beneath the patient. The Standard Lead-Lined Treatment Couch for deep therapy was provided with two treatment ports, one on the top, the other in the front: by turning the x-ray tube 45° on its major axis, two patients could be treated simultaneously with a loss of only about 15 per cent in dose rate. Since at that time most deep therapy sessions lasted an hour or so, this represented a significant gain in time.

A unique development of Standard's was the Limited Capacity Safety Transformer, used to minimize electrical hazards during fluoroscopy and therapy.

This was later available in a combination transformer, as described in a leaflet of the Standard Type "H" 125 pKv machine (printed in March, 1929). There were two primary windings on its transformer, one designated as Full Capacity and used for radiography, when high intensity currents were needed. Due to the size

The Story of the "Standard"

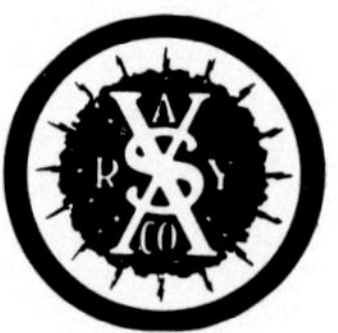

Standard X-Ray Co.
Throop, Harrison & Congress Sts.
CHICAGO
1920

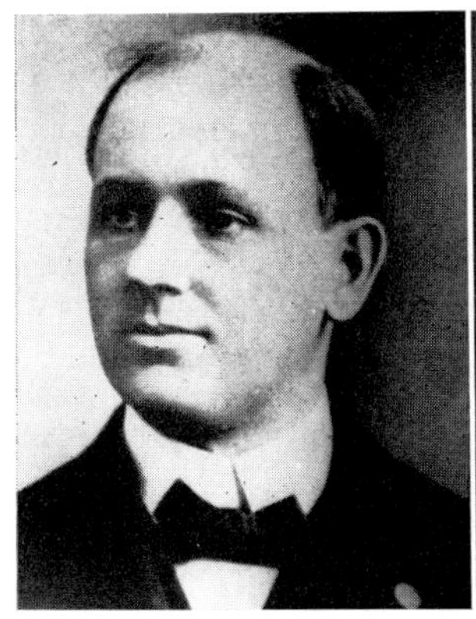
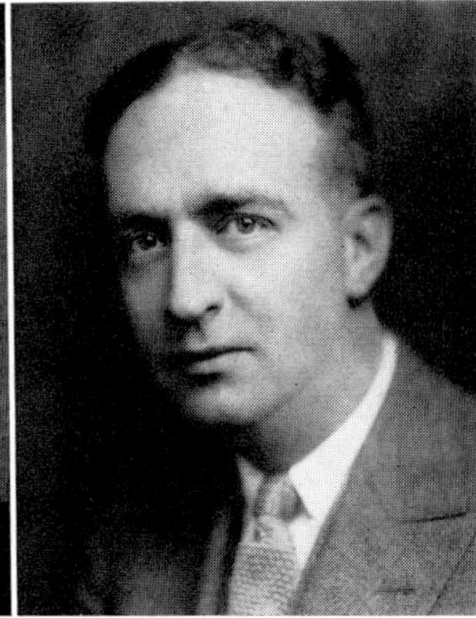

Courtesy: Byron Hess

Rome Wagner and Bill Hettich. In many ways, the Standard X-Ray Company may be regarded as the continuation of the Wagner Co. (the intervening bankruptcies notwithstanding). After Bill Hettich's death, his son-in-law – Arthur Frederick Albert, Sr. – became and still is the president of Standard, but he was adamant against having his portrait reproduced.

BULLETIN No. 8

X-RAY

and

Electro Therapeutic Apparatus

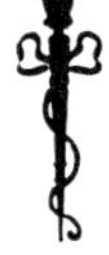

Manufactured by

THE WM. HETTICH CO.

19 West Lake St.

CHICAGO, ILL.

Successors to

THE R. V. WAGNER CO.

Mica Plate Static Manufacturers

and position of the other (the Limited Capacity) winding, great magnetic leakage took place in the high tension transformer as soon as the current from it increased. It was so designed as to operate efficiently only on currents of eight milliamperes or less: beyond that point, leakage became excessive with very slight increases of current. The leakage kept the output of the transformer below practical danger from electrical shock (*i.e.,* from drawing a current very much higher than 8 ma when shorting the secondary of that transformer). A spectacular way of demonstrating this (all of them from Hettich on down through Landauer and Byron Hess were doing it) was to touch the open secondary with the machine in operation, and smile while doing that. But then came along the high-tension cables. Even though these cables were not used routinely until after passing of the Golden Age, eventually the Limited Capacity Safety Transformer lost its reason for existence.

From various viewpoints a most outstanding piece of equipment was the Standard Deep Therapy Tilting Tube Container, a creation of the (previously mentioned) W. C. Dee.

This was another way of obtaining practically shockproof apparatus without submerging the whole thing in oil. The tube was encased in a grounded container, the width of which exceeded the length of available deep therapy tubes. A fan provided air circulation around the tube. It had been so well designed (with a huge lead counterbalance) that it did not have to be bolted down to the floor. Its center of gravity was low, and

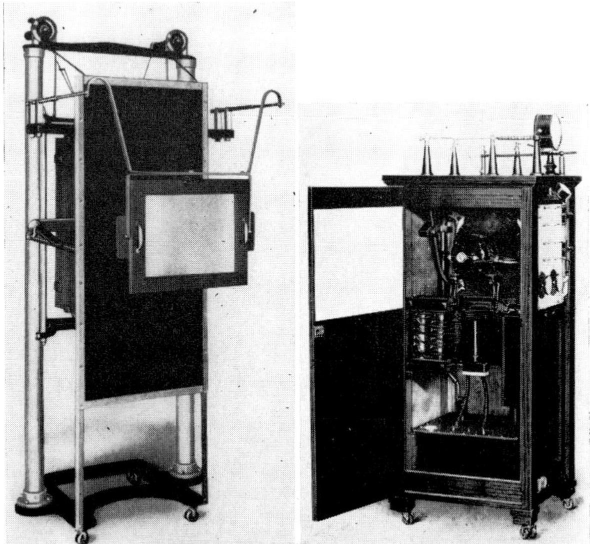

Courtesy: Byron Hess.

Standard Vertical Fluoroscope. This model was first advertised in 1921. The "cabinet" on the right is Standard Interrupterless Transformer. This was one of the company's bestsellers (1919).

none of these units had ever been known to tip over. This masterpiece was also financially successful (by the standards of that era), and several dozens of it were sold — Willis Manges had one of the first units installed in his department. But Bill Dee was just as head-strong as Bill Hettich, and two spiders cannot stay on one web. Dee resigned from Standard, went to GE as sales manager, and thus departed the field of x-ray design.

The first time I heard about Dee was from Robert Stern Landauer, who is the physicist of the Department of Radiology in Cook County Hospital.

In Illinois, Indiana, and Iowa, Landauer was the first (for many years the only, and today the most respected) calibrator of x-ray equipment, as well as all-around adviser on radiation protection and related problems. In the early 1920s Landauer was working for Standard, and he remembers Dee's phenomenal ability as a designer of x-ray equipment, especially because Dee never had any formal training in engineering. But then, only common people require a diploma to prove that they have reached a certain standard of achievement. Those who are really outstanding need no "sheepskin" to demonstrate their capabilities in the chosen field.

Dee designed the tilting tube container, and built a

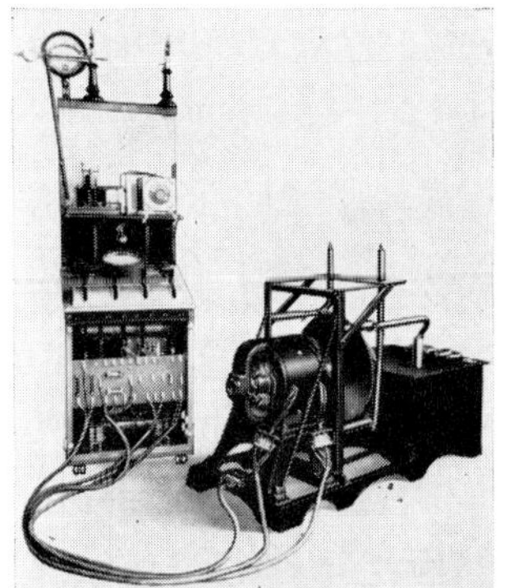

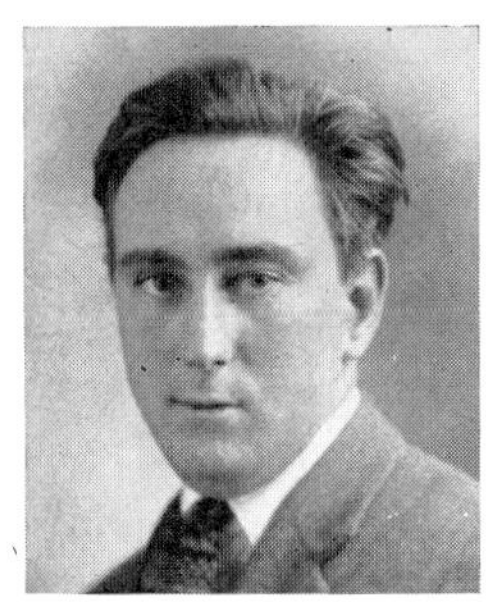

ROBERT LANDAUER, SR.
Courtesy: Byron Hess.

STANDARD'S DISC-TYPE RECTIFIER (1921). Note the spintermeter next to the milliamperemeter on the very top. The portrait is of young ROBERT STERN LANDAUER, SR.

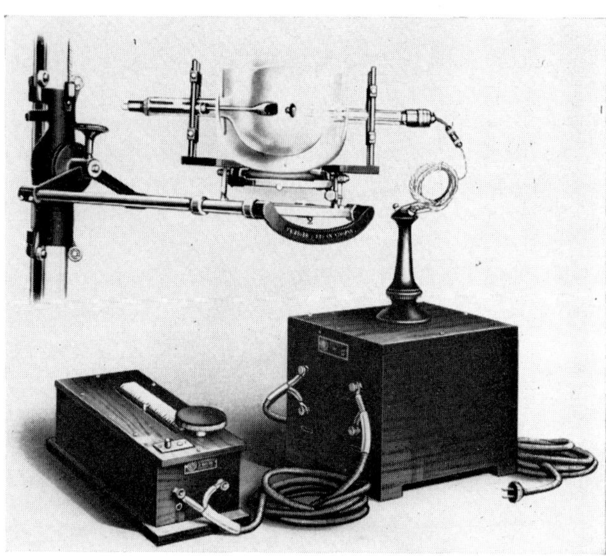

Courtesy: Byron Hess.

STANDARD THERAPY UNIT (1918). Note slender anode stem of the Coolidge tube; the protective lead glass bowl; and the timer, that contraption next to the transformer.

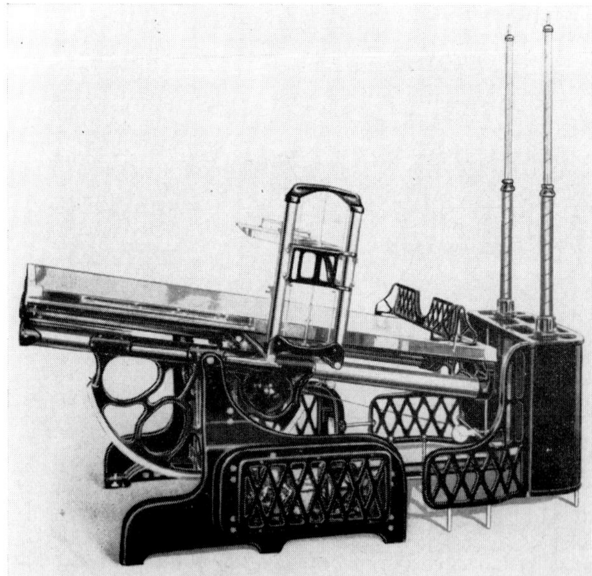

STANDARD LUXURY TABLE (1928). Cast-iron legs, reclining motorized, and overall classic lines.
Courtesy: Bob Landauer.

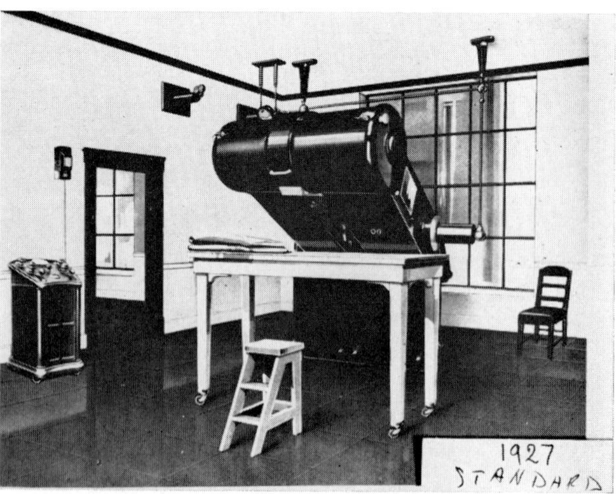

Courtesy: Byron Hess.

TILTING THERAPY TUBE. Standard's Deep Therapy Tilting Tube Container was the creation of Bill Dee, implemented by Bob Landauer.

pilot model just before resigning. This left Landauer to struggle with the menial details. The container had also a "filter case guarding the port in the shell, through which rays emerged." One of its main advantages, also due to the excellent balance, was the ease (finger pressure) with which it could be positioned for treatment. Besides, it was undoubtedly shock-proof.

Landauer earned his PhD at the University of Chicago in 1920 – his dissertation on *Tri-Atomic Hydrogen* (1922) appeared first in three installments in the *Journal of the American Chemical Society* (the first installment in May, 1920, and the others in March and November, 1922). He started with Standard in 1921 and became immediately interested (among other things) in the design and construction of an x-ray measuring instrument to be used principally for the determination of depth doses (there was at that time no widely accepted unit of quality such as the roentgen). The first instrument designed by Landauer was an integrating type of the generic name Ionto-quantimeter. His final version, the 1929 Standard Roentgenometer, had a large ionization chamber, connected by a cable to a large meter. This was again a very successful item on Standard's sale list.

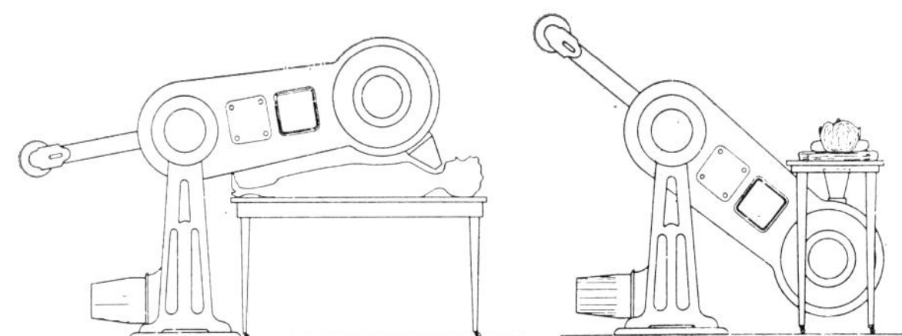

Tilting Therapy Container. It was so well counterbalanced that it could be moved with fingertip pressure; it was never bolted to the floor, and yet none ever fell.

Price-wise, Standard was usually quite competitive. In 1920 the Standard interrupterless transformer, complete with ma-meter, polarity indicator, and cord reels (for 220 volts A.C., 60 cycle) cost $650.

The same, in a deluxe model (Type B) was $790. During the 1920s the Standard X-Ray Screen, hinged to the cabinet, was $40; a Standard Stereo-Tubestand with lead glass screen and one Standard Diagnostic Box (viewbox) $30; and the Standard Stereoscope $95 (while the respective Wappler or Keleket Stereoscope

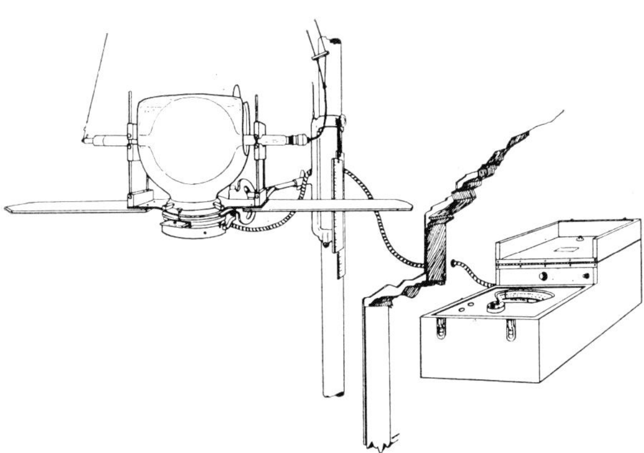

Standard Roentgenometer. Bob Landauer's creation.

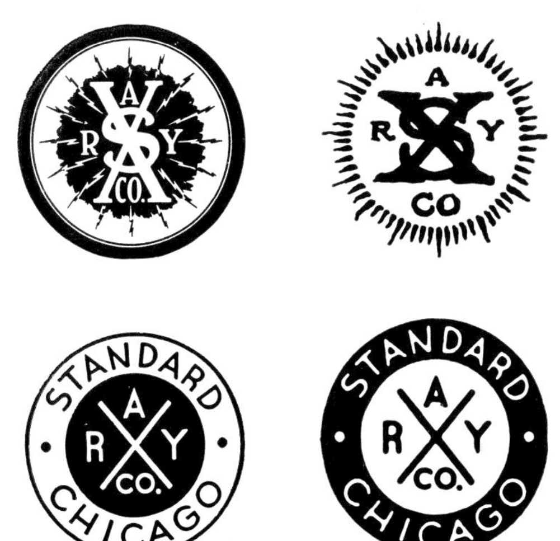

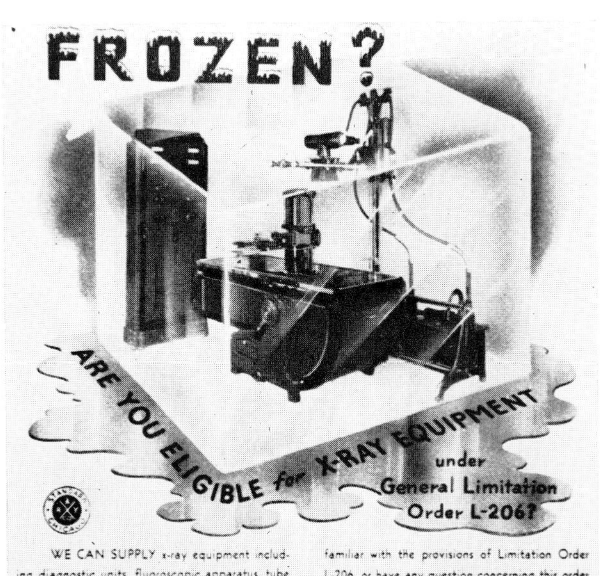

Standard WWII ad. There are always some people who can (know how to) get around the most freeze-proof limitations.

was $150). A complete set of overhead connections, consisting of high-tension insulators, turnbuckles and boards, hoops, wires, etc. was only $20. The Standard Tube Rack for four tubes cost $5. The Coolidge Tube Transformer and Controller was $70; the Coolidge Tube $125; while the 7″ Coolidge Tungsten Target Transformer (valve) Tubes sold for $38.50 each. A Standard Portagraph (portable) was $790; a flat top Bucky diaphragm for 11x14″ films $175; the same for 14x17″ films $260. A Standard Hand Timer with spring mechanism was $53; a motor driven Standard Timer with range from 1/20 to 25 seconds was $175. Another popular item was the Standard Vertical Stereoscopic Cassette Changer, with magnetic release, which sold for $385, while the compression band and winding attachment for the same required another $25.

By far the best known item from Standard's line was their pre-World War II 220 kvp therapy machine, with the tube container supported by one heavy column.

These units were staunchly built, almost indestructible: two of them have been in continuous usage for over 20 years at Cook County Hospital, and are still in good operating condition.

OTHER MANUFACTURERS

Herman George Fischer (1879-1950) — formerly vice-president in charge of all manufacturing operations of the (electrotherapeutic) Sam J. Gorman Co., of Chicago — began to manufacture x-ray equipment under his own name in 1910. The firm was incorporated in 1914 as H. G. Fischer & Co., of which he was president until 1945 when he became board chairman for the balance of his life. At that time his son, Warren George Fischer, took over the firm's presidency. During World War II, the Fischer Co. was located on Wabansia Ave., near Western, where they made mobile dental x-ray units, and units for the services. In 1948 they built and moved into a new plant located in Franklin Park, and have since continued to expand.*

Carl Frederick Dick was a physician who originally practiced in Indianapolis. He became interested in the commercial aspects of radiology, and acquired an x-ray dealership in Indianapolis, first as a Scheidel-Western, then as a Keleket representative. Thence Dick moved to St. Louis and established the St. Louis Supply Company in 1918. In August of 1923 the firm was incorporated as the Dick X-Ray Company with Dick as salesman, while the chief engineer was Ludwig Carl Niedner. At the time they had a franchised Keleket dealership.

Soon the Dick Company expanded to include in its territory seven midwestern states — Missouri, Illinois, Indiana, Kentucky, Tennessee, Arkansas, and Mississippi. Because of the geographical location of its trade area, Dick incorporated in its letterhead a device consisting of a map of the seven states, on which was super-imposed a heart, with the slogan "we serve the heart of America."

During World War I, Frank R. Eltinge — formerly a sales manager for the Defender Dry Plate Co. at Wayne Junction in Philadelphia — started in business as the American Vacuum Glassware Co., with a glassblower named Crozier as partner. They repumped and reconditioned gas tubes, which was then a good business. With the advent of the Coolidge tube, this phase of their activities was discarded, and x-ray plates and

*This information was courteously offered by their publicity expert, Mr. Maurice Henry Sanford.

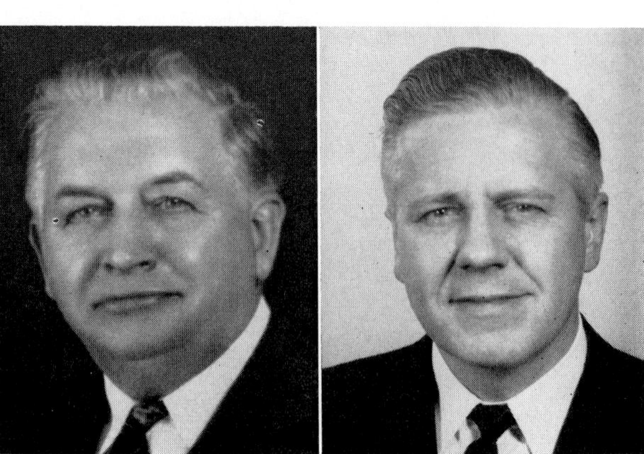

Herman Fischer and Warren Fischer

accessories became the bulk of their sales. The name was then changed to American Vacuum Co.

In 1933 Wm. J. Hogan – former Philadelphia manager of Keleket – joined Eltinge as a partner, and the name was changed to Franklin X-Ray Corporation. In 1935 Eltinge agreed to sell his interests in the company if Charles W. Smith, then Eastman Kodak's representative in Philadelphia, would join the firm. This was done, and in 1939 Eltinge was paid in full. Thereupon Hogan and Smith formed a partnership as Franklin X-Ray Company. They were primarily distributors for Standard in Philadelphia, but produced also their own equipment, especially the well known skull stand.*

A Chicago firm was founded in the early 1920s by the Mattern brothers, who both died in an accident on Lake Michigan. The business was then taken over by Charles Freeman, Sr.

*In 1946 Charles W. Smith sold his interest in Franklin, and in 1959 organized the Pennsylvania X-Ray Corporation, which sells mainly accessories and films.

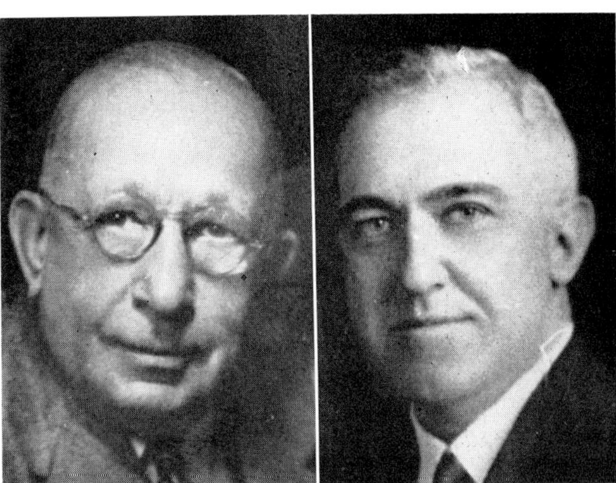

DICK AND NIEDNER. The physician Carl Frederick Dick (with glasses) founded the Dick X-Ray Company. His long-time chief-engineer was Ludwig Carl Niedner. Although independent to some degree, the Dick X-Ray Co. was first a Keleket, is now a Westinghouse dealer.

THE DICK X-RAY COMPANY

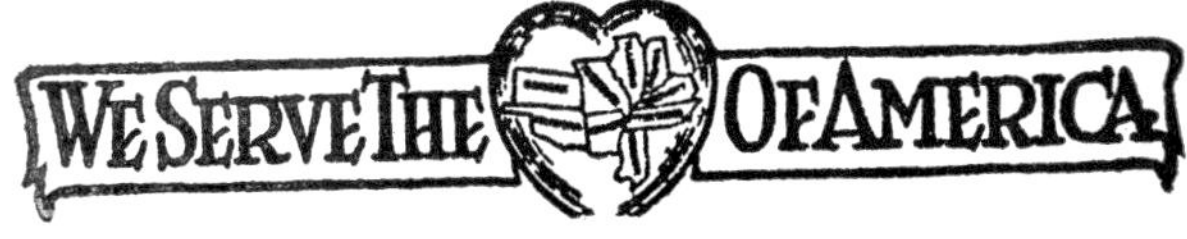

X-Ray Tubes - - - - Supplies
Equipment

American Vacuum Company

F. R. Eltinge, Manager

1011 Chestnut Street Philadelphia, Pa.

Radiology 1928

The Mattern Company had always concentrated on such items as had stood the test of time (with other firms). One of their better models was (and is) called Medalist. As time went on, after several episodes of bankruptcy, they became the wholly owned subsidiary of an electronics firm from California, with headquarters in Chicago (Land-Air). This transaction, made for purposes of diversification, has since been altered.

Universal Vacuum Products was started in 1929 by J. J. Heger (formerly with Ray Machlett at the ill-fated Rainbow), A. E. Begole (disillusioned with Acme), and A. Schoententaur (a glassblower). They commenced operation in Heger's basement at 4047 North Kildare in Chicago, making experimental cathode x-ray tubes for industry and ultraviolet burners for electrotherapists. And they repaired damaged x-ray tubes, of foreign manufacture. In 1931 they moved to larger quarters on Irving, Milwaukee, and Cicero. In 1933 they moved into a three level building at 1800 North Francisco Ave. in Chicago, and began producing their own tubes and small x-ray transformers. They gradually expanded and in 1941 they opened another plant on Milwaukee Ave. In 1947 Merton Moss, an electrical engineer who started and operated Moss X-Ray and Equipment Co., bought one half interest (subsequently the other half) in the company, which had changed its name to the one currently held, Universal X-Ray Products.

In 1934 J. Loyal Worden organized the Continental X-Ray Co., and started the manufacture of x-ray transformers and controls. The firm was incorporated in 1936 by J. L. Worden, P. C. Worden, and J. D. Worden, and has remained to this day under the same management.

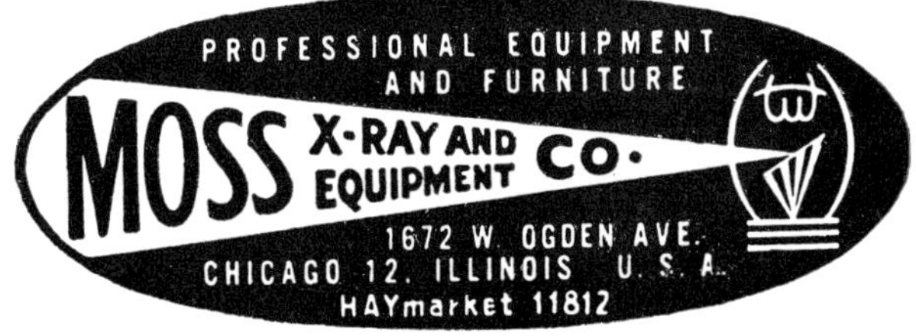

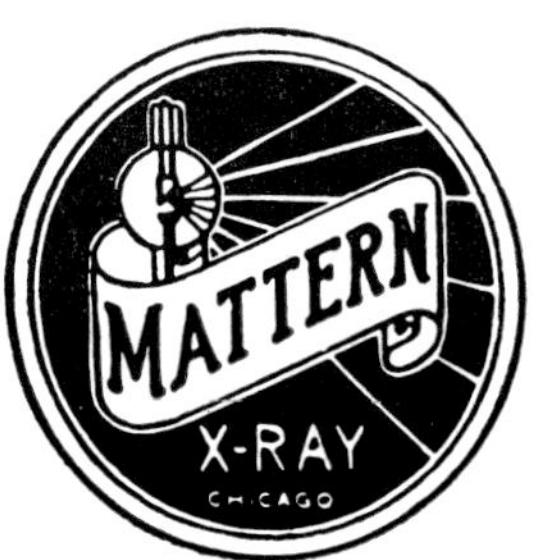

At one time or another, each and every one of these firms built certain pieces of equipment which were excellent. But then, anything that has moving parts, will eventually get out of order. Therefore x-ray equipment is only as good as the service you get on it. This truism has not been sufficiently emphasized because even now many people give more importance to initial price than to quality or availability of service, on that particular brand and in the geographic area under consideration.

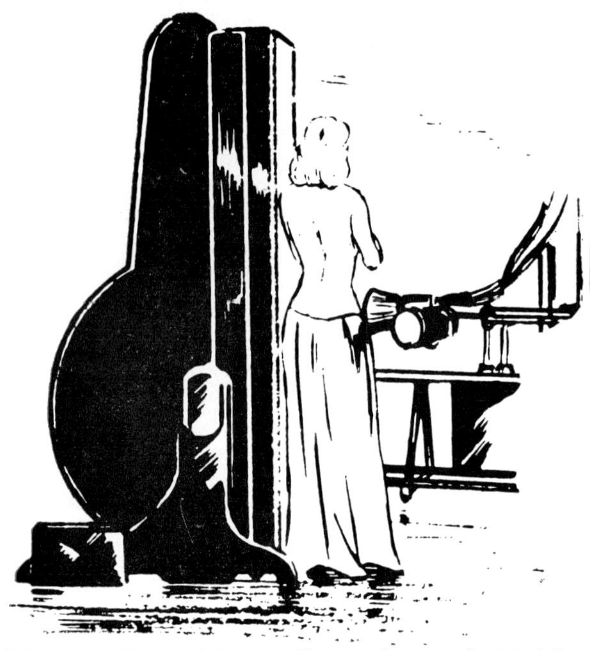

MATTERN TABLE MODEL. Shape of an early Medalist.

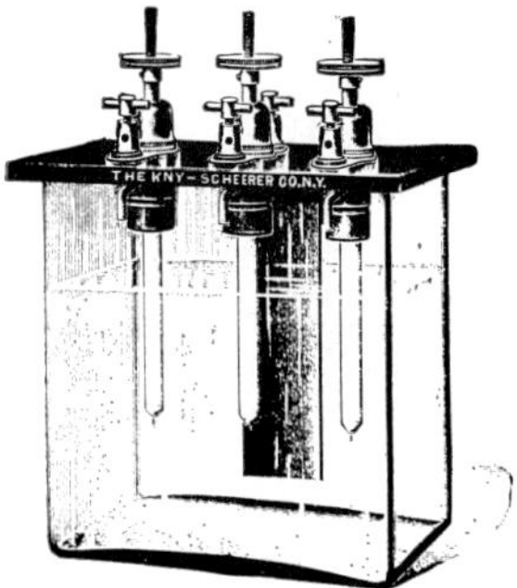

Electrically Heated
Hot-Air Apparatus

For Hyperaemic Treatment

Devised by
Dr. D. Tyrnauer, Karlsbad

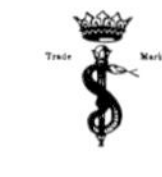

The Kny-Scheerer Company
404-410 West 27th Street
Corner Ninth Avenue
New York

KAYESS PRODUCTS. The Kny-Scheerer Corporation of America made and sold a variety of apparatus, including the Wehnelt electrolytic interrupter, later an interrupterless machine, all sorts of darkroom accessories (the all-aluminum x-ray cassette), as well as physiotherapy equipment, for instance a hot gas-forming contraption.

KNY-SCHEERER

The Kny-Scheerer Company, located in New York City at 404-410 West 27th Street, manufactured a diversified line of electro-medical equipment, from electrically-heated hot-air devices to Wehnelt electrolytic interrupters, and from all sorts of physiotherapy apparatus to the Kayess All Aluminum X-Ray Cassettes. The latter were advertised in 1922 from the firm's new location at 56 West 23rd Street: these metal cassettes had obvious advantages, "no wood to warp or crack open at the corners." Of interest are also the firm's trade-marks, one with a crowned single snake (date: 1914); the other, from their euphonicized initials — Kayess — appeared after World War I.

LIEBEL-FLARSHEIM*

George Henry Liebel (1891-1934) began to manufacture electrical equipment before 1917, when Ed-

*Most of this information was offered by Mr. John Thomas Johnson, currently Sales Manager for Liebel-Flarsheim.

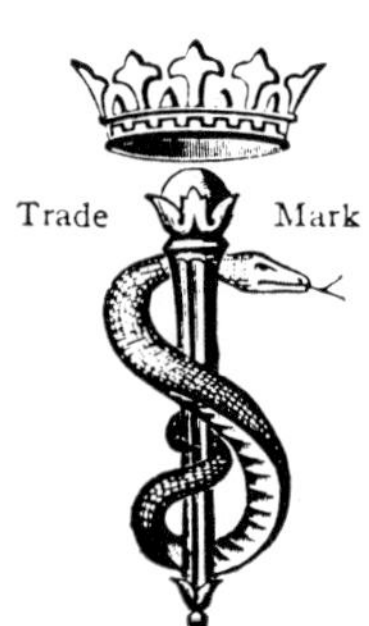

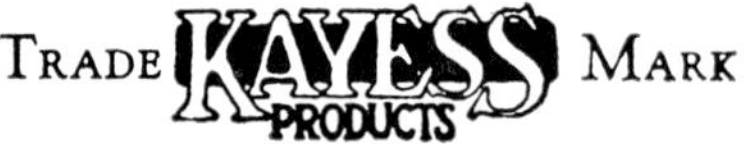

X-RAY EQUIPMENTS
AND HIGH FREQUENCY
APPARATUS *and* ACCESSORIES

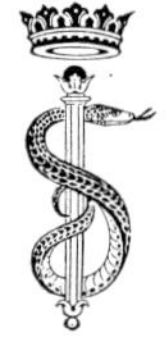

Catalogue No. 15

The KNY-SCHEERER COMPANY
MANUFACTURERS
404-410 WEST 27th STREET
NEW YORK

win Simon Flarsheim (1894-1948) joined him to form the Liebel-Flarsheim Company. It was incorporated in 1917 with Liebel (president), Flarsheim (vice-president and treasurer) Mrs. Flarsheim (vice-president), and Mrs. Liebel (secretary).

They employed at that time six people besides the officers, and were located on Vine St. in Cincinnati, with only 1500 sq. feet of usable floor space. Liebel was the salesman, Flarsheim, the engineer. In 1918, they moved to 410 Home St. into 15,000 sq. feet. There they manufactured x-ray apparatus, treatment timers, hypodermic needles, stethoscopes, and the well known Bovie electro-surgical unit. By 1928, they had moved to Third and Plum Streets.

In 1934, Liebel, who was flying his own plane, went to Cleveland to see Ed Goldfield. Liebel was going to New York and he invited Goldfield to come with him, but the weather was not too good, and Goldfield declined urging Liebel to take the train. Liebel flew anyhow and made it but on his return trip from New York to Cincinnati, he got lost in bad weather, ran out of fuel and was killed in the crash.

Flarsheim took over the presidency and the firm continued to prosper. In 1938, Flarsheim had the first of a series of heart attacks which forced him into semi-retirement. At his official retirement, in 1945, his wife became president of the company, and John F. Otto, its previous sales manager, was named vice president and general manager.

The Liebel-Flarsheim Co. concentrated its efforts on a few well known items including moving and stationary grids, timers, the Hugh Young Urologic Table, and the only (American) Kymograph. Unfortunately, as the Atomic Phase was setting in, because of the lack of demand they discontinued producing the Kymograph, about the time when they became a wholly owned subsidiary of the Ritter Company.

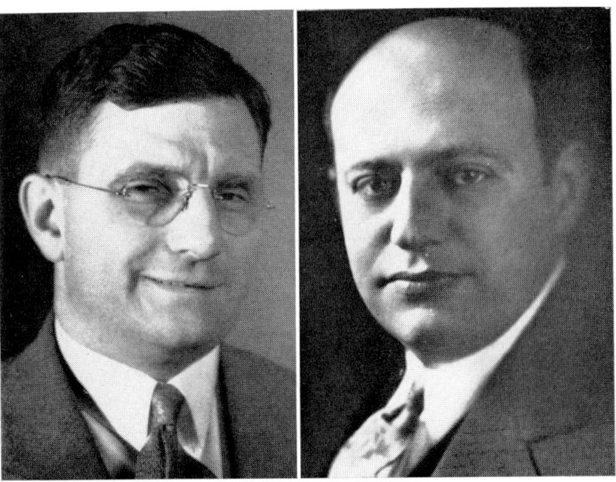

Courtesy: Liebel-Flarsheim Company.

LIEBEL AND FLARSHEIM. George Henry Liebel (1891-1934) and (on the right) Edwin Simon Flarsheim (1894-1948) founded the firm which perpetuates their names.

KELEKET

A famous "x-ray company" was once located in Covington (Kentucky), facing Cincinnati across the Ohio River.

One of its two founders was John Robert Kelley, who studied electricity in the district and grade schools of

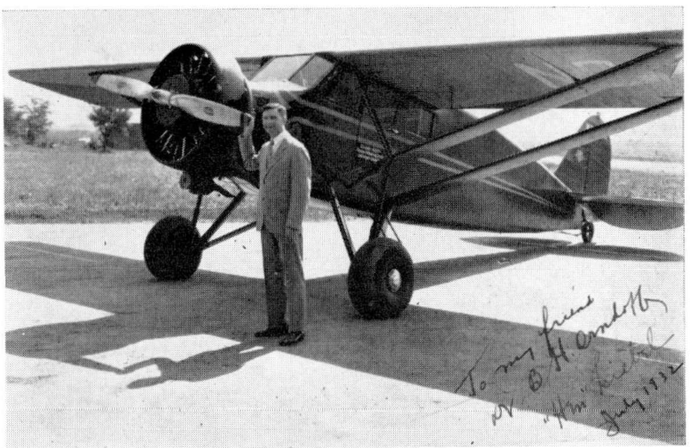

Courtesy: Ben Orndoff.

LIEBEL AND HIS PLANE. Liebel was an ardent aviation enthusiast. His ship, a Stinson Junior, built in the late 1920s, was registered as nr. 6274. The plane's home base was the Lunken Airport, southeast of Cincinnati on the Ohio River. Navigation aids had not yet come into general use, airports were then few and far apart. On a return flight from New York, Liebel lost contact with his landmarks, ran out of fuel, and died in the ensueing crash.

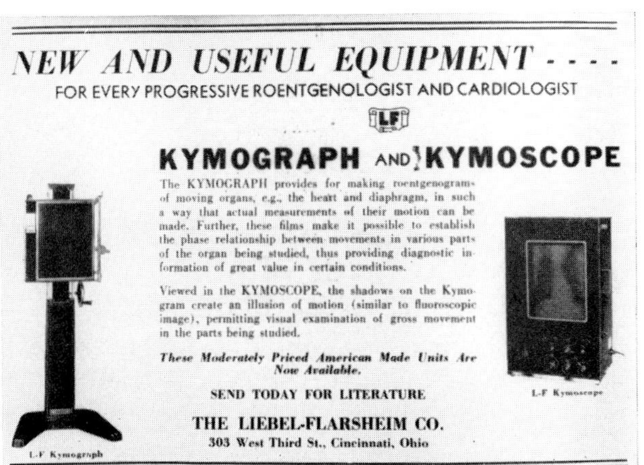

L-F's KYMO. Lack of demand forced discontinuation of this research tool long before cinefluorography made it (almost) obsolete.

Gyles County in his native (small) town Thessalia (Virginia). He moved to Boston, and became salesman for an electro-surgical firm. After Röntgen's discovery he tried to interest that firm in producing x-ray apparatus, but they turned him down. He went to New York City, applied (unsuccessfully) for a job with Waite & Bartlett, then went to Cincinnati where he represented Scheidel-Western.

Albert B. Koett* was born in Weimar (Germany), attended there a technical night school, spent one year in traveling through France, Spain, and Italy, and came to America in 1897. He was first employed as a cabinet maker, with wood-carving and sculpture as sidelines. After naturalization and marriage, Koett decided to "go West" and settled in Covington (Kentucky), where he worked for the Wurlitzer (Musical Instrument) Co. In his spare time he experimented with coils.

The exact date of the founding of Keleket is shrouded in the legends woven by subsequent copywriters. Shortly after Kelley met Koett they decided to go in business together. In 1903, they set up shop in a small shed in the backyard of Koett's cottage.

The first thing they built was a motor-driven rocker for shaking the trays in which x-ray plates were being developed. It was later called the titubator, and manufactured well into the 1920s. Some of the larger models

*Richard Perkins Kincheloe, Sr., a life-long Keleket distributor for Colorado, Oklahoma, Texas, and Louisiana—located in Dallas (Texas)—told me that Koett's middle initial was inserted only to conform with American tradition; it came from the name of his wife, Blanche Koett. Mr. Kincheloe provided also early Keleket literature, and several historic glossies.

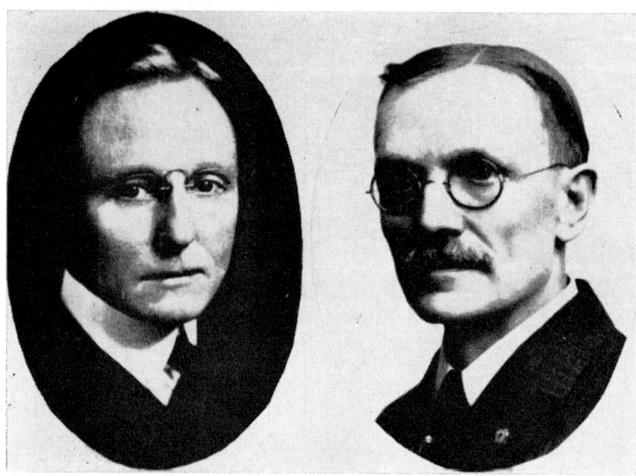

KEL-E-KET. John Robert Kelley (1869-1931), native Virginian, dynamic salesman, and born civic leader and – on the right – the German-born master-mechanic Albert B. (for Blanche, his wife's name) Koett (1876-1954), founded the Kelley and Koett Company around 1903 – it became operational in a small shed behind Koett's cottage in Covington (Kentucky).

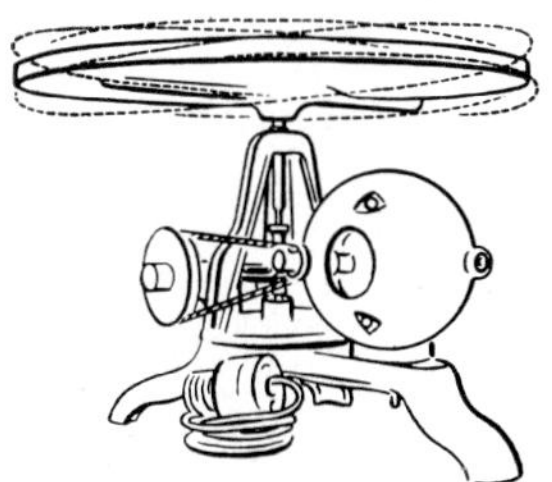

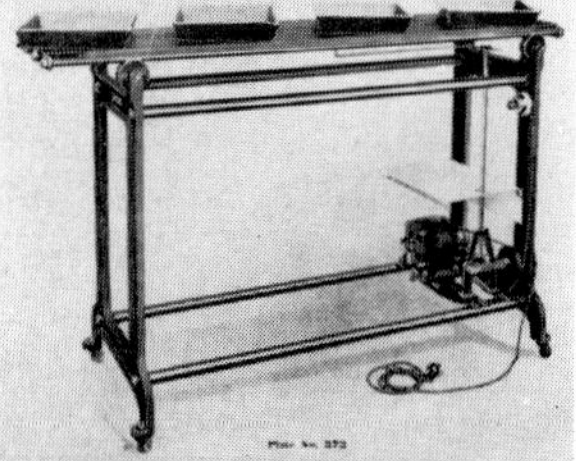

KELEKET'S TITUBATORS. The primitive model on the left (first product marketed by Keleket in 1903) seems puny by comparison with the large-sized contraption of the early 1920's.

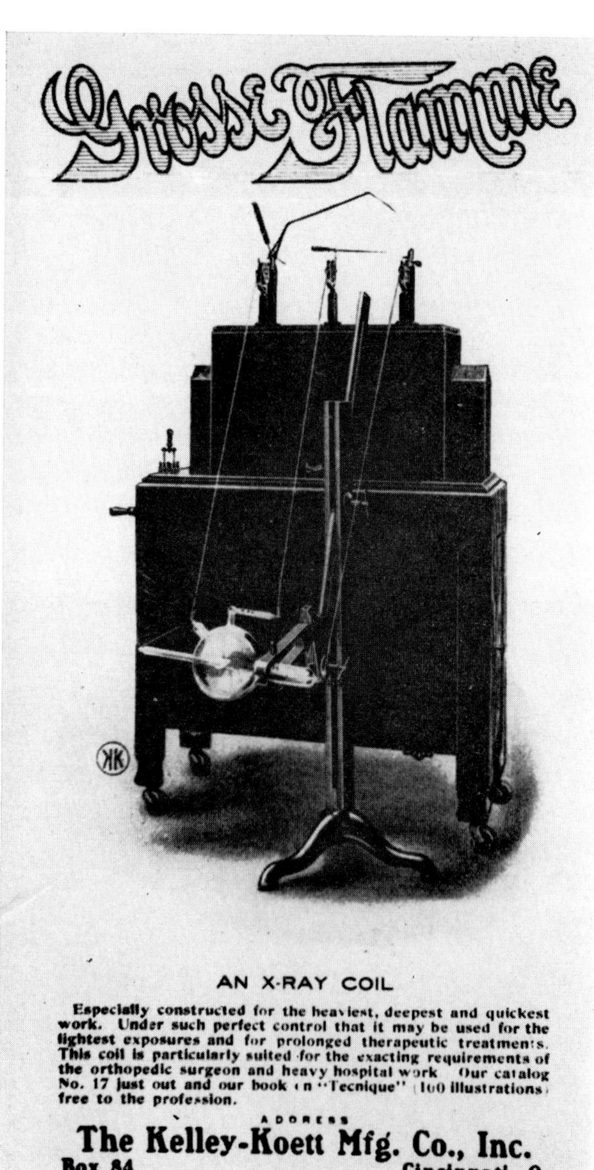

accommodated as many as four trays at a time.

The second item in production was a greatly improved wooden tube holder, selling for $10.00. The third was a compression diaphragm, similar to that of Albers-Schoenberg. Next came a table, and slowly their business picked up.

In 1907, they made their first x-ray coil, which produced a 12″ spark and drew from Koett the (German) exclamation *Grosse Flamme!* It simply means "big flame," but the term seemed very appropriate and was adopted as the name of their then new x-ray "generator." A circus came to Covington, and an elephant was suspected of having swallowed a diamond ring. Kelley was called in to investigate, and Kincheloe remembers seeing in the newspaper a photograph of the elephant on its side, Kelley with a Grosse Flamme coil, and a gas x-ray tube in a wooden tube holder.

An original Grosse Flamme is now on exhibit in the Smithsonian in Washington (D.C.). Incidentally, Ed Goldfield's very first repair job was a Grosse Flamme. He "fixed" it, but then caught a *kleine Flamme* (small spark) in the knee – it did not hurt as much as it scared. He stumbled, and the noise attracted the physician's secretary (female, blonde, young, and pretty) who came in to find Ed sitting on the floor, a bit stunned and certainly embarassed, but otherwise unharmed.

Keleket's plant, located at Fourth and Russell Streets in Covington, was completed in 1917. This information is from an old Keleket advertisement, but Kincheloe, Sr. thinks the building was already in operation when he came in 1914 to work for Keleket as

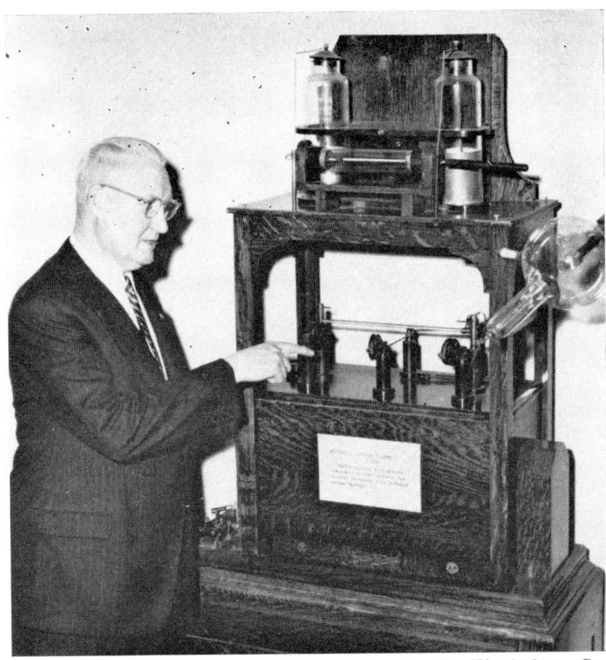

Courtesy: R. P. Kincheloe, Sr.

SMITHSONIAN'S GROSSE FLAMME. One of Keleket's original models of the *Grosse Flamme* coil (first marketed in 1907), on exhibit in the Smithsonian Institution in Washington (D.C.), is viewed by George Edward Geise, one of Keleket's presidents, who died in 1954.

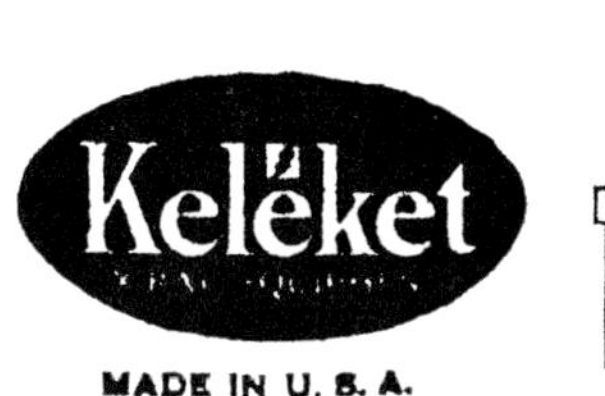

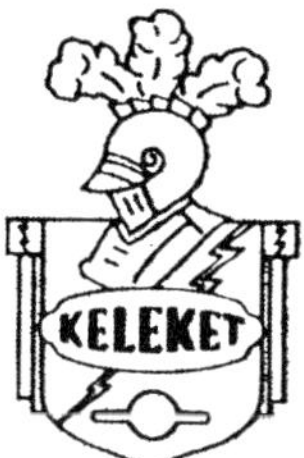

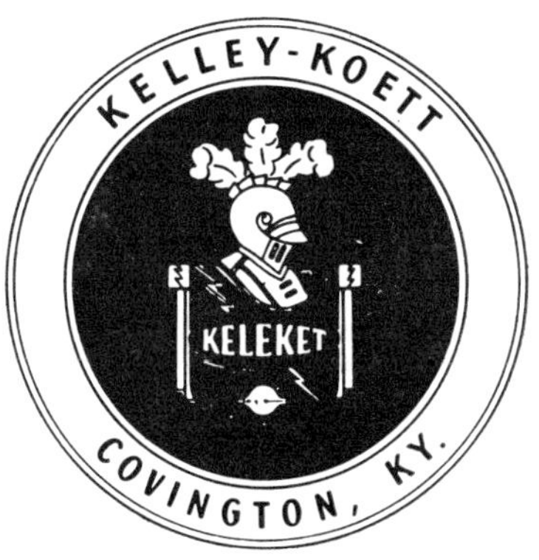

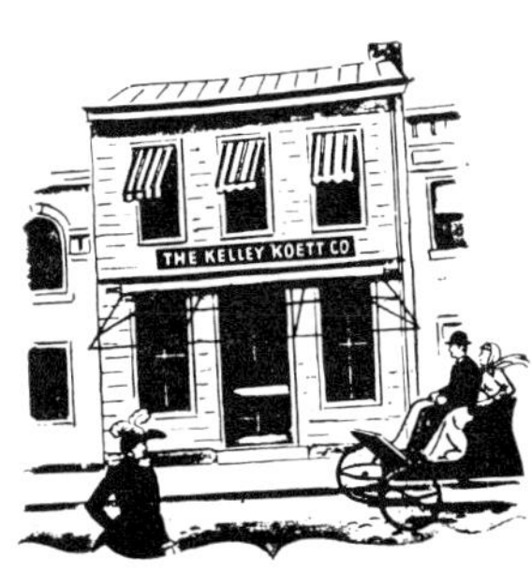

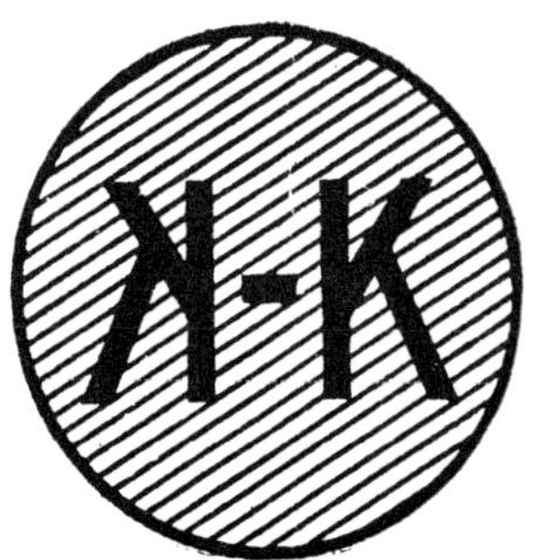

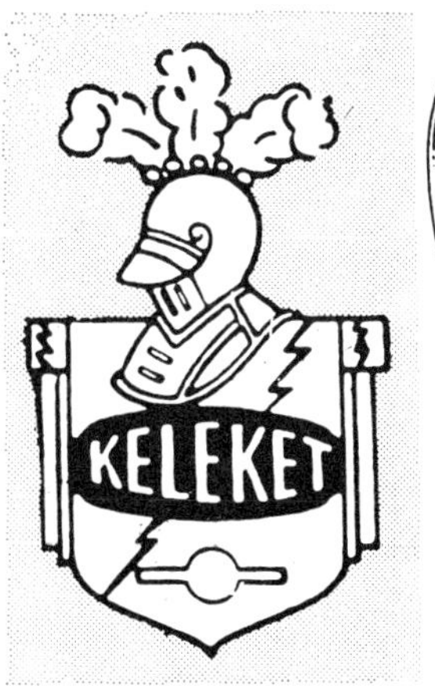

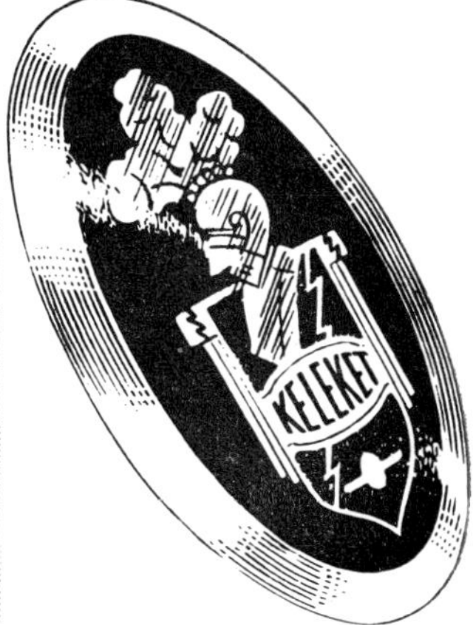

chief engineer. In 1919 Kincheloe went to Dallas as a Keleket distributor, and was quite successful at it, being currently also the representative for Continental and Liebel-Flarsheim. Dick Kincheloe, Jr., a graduate electrical engineer like his father, is presently the second-in-command.

During World War I, 83 per cent of Keleket's entire production was for the government. Indeed, in the U. S. Army X-Ray Manual of the time, numerous illustrations are of Keleket designs, adopted as standards. Hundreds of portable horizontal fluoroscopic tables known as the "Standard United States Army Table" were built. A special ARRS committee had approved the design. While Army red tape held up the order, Kelley — a very patriotic man — ordered production to continue. That order never came, but the tables sold quite well to Civilian purchasers.

The famous No. 6 metallic tubestand, built early after the titubator, incorporated a large pulley, placed

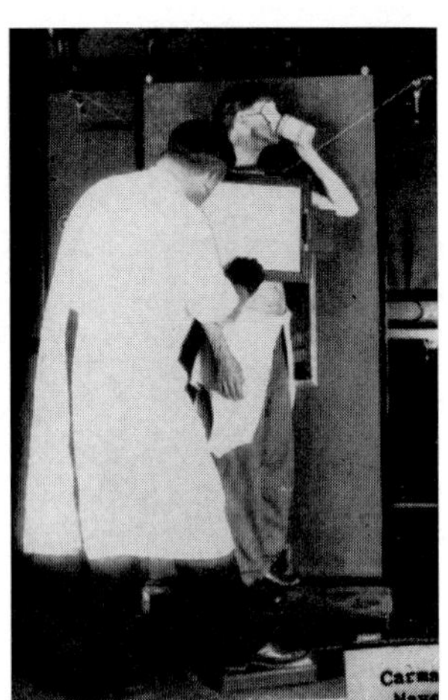

CARMAN AT THE FLUOROSCOPE. Russell Daniel Carman (1875-1926), chief-radiologist at the Mayo Clinic in Rochester, Minnesota, is shown during examination of the esophagus. The machine is a Keleket. Carman laid the groundwork for modern gastro-intestinal fluoroscopy: he is remembered for the eponymic meniscus sign in malignant gastric ulcer (we know today that such meniscus may also be found around benign craters). Carman was in the process of accumulating for publication a series of cases of gastric carcinoma when he himself was found to have an inoperable malignancy of the stomach.

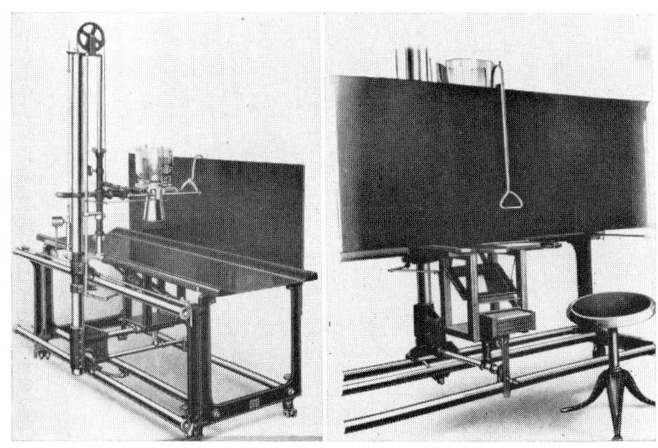

KELEKET SERIAL FLUOROGRAPHIC TABLE. The design was adapted from an idea of Lewis Gregory Cole. Note the oversized pulley on top of the rail-mounted tubestand, and mirror-viewing of the fluoroscopic screen.

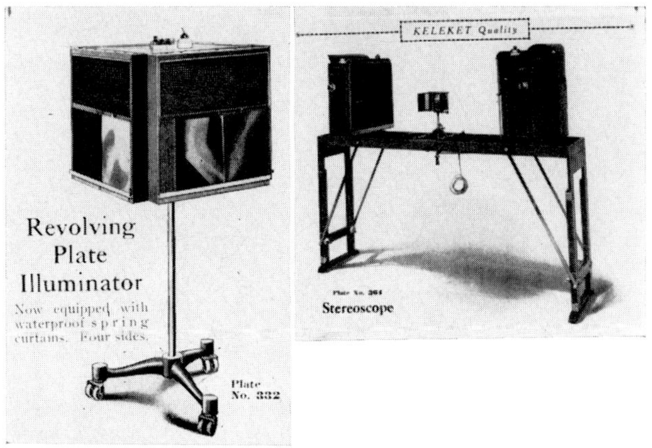

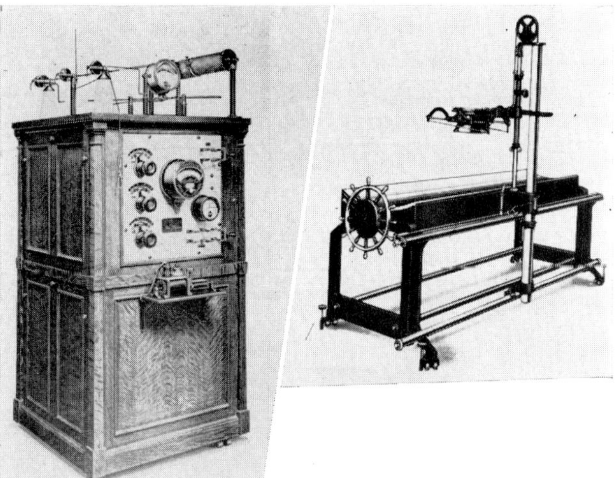

KELEKET LANDMARKS. The constant potential magnetically-controlled interrupterless transformer (shipping weight 1800 lbs.) was rated at 80 kvp and 200 ma. The revolving radiographic table (a Carman design) permitted stereoscopic as well as Bucky diaphragm work with a minimum of adjustment; the diaphragm was connected to the tubestand, so that centering was easy as opposed to the then common way of moving the patient, which was still simpler than trying to align separately the tube and the hidden diaphragm. That diaphragm contained both a flat and a curved set of grids, and both of these were activated by one motor, so that either of them could be used as desired, simply by revolving the table top on its longitudinal axis.

on top to carry the wire for the counterweight. That pulley remained a typical feature of their equipment, indeed Keleket may have been the last manufacturer to hide it behind a cast hood.

Keleket's old trademark had two letters K (like the Kiwanis K), of which the left was seen as in a mirror. Then they introduced the armored knight in various projections, black-on-white and white-on-black, with and without x-ray tubes: finally, they "tilted the coin."

Kelley was a distinguished gentleman, very polished, excellent "mixer" (and esteemed local politician), who had many personal friends in the medical profession. This is why Carman became a Keleket man (just as Lewis Gregory Cole was a Waite & Bartlett man, and Jimmy Case a Victor fan): to this day, the Mayo Clinic shows a certain preference for Keleket equipment. Contrary to Kelley the salesman, Koett the engineer remained most of the time in the background.

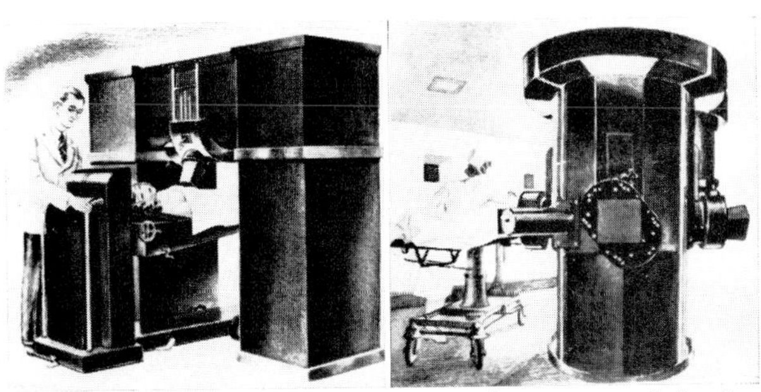

KELEKET THERAPY EQUIPMENT. The unit at left delivered up to 400 kvp, the one on the right, installed at Miller Hospital in St. Paul, Minnesota, was rated at 1.2 mev.

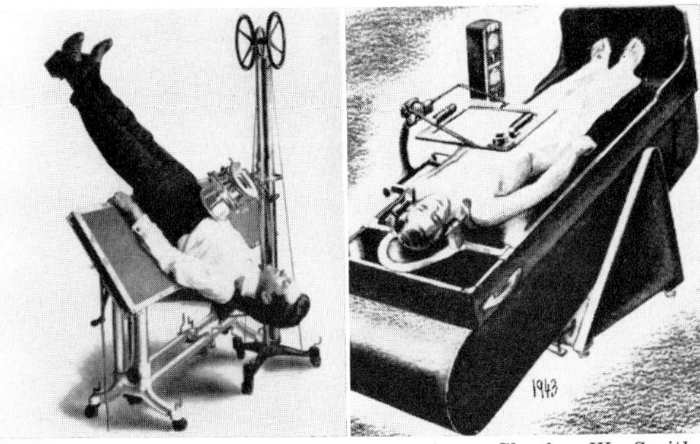

Courtesy: Charles W. Smith.

KELEKET TILTING TABLES. Keleket copywriters go back to 1943 when they claim the first 30° Trendelenburg table in the industry. I found in Charlie Smith's collection of old catalogs (it had been in Pfahler's possession) a leaflet with this 1907 tilting stereoscopic unit. One needed gymnastic skill and vigor to cooperate for the head-down position, but there it is, and it is unbeatable as far as chronologic first is concerned. Its practical value at the time (even today) is debatable – except for a few, seldom encountered circumstances.

A few other memorable Keleket items were the Hickey Universal Sectional Cone, the Keleket single disc rectifying unit for alternating current, their characteristic black marble switchboard with the kv-meter protruding from the back panel, and the mobile and portable models with the immutable pulley.

A unique Serial Fluorographic Table was adapted from Lewis Gregory Cole (who infrequently cheated on W & B): it had a steel plate as a protective shield for the operator. The fluoroscopic image was viewed through a mirror, so that the primary beam could not possibly strike the radiologist.

They had a Revolving Radiographic Table (designed by Carman), with two Bucky diaphragms, one flat, the

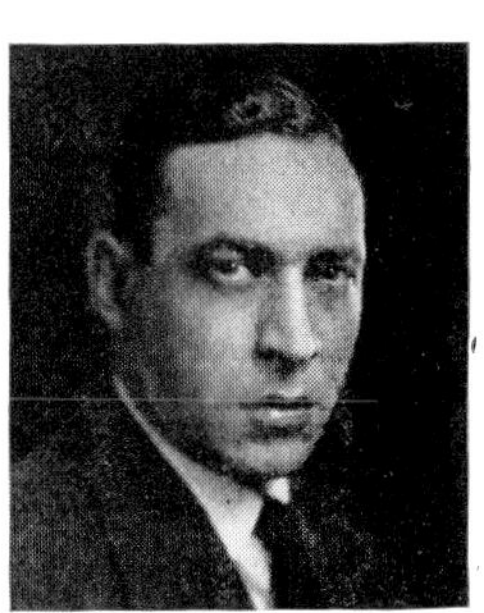

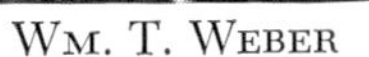

WM. T. WEBER

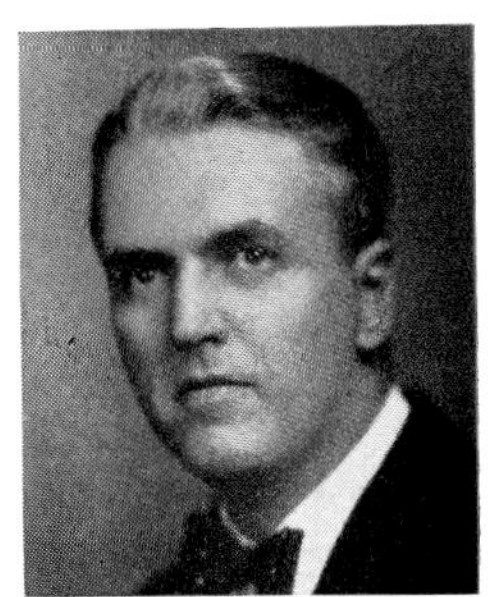

WILBUR STANLEY WERNER

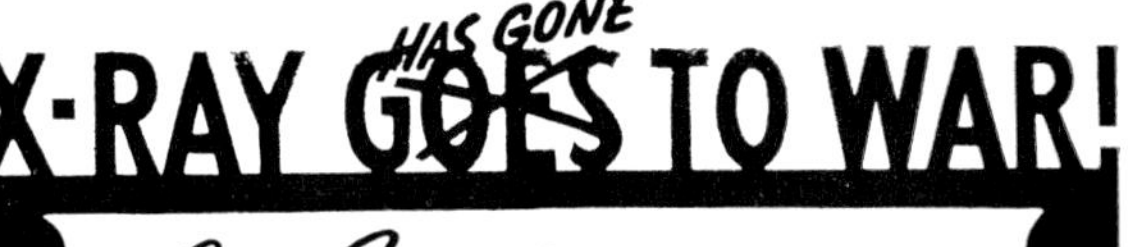

Just Suppose— ALL YOUR X-RAY EQUIPMENT BROKE DOWN Tomorrow!

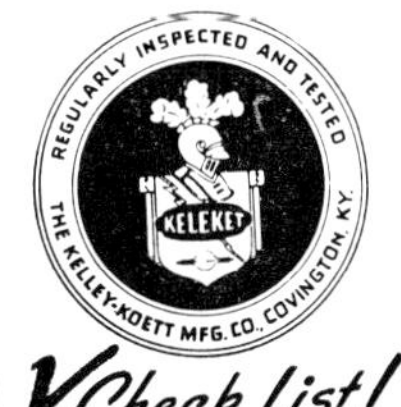

✓Check List!

A few of the important parts of your units that will be regularly checked—both electrically and mechanically.

✓ Controls
✓ Transformer
✓ Aerial System
✓ Tubes
✓ Bucky
✓ Tube Stand
✓ Insulation
✓ Calibration
✓ Darkroom Equipment
✓ Wiring
✓ Switches
✓ Cables

IT'S possible, but not probable. Yet, if only one of your units were out of order, your service would certainly suffer and emergency patients might be neglected.

Sound advice to all owners of X-ray apparatus is to take the best possible care of your equipment. It will have to last a good long time because it is difficult—practically impossible—to obtain any new X-ray units for the duration.

You can, however, prolong the life of your present units and keep them operating at top efficiency through use of KELEKET'S Conservation Plan, now available to you regardless of the age of your equipment.

This wartime KELEKET service provides a periodic inspection of every part of every unit and accessory—both principal and auxiliary equipment. This is not just a cursory inspection, but the most complete and thorough check-up plan yet devised for the accurate checking of the electrical and mechanical systems and the expert testing of therapy and radiographic performance.

Communicate at once with the nearest KELEKET office, or write to us direct to arrange for these vital periodic inspections of your equipment.

THE KELLEY-KOETT MFG. CO., 203-11 W. Fourth St.
Covington, Ky.

Service Engineers in 64 Cities

KELEKET X-RAY CONSERVATION PLAN

PIONEER CREATORS OF QUALITY X-RAY EQUIPMENT SINCE 1900

other curved. These were mounted on opposite faces of one table, and either could be brought "up" for utilization. One of Kincheloe's first jobs at Keleket was to design a "generator" with autotransformer control especially for the Coolidge tube. That autotransformer control precluded the use of gas tubes. Kelley had faith in the hot cathode tube, despite the large focal spot size of early models, and other initial drawbacks. The rail mounted tube stand was another typical Keleket feature. They also used magnetic shifts for stereoscopic work, and constructed a number of special devices such as Carman's Orthodiagraphascope, and Kieffer's Laminagraph.

In 1920 they came out with a constant potential x-ray generator, used for both therapy and diagnosis. They also claimed to have initiated the development of fixed milliamperage, and auto-transformer control, the electronic* radiographic timer, the two way tilting diagnostic table, a telescopic tube carriage, a 1.2 mev therapy unit, and a self-contained 400 kvp therapy generator. Incidentally, one of the latter units is still in operation, after a quarter of a century, in Ottawa (Illi-

*Keleket's copywriter used the term "electronic timer" rather loosely: both Ed Goldfield and Bob Landauer objected to it. They agreed that, during the Golden Age of Radiology, Keleket developed an electro-mechanical-timer which interrupted the entire primary current, *i.e.,* it did not operate through a relay or contactor, and in this respect it was novel. Because it was driven with a synchronous motor, it was reasonably accurate. It certainly had no tubes, and therefore the word electronic timer should not be used for it. The consultants objected to several other manufacturers' claims, but not all their objections could be included in this text. To this particular objection, Kincheloe replied that said Keleket timer — accurate down to 1/120 sec. — was not truly electronic, it was rather noisy, and it cost $500 but it worked.

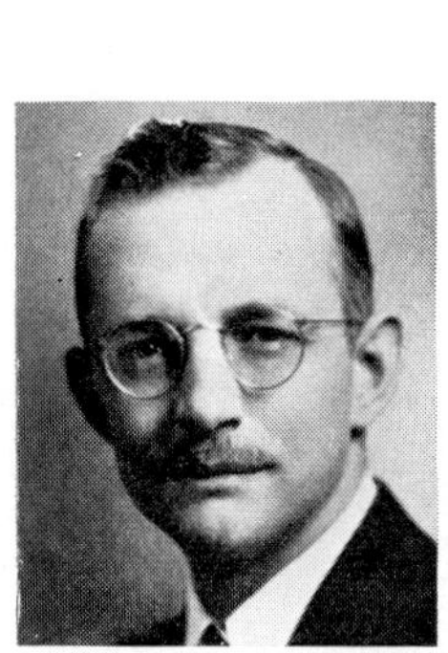

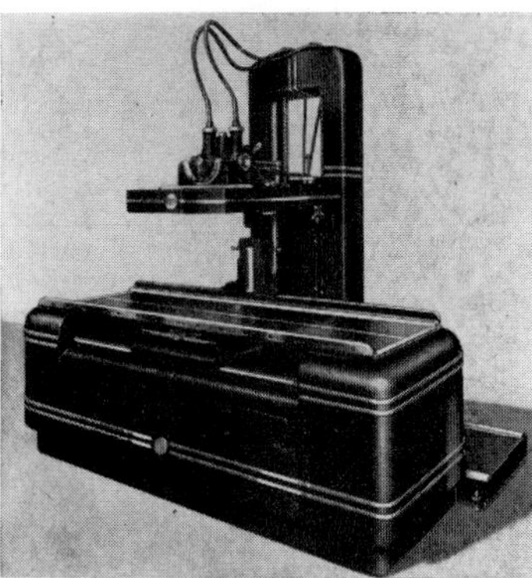

JEAN KIEFFER AND HIS KELELET LAMINAGRAPH.

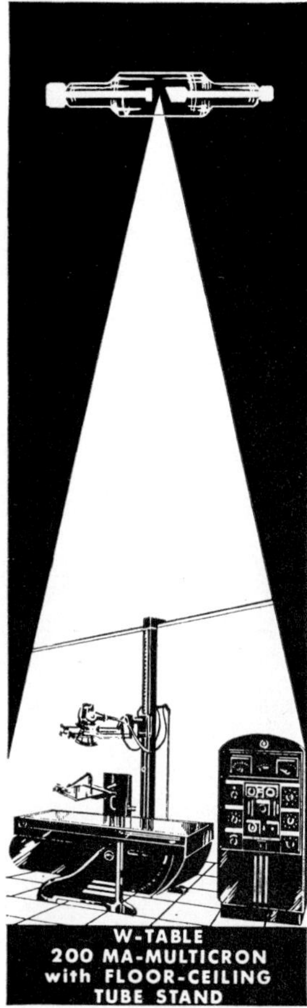

KELEKET'S "ULTIMATE IN X-RAY" (1943). Their copywriter recognized the inevitable obsolescence in the first sentence of the attached advertisement: "If there is such a thing as a last word in x-ray equipment . . ."

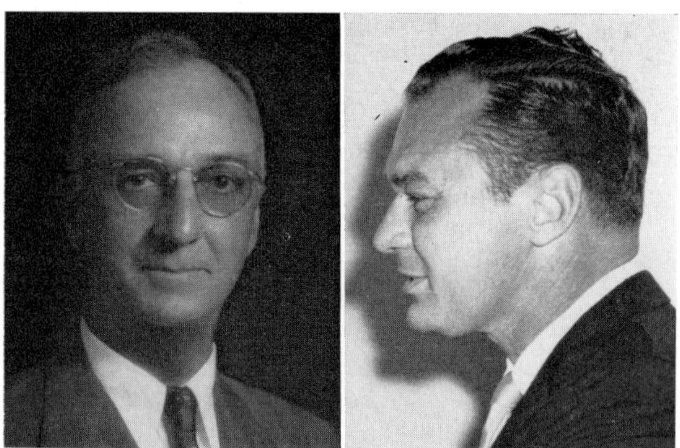

RICHARD PERKINS KINCHELOE, SR. AND JR.

THE KELLEY-KOETT MFG. CO.

INCORPORATED

203 WEST 4TH STREET, COVINGTON, KENTUCKY, U. S. A.

"The X-ray City"

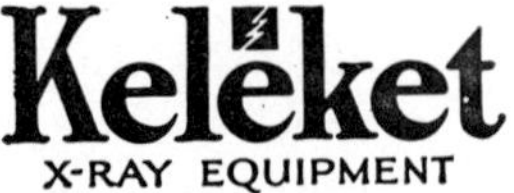

Advertisements please mention The American Journal of Roentgenology nois) at the private office formerly owned by Pettit, now operated by his former associate, Ralph Bailey.

The Kelley-Koett Manufacture Company, as it was first called, was operated until 1905 as a sole owner Kentucky corporation. In 1905 it was incorporated under the laws of the state of Ohio. Kincheloe recalls that in 1928 there were Four Big Keleket dealers: Dick (St. Louis), Engeln (Cleveland), Kotraschek (New York City), and Magnuson (Omaha). The tilting table had come into general use, and the Big Four asked Kelley to include such a table in his production line. He refused, whereupon all four resigned.

After Kelley's death in 1931, G. Ed. Geise became Keleket's president, being followed in 1934 by a distinguished and very efficient as well as personable electrical engineer, Wilbur Stanley Werner (1895-1939), a Covington boy who had made good, but died unexpectedly of pneumonia while attending a conference in Milwaukee. In 1937 the Ohio river flooded the area: water stood 7 feet high inside the Keleket factory at Covington. In 1941 Keleket was purchased by Philip Meyers, a successful dress manufacturer in Cincinnati, thus Adolph A. Feibel became Keleket's president.

Then, in 1951, Tracerlab bought out Keleket, and the plant "moved" to a Boston suburb. In its heyday, though, Keleket could rightfully claim to have put the K in Covington. They had also coined a new (now obviously obsolete) nickname for Covington, "their" first town, that of "X-Ray City."

VICTOREEN

The Fricke-Glasser X-Ray Dosimeter was developed by German-born Otto Glasser, who first briefly calibrated therapy machines in Baltimore, then worked as a full time physicist for the Cleveland Clinic; and by Robert Elmer Fricke, a radiotherapist at Mayo's. In his book, Glasser gives the date of 1929 for the condenser dosimeter (developed by him together with U. V. Portmann and Valentin B. Seitz), which has generally become known as the Victoreeen condenser r-meter.

John Austin Victoreen was a very talented wireless telegraph enthusiast. He had a third floor shop, amateur radio station, photography lab, and general experimental headquarters, and this is where he began to assemble the dosimeter in 1925. The Victoreen Instrument Company was officially formed in Cleveland Heights in 1928, and soon thereafter incorporated. Concurrently there existed a Victoreen radio and radio parts business, but that was not so successful, although he put out an excellent super-heterodyne receiver.

The Victoreen dosimeter — the Condenser R-Meter — became world famous. Its earliest trademark was a balance suspended from a V of which the right leg was longer — this oversized V-limb has survived to this day, but Victoreen is no longer with that company, he has his own laboratory in Colorado Springs. John Victoreen is a very resourceful electronics man with original ideas, for instance he aimed to build a hearing aid which — contrary to accepted misconceptions — was not going to be as small as feasible; it was to give as natural (as "hi-fi") a reproduction as modern electronics could make it.

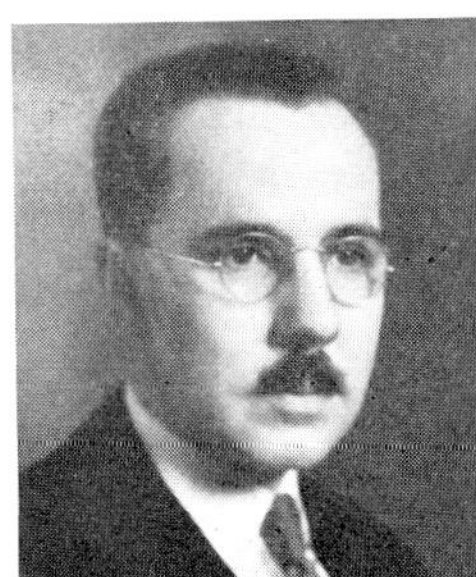

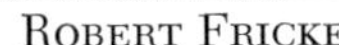

ROBERT FRICKE

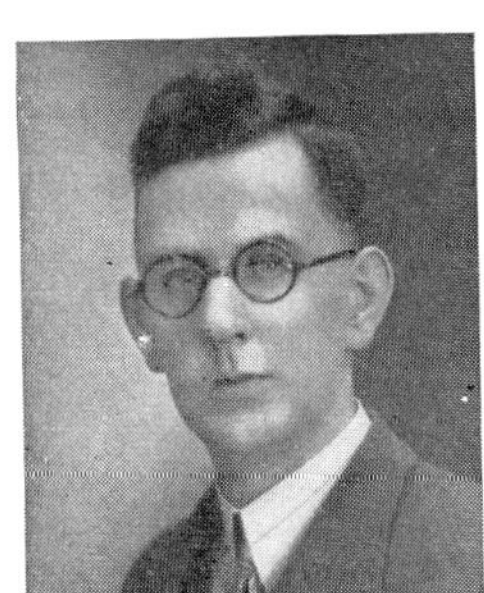

OTTO GLASSER

RADIOLOGY SEPT. 1928

PRACTICAL---FLEXIBLE

for total dose and intensity

THE FRICKE-GLASSER X-RAY DOSIMETER

Calibrated in the R Unit as recommended by the U. S. Bureau of Standards and the Standardization Committee of the Radiological Society of North America.

Eliminates the possibility of X-Ray burns. Eliminates uncertainty due to fluctuation in primary potential. Makes the treatment more simple and accurate.

An American made instrument

Send for free descriptive literature

THE VICTOREEN INSTRUMENT COMPANY

2825 Chester Avenue -:- CLEVELAND, OHIO

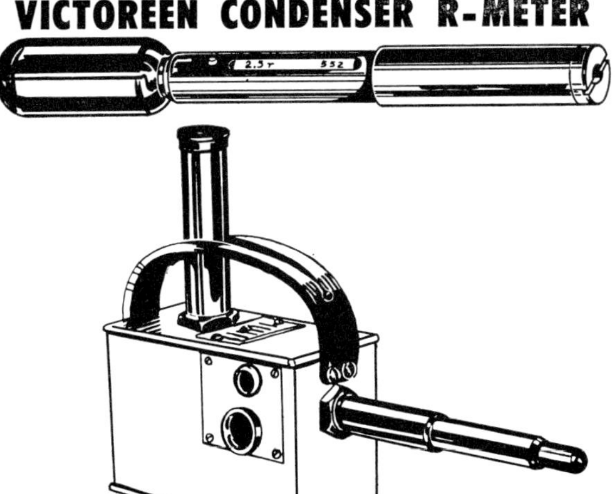

THE VICTOREEN INSTRUMENT CO.

In the early 1940s the Victoreen Company worked with the University of Chicago on the design of the detection apparatus used in conjunction with the Fermi pile. In 1945 the Victoreen Company provided 95% of the instrumentation needed for the Bikini bomb test. This is why today they bill themselves (rightfully so) as the world's first nuclear company.

POWERS

In 1931, the Queensboro (New York) Tuberculosis and Health Association wanted to "do something about eradicating tuberculosis." They considered tuberculin testing and chest x-ray surveys of about two thousand children each year, for four years. To launch the project they could allocate only $6,000 – perhaps enough for one thousand conventional chest x-ray examinations on celluloid film. This seemed like a nice step forward, but one thousand children would be too small a number on which to base significant conclusions. Five or ten thousand examinees sounded much better, and periodic films of the apparently healthy were also considered "essential for the rapid control of tuberculosis in this country" (the quotation is from Jay Arthur Myers of Minneapolis, and was told in May, 1931 to the physician Charles S. Prest. Such statements were fallacious, tuberculosis was declining for decades, *cf.*, the *Arcana of Tuberculosis* in the *American Review of Tuberculosis* of August, 1958). Thereupon the Queensboro anti-tuberculous leaders wondered if there were or if there could be devised a method to make x-ray examinations less expensive.

The dilemma was that simple: more money or cheaper examinations! Henry E. Wright (the president of the Queensboro Tuberculosis Assn.), who lived at Douglas Manor (New York), took the matter up with his friend and neighbor, Frank Thomas Powers (1882-1948). The latter was the most inventive among three brothers who owned and operated a photo-engraving firm called the Powers Chemco Co.

Powers used a roll of 14″-wide photographic paper* and succeeded in obtaining acceptable views of the chest. On July 13, 1931 the Queensboro Tuberculosis Assn. appropriated their $6,000 for an x-ray program. It was to start in the Fall and screen 35,000 children, or as many as could be done with that money.

On October 22, 1931 a trial run was performed with 35 first graders from the Public School in Little Neck (Long Island). Views on film will always be of superior diagnostic quality than films on paper. For *screening* purposes, however, "paper pictures" of the chest may be made almost as satisfactory as those on celluloid.

Officially, the era of scheduled mass x-ray programs was ushered in on November 30, 1931 with a line of children from Public School no. 90 in Richmond Hill

*It is not generally known that in the *Kodak News* of December, 1896 appeared the following ad: "Eastman's X-Ray Bromide Paper takes the place of plates in radiographic work." Knott also sold paper for regular radiography but paper never became more than a half-way acceptable substitute for x-ray films.

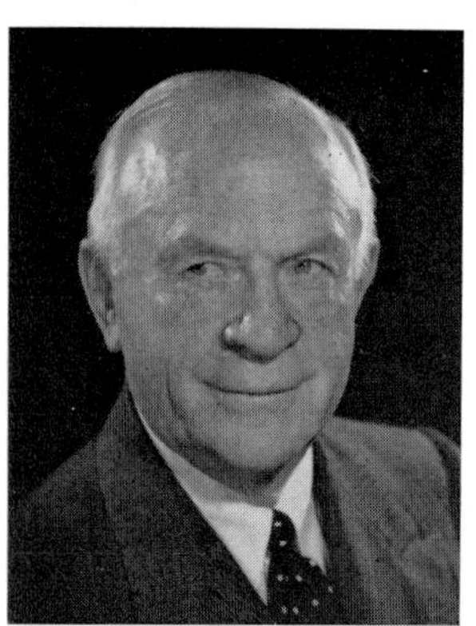

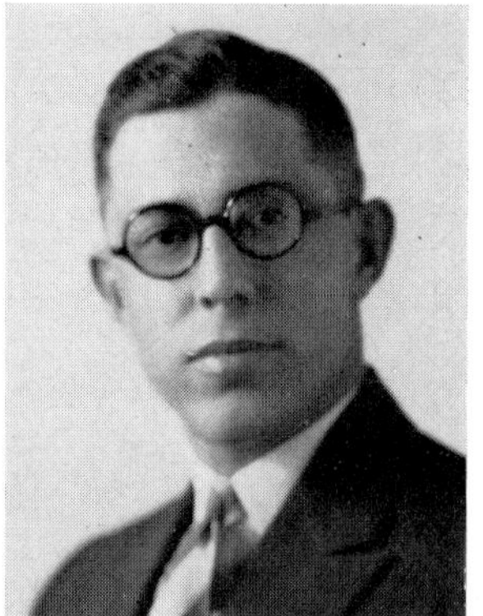

Courtesy: Joseph Dioguardi. *Courtesy: William J. Dee, Jr.*

FRANK THOMAS POWERS (1882-1948). An inventive photo-engraver from New York City who was the first to make photographic paper-roll radiography practical as a tool for mass chest surveys. The man with glasses is WILLIAM CHRISTOPHER DEE (1890-1935). Although lacking a formal education, Dee was one of the most imaginative and effective American designers of x-ray equipment. He worked first for Engeln, then for Bill Hettich at Standard, finally for GE in Chicago (where he died of carcinoma of the liver). Among the machines he built were an unusually well protected (Engeln) Dental Unit, and the (Standard) Tilting Therapy Container.

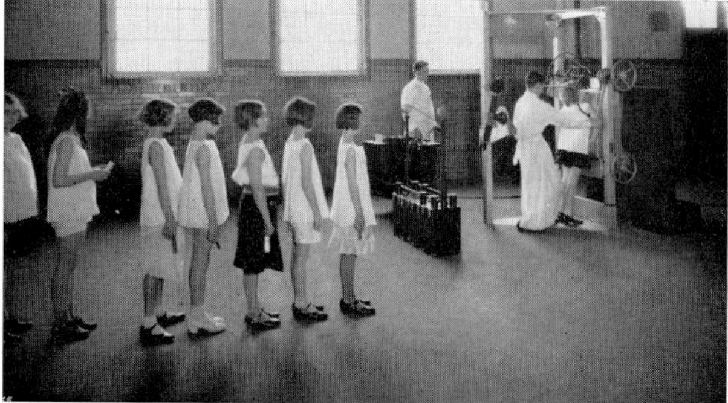

NOVEMBER 30, 1931. On that day, at Public School No. 90 in Richmond Hill (Long Island, New York), a line of children formed before the x-ray equipment provided with an x-ray paper-roll: two pictures per minute at seventy-five cents each!

(Long Island). The average take was two "pictures" per minute, the cost about 75¢ per "picture." After the death of Powers, the company continued under changed ownership* The radiation scare (which accompanied the installation of the Atomic Phase) has inevitably curtailed the mass survey activities of the Powers Company.

INTERMEZZO

In the early 1920s the short-lived General X-Ray Company, located in the Park Square Building in Boston, marketed several "electrologic" specialty items including the Type A-27 "Morse" Wave Generator (a "muscle exciter"), and the G-X Galvanic-Faradic Plate.

At about the same time, the R-B Company of Minneapolis produced a spotfilm device called the Serialograph.

The Rogers Electric Laboratories and Co., at 2015 E. 65th St. in Cleveland, made a bedside x-ray unit for surgical as well as for dental use.

ENGELN

Another milestone in American x-ray history was the Engeln Electric Co., located from 1918 to 1923 at 4601 Euclid Ave., then at 30th & Superior in Cleveland.

The *Engeln X-Ray Special*, their promotional periodical, carried such gems of advice as "a man who believes in ghosts has no trouble in seeing them" or "confidence is an asset, but over-confidence is a liability." Others were not quite as "specific", for instance, "don't try to do everything – let posterity solve some of the problems," and "fishing is always good five miles farther on."

Following are a few reminiscences from the pen of Ed Goldfield:

"Henry Engeln was the first around Cleveland to enter the x-ray and electro-medical field. His company went through bankruptcy once or twice, and then started again in 1918. I had been trying to join them for about 8 years. They offered me sales work, but I wanted to be in on the design and manufacture of x-ray equipment. I became their seventh employee on December 23, 1918. Within three or four months, I was given charge of their (then small) shop. Within a year I was placed in charge of design and production, and continued in that capacity until the merger with Acme in 1929. By then, the Engeln factory employed 200 people."

"In 1923, the plant was moved to Superior and 30th and had the first floor of the building. Later it took part of the second floor. When I joined them, their engineering was in the hands of Wm. C. Dee. I took over when Engeln transferred Dee to Chicago to open there a sales territory. Mike Hoban was then put in charge over Dee, as a result of which Dee left Engeln for a better job with the Standard X-Ray Co."

"In the early 1920s, Henry Engeln owned 25 per cent interest in the Standard X-Ray Co., and was selling some of their equipment. He also sold Wappler equip-

*The portraits of Powers and of the historic moment of the first survey were graciously provided by Mr. Josef Dioguardi of the Powers X-Ray Service, located in Glen Cove (New York).

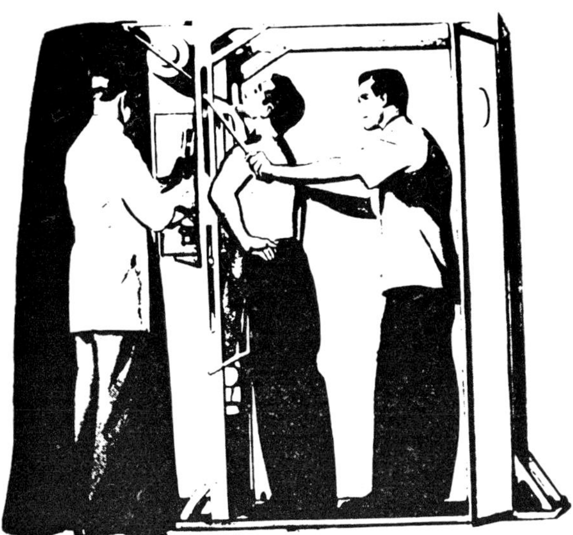

Group Radiography

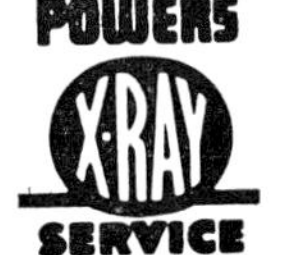

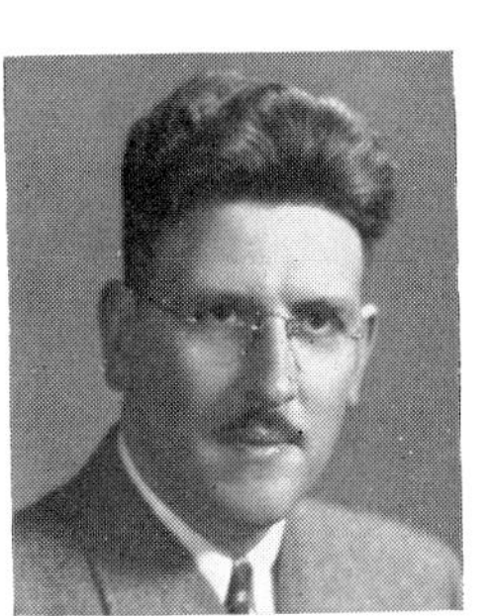

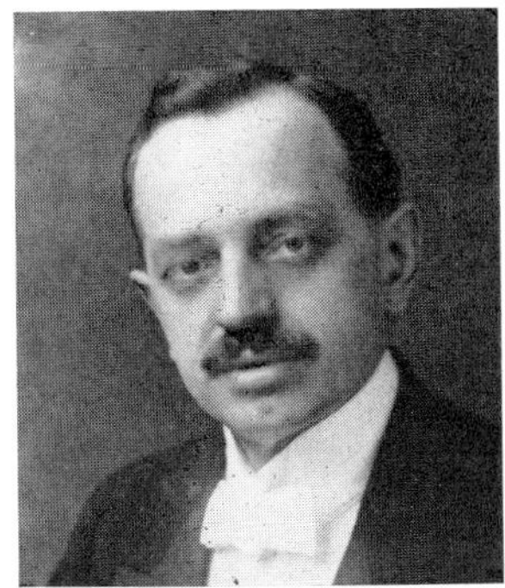

Courtesy: Ed Goldfield.

John Victoreen and white-tied Henry Engeln.

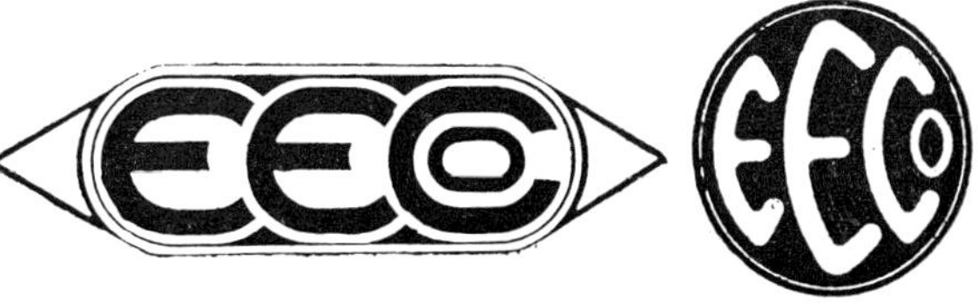

ment. Later, he entered into an agreement with Keleket, whereby Engeln would build small devices and accessories (for instance, the Engeln Grier Head Rest, and the Engeln Cassette Tunnel Changer), and Keleket would make the larger equipment."

"Before the agreement with Keleket in 1918, Engeln built the first all-metal dental units and the first all-metal bedside unit. Both of these were constructed around hot cathode tubes. Engeln built also the first tubular high tension system and the first high tension switch. All these (and several other) developments were the work of Dee, although I did come early enough to make some contributions* to their design. I also produced the parts and assembled the first of these devices before they were delivered."

"Another development which Dee and I created was a better illuminator (viewbox). Until then, all illuminators made use of incandescent bulbs. We developed single illuminators 5 or 6 feet long, containing Cooper-Hewitt tubular (mercury vapor) lamps. While the color was ghastly, the distribution of light was very even."

"About 1920, Dee and I read an article on the Bucky diaphragm. Although the description was vague and gave no manufacturing instructions, Dee and I set out to build one. I made our first grid from one piece of wood in which slots had been made with parallel saw-cuts not quite through it. The wood could then be readily curved to the desired radius. The saw-cuts provided a place to drop the strips of lead, but the lead was so thin that it curled in the slots. U-shaped pieces of cardboard were formed, the lead was placed in the pockets, and the whole combination was slipped into the wooden slots. Our first grid was very satisfactory but later a much better method was developed. It consisted of building the Bucky from alternate wooden and lead strips, to increase accuracy, firmly secure the

*A reliable informer told me that Goldfield (a mechanical genius in his own right) has always been very modest about his own contributions. Even when he stressed that this or that contraption was the result of teamwork, it usually had been his own idea, developed in off-hours in the small shop in the basement of his home. He would then bring a rudimentary model to the plant, and have the "team" improve on it.

CATALOG
of
X-RAY ACCESSORIES
AND
SUPPLIES

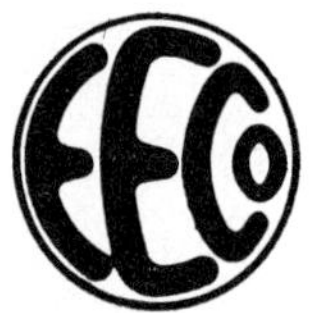

THE ENGELN ELECTRIC COMPANY
HOME OFFICE AND FACTORY
4601-11 Euclid Avenue Cleveland, Ohio

Branches

New York City
127 E. 23rd Street
Detroit
845 D. Whitney Bldg.
Chicago
30 E. Randolph St.
Los Angeles, Cal.

Toronto
203 Hobberlin Bldg.

Philadelphia
20 So. 20th Street
Pittsburgh
617 Fulton Bldg.
Portland, Ore.
319 Morgan Bldg.
Cincinnati, Ohio

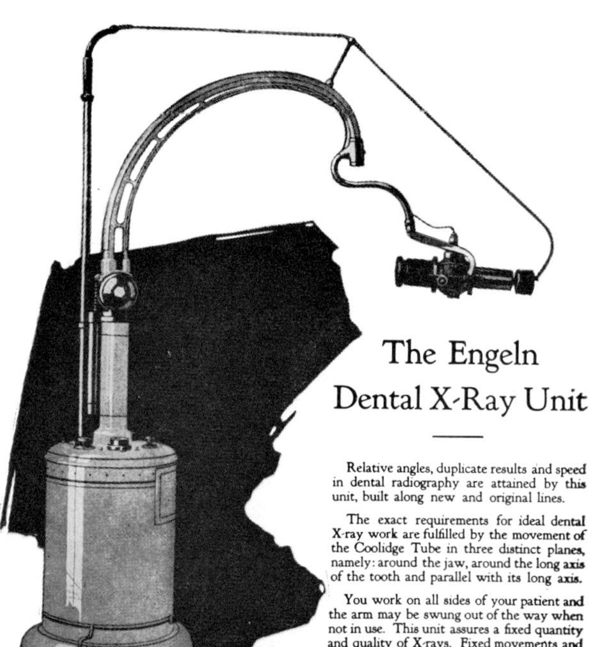

THE ENGELN ELECTRIC COMPANY
HOME OFFICE AND FACTORY
Euclid Avenue at 46th Street CLEVELAND, OHIO
BRANCHES:
PHILADELPHIA
16 South 17th Street
PITTSBURGH
617 Fulton Building
DETROIT
845 David Whitney Bldg.
BUFFALO, N. Y. SCHENECTADY, N. Y.

DEE'S DENTAL DESIGN. Dee's solution was both simple and effective against electrical hazards. In the *History of Radiodontia,* Raper recalls that in 1920 C. L. Cope, an alumnus of the class of 1917 of the Indianapolis School of Dentistry, lost his life in an electrical accident while exposing dental radiographs. The cause of death was attributed to "tonic spasm of the heart" (ventricular fibrillation?) and explained by the fact that one of the electrodes came very close to the dentist's heart.

lead, and make it more practical to build various ratios of thickness to height of the strips."

"The grid was moved with a spring. Its speed was controlled at first through an air-check but this resulted in a bounce which tended to produce grid lines. One day I observed how very smoothly a door closed from the action of an oil-check. We adapted such a door check to our Bucky diaphragm and this eliminated the bounce. Over 700 were produced before we had to improve the model. Even then we used the same simple fluid door check. We produced this Bucky diaphragm for over one year and a half before competition started. Some of our competitors made the mistake of coming out with an air check, but eventually everyone had to go to the oil model. I still have at home one of these original Engeln *Bucky motors.*"

"The first unit design in x-ray apparatus was originated in Engeln equipment. In the mid-1920s, the Engeln Company no longer represented Wappler or Standard, and there were hard feelings between Engeln and Keleket, so we set about to develop a complete line of major x-ray apparatus. Only one of our generator was not of the double disc type. That one was built with oil immersed valve tubes on a license from Waite, Jr., and it proved to be very successful. I understand some of these units are still in operation, although they were produced in 1927 and 1928."

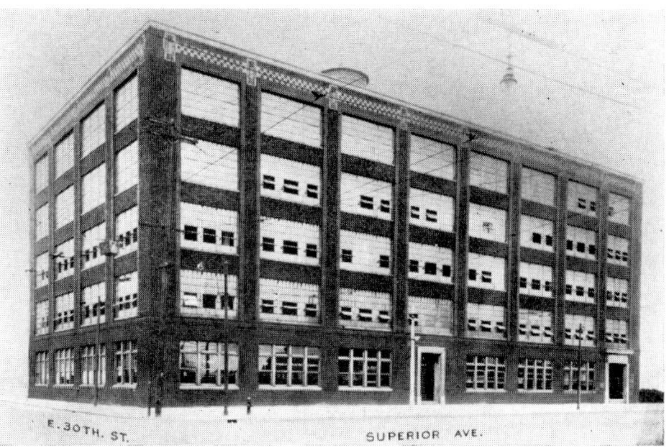

Courtesy: Picker Archives

THE FIRST PLANT. This had been Engeln's old plant. After the debacle of the American X-ray Corporation, when Picker formed the Waite Manufacturing Division in Cleveland, Ed Goldfield arranged to move into this abandoned building, bought out the old machines, and re-placed them in their previous locations, using the same bolt holes in floor and ceiling.

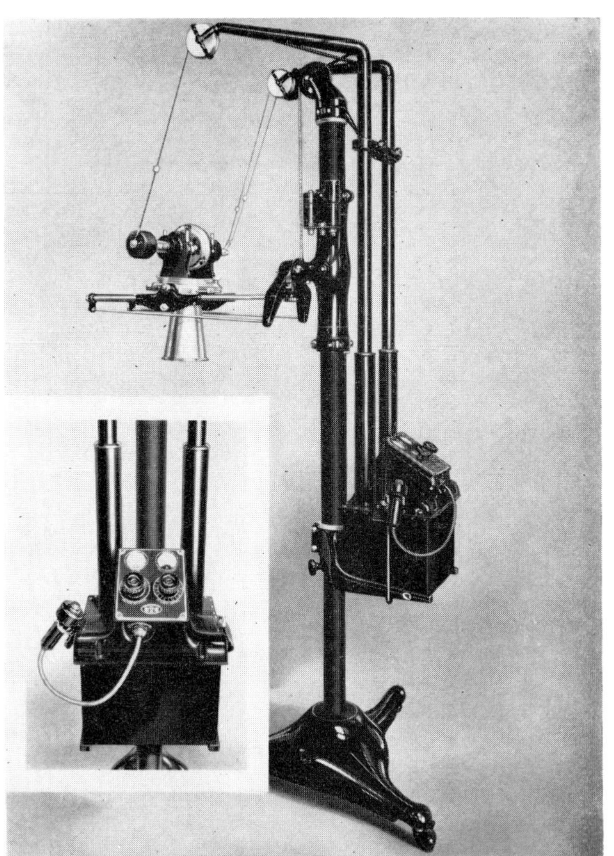

Courtesy: Ed Goldfield.

ENGELN SIMPLEX. A mobile unit, also available as a portable. The insert shows the controls.

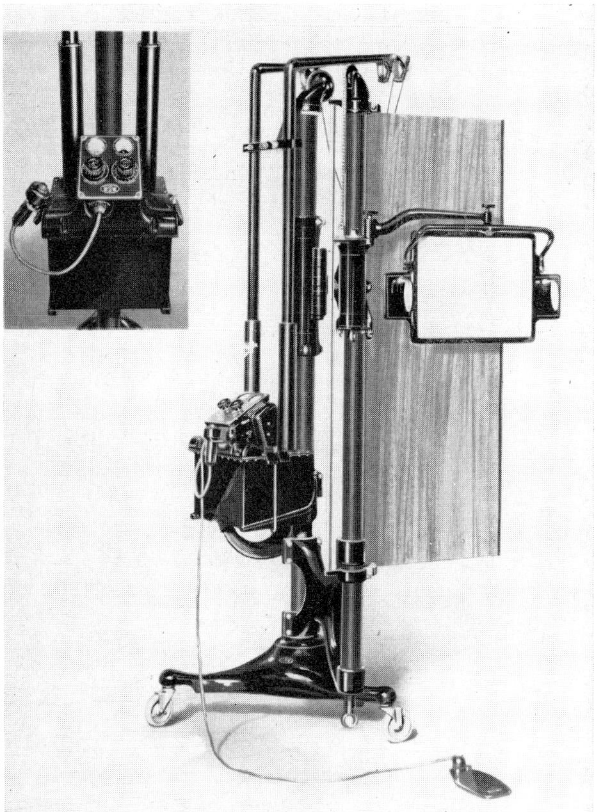

Courtesy: Ed Goldfield.

ENGELN DUPLEX. An upright fluoroscope made from the SimpleX (same controls), with the addition of a wooden board, and a screen.

Perhaps the most popular Engeln equipment — meaning the one with the largest production — was a tryptich, the first of which was called SimpleX, a portable tubestand with carrying case (its twin was a mobile unit). Next largest was the DupleX, advertised as an upright fluoroscope. It came also in a more expensive version, with a tilting table. The largest in this series, the TripleX, had a Bucky in the slot of its tilting fluoroscopic table.

These (Goldfield creations) were the first American set of low-cost, self-contained, all-metal, office-type x-ray units ever to be placed on the market. They came out in 1926, and became a rousing success. Just before the merger, in 1929, business was so good that Engeln maintained sales offices in several cities in the USA.

BUCKY-POTTER

At this point, a digression will be inserted, in an attempt to do justice to the "who, how, and when" questions related to the introduction and improvement of the anti-scatter diaphragm. This device is today absolutely indispensable for the practice of diagnostic radiology. It brought in the Golden Age of Radiology, on a par with Snook's rectifying switch, Caldwell's tilting table, Eastman's duplitized film, and Waite's oil-immersion principle, if not quite on a level with Coolidge's hot cathode x-ray tube.

The roentgen pioneers realized quite early that something beclouded the abdominal plates. They called that something "extra-focal rays," "glass-wall rays," "inverse currents," etc.

Albers-Schoenberg was the first who used circular, square, and other simple (later lead-lined) diaphragms, and was also the first who compressed bulky parts.

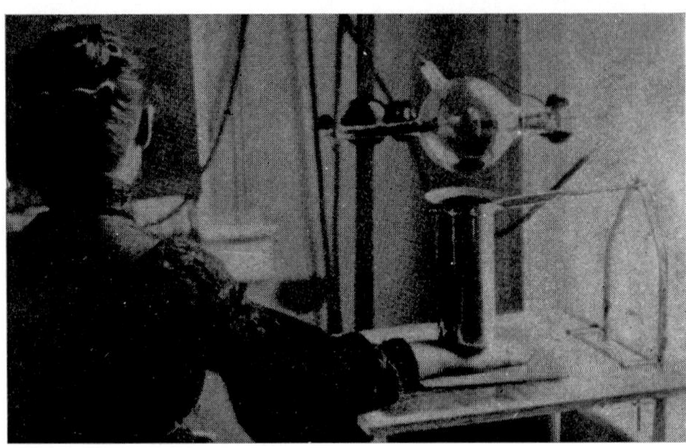

Beck's "diaphragm." Carl Beck (1856-1911), a surgeon from New York City, captioned this illustration as follows: "Skiagraphing hand by the aid of Author's diaphragm".

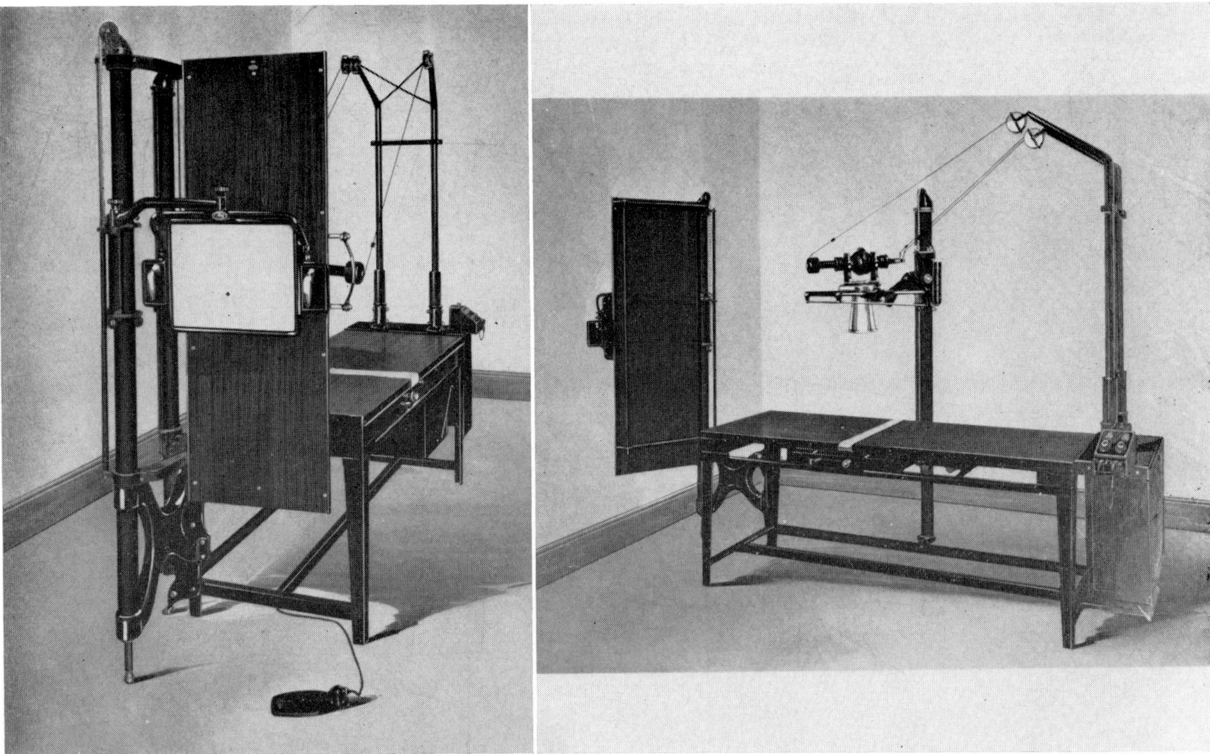

Engeln TripleX. Same machine as the SimpleX, with added table and fluoroscope, in an arrangement intended for generalists.

Hickey designed special "cones" (this seems to be where that term originated) to increase the efficiency of the procedure.

Pirie's "moving-slot" diaphragm – described in the *American Journal of Roentgenology* of September, 1913 – consisted of a transverse slot, cut into a flat piece of lead, interposed between tube and patient: during the exposure, the slot was moved in such a way that the narrow x-ray beam covered the plate in succession, from top to bottom. Lewis Gregory Cole added a second flat lead piece with a similar, though larger, slot (the "double-slot" method) moving between patient and plate, to protect the latter from any but the intended x-ray beam.

Coolidge's "hooded target" was a metal shield placed about the focal spot, for the reduction of "extra-focal" rays.

As Hollis Potter put it — in the *History of Diaphragming Roentgen Rays,* published in the *American Journal of Roentgenology* of March, 1931 — all these devices, while undoubtedly helpful, reduced fog only because they circumscribed, or otherwise limited, primary x-ray beam.

The crux of the problem — reduction of the amount of secondary x rays — was first attacked by Gustav Bucky* (then in Germany), who began experimenting around 1909 with a stationary honeycombed grid-diaphragm *(Gitter-Blende),* described by him in the (British) *Archives of the Roentgen Ray* of June, 1913. Bucky obtained also in 1913 a German patent on the matter.

*Died February 19, 1963.

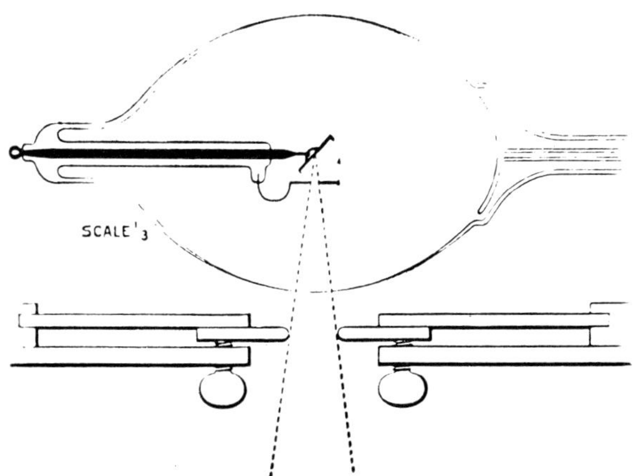

ROLLINS' "INTERNAL DIAPHRAGM" TUBE. This illustration appeared under the title *Roentgen Light Notes* in the *American X-Ray Journal* of July, 1899. Its author, William Herbert Rollins (1852-1929), was a Boston dentist who made very many pioneering contributions to x-ray technic. Incidentally, the ⅓ scale no longer applies.

Potter had noticed Bucky's original communication, and decided to work on the grid diaphragm in the hope of making it practical for routine clinical use. In its original form, Bucky's device was not only cumbersome: the criss-crossed lines which it left on the plate obscured most of the findings, and were so bothersome that the procedure never became popular. Potter decided to move the grid(s) he built, which would (tend to) make them invisible on the plate.

At the February, 1915 meeting of the Central Section of the ARRS, Potter showed his first model, a movable tubular grating. He described it in the *American Journal of Roentgenology* of March, 1916. At the 1916 meeting of the ARRS in Chicago, Potter had a likewise movable, circular disc grid, with strips placed radially. Finally, at the February, 1917 meeting of the Central Section of the ARRS in Cincinnati, Potter demonstrated his first movable, parallel-strip curved grid. After that meeting, Caldwell came to Chicago; Potter had a long session with him, and explained to Caldwell, in detail, all the progress he (Potter) had made. Next day Potter wrote to Caldwell, and asked him point blank how far he (Caldwell) had gone in his experimentation with the Bucky principle. Caldwell's reply is herein reproduced *in-toto,* also because it sheds light on the trials and tribulations of other past (and perhaps present as well as future) "x-ray inventors."

March 8, 1917

Dr. Hollis Potter
1410 Peoples Gas Bldg.
Chicago, Illinois
Dear Doctor:

In answer to your letter of February 27th., which reached me only a day or two ago, I have to say that immediatly after the publication of the Bucky apparatus, I conceived the idea of moving the screen to get

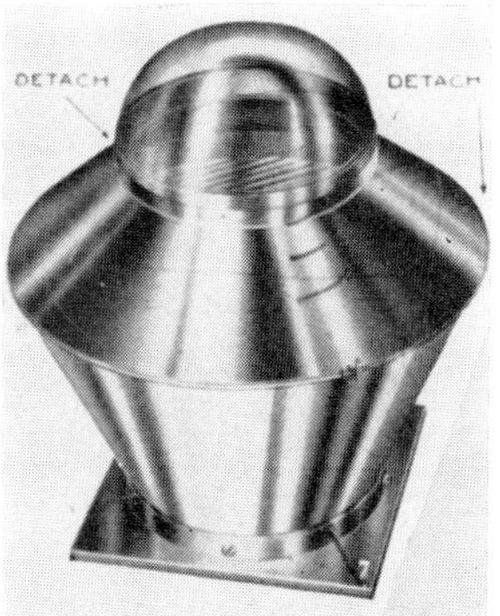

HICKEY'S "UNIVERSAL CONE." Preston Manasseh Hickey (1865-1930), a Detroit Ear, Nose and Throat man who became professor of radiology at Ann Arbor (Michigan), designed this "cone" and coined that name for it. This illustration is taken from a Keleket catalog of 1920.

rid of the shadows of the grid, and did a little experimenting in this direction. At the same time, I looked up the patent question and found that Bucky himself had described about every means of moving the screen for this purpose. I found also that there was a German patent but I send you herewith a copy of Bucky's United States patent, application for which was filed February 3, 1914, and of my patent, application for which was filed October 12, 1915. You will see that my patent refers to a time switch in connection with an automatic device for moving of Bucky screen through a very small space. So far as my patent is concerned, it has no relation whatever to your work. The Bucky patent probably covers everything that you have done.

I think that these patents need not deter you in the least from any experimentation you wish to do if you care to repeat work that has already been done. It is so easy to find out from the patent office what has been done in such a case that I think we should really investigate this before publishing work as our own.

I am just a little sensitive over the criticism that has been made in regard to patents granted to me. Most of this criticism I think is due to ignorance, but some of it seems to be malicious. About all the patents have ever done for me is to establish a date and to give proof of priority. I have felt that anything upon which the patent office would allow me a patent, was very likely original with me. In a great many instances the patent office has informed me that devices which I supposed were new and original with me, were really very old.

There is no money to be made out of patents on such x-ray devices. One does not even recover the cost of doing the development work and experimentation. Theoretically, at least, one benefits his colleagues by patenting anything useful that he may develop, because he is then able to insist that any maker who undertakes the construction of these devices shall make them well and also because it should be easier to induce a maker to manufacture a patented article, the sale of which he cannot (*sic*) control. The insinuation that has sometimes been made, to the effect that one patents such a device for the sake of preventing his colleagues from using it in order to accumulate wealth by taxing his colleagues for royalties, is of course absurd. One's colleagues seldom appreciate the amount of labor and expense necessary to develop even a simple device to a point where it can be manufactured.

Yours very truly,
(signed) E. W. Caldwell

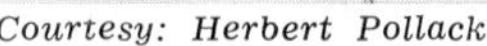
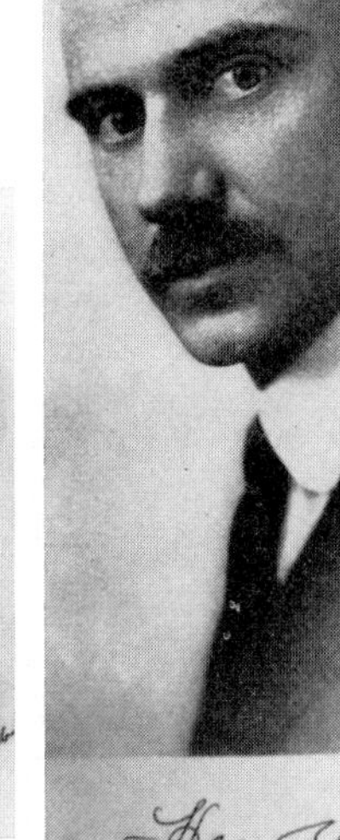

Courtesy: Herbert Pollack.

Gustav Bucky. This drawing of the inventor of the grid was executed by Helmuth Nathan, and autographed by the subject. The original is in the Hall of Fame of the ICS. On the viewer's right is the young Hollis Elmer Potter. Better known is his portrait with the sailor captain's cap (Potter was very proud of his yachting records); this photograph is from the time when he moved Bucky's grid into celebrated usefulness.

Potter was dismayed by Caldwell's reply; all three of them (Bucky, Caldwell, and Potter) had advanced along similar pathways, up to a point. Until then, Potter had never heard that Bucky had conceived the idea of making the grid invisible by movement, and had only heard rumors that Caldwell was working on Bucky's principle. In his disillusionment, Potter decided that it would be unfair to speak or write further on the grid diaphragm until the close of the war. Bucky should then be given opportunity to show what he had achieved in practical apparatus, and Caldwell should also be allowed to produce his models.

Bucky's American patent contained the following sentence: "The velocity of the drive must be such that the walls of the grid will not cast a visible shadow upon the photographic plate or upon the fluoroscent screen." To Potter it seemed that Bucky's patent was couched in terms broad enough to cover almost anything — and

THE AMERICAN JOURNAL OF ROENTGENOLOGY
January 1922

BRADY'S POTTER-BUCKY DIAPHRAGM

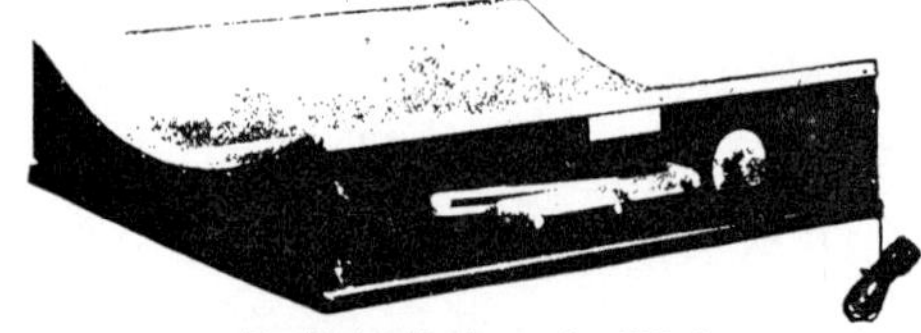

For Finest Radiographic Work

We placed the first Bucky diaphragm on the market months ahead of other firms. Some of the first twelve are still in use by prominent roentgenologists. The many hundreds of satisfied users are our best "ads."

We claim to have the smallest, neatest and most accurate Potter-Bucky on the market. Electrically welded frame and base, with metal construction, make it practically indestructible. Takes all makes of cassettes up to 17 x 17. Operates in horizontal or vertical position. Exposures range from 1 to 90 seconds. Distance from 16 to 40 inches. Does stereoscopic work in either direction. Electric light signal device indicating when grid is moving, free if desired.

yet the Austrian Patent Court later ruled that Bucky's claim covered only the honeycomb type of construction described at length in his patent.

Caldwell also favored a crossed grid, moved in linear direction. The "start-and-stop" device was combined with an arrangement for closing the x-ray circuit at "start" and opening it at "stop."

Potter "never having seen a patent or talked to a patent lawyer, and not caring to become educated regarding them" turned to other lines of experimentation. Every so often, though, he reverted to the problem of perfecting the smooth action of the parallel slotted grid apparatus. In his history, Potter specifies that "it was Carl Lundberg, an assistant supplying vacancies during the war, who superintended much of the building of the first 14″ by 17″ model equipped with an oil dash-pot for smoothly regulating the motion." That model was shown in February, 1919 at the meeting of the Central Section of the ARRS in Chicago. After that meeting, on February 22, 1919, Potter consulted Henry Engeln about building a special table to accommodate the unit. Engeln rounded up a number of ARRS members whose trains were not yet due, and they stayed over for a private demonstration, which took place in Potter's office the following morning.

Immediately after the armistice, Coolidge and Carl Darnell made a survey of x-ray apparatus used in Central Europe, and reported that Bucky had made no improvements on his original model. The only such device in use was a fixed cross-grid grating which Albers-Schoenberg had mounted on his fluoroscope. Caldwell had died, and Potter felt that he was reaching a position where it began to look as if something was being withheld from the profession. He took from his shelves the paper given at Cincinnati in February, 1917, "smoothed" it out, and had it printed in the *American Journal of Roentgenology* of June, 1920. At the next meeting of the ARRS in Minneapolis (September, 1920), George Brady demonstrated the first commercially produced model of the Bucky-Potter diaphragm. The practical value of the device was easily shown: plates of the abdomen made with the grid were so much "cleaner." The scientific "proof of the pudding" was adduced in the Research Laboratories of Eastman-Kodak in Rochester (New York) by Rex Wilsey, a physicist who studied the amount of scattered radiation absorbed by grids: his findings were published in a series of classic papers, the first of which appeared in the *American Journal of Roentgenology* of January, 1922.

In that same issue Liebel-Flarsheim advertised a table built to accommodate a curved model of Bucky-Potter grid, from one of the three brands which were then dominating the market: Brady, Engeln, and Victor. Actually, Brady never built a piece of equipment himself: he had them made, and only sold them with his

AJR January, 1922

name, as he did with the famous Paragon X-Ray Plates.

In the early 1920s, several others began making Bucky-Potter grids, for instance Violi in Boston. Today, it is a highly specialized manufacturing process, requiring a great deal of technical know-how.

In the obituary, prepared for the *Journal of the ICS* of September, 1963, Herbert Pollack wrote: ". . . (Bucky), a truly great scientist and radiologist, failed to receive in this country the recognition and honor that were due to him." In 1960 the late Senator Estes Kefauver became interested in introducing a private bill in Congress to honor Gustav Bucky on the latter's eightieth anniversary, but nothing came of it.* At the end of World War I, under the War Reparations Law, the USA Government confiscated about 1200 German patents: on that occasion, Bucky's patent was sold to the Chemical Foundation. It has been estimated that until that original antiscatter diaphragm patent ran out in 1933, about $4 million should have been paid to Bucky in royalties. He never got a penny of them.

In one of his letters, Gustav Bucky wrote: "I emigrated to the USA in 1923. Being a newcomer, I did not want to start a controversy on priorities. My patents contained all the ideas ever built into the antiscatter diaphragm, except for minor constructive features. In spite of this fact, Potter's name always appears in connection with mine as co-inventor."

Gustav Bucky's inventiveness was not restricted to the antiscatter device. As an expert photographer, he patented an automatic color camera, which was being sold by the Coreco Co. of New York City. And Bucky developed with the mathematician Albert Einstein a Light Intensity Self-Adjusting Camera (US Patent 2,058,562 filed December 11, 1935), in which the lens aperture is automatically set by a photoelectric cell. As soon as that patent expired in 1953, several camera manufacturers began to market models with that feature. And Gustav Bucky is, of course, the man who developed, beginning in 1925, the treatment of superficial lesions with ultra-soft x radiation, the so-called Grenzstrahlen-Therapy.

In 1923 Bucky became the seventh physician to be granted — without examination — a license to practice medicine in the state of New York. In 1930 he departed for Berlin, having been offered the directorship of the radiologic department in the Rudolf Virchow Krankenhaus. In 1933 Hitler came to power, whereupon Bucky, being Jewish, preferred to return to the USA. He was a good personal friend of Albert Einstein. The families spent summers together, and Gustav Bucky was the attending physician at Einstein's terminal illness. In 1952 Einstein, who disliked making public appearances, did testify in a federal court in behalf of Bucky in a patent infringement suit. Gustav Bucky (1880-1963) died in New York City, of melanoma.

In summing up, "trailblazer" credit for discovery of the antiscatter device belongs to Bucky, and to no one else. Caldwell was in this matter an innocent bystander (not counting the invectives). Potter deserves more than "hitchhiker" credit because he popularized the procedure. In fact, the Bucky principle had been abandoned in its native Germany years before the perfected Potter grid began "moving" in 1918 in the United States. In proper eponymic usage (if eponymic usage is proper), the device ought to be called the Bucky-Potter grid.

*A copy of the memorandum, prepared on that occasion, and related documents were graciously placed at my disposal by Gustav Bucky's son, Peter Arthur Bucky, who is selling x-ray equipment (Bucky International, Inc. of New York City).

ACME

The defectors from Victor formed the Acme X-Ray Co., located at 341-351 West Chicago Ave., almost within walking distance from Victor's plant. Their first sales gimmick was the Acme Coronaless Overhead System, well described in *Roentgen Accessories* (a promotional leaflet issued by Acme).

At the first scientific meetings after the karyokynesis between Victor and Acme, the equipment shown by these two manufacturers was almost identical (on some of the pieces even the pattern numbers were the same). Obviously, many original patterns had been "liberated" at the time of the split. Such incongruities were not

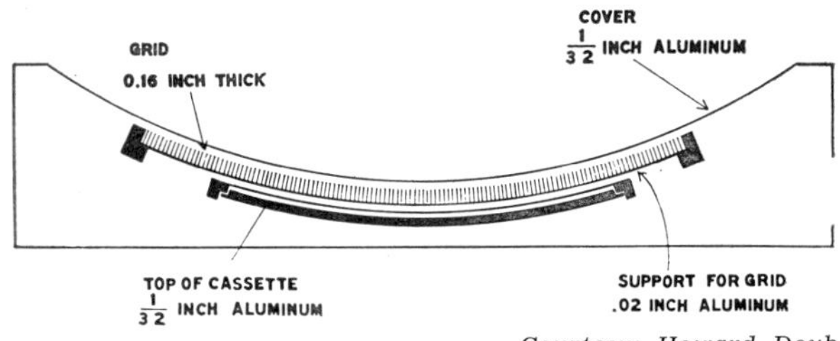

Courtesy: Howard Doub

REX WILSEY'S CURVED GRID. This sketch appeared in *Radiology* of September, 1923.

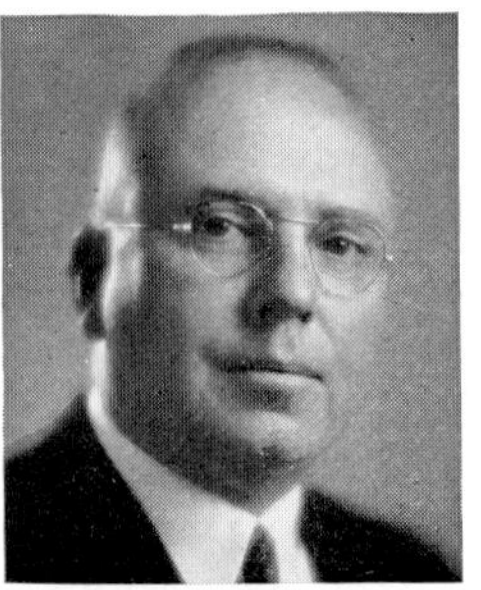

REX WILSEY

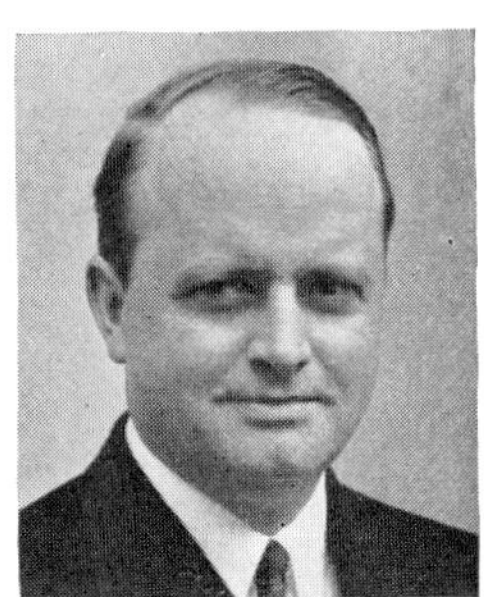

MONTY MORRISON

likely to create a respectable corporate image in the mind of prospective customers.

At 326 Broadway, in New York City, was located the International X-Ray Corporation. Their advertising slogan was the Precision X-Ray Apparatus, claimed to be the only equipment in existence with non-corona producing constant form of rectification, having a Crest* Kilovolt Meter for continuous, direct measurement of its secondary potential.

The Acme and the International merged, and so did their promotional semantics. After the symbiosis, the Acme International used both terms, "Precision Transformer" as well as "Coronaless."

*An acute disagreement raged between Monty Morrison and the remainder of the American X-Ray Industry over the use of the term "crest kilovolts" *vs.* "peak kilovolts." Morrison preferred and promoted "crest," but today very few people—if any at all—have so much as heard about the controversy. *Vae victis!* The losers are "always" (historically) wrong.

WRITTEN FOR

ROENTGENOLOGISTS

BY

MONTFORD MORRISON

Consulting Engineer

ACME-INTERNATIONAL X-RAY COMPANY

MEMBER

American Institute of Mining and Metallurgical Engineers
American Institute of Electrical Engineers
American Society of Mechanical Engineers
American Electro-Chemical Society
Illuminating Engineering Society
American Mathematical Society
Western Society of Engineers
Institute of Radio Engineers
American Chemical Society
American Physical Society
And others.

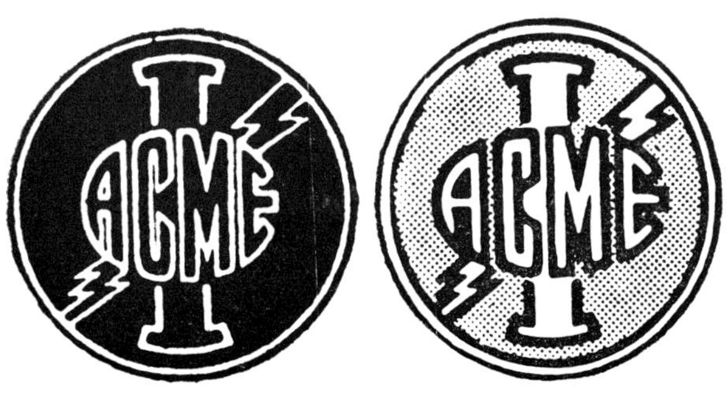

They issued a Bedside Unit, called the Five-Thirty, in which five meant inches of spark and thirty meant 30 ma. They had also a Six-Sixty, meaning 60 ma and 6″ of spark, equivalent to about 100 kvp.* They built in 1928 a Precision Fluoroscopic Unit, with an optional ortho-diagraphic attachment. Their Deep Therapy Tubestand (sold also through Picker) was of the drum type and stationary: positioning of the patient was done by moving the table.

Acme International had also overseas outlets. Their representative in Brussels (1, Rue de Loxum) was E. Fueter, as advertised in the *Journal de Radiologie* of 1923. In Milan their agents were the Iten Co.

The driving force at Acme was Montford Morrison, a very capable engineer, but perhaps a bit too willing to exaggerate the promotional aspects of the trade. As an exemplification may be recalled the way in which he

*Byron Hess called the Six-Sixty the most over-rated equipment he had ever seen.

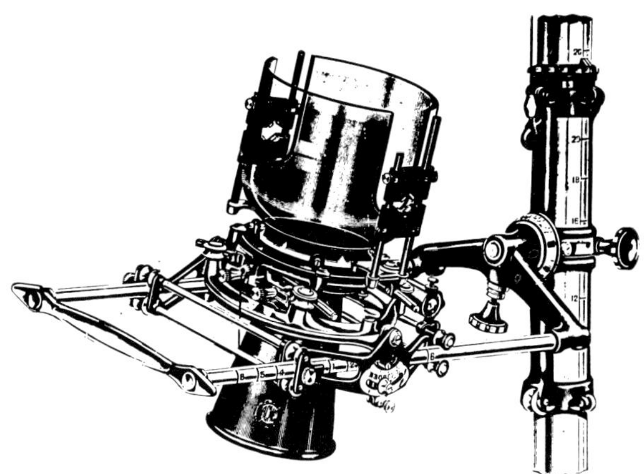

ACME TUBESTAND. In a Waite & Bartlett catalog of the 1920's appeared this picture of the cone with lead-glass open bowl ready to receive a tube.

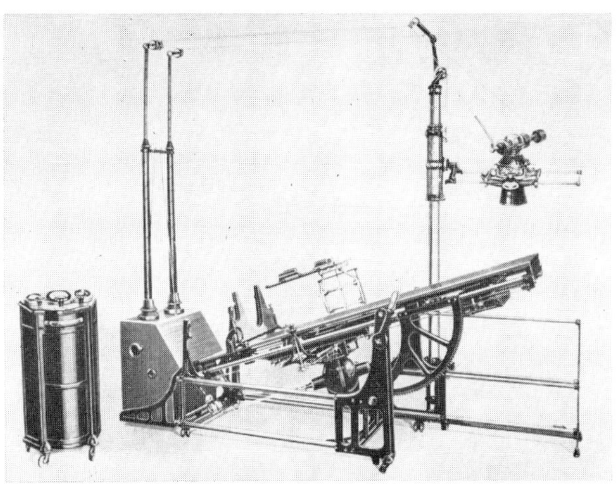

ACME INTERNATIONAL UNIT

listed as titles his membership in various trade organizations.

Acme's sales manager was "Hooknose" BeGole, well remembered in Chicago x-ray circles for his dynamic salesmanship combined with jovial personality.

THE BIG MERGER

In 1920, GE had "looked over" the Engeln Co. Nothing came of it because Engeln was not sufficiently diversified (by comparison Victor produced not only x-ray apparatus, but all sorts of electrical equipment). In 1924, Engeln became "engaged" to Standard. They issued advertisements under the combined name of Standard-Engeln X-ray Co., but then they "disengaged" and their union was never consummated. Finally, in 1929, Engeln and Acme International united and became the American X-Ray Corporation.

Here will be inserted another quotation from a letter written by Ed Goldfield:

"We (Engeln) had a full x-ray line at the time of the merger with Acme-International and we were in the best financial state that we had ever been. I was invited to go along in the merger, but I felt it would hurt my future if the company failed and this I predicted would happen. The new company had agreed to take over the Engeln sales organization, while most of the Engeln line was soon abolished. I did not believe that Engeln salesmen could be successful in selling 'old' Acme equipment. I was proved a bit wrong: the American X-Ray Company failed in eight months instead of in one year as I had predicted."

Monty Morrison would have made an expert patent attorney. He was a brilliant man but brought no great contributions to the design of x-ray equipment, or to the advancement of the art.

In the 1918 *AMA Directory* Morrison (who was not a physician) inadvertently appears listed among the medical x-ray specialists in Chicago: the address given is that of the Victor Company. During his years with Acme and American X-Ray Company, Morrison and associates worked on a series of x-ray tubes. He was a good salesman, and convinced the executives of the Westinghouse Company to manufacture these tubes, which were not conventional in shape, size, or bulk. One of these tubes was nicknamed the "bomb."

In the quest for data on Morrison, I succeeded to get in touch with Joseph Denny who is living in Ocean City (New Jersey) since his retirement of ten years ago. This is what he answered:

"I was associated with Monty Morrison since the first big merger of x-ray companies in 1916. Monty was "quite a reader," especially of foreign magazines and books pertinent to the electrical art. He was also what one would term "quite a joiner," being member of so many societies that he had a special vest adorned with buttons, badges, medals, and other membership identifications — there must have been at least fifty items on that vest. He was also "quite a gourmet," and as I was inclined along the same line we had many nights together preparing and serving our favorite foods and wines.

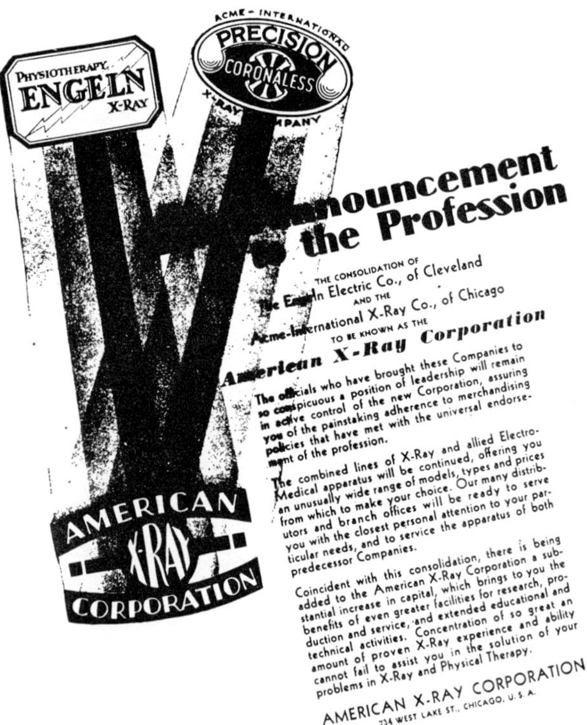

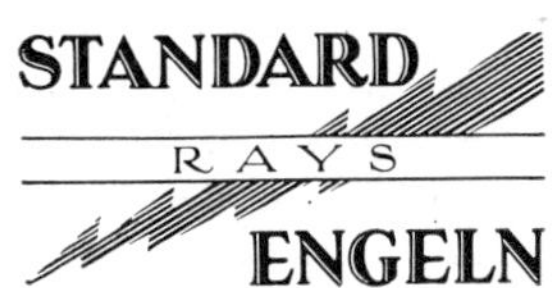

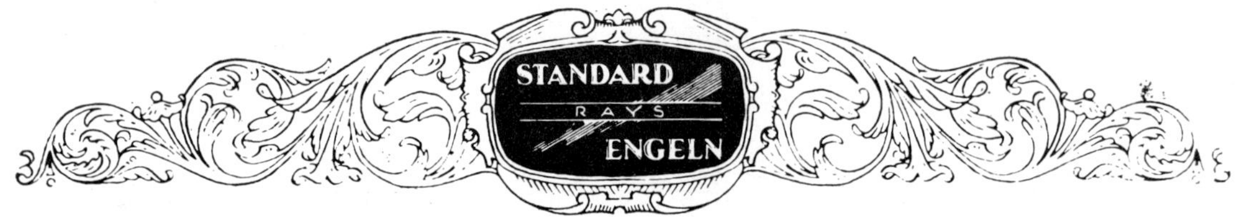

"In 1916 the Victor X-Ray Company was formed by merger of the Victor Electric Company, Scheidel-Western, Snook-Roentgen, and Macalaster-Wiggin. Monty was the chief engineer at Scheidel-Western. I was connected with Snook. Monty left Victor to go to International X-Ray (in New York City) and I joined him, he was chief-engineer and I was general manager at International. Then Acme and International merged, next Acme-International and Engeln merged, finally American X-Ray Co. was taken over by Westinghouse. Monty and I went through three mergers. The last contact I had with Monty was in the early 1940s when he was doing consulting work, and living in Montclair (New Jersey).

"You state you would be interested in old catalogs, photographs, and literature – well I had a wonderful collection, but I gave them to Monty for his library in about 1935. If you locate his library, you would sure hit pay dirt.

"About the"bomb" tube that Monty had some patents on – I forget what it was officially called, but it looked like a bomb, so that is what we referred to it as. The "bomb" was a therapy tube."

At this point another quotation from a letter by Ed Goldfield follows:

"Before me in my desk drawer are reminders from the past – stock certificates acquired while I was as-

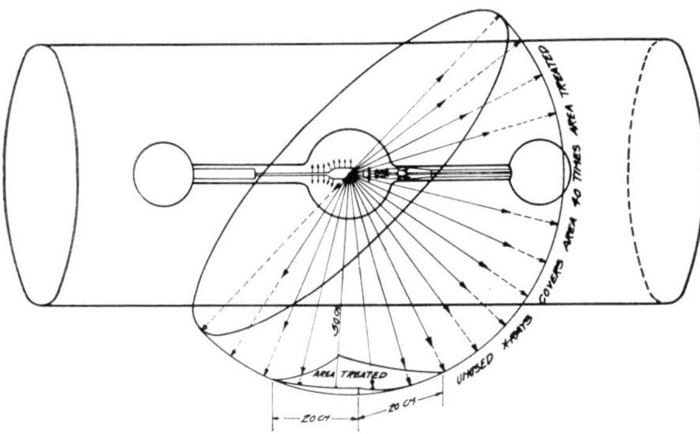

Cover for Monty's "bomb" of 1923.

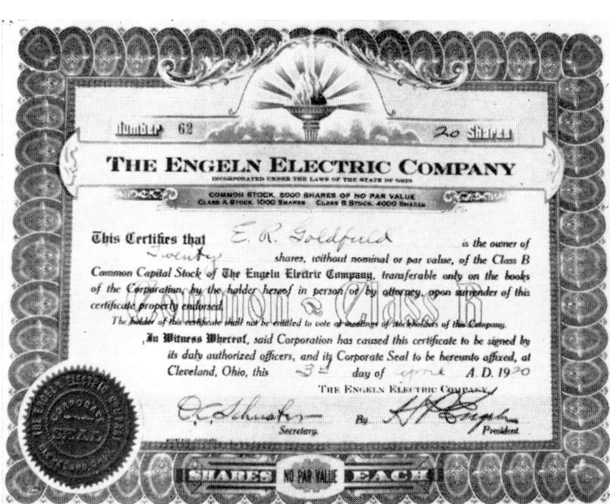

Number 62 20 Shares

THE ENGELN ELECTRIC COMPANY

INCORPORATED UNDER THE LAWS OF THE STATE OF OHIO

COMMON STOCK, 5000 SHARES OF NO PAR VALUE
CLASS A STOCK, 1000 SHARES CLASS B STOCK, 4000 SHARES

This Certifies that E. R. Goldfield is the owner of Twenty shares, without nominal or par value, of the Class B Common Capital Stock of The Engeln Electric Company, transferable only on the books of the Corporation, by the holder hereof in person or by attorney, upon surrender of this certificate properly endorsed.

Common Class B

The holder of this certificate shall not be entitled to vote at meetings of stockholders of the Company.

In Witness Whereof, said Corporation has caused this certificate to be signed by its duly authorized officers, and its Corporate Seal to be hereunto affixed, at Cleveland, Ohio, this 3d day of April A.D. 1920

THE ENGELN ELECTRIC COMPANY

Secretary. By President

SHARES NO PAR VALUE EACH

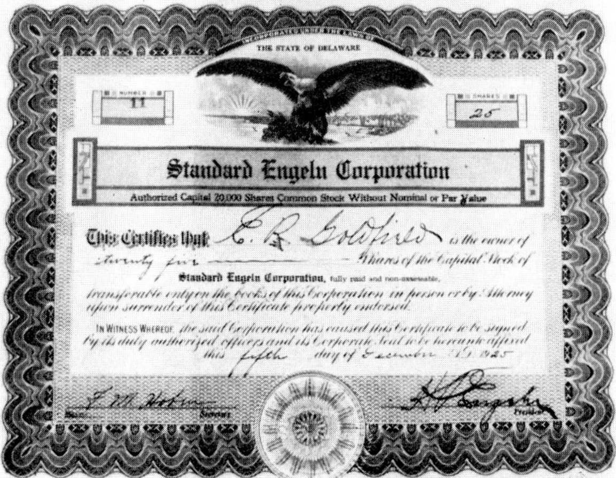

THE STATE OF DELAWARE

NUMBER 11 SHARES 25

Standard Engeln Corporation

Authorized Capital 20,000 Shares Common Stock Without Nominal or Par Value

This Certifies that E. R. Goldfield is the owner of twenty five Shares of the Capital Stock of Standard Engeln Corporation, fully paid and non-assessable, transferable only on the books of this Corporation in person or by Attorney upon surrender of this Certificate properly endorsed.

In Witness Whereof the said Corporation has caused this Certificate to be signed by its duly authorized officers and its Corporate Seal to be hereunto affixed this fifth day of December A.D. 1925

Secretary President

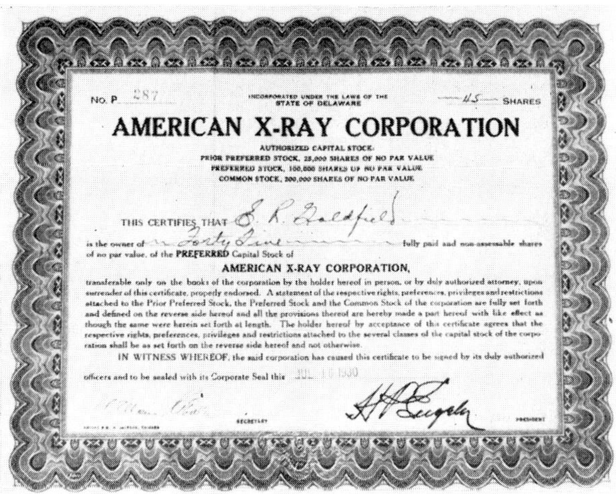

No. P 287 INCORPORATED UNDER THE LAWS OF THE STATE OF DELAWARE 45 SHARES

AMERICAN X-RAY CORPORATION

AUTHORIZED CAPITAL STOCK:
PRIOR PREFERRED STOCK, 25,000 SHARES OF NO PAR VALUE
PREFERRED STOCK, 100,000 SHARES OF NO PAR VALUE
COMMON STOCK, 200,000 SHARES OF NO PAR VALUE

THIS CERTIFIES THAT E. R. Goldfield is the owner of Forty Five fully paid and non-assessable shares of no par value, of the PREFERRED Capital Stock of

AMERICAN X-RAY CORPORATION,

transferable only on the books of the corporation by the holder hereof in person, or by duly authorized attorney, upon surrender of this certificate, properly endorsed. A statement of the respective rights, preferences, privileges and restrictions attached to the Prior Preferred Stock, the Preferred Stock and the Common Stock of the corporation are fully set forth and defined on the reverse side hereof and all the provisions thereof are hereby made a part hereof with like effect as though the same were herein set forth at length. The holder hereof by acceptance of this certificate agrees that the respective rights, preferences, privileges and restrictions attached to the several classes of the capital stock of the corporation shall be as set forth on the reverse side hereof and not otherwise.

IN WITNESS WHEREOF, the said corporation has caused this certificate to be signed by its duly authorized officers and to be sealed with its Corporate Seal this JUL 10 1930

SECRETARY PRESIDENT

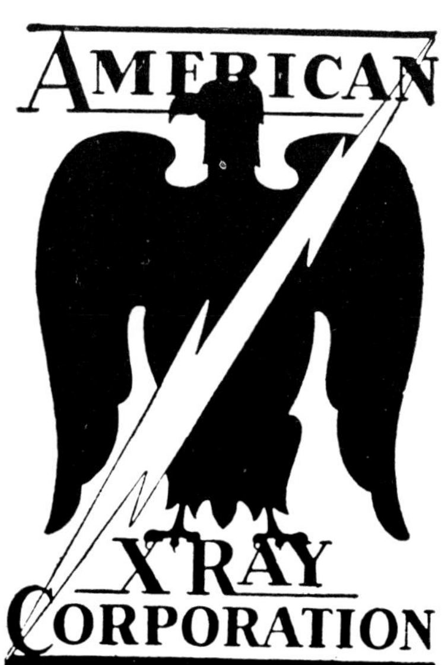

sociated with Henry Engeln. First are stocks of the Engeln Electric Company, then certificates in the name of the (never materialized) Standard Engeln Company, and finally the fancy papers issued by the American X-Ray Company. At about that time the stock market crashed, and the American X-Ray Company (which had taken over the responsibility for all this stock) went broke: The stock certificates were later retired at two dimes to the dollar. I chalked it up as experience gained. I want to make it clear, though, that there had been nothing dishonest, it was simply the beginning of the Big Depression. Nor am I angry; my association with the Engeln Company gave me the necessary technical background for what I was later to achieve in Cleveland."

WAPPLER

German-born Frederick and Reinhold Wappler came to this country when they were about 20 years old. Wappler & Fayer was the name of a firm, established in Manhattan in 1897, for the repair of electric instruments. It went through several changes of name, and became in 1901 the Wappler Electric Controller Co., which for many years was one of the most respected names in the American x-ray industry.*

In 1910 they advertised an interrupterless machine with 7½″ spark and "phenomenal speed, mildest as well as heaviest out-put, up to 200 ma and over," claimed also to be "easiest on x-ray tubes" through its peculiar wave form. In 1916, the same equipment was called the King Model and came with Coolidge tubes. By that time, Wappler had also a branch office at 1871 Ogden Ave. in Chicago, and representatives and service stations in Newark, Philadelphia, Pittsburgh, Cleveland, Detroit, Toronto, Tacoma, San Francisco, and Los Angeles. The Wappler plant and headquarters were then on Long Island (New York.)

In 1924 the Wappler Co. brought out the first American made transformer with hot cathode kenotron rectifiers (Imboden).

Following are excerpts from letters by Joseph Burns, Sr.:

"I was personally acquainted with Frederick Wappler, president of the Wappler Electric Controller Company, and with Reinhold Wappler, president of the American Cystoscope Makers, Inc. (ACMI). Both companies were at one time located at 160 Harris Ave. in Long Island City.

"The Wappler Electric Co. required most of the space in the building, while the ACMI had the top floor. Wappler and their distributors had exclusive sales and distribution of ACMI products.

"Both Wappler brothers were excellent mechanics. The cystoscope in its present form (especially the re-

*The information herein contained was obtained through the obliging (though a bit reluctant) courtesy of the Wappler family. One of them is Bert Carl Wappler (Frederick's son), whose firm — Wappler, Inc., manufacturer of electronic, medical, dental, and other equipment — retired from the trade in 1958. The other is Reinhold D. Wappler, the first Reinhold's grandson, currently one of the officials of the American Cystoscope Makers.

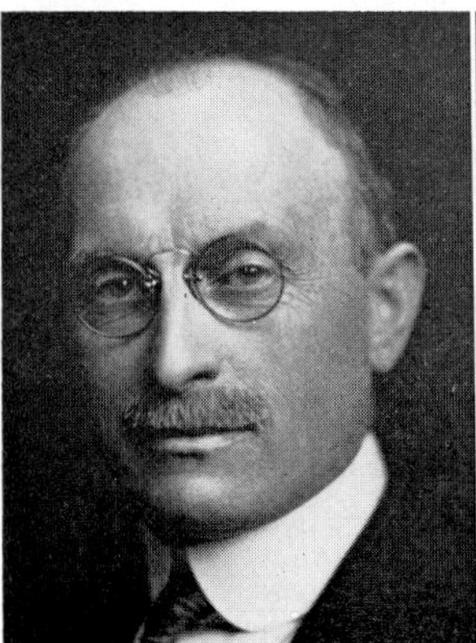

FRED WAPPLER

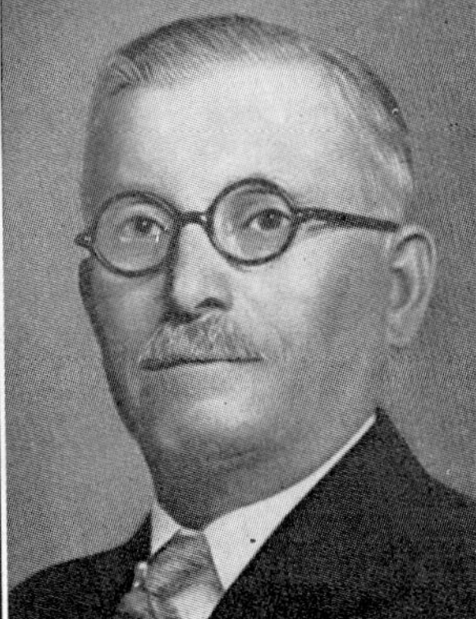

REINHOLD WAPPLER

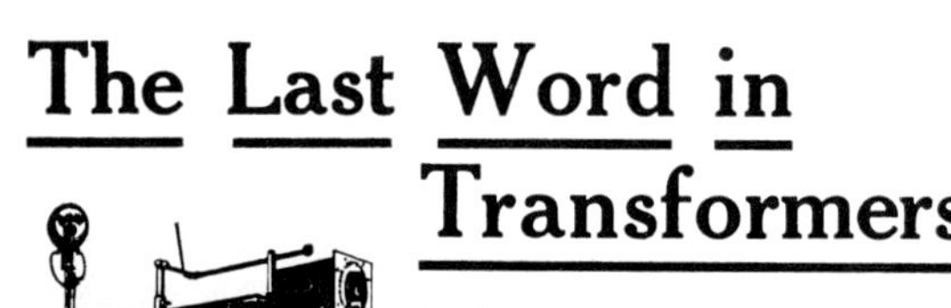

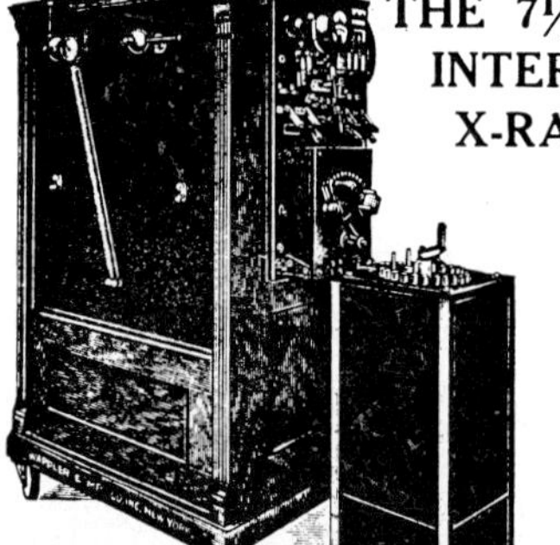

THE 7½ KILO-WATT INTERRUPTERLESS X-RAY MACHINE

Five years of careful and scientific development have produced this **Marvel of Efficiency.**

Qualified experts have recorded their praise of its correct Engineering, Electrical principles and its highest grade of workmanship.

Phenomenal Speed—mildest as well as *heaviest output.* ½ to 200 milliamperes and over.

Flexibility of control and range.

Fluoroscopic as well as **Radiographic.**

Easiest on X-Ray Tubes, through peculiar wave form.

Produces widest range of contrast on plates.

And We are Ready to Prove It

Manufactured in Sizes From 1 Kilo-Watt Up

Write for Catalog and Details

Wappler Electric Man'fg Co., Inc.

173-175 E. 87th STREET NEW YORK

sectoscope) owes much to Reinhold's personal endeavors. And Fred was just as able and willing to perform in his workshop. I remember being in the factory when Dr. Walter E. Dandy, the neurosurgeon from Johns Hopkins, came and asked for a special electrode which he wanted to use in a brain operation with one of Wappler's early "bloodless knives" (diathermy). The three of us went into the factory, and Fred machined the electrode while Dandy was describing it. The piece was subsequently used with success.

The Wapplers made frequent trips to Europe. They were personally acquainted with Röntgen, Einstein, and Bucky. On their trips they picked up ideas as well as men. C. Fayer was Wappler's chief engineer. Fayer's daughter was an electrical engineer, also on Wappler's payroll. The Kelly Clinic on Eutaw Place in Baltimore – known to contain at the time the world's largest private collection of radium – wanted a physicist to do their calibrating and similar jobs, I communicated with the Wapplers, who promised to do their best. The man they convinced to come to Baltimore from Germany was a tall, lean, and lanky physicist by the name of Otto Glasser. Arthur Mutscheller came to America to work as a physicist for Wappler.

WAPPLER

"Among Wappler distributors I remember Charles Kehlenbach in Boston, George Wm. Finegan in Rochester (New York), William Weber in Philadelphia,

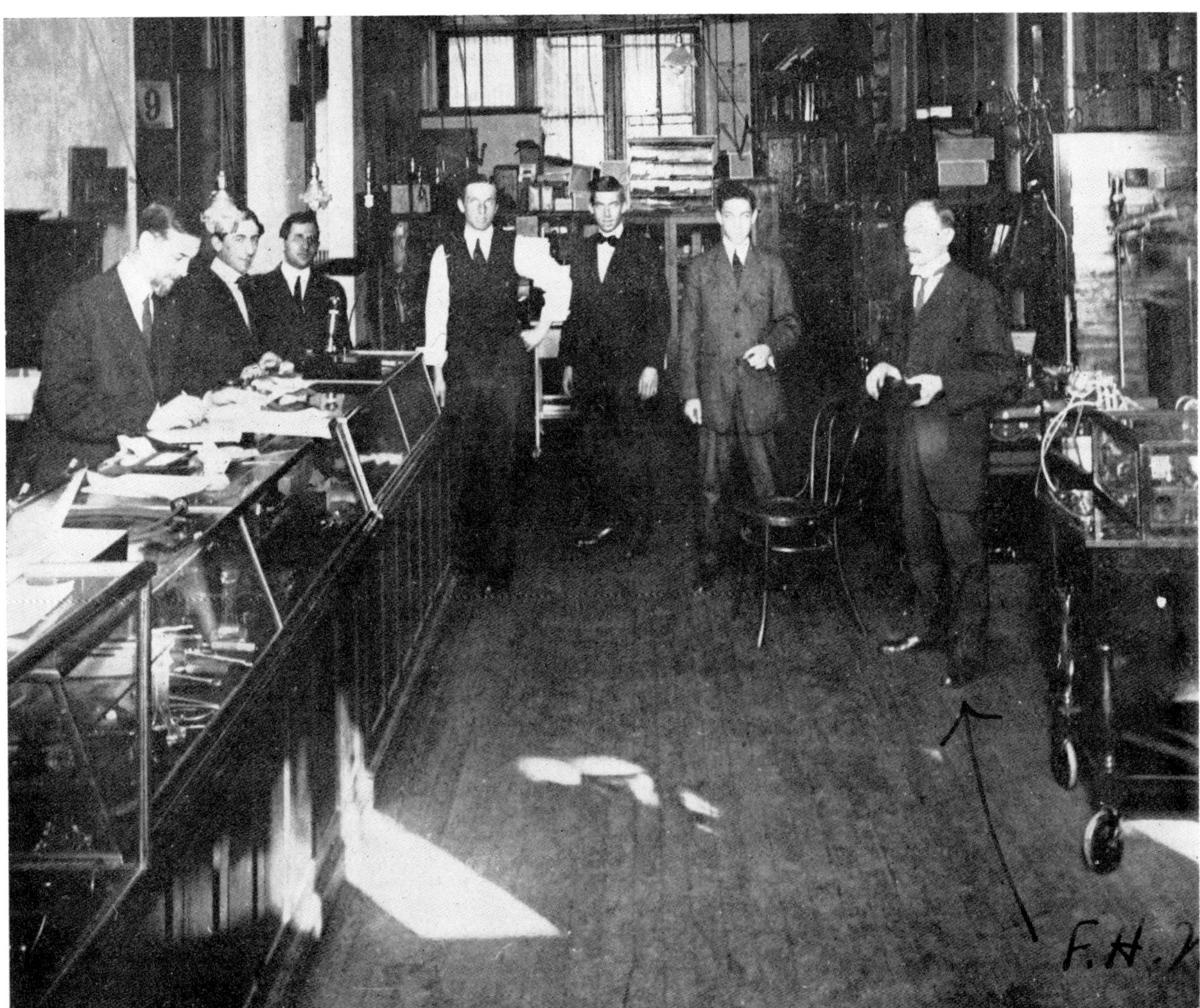

Courtesy: Bert Wappler

WAPPLER ELECTRIC CONTROLLER COMPANY, while at 173-175 East 87th Street in New York City. Balding Fred Wappler stands at far right. Counterclockwise are Wm. Weber (who was then an errand boy, but later became Keleket's sales manager); Harry Ernst, a salesman; Leo Kotraschek, Wappler's general manager; S. Freifeld, the bookkeeper; Martin Krongoldt, a salesman; and W. W. Hoag.

Kronenberg in Baltimore, Schoeck in Atlanta, J. U. Christ in Cleveland, Dodge in Detroit, Magnuson in Omaha, and Pengelly in Minneapolis (and Milwaukee).

"Early in 1930, while in Roanoke (Virginia), I heard rumors of a sale. Inquires with Wappler headquarters (I was then with Kronenberg) brought only a denial. But the deal had been made, and Westinghouse purchased Wappler Electric Controller Co. about June 15, 1930. Reinhold owned stock in Wappler Co., but Fred held controlling interest (the situation was reversed as far as ACMI was concerned). Fred had sold out to Westinghouse against Reinhold's advice and explicit desire. I remember being at the AMA convention in Detroit in June of 1930 when I saw with astonishment how the Wappler brothers (always so friendly to each other) turned their heads in opposite direction during a fortuitous encounter. The resulting family feud may still be in effect. Reinhold's son, Frederick C. Wappler, changed his business cards to read F. Charles Wappler.

"The ACMI, released of its agreement with Wappler for distribution, made better marketing arrangements, prospered, and is today one of the world's leading firms in its field. Incidentally, there is a close co-operation between ACMI and the C. R. Bard Co., makers of catheters: well known among radiologists is the Bardex retention catheter for barium enema."

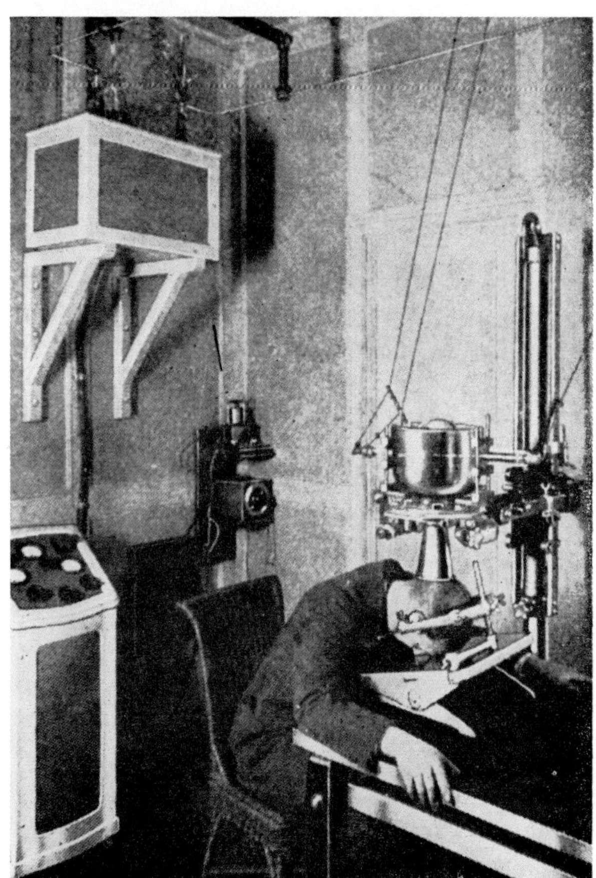

Courtesy: Bert Wappler

WAPPLER'S MONEX IN 1927. Wappler introduced valve-rectification to this country (with Müller kenotrons). His diagnostic models were called Monex, Diex, and Quadrex, and had the kenotrons "hidden" to permit fluoroscopy. The Monex was also usable for superficial therapy, the Diex for intermediate therapy. A unit, built for therapy only, was called the Quadrocondex.

At the time of the sale to Westinghouse, Fred Wappler's company had 300 employees, working in the Long Island City plant, which had been built in 1917, at 21-16 43rd Ave. After the merger, Fred was elected president and treasurer of the Westinghouse X-Ray co., a prosition from which he retired three years later. In the last two decades of his life he was active in voluntary hospital work, and other charitable occupations.

AXC + W = W

It is not generally known that Westinghouse sold x-ray tubes long before 1930: as far back as 1914 they advertised in the *Journal de Radiologie* a Westinghouse X-Ray Tube (gas), the so-called Intensive Model. It was manufactured with Cooper-Hewitt help.

GE had been very successful with its Victor diversification, and Westinghouse was quite desirous to follow in their footsteps. In 1930 the Big Depression had reached its height, but was still growing in depth. It seemed like a propitious time to acquire a production line of x-ray equipment for their tubes. They purchased the faltering American X-Ray Corpora-

Ampoules à Rayons X

WESTINGHOUSE

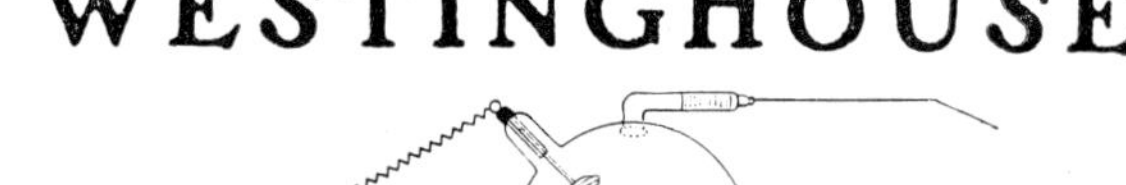

MODELE INTENSIF

ANTICATHODE EN TUNGSTEN

(Demander également nos Tubes à platine et à eau)

DES MILLIERS FOURNIS AUX ARMEES ALLIEES

LIVRAISON IMMEDIATE

(Se trouvent dans toutes les Maisons électro-médicales)

DEMANDER NOTRE TARIF 1077 1915

THE WESTINGHOUSE COOPER HEWITT C° Ltd

Adresse télégr. HEWITLIGHT — **SURESNES** (PRÈS PARIS), 11, rue du Pont — Téléphone : Wagram 86-10 tion, and at the same time Wappler's plant. Everything worthwhile was moved to Westinghouse's (Wappler's former) location at Long Island.*

Wappler had used in a few advertisements a W. Westinghouse's own emblem (introduced about 1905), a "bolder" capital W, underwent several changes. It has lately been stylized into a sort of crown.

*The job of president of the American X-Ray Company was given to Millard B. Hodgson, who was then Eastman Kodak's "medical" sales manager, had many friends in radiology, and whose excellent article was published in the *American Journal of Roentgenology* in March of 1920. Joseph Burns recalls receiving a circular from Hodgson, while at AXC, vowing to end the "horse-trading" stage in the American x-ray industry. Hodgson, and his career, went down with the AXC. He later got a position as a clerk in Washington (D.C.), where he was still living when Goldfield last heard of him. Hodgson's brilliant future at Eastman had been destroyed by his acceptance of the offer to act as a figurehead for Engeln and Morrison. After the failure of the American X-Ray Co., Morrison worked for Westinghouse's Long Island branch, then went to Canada and when last heard of, was somewhere in New Jersey. Engeln became a salesman of electromedical equipment, and died in 1942.

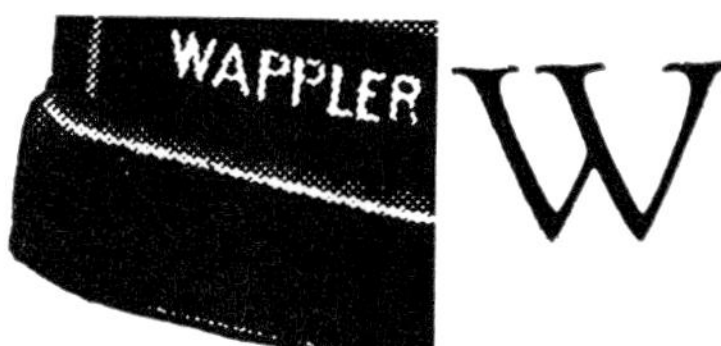

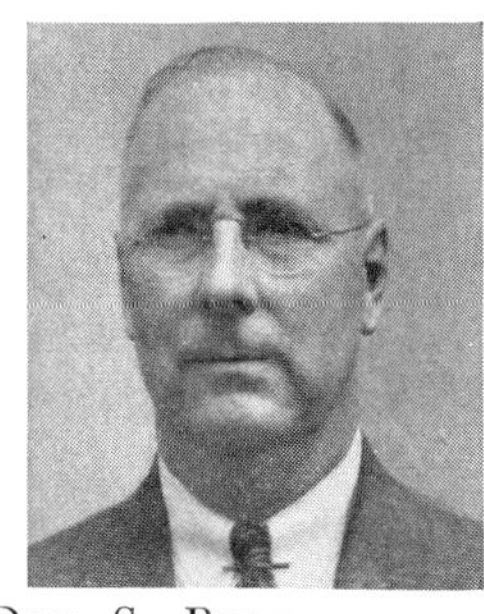

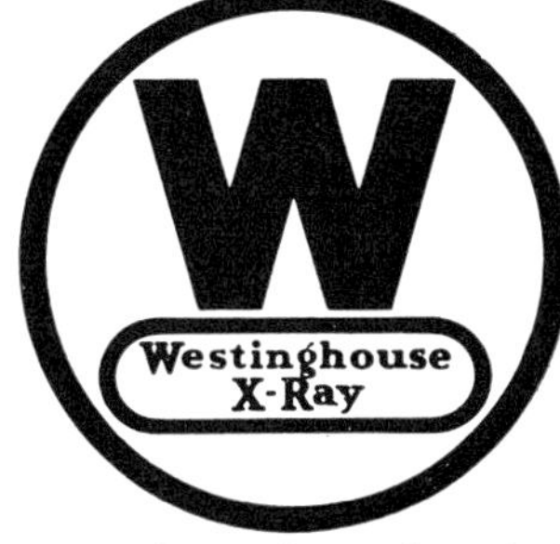

DON S. BROWN was vice-president, formerly of the Wappler Electric Controller Co., then of the Westinghouse X-Ray Co. And Wappler's "skinny" advertising initial was replaced by Westinghouse's "bolder" W.

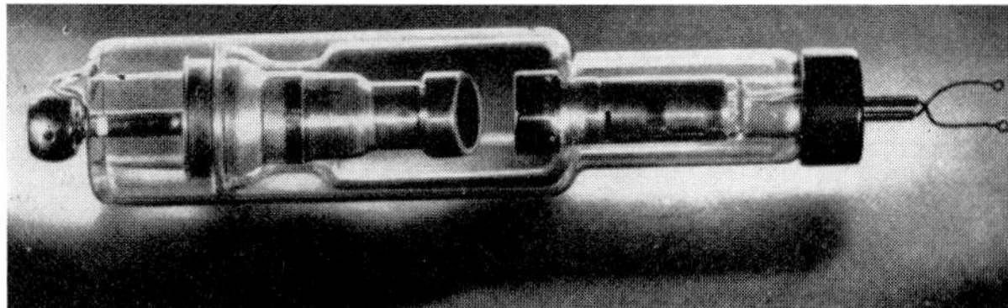

WESTINGHOUSE THERAPY TUBE. This double wall envelope tube was probably one of the best tubes among Westinghouse's entire production. Also well-remembered is their "angulated" dental tube.

Westinghouse claims to have been the first to build x-ray protection inside the tube in the form of a chrome shield, the first to make radiographic tubes free from stem radiation, the first to use Pyrex glass, the first to establish a system of tube ratings and accurately standardized focal spot sizes and limitations, the first to establish hot cathode tube ratings, the first to build an x-ray tube operated at voltages below 10 kVp, the first to develop the heavy anode so as to eliminate the need for water cooling, and the first to bring out a shock-proof high power therapy tube.*

*These statements have been reproduced *verbatim* from Westinghouse literature, and are herein reprinted without necessarily subscribing to their correctness. Ed Goldfield questioned what was meant by the wording "shock-proof x-ray tubes." He wrote to me: "If burying a GE XPT tube in a complete metallic enclosure, and introducing for the first time the flexible shock-proof cables with attractive outer covers or jackets (under which was a grounded, flexible metal sheath) means making a shock-proof x-ray tube, then this is what Picker first presented in Milwaukee in the year 1933."

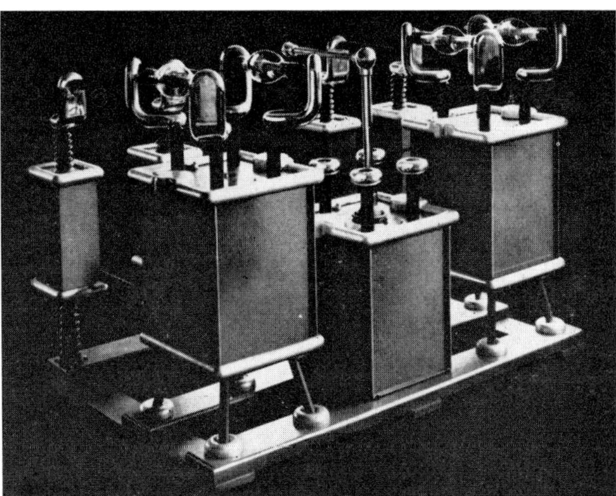

WESTINGHOUSE QUADROCONDEX (1936). Condenser therapy unit in square assembly.

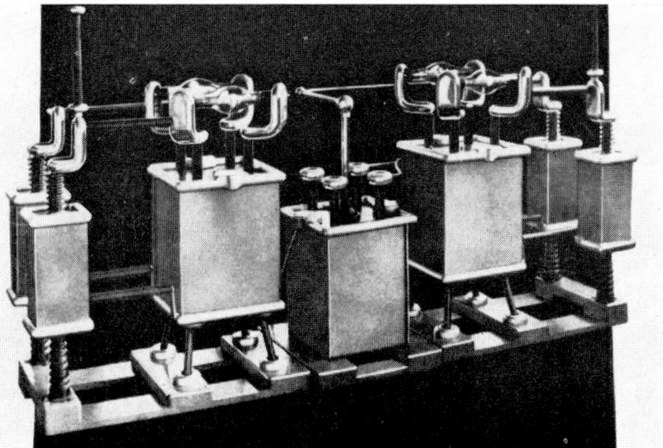

WESTINGHOUSE QUADROCONDEX (1936). Long assembly breaking through the picture's confines.

After the end of the Golden Age of Radiology, Westinghouse discontinued the manufacture of x-ray tubes. Among those that they had on the market, several were outstanding, such as the Double-Wall Envelope Deep Therapy Tube.

A famous Westinghouse x-ray apparatus, taken over from Wappler, was the Quadrocondex, a very elaborate and exquisitely photogenic constant po-

WESTINGHOUSE FLUOROSCOPE (1932). In the Golden Age of Radiology one r (1000 milliroentgens) of daily total body radiation was regarded as a "tolerance dose." This is well exemplified in the aide's total disregard for secondary radiation.

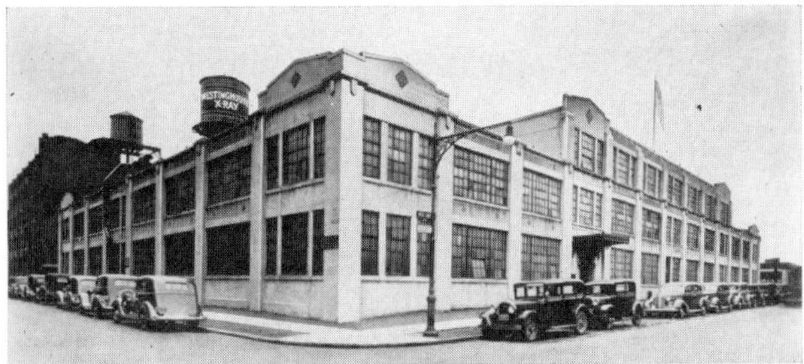

Courtesy: Westinghouse.

LONG ISLAND CITY PLANT. This was Wappler's former plant, shortly after its purchase by Westinghouse.

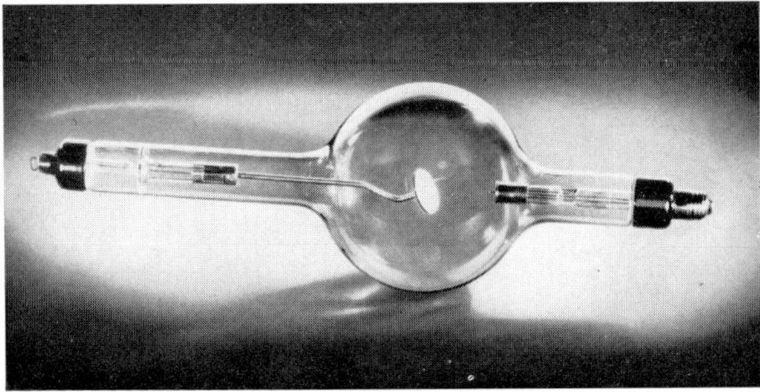

Courtesy: Westinghouse.

WESTINGHOUSE DEEP THERAPY TUBE. Air-insulated mode, manufactured in late 1920's.

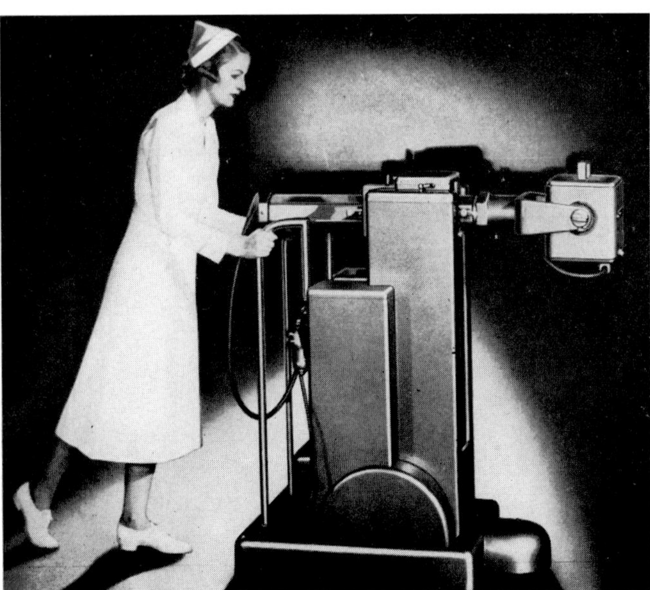

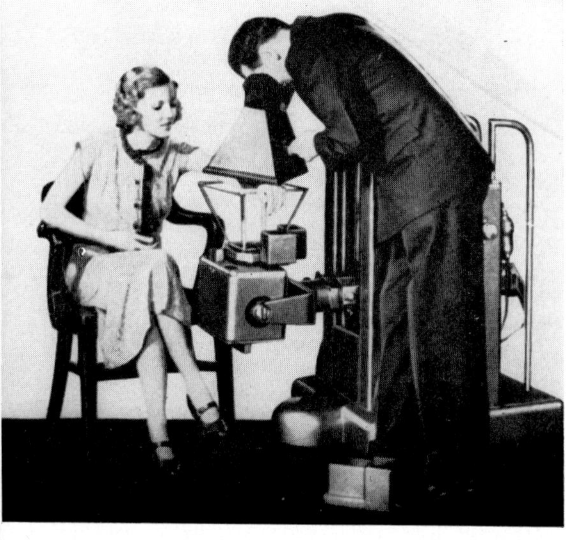

WESTINGHOUSE DIADEX (1936). This mobile unit was also advertised as offering an easy way of fluoroscoping in the emergency room.

tential machine for deep therapy. Classic styling was also achieved in their Diadex Mobile Unit of 1936; it was available as a portable unit, or as an office machine.

At this point, after several detours, information on Westinghouse was obtained from their unofficial historian, Harry Jay DePriest. Following are excerpts from his letters:

"The development of the Westinghouse X-Ray Division has been typical of the growth of American industry in general. Within twelve years after the purchase of the Wappler plant in Long Island City, the facility had been outgrown. In order to find more room for expansion and to become more closely allied with Westinghouse Electronic activities, the operation was moved to Baltimore in 1942. But war came, and the Baltimore factory became a very active center for the manufacture of radio transmitters and radar equipment – thus the X-Ray Division had to be fit into much less space than was available at Long Island City. With file space at a premium, much of historic interest was eliminated, which makes it difficult to trace certain things.

"The parent company was interested in x-ray tubes, so much so that when the X-Ray Division was organized, it was placed under the supervision of Westinghouse's Lamp Company, and remained that way until the X-Ray Division merged with the Westinghouse Electronics Division in 1941. Tubes were manufactured in the Bloomfield (New Jersey) Lamp Company Plant, and we kept pace by manufacturing various types of shock-proof tubes until World War II.

"I have been unable to learn anything about the French advertisement of 1914 for Westinghouse x-ray tubes. It is not impossible that these tubes were manufactured in Belgium under some license arrangement. I rather imagine World War I wiped out this business in short order and that it was never revived.

"The first actual Westinghouse x-ray tube was a dental unit developed and manufactured at the Bloomfield Works in 1921.

"This was a profitable venture and resulted in the development of a medical tube shortly thereafter. The Acme-International Therapy tube was developed around 1926. I can find no record of the therapy tube

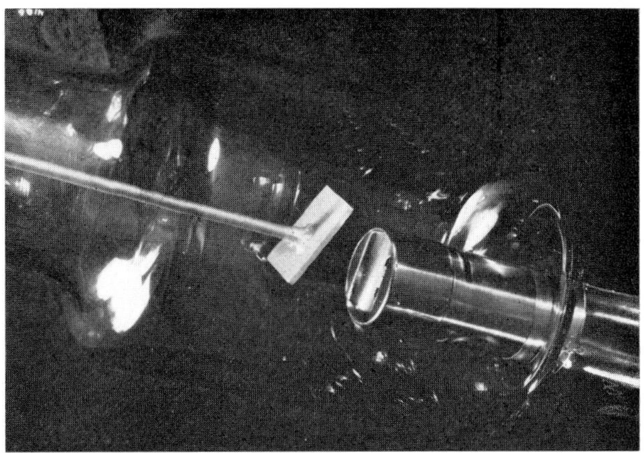

Courtesy: Westinghouse.

WESTINGHOUSE MICRONEX TUBE. For milli-second exposures, this tube is often operated at twenty-five-hundred amperes, is said to have been energized at six thousand amperes.

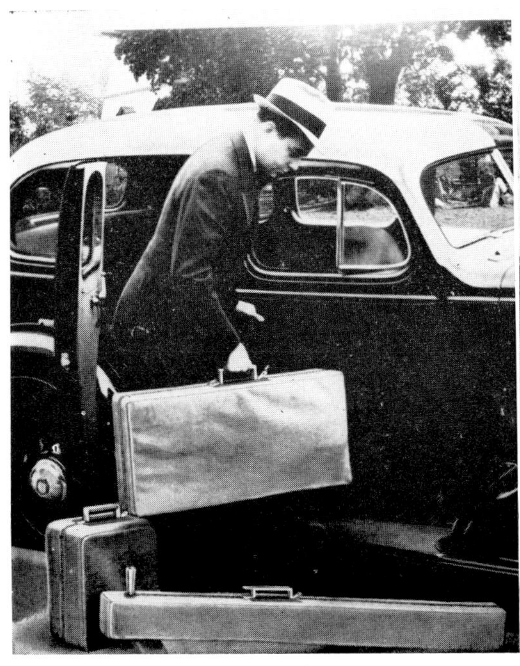

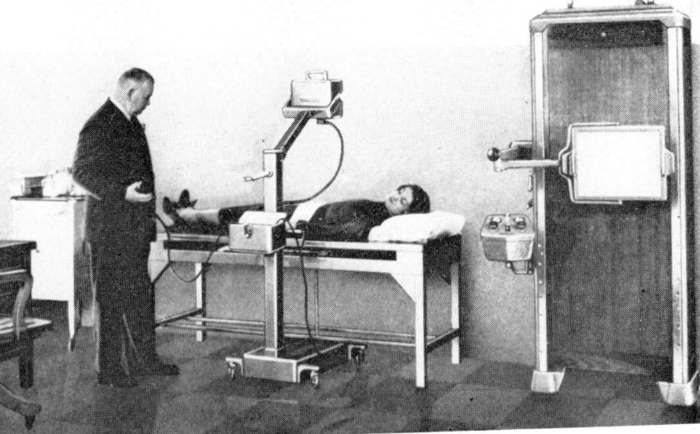

WESTINGHOUSE PORTABLE (1938). The same Diadex came also as a portable, and could be used in the office for varied radiographs, although one would question the wisdom of employing a 20 ma unit for abdominal Bucky-Potter views.

you describe ("the bomb"), but imagine it must have been built as what we call a "customer order development." We follow this practice today in many areas.

"The Bloomfield Lamp Works produced many types of interesting tubes, the most sophisticated of which to my way of thinking was the Micronex Unit. This tube was developed by Dr. Charles Slack. It was a cold cathode type, but its rating was astounding. The exposure factors are given in the attached bulletin, and the 2500 amperes is not a misprint. I have heard of this tube being operated at 6000 amperes for one millisecond. I believe a number of these units are in operation at government installations, but Westinghouse has released the manufacture of the tube to another organization.

"At the beginning of World War II "Emergency" decision was that if you manufactured a number of models of a certain item the government stipulated that we decide on which one we could do the best job and concentrate on that. We had the choice of tubes or apparatus, and as tubes were naturally limited, the decision was to go to apparatus, and we had to select certain x-ray equipment models, discontinuing others. Because of this decision of the government, Westinghouse concentrated on x-ray equipment orders, and kept tube manufacturing schedules to the minimum. Machlett, being an exclusive tube manufacturer, concentrated on x-ray tubes and Westinghouse became purchaser of Machlett products.

"A relatively mild effort was made to get back into the x-ray tube business after World War II. The Electronics Tube Division was built at Elmira (New York), and what few x-ray and valve tubes Westingtouse was continuing to produce were moved from Bloomfield to the new plant. Then came television and image intensification. While the latter are small volume as compared with all the various tubes needed for television cameras and receivers, they did compete successfully with other tubes for factory space, and the x-ray tube was one loser in this competition.

"We do not manufacture all x-ray items we sell. For instance, we do not manufacture Bucky diaphragms. In our therapy line, we obtain from outside suppliers stretcher units and therapy treatment tables.

"Westinghouse has quite a tradition in therapy equipment. When the AXC and Wappler interests were acquired, all their employees who wished to join us, received seniority rights as Westinghouse employees. There were many specialists in therapy equipment among them, and they continued to improve on the design of the Quadrocondex, which for many years

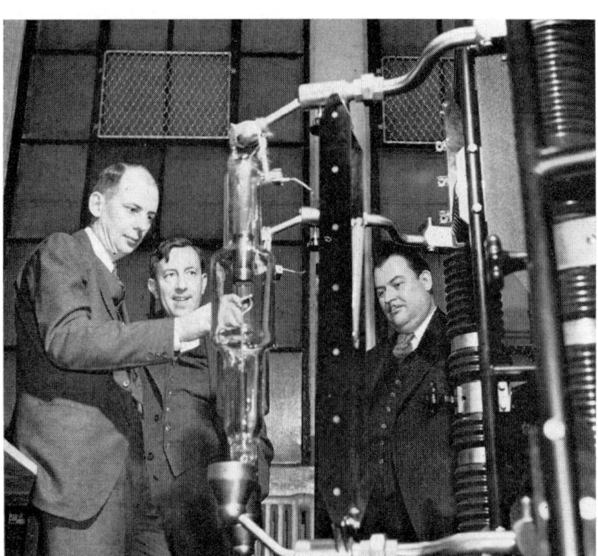

Courtesy: Westinghouse.

Charles Slack and the micronex. Balding Slack points to a feature of the tube which had three electrodes, one an anode, then a cold cathode, and finally an auxiliary cathode. The cold cathode is of the field emission type. In operation, high voltage is applied between the two cathodes, causing a metallic arc to form in the space between them, thus creating a source of electrons. Instantaneously after commencement of the initial arc, a flow of electrons is transferred to the anode and x rays produced. The method was used for high-velocity x ray examinations, such as bullet impact. Today, the field emission principle is used in machinery marketed by a company of this name in McMinnvile (Oregon).

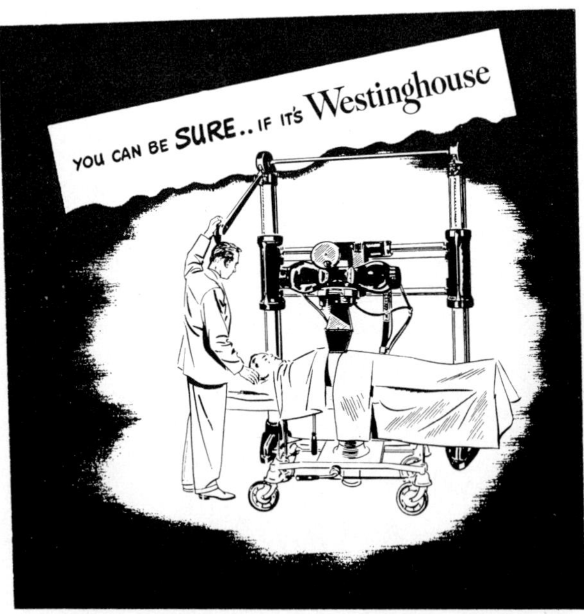

Courtesy: Westinghouse.

Quadrocondex (1944). Note power-assist activated by operator. The stretcher could be cranked into raising separately each of three sections (for head, trunk, and legs).

had an excellent sales record. It has now been superseded by the Coronado."

At this point will be inserted excerpts from a recently received letter, written by Julius Lempert, currently one of the technical executives of the Research and Development Center (Pittsburgh) of the Westinghouse Electric Corporation:

"Westinghouse activities in the x-ray tube field started in the Westinghouse Lamp Division in Bloomfield (New Jersey) in 1924 with a line of improved internally shielded x-ray tubes.

"In 1929 a thin window (4-10 micron) was developed, which became the first Lenard ray tube that could be sealed off (Patents 1,735,302 and 1,961,715).

"In 1930 were issued a line of light and deep therapy tubes incorporating for the first time a large diameter anode and a large ring-shaped focal spot, permitting increased x-ray output. This was the first type to operate stably on a constant potential power supply. It also inaugurated *W* production of x-ray tubes (WL311, WL312).

"Also in 1930 Westinghouse introduced hard glass bulbs instead of the soda lime glass previously in use, a feature later adopted by all other tube manufacturers.

"In 1931 Westinghouse pioneered the Grenz Ray tube (soft x rays for dermatologic applications) with thin glass re-entrant window (Patent 1,942,007). In the same year was inaugurated the first line of x-ray tubes in the USA (WL617 was the very first) for radiography incorporating internal shielding and line focus design. In this tube the x rays emerged from the end of the tube, which simplified internal shielding. The design of this line incorporated the focal spot progression where each successive projected spot size was two times the area of the smaller spot size: 1.5, 2.1, 3.0, 4.2, and 6.0 mm (Patent 1,992,975).

"In 1932 was developed the first high speed condenser discharge unit with a specially designed triode as the trigger or switch tube for initiating the radiographic exposure. It permitted short time "heart-arresting" radiography (Dynex line) without the necessity of high current input to the transformer. These units became portable, and could be plugged into any wall outlet (Patents 2,010,052; 2,072,993; 1,929,155 and 2,129,383).

"In 1934 Westinghouse introduced the line of oil-immersed radiographic x-ray tubes mounted in heads and connected to the power supply by shock-proof cables (Patents 2,089,079 and 2,129,387). The high-powered x-ray tube WL340 for deep therapy incorpo-

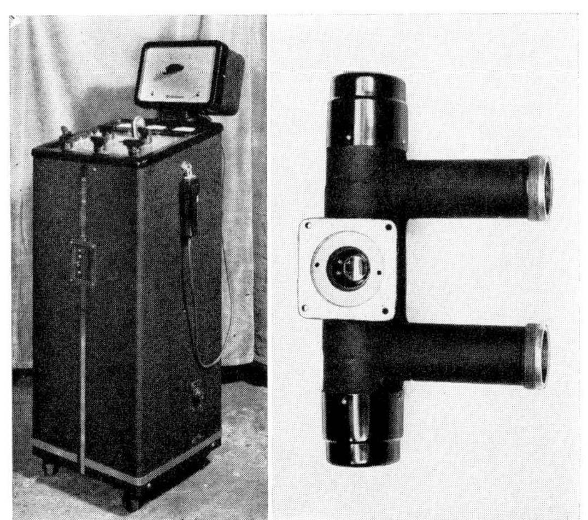

Courtesy: Westinghouse.

WESTINGHOUSE MATERIAL. The 200 ma pedestal control is of World War II vintage; several hundreds are still in use around the globe. The XFEP-1012 was one of the early shock-proof and ray-proof tubeheads, first built in 1938.

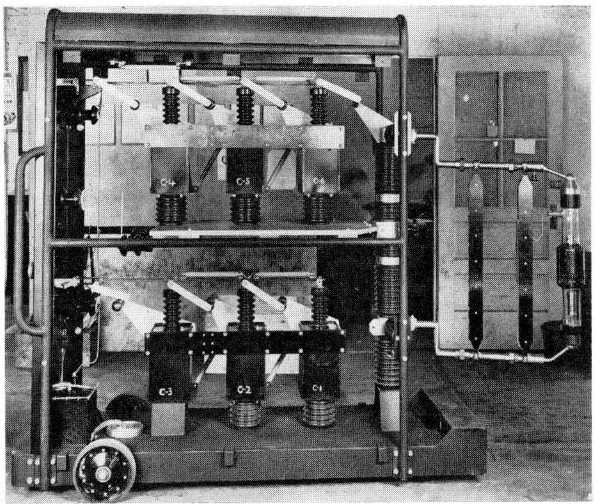

Courtesy: Westinghouse

SURGE "GENERATOR" FOR MICRONEX TUBE

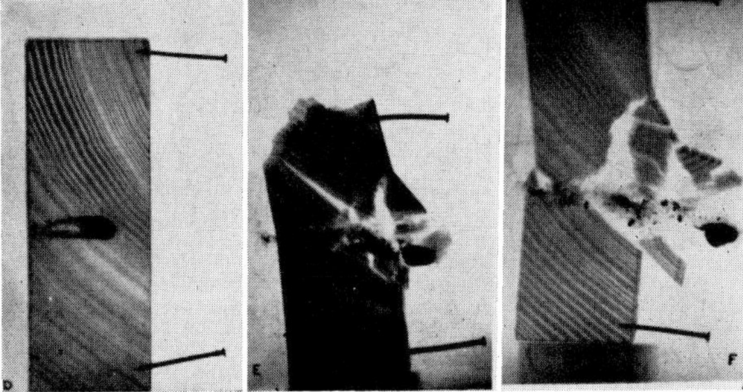

Courtsey: Westinghouse

MICRONEX RADIOGRAPHS OF BULLETS IN FLIGHT. Note "explosion" of wooden block at right. Similar studies were performed to evaluate bullet damaging effects, *cf.*, section on *Mechanism of Wounding* by E. Newton Harvey *et al.*, in the *Medical History of World War II* published by the Surgeon General of the U.S. Army rated a shock-proof design which had a removable oil spreader in its forced-oil-cooling system.

"In 1935 lead-impregnated plastic housings were built for the radiographic tubes in the WL365-8 line, which gave better radiation protection (Patent 2,063,329). The same year were introduced massive copper anodes (WL370-3) for increased exposure ratings, and double focus tubes.

"In 1937 came out small, self-rectified radiographic tubes (WL349, WL353), which could be inserted in a compact housing, together with their power supply, thus making them both shock-proof and ray-proof.

"In 1938 the life of WL340 tubes was improved by a force-oil-turbulence cooling system (Patent 2,277,430).

"In 1939 Westinghouse developed the first high speed x-ray tube (micronex) utilizing a suitable Marx Condenser discharge circuit in which exposures of a microsecond and a tenth of a microsecond could be achieved. This permitted x-ray "flash photography" of explosions, bullets in flight, and other fast moving phenomena, and proved to be an invaluable tool in studies of projectile penetration in solids (Patents 2,311,705; 2,409,716 and 2,349,468).

"In 1945 Westinghouse built the first compact (which were also the first cable-connected) 250 kvp constant potential x-ray tubes, the WL381 small spot industrial, and the WL395 therapy tubes.

"In 1946 was developed the millinex high speed x-ray tube, used by the Army Ordinance for x-ray movies.

"The image intensifier patents (2,456,968 and 2,555,545) of 1948 will be mentioned elsewhere.

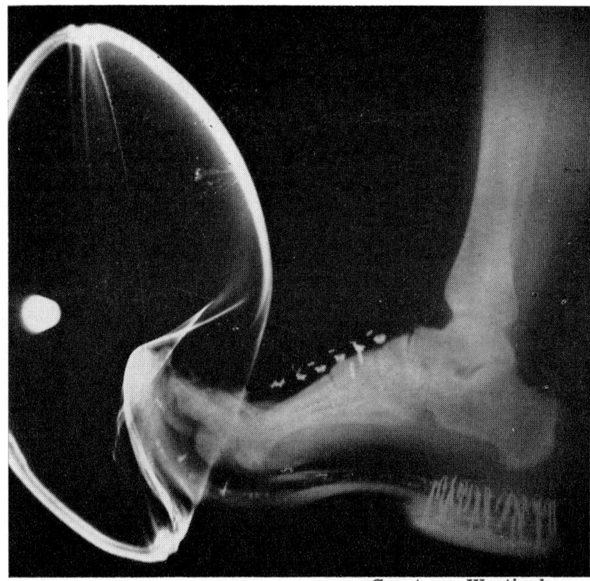

Courtsey: Westinghouse

MICRONEX RADIOGRAPH OF FOOTBALL KICK. The supposedly rigid ball is quite deeply indented before it "takes off."

"Finally, in 1950, was introduced the Westinghouse x-ray thickness gauge for controlling thickness of rolled sheet (Patent 2,669,662).

"This chronological outline was borrowed from "Westinghouse Developments in the Electronics Field," a report written in March of 1959 by H. F. Dart.

"Turning now to the people connected with Westinghouse x-ray tubes, I shall first mention Charles Morse Slack – presently retired – who was in charge of x-ray research work at the time the micronex and the surge gentrator were developed. He published, among other papers, with Louis F. Ehrke (1902-1955) a description of the field emission x-ray tube in the *Journal of Applied Physics* of February, 1941, and a discussion of radiography at high speed in *Electrical Engineering* of September, 1941.

"Norman Carl Beese, at present with Westinghouse Lamp Division, wrote a classic paper on the focusing of electrons in an x-ray tube, which appeared in the *Review of Scientific Instruments* of July, 1937.

"William Harold McCurdy managed the x-ray tube engineering work since 1932. When he was made manager of electronic engineering in 1937, John Hamley Findlay replaced him in the previous job. From 1944 until discontinuance of production of x-ray tubes, Joseph Lempert was in charge of the x-ray tube development section."*

A list of Westinghouse "firsts" will be found in the next chapter, because most of it is concerned with Atomic Phase items. Among the earlier titles are a tilting fluoroscopic table using shockproof tubes; the constant potential therapy at 250 kvp; micronex superpower radiographic unit for microsecond timing; high voltage trigger tube; condenser discharge radiographic generator; first use of valve tube rectifiers; and the first commercial phototimer.

The phototimer consists of a photo-multiplier tube connected to appropriate electronic circuits, designed

*Lempert wrote the chapter on "Industrial X-Ray Tubes" in Wiley's *Industrial Electronics Reference Book* (1948).

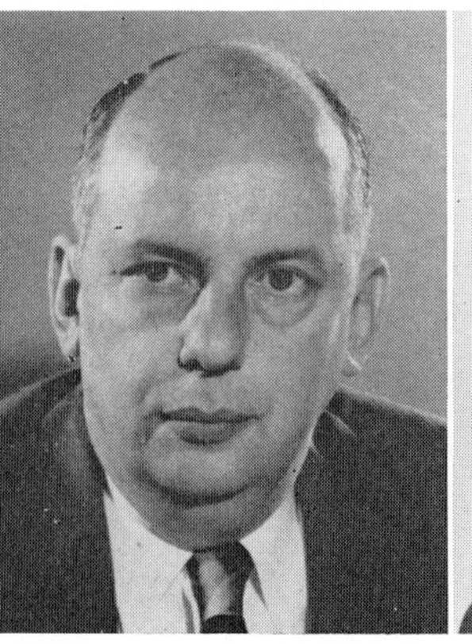

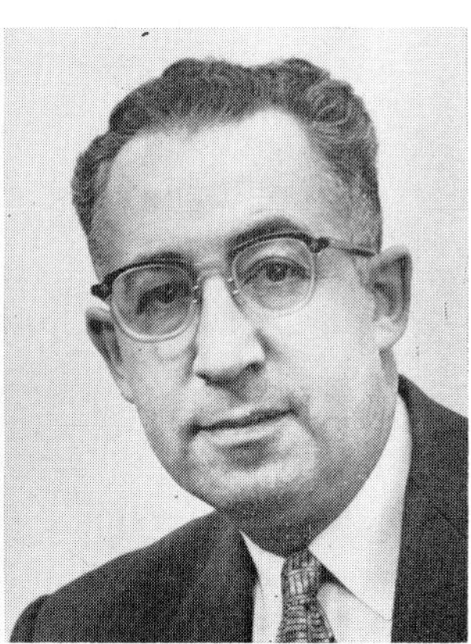

Courtesy: Westinghouse

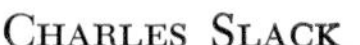

CHARLES SLACK JOSEPH LEMPERT

to cut off the radiographic current (automatically) as soon as a pre-determined exposure has been received by the film. In this way an average film density (blackening) can be duplicated, within reason, regardless of the patient's thickness. The first phototimer was built by Russell Hedley Morgan, who is now professor of radiology at Johns Hopkins.* Morgan developed the

*It was built on the basic fact recognized in Germany in 1923 by Heinrich Franke: there is on every film a so-called dominant area, the darkening of which is proportional with the average darkening, and general appearance of the entire film.

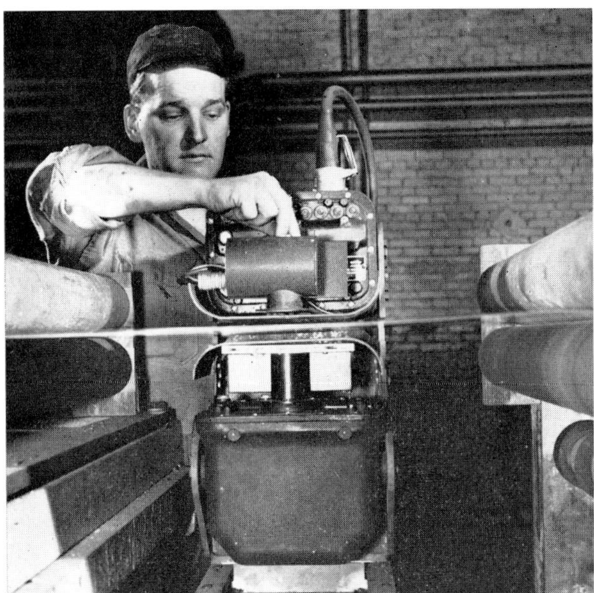

WESTINGHOUSE X-RAY THICKNESS GAUGE

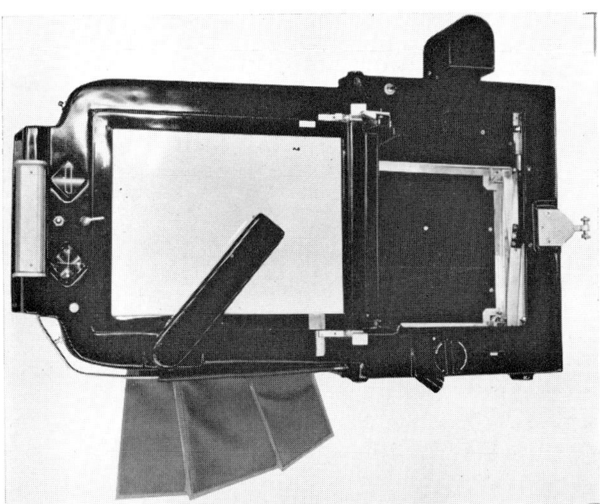

Courtesy: Westinghouse.

WESTINGHOUSE PHOTOTIMER ON SPOTFILM (1948). This is based on the Russell Morgan principle. The sensing unit is contained in the movable arm, which also activates the cassette carrier.

phototimer while he was the resident of Paul Chesley Hodges, at the time professor of radiology in the University of Chicago.*

PHILIPS

The Philips Metalix Corporation was established in Mount Vernon (New York) in 1933. Its first activities were concerned with medical x-ray equipment. In 1937 the company began to sell also table model Diffraction Units and cameras.

In 1940, a new line of x-ray transformers and cameras went on the market, and in 1945 that stained glass window was produced on the fiftieth anniversary of Röntgen's discovery. In the interim, World War II had created a heavy demand for quartz crystals to control the frequency of radio communication systems. This led to the development of the Norelco Crystal Analysis Unit in 1941: it is an application of x-ray diffraction to the quick determination of the "axis and atomic planes;"

*Hodges is now a visiting professor of radiology on Taiwan (Formosa). He had held a similar position in the early 1920s in Peking under a grant of the Rockefeller Foundation.

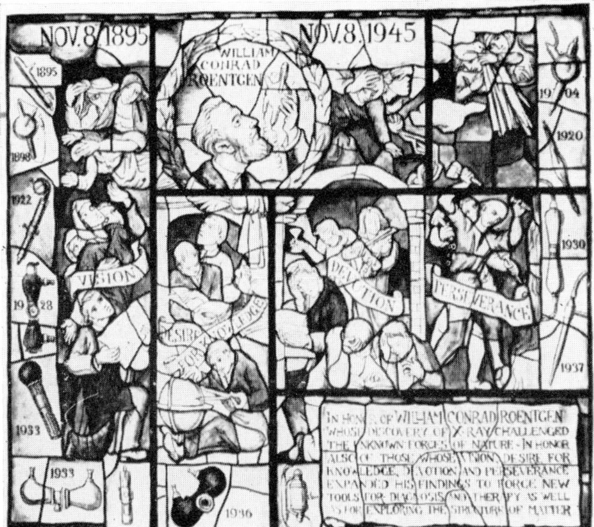

RONTGEN WINDOW. Commissioned by the Philips Company, this stained glass composition was executed by Joep Nicolas. It is inscribed, "In honor of William Conrad Roentgen, whose discovery of x-ray challenged the known forces of nature . . .". Röntgen's face is quite "stylized" (hard to recognize if it were not specifically identified), but the various models of Philips Metalix tubes are unmistakably displayed, which is, of course, quite legitimate in an advertisement. The date of the discovery is given as November 8, 1895, which is correct to the best of current knowledge.

such determination is so important because then the quartz can be sawed into accurately gauged wafers.

Incidentally, the name Norelco is no abbreviation, indeed it meant nothing. It was picked from the suggestions submitted by various employees. Now it has acquired the respectable status of a trade-mark.

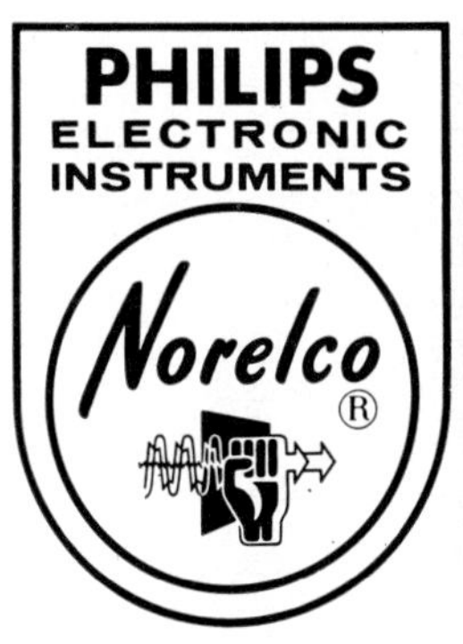

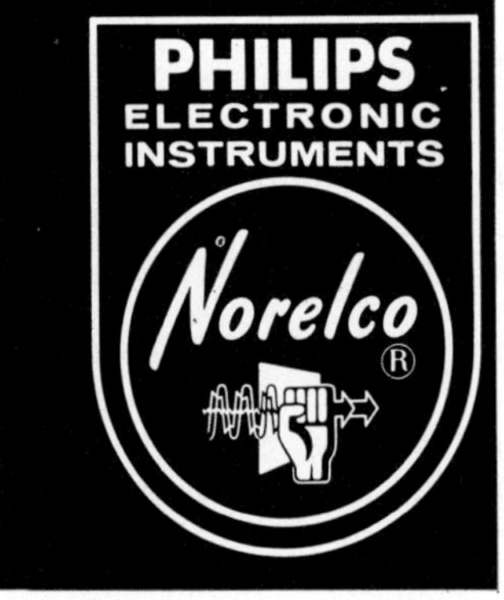

The North American Philips Co. came into being in January, 1942 with headquarters at 100 East 42nd Str. in New York City. A few months later the company acquired a plant in Dobbs Ferry (New York) and began manufacturing medical and industrial x-ray tubes; medical, diffraction, and industrial radiography equipment; as well as strictly non-medical items. In 1944 Philips introduced the first analytical x-ray instrument that did not require cameras or films: it was called the Norelco Geiger Counter X-ray Spectrometer,

NORTH AMERICAN PHILIPS COMPANY, INC.
750 S. FULTON AVENUE, MT. VERNON, N. Y.

Foremost in X-ray progress since 1896

COPYWRITER'S CONTRIBUTION. I have pondered over, though I have not understood, what is meant by the reference to 1896.

Medical X-ray Apparatus

PHILIPS METALIX

NORTH AMERICAN PHILIPS COMPANY, INC.
DEPT. R-5, 100 EAST 42ND STREET, NEW YORK 17, N. Y.
IN CANADA: PHILIPS INDUSTRIES LTD., 1203 PHILIPS SQUARE, MONTREAL

THE AMERICAN JOURNAL OF ROENTGENOLOGY

Seed X-Ray Plates and Films
at Prices Never Offered Before

X-Ray Tubes of Every Make

Sizes	List Price	Our Net Price Per Doz.	No. Doz. in Case
5 x 7	$1.10	$ .89	20
5 x 8	1.25	1.01	20
6½ x 8½	1.65	1.34	12
8 x 10	2.40	1.94	10
10 x 12	4.20	3.40	3
11 x 14	6.00	4.85	3
14 x 17	9.00	7.27	2

Our net price applies to orders of case lots only

Dental Film

Sizes	List Price	Our Net Price Per Doz.
1¼ x 1⅝	$ .50	$ .40
1½ x 2¼	.85	.68
2¼ x 3	1.75	1.40

Chemicals of Standard Quality

OUT-OF-TOWN ORDERS SOLICITED

JAMES PICKER
X-Ray Supplies
MADISON AVENUE AND 101st STREET : : : NEW YORK
Phone: 7569 Lenox

1916

known today as the Norelco Diffractometer. With it, diffraction data could be directly read on meters, or on a chart, an obvious improvement over the computations previously required.

Most of the medical x-ray equipment sold by the North American Philips Company was manufactured at Eindhoven (Holland) and imported from their parent organization, the (Dutch) Philips. Their outstanding products during the Golden Age of Radiology were the two models of x-ray tubes, the Metalix (since 1925) and the Rotalix (since 1929).

PICKER

James Picker, born in 1882, started out in business as a graduate pharmacist, then enlarged this activity to surgical supplies, and in 1909 began furnishing x-ray plates and accessories as part of his surgical supply business. In 1914, he gave up the pharmaceutical and surgical supply end of the business and devoted himself entirely to x ray. About that time he coined the slogan "in business to serve doctors." In 1915, he introduced the first printed price list for x-ray accessories and supplies. At the same time he initiated the policy of shipping the wares on the same day the order was received.

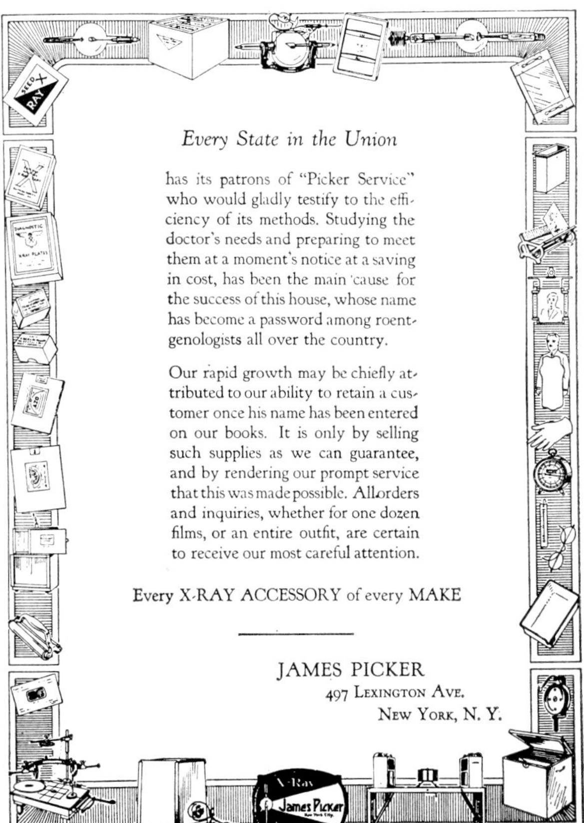

In 1916, at Madison Ave. and 101st Str. in New York City, Picker was selling "x-ray tubes of every make and chemicals of standard quality, at prices never offered before." The ads offered also "films 14x17" list price $9.00, our net price per dozen $7.27." Discount houses are not a recent innovation.

Later on, the firm moved to 497 Lexington Ave. In 1918 it was incorporated as James Picker. In 1921, the name was changed to Picker X-Ray Corporation. It remained for many years a closely-knit family-owned enterprise, and a very efficient management made it prosper right through the Depression.

Picker was always willing to get involved in goodwill gestures. In 1919, double-emulsion films became available, and soon replaced the glass plates. But the films were highly flammable, and in 1925 Lewis Gregory Cole had a serious fire in his office. Thereupon Picker tried to convince Eastman-Kodak to produce safety base film, on which they had been working for some time, but it was not ready. After the disastrous Cleveland hospital fire of 1930, caused by ignited x-ray film, Picker imported safety film from Pathé in Paris (France), but that was inferior in quality to the non-safety Eastman film. One month after the Pathé films had arrived, Eastman came out with safety film of good quality. Picker replaced the inferior quality Pathé on the physicians' shelves with new Eastman film at no charge. He took a loss, but gained considerably in stature.

In the meantime the Picker organization was moving, after having absorbed Cooper & Cooper – on that occasion Ivor (Dave) Bennett came into the Picker firm. In 1923, Picker became the Acme dealer for the New England territory. Wappler had presented the first self-rectified transformer in 1917, and by 1926 (after GE

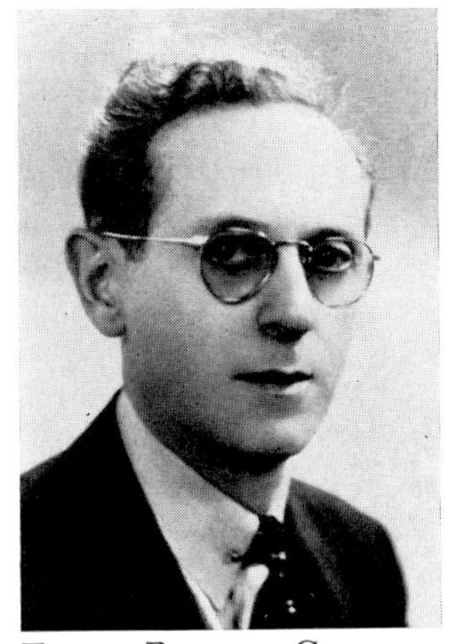

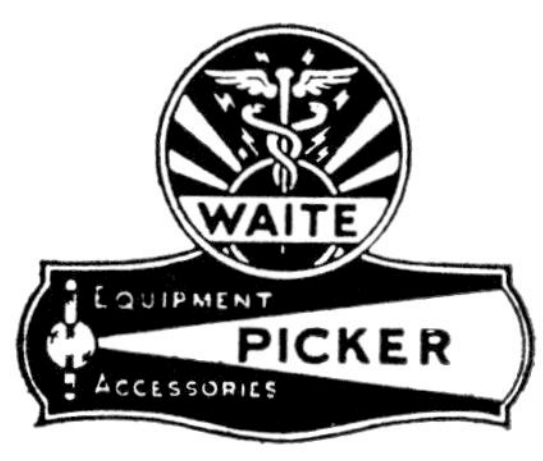

Edwin Russell Goldfield. A typical Golden Age of Radiology representative, superb designer of x-ray equipment, and excellent organizer, Ed Goldfield is shown here at about the time when he started to organize (create) the Waite-Picker Manufacturing Division in Cleveland.

had put out hot cathode kenotrons) they came into general use. Throughout 1927 and 1928, Picker tried unsuccessfully to convince Acme to develop and produce equipment with valve-tube rectification. In the meantime, in 1928, the patent for the immersion of valve-tubes in oil was issued to Harry Waite of Waite & Bartlett. In 1929, Picker gave up the Acme dealership and entered into negotiations with W & B, whose business he purchased. At the time, W & B was manufacturing a crude, enclosed upright fluoroscope, called "Coffin." This, and rectification with oil-immersed valves were some of the equipment produced in the first years after taking over the W & B.

Here shall be inserted another quotation from a letter by Ed Goldfield:

"After the merger of Engeln and Acme, the Engeln factory was dismantled. I tried to convince Mr. Picker to start a plant in Cleveland to manufacture x-ray apparatus under the Picker name, only to learn that ten days earlier Picker had purchased controlling interest in the Waite & Bartlett Co."

"Consequently I started alone, and in spite of the Depression I was doing fairly well – considering the circumstance, it may be said remarkably well. But I needed more money for expansion, and – more important than money – I needed the association with the experience and knowledge in the field of merchandising, found only in a larger organization. I felt that with assistance I could design and produce excellent equipment. Eight months later, when Mr. Picker re-opened the issue, I was glad."

"After some discussions, Picker allowed me to start the Waite Manufacturing Division at Superior and 30th, where Engeln had been located. This was quite a thrill because I went to the then defunct American X-Ray Company (actually to their 'successor,' Westinghouse), and bought from them prized machinery, which they had dismantled and taken out of the Engeln factory. I re-installed it at Superior and 30th, utilizing the same bolt holes in ceiling and floor. The 'wise guys,' who had put this merger through, were now out of business. It was during the world's worst depression, but with the financial support of the Picker organization, and with the moral guidance of Harry Waite, we embarked confidently on a new, thrilling adventure."

As a matter of fact, Edwin Russell Goldfield, a Cleveland lad of pure German ancestry, was an 'old hand': he had been in the "electric" field since 1911. Ed Goldfield opened Picker's Cleveland plant, and was — from the beginning — its general manager.

Picker did not maintain the Long Island plant of Waite & Bartlett for a very long time. But x-ray accessories continued to be manufactured in a New York location. The Cleveland plant produced Picker's big equipment; as they expanded, the plant was moved to larger quarters, at 17325 Euclid Avenue, still in Cleveland.

In its days of glory, Victor had accumulated a brilliant staff by hiring men formed elsewhere. Conversely, most of the Picker people in Cleveland had worked their way through the ranks. This made for a more homogeneous staff, and less turnover. It also makes selection more difficult when one wants to mention their outstanding staff members. Only a few names (among the many who would have deserved it) can be listed here.

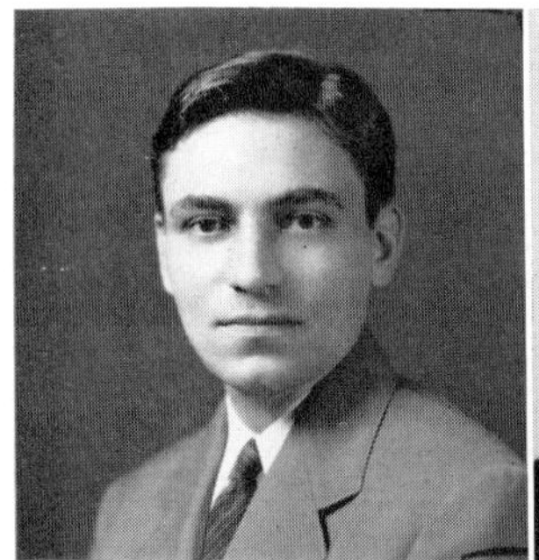
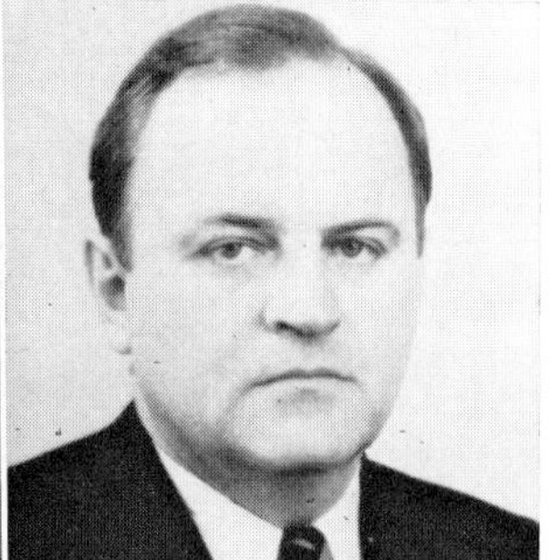

Courtesy: Picker Archives

PICKER EMPLOYEES. Robert Joseph Stava (left) was a mechanical engineer who joined Picker in 1934 and stayed on until his death in 1953. Caperton Braxton Horsley was with Engeln from 1927 until 1929, and with Picker from 1931 through 1937; he developed with Goldfield and patented the first saturable core capacity type of static stabilizer used in the x-ray industry, for filaments in hot cathode tubes.

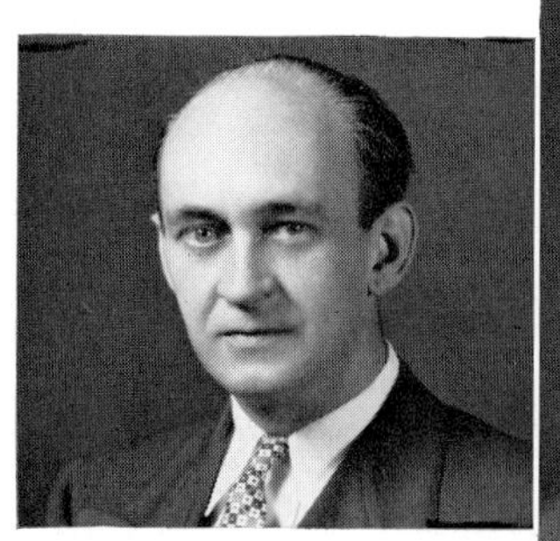
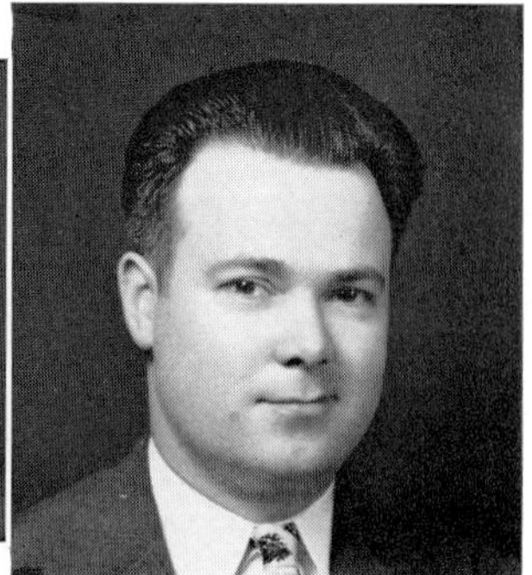

Courtesy: Picker Archives

PICKER EMPLOYEES. Edward Borchard Graves (left) was an electrical engineer with Keleket from 1922 until 1936 when he joined Picker, and worked his way up to director of engineering. Jack Ball came in 1939 to Picker, and became chief electrical engineer.

There was for instance Robert Joseph Stava, who joined the Cleveland plant in 1934 as a mechanical engineer and stayed on until his death in 1953. Edward Borchard Graves was an electrical engineer with Keleket from 1922 until 1936, when he joined Picker and became director of engineering.

Caperton Braxton Horsley was with Engeln as a sales and serviceman in Pittsburgh. Because of his engineering degree he was brought into the Engeln factory around 1927, and remained there until it closed in 1929; he joined the Picker factory in 1931, and stayed until 1937. For Coolidge's tube, Victor brought out the Kearsley stabilizer: it was a vibrator model and thus had to be cut out for the fastest, highest ma exposures, which was a disadvantage. Horsley and Goldfield developed and patented the first *static stabilizer* used in the x-ray industry (saturable core capacity type). This stabilizer is now produced by many companies outside the x-ray industry and is generally known as a Line Voltage Stabilizer.

Another young man, Ralph Clarence Schiring, who joined the company in 1931 as a mechanical engineer, was appointed president of the Waite Mfg. Division in 1958.

The first piece of apparatus built in 1931 at the Picker plant in Cleveland was an enclosed vertical fluoroscope. It was completely shock-proof and provided a greater degree of radiation protection than the fluoroscopes of that day. It had been designed before shock-proof tubes and shock-proof cables were available. Apparatus could be made electrically safe by enclosing it in a grounded "cover-all." The model was very well received, indeed, less than two years after its appearance on the American market, open exposed fluoroscopes had become a thing of the past. Actually, Waite and Garretson originated the idea, and marketed 2½ years earlier an equally safe, enclosed fluoroscope. It was not very attractive (nickname: the Coffin), but it conveyed the same idea of safety. At the time, though, the x-ray industry was not scared of W & B, a small company. By contrast, the industry reacted strongly when it faced competition from the aggressive Picker sales organization.

The first all-flexible, shock-proof, counter-balanced, tubestand therapy equipment developed by the Picker Corporation was installed at the University of Iowa in 1933. The unit was air-insulated and oil-cooled under pressure. It operated at a maximum of 200 kVp at 25 ma. The tube (Coolidge's XPT) was one of the

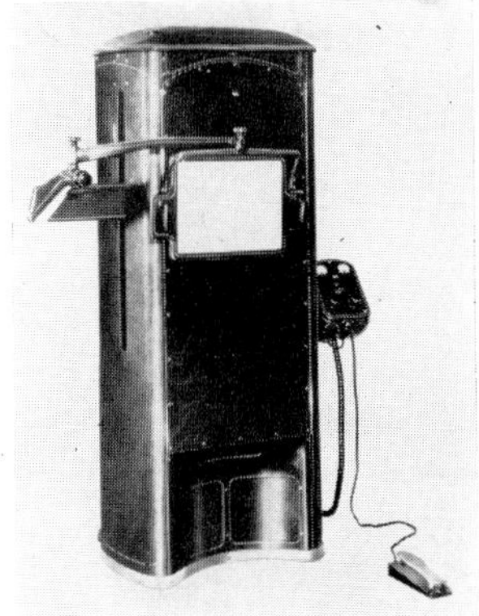

Courtesy: Picker Archives

PICKER FLUOROSCOPE. Earlier version, just as enclosed, had been issued by Waite and Garretson, but the Picker model (designed in 1931) was really successful.

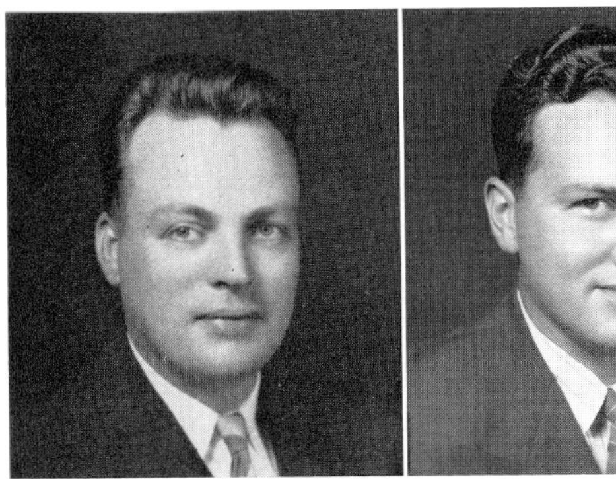

Courtesy: Picker Archives

PICKER EMPLOYEES. George Edward Maxim (left) started with Picker in 1931, and his outstanding contribution has been the liaison between the plant, the user, and the serviceman. Ralph Clarence Schiring joined Picker in 1931 as a mechanical engineer, and was appointed in 1958 president of the Waite Manufacturing Division.

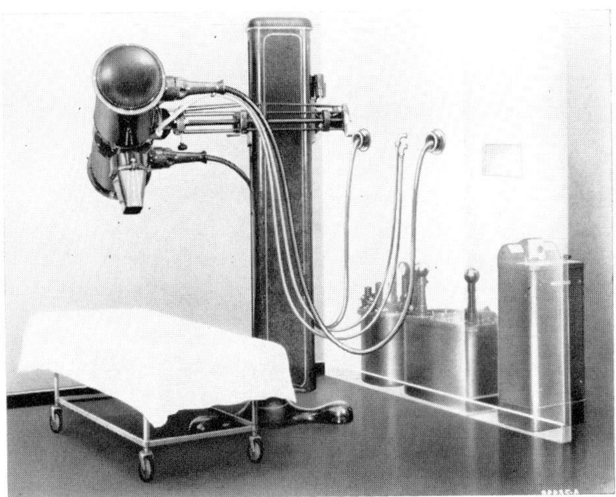

Courtesy: Picker Archives

PICKER THERAPY UNIT. First all-flexible, shockproof, counterbalanced tubestand type, 220 kvp treatment equipment installed at the University of Iowa, in 1933.

finest therapy tubes ever made: it lasted very often in excess of 6000 to 7000 hours.

In 1934, was developed a bi-plane fluoroscopic table intended for bronchoscopy, provided with two shock-proof heads. It was ahead of its time and did not sell too well.

The first full-ranged synchronous motor-driven timer was made by the Cleveland Picker Division. This timer covered both the long and the short range. The latter included also a time-proving device. The long range covered exposures from 1/20 to 2½ seconds and the short range from 1/120 to 1/5 of one second.

Spotfilm units were quite popular in Europe, especially in Germany, decades before they were accepted in the United States. The first table-supported counterbalanced serialograph, produced in this country, was made by Picker in 1939. It permitted a single (full film) exposure, two (one-half) exposures, or four (one-quarter-film) exposures. It was attached to the first motor-driven tilting table produced in the Cleveland Picker Plant.

About 1939, the Long Island plant of the former Waite & Bartlett Co. was condensed to a small shop above the offices of the Picker X-Ray Corporation at 300 Fourth Ave. in New York City, in order to provide employment for about a dozen of the older members of the W & B work staff. After that shop was closed, production of the dental machine was moved to Cleveland.

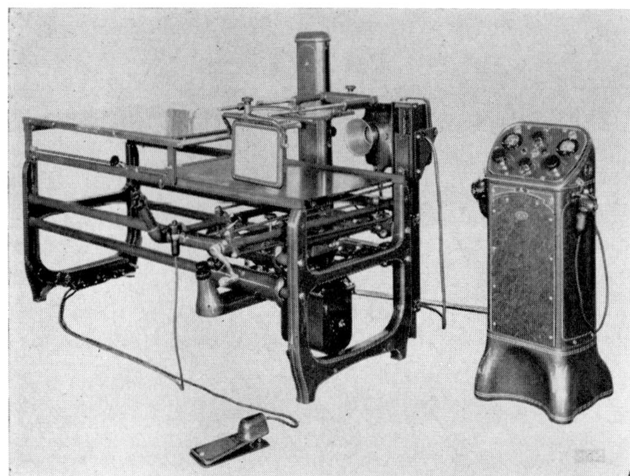

Courtesy: Picker Archives

PICKER BI-PLANE FLUOROSCOPE. Intended for bronchoscopy, this table was developed in 1934.

A few additional quotations from letters by Goldfield:

"GE, through their sales organization, suggested that we develop a 400 kvp therapy machine to help justify the fact that they were working on a 400 kvp therapy tube. We spent a tremendous amount of time and money developing a completely self-contained, fully motor-driven 400 kvp unit. We took it to the first convention to show the end result of our efforts, but this proved to be a mistake. The real end result was that we were told we could obtain one 400 kvp therapy tube from GE, and no more than one. Therefore the entire development cost had to be written off."*

*Later on, GE came out with its own 400 kvp deep therapy "bomb."

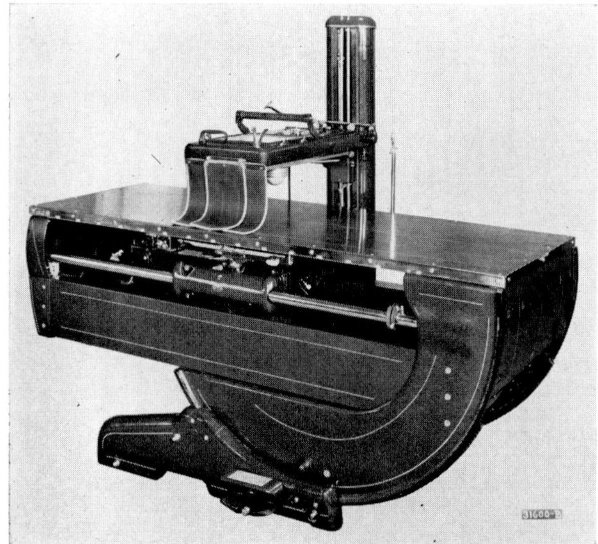

Courtesy: Picker Archives

PICKER SPOTFILM UNIT. First American counterbalanced serialograph (1939).

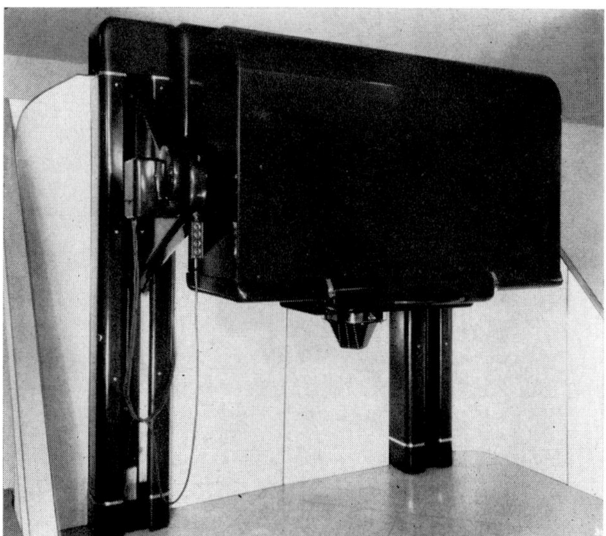

Courtesy: Picker Archives

PICKER 400 KVP UNIT. The girl that has never been kissed.

Another quotation from Goldfield:

"Two devices stand out in my recollection for having been in production for especially long periods of time. One is a handtimer designed by Liebel-Flarsheim; it has been produced in greater total numbers than any single item except x-ray tubes. The other is Picker's Century Table, originated in 1937. Its production (with none but minimal changes) has continued to this very day, and it is still fairly popular. It had its birth one evening in my basement: I took three pieces of 2x4 lumber, and nailed them together. The following morning I brought them into the conference of the Engineering Department of our plant, and demonstrated the principle of an arm that might support an x-ray tube, and at the same time could readily swing over as well as under the x-ray table. Single tube x-ray tables had been built by many companies prior to this but in every instance it was difficult to get the tube from under the table and position it above or vice-versa. In some of the competitive models, a mechanic was needed to make the change-over. The Picker Century is still (after so many years) the simplest and easiest with which to change from fluoroscopy to radiography."

The Long Island plant of the Waite & Bartlett Co., and later Picker's Cleveland factory were the only ones to produce three-phase x-ray apparatus in the United States. Its greater cost made it finally prohibitive. As

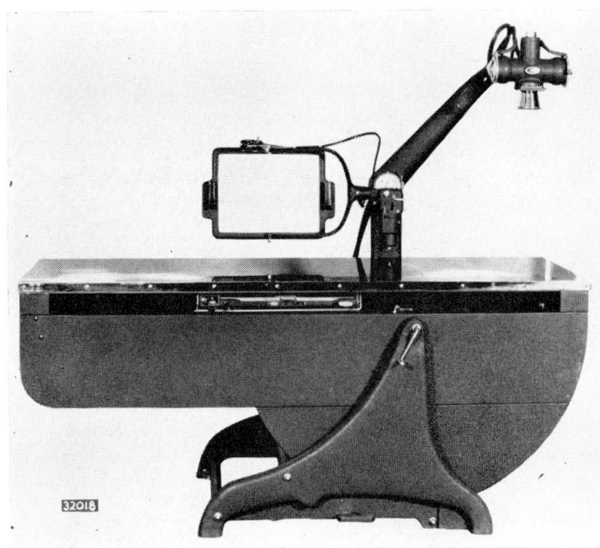

Courtesy: Picker Archives

PICKER CENTURY TABLE. First practical over-and-under-the-table, single tube unit, first designed in 1937, still in production.

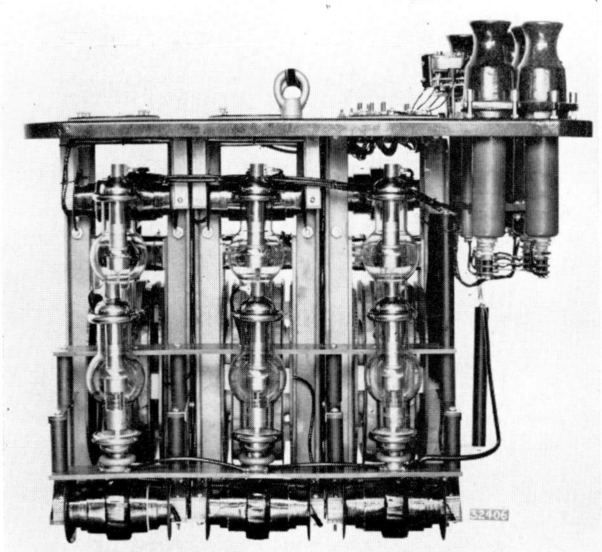

Courtesy: Picker Archives

PICKER'S TRIPHASIC GENERATOR. Innards of the only American-made triphasic x-ray transformer.

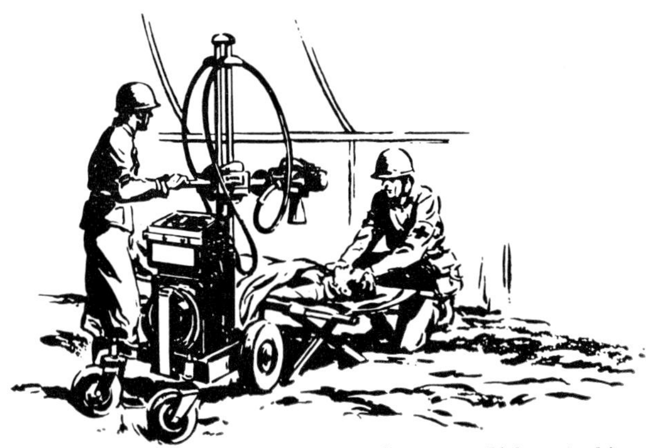

Courtesy: Picker Archives

PICKER ARMY FIELD X-RAY UNIT. In action.

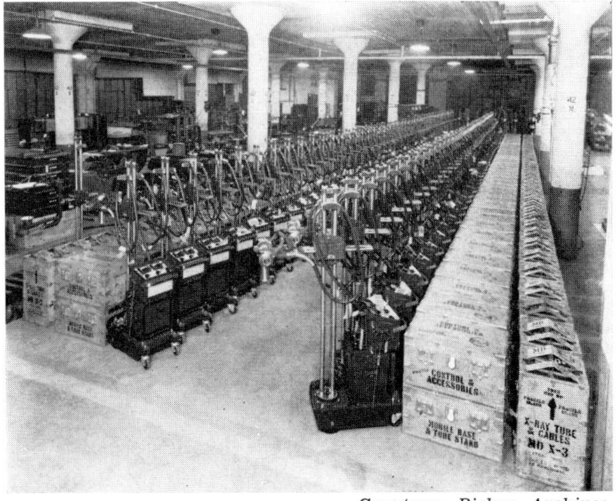

Courtesy: Picker Archives

FIRST 100 FIELD UNITS. These were sent to the USSR.

produced in Long Island it was a multiple tank device. In Cleveland it also included a 2 or 3 way oil-immersed high tension switch. It was produced until the war when the storage of material forced its "temporary" discontinuance, which is still in effect.

Undoubtedly, though, Picker's most "popular" piece of equipment was the Army Field X-Ray Unit of which Picker was the sole supplier during World War II. The first 100 pieces of this model, made in a big hurry, were sent to the USSR. Later the Field Units were commonly flown to their destination as they came in three boxes, weighing 390 lbs., with the dimensions about 3x3x4 feet.

This Army Field X-Ray Unit had been developed by Goldfield and his staff in following the specifications established for the Army by the then Major Alfred de

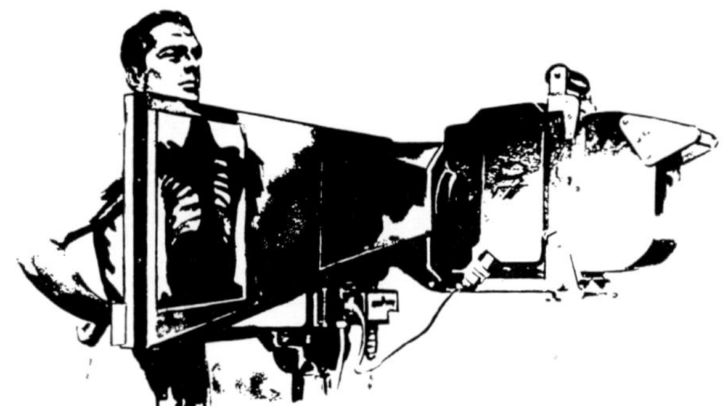

Courtesy: Picker Archives

PICKER PHOTOFLUOROGRAPHIC UNIT. Schematic view of the screen which forms the base of the pyramid.

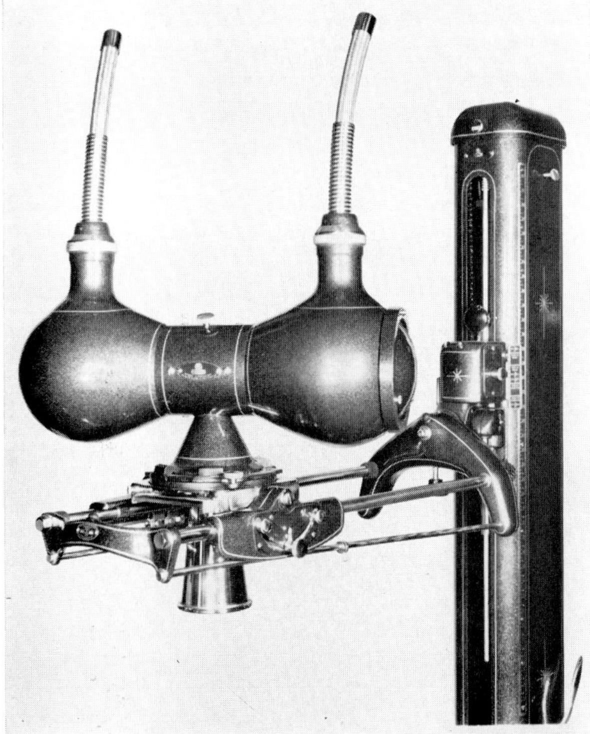

Courtesy: Picker Archives

PICKER SHOCKPROOF HOUSING. This was insulated with air (rather than oil), and the tube could be replaced by removing the cover at the end of the housing.

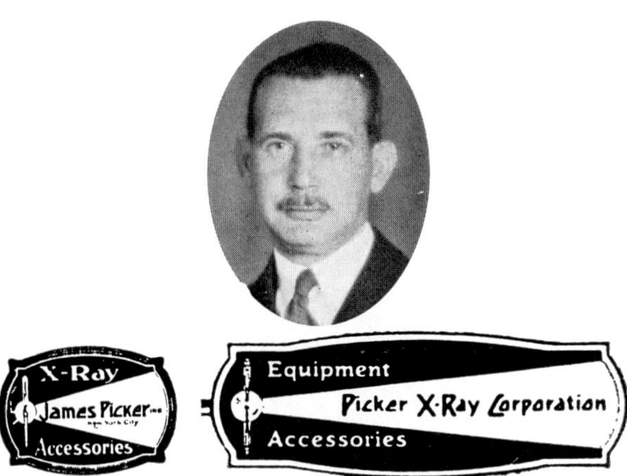

JAMES PICKER (1882-1963), being a Russian-born immigrant — in a gesture of gratitude toward his adoptive country — donated to the US Treasury the profits made by his firm during World War II. After that war, the Picker Company forged (at least temporarily) ahead of GEX-RAY, which had held the lead in the American x-ray business since the Victor merger of 1916. The Picker spirit and competition caused also other, perhaps less tangible, changes in the x-ray industry. For his contributions, the ACR gave James Picker a special award of honor.

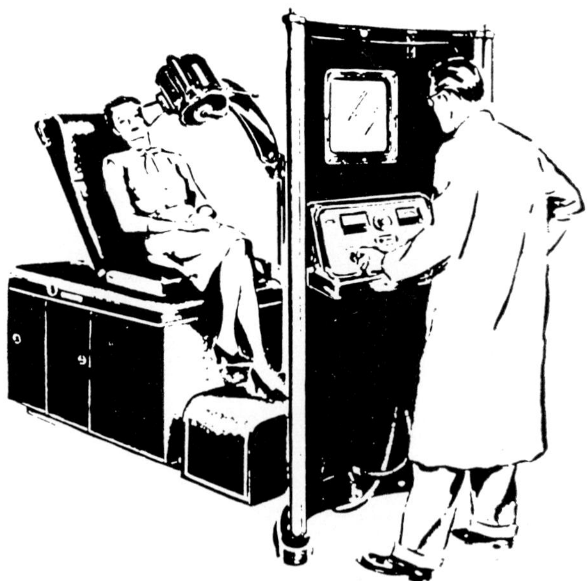

Courtesy: Picker Archives

PICKER ZEPHYR. First American shockproof 125 kvp therapy unit, using a special tube developed for this unit by Machlett.

Lorimier. The Picker plant furnished the actual x-ray equipment; Liebel-Flarsheim the grids; Buck the dryer and loading-bin combination; D. W. Owen & Sons the gasoline powered, 2500 watts, x-ray field generator; Westinghouse the darkroom processing unit; and Westinghouse, as well as H. G. Fischer & Co. the mobile table units for field fluoroscopy. For the production of the Army Field X-ray units, the Picker Corporation received a production award E on August 28, 1942, commemorated in a privately printed book, of which only a few copies remain.

Following is a list of "Picker Firsts," compiled by one of their engineers (B. G. Meyers) on November 21, 1961. It is herein printed without necessarily subscribing to it:

1. First completely safe shockproof x-ray apparatus.
2. First shockproof therapy tubestand.
3. First to immerse rectifying valve tubes in dehydrated oil in the same tank with the high tension transformer.
4. First shockproof vertical fluoroscope.
5. First shockproof high tension cables.
6. First impulse timer.
7. First single tube self-contained x-ray unit for radiography and fluoroscopy.
8. First motor-driven serialograph.
9. First integrated full-scale phototimed x-ray control apparatus (V9).

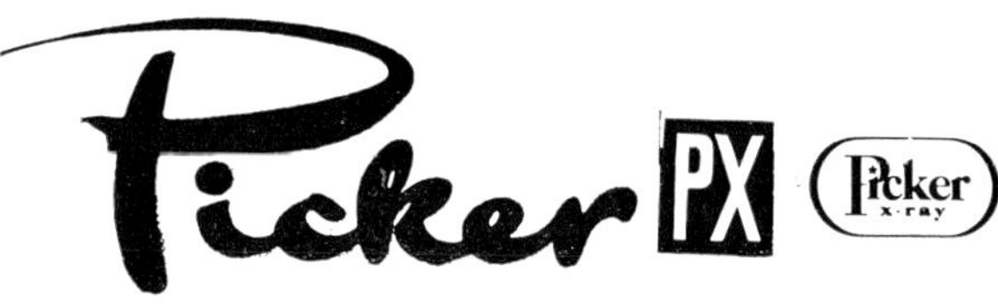

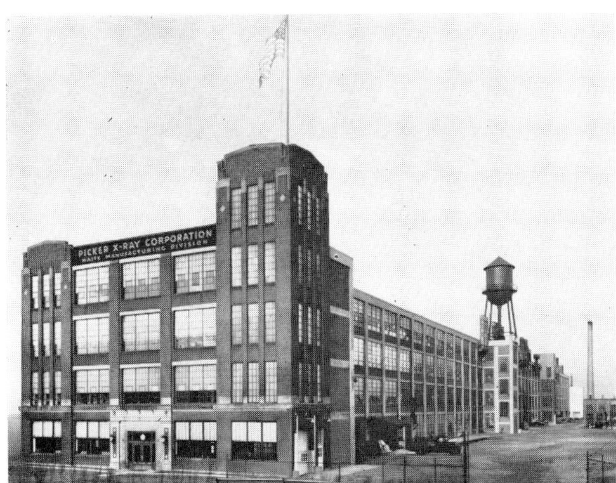

Picker's Plant In Cleveland

All x-ray equipment developed for operating room use are Picker firsts including:

10. First explosion-proof film illuminator.
11. First low-power x-ray mobile unit.
12. First tube unit for permanent O.R. installation.
13. First high-power x-ray mobile unit.

Following first in x-ray diffraction.

1. First biplane diffractometer.
2. First diffractometer with integral tube unit.
3. First diffractometer with full circle omega motion.
4. First diffraction equipment with leakproof shutters permitting variable take-off angles.
5. First monitor type x-ray diffraction control.

On April 1, 1949 — as the Atomic Phase was well on its way — Ed Goldfield, as typical a Golden Age of Radiology man as any, decided to retire, and make place for younger talents. A series of rumors were circulated regarding the alleged causes of that early retirement: I checked them out, and interviewed the main actors, and I speak with authority when stating that there was really nothing else behind it. Ed Goldfield simply wanted to make place for younger men, for Atomic Phase executives. He is still very much connected with and appreciated by the Picker organization. He is now an elder consultant, and part-time historian, comes regularly to the plant, and to conventions, but no longer in an "active" way.

The Picker Company is no longer exclusively owned by the Picker family (their controlling stock is in the hands of a financial concern, the CIT), but Picker's son Harvey, who spent his wartime in the Research Electronic Lab of the U. S. Navy, runs the company as its current chief executive. The former chief, James Picker,* established the (completely independent) James Picker Foundation for Radiologic Research, placed under the guidance of the National Research

*Died May 29, 1963.

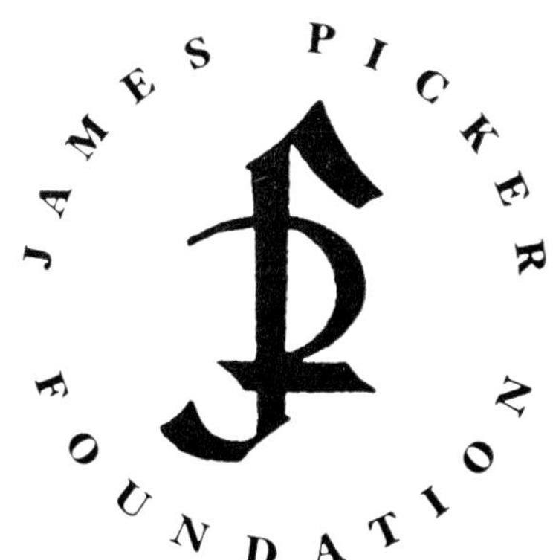

Council. For his many contributions to radiology, the American College of Radiology conferred on James Picker a special Award of Honor.

RECAPITULATION

The following "Outline of the X-ray Industry" arrived in the mail after completion of the manuscript. It is inserted at this point also because its author's activity in the x-ray industry spans six decades. His remarks recapitulate some of the things discussed in this chapter.

The author of this "outline" is Leo Carl Kotraschek, who joined the x-ray industry in 1904 as an apprentice of the Wappler Electric Controller Company, working sixty hours per week for $3.00 per week, with 50 cent raise promised for each ensuing six months. As he learned the trade, he decided to go to night school, and earned a degree in Electrical Engineering at Cooper Institute in New York City, whereupon he was made Wappler's general manager. In 1916, Kotraschek resigned, and became a franchised Keleket dealer. But, as he recalls, "Keleket was always in some sort of financial difficulties," so in 1940 he joined Picker as sales manager, and stayed in that position for eleven years. Then Philips made him a better offer and in 1951 he became general manager for the North American Philips Company, a position which he held until his retirement in 1957. Thereafter he went to Clearwater (Florida) where he again opened a small x-ray consulting business. Following is the text of Kotraschek's *Outline of the X-ray Industry.*

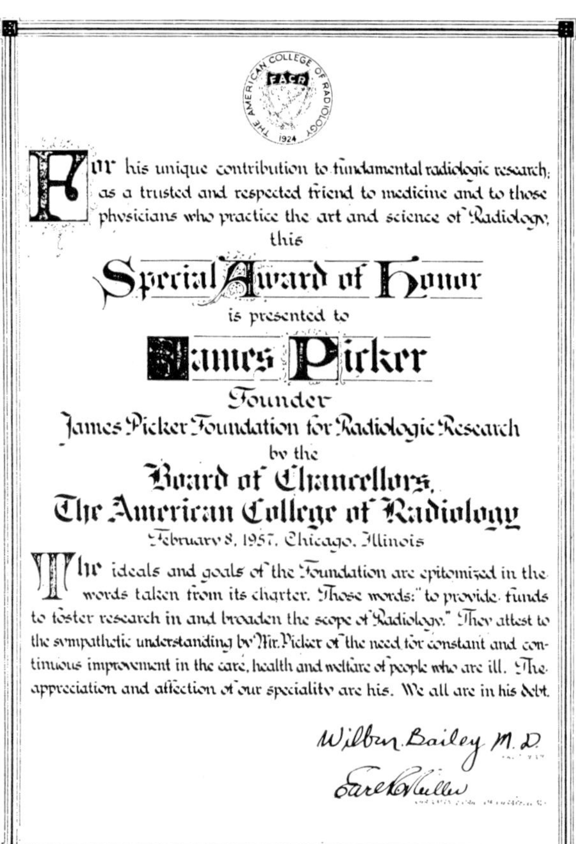

THE AMERICAN COLLEGE OF RADIOLOGY
FACR
1924

For his unique contribution to fundamental radiologic research; as a trusted and respected friend to medicine and to those physicians who practice the art and science of Radiology,

this

Special Award of Honor

is presented to

James Picker

Founder

James Picker Foundation for Radiologic Research

by the

Board of Chancellors,
The American College of Radiology

February 8, 1957, Chicago, Illinois

The ideals and goals of the Foundation are epitomized in the words taken from its charter. Those words: "to provide funds to foster research in and broaden the scope of Radiology." They attest to the sympathetic understanding by Mr. Picker of the need for constant and continuous improvement in the care, health and welfare of people who are ill. The appreciation and affection of our speciality are his. We all are in his debt.

Wilbur Bailey M.D.

Earl E. Miller

"The development of electrical and mechanical improvements in x-ray apparatus was a slow process. I feel that the radiologic fraternity owes a debt of gratitude to the host of x-ray salesmen, the detail men, and service men, as they were during all that formative period the disseminators of news, techniques, and development, being at the same time good listeners to boot.

"One of the early sources of high voltage for the production of x rays was the static machine. It was either rotated by hand crank or a direct current motor. The output was in the order of 100 kvp at 0.5 to 1.0 ma. It took minutes of exposure for a hand, and perhaps 20 minutes or longer for a hip. The static machine was temperamental; and quite sensitive to humidity. A large bowl of calcium chloride, or a kerosene lamp, placed in the same cabinet, helped to absorb the moisture. These machines were mostly used for electrotherapy, therefore many early electro-therapists became roentgenologists. One of the earliest manufacturers of static machines was the Galvano-Faradic Manufacturing Company, which became Waite and Bartlett, then Waite X-Ray, after which it was finally absorbed by Picker.

"Another way to energize the early gas x-ray tubes was the Ruhmkorff coil, in a sense an open core transformer, suitable only for direct current power supply. The electrolytic interrupters were quite noisy, and the

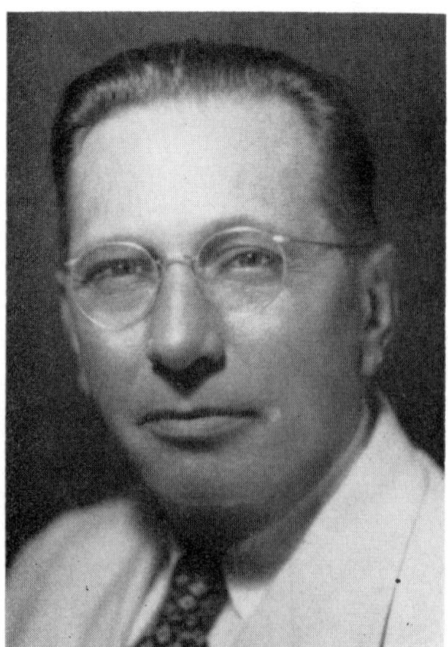

LEO CARL KOTRASCHEK

sulphuric acid produced intolerable fumes. It also leaked on carpets, and floors were ruined. Then came the mercury turbine interrupter, and all sorts of mechanical rotary interrupters. Output and power were increased to about 200 kvp to 20 ma.

"X-ray tubes in the gas era were quite unreliable. The thin platinum face of the anode had a low melting point, therefore soon copper backed anodes were built to remove the heat, and there were tubes built with various sizes of focal spots; in a given case the selection was usually based on the degree of vacuum, meaning a soft, medium, or hard tube, corresponding to a low, medium, or high penetration. And when tubes became too hard, they could be used for therapy. In New York City, aside from Machlett, one of the early manufacturers of gas x-ray tubes was Oscar Boehm. Despite the often personalized service, the quality of x-ray tubes varied widely even within the production of one manufacturer. There was then a standard joke among salesmen, offered whenever a customer voiced too many complaints against one particular tube. The suggestion for "curing" that particular tube was to wrap it in a towel, place it for fifteen minutes in a hot oven, then remove it and finally hit it sharply with a hammer.

"A great awareness of skin damage from roentgen irradiation occurred at a very early time. Protection soon became a problem and lead screens were introduced before the turn of the century. There were also electrical hazards, leakage and corona formation were great. Lead glass shields, looking like a round fish bowl, were devised, with the anode and cathode stems sticking out from the sides. Therapeutic tubes were made of lead glass with a flint glass window, such as used in the Piffard tube and in the Geissler tube. the latter had a glass handle, allowing it to be held against the lesion treated, which is the way contact therapy was born. More rigid tubestands were required for stability and adjustment. Keleket developed the best tubestand at that time. Erect fluoroscopes made their appearance before 1910, but were large cumbersome structures.

"A variation of the coil was Nicola Tesla's high frequency system to produce high voltage, with condensers so that no iron core was necessary. The energy was limited but the weight was low and the design compact. The suitcase workshop and cabinet styles were promoted, and this became the first portable unit.

"Clyde Snook in Philadelphia developed the synchronous rotating rectifying switch to convert the alternating current to high voltage direct pulsating current. A similar device was manufactured by Kny-Scheerer in New York City. As these machines were shown at a convention of the New York Electrotherapeutic Society, I remember how enthused were both my boss, Fred

x Mr. Chas Fayer
xx Scroud
Top floor of Wappler
Electric Controller Co.
177 E. 87 St. 1903

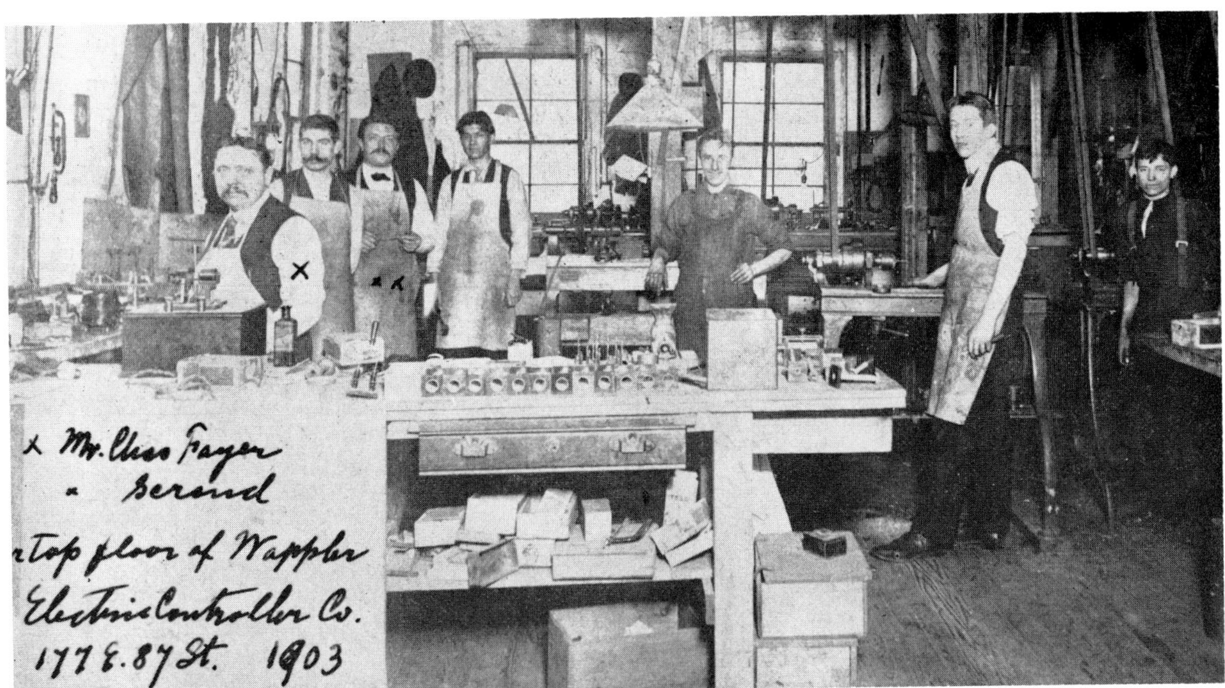

Courtesy: Bert Wappler

WAPPLER'S SHOP IN 1903. Charles Fayer (his title at the time was "general designer") is on the far left. Next are Zemich and Scroud. Joseph Kodlec completes the quartet at left. Leo Kotraschek could not identify any of the others. I thought the tall lad on the right was young Kotraschek himself, but this photograph was made one year before he joined the firm.

Wappler, and I. He suggested that we investigate and at night we opened up the cabinets and sketched out the design. From this we developed the single disc rectifier.

"During that time, little was known of the physical factors involved in the production of x-radiation. The ma-meter was of course used. Penetration was judged in many ways, for instance from the appearance of the greenish color of the ionized gas in the x-ray tube. Various forms of aluminum penetrometers were available, notably the Benoist, but they would have to be radiographed in advance. While the tube was being operated, the spark gap was gradually closed until a spark jumped. Its length, measured in inches, was used to indicate the quality of the radiation.

"In therapy, the dose was judged by exposure of the patient's back or forearm through protected small holes in the sheet lead. A different length of time was given for each hole so that the subsequent skin reaction was determined by the degree of redness produced, and classified as first, second, and third degree erythema.

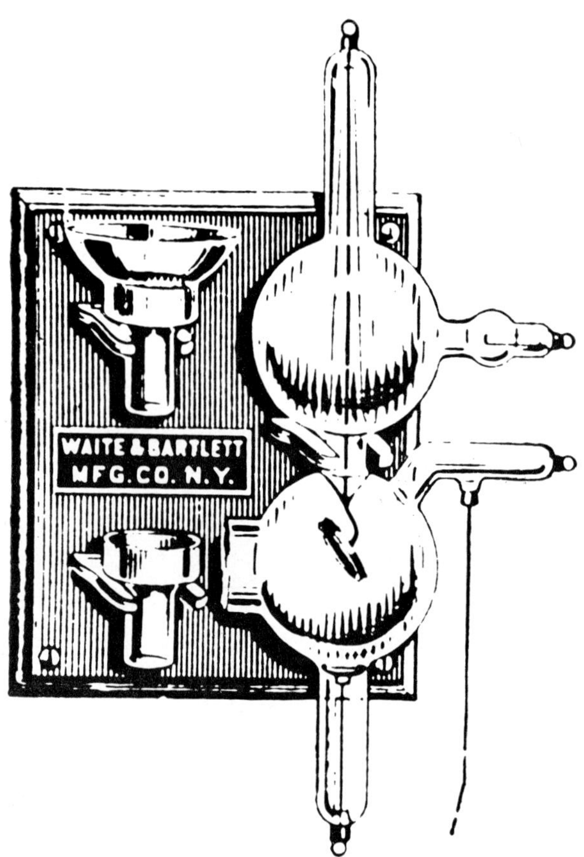

PIFFARD'S "SAFETY" THERAPY TUBE. Its bi-loculated shape is typical. The two lead glass cups are Robert Machlett (II)'s own addition: either the wide or the narrow port could be delineated by using one or the other. The rack is a Waite & Bartlett creation.

Only later came the chemical methods such as Sabouraud's pastilles.

"The "interrupterless" was quite noisy, the controls were live (that is exposed switches as well as exposed high voltage), but it had more power than the x-ray tubes could use. To reduce noise and size I developed a small synchronous motor set. Most of the manufacturers went into the "interrupterless" business and each of them made terrific claims for their product. During the years there were many patents issued on different improvements but none to my knowledge was adequately validated. GE served notice on Wappler for infringement on their Lemp patent, a rotating rectifier. Wappler was enjoined, but I denied infringement on the basis that their claim was that a spark gap must be maintained in the rectifier at all times during rectification. I inserted bronze wire brushes and thus avoided the patent.

"One was supposed to obtain the best results with a Snook and a Coolidge tube. Waite and Bartlett made a cross arm, similar to the Snook, but Wappler stuck to the single disc rectifier and so did Keleket. The Standard Company came into being with a disc and so did Campbell. Competition was furious but results obtained by all machines were about the same, A ridiculous selling point was claimed by Standard who considered their machine better because the controls were exposed in the rear of the cabinet, with all the switches "cooled" by the wind of the revolving disc. Waite had a simple selling slogan, "our machine needs no service, anybody can install or repair it with pliers and screwdriver." The Scheidel-Western Company promoted the sale of both a coil and mechanical rectifier, saying that two machines should be bought, the coil for fluoroscopy because the wave form gives a better image, and a rectifier for radiographic work.

"The Coolidge tube was a tremendous improvement but it was very amusing to hear all the claims made for it. "Hip in a second" was a prevailing expression. The Coolidge tube had a slight drawback because of

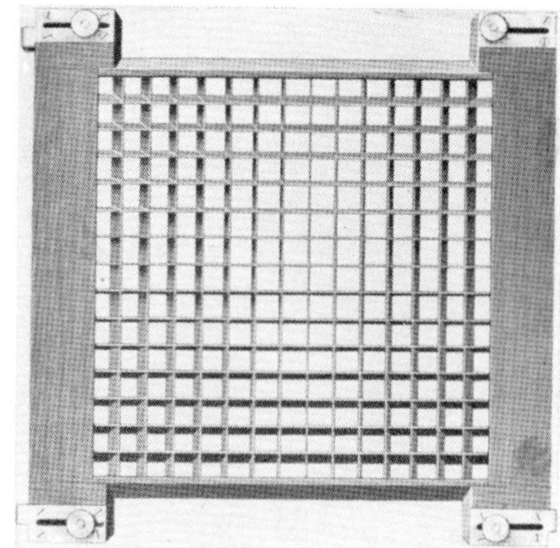

Courtesy: SRW Archives

BUCKY HONEYCOMB GRID (1913), manufactured by Siemens & Halske.

the full tungsten anode which caused much scatter. In the beginning, the resistor for the tube filament was varied with a long fish pole.

"Snook brought from Europe some of the first intensifying screens, a German product. Snook then began to manufacture screens, for which he employed a young chemist, Carl Patterson. His first product for Snook was a "Lagless" screen. Later Patterson, with Fred Reuter, created his own firm called the Patterson Screen Company.

"Just before World War I, R. Wappler brought from Germany a device shaped like an egg crate formed from square lead grids. He told me that was a grid to reduce scatter. It was built by Siemens following a design by Gustav Bucky. In the matter of Bucky grids, Wappler missed the boat by delayed action. Caldwell developed and patented a moving grid with parallel strips and one in a spiral. The Geo. W. Brady Company of Chicago produced a curved grid, actuated by a gravity drop weight to provide uniform motion. Hollis Potter collaborated with Brady in the investigation of grid efficiency with respect to design in ratios of spacing, lead thickness and depth ratio. Then Engeln of Cleveland marketed a curved Bucky actuated by a door check. Victor and several others got into the act. When flat grids were developed, competition had a field day extolling the virtues of curved *vs.* flat models. Keleket took the bull by the horns and made a flip-flop table, revolved about its long axis, having both flat and curved grids. Finally Liebel-Flarsheim in Cincinnati entered the field and stayed to this day as the leading manufacturer of grids.

"There were many improvements in the design of interrupterless transformers. Sinclair Tousey of New York City introduced the multiple phase unit. Snook himself made a triphasic in the hope of producing more energy per unit time but it did not last very long. Frank Rieber, a young engineer in California, built the oil-immersed rectifier which cleared up the noise problem but it introduced new problems in that the high speed churning emulsified the oil and the insulation was destroyed. This was the end of the oil-immersed rectifier.

"It was quite a problem to shock-proof the control switchboard. I remember an amusing experience which I had with a live control. A radiologist had asked me to calibrate his therapy unit with Sabouraud pastilles, which I did. I timed by laying my watch on a safe clear space on the horizontal control. Later in the day he called me frantically that the machine had blown up. I rushed over and found all of the switches melted. "Leo," he said, "I did exactly as you did, I laid my golden watch and chain on the switchboard, and when I turned the machine on, the whole thing blew."

"As a safety measure, the control panel was covered with glass plate, handles and knobs protruding, then recessed below metal panels. Later spark gaps were eliminated and replaced with kilovoltmeters to read the voltage applied to the primary of the transformer. In all of the apparatus the voltage control was accomplished by means of a resistance rheostat. It was an unstable affair, so I developed the auto-transformer control for voltage regulation. The ma-meter was positioned in the high-voltage circuit. It had a switch to change from low scale to high. Many a user got a bad shock by forgetting the high voltage was on, while attempting to change the switch or point too closely at the meter. So I put a string on the switch.

"In the beginning, as an aerial conductor of high voltage across the room, wire was strung on insulators, with automatic take-up reels fastened and connected to the tube. There was much leakage and corona formation, bothersome in the dark. Bill Dee of Engeln developed the tubular aerial system of ¼″ copper tubing, then incapsulated the reels. This reduced both leakage and corona to acceptable levels.

"Radiographic techniques were empirical, with varying time and set kvp values. To improve the work, W. W. Mowry and myself undertook a long study and many tests. We developed the penetration per part technique. Two times the thickness plus 27 gave the minimal kvp for adequate penetration. Fixed mas values were assigned to the various regions of the body for proper density of film, a technique which is still in use to this day.

"Not satisfied with things as they were going, R. Wappler visited Mueller in Hamburg, and saw the first electronic tube valves in operation. These were high voltage rectifiers. He came home with a set, and proceeded to manufacture the first single half-wave, valve-rectified x-ray generator, called the Monex. Its most important feature was the absence of noise. Competition set up a howl, "it won't last long!" "critical glass wear!," "filament failure!," etc. Wappler's sales increased so fast that competition had to fall in line. Then followed the full-wave valve circuits, utilizing four valves in bridge circuit. GE began making valve tubes. Another era was born, valve rectification in air. We had silent machines. Harry Waite had GE make shorter valves for him, and immersed them under oil in the same tank with the transformer. This was the beginning of oil-immersed valve rectification.

"Harry Waite had developed the oil-immersed tube and transformer in a single tank. This was after World War I. A young doctor Middleditch figured that Waite's design might develop into a shock-proof as well as ray-proof x-ray tube. He found some guttapercha rubber cables which would hold the voltage. By putting this 30 ma tube in a lead-lined casing under oil, with suitable entrance terminals for the cables, the first shock-proof and ray-proof tube was born. Thereupon it was found that the glass envelope of a tube could be considerably shortened for oil immersion and a whole new line of x-ray tubes evolved.

"Lilienfeld came over from Austria, with his development of a cold cathode tube in which the source of electrons was a point. Under high voltage stress, it ejected electrons, which was known as the Lilienfeld effect. I experimented with this tube. It was a ticklish affair. Green and Bauer tried to manufacture it but without success. Then came Mueller of Hamburg with the line focus tube, with the so-called Metalix type. Dealers started to import these tubes but were blocked by GE with injunctions and stoppage at the ports, because of alleged infringement. So we took steps to bring them through Canada. The tubes were an immediate success and line focus tubes are with us to this day.*

"Members of the RSNA, under the prodding of Eddy Ernst of St. Louis, were up in arms because of GE's action and their high cost of tube replacement. The ultimate result was that a protective corporation was formed and financed to fight the GE patent through a lawsuit pending against Lee De Forrest of California on radio tubes. The upshot was a decision that the main point at issue was a patent on a degree of vacuum. This was judged unpatentable. That opened up the market for Mueller tubes. GE then offered an elliptical focus tube as being better, but ultimately came out with a line focus. About the time or shortly before Coolidge's patent ran out, young Ray Machlett started manufacturing line focus tubes, and so did Universal X-ray and Eureka in Chicago.

"After the advent of the Coolidge tube, with its storage battery filament source, the insulated step-down transformer was developed to serve as the source of voltage for the filament. Through its primary the voltage could be regulated at the control stand. An inherent fault was the variation in ma, caused by the line voltage fluctuation. Frank Rieber corrected this by the design of a magnetic stablizer which supplied constant voltage. GE and Waite came along with vibrating elements. The magnetic won out and is used to this day.

"Around 1929, Philips of Holland came out with their Rotalix, the first rotating anode tube. Philips had a strong patent. The Eureka of Chicago was licensed to produce it. Then the shock-proof and ray-proof (encased) variety came along and GE as well as Machlett came to make them but Philips received $5.00 of royalty per tube.

"Vertical fluoroscopes became a fad at the end of the 1920's and were sold by the carloads at a low price of $695.00. The 30 ma radiator tube made all these possible. The shock-proof tubes created simple tilt table combinations, and also vertical fluoroscopes, wherein the tube could be rotated away from the rear, and used over a table. Portable shock-proof units were in demand. Many of the users became so interested that they took postgraduate courses in radiology.

"The technical work, done by Mowry and myself on the penetration-per-part technique, led us to have Keleket build a machine embodying these principles. The kVp selector was calibrated in terms of centimeter thickness (of the patient's part). The mas-timer, electronic in action, could be set to the region of the anatomy which was to be radiographed at specified distances. The machine could be compensated for losses at 33-100-200 ma. There was to be no ma-meter, no volt meter, except a line compensator device. The figure of 33 ma was chosen because it was ⅓ of 100 ma. The

RADIOLOGY NOV. 1929 xiii

MULLER METALIX X-RAY TUBES

LINE FOCUS

CROSS SECTION OF A MULLER HELIUM FILLED METALIX X-RAY TUBE

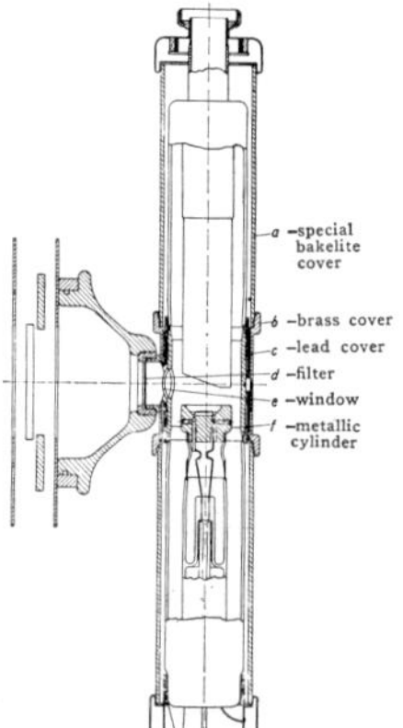

The X-Ray diagnostician NOW insists on having films before him in his stereoscope which are not only uniform in quality but which show the maximum degree of definition and detail. A life may be hanging in the balance and a poor radiograph may be the cause of an error in making a diagnosis.

Do not blame the film, the X-Ray generator, the technique, or the technician. It is more than likely that the technician is forced to work with a tube which has long been worn out, or which was not efficient to begin with.

Muller X-Ray tubes added to your equipment will permanently eliminate the cause of most of the indifferent work exhibited today. New standards of quality in Radiographs were instantly established all over the world, with the advent of MULLER LINE FOCUS X-RAY TUBES.

The men who have used Muller Tubes can quickly tell you of their many points of superiority as well as economy in operation. There are Muller tubes for every purpose. Incorporated in their construction are many exclusive patented features.

An importing service on foreign made technical apparatus of all kinds has been available for many months through the trained organization representing

THE WALLER MULLER COMPANY

Importers---Brokers

6331 Hollywood Boulevard **Los Angeles, California**

Foreign Office: 72 Neuerwall, Hamburg, Germany

Chicago Offices: Now being opened

*Harry DePriest stated that the first x-ray tube built by Westinghouse was a dental model, made at the Bloomfield plant, in 1921. I asked Zed Atlee whether he had ever seen a Westinghouse tube in the 1920s, or whether this meant 1931. Atlee's answer was: "In 1931 I first saw and tested a Westinghouse x-ray tube. It was a right angle dental air-insulated type like GE's RA. Westinghouse claimed their tube was filled with neon, to get around the Coolidge patent. I was able to prove that the gas was cleaned up with operation so that in effect it was a high vacuum tube. You will recall that the Europeans claimed helium filling avoided this patent (Coolidge's vacuum tube), which was a farce, too, as we know today that helium goes through glass walls like a sieve."

technique was standardized for par-speed screens. The operator selected the area with the proper cone, set the timer to the anatomical part, measured the thickness, and checked (compensated) the line voltage, after which he could press the button. There was a density control for adjustment of age correction or screen speed or kvp change. This was the first really automatized control. At a showing of this unit, we were condemned by the radiologic profession for making it possible for anyone to take "pictures." Leopold Jaches was quite critical, and emphatically so. All I could reply was that I did not know radiologists as being picture makers; in my understanding they were supposed to be diagnosticians!

"After World War I, the progress made in Germany in matters of deep therapy awakened the interest of American radiologists. Friedrich Dessauer, who recently died at 81 with radiation damage, was one of the prime movers of therapy in Germany. Holfelder investigated depth dose intensities. So the American manufacturers had to create 180 to 200 kvp transformers. They simply enlarged the mechanical rectifiers, and GE had to build Coolidge tubes three feet long to take the voltage in air. Lead glass shields had to be doubled in thickness. Rooms became sealed vaults of ¼″ lead. Shock-proofing did not exist then. Mechanical disc rectifiers were made with 36″ discs. Snook rectifiers had six feet long cross arms. Tubestands were made with long wooden arms. There were no dose meters. The noise was terrific but we "muddled" through. Multiple port techniques were developed. All the glassware in the x-ray room became colored and tinted from radiation, brown, light brown, purple. This effect caused American Optical to use a similar method to tint eye glasses.

"The protection problem and the scatter to the patient caused the placing of lead-rubber blankets over the patient, above and below the field treated. Then came large wooden tanks, lined with ¼″ lead, in which the tube was mounted. To make positioning and angulation possible, large iron drums lined with lead were designed. These could be rotated on their long axis. They were mounted on tubular legs, spaced apart to permit patient positioning. The manufacturers at that time were Acme International and Wappler. Noise was eliminated when valve tubes came to be used. The valves were mounted on top of the transformer in air. Then came valve tubes under oil, introduced by Waite. He gained possession of the Villard patent through Jack Binns, the first ham radio operator in this country. The Villard circuit was a voltage doubling affair with condensers.

"Westinghouse entered the x-ray field by absorbing Wappler, Acme-International, and Engeln. Many of the key men were eliminated, one of the most notable of these being Ed Goldfield from Engeln. Goldfield was a promising young engineer of unusual ability. He then worked in Picker's new plant in Cleveland. Since GE had available only the air insulated therapy tube, Goldfield designed the first flexible ray-proof and shock-proof therapy tubestand. GE and Keleket followed suit. With the advent of shorter tubes due to oil immersion, a smaller therapy head was developed. In the cooling aspect, not only was the oil forced through the anode, but through the entire head. Insulated oil lines eliminated the need to insulate the cooler. Dr. McEuen of Jacksonville called the manufacturer's attention to his patent on this system of cooling, and made satisfactory financial arrangements with all of them. So therapy equipment finally became stabilized.

"A few of the other matters of interest will be mentioned. GE entered the x-ray industry shortly after the introduction of Coolidge's hot cathode tube. The merger was finalized at a meeting held in New York City, after which the name brands of the merger companies went out of existence.

"The International X-Ray Co. of New York City became interested in a special rectifier, developed by Monty Morrison in Chicago. It was called a toroid, as it resembled revolving sausages. The toroid rectifier suppressed most of the corona discharge, but favored surges. The theory was that, with spherical surfaces commuting the high voltage, one could rectify only the peaks or crests of the voltage wave. Thereupon International combined with Acme of Chicago and launched a valiant promotional bally-hoo to sell the world on this "new" theory. In my opinion the radiographic results were no better but they did quite a lot of business. A competitive situation developed between Acme with their toroid, and GE with the Snook, based on GE's slogan, "The Coolidge tube loves the Snook, because these tubes were pumped while being operated from a Snook rectifier."

"Prior to 1930, gastro-intestinal work was done in the Cole serialographic manner or by means of a four-exposure tunnel placed on fluoroscopic table. The patient was positioned over the tunnel aperture with the fluoroscopic screen, and then four exposures were made. Around 1930, fluoroscopic compression techniques in the erect position were developed in Germany and Austria. They devised small magazines with about 6 cassettes, each 4x5″ in size. Successive shots were made by a trigger release. Then followed the drop type magazine, hung in the rear of the fluoroscopic screen. A cassette would be dropped into position, exposed, and finally dropped into a container. In America, Frank Scholz in Boston, working together with Dr. Schatzki, finally made a satisfactory spotfilm device.

"After the Bucky grid became well known in this country, Engeln induced Bucky to immigrate to the U.S.A. in the hope of obtaining the sole rights to his grid. Engeln manufactured such grids as well as Brady,

Victor, and others. The patent squabble was never settled but some royalties were paid. The Caldwell patent interferred. Bucky decided to remain in this country and opened up a practice in New York City. He came to see me at my place of business, at the time when I was a Keleket dealer. We sat down to complete a list of what he wanted, then he looked over my display, but we did not agree on money matters, and Wappler finally got the order.

"Caldwell was one of the most progressive of the early radiologists in the east. Aside from originating many techniques in skull and chest radiography, he had a fully equipped machine shop, where with the help of a good mechanic (Parsarolli) he developed many accessories and cones. He built his own tubestands of wood with worm-gear adjustments. He built one of the earliest tilt tables of wood and metal, incorporating a motor drive. Before electronic valve tubes were invented, Caldwell sought to improve gas valves. He had the idea before anyone else, and immersed these valves in oil with the transformer, for full wave operation. One Sunday he had me help him, and I was interested, to test such a unit. I had on my gray checked Sunday suit, when the valves exploded and showered me with oil. Caldwell will always be remembered as one of the brightest lights among x-ray pioneers.

"Another memorable person was Lewis Gregory Cole, a staunch friend of Harry Waite, for whom they named their "Cole Golden Flame." Cole had a very elaborate fluoroscopic table in which protection was achieved by having the operator sit behind a steel plate, looking at the screen through a mirror. This machine was marketed by Keleket. He improved his spot-film device to the point where he could later take moving pictures of the passage of contrast material through the gastro-intestinal tract. One such moving picture was being offered to the radiologic profession through the good offices of Picker. Cole was also very interested in tuberculosis, and I remember a case of miliary which he followed by serial films until the then inevitable end. It is a grizzly sensation to be aware of impending death. I will always remember Pop Cole calling me on the phone to say, "Leo, please come up to see me, I have carcinoma of the prostate, and cannot last very long." I answered the call, and that turned out to be, indeed, my last visit with him."

TECHNICAL EXHIBITS

A compendious view of the American x-ray industry can be gleaned also from the accounts of the exhibits presented by the various manufacturers at the scientific meetings.

Following is Trostler's description of the commercial stands planned for the meeting of the RSNA in Rochester (Minnesota) on December 3-7, 1923. It appeared in *Radiology* of December, 1923 and is herein reprinted with the gracious permission of the Radiology Publishing Company.

"The Commercial Exhibit at the Rochester meeting bids fair to exceed any of those shown at previous meetings. It will be held on the ground floor of the First Methodist Church at Rochester.

"It has been the main effort of the writer to bring together as many of the manufacturers of apparatus as possible at these exhibits. The educational value of such exhibits cannot be overestimated. The opportunity for the visiting physicians to compare the different makes and types of apparatus side by side, and to become acquainted with the different arguments of the respective salesmen, dealers, and manufacturers, is of inestimable value. Aside from this, the opportunity given the manufacturers to display their wares makes it worth while for them as well as for us.

"We have purposely refused the sale of large areas of space to one or more manufacturers, deeming it of greater benefit to all to have a large number of exhibitors, rather than a few large exhibitors.

The Exhibitors

"Acme-International X-Ray Company, of Chicago, will show in spaces 14, 15, and 16 a complete line of "Precision Type" Roentgen apparatus. This will include several of their generators, incorporating the "rectifier with sphere gap characteristics," the Deep Therapy tube stand with protective cylinder, and the "Precision Type" Magnetic Sphere Gap. The latest addition to their line, the Vertical Stereo-Plate Changer, will also be exhibited.

"George W. Brady & Company will exhibit in space 26 a number of new items, among which is their Potter-Bucky Diaphragm with a number of new features, including an attachment for operating the time switch, making the exposures automatically from one-half sec-

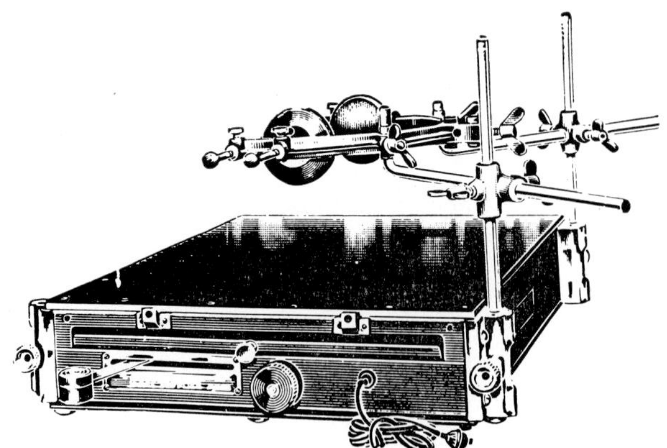

Courtesy: Dave Bennett.

FLAT BUCKY POTTER. This 11x14″ flat top was featured in a Picker catalog of the early 1920's. It was manufactured by Geo Brady and sold for $197.00.

ond up. They also will have a new type of Fluoroscopic Bucky Diaphragm with curved screen, and measuring devices for indicating the proper dosage of x-ray treatments, with a working demonstration of same. They will also show a combination Bucky and Fluoroscopic Table. George will be on hand (with a supply of pencils, of course).

"Buck X-ograph Company, of St. Louis, will occupy space No. 23 and aside from the usual exhibit of Dental Films, Developing Chemicals, etc., will show X-Ograph Contact Cassettes and X-Ograph Ultra-Rapid Durable Intensifying Screens—a combination worthy of your careful consideration.

"The Raper Angle Meter will also be shown. This is a new and useful instrument for indicating the radiographic angle of the teeth. This is something which should not be overlooked. The exhibit will be in charge of Mr. Buck.

"In space number 9, the Burdick Cabinet Company, of Milton, Wis., will display their new quartz lamp which makes possible the establishment of the mercury vapor arc without tilting of the burner, preventing mechanical shock, adding to burner life and establishing the arc stream at full efficiency in from two to three minutes rather than the twelve to fifteen minutes previously required. It is so constructed that raising or lowering over the treatment table, rotation in any horizontal plane, and effortless horizontal movement permit perfect adaptation to every possible treatment requirement with the minimum of effort. New models of the Burdick Deep Therapy Lamps will also be shown as well as a complete line of Infra-red Generators.

"Cameron Electro-Diagnostic and Surgical Specialties will be exhibited in space number 7, by the Cameron Surgical Specialty Company, of Chicago. A number of new and improved instruments developed during the past year will have their first demonstration to the medical profession during this meeting. Among the specialties to be demonstrated are Cameron's Electro-Cautery for major surgery, Cameron's Surgilites, and the improved Cameron's Electro-Diagnosto-set.

"The Jno. V. Doehren Company, of Chicago, in space 24, will exhibit a general line of X-ray accessories, especially the well known Gehler-Folie intensifying screens. The exhibit will be in charge of John Doehren, who will be glad to meet old friends and make new ones.

"The exhibit of the Eastman Kodak Company, in space numbers 5 and 6, will consist of two general divisions, x-ray and clinical photography. Representative negatives made on the new Super Speed X-ray films will be displayed, as well as accessories for handling the films.

"In the field of clinical photography, various routine cases which illustrate the value of photography will be shown.

"The new Cine-Kodak, which is made for amateur motion pictures, will also be displayed. The exhibit will be under the charge of Mr. Millard Hodgson.

"The Engeln Electric Company, of Cleveland, Ohio, will exhibit, in space number 30, a general line of roentgen accessories, their fluoroscope unit and dental unit. Henry Engeln will be in charge.

"H. G. Fischer & Company, of Chicago, in space No. 33 will show apparatus for medical and surgical diathermy, specializing on their Portable Type "G," which they claim to be the most efficient and adaptable apparatus of its kind on the market, because it is light in weight, easily portable, has plently of capacity, and is reasonable in price. They also will show one of their new Style "FO" Senior combination Physiotherapy Cabinets. This outfit is equipped with the new type Kolischer Spark Gap, which they believe is the only gap with which the real sedative diathermic technique may be employed.

"The French Screen Company, of Detroit, Mich., in space number 8, will exhibit the French Intensifying and Fluoroscopic Screens. They say that "the Radiologist should select his screens as the surgeon does his knife – nothing but the best possible – rather than risk his reputation upon price or sales talk."

"Space number 21 will be occupied by the Hanovia Chemical and Manufacturing Company, of Newark, N. J., who will give an actual demonstration of the therapeutic quartz lamps, the Alpine Sun, and Kromayer. They will also show the new addition to their quartz light family, the Luxor Patient's Model Quartz Lamp. This lamp enables all patients, because of its low cost, to be benefited by the use of this modality. The lamp being simplified in construction, contains the burner and furnishes the rays the same as the Alpine Sun Lamp.

"Horlick's Malted Milk Company, of Racine, Wisconsin, will exhibit in space number 11. They will demonstrate the new Model Six Dumore Mixer, "Horlick's," which they claim is the best electric mixer of its kind on the market, and greatly facilitates the preparation of Horlick's Malted Milk with barium sulphate, which is considered by many the best medium for opaque meal in roentgenologic diagnosis. Samples and litera-

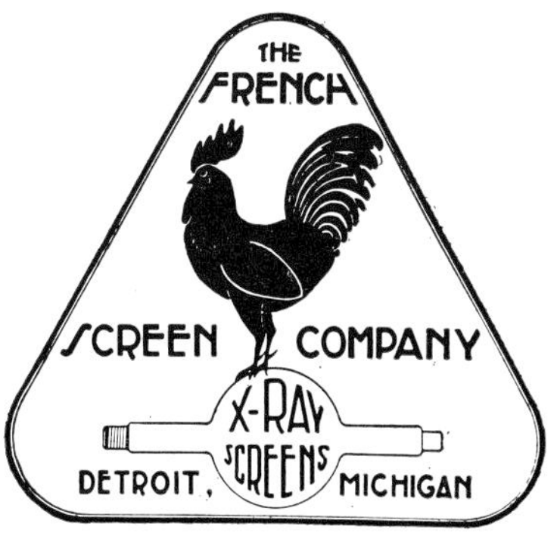

ture will be supplied, and "smiling Dr. Hobart" will be pleased to answer all questions.

"The Kelley-Koett Manufacturing Company, of Covington, Kentucky, will show, in spaces 31 and 32, a number of new devices that will be novel and entirely different from anything shown before. Mr. J. Robert Kelley will be in charge, and this firm assures us that a number of surprises are in store for the visitors to this exhibit. They promise that they will have one of the best exhibits they have had at any meeting in years.

"The Liebel-Flarsheim Company, of Cincinnati, O., will occupy space number 29, and exhibit two models of their Dynelectron – the model P Dynelectron for electro-coagulation, desiccation work, and high frequency current for medical diathermy and autocondensation; the model K Dynelectron, a recent development, intended for use by the specialists who require electro-coagulation and desiccation modalities only. The exhibit will be in charge of Mr. G. H. Liebel.

"The Middlewest Laboratories Company, of Chicago, in space 10, will feature the Metabolimeter and accessories for making basal metabolic rate determinations. Demonstrations will be made on normal subjects, and the complete test followed through to the final result will require a total of less than five minutes. Clinical applications of the test will also be discussed for those unfamiliar with the subject. Dr. Harry Jones will be in charge.

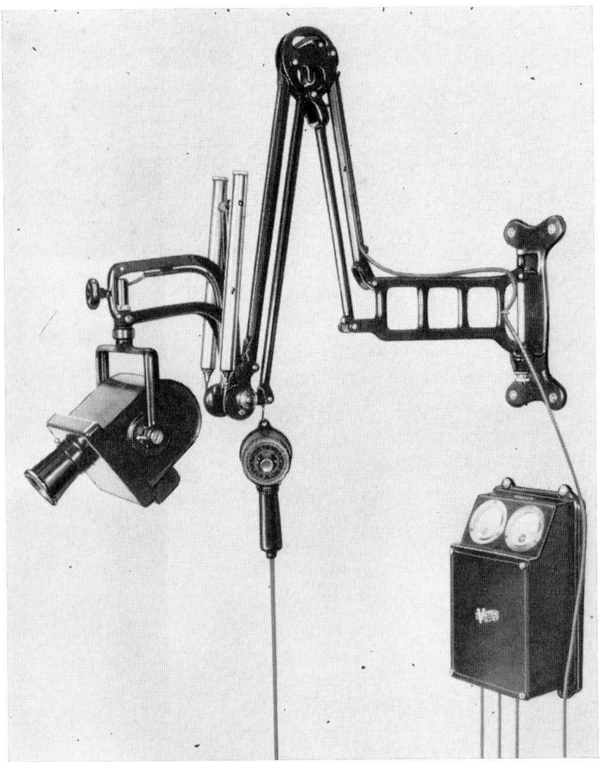

Courtesy: GE Archives.

GE's CDX. This is how Coolidge's first self-contained, oil-immersed, shock-proof dental unit looked. It was placed on the market in 1921.

"The National X-ray Screen Company, of Chicago, will occupy space No. 13, and will exhibit a series of films of unusual cases, made with the aid of National Intensifying Screens.

"The Patterson Screen Company, of Towanda, Pa., occupying space number 28, will exhibit the Patterson Cleanable Intensifying Screen, and demonstrate the manner in which the surface of this screen resists dirt and soil. They will also show the Patterson Fluoroscopic Screen and the Patterson Operating Fluoroscope. Mr. Carl V. S. Patterson will be in charge of the exhibit.

"James Picker, of New York City, will occupy space number 17. He will exhibit a general line of x-ray accessories and supplies for the radiologist. He will also show some of the smaller apparatus produced by the Acme-International X-ray Company.

"In space number 22, the Radium Chemical Company, of Pittsburgh, Penn., will display various new clinical applicators in connection with the use of radium, and the clinical and operator's applicators to be used in connection with radium emanation. The radium emanation is a new service available to physicians. Mr. Fordyce will be in charge.

"In spaces 18, 19, and 25 the Standard X-ray Company, of Chicago, will exhibit a new High Voltage Transformer, and a new type Combination Radiographic, Fluoroscopic Tilt Table showing many improvements. This is a new offering over any of the present types of apparatus now obtainable. They say that their exhibit should prove very interesting to the profession. Mr. Hettich ("Bill") will be in charge.

"In space number 12, the Sweet-Briar Laboratories, of Pittsburgh, Penn., will have a very interesting exhibit showing some of the methods used in the production of Sweetbriar Waterproof Intensifying Screens; as well as films demonstrating results obtained with the aid of Sweetbriar Screens.

"Victor X-ray Corporation, of Chicago, will exhibit, in spaces 1, 2, 3, and 4, the new Victor CDX unit, an oil immersed dental machine that is so compact in construction that it takes up a minimum amount of space, and is so easily operated that it is unquestionably one of the most distinctive and radical changes that has been made in the perfection of x-ray equipment in several years, according to their statement. They will also exhibit the Snook Special Combination Deep Therapy and Diagnostic unit. In addition, other apparatus will be available for inspection of those in attendance. A considerable part of their space will be devoted to the display of radiographs produced by their educational department.

"Wappler Electric Company, of Long Island City, New York, will exhibit in space number 20, some recent developments in x-ray apparatus, and promise some instructive and interesting information in regard to the physics of deep x-ray therapy. Dr. A. Mutschel-ler, physicist of the Wappler Research Laboratory, will be present and glad to discuss deep roentgen therapy with the visitors."

COMMENTS BY THE EXPERTS

The galley proofs for this chapter were submitted to several additional senior x-ray advisers. Richard Kincheloe, Sr. offered more material on Keleket, and Charles Smith more on Queen and on Franklin — all that was incorporated in the final text. Leo Kotra-schek thought there was not enough on Wappler (this has since been corrected), and too much on Westing-house.

Zed Atlee pointed out that while there was a wealth of details on Westinghouse, too little was said about the x-ray tube history made between 1929 and 1946 at GE's Research Laboratory under the direction of E. E. Charlton.

Atlee also deplored the lack of information on several x-ray tube makers such as Quality in Beloit (Wiscon-sin) where it was located; on several equipment manu-facturers, such as Newman, Humphries, and Peerless; on "shoefitting x-ray makers," such Adrean and Primex; and on dental x-ray manufacturers, such as Ritter, Weber, S. S. White, Grenz-Ray Corp., and X-Cel X-Ray.

In the category of omitted names – in this respect no text could ever be "complete" – Atlee mentioned that Loyal Worden, the founder of Continental, was also one of the founders of Eureka. Dunmore Dunk, the engineer who made Eureka successful, had previously worked for GE. And R. L. Sweeny (now chief-engineer at Standard) started out at GE under Charlton. Jim Craig (now chief-engineer at Profex) started out with Mattern.

I invited Atlee to write a few pages on these omis-sions, and he gave it some thought, but no such pages arrived before the deadline for returning the galley proofs to the printer.

The proofs were also seen by Joe Burns, Sr., who provided the additional material on Wappler. Joseph Arthur Burns, Sr. had been with Kronenberg X-Ray & Supply Co. since 1921, and with Westinghouse X-Ray Co. from 1930 until his retirement in 1957 as their manager for supplies and accessories.

Burns prepared for me a flock of pages with amus-ing or unusual experiences, accumulated in his decades of x-ray life. He had sold x-ray equipment even to a famous "psychic healer" (*i.e.*, quack); to a physician who was later accused of having murdered his wife, but continued to send in his installment payments using the jail as return address; and to a man-and-wife team of physicians, doing missionary work in the mountains of North Carolina (the wife became the 1951 USA mother-of-the-year). A good salesman is always on the alert, as new prospects may turn up anywhere: Burns learned in church of the x-ray needs of the cancerologist Joseph Colt Bloodgood, and soon clinched the deal. One of Burns' luckiest salesmen, John James Jones

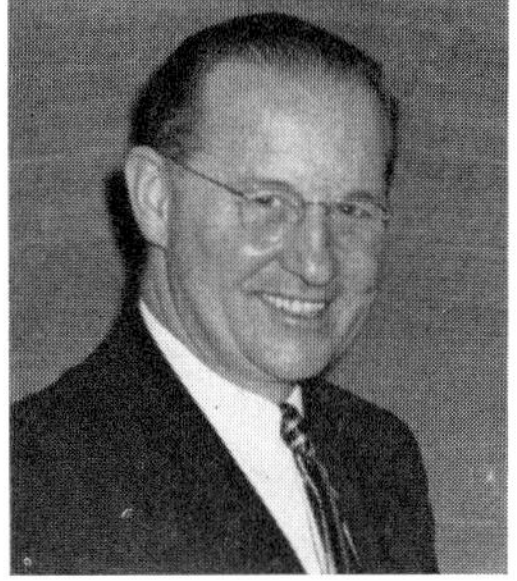

Charles W. Smith

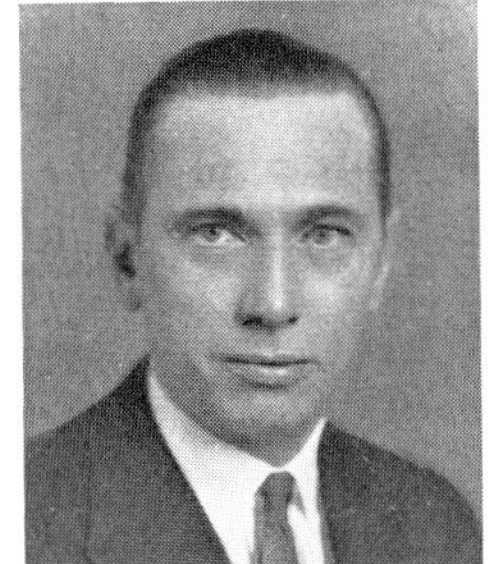

Leo Kotraschek

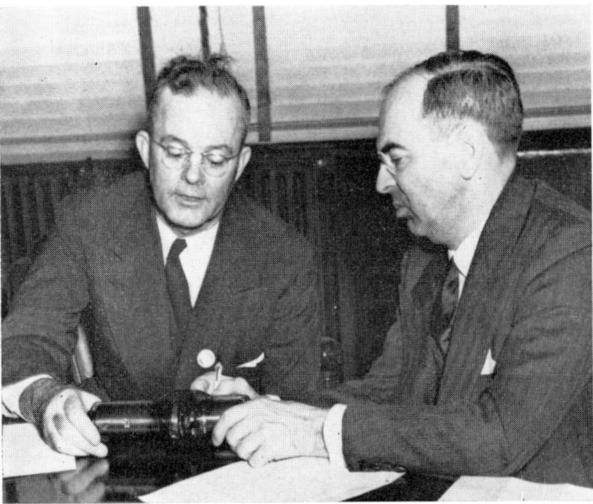

Courtesy: GE Archives

E. E. Charlton and John Clough

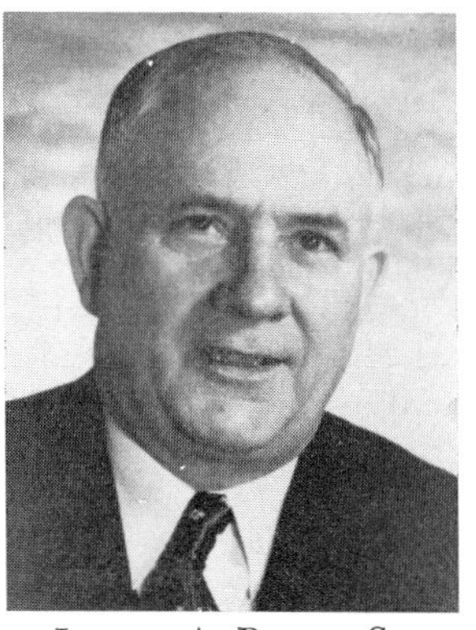

Joseph A. Burns, Sr.

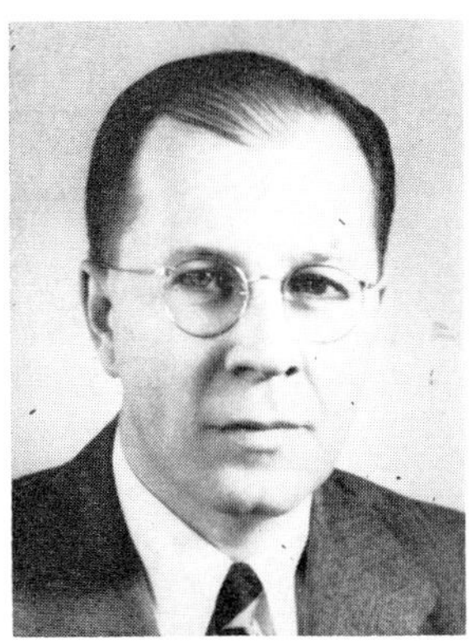

Zed J. Atlee

Cox,* slept undisturbed through the night with open window and wide open door, while a murder was committed in the adjoining hotel room (there ensued a famous trial, at which he was a witness). Following are excerpts from letters by Burns:

"I joined Kronenberg by answering a want ad in 1921. The Kronenberg X-Ray & Supply Corporation had been founded with varied financial support by a physician, J. B. Kronenberg. They held distributorships for Wappler, for two quartz lamp makers, and for Eastman Kodak, but the business was being operated at a loss. In 1922 a "re-organization" resulted in my promotion to general manager, and in a few years I succeeded to turn out tidy profits. The physician-founder and his non-physician brother then experimented with a coffee substitute, and moved to other towns.

"At the time, our source of supply for lead gloves and aprons was in Scotland. For better handling, several companies pooled their orders, and had shipments made directly to the George W. Brady Co., for redistribution to us and others in the pool.

"In the 1920s a three-compartment, five-gallon soapstone tank made in Alberene (Virginia) cost $50 fob. In the summer time, a goodly supply of ice had to be on hand in the x-ray place, to help cool the solutions and wash water. In the winter there were cracked tank walls, and long delays in shipping replacements. That was before bakelite tanks with metal inserts became available.

"There had been talk about shock-proof x-ray equipment, for instance, Wm. F. Healer, then chief-radiologist at Georgetown University Hospital, experimented with various hook-ups. In June, 1928 – while on the train headed for the AMA convention in Minneapolis – W. S. Kendrick (GE's x-ray sales manager) told George Brady, Henry Engeln, and myself that on the following day they were going to unveil a special piece of equipment. It turned out to be the first shock-proof tubehead, a bit heavy and a bit too bulky, though undoubtedly a forerunner in safety.

"In date of January 21, 1930 I sent the following letter to P. J. Murley, who was then manager of Wappler's: 'In times gone by, we have heard of the Picker Company buying Waite & Bartlett, and later on they purchased the controlling stock in Keleket. Of course, once upon a time they owned International (here Murley noted in pen *Oh !?!*), but it is apparent that International was a bad investment and they turned International down cold. The latest reports in the State of Virginia are to the effect that Picker has purchased heavily in Wappler stock and also that the Wappler Company has contracted to manufacture double disc mechanical rectified x-ray machines for Picker exclusively. It seems that all of the doctors in Roanoke that our representative called upon last week informed him of this transaction. Of course, if Picker is going to line up with Wappler, naturally we do not want to knock Picker, therefore we would appreciate your advising us just what the situation is so that we may be in a position to reply to these statements when necessary.' Murley's pencilled reply on the bottom of the letlet was *'Nothing but a lot of old scrub-woman's idle gossip. Or—in plain language—a bunch of damned lies with no foundation whatever. PJM.'*

"My duties as Kronenberg's general manager required regular trips to the Wappler plant. When in New York City, it was customary for me to call also on Eastman Kodak's offices, and on James Picker. The latter was a real business man, always impressive, with long draperies in the background, and an elegant desk. He came to all x-ray meetings, and was very friendly to potential customers and competitors alike (even competitors might turn into customers). He explained to me that discounting bills paid before the 10th of the following month meant he could use the customer's money to pay for the transaction. It also meant that customer's money could be turned over ten to twelve times a year, all the while turning in a nice profit.

"In June, 1930 Westinghouse purchased the Wappler Co., and by September, 1930 it became evident that Kronenberg faced the choice of being purchased by Westinghouse, or finding some competitive line to sell. Purchase was decided upon, and I became the manager of Westinghouse's Baltimore branch.

"Liebel-Flarsheim made Young Urologic Tables, named after Hugh Hampton Young, the famous urologist at John Hopkins. I had known him for many years. In 1945 I went to see him about the foreword to a bulletin on the Young Table, being issued by Westinghouse (as a Liebel-Flarsheim distributor). That was the last time Young's signature was used—as of July 28, 1945. He died in August, 1945.

"Two other physicians stand out in my memory. John William Pierson (1883-1960) followed in 1933 in Frederick Baetjer's position of chief-radiologist at Johns Hopkins. In 1947 Pierson was in turn succeeded by Russell Morgan. The other physician I so well remember was the "sportsman" Charles (Buck) Waters (1890-1961). He co-authored a book on bone diagnosis (with Baetjer), and one on urologic roentgenology

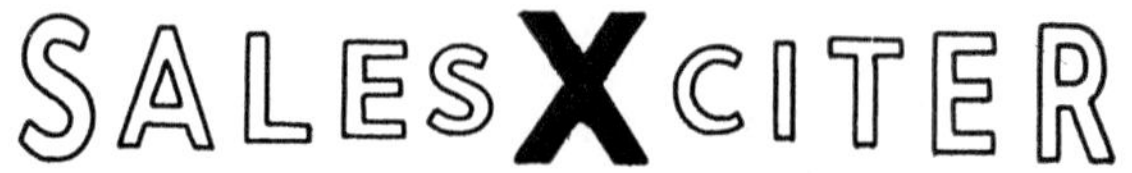

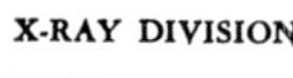

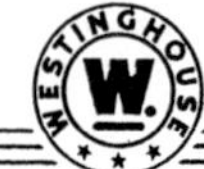

*He was known as Jay Jay, or Triple Jay. His business often came on a platter, almost without work, because of his easy-going personality. Triple Jay's favored saying was, "God always protects children, drunks, and x-ray salesmen."

(with Young), and co-edited the Year Book of Radiology. He is best remembered for the Waters' view for the demonstration of paranasal sinuses.

"I would like to emphasize that most of my success was due to my associates, especially during the period 1921 through 1942. That group of young people under my jurisdiction not only secured the business which made our operations profitable. They also followed things up by giving the customers the best possible service. This was in line with my business philosophy that the most important asset is a satisfied customer!"

CONCLUSION

This presentation terminates with the advent of the Atomic Phase. Regarding design of x-ray apparatus, the new phase did not materialize until at least one decade after the moment when Fermi initiated the first chain reaction at Stagg Field in Chicago. That was simply due to the time lag needed for designing new models of x-ray equipment after materials became again available following the end of the hostilities.

In 1950, the Calculex Company of Dallas (Texas) advertised an X-Ray Exposure Meter, which they claimed was a "must" in every x-ray department, as it was supposed to save time, film, and tubes. Somehow it must not have caught on, and the ads disappeared from the journals. Their advertising copy is of interest because it carries, in alphabetical order, the names of seven x-ray companies billed in 1950 as the major firms in the American X-Ray Industry. The second through the seventh of these firms (GE, Keleket, Mattern, Picker, Standard, and Westinghouse) are still in existence, although two of them (Keleket, Mattern)

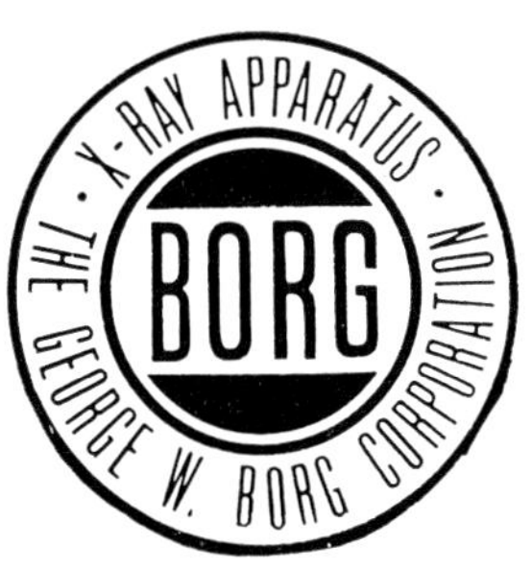

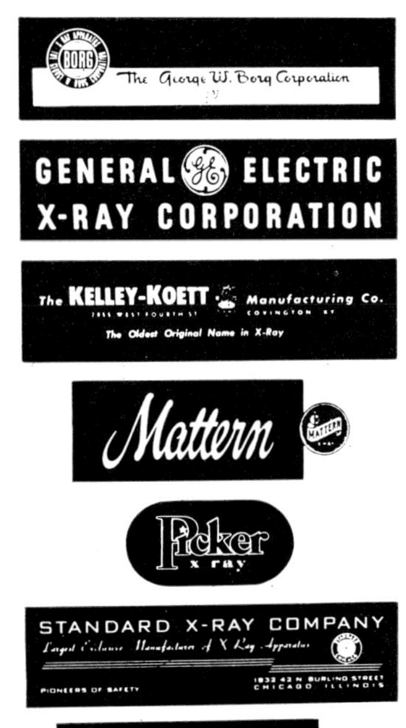

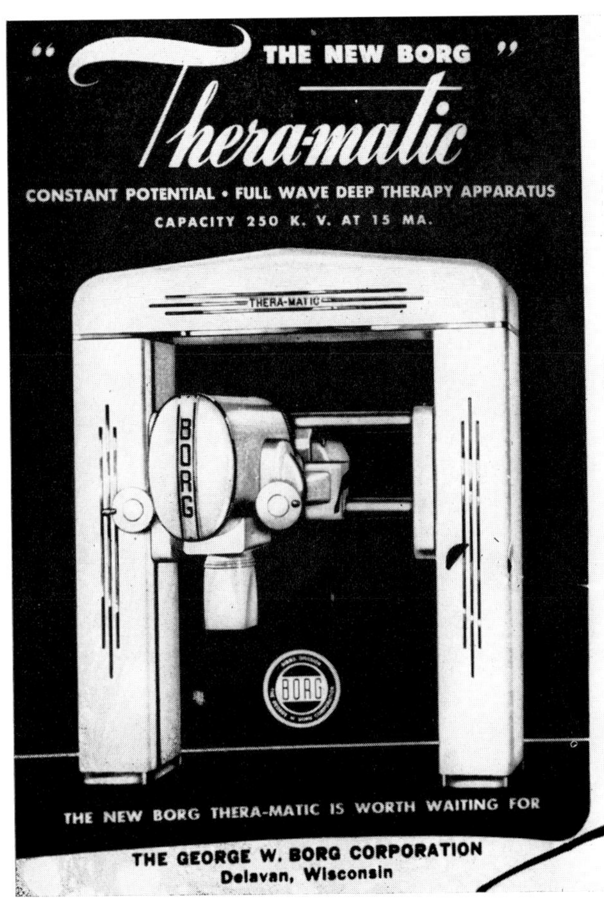

under "strange" flags. As a matter of fact, only four of these six (GE, Keleket, Picker, and Westinghouse) have nationwide service organizations.*

Ironically, the first name on the Calculex list, the George W. Borg Company of Delavan (Wisconsin) is no longer with us. It had been created because during World War II there accumulated a significant backlog of orders on x-ray equipment. As soon as the "big four" in the American x-ray industry resumed peacetime production, Borg went broke. And yet, Borg equipment had been both well built and pleasantly styled, such as the Theramatic, a 250 kvp, 15 ma treatment apparatus. Incidentally, their former chief engineer, Max Lee, passed away in 1961.

Toward the end of the Golden Age of Radiology, technologic developments in the x-ray industry had reached a level at which small firms were hard put to survive. Large facilities and large lay-outs became necessary just to keep up with new models brought out by the competition, let alone to improve on existing designs. In the Atomic Age only "big business" would seem to have a permanent place in the highly competitive x-ray field. This does not include the manufacture of certain x-ray accessories, nor of special tables.

The Scripture (*Ecclesiasticus* 38, 24) teaches, "The wisdome of a learned man cometh from opportunity of leisure; and he that hath little business shall become wise . . . ," presumably from too much leisure. The solution is to turn the little business into (or affiliate it with) a big business. That failing, "he" ought to have sufficient wisdom to look for a new job before his leisure turns into full idleness.

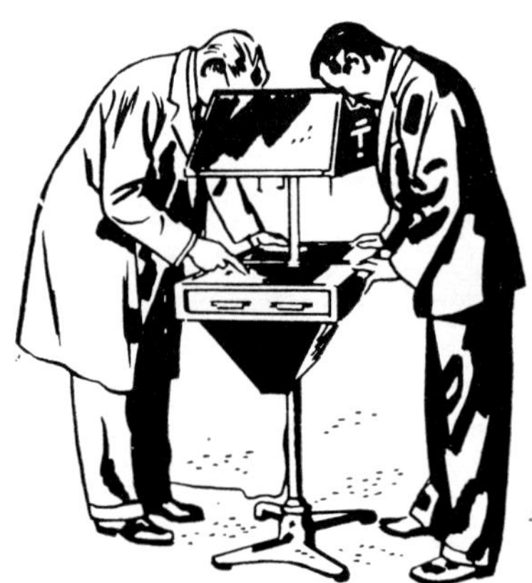

Twin Stereo Viewer

*This needs some qualifications: Keleket's outlets have been "affected" to some extent by the changes in ownership of the mother company; Westinghouse is represented in seven mid-western states by the semi-independent Dick X-Ray Company; in Oklahoma by Merkel X-Ray Company, and in Minnesota by Pengelly X-Ray Company.

Chapter 3

FROM X-STRAHLEN TO RADIO(BIO)LOGY. A SEMANTIC TREATISE ON HISTORIC PRINCIPLES

For words, like Nature, half reveal
and half conceal the soul within
ALFRED TENNYSON

In the *Golden Bough* (1890), Sir James George Frazer (1854-1941) emphasized that superstitions related to the magic of names have always played a significant role in the primitive folklore of savage tribes. The main (i.e., the true) name of an individual was often taboo, except when used in domestic or otherwise private ceremonies. Its invocation in public, before strangers, was prohibited. For purposes of appellation, several aliases or surnames (*i.e.*, false names) were selected, preferably from "foreign" tongues. To these were added designations derived from certain traits of, or feats performed by, the bearer, or from his occupation, (*i.e.*, trade names). The result may have been colorful, but just as confusing to the uninitiated as its modern counterpart, our "scientific" medical nomenclature.

THE NEW (UNKNOWN) KIND OF RAYS

In the final decades of the 19th century it became fashionable to investigate the fluorescence caused by cathode rays. Here and there an investigator would complain of the "darkening" of photographic plates stored on the table on which cathode ray experiments were in progress — as if the plates had been defective or the black paper seal had not protected the light-sensitive material. Several highly qualified investigators, Crookes, Goodspeed, Lenard, had witnessed such occurrences, but they paid no attention to them. In the *Electrical Engineer* of March 11, 1896 Wilbur Morris Stine (1863-1934), a physicist from New York City, admitted frankly that he had given no importance to those "accidents." Such "darkening of the plates" came to be regarded as an inevitable incident in cathode ray experiments. As acknowledged also by Edgar Ashworth Underwood in the *Journal of the Canadian Medical Association* of January, 1946 — Wilhelm Conrad Röntgen was the first who grasped the significance of such penetration through opaque material.

This alone would have sufficed to qualify Röntgen as a scientific "pathfinder" yet, in addition, he described in a magistral manner the physical characteristics of that penetrating agent. In his very first paper — to stress the enigmatic nature of the phenomenon which he had discovered — Röntgen combined *X*, the algebraic symbol for unknown, with *Strahlen*, the German word for rays (from cathode rays), and called the new agent (i) *X-Strahlen*. Because of Christmas vacation, the first of Röntgen's three re-

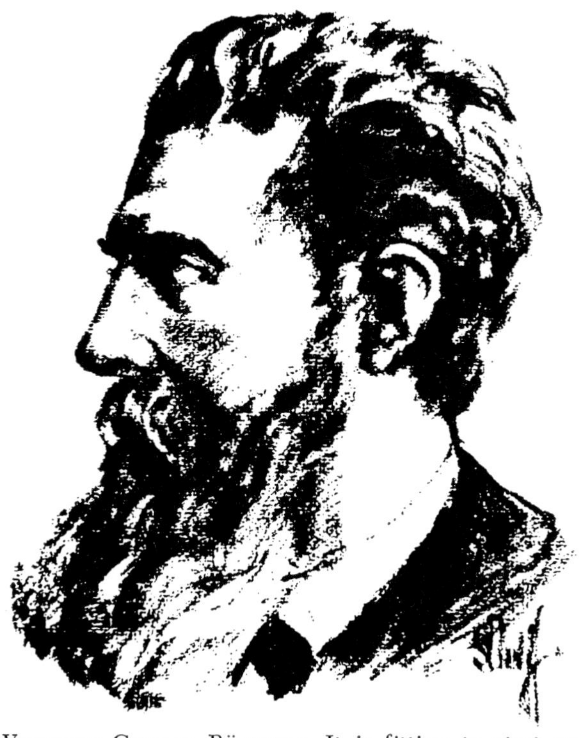

WILHELM CONRAD RÖNTGEN. It is fitting to start an etymologic history of radiology by paying homage to "papa" Röntgen, meaning at least one inedite portrait. This drawing was executed in 1933 by one of Ben Orndoff's daughters, now living in California, Sarah Orndoff Bohmke. The portrait had been commissioned to provide a not as yet published image of Röntgen for the exhibit of the American College of Radiology at the World Exposition (today the Chicago Museum of Science and Industry). People who had met Röntgen declared that the portrait is an excellent likeness. The drawing adorns a wall in Ben Orndoff's office, and he graciously consented to have it reproduced.

ports was not actually read before an audience. It was, however, printed as if it had been delivered on December 28, 1895 before the Physical and Medical Society of Würzburg. It made world news, and within a few weeks an evergrowing cohort of scientific "hitchhikers" began to widen the newly opened trail.

X-STRAHLEN TRANSLATED

Röntgen's experiments were reproduced at the Hôpital Trousseau in Paris by Paul Oudin (1851-1923), who was to become both a pioneer radiumtherapist* and a radiation fatality. The French text of

*A German medico-biographic dictionary credits Oudin with having introduced radium therapy in gynecologic practice. In this respect, uncontested priority belongs to the *Light Energy* (1904) therapist Margaret Abigail Cleaves (1848-1917) of New York City, who described in the October 17, 1903 issue of the *Medical Record* how she had inserted radium into the uterine cavity of a patient with carcinoma of the cervix.

LIGHT ENERGY

Its Physics, Physiological Action and Therapeutic Applications

By

MARGARET A. CLEAVES, M.D.

Fellow of the New York Academy of Medicine; Fellow of the American Electro-Therapeutic Association; Member of the New York County Medical Society; Fellow of the Société Française d'Électrothérapie; Fellow of the American Electro-Chemical Society; Member of the Society of American Authors; Member of the New York Electrical Society; Professor of Light Energy in the New York School of Physical Therapeutics; Late Instructor in Electro-Therapeutics in the New York Post-Graduate Medical School

WITH NUMEROUS ILLUSTRATIONS IN THE TEXT AND A FRONTISPIECE IN COLORS

"But if darkness, light and sight be separate and independent one of the other, then if you remove light and darkness, there is nothing left but void space."—*Buddhistic Sutra.*

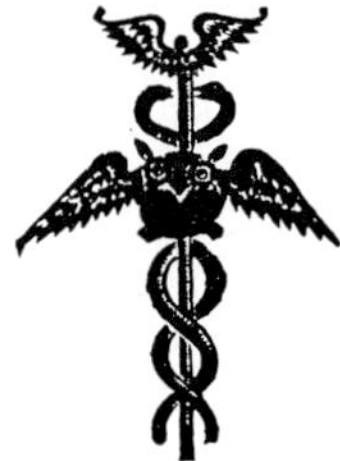

NEW YORK
REBMAN COMPANY
10 WEST 23D STREET, COR. 5TH AVE.

LONDON AGENTS
REBMAN LIMITED
129 SHAFTESBURY AVENUE, W. C.

1904

their communication of January 20, 1896 to the *Académie des Sciences* contained the German term *X-Strahlen.* In France, the common form was (and is) the translated *rayons X* as used by another Gallic pioneer André Broca (1863-1925) in the February 2, 1896 issue of *Gazette Hebdomadaire de Médecine.* Enrico Salvioni (1863-?), an experimental Italian physicist reported on *raggi X* to the Accademia Medico-Chirurgica in Perugia on February 5, 1896. Corresponding translations were utilized in this country by the astronomer Edwin Brant Frost (1866-1935), and in Russia by the physicist Prince Boris Borisovich Golitsyn (1862-1916). The term x-rays was adapted into practically all languages, for *instance* in Japanese it sounds something like *ekkusu-kosen.*

In England, Frederick Thomas Trouton (1863-1922) – whose eponym graces a law of molecular heat – modified the word to (ii) *x-radiation* (*Nature* of October 8, 1896), a form in which it has remained popular to this day among therapists and physicists (although some, like Roberts Rugh and Erika Grupp of Columbia University, prefer *X-irradiation*).

A slightly different version, *x-radiance*, was promoted by David Littlejohn (1876-1953) in the November, 1898 issue of the *Journal of Osteopathy.* He was a physician – M. D. 1897, Medical College, St. Joseph (Missouri) – who taught "X-Radiance and Sanitary Science" in the Osteopathic School in Kirksville (Missouri). Subsequently he founded (with his two brothers, John Martin Littlejohn and James Buchan Littlejohn) the Chicago Osteopathic Hospital, but soon he separated from them and turned to Public Health and numberless peregrinations.*

In his *Radiologic Glossary* (1960),** and in the editorials in *Radiologic Technology* of July, 1963 and in the *Yellow Journal* of September, 1963, Lewis Elmer Etter emphasized that the "orthographically correct" form, when used as a noun, contains no hyphen, x rays, x radiation. This is the spelling found in some of the early publications (for instance in Morton's paper in the June, 1896 issue of *Dental Cosmos*). It is also the spelling accepted in the Merriam-Webster. And yet, the "proper" terminology (name!) and its "correct" spelling are determined, not by academic desirability, but by the degree of public acceptance. Periodically, dictionaries are revised to conform to popular preferences. So far, the majority seemed to prefer the hyphen in x-rays, but in this matter I refuse to yield to the majority. In my text x rays, as a noun, will not ap-

*In 1916, we find him in Bridgman, in 1923 in Bluefield, in 1936 in Charleston (all in West Virginia), in 1940 in Sault St. Marie (Michigan), and in 1950 in Dearborn-Eloise (also in Michigan).

***Glossary of Words and Phrases Used in Radiology and Nuclear Medicine* — Charles C Thomas, Springfield, Ill. 1960.

pear hyphenated, except in other languages (the hyphenated form is correct in German), in quotations, or – *horribile dictu* – by mistake.

The eponymic (iii) *Röntgen rays,* evidently a variation of Röntgen's rays (which had been suggested by Kölliker) — similar forms being in Spanish *rayos Röntgen,* in Italian *raggi del Röntgen* or *radiazioni Röntgen,* in French *rayons de Röntgen, etc.* — can be found in very early reports, as in France (Lannelongue and Oudin), in this country (Pupin), in Czechoslovakia (Pick), in Italy (Battelli and Garbasso), in England (Davidson), in Russia (Piltchikoff), and in Peru (Matto). Even the eclectic *Röntgen'schen X-Strahlen* was to be encountered, not only in Germany (Winkelmann and Straubel), but also — in translation — in the USA (Goodspeed), in the Netherlands (Wertheim-Salomonson), in Cuba (Ragúes), in Denmark (Riis) and in Greece (I. E. K.).

These references are easily found in the *Index Catalogue.* The Greek article, published on March 14, 1896 in the *Galynos* (Athens) was re-inspected with the help of Emanuel Samouhos, a radiologist of Greek extraction, who lives in Ohio. The name hidden behind the initials I. E. K. was identified for us by K. B. Kotoulas (the current general secretary of the Greek Radiological Society). I. E. K. was Ippocrates Epaminonda Karavias, assistant professor of Pharmacology and Therapeutics in the University of Athens, and editor of the *Galynos* at the turn of the century.

MORE RAYS

Among the surnames selected, several were based on the idea that the new agent was akin to rays. In London the physicistical "dimensionist" Alfred William Porter (1865-1939) classified the new agent among (iv) *actinic rays, cf., Nature* of February 6, 1896. The tautology is blatant: in Greek *aktys* means ray. Thus the combination is something like "rayic ray" but even the latest 'Supreme Authority,' the unabridged 3rd edition of the Merriam-Webster Dictionary carries the word and applies it to all those rays which exhibit actinism (photo-chemical effects), such as blue and violet in the visible spectrum, ultraviolet beyond it.

In the *Electrical Engineer* (New York) of February 19, 1896 Park Benjamin (1849-1922), editor of Appleton's *Cyclopaedia,* suggested adoption of the nickname (v) *tithonic rays.*

The name comes from the mythological Tithon (the aging and decrepit husband of Aurora, a morning goddess assigned to open the rising sun's oriental gates) and signifies light rays of a sort. The term tithonic rays had been created by John William Draper (1811-1882), a radiation precursor who in 1850 became the president of the Medical School of the University of the City of New York. Draper presented a full slate of vocables, which to him were both "musical in an English ear" and etymologically enticing: tithonoscope, tithonometer, tithonography, tithonic effect, diathitone-

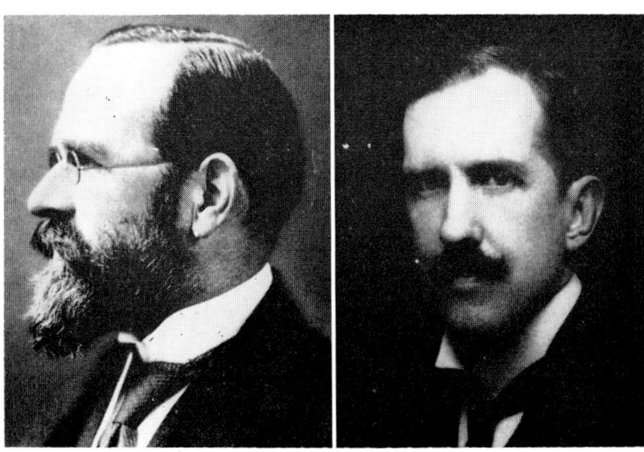

ALFRED PORTER AND C. E. S. PHILLIPS

LA

FOTOGRAFÍA ASCÉTICA

POR MEDIO DE LOS RAYOS RÖNTGEN

FOTOGRAFÍA DE LO INVISIBLE

Teoría – Procedimiento – Aplicaciones

POR

JULIO CANALEJO Y SOLER

FOTÓGRAFO

Edición ilustrada con grabados

BARCELONA

SALVADOR MANERO BAYARRI—EDITOR

27 y 29. Calle de la Universidad, 27 y 29.

scence, tithonicity, tithonotype, detithonizing power, etc. Some of his sentences (written before 1844) foreshadow things to come: "A large number of bodies obstruct the radiation of the tithonic rays so that apparently shadows will remain on a sensitive plate . . ." Other passages can be interpreted (with some leniency) as referring to the existence of what is known today as gamma radiation in sunshine. The latter quote appears in the second edition of his treatise *(Forces Which Produce the Organization of Plants)* on the same page on which, to complete the premonition, the binder's signature is the Roman numeral ten, that is *X* (p. 161).[*]

At the *Académie des Sciences* in Paris, Pierre Picard paraphrased Röntgen by referring to (vi) *rayons obscurs* while François Pierre Le Roux (1832-?)[†] proposed the euphonious (vii) *radiations hyperdiabatiques,* which is merely a transliteration from the Greek, and means overpenetrating rays. In this category can be found also two German entries, (viii) *Kraft-Strahlen* (power rays) and (ix) *Aether-Strahlen* (ether rays), both taken from a cursory mention by Büttner and Müller.

THE INVISIBLE LIGHT

Another series of appellations stemmed from the similarity of effect on silver salt emulsions, known to be sensitive to the rays of "invisible" light, hence the designation (x) *invisible light.*

In a nostalgic vein, O'Hara, who had been in this field since the very year 1896, recited (in May-June 1932 in *Radiography and Clinical Photography*) some memories about the Brethren of the Invisible Light.[‡]

Other samples of early radiation slang can be found in the same reference. Most of these pioneers were so tough that their canary birds sang bass, for instance when Rome Vernon Wagner (1869-1908) was "cooked" for "sleeping with the tube," he refused to yield to self-pity, and boasted of still having one finger left to wrap around a cigarette.

Its reverse was "photography of the invisible" — quoted from Morton (*Electrical Engineer,* February 5, 1896): in his printed title Crookes was misspelled Brookes — or "photography of the unseen" (by Van Rensselaer, in the *Albany Medical Annals* of the same month).

In the beginning, this created an editorial confusion (*Electrical Engineer,* January 29, 1896) with the "etheric (cold) lighting" of Daniel McFarlan Moore (1869-1926). Denshaw, an otherwise unidentified disciple of Zoroaster, recognized the "unknown light" (meaning Röntgen's penetrating agent) as one manifestation of what had been known to "Eastern scientists" as "astral light" or the seventh dimension of matter (see the very first page of the first issue of *Laryngo-*

[*]In this same category enter the odic or odylic rays of Baron Karl von Reichenbach, mentioned in the first chapter.

[†]LeRoux and LeBon were identified with the courteous assistance of Mr. Pierre Gauja, the secretary-archivist of the Paris Academy of Sciences. No information was available on Pierre Picard.

[‡]Since revolutionary feelings ran fairly high during the lean Depression days, a frustrated radio-fellow must have coined the short-lived slogan: *Brethren of the Invisible Light, Unite!*

APPAREILS ET USTENSILES POUR
Expériences avec les rayons X
de Röntgen
— (PHOTOGRAPHIE DE L'INVISIBLE) —
RICHARD, CH. HELLER et Cie
Fabrique d'Appareils d'électricité médicale et industrielle. 18, cité Trévise, PARIS
Nous demandons, à cause des nombreuses commandes, un délai de livraison de 8 à 10 jours. — CHARGE DES ACCUMULATEURS A FORFAIT

NOTES

ON

X-LIGHT

BY

WILLIAM ROLLINS

BOSTON, MASSACHUSETTS
MCMIV

scope of July 1896). Better yet, an amateur astrologist, the homeopathically famous Egbert Guernsey (1823-1903) of New York – a physician immortalized by Bret Harte – applied such terms as the "cathode rays of clairvoyance" and the "all-seeing light."*

The French physician, sociologist, and physicist Gustave Le Bon (1841-1931) included the penetrating rays among the components of the (xi) *black light.*

The English authority on electro-magnetism, Silvanus Phillips Thompson (1851-1916), thought at first that the x rays were (xii) *ultraviolent sound,* a contention supported by Edison. The term (xiii) *Röntgen light* was apparently first printed in Italian, as the title of an abstract by Bartorelli in the *Settimana Medica dello Sperimentale* of February 1, 1896. The German translation, *Röntgenlicht,* was occasionally employed, as in the paper of (the Viennese) Moritz Benedikt, in *Deutsche Medic. Wchschft* of June 5, 1902. It was later used also by American authors, for instance by Francis Williams. In 1906, in the *Russky Vrach* (Petersburg), Y. V. Zelenkovsky printed several installments of a paper concerning the treatment of trachoma with Becquerel's light (radium)! The "official" terminology, found both in the Czarist and in the Sovietic versions of their *Enzyklopedya* is *rentgenovsky luchy,* meaning roentgen rays. The Russian term for rays sounds somewhat like *luce,* the Italian word for light.

The weird combination (xix) *x-light* must have appeared around the turn of the century. In the August, 1896 issue of the *International Dental Journal,* the inventive Boston dentist William Rollins (1852-1929) published a paper entitled conventionally *"Oral Röntgen-Photography."* In 1903 when he reprinted (at the Cambridge University Press) his earliest papers in the limited and now very rare edition of the comprehensive *Notes on X-Light,* he changed the titles from their original wording so as to conform with that "novel" terminology. In October, 1902 in the *American X-Ray Journal,* Clarence Edward Skinner supported this nickname which disappeared nonetheless from common American usage before 1910.

*The original source of Bleyer's quotation — from the *New York Medical Times* of February, 1896 — was unearthed by Miss Gertrude Louise Annan, the scholarly chief-librarian of the New York Academy of Medicine.

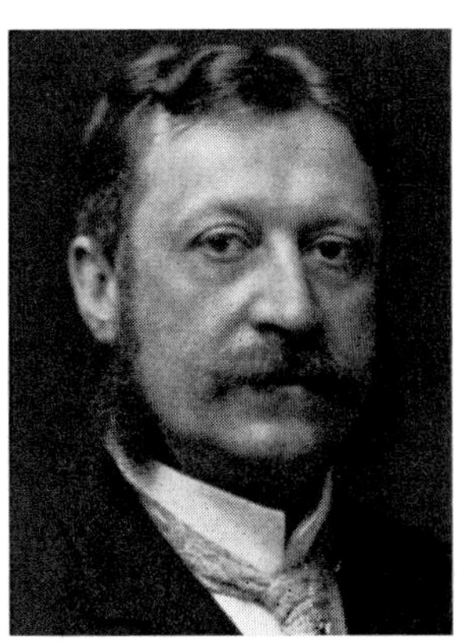

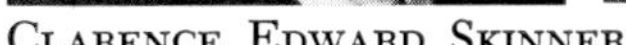

Clarence Edward Skinner

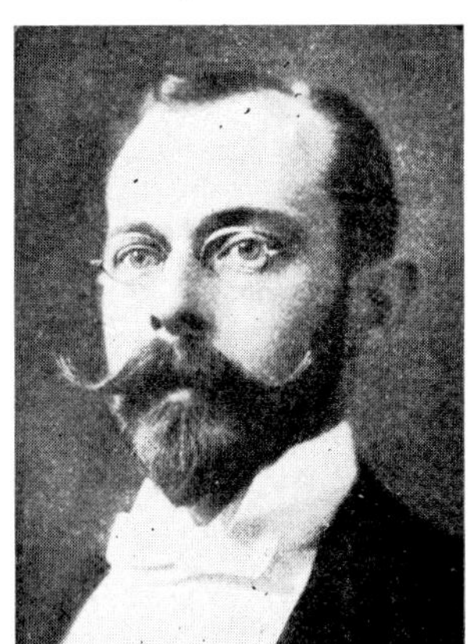

Carl Beck

THE NEW METHOD

The term *Rontgen'sche Methode* was used by the psychiatrist Moritz Jastrowitz (1839-1912) before the Berlin Medical Society on January 20, 1896. Very soon, though, terms more specific than this somewhat vague "method" were introduced. The study of the cathode rays recognized two modalities: visual inspection of a cardboard coated with a fluorescent substance* (screen), and recording on photographic plates. Both procedures were in current use long before Röntgen's heyday, indeed the frustrated Philipp Lenard (1862-1947) had excelled in their physicistic manipulation.† Both procedures were subsequently adopted for, and improved in, experiments with the new penetrating agent. By way of nomenclature, when the screen image was viewed, the suffix *-scopy* (from the Greek σκοπεἰν, to inspect) was added, while *-scope* indicated the apparatus needed for this purpose.

The trochoscope (from τροχεἰν, to turn) is a table used only in horizontal position; its special feature is the possibility to rotate the under-the-table tube on its longitudinal axis; according to Grashey, the first model of this table was built by O. Sommer in Vienna in 1902, following the specifications of Holzknecht and Robinsohn.

In 1912, Eugene Wilson Caldwell built the first motor-driven continuous tilting table. In 1923 Hubert Kress, an engineer at the German firm Veifa, called *Klinoskop* his improved version of Caldwell's reclining table.‡

The (herein transliterated) encyclopedic Russian term *defektoscopy* means screening of processed industrial parts to detect flaws in manufacture. The suffix has also other connotations in radiology for instance the negatoscope is a synonym for viewbox.

The osteoscope of the New York surgeon Carl Beck (1856-1911) was a shadowmeter used to test the

*Pentadecylparatolylketon.

†In *Nature* of April 2, 1896, J. Joly (of Dublin) eponymized the then new agent as Lenard-Röntgen's rays.

‡In British usage the x-ray table, especially for purposes of therapy, is called a couch. In Italy, it was sometimes referred to as a bed *(letto).*

"hardness" of a gas tube (*New York Medical Journal,* November 28, 1903). It consisted of the dried bones of a forearm and hand, fastened to a sheet of pasteboard. The contraption was intended as a stand-in for the operator's hand. In the beginning it was common practice to view one's own hand on the screen (a few were still doing it in the 1940s): "black" bones indicated a poor vacuum, *i.e.,* "soft" radiation, while the desirable condition was a pleasantly grayish shade.

A modern creation is the term *autofluoroscope* (meaning scintillation camera). It was made up by Merrill A. Bender of the Roswell Park Memorial Institute in Buffalo (New York). The term autofluoroscope was first published in an abstract in the *Journal of Nuclear Medicine* of April, 1960.

In the *American Medical Journal* of June, 1896 Monell referred to the fluoroscope as *Röntgen's spectacles.* This might have been a transposition of Séguy's *lorgnette humaine.* In my files the latest reference in this respect is F. Schopf's *Röntgenbrillen* in the *Wiener Klinische Wochenschrift* of 1907.

The suffix *-graphy* (from the neo-Greek suffix γραφία, written presentation) pertained to the exposing of plates. (It was used in the *Electrical Review* of February 19, 1896). The now rarely employed Italian term *igografia* (Amisano and Reale) meant systematic roentgen examination of apparent healthy individuals.

Initial "graphic" inadvertencies were inevitable. The surgeon Franz Koenig (1832-1910) reproduced in the *Berliner Klinische Wochenschrift* of February 17, 1896 paper prints made from roentgen glass negatives of an amputated sarcomatous tibia, and called the procedure *Durchleuchtung,* meaning translumination. The latter is today – but apparently was not then – the accepted German term for screen examination. Conversely, the Scottish oto-rhino-laryngologist John Macintyre (1857-1928) concealed under the title *Roentgen Photography* (*Nature,* May 16, 1896) a discussion of screen findings and hopes.

The abbreviation *Pediagraphy,* found in Du Pont X-Ray News nr. 12, is a contraction of pediatric radiography. *Reprography* means the reproduction of documents (papers, etc.) by any means available (heat transfer, silver transfer, microfilming, etc.): The first International Congress for Reprography took place in Köln (Germany), October 14-19, 1963.

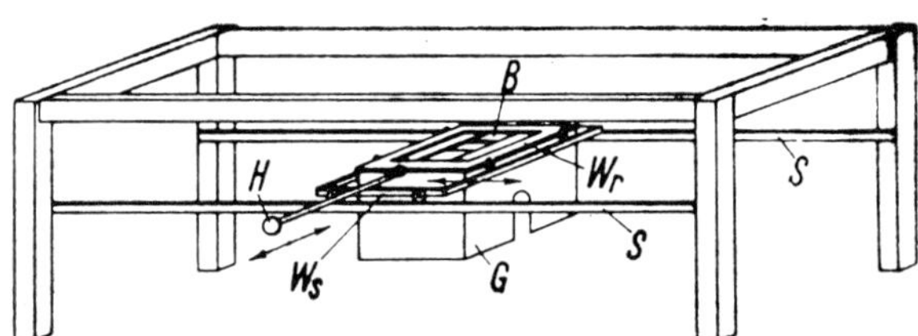

Courtesy: George Thieme Verlag, from Albers- Schönberg's Röntgentechnik, edited by Grashey in 1941.

SOMMER'S TROCHOSKOP. The handle *H* is co-axial with the center beam, and permits activation of the shutters *B,* as well as motion of the diaphragm and tube carrier *G* along the rails S. Gilmer (from Reiniger, Gebbert & Schall), instead of moving the carrier, mobilized the table top (patient and all) on roller bearings, thus preceding by decades the principle of the Swedish table Koordinat.

PREFIXES

Whereas the suffixes -scopy and -graphy were widely and definitely accepted within a few months, considerable variation occurred in the choice of the prefix. The following list of such prefixes is admittedly incomplete, since it contains only such titles as could be substantiated by at least one quotation from a printed source.

1. *Actino-* (from ἀκις, ray). On March 14 1896 the form actinography was regarded by the *British Medical Journal* as a "thoroughbred term." The corresponding term *Aktinoskopie* was actively but unsuccessfully promoted by the German internist Emil Grunmach (1848-1919). Stedman's Medical Dictionary, ed. 16 (1946) carries actinocinematography as a synonym of radiocinematography.

2. *Bio* (from βίος, life). Although meaning anatomic demonstration *in-vivo* (non-destructive testing!) the term biography, mentioned in Gocht's *Lehrbuch* (1898) would have been utterly confusing. The (American) biograph was an early motion picture projector, while in England, once upon a time, a moving picture theatre was called a bioscope.

3. *Catho-, catholo-* (from κάθοδος, way down). Initially, the new agent was regarded as just another type of cathode rays, therefore the terms cathography, cathode photography, and cathodography were quite commonly employed (*Terminology,* in the August 1896 issue of the *Albany Medical Annals*). In fact, the second but not the latest edition of the Merriam-Webster

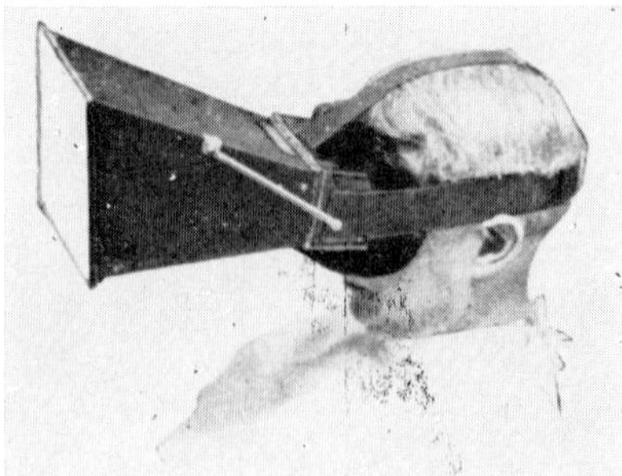

SURGICAL CRYPTOSCOPE. This model was sold by (and is herein reproduced from a 1920 catalog of) Waite & Bartlett.

lists even cathodegraphy and cathodography (in the sense of radiography). Elihu Thomson's demonstration that roentgen rays are *anodic not cathodic* (*Electrical Engineer* of March 25, 1896) may have slighted the fortunes of this prefix. Neither cathoscopy, nor cathodoscopy could be located in print.

4. *Crypto-* (from κρυπτός, hidden, secret). Cryptography was never employed in connection with roentgen procedures (although it would certainly qualify for some of the gems issued as reports to referring clinicians). Salvioni coined the word *criptoscopio* for the screening device which he first presented at Perugia, and three days later (on February 8, 1896) to the Rome Medical Society. The word *criptocrosi* originated with the Garibaldian physicist Antonio Róiti (1843-1921), and meant "colorization", *i.e.*, identification of a spectrum of different "colors" (wavelengths) within the roentgen beam.*

The term *criptocrosi* derives (somehow) from the Greek χρῶμα which means color, and from the "hiding" *krypto* — the combination refers to the existence of "hidden colors" in x radiation.

A more complex German derivation was the *Krypto-skiaskop* of H. E. Schmidt, a hooded screen. Even today, cryptoscope means a pyramidal or conical casing in which the (inside) "base" is a fluorescent screen, while the "apex" is cut off to provide an opening for the eyes. The device is hand-held, or lighter versions are strapped to the observer's head. The appliance is hopelessly obsolete by any standards of radiation protection.

5. *Dia-* (from δυά, through, across). This prefix suggested by Levy, was obviously intended to express the penetrating quality of the new agent.

*A printed reference for the term *criptocrosi* was graciously located by Mrs. Doralee Agayoff, from the Reference Unit of the NLM in Washington (D.C.). This particular paper by Róiti can be found in the *Atti della Reale Accademia dei Lincei (Memorie della Classe Scienze Fisiche)* ser. V, 20:131-142 (July 30) 1896. The unwary bibliophilic neophyte—who may want to look it up for himself—is herewith cautioned that even though Róiti's presentation date was well in mid-1896, his paper appeared in a volume which on the outside has the year 1895.

Max Levy was an engineer with the AEG (*Allgemeine Elektrizitäts-Gesellschaft*) in Berlin. He later went in business for himself as a roentgen manufacturer. He made significant contributions to roentgen technology, for instance he favored double-coated films, but — unlike another roentgen pioneer, the physician Max Levy-Dorn (1863-1929) — somehow never qualified for inclusion in Wininger's Jewish National-Biographie. Max Levy also helped to popularize the use of celluloid base, as described by Nicholas Brunner in a communication to the 1st International Congress of Medical Electrology and Radiology (1900).

Both terms, diagraphy as well as diascopy, were quite often encountered in the early times (Dumstrey and Metzner).

Objections were raised because of possible confusion with the *Diaskop* of the German dermatologist Paul Gerson Unna (1850-1929), which was a plate of glass pressed against the skin to expel the blood from the part examined, showing then anatomic (not functional) changes.

The famous cardiologist Friedrich Moritz (1861-1938) called *Orthodiagraphie* (*Münchener Medizinische Wochenschrift,* July 17, 1900) the marking with wax pencil on the fixed screen (later transfered to paper) of the outlines of the examined organ (in this case, the heart), traced with the help of a closely collimated central beam from a movable roentgen tube. The procedure was at one time widely used in Europe. Bouchacourt (in Bouchard and Guilleminot's *Traité de Radiologie Médicale* of 1900) labeled it *endodiascopie.*

Fabrik elektrischer Apparate

BERLIN N. **Dr. Max Levy** Chausseestr. 2a.

Specialfabrik für Röntgen-Apparate. 373

Preisliste kostenfrei. Vertreter gesucht.

LEVY'S FIRST AD. This box appeared in the *Wiener Medizinische Wochenschrift* in February, 1897. In later advertisements, Max Levy referred to his plant as the oldest *Röntgenfabrik,* presumably meaning the oldest enterprise devoted to the manufacture of roentgen apparatus (the distinction is hazy because he was also making coils and other machinery for electro-therapy).

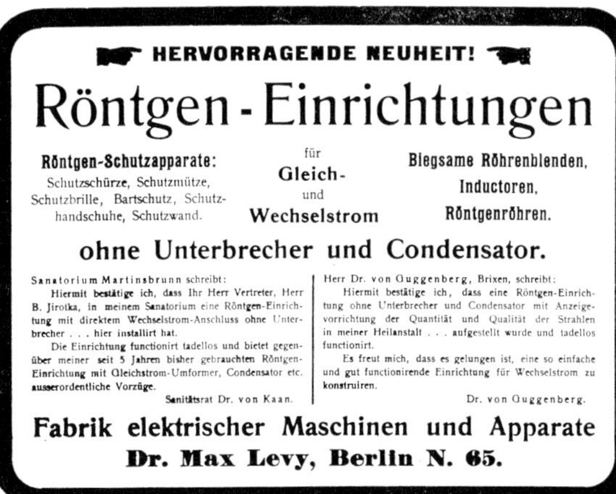

ROENTGEN INSTALLATIONS. This ad (from the *Fortschritte auf dem Gebiete der Röntgenstrahlen* of 1907) describes as a novelty an x-ray machine with neither interrupter nor condenser, presumably with a rotary switch. The claim of "*älteste* (oldest) *Spezialfabrik für Röntgen-Apparate*" did not appear until about 1910.

The Italian *diafanoscopio* — another tautology, because the Greek δυαφανής conveys the idea of showing through — is a viewbox. The corresponding term in English (diaphanoscope) means the same thing, but is used mostly (only?) by photographers.

6. *Electro-* (from ἤλεκτρον, the amber which gives sparks when rubbed). The relationship between (static) electricity and x rays need no explanation. The term electrography (in the sense of radiography) was not uncommonly used in 1896, and was still carried with this meaning in the Merriam-Webster of 1950. In a London newspaper (which is printed today as the *News Chronicle*) appeared the following notice: "Mr. Stanley Kent photographed, shadowgraphed, electrographed, or radiographed — for the proper verb is still undetermined — a fractured finger at St. Thomas's Hospital." This occurrence took place on February 13, 1896, but for some unexplained reason was reported only two weeks later (*Daily News,* London, February 29, 1896).

The complicated form electroskiagraphy was too much of a preciosity to the *British Medical Journal.* The corresponding term electroscopy proved inconvenient due to outright interference with the well known instrument for measuring electrical charges.

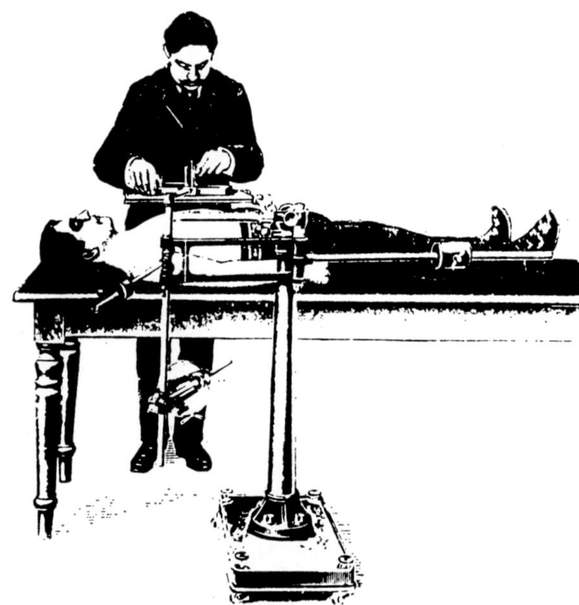

GRUNMACH'S ORTHODIAGRAPH. This version was designed by Emil Grunmach, and marketed by the AEG (Berlin). It came without the table, which was a common piece of furniture. After removal of the table, the tube-carrier (connected to the pencil carrier) and the "independent" screen could be raised for upright orthodiagraphoscopy. Keleket built (from specifications furnished by Russell Carman) a similar device, but only for examination in the erect position, called the Diagraphoscope. A conventional vertical fluoroscope made by the British firm Dean was called a Diascope.

7. *Fluoro-* (from the Latin *fluere,* to flow, but the actual derivation is from fluorescence.)* The term fluoroscope was introduced by Edison and is recognized today as an Americanism — *cf.* Mitford Mathews' *Dictionary* (1951) — perhaps because of the attending publicity: the imagination of the contemporaries was fired by the possibilities derived from being able to "watch the innards of the living body" (*American Journal of Photography,* April 30, 1896). As a matter of fact, the great virtuosi among the pioneers were fluoroscopists. The slightly different fluor*e*scope (Francis Williams) was rarely used.

At this point may be mentioned two terms of uncertain origin. The first is *iriptoscopio* (possibly derived from the Latin *reptare,* to creep, conveying the idea of subreptitious passage of the penetrating agent), taken from a Peruvian author, David Matto (*Cronaca Médica,* June 15, 1896). The other is *iristoscope* (perhaps a barbarous usage of the name of the rainbow goddess; if so it should have been iridio-scope, a term cited in Kolle's book on *X-Rays* (1898).

A laryngologist of the Metropolitan Opera, Julius Mount Bleyer (1859-1915) was well versed in electrotherapy, in fact so well that he actually helped in the construction of the "hot seat," the electric chair of the State of New York. Bleyer constructed also a set-up in which the shadows cast on the fluoroscopic screen could be photographed, and labeled this contraption (improperly) a photofluoroscope. The principle was later (re)discovered and, with better screens and faster emulsions, it became a chest survey method,

*The colored luminosity produced in certain transparent substances by the action of ultra-violet (or other types of) radiation was called by Sir John Frederick Wilhelm Herschel (1792-1871) *epipolic dispersion.* In a famous monograph (*Philosophical Transactions,* May 27, 1852) Sir George Gabriel Stokes (1819-1903) replaced this name with *dispersive reflexion,* but added—in the footnote on page 479—"I confess I do not like this term. I am almost inclined to coin a word, and call the appearance fluorescence from the fluor-spar as the analogous term opalescense is derived from the name of a mineral." The fortune of this term, although it originated strictly as a passing fancy, is not unusual in word lore.

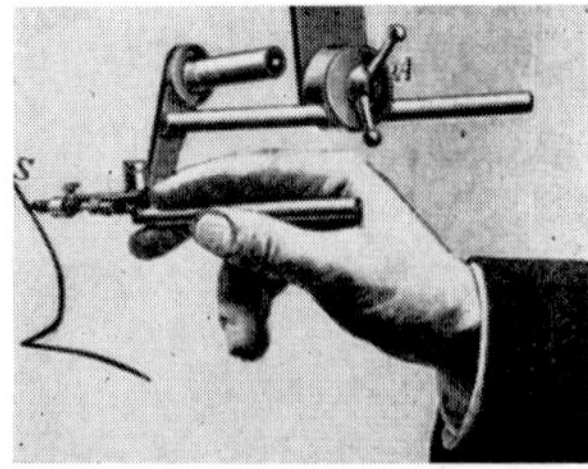

MOVING (BEAM) PENCIL. Orthodiagrapher's hand negotiates the curve around the apex of the heart.

known today under several names, including that of photo-fluorography, or simply fluorography. In the days of the pioneers, however, fluorography was synonymous with radiography (a term which, as it shall be seen, is older than roentgenography). Even today, fluorography is a confusing word because it also means to write or draw on glass with hydrofluoric acid.

8. *Ixo-* (from the German pronunciation of the letter X, *i.e.*, *Ix*). The only entry available is *Ixographie* (Büttner and Müller); it was never widely used.

9. *Phosphoro-* (from φωσφόρος, lightbringer). There is a single entry, the phosphoroscope, a term proposed by Michael Idvorsky Pupin (1858-1935), the Serbian immigrant who became professor of physics in Columbia University (*Electricity*, April 1, 1896). Phosphotography was an editorial term (*Electrical Engineer*, February 5, 1896) for a secret method of "Photographing and seeing in the darkness" (using the infra-red spectrum) devised by Georges d'Infreville, who thought he was working with ultra-violet radiation.

10. *Photo-* (from φῶς, light). Very early references call the roentgen method either "photography of the inside of the body" as in the first Italian article on the subject (Regnani), or "photography through opaque bodies," as in an American editorial (*Electrical Engineer*, January 29, 1896), or simply "new photography", as in the report of the first clinical roentgenogram produced by Cox in Canada.

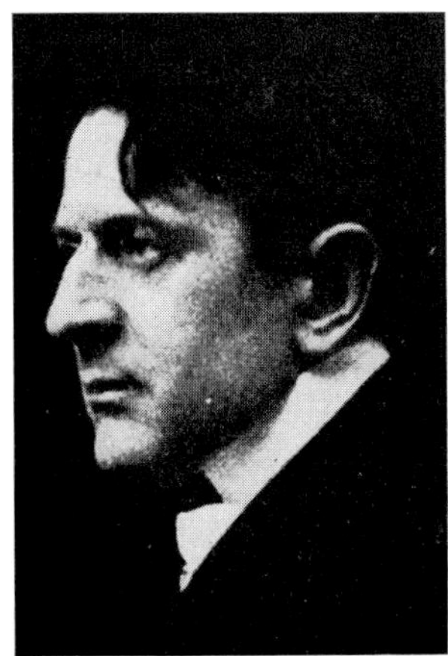

Julius Mount Bleyer. Operatic laryngology, photo-fluoroscopy, and the ultimate in electro-therapy.

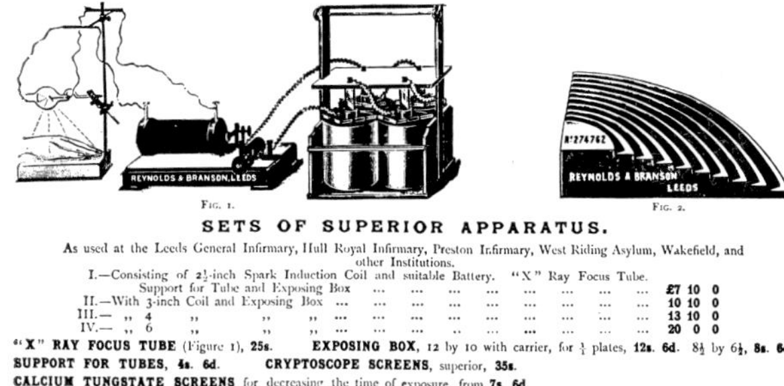

The New York gastro-enterologist Max Einhorn (1862-1953) – known for his eponymic duodenal tube – made several grotesque attempts to visualize the stomach without using roentgen rays. He called the method *radium photography:* the patients ingested the "radiodiaphane" (which in this case was a capsule containing fifty milligrams of "pure radium bromide"), and were then placed in prone recumbency with a photographic plate under the epigastrium, for an hour or two of exposure, after which the capsule was withdrawn and the plate developed. The reproductions (*Archives of Physiological Therapy*, September 1905) exhibit a diffuse, nebulosa-shaped darkening, hardly diagnostic of anything but the presence of a sizable source of both penetrating and ionizing radiation.

Einhorn's stark exploit (not at all unusual for the year 1905) shows that in x-ray nomenclature, the suffix *-graphy* stems from its close relationship with photography. Similarly, cathode photography became cathodography, then cathography. An excep-

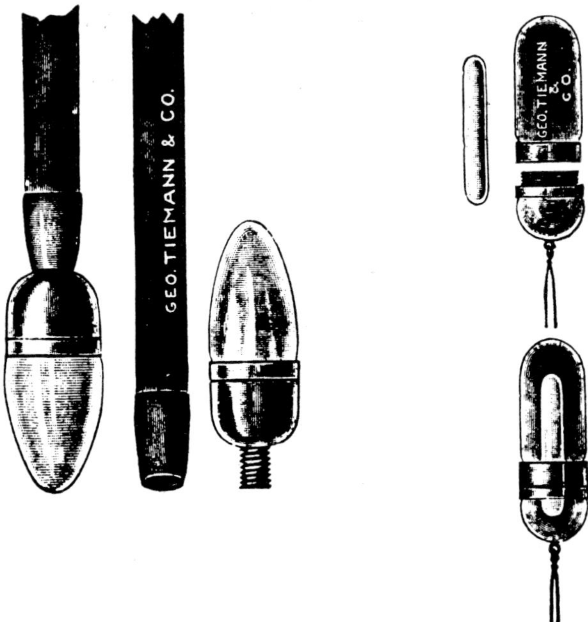

Radium receptacles. These drawings (from Margaret Cleaves' *Light Energy* printed in 1904) show at left the rounded receptacle for the stomach, at right the oval shape used for esophagus as well as for the rectum (one wonders what methods of cleansing and sterilization were used at the time).

tion to this type of contractile derivation is the (chiropractic) spinography, which is not an abbreviation of spinal photography.

Innocent souls might be guiled into the contumelious belief that spinography was derived from (or grew its king-size 14x36 inch plates after ingestion of) *spinogre,* the Old English name for spinach: such a malicious presumption is akin to slander! To be sure, the elegant vocable spinography was unfamiliar to the Davenport (Iowa) grocer Daniel David Palmer (1845-1913), who in 1895 turned from the artful (but somehow unprofitable) magnetic healing to the prosaic (but how lucrative) chiropractic thrust. This hit, called *napra* in the Czech folklore (whence the Chicago naprapaths) was said to reduce alleged cervical vertebral subluxation(s), and thus reliever the pressure which had impaired nervous flow.

Andrew Taylor Still (1828-1917) devised osteopathy some time after 1865 (1867?), and moved in 1875 to Kirksville (Missouri) which is only 150 miles from Davenport. This is why vilifying vituperators, such as Louis Reed (*The Healing Cults,* 1932), have dared to imply that chiropractic was no more than a relabeled part of osteopathy. In August, 1897 the *Journal of Osteopathy* began to copyright its issues, and explained that this was done because Palmer, Sr., along with other "fakeopaths," had been borrowing too much from their pages.

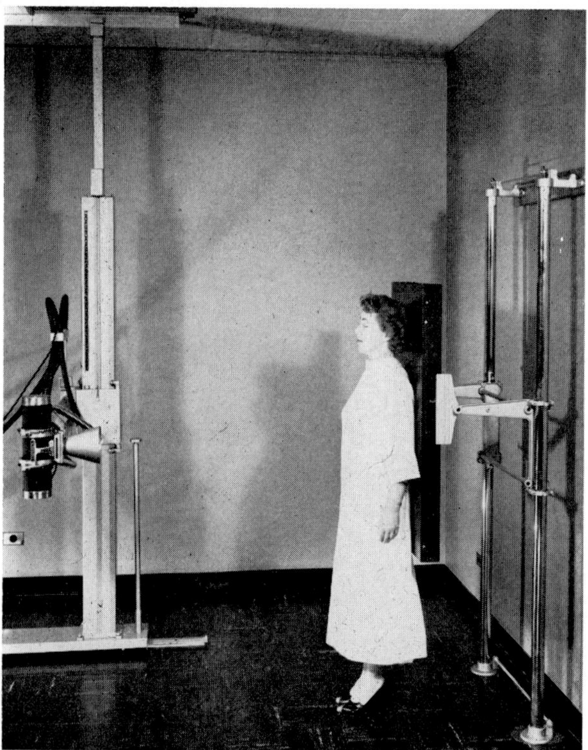

Courtesy: H. G. Fischer & Co.

MODERN CHIROPRACTIC EQUIPMENT. 14x36″ cassette holder and wedge filter on the tube.

The irreverent Mencken had discovered in an Act of the Legislature of South Carolina (1938) a definition of osteopathic practice, said to consist "principally in the correction of all structural derangement by manipulative measures, including physio- and electrotherapy, minor surgery, diet, hygiene and obstetrics." After deleting dogmatic deviations (such as ill-advised attempts to manipulate meningitis, multiple myeloma, or megacolon*), osteopathy still retains several effective procedures, heretofore "unknown" to orthodox medicine. In an answer published in the *Journal of the AMA* (December 24, 1960) Edward Lyon Compere, professor of orthopedics in Northwestern University, affirmed that osteopathic manipulations can "loosen up tension on articular facets in the spine," but specified that "exactly what is accomplished by these manipulations, no one has ever explained." I have seen instances of protruded intervertebral disc(s) suddenly relieved of pain by a relatively simple osteopathic manipulation. Most of the adversity of the medical profession comes from the fact that some of the older osteopaths still in practice are ready to "manipulate" everything from adenoids to hemorrhoids. By contrast, the younger generations of osteopaths receive theoretical and practical training comparable to that offered in recognized medical curricula, and regard the manipulations rightly as just another form of physical therapy. I have never understood why osteopathic manipulations are not being made a part of the curriculum in (orthodox) medical schools!

An old osteopathic tenet (perfect health depends on a perfect circulation . . . in every tissue of the body")† held that the "lesions" caused also circulatory disturbances. To prove this "ideologic" point, Still purchased in the spring of 1898 a "ten plate Van Houten and Ten Broeck static machine" for the American School of Osteopathy. The job to run the apparatus fell to William Smith (1862-1912), who was teaching Anatomy, Symptomatology, and Obstetrics at Kirksville, and who thus competed with David Littlejohn for the title of first osteopathic radiologist. Smith went to work and injected vessels (post-morten) with "Chinese vermillion" (bi-sulphuretted mercury) added to beeswax, and obtained *angiographic* prints which were published in December, 1898 in the *American X-Ray Journal,* together with a photograph showing the machine, the anatomic table with the dead woman's body, two assistants, and the heavily mustachioed author.

---

*The method has certain (obvious) merits in megalomasty.

†This is quoted from Emmond Rutledge Booth's *History of Osteopathy* (Ed. 2, Cincinnati, 1924). That text cites Bacon's "He who will not reason is a bigot; he who can not reason is a fool; and he who dares not reason is a slave."

In the *Journal of Osteopathy* of February, 1907 appeared an "interview" with the same William Smith who declared having proved, by "skiagraph," that embalming fluid unquestionably permeated the lungs.

Jamaica-born Smith was a colorful figure, licentiate of the Royal College of Surgery (Edinburgh 1888) and of the Faculty of Physicians and Surgeons (Glasgow 1889) — who came to this country in 1892. Before (1893-1896) and after teaching at Kirksville, Smith was in private practice in Kansas City, and then in St. Louis. After 1907 he returned to Europe, and died in Dundee, Scotland.*

*Some of this information was courteously provided by Mr. F. M. Walter, Assistant Dean of the Kirksville College of Osteopathy and Surgery.

The development of radiology among osteopaths paralleled their gradual approach toward orthodox medicine. In 1938, appeared a text by Frederick A. Long and Paul T. Lloyd, from the Departments of Research and Radiology in the Philadelphia College of Osteopathy: based on twenty "normal" and sixty "pathologic" cases, they studied the effect of manipulation on vertebral motion, and they correlated roentgen and palpatory findings. Today there are "approved" residencies in osteopathic radiology, at the end of which the candidates submit to examination, and are then granted a certificate by the American Board of Osteopathic Radiology. This has not failed to raise their standards.

The originator of the chiropractic cult, Palmer, Sr., remained a "clinical purist" to the very end. But his

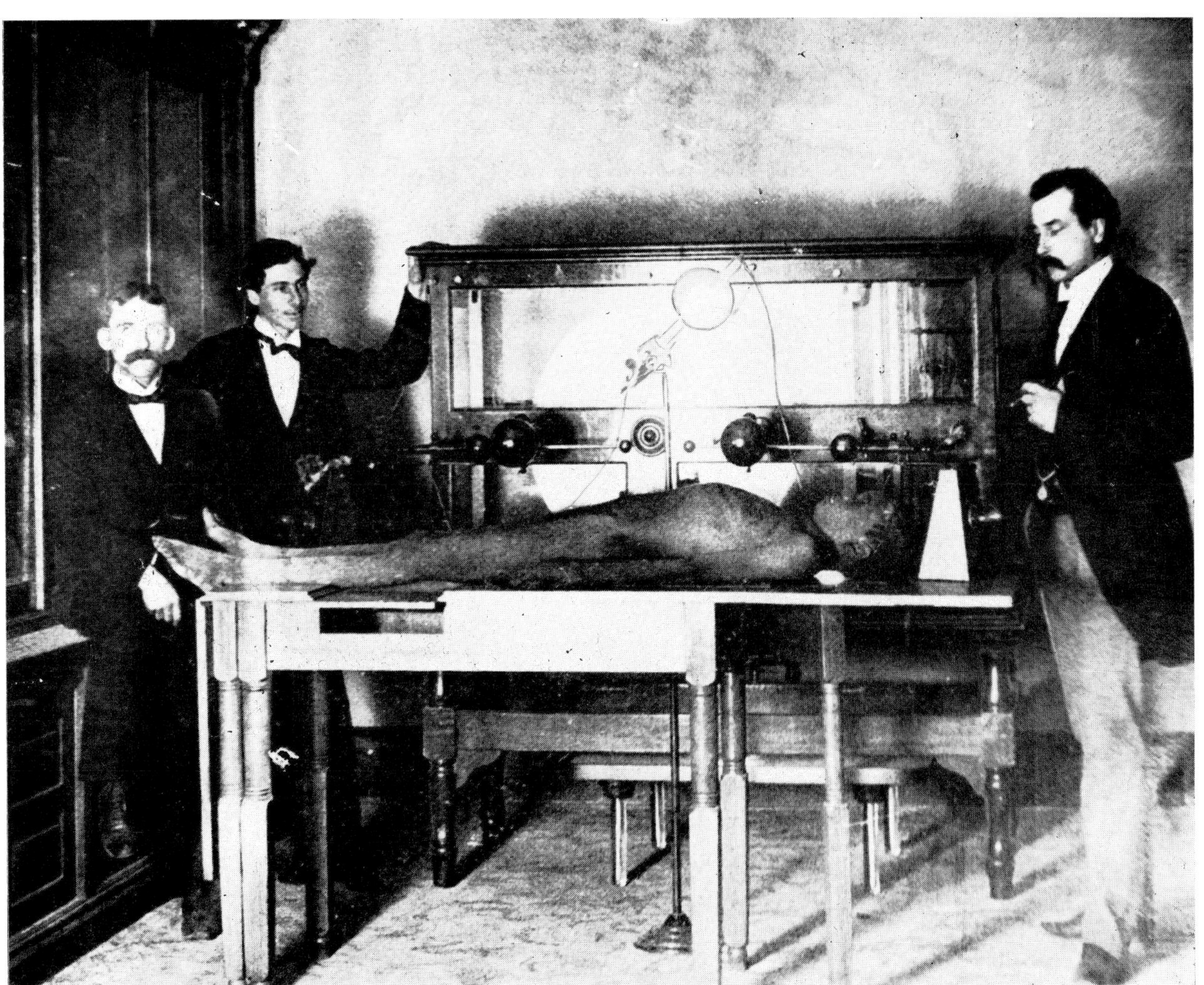

OSTEOPATHIC ROENTGEN PIONEER. William Smith, the cigar-smoking figure on the right, has just put down the cryptoscope with which he had checked the hardness of the tube mounted on the face of the 10-plate Van Houten & Ten Broeck machine. Locale: American School of Osteopathy in Kirksville (Missouri). Year: 1898. Subject female cadaver. Procedure: angiography.

son, Bartlett Joshua Palmer (1881-1961), introduced the roentgen method to chiropractic: in 1910 he purchased the first "machine" for their school, and soon thereafter patterned the word spinography as a counterpart to shadowgraphy (Ernest Archibald Thompson, 1923). Ever since, the "Chiropractic Fountainhead" (nickname for the Davenport school) has tried to maintain its "lead in spinography" (Percy A. Remier, 1957), despite the advances of "foreign" proselytizers (Lars Sandberg, *Atlas and Axis,* Stuttgart 1955), "mixers," and other competitors, including the naprapaths.

Modern terms continue to be formed with -graphy, for instance gammagraphy is a very comprehensive (catch-all or wastebasket?) type of vocable. It is supposed to cover every kind of recording (pictorial display") obtained with the help of gamma rays. As it stands today, *autoradiography* or *radioautography,* even when produced with bastard Brems-Strahlen, fathered by some low grade beta emmiter, always qualifies in this category.

In 1959 Fritz Kaindl, Kurt Polzer, and Felix Schuhfried, published at Darmstadt a book entitled *Rheographie,* meaning a study of peripheral blood flow. The same year, in Paris, T. Paniol authored a text on *gammaencephalographie:* he calculated the speed of circulation through the brain by tracing isotopes with scintillation counters. Still in 1959, in Vienna, it was called *Radiozirkulographie by O. Eichhorn.* In the *Minerva Nucleare* of February, 1960 Fieschi termed it *radioencefalografia.* On May 23, 1960 the *Medical Tribune* published the photograph of an exhibit on Cerebral Radiorheography prepared by Wilhelm Henry Oldendorf, a Los Angeles neurologist versed in electronics: his method (using radioiodine-labeled Diodrast) is described in the *Transactions of the Institute of Radio Engineers* of July, 1960. The vocable, derived from the Greek ῥέος, which means steam, must have caught on because Fritz L. Jenkner published in 1962 a book entitled *Rheoencephalography.*

As to the problem of differentiating between roentgen procedures and photography, one merely has to refer to the wavelength of the electro-magnetic radiation employed (in this respect, reinforcing screens are only a "power-assist"). In the early days, the roentgen method was regarded by most people as a sort of

WILLIAM SMITH, M. D.

Licentiate of the Royal Colleges of Physicians and Surgeons, Edinburgh, and of the Faculty of Physicians and Surgeons, Glasgow.

DIPLOMATE IN OSTEOPATHY,

1411-12 MISSOURI TRUST BLDG.,

7th and Olive Sts., St. Louis.

OFFICE HOURS:
9 to 12 and 1 to 4.

RESIDENCE:
3949 WASHINGTON BOULEVARD.
(By Appointment Only.)

Twelve Years in Regular Medicine, (1880-1892.)
Ten Years as Teacher and Practitioner in Osteopathy.

MY TEN YEARS IN OSTEOPATHY.

JULY, 1892—MARCH, 1893. KIRKSVILLE, MO.
Taught first class in first school in the world.
MARCH, 1893—1895. KANSAS CITY.
430-434 Ridge Bldg.
1895—1900. KIRKSVILLE, MO.
Teaching in Dr. Still's School, Anatomy, Osteopathy, Diseases of Women, Midwifery and Symptomatology.
1900—
President of the Atlantic School of Osteopathy, Wilkesbarre, Pa.
1901—JUNE, 1902.
Medical Schools in France, Germany, Belgium, England and Scotland.

Osteopathic Advertisement, herein reproduced from the September, 1902 issue of the *American X-Ray Journal.*

epiphotography (Grashey) — from ἐπὶ, upon, in addition. It took many years and considerable effort to get the message across that diagnostic radiology is a complete departure from photography. Apparently, a few people were not home when the messenger called.

1. *Pycno-* (from πυκνός, thick, dense). Both *Pyknographie* and *Pyknoskopie* were suggested by the Erfurt neurologist Oskar Büttner (1863-1923),* but received only scant attention from other authors (Gocht).

12. *Scia-, scio-, skia-, skio* (from σκιά, shadow). The Athenian shadow painter Apollodorus Skiagraphos (5th century B. C.), an innovator in chiaroscuro and perspective, is said to have originated the art of silhouette drawing. In 1801, the Swiss illustrator Johann Heinrich Füssli (1742-1825) defined skiagrams (silhouette pictures) as outlines of shades without any other addition of character or feature but what the profile of the object thus delineated could afford. Many of the early roentgen plates were underexposed and underpenetrated, while additional loss of detail occurred during printing, or transfer to the slide for projection (not to speak of half-tones). The final stage exhibited seldom more detail than the bare outlines of the bones, hence the appellations derived from the Greek word for shadow were apparently in order.

In the *New English Dictionary on Historical Principles,* the philologist Harry Bradley (1845-1923) found that by comparison with other English words having Greek etymons, the root scia- or scio** would have been the "proper" transliteration. He also added that by 1910 skiagraphy (rather than sciagraphy) had become the "universally adopted term for the production of x rays." This was a case of wishful thinking (even after reducing the universe to that of the English-speaking world) because neither skiagraphy, nor any of its derivated terms are to be found in the 1913 edition of the American *New Century Dictionary and Encyclopedia.* This "omission" was apparently neither unintentional, nor unique for American circumstances, as there exist entries dated 1896 for all four roots, such as sciascope (Thompson and Anthony), sciagraphy (Stine), sciography (Sachse), and skiography (Rowland).

The word skiascopy was introduced (*American Journal of Medical Sciences* of March, 1896) by William Francis Magie (1858-1943), professor of physics at Princeton, but he did not use it in his first communication (*Medical News* of February 15, 1896).

In the March, 1899 issue of the *Philadelphia Monthly Medical Journal* appeared the famous paper *Skiascopy of the Respiratory Organs.* In it (the eminently practical radiologist from Kalamazoo) Augustus Warren Crane (1868-1937) described an accurate skiameter, and emphasized that by studying differences in density on either or both screen and plate, one gains much more information than from the mere contours. Crane's contribution carried so much significance that the main body of his paper was reprinted by Hickey in the September, 1916 issue of the *American Journal of Roentgenology.* The term itself never really caught on, perhaps because it provoked the ire of the opthalmologists, who wanted to monopolize it in conjunction with their similarly named keratoscope (*Philadelphia Medical Journal,* May 13, 1899).

Nor did the vocable skiagraphy ever gain universal acceptance, but in the first decade after Rontgen's discovery it was fairly often encountered in both British and American publications. The pathologist Henry Ware Cattell (1862-1936) used it in the first article on roentgen rays originated in Philadelphia (*Medical News,* February 15, 1896). In 1907, it became part of the title of a famous study on the (*Skiagraphy of the*) paranasal sinuses in the second issue of the *American Quarterly of Roentgenology,* from the pen of the radiologist of Bellevue Hospital in New York, Eugene Wilson Caldwell (1870-1918).

In the *Chicago Medical Record* of April, 1903 Edmond Moras described how to transpose a (negative) x-ray plate onto a (positive) photographic plate, from which a (negative) paper print could be obtained. The procedure was called photo-skiagraphy, because it appeared to be a combination of photography and skiagraphy.

The word skiagraphy is now obsolete (since before World War I), but its root is sometimes recalled for incidental duties, as in the name of proprietary preparations*, or in fancy medical slang, e.g., skialytic (*Dorland's Medical Dictionary*) is that which eliminates

*These biographic dates were obligingly forwarded in a personal communication by Mr. Wiegand, director of the Municipal Archives in Erfurt (Germany).

**In Elizabethan England, *sciographie* or the *art of shadowes* was the practice of finding the hour of the day or night by checking the shadow of the sun, moon, or stars upon a dial for which reason it was also called the *art of dialling.*

*Merck's *Skiabaryt,* a sweetened and sticky (tragacanth!) mixture of barium sulphate and chocolate, and the European (?) *Skiagenol* (20% iodinated oil) are now "defunct," but Winthrop's *Skiodan* (Methiodal sodium) is still on the market.

or destroys the shadows by some form of lysis: the pulmonary infiltrate-dissolving property of antibiotics (or of roentgentherapy when the infiltration is lymphomatous in nature) might fit in this class. At times, the entire word skiagraphy is summoned from the shrines of obsolescence as when Leo Henry Garland, the professor of Radiology at Stanford, had to clarify some etymologic difficulties encountered in court proceedings (*California Medicine* of November, 1957).

13. *Scoto-, skoto-* (from σκότος, dark). This root was suggested in the British Medical Journal, March 14, 1896, by the encyclopedic classicist and longevous magistrate Sir Alfred Wills (1828-1912). Both scotography (Gocht) and skotography (*Albany Medical Annals*) have authenticated entries.

The kinetoskotoscope (just a fancy name for fluoroscope) was conceived on the observation — confirmed also by recent cine-studies — that motion brings out certain small details, which could not be (properly) detected in the stationary image. The author, who was so anxious about priority rights as to put down the date when he first accomplished this idea (February 1, 1896), was a mystery man, by name of Edward Pruden Thompson (*Electrical Engineer*, March 5, 1896). He claimed membership in both the American Society of Mechanical Engineers, and in the American Institute of Electrical Engineers (AIEE). Upon inquiry, the Mechanical Engineers stated that they could find no such name in their files. The AIEE* located Thompson in their yearbooks. He had been elected to associate membership on April 15, 1884, was transferred to member grade on December 3, 1889, and resigned in good standing as of March 21, 1916, at which time he was a retired patent attorney. The *New York Times* annuals were perused, and inquiries were sent to the Bar Association, the Historical Society, and Academy of Medicine, and other institutions in New York, to no avail. One generation ago (in Glasser's *Science of Radiology*) Williams Albert Evans, Sr. (1876-1940), of Harper Hospital fame in Detroit, deplored the fact that there was no information whatsoever on Thompson, who had compiled abstracts of early experimental x-ray work. Thompson's 1896 text, *Roentgen Rays and Phenomena of the Anode and Cathode* is a fairly reliable source for the dating of contributions by other authors.

*Through the obliging courtesy of Mr. G. E. Herrmann, manager of the New York office of the AIEE.

COMPOSITION ANTI X
du Docteur ANGEBAUD

La CUPULE du Docteur ANGEBAUD, connue dans le monde entier, est:
1° La **plus opaque aux Rayons X**: 10 m/m d'épaisseur de cette composition équivalent à 2 m/m de plomb.
2° **Incassable, opaque à la lumière, la plus légère**, d'un **superbe aspect**, **maniable**, pouvant se **scier**, se **découper**, se **sculpter**, se **visser**, s'**adapter** à n'importe quel **Modèle de Pied Radiologique.**
3° **Très isolante** à basse tension et suffisamment à haute pour être utilisée aux plus fortes intensités et sur les **Installations les plus puissantes.**
Cette **composition** est variable dans sa forme: cupules, panneaux, écrans, meubles, etc., etc.

Appareils Anti X du Docteur ANGEBAUD, 9, rue d'Orléans, Nantes. - TÉL.: 1-283

14. *Shadow-* (from the Old English *sceadwian*). An editorial writer of the *British Medical Journal* remarked that "shadowgraphy (as a vocable) is an impossible monster." And yet, its precursor, the extended form shadow photography (*Electrical Engineer*, February 19, 1896), was likewise less ephemeral than one could reasonably expect.

15. *X ray-* (From the German X-Strahlen). The combination x-ray photography became x-raygraphy, and finally the clumsy raygraphy (G. W. Colles, Jr., *Electrical Engineer* of March 4, 1896), but neither lasted very long.

Most of the terms made up with above listed fifteen roots were all but gone from common usage by the end of the year 1896. Many of them are still carried in the larger dictionaries, as in the "international 2nd unabridged" editions of both the Merriam-Webster and the competitive World Webster.* From the over-modernistic 3rd edition of the Merriam-

*The similarity of title between these dictionaries stems from the fact that the good old name of Noah Webster (1758-1843) cannot be copyrighted.

DIE RÖNTGOGRAPHIE

IN DER

INNEREN MEDICIN.

HERAUSGEGEBEN VON

PROFESSOR **H. v. ZIEMSSEN** UND PROFESSOR **H. RIEDER**
IN MÜNCHEN.

50 TAFELN MIT TEXT.

WIESBADEN.
VERLAG VON J. F. BERGMANN.
1902.

ROENTGOGRAPHY

IN

INTERNAL MEDICINE.

EDITED BY

PROFESSOR **H. v. ZIEMSSEN** AND PROFESSOR **H. RIEDER**
IN MUNICH.

50 PLATES WITH TEXT.

WIESBADEN.
J. F. BERGMANN.
1902.

Webster (1961)* many of these antiquated vocables have been deleted by their "expert in Radiography" Herman Eastman Seemann, a physicist with Eastman Kodak.

ROENTGENO- AND RADIO-

In January, 1896 the orthopedic surgeon Carl Thiem (1850-1917) of Cottbus in Germany proposed another eponymization of Röntgen's name by calling the new procedure *Röntgographie* (Gocht). On February 14, 1896 (in *Science*) Arthur Willis Goodspeed (1860-1943), professor of physics in the University of Pennsylvania, suggested the term radiography. In the ensuing thirty years these two prefixes (the eponym and radio-) competed bitterly for etymologic supremacy. Eventually, the struggle reached political levels, and at times acquired noticeable chauvinistic undertones, only to confirm Bacon's thought: "Men believe that reason governs their words; but it often happens the words have power to react on reason!"

*In *Horizon* of July, 1963 Lincoln Barnett asks, "Who is behind the assault on English? The Bible and Webster are mutilated, the new poets must be decoded, correct speech itself is 'undemocratic.' The ad men debase the language consciously and admit it; but do the 'look-say' teachers, the government jargon-makers, and the pedants of social science know the harm they do?" A few sentences will be quoted from his beautiful answer (Alfred A. Knopf, Inc. is publishing it as a book, *The Treasure of Our Tongue*): "Not even the most embittered critic of the huge dictionary (Merriam-Webster, ed. 3), that has become the hostage of Structural Linguistics, has ever contended that the English Language is static or will ever be. . . But the written word is the brake on the spoken word. The written word is the link between the past and the future. It demands precision if it is to be the carrier and container of all that is precious in human thought. And along with precision it can be invested with elegance."

It was simple to pronounce Röntgen rays, but in combination, the eponym became a problem. An amateurish wordmonger, possessed by the abbreviating demon, compounded the (difficult to pronounce) triad of consonants *-ntg-* into the tetrad *-ntgr-* as in *roentgram*. The British magazine *Photography* flirted with the term Röntography — sporting the Germanic ö as in the 5th (1909) edition of Dorland's dictionary — but the *British Medical Journal* objected, for fear it might soon be corrupted to Runtography. By the turn of the century, roentgeno- emerged as the preferred (but not yet universally accepted) spelling of the eponymic prefix. At Wiesbaden, in 1901, H. von Ziemssen and Hermann Rieder edited the first issue of the short-lived periodical *Die Röntgographie in der Inneren Medizin.*

The term *radiologie* was coined in 1896 by Antoine Béclère* (1856-1939), the respected "father" of radiology in France. On Sunday, November 6, 1897, at 10 a.m. Béclère started a weekly *Conference de Radiologie* at *Hôpital* Tenon.

*This information comes from his daughter, Miss Antionette Béclère, one of the founders and current Secretary of the Centre Antoine Béclère for International Radiology in Paris.

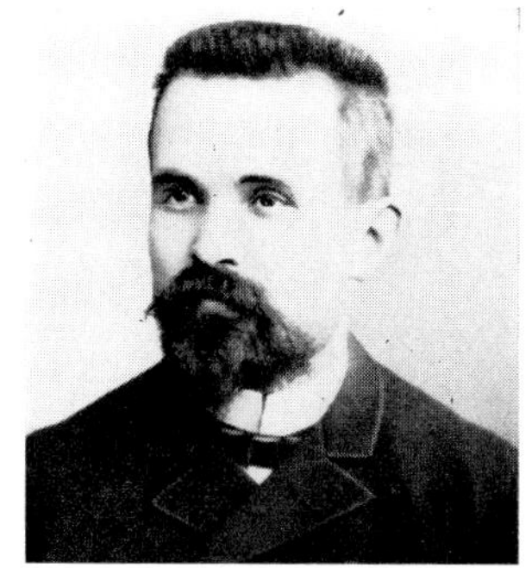

ANTOINE BÉCLÈRE. The father of French radiology, shown here a few years before the announcement of Röntgen's discovery. Béclère coined the word *radiologie*.

Mars 1897: 1er Enseignement de la radiologie médicale

HOPITAL TENON

2ème Session

RADIOSCOPIE MÉDICALE

Le Docteur A. BÉCLÈRE, médecin de l'hôpital Tenon, commencera le Dimanche 6 Novembre, à 10 heures du matin, et continuera les dimanches suivants à la même heure, en son laboratoire, une nouvelle série de Conférences et d'Exercices pratiques :

A 10 *heures*. — CONFÉRENCE DE RADIOLOGIE (Les rayons de Röntgen : moyens de production, modes d'emploi, applications au diagnostic médical).

A 10 *h*. 1/2. — PRÉSENTATION ET EXAMEN RADIOSCOPIQUE DES MALADES

There were no euphonic problems with the prefix radio-, which acquired many followers, both in and outside France. On February 17, 1896, Antoine Henri Becquerel (1852-1908) communicated to the *Académie des Sciences* his discovery of *radiations phosphorescescentes* emitted by uranium ore. Before the same forum, on July 18, 1898, Pierre Curie (1859-1906) and Marja Sklodowska Curie (1867-1934) introduced the term *activité radiante,* then *radio-activité.* This connotation of the prefix radio- (*i.e.,* its relationship to radioactivity) contributed considerably to the acceptance of the term *radiologie.*

In 1900 the first *Congrès International d'Électrologie et de Radiologie Médicales* convened in Paris. In 1904, the *Traité de Radiologie Médicale* — 1100 pages — —was published under the direction of Charles Jacques Bouchard (1837-1915) with Hyacinthe Guilleminot (1869-1922) as secretary.

Meanwhile, *radiographie* and *radioscopie* became the accepted terminology not only in France (Nemirovsky), and in Holland (J. E. Stumpff), but also (appropriately transliterated) in practically every country having a Romanic language, for instance in Rumania (G. T. Michaescu), in Italy (*cf.,* the

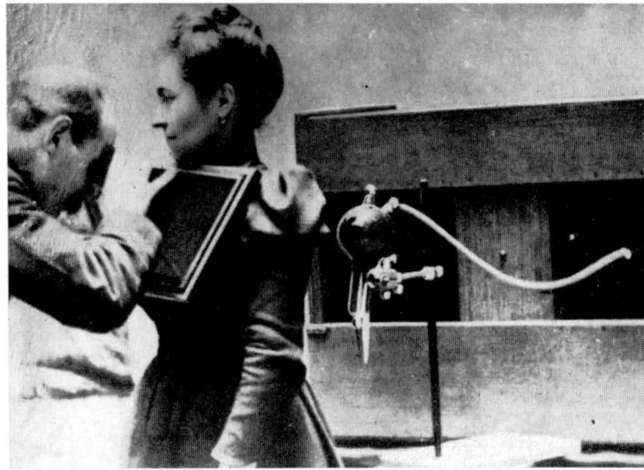

Courtesy: Centre Antoine Béclère.

FRENCH FLUOROSCOPY. Cryptoscopy at Hôpital Tenon in Antoine Béclère's department in 1897.

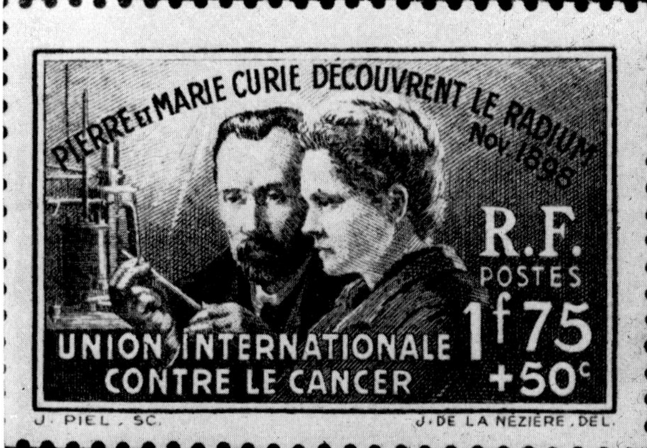

RADIUM REVEALERS. Pierre Curie and his wife Marja Curie (*née* Sklodowska) isolated radium from *Pechblende* (Czech uranium ore), and coined the term radioactivity. The stamp is from Stan Bohrer's collection.

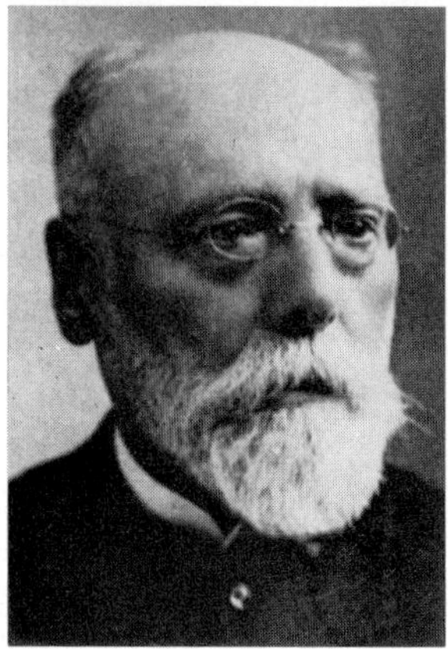

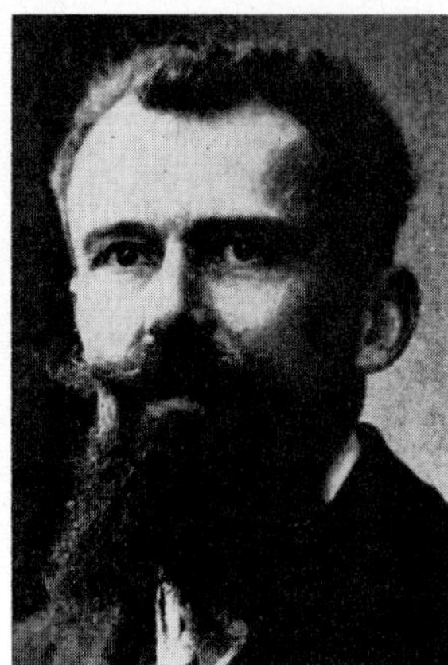

TREATISE EDITORS. Charles Jacques Bouchard directed publication of the first French treatise of radiology, and is also remembered for having described the roentgen appearance of pulmonary (tuberculosis) cavities. On the right is Hyacinthe Guilleminot who was the secretary-editor of that radiologic treatise.

VOL. II.—NO. 1.] JULY, 1897. [PRICE 4/- or $1.

ARCHIVES

— OF —

THE ROENTGEN RAY

(*Formerly* ARCHIVES OF SKIAGRAPHY).

EDITED BY

W. S. HEDLEY, M.D., *M.R.C.S., in charge of the Electro-Therapeutic Department, the London Hospital.*

SYDNEY ROWLAND, M.A., *M.R.C.S., etc.*

EDITORIAL COMMITTEE.

MACKENZIE DAVIDSON, ESQ., LONDON.
JOHN MACINTYRE, M.D., GLASGOW.
THOMAS MOORE, ESQ., F.R.C.S., LONDON.
W. J. MORTON, M.D., NEW YORK.
CAMPBELL SWINTON, ESQ., LONDON.
LYNN THOMAS, ESQ., CARDIFF.
R. NORRIS WOLFENDEN, M.D., LONDON.
SILVANUS THOMPSON, D.Sc., F.R.S., LONDON.
W. WHITE, M.D., PHILADELPHIA.

London:

THE REBMAN PUBLISHING COMPANY, LIMITED,

11, ADAM STREET, STRAND.

AMERICAN AGENT: W. B. SAUNDERS, 925, WALNUT STREET, PHILADELPHIA, PA.

AUSTRALIAN AGENT: ANDREW BYRNE, ST. KILDA, MELBOURNE.

1897.

radiolimitatore of C. Luraschi), and in Argentina (Carlos Heuser).

TRAIL OF TWISTED TITLES

In the field of radiology, the mastheads of all publications, and the titles of all of the associations have been influenced by the etymologic anatagonism between x ray, the root radio- and the eponymic forms.

The first journal devoted exclusively to the specialty appeared in May, 1896 in London as the *Archives of Clinical Skiagraphy*. It was edited by Sidney Donville Rowland (1872-1917); he had been at Downing College (Cambridge) and was then a Shuter Scholar at St. Bartholomew's Hospital, but had not yet sat for his "Finals" (as detailed by Montague Horace Jupe in *Clinical Radiology*). Rowland was at the time "special commissioner" to the *British Medical Journal* for the "new photography," and "qualified" in April, 1897 albeit he did not "register" (as a physician) until 1914.

In the *British Medical Journal* of February 22, 1895 Bertram Leonard Abrahams (1870-1908) mentioned that one of his patients was skiographed at Rowland's office. Rowland's *Archives* contained many prints made by Rowland himself, including one of the skull, trunk, and upper limbs of a "fully grown child aged three months." With the fourth issue, the *Clinical* was deleted from the title, it became *Archives of Skiagraphy*. That fourth issue, dated March, 1897, contained a small notice:

BRITISH BEGINNINGS

"A Skiagraphic Society has been formed in London by some of the leading men interested in the study of the X Rays, both in their medical and scientific application. That such a combination is greatly needed is recognized by all those engaged in working at the subject. All interested are requested to communicate with D. Walsh, 5 Pump Court, Temple, E. C."

This announcement led to a preliminary reunion (*cf.*, Vesey in July, 1904 in the *Journal of the Röntgen Society*), the protagonists being three physicians, Fenton, Harrison Low, and Walsh. They had met at the Medical Defence Union (20 King William Street, Strand, W. C.) on March 18, 1897 and had decided on the name "The X-Ray Society."

The name was changed* and the first general meeting of "The Röntgen Society" convened on June 3, 1897 at 11 Chandes Street at the Medical Society. The first slate of officers (as listed by Russell John Reynolds in *Clinical Radiology* of April 1961), consisted of president: S. P. Thompson; vice-presidents: Dawson Turner Ferrier, J. H. Gladstone, John Macintyre, C. E. Mansell-Moullin, and Fletcher Moulton; council: F. Fenton, J. M. Davidson, Rowland, Campbell-Swinton, J. J. Vesey, W. Webster, R. Norris Wolfenden, and Snowdon Ward; treasurer: T. Moore; and secretary: David Walsh.

Walsh became the author of the *Röntgen Rays in Medical Work*, first published in 1897, and reissued in at least four British and three American editions.

*The name X-Ray Society was rejected, presumably because of possible confusion with the British *Ray Society*, founded in 1844 to honor John Ray or Wray (1625-1705), the English "father" of Natural History.

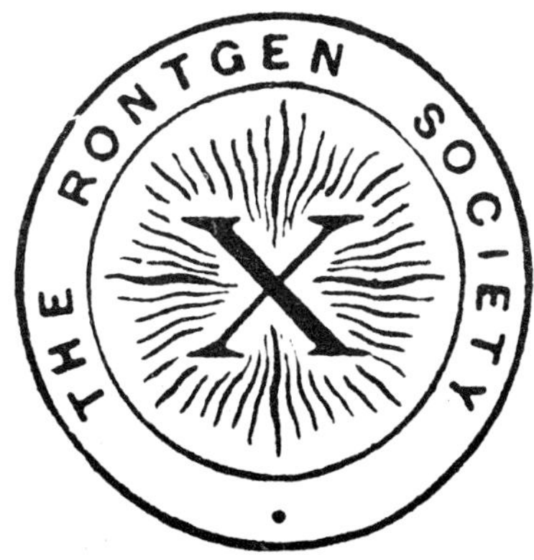

THE RONTGEN RAYS IN MEDICAL WORK

BY

DAVID WALSH, M.D. EDIN.

PHYSICIAN WESTERN SKIN HOSPITAL, LONDON, W.

LATE HON. SEC. RONTGEN SOCIETY, LONDON

PART. I.—APPARATUS AND METHODS

RE-WRITTEN BY

LEWIS JONES, M.D. CANTAB., F.R.C.P.

MEDICAL OFFICER IN CHARGE OF THE ELECTRICAL DEPARTMENT OF ST. BARTHOLOMEW'S HOSPITAL

PART II.—MEDICAL AND SURGICAL

(BROUGHT UP TO DATE WITH AN APPENDIX)

THIRD EDITION

NEW YORK

WILLIAM WOOD & COMPANY

MDCCCCII

In July 1897, the *Roentgen Society* adopted the *Archives* as its official organ but the title was changed to *Archives of the Röntgen Ray*, Rowland was demoted to second in command, and the electrotherapist William Snowdon Hedley became the chief editor.

The first formal meeting of the (British) Roentgen Society was held on November 5, 1897 at St. Martin's Tower. According to the computation of Cuthbert Andrews (see his Presidential Address delivered at the British Institute of Radiology on October 15, 1951), there were 432 persons mentioned by name as being present at that meeting, only forty-seven of them physicians. The presidential address was given by a teacher of Experimental and Applied Physics, Sylvanus Phillips Thompson* (1856-1919).

Not long thereafter, both Rowland and Hedley were replaced (by Thomas Moore and Ernest Payne). Rowland faded out of radiology and (for the remainder of his life) into bacteriology. Hedley switched (with Margaret Cleaves and others) to the *Journal of Physical Therapeutics* (published in London since 1900) which — in response to the French etymology — was renamed in 1902 *Medical Electrology and Radiology:* it merged in 1907 into the *Proceedings of the Royal Society of Medicine.*

*In Thompson's biography (1920), written by his daughters, it is told that in February 1896 Thompson found that where uranium salts were used, an effect was obtained through a sheet of aluminum (impervious to x ray). He wrote a letter to Sir George Stokes, president of the Royal Society, but it soon turned out that Becquerel had already announced the "new radiation" which was to lead to the discovery of radium.

The (British) Roentgen Society was at that time much more representative of physics than of medicine and in 1902 several pioneer medical radiologists formed the Electrotherapeutic Society which in 1905 became the Electrotherapeutic Section of the Royal Society of Medicine.

ARRS ARISING

The *American X-Ray Journal* was started in May 1897 by Heber Robarts (1852-1922), at his office located at 2914 Morgan Street in St. Louis. In the April 1900 issue of that journal appeared the following notice:

"Pursuant to a call by Dr. J. Rudis-Jicinsky of Cedar Rapids, Iowa, for a meeting of a number of workers with the x-ray to convene at the office of the *American X-Ray Journal,* St. Louis, March 26, 1900, the *Roentgen Society of the United States* was organized. Officers: president, Dr. Heber Robarts, St. Louis, Missouri; Dr. J. Rudis-Jicinsky, Cedar Rapids, Iowa, secretary." The *Western Electrician* of April 14, 1900 mentioned that, by unanimous vote, Nikola Tesla was elected the first honorary member.

On November 24, 1900 the *Western Electrician* carried the last call to manufacturers of x-ray apparatus to exhibit at the first meeting of the Roentgen Society, to be held in New York the following month. Chairman of the Committee of Arrangements was Samuel Howard Monell (1857-1918), whose address

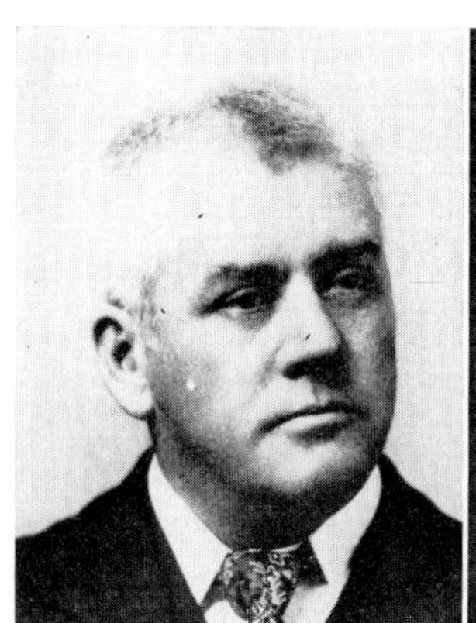

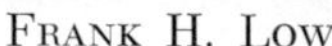

FRANK H. LOW

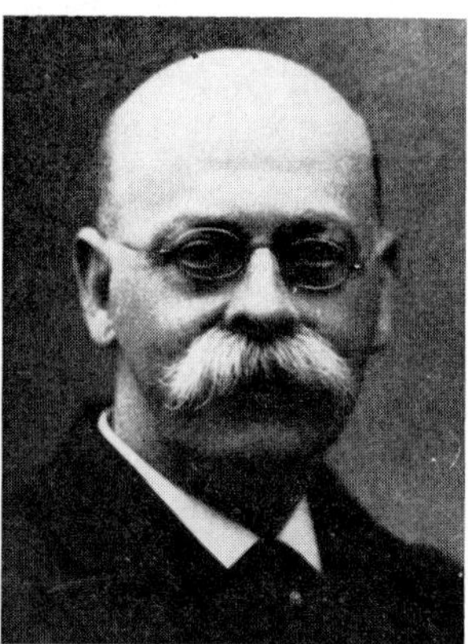

JOHN J. VESEY

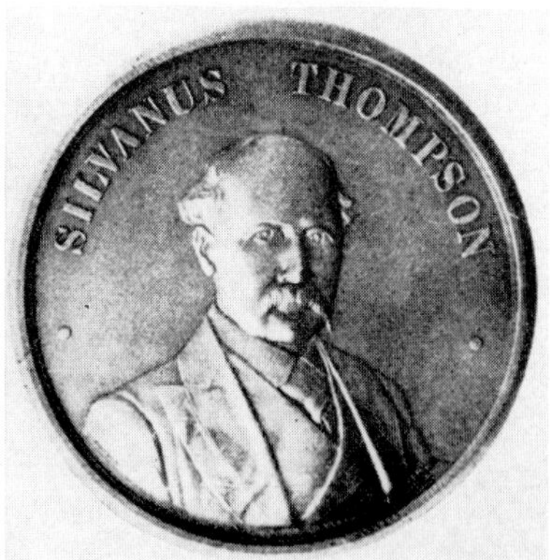

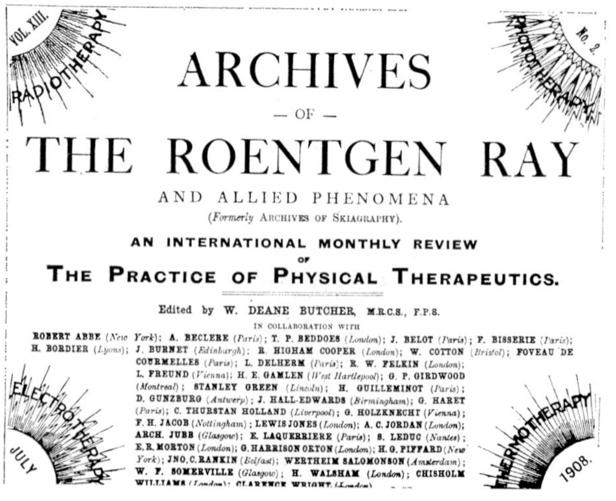

VOL. XIII. RADIOTHERAPY — No. 2. PHOTOTHERAPY

ARCHIVES

— OF —

THE ROENTGEN RAY

AND ALLIED PHENOMENA

(Formerly ARCHIVES OF SKIAGRAPHY).

AN INTERNATIONAL MONTHLY REVIEW OF THE PRACTICE OF PHYSICAL THERAPEUTICS.

Edited by W. DEANE BUTCHER, M.R.C.S., F.P.S.

IN COLLABORATION WITH

ROBERT ABBE (*New York*); A. BECLERE (*Paris*); T. P. BEDDOES (*London*); J. BELOT (*Paris*); F. BISSERIE (*Paris*); H. BORDIER (*Lyons*); J. BURNET (*Edinburgh*); R. HIGHAM COOPER (*London*); W. COTTON (*Bristol*); FOVEAU DE COURMELLES (*Paris*); L. DELHERM (*Paris*); R. W. FELKIN (*London*); L. FREUND (*Vienna*); H. E. GAMLEN (*West Hartlepool*); G. P. GIRDWOOD (*Montreal*); STANLEY GREEN (*Lincoln*); H. GUILLEMINOT (*Paris*); D. GUNZBURG (*Antwerp*); J. HALL-EDWARDS (*Birmingham*); G. HARET (*Paris*); C. THURSTAN HOLLAND (*Liverpool*); G. HOLZKNECHT (*Vienna*); F. H. JACOB (*Nottingham*); LEWIS JONES (*London*); A. C. JORDAN (*London*); ARCH. JUBB (*Glasgow*); E. LAQUERRIERE (*Paris*); S. LEDUC (*Nantes*); E. R. MORTON (*London*); G. HARRISON ORTON (*London*); H. G. PIFFARD (*New York*); JNO. C. RANKIN (*Belfast*); WERTHEIM SALOMONSON (*Amsterdam*); W. F. SOMERVILLE (*Glasgow*); H. WALSHAM (*London*); CHISHOLM WILLIAMS (*London*); CLARENCE WRIGHT (*London*)

ELECTROTHERAPY — JULY — THERMOTHERAPY — 1908.

was given as 43 East 42nd Street in New York City. The meeting place had been changed from the Academy of Medicine to Hotel Victoria and they boasted of three thousand square feet of commercial exhibits with 234 volt direct power circuit. At the last moment, the meeting place was again switched.

They actually met at the Grand Central Palace (New York) on December 13-14, 1900. Committee reports and other business matters were transacted on Thursday morning and in the afternoon the scientific session started. Among the papers presented were the following:

J. N. Scott (Kansas City): Development of the x-ray plate.

C. E. Kells (New Orleans): Applications of roentgen rays to dentistry.

F. Wesley Sells (Murray, Ia.): The first legal victory of the x-ray shadow as seen by the Iowa Jury.

E. A. Florentine (Saginaw, Mich.): A review of x-ray "burns."

Wm. Rollins (Boston, Mass.): X-light apparatus for physicians in the country.

Carl Beck (New York City): On diagnosticating osteitis, osteomyelitis, and osteosarcoma by the roentgen rays.

S. H. Monell (Brooklyn): Monell position finder for centering skiagrams.

S. H. Monell (Brooklyn): Monell x-light standardizing gauge and fluoroscope test.

S. H. Monell (Brooklyn): Monell distortion landmark for x-ray negatives.

J. M. G. Beard (Fruita, Colorado): Practical work with the static machine and vacuum tube.

Rudis-Jicinsky (Iowa): The electrochemic action of the x-ray in tuberculosis.

Weston A. Price (Cleveland): Skiagraphy in oral and dental surgery.

J. M. Bleyer (New York): Demonstration of the Mount Bleyer electro-arc chromoline for the treatment of tuberculosis by colored light rays.

Prof. A. Tripier (Paris): Indications for general Franklinization.

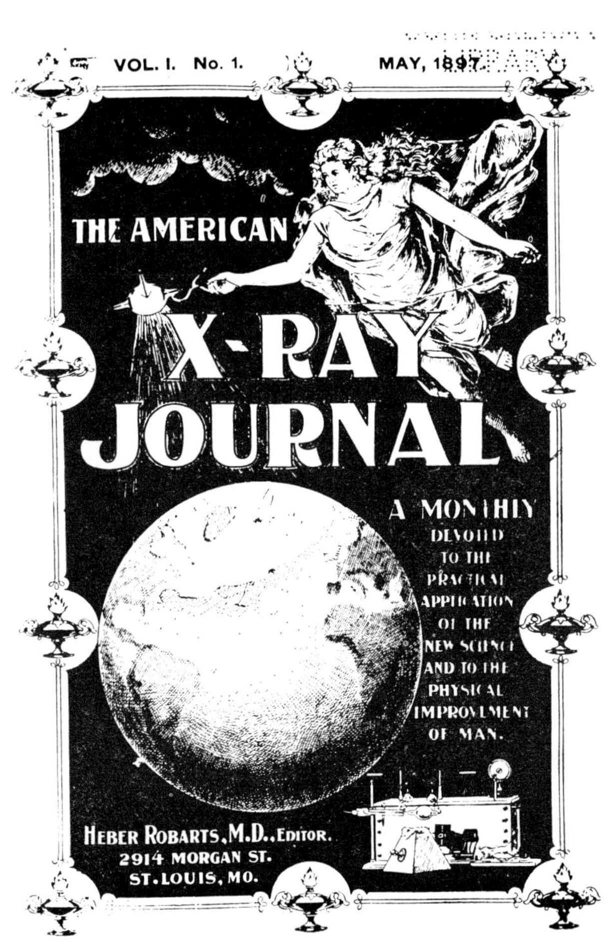

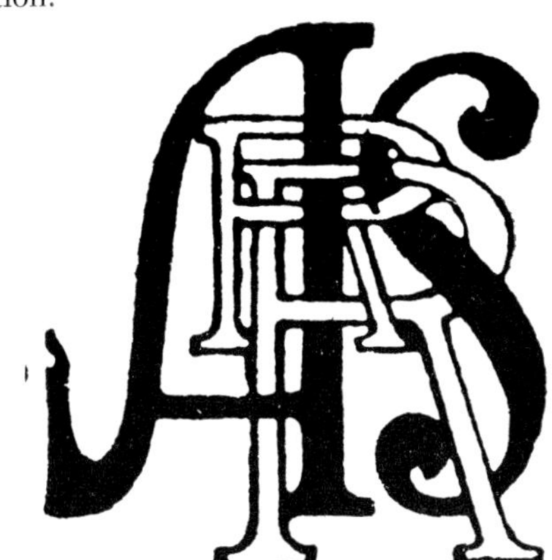

FIRST SEAL OF THE ARRS.

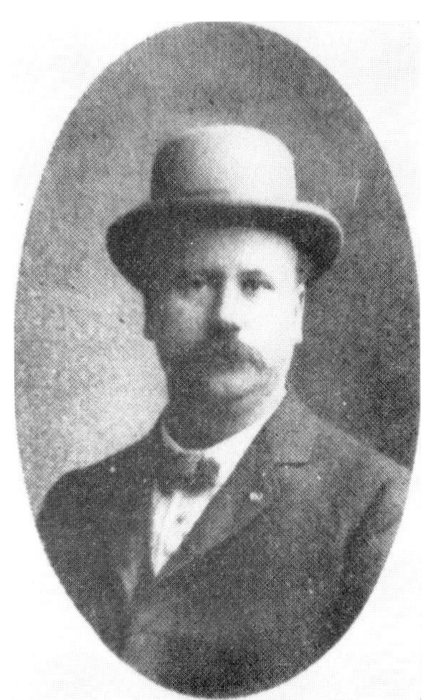

HEBER ROBARTS

L. A. Weigel (Rochester, New York): Standard fixtures in skiagraphy and how they may be obtained.
L. A. Weigel (Rochester, New York): Stereoscopic skiagraphy.
Mihran Kassabian (Philadelphia): The technique of x-ray work.
W. C. Fuchs (Chicago): Technique of skiagraphy.
H. Westbury (Harrison, New Jersey): General observation on Crookes tubes.

Application Blank.

ROENTGEN SOCIETY OF THE UNITED STATES.

APPLICATION FOR MEMBERSHIP.

I hereby make application for membership in the Roentgen Society of the United States.

Signed ....
Full name.

P. O. Address ....

$5.00 must accompany each application. There is no initiation fee. The official organ, "THE AMERICAN X-RAY JOURNAL," free. Send this slip with enclosure to Treasurer and Secretary:

DR. J. RUDIS-JICINSKY,
Cedar Rapids, Iowa.

July 1900

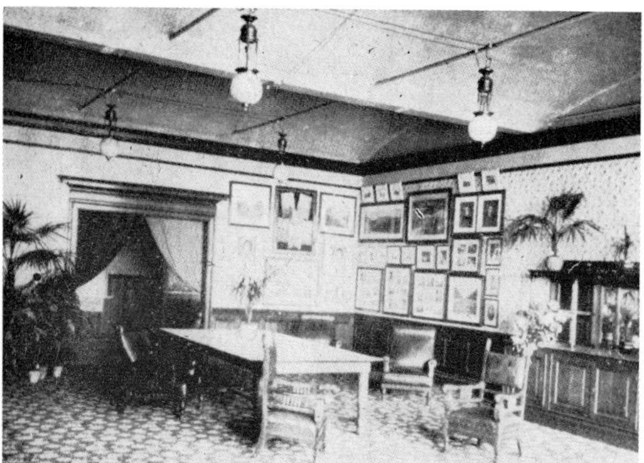

FIRST AMERICAN ROENTGEN CONVENTION. On December 13 and 14, 1900, at the Grand Central Palace in New York City took place the first meeting of the Roentgen Society of the United States (so named before it changed to ARRS). This room was "filled with exhibits," a similar one was "seated for 230 members and spectators. A total of 150 people attended the meeting, eighteen of them being members of the Roentgen Society of the USA.

G. P. Girdwood (Montreal): Stereoskiagraphy.
E. W. Caldwell (New York): A demonstration of electrolytic interrupters.
Prof. Elmer Gates (Chevy Chase, Md.): Amplifying and parallelizing x-rays.
Jos. Hoffmann (Vienna): X-ray in Lupus vulgaris.

The story of the ARRS had been summarized in *Science of Radiology* (1933) by Edward Holman Skinner, Jr. (1881-1953) of Kansas City. The latter's account served as material for a similar paper by Arthur Wright Erskine (1885-1952) of Cedar Rapids, published in the November 1945 (anniversary) issue of *Radiology.* By contrast, sentimental name-calling *(Lest We Forget)* and philosophic interpretations ("discovery of radioactivity changing a fixed and predictable world into permanent flux") pervade the sketch by Arthur Carlisle Christie (1879-1956) in the July 1956 (anniversary) issue of the *American Journal of Roentgenology.*

For the Golden Anniversary meeting of the ARRS in St. Louis in 1950, Charles C Thomas published 1100 copies of a historical booklet. The first article in the booklet was by Edward Skinner. He stated that that memorable first meeting in New York City in 1900, there were eighteen ARRS members among a total of 150 participants, including manufacturers. Skinner also mentioned that he had not uncovered anything in the way of a program prior to 1901 (this is why I have reproduced above the name and titles of the communications to that 1900 meeting). Skinner continued: "If one will read the first Presidential Address (by Robarts in 1900, reprinted in said historical booklet) he cannot escape some understanding of the

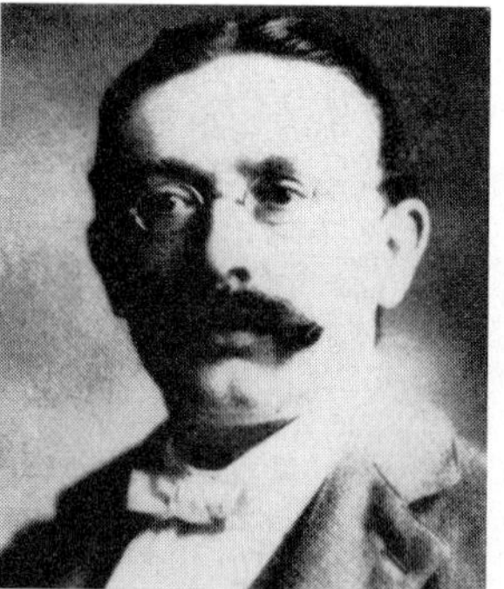

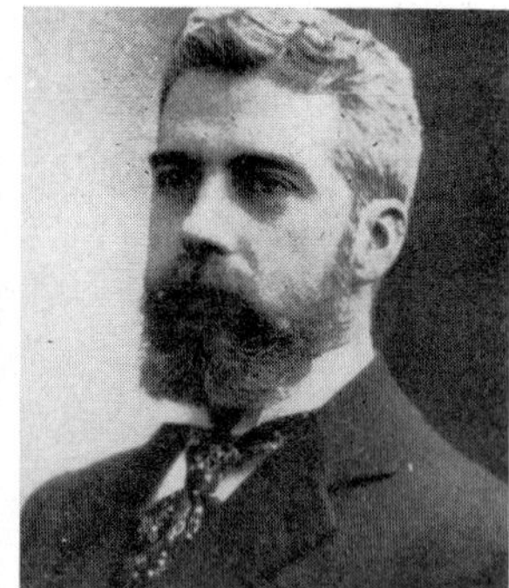

JOHN RUDIS-JICINSKY (with spectacles) practiced for some time in Cedar Rapids, went during World War I to Serbia, then returned to his native Chicago. He was ARRS's first secretary. More colorful was ARRS's first chairman of the Committee for Local Arrangements, SAM HOWARD MONELL. Brooklyn roentgen pioneer who, in 1896, attempted (unsuccessfully) to create a roentgen society in New York City, wrote extensively on "para-electric" subjects (including several books), had a thriving electrologic and x-ray practice, but "cryptoscoped" too often, and died as a radiation martyr.

desperate plight in which Dr. Robarts seemed engulfed with electrotherapists to the left of him, jealous x-ray neophites to the right of him, up-start manufacturers in front of him, and colleagues at home pulling his coat tails."

In that Presidential Address, Robarts indicated that early in 1896, Monell had unsuccessfully proposed the formation in New York City of a Roentgen Society.

A SYSTEM OF INSTRUCTION

IN

X-RAY METHODS AND MEDICAL USES OF LIGHT, HOT-AIR, VIBRATION AND HIGH-FREQUENCY CURRENTS

A PICTORIAL SYSTEM OF TEACHING BY CLINICAL INSTRUCTION PLATES WITH EXPLANATORY TEXT. A SERIES OF PHOTOGRAPHIC CLINICS IN STANDARD USES OF SCIENTIFIC THERAPEUTIC APPARATUS FOR SURGICAL AND MEDICAL PRACTITIONERS

PREPARED ESPECIALLY FOR THE POST-GRADUATE HOME STUDY

OF

SURGEONS, GENERAL PHYSICIANS, DENTISTS, DERMATOLOGISTS AND SPECIALISTS IN THE TREATMENT OF CHRONIC DISEASES, AND SANITARIUM PRACTICE

BY

S. H. MONELL, M.D.

NEW YORK

Professor of Static Electricity in the International Correspondence Schools; Founder and Chief Instructor of the New York School of Special Electro-Therapeutics; Member of the New York County Medical Society; Member of Kings County Medical Society; Charter Member of the Roentgen Society of the United States; Formerly Editor of the Electro-Therapeutic Department of the Medical Times and Register, 1894–8; Author of "The Treatment of Disease by Electric Currents," "Manual of Static Electricity in X-Ray and Therapeutic Uses," "Elements of Correct Technique," "Rudiments of Modern Medical Electricity," etc., etc.

NEW YORK

E. R. PELTON, PUBLISHER

19 EAST SIXTEENTH STREET

All rights reserved

X-RAY INSTRUCTION.

The Brooklyn Post-Graduate School of Clinical Electro-Therapeutics and Roentgen Photography.

THE BEST CROOKES' TUBES ARE USELESS UNLESS YOU KNOW HOW TO OPERATE THEM PROPERLY.

High-class work is both simple and practical. Fine effects with short exposures only require reasonable skill.

The art of selecting and manipulating Crookes' tubes to secure *maximum x-ray effects* can be acquired by every physician, and is successfully taught in a single object-lesson of about two hours. Effects demonstrated are described in "Crookes' Tubes and Static Machines," *Medical Record*, February 6, 1897, and "A Study of Maximum X-Ray Effects with the Static Machine," *Medical Record*, June 26, 1897, and also set forth in full in my book. Instruction in this branch is intended to aid the many who have spent considerable time and money in the difficult attempt to acquire experience alone.

Hours for x-ray instruction arranged by special appointment. X-ray photography. Address all communications to

S. H. MONELL, M. D.,
865 Union Street, BROOKLYN, N. Y.

In writing to advertisers mention The American X-Ray Journal.

FOURTH ANNUAL ANNOUNCEMENT NEW YORK SCHOOL

—OF—

Special Electro-Therapeutics

S. H. MONELL, M. D., Director.

No. 45 East 42d Street, - - - New York City.

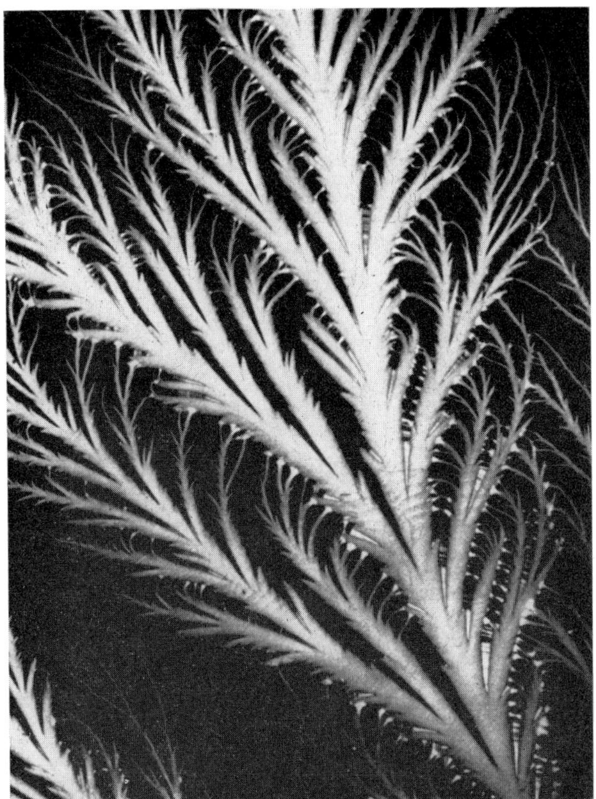

MICRO-LIGHTNING. This illustration from one of Monell's books was therein called "positive phase of electrical energy." It is from an 18x22″ photograph, one of fifty different electric discharges produced by Kinraide (of Boston) with his coil (sold by Meyrowitz of New York City). Writes Monell: "without question they (the 50 photographs) furnished the most striking, unique, and magnificent record of electrical discharges ever made. They would have astonished Faraday beyond words."

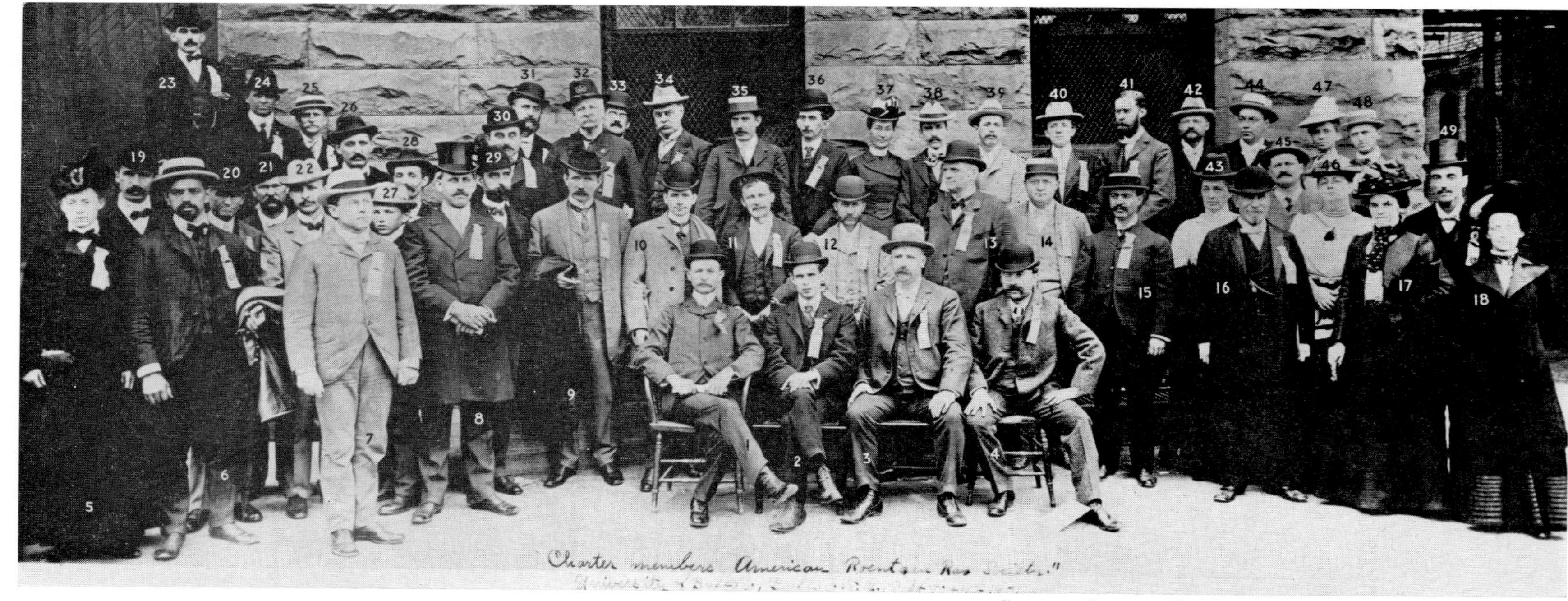

Courtesy: Eastman Kodak

ARRS Meeting, held on September 10-11, 1901 in Buffalo (New York). The following could be identified: 1. Weston Price, D.D.S., Cleveland; 2. E. A. Florentine, M.D., Saginaw (Michigan); 3. Heber Robarts, M.D., St. Louis; 4. J. Rudis-Jicinsky, M.D., Cedar Rapids; 5-6 Henry Engeln & wife, Cleveland; 8. Henry Hulst, M.D., Grand Rapids (Michigan); 10. John McIntosh, Chicago; 15. Mihran Kassabian, M.D., Philadelphia; 25. Augustus W. Crane, M.D., Kalamazoo (Michigan); 26. G. G. Burdick, M.D., Chicago; 32. H. E. Waite, M.D., New York; 37-38. Ed Jerman and wife, Indianapolis; 44. Preston Hickey, M.D., Detroit.

Sam Monell had many ideas which became successful only when other people re-discovered them. Thus, at that very first meeting in New York City, Monell became the chairman of the Committee on Standards of Nomenclature in X-Ray Work and published a *Letter* to this effect in the *American Electrotherapeutic and X-Ray Era* of August 15, 1901.

Monell's fertile imagination was also demonstrated in his many books. There appeared for instance his *System of Instruction in X-Ray Methods* (which for some strange reason – perhaps creditors – was copyrighted in 1902 in the name of F. W. Monell). In 1933 Evans, Sr. expressed a very poor opinion of that book by Monell, mainly because of its second half, which was devoted to Hot-Air Therapy, Vibration Massage, and High-Frequency Currents. It contained also a photograph of Monell himself undergoing "tissue-oscillating" of the calves. The procedure was alleged to be tonic, derivative, warming, nutritional, muscular, analgesic, and so on depending on the indication. In the first half of the same book, Monell is shown performing various fluoroscopic procedures without the slightest protective measures. Indeed, his name is inscribed on the obelisk of roentgen martyrs in the St. Georg Hospital in Hamburg. But he is not included in Percy Brown's book of martyrs. Could that be because of Monell's activity as the owner and operator of the New York School of Special Electrotherapeutics, and for his having promoted correspondence courses in radiology? On the other side of the ledger remains the unquestionable fact that Monell was one of the pioneers, devised many original arrangements of apparatus for x-ray technics, and – according to Trostler – Monell had been the "first to diagnose" an osteosarcoma on October 17, 1896.

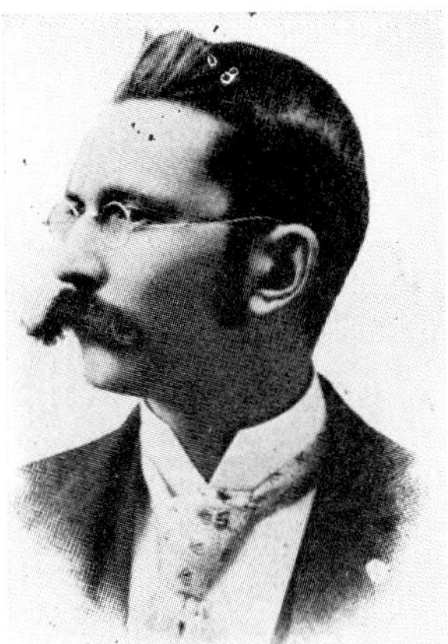

RÖNTGEN QUACK I. This is the portrait of "Prof. W. O. Horner of Cleveland, Tennessee," as it appeared in the *American X-ray Journal.*

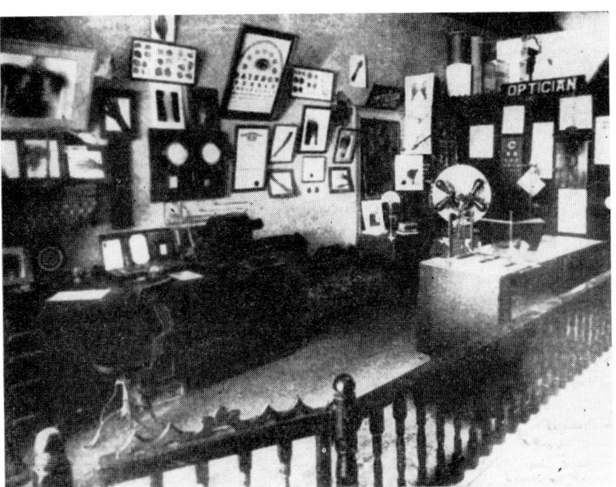

HORNER'S OFFICE. Note the sign optician, the coil, and the x-ray prints on the wall.

At the meeting in New York City in 1900, the name of the Society was tentatively (and then definitely) changed to American Roentgen Ray Society. The point was to "cover" also the Canadian members. The next meeting was set for Buffalo (New York). Again, Robarts was elected president, but he refused to accept the office, and later resigned his membership.

The St. Louis

X-Ray Laboratory

Is owned and managed by

MR. M. E. PARBERRY, M. E.

Member of the Roentgen Society of the United States.

THE appointments of this Laboratory are as nearly complete as professional skill can accomplish. The static machine is of the highest grade and type and the coils are of the most recent designs. There are indications for the use of two designs of coils depending upon penetration and shadowing, which in each case must be selected. Likewise the static machine comes in requisition for another class.

One coil is equipped with an independent multiple vibrator, an interlocking switch, a fuse block, series and parallel spark gaps; and it may run on the 110 volt direct current circuit, 110 volt alternating current circuit, seven cells of storage battery, 14, 40, 70 volts, either its own or mechanical break, the electrolytic break or any outside break of the mechanical or mercurial type. The automobile service is a convenience to physicians where it is found impracticable to move the patient from home or from hospital.

The experimental stage of the x-rays has passed and physicians now ask for clearer definition and proof of the accuracy of the picture shown. These two requisites are here accomplished. The aim is to reach as near scientific perfection as can be done and to offer to the medical profession a correct system indisputable in many cases and in others corroborative evidence. We have done work for more than 200 physicians, but desire to enlist the patronage of all doctors both in and out of the city. No delay will occur when called to outside towns.

Our work includes pictures of the hip joint, stone in the kidneys, gall stones, tumors, abscesses and other work that formerly proved so difficult or impossible.

We cordially solicit personal inspection of our work by physicians and surgeons.

M. E. PARBERRY, *Manager.*

Chemical Building.

The reason was (allegedly or apparently) the large number of non-medical members in the Society.

Information on Robarts can be found in the obituary notice written for the *American Journal of Roentgenology* of October 1922, in the *Backward Look* of Fred O'Hara in the May-June, 1932 issue of *Radiography and Clinical Photography,* and in the biography included in Percy Brown's roentgen-martyrologue.

After graduation from Missouri Medical College in St. Louis (1880), Robarts established himself in Belleville (Illinois), and was also Surgeon for the Great Northern Railroad. After Röntgen's discovery, he moved to St. Louis and opened an "x-ray office," where Fred O'Hara was his assistant for seven years. For the publication of the *American X-Ray Journal,* Robarts had founded also the American X-Ray Publishing Co.* with offices next door to his medical office on the third floor of the Chemical Building (8th and Olive Sts., in St. Louis).

*After World War I, there existed a firm by the same name in New York City; it published for instance the *Principles and Practice of Roentgenological Technique* (1920) by I. Seth Hirsch.

Lupus, Rodent Ulcers,

Skin Cancers

—and—

Open Malignant Sores.

FOR the treatment of such diseases we have completed all the necessary details when the patients are brought or sent to this Laboratory by their physician or surgeon.

We appeal to doctors only for these cases, and for such that are either non-operative, or in the judgment of the attending physician, a case for the x-rays.

These open sores require a continuous radiation of 10 minutes daily for some 30 days. The question of recovery of these cases by the x-rays is not in dispute. We keep the doctor informed of the progress of the case and, when convenient for him, urge his personal observation while the case is under treatment.

The management of the

St. Louis X-Ray Laboratory

is and will continue to be wholly ethical with its dealings with the profession.

We invite inspection.

300 Chemical Building, Eighth and Olive Sts.

Call or write for fuller particulars.

1899

In 1931, Skinner, Jr. had deprecatory words for the quality of the material in the *American X-Ray Journal.* In fact some of the advertisements and many of the articles which it printed are unacceptable by present-day standards. But a proper judgment cannot be rendered without considering the time and place of publication. When so qualified, Robarts' pioneering work in bringing out the *American X-Ray Journal* remains an important and valuable page in the history of radiology.

It seems that around 1905, under the influence of Girdwood, Goodspeed, Beck, Kassabian, Pfahler, and Leonard, to name only a few, the ARRS purged itself of undesirable elements (including Monell), and thus acquired respectability. We use the word undesirable on purpose because in actual life there are no true saints and villains, most persons have some good and some evil traits. The "rejects" from the ARRS retreated into what was later called the Society of Electrotherapists — and Robarts sold them his property rights in the *American X-Ray Journal.* Afterwards, his main interest centered on radium therapy. He wrote on the effects of "radium light" in several installments in the 1903 volume of the *American Journal of Surgery and Gynecology* (St. Louis). He printed privately (Nixon-Jones, St. Louis, 1909) a relatively brief Platonic dialogue, entitled *Practical Radium:* this dialogue is assumed to occur between Robarts (Dr. Radium) and an imaginary pupil (Dr. Interrogator). It is (unintentionally) quite entertaining.

As a result of prolonged exposure, Robarts developed radiation dermatosis, then malignancy, and died with generalized carcinomatosis. Unbearable pain made him

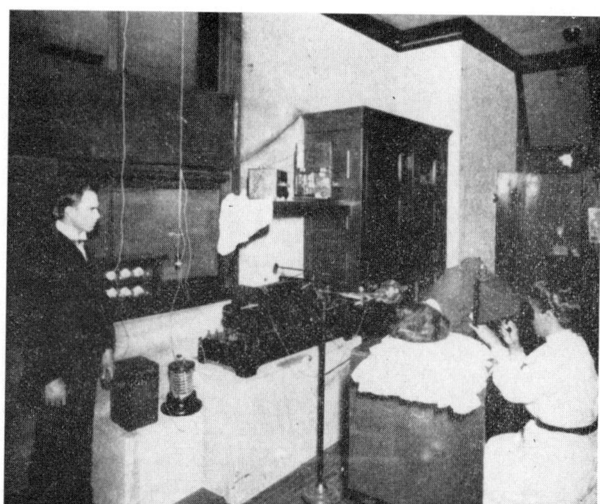

PARBERRY AS EDUCATOR. This is Parberry's office while a student is being instructed in the use of the Dennis Fluorometer.

come to Chicago (that was about two weeks before his death). He asked Orndoff to do something, but no mutilating surgery (amputation of a "shoulder") seemed advisable in the presence of widespread carcinoma. The "patient" could not be told the entire truth, and Robarts left Chicago with the impression that he had been "let down" by timorous colleagues. Orndoff's judgment and decision had been correct and yet, to this day, he remembers with a feeling of (absolutely unjustified) guilt the sad look of disappointment and despair on the face of Robarts when his request for surgery had to be turned down.

John Rudis-Jicinsky (1865-1921) was a graduate of the University of Illinois (1896). He practiced for some time in Cedar Rapids, Iowa, then returned to Chicago. In World War I he volunteered for service in Europe, and published in the February 15, 1917 issue of the *New York Medical Journal* his experiences with "x-ray service" in Serbia. After his initial organizing activity in the ARRS, Rudis-Jicinsky remained just a rank-and-file member (which is more than could be said of either Robarts or Monell).

The first issue of *Electrotherapeutic and X-Ray Era,* published in June 1901, was edited by Julius Silversmith. The second and third issues, edited by J. O. M. Hewitt, were entitled *American Electrotherapeutic and X-Ray Era.* Beginning with the fourth issue, the name was again changed — presumably due to French influence — to *Archives of Electrology and Radiology.* The editors for 1902-1903 were C. H. Treadwell and F. W. Butterman,* and in 1904 the editorship went to Clarence Edward Skinner, Sr. (1868-1937),* the radiotherapist trans-*Ray Journal* into the *American Journal of Progressive Therapeutics* (final fadeout: 1906). The casualty planted from the East to Kansas City, who consolidated the Era with the remnants of the *American X-*

*Among these four, only Charles Humphrey Treadwell (1871-1918) of Chicago was identified as a physician by Miss Patricia Corinne Witt, of the Records Control Unit of the American Medical Association (AMA). Miss Witt also provided data on many other American physicians listed in the text.

*Skinner was involved in several publicistic ventures, for instance he edited the first four volumes of the *Archives of Physiological Therapy* which then, by putting the cards on the table, merged into the *Journal of Inebriety.*

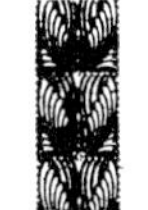

Patients received between the hours of
9 A. M. and 3 P. M.

OFFICE AND LABORATORY
OF
Dr. Heber Robarts

301 Chemical Building,
8th and Olive Streets,
PHONE, B 4. ST. LOUIS.

BETWEEN the hours of 10 A. M. and 12 M., (Sunday excepted) physicians may call at my Laboratory and arrange hours for instruction in x-ray diagnosis and x-ray therapy. Physicians taking instruction, can see patients under treatment, with cancer lupus, rodent ulcers, neuralgias and those diseases rebellious to medicine, or inoperable.

When not convenient to come, correspond with me at above address.

HEBER ROBARTS.

Late President of the Roentgen Society of America; Editor, American X-Ray Journal; Formerly Surgeon to Illinois Central R. R., N. P. R. R., etc., etc.

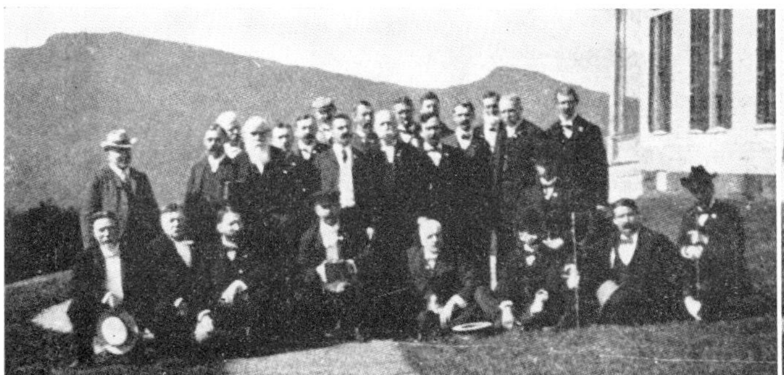

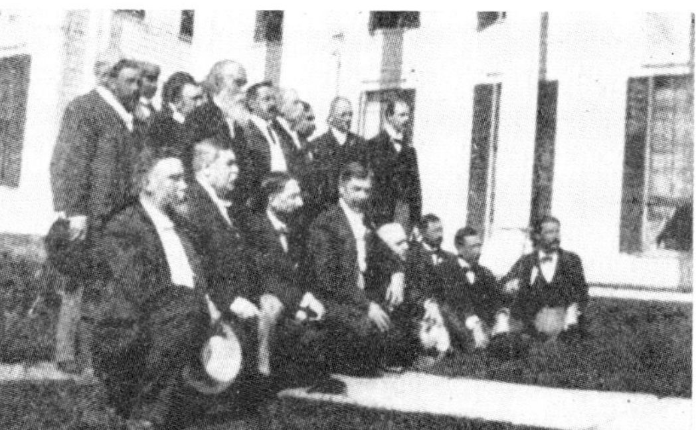

FELLOWS OF THE ETA. Antero-posterior and right lateral of the Electro-Therapeutic Association meeting at Hotel Kaaterskill in the Catskill Mountains (New York) on September 4, 1902.

(merger) and fatality rates of specialty journals had always been fairly tall, *e.g.,* the ambitious weekly folio of Edmond de Bourgade la Dardye — *Les Rayons X* (Paris) — lasted only from February 5, 1898 to April 22, 1899, perhaps because at that time the recognized radiologic journal in France was the *Archives d'Électricité Médicale.*

TEUTONIC RÖNTGEN TERMINOLOGY

The first issue of the *Fortschritte auf dem Gebiete der Röntgenstrahlen* (Hamburg) appeared in September 1897, its editors being Heinrich Ernst Albers-Schönberg (1865-1921) and his office partner and friend Georg Deycke* (1865-1940). The *Berliner Röntgenvereinigung* was created on March 18, 1898. In the *Fortschritte* of December 29, 1903, the *Berliner Röntgenvereinigung* issued an invitation to a pro-

*The following year, Deycke-Pasha joined the Faculty of the Imperial Ottoman (teaching) Gulhane Hospital, and thereby introduced the clinical roentgen method into Turkey.

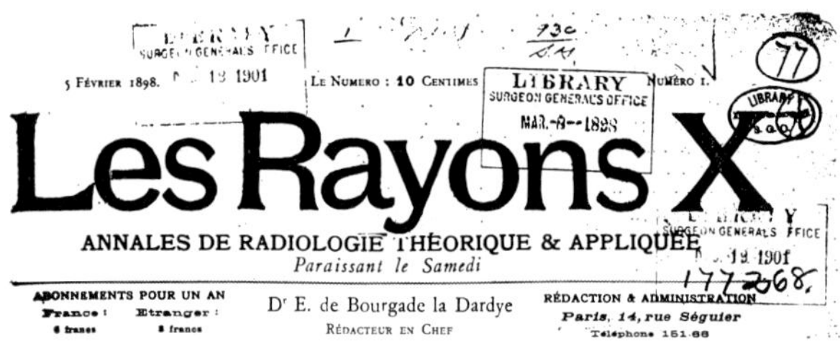
5 Février 1898. | Le Numéro : 10 Centimes | Numéro 1.

Les Rayons X

ANNALES DE RADIOLOGIE THÉORIQUE & APPLIQUÉE

Paraissant le Samedi

ABONNEMENTS POUR UN AN — France : 6 francs — Etranger : 8 francs

Dr E. de Bourgade la Dardye, Rédacteur en Chef

RÉDACTION & ADMINISTRATION — Paris, 14, rue Séguier — Téléphone 151.68

Fortschritte

auf dem Gebiete der

Röntgenstrahlen

Unter Mitwirkung von

Geh. Med.-Rat Prof. Dr. v. **Bramann** in Halle, Prof. Dr. v. **Bruns** in Tübingen, Geh. Med.-Rat Prof. Dr. **Curschmann** in Leipzig, Geh. Med.-Rat Prof. Dr. **Czerny** in Heidelberg, Prof. Dr. **Deycke** in Constantinopel, Prof. Dr. **Forster** in Bern, Dr. **Gocht** in Halle, Prof. Dr. **Grunmach** in Berlin, Prof. Dr. **Henschen** in Upsala, Geh. Med.-Rat Prof. Dr. **Hoffa** in Berlin, Dr. **Holzknecht** in Wien, Prof. Dr. **Kölliker** in Leipzig, Prof. Dr. **Krause** in Berlin, Oberarzt Dr. **Kümmell** in Hamburg, Stabsarzt **Lambertz** in Metz, Oberarzt Dr. **Carl Lauenstein** in Hamburg, Prof. Dr. **Lenhartz** in Hamburg, Prof. Dr. **Lennander** in Upsala, Prof. Dr. **Oberst** in Halle, Geh. Med.-Rat Prof. Dr. **Riedel** in Jena, Prof. Dr. **Rumpf** in Bonn, Generalarzt Dr. **Schjerning** in Berlin, Prof. Dr. **E. Schiff** in Wien, Prof. Dr. **F. Schultze** in Bonn, Oberarzt Dr. **Sick** in Hamburg, Geh. Reg.-Rat Prof. Dr. **Slaby** in Charlottenburg, Generalarzt Dr. **Stechow** in Hannover, Prof. Dr. **Voller** in Hamburg, u. Dr. **Walter** in Hamburg

herausgegeben von

Dr. med. Albers-Schönberg

Sechster Band

Hamburg

Lucas Gräfe & Sillem

(Edmund Sillem)

1902—1903

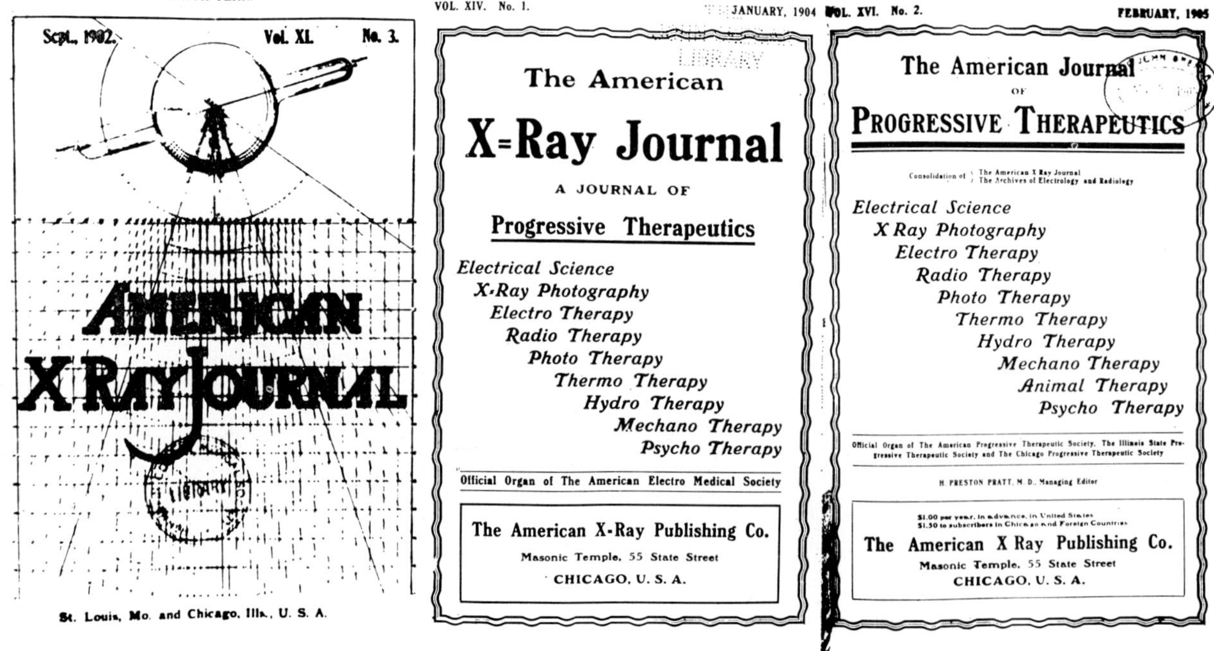
SIXTH YEAR.

Sept. 1902. Vol. XI. No. 3.

AMERICAN X RAY JOURNAL

St. Louis, Mo. and Chicago, Ills., U. S. A.

VOL. XIV. No. 1. JANUARY, 1904

The American

X=Ray Journal

A JOURNAL OF

Progressive Therapeutics

Electrical Science
X-Ray Photography
Electro Therapy
Radio Therapy
Photo Therapy
Thermo Therapy
Hydro Therapy
Mechano Therapy
Psycho Therapy

Official Organ of The American Electro Medical Society

The American X-Ray Publishing Co.
Masonic Temple, 55 State Street
CHICAGO, U. S. A.

VOL. XVI. No. 2. FEBRUARY, 1905

The American Journal of

PROGRESSIVE THERAPEUTICS

Consolidation of The American X Ray Journal / The Archives of Electrology and Radiology

Electrical Science
X Ray Photography
Electro Therapy
Radio Therapy
Photo Therapy
Thermo Therapy
Hydro Therapy
Mechano Therapy
Animal Therapy
Psycho Therapy

Official Organ of The American Progressive Therapeutic Society, The Illinois State Progressive Therapeutic Society and The Chicago Progressive Therapeutic Society

H. PRESTON PRATT, M. D., Managing Editor

$1.00 per year, in advance, in United States
$1.50 to subscribers in Chicago and Foreign Countries

The American X Ray Publishing Co.
Masonic Temple, 55 State Street
CHICAGO, U. S. A.

posed *Röntgenkongress* combined with a *Röntgen-ausstellung* (roentgen exhibit); the invitation was signed by Eberlein (president), Immelmann (secretary), Cowl (treasurer), Albers-Schönberg and Rieder (corresponding members).

That first Röntgenkongress met in Berlin from April 30 through May 3, 1905. *The Ehrengast* (guest of honor), Röntgen, snubbed the meeting and did not attend. The Honorary President, a famous surgeon, Ernst von Bergmann (1836-1907) was absent because of illness. Nevertheless, the meeting was extremely successful, in part because of the exhibits (Cowl was chairman of that committee). Moreover, on May 2, 1900 was born the *Deutsche Röntgen-Gesellschaft,* its founders being Albers-Schönberg (40 years old at the time), Cowl (50 years), Eberlein (35 years), Gocht (36 years), Grashey (29 years), Immelmann (40 years), Köhler (31 years), Rieder (47 years), and Walter (43 years).

On the occasion of the 37th *Röntgenkongress* (München, October 16-19, 1955), which was also the 50th anniversary of the German Roentgen Society, its historiographer* the internist Bernhard Kurt Walther prepared scholarly biographies of the founders, printed in the October 1955 issue of *Röntgen-Blätter.*

Albers-Schönberg was originally trained as a gynecologist. He entered the field soon after the announce-

*Could it be that the semantic difference between historian and historiographer is simply *(wie sich das der kleine Moritz schon vorstellt!)* that the historiographer really writes history while the historian only promises to do so at some later time?

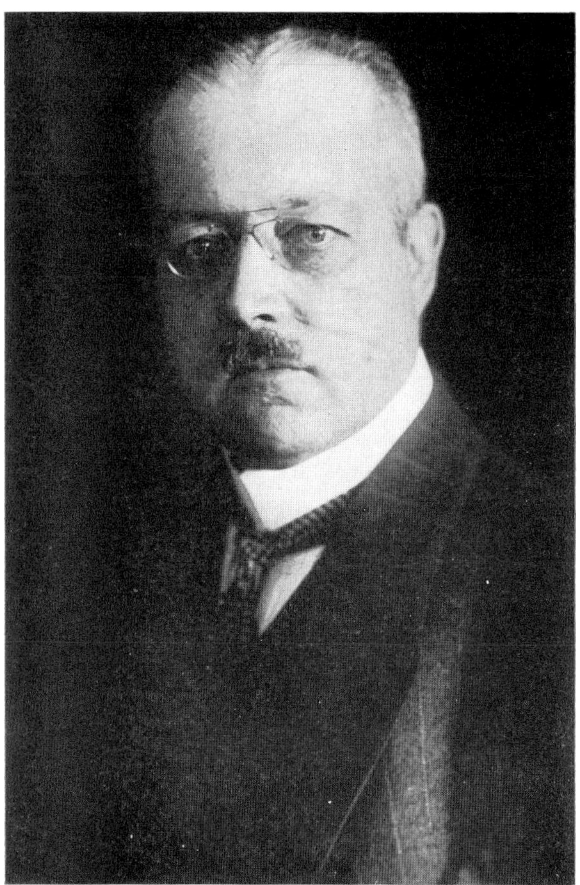

Courtesy: Röntgen-Blätter & Girardet-Verlag

HEINRICH ALBERS-SCHÖNBERG

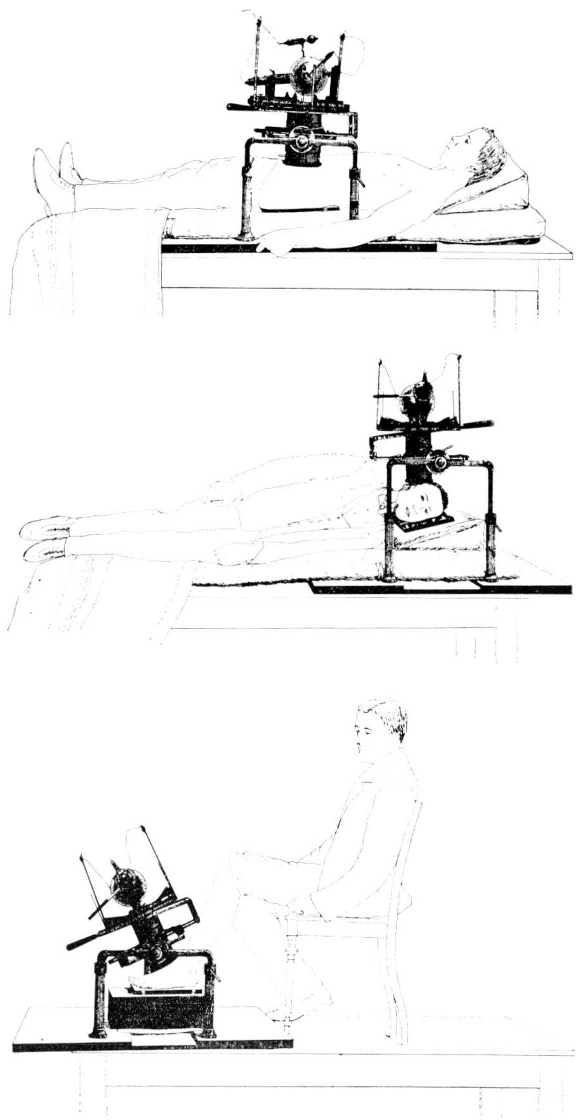

ALBERS-SCHÖNBERG'S KOMPRESSIONS-BLENDE. It was really a cylinder, although today many refer to it as a cone (a term coined by Hickey, who preferred that geometric shape). These sketches are reproduced from ed. 1 of his *Röntgentechnik.* The tube was used not only as a compression device, but also to limit the beam in the radiography of other parts of the body.

ment of Röntgen's discovery, and is regarded as the first German physician who devoted all his time to the new specialty *(Facharzt für Röntgenologie).* In February 1897, he opened with Deycke the first *Privat-Röntgen-Institut* (on *Klopstockstrasse,* in Hamburg). In 1904, he came in official capacity to the International Exposition in St. Louis, and received two gold medals for his scientific exhibits. In March 1905, he opened the *Röntgenabteilung* (Roentgen Department) at the St. Georg Hospital (Hamburg). He described "marble bone disease" which carries his eponym. Albers-Schönberg made many technical contributions, the best known of which is his compression cone (he had close connections with the firm Richard Seifert & Co. of Hamburg), and in 1903 he brought out the first edition of his famous *Röntgentechnik.* His numerous publications included both experimental and clinical work in roentgen therapy. In 1908, Albers-Schönberg developed his first *Roentgenkarzinom* on the right middle finger. He died thirteen years later, after many mutilating operations, which did not prevent the ultimately generalized malignant metastases. His name is inscribed on the obelisk of the *Röntgenmärtyrer* in the garden of St. Georg Hospital. As a distinguished *Bürger* of the *freie Hansestadt* Hamburg he was not only dynamic and dependable but always dignified.

Walter Cowl (1854-1908) was a native of New York City where he studied and was licensed to practice medicine. He had a cardiac condition and therefore in 1885 he decided to go to Berlin. He wanted to work in the *Physiologisches Institut,* and did just that until his coronary death. His first work in the roentgen field dates from April 24, 1896 when he addressed the Physiologic Society in Berlin (the text was published in the *Deutsche Medicinische Wochenschrift* of May 14, 1896).

Richard Eberlein (1869-1921), was a veterinary surgeon in Berlin, and one of the pioneers in the utilization of the roentgen method in animals. He was regularly re-elected as president of the *Berliner Röntgenvereingung* up to the time of his death (due to a carbuncle on a background of diabetes). He was also the active president of both the first and the second Röntgenkongress.

Hermann Gocht (1869-1938), an orthopedic sur-

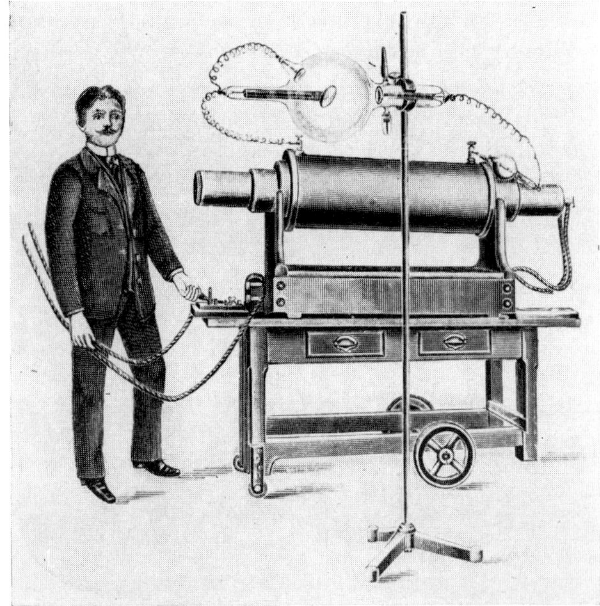

ALBERS-SCHÖNBERG AND HIS "BIG" TUBE. The German *Altmeister* is shown with a king-sized Gundelach *Dauerröhre.* Its huge glass bulb preserved the vacuum for a longer time than other tubes, and it worked fine with either mercury or Wehnelt interrupters, but it needed a *Ventil* (kenotron), shown on the viewer's right side of the coil.

Die Röntgentechnik

Lehrbuch für Ärzte und Studierende

von

H. Albers-Schönberg

Dr. med.

Mit 85 Abbildungen im Text und 2 Tafeln

Hamburg

Lucas Gräfe & Sillem

(Edmund Sillem)

1903

DIE RÖNTGEN-LITERATUR

Gesammelt von Professor Dr. Hermann Gocht

geon, who had opened on March 20, 1896 the first *Röntgeninstitut* in Hamburg (at Kümmel's *Klinik* in the Eppendorf Hospital), suffered early radiation damage to his hands. After a nephrectomy, performed in 1899, he switched completely to orthopedics and became one of the leading specialists in that field. He did not neglect roentgenology and was the Editor of the monumental fifteen volumes of *Röntgenliteratur* (1911-1934).

Shortly before his death, Gocht wrote to Köhler, and included a poem in which he described the radiation damage to his fingers. It included the following verses:

Ach ich bin so traurig,
Meine Hände, Finger
Röntgenrisse hiessen
Haut and Nägel schwinden,
Röntgenwunden liessen
Keine Ruhe finden!*

Rudolf Grashey (1876-1950) was trained as a surgeon. In October 1902 he took over the Roentgen Department attached to the Chair of Surgery in the University of Munich. One of his first endeavors was to bring the x-ray tube into the operating room and this is why he created the *Monokelkryptoskop*. He became the all-time expert in foreign body localization (his monograph *Steckschuss und Röntgenstrahlen* was published by Thieme in 1940). He was also the author of the beautiful *Atlas Typischer Rontgenbilder vom Normalen Menschen* (1905) and *Atlas Chirurgisch-Pathologischer Röntgenbilder* (1908). In 1921, after the death of Albers-Schönberg, Grashey took over the editorship of the *Fortschritte*. On January 23, 1929, he became *Ordinarius für Röntgenologie* (regular professor of roentgenology) in the University of Köln. Those were his happiest years until 1944 when Allied bombing destroyed both his place of work and his home. Somehow he "travelled" to Berlin (mostly on foot) and worked there at the Charité until a few months before his myocardial death.

Max Immelmann (1864-1923), director of (his own, private) *Medicomechanisches Institut mit Röntgenlaboratorium* in Berlin (West, Lützowstrasse 72) was for many years the secretary of the German Roentgen Society. He published more than 50 papers, including several monographs, one of them on uro-genital roentgenology. As early as April 4, 1898, he presented to

*Translation: I am so sad, roentgen tears in my hands and fingers caused skin and nails to disappear; roentgen wounds let me find no peace!

Courtesy: Röntgen-Blätter & Girardet-Verlag
WALTER COWL

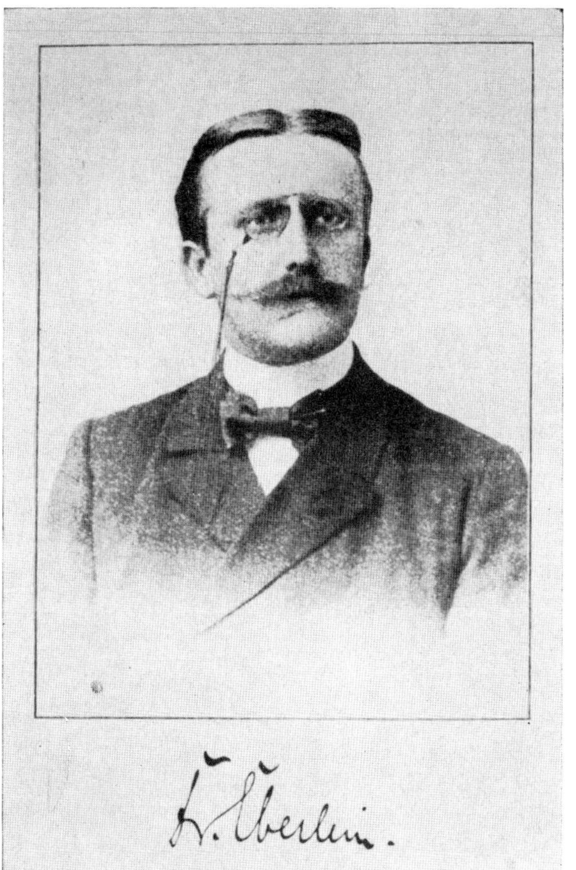

Courtesy: Röntgen-Blätter & Girardet-Verlag
RICHARD EBERLEIN

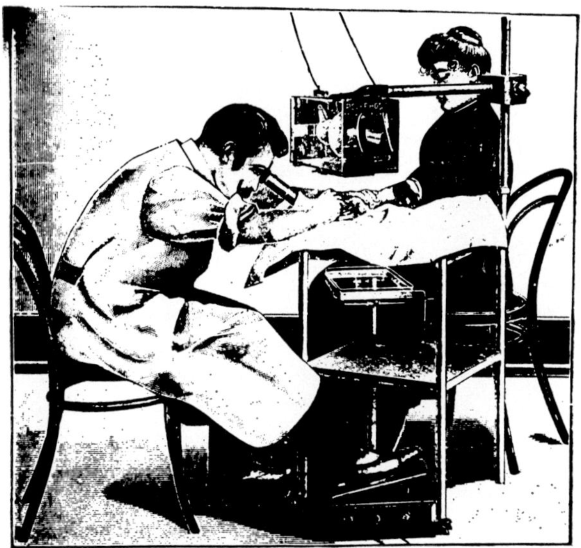

ORTHODIAGRAPHIC LOCALIZER. Drawing of young Grashey locating a foreign body in the patient's hand. Such bushy hair did not stay with him for very long. The roentgen outfit was manufactured by Polyphos in München.

the *Berliner Röntgenvereinigung* a case of aneurysm of the aortic arch, demonstrated with roentgen rays. He reported in the *Berliner Klinische Wochenschrift* of May 1905 on the first Röntgenkongress: 62 roentgenologists and 32 commercial firms had participated and 21 state institutions (German and others) had been represented at the meeting. But Max Immelmann was perhaps best known for his practical book for x-ray technicians written together with Robert Fürstenau and Johannes Schütze), *Leitfaden des Röntgenverfahrens für das Röntgenologische Hilfspersonal,* of which the first edition appeared in 1914, the fourth in 1923. He founded shortly before his coronary death the technical publication *Röntgenhilfe* which was later continued by his son Kurt Immelmann under the title *Zeitschrift für Röntgenologie.*

Alban Köhler (1874-1947), located most of his life in Wiesbaden, had his first episode of *Furor roentgenologicus* in 1899, when he began to produce the then customary plates of foreign bodies and fractures. His *magnum opus* was the *Lexikon des Normalen und Anfänge des Pathologischen im Röntgenbilde,* of which the first edition appeared in 177 pages in Hamburg in 1910; the eighth edition in 1943, had 809 pages. New

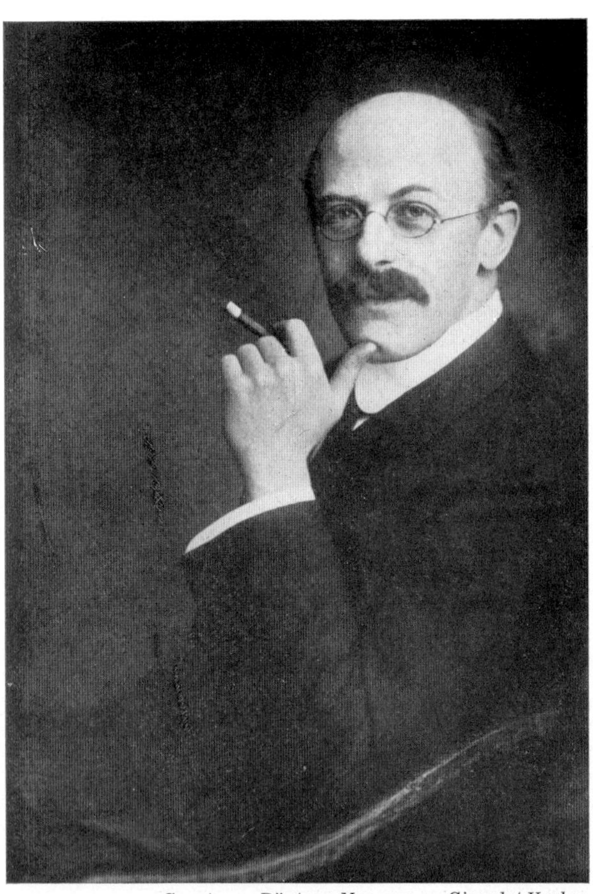

Courtesy: Röntgen-Museum & Girardet-Verlag

RUDOLF GRASHEY

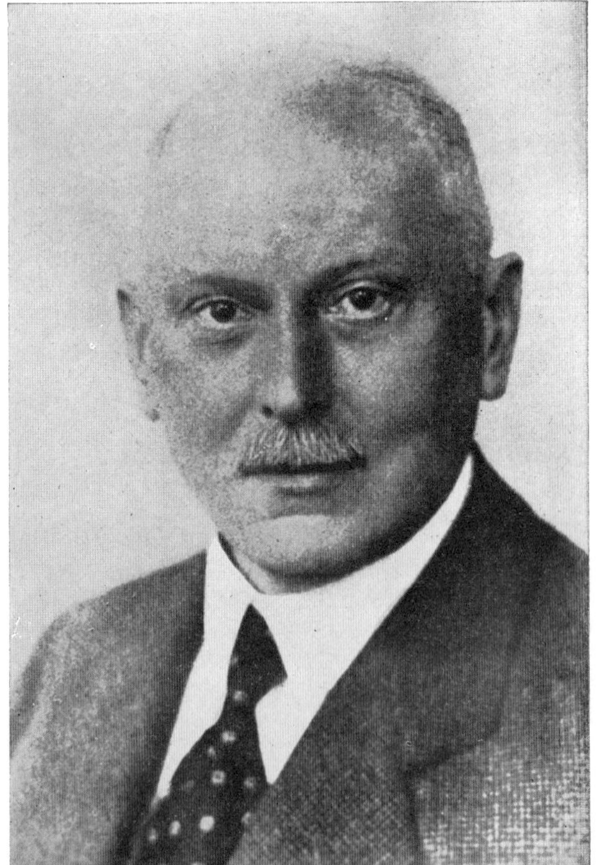

Courtesy: Röntgen-Museum & Girardet-Verlag

MAX IMMELMANN

editions are still being prepared and it seems to keep on growing. Köhler was also one of the developers of teleroentgenography (the term was actually coined by Grashey), and his eponym graces two sites of aseptic necrosis (Köhler I is in the tarsal navicular, Köhler II in the second metatarso-phalangeal joint).

Hermann Rieder (1858-1932) lived most of his life in Munich. He published in September, 1904 in the *Münchener Medizinische Wochenschrift* the famous *Radiologische Untersuchungen des Magens und Darmes beim lebenden Menschen,* in which he reported actual visualization of the upper gastrointestinal tract, after ingestion of food mixed with bismuth salts. In München, Grashey was the bone roentgenologist, while Rieder remained the internistic roentgen specialist, for instance Rieder described in 1910 the silent (tuberculous) cavity.

The last of the founders of the German Roentgen Society was also the most longevous, the *Röntgenphysiker par excellence,* Bernhard Walter (1861-1950), who lived most of his life in Hamburg. Although not a physician, he was intimately connected with the development of medical roentgen apparatus, and as a personal friend of Albers-Schönberg, he collaborated in the publication of the *Röntgentechnik.* Two years after Walter became professor emeritus in the University of Hamburg, he published his *Physikalische Grundlagen der Medizinischen Röntgentechnik* (1926). He was so well known that the suicidal Swiss creator of the half-value-layer, Theophil Christen (1873-1920), proposed as a unit of measurement the *Walter* (one milliampere times one second, divided by one square centimeter –

$$\frac{\text{ma x sec.}}{\text{cm}^2} = \text{W}).$$

At that first Röntgenkongress, a Committee on Terminology was appointed, under the chairmanship of Albers-Schönberg. All the founders were in it with the exception of Cowl, perhaps because he was "foreign-born." The committee decided on a clean sweep: Röntgen's eponym would be used as a prefix for all specialized vocables related to the procedure. Their exemplification included nine nouns, from *Röntgenologie* and *Röntgenoskopie* to *Röntgenographie* and *Ortho-Röntgenographie,* and one verb, *röntgenisieren* (which in actual usage became *röntgen,* with the somewhat indigestible form *geröntgt*).

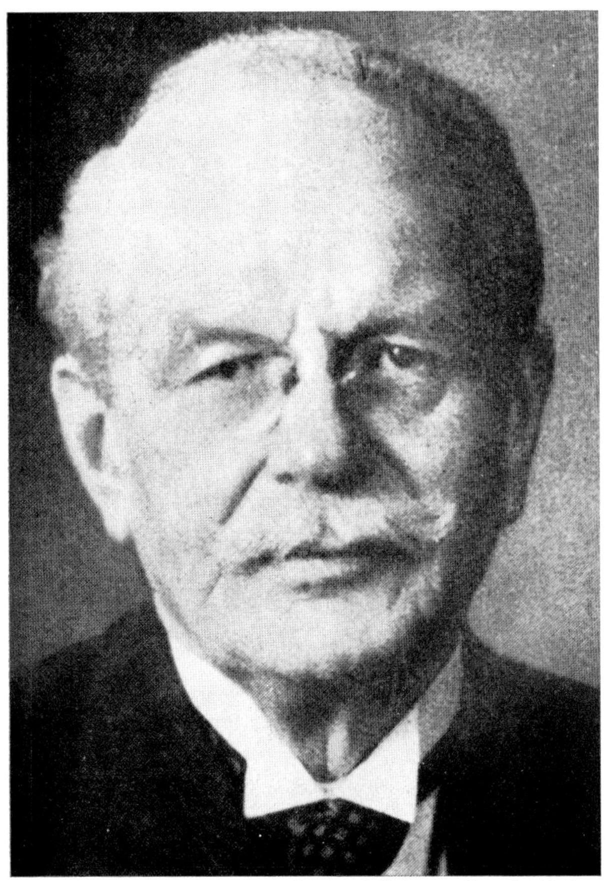

Courtesy: Röntgen-Blätter & Girardet-Verlag
ALBAN KÖHLER

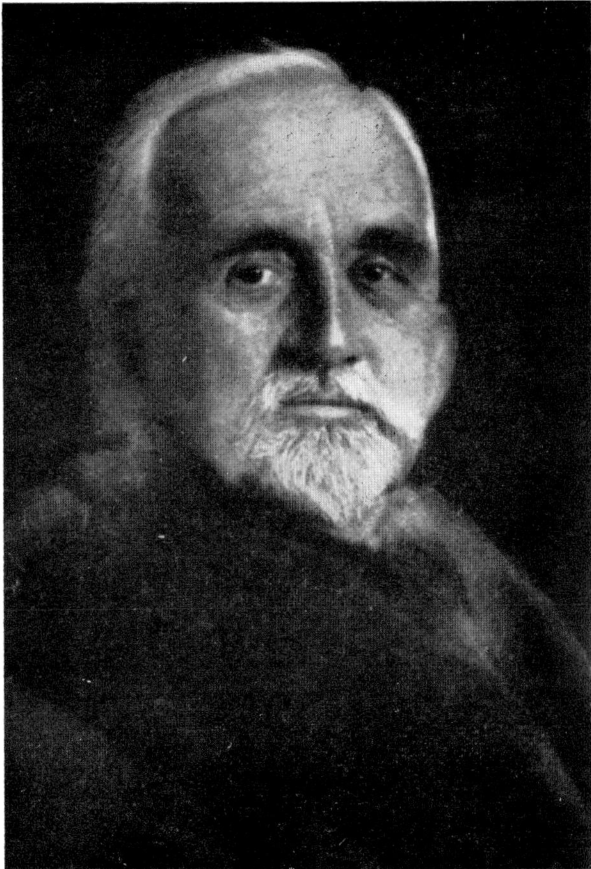

Courtesy: Röntgen-Blätter & Girardet-Verlag
HERMANN RIEDER

The committee's resolution was unanimously approved in the first plenary session of the German Roentgen Society held on May 2, 1905, and it was printed in the next issue of the *Fortschritte.*

This occurrence received little more than scant notices in London (under the title *Nomenclature* in *Nature* of July 27, 1905, and under the same title in the August, 1905 issue of the *Archives of Roentgen Ray*). The official British delegate to the *Röntgenkongress,* the dermatologist William Deane Butcher never so much as mentioned this semantic episode in his printed report of the proceedings (*Journal of the Roentgen Society* of July, 1905).

And yet the Germans meant business, *viz.,* Grashey, who had presented a *Peridiaskop* at the meeting (as recorded by Immelmann) renamed it *Periröntgenograph* before it was published in the *Verhandlungen* (transactions) *der Deutschen Röntgen-Gesellschaft.* By and large, the roentgen terminology became at once the accepted standard throughout Central Europe. There were a few defectors — even these "sinned" only on certain occasions — such as Franz Maximilian Groedel (1881-1951), the Wiesbaden cardiologist (on page 8 in his otherwise properly labeled *Orthoröntgenographie* of 1908) who subsequently resettled in New York, or the Prussian urologic internist Rudolph von Jaksch-Wartenhorst (1855-1947), who in this case was merely an outsider (*Zeitschrift für klinische Medizin,* 1907).

Another "offender" was Béla Alexander (1857-1916) of Késmark, later professor of roentgenology in Budapest; in his case it was not unexpected because he had been a gentlemanly but controversial figure ever since he introduced without divulging the way in which he had executed his "plastic plates" (contact exposures made from superimposed negatives and positive transparencies, giving an impression of bas-relief).* Subsequently, Alexander sustained irreparable radiation damage while attaining quasi-perfection in the fluoroscopy of carpal bone motion.

Perhaps the transient general deterioration in Germany at the end of World War I (when they began to utilize newsprint also in medical journals) could explain the slip-up by which Max Frankel published in December, 1918 in the *Fortschritte a* paper entitled *X-Strahlen im Kampfe gegen die Tuberkulose.* It is however completely unexplainable why Immelmann himself published in Sommers' *Röntgentaschenbuch* of 1918 an article called *Radiologische Darstellung von Fistelgängen.*

*A similar method of superimposing positives and negatives was more recently proposed by Ziedses des Plantes under the name of *subtraction.* The latter is of value in the evaluation of changes that occur between several examinations, for instance in fractures. It is even more helpful in contrast procedures, especially in cardiac, aortic, and cerebral angiography.

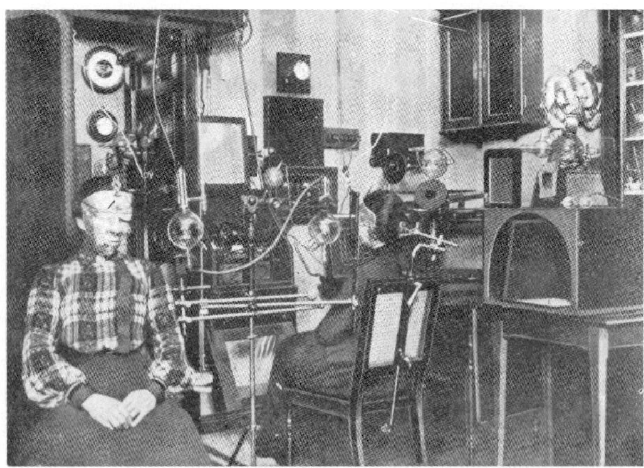

Courtesy: C. H. F. Mueller.

RIEDER'S OFFICE (ABOUT 1900). Two patients receive roentgen therapy from two different tubes connected in series with one induction coil.

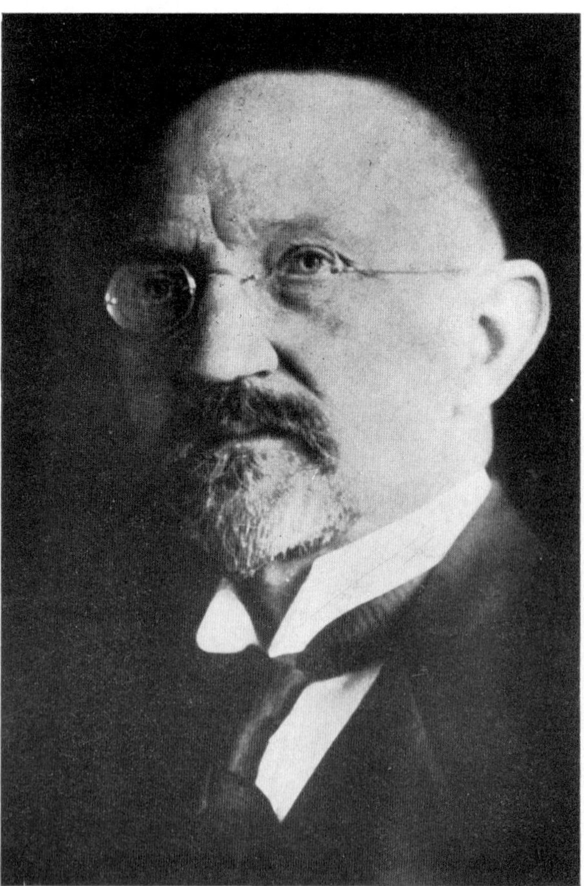

Courtesy: Röntgen-Museum & Girardet-Verlag

BERNHARD WALTER

Prior to the Röntgenkongress the Viennese (who often enjoyed spicing their professional talks with French or Latin vocables) were sold on the radio-root. After the eponym was put through, the Viennese became chronic offenders of the roentgen edict. One of Holzknecht's classics of 1908 was entitled *Radiologische Diagnostik*. A booktitle of Freund's of 1916 contained the words *Radiologische Fremdkërperlokalisation*. In 1920 Konrad Weiss published in the *Wiener Medizinische Wochenschrift* in several installments a paper on *Teleradiologische Vergleichsaufnahmen*.

Aus der III. medicinischen Universitätsklinik
des Hofrathes Prof. L. v. SCHRÖTTER in Wien.

ATLAS
der
Radiographie der Brustorgane
von
DR. MAXIMILIAN WEINBERGER,
klinischem Assistenten.

WIEN und LEIPZIG.
Verlag der k. u. k. Hof-Verlags-Buchhandlung Emil M. Engel.

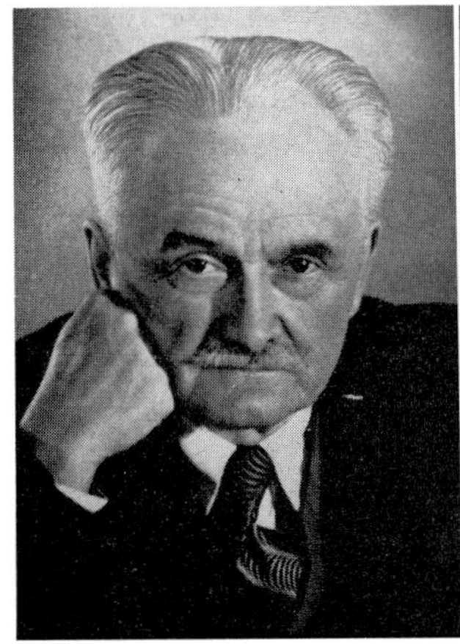

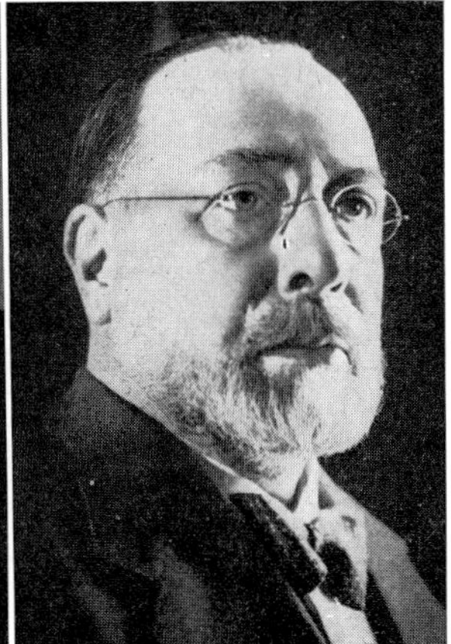

Courtesy: Georg Grössel - Agfa.

FOREIGN FANS OF THE ROENTGEN PREFIX. J. A. C. Belot of France and bespectacled Cesar Cómas y Llabería of Spain.

GRUNDRISS
DER
GESAMMTEN
RADIOTHERAPIE
FÜR
PRAKTISCHE ÄRZTE
VON
DR. LEOPOLD FREUND
IN WIEN.

MIT 110 ABBILDUNGEN UND 1 TAFEL.

URBAN & SCHWARZENBERG
BERLIN N., FRIEDRICHSTRASSE 105b
WIEN I., MAXIMILIANSTRASSE 4
1903.

DOTT. I. VALOBRA
Medico dell' Ospedale Mauriziano Umberto I di Torino

ELEMENTI
DI
Röntgenologia Clinica
(Tecnica - Diagnostica - Terapia)

Con 95 Figure intercalate nel testo e sei Tavole

PREFAZIONE
DEL
Prof. CAMILLO BOZZOLO
DIRETTORE DELLA CLINICA MEDICA GENERALE DELLA REGIA UNIVERSITÀ DI TORINO.

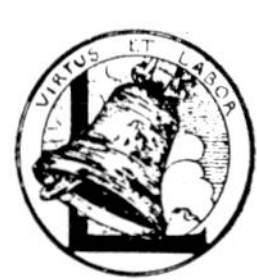

TORINO
S. LATTES & C., Librai-Editori
Via Garibaldi, 3 (Piazza Castello)
FIRENZE: R. BEMPORAD & FIGLIO - BOLOGNA: Ditta NICOLA ZANICHELLI.
1908

The impact of the first Röntgenkongress was felt also in France, Spain and Italy.

Having been to Berlin in 1905, Joseph Antoine Charles Belot (1876-1953) was also expected to "go to Canossa," indeed he published in 1906 in the *Fortschritte* a progress report on *röntgenologie* in France. Actually, in the same year in which the Röntgenkongress was held, Laquerrière and Delherm had come out in the *Archives d' Électricité Médicale* with an item on röntgenisation. In Spain the pioneers Cesar Comás y Llabería (1874-1956) and his cousin Augustin Prió y Llabería (1873-1929) had discussed on March 3, 1904, in the *Revista de Medicina y Cirurgia* (of Barcelona) the medico-legal applications of *röntgenologia.* This was before the Röntgenkongress (Comas y Llaberia was one of the participants), but as late as 1918 a Barcelona booktitle, by R. Torres Carreras contained the word *semiología rontgenológica.*

In Italy, until 1905, *radioscopia* and *radiografia* were the terms commonly used, as in the classical lecture held on June 14, 1897 by Eduardo Maragliano (1849-1940), professor of internal medicine in the University of Genova and founder of the *Scuola Elettroradiologica Genovese.**

*An historical volume by this name, edited by Pietro Amisano and Lucio Reale, was graciously sent to me by Prof. Alessandro Vallebona (pupil of and academic heir to V. Maragliano). Among Vallebona's contributions is the thorough *Trattato di Stratigrafia* (1952), in which all sorts of body section procedures are described, including the transverse variety.

His son, Mario Vittorio Maragliano (1878-1944), reported to the second International Congress of Physiotherapy (Rome, 1907), on *Progressi della Röntgen-*

TRANSACTIONS

OF THE

AMERICAN ROENTGEN RAY SOCIETY

THIRD ANNUAL MEETING

CHICAGO, ILL.

DECEMBER 10 AND 11, 1902.

LOUISVILLE
Courier-Journal Job Printing Co.
1903

Рентгеновскій Вѣстникъ

Въ журналѣ принимаютъ участіе слѣдующія лица:

Dr B. Alexander [Венгрія]. **Dr Albrecht** [Берлинъ]. **Dr P. Bade**—[Ганноверъ]. **Dr A. Beclere**—[Парижъ]. **Dr F. Braun** [Страссбургъ]. **Dr E. C. Главче** [Одесса]. **Dr A. И. Гешелинъ** -[Одесса]. **Fr Dessauer** [Ашафенбургъ]. **Dr L. Freund** [Вѣна]. **Dr R. Friedländer** [Висбаденъ]. **Dr H. Gocht**—[Галле]. **Dr P Haglund** [Стокгольмъ]. **Prof. Dr Hammer** [Гейдельбергъ]. **Prof. Dr A. Hoffmann** - [Диссельдорфъ]. **Dr G. Haret** [Парижъ]. **Dr G. Holzknecht** [Вѣна]. **Prof. Dr Hildebrand** - [Марбургъ]. **Dr Immelmann**—[Берлинъ]. **Dr П. М. Каменецкій** [Одесса]. **Prof. Dr P. Krause** [Бреславль]. **Doz. Kienböck** [Вѣна]. **Prof. Dr E. Lassar** [Берлинъ]. **Dr M. Levy-Dorn** [Берлинъ]. **Dr К Ч Пурицъ** – [Одесса]. **Dr I. Robinsohn** [Вѣна]. **Dr З. Л. Шапиро** [Одесса]. **Prof. Dr A Voller** [Гамбургъ].

Редакторъ **Проф. П. А. Вальтеръ.** Редакторъ-Издатель **Д-ръ Я. М. [illegible]**

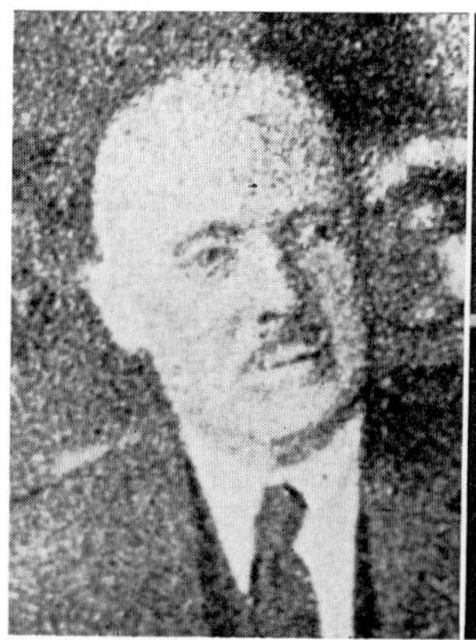

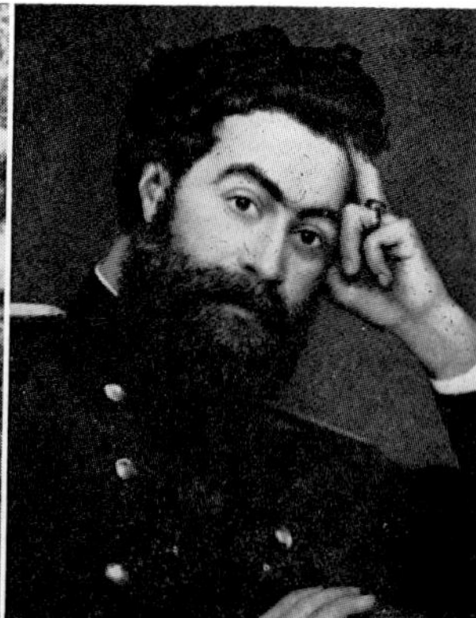

RUSSIAN ROENTGEN PIONEERS. Yasha Rozenblatt lived in Odessa, a city which was in the war zone during World War II; many archives had been destroyed, and no portrait of Rozenblatt could be located; finally this reproduction from a newspaper of 1922 was unearthed for me by Boris Mikhailovich Shtern, who teaches radiology in Leningrad. The portrait of bearded Ivan Tarkhan-Mouravov is from Agfa's files.

ologia. He was at that time head of the *Instituto Röntgenologico* which in 1913 became the *Cabinetto Radiologico.* During the 1907-1912 period, the eponymic prefix was fairly often encountered in Italy – as in Iona Valobra's *Elementi di Röntgenologia Clinica* of 1908 – though rarely in France. Even this sporadic popularity vanished with the beginning of World War I.*

The roentgen prefix made more important and more lasting gains in the U.S.A.† and in Russia. After the resignation of Robarts and the attendant upheavals, the papers presented at the annual meetings of the ARRS were printed intermittently from 1902 to 1911 in the *Transactions of the ARRS.* The official U.S.A. delegate to the *Röntgenkongress* had been the Philadelphia surgeon Charles Lester Leonard (1861-1913). After his return the wheels began to spin and in October, 1906, under the editorship of Preston Manasseh Hickey (1865-1930), a former Detroit Ear, Nose, and Throat specialist who subsequently taught radiology at Ann Arbor, appeared the official organ of the ARRS, the *American Quarterly of Roentgenology.*

Its shorter-lived Russian counterpart, the *Rentgenovski Viestnik* was issued for the first time in July, 1907 in Odessa by P. A. Valter and Yasha M. Rozenblatt (the latter operated a Bacteriologic Institute when he came to the 1905 Röntgenkongress; when he returned to the 1907 Röntgenkongress he gave his title as director of the Bacteriologic and Roentgen Institute, a private venture). Aside from these "bourgeois" endeavorers, the Russian roentgen pioneers included an aristocratic physiologist, *Kniaz* Ivan Romanovich Tarkhan-Mouravov (1846-1908) who had also been to Berlin in 1905.

AMERICAN ETYMOLOGIC ORDINANCE

Prior to World War I, American medicine nurtured a more or less outspoken respect for the German professors, an attitude which permeated all levels of the profession. This may be why organized medicine demanded more in the way of recognition than the implication coming from the title of a journal. Consequently — as stated in Pancoast's editorial of September, 1919 in the *American Journal of Roentgenology* — the AMA brought considerable pressure on the ARRS to "legalize" the German terminology. The "hatchet man" selected to do the job was Frederick Carl Zapffe (1873-1951), a Milwaukee-born physician from Chicago, who soon became the chairman of the ARRS Committee on Nomenclature: the other two members were recognized specialists, Percy Brown (1875-1950) and David Ralph Bowen (1872-1939). Their preliminary report, printed in September, 1913, in the *American Quarterly of Roentgenology,* underwent subsequently several significant corrections.

In the draft (presumably Zapffe's own work) roentgenography appeared as the specialty in medicine which makes use of the roentgen ray, with roentgenology as the study of this agent. Another inadvertency was the definition of roentgen-fluoroscopy (fluoroscopic examination with roentgen rays as a source of light). In the corrected edition, roentgenology had become the study and practice of the roentgen ray, while roentgenography was not specifically included (except for the verb to roentgenograph). Roentgenoscopy emerged as the accepted term, and the whimsical neo-German verb *röntgenisieren* was added in the transliterated form to roentgenize. The fastidious vocables roentgenism and roentgenization – seldom if ever spontaneously employed, either before or after publication

*As a matter of fact, the prefix roentgeno- never quite disappeared from either the French, the Italian, the Spanish (including the South American) nomenclature. In 1959 appeared in Torino (Italy) the book *Roentgencraniologia infantile* by Giancarlo Lischi and Giuseppe Menichini (Edizioni Minerva Medica).

†In his textbook on *Roentgen Rays and Electrotherapeutics* (Lippincott, 1907), Mihran Kassabian wrote under the heading *Skiagraphy, Synonyms, Definition and Nomenclature*: "Skiagraphy (Röntography, Shadowgraphy, Ixography, Electrography, Skotography, Kathography, Fluorography, Actinography, Radiography, Diagraphy, Skiography, Pyknoscopy, New Photography, and Electro-Skiagraphy) is the art of photographing shadows on sensitive plates by means of transmitted light. The Röntgen Congress in Berlin on May 2, 1905 adopted a uniform nomenclature for the use of the Congress and for expression in writing. The following terms will be used in the future: Röntgenology, Röntgenoscopy, Röntgenography, Röntgenogram (Röntgen negative, Röntgen positive, Röntgen diapositive), Ortho-Röntgenography, Röntgentherapy, Röntgenizing. I present this new nomenclature, but I can hardly endorse it. I believe that the word "skiagraphy" and its modifications are more easily pronounced, more general, and more euphonious." *Dixit et salvavit animam suam!*

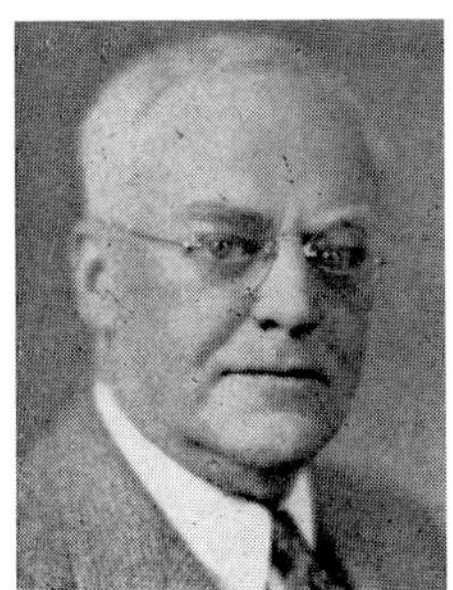

Courtesy: Association of American Medical Colleges
FRED ZAPFFE

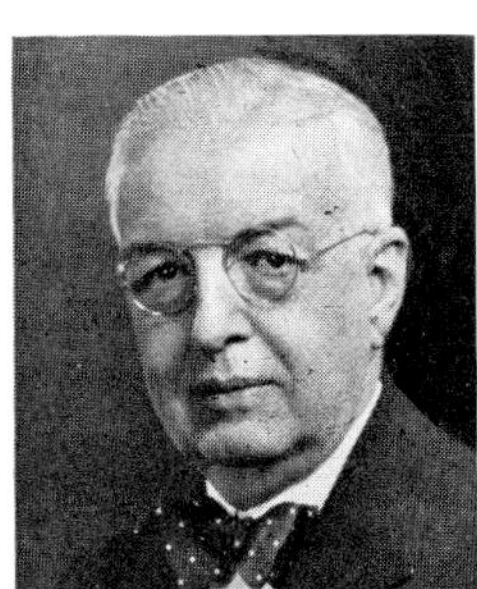

Courtesy: Ben Orndoff
DAVID BOWEN

THE AMERICAN ROENTGEN RAY SOCIETY, (12TH ANNUAL CONVENTION) RICHMOND, VA. SEPT. 20-23, 1911

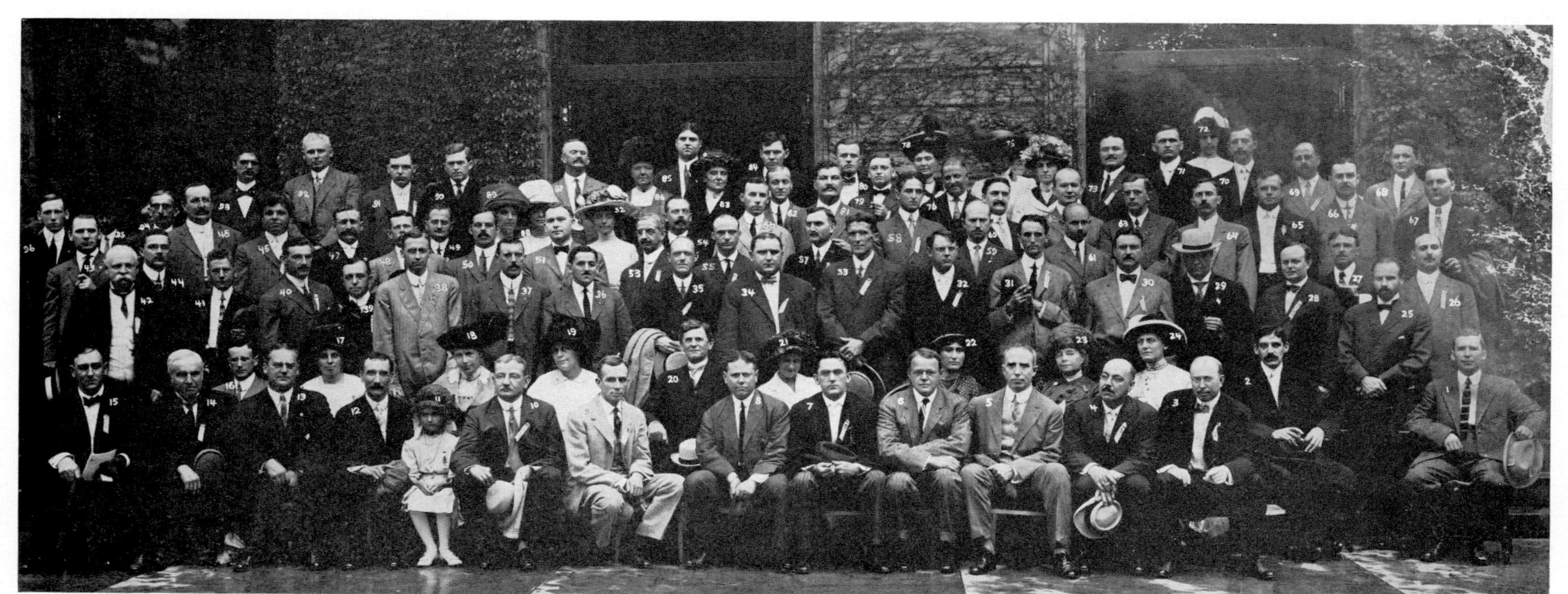

Courtesy: Eugene Percival Pendergrass. Plate courtesy of the W. B. Saunders Co.

1 F. L. Andrews, Pittsburgh, Pa. (**N. M.)
2 Russell H. Boggs, Pittsburgh, Pa.
3 E. W. Caldwell, New York
4 P. M. Hickey, Detroit, Mich.
5 G. E. Pfahler, Philadelphia, Pa.
6 H. K. Pancoast, Philadelphia, Pa.
7 Chas. F. Bowen, Columbus, O.
8 F. H. Baetjer, Baltimore, Md.
9 Percy Brown (President), Boston, Mass.
10 C. L. Leonard, Philadelphia, Pa.
11 G. C. Johnston's daughter
12 Geo. C. Johnston, Pittsburgh, Pa.
14 G. M. Steele, Oshkosh, Wis.
15 A. L. Gray, Richmond, Va.
17 Mrs. Geo. C. Johnston, Pittsburgh, Pa.
18 Mrs. H. K. Pancoast.
20 D. C. Richardson (Mayor), Richmond.
21 Miss Richardson, Richmond.
23 Mrs. G. M. Steele, Oshkosh, Wis.
24 Mrs. H. W. Dachtler, Toledo, O.
25 A. Holding, Albany, N. Y.
26 G. C. Chene, Detroit, Mich.
28 L. Jaches, New York.
30 W. H. Stewart, New York.
31 Thos. A. Groover, Washington, D. C.
32 J. H. Selby, Rochester, Minn.
33 C. E. Coon, Syracuse, N. Y.

35 R. Hammond, Providence, R. I.
36 Sidney Lange, Cincinnati, O.
37 W. H. Eagar, Halifax, N. S.
38 A. J. Quinby, New York City.
39 W. F. Manges, Chicago, Ill.
40 E. H. Skinner, Kansas City, Mo.
41 Jno. Mackintosh, Chicago, Ill. (**N. M.)
42 H. E. Waite, New York.
44 D. D. Tally, Richmond, Va.
45 J. W. Frank, Philadelphia, Pa.
46 M. Hagopian, Philadelphia, Pa.
47 A. J. Abell, Syracuse, N. Y.
48 Chas. Hazen, Richmond, Va.
49 E. R. Rasely, Uniontown, Pa.
50 T. S. Stewart, Philadelphia, Pa.
51 E. G. Meter, Reading, Pa.
52 Mrs. C. E. Skinner, New Haven, Conn.
53 D. R. Bowen, Philadelphia, Pa.
54 C. E. Skinner, New Haven, Conn.
55 H. E. Potter, Chicago, Ill.
57 L. T. LeWald, New York.
58 H. W. Dachtler, Toledo, O.
59 J. T. Case, Battle Creek, Mich.
60 H. T. Edwards, South Bethlehem, Pa.
61 Lewis Gregory Cole, New York City.
62 H. M. Imboden, Clifton Springs, N. Y.
63 H. W. Van Allen, Springfield, Mass.

Photo by Foster, Richmond

64 G. W. Grier, Pittsburgh, Pa.
65 G. H. Stover, Denver, Colo.
66 J. S. Janssen, Milwaukee, Wis.
67 A. G. Magnuson, Chicago, Ill.
68 Mr. Howe, Chicago, Ill. (**N. M.)
69 T. D. Rupert, Geneva, N. Y.
70 L. R. Corman, Rochester, N. Y.
72 Mrs. L. R. Corman, Rochester, N. Y.
73 H. C. Snook, Philadelphia, Pa.
75 Mrs. T. S. Stewart, Philadelphia, Pa.
76 H. Green, Hartford, Conn. (**N. M.)
78 Mrs. C. L. Leonard, Philadelphia, Pa.
80 J. H. Edmonson, Birmingham, Ala.
81 Wm. Painter, Minneapolis, Minn. (N. M.)
82 Albertus Cotton, Baltimore, Md.
83 Mrs. Alburtus Cotton, Baltimore, Md.
85 J. W. Hunter, Jr., Norfolk, Va.
86 Mrs. R. Hammond, Providence, R. I.
88 T. C. Turley, Chicago, Ill.
89 Miss A. H. Brindley, Chicago, Ill.
90 G. W. Holmes, Brookline, Mass.
91 Leonard Reu, Buffalo, N. Y.
92 E. G. Wilkinson, N. Y. (**N. M.)
93 W. S. Newcomet, Philadelphia, Pa.
94 J. W. Adair, Marion, O.
96 H. E. Ashbury, Baltimore, Md.

**N. M. Non Member.

of this ordinance – were displayed both in the preliminary and in the final versions.

Zapffe presented the definitive edition to the ARRS in the morning session of October 3, 1913 — during its 14th annual meeting, held in Boston. Caldwell motioned acceptance of the report, and George Edward Pfahler (1874-1957) seconded — both had been to Berlin in 1905, and both were members of the German Roentgen Society. The ARRS was mourning the death of Leonard — who had been a staunch defender of the roentgen nomenclature — and no objections were raised. The resolution was passed by voice vote, and the secretary was instructed to notify the important medical magazine editors and other pertinent individuals. The terminologic slate (thirteen vocables) was a bare variant of the German communiqué of 1905, and acknowledged that henceforth also in the USA, roentgen- (or roentgeno-) were to be the only approved prefix(es) for the coinage of words in this specialty.

At the same meeting of the ARRS, the *Quarterly* became the (yellow-coated) *American Journal of Roentgenology,* and Zapffe stayed on as Associate Editor, but not for long. His task was completed. As a genuine organization man, Zapffe returned to the AMA for other assignments (he became and remained for many years the secretary of the Association of American Medical Colleges). Zapffe authored a successful textbook on Bacteriology. Careful search revealed neither radiologic publications, nor evidence of any other relationship between Zapffe and radiology, except for that unique, triumphant episode. It had been a solid victory indeed. The ARRS was then setting both ethical and professional, as well as scientific standards in the specialty, and its etymologic ordinance carried significant weight.

The American Journal of Roentgenology

Edited by P. M. Hickey, M. D.
Associate Editor, F. C. Zapffe, M. D.

VOL. I New Series November, 1913 No. 1

Memorial
To
Charles Lester Leonard, A. M., M. D.

Poetry . . . Esther Morton Smith
Resolutions
Portrait
Radiography of the Stomach and Intestines—A Report Prepared by Charles Lester Leonard for the Section on Radiology of the XVIIth International Congress of Medicine, London, 1913
Bibliography
Biography
Contributions to Medical Literature by Charles Lester Leonard, M. D.

Published by
The American Roentgen Ray Society

At that time the profession was quite willing to use the German roentgen nomenclature. Two of the largest local specialty societies, both organized before the ARRS ordinance, conformed to its provisions. The Chicago Roentgen Society was created in 1913 following a meeting of eight physicians in the office of Hollis Potter. The seal of the society is more conciliatory towards less orthodox semanticists than its sole title would indicate.

The New York Roentgen Society was formed one year earlier. Its first Minute Book opens with the statement:

"At an informal dinner at the New York Club on April 3, 1912, which was attended by Doctors William H. Stewart, L. Jaches, Edward Leaming, Percy Brown, G. M. MacKee and E. W. Caldwell, the desirability of a local society of roentgenology was discussed and it was decided it would be advisable to call a formal meeting of the organization."

The same persons, with the addition of another physician (Busby) met on June 18, 1912 at MacKee's residence. Percy Brown, who lived in Boston, was elected a non-resident member, the other six became charter members. The society was legally incorporated on July 6, 1912.

The first president was Edward Leaming, with MacKee the first secretary-treasurer. The next resident

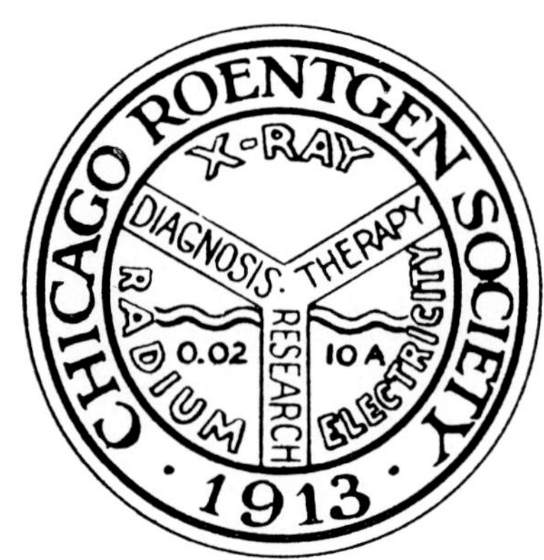

members were Imboden, Remer, and Law, elected March 11, 1913; L. T. LeWald, December 15, 1913; and Charles Eastmond, December 7, 1914. An eight point Code of Ethics was adopted at the second meeting on June 24, 1912. It had been formulated by Leaming, and is regarded as being fully valid today:

1. The Code of Ethics for practitioners of the medical Association is to be the standard.

2. The Roentgenologist being a consulting diagnostician should only reveal his findings to the attending physician or surgeon who has referred the case to him and not to the patient except with the specific request and permission of such attending.

3. It is to be considered unwise to accept as a patient anyone not sent by a reputable physician or surgeon unless such patient be personally known to the Roentgenologist or referred by a well-known mutual friend.

4. It shall be unethical to advertise by circulating either the medical profession or the laity with price lists, description of office facilities and apparatus, etc.

5. It shall be unethical to claim superiority in diagnosis or treatment due to some secret method or apparatus or improvement in existing methods or apparatus held to be known only to the claimant.

6. It shall be unethical to advertise by signs stating the medical specialty-practice, or statements of one's specialty, in the public press, in lists of telephone subscribers, or in the City, State, and National directories printed for general public use.

7. It shall be considered unwise to provide the patient or his or her relatives or friends with radiographs taken for diagnostic purposes.

8. Each radiograph may bear some statement in writing or by printed label or both, indicating it to be the property of the radiologist who was responsible for its production.*

Eugene Wilson Caldwell (1870-1918) whose name looms large in the history of roentgen pioneers, was an electrical engineer, and in the basement under his office he maintained an experimental shop.*

It is interesting to note in the minutes of the meeting of the New York Roentgen Society of March 17, 1915 that "Coolidge showed a small tube which would be appropriate for treatment or fluoroscopy and which would accommodate about 4 ma with a backup of about 7." Coolidge stated that he had brought this tube down to Caldwell's office to "try it out." At the meeting of May 17, 1915, Coolidge was elected an honorary member and so was J. S. Shearer, professor of Physics in Cornell University. The *X-Ray Manual* used in World War I was largely the work of Shearer and Caldwell. The Annual Lecture of the ARRS in the memory of Caldwell is well known.

Another well known member of the New York Roentgen Society was Leopold Jaches (1874-1939), beloved by all. He had a degree in law and was quite expert in problems of policy and legal matters. He is also remembered for his co-authorship in a textbook on *Chest Roentgenology*.

Among the honorary members of the New York Roentgen Society there may be mentioned: Gösta Forssell, his successor Elis Berven (both from Stockholm), and Fedor Haenisch from Hamburg. The latter un-

*This information and their Code of Ethics was graciously provided by Dr. Ramsay Spillman, historian of the New York Roentgen Society, through the obliging courtesy of Maxwell Herbert Poppel, professor of Radiology in New York University Medical School.

*Caldwell's associate, Harry Imboden recollected in 1931 about the fact that Caldwell had constructed a nine phase high tension alternating current generator. Rectification was done with gas valve tubes, provided with an automatic regulator. The results were not satisfactory because of the instability of the valves.

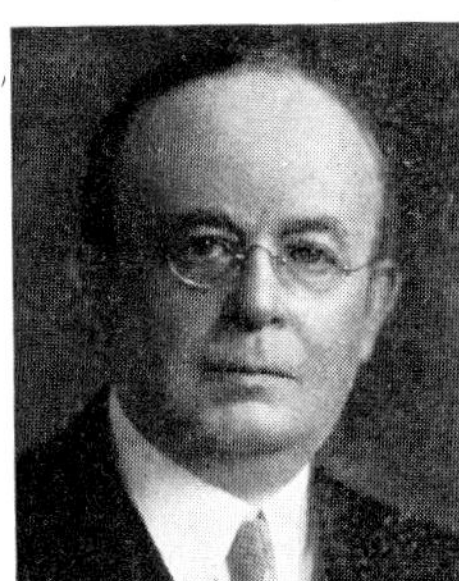

LEOPOLD JACHES

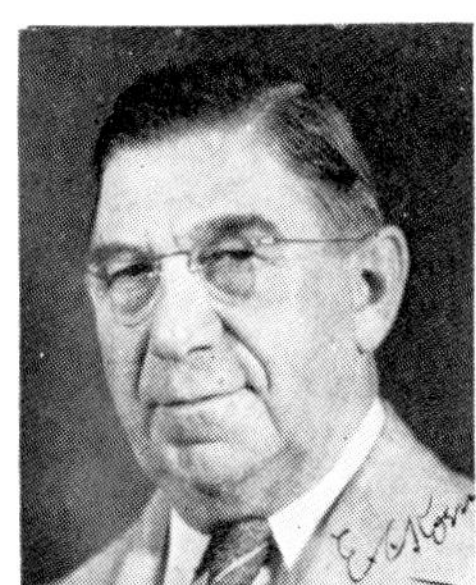

E. C. KOENIG

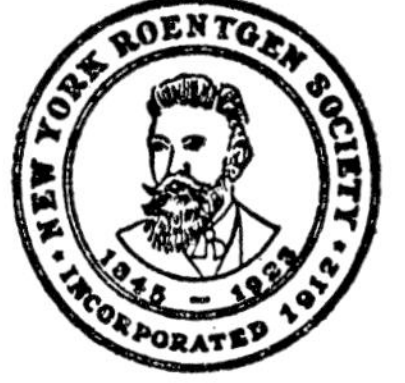

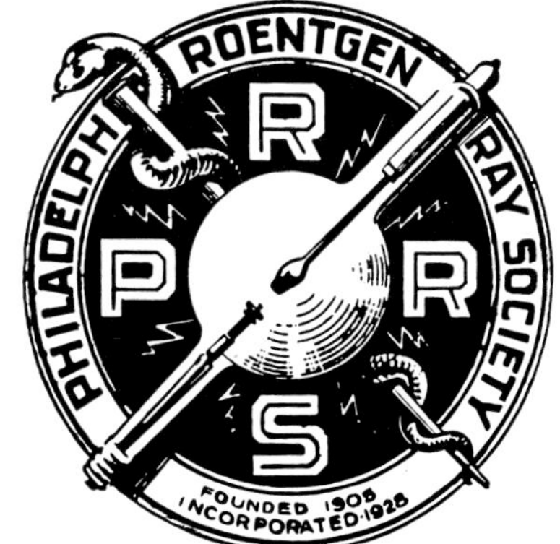

complainingly underwent untold hardships when Hamburg was bombed during World War II.

In its early days, the New York Roentgen Society chose to be very restrictive in its membership. In the past few years, with the great increase in the number of radiologists, they decided to expand their membership and also to increase the amount of material presented at the meeting. A popular feature of the larger meetings is the competition among residents in radiology for a monetary prize given to those who show ability in the recognition of pathology on the films presented.

The Code of Ethics of the New York Roentgen Society reveals quite clearly what they were fighting in 1912. It also shows that they used not only the term roentgenologist, but radiologist and radiograph as well. After the ARRS ordinance, however, when the New York Roentgen Society edited and published a periodical, it was dutifully christened *American Atlas of Stereoroentgenology.*

In its brief lifespan (1916-1920), the *Atlas* used only pasted-in positive prints, many of which convey a truly artistic impression due to the harmonious distribution of highlights and shades. One of the protagonists in this venture was Edward Charles Koenig (1877-1949), a radiologist of whom it was said that he literally lived and died in the Buffalo (New York) General Hospital.

If not the largest, the Philadelphia Roentgen Ray Society is certainly America's oldest "municipal" radiologic association.

George Pfahler wrote its history for the period 1899-1920 in the *American Journal of Roentgenology* of January, 1956. For the same issue, Ralph Bromer prepared the period 1920-1954.

In their book of Minutes* the first three pages are typed, then in longhand until 1924. The type of those first three pages is of relatively recent origin, so that one may rightfully question the authenticity of the initial minutes.

According to those minutes, the organizational meeting was held on February 2, 1905, present being Mihran Kassabian, Charles Leonard, Mason McCollin, Bill Newcomet, Henry Pancoast, George Pfahler, H. H. Riddle, John Shober, Homer Snook, Henry Stelwagon, Thomas Stewart, and Bill Sweet. Leonard, who had taken the initiative and in whose place the meeting was held, acted as chairman, Snook as secretary. The statutes limited active membership to fifteen. New members had to be elected unanimously (secret ballot; candidates announced one month prior to election; ballot by proxy permitted). One of their first resolutions was not to furnish refreshments at their meetings.

On the second page are listed the same names as being active members, except that Kassabian, Riddle, and Shober are crossed out. Could that mean that that second page was revised after Kassabian's death in 1910?

FIRST INTERNATIONAL CONGRESSES

The French, Italians, and British never ceased to employ the term x rays, for instance J. H. Gardiner, the editor of the *Journal of the Roentgen Society,* published in May, 1909 his valuable contribution to the history of x-ray tubes. At the same time the prefix radio- and especially the term radiology continued to accrue territorial gains outside of Central Europe. Electrology started instead on a downhill course, and when not altogether dropped, was demoted to second place.

The first *Congrès International d'Électrologie et de Radiologie Médicales* was held in Paris from July 27 through August 1, 1900, under the presidency of E. Doumer, the secretary being Moutier. They met again as follows:

Bruxelles (1904): P. Dubois, M. Schnyder
Milano (1906): C. Bozzolo, Luraschi

THE JOURNAL

OF THE

RÖNTGEN SOCIETY.

EDITED BY

J. H. GARDINER. F.C.S.,

WITH THE CO-OPERATION OF

J. MACKENZIE DAVIDSON, M.B.
A. W. ISENTHAL, F.R.P.S.
PROF. HERBERT JACKSON, F.I.C., F.C.S.
F. HARRISON LOW, M.B.
J. MACINTYRE, M.B.
C. W. MANSELL MOULLIN, M.A., M.D., F.
ERNEST PAYNE, M.A.
C. E. S. PHILLIPS.
J. J. VEZEY, F.R.M.S.
H. SNOWDEN WARD, F.R.P.S.

Communications for the Editor to be addressed to 19. Hanover Square, London, W.

VOLUME I.

1904–1905.

PRINTED AND PUBLISHED FOR THE RÖNTGEN SOCIETY
BY WERTHEIMER, LEA & CO., CLIFTON HOUSE, WORSHIP STREET, FINSBURY, E.C

*Graciously offered for inspection, by means of photostats, through courtesy of its current secretary, Antolin Raventos.

Amsterdam (1908): Wertheim-Salomonson, Gohl and Myers
Barcelona (1910): Cicera Salse, Comas Llabería
Praha (1912): Jellinek, E. Slavic
Lyon (1914): J. Renaud, J. Cluzet

In 1911, when Francisco Dominguez y Roldán (1864-1942), the only official Cuban delegate to the Congress in Barcelona, reported to his own government, the title was reversed to *Congreso de Radiología y Electrología Médicas.* The 1914 meeting, to which one of the *rapporteurs* had been the Swiss editor of *Röntgen-Taschenbuch,* Ernest Sommer (1872-1938) of Berne, was disrupted by the outbreak of World War I.

Most of the therapists were closely connected with electrology, for instance in France, Jean Alban Bergonié (1857-1925), an editor of the *Archives d'Électricité Médicale,* in Great Britain Dawson Turner (1857-1928) of the Royal Infirmary in Edinburgh, and G. R. C. Lyster (1860-1920) of the Middlesex Hospital in London, in Austria Leopold Freund (1868-1943) and Robert Kienböck (1871-1954), in Sweden Tage Sjögren and Thor Stenbeck, in this country W. J. Morton and Piffard, and so on. A *Congrès International pour l'Étude de la Radiologie et de l'Ionisation* convened in Liège in September of 1905, the second in Bruxelles was in September of 1910, with a slight change in the title (. . . *de la Radiologie et de l'Électricité*). The third meeting, scheduled for 1915, never materialized. At these conventions, most of the participants came from Belgium, France, and the Netherlands.

The *Société Belge de Radiologie* was founded in August, 1906 by nineteen physicians. The first slate of officers comprised De Nobele (president), Klynens (vice-president), Bienfait (secretary) and Hauchamps (treasurer). Before the year was over they had fifty-five members, and decided to issue a *Bulletin* which was started in January 1907 under the title *Journal Belge de Radiologie* (De Nobele was its first editor): in one of its earliest numbers appeared the pioneering article on pneumoarthrography of the knee by Kaisin of Floreffe. The title of their journal has varied, and for some time it carried the subtitle *Annales.* The Belgian Society of Radiology and Electrology had, at the latest count, about 450 members.

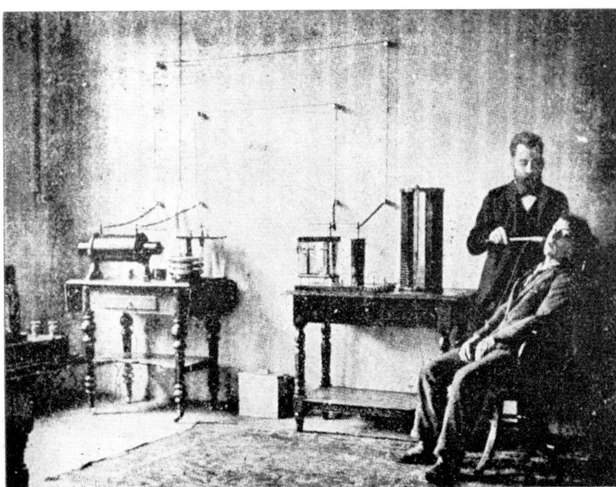

LEOPOLD FREUND. "Electrifying" a patient in 1900.

SIRM

Beginning in 1911, in Italy, preliminary meetings were held in which participated Bertolotti, Busi, Maragliano, Perussia, Parola, Ponzio, and Tandoja. The *Societa Italiana di Radiologia Medica* (SIRM) was declared founded at the first formal organizational meeting, held on January 5, 1913, in the Library of the *Ospedale Maggiore* in Milano. At that time, they also elected their honorary president, Augusto Righi.

Their first *Congresso* took place in October 1913 in the Radio-Phototherapic Section of the Dermato-Syphilopathic Department of the same *Ospedale Mag-*

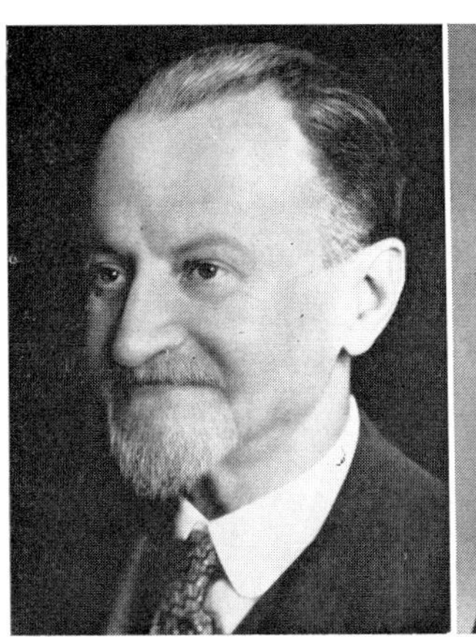

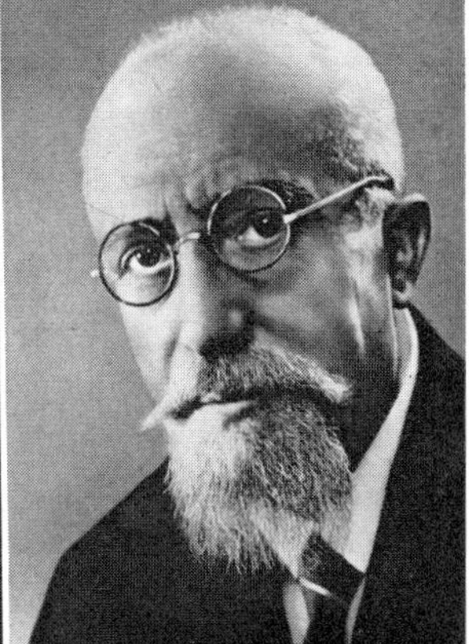

Courtesy: Georg Grössel - Agfa.

BELGIAN ROENTGEN PIONEERS. E. Henrard and bespectacled L. Hauchamps.

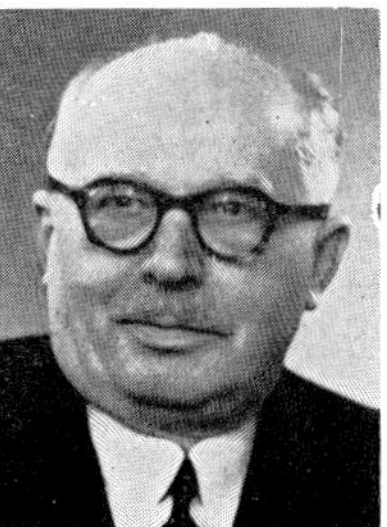

ZEPHIR GOBEAUX

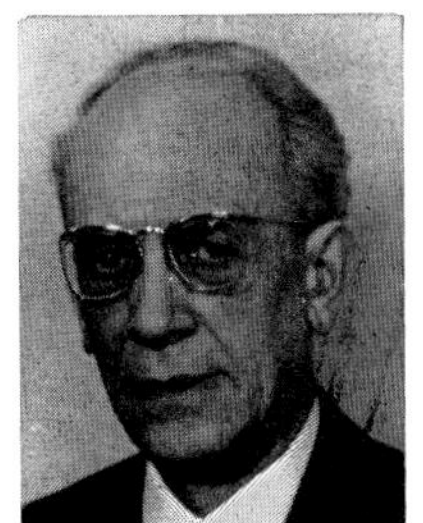

FREDERIC DE WITTE

giore, at nr. 9 on *via* Pace in Milano (president: Luigi Parola, secretary: Perussia).

Their second national meeting took place in 1914 in Bologna, under the presidency of Aristide Busi. The Secretary was Mario Ponzio (1885-1956) who remained the perpetual secretary-treasurer of the SIRM. He was *professore ordinario* in the University of Torino. His radiation death was barely delayed by numerous mutilating interventions, which included disarticulation in the left gleno-humeral joint and amputation of the right hand.

The papers read in their annual meetings are published in *Rendi-conti* of the *Congresso Italiano* (since 1936 *Nazionale) di Radiologia Medica.* In charge of the publication for the first meeting was Felice Perussia (1886-1959). He fulfilled his task so well that they designated him to become the editor (actually the founder) of their official journal, the now venerable *Radiologia Medica,* first issued in 1914. Perussia, who was also professor of Radiology in the University of Milano, remained the editor until his death. He was succeeded in both jobs (professorial as well as editorial) by the "radio-oncologist" Arduino Ratti, while his own son, Aldo Perussia, continued as editorial assistant of *Radiologia Medica.*

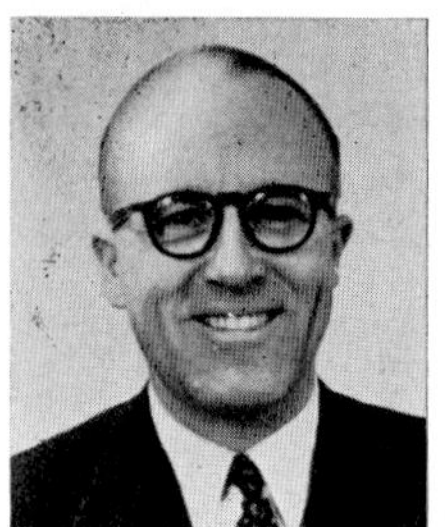

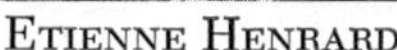

ETIENNE HENRARD

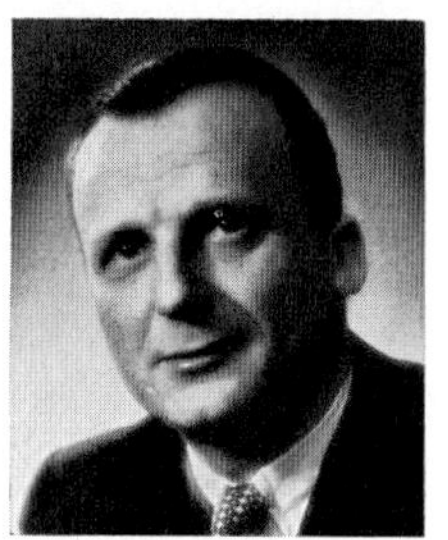

SIMON MASY

Vol. XLVI GENNAIO 1960 Fasc. 1

LA RADIOLOGIA MEDICA

RIVISTA MENSILE

ORGANO UFFICIALE della SOCIETA ITALIANA DI RADIOLOGIA MEDICA

Redazione: Via Comelico, 2 — Amministrazione: Corso Bramante 83 TORINO

PROF. FELICE PERUSSIA

16-XII-1885 - 18-XII-1959

Courtesy: Arduino Ratti, editor of Radiologia Medica.

EDITOR EULOGIZED. Felice Perussia was editor of *Radiologia Medica* from the journal's inception in 1916 to the day of his death. It is fitting to bring his portrait together with the masthead of his publication, as it paid tribute to its founder.

RADIOLOGIE IN FRANCE

There existed a *Société Francaise d'Électrothérapie* which printed since 1893 a *Bulletin Officiel:* after Röntgen's discovery they simply added to their name the words. . . *et de Radiologie Médicale.*

The earliest organizational meetings of the French Radiological Society took place in November 1908 at Béclère's residence, but the first official session of the *Société de Radiologie Médicale de Paris* was held in January 1909. Their first *Bureau* consisted of Béclère (president), Guilleminot (vice-president), Haret (general secretary), P. Aubourg (treasurer), and the Publication Committee, composed of Belot, René Ledoux-Lebard and Lenglet. Haret became the editor of their *Bulletin et Mémoires de la SERM de Paris.* In 1912 they expanded to give nation-wide (French) coverage, and the name was changed to *Société de Radiologie Médicale de France.* In 1945

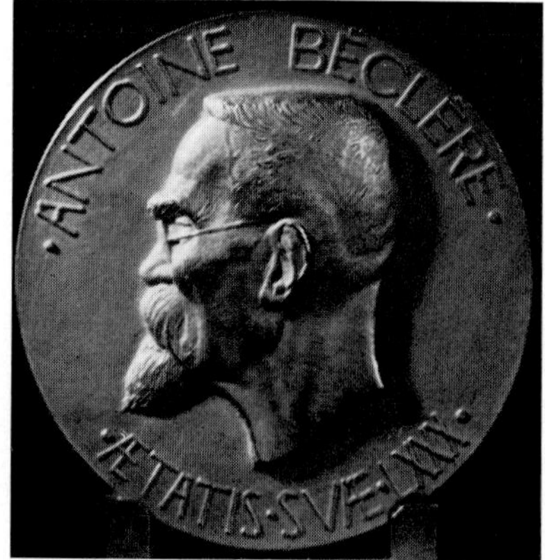

Courtesy:* Centre *Antoine Béclère.

BÉCLÈRE GOLD MEDAL. Issued on the 80th birthday of Antoine Béclère, and given since then to meritorious individuals in the field.

they absorbed the above mentioned Electrotherapeutic Society, at which time the current name was adopted: *Société Française d'Électro-Radiologie Médicale.*

The actual founder of the Society was the Grand Old Man of French Radiology, the longevous Antoine Béclère (1856-1939), in his time one of the best known, most colorful, and universally esteemed among the world's radiologists. In 1897 (with Oudin and Barthélemy), he reported the *radiodiagnostic* of an aneurysm of the aortic arch. In 1899, he studied carefully and offered pertinent advice regarding dark adaptation prior to fluoroscopy. In 1902, he introduced Holzknecht's quantitometer into France. In 1904, he published a 12° on the Radio-Diagnosis of Internal Diseases. In 1905, he described the extreme radiosensitivity of seminoma. The many honors bestowed upon Béclère did not affect his ways of life; after the official retirement, he continued to work, thus at seventy-five years of age he resumed research on "immunity" in cancer (he believed in the infectious origin of certain tumors): the very last time he walked out of his house was to procure material for immunologic experiments.

One of Béclère's pupils was Georges Haret (1874-1932). He served as first editor of the *Bulletins et Mémoires,* but is better known for his researches in the therapeutic aspect of the new specialty. Haret had many original ideas, for instance he attempted to introduce radium ions into the body by iontophoresis.

Another of Béclère's pupils who must be mentioned, was François Jaugeas (1880-1919), who first became known for the translation of Grashey's *"Normal Atlas."* His thesis on the use of x rays in the diagnosis and treatment of acromegaly (1909) was at the time a novel subject. His most successful work remains the *Précis de Radiodiagnostic,* first issued in 1913. During a fluoroscopy performed at the American Hospital in Paris, Jaugeas touched inadvertently a live overhead wire, and was fatally electrocuted.

The one name longest identified with the French Radiological Society was that of André Dariaux (1881-1960), who had been its general secretary for over a quarter of a century. Dariaux was the associate and friend of Haret, with whom (and with Jean Quénu) he had brought out the beautiful *Atlas de Radiographie Osseuse* (1927). In 1928 failing health (due to prolonged radiation exposure) forced Haret to resign the job of secretary general of the French Radiological Society. Haret was succeeded by Dariaux. During the latter's tenure, the creation of provincial branches of the Society was encouraged (today they have eight of these), the merger with the electrotherapists was brought about in 1945, and with Belot, Dariaux founded the *Congrès des Médecins Radiologistes et Électrologistes de Culture Latine* (their fifth meeting

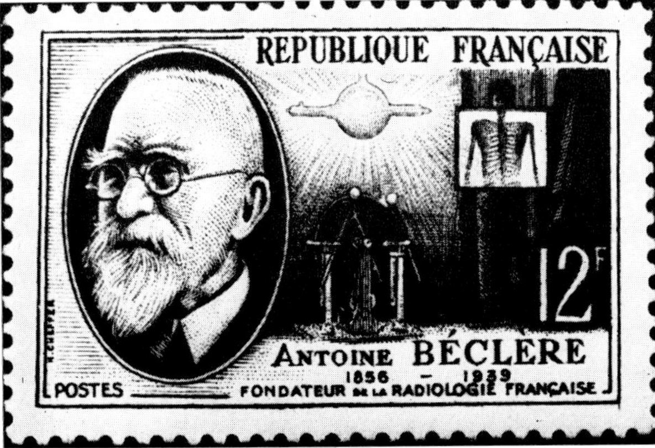

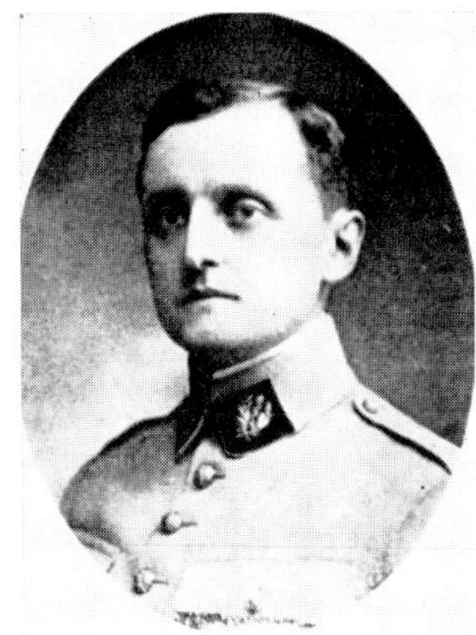

FRANCOIS JAUGEAS. One of the better known electromartyrs.

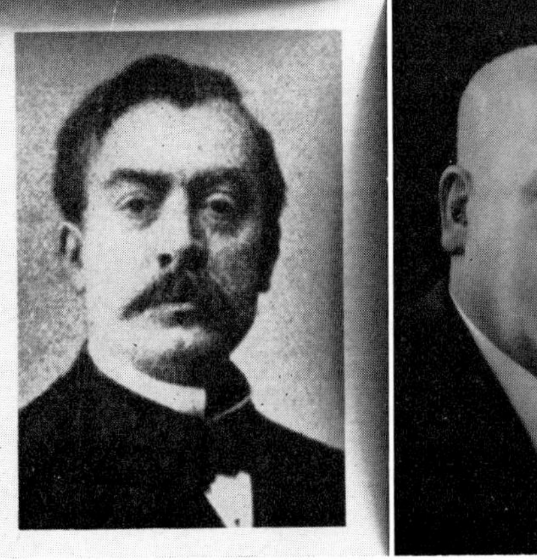
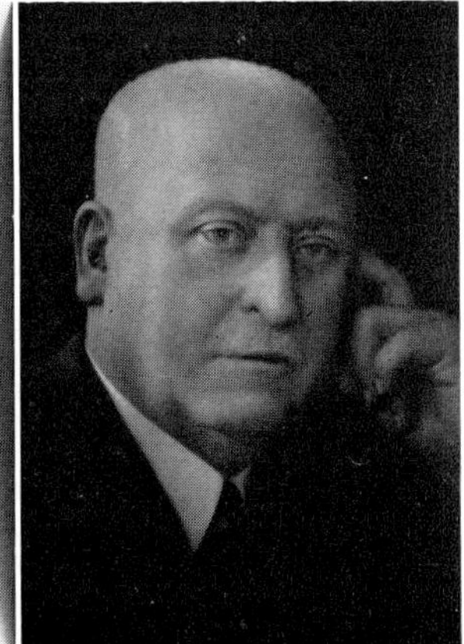

GEORGES APOSTOLI & LOUIS DELHERM.

JOURNAL DE RADIOLOGIE ET D'ÉLECTROLOGIE

was held in Paris in July 1961). Dariaux's successor and eulogist, Charles Proux, is continuing in his footsteps.

In 1914, only a few months before Sarajevo, appeared the first issue of the official journal of the French Society of Radiology, the *Journal de Radiologie et d'Électrologie* (Editor: Belot). Only a few months after Sarajevo, England and Germany were at war, and the *British Archives of the Roentgen Ray* — edited at the time by George Alexander Pirie (1863-1929) — became the *Archives of Radiology and Electrotherapy.*

RENTGENOLOGYA IN RUSSIA

In Czarist times, Russian roentgen achievements paralleled those of other countries. Before the end of 1896, I. F. Kotovich had addressed a Convention of Military Physicians in Moscow on the subject of "Roentgen's X-Light" and its utilization in medicine.

Most of the material for this section was collected from articles written or edited by Samuel Aronovich Reynberg, who teaches radiology in the Post-Graduate Medical Institute in Moscow. Reynberg's achievements are numerous: among his hundreds of pupils, twenty-one have become professors of radiology in various sections of the Soviet Union; his personal bibliography exceeds 250 titles in eleven languages, comprising both diagnosis (his specialty field is chest diseases) and therapy (particularly "roentgen-biology"); his "spare time" is devoted to the history and philosophy of radiology. Reynberg's 65th birthday anniversary was feted in April 1962.

During the Russo-Japanese War, in the battle at Tshushima Straits (May 27-29, 1905), V. S. Kravchenko, the Chief Surgeon of the cruiser "Aurora," reported that of eighty-three wounded sailors, forty were examined with roentgen rays installed in the ship's infirmary. After the battle, "Aurora" pulled into Manila Harbor.

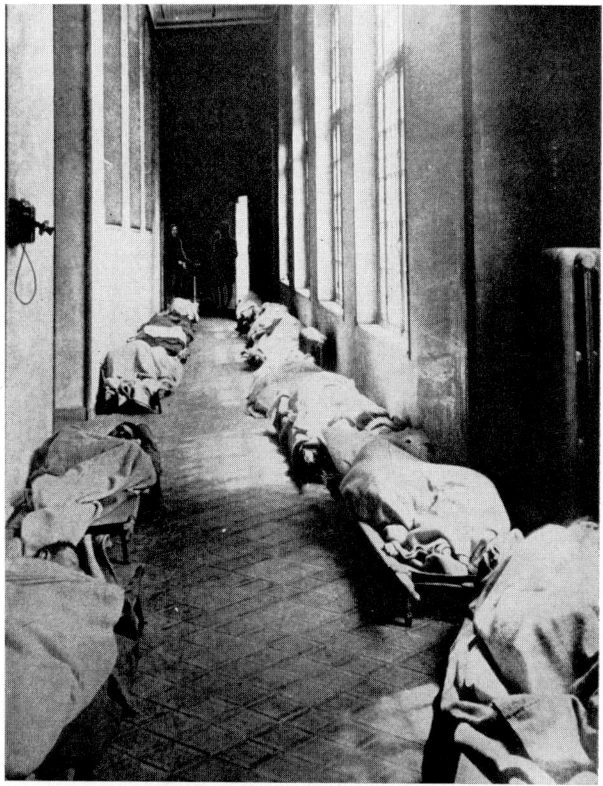

EN ROUTE TO THE X-RAY ROOM. This was the caption used by the *American Journal of Roentgenology* when it reproduced this picture of the corridor of a French castle, transformed into an Army hospital, during the "Great War" (to many of its veterans it remained "the" War).

ОЧЕРКИ
РАЗВИТИЯ
МЕДИЦИНСКОЙ
РЕНТГЕНОЛОГИИ

50
лет
РЕНТГЕНОВЫХ ЛУЧЕЙ
В МЕДИЦИНЕ

ПОД РЕДАКЦИЕЙ
С. А. Рейнберга
УЧЕНЫЙ СЕКРЕТАРЬ СБОРНИКА
Е. А. Лихтенштейн

ГОСУДАРСТВЕННОЕ ИЗДАТЕЛЬСТВО
МЕДИЦИНСКОЙ ЛИТЕРАТУРЫ
Медгиз · 1948 · Москва

Courtesy: Fedor Krotkov.

REYNBERG-EDITED RUSSIAN ROENTGEN-HISTORY. With contributions by many authors, this volume was prepared for the fiftieth anniversary of Röntgen's discovery, but postwar difficulties delayed printing until 1948.

The stationery x-ray equipment on one of the American ships was transiently out of order. As Russo-American relations were very friendly in the wake of Teddy Roosevelt's mediation offer which led to the Russo-Japanese Peace Treaty at Portsmouth – Kravchenko offered his equipment to be used on American sailors.*

In 1906, at the Pirogov Institute, P. N. Vinogradov reported on the utilization during the Russo-Japanese campaign of "roentgen cabinets" by the ground forces in Manchuria. There was seldom electrical power available, so they had to utilize very often hand-operated generators.

Roentgen experiences accumulated during the Balkan War of 1912-1913 were reported by M. E. Shmighelsky. Also from that time date the contributions on the wave properties of roentgen rays; that work had been done in the Institute of Physics of Peter Nikolaevich Lebedev (1866-1911), renowned for having proved the existence of pressure of light on bodies.

Two other names shall be mentioned. The first is N. N. Cherkassov, an extremely talented physician and neuro-pathologist from Moscow, who developed in his own laboratory many improvements, for instance a rotary switch; he never published anything and remained therefore largely unknown. The other name is that of the brilliant S. P. Grigoriev (1878-1924), who practiced for twenty years in Kharkov; he was mainly an internistic roentgenologist; after the revolution he came to this country and died of typhus in the Oak Park (a Chicago suburb) Hospital; the autopsy, performed by another immigrant from Kharkov, the pathologist Eugene Constantine Piette showed findings which suggested that "chronic exposure to radiation had lowered body defenses" and in Piette's opinion Grigoriev was a roentgen martyr.

In Russia, the first comprehensive roentgen monograph, including both diagnosis and therapy, was published in 1906 in Moscow by D. F. Rieshetillo. During World War I a Roentgen Commission was formed in Kiev through private initiative; they collected 80,000 rubles from which *rentghen kabinets* were purchased for both civilian and military uses; they also issued their official organ, the *Izvestja Kievskoye Rentgenovskye Kommissye.*

Prior to World War I there were in Kiev only three hospitals with x-ray installations. In September, 1914 was organized the so-called Commission for roentgen assistance to the war wounded. It had support from charity as well as from official institutions: by January, 1916 a total of eighteen new x-ray installations had been placed in hospitals in Kiev. The number rose to twenty in January, 1917, when the cumulated number of x-ray examinations in Kiev had exceeded 50,000. One of these twenty installations was mounted as a mobile unit on a horse-drawn carriage (with its 2 kw motor-dynamo combination). Six other horse-drawn mobile units were given by the Commission to the Russian Army for use behind the front lines, and one other mobile unit was installed in two railroad cars. The Commission created a repair center in Kiev which, before the end of 1917, handled more than 500 x-ray tubes (they were first Müller tubes, soon replaced by Fedoritzky tubes made in Petersburg, finally by a then new type, called Coolidge). The newsletter (*Izvestja*) of this Commission was issued every month in twenty-four pages, beginning in 1915. The Kievskoye Rent-

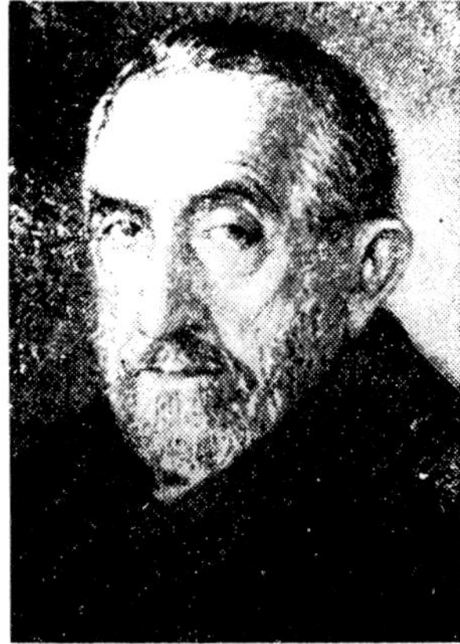

Courtesy: Georg Zedguenidze.

Orest Danilovich Khvolson. Russian roentgen pioneer, remembered also for having translated (into Russian) Röntgen's first paper, and for having been absent from the first Russian roentgen-congress.

*This information was submitted to the National Archives in Washington, (D.C.) who searched their documents and reported that the Russian ships "Aurora," "Zemtchug," and "Oleg" came into Manila Harbor on June 4, 1905 and were interned for the remainder of the duration of the Russo-Japanese War (they left Manila in October 1905). The US ship "Solace" was anchored near Cavite, P.I. (a short distance from Manila) from June 13 to June 27, 1905, but it had previously been reconverted to a Navy Transport.

An inquiry was also sent to Rear Admiral Allan Simpson Christman (Medical Corps), currently Deputy Surgeon of the US Navy. Their records indicate that 58 patients were then removed from the three Russian ships to the US medical installation at Canacao. After 1898, x-ray equipment in Naval stationary installations was of the Oscar Wiezerhold make and records show that in 1905 steps were taken to begin replacing worn equipment (a collection of x-ray tubes used since the early times is preserved at the US Naval Medical Center in Bethesda). Dr. Christman also mentioned that in 1905 two Navy Surgeons, William Clarence Braisted (1864-1941) and Raymond Spear (1873-1937), visited Japanese and Russian military and naval installations and reported that there were six hospital ships attached to the Russian squadron at Port Arthur. They were converted passenger ships, maintained to a considerable degree by the strong Russian Red Cross Societies, and each of these ships had a roentgen ray apparatus installed. On the Japanese hospital ship "Kobe Maru" (a specially fitted transport) there was Siemens-Halske x-ray equipment.

genovskye Kommissye wrote a page of dedication in Russian roentgen history.

The first all-Russian Svyezed (meeting) of roentgenologists assembled in Moscow, amid political turmoil, in mid-December 1916. Its honorary presidency went to Serghei Petrovich Feodorov. The seats on the dais were occupied by Lazarev, Yanovsky, Krasnobaev, Budinev, Nemenov, Luter, and Uspensky while the (active) president was N. E. Egorov, who had produced the first roentgen plate in Russia. Two of the better known absentees were Orest Danilovich Khvolson (1852-1934) and Grigoriev. The scientific

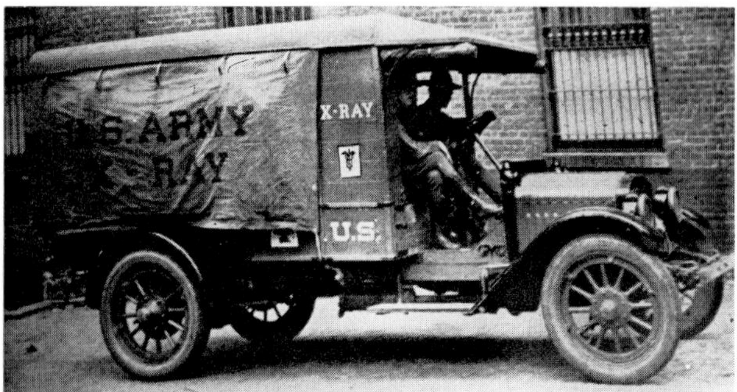

X-RAY CAMION. World War I x-ray truck: note the twin-winged snakes.

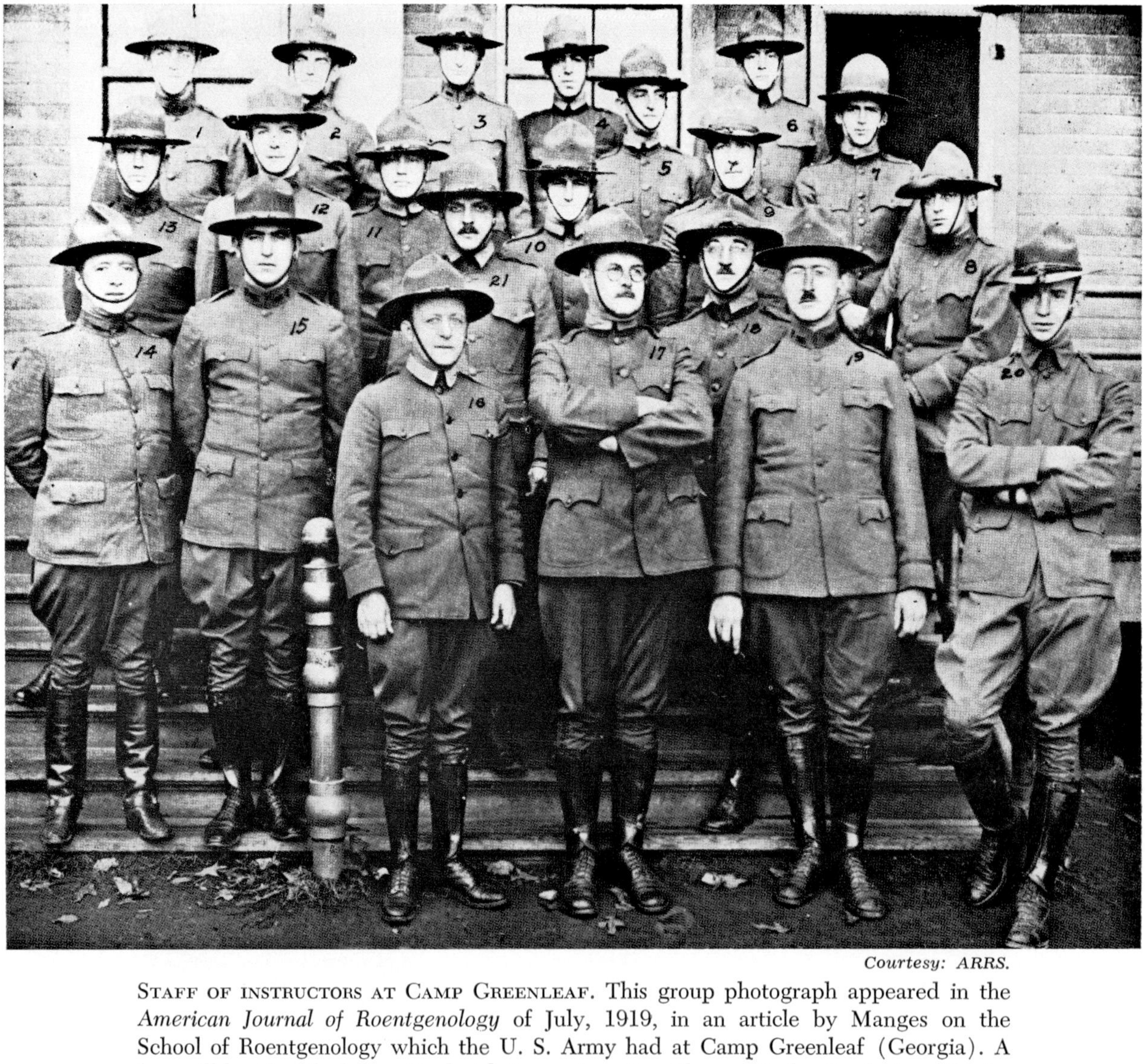

Courtesy: ARRS.

STAFF OF INSTRUCTORS AT CAMP GREENLEAF. This group photograph appeared in the *American Journal of Roentgenology* of July, 1919, in an article by Manges on the School of Roentgenology which the U. S. Army had at Camp Greenleaf (Georgia). A few will be identified: 3 – Frederick Oscar Coe; 7 – Thomas Burke Bond; 8 – Charles Alexander Waters; 13 – Henry Janney Walton; 14 – Edward Smith Blaine; 15 – Frank Edward Wheatley; 16 – Willis Fastnacht Manges; 17 – William Holmes Stewart; and 18 – James Jay Clark.

sessions were successful, and well attended. As the meeting was in progress, special newspaper editions announced the murder of the hypersexed monk, Rasputin. Before adjourning, the first all-Russian roentgen congress decided to meet again after one year, in December 1917, but they had to wait longer than that: on October 24, 1917, the (Bolshevik) Revolution set Russia on fire.

PERIODS IN UNIVERSAL RADIOLOGIC HISTORY

The History of Radiology comprises three fairly distinct periods, separated by World Wars I and II: (a) the *Era of the Roentgen Pioneers* was followed by (b) the *Golden Age of Radiology,* while the present time may well be called (c) the *Atomic Phase.* In this context the wars were more than simple chronologic dividers. For one thing, at least in the USA, a large number of physicians received specialized training during their tours of duty in the Armed Forces.

UNITED STATES ARMY

X-RAY MANUAL

AUTHORIZED BY THE SURGEON-GENERAL OF THE ARMY

Prepared under the Direction of the Division of Roentgenology

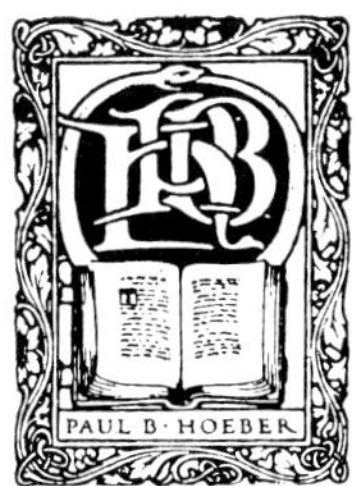

[219 ILLUSTRATIONS]

NEW YORK
PAUL B. HOEBER
67-69 EAST 59TH STREET
1918

In 1918, the Division of Roentgenology of the US Army issued its first *X-Ray Manual,* published by Hoeber. Among the (unnamed) authors of this manual was the Terre Haute radiologist Harold Jesse Pierce. In this country, the teutonophobia created by World War I may have contributed to the terminologic changeover which took place during the early 1920s.

WESTERN ROENTGEN SOCIETY

The ARRS never strove to accumulate a large membership. Quite the contrary, it wanted to be the honor society of a carefully selected elite. Toward the end of the Era of the Roentgen Pioneers, the East held the balance of power in the ARRS. The Industrial Revolution had for several decades replaced the no longer advancing frontier. The Midwest was up-and-coming, and graduates from Cincinnati, from Ann Arbor, from St. Louis, from Chicago were beginning to gain national stature. They had fewer ties with Europe, and they had less inherent respect for established Eastern authority.

In the summer of 1915, in St. Louis, Fred Summa O'Hara (1876-1950) — the former amanuensis of Heber Robarts — met with several friends in Miles Titterington's office (formerly occupied by Russell Daniel Carman) on Olive Street. They decided to create a regional association of roentgen ray workers. With the monetary help of George W. Brady invitations were sent into Missouri, Illinois, and Iowa, and the first organizational meeting was held on Decem-

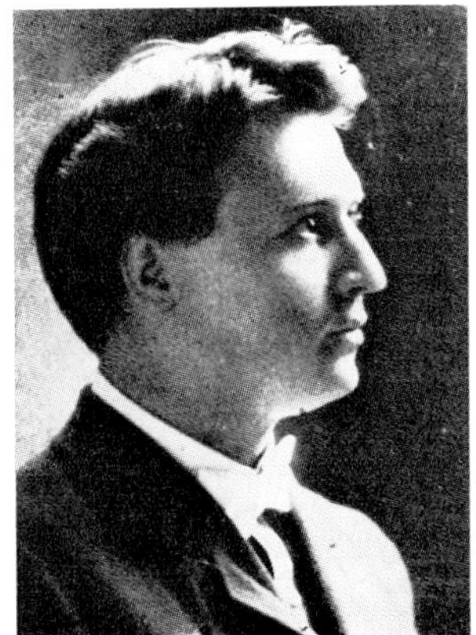

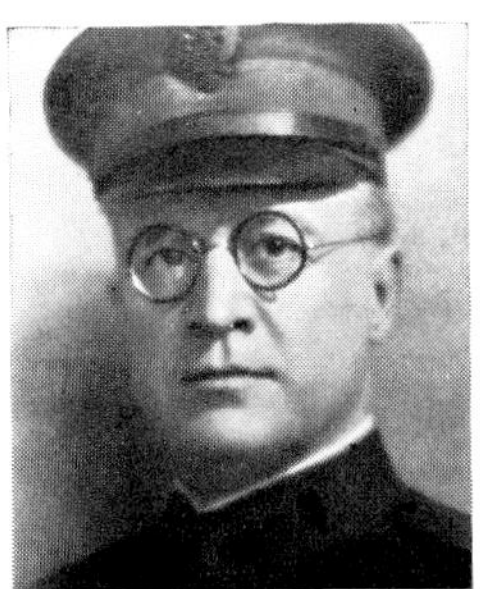

FRED SUMMA O'HARA. Founder and first president of the Western Roentgen Society (which then became the RSNA). O'Hara had been the associate of Heber Robarts at the time when Robarts founded the ARRS in his office in St. Louis. The Western Roentgen Society was founded in the same way in a private x-ray office, that of Miles Titterington in the same city of St. Louis. Both portraits show O'Hara, one at the turn of the century, the other during World War I.

ber 15-16, 1915, at the Hotel Sherman in Chicago with about thirty (charter) members present. O'Hara was elected president of this new organization, called the *Western Roentgen Society* (WRS).*

In the words of Arthur Wright Erskine (in the November, 1945 issue of *Radiology*), the motive for founding the WRS was as follows: "Probably the most compelling reason for forming a new society was the firm belief held by its founders that there should be a place in organized radiology for young men, who should be encouraged to develop within the organization. . . . The founders and the older members of the RSNA have been proud of the fact that no member, regardless of his obscurity or the modesty of his attainment, has ever been denied the right to raise his voice in either the scientific or the executive sessions of the society."

This sounds very good, and is true, but a number of qualifications are certainly in order. Recently the scientific sessions are crowded with so many papers that there is little if any time left for discussions from the floor. As for business meetings, the large majority of RSNA members have never attended a single one of the society's executive sessions. They prefer to "let George do it," which goes hand in glove with the existence of a committee of 'king-makers," who decide who is going to be the next president, secretary, and so on down the line. That single slate of officers is then presented before the so-called quorum (usually between two and three per cent of the total membership); as soon as that single slate has been read, nominations are closed by motion. To prevent any possible "inadvertencies" – meaning surprises from the floor – nominations are offered at one business meeting, but are not voted upon until another day. The same system is in use in most if not all American medical (and other

*In the morning of May 12, 1961, in the plush lobby of the Broadmoor in Colorado Springs, Edwin Charles Ernst (of St. Louis) was reminiscing about the 1915 meeting of the ARRS in Atlantic City. He told me that he had sat across a bar table from Willis Fastnacht Manges when he (Ernst) asked Manges point-blank whether he (Ernst) and O'Hara would or would not be accepted as members of the ARRS. Manges was politely evasive (actually, as soon as Manges became president-elect of the ARRS in 1917, he had Ernst elected to membership; O'Hara proudly refused). Thereupon, Ernst raised his glass and toasted to the *Western Roentgen Society* adding, "we will get our own members."

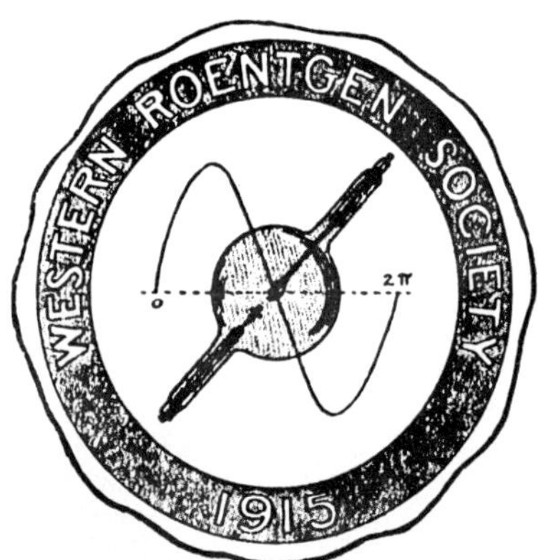

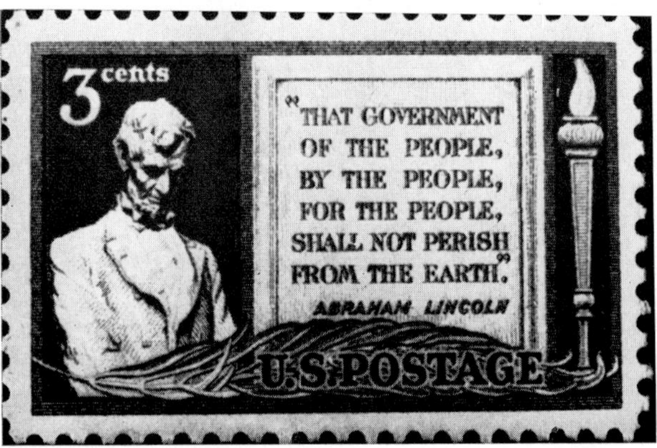

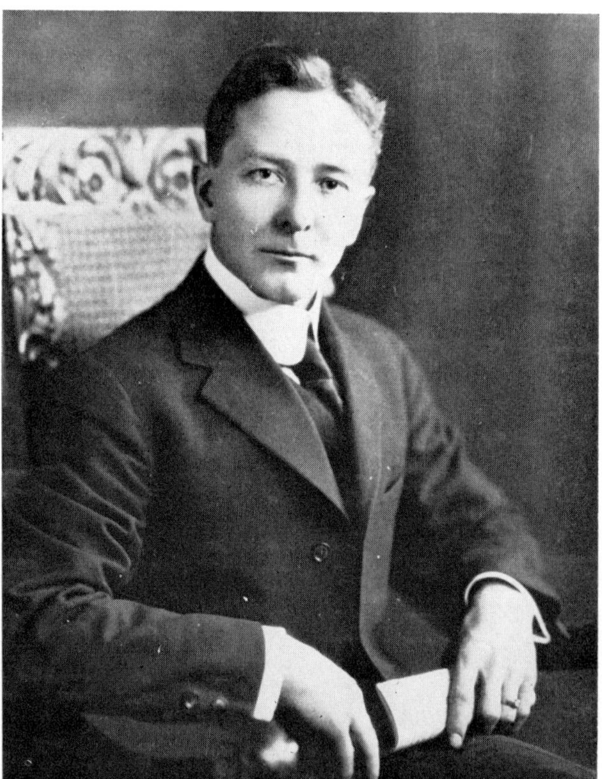

Benjamin Harry Orndoff. This photograph shows him about the time when he became president-elect of the Western Roentgen Society. Antoine Béclère coined the word *radiologie;* Orndoff made it popular in the USA by inserting its root into the name of the RSNA (and in that of its official journal). Later Orndoff played an important role in the creation of the American College of Radiology.

scientific and professional) organizations. It is admittedly imperfect but, as long as the membership refuses active participation in organizational functions (*faute de mieux, on couche avec sa femme*), no better system can be devised, and this one will have to do.

JOURNAL OF ROENTGENOLOGY OR OF RADIOLOGY

The WRS president for 1918 was a bright young lad from Chicago, named Benjamin Harry Orndoff. In a caucus held at the Congress Hotel, he emphasized the need of the growing WRS for an official mouthpiece, and was promptly offered the editorship of this prospective journal. He declined the privilege, bestowed it upon Bundy Allen (1885-1935), then of Iowa City, and retained for himself the associate editorship. The first number of the *Journal of Roentgenology* was issued in May, 1918. At the end of the same year, during the annual convention of the WRS, held at the Sherman Hotel, it was shown that the WRS roster of 472 members covered thirty-eight states in the Union. This called for a modification of the obviously regional name. It was Orndoff's idea — he has preserved the minutes of that session — to use the adjective radiological, as being more comprehensive, and on November 22, 1918 the name *Radiological Society of North America* (RSNA) was adopted. Nevertheless, the old name (WRS) was maintained on the journal's masthead for another year (1919), as the opposition connived frantically to force a reversal of the decision. In his stern struggle, Orndoff received indirect support from the ARRS which objected to the title *Journal of Roentgenology* because of possible confusion with the name of its own organ.

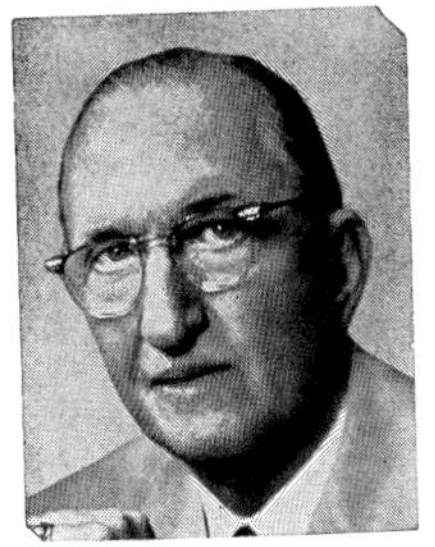
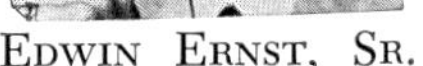

EDWIN ERNST, SR.

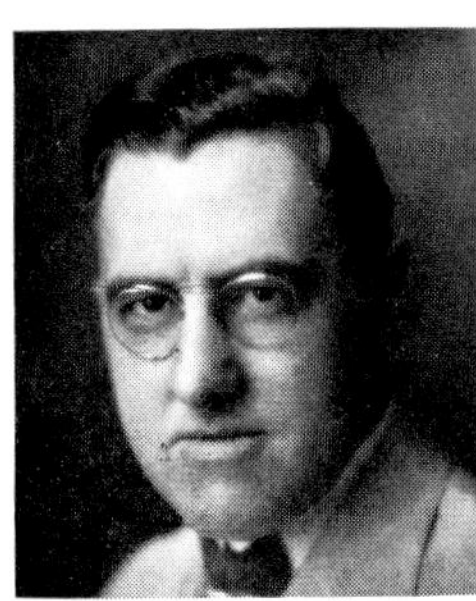

BUNDY ALLEN

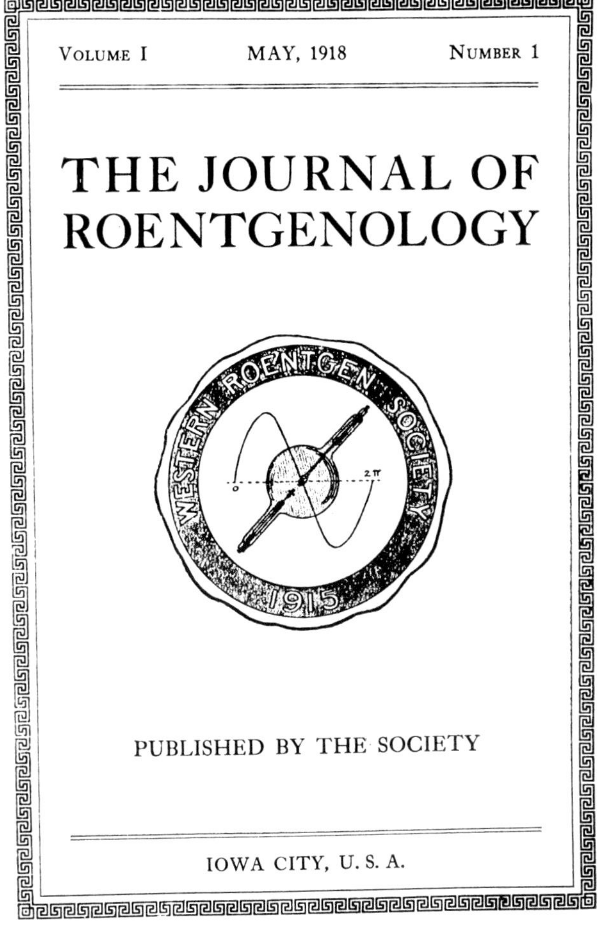

VOLUME I MAY, 1918 NUMBER 1

THE JOURNAL OF ROENTGENOLOGY

PUBLISHED BY THE SOCIETY

IOWA CITY, U. S. A.

It was legally impossible to copyright either the term *journal* or *roentgenology*, but much personal resentment resulted nonetheless. Ben Orndoff was repeatedly warned by Edward Smith Blaine not to waste time and effort ever to apply for admission to ARRS membership. But a few years later it so happened that Carman (who was one of Orndoff's personal friends) acceded to the ARRS presidency. Carman was the only one who held the highest office both in the RSNA and in the ARRS. As soon as elected, Carman personally shouldered Orndoff's application past the ARRS Executive Committee. It was one of the last things Carman did because he died in that same year of 1926 without completing his term in office. Almost all who were involved on the ARRS side in that wrangle have passed on. This footnote to history might have been

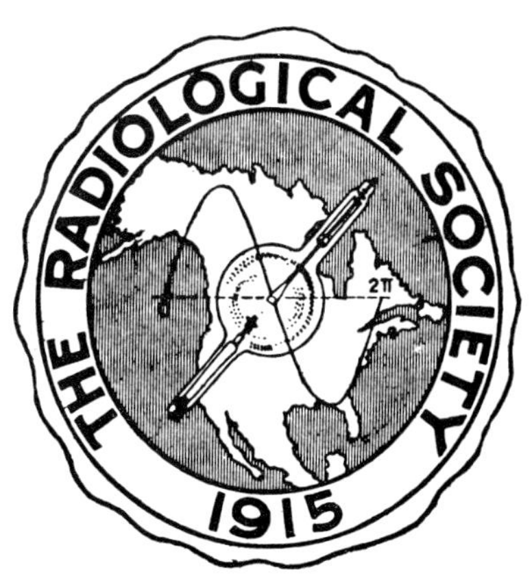

The Radiological Society of North America
Ninth Summer Meeting
Hotel Sherman, Chicago, June 6, 1924.
KAUFMANN & FABRY CO.
CHICAGO

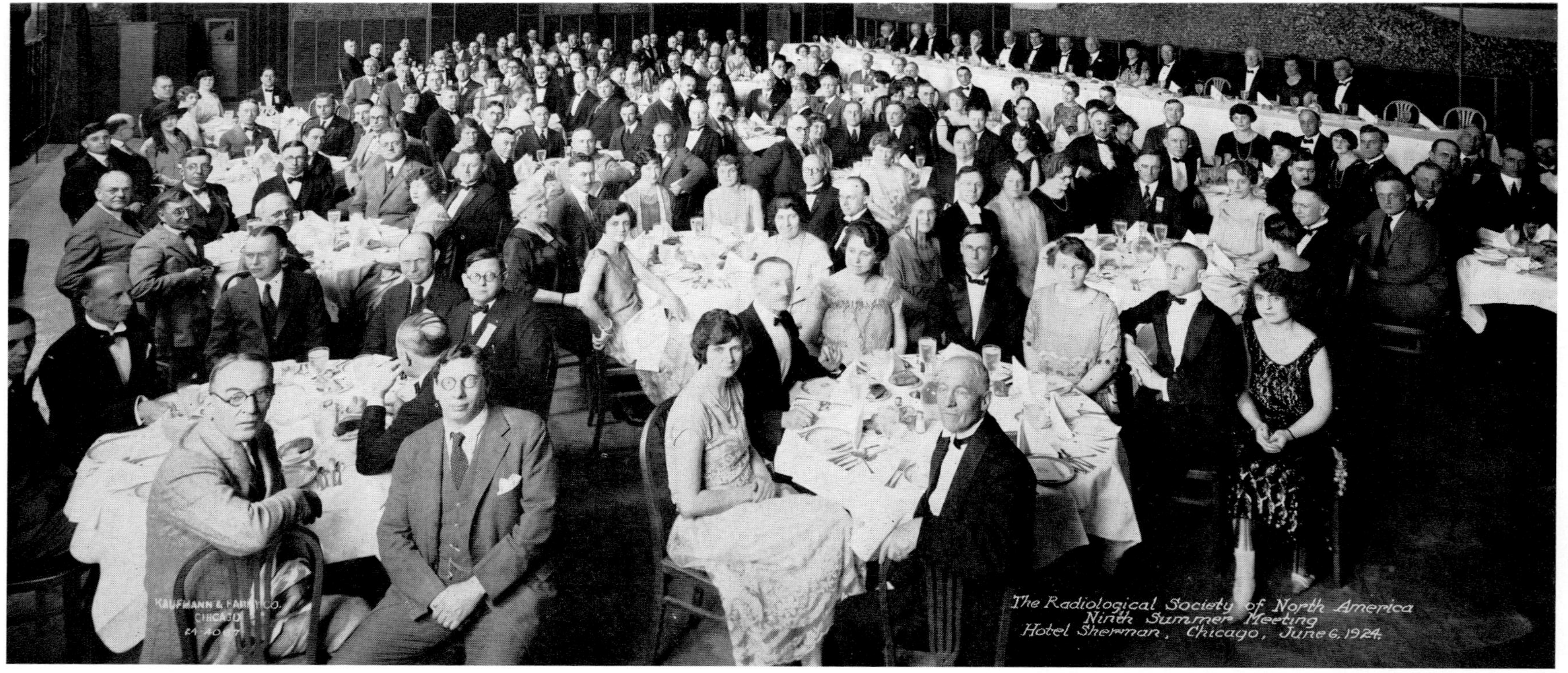

Courtesy: Ben Orndoff.

RSNA SUMMER MEETING (1924). For many years both the ARRS and the RSNA held not only national annual conventions, but also regional, at times even quarterly meetings. This one took place in Chicago at the very time when the Tyler lawsuit was in process. Byron Jackson is the bespectacled, half-turned figure in left foreground. The gray-haired, half-turned figure in center foreground is that of Castellin, an x-ray technician originally trained by the Beck brothers. Clockwise around the table from Castellin is Miss Kempton, an Orndoff aide (she became later one of the officials of the Bahai Temple, an interdenominational religious group). The other three men at that table were Oliver McCandless, Warner Watkins, and Bill Culpepper (a former World War I aviator, who earned a medical degree, was trained as a radiologist by Orndoff, and is now in semi-retired radiologic practice in Pinckneyville in Southern Illinois). Directly behind Watkins is white-tied and tail-coated Orndoff with his charming but usually retiring wife (they have five children and many grandchildren). The monocled lady is Maude Slye (who was the first to prove the existence of a genetic factor in experimental neoplasia in mice); she had come as Orndoff's guest. Several of the other beautiful ladies at these two tables were from Orndoff's group. He always liked to have a number of good-looking nurses and technicians at his office, and they appeared at many of his social functions. The "casualty-rate" (loss through marriage) was fairly high, but a few of the original group are still with him, and new ones have joined, all helpful, all willing, all efficient, and all good-looking. The people on the dais (from the viewer's right) include Arthur Erskine (who was then president-elect of the RSNA), George Pfahler, William Pusey, Rollin Stevens, James Case, and Augustus Crane (four of the men are not identified, the four ladies are wives of the aforegoing).

deleted from our text. But then – in the words of the freed Punic slave Publius Terentius Afer (190-150 B.C.) – *Homo sum: humani nihil a me alienum puto!* Pettyness and trivia are indelible aspects of human nature, and have often altered the course of events. In writing (or in reading) history, I prefer prosaic reality to dithyrambic overtones.

Finally, the first issue of the *Journal of Radiology* appeared in January, 1920, and it carried the new emblem, with the new name of Radiological Society of North America (RSNA).

RADIUMOLOGY

The flow of time deposits a blurring veil over the details of many a memory. This is why quite a few historical papers of the "remembrancer" type often retained no more significance than unsubstantiated rumors. Not so the beautiful Janeway Lecture which James Thomas Case (1882-1960) delivered on April 8, 1959 in Hot Springs (West Virginia) before the American Radium Society.

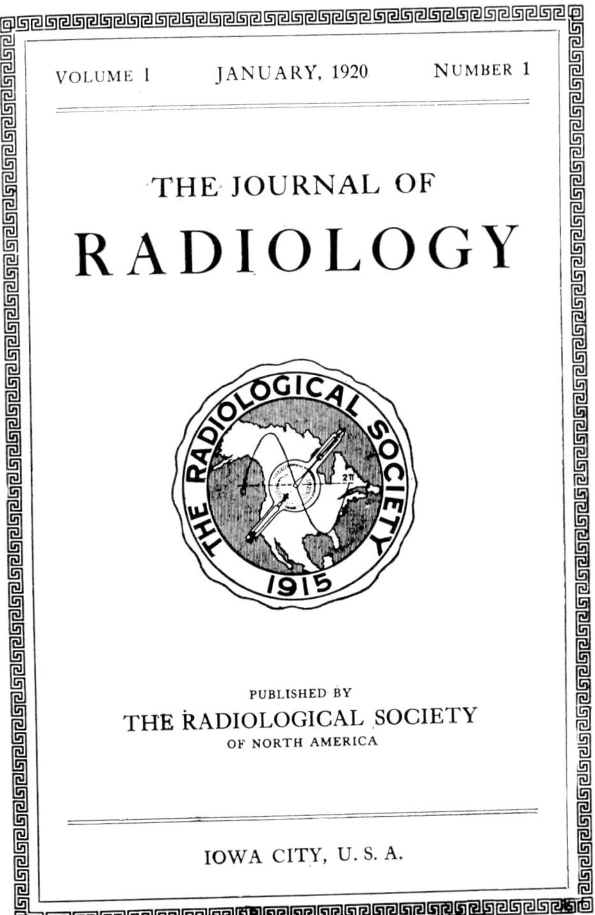
VOLUME I JANUARY, 1920 NUMBER 1

THE JOURNAL OF

RADIOLOGY

PUBLISHED BY
THE RADIOLOGICAL SOCIETY
OF NORTH AMERICA

IOWA CITY, U. S. A.

There is a secret ingredient with which such reminiscences can be made historically valid. One must substantiate the statements with dated references – and in this Case has always been a consummate master. His earliest "x-ray work" was performed in the Battle Creek (Michigan) Sanitarium until 1912 when he went to Chicago as a lecturer in radiology at Northwestern Medical School, and at the same time opened a very successful private office in the Chicago Loop. In 1915 Case became full professor of radiology, and stayed on until his retirement in 1947, then moved to Santa Barbara (California). He remained there until the spread of colonic carcinomatosis forced him out of this transient habitat, and into the history of radiology.

Case's first longer publication was an *Atlas of Stereo-Roentgenology of the Digestive Tract* (1913). He edited the *American Journal of Roentgenology* from October, 1916 through July, 1918. He published about 200 articles on everything radiologic, from diagnosis and therapy to ethics and bibliography. In this country, Case became best known to the younger generation of radiologists for having edited the translations of Schinz's *Textbook* and of Köhler's *Borderlands.* He was even more popular in Spanish-speaking countries, because of his familiarity with the language and the many personal contacts. At the sixth Inter-American Congress of Radiology in Lima in 1958, he was given a silver platter by radiologists from South of the Border, who called him their (unofficial) Ambassador of Radiology.

Preliminary arrangements for the creation of a Radium Society were made at the AMA meeting in Detroit in June 1916, by a physicist (Charles H. Viol) and by a physician (William H. Cameron) both associated with the Radium Chemical Company of Pittsburgh.

By that time, phony advertisements, such as "nature's gift to man, *radiumite*" (Case), and stunts like the "radium dinner" at the Massachusetts Institute of Technology (described by the reporter C. Moffett in January, 1903 in *McClure's Magazine*) were mostly a thing

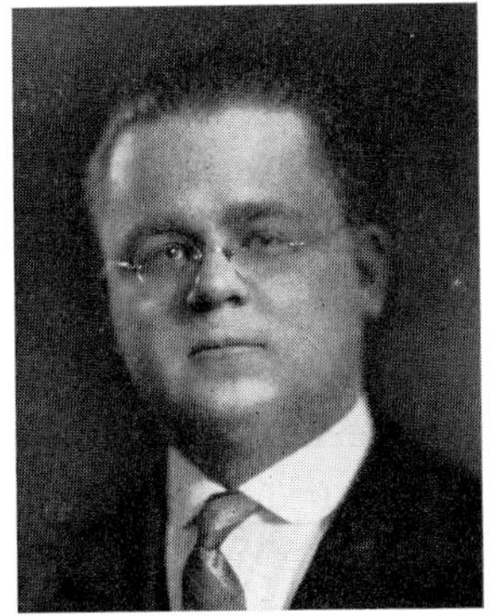
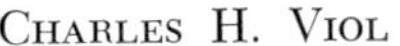
CHARLES H. VIOL

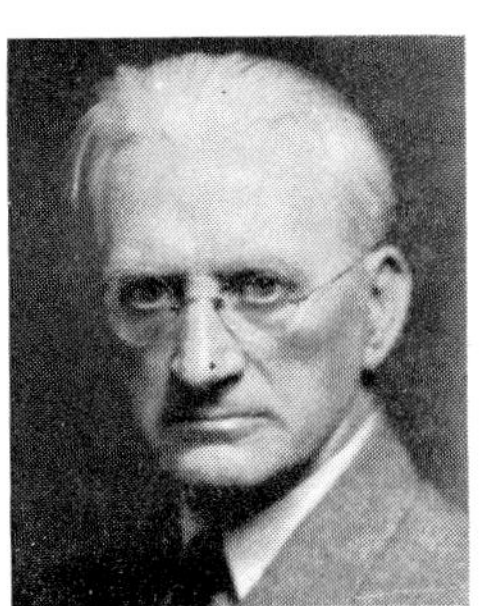
WM. H. CAMERON

of the past. Ernest Sommer's first edition of *Emanations* had appeared in München in 1908; the *Radiumthérapie* of L. Wickham and P. Degrais first issued in Paris in 1909, had been re-edited and translated; the previously mentioned Rieshetillo had printed his *Radiy* in St. Petersburg in 1910, and his compatriot E. S. London had published a text on radium in Leipzig in 1911; in London in 1911, Dawson Turner authored a similar manual, while in Wiesbaden were published in 1912 a *Grundriss* (with contributions by S. Löwenthal and F. Gudzent), and in 1913 a *Handbuch* (with contributions by E. F. Brashford and Becquerel); in Philadelphia in 1914 appeared *Radium and Radiotherapy* by William Stell Newcomet. And one year earlier had been issued in Bonn the *Radium als* (as) *Kosmetikum* by A. Dreyer.

Becquerel was the first to notice the biologic effects of radium. He had carried a glass tube containing radium salt in his vest pocket, and found a "burn" on the skin underlying the "radium pocket." Pierre Curie deliberately produced a similar reaction on his arm, which led to animal experiments and then to the suggestion that radium could be used in treating certain skin conditions.

The radium physicist Edith Hinckley Quimby recalled in December, 1948 in the *American Journal of Roentgenology* that the first radium for medical use was loaned by the Curies to Danlos, at Hôpital St. Louis in Paris. In 1906 Wickham and Degrais established their center for radium therapy, with Dominici in charge of the clinical work.

In this country, several physicians obtained small quantities of radium at a very early date; for instance, Francis Williams and William Rollins in Boston. Robert Abbe of New York City was the first to implant radium directly into a tumor in 1905. Intracavitary radium in treating carcinoma of the cervix had been pioneered by Margaret Cleaves in 1903. Independently, Alexander Graham Bell wrote his letter in which he suggested that radium be implanted directly into malignant tumors.

The *American Radium Society* (ARS) was formally organized at the Rittenhouse Hotel in Philadelphia on October 26, 1916. There were a total of twenty charter members (listed by Case), of whom only one was alive at the time of this writing — D. T. Quigley of Omaha. The officers elected were W. H. B. Aikins of Ontario, president; R. H. Boggs of Pittsburgh, vice-president; H. K. Pancoast of Philadelphia, secretary; and R. E. Loucks of Detroit, treasurer. Other important charter members (aside from Viol, Cameron, and Case) were Henry Schmitz and Frank E. Simpson of Chicago, and the "father" of interstitial radium therapy in this country, Robert Abbe from New York City.

A comprehensive work on the history of radium has yet to be written, but there are several excellent sources of information, one of which is the above cited lecture by Case. Edith Quimby has assembled important material on the subject. At the 1961 meeting in Pittsburgh of the Society of Nuclear Medicine, Asa Seeds and Richard Peterson had an exhibit on early "radium manufacture" in the USA. Fragmen-

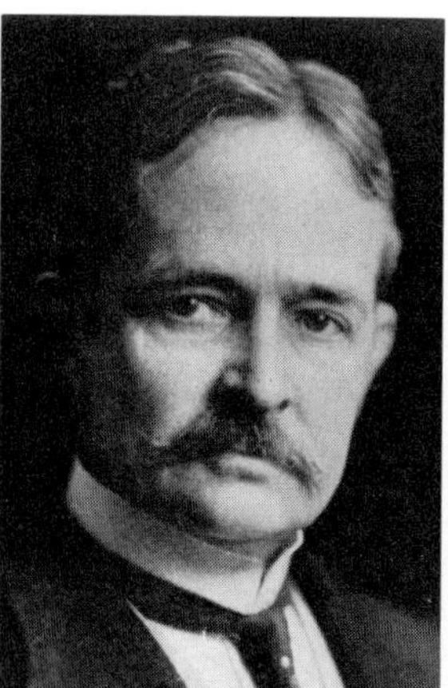

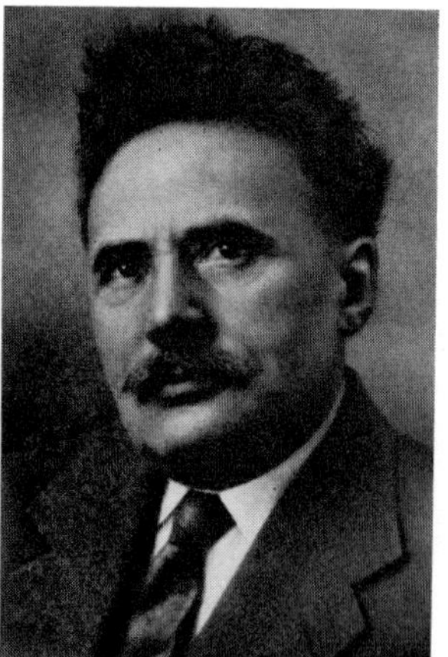

Courtesy: NLM

RADIUM PIONEERS. Robert Abbe (on the viewer's left) in 1905 in New York City was the first to implant radium directly into a tumor. E. S. London in Russia started autoradiography in 1904: he subjected a frog to emanation, then placed the frog on a photographic plate and obtained a faint image.

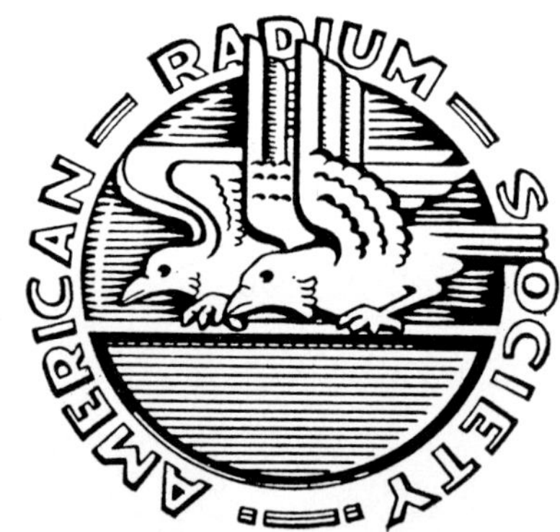

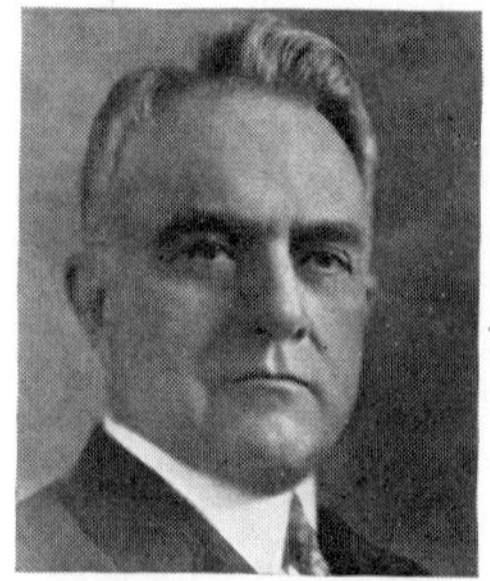

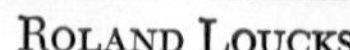

ROLAND LOUCKS

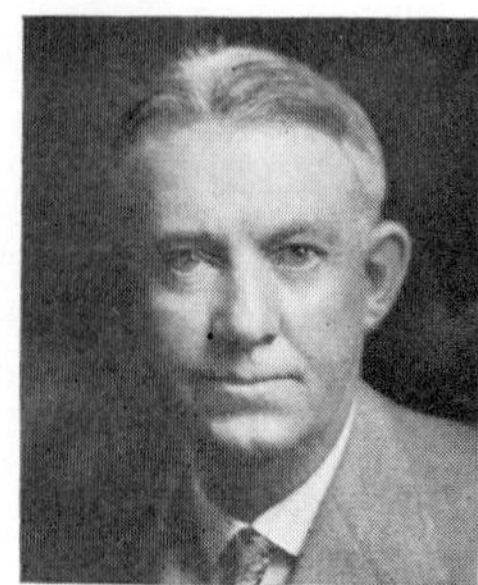

DANIEL QUIGLEY

tary data can also be found here and there in the medical literature.

The first preparations of nearly pure radium salt were put on the market by Giesel of the Chininfabrik Braunschweig, selling radium bromide at one English pound per milligram; the price later went to 12 times that, but the firm never really made a business of radium supply. The Curies decided not to patent their process, or take any material benefit from their discovery. The idea of a "radium factory" was first conceived in Paris by Armet de Lisle; with the technical help of the Curies he started such an enterprise in 1902, to supply early French demands. Armet de Lisle founded in 1906 a laboratory for clinical study, and provided it with radium; he also subsidized the French journal *Le Radium.*

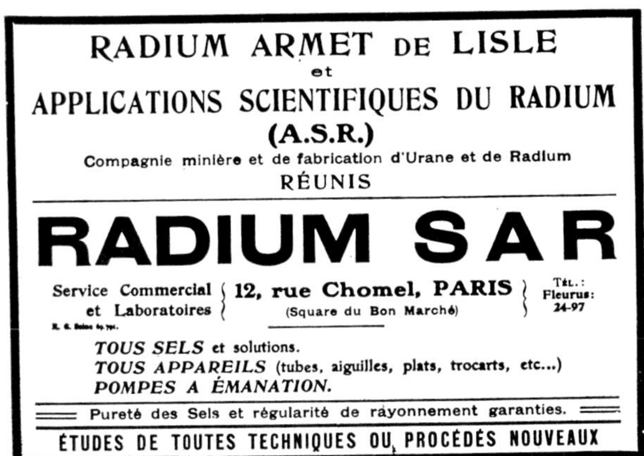

Armet de Lisle in late 1920's. As shown in this ad of 1928, they had to merge to keep afloat, the reason being the same as for the American radium firms — competition from the Congo!

Other extraction plants were established in Europe. The source of their ore was at first Bohemian pitchblende, of which the Austrian government had made a monopoly. Then radium was discovered in a Colorado ore, called carnotite, and for a while this ore was shipped to Europe.

In late 1902 — months before Marie Curie's thesis was completed — Stephen T. Lockwood of Buffalo (New York) wrote to Pierre Curie inquiring about the procedure for separating radium from uranium ore. The Curies replied in January, 1903 giving complete details of their process.

Radium from American ores was initially obtained as a by-product of mining for copper or vanadium, Carnotite was being mined since 1903 by James H. Lofftus in Richardson (southeastern Utah), and since 1905 by James H. McBride in the Paradox Valley (Southwestern Colorado). Domestic production of carnotite rose sharply about 1911, and continued active until 1922. It required starting with from 200 to 300 tons of car-

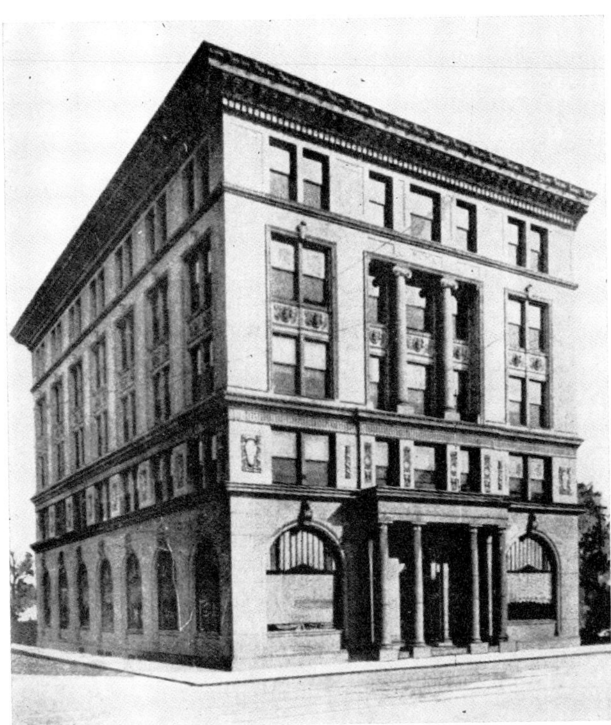

Radium rampart. Radium Research Laboratory and headquarters of the Standard Chemical Company and the Radium Chemical Company, at Forbes Street and Meyran Avenue in Pittsburgh; this is where, in 1913, was started the first commercial production of radium in America; by 1921 over 71 grams of radium had been refined there, which was more than half the world's entire production at that time.

RADIUM
STANDARD CHEMICAL CO.
U. S. Bureau of Standards Measurement.

Radium element content and delivery guaranteed

Radium Chemical Company
Pittsburgh, Pa., U. S. A. 1916

RADIUM

A Monthly Journal Devoted to the Chemistry, Physics and Therapeutics of Radium and Other Radio-Active Substances

Published by THE RADIUM PUBLISHING COMPANY
Forbes and Meyran Avenues, Pittsburgh, Pa.

Vol. I — APRIL, 1913 — No. 1

notite ore to refine one gram of radium. The price of radium was then about $120,000 per gram. As soon as less expensive sources for ore were found, mining for uranium in the U.S.A. was almost discontinued until 20 years later, when the Atomic Phase gave it renewed impetus.

An inmportant document for the history of radium is the *Souvenir,* originally prepared by Stephen T. Lockwood, and given in 1922 to Marie Curie who was then visiting the USA. The *Souvenir* was a document, entitled *Radium Research in America,* some of it typewritten, interspersed with printed parts, containing mainly two periods: 1902, when Lockwood first explored radium production, and 1914 when he testified before a Congressional Committee. To this he added a post-scriptum dated 1939. The whole thing, bound in silk and limp leather, was deposited in (and is preserved by) the Buffalo (New York) Society of Natural Science. Another copy is in the Buffalo Public Library, and one in the National Library of Medicine.

Lockwood established the Rare Metals Reduction Company in Buffalo (New York) which produced mainly vanadium and uranium oxides between 1906 and 1910. At the time the quantities of carnotite available were too small to make refining profitable. Before discontinuing his operation – on March 2, 1909 – Lockwood had a long interview with a confidential agent of Joseph M. Flannery (1867-1920) of the American Vanadium Company, in which Lockwood pointed out the advantages of using carnotite instead of roscoelite as a source of vanadium.

In 1911, Flannery organized the Standard Chemical Company in Pittsburgh for extraction of uranium and refining of radium from carnotite, and the latter operation was started in 1914 under the name Radium Chemical Co. They published the journal *Radium* (edited by Viol and Cameron).

In 1914, Howard Kelly (a gynecologist) and James Douglas (an engineer, formerly with the Phelps Dodge Corporation) established the National Radium Institute. This Institute, in a joint venture with the US Bureau of Mines, mined carnotite in the Paradox Valley, pro-

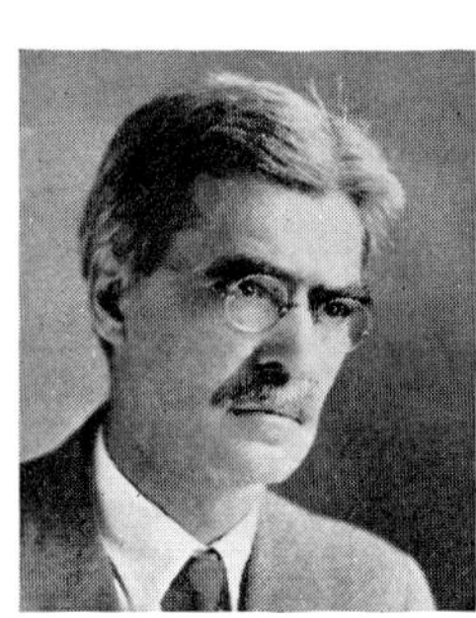

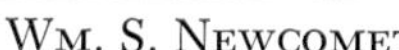

Wm. S. Newcomet

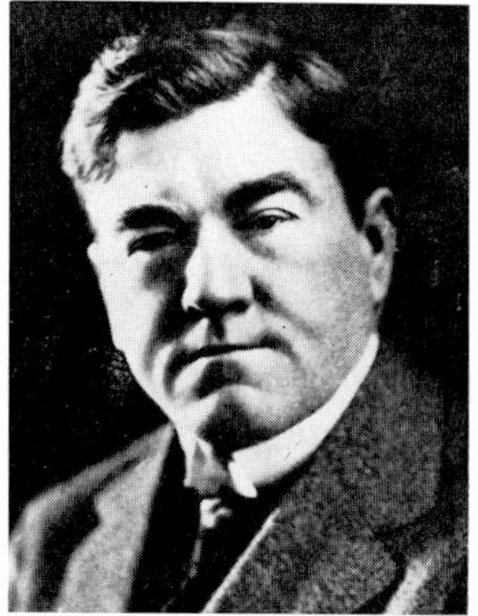

Joseph M. Flannery

cessed the ore, and refined radium in Denver. During its existence it produced between eight and nine grams of radium, most of which was divided between Kelly and the Memorial Hospital in New York City.

In 1915, the Radium Company of America (as a subsidiary of the Standard Chemical Co.), started refining operations at Canonsburg (Pennsylvania). Other companies appeared, such as the United States Radium Corporation (formerly the Radio-Chemical Corporation) and the Radium Emanation Corporation, both in New York City; the W. L. Cummings Chemical Co. in Philadelphia; and, of course, the Radium Company of Colorado in Denver.

Prior to 1914, the total radium production in the USA did not exceed three grams: in 1915 it rose to fifteen grams. Until 1922, about 80 percent of the world's supply of radium was produced in the USA. Then cheaper and richer uranium ores were discovered in Katanga Province in the Belgian Congo, which reduced the cost of radium to about $70,000 per gram. Ores that were even richer in uranium, and easier accessible, were found near the Great Slave Lake in Canada; this brought the radium price down to $35,000 per gram. It reduced USA radium production to nil. With the large scale refining of uranium in the past two decades, the price of radium on the international market has declined to about $20,000 per gram. The present 1960 USA stock of radium is estimated to be in excess of 1500 grams.

Radium was first imported to America for medical therapy in 1904. Stephen Lockwood brought from England and presented five milligrams of radium to the surgeon Roswell Park of Buffalo. Abbe, senior surgeon of St. Luke's Hospital in New York City, and Howard Atwood Kelly, professor of Gynecology at Johns Hopkins, both obtained small amounts of radium

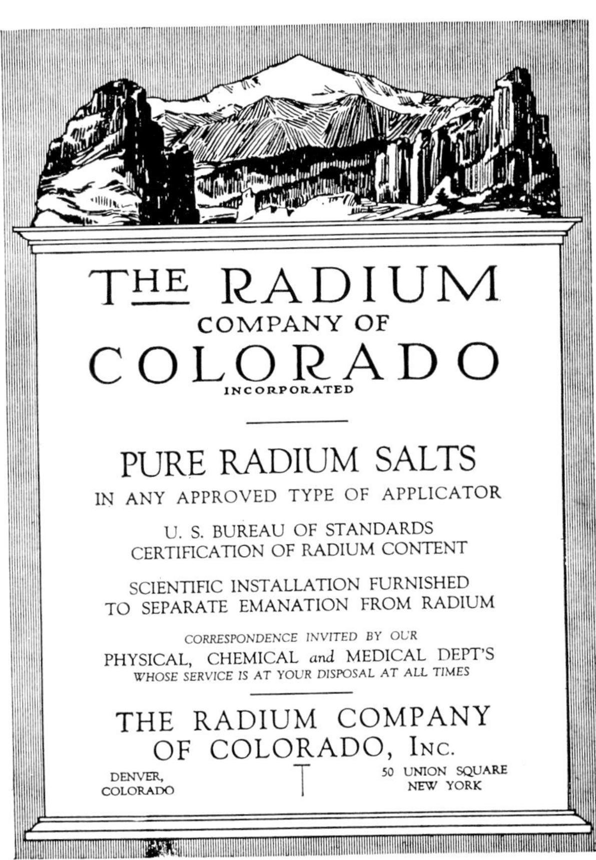

Radium Chemical Company, Inc.

FORBES and MEYRAN AVENUES — Pittsburgh, Pennsylvania, U.S.A.

Seuls Agents de vente pour les produits de Radium

de la Standard Chemical Company, Inc.

de Pittsburgh, Pennsylvania, U. S. A.

LES PLUS GRANDS PRODUCTEURS DE RADIUM DU MONDE

La production totale depuis 1913-1920 dépasse 128 grammes de cristaux de Bromure de Radium purs ($RaBr_2 2H_2O$)
La production pour l'an 1920 dépasse 32 grammes de cristaux de Bromure de Radium purs ($RaBr_2 2H_2O$)

Nous avons fourni le gramme de Radium offert à Mme M. Curie,
par les Dames des États-Unis

Vente garantie de tous les sels de Radium

Mesures certifiées exactes par le Bureau de Standardisation des Etats-Unis et basées sur l'étalon international du Radium.
La Standard Chemical Company garantit que moins de 0,2 pour 100 du rayon Gamma est dû au Mésothorium, Radiothorium, ou à des produits autres que le Radium et ses dérivés.

Littérature et prix sur demande

ADRESSE TELEGRAPHIQUE : RADIUM, PITTSBURGH, PENNA, U. S. A.

Courtesy: Masson & Cie.

AT THE TOP OF THE HEAP IN 1921. Ad appearing in the *Journal de Radiologie et d'Électrologie* in 1921 states that Radium Chemical Co. is the sole distributor for the Standard Chemical Co., world's largest producer of radium (total production 1923-1930 being over 128 gr.; over 32 gr. in 1920 alone); they furnished the gram of radium graciously offered by the *Dames* of the U. S. A. to Madame Curie during the latter's visit to this country.

RADIUM BELGE

(Union minière du Haut Katanga)
10, rue Montagne du Parc, **BRUXELLES**
Adresse télégraphique : RABELGAR-BRUXELLES

Sels de Radium, Tubes aiguilles et Plaques
Appareils d'émanation, Accessoires

LABORATOIRE DE MESURES -:- ATELIER DE CONDITIONNEMENT -:- FACILITÉS DE PAIEMENT -:- LOCATIONS A LONGUE DURÉE

FRANCE ET COLONIES
Agent général : « Cuivre et Métaux rares », 54, *Avenue Marceau*, PARIS (8e).
EMPIRE BRITANNIQUE
Agents généraux : Messrs. WATSON and SONS Ltd (Electro-Médical), 43, *Parker Street* (Kingsway), LONDON.
SUISSE
Agent général : M. Eugène WASSMER, Dr. Sc., Directeur du Radium Institut Suisse S. A., 20, *rue de Candolle*, GENÈVE.
ESPAGNE
SOCIEDAD IBÉRICA de CONSTRUCCIONES ELÉCTRICAS, Barquillo 1, Apartado 990, MADRID (CENTRAL).
JAPON
Agents généraux : MM. SUZOR et RONVAUX, *Post Office Box*, 144, YOKOHAMA.
ITALIE
Agent général : M. EINARDO CONELLI, 8, via *Aurelio Saffi*, MILAN (17).
ALLEMAGNE
RADIUM CHEMIE AKT GES. — Wiesenhuttenplatz, 37, FRANCFORT-sur-MEIN.

SIC TRANSIT GLORIA MUNDI. Only a few years later, the leader in radium production was the Belgian Congo, and this ad from the *Journal de Radiologie et d'Électrologie* of 1926 shows that agencies of the Radium Belge, including the (British) Watson & Sons, spanned the globe.

from Paris, which is how they became acquainted with the "subtle power" of radium (Abbe).

Marie Curie had discovered that radium gave off a radioactive gas which she called Emanation (it is now called radon). This has all the biologic effects of radium, and it began to be employed in therapy. The precious radium (at $120,000 per gram) could be kept in a safe, with no danger of loss, theft, or breakage, and the gas regularly drawn off.

Quimby relates that Kelly had obtained in 1908 a small glass tube containing a few milligrams of radium. In 1909 – after Wickham's visit to New York City – Kelly and his associate Curtis Burnam were determined to set up a clinical program of radium therapy. In 1911, they acquired 130 mgm. in an apparatus for emanation extraction, and nearly 100 mgm. in metal tubes (for gynecologic purposes). The emanation (in solution, "radium water") was used to treat arthritis and gout. In 1912, Kelly and Burnam received another 200 mgm., and then they made a contract with the Austrian government for one gram to be delivered in 1913. That contract was never fulfilled; the rapidly increasing demands by German and Austrian clinics absorbed the meager Austrian supply.

By 1914, Abbe had acquired 340 mgm. of radium, and Kelly had one gram. Kelly was so enthusiastic about the future of radium therapy that he invested over

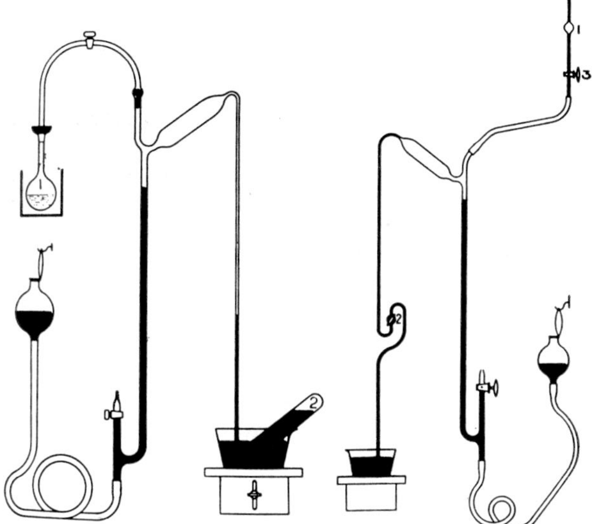

Courtesy: Lea & Febiger.

EARLY EMANATION EXTRACTER. On the left apparatus for pumping off and collecting emanation, on the right a combined pump and device for concentrating the emanation by liquid air (from C. W. Allen's book published by Lea & Brothers in New York City in 1904).

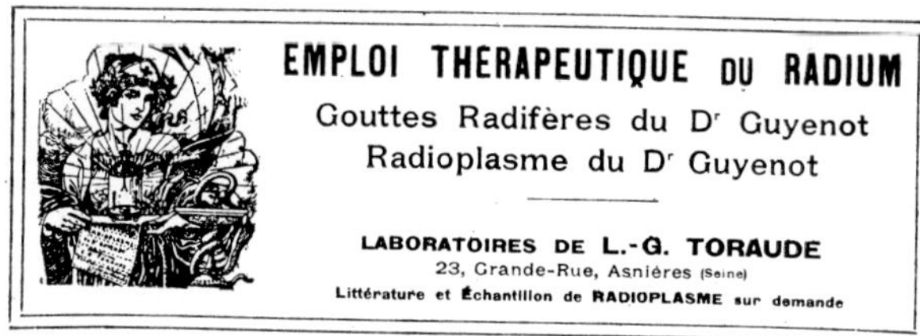

FANCY USE OF RADIUM. Ad of 1917 showing a nurse carrying an electroscope on a platter. The purpose was to sell radium water."

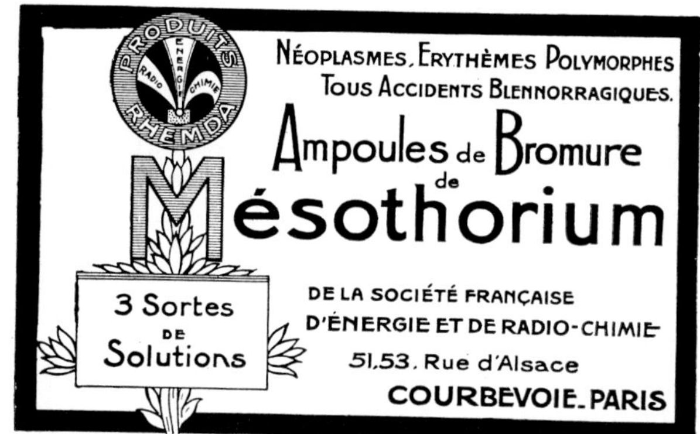

NEISSERIAN ANTIDOTE. Neoplasia, polymorphous erythema, and all gonorrheic accidents are purported as indications for the administration of mesothorium bromide (1920).

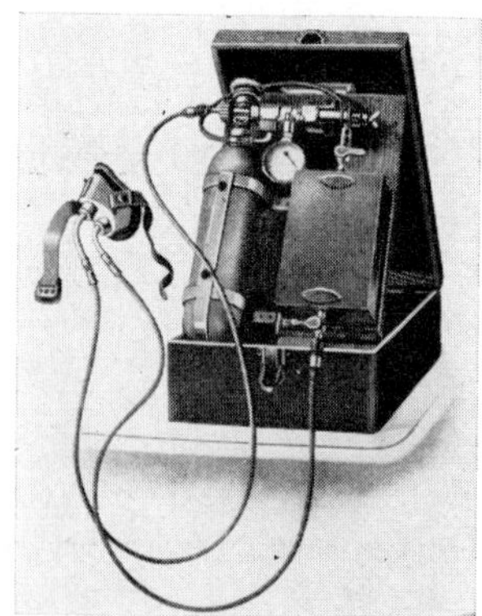

BRITISH EMANATION INHALER. Apparatus for inhalation of radium emanation and oxygen, built and sold by Radium, Ltd. around 1907.

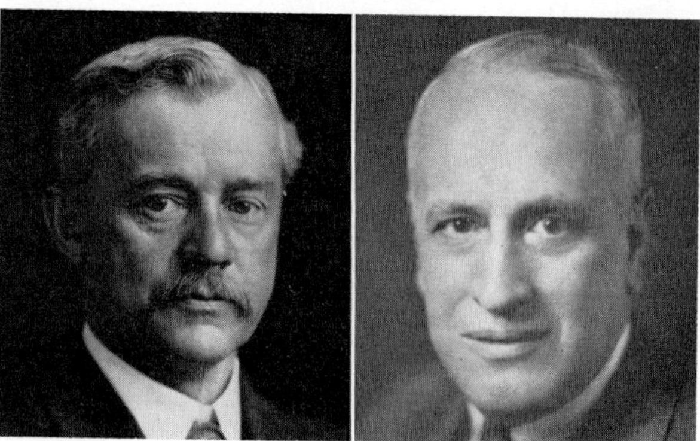

HOWARD KELLY CURTIS F. BURNAM

$500,000 of personal funds in building up USA sources, with the hope of acquiring the estimated minimum five gram needed for a radon plant. At the time radium salts were used also as radioactive waters by mouth, in intravenous injection, and in larger amounts applied for short intervals as plaques.

Kelly's biography was the subject of the Presidential Address of R. W. Te Linde before the American Gynecological Society. It was printed in the *American Journal of Obst. & Gynec.* of November, 1954. Kelly was not only the very famous surgeon who gave freely of his services to the poor, and charged tremendous fees to the rich. Kelly loved nature intensely, and was an excellent swimmer, diver, and canoeist. His interest in mineralogy prompted him to become involved in radium. Kelly was very fond of snakes; there were always several of them running freely in his house. Being deeply religious (and yet religion never interfered with his scientific endeavors – there was an airtight separation between these two in his mind), Kelly spearheaded a campaign to do away with Baltimore's red light district. He strove to rehabilitate "those" women, even invited them to his own home. A prominent British surgeon, while visiting at Kelly's, was placed between two of these girls at the dinner table. During the meal the conversation turned to the snakes that were crawling under the table. One can understand the poor man's feelings, with snakes at his feet, and a harlot at each elbow.

Kelly died in 1943 at 85 years, only a few hours before his wife. All but one of their nine children were present at the double funeral. I corresponded with that ninth child, Edmund Kelly, a physician who practices in Baltimore. He wrote: "I did not return from the war until three years after my father's death, and found that most of his papers I would have kept had already been preempted. Then in 1952 his clinic burned down, at which time all pictures pertaining to the early days were destroyed. My father was very interested in radium, having made the first successful treatment of carcinoma of the cervix uteri in 1904. He gathered a total of about 5½ grams of radium. I am enclosing (for reproduction) a portrait of my father, which shows him in 1914 at the height of his career."

In 1912 Howard Kelly said (in his Presidential Address before the American Gynecological Society): "Accordingly as we remember others so those yet to come will remember us. If we live only for the present and for our own age and reject the past because of imperfections, so in turn will we ourselves as surely be forgotten and despised as the centuries roll over our dust."

In 1916, Kelly got Sir Ernest Rutherford's co-operation for building a radon extraction plant. It was a modification of that devised by William Duane (published in 1915 in the *Physical Review*). Rutherford's technician, Landsbury, brought it to Baltimore and set it up. A former student of Rutherford's, the physicist Fred West, came from Buffalo to take charge of its operation. It was in use continuously until 1959. By that time leaks and increasing stringency of AEC regulations made it necessary to cease its operation. The contaminated apparatus and glassware had a decent sea burial off Hampton Roads (Virginia).

Recent American radon plants are of the semi-automatic variety, developed in the early 1920s by Failla. Kelly once stated that the initial supply of radium for the Memorial Hospital (where Failla made his momentous contributions to radiumology) came from his joint venture with the U. S. Bureau of Mines, at the sale price of one dollar.

The advantages of intracavitary and interstitial applications of radium were recognized from the very

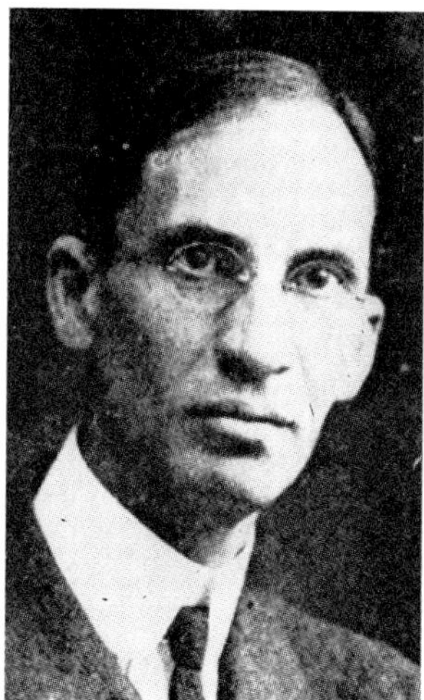

HENRY H. JANEWAY

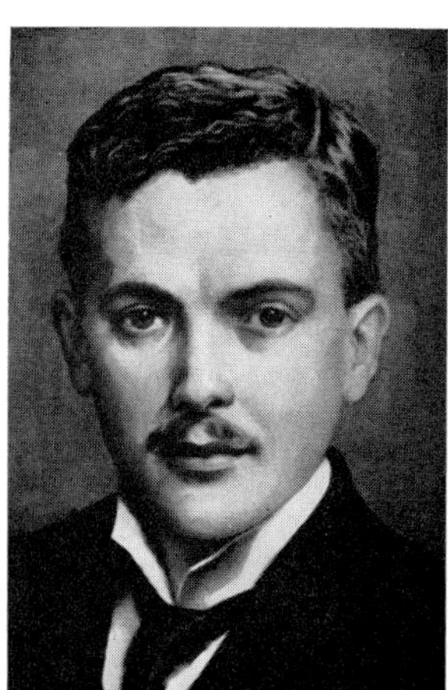

W. C. STEVENSON

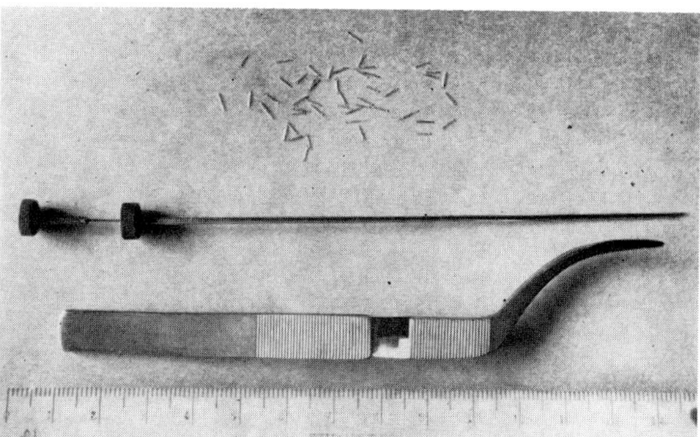

Courtesy: Leonidas Marinelli.

JANEWAY'S "BURIED EMANATION." Glass seeds, containing "emanation" (radon), were inserted into malignant tissues by means of the hollow steel needle and plunger. No attempt was made to remove these seeds, because they became "extinct" after a few weeks. This illustration is from a paper called Radium – The Supreme Marvel of Nature's Storehouse, by G. F. Kunz and G. Failla, published in *Natural History* of May, 1921.

beginning. The short distance, and the rapid fall-off of intensity were turned into assets. The bulky containers of early times were quite satisfactory for intracavitary situations, as in gynecology, but not very satisfactory for direct implantation into tumors.

In 1914, Stevenson and Joly of Dublin (Ireland) developed a method of collecting radon in fine glass tubes, which they then placed in hollow metal needles for insertion into (and later withdrawal from) tumors. With only a few radon plants in operation, this procedure did not become too popular, but it stimulated the production of "radium needles," using pure radium sulfate tightly packed in steel or platinum needles.

In Paris, Dominici had utilized metal tubes to hold his glass tubes of radium salts. In this country Dominici tubes were widely used in gynecologic applications. In 1915, the Harvard radio-biophysicist William Duane (1872-1935) collected emanation in a very fine capillary glass tube, which was then divided into pieces 3 or 4 mm. long. These could be implanted directly into the tumor by means of a small trocar, and allowed to remain there permanently. Radon decayed at the rate of about 16 per cent per day of the amount present; it was effectively gone before the end of one month. The glass, being inert, could be left in place indefinitely.

In 1933, the American Radium Society — through the efforts of its president for that year, Burton James Lee — established a yearly Memorial Lecture, dedicated to the memory of Henry Harrington Janeway (1873-1921), one of the pioneers of radium therapy. Janeway had joined the ARS as a member

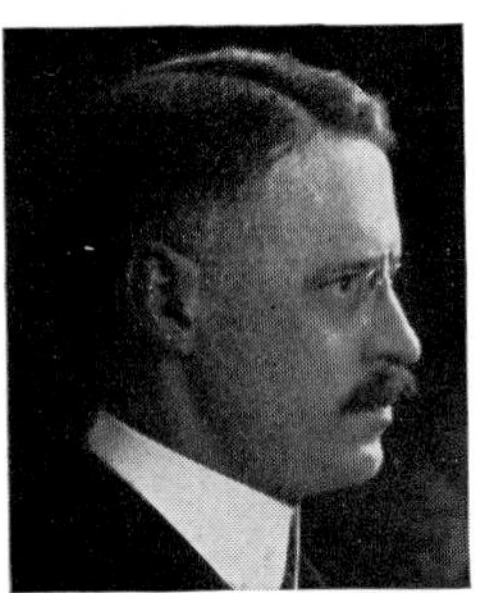

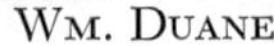

WM. DUANE

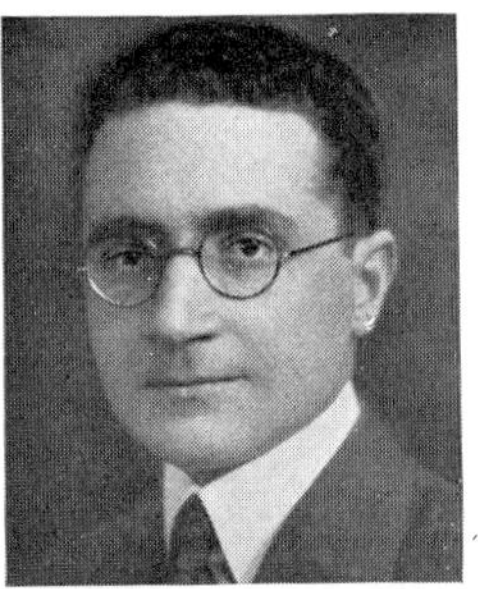

GIOACCHINO FAILLA

To The Credit and Prestige

— of the *SURGEON*

RADIUM Is Being Used To Successfully Treat

The Following Non-Malignant Conditions

GENERAL SURGERY

DEEP LESIONS	SUPERFICIAL LESIONS
HYPERTHYROIDISM	ANGIOMA
LYMPHADENITIS, CHRONIC	PAPILLOMA
HODGKIN'S DISEASE	POLYP
CIRSOID ANEURYSM	NAEVUS
ACROMEGALY	LUPUS VULGARIS
HYPERTROPHIED THYMUS	CONDYLOMA ACCUMINATUM
LEUCAEMIA	TUBERCULOSIS, ULCERATIVE
SPLENOMEGALY	XANTHOMA
SPLENIC ANAEMIA	LEUKOPLAKIA
ARTHRITIS, CHRONIC	BLASTOMYCOSIS
ARTHRITIS DEFORMANS	KELOID
ACTINOMYCOSIS	

Write our Nearest Office

Our complete service includes co-operation with the physician to the end that he may as quickly as possible acquire a first-hand knowledge of the technique and dosage of radium therapeutic application.

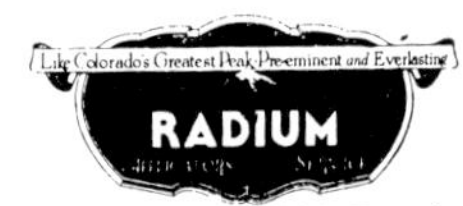

THE RADIUM COMPANY OF COLORADO

PRINCIPAL OFFICES - LABORATORIES

RADIUM BUILDING DENVER, COLORADO

BRANCH OFFICES

SAN FRANCISCO 582 MARKET ST. · CHICAGO PEOPLES GAS BLDG. · NEW YORK 50 UNION SQUARE

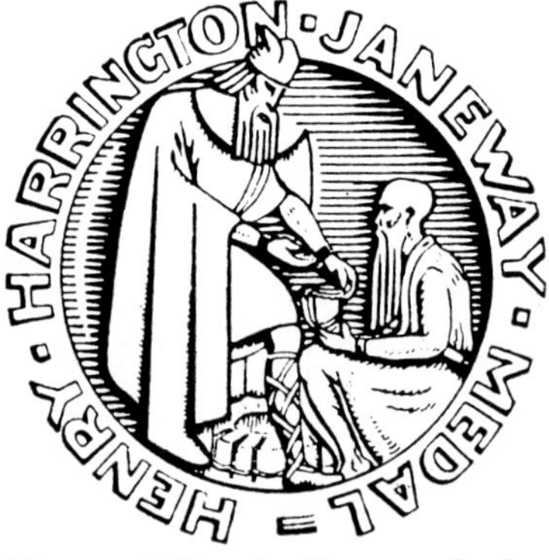

ARS GOLD MEDAL. Odin, the Norse god who had power over precious minerals, is seen giving one of his eyes to the sitting giant Mimir in pawn for a cup of the water of wit and wisdom. This symbolizes the physical sacrifice of radiation-damaged pioneers. The reverse of the medal shows Odin's two ravens, Hugin (thought) and Munin (memory), flying around in daylight so that in the evening they could perch on Odin's shoulders and tell him what was going on in the world. The encircled drawing of these two extra-special news services serves also as the mandala of the ARS.

Results obtained in Tubercular adenitis with radium justify the assertion that this condition may be controlled without surgical interference.

RADIUM CHEMICAL CO.
PITTSBURGH, PA.
NEW YORK BOSTON CHICAGO

in 1917, shortly before the publication of his book (with Benjamin S. Barringer and Gioacchino Failla): in that book he detailed their experiences at the Memorial Hospital with the treatment of oral cancer by using "buried emanation" (glass radon seeds permanently imbedded in tumor tissue).

The Curies had observed that there were three types of "radiation" emitted by radium, but their nature was understood only later. Lord Rutherford at the Cavendish Laboratory in Cambridge identified before 1899 the two types of "radium rays" called alpha and beta. Almost immediately afterwards, Villard in Paris discovered the gamma rays, and before the turn of the century most of the characteristics and properties of these three types of energy emission had been studied.

Some of these "rays" were more penetrating, others could be stopped by paper or by thin sheets of metal. Among those which were non-penetrating, one type was only slightly deviated by a magnet, and those were called alpha-rays. The non-penetrating variety susceptible to magnetic deviation received the name of beta rays. Finally, there were the highly penetrating gamma rays. Today instead of alpha rays we speak of alpha particles or helium nuclei, while the term electrons appears preferable to beta rays.

Duane had intended to utilize beta rays in his glass tubes. When Janeway "buried" emanation glass tubes into the tumor he obtained very good results but there was intense necrosis produced around each seed by

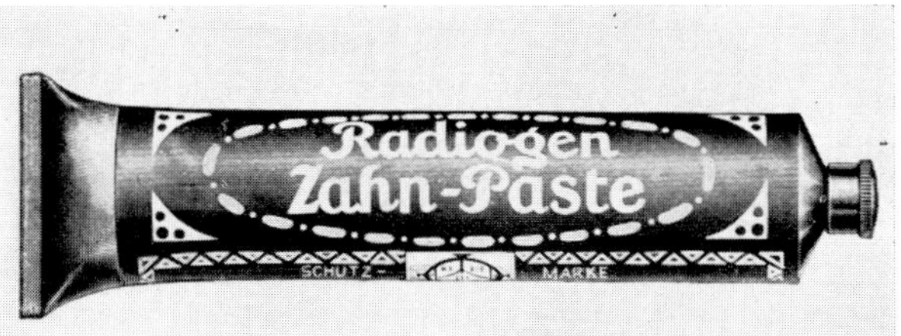

Courtesy: Charles W. Smith.

RADON TOOTHPASTE. This brand was marketed around 1920 by the Allgemeine Radiogen-A.G. of Berlin. It contained radium, and would release emanation as the teeth were brushed. Activity was allegedly constant. It was said to reduce the decomposition of alimentary residues, and thus prevent the deposition of "dental stone."

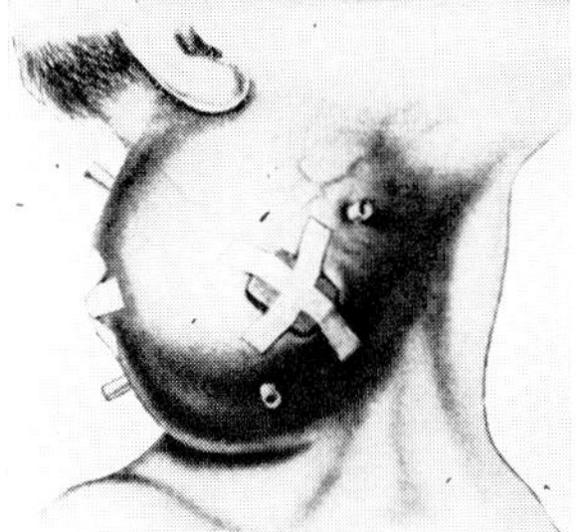

Courtesy: Baillière & Co.

INTRATUMORAL IRRADIATION. This picture is from Wickham & Desgrais' *Radiumthérapie,* published by J. B. Baillière in Paris in 1909.

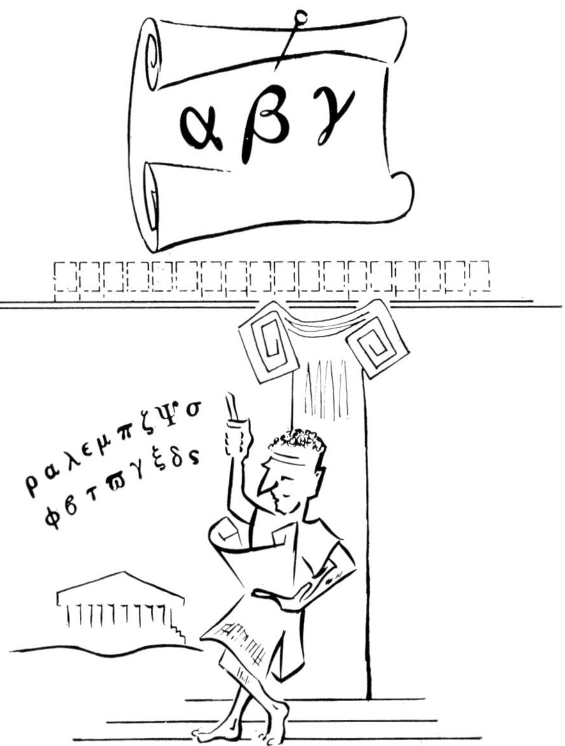

Courtesy: Robert Sulit's PORACC.

THERE IS A GREEK WORD (OR LETTER) FOR IT. The metaphysic bases of the atomistic theory were proposed by Leucippus (5th century B.C.), and developed by the "laughing philosopher" from Abdera, Democritus (4th century B.C.). The two rows of letters are subatomic particles.

Francis H. Williams

Zoe A. Johnston

E. T. Leddy

Harry H Bowing

Rutherford

Hugh H. Young

W. D. Coolidge

B. S. Barringer

A. H. Pirie

Clarence F. Ball

Howard A Kelly

Edwin C. Ernst

Albert Soiland

James T Case

George T Pack

Henry Schmitz

Douglas Quick

William S. Stone

James J. Duffy

Rollin H Stevens

William T Watson

Burton J Lee

Norman Treves

Curtis F Burnam

G. Allen Robinson

G. Failla

James Ewing

Sanford Withers

Herman L. Kretschmer

Bernard H Schreiner

Isaac Levin

Frank E Adair

Chas L Martin

Orville N. Upland

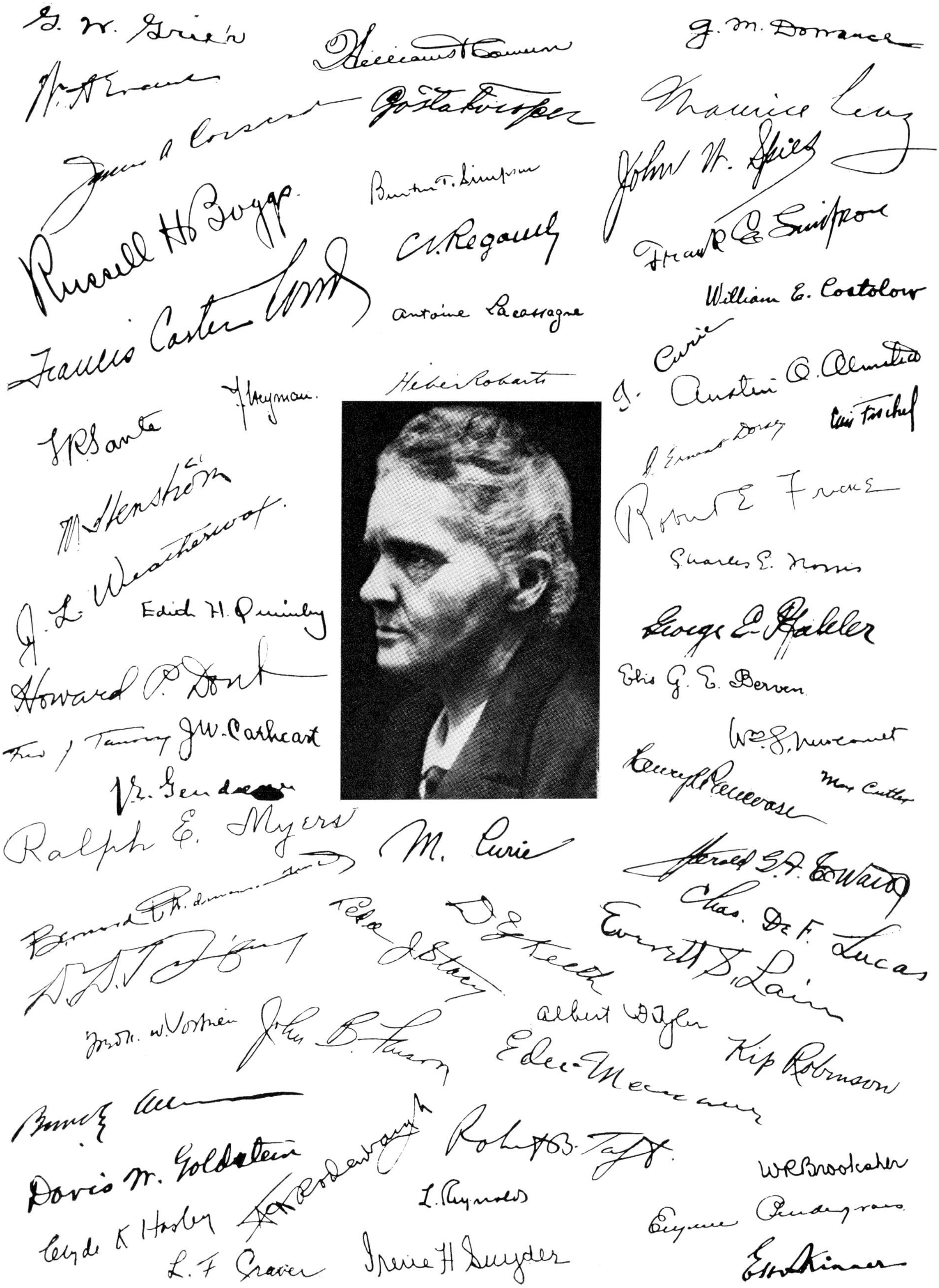

the beta rays. This caused severe pain for a considerable time. Contrary to Duane's idea, the gamma rays were those which gave therapeutic benefit. In France and England beta rays were filtered out with small platinum needles, but these had to be removed at the end of the procedure (because they contained radium).

Arthur Heublein, a physician from Hartford (Connecticut) wanted to place the glass needle in the tumor and then cover it with bismuth paste. The idea was very good but the method was much too difficult and unreliable.

Failla (Janeway's physicist) decided to develop a filtered seed. After trying various schemes (including lead glass) he had the idea of using pure gold capillary tubing, which was very soft and self-sealing when cut with dull pliers. The gold seeds were immediately adopted by many radiotherapists, and are still widely used.

Improvement in the clinical use of radium has always been the result of cooperation between physicians and physicists. French physicians were helped by the Curies and Becquerel, English physicians by Rutherford and Soddy. In this country Duane, later Failla and his group at the Memorial Hospital in New York City, Weatherwax at the Philadelphia General Hospital, Glasser at Cleveland Clinic, and Stenstrom at the State Institute in Buffalo, have provided significant contributions. Among the clinicians, aside from Janeway, and Abbe and Kelly before him, Barringer, Bailey, Quick, and Stone should be mentioned at Memorial Hospital, Leddy and Widmann in Philadelphia, Portmann at the Cleveland Clinic, and Gaylord and Schreiner in Buffalo. A truly representative list would be much longer, because Pancoast, Pfahler, Clark, Bowing, Withers, Grier, and so many others are just as entitled to at least a cursory mention.

In institutions with small amounts of radium and no radon plant, interstitial needles were employed to a larger extent. In this country the needles available until quite recently were rather strong. In England and France comparatively much weaker needles were used. An American pioneer in low intensity needles was Charles Martin from Texas. Lately, in the USA most hospital radon plants have been abandoned, the radium was put into tubes and low intensity needles, while commercial suppliers provide radon seeds whenever needed.

Quimby believes that gynecologic treatment still accounts for the greatest radium use in this country. Several systems of intrauterine radium distribution have been worked out, here and abroad, for instance the Manchester, Paris, and Stockholm techniques. Edwin Ernst from St. Louis has been particularly persistent and successful in perfecting a satisfactory applicator for this purpose.

The Janeway Memorial Lecture has brought many significant historic contributions from the medalists selected. The very first one, the oncologist James Ewing (1923), and the previously mentioned Curtis Burnam (1936) discussed early experiences with radiation therapy. Henry Schmitz (1938) and Frederick

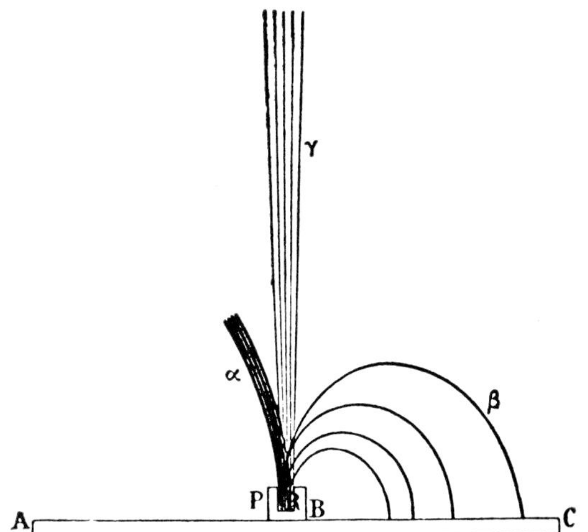

ALPHA, BETA, AND GAMMA. This representation goes back to around 1900, perhaps to the Curies. It is herein reproduced from Cleaves' *Light Energy* (1904). P is a lead block which contains radium, AC a photographic plate, and a uniform magnetic field is established around the receptacle P. Alpha particles are helium nuclei, beta "rays" are electrons, and gamma rays are today regarded as electro-magnetic radiation.

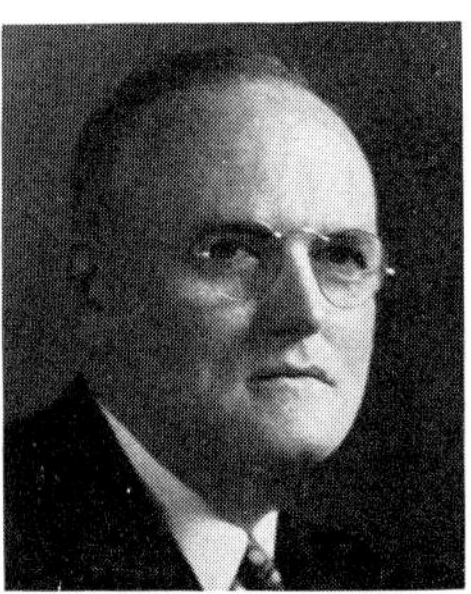

JAMES WEATHERWAX

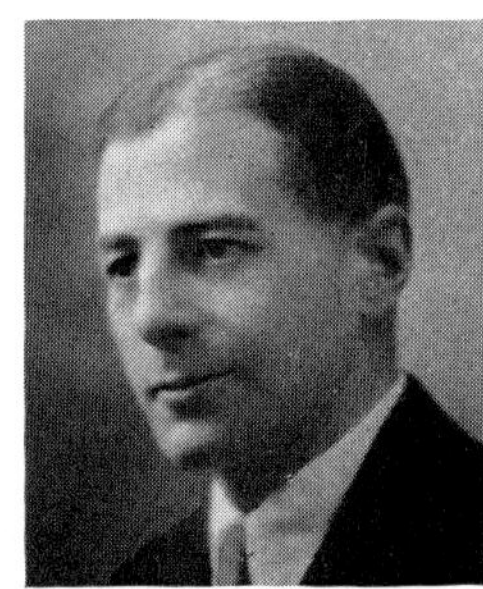

WM. STENSTROM

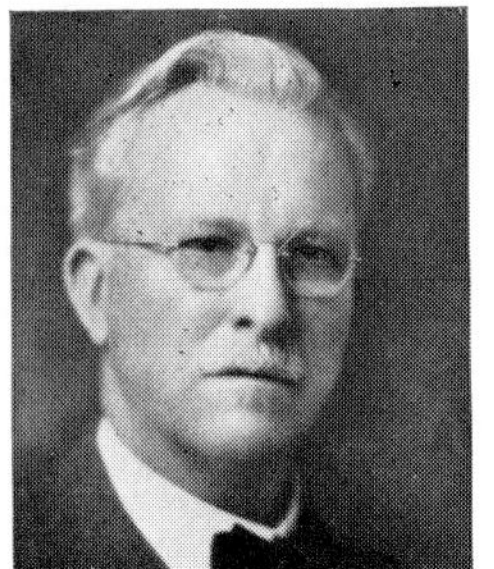

JAMES MARTIN

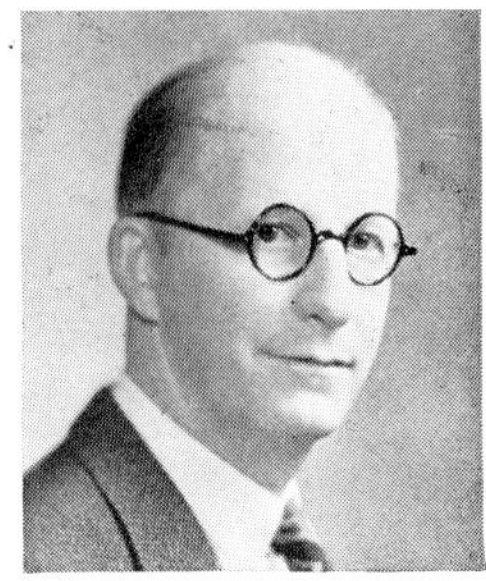

CHARLES L. MARTIN

O'Brien, Sr. (1946) presented retrospective reviews of the treatment of carcinoma of the cervix.

I received from the Radium Chemical Company (New York City) two pages with signatures, surrounding the portraits of Janeway and Curie. The only reference in their files called it the "Janeway-Curie" banquet. The signatures are a representative sample of the best known names in American radiology, with a few notable foreigners to boot. The disparity in ages made it impossible for all these people to have met at a dinner – after all Janeway died in 1921. I asked Howard Doub (who is the historian of the RSNA) and this is what he replied: "These signature pages were given out at the banquet of the ARS in Kansas City (Missouri), in 1936 by Edward Skinner, who was chairman of the local committee. I am absolutely sure that I did not sign my name to anything having these two photographs. Ed Skinner wrote and asked if I would send him my signature on a piece of white paper. I am sure he did that to all the other people and then randomized the signatures and reproduced the pages for that meeting." Even so, it is invaluable for the historian, which is why I reproduced it – for "safe-keeping."

Université de Paris

Institut du Radium

1, rue Pierre Curie. Paris V.

Téléphone { Pavillon Curie – Gobelins 14.69
Pavillon Pasteur – Gobelins 45.75

Feuille d'applications pour le tube d'Émanation du Radium N° 18/D contenant 55,2 millicuries le 20 Mars 1919 à 16 H dans l'étui-filtre n° 13 en or d'épaisseur 1 m/m

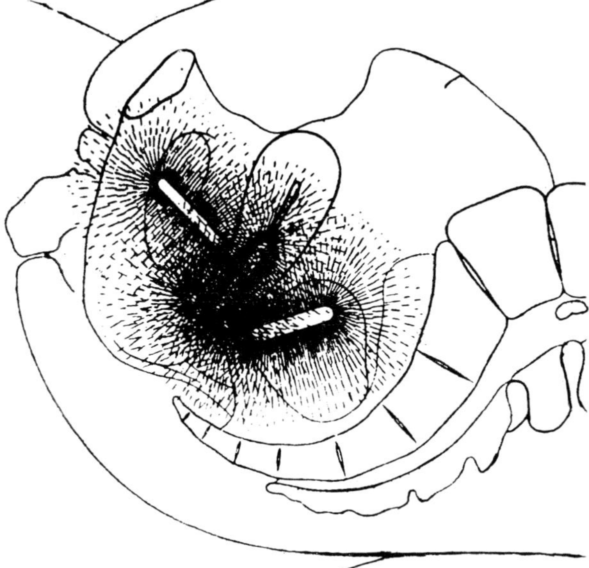

Courtesy: *Journal de Radiologie et d'Electrologie and Masson & Cie.*

EARLY BELGIAN RADIUM APPLICATION. This drawing appeared in a paper by P. de Backer (of the University of Gand) published in January, 1923. It shows radium tubes inserted in the vagina, in the rectum, in the urinary bladder, and in the uterine os, all for a carcinoma of the cervix. This is how experience in necrotizing dosages was gained before we arrived at today's well established techniques.

In 1910, the surgeon John Berg founded the Radiumhemmet of Stockholm with sixteen beds, a single x-ray machine and 120 mg. of radium. A radium center had been established at Trieste in 1904, while in 1903 (according to the London *Lancet* of November 14, 1903) a quantity of "pure radium" had been given to the Cancer Hospital on Fulham Road in London. Since then various institutes, devoted (mainly) to radium therapy, were developed from Paris to Belo Horizonte (Brazil), from the Charite in Berlin to San Sebastian in Spain, and from the Holt Institute in Manchester to the one in Queensland (Australia).

Both radium and radium therapy were "born" in Paris. In 1901, Danlos and Block used radium for the treatment of lupus at Hôpital St. Louis. Wickham and Degrais opened their Laboratory in 1906 and, soon thereafter, Wickham first employed *filters* with radium to modify the dosage in the deeper tissues: to make a filter he wrapped cotton wood in goldbeater's skin and in layers of aluminum. Wickham also originated crossfiring in radium (he treated sciatic pain in this manner in 1905). Perthes had employed crossfiring with roentgen rays in 1904.

The Institute of Radium in Paris was proposed in 1909 but did not open until a few months before the outbreak of World War I. No work was done from 1914 to 1918. During the war, Regaud recruited Coutard, Lacassagne, Roux-Berger, Monod, and Pierquin, who

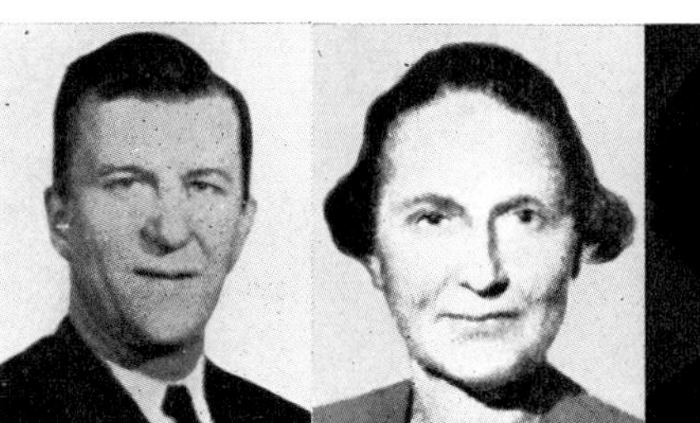

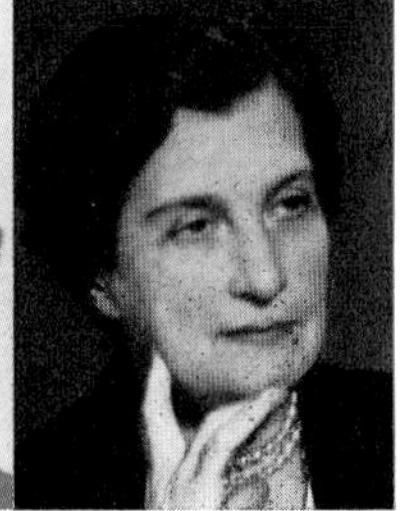

BERNARD PIERQUIN JULIETTE BAUD SIMONE LABORDE

became the nucleus of the Institute. There were trainees even before that time; for instance, William Duane had been the assistant of Pierre Curie (until the latter died in a traffic accident in 1906), and then Duane became the assistant of Marie Curie until 1913. Several of the students who had come to Paris from foreign lands made contributions to the development of radium therapy. Alfonso Esguerra Gomez from Bogotá was assigned to find a paste that could be molded to the shape of the patient's face in order to support the radium sources at fixed distances from the skin. He came up with a mixture of paraffin, beeswax, and sawdust which Regaud called "pâte Colombia." Juan Angel del Regato worked with Regaud as they attempted in 1933 to use (rather unsuccessfully) radium packs. Regato is now a famous radio-oncologist, while Alfonso teaches physiology in Cali (Colombia).

Jimmy Case related the following anecdote: Regaud and Lacassagne used to bicycle to the hospitals in Paris with a lead box containing those few milligrams of radium which they used to perfect the technics now universally adopted. Regaud usually had a return ride offered him by one of the professors, while Lacassagne bicycled back to the Institute of Radium pulling Regaud's bicycle by the hand to have it ready for the next expedition.

In 1911 in London, Finzi assembled for a millionaire patient an applicator containing over 600 mg. of radium. In 1914, Cameron prepared, for the treatment of a carcinoma of the breast, a pack containing 1020 mg. of radium in tubes of varying amounts applied at a distance of 5.5 cm. from the skin, screened with 0.5 mm. silver and 1.0 mm. brass. Therefore a radium surface pack was considered to mean one to four grams of radium element (or its equivalent in radon), divided into 50 or 100 mgm. tubes, arranged in a somewhat regular form, at times circular. The Mallet-Coliez apparatus consisted of three sources, supported by a semicircular frame. Multiple, concentrically distributed units made up the ceiling-suspended Sluys-Kessler apparatus. The entire amount of radium was placed in one container, at a distance of 3-10 cm. from the skin, by Regaud and Ferroux, who also coined the term telecurietherapy. Simone Laborde's apparatus, suspended from a ceiling rail, was the forerunner of today's cobalt units. Failla's design for teleradium appplication was similar to Laborde's, but the container could be positioned over either of two tables, separated by heavy lead shielding, so that the next "customer" was being set up, while the previous one was being treated. All such machines were home-made, as those of Forssell

Les Laboratoires
BRUNEAU et Cie
17 Rue de Berri
Paris VIIIe
Tel-Elysées 61-46 / 61-47

Appareils plastiques de Curiethérapie
PATE COLOMBIA
FORMULE DE L'INSTITUT DU RADIUM DE L'UNIVERSITÉ DE PARIS
Appareils plastiques moulés — Plaques rectangulaires
Plaques d'éloignement et tous accessoires

Traitements postradiothérapiques
PAREMANOL BRUNEAU
Radioépidermites — Radiodermites
Echantillons et Littérature sur demande

R. C. Seine 31.381.

THE AMERICAN JOURNAL OF ROENTGENOLOGY
Editor, H. M. Imboden, M.D., New York

VOL. VIII (NEW SERIES) APRIL, 1921 No. 4

THE INTRALARYNGEAL APPLICATION OF RADIRM FOR CHRONIC PAPILLOMATA*
By PRESTON M. HICKEY, M.D., F.A.C.P., F.A.C.S.
DETROIT, MICHIGAN

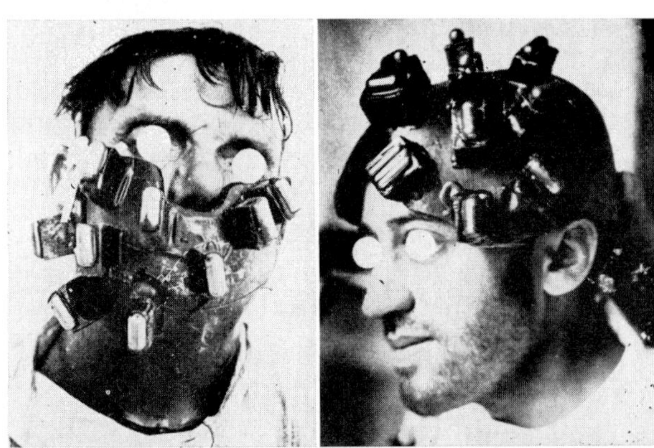

Courtesy: Radium Chemical Company.

Radium surface packs. Cervico-mandibular wax mould with imbedded radium containers, and helmet applicator for intracranial tumor.

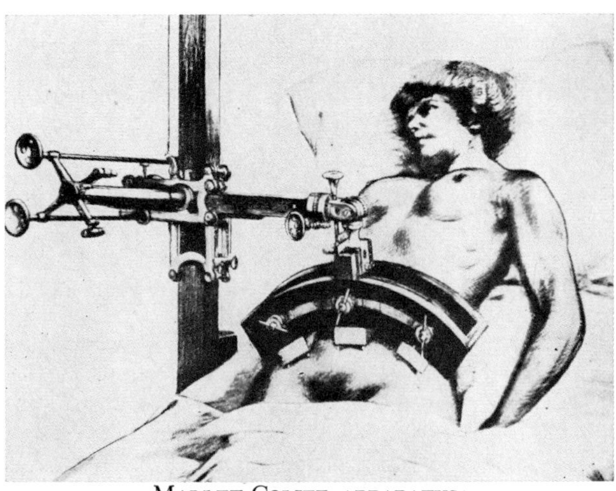

Mallet-Coliez apparatus.

and Berven in Stockholm, Max Cutler in Chicago, or Albert Soiland in Los Angeles.

At the Roosevelt Hospital in New York City, Douglas Quick accumulated interesting clinical experience with a super-radium bomb of fifty grams (distributed on a special multi-source unit, devised by Failla). All these were dwarfed (and therefore superseded) by the advent of teletherapy units using radioactive isotopes.

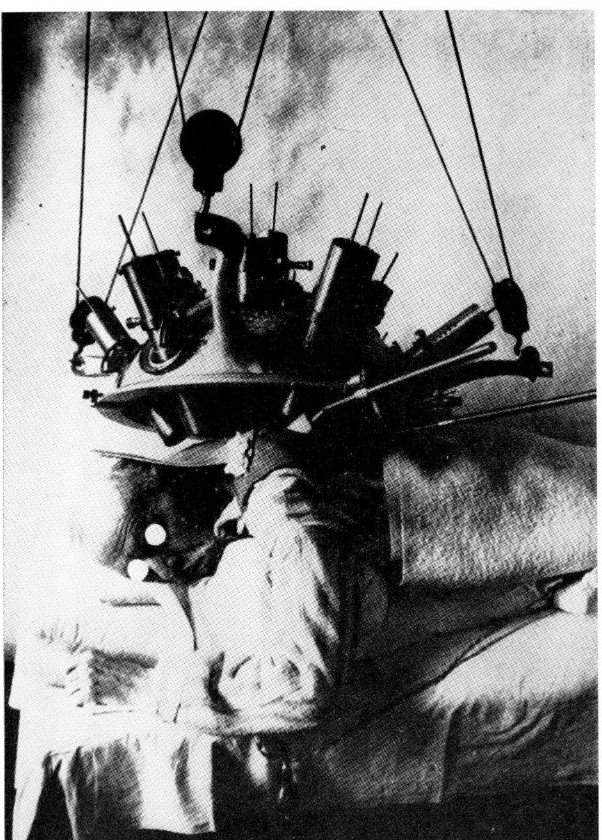

SLUYS-KESSLER APPARATUS.

The Golden Age of Radium Therapy arrived only after the establishment of methods by which dosage could be calculated and duplicated with some degree of accuracy.

The first international radium standard had been prepared by Marie Curie after the Austrians made one for their own consumption. The determination of dose of radium radiation in terms of roentgens was more difficult. Today it is accepted that a point source of radium, filtered by 0.5 millimeter of platinum, delivers 8.4 roentgens per hour at a distance of one centimeter. Due to the very penetrating nature of the secondary rays from a radium source, the standard ionization chambers which had been developed for 200 kvp roentgen rays were unsuitable. Calibrated thimble chambers gave discordant results. It became evident that the basic measurements ought to be made in very large open spaces. Failla and Marinelli (at Memorial Hospital in New York City) and Friedrich (at the University of Berlin) studied this problem. Friedrich finally made use of an armory 100 x 50 x 22 meters in size to achieve unequivocal results. After determining the necessary amount of air, it was evident that the same result should be obtained with the same amount of compressed air. Pressure chambers up to 50 atmospheres were tested, and they gave satisfactory results. The final step was to replace air by an "air-equi-

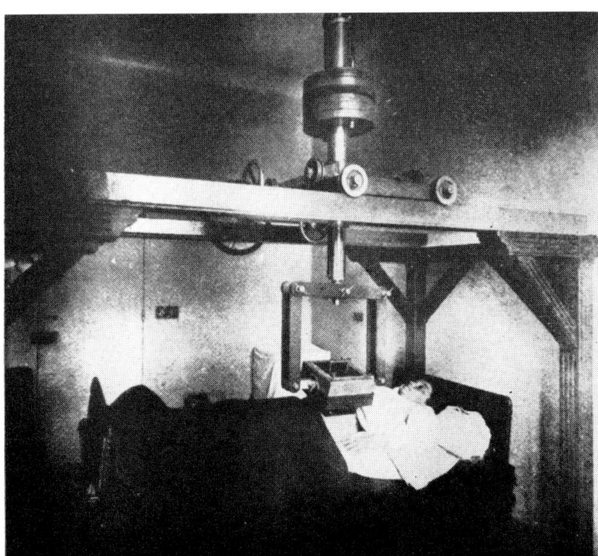

REGAUD-FERROUX APPARATUS.

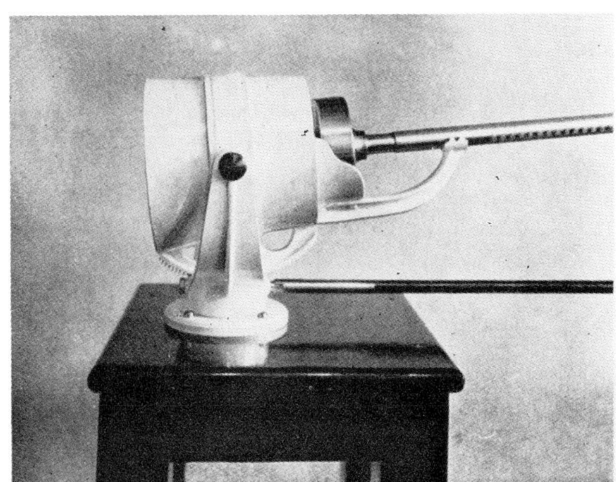

RUSS 2.5 GM RADIUM RECEPTACLE (1922). Marshall Brucer told me that after World War I, in England, Sidney Russ collected the radium accumulated by the Royal Air Force (presumably for use on instrument faces), and combined it into a potent irradiator. This illustration is from one of Brucer's slides, left at Oak Ridge (Tennessee).

valent" solid, and use a sufficient thickness of this to make thimble-type chambers.

Knowing the output of one milligram of radium, it is possible to calculate the expected radiation from a given radium content, taking in consideration the geometrical size and shape of the source, and its filtration. The study of distribution of radiation within the tissues for a particular distribution of sources is much simpler than if large series of measurements had to be made in suitable phantoms with adequate ionization chambers. In fact, the latter would be an almost impossible procedure.

Even before the actual output of a radium source in roentgens had been established, Edith Hinckley Quimby started a long series of studies on relative amounts of radiation delivered at different points by groups of radium sources. The relative numbers were readily converted to roentgens when a standard value became available. These studies had been carried out first at Memorial Hospital in New York City, and later at the College of Physicians and Surgeons. This was Quimby's most lasting contribution, and for this she was elected to give the Janeway Lecture in 1940: her

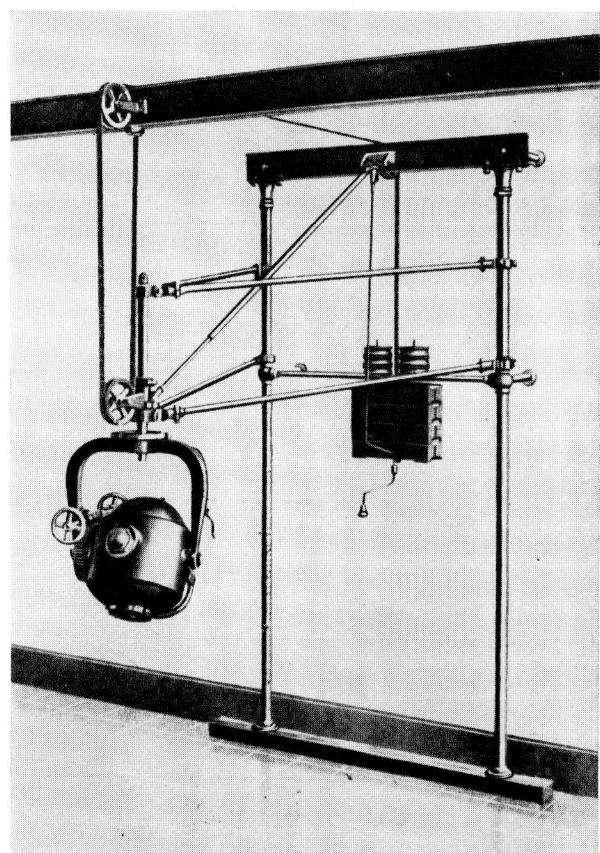

Courtesy: *Radium Belge.*

SIMONE LABORDE APPARATUS. The resemblance with a deca-curie Cobalt unit is striking.

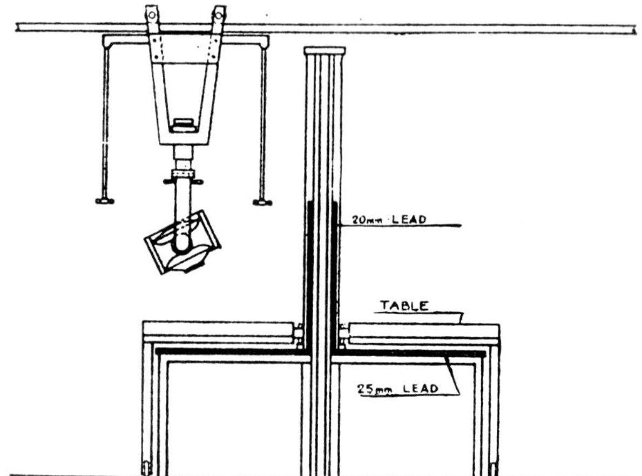

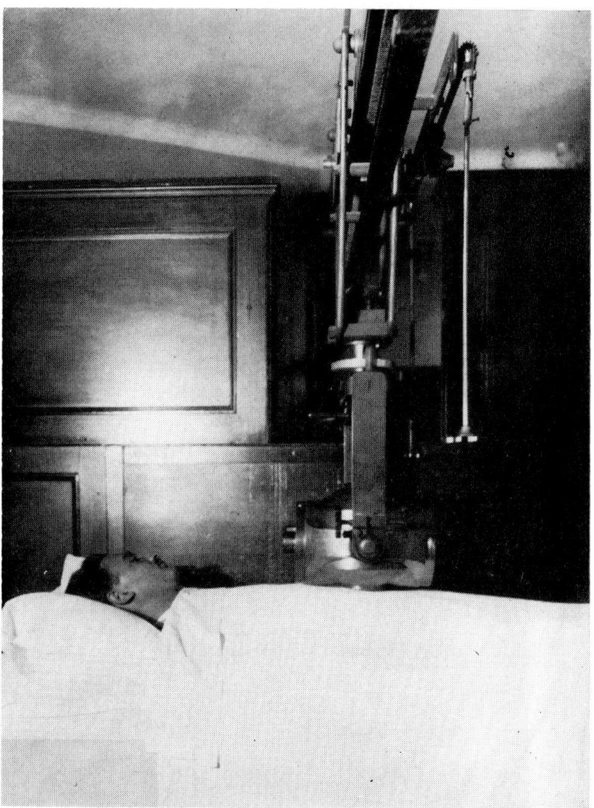

Courtesy: *Leonidas Marinelli*

FAILLA'S 4 GRAM RADIUM PACK. Two adjoining rooms at Memorial Hospital in New York City were separated by a heavily leaded wall. Failla's pack was unique as regards the large thickness of protective lead, the device for "turning off" the radiation beam while the pack was being adjusted, the method of raising and lowering the heavy container, and the provision of two adjacent rooms in which the pack could be used alternately. It was described in the *American Journal of Roentgenology* of August, 1928. Incidentally, the term radium pack was coined by Janeway around 1914.

subject was *Specifications of Dosage in Radium Therapy*. It may be mentioned that Paterson and Parker at Manchester (England) developed a system of dosage determination which came into widespread use. Important contributions to the development of radium therapy were also made by Sir Stanford Cade in England, Stevenson in Ireland, James Heyman in Sweden, Paul Lazarus in Switzerland, M. A. Bioglio in Italy, P. G. Mesernitsky in Russia, F. Gudzent in Germany, and Harry H. Bowing and Robert E. Fricke in this country.

The hazards related to the handling of radium became known at an early date. When Burnam went to Vienna to bring 200 mg., he carried for a few hours that amount of radium in a thin lead wrapping in his overcoat pocket. Within twenty-four hours he developed acute nausea: the subsequent skin "burn" took weeks to heal. By that time fifty-four cases of malignant tumors due to roentgen rays had been reported, and it soon became evident that radium rays were just as dangerous. Viol, the chief-chemist of the Standard Chemical Co., died of radiation-induced malignancy.

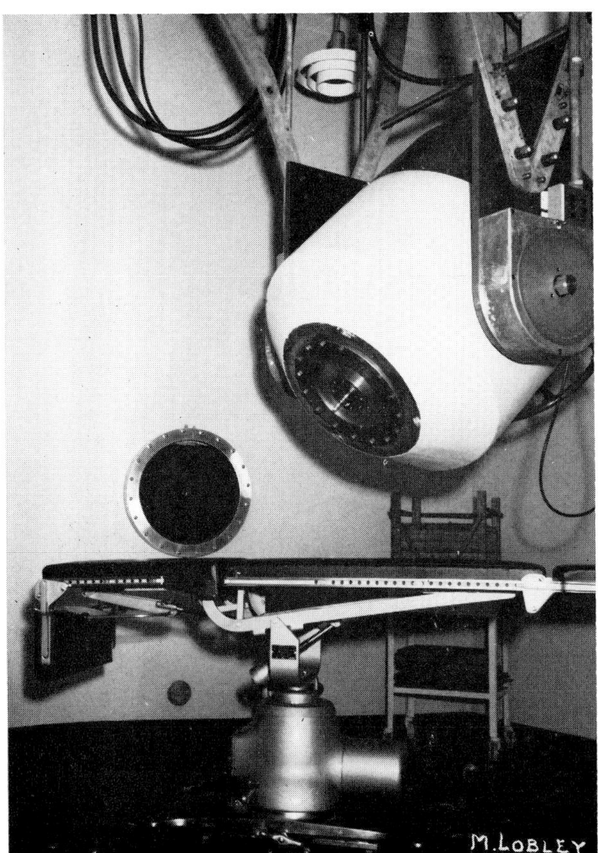

Courtesy: Patricia Failla.

FAILLA'S 50 GRAM RADIUM-BOMB. It was designed and built for Douglas Quick at the Roosevelt Hospital in New York City, for the Henry H. Janeway Clinic for Therapeutic Radiology.

There have been fairly numerous similar instances in both medical and technical personnel. There have been also cases of profound and sometimes fatal anemia:

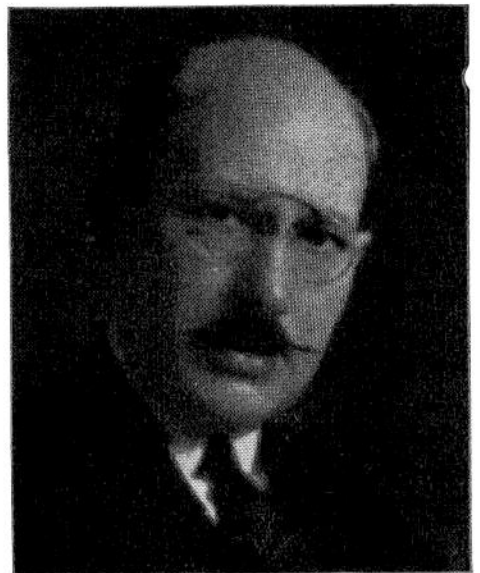

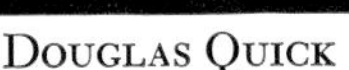

DOUGLAS QUICK

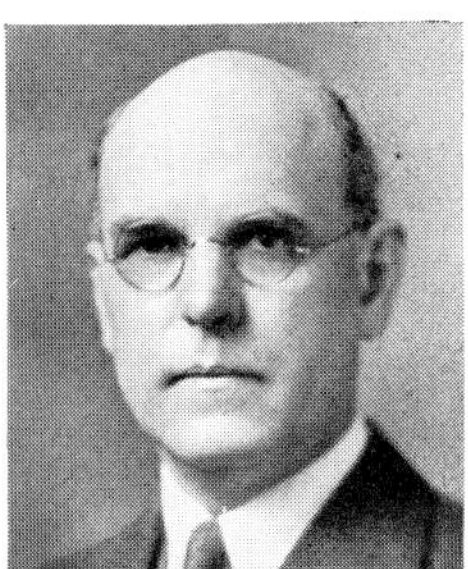

HARRY BOWING

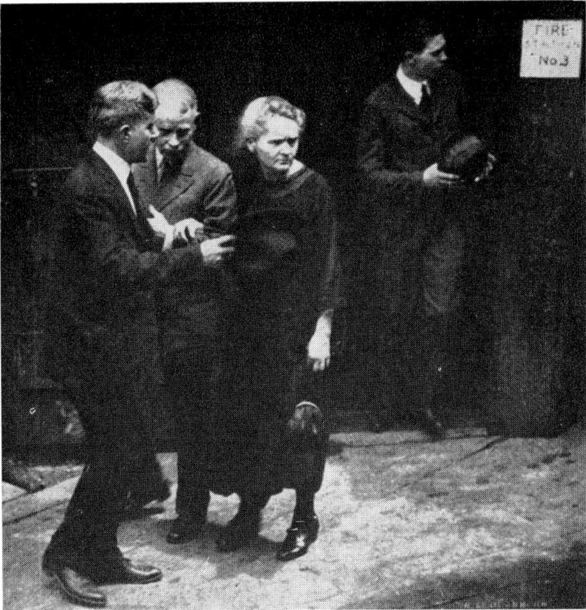

Courtesy: James Ernest Breed.

MARIE CURIE'S AMERICAN GRAM OF RADIUM. Mrs. Meloney, editor of the *Delineator* (New York) conceived the idea of launching a collection for one gram of radium, to be offered to Mme Curie. For that purpose, Marie Curie visited the United States, with stops in Pittsburgh, Chicago, the Grand Canyon, and Washington (D.C.), where President Harding – in behalf of the women of the U. S. A. – presented her the gram of radium on May 20, 1921. The gram of radium (purchased from the Standard Chemical Company for $120 thousand) came in a lead safe, with a golden key. The photograph shows Mme Curie inspecting the extraction plant of the Standard Chemical Company in Canonsburg (20 miles southwest of Pittsburgh). She holds the arm of James Gray (a lawyer who was then president of the Standard Chemical Co.), while L. F. Vogt, the plant manager, offers explanations. The unidentified gent coming out of the plant must have been a football player.

GUSTAVE LOREY, PHOTOGRAPHER.
20TH ANNUAL MEETING
THE AM. ROENTGEN RAY SOC'Y.
SARATOGA SPRINGS, N.Y.
SEPT. 3RD TO 6TH 1919

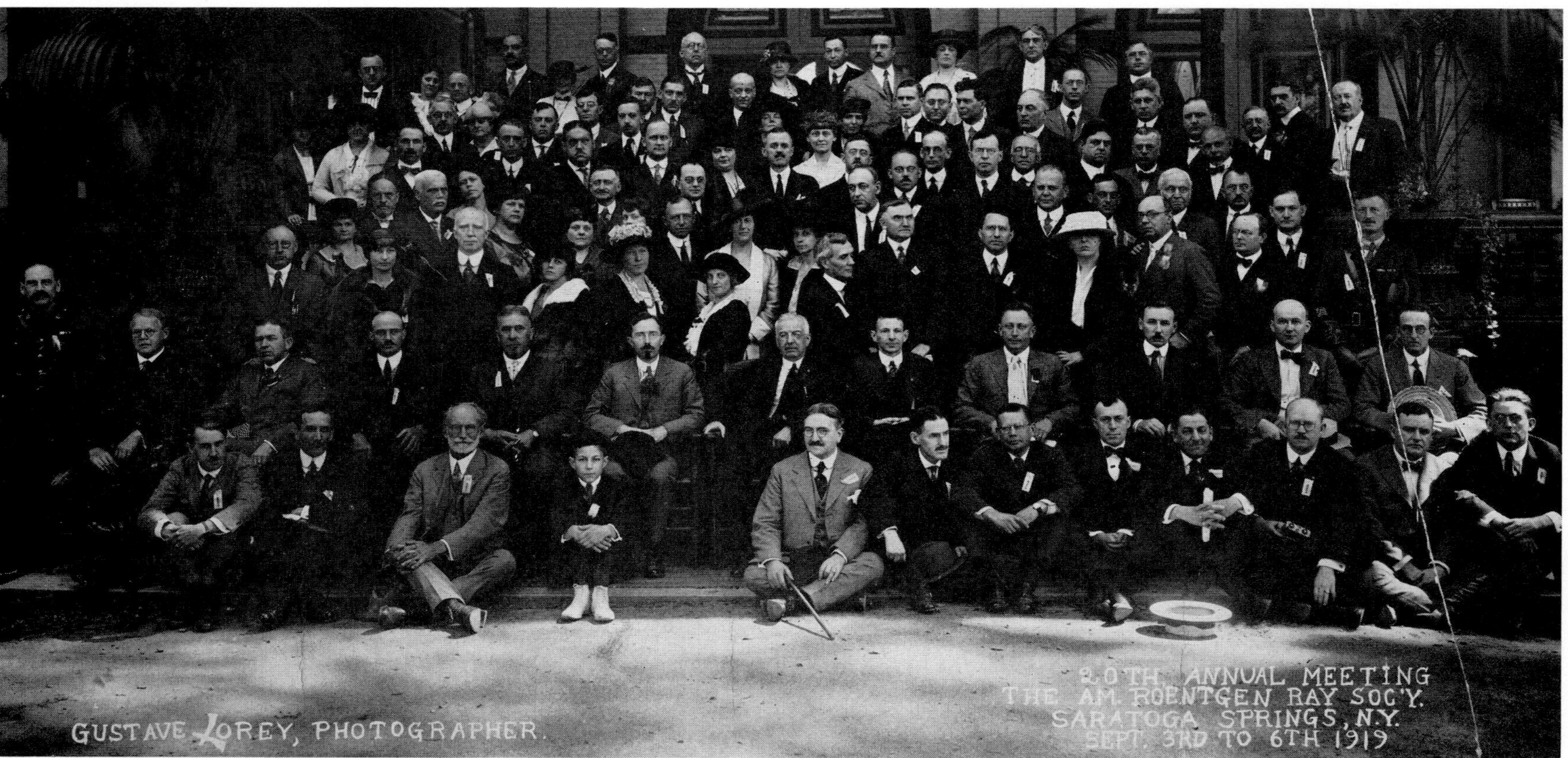

Courtesy: Mrs. Emma Brady.

ARRS IN SARATOGA SPRINGS (1919). The original picture had been given to me by the widow of George Brady, and many of the participants were identified by two other x-ray widows, Mrs. Wm. H. Stewart and Mrs. Eugene W. Caldwell. This was a very important meeting, and both Orndoff and Percy Brown attended it, but are not in the photograph. In the front row, the third from the left is white-bearded Augustus Crane. In symmetrical position (third from the right) is James Case. Right behind Case sits Imboden. In that same second row, two seats from Imboden is white-tied Albert Soiland, next to a very young-looking Coolidge. Still in the second row, the second from left is Pancoast, the fourth is Hollis Potter, the sixth is Grier. In the third row, third from the left is white-haired George Pfahler with his wife (they were married in 1918). In the same third row, standing at the extreme right is uniformed Pirie, while the fourth from the right is baldy, bespectacled Preston Hickey; in the same row, further to the left is Manges, flanked by six women. Balding, gray-haired, and goateed Lewis Gregory Cole is seen in the fifth row, extreme right. In the last row, white-dressed Mrs. Stewart stands between her mustachioed husband and white-tied Fred Law. The hirsute head of Rollin Stevens projects over Mrs. Stewart's left arm. Hickey is between Jaches and white-hatted Yon Poswik. Shearer (with walking stick) sits in mid front row.

thus there is little doubt that Madame Curie's long illness and death could be attributed largely to the radium with which she worked so long.

The radium dial painters of the 1920s were the first group of people chronically exposed to potentially lethal doses of radioactivity. The idea to make instrument faces visible in the dark by painting them with a radium or thorium compound originated with Austrian-born Sabin A. von Sohocky (1882-1926), who received medical training in Moscow, then spent wartime in Germany. This is why the procedure was first used on German submarines during World War I.

After the war von Sohocky came to this country, and became the technical director and eventually the president of the U. S. Radium Corporation. The firm began to produce luminous watch dials. The actual painting of the dials was done by female employees, who applied the substance with fine brushes. To keep the brushes well pointed, the girls used to moisten the brushes with their lips. Most of the thus ingested bone-seeking radium never left their bodies, and soon the mortality rate among these dial painters reached unusual proportions. The plant was located in Orange (New Jersey), and Harrison Martland, the medical examiner for Essex County became suspicious. Then, in 1924, he read in an article by Theodor Blum (in the *Journal of the American Dental Association*) a footnote about "radium jaw," the osteomyelitis caused by ingestion of radium.

Harrison Martland spent twenty years in studying the radium dial painters. Some of his papers on the subject are classics, such as those in the *JAMA* of February 9, 1929 and in the *American Journal of Cancer* of October, 1931. His endeavors are being continued by several groups of investigators, under AEC grants. Estimates of the total number of "radium ingestors" exceed one thousand individuals. As it happened, Harrison Martland was the attending physician of von Sohocky, and signed the latter's certificate of death – from aplastic anemia due to the accumulation of radium in the deceased's body.

Much more common than fatalities have been fingers damaged from carelessness or foolhardiness in handling tubes and needles, preparing applicators, and making implantations. It had been said that in most radium procedures over-exposure is inevitable, but detailed monitoring of careful operations has shown that this is seldom the case.

Failla became concerned with radiation safety, and devoted much time and thought to development of adequate storage safes, shielded handling tools, remote-controlled operations, and general good practice. At present there are well protected radium preparation rooms in most hospitals in this country. A very ingenious storage case was built in concrete by Landauer for the Radiation Department in Cook County Hospital in Chicago. It must be realized though, that no amount of good equipment can compensate for carelessness or ignorance.

During the third meeting of the ARS, at the Palmer House in Chicago, on June 10, 1918, the decision was

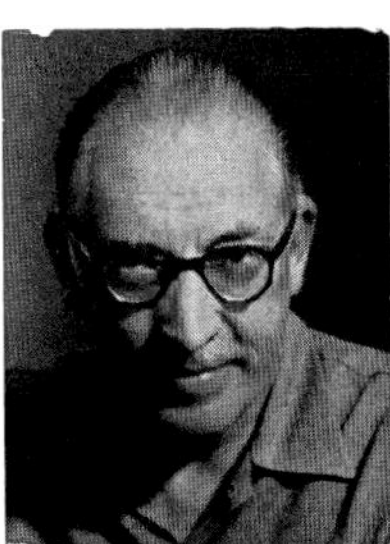

Robert Coliez

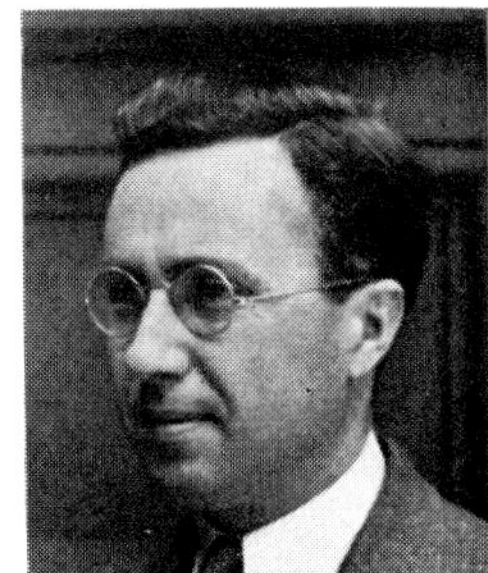

Leonidas Marinelli

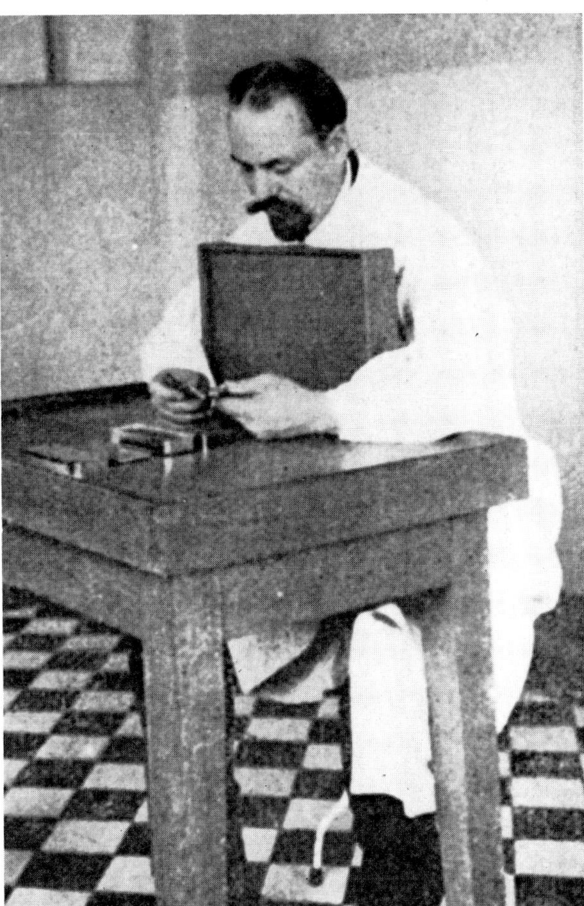

Courtesy: Masson & Cie.

Protective lead shield. At the Institut du Radium of the University of Paris, in 1919, A. Félix hugs the wood-covered lead shield mounted on an extra-heavy table with built-in lead sheets for the operator's gonads. This picture appeared in the *Journal de Radiologie* of February, 1921 wherein Felix calls himself a *radiumlogiste opérateur.*

made to publish their *Proceedings* in the *American Journal of Roentgenology.* To externalize this fact, at the following ARRS meeting held in September, 1919 in Saratoga Springs (New York), Case motioned to have the words *and Radium Therapy* added to the title of the yellow journal. The motion was carried, but the Executive Council of the ARRS hesitated to implement it, partly because of the Philadelphia Quaker and respected magister Henry Khunrath Pancoast (1875-1939), who went on record in a clearly anti-Teutonic, but otherwise somewhat ambiguous editorial (printed in the *American Journal of Roentgenology* of September, 1919), in which he praised certain advantages of the radio-prefix. As a matter of fact, in the first decade of the 20th century, the term "radiologic" had been used quite often in a sense which included only the therapeutic applications of (any kind of) radiant energy.*

As an example, the New York dermatologist and pioneer therapist Henry Granger Piffard (1842-1910) — better known for his eponymic x-ray tube — in mentioning "radiologic misinformation," referred in harsh words in the *Medical News* of April 23, 1905, to early gems of therapeutic literature: ". . . that some of these articles are dictated by vanity is extremely probable; that others are potboilers pure and simple is undoubted; while still others give one the impression of being deliberate and intentional fakes."

The tongue-twister *radiumlogia* was used in Italian to indicate everything (both physics and medical ap-

*In the *American X-Ray Journal* of May, 1903 the term radio-praxis refers to the 25 years of experience accumulated by Piffard in treating lupus with the sun ray. The first chapter in Charles Warrenne Allen's *Radiotherapy and Phototherapy* (Lea Brothers & Co., 1904) is entitled *General Considerations upon Radiology* but the term radiology never again appears in that book, except in the table of contents.

Courtesy: Pfizer Co.

THE X-RAY WIDOW. This drawing, like a composite likeness, reminds me of some of the lovely ladies who have managed to survive their x-ray spouses. Elizabeth Caldwell (Eugene's widow), who is an excellent driver and is not afraid of taking her car alone from New York City to Tucson, is quite a beauty. Only she must have walked bare-headed through some (untimely) blizzard, and neglected to wash the snow out of her hair.

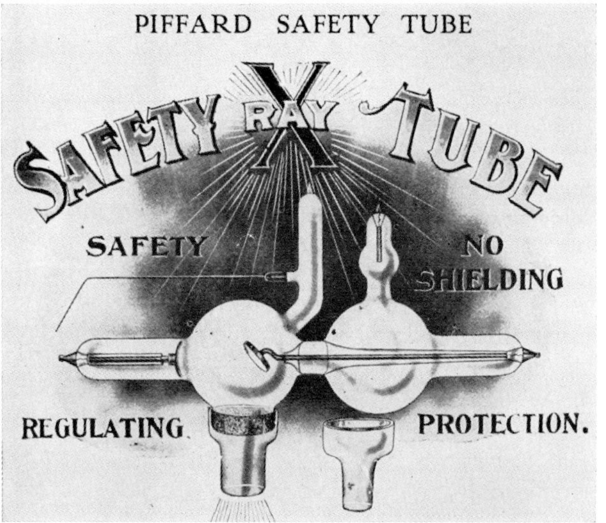

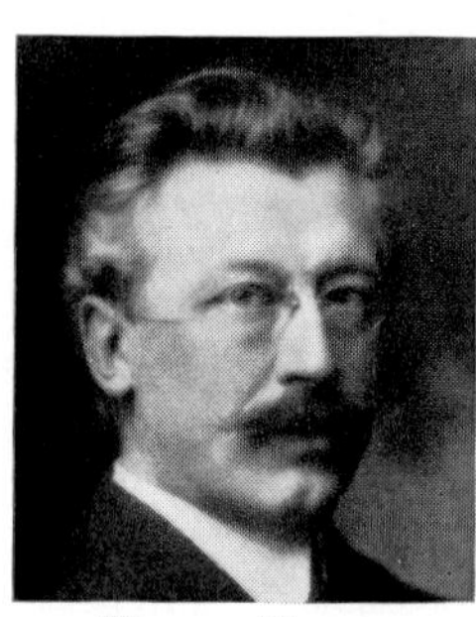

HENRY HULST

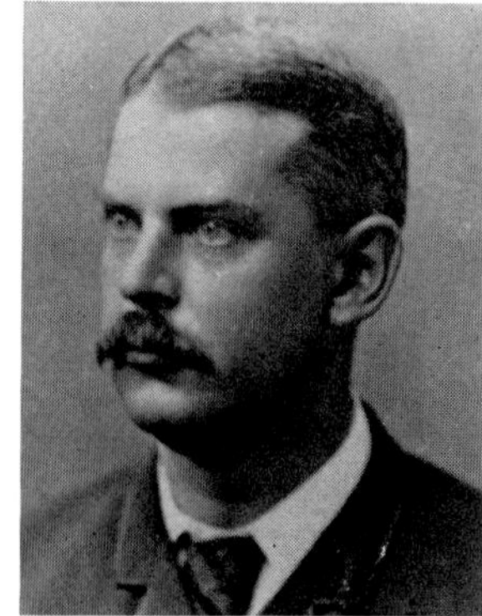

HENRY PIFFARD

plications) related to radium. In 1913, at the first meeting of the SIRM in Milano, the commercial exhibits were called *Mostra d'Apparecchi di Röntgen e di Radiumlogia.* As late as 1922, in the *Gazette des Hôpitaux,* Simone Laborde used in French the term *radiumlogie.* Of course, Pancoast never mentioned the barbarous transliteration radiumlogy; in his sibylline circumlocutions, he seemed to suggest that the words radiology and radiation therapy were synonymous. In that case, the proper title should have been *American Journal of Roentgenology and Radiology,* rather than *American Journal of Roentgenology and Radium Therapy.*

SOVIETIC SOLUTION

It is hard to believe that Pancoast's editorial suggestion was read, let alone heeded in the Soviet Union. A few months later, in 1920, appeared in Petrograd (as St. Petersburg had been renamed at the beginning of World War I) the *Vestnik (herald) Rentgenologii y Radiologii.* It has remained to this day the main Sovietic specialty journal in this field.

ВЕСТНИК
РЕНТГЕНОЛОГИИ
И
РАДИОЛОГИИ

ЖУРНАЛ ГОСУДАРСТВЕННОГО РЕНТГЕНОЛОГИЧЕСКОГО И РАДИОЛОГИЧЕСКОГО ИНСТИТУТА

ОТДЕЛ
МЕДИКО-БИОЛОГИЧЕСКИЙ
РЕДАКТОР М.И.НЕМЕНОВ

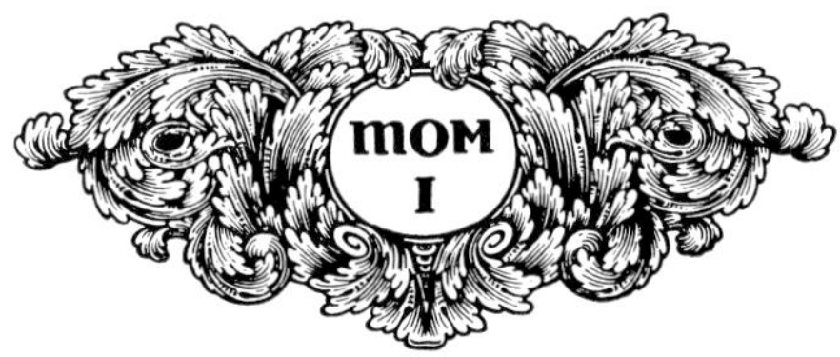

ВЫПУСК
1—2

ГОСУДАРСТВЕННОЕ ИЗДАТЕЛЬСТВО
ПЕТЕРБУРГ
1920

VIRGINAL VESTNIK. The very first issue of the oldest Soviet radiological organ is not available at the NLM, nor at John Crerar, or at the NYAcademy of Medicine. This historic title page was obtained through courtesy of Georg Zedguenidze.

Political upheavals are often punctuated by semantic re-adjustments. The first editor of the *Vestnik* was Mikhail Isaevich Nemenov (1880-1950), who founded and was both the organizer and the first director of the Gosudarstvennoye (public) Rentgen Institut in Petrograd. The building – which had previously housed a homeopathic hospital – had been selected by Nemenov, and "approved" by no lesser power than Anatol Vasilievich Lunachiarsky (1872-1928), the bellicose revolutionary who was then a sort of governor of the town.

In 1920, Nemenov obtained permission to change its name to Institute of Roentgenology and Radiology, which coincided with the appearance of the first issue of the *Vestnik.* The name of the institute remained unchanged until well in the Atomic Phase when it expanded into the Institute of Roentgenology, Radiology, and Oncology (which was in keeping with a general trend in connecting cancer therapy with radiation centers).

Also in 1918 was created in Petrograd the (nonmedical) Physical and Technical Roentgen Institute. Its first director was Abram F. Joffé (1880-1960), who was to attain fame as an expert in solid state physics. The Ukrainian Roentgen Academy was organized in Kharkov in 1920, the first Moscow Roentgen Institute was opened in 1924 by their Ministry of Health. Similar institutions were subsequently created in Kiev, Rostov-on-the-Don, Voronejh, Baku, etc. The Institute in Odessa was directed by the previously mentioned Yasha Rosenblatt (1872-1928), who was to die

ANNALES
DE
ROENTGENOLOGIE
ET
RADIOLOGIE

Journal de l'Institut d'Etat de roentgénologie et radiologie à Pétersbourg

Rédacteur en chef
Prof. M. Nemenow

TOME
I

Edition d'Etat
Pétersbourg
1922

ANNALES
DE
ROENTGENOLOGIE
ET
RADIOLOGIE

Journal de l'Association de Radiologie de l'URSS et de l'Institut d'Etat de Radiologie à Léningrad

Rédacteur en chef
Prof. M. Némenow

TOME
III

FASC. I

Paris
Les Presses Universitaires de France
1928

Courtesy: John Crerar Library.

MASTHEAD MODIFICATIONS. The *Vestnik* had for some time a French edition, appearing at irregular intervals. The first volume was printed in 1922 in Petersburg, the third and last in Paris in 1928.

of generalized, radiation-induced carcinomatosis. He kept on working to the very last, even after amputation of the left arm.

A foreign edition of the *Vestnik* was published at irregular intervals – 3 volumes in 1922-1928 – in Petrograd (the imprint changed in 1924 when the city was re-christened Leningrad) and in Paris under the title *Annales de Roentgenologie.* In his time, Nemenov was one of the most respected roentgen specialists in Soviet Russia (he is in their encyclopedia).* After 1930 he taught in the Kirov Military (medical) Academy.

At several of the above mentioned roentgen institutes, experimental workshops were established between 1922 and 1924. In 1928, the shop in Leningrad Institute was re-organized as a roentgen plant, and named "Burevestnik." In Kiev, the roentgen plant (1930) was named "Rentok." The largest of these plants was organized in 1930 in Moscow; there, in 1926, when it was still a workshop, V. A. Vitka developed his well known wiring diagram. In Leningrad is located the "Elektro-Vakuum" factory "Svetlana," which in 1946 had reached a yearly production of about 12,000 x-ray tubes and valves. Regular imports of x-ray equipment into the Soviet Union ceased about 1932.

In a review of roentgen engineering in the Soviet Union published in the 1956 Sovenir Number of the *Indian Journal of Radiology,* V. V. Dmokhovsky (from the Moscow Roentgen Plant) indicated that since 1937 there is governmental licensing of models of newly proposed equipment, prior to issuing the approval for beginning of production. Their first dosimeter came out in 1932 (L. R. Broksh and Y. L. Shekhtman) from which about a dozen models have evolved. In 1935, G. A. Zhegalkin investigated film sensitometry as a possible gauge of quality. This became feasible after Dmokhovsky established in 1947 that the intensity of irradiation behind the human body is proportional to the fifth power of the kilo-

*Orndoff, who met him at some of the ICR meetings, remembers Nemenov as very friendly and polite, but always reserved and dignified.

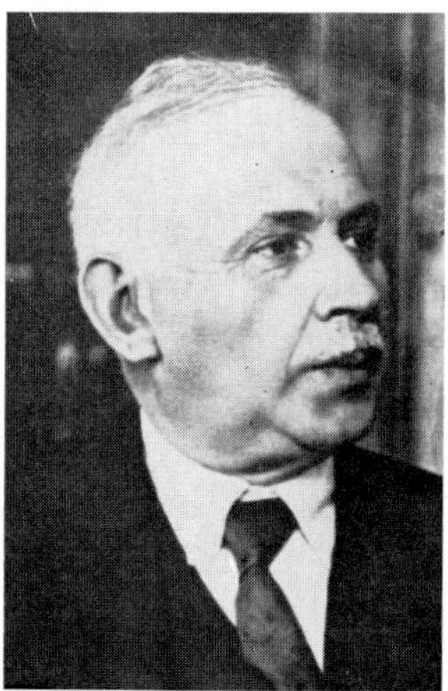

Mikhail Isaevich Nemenov. "Father" of Sovietic radiology, organizer of their first (and for many years the most important) radiologic center (in Leningrad) and long-time editor of the *Vestnik Rentgenologii i Radiologii,* their oldest specialty journal in the field.

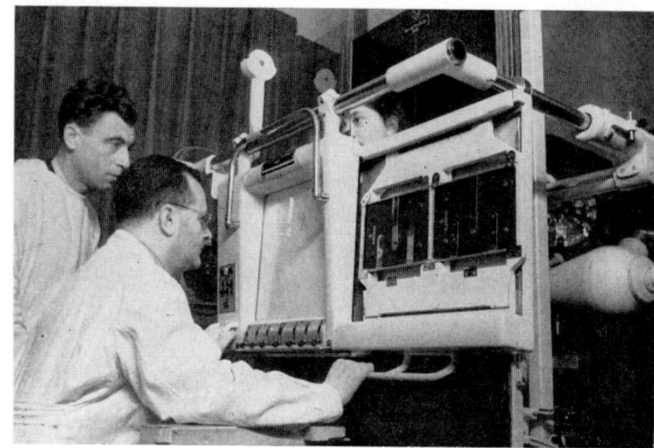

Courtesy: Sovfoto.

Fluoroscopy in the Soviet Union. In the late 1920's, seated Sam Reinberg is teaching one of his residents. The machine is a (German) Sanitas Noveloskop.

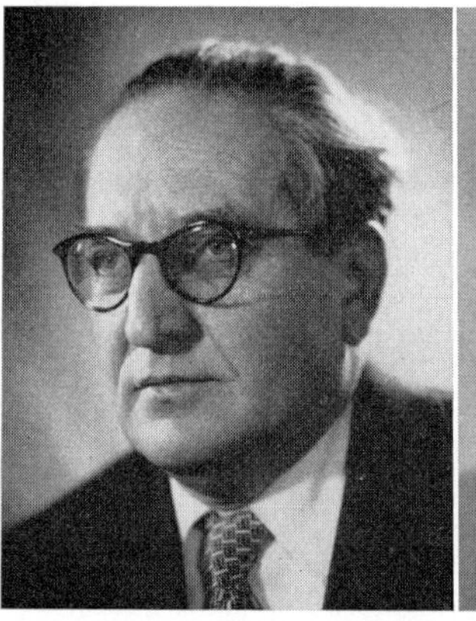

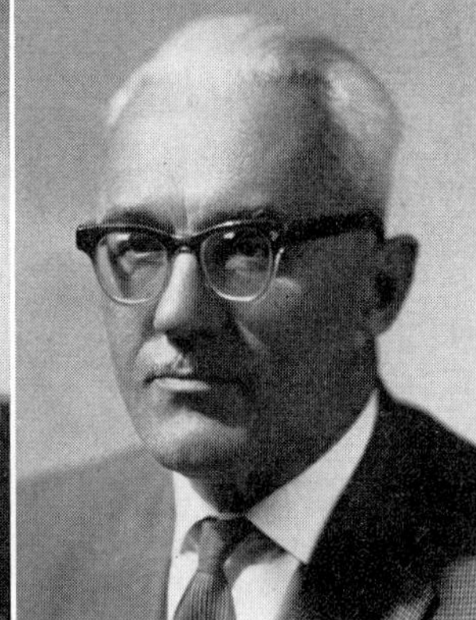

Courtesy: Georg Zedguenidze.

Sovietic roentgen-intelligentsia. Vladimir Vladimirovich Dmokhovsky (left) is the jovial director of the roentgen plant in Moscow. Yuri Nikolaevich Sokolov is the snappy editor of the *Vestnik* (Nemenov's successor). Dmokhovsky has the equivalent of a PhD degree, Sokolov is professor of radiology at one of Moscow's schools, and both are not only competent in their fields but also conoisseurs of the Sovietic x-ray literature in their respective domain. They are typical representatives of the new class of technicians who, next to the top-flight politicians, hold the balance of power in the Soviet Union.

voltage employed. A lady-engineer, Y. A. Chizhunova, found in 1954 that x-ray tubes operated horizontally lived longer than if they are placed vertically with the anode downwards; the explanation is that a bottle-neck prevents oil circulation with resulting lesser cooling of the anode.

In the same 1956 *Indian* souvenir number, Y. N. Sokolov of Moscow, the current editor of the *Vestnik,* offered a brief survey of Sovietic "roentgenodiagnostic" trends. The need for a scientifico-materialistic perspective of the universe is stressed, and the blessings derived from the October Revolution are dutifully mentioned. Having thus presumably appeased the powers-that-be, it then appears that Sovietic radiologists worry about the usual things such as the rising incidence of bronchogenic carcinoma, the differential diagnosis of fibrous dysplasia (or of rigid gastric antrum), and the comparative value of (the almost discarded) roentgen-kymography *versus* roentgenometry in roentgeno-cardiology. In fact, the names of their state-fabricated opaque media — cardiotrast, bilitrast, bilignost, iodolipol — have a familiar ring, as they are formed with the same roots utilized in the West.

DANSK
RADIOLOGISK SELSKAB'S

FORHANDLINGER

1926

Redigeret af
Selskabets Sekretær
Leif Arntzen.

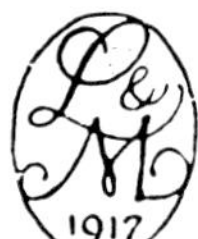

LEVIN & MUNKSGAARDS FORLAG
NØRREGADE 6 - KØBENHAVN
MCMXXVII

SCANDINAVIAN SCOFF

On November 21, 1960 Poul Flemming Móller delivered a commemorative address on the 40th anniversary of the creation of the *Dansk Róntgenologisk Forening.* His subject was of course the history of the specialty in Denmark. He mentioned their earliest pioneer, Lauritz Johannes Mygge (1850-1935), who in 1921 had published in *Ugeskrift for Laeger* his *Erindringer* (reminiscences) with røntgenstråler. He listed also Carl Christian Riis (1865-1938), who had worked with a *røntgenapparat* since 1897, the therapist Severin Nordentoft (1866-1922), who became known for his *røntgenbehandling* (treatment) of cancer of the cervix, and Johann Friedrich Fischer (1868-1922), who until his radiation death had been the director of three *róntgenklinikker.* At the very first scientific meeting of their society, held on March 4, 1921 at the Rigshospitalet in Copenhagen, Flemming-Móller gave a paper on the *røntgenundersøgelse* (examination) of ileocecal tuberculosis.

Such a compelling roentgen tradition nothwithstanding, the name of *Dansk Róntgenologisk Förening* was replaced by the (scientific) *Dansk Radiologisk Selskab* and the (professional) *Organisationen af Danske Radiologer.**

There is an explanation for this change of heart. At first, a "call-to-arms" was issued by the radiologist of Oslo's Rikshospitalet, Severin Andreas Heyerdahl. Thereupon, on July 2, 1919, in Oslo, delegates from the four Scandinavian countries assembled in Oslo and founded a common society, called *Nordisk Förening for Medicinsk Radiologi.* With Gösta Forssell as editor, the first number of *Acta radiologica* (one radio-journal for all Scandinavian countries) appeared on July 25, 1921. The first *Nordiske Ra-*

*This information, the portraits herein reproduced and other documentation, have been graciously provided by Carl Einer Gudbjerg (from the Rigshospitalet) who is currently the editor of *Dansk Radiologisk Selskab Forhandlingar.*

ACTA RADIOLOGICA

EDITA PER SOCIETATES RADIOLOGICAS
DANIÆ, FENNIÆ, NORVEGIÆ ET SUECIÆ

VOL. I FASC. I 25: VII 1921 N:o 1

diologkongres convened in 1921 in Copenhagen, under the presidency of Johann Fischer.

In 1955, after receiving the Gold Medal of the Centre Antoine Béclère in Paris, Elis Berven spoke the following words (in excellent French, reproduced herein in the "official" translation):

"The history of Sweden is that of her Kings. With the same certainty one could say that the history of Swedish Radiology is that of Gösta Forssell, the recognized 'father' of Swedish Radiology."

The *Svenska Radiologisk Föreningen* was founded in 1907 during a luncheon, offered by the Swedish x-ray manufacturer Bror Järnh to the following "founders": F. von Bergen, I. Bagge, P. Haglund, G. Holm, G. Forssell, and T. Sjögren. Their organization had mainly economic purposes, for instance a committee of three (Bagge, Forssell, and Sjögren) issued on September 6, 1907 a "Medeltaxa" or price schedule for roentgen services. On May 8, 1919 Forssell invited the outstanding Swedish radiologists to create also a scientific society. The organizational meeting took place on May 17, 1919 at 7:00 P.M. in the Serafimerlasarettet (a Stockholm hospital) with 37 participants: aside from the above "founders" there came Berven, Heyman, Åkerlund, Torbern Klason (who was to prepare in 1959 the brief historical account of their society), Lundberg, Schonander, Edling, and Hugo Laurell. After some discussion of possible titles, the name adopted on the recommendation of Forssell was *Svensk Förening för Medicinsk Radiologi,* the idea being to include also the electrotherapists and the physiotherapists. Forssell, Berven, and Heyman became (in this order) the first president, secretary, and treasurer.

Gösta Forssell (1879-1950) was a pupil of Thor Stenbeck (the "first" Swedish radiologist), and had assisted the latter in the first "cure" of a skin carcinoma in 1899. Forssell was above all an excellent organizer. As the Radiologist of Serafimerlasarettet he insisted on centralizing all the x-ray equipment into a single department and this became a trend throughout the

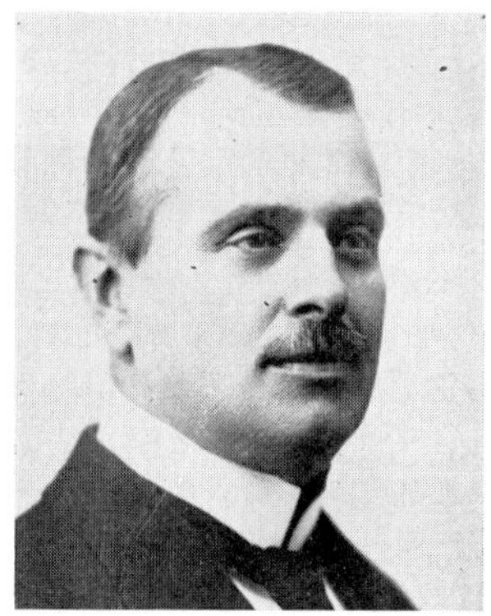

Courtesy: Carl Gudbjerg

JOHAN FREDERIK FISCHER. One of the most representative of roentgen pioneers in Denmark, who was president of the first *Nordiske Radiologkongres* which met in Copenhagen in 1921. Fischer died as a radiation casualty.

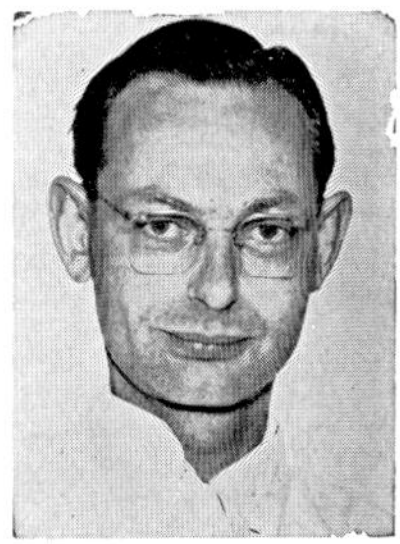

C. E. GUDBJERG

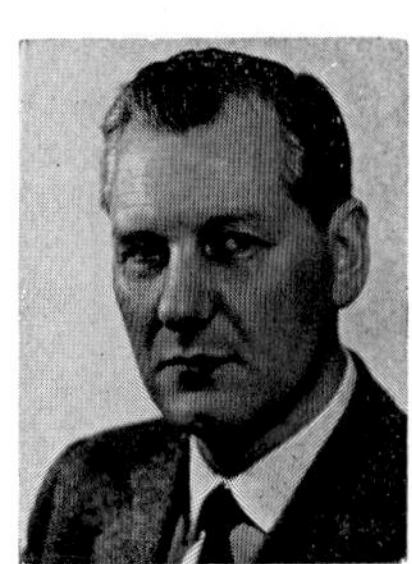

SVEN HULTBERG

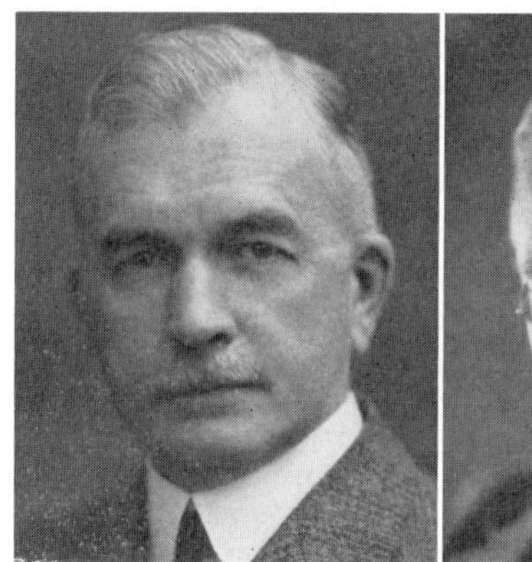

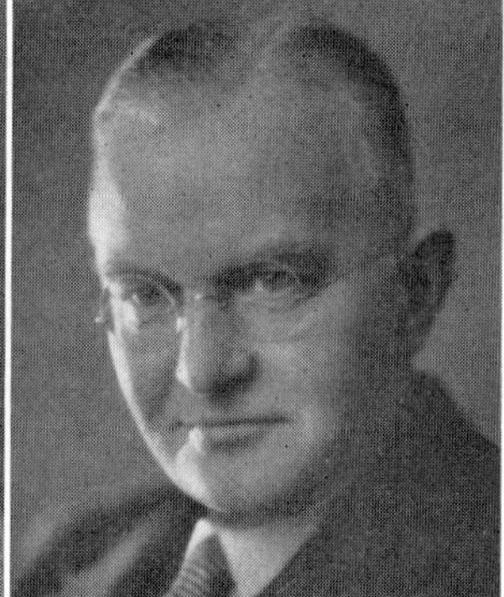

Courtesy: Ben Orndoff

LARS EDLING AND (BESPECTACLED) ÅKE AKERLUND

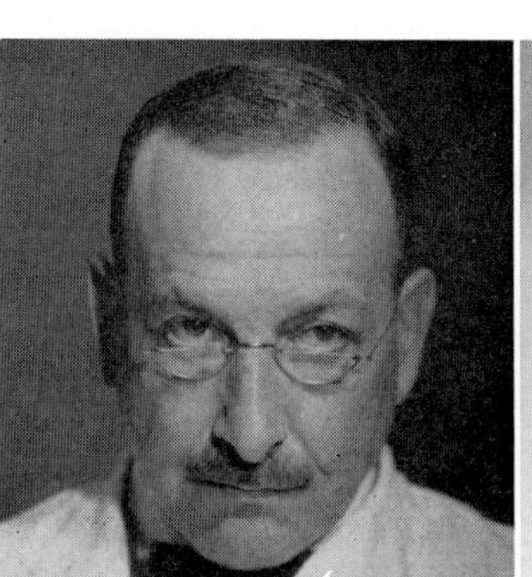

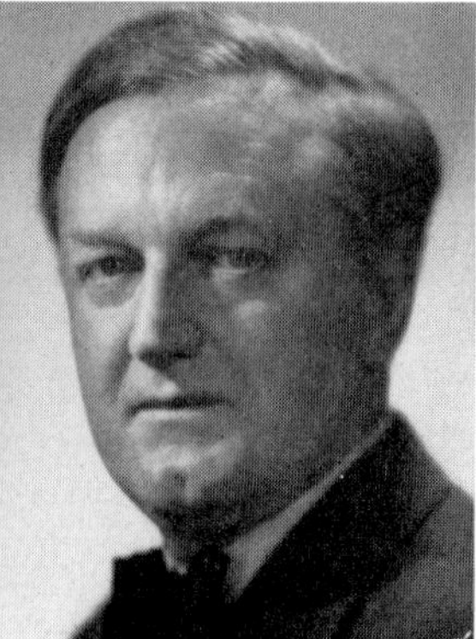

Courtesy: Ben Orndoff

JAMES HEYMAN (WITH SPECTACLES) AND ERIK LYSHOLM

Golden Age of Radiology.* In 1911 he designed the new x-ray department built at the Serafimerlasarettet, and it became a model copied by many, both in and outside Sweden. During his lifetime, Forssell published about 200 articles on both diagnosis and therapy. He advocated and achieved the separation of radiology into two subspecialties. In 1936 he created at the Karolinska Institutet a professorial chair for radiodiagnosis and another one for radiotherapy (later on, two more disciplines were to receive similar recognition, radiopathology and radiophysics.† There is in the Radiumhemmet (which, as a result of the Jubilee Fund, is once again part of the Karolinska) a Forssell Memorial Room which contains his books, diplomas, medals, other personal belongings, portraits, and sculptures: it serves as a permanent memento of a good man!

Two among Forssell's pupils became well known in their own rights. Eric Lysholm (1892-1947), his successor at Serafimerlasarettet, may be regarded as one of the founders of neuroradiology (he is best known for his eponymic skull unit). The other, who became also Forssell's eulogist, was Åke Åkerlund (1887-1958): he left two books (one on craters in the duodenal bulb) and eighty papers, and was one of the founders of pediatric radiology. James Ernst Heyman (1882-1956) gave his name to the well known intra-uterine applicator. Elis Berven was the long time (now retired) director of the Radiumhemmet: as his successor Hultberg remarked, the history of the Radiumhemmet is the history of Berven. Sweden's contribution to the science of radiology exceeds, both in quality and in quantity what one could reasonably expect from a country of that size: after all, even today, there are only about 350 radiologists in Sweden. Incidentally, the name of the Swedish ACR is Radiologförbundet.

*During the Atomic Phase, decentralization of x-ray departments in large hospitals is again becoming popular. Actually, with the communication problems inherent in a 2,500 bed hospital, it is difficult to deny separate x-ray departments to a 500 bed Pediatric Unit or to a 250 bed Gastro-Enterologic Service.

†Beginning with 1962, *Acta Radiologica* comes in two separate editions, one for diagnosis, the other for therapy. This brings up the problem where to pigeon-hole a paper that envisions both the identification and the treatment of a disease (which they would prefer to publish in the monograph series, anyway). More difficult would be a review of the use of one radioisotope utilized for both diagnostic and therapeutic aims.

In Finland, the first x-ray equipment was installed in 1900 in the surgical out-patient department of the University Hospital in Helsinki. The Finnish Society of Radiology was formed on September 23, 1924 upon the initiative of G. A. Wetterstrand, and was registered in 1930. By 1954, when S. Mustakallio became president of the Society, there were 101 members.

As in the other Scandinavian countries, there are in Norway two separate organizations of radiologists, one for economic purposes (to which they refer, perhaps jokingly, as their trade-union), the other for scientific pursuits, called Norsk Forening for Medicinsk Radiologi. It was formed in 1920, the first president being the previously mentioned Heyerdahl, with Schiander as the first secretary.*

*These details were graciously offered by the current secretary of the Norwegian Radiologic Society, Dr. Aksel W. Johannessen. He mentioned that the records of the society's early years have been lost during the war years.

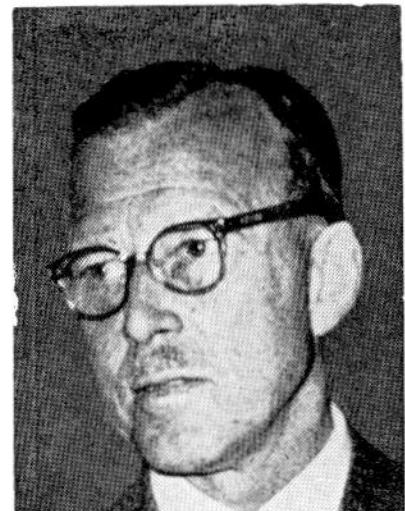
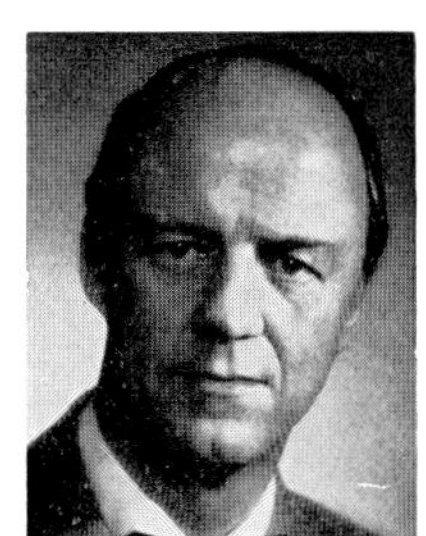
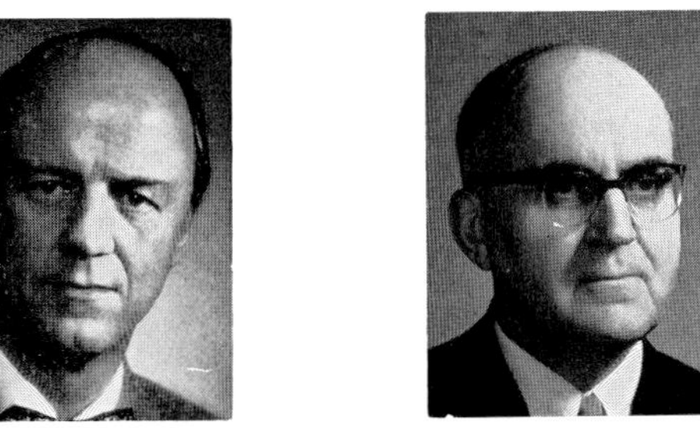
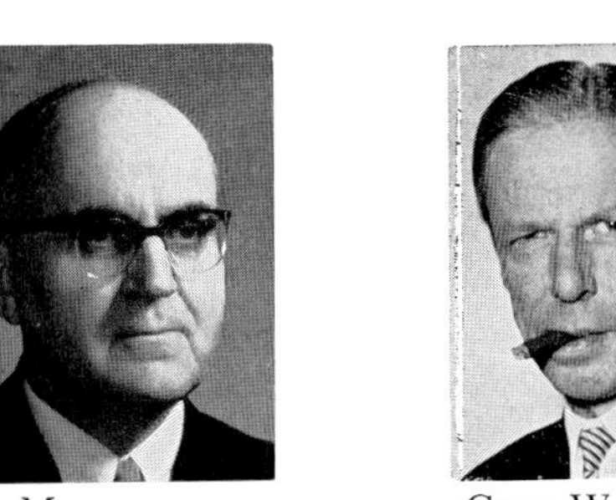

FOLKE KNUTSSON NILS EDLING S. MUSTAKALLIO CARL WEGELIUS

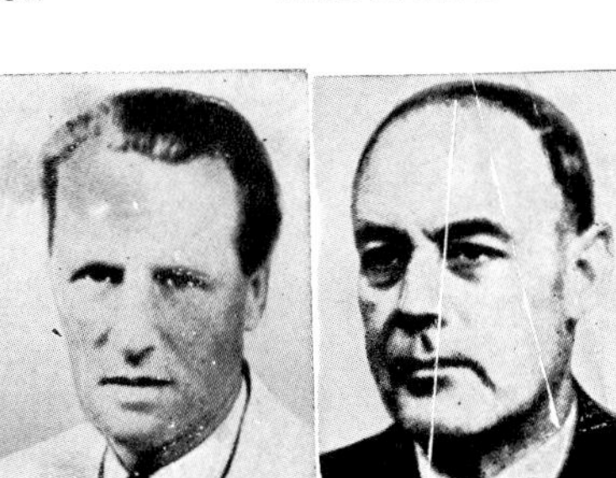
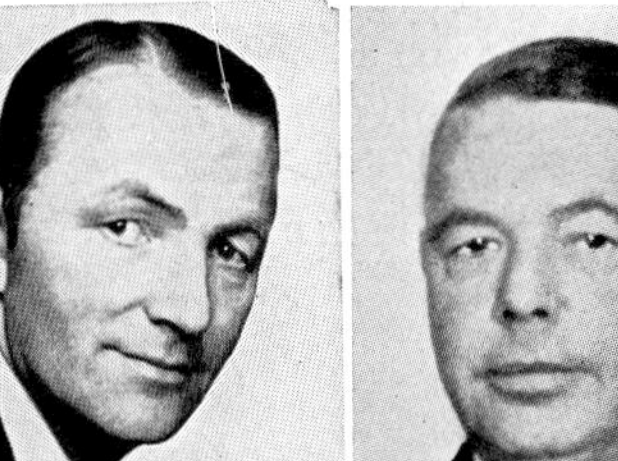
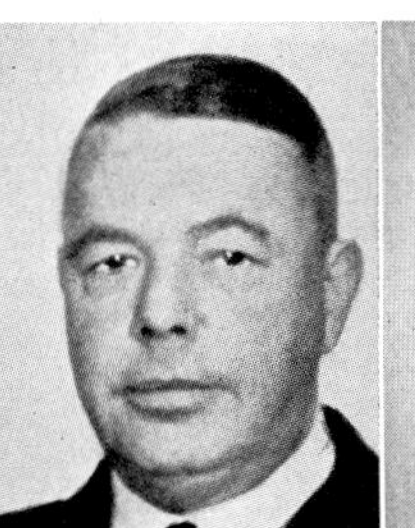
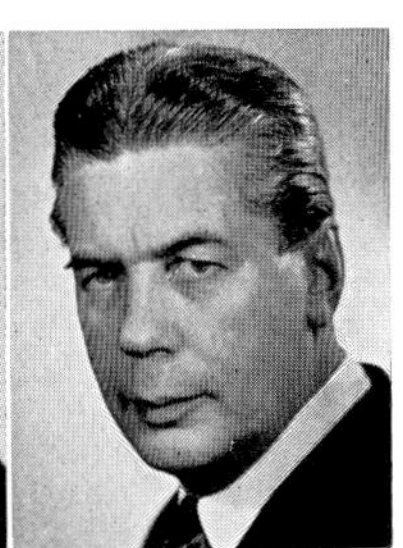
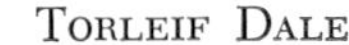

BO LINDELL FRIMANN-DAHL ROBERT THORAEUS TORLEIF DALE SIGVALD BAKKE SÖLVE WELIN

Whatever the official explanation, the Scandinavian decision to switch to "radiologic titles" was at least in some way related to the fact that such a terminology was favored in the countries victorious in World War I (especially England and France).

BEGINNING OF THE GOLDEN AGE

In the year 1920 appeared the exquisitely illustrated text by Frederick Manwaring Law (1875-1947), on the *Roentgenologically Considered Mastoids.* The princeps edition, with pasted-in positive prints (but not the second printing, in which reproductions were used) is now a collector's item, rarer than many incunabula. It was the first volume in a monographic serial, sponsored by the ARRS, edited by Case, and therefore appropriately named *Annals of Roentgenology.*

The *Annals of Roentgenology* were published by Paul Benedikt Hoeber, Sr. (1883-1937), who was also the publisher of the famous (never since duplicated)

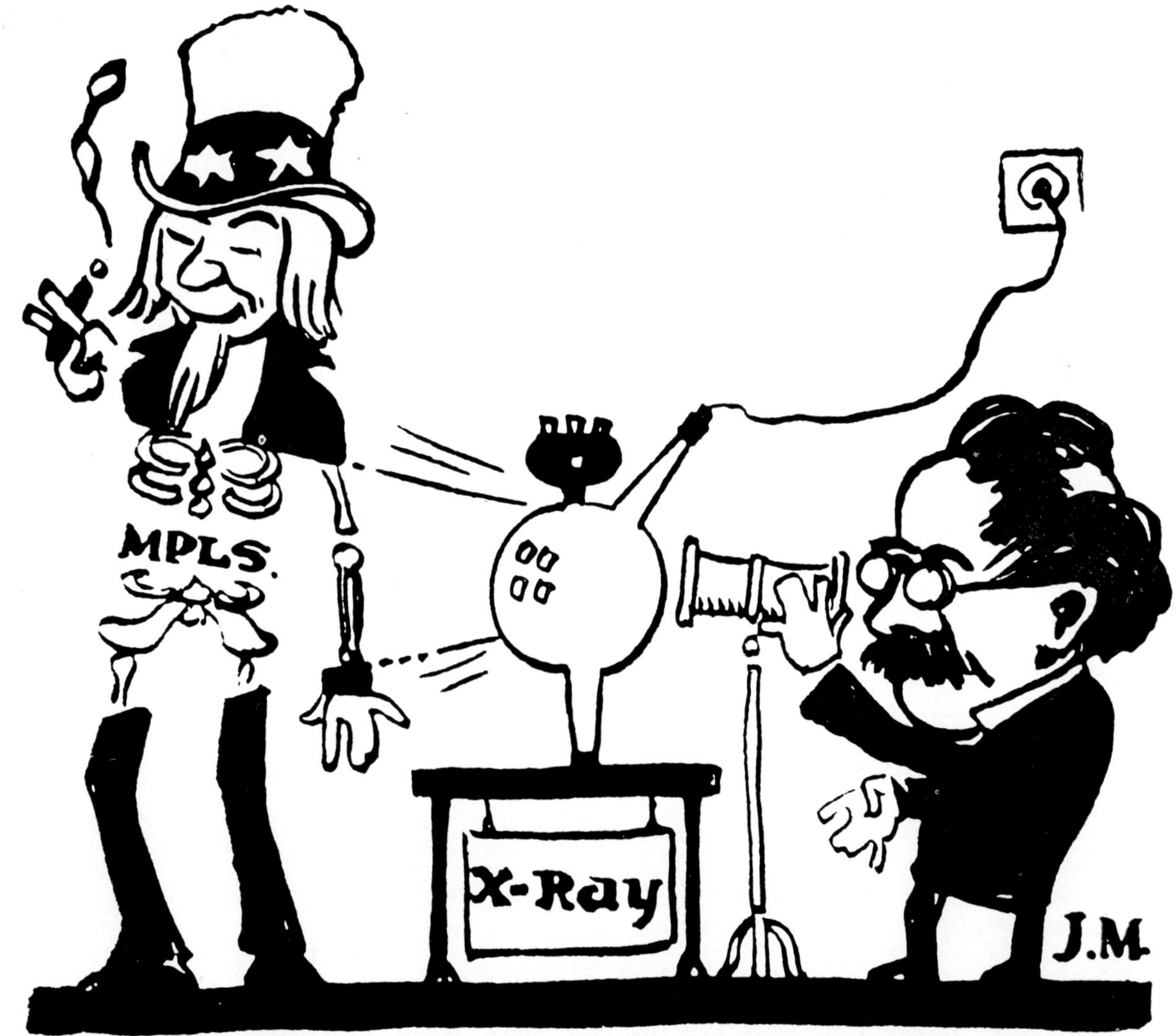

COME TO MPLS! This is from a poster inviting members and guests to the annual meeting of the ARRS in 1920 in Minneapolis – which is the MPLS located ("localized") by the shadowgazer who is searching Uncle Sam's innards. At that meeting, presided over by James Thomas Case, the first commercially produced Bucky-Potter diaphragm was shown by George Brady; Coolidge's tube was beginning to replace (displace) the gas models; Caldwell's tilting table was being manufactured by Campbell; and Eastman had started to duplitize film. In many ways this meeting of 1920 marked the passing of an era: by the same token, this cartoon symbolizes the transition from the *Era of the Roentgen Pioneers* to the *Golden Age of Radiology.*

Famous Physicians at X-Ray Congress

TWO HAIRY ONES FROM MICH:
DR J G VAN ZWALEWENBURG, UNIVERSITY OF MICHIGAN
HE REPRESENTS THE SOCIETY IN THE NATIONAL RESEARCH COUNCIL
DR. A. W. CRANE, OF KALAMAZOO, FORMER PRESIDENT AMERICAN ROENTGEN RAY SOCIETY
DR. JAMES T. CASE, PRESIDENT, OF BATTLE CREEK, MICH.
DR. CASE HAD CHARGE OF X-RAY WORK WITH OUR ARMY IN FRANCE
DR. A. H. PIRIE, OF MONTREAL. HE WAS WEARING DANCING PUMPS
DR. GEORGE E. PFAHLER, OF PHILADELPHIA, PAST PRES.
DR J. M. MARTIN, OF TEXAS, "HIGHEST MEDICAL AUTHORITY OF HIS STATE—ABOUT 6 FT. 5 IN.
DR. COOLIDGE, OF SCHENECTADY, N. Y., INVENTOR OF THE "NEW" X-RAY TUBE, ABOUT EIGHT YEARS AGO

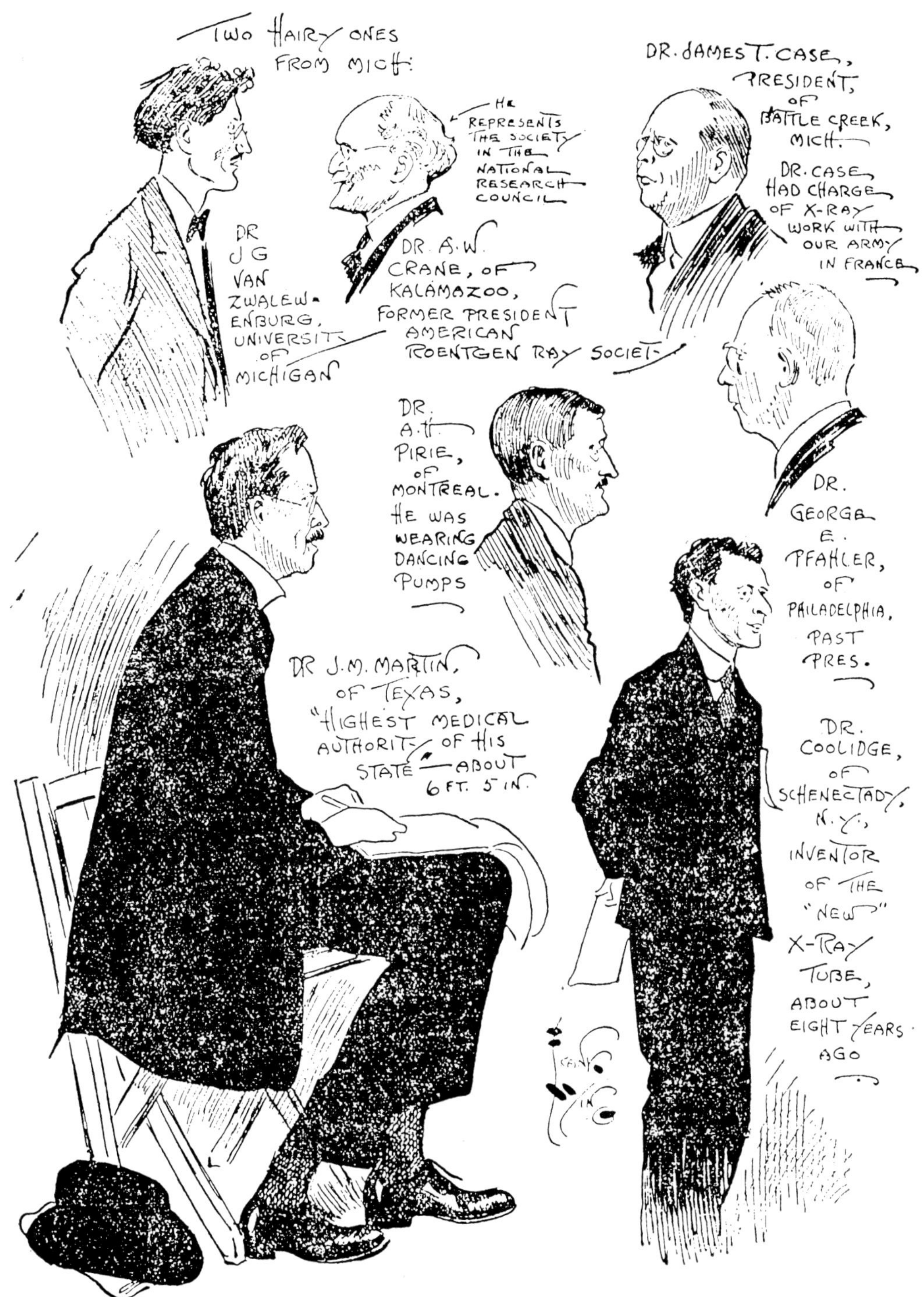

World's Greatest Doctors Here for Roentgen Ray Convention

session yesterday those attending the convention were the guests of the Hennepin County Medical society for an automobile trip to points of interest in the city.

In the evening they attended a din-

Annals of Medical History. This bookman and his elegant bookplate did much for American Radiology in general, for the ARRS in particular. As a result, he was one of the few non-medical people honored with an obituary notice in the yellow journal (of October, 1937), signed by one of its former editors, Arthur Carlisle Christie (1879-1956). Hoeber's financial reward was not commensurate with his other achievements, and two years before his death, Paul B. Hoeber, Inc. became (and has remained to this day) a part of Harper & Brothers.

The Golden Age was creeping up, and the ARRS had to make a decision about changing the title of their journal for the semantic inclusion of the ARS. Its editor at the time, Harry Miles Imboden (1878-1951), reprinted in the name of the Executive Council the old etymologic ordinance of 1913 in the December, 1922 issue. This was allegedly done for the benefit of the many newcomers to the roentgenologic fraternity. With the ensuing issue of January, 1923 (volume 10) the name on the frontispiece was changed to *American Journal of Roentgenology and Radium Therapy.*

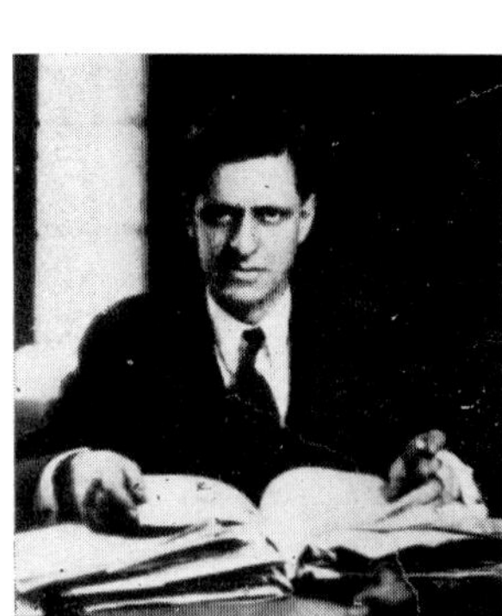

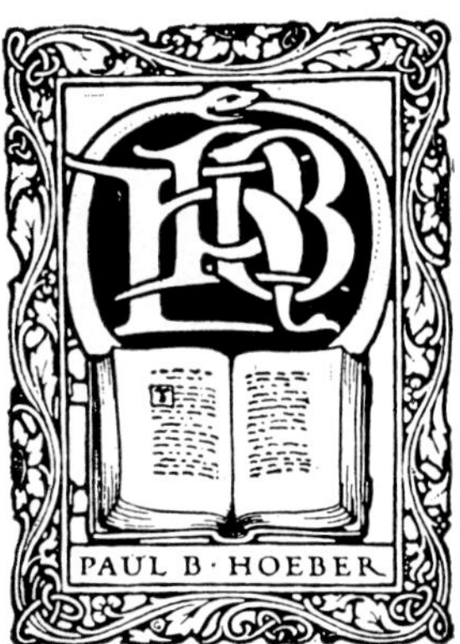

Courtesy: New York Academy of Medicine.

HOEBER, SR. AND HIS BOOKPLATE. According to P. B. Hoeber, Jr., this is the only portrait extant of Paul Benedict Hoeber, Sr. and is herein reproduced from the obituary in the *Annals of Medical History.* Hoeber, Sr., may be regarded as this country's first "radio-publisher." He deserves credit also for many other "bookish" accomplishments, herein symbolically memorialized by reproducing his bookplate. While snake-eating snakes are not uncommon, a snake that would swallow its own tail occurs mainly in fables — possibly also in the publishing business. Publishers who, like Hoeber, Sr., place the excellence of their products ahead of solid business appraisal, terminate — so to speak — by catabolizing their own financial substance which, evidently, is a very sad postscript to the devious ways of human endeavor.

SECTION ON RADIOLOGY OF THE AMA

In the afternoon of June 23, 1923 a therapist from Los Angeles, Albert Soiland (1873-1946), presented to the AMA Convention in San Francisco a resolution calling for the creation of a "Section of Radiology." The ARRS objected editorially in April, 1924, and wanted the name changed to "Section of Roentgenology and Radium Therapy," but the tide went against them: Pancoast's famous first communication on his eponymic (superior sulcus) tumor was read before the "Meeting of Radiology of the Section of Miscellaneous Topics" at the 75th Annual Meeting of the AMA in Chicago in 1924. The Section on Radiology of the AMA was officially inaugurated in 1925. It started out with its own *Transactions,* but this publication was discontinued after the very first issue.

TRANSACTIONS OF THE

SECTION ON

Radiology

of the
American Medical Association
at the Seventy-Seventh Annual
Session, held at Dallas, Texas,
April 19 to 23, 1926

AMERICAN MEDICAL ASSOCIATION PRESS
CHICAGO: NINETEEN HUNDRED TWENTY-SIX

CIVIL WAR WITHIN THE RSNA

Meanwhile, the RSNA was engaged in a "civil war, testing whether that *society,* or any *society* so conceived and so dedicated, can long endure" without having the right to manage, control, and publish its own journal, or without the privilege to expel (under terms provided in the By-Laws) a member who transgresses the rules of conduct. As the first journal of the RSNA was being organized, Orndoff wanted to avoid the initial financial handicaps incurred under similar circumstances by the American College of Physicians and the American College of Surgeons (ACS).

If Franklin Henry Martin (1857-1935), a gynecological surgeon from Chicago, had been elected president of the AMA, certain events might never have taken place. But he was turned down, and in anger decided to form his own organization: this is how the ACS was founded. Then Martin started in 1905 the now famous and flourishing *Surgery, Gynecology, and Obstetrics.* For the latter purpose (*i.e.,* to facilitate the separation of financial responsibilities) an "independent" Surgical Publishing Company was created. If Max Thorek (1880-1960), a surgeon from Chicago, had been accepted as a member of the ACS, certain events might never have occurred. But he was turned down, and in anger decided to form his own organization: this is how the International College of Surgeons (ICS) was founded. The ICS is currently the largest association of surgeons in the world, and prints its own *Journal of the ICS.*

But splinter groups will flourish only if they fulfill a definite need. In the *American Journal of Roentgenology* of February, 1920, Preston Hickey mentioned the existence of an Inter-Allied Roentgenological Club, intended to facilitate the furtherance of international post-graduate instruction. The first section formed was the English Roentgenologic Club with Sir Archibald Reid as president, and Robert Knox as secretary. The corresponding American organization had Hickey as president, and William Holmes Stewart as secretary. The French section was in the process of formation, and the entire Anglo-French-American group was to have met in the fall of 1920, but nothing ever materialized.

Instead, during the September, 1920 meeting of the ARRS in Minneapolis was organized the American Association of Military Roentgenologists with A. C. Christie as president; Pancoast as vice-president; and Francis Frank Borzell as secretary.

I wrote in 1960 to Borzell to ask what happened to the association, and this is what he answered: "The gatherings we had were pleasant, and, as usual with such organizations, derived their sustenance from memories. I suspect that as our capacity for Scotch (or, at the beginning, boot-leg Gin) diminished, our interest also waned, and finally like old soldiers just faded away. So did the Association!"

Irvin Hummon founded the Lambda Rho Honorary Radiological Fraternity in 1924, and was president of its first (alpha) chapter. Another (beta) chapter was formed in Wisconsin, but the organization did not gain the wide acceptance needed for survival. Lambda Rho withered slowly, and disappeared about 1934.

The RSNA had incurred losses in the first two years of publication of its *Journal.* Therefore, during the December, 1920 meeting at the Palmer House (Chicago), a Radiological Publishing Company was formed, and various members subscribed stock in this non-profit organization. Somehow, Albert Franklin Tyler (1881-1944), clinical professor of radiology at Creighton, and radiologist of Immanuel Hospital in Omaha, acquired controlling interest in the company.

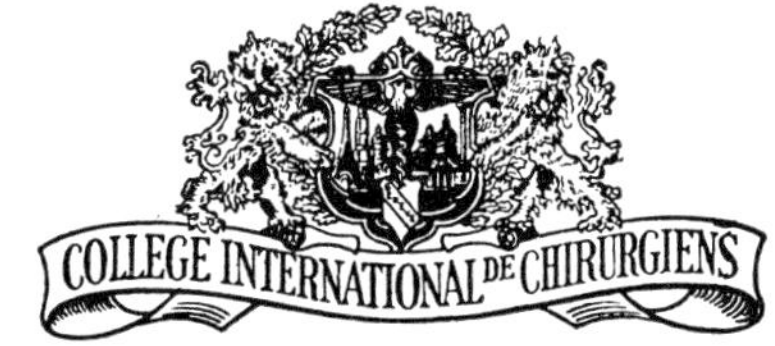

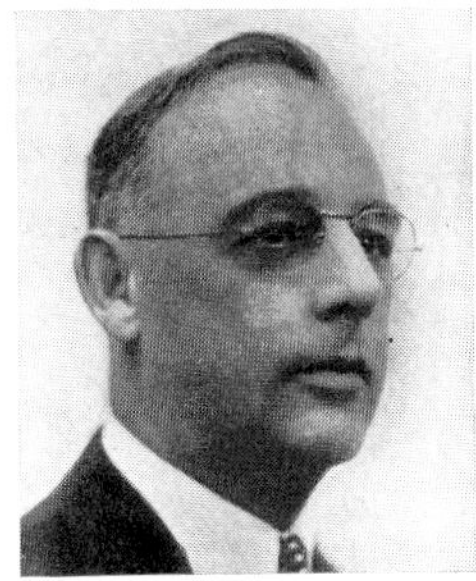

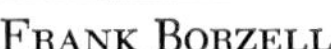
FRANK BORZELL

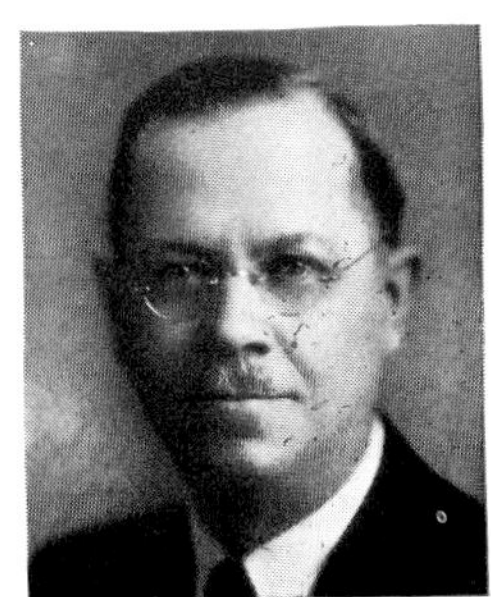
ALBERT F. TYLER

He became editor of the *Journal* and the offices were moved to Omaha. He acted more and more independently, RSNA directives were disregarded, and repeated conferences led only to name-calling.

A serious decision had to be made. The RSNA statutes were modified to allow for the creation of a remodeled (and this time adequately safe-guarded) Radiology Publishing Company. Tyler was expelled from the RSNA, and a brand new (and to this day gray-covered) journal came into being: the first number of *Radiology* appeared in September 1923 under the editorship of Maximilian John Hubeny (1880-1942), who for many years also graced the position of chief-radiologist of Cook County Hospital in Chicago.

Tyler continued to issue the *Journal of Radiology* with the same by-line "published for the RSNA," and sued the 1923 slate of RSNA officers, including its president, Russell Daniel Carman (1875-1926) of the Mayo Clinic. On April 21, 1924, in District Court at St. Paul (Minnesota), Judge R. D. O'Brien absolved the defendants (the officers of the RSNA, and J. R. Bruce, business manager of *Radiology*) of any wrongdoing, and both the RSNA and its officers recovered their costs of litigation. The April, 1924 issue of the *Journal of Radiology* was the last one "published for the RSNA." Beginning with the May, 1924 issue, Tyler was listed as managing editor. He had lost an invaluable sponsor, but (as we shall see) he was already searching for a replacement.

Another delicate (*i.e.*, embarrassing) episode in the life of the RSNA came in 1929 when it accepted a subsidy from a non-profit organization, called the Chemical Foundation. The latter was controlled by the noted cancerologist Francis Carter Wood (1869-1951), who was the pathologist of St. Luke's Hospital in New York City. The Foundation's business manager was William Buffum, who also managed Wood's *American Journal of Cancer*. In 1931 Wood became president-elect of the RSNA — he was a recognized researcher in the roentgen field, and his classical investigations into the biologic effectiveness of different wavelengths (1924) were repeated and extended in "his" Columbia University Cancer Institute by his

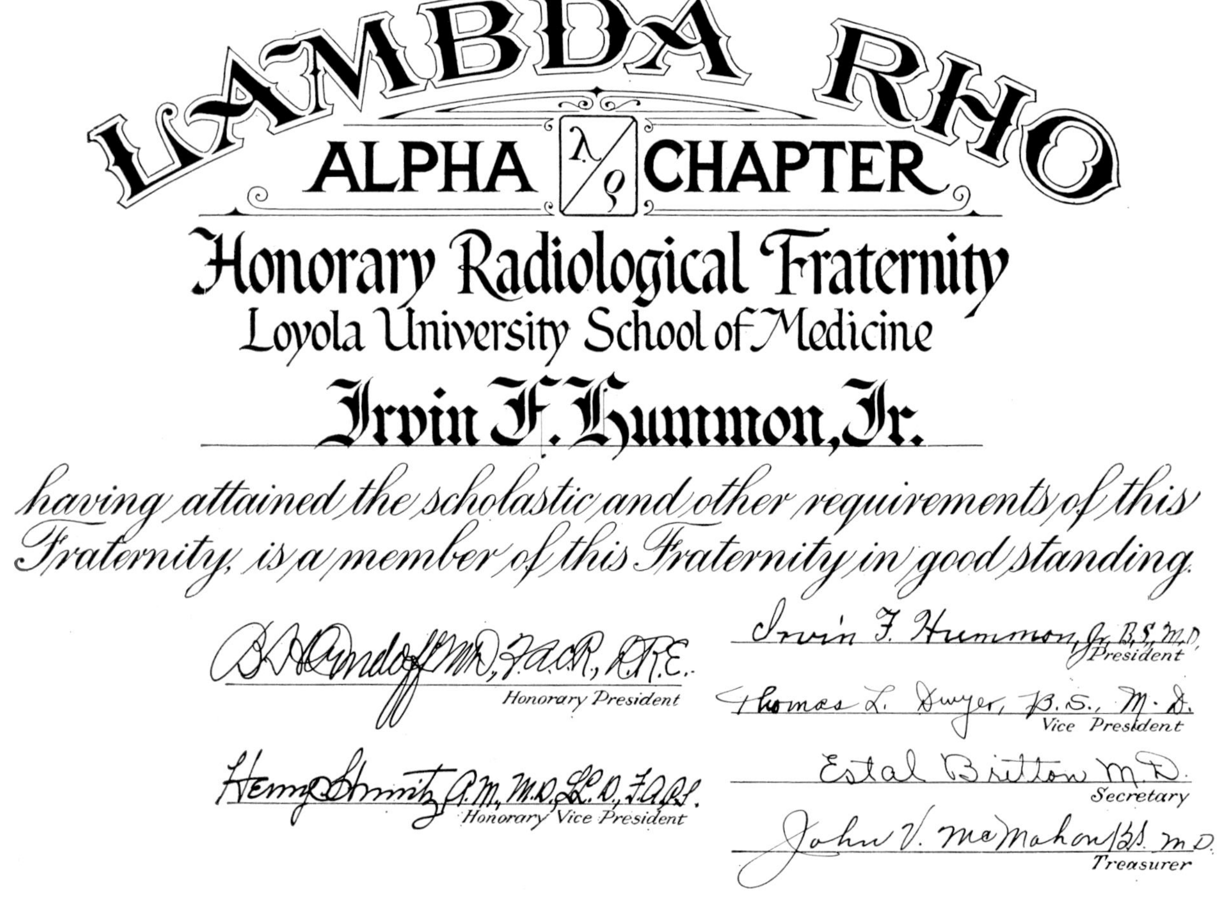

LAMBDA RHO
ALPHA λ/ρ CHAPTER
Honorary Radiological Fraternity
Loyola University School of Medicine

Irvin F. Hummon, Jr.

having attained the scholastic and other requirements of this Fraternity, is a member of this Fraternity in good standing.

B. H. Orndoff M.D., F.A.C.R., R.T.E. — Honorary President	Irvin F. Hummon, Jr. B.S. M.D. — President
Henry Schmitz A.M., M.D., LL.D., F.A.C.S. — Honorary Vice President	Thomas L. Dwyer, B.S., M.D. — Vice President
	Estal Britton M.D. — Secretary
	John V. McMahon B.S. M.D. — Treasurer

associates. One of the latter was Charles Packard, who is now a Trustee of the Marine Biological Laboratory in Woods Hole (Massachusetts). During Wood's term of office, a request was made for changes in the By-Laws, intended to give the Chemical Foundation control over the RSNA. The move was implemented by the threat to cut off the subsidy to *Radiology*. For one who knows the strength and wealth of today's RSNA, it is hard to believe that they could ever have placed themselves in such a situation. But had they not acted wisely and severed at that time all relationship with the Chemical Foundation, the RSNA might never have achieved its present position.

AMERICAN COLLEGE OF RADIOLOGY

On June 26, 1923 — during the previously mentioned AMA convention in San Francisco — Albert Soiland arranged a meeting of twenty-one prominent radiologists, and there the *American College of Radiology* (ACR) was born. The first convocation and assembly of the ACR was held in Chicago on June 11, 1924.*

The original slate of officers consisted of George Pfahler – president; Henry Schmitz – vice-president; Soiland – executive secretary; Orndoff – treasurer; Isadore Simon Trostler – historian; and Carman – chairman of the Board of Chancellors. Chancellors were Lloyd Bryan (1884-1946), Edwin Charles Ernst, Sr., Arial Wellington George (1882-1948), Amedée Granger (1879-1939), Leon Theodore LeWald, Gordon Earle Richards (1885-1949), William Walter Wasson, and William Warner Watkins (1883-1956). President-elect was William Holmes Stewart (1868-1954) of New York City.

Albert Soiland (1873-1946) was born in Stavanger (Norway), and graduated in 1900 from medical school in Southern California. While he dabbled with many subjects in the field of radiology, his main interest concerned the therapeutic applications of both radium and x rays. He was a man of wit, and had also semantic preoccupations: in his article on *Radiophobia and Radiomania* in the *American X-Ray Journal* of October, 1903 Soiland defined radiomaniacs as those who at the slightest provocation will make (extreme) therapeutic use of x rays. Soiland founded, and was for many years the director of, the Los Angeles Tumor Institute.

*Mr. William Charles Stronach, the executive director of the ACR, and his staff (especially Miss Jewel Pruett) have collected many of these data. Interesting information was also furnished by Mr. Hugh Nehemiah Jones, who until recently was director of public relations of the ACR.

ROENTGENOTHERAPY

BY

ALBERT FRANKLIN TYLER, B.Sc., M.D.

PROFESSOR OF CLINICAL ROENTGENOLOGY JOHN A. CREIGHTON MEDICAL COLLEGE; ATTENDING ROENTGENOLOGIST ST. JOSEPH'S HOSPITAL, BISHOP CLARKSON MEMORIAL HOSPITAL, FORD HOSPITAL, IMMANUEL HOSPITAL, DOUGLAS COUNTY HOSPITAL, AND LORD LISTER HOSPITAL, OMAHA, NEBRASKA; MEMBER AMERICAN ROENTGEN RAY SOCIETY; FELLOW AMERICAN MEDICAL ASSOCIATION, ETC.

WITH 111 ILLUSTRATIONS

ST. LOUIS
C. V. MOSBY COMPANY
1919

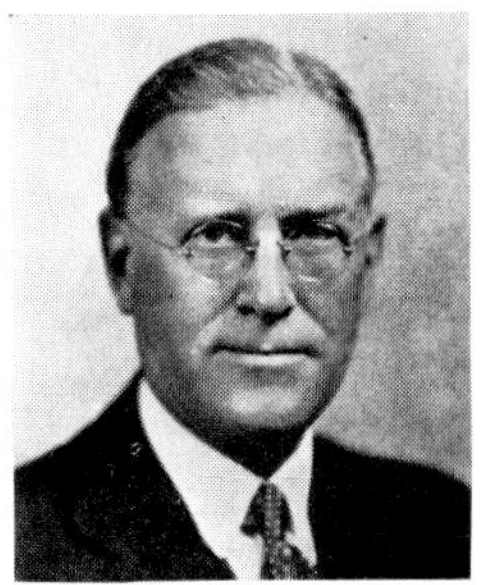
FRANCIS CARTER WOOD

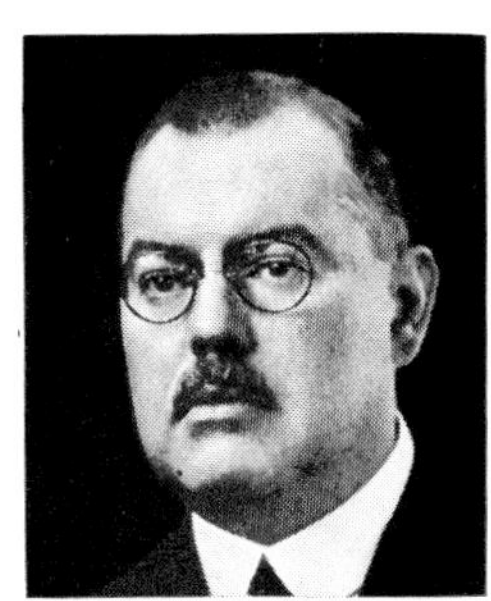
AMEDEE GRANGER

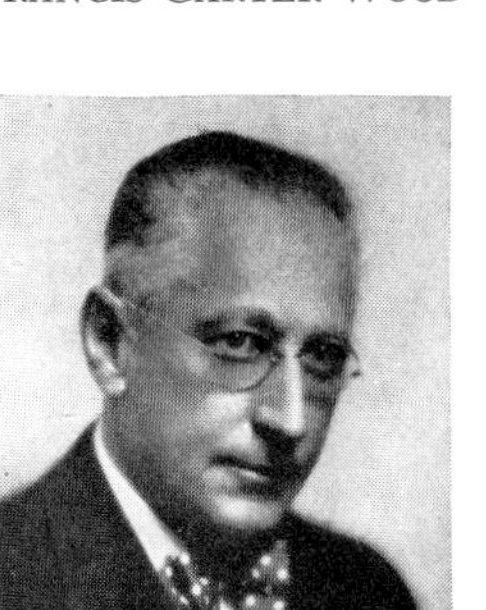
ALBERT SOILAND

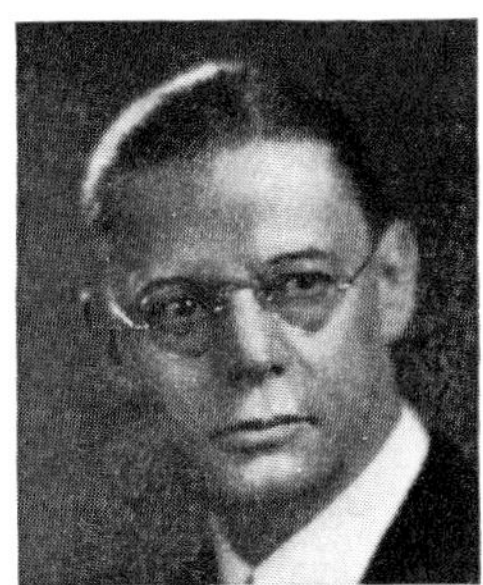
HENRY SCHMITZ

He enjoyed varied extramedical activities, for instance in *Radiology* of September, 1923 appeared the notice that Soiland, admiral of the Southern California Yacht Club, is aboard his yacht, Viking IV, on a cruise to Honolulu. He accumulated considerable experience as a court witness in cases involving radiation injury. As a former president (1926) of the American Radium Society, he contributed the idea for the face of the Janeway Medal, symbolic of the physical impairment paid, as a price for wisdom, by the many radiation casualties. In his testament, Soiland requested that his ashes be returned to his native Norway, and scattered in the fjord near the place of his birth.

AMERICAN COLLEGE OF RADIOLOGY AND PHYSIOTHERAPY

Soiland's call for the ACR was published in that very first (September, 1923) issue of *Radiology*. In October, 1923, in the *Journal of Radiology,* appeared a lengthy editorial which purported that on September 18, 1923 had been created in Omaha the *American College of Radiology and Physiotherapy* (ACRP), an obviously competitive and clearly "paternalistic" organization. Its first act had been to "recognize" twenty-six (grass-root) organizations, with the avowed intention to provide them with "guidance" and other types of protection. Some of these organizations will be mentioned because of the possibly significant relationship between their geographic location and the etymologies used in the respective titles.

There were X-Ray Clubs in Iowa and Milwaukee, and a Detroit Radium and X-Ray Society. Roentgen Ray Societies (aside from the ARRS) existed in Chicago, New England, New York, on the Pacific Coast, in Central Pennsylvania, and in Philadelphia. Radiological Societies (aside from the RSNA) were in Canada, in Central Illinois, and in Missouri. Combined Radiological and Physiotherapy Societies had (allegedly*) been formed in Iowa, Nebraska, South Dakota, and Utah. Protective coverage was also offered to the American

*An inquiry was sent to the secretary of the *Iowa Radiological Society,* James Thompson McMillan III, a (Minnesota-born and bred) radiologist from Des Moines: he replied that the Iowa X-Ray Club held its first meeting in Iowa City on June 12, 1920, and that the current name was adopted on April 27, 1953, but he knew of no connection with any *Physiotherapy* organization. A query was also sent to Joseph Franklin Wepfer in Milwaukee who replied that the *Milwaukee X-Ray Club* went out of existence around 1908, while in 1923 was formed with John Edwin Habbe the *Milwaukee County Radiological Society,* which in January, 1929 changed its name to the current *Milwaukee Roentgen Ray Society.*

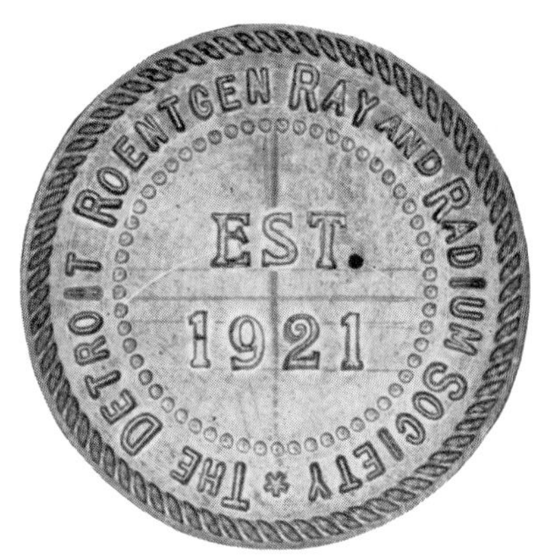

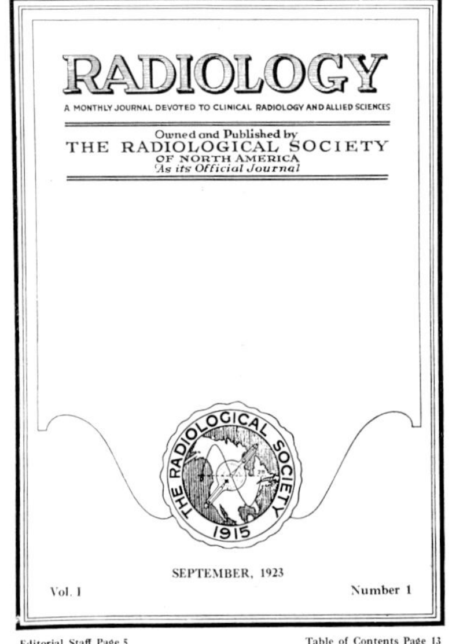

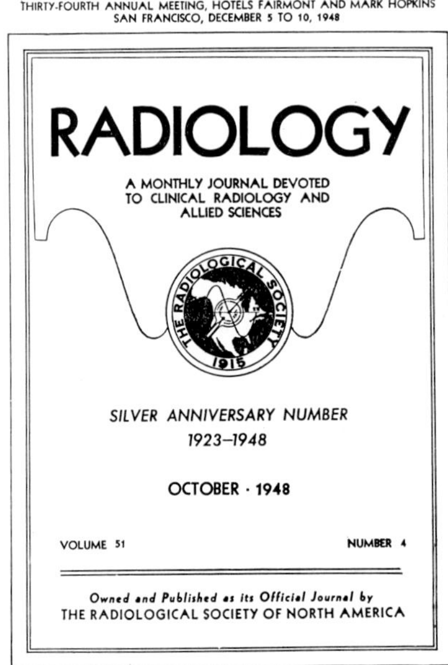

VOLUME 79 NUMBER 1 July 1962

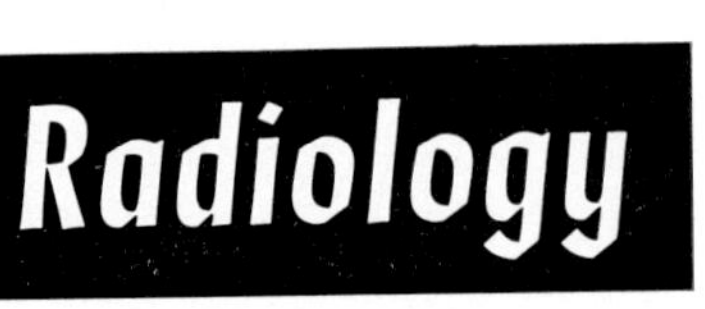

a monthly journal devoted to

clinical radiology and allied sciences

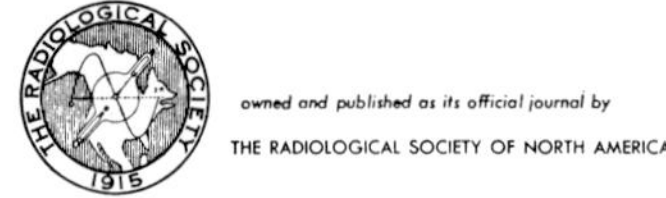

Forty-eighth Annual Meeting / Palmer House, Chicago / November 25–30, 1962

Society of Dental Radiographers (which at that time did not mean dental x-ray technicians.)

The first large-scale meeting of the ACRP was scheduled for December 3-7, 1923 in Rochester, Minnesota – under the presidency of Samuel Beresford Childs (1861-1939), a (formerly tuberculous) New Yorker who had made good in Denver. They selected Edwin Atkins Merritt (1880-1946) for their president-elect, but the driving force was the secretary-treasurer Roy W. Fouts (1885-1951),* radiologist of Lord Lister Hospital in Omaha from 1923 to 1936.

At the organizational meeting, the inaugural presidential address – printed in the *Journal of Radiology* right after the editorial – had been given by C. L. Mullins, a general practitioner and part-time electrotherapist from Broken Bow (Nebraska). Merritt – partner in the famous triumvirate of private radiologists, Groover, Christie, and Merritt of Washington (D.C.) – did not appear very prone to accept the presidency. And Arthur Ulderic Desjardins, who was to become Carman's heir at Mayo's, wryly commented in December, 1923 in *Radiology* on the benefits which could be derived from reducing, rather than increasing, the number of specialty organizations.

*All efforts to find Fouts' middle name failed. Neither the AMA, nor any of the other directories give more than the initial. The professor of radiology in Nebraska University, Howard Beeman Hunt, did not know it, none of the former associates and colleagues of Fouts in Omaha knew it. And it was not found in the records of Fouts' own *alma mater,* the University of Illinois.

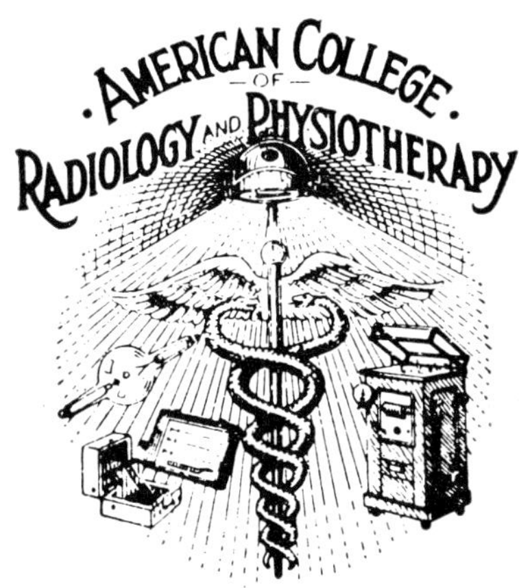

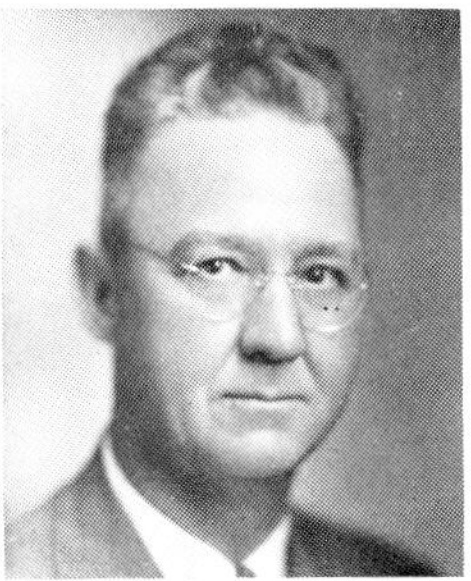

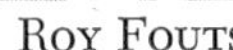
ROY FOUTS

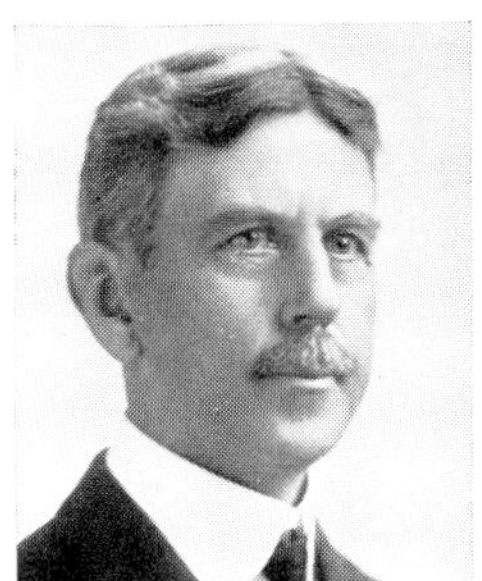
SAMUEL B. CHILDS

The ACRP continued nonetheless to hop, skip, crawl, and fumble for another two years until their official organ, the *Journal of Radiology* passed away, while preserving to the bitter end its forceful subtitle, *Journal of Ideas and Ideals!* The final idea (in the closing 1926 issue) was to drop the word Radiology from the title of the ACRP: it became the American College of Physiotherapy, and soon thereafter the respectable American Congress of Physical Therapy. Fouts continued as the latter's secretary and became vice-president of the AMA in 1948, proving that "active" people are always in demand.

The American Congress of Physical Therapy continued to publish the former *Journal of Radiology* under the title *Archives of Physical Therapy, X-Ray, Radium* (1926-1937). It was absorbed by the *Archives of Physical Therapy,* which had superseded the *American Journal of Electrotherapeutics and Radiology* (1916-1925), itself an outgrowth of the *Journal of Electrotherapeutics* (1890-1901) and *Journal of Advanced Therapeutics* (1902-1915). The then reinforced *Archives of Physical Therapy* (1938-1944) became the *Archives of Physical Medicine* (1945-1952) and – as its territory was gradually delineated – it changed its name in 1953 to *Archives of Physical Medicine and Rehabilitation.*

RADIO- IN GERMANY

The *Golden Age* had caused many changes. The Germans condescended to issue in Berlin four volumes of an export item for Spanish-speaking countries, the *Revista de Radiologia-X,* with the educational subtitle *Revista de Roentgenologia.* In Frankfurt-am-Main and Leipzig appeared 20 volumes of a monographic series called *Radiologische Praktika* (1924-1933). During the Era of the Pioneers, Albert E. Stein (1875-?)* had edited ten volumes (1910-1919) of the *Zentralblatt für Röntgenstrahlen und Verwandte Gebiete* (related domains). It was re-issued by the German Roentgen Society during the Golden Age in 1926: the editor was Karl Frik, and the name was also changed, to *Zentrablatt für die Gesamte* (entire) *Radiologie.* It was discontinued in 1944, and re-started in 1952.

The *Radiologische Rundschau* (panorama) appeared first at Münich in 1932 as the official organ of the Bayrische Gesellschaft für Roentgenologie und Radiologie (patterned after the Sovietic terminology,

*No biographical information is available on Stein, who lived in Wiesbaden, and was undoubtedly one of the recognized German roentgen pioneers.

used at that time also in Czechoslovakia). It was being published by the Karger Verlag, located in Berlin. When Hitler came to power, Karger had to move to Switzerland, and the title of the *Radiologische Rundschau* became the subtitle of the (internationalized) *Radiologia Clinica*, which is still appearing in Basel, where it was edited by the regretted Max Lüdin, who died in 1961.

Another quadrilingual periodical, the *Radiologica* (Berlin, 1937-1940) had four subtitles, the one in Ger-

„Radiologische Praktika"

Herausgegeben von

Prof. Dr. **W. Alwens**, Frankfurt a. M., Prof. Dr. **Fr. Dessauer**, Frankfurt a. M., Prof. Dr. **R. Grashey**, München, Dr. **P. Happel**, Frankfurt a. M., Prof. Dr. **R. Kienböck**, Wien, Primarius Dr. **W. Frh. v. Wieser**, Wien

Band I

(II4 des Themenverzeichnisses)

Ein Verzeichnis der vorgesehenen **Praktika**-Bände befindet sich am Schluß des Buches

Verlag von Keim & Nemnich
Frankfurt a. M.
1924

Zeitschrift
für medizinische
Elektrologie und Röntgenkunde

Begründet als Zeitschrift für Elektrotherapie
von **Dr. Hans Kurella.**

Unter Mitwirkung

der Herren: Geh.-Rat Prof. Dr. BERNHARDT, Berlin, Prof. Dr. BONHOEFFER, Breslau, Prof. Dr. BORUTTAU, Berlin, Prof. Dr. L. BRAUER, Marburg i. H., Dr. TOBY COHN, Berlin, Prof. Dr. CZERNY, Breslau, Prof. Dr. de la CAMP, Freiburg, Geh.-Rat Prof. Dr. ERB, Heidelberg, Privatdozent Dr. FRANKENHÄUSER, Berlin, Privatdozent Dr. L. FREUND, Wien, Geh.-Rat Prof. Dr. GARRÈ, Bonn, Dr. GOCHT, Halle a. S., Dr. W. S. HEDLEY, London, Prof. Dr. HILDEBRANDT, Marburg, Dr. J. L. HOORWEG, Utrecht, Prof. Dr. JAMIN, Erlangen, Prof. Dr. JENSEN, Breslau, Prof. Dr. KLINGMÜLLER, Kiel, Dr. KÖHLER, Wiesbaden, Privatdozent Dr. LADAME, Genf, Dr. LAQUERRIÈRE, Paris, Dr. LEONARD, Philadelphia, Prof. E. LEXER, Königsberg i. Pr., Prof. Dr. LUDLOFF, Breslau, Prof. Dr. LUMMER, Breslau, Prof. Dr. von LUZENBERGER, Rom, Geh.-Rat Prof. Dr. MORITZ, Straßburg i. E., Dr. O. MUND, Görlitz, Geh.-Rat Prof. Dr. NEISSER, Breslau, Oberarzt Dr. NONNE, Hamburg, Prof. Dr. REMAK, Berlin, Prof. Dr. RIEDER, München, Prof. Dr. RUMPF, Bonn, Prof. Dr. WERTHEIM-SALOMONSON, Amsterdam, Prof. Dr. SCHATKIJ, Wien, Prof. Dr. SCHIFF, Wien, Privatdozent Dr. SCHÄFER, Breslau, Prof. Dr. SCHOLTZ, Königsberg, Geh.-Rat Prof. Dr. STINTZING, Jena, Geh.-Rat Prof. Dr. von STRÜMPELL, Breslau, Prof. Dr. WINDSCHEID, Leipzig, Dr. ZANIETOWSKI, Krakau, Geh.-Rat Prof. Dr. TH. ZIEHEN, Berlin, Dr. A. ZIMMERN, Paris

redigiert von

Prof. Dr. Paul Krause und **Prof. Dr. Ludwig Mann**
Direktor der mediz. Poliklinik in Jena — Privatdozent für Neuropathologie in Breslau

10. Band.

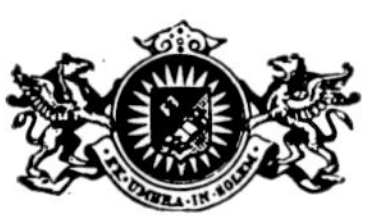

Leipzig 1908
Verlag von Johann Ambrosius Barth
Dörrienstraße 16.

Année 1914 **THESE** N°

PRÉSENTÉE POUR
LE DOCTORAT DE L'UNIVERSITÉ DE PARIS
(MENTION MÉDECINE)

PAR

Mlle Sophie FEYGIN
Née à Lodz, le 15 mars 1883
Externe des Hôpitaux
Médaille de bronze de l'Assistance publique

DU CANCER RADIOLOGIQUE

Président : M. HUTINEL, *professeur*

PARIS
LIBRAIRIE MÉDICALE ET SCIENTIFIQUE
JULES ROUSSET
1, rue Casimir-Delavigne, et rue Monsieur-le-Prince, 12
1914

Aus dem Samariterhause zu Heidelberg

KASUISTISCHER BEITRAG ZUR FRAGE DES RÖNTGEN-CARCINOMS

INAUGURAL-DISSERTATION
ZUR ERLANGUNG DER DOKTORWÜRDE DER
HOHEN MEDIZINISCHEN FAKULTÄT
DER
GROSSHERZOGLICH BADISCHEN RUPPRECHT-KARL-UNIVERSITÄT ZU HEIDELBERG

VORGELEGT VON
ANTON TILLING
AUS LÜTKENBECK

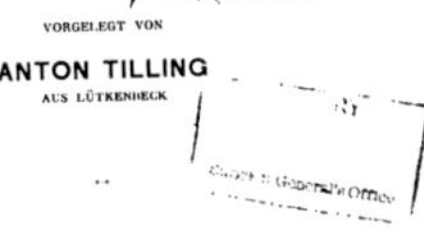

DÜSSELDORF
VERLAG W. GIRARDET
1915

FORTSCHRITTE AUF DEM GEBIETE DER RÖNTGENSTRAHLEN

Organ der Deutschen Röntgen-Gesellschaft und der Röntgenvereinigung in Budapest

BEGRÜNDET VON HEINRICH ALBERS-SCHÖNBERG
HERAUSGEGEBEN VON
RUDOLF GRASHEY-KÖLN

GEORG THIEME · VERLAG · LEIPZIG

man began with *Internationale Zeitschrift für Photobiologie und Biophysik.* The name was later changed to *Fundamenta Radiologica.*

Usually, though, recognized and other Germanic etymologies prevailed, as in the perennial *Strahlentherapie* (which, at its start in 1912, was tri-headed, but only two heads survived), in the *Ergebnisse der Medizinischen Strahlenforschung* (first issued in 1925), and the short lived *Röntgenkunde in Einzeldarstellungen* (translatable as roentgen science in monographs) begun in 1928. The *Röntgenpraxis* (1929) was a supplement to the *Fortschritte* with which it later merged. Above all, though, there existed in Germany since 1905 a famous tube factory with the provocative title Radiologie GmbH, and it stayed in business until Allied bombers destroyed it during the Berlin air raids.

HANDBUCH DER RADIOLOGIE

UNTER MITWIRKUNG VON

Prof. Dr. A. BESTELMEYER-GREIFSWALD, Prof. Dr. P. DEBYE-GÖTTINGEN, Prof. Dr. A. EINSTEIN-BERLIN, Dr. L. FÖPPL-WÜRZBURG, Prof. Dr. E. GEHRCKE-BERLIN, Prof. Dr. H. GEITEL-WOLFENBÜTTEL, Prof. Dr. A. HAGENBACH-BASEL, Prof. Dr. W. HALLWACHS-DRESDEN, Prof. Dr. H. A. LORENTZ-LEYDEN, Prof. Dr. E. MARX-LEIPZIG, Prof. Dr. G. MIE-HALLE, Prof. Owen W. RICHARDSON-LONDON, Prof. Dr. E. RIECKE-GÖTTINGEN †, Prof. Dr. E. RUTHERFORD-MANCHESTER, Prof. Dr. R. SEELIGER-GREIFSWALD, Prof. Dr. A. SOMMERFELD-MÜNCHEN, Prof. Dr. H. STARKE-AACHEN, Prof. J. S. TOWNSEND-OXFORD, Prof. Dr. W. WIEN-WÜRZBURG, Prof. Dr. P. ZEEMAN-AMSTERDAM

HERAUSGEGEBEN VON
DR. ERICH MARX
A. O. PROF. an der UNIVERSITÄT LEIPZIG

BAND V

LEIPZIG
AKADEMISCHE VERLAGSGESELLSCHAFT M. B. H.
1919

Fürstenau - X - Ray - Tubes

Fürstenau-Intensimeter and Accessories

Eppens Intensifying Screens

Distributed by
Paul Luck[illegible]h
[illegible] East 2[illegible] St.
New York City

RADIOLOGIE
Fürstenau, Eppens & Co.
Berlin W 35

Issued August 1921

RADIOLOGICA

Internationale Zeitschrift für Photobiologie und Biophysik Strahlenmedizin und Photochemie	Revue internationale de photobiologie et biophysique radiologie médicale et photochimie
International Journal of Photobiology and Biophysics Medical Radiology and Photochemistry	Rivista internazionale di fotobiologia e biofisica radiologia medica e fotochimica

Unter besonderer Mitwirkung von

A. AIMES-Montpellier, ALMEIDA E SÁ-Lissabon, W. R. G. ATKINS-Plymouth, H. L. J. BÄCKSTRÖM-Stockholm, E. et H. BIANCANI-Paris, E. BRUNER-Warschau, K. BÜTTNER-Kiel, JANET H. CLARK-Baltimore, G. CHARRIER-Bologna, W. W. COBLENTZ-Washington, W. CZUNFT-Budapest, N. DHAR-Allahabad, CH. DHÉRÉ-Freiburg (Schweiz), B. M. DUGGAR-Madison, J. EGGERT-Leipzig, W. FRIEDRICH-Berlin, C. FUNK-Müncheberg, G. GATOSCHI-Bukarest, J. GHOSH-Dacca, J. GROBER-Jena, J. GUNZBURG-Anvers, M. D'HALLUIN-Lille, H. M. HANSEN-Kopenhagen, W. HAUSMANN-Wien, H. HAVLICEK-Schatzlar, F. HERČIK-Brünn, PAULA HERTWIG-Berlin, V. HESS-Graz, M. JÖRG-Buenos Aires, P. JORDAN-Rostock, E. KNAPP-Müncheberg, W. KOLLATH-Rostock, F. M. KUEN-Wien, A. LAMBADARIDIS-Athen, H. LANGENDORFF-Freiburg i. Br., R. LATARJET-Lyon, F. LINKE-Frankfurt a. M., H. LUNELUND-Helsingfors, J. MAISIN-Louvain, H. MEYER-Bremen, J. MEYER-Paris, G. MIESCHER-Zürich, J. MÖLLERSTRÖM-Stockholm, W. MÖRIKOFER-Davos, G. MOURIQUAND-Lyon, M. NAKAIDZUMI-Tokio, Y. NAKASHIMA-Fukuoka, H. PASCHOUD-Lausanne, A. PETRIKALN-Riga, H. PFLEIDERER-Kiel, A. PIRES DE LIMA-Porto, M. PONZIO-Torino, O. RICHTER-Brünn, O. RISSE-Berlin, J. SAIDMAN-Vallauris, F. SCHEMINSKY-Wien, A. SCHÖNBERG-Cairo, MONA SPIEGEL-ADOLF-Philadelphia, E. STENGER-Berlin, A. STÜHMER-Freiburg i. B., T. SWENSSON-Stockholm, N. W. TIMOFÉEFF-RESSOVSKY-Berlin, F. VOLTZ-München, P. WELS-Greifswald, A. VAN WIJK-Eindhoven

herausgegeben von

H. JAUSION-Paris, J. PLOTNIKOW-Zagreb, H. SCHREIBER-Berlin

ERSTER BAND

Mit 81 Figuren im Text und auf 3 Tafeln

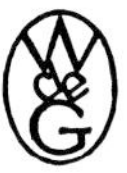

BERLIN und LEIPZIG 1937
WALTER DE GRUYTER & CO.
vormals G. J. Göschen'sche Verlagshandlung / J. Guttentag, Verlagsbuchhandlung / Georg Reimer / Karl J. Trübner / Veit & Comp.

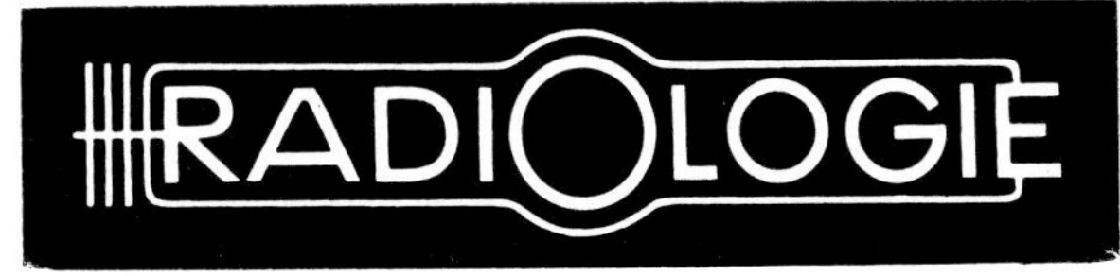

BRITISH INSTITUTE OF RADIOLOGY

Non-medical members prevailed in the (British) Roentgen Society. This is why in 1902 pioneer medical radiologists formed the Electrotherapeutic Society which developed in 1905 into the Electro-Therapeutic Section of the Royal Society of Medicine. In

1917, when a Cambridge University Diploma in Medical Radiology and Electrology (DMRE) was proposed, there was no medical body to inaugurate and sponsor the teaching in London. Therefore a new and purely medical society was formed, from the medical members of the Roentgen Society and members of the afore-mentioned Electro-Therapeutic Section. This new society, the British Association for the Advancement of Radiology and Physiotherapy, was incorporated in 1921, acquired 32 Welbeck Street (London, W. 1) as its home in 1922, and in 1924 changed its name to the British Institute of Radiology. In 1927 it was amalgamated with the Roentgen Society under the present title of British Institute of Radiology incorporated with the British Roentgen Society (BIR).

In 1918, the *Archives of Radiology and Electrology* was adopted as the official organ of the BIR. In 1923 the *Archives* became the property of the BIR and in January, 1924 the BIR altered that title to *British Journal of Radiology* (BIR Section). At the same time the *Journal of the Roentgen Society* was renamed *British Journal of Radiology* (Roentgen Society Section), and the two sections of the *Journal* were published concurrently by the two bodies concerned until the end of 1927. At that time, the two journals merged and in January, 1928 began to appear as the unique *British Journal of Radiology.*

Among the former presidents of the BIR should be mentioned Sir James Mackenzie Davidson (1857-1919), a former opthalmic surgeon in Aberdeen. He was one of the British roentgen pioneers, and became particularly well known for his method of roentgen-stereoscopic localization of foreign bodies, especially in the orbit. After him is named the Library of the BIR, and they have since 1920 a Memorial Lecture in his name.

Another president of the BIR was John Macintyre (1857-1928) – Kurt Walther published a delightful biography of Macintyre (with portrait) in the January, 1958 issue of *Röntgen-und Laboratoriumpraxis* – a laryngologist in Glasgow, best remembered for having pieced together in May, 1896 the first "cinematographic" film of the movement of the leg of a frog. Macintyre never practiced radiology professionally.

Sir Herbert Jackson (1863-1936) introduced the curved cathode x-ray tube, which he declined to patent;

BRITISH INSTITUTE OF RADIOLOGY & RONTGEN SOCIETY

The BRITISH JOURNAL OF RADIOLOGY

NEW SERIES, VOL. I. JANUARY, 1928. NO. I.

ADDRESS AT THE AMALGAMATION OF THE RÖNTGEN SOCIETY AND THE BRITISH INSTITUTE OF RADIOLOGY, NOVEMBER 17th, 1927.

By SIR HUMPHRY ROLLESTON, Bart, K.C.B., M.D., Regius Professor of Physic in the University of Cambridge, President of the British Institute of Radiology

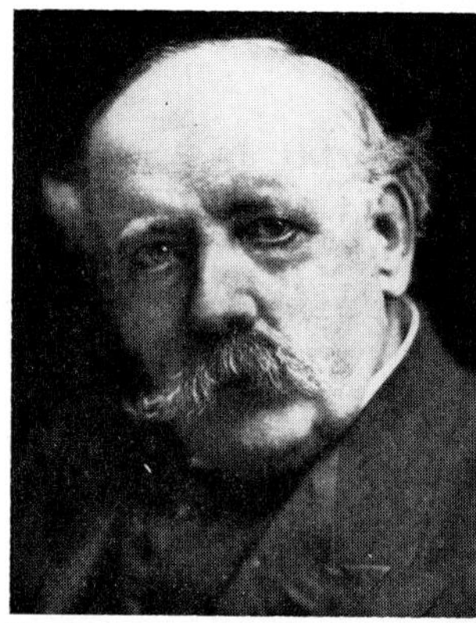
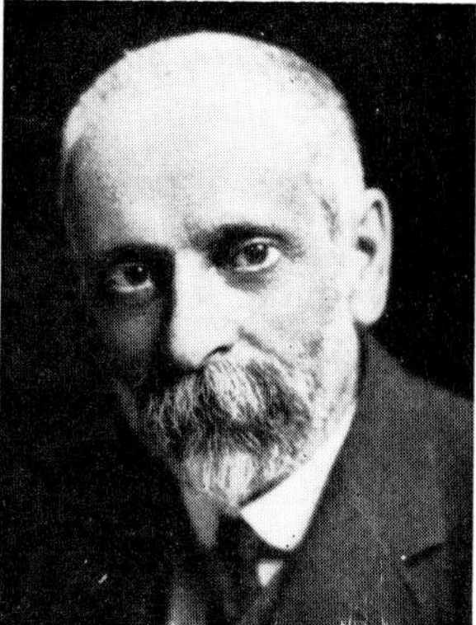

EDITORS OF THE BIR: William Deane Butcher and (goateed) James Gardiner.

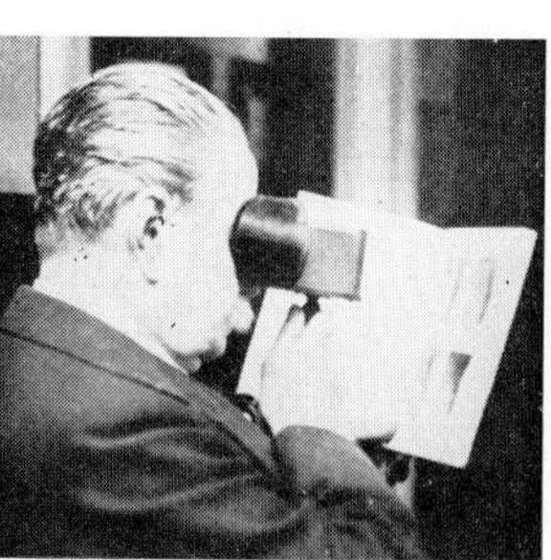
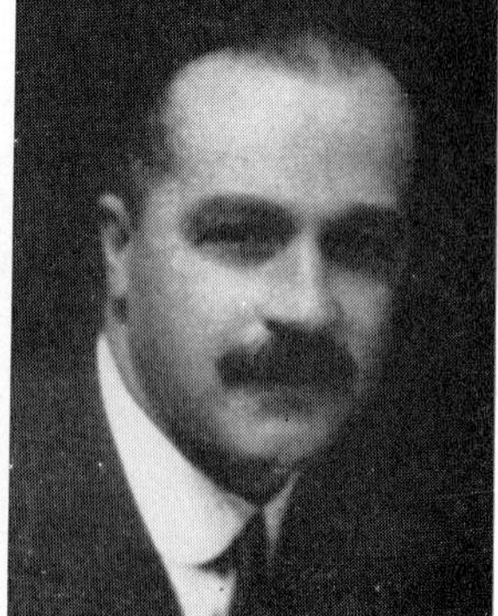

SIR JAMES MACKENZIE DAVIDSON. Looking at his stereoscopic (rather, sterreographic) achievement. The other portrait is of ALFRED ERNEST BARCLAY.

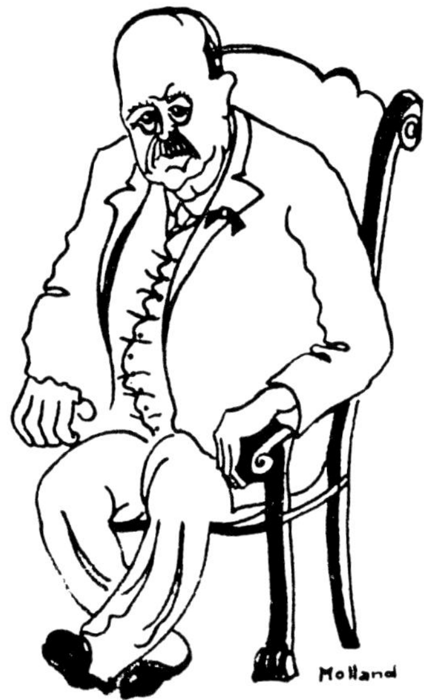

THURSTAN HOLLAND

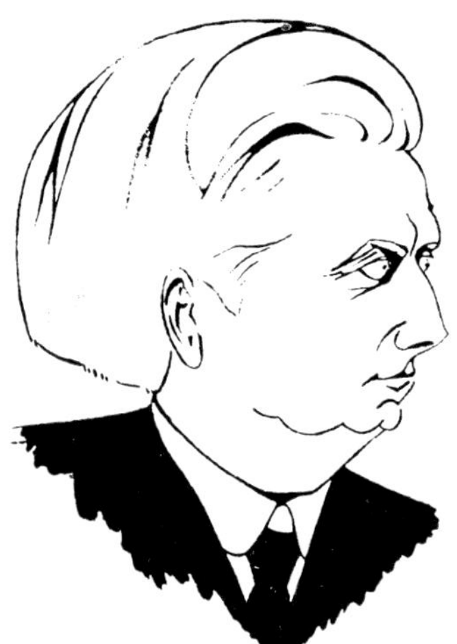

GÖSTA FORSSELL

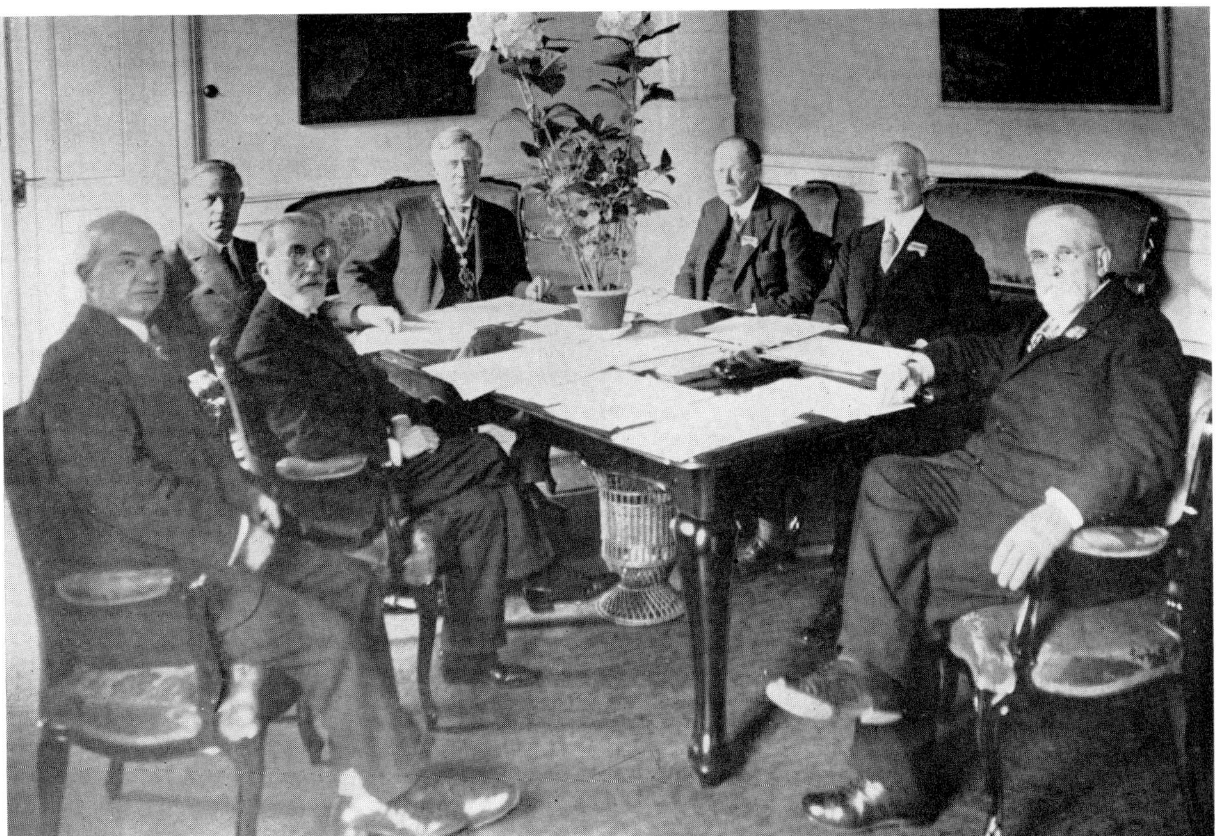

Courtesy: Centre Antoine Béclère.

EXECUTIVE COMMITTEE OF THE 2ND ICR (1928). As it met in Stockholm, chairman was Gösta Forssell (Sweden) seated at the head of the table in line with the door. Clockwise around the table are Thurstan Holland (U K), George Pfahler (U S A), then Antoine Béclère (across from Forssell). Next is Martin Haudek (Austria) – remembered for his ulcer niche – Pasquale Tandoja (Italy), and Walter Friedrich (Germany) – known for his groundbreaking research into the dosimetry of radiation.

during World War I he contributed significantly to the chemistry of lens glass, for which he was knighted. Another president, Charles Edmund Stanley Phillips (1871-1945), an amateur physicist who never went to college, contributed his share to "x-ray science," including a very early bibliography, published in the *Electrician Series* (1897).

The BIR awards also an annual prize in the memory of Alfred Ernest Barclay (1877-1949) who worked at the Manchester Royal Infirmary, taught thereafter in Cambridge in connection with the D.R.M.E., and finally was associated with the Nuffield Institute for Medical Research. He was a very astute investigator and published beautiful papers on gastro-intestinal diagnosis, cineradiography, and microradiography. Barclay had many friends in this country, especially among those stationed in England during World War II.

Robert Knox (1867-1928), another former president of the BIR and editor of the *British Journal of Radiology,* was instrumental in organizing after World War I the first International Congress of Radiology (ICR) held in London in 1925. At the 2nd ICR in Stockholm (1928) the BIR presented a presidential badge and chain of office for the perpetual use of future presidents, the names of whom

Antoine Béclère

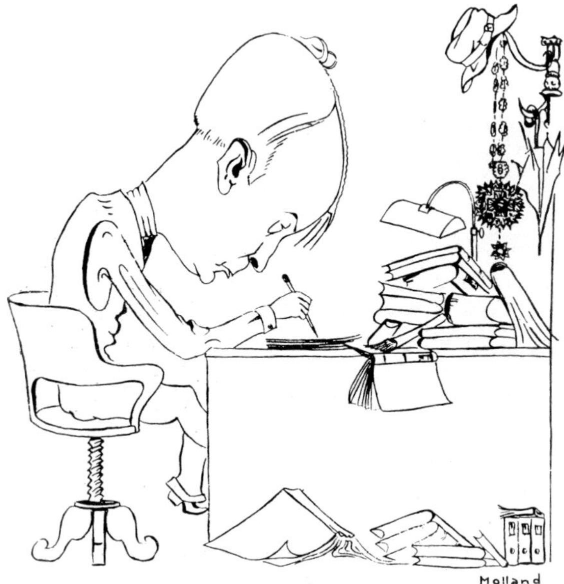

Hans Schinz

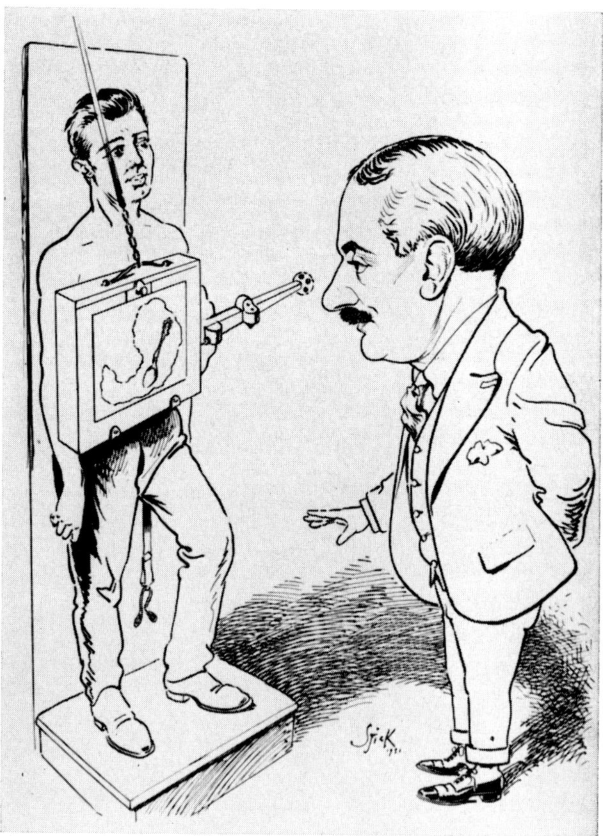

René Ledoux-Lebard. The secretary-general of the 3rd ICR (Paris) was a renowned diagnostician, and this cartoon was produced during and for the occasion of that ICR (it is from Prof. Ben Orndoff's collection, as are several other items, some of which inadvertently may not have been so labeled).

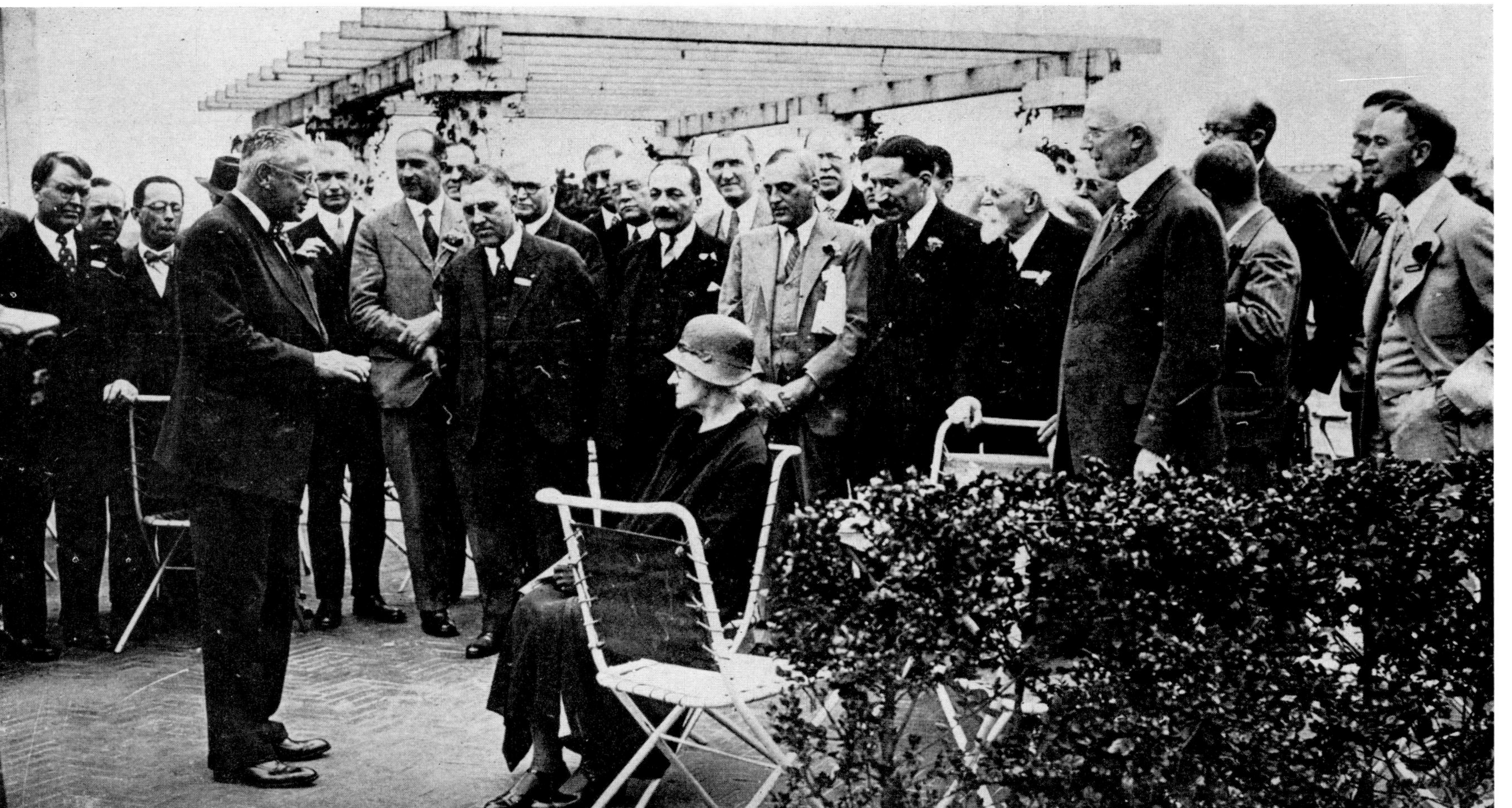

Courtesy: Ben Orndoff.

ACR Conference during the ICR in Paris (1931). One of the functions of the "old" ACR (continued by the "new" ACR) was to hold festive convocations during the successive meetings of the ICR – for which Garland referred to the ACR as the cape-and-gown society of senior radiologists. Here Albert Soiland is honoring Marie Curie with the ACR's Gold Medal. Bespectacled Elis Gustav Berven projects to the viewer's left of Soiland, while Severin Heyerdahl's face seems contiguous with Soiland's. Next to Heyerdahl stands Barclay, partly covered by Bundy Allen; further to the right is René Ledoux-Lebard with his black mustache. Between Allen and Lendoux-Lebard appear three heads, Leon LeWald, W. E. Chamberlain, and Fedor Haenisch. On the viewer's right side of Ledoux-Lebard is the head of Eddy Ernst, then Charles Waters (with hands clasped in front), whose head partly obscures that of Thurstan Holland. The very black mustache of Jacques Forestier contrasts with the white beard of Antoine Béclère, next to whom stands another white-headed figure, George Pfahler. At the far right is Ben Orndoff, who had made all the arrangements for this ceremony, and who was to give a belated account of it (more than a quarter century after it had occurred) in *Radiology* of November, 1958.

are (and will continue to be) engraved on the chain. At the 6th ICR in London (1950) the BIR donated a congress bell, the appropriate number of strokes on which should open and conclude future congresses. At the 10th ICR in Montreal (1962) the Canadian Radiological Society started a golden ICR book in which are being inscribed important names, dates, and other information related to future ICR assemblies.

The following meetings of the ICR were held between World Wars I and II. The names are those of the respective president and secretary:

1. London (1925), Charles Thurstan Holland and Stanley Melville.
2. Stockholm (1928), Gösta Forssell and Axel Renander.

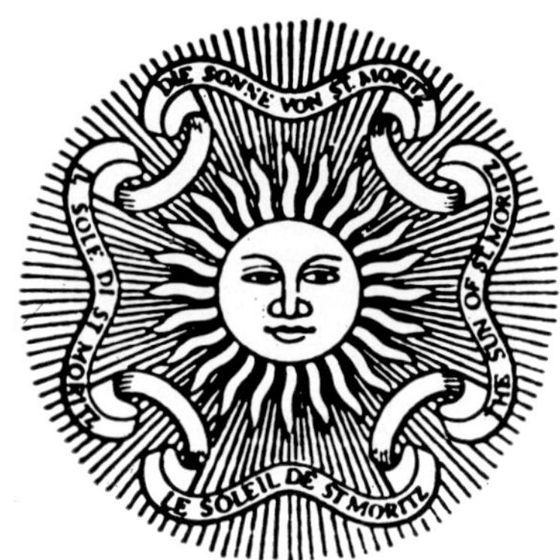

Pseudo-seal of the 4th ICR. This advertising mandala was the only emblem-like item reproduced in the books of the 4th ICR, and only one time, at the very end of the last volume. Since it contains the sun, it is not at all inappropriate as a radiologic symbol, and may be considered as the precursor of the ICR seals.

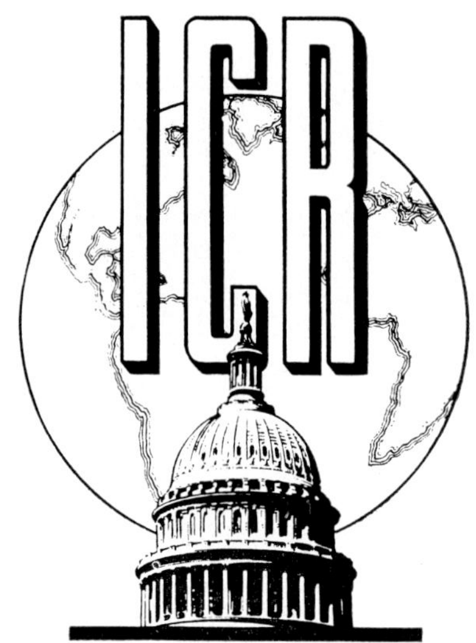

Seal of the 5th ICR. The ICR seals were inaugurated with this design (the idea was Orndoff's who, in 1933, had a beautiful symbol made for the American Congress of Radiology). Ever since, a seal is prepared for each succeeding meeting of the ICR.

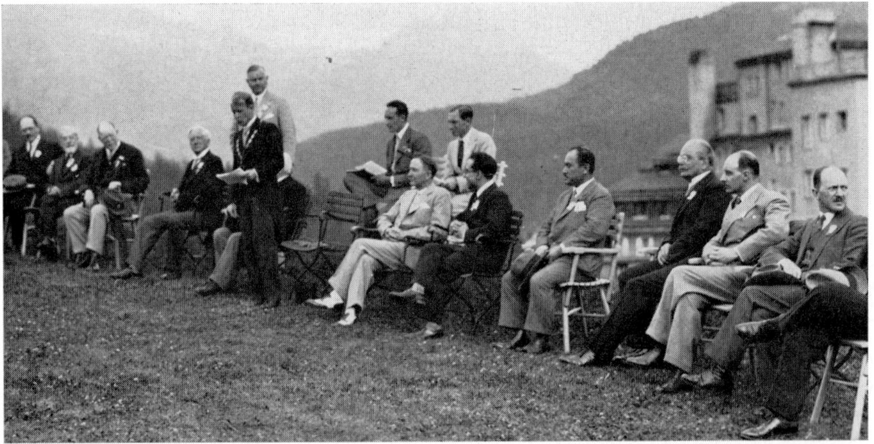

Courtesy: Ben Orndoff.

Open-air amphitheatre at 4th ICR. After three days in Zürich the 4th ICR moved to St. Moritz where many of the sessions were held outdoors. The white-bearded figure far to the left is Tandoja, next to him is Thurstan Holland, then white-haired Forssell and Schinz (wearing the president's chain). Behind Schinz stands Hans Walther (secretary of the 4th ICR). The relaxed Orndoff has a light suit and brown and white shoes, and next to him sits the chairman of the Spanish delegation, Heliodoro Tellez-Plasencia. The elegantly black-suited, mustachioed, and bespectacled Alban Köhler, and (on the far right) Alfred Ernest Barclay (Great Britain) who is looking the other way.

3. Paris (1931), Antoine Béclère and René Ledoux-Lebard.
4. Zürich (1934), Hans Rudolf Schinz and Hans E. Walther.
5. Chicago (1937), Arthur Carlisle Christie and Benjamin Harry Orndoff.

At this point will be inserted a bit of behind-the-scenes history. Orndoff headed the American delegation at the fourth ICR. He noted that the Scandinavian group under Gösta Forssell "wavered" and seemed willing to vote for Berlin as the next meeting place. Thereupon Orndoff agreed with his good friend Pasquale Tandoja (head of the Italian delegation) that if Italy and other South-European states would vote for Chicago, the next time around it was going to be Rome.

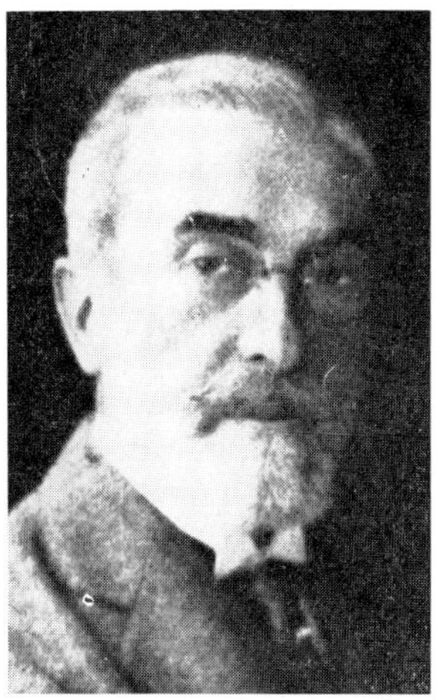

Courtesy: Prof. Arduino Ratti.

Pasquale Tandoja (1870-1934). Italian radiologist who would have been ICR president if it had met in Italy during his lifetime. I hope Tandoja's name will be remembered during the proceedings of the next ICR, to be held in Rome in 1965.

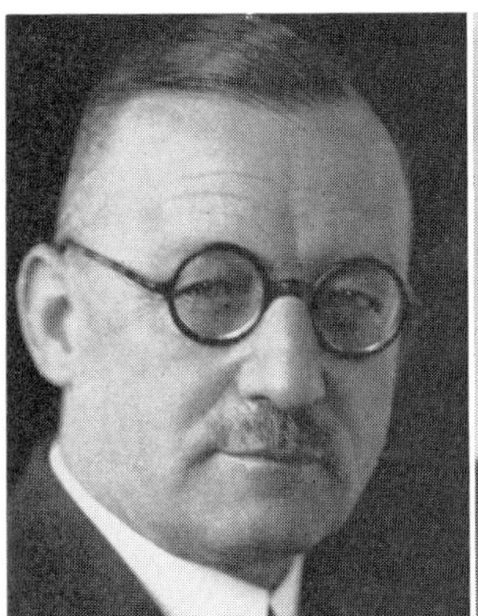

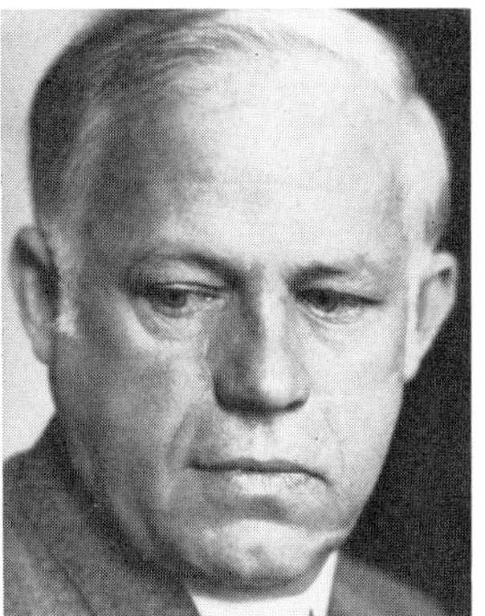

Courtesy: Ben Orndoff

German Roentgen Brass. Karl Frik and (white-haired) Walter Friedrich would have been the president and secretary of the ICR, if it had met in Berlin in 1940.

X光線

レントゲン光線

X線科学

レントゲン科学

放射線科学

Japanese radio-ideographs. This is how the Japanese write various radiologic terms. In their written language are used many Chinese ideographs, with added syllabic *kana* characters, to denote Japanese inflections. The *kana* sillabary (48 phonetic signs) has two versions, the *katakana* and the more complicated *hiragana*. The first row – transliterated *ekkusu-kôsen* (meaning x-ray) – begins with the Latin letter X (they have no corresponding sign), and ends with the Chinese character for ray (which can also be found in all but the fourth row). The second row – transliterated *Rentogen-kôsen* (meaning Röntgen's ray) – starts with Röntgen's name in *katakana* symbols. The third line – transliterated *ekkusu-senkagaku* – begins again with the Latin X, continues with the Chinese ideograph for ray, and ends with two ideographs which signify scientific discipline: it all adds up to "x-rayology." In the fourth line there is a similar ending, but it comes after Röntgen's name in *katakana* – transliterated *rentogen-kagaku* (meaning roentgenology). The last row contains only Chinese ideographs, among which we can by now identify the last three (ray and science); it begins with the ideographs for the sense of medical; the whole thing can be transliterated as *hosha-senkagaku*, and means medical radiology. The brushwork was obligingly performed – especially for this book – by a Japanese friend of mine, Prof. Masaaki Nishida, who teaches Somatologic Esthetics (Art Anatomy) in the Tokyo University of Arts.

Chicago made it, but Tandoja died only weeks later. Orndoff, true to his promise, came out strongly in favor of having the 6th ICR in Rome. In Chicago the vote went against him, and Berlin was selected so that the following president of the ICR was to have been Karl Frik. But in 1940 World War II was in full swing, and no ICR meeting was held until 1950.

A short digression is in order to specify that there was no official seal for the ICR held in Switzerland in 1934. And yet, on the very last page of the very last volume of their proceedings, and only there, was reproduced the "sun of St. Moritz," perhaps as a melancholy reminiscence of the passing of heliotherapy. The first official seal of any ICR was created by Orndoff for the Chicago meeting of 1937. Ever since, a special seal was designed for each successive ICR.

MORE RADIO

Throughout the Golden Age, the German roentgen terminology was solidly entrenched, not only in the Soviet Union and in Central Europe, but also in the USA. Actually, all the etymologies had circled the globe, thus in the eclectic Japanese there is a term for roentgenology, which sounds like *rentogenkagaku,* another for radiology, *hoshasenkagaku,* and the peculiar form *ekkususenkagaku* (x-rayology).

There were several Japanese publications in the field. The most important was the *Nippon Rentogen Gakkai Zasshi,* edited by Omasa Saito; it appeared since 1924 with a bibliographic supplement, the *Rentogengaku Nippon Bunken.* An excellent bibliographic survey of Japanese radiologic literature was published in 1931 in German by Koichi Fujinami (1880-1942), professor of radiology in Keio University (Tokyo).

In Latin America, the prefix radio- was uncontested champion. When Carlos Vieira de Moraes pub-

REVISTA

DE LA

SOCIEDAD ARGENTINA DE RADIO Y ELECTROLOGÍA

(CRÓNICA DE SESIONES)

Publicación de la Asociación Médica Argentina

TOMO I

BUENOS AIRES

DIRECCIÓN Y ADMINISTRACIÓN: SANTA FE, 1171

1925

ARCHIVIO

DI

RADIOLOGIA

DIRETTO

dal prof. CARLO GUARINI

ANNO I. MARZO - APRILE 1933 N. 2

NVNTIVS RADIOLOGICVS

SCRIPTA AD REM PERTINENTIA RECENSET

DIRETTORE

ARISTIDE BVSI

ROMA

REDATTORI CAPO

PROF A SALOTTI — SIENA

PROF L TVRANO — ROMA

STABILIMENTO TIPOGRAFICO COMBATTENTI - SIENA

lished in 1935 in São Paulo (Brazil) a study of cardiovascular dynamics based on the roentgenkymography of Pleikart Stumpf, he rechristened it *radiokymographia*.

In 1925, appeared in Buenos Aires the *Revista de la Sociedad Argentina de Radio- y Electrologia*, in Bruxelles the *Radiologie et Chirurgie*, and in Naples the *Archivio de Radiologia*. Similarly authenticated entries are dated 1932 in Brazil, the *Revista de Radiologia Clinica* (Porto Alegre), 1933 in Italy, the *Nuntius Radiologicus* (Siena), and 1937 in Yugoslavia, the *Radioloski Glasnik* (voicer).

As a political entity, Yugoslavia appeared on the maps only after World War I. In Croatia (which was then under Austro-Hungarian rule), the first professional article dealing with x rays was published in the medical periodical *Liecnicki Viestnik* of February 15, 1896. In 1905, M. Cackovic produced the roentgen plates of single bones of the fossil *Man of Krapina* for reproduction in an anthropologic study. The Yugoslav "father" of Radiology was Laza Popovic, appointed in 1922 extraordinary and in 1931 ordinary professor of roentgenology in Zagreb. In 1923, Popovic authored their first specialty manual, called *Klinicka Rentgenologija*. Popovic was also editor of the above mentioned specialty journal, which in 1940 changed its title to *Jugoslavenski Radioloski Glasnik*, but only a single issue came out under this name, because of World War II. There existed in Zagreb a Medical Roentgen Society since 1927: on October 16, 1936 it was organized as the Section for Radiology, Electrology, Physical Therapy and Balneology of the Medical Association of Croatia; its first and long-time secretary was S. Kadrnka. Its first president, B. Bressan, became a radiation casualty.

RADIOLOŠKI GLASNIK

REVUE DE RADIOLOGIE YOUGOSLAVE

JUGOSLAVISCHE RADIOLOGISCHE RUNDSCHAU

REVIEW OF YOUGOSLAV RADIOLOGY

REDAKTOR I EDITOR:

PROF. DR. LAZA POPOVIĆ, ZAGREB

COLABORATORES:

Dr. A. ST. GANEV, VARNA; Dr. G. KOŽUHAROV, SOFIJA; Dr. ANG. NIKOLAJEV, SOFIJA; Prof. dr. A. SAHATČIJEV, SOFIJA; Dr. G. TENČEV, SOFIJA; Doc. dr. BEHOUNEK, PRAHA; Dr. FORT, PRAHA; Prof. dr. GRUSS, Praha; Doc. dr. J. KRAL, PRAHA; Dr. MATOUŠEK, PRAHA; Doc. dr. F. V. NOVAK, PRAHA; Prof. dr. OSTRČIL, PRAHA; Doc. dr. POLLAND, PRAHA; Prof. dr. SAIDL, PRAHA; Doc. dr. V. ŠVAB, PRAHA; Doc. dr. TOMANEK, PRAHA; Dr. T. ALKIEWICZ, POZNAN; Doc. dr. A. ELEKTOROWICZ, WARSZAWA; Dr. J. KOCHANOWSKI, WARSZAWA; Prof. dr. K. MAYER, POZNAN; Dr. M. WERKENTHIN, WARSZAWA; Doc. dr. W. ZAWADOWSKI, WARSZAWA.

BROJ 1 IZLAZI TROMJESEČNO GOD. 1937

On September 3, 1918, Nemirovsky and Tilmant presented to the Academy of Medicine in Paris drawings of the *Aero-Radio-Chir*, the radio-surgical airplane (their paper was abstracted both in the *AMA Journal* and in the *American Journal of Rentgenology*).

In France the radio-prefix had penetrated deep into the vernacular. In a French novel called *New York* (written by the obscure Valentin Mandelstamm), published in *l'Illustration*, there appeared on November 4, 1922 (on page 59) a stylistic gem in which the heroine (Gladys) was said to be as fascinating as if she were to emit *des particules radio-attractifs!*

RADIOLOGY = DIAGNOSIS?

The term radiology never meant the same thing to all people. On an etymologic basis, *Radiology* can be defined as the *study of both the medical and the non-medical aspects of all forms of radiant energy*, whether corpuscular, electro-magnetic, or others. The correctness of this generic meaning is acknowledged

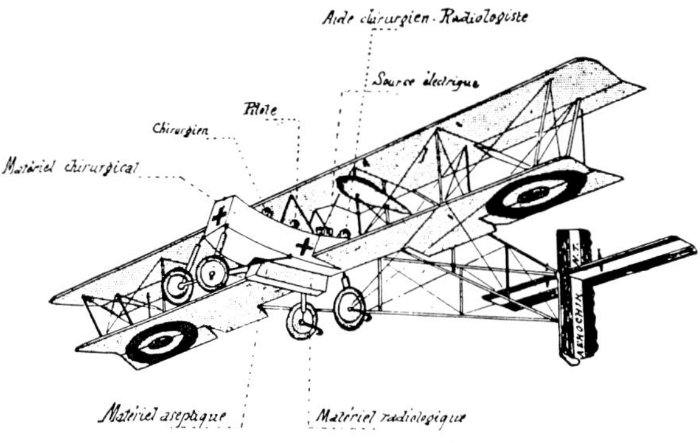

L'avion radio-chirurgical « Aérochir. (1) »,

par

M. A. NEMIROVSKY,	M. TILMANT,
Ingénieur-constructeur, Chef des laboratoires radiologiques aux hôpitaux Espagnol et Russe.	Médecin aide-major de 1re classe, affecté à la mission médicale du major STRONG de l'U. S. Army.

(Projet déposé au Ministère des Inventions le 21 février 1918.)

Courtesy: Bulletin de l'Académie de Médecine, Paris.

AERO-RADIO-CHIR. Radio-surgical airplane, designed by Nemirowsky and Tilmant for the famous (French) Escadrille Pozzi: a single-engine bi-plane which seated three (pilot, radiologist, and surgeon), and carried mobile x-ray apparatus (transformer with interrupter, power provided by airplane engine) as well as gear for emergency surgery (instruments, sterilizer, operating table).

in the (French) Larousse Medical Dictionary of 1952: they specify though, that such correctness notwithstanding, it is the accepted tradition in France to employ the word *radiologie* (and its derivatives, such as *radiologique*) only in connection with medical matters pertaining to *rayons X*. Some authors are more restrictive, and use it only in the sense of diagnostic roentgenology, even though this particular meaning is covered in French and Italian scientese by the term *radio-diagnostic*.

One is not surprised to find the same restricted meaning in the *Tratado Practico de Radiología* first published in 1920 in Buenos Aires by Carlos Heuser. As a matter of fact, there are instances when this narrow sense occurs in the English language. On October 17, 1919, in the *Proceedings of the Royal Society of Medicine,* Albert Ernest Barclay contrasted "radiology" (meaning diagnosis) and "x-ray therapy." Then there is the famous, strictly diagnostic text *Radiology of Bones and Joints* by James Frederick Brailsford, first printed in 1934.

The same restricted meaning of radiology appears in the title of a Turkish diagnostic textbook (*Tibbi Radyoloji*), by Ahmet Tevfik Berkman, published in 1939. Actually, they have used also the Germanic terminology, for instance the term *Röntgen-Diagnostick* appeared in a technical primer issued by V. Yener in 1955. The Turkish Radiological Society, *Türk Radyoloji Cemiyeti,* was founded in 1924. Its official journal, *Türk Radyoloji Mecmuasi,* first issued in 1955, was founded and edited by Muhterem Gökmen, professor

VICHY SAISON Mai à Octobre

ÉTABLISSEMENT THERMAL

BAINS, DOUCHES, PISCINES, MASSAGES

THERMOTHÉRAPIE: Air chaud, Bains d'Air chaud, Bains de Lumière

MÉCANOTHÉRAPIE COMPLÈTE

RADIOSCOPIE, RADIOGRAPHIE

RADIOTHÉRAPIE

ÉLECTROTHÉRAPIE COMPLÈTE

Courants galvanique, faradique, galvano-faradique, sinusoïdal, Électricité statique, Franklinisation hertzienne

HAUTE FRÉQUENCE

Auto-conduction ·:· Lits condensateurs ·:· Diathermie

CURE DE L'OBÉSITÉ par la Méthode du Professeur BERGONIÉ

TRAITEMENT SPÉCIAL des Maladies de Foie, Estomac, Goutte, Diabète, Arthritisme.

HOTEL RADIO HOTEL DE RÉGIME RESTAURANT DE RÉGIME

sous la Direction Médicale du Docteur DAUSSET, de Biarritz.

Radio-Hotel in Vichy. Vichy, a famous hot-water spa in East-Central France, advertised in 1923 this polyvalent diagnostic treatment center, intended mainly (but by no means exclusively) for clients from foreign lands. Although broadcasting was already in full bloom, the term *radio* seemed more suggestive of radiology, or else it would not have been used in the title of this establishment.

INSTITUT du RADIUM et de la RADIOLOGIE

58, Av. Malakoff. Paris · Tél Passy 22·37

LOCATION D'APPAREILLAGES de RADIUM & RAYONS X AUX MÉDECINS RADIOTHÉRAPEUTES

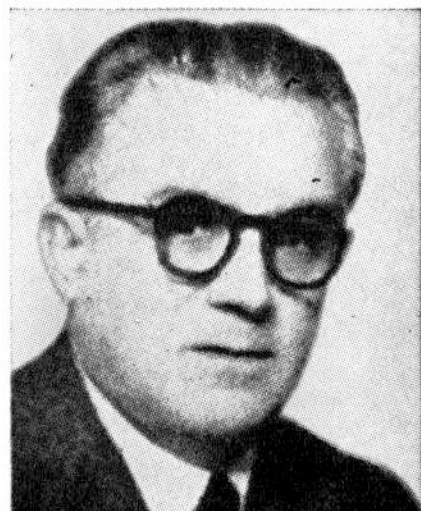

Tevfik Berkman

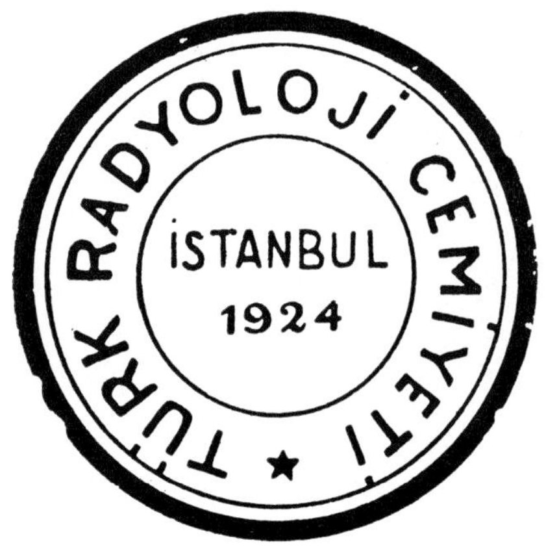

of radiology in the University of Istanbul (who has also written a brief history of their Society).

In this country since the advent of the *Golden Age,* the term radiology carried an all-encompassing sense. Even this general sense was at times exceeded, for instance the *Radiological Review,* a periodical started in Quincy (Illinois) in September-October, 1924 often carried non-radiological items. It underwent several mergers and rechristenings, and is still published now and then as a supplement to the *Mississippi Valley Medical Journal.* Several other supplements appeared in this country, the best known of which was the pre-World War I *Supplement on Roentgenology* of the *Interstate Medical Journal* (St. Louis).

Today's lavishly illustrated but irregularly published *Medical Radiography and Photography,* issued by the Eastman Kodak Co. was called the *X-Ray Bulletin* from 1925 to 1930. Until 1946 it was renamed *Radiography and Clinical Photography* (it has now a dental version as well as Spanish editions).

The *Revista de Radiología y Fizioterapía* (Chicago, since 1934) was a GE house organ: both in its title and in its contents, the radiology-equivalent terms were used in the Latin-American sense.

PORTUGAL

In Lisbon, the first specialty monograph was published in 1897 by the photographer A. Bobone: it was really an advertisement for the work done at his own private "X-ray Laboratory" opened the year before. In 1897, Carlos Santos, Sr. and Vergilio Machado (both of them physicians) had their own X-ray offices, and so did Araujo e Castro in Oporto. In 1900, Leite opened his private "X-ray Clinic" on the island of Madeira.

The Sociedade Portuguesa de Radiologia was founded in June, 1931. Its first meeting was held on January 28, 1932. Its first president was the previously mentioned roentgen pioneer, Carlos Santos, Sr. The first secretary was Bénard-Guedes, who had given the first formal courses in radiology in the University of Lisbon in 1924. Since 1932 they published the *Boletim da Sociedade Portuguesa de Radiologia Medica.* It was discontinued in 1950 when an arrangement was made with Carlos Gil y Gil's *Radiologica-Cancerologica.* This was in line with the friendly relationship between Portugal and Spain, also shown in the Congreso Luso-Hispano de Radiología – the first such combined meet-

TÜRK

RADYOLOJİ MECMUASI

ÜÇ AYDA BİR ÇIKAR

VOL : 1 — SAYI : 1 EKİM : 1955

İÇİNDEKİLER

Prof. Dr. Muhterem GÖKMEN	3	Başlarken
Prof. Dr. A. Tevfik BERKMAN	5	Hemangioma «Kan Mamarı Tümörlerinde» Radiotherapie
Prof. Dr. Muhterem GÖKMEN	20	Bir Gastro-Bülber Fistül Vak'ası
Dr. İsmet SAYMAN	22	Dal Bloklarının Ve Koroner Ensüffizanslarının Kimografi İle Tâyini
Doç Dr. Ahmet ATAKAN	27	Alber Schönberg'in Mermer Kemik Hastalığı
Cal. E. Gudbieig — Tercüme —	31	Bronchiectasis - Dextrocardia - Sinusitis - Bronchiectasis'in Etiolojisine Dair

Sahibi: Türk Radyoloji Cemiyeti adına Prof. Dr. Muhterem GÖKMEN — Yazı İşleri Müdürü: Dr. Saim Aykın — Türk Radyoloji Mecmuasında çıkan yazılar Yazı İşleri Müdürlüğünden müsaade almadan ibtibas edilemez. Sayısı 2 lira. İdarehane: Babıali Caddesi Zeki Bey Ap. No. 2 - Cağaloğlu — İstanbul — Telefon: 20037

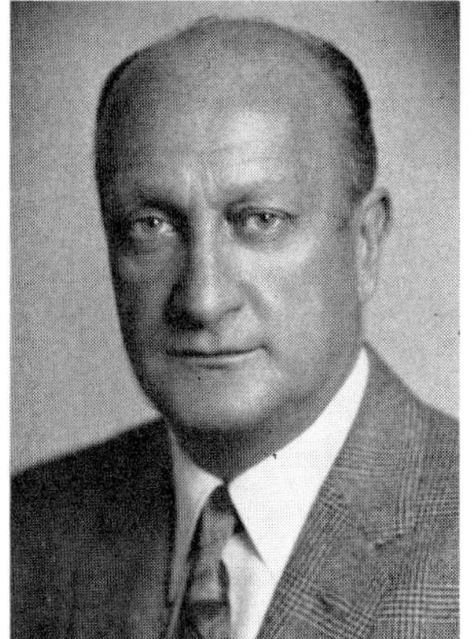

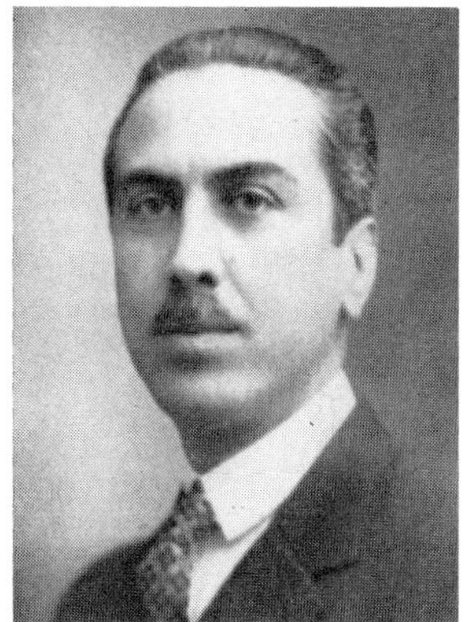

MUHTEREM GÖKMEN. Founder and editor of the official organ of the Turkish Radiological Society, Gökmen has a teaching appointment in the University of Istanbul. FRANCISCO BENARD-GUÉDES (on the viewer's right), of Lisbon (Portugal), was the first president of the first *Luso-Hispano* radiologic congress (1950).

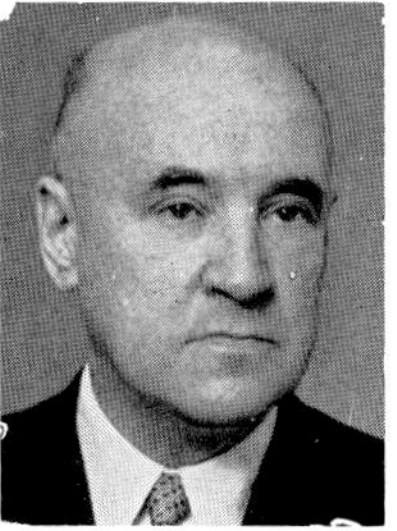

CARLOS SANTOS, JR.

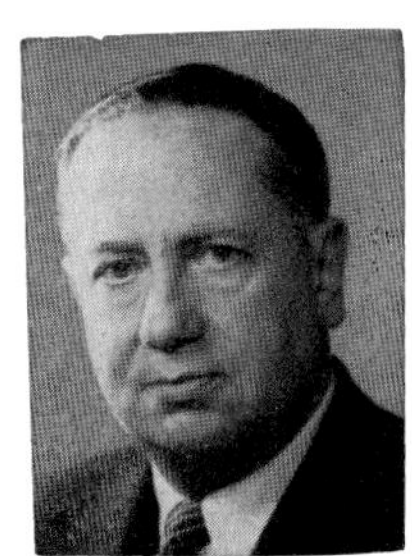

ALEU SALDANHA

ing being held in 1950 in Lisbon (President. Bénard Guedes).

The most significant Portuguese contribution to the science of radiology was *in-vivo* visualization of vessels with contrast materials. In 1927, Egas Moniz introduced cerebral angiography. In 1929, Reynaldo dos Santos expanded to arteriography of the abdominal aorta and its branches. In 1930, Hernani Monteiro, Alvaro Rodrigues, Sousa Pereira and Roberto Carvalho (from Oporto) explored the lymphatic system. In 1931, Lopo de Carvalho reported on angiopneumography and Cid dos Santos investigated the venous system. Among the younger generation, Carlos Santos, Jr. worked out the cholecystometry and microlocalized radiotherapy while Ayres de Sousa performed unusual angiographic studies by using microscopic and kymographic techniques. The latter wrote also a *History of Portuguese Radiology.*

Among the following five names of Portuguese radiation martyrs, Carlos Leopoldo dos Santos (1864-1935), Joaquim de Sousa Feyo e Castro (1877-1937), Joaquim Roberto Carvalho (1893-1944), Jose Casimiro Carteado Mena (1876-1949), and Adolfo Pinto Leite (1881-1933), only the third and the fourth are listed on the memorial stone in St. Georg Hospital in Hamburg.

U. S. RADIO— GOES LEGIT

In the mid-1920s the term radiology and many radio-derivatives had come into common usage in this country. And yet, whenever the AMA was queried about the propriety of such usage, the respondent would invariably point out that the etymologic ordinance of the ARRS of 1913 (reprinted in 1922) prohibited any root except the roentgeno-prefix. It was high time to give legal recognition to this linguistic concubinage, if only to legitimize its semantic offspring. The task was assigned to a Subcommittee on Nomenclature, consisting of Pancoast, Failla, and Watkins. They were appointed by T. A. Groover during his term as chairman of AMA's Section on Radiology.

In 1916, Thomas Allen Groover (1877-1940) entered into a partnership with A. C. Christie, and in 1919 Edwin Atkins Merritt (1880-1946) joined them as the third man. Today the partnership still goes under the name of Groover, Christie, and Merritt but the senior man is Fred Oscar Coe. The mastermind had been

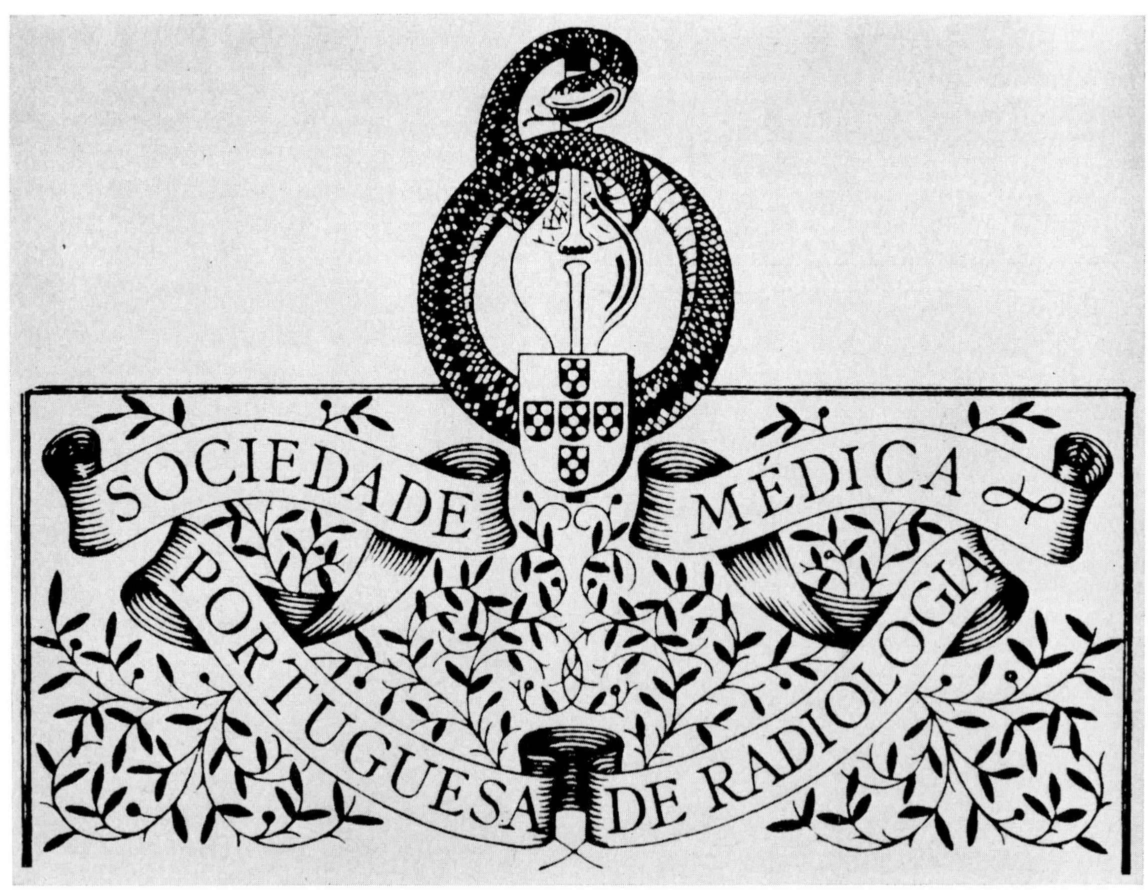

Groover, (by Orndoff's testimony) one of the best all-around organizers American radiology ever had. Christie was a forceful personality, well suited to become a figurehead, while Groover preferred the role of gray eminence. At the time he appointed above Subcommittee, Groover had already had his left forearm amputated (in 1926); he died a stoic death from radiation-induced generalized carcinomatosis.

The Subcommittee's Report was presented to the Section on June 15, 1928 during the AMA's 79th Annual Meeting in Minneapolis. It was accepted, went through channels, was sanctioned, and printed in the official organs of both the AMA and the RSNA (but not in that of the ARRS).

The Report (as published in the *AMA Journal* of September 29, 1928) contained in essence the "official" terminology accepted to this day, for instance it suggested that roentgenology be regarded as part of radiology. It discarded the vocable ray from the combination roentgen ray (roentgen examination rather than roentgen ray examination), decapitalized the eponymic prefix (roentgen in place of roentgenologic or roentgenological). It also discouraged the use of the term radiotherapy as being too vague, recommending either roentgen therapy or radium therapy, whichever applied.

It placed the term fluoroscopy on a par with roentgenoscopy. It asked that the term x ray be used in its singular form as an adjective (x-ray tube), and in the plural only to denote the physical agent (x rays). It also requested that the verb x-ray be deleted from the vocabulary. Actually, undue limitations had been attached to the term radiology by defining it as "the broad subject of the medical use of roentgen rays in diagnosis and treatment, and of radium in treatment."

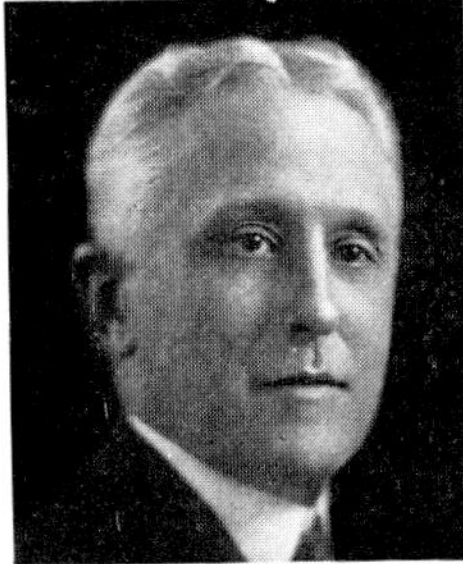
Thomas Groover

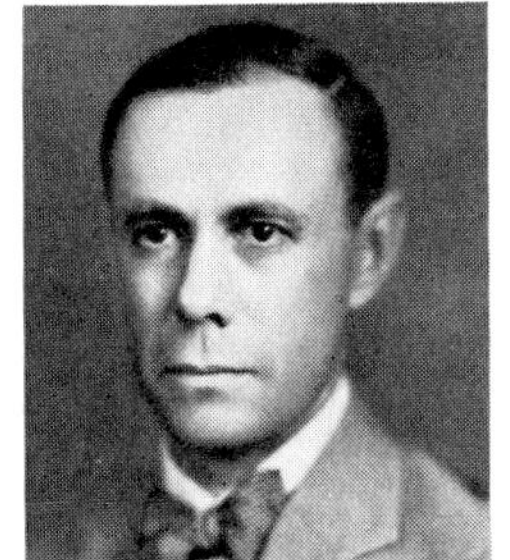
Wm. Warner Watkins

ANOTHER AMERICAN ETYMOLOGIC EDICT

A few years later, in an effort to promote numerically classified terminology, the American Standards Association convoked a Sectional Committee on Electrical Definitions (sponsored by the AIEE). Its Subcommittee No. 13 — Radiology — was under the chairmanship of Morton Githens Lloyd (1874-1941), a physicist from the National Bureau of Standards (NBS) in Washington. The members of this Subcommittee were (in the alphabetical order listed in their report) Christie; Desjardins; Failla; the Tulane professor of radiology (and former editor of *Radiology*) Leon John Menville (1882-1951); the electrical engineer Montfort Morrison*; the Stanford professor of radiology Robert Reid Newell† and Pancoast.

The Subcommittee issued first a provisorial (*Radiology* of October, 1931) and then (*Radiology* of May, 1932) a final communiqué. The comprehensiveness of the term radiology was extended to where it became the "branch of science that relates to roentgen rays, radium rays, and other high frequency rays." The text contained several other dyspeptic sentences,

*At the time of the meeting of Subcommittee No. 13, Morrison was manager of Westinghouse's X-Ray Plant in Long Island City, Mr. Herrmann from the American Institute of Electrical Engineers (AIEE)) found in their records that Morrison was born in 1883, became a member of the AIEE in 1919, and held this membership until 1938; at the time they last heard from him he was a "consulting engineer" residing in Upper Montclair (New Jersey).

†In *Radiology* of May, 1939 Newell committed to paper his personal exercise in semantics by offering several very logical, but exotic sounding (and never accepted) terms such as *rhegma, rhothion, kludon, plem,* and *aith.*

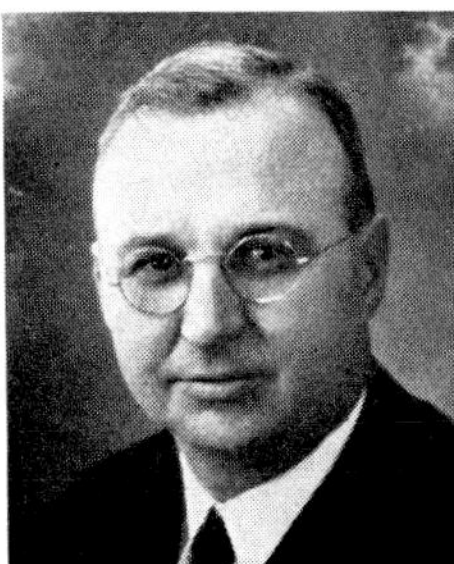
John Pierson

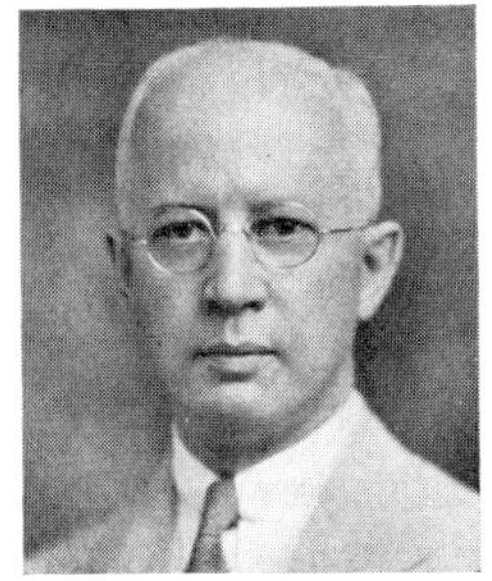
Arthur Desjardins

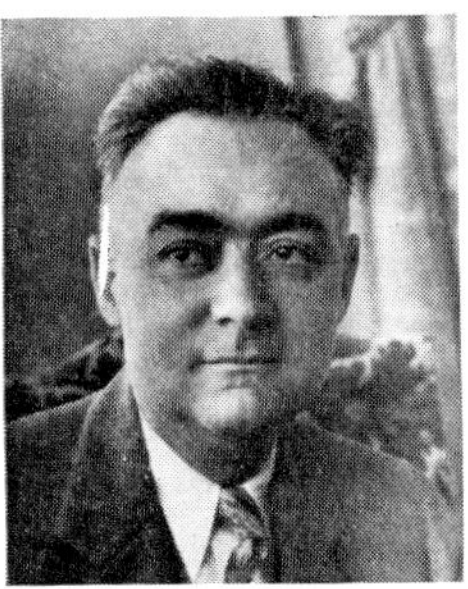
Lloyd Bryan

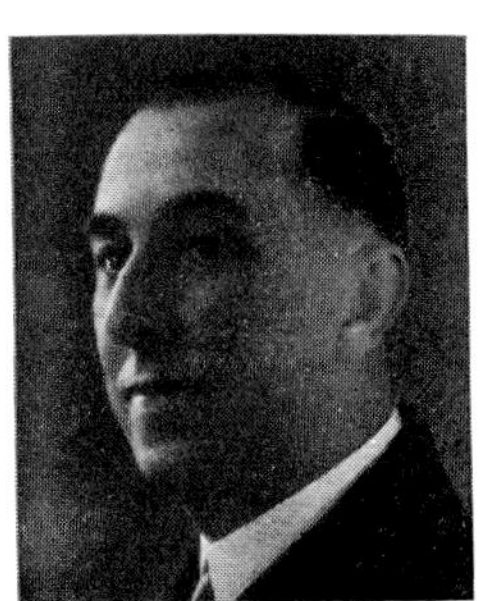
Leon Menville

viz., "radiography is the art of producing radiographs." As with so many etymologic edicts (which should never be issued except to ratify existing situations), time and continued usage have (and decide upon) the final word(s).

CANADIAN CONSOLIDATION

Listings of specialty societies (both domestic and others) are now regularly printed in *Radiology*, as well as in the *American Journal of Roentgenology*. The first such listing appeared in the latter in 1925, carrying the Scandinavian groups (erroneously) as Roentgen Societies, and Radiologic Associations (correctly) in Cleveland, in Central Illinois, and in Canada. It included the mention that the early Canadian Radiologic Society had its "next" annual meeting scheduled for June 22-26, 1925 in Regina (Saskatchewan) with E. C. Brooks of Montreal as secretary. A recent inquiry with the keeper of the current Canadian radiologic archives revealed that they had no records of those (pre-historic?) meetings.

Orndoff offered for publication an inedited group photograph of the 3rd annual meeting of the Canadian Radiological Society, held on June 23, 1922. This would indicate that their first meeting was in 1920, after the death in 1917 of the "first" Canadian radiologist, Gilbert Prout Girdwood (who was president of the ARRS after Heber Robarts, in 1902). Other Canadian roentgen pioneers who do not appear on that group photograph were W. A. Wilkins, and W. H. Dickson.

In bi-lingual Canada the development of radiology was dichotomous, at least in the beginning. The non-medical pioneers (mentioned in the first chapter) were Cox from Montreal, and Laflamme from Quebec. The French-Canadians gravitated toward France, thus during Christmas of 1895, at the time Röntgen's discovery was first printed, Charles de Blois and Henri Lasnier

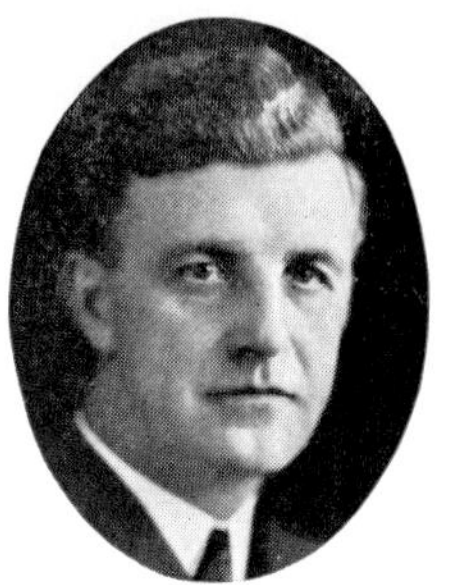

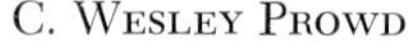

C. Wesley Prowd

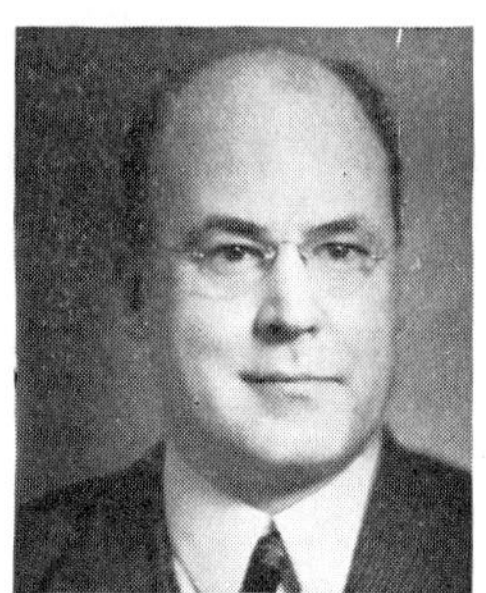

W. Herbert McGuffin

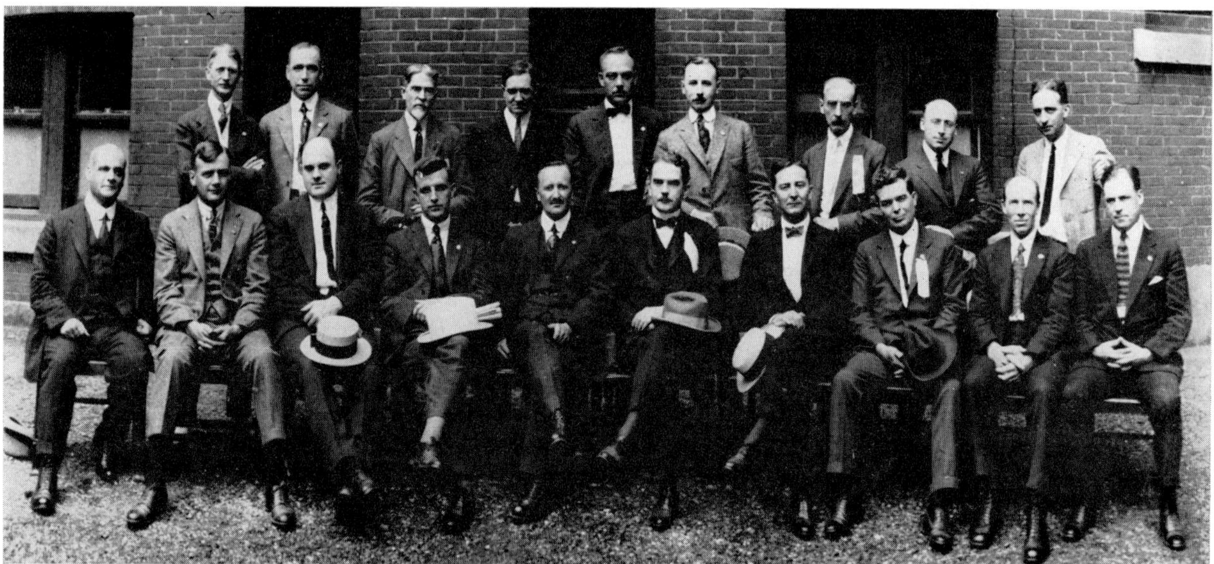

Courtesy: Ben Orndoff.

Canadian Radiological Society meeting of 1922. *Upper row* (beginning from viewer's left): C. M. Henry, Regina (Sask.); H. H. Murphy, Victoria (B. C.); E. C. Jerman, Chicago; George W. Brady, Chicago; Frank A. Smith, Winnipeg (Man.); Frank S. Bissell, Oakland (Calif.); W. S. MacDonald, Winnipeg, (Man.); R. Michaud, Moosejaw (Sask.); and William G. Hettich, Chicago. *Lower row*: C. H. Burger, Winnipeg (Man.); J. C. McMillan, Winnipeg (Man.); L. K. Poyntz, Portland (Ore.); C. Wesley Prowd, Vancouver (B. C.); L. J. Carter, Brandon, (Man.); Gordon E. Richards, Toronto; B. H. Orndoff, Chicago; Rollin H. Stevens, Detroit; A. E. Walkey, Hamilton (Ont.); and W. H. McGuffin, Calgary (Alberta).

were guzzling champaign* at the Hotel des Balcons in rue Casimir-de-LaVigne in Paris. After his return, De Blois established his practice in Trois-Rivières at the confluence of the Saint-Laurent and Saint-Maurice rivers in Québec Province, where he installed the first radiographic equipment in 1900. He went back to Paris in 1902, 1908, 1917, 1927, and 1930, to continue his specialization in hydro-therapy, electro-therapy, as well as radiology.

Henri Lasnier, after leaving Paris, stayed for two years as house surgeon in a London hospital, and returned to Canada in 1900, becoming the radiologist of St. Justine Hospital in Montreal. He had bought for $30.00, and brought with him a portable x-ray outfit made by Gaiffe. He used it to open an office at 143 Rue St. Denis in Montreal.* This is where he became well known for performing the radiographic examination of the fractured patella of the Hon. Perodeau. Lasnier also saw the giant (7′2″) Beaupré, who wanted to know whether his epiphyses had closed (they were). During World War I, Lasnier served as a radiologist with the British Army, first in Malta, then in London. Back in Canada, he established himself in Quebec where he practiced both radiology and "versificated political name-calling." He is remembered mostly because of *Les Rayons X*, a periodical devoted to Electro-Radiology, of which he issued seven numbers in 1910.†

*Gobbling or gulping down might also cover the sence of the French term *sablant* used in the History of French-Canadian Radiology in the January, 1959 issue of the *Union Médicale* by Louis-Philippe Bélisle of Montréal. Docteur Bélisle graciously offered also other documentary material for this book.

*This information as well as the graphic proof came from Dr. O. Raymond of Montreal.

†Only two sets of the (Canadian) *Les Rayons X* are known to be in existence. One set is preserved at Laval in Quebec City, the other set (of which the first number is missing) was donated by the widow of Dr. Edmour Perron to the French-Canadian Electro-Radiological Society.

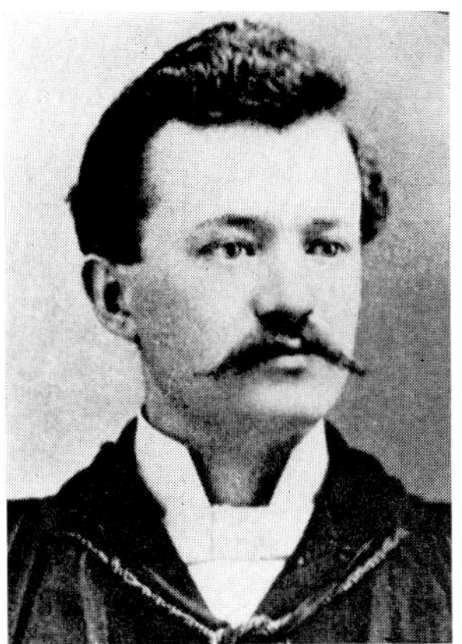

Courtesy: O. Raymond.

Henri Lasnier at graduation (1895). This Canadian roentgen pioneer is remembered for his x-ray laboratory on rue St.-Denis in Montreal, and for having issued the first Canadian radiologic specialty journal, *Les Rayons X*, of which seven issues were printed before it went out of existence in 1910.

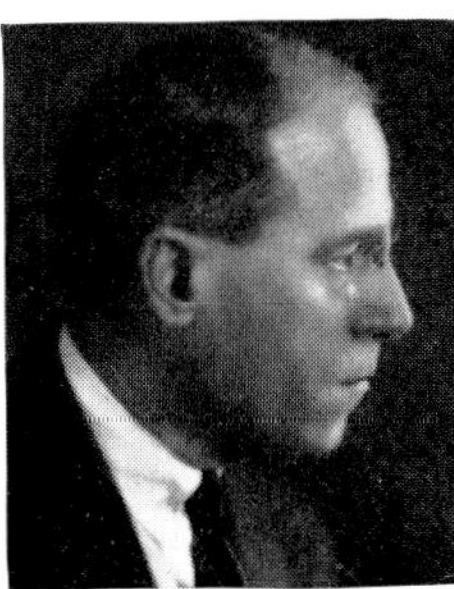

J. Edmour Perron

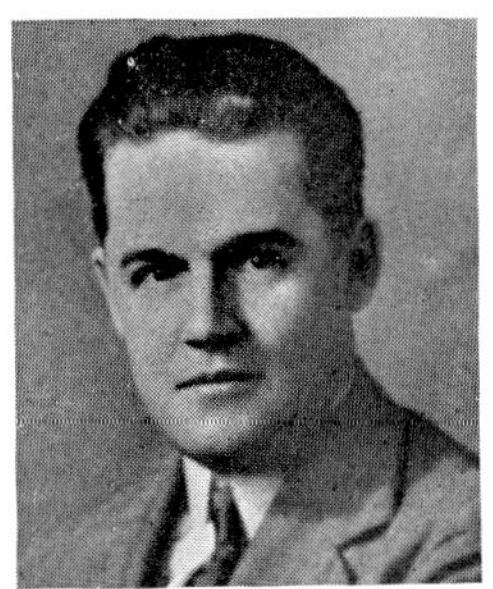

Albert Comtois

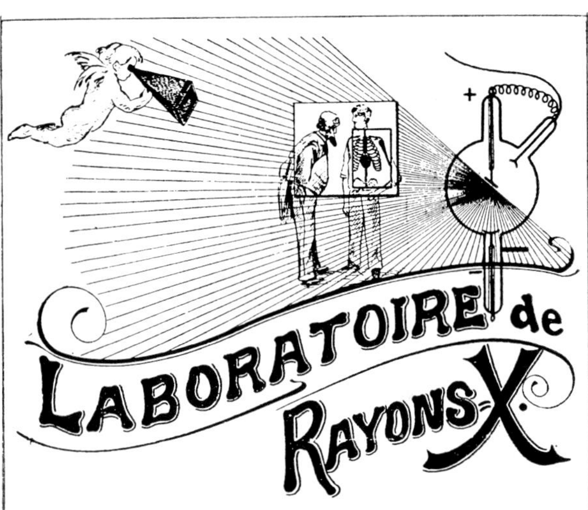

Courtesy: O. Raymond

Radiologic Office Handbill. The sketch showing a fluoroscopy is from an advertisement by Radiguet & Massiot.

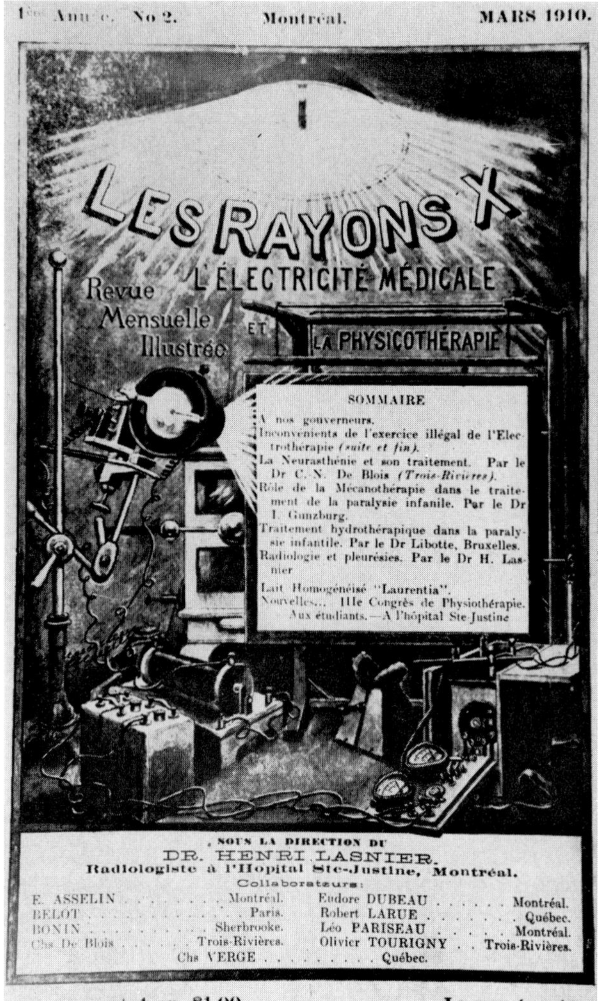

1re Année. No 2. Montréal. MARS 1910.

LES RAYONS X
Revue Mensuelle Illustrée
L'ÉLECTRICITÉ MÉDICALE ET LA PHYSICOTHÉRAPIE

SOMMAIRE

A nos gouverneurs.
Inconvénients de l'exercice illégal de l'Electrothérapie *(suite et fin)*.
La Neurasthénie et son traitement. Par le Dr C.-N. De Blois *(Trois-Rivières)*.
Rôle de la Mécanothérapie dans le traitement de la paralysie infanile. Par le Dr I. Gunzburg.
Traitement hydrothérapique dans la paralysie infantile. Par le Dr Libotte, Bruxelles.
Radiologie et pleurésies. Par le Dr H. Lasnier
Lait Homogénéisé "Laurentia".
Nouvelles... IIe Congrès de Physiothérapie. Aux étudiants.—A l'hôpital Ste-Justine

SOUS LA DIRECTION DU
DR. HENRI LASNIER.
Radiologiste à l'Hopital Ste-Justine, Montréal.
Collaborateurs:

E. ASSELIN . . . . Montréal. Eudore DUBEAU . . . . Montréal.
BELOT . . . . Paris. Robert LARUE . . . . Québec.
BONIN . . . . Sherbrooke. Léo PARISEAU . . . . . Montréal.
Chs De Blois . . . . Trois-Rivières. Olivier TOURIGNY . . Trois-Rivières.
Chs VERGE . . . . Québec.

Abonnement, 1 an, $1.00 Le numéro, 10c.

COLLECTOR'S ITEM. Cover of the 2nd of seven issues of this first Canadian radiologic journal. It is reproduced from a photostat contributed by Robert Lessard, radiologist at Hôtel-Dieu in Quebec City and *archiviste* of the Société Canadienne Française d'Electro-Radiologie. Miss A. Beaulieu, from the Bibliothèque Générale of Université Laval sent me the photostat of the very first issue, but the Lessard copy had more details on it.

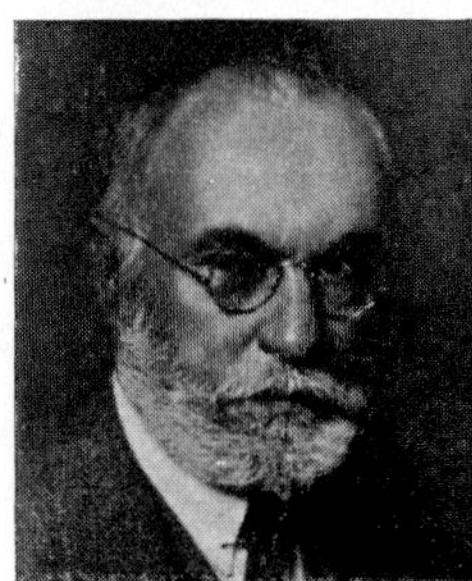

LEO PARISEAU

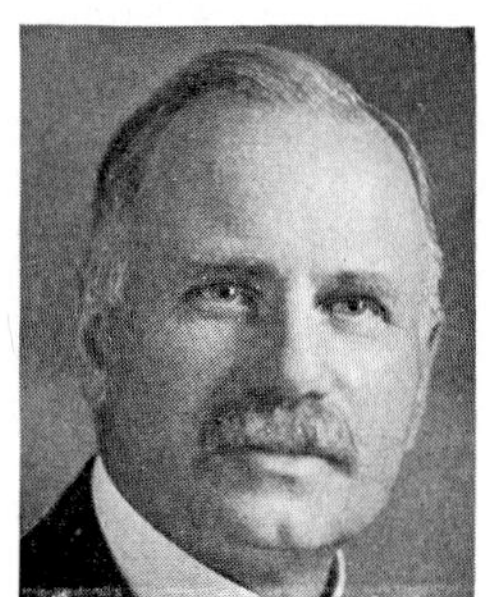

LEGLIUS GAGNIER, SR.

Pariseau, Gagnier, Sr., and Perron are the true founders of the *Société Canadienne-Française d'Électrologie et de Radiologie Médicales.* The idea came up between Pariseau and Gagnier in 1927 during a trip to Europe. They discussed it with several other Canadian radiologists. Among the latter, Perron was the most helpful, and the Society was officially created on May 22, 1928. It is still in existence.

The fighting erudite and bearded non-conformist Leo Pariseau (1882-1938) was for twenty years (until 1938) the *electro-radiologiste* at Hôtel-Dieu in Montréal (he was succeeded by Albert Jutras). Pariseau was the Society's first president and he designed its seal.* Léglius Gagnier, Sr. who had trained with Béclère and Jaugeas in Paris, opened his own electro-radiologic *clinique* in the same rue St. Denis in Montréal where Lasnier had his place; Gagnier is remembered as a short, white-haired, very dignified and respected, amiable gentleman who became the Society's first secretary. Jean-Edmour Perron (1888-1954) was the professor of radiology in Université Laval, a ("delightfully absurd") bibliophile, who became president after Pariseau, in 1932. The other four official founders were Joseph Ernest Gendreau (1879-1949) Origène Du-

*The seal is herein reproduced through courtesy of their archivist, Dr. L. I. Vallée.

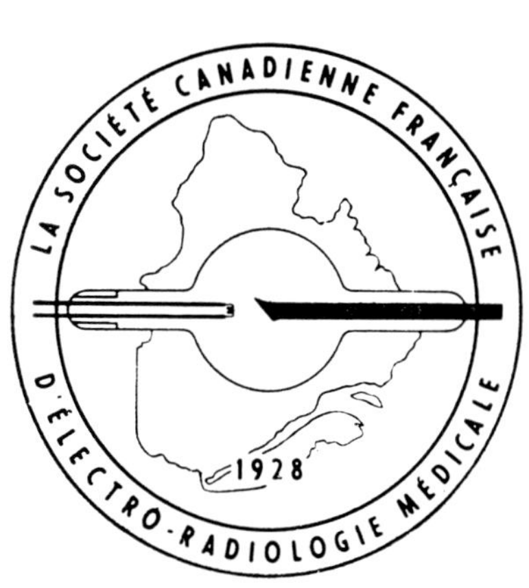

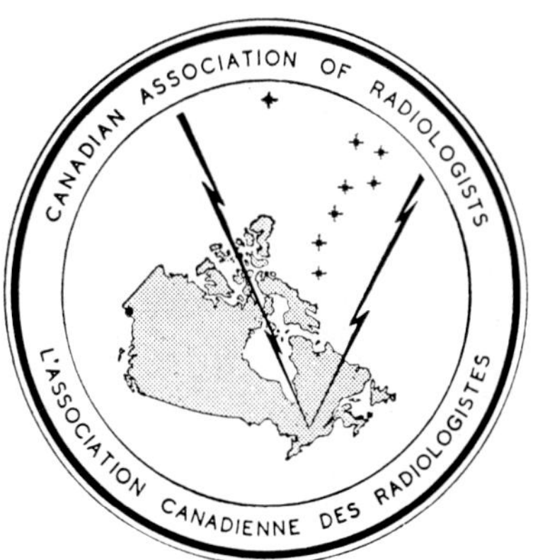

fresne, Albert Comtois, and Alfred Rosario Potvin (Perron's eulogist).

Girdwood's successor at the Royal Victoria Hospital in Montreal was the witty Scotsman Alexander Howard Pirie (that position is held today by Carleton Barnhart Peirce, the professor of radiology in McGill). Perhaps the best known and most respected Canadian radiologist was Gordon Earle Richards (1885-1949), radiotherapist at Toronto General Hospital and at the Ontario Cancer Institute.

Richards founded on January 4, 1937 the bi-lingual Canadian Association of Radiologists-Association Canadienne des Radiologistes. The first meeting was held in the Toronto General Hospital. The first executive officers of the Association were: president, W. A. Jones of Kingston; vice-president, J. E. Gendreau of Montreal; and secretary, A. C. Singleton of Toronto. In 1948 they were incorporated and established national headquarters in Montreal.* The Association is today the representative body of Canadian radiology.

*This information was graciously provided by Dr. Robert G. Fraser, their current honorary secretary-treasurer.

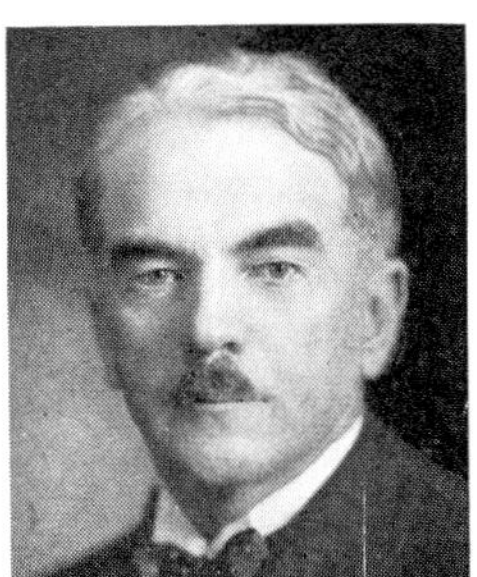

Gordon Richards

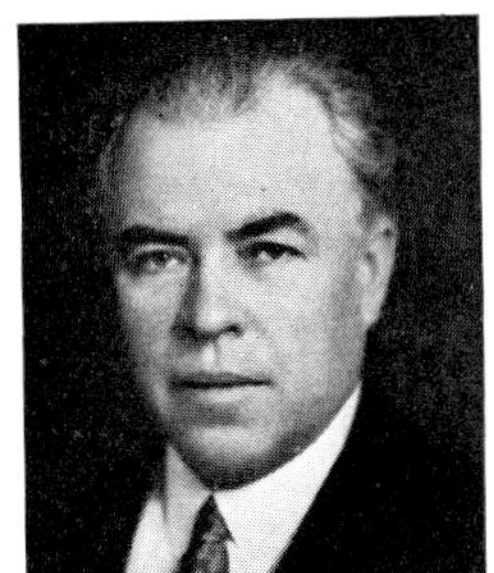

Joseph Gendreau

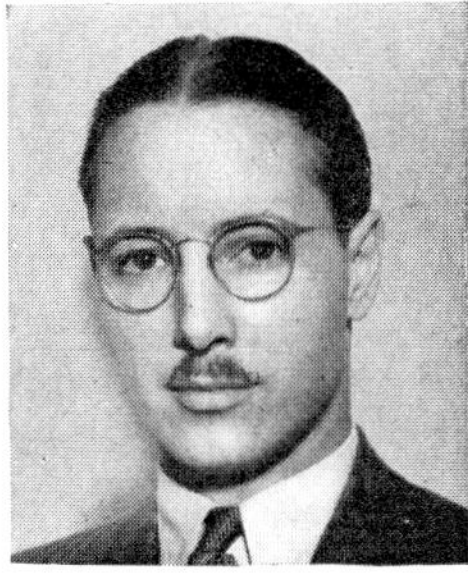

Arthur Singleton

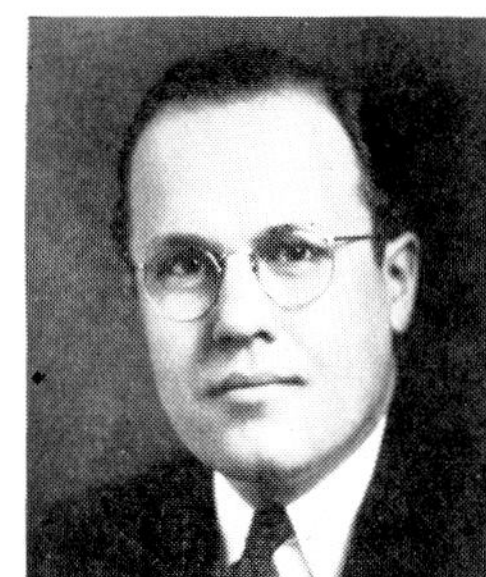

Carleton Peirce

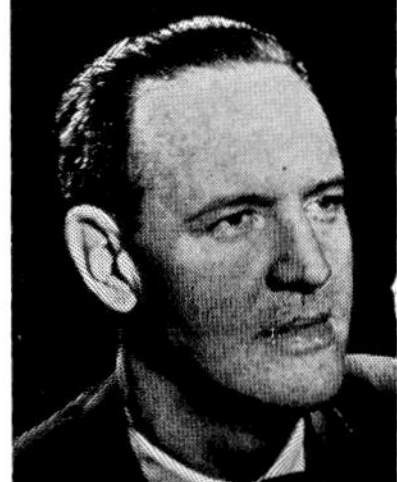

Robert Fraser

BACK TO THE FINISHED PRODUCT

In the *American Journal of Photography* of March 1896, its editor and masonic historian Julius Friedrich Sachse (1842-1896) gave a second-hand account of a miraculous revival credited to Röntgen's rays:

"A drowned mouse was laid upon a plate-holder under the rays, and after a short exposure, the mouse came to life and scampered off, merely leaving the *shadow* of its skeleton impressed upon the plate within the holder."

This little tale does not qualify for an inscription on a hollow pillar, but it is adequate as an introduction to the listing of the many vocables employed at one time or another to name those "electric shadows" (Silvanus Thompson) which Sachse called either photo-sciograph or, simpler, sciograph. The Philadelphia surgeon William Williams Keen (1837-1932) favored the term skiagraph. The historian of American Homeopathy, William Harvey King (1861-1942) from New York City, preferred the form skiograph, while Harry Tetrell wanted to use instead skiagram (Hickey).

In *Electricity* of February 19, 1896 appeared the editorial *After Roentgen What?* They acknowledged the then current inability to find a suitable term for what was called with the abominable name shadowgraph: no less abominable forms were cathodograph, kathodograph, skotograph, kinetoskotoscope, electrograph, and radiograph. The latter was the choice of another editorial writer, who (also on February 19) published his opinions in the *Electrical Review*.

The controversy continued and in date of March 21, 1896 the *Electrical World* repeated the editorial pun of the *British Medical Journal* of March 14, in the headline *Wanted, a Name*. The *Electrical World* called shadowgraph a mongrel word, observed that skotograph, scotograph, and sciagraph were tinged with pedantry, declared x-ray absolutely inexcusable, regarded radiograph as a derivation of photograph, and finally requested the readers to send in their opinion(s) of what word ought properly be used. A few notabilities replied spontaneously, others were admonished by letter, or by direct contact. A total of thirty-eight answers were printed on April 4 and April 11, 1896 in the same *Electrical World*. Four people (including Nikola Tesla) declined comment, nine voted for the term radiograph, the others preferred one or more among an assortment of oddities:

Frederic C. Whitmore (Philadelphia) wanted silhougraph; Henry A. Bumstead of the Sheffield Scientific School (New Haven) rejected X-gram; Louis Bell (Boston) called everything (except x-ray picture) barbarous and sophomoric; A. F. McKissick of Alabama Polytechnic Institute (Auburn) was delighted with Röntgraph, which W. F. Magie found hideous; C. F. Brackett of Princeton College contended that skiasmagram (meaning shadow-picture) would be just perfect; Alex Roy (Toronto) selected ethergraph; Reginald Fessenden (Pittsburgh) came up with Lenardograph; and F. L. Woodward of Harvard had the combination electro-sciagraph.

Several respondents plugged their previous choices, for instance Edison went for fluorograph; Magie for skiagraph; Max Osterberg of Columbia College (New York) for skotograph; and A. W. Wright of Yale for cathode (or Röntgen) pictures. Finally Arthur Goodspeed indicated he had coined the term radiograph on February 7, 1896, had published it in *Science* of February 14, and had learned that Dr. Lodge – he meant Sir Oliver Joseph Lodge (1851-1940) – had suggested the same term a few days later.

The suffix–gram, -gramm, or -gramme (from γραμ, that which is written) enters in combined forms meaning that which is drawn or recorded (or written, etc.), as in program (programme), or malignogram.*

One of the meanings conveyed by the suffix -graph (from drawing, writing) is similar to that of -gram, *e.g.*, photograph or autograph. In addition, to confuse the issue thoroughly, the words ending in -graph carry also an active sense of that which writes or draws, and are often used as names of instruments which write, draw, or record, such as the chronograph.

*In the late 1920s the German-born pathologist of Mercy Hospital in Chicago, Wilhelm Carl Heinrich Hueper, who is now an oncologic environmentalist in Bethesda (Maryland), established a set of nine outstanding histologic traits of tumor activity: these features could be expressed in figures (malignancy index), or plotted on paper (malignancy graph), in which case the typical carcinomatous appearance would constitute a malignogram.

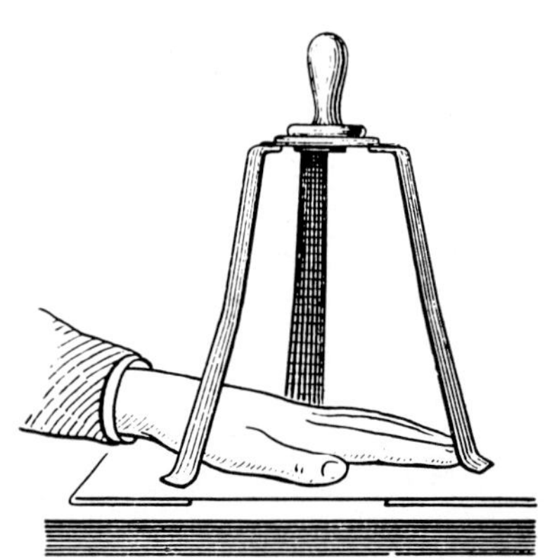

Radiumgraph (1908). The radium source is in the "handle" on top of the tripod, while the hand rests on the black-paper-sealed plate.

To exemplify, one may refer to the Animagraph, which is the table for small animal radiography, currently manufactured by the Campbell X-Ray Corporation. A Shadograph is a small animal balance put out by the Exact Weight Scale Company of Columbus (Ohio). The Radigraph is a scintillation counter with pulse height analyzer from the Nuclear Corporation of America. The Rotatograph is called a transverse body section apparatus of Japanese extraction.*

Gastrografin is the registered name of iodinated contrast medium for gastro-intestinal examinations (Squibb). All these "graphic" names have printed entries dated after 1960 except for one from a Dupont advertisement, which appeared in July 1940 on the inside front cover of the *Ontario Radiographer*; in it x-ray shadowgraph is called the roentgenogram of a painting.

Before World War II, a serial filmer was called a rapidograph, but the term is now obsolete.

Either or both -gram or -graph were used with most of the prefixes listed earlier in this chapter (from actino- to x-ray), including x radiograph in the *American Electrician* of June, 1896,† the tongue-twister raygraph (*Electrical Engineer,* of February 12, 1896) and inductogram (Gould's *Medical Dictionary,* 1941). In the *Philosophical Transactions* of February 20, 1840 Sir John Frederick William Herschel (1792-1871) — who was also the first to use the terms "positive" and "negative" for photographic images — had called a self-registering photometer an actinograph; this did not prevent Emil Grunmach (1848-1919) from coining the word *Aktinogramm* (for roentgenogram) and to use it as late as 1914 in the title of his *Atlas.*

Some of the "coiners" had a feeling of ownership for their creations, for instance in the *American X-ray Journal* of January 1900 the physicist and theosopher Elmer Gates (1859-1923) of Chevy Chase (Maryland) denied everybody else the right to use electro-graph for

*Described by S. Takahashi and T. Matsuda in *Radiology* of January, 1960.

†The title is *X Ray Foolery,* and the text purports that at Vanderbilt University "A Röntgen tube was kept a half inch from a patient's head for an hour in an attempt to obtain an X radiograph and several weeks later the spot on the head opposite the place of the tube became bald."

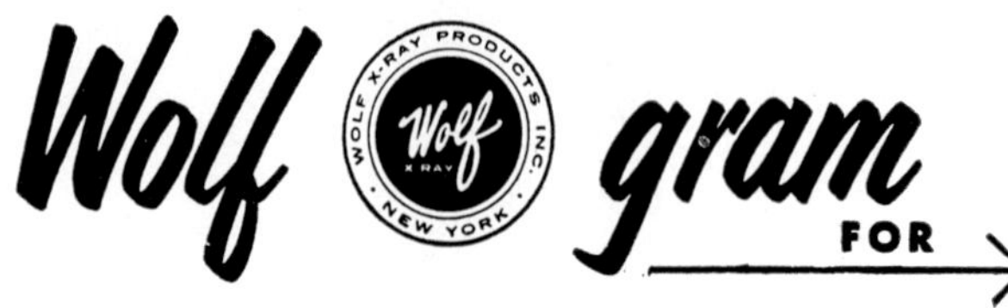

anything but his own type of photographs of electric sparks.

The confusing term radiogram (intended to mean roentgenogram) was used on October 26, 1902 in the *Wiener Klinische Rundschau* by Robert Kienböck 1871-1954); in the Czarist *Enzyklopedia* of 1905; in July 1911 in the *American Quarterly of Roentgenology* by George Henry Stover (1871-1915); and in 1921 by Robert Knox (1867-1928), who at the time was president of the British Röntgen Society.

Variants can also be cited. In 1906 Edward Warren Hine Shenton (1872-1955) of Guy's Hospital fame called viscerograms the sketches of abdominal organs made from either fluoroscopy or plates.* In the *Deutsche Medizinische Wochenschrift* of February 29, 1912 Max Levy-Dorn (1863-1929) gave the details of repeated exposures of a movable organ on one plate, aimed to evaluate the extent of motion: he christened the result *Polygramme,* for instance he showed *Diplogramme* of the stomach.

A modern mutant of the same suffix is the *Wolfgram,* a promotional newsletter issued by Wolf X-Ray Products, a Brooklyn firm which sells accessories.

In 1915, a few hard-boiled (radio) hams published in Elmira (New York) three issues of a periodical entitled the *Radiogram.* In January 1920, the *Radio Officers Union* of London started their official organ named the *Radiograph,* and it took eighteen months of confusing references to make them change this title to the more appropriate *Signal.* For the records it must be specified that as far back as April of 1881, in the *Journal of Science,* radiograph was called an apparatus designed to inscribe the duration of sunshine.

*Later, Shenton published a *Descriptive Atlas of Visceral Radiographs* with Alfred Pilkington Bertwistle. In August 1924 the latter described in the *Canadian Medical Association Journal* a crude masking technic by which he obtained silhouette radiographs.

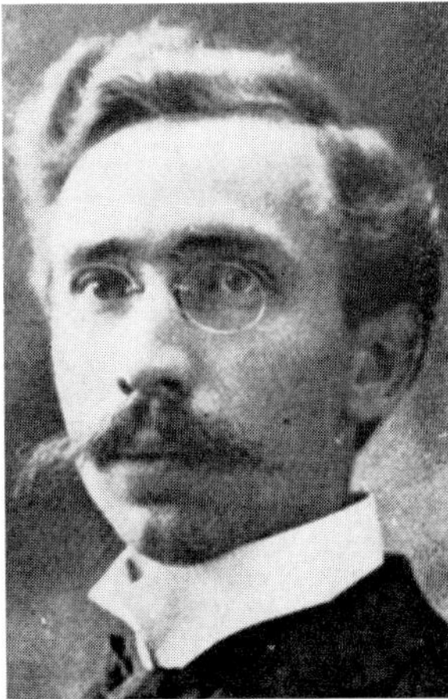

FREDERICK STRANGE KOLLE. A plastic surgeon who wrote *Röntgenogram Ethics* (an article in the *American X-Ray Journal* of March, 1898). He also authored *The X Rays,* a book of 191 pages, published by J. S. Ogilvie (New York City) in 1898.

While the terms Röntgraph and Röntgenograph were not uncommonly used, in this country, the earliest entry for the word Röntgenogram is in March, 1898 in the *American X-Ray Journal:* the author who used it was a German-born plastic surgeon from New York City, Frederick Strange Kolle (1871-1929). The word roentgenogram was officially and repeatedly blessed, by the ARRS in the teens, by the AMA and RSNA in the twenties, and by the National Bureau of Standards in the thirties. Lloyd's committee went so far as to "deprecate" the use of all other terms (skiagram, skiagraph, radiogram, and radiograph) anl declared that roentgenogram and curiegram (record produced on plate, film, or paper by the action of radium) covered all the needs.

To set the record straight, in the 1961 bibliographic listings of the National Library of Medicine the preferred term is radiography, while roentgenography carries only a cross reference to the former, Moreover, in colloquial medical language roentgenogram is regarded as a preciosity. The term curiegram was never common, and is practically obsolete, in popular usage one will encounter either autoradiograph or radioautograph.

X-RAY PICTURES

As previously pointed out, roentgenography is a contraction of roentgen photography and therefore roentgenogram derives in more than one way from roentgen photograph. This kinship has caused many difficulties in the past, and many of them resulted in etymologic convulsions.

The very earliest terms were unabbreviated combinations such as x-ray photograph, or shadow photograph, if not outright photograph, or photogram, as in the *Atlas Klinisch Wichtiger Rontgen-Photogramme* published in 1900 by the Prussian surgeon Anton von Eiselsberg (1860-1939). In many languages the colloquial term for roentgenogram is even today derived from the respective word for (photographic) snapshot, as the Russian *snimok,* or the Hungarian *kép.* In Italian it comes from the word for plate, *lastra,* which originally meant polished stone. In French it is a feminine abbreviation, *la radio.* In German, the *Röntgenbild* has always been, and still is, an honorable term; but in this country its literal translation, roentgen picture, and a more popular derivation, x-ray picture – used in the *AMA Journal* on November 6, 1897, by the dignified Boston internist Edward Aloysius Tracy (1863-1935) – is outlawed since 1913.

Even ethical practitioners continued for a long time thereafter to use odd terms – "x-ray plates" appeared in March, 1925 in *Northwestern Medicine* – because they were unaware of (or unconcerned with) their implication. At the time, the ARRS was making strenuous efforts to excommunicate the term x-ray picture.

In those years radiology was striving hard to gain acceptance as a recognized medical specialty. There were, however, a conspicuous number of "x-ray laboratories," manned by lay practitioners, who operated on the assumption that the interpretation of their "x-ray pictures" was just as simple and as obvious as that of any "other" photograph. By contrast physicians who specialized in this field would perform roentgen examinations, and expose only such plates as they deemed necessary for that particular patient (which is as it should be).

James Thomas Case was perhaps one of the most articulate exponents and violent fighters for that cause, as shown in his discussions of the matter at the 1915 meeting of the ARRS in Atlantic City. The same viewpoint appeared well documented in the *Illinois Medical Journal* of November, 1916 signed by Edward Smith Blaine (1882-1958), who for some time was both the radiologist of Cook County Hospital and the secretary of the Chicago Roentgen Society. The problem had to be repeatedly aired, for instance the Brooklyn student of radiologic economics, Frederick Esterbrook Elliott, was the main cog in the publication of the periodical *Roentgen Economist* (1933-1938), which was really an attempt to put harder (and perhaps more lasting) covers around the *Bulletin* of the (ephemeral) New York Society of AMA Approved Roentgenologists. Elliott, who died in 1963 at 81 years of age, is remembered as the founder of Blue Shield (a voluntary insurance for prepayment of medical fees), and for his pungent prose.*

Some of the lay laboratories were still in existence in 1962 but it seems that by a peculiar twist of fate, they have to go as a result of the radiation laws, enacted by various state legislatures. The standard stipulation is that only licensed practitioners of the healing arts may use ionizing radiation on human beings, and then only for diagnostic or therapeutic purposes.

Outside of the United States, much less importance was attached to the terminology *x-ray laboratory*, for instance, Holzknecht had a *Röntgenlaboratorium* in the *Allgemeines Krankenhaus* in Vienna. Actually, the term more often used in German is *Röntgenabteilung* while in England it is the *X-Ray Department*, in France the *Section de Radiologie* (in times past they called it *Laboratorie Radiologique*).

There are close connections between radiology and photography, for example John F. Hall-Edwards (1858-1926) of Birmingham was not only a brilliant radiologist but also a world famous photographer, whose one-man shows were exhibited from London and Sydney to New York and Calcutta.

The German expert in *Röntgenphotographie*, John Eggert was quite successful with his specialized technical manual, called *Einführung* (ed. 7, 1951), whereas the *Anleitung*, a similar item by Paul Knoche never went beyond the first printing (1925). The corresponding, much more elaborate (990 pages) British counter-

ROENTGEN
ECONOMIST

Survival is not dependent upon strength, wealth or education. It depends upon the awakening each morning to an appreciation of change and the adjustment to the new environment.

VOL. III., NO. 2 — *Annual Subscription Three Dollars Thirty Cents Per Copy* — NOVEMBER, 1935

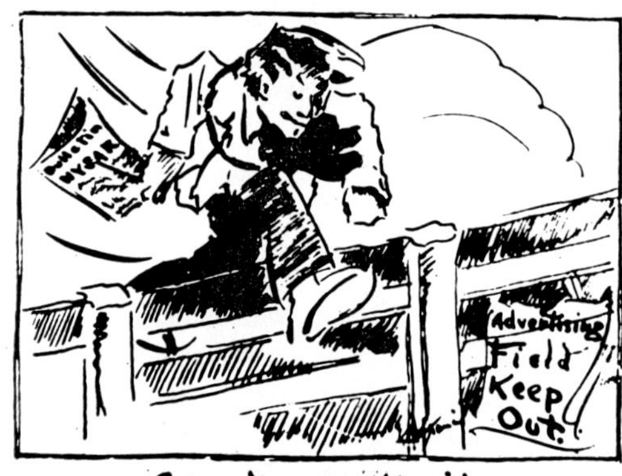

Can he make it
to
BULLETIN
NEW YORK SOCIETY
A. M. A.
APPROVED ROENTGENOLOGISTS

HE MADE IT . . . FOR A SHORT WHILE. This very rare item is herein reproduced through the graceful assistance of the New York Academy of Medicine. The *primum movens* of the *Roentgen Economist* was Frederick. Esterbrook Elliott, a Brooklyn radiologist. In subsequent issues, the *Roentgen Economist* accepted advertisements, but even so they could not "make it" for very long.

*Quotation (from the *Long Island Medical Journal* of July, 1928): "Most hospital x-ray departments are located in the basement, not far from the morgue. The cancer patients stop in for diagnosis as they go by."

part is T. A. Longmore's *Medical Photography, Radiographic and Clinical* (ed. 5, 1955), while Lehman Wendell's *Systemic Development of X-ray Plates and Films* (St. Louis, 1919) was never reprinted.

The excellent (British) *Positioning in Radiography* (ed. 5, 1955) by Kathleen C. Clark cannot very well compare with the monumental (American) *Atlas of Roentgenographic Positions* (ed. 2, 1959) by Vinita Merrill.

Also significant are the titles of known technical texts for instance *X-rays* (ed. 7, 1956) by (the fairly British) William Edward Schall, son of the third founder of the German firm Reiniger, Gebbert and Schall. A. C. Christie, just before joining the ARRS in 1916, had issued the first edition of his *X-ray Technic,* while the now classic *Modern X-Ray Technic* by Eddy Clifford Jerman (1865-1936) came out first in 1928. Darmon Artelle Rhinehart (1887-) never changed the title of his *Roentgenographic Technique* (ed. 4, 1954) but Le Roy Sante's *Manual* was first called *Radiological Technique,* while it is now (ed. 20: an all-time record) the *Roentgenological Technique.*

RADIOGRAPH (RE)DEFINED

The peculiar pastime of searching for a proper definition of the radiograph (roentgenogram) might stem from the same desire to prove that it was *not* a photograph.

One of the earliest (*American X-Ray Journal* of April, 1903) was offered by the Philadelphia electroradiologist Mihran Krikor Kassabian (1870-1910), to whom it meant "keeping the shadow, permanently, on sensitive plates." In 1904, in the *Journal of the Michigan Medical Society,* Preston Hickey defined the "radiograph" as "the record of the density of objects interposed between an energized Crookes tube and the plate" (the atomic numbers had not yet come to the fore). In March 1916, in the *American Journal of Roentgenology,* the New York dentist Rodrigues Ottolengui (1861-1937)* insisted that the "radiograph is not a picture of disease. It is a record only of the varying resistance to the passage of the ray offered by the parts pictured."

In 1921, the British physicist Alice Vance Knox defined it as a "shadow-picture of the structures lying in different planes reproduced as a flat surface . . . (adding that) it is not a photograph, although the positives have to be printed on paper." In the ARRS ordinance of 1913 the roentgenogram (was) the shadow picture produced by the roentgen rays on a sensitized plate or film. By comparison, a definition of 1956 (in Simon Kinsman's *Radiological Health Handbook*) calls the radiograph a "shadow image on photographic emulsion by the action of ionizing radiation, the image being the result of the differential attenuation of the radiation in its passage through the object under examination." It is undoubtedly longer, but does it cover xerography?

In the Unabridged Merriam-Webster (ed. 2, 1950) the roentgenogram was defined as a "photograph made with X rays." Their terse interpretation was in conflict with the chiropractors, because in 1923 Palmer, Jr. had said:

"Spinographs are not photographs. A photograph is a graphic recording of that which is superficial to the object being pictured. A spinograph is a graphic recording of that which is deeply imbedded in the object being spinographed."

In Gould's Medical Dictionary (ed. 5, 1941) a spinograph is "an x-ray picture of the spine." In the latest edition of Gould's, in which the spinograph has become a "radiograph of the spine," its next of kin, the spinogram is regarded as a synonym to myelogram. Alas, the Oxonian philosopher Thomas Hobbes (1588-1679) was quite right in stating that "words . . . are wise men's counters — they do but reckon by them — but they are the money of fools!"

AMERICAN BOARD OF RADIOLOGY

The extremely successful (and quite international) *American Congress of Radiology,* which convened in

*Biographic information on Ottolengui, Kolle, and Einhorn was provided through courtesy of Mr. James John Heslin, chief-librarian of the New York Historical Society.

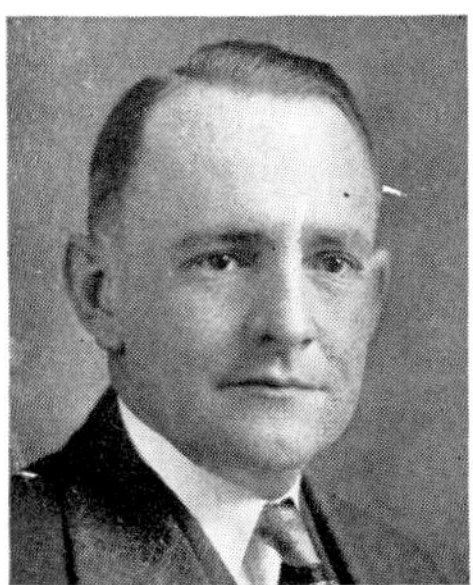

DARMON RHINEHART

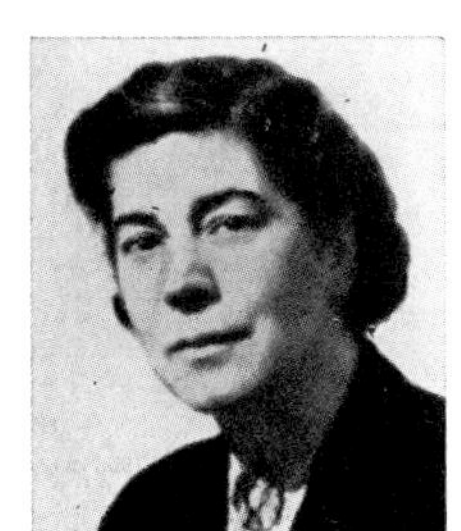

KATHERINE CLARK

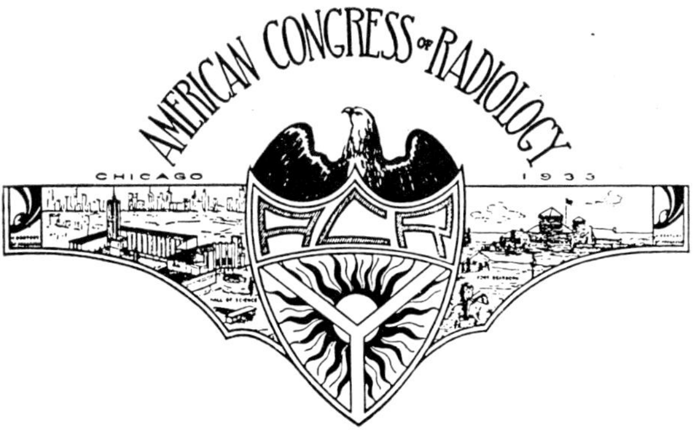

Chicago on September 25-30, 1933, was in many ways a turning point. For its secretary, Benjamin Harry Orndoff, who also chaired the Executive Council and was thus, virtually, its organizer, it constituted a rehearsal for the ICR of 1937. It gave undisputed recognition to the new radioterminology, as in *Science of Radiology,* a commemorative volume

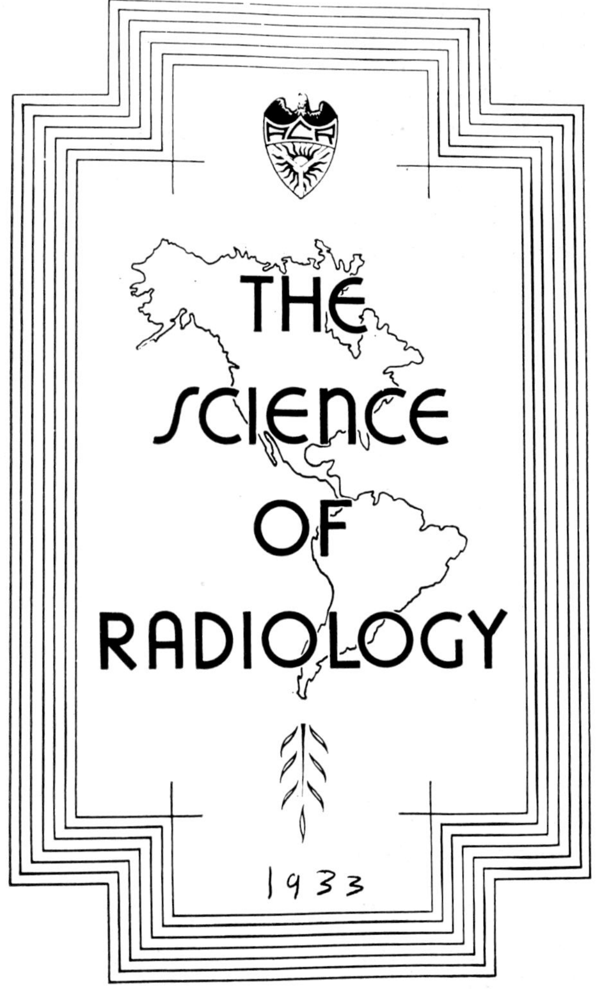

CLASSIC FRONTISPIECE. This beautiful design introduces the historic summary of radiologic science, prepared for the occasion of the American Congress of Radiology in 1933. Ben Orndoff set forth the aims and objects of this volume, Byron Hubbard Jackson (as chairman of the Committee on History and Education) expanded the original idea of a small booklet to a wider scope, and the editorship of the volume went to Otto Glasser (a member of that Committee). *Science of Radiology* was published by Charles C Thomas, then a comparative newcomer (his publishing house was started in 1927). The book became a classic, is long out of print, and Lewis Etter is now in the process of preparing an up-dated second edition.

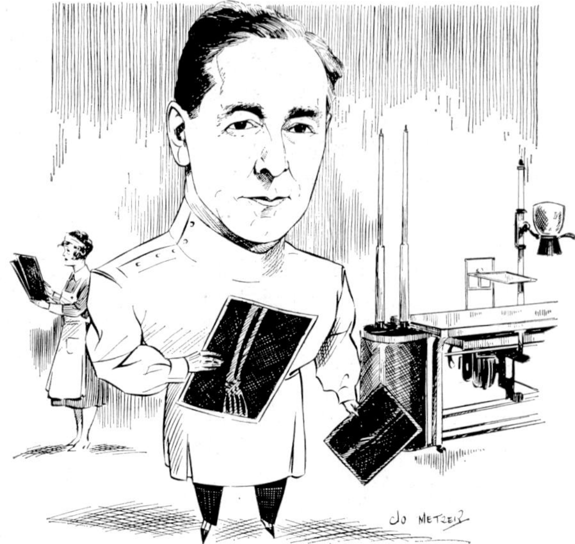

BENJAMIN HARRY ORNDOFF. Cartoon executed by Jo Metzer at the height of Orndoff's career, during the meeting of the American Congress of Radiology in 1933.

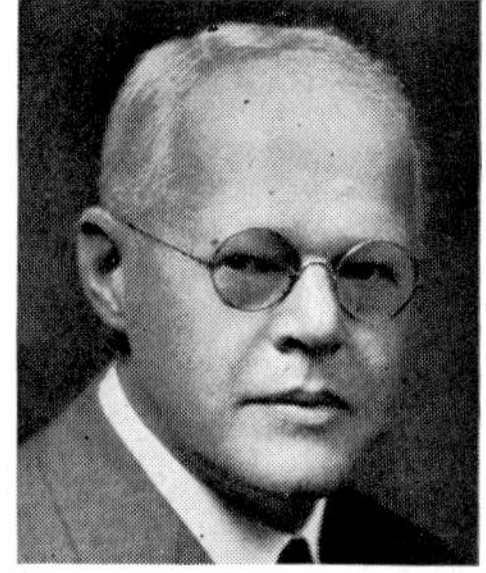

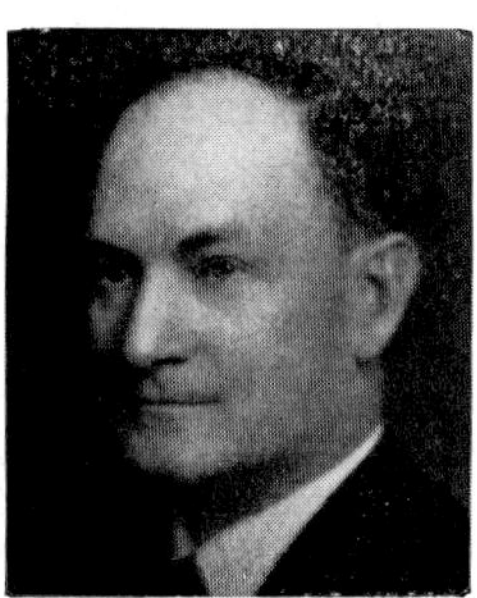

HENRY PANCOAST A. C. CHRISTIE

PANCOAST was president of the American Congress of Radiology (1933), Christie was president of the International Congress of Radiology (1937), both held in Chicago at the Palmer House.

THE AMERICAN BOARD OF RADIOLOGY
INCORPORATED
IN THE
DISTRICT
OF
COLUMBIA
1934

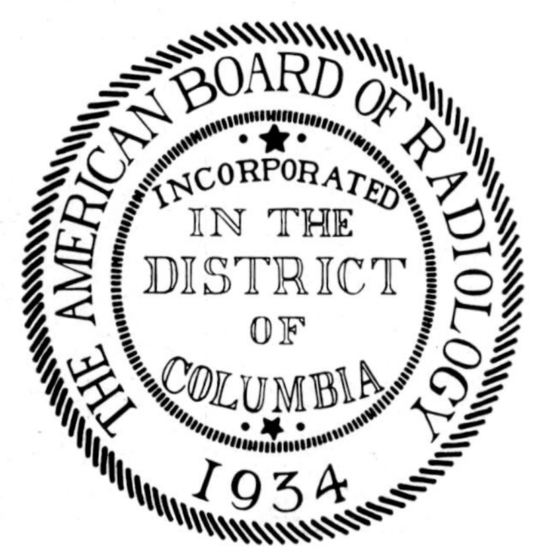

AMERICAN CONGRESS OF RADIOLOGY
PALMER HOUSE CHICAGO SEPT. 25. TO 30. 1933
CHICAGO
WORLDS FAIR
1933
KAUFMANN-FABRY
OFFICIAL PHOTOGRAPHERS
33-4077

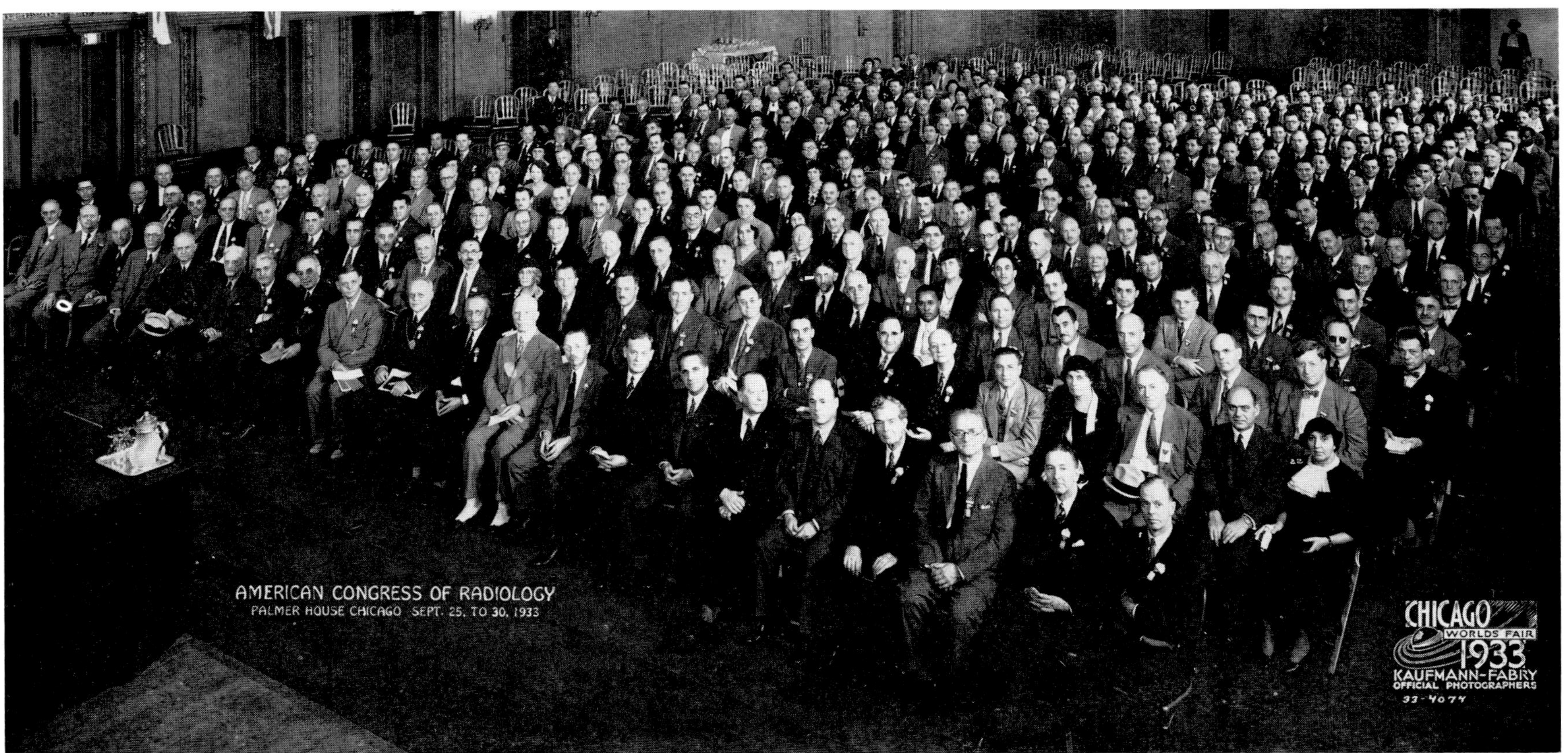

Courtesy: Ben Orndoff.

PFAHLER'S PICTURE. George Edward Pfahler labored assiduously for several days to make the necessary arrangements, and his efforts resulted in this historic record, with the Grand Ballroom of the Palmer House (Chicago) as a background. In the front row (beginning from the viewer's right) is Kenneth Allen, then Ben Orndoff, Alden Williams, Rollin Stevens, W. H. McGuffin, Carlos Heuser, J. A. Saralegui, Wm. A. Evans, Sr., George Grier, George Pfahler, Albert Soiland, Henry Pancoast, Henry Schmitz, Byron Jackson, John T. Murphy, Wm. Cameron, John McReynolds, Hugh S. Cumming, Frank Dunn, James Case, and Frank Keichline. Behind Case (second from the left in second row) is Willis Manges, behind Dunn is Paul Hodges, behind and between Schmitz and Pancoast is Harvey Ward van Allen. The Negro in the third row right is John Lawlah, behind Lawlah is Mrs. Percy Brown, sitting next to her white-haired husband. Behind Mrs. Brown is Herman Lemp, behind Percy Brown is young Robert Newell. Behind van Allen is J. Edmour Perron, next to Perron (to the viewer's left of Perron) is Albert Comtois, and next to Comtois is Clyde Snook.

(1933), edited by Otto Glasser, the physicist of the Cleveland Clinic, better known as Röntgen's biographer. Finally, it helped to create a powerful, new instrument, the *American Board of Radiology* (ABR).

H. K. Pancoast presided over the Section on Radiology (at the AMA Convention in New Orleans) during the morning session of Friday, May 28, 1932 when A. C. Christie sponsored a resolution which called for the formation of an "American Board of Radiologic Examinations." The initial organizational meeting of the ABR convened on September 28, 1933 at the Palmer House in Chicago (during the Congress), but the first real convocation was held on January 27-28, 1934 in Washington (D.C.) when the current name was adopted. Its first president was Pancoast, and an all-Eastern Committee was delegated to write the By-Laws: Willis Fastnacht Manges (1876-1936) from Jefferson Medical College; A. C. Christie; and John William Pierson from Johns Hopkins. And yet, the spirit of the ABR was molded by its long-time secretary, educator *par excellence* of American radiology, Byrl Raymond Kirklin (1888-1957) of the Mayo Clinic, also remembered for his contribution to the roentgen study of the gastrointestional tract. The current secretary of the ABR is H. D. Kerr, a former radiotherapist from Iowa City.

ACR INVIGORATED

During the Era of the Roentgen Pioneers, the ARRS had dominated the "x-ray scene." In the Golden Age of Radiology, this role was filled by the RSNA. In the Atomic Phase, the guiding function went to the ACR, but only after being properly conditioned for the job by an efficient coach, William Edward Chamberlain, who was at the time professor of radiology in Temple University (Philadelphia).

In 1937, the Board of Chancellors of the ACR proposed, and the ARRS, RSNA, and ARS cooperated in the creation of an *Inter-Society Committee for Radiology,* which was to concern itself with economic, ethic, and other professional problems. Each of the four groups (which used to be interchangeable at the top) agreed to name the same delegates to this Committee: A. C. Christie; Edward Holman Skinner (1881-1953) of Kansas City; and Lowell Sidney Goin of Los Angeles. This committee hired a full-time executive secretary, Mac Fullerton Cahal. At that point the old ACR "died" and the functions of the Inter-Society Committee were taken over by the new ACR, which then changed grad-

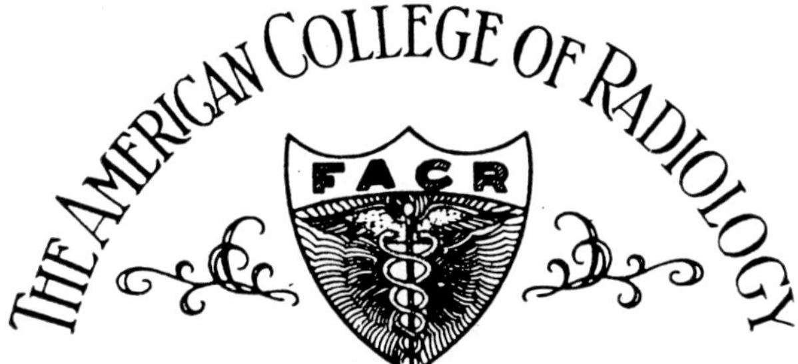

SIGN OF THE "OLD" ACR. Note the twin-serpented caduceus!

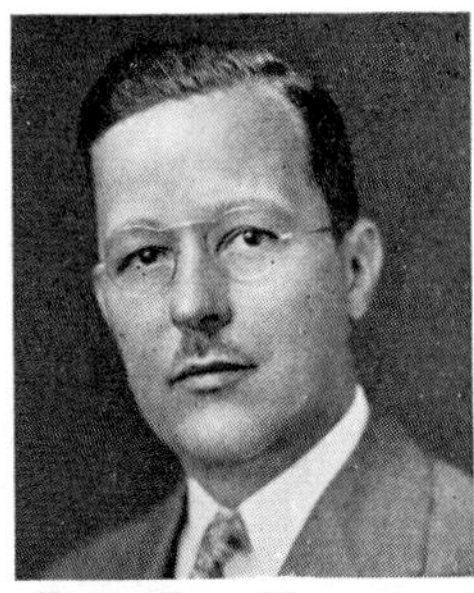

BYRL RAY KIRKLIN

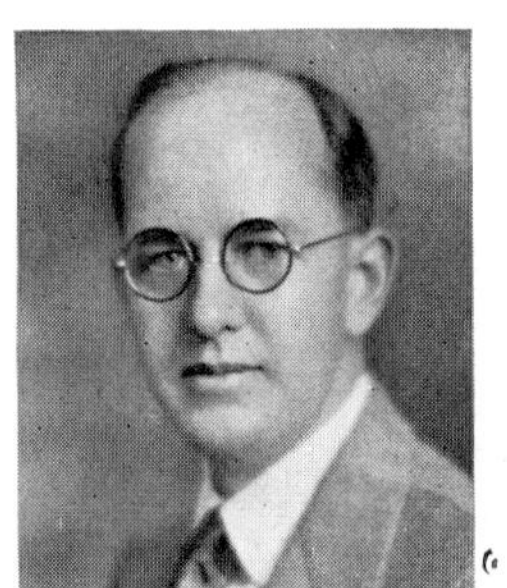

H. DABNEY KERR

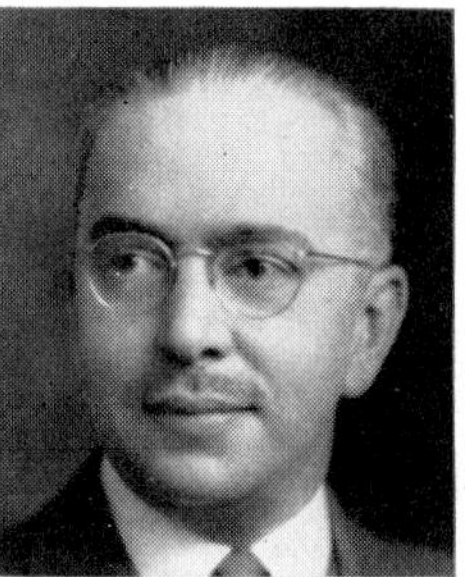

LOWELL GOIN

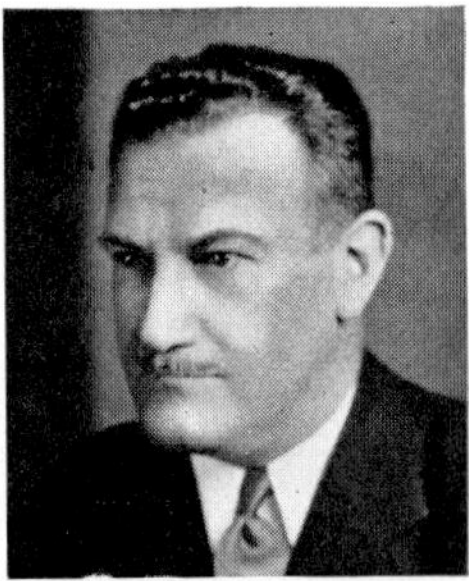

E. H. SKINNER

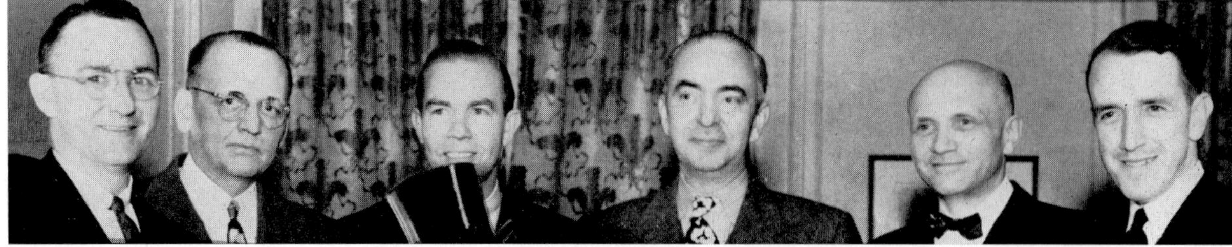

Courtesy: Mac Cahal

ACR MEETING (1944). From Left to right are Gene Pendergrass, Lewis G. Allen, Mac Cahal, Lowell Goin (hypermnemonic raconteur and official toastmaster for that occasion), Ross Golden, and Henry Garland.

ually into today's aggressive, business-like association, truly representative of organized American Radiology.

People often join professional organizations in the hope that membership will confer status. At that stage the neophyte is quite willing to give time, but nobody wants him. By the time he has "arrived," he is seldom inclined to spend a lot of time on organizational matters. But he usually enjoys the feeling of "security" engendered by associating with his peers at periodic intervals. Obviously, members will bring into the organization their good as well as their bad habits. Some feel that the periodic meetings offer the perfect excuse for sacrificing to Bacchus. Tee-totaler Orndoff told me that Albert Soiland and Ed Skinner were quite prone to indulge in such libations. There existed for some time within the ACR a subgroup, called the AOABF (Accidental Order of Alcoholic Bull Festers), which convened at the time of the ACR meetings, providing a good time for its (highly selective and restricted) membership.

During the period 1923-1930 Albert Soiland was the executive secretary of the ACR, and the ACR offices were at the Los Angeles Tumor Institute. B. H. Orndoff was executive secretary from 1931 to 1936 when he assumed the presidency of the ACR. At that time Edward Leland Jenkinson, a Chicago radiologist, became executive secretary. In 1939 Jenkinson was succeeded by Cahal as the ACR was consolidated with the Inter-Society Committee. Cahal did an excellent job.*

At this point it seemed desirable to insert the recollections of some who had helped in changing the ACR into what it is today. I tried several times to contact Ed Chamberlain, but he remained true to his reputation of never answering the first five letters. Others were kinder to our endeavors. First arrived the *Reorganization at the ACR* by Ross Golden. He wrote:

"The ACR was founded in 1923 as a purely honorary organization. Leon Menville, a charter fellow, told me that one of the objectives was to give prestige to well qualified radiologists when testifying in a Court of Law. I wonder how important this element of prestige really was; it was not very important in the eastern part of the USA. In 1934 the American Board of Radiology was established, and became the arbiter of the radiologist's professional competence. As a purely honorary organization, the ACR was then criticized as being useless. With its impressive title, the ACR at least represented our specialty among similar American medical organizations, such as the College of Surgeons, of Physicians, and so on.

"In the 1930s radiology changed considerably. Medical economies became very important as more and more hospitals attempted to get more and more income from their x-ray departments by reducing the income of the respective radiologist. This convinced many of the leading radiologists that closer attention must be given to economic factors. To this end the Inter-Society Committee was planned in 1936. Its three members, Christie, Goin, and Skinner, were all engaged in the private practice of radiology. The committee's expenses were paid by the four sponsoring societies, the ACR, ARRS, RSNA, and ARS. An able secretary, Mac Cahal, was employed, and he opened an office for the committee in 1937.

"The majority of radiologists approved of the Inter-Society Committee. A few well known and highly articulate men believed it was not necessary, and vigorously opposed it as a waste of money. Next we became convinced that, if properly reorganized, the ACR should be able to take over the work of the committee. This is when Ed Chamberlain was persuaded to accept the chairmanship of the Board of Chancellors of the ACR.

"To broaden the base of the ACR, a way had to be found to increase its membership. The original By-Laws stipulated that total membership in the ACR must not exceed one hundred radiologists. Later on tremendous pressure was exerted on ACR officers, until the "one hundred barrier" was broken around 1930, but even in 1936 the ACR had only 192 members, *i.e.*, fellows. One of the severest critics of the Inter-Society Committee suggested that the ACR should include not only eminent leaders in radiology, but all diplomates of the Board of Radiology. Because many of the older men regarded ACR fellowship as a very high honor, it would obviously be offensive to them to invite young diplomates to become fellows. Furthermore, these young men could not very well afford to pay the dues of fellowship.

"To solve this problem, a Standing Committee on Constitution and By-Laws was appointed with Ross Golden as chairman. A dual membership plan was evolved. The fellows could retain the honorary status they already had. The diplomates became eligible for membership at about two-fifths of the dues being paid

*The dynamic Mac Cahal is now the very successful executive director and general counsel of the American Academy of General Practice (Kansas City).

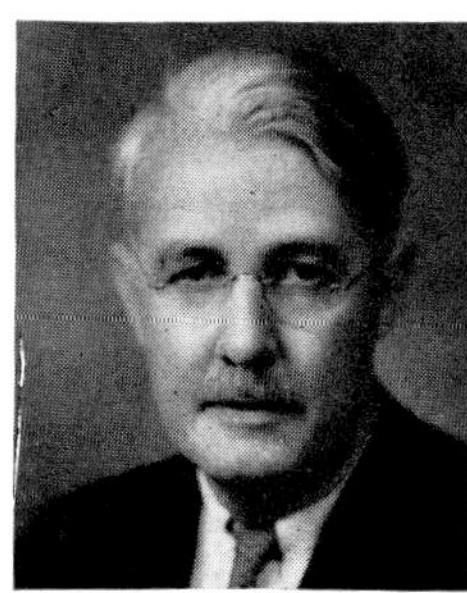
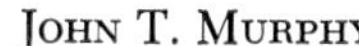
JOHN T. MURPHY

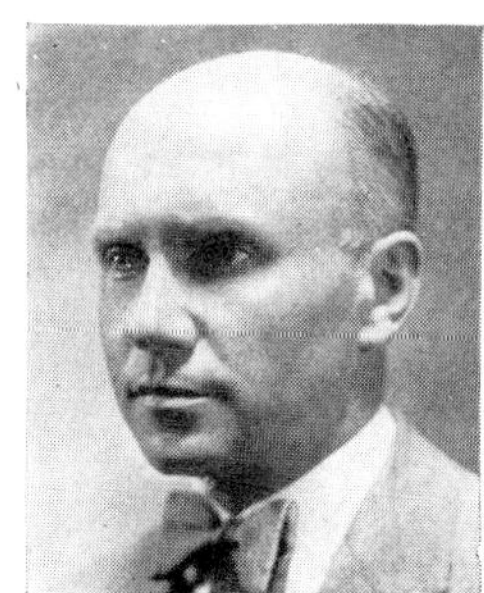
ROSS GOLDEN

by fellows. Only fellows were eligible for nomination as officers (including chancellors). All members and fellows were eligible to vote, and to serve on commissions and committees. After ten years of membership, the member became eligible for fellowship. The formula was adopted, and resulted in the steady growth of the ACR. At the latest count, total ACR membership was hovering around the six thousand mark."

Ross Golden was, indeed, quite correct in judging that he who has the most members will set standards for, and speak in the name of, the specialty. Another valuable document was received from Mac Cahal. With a degree in journalism, and a doctorate in law, he had gone to work as executive secretary for the Sedgewick County Medical Society. As a consultant to the Kansas Medical Society, Cahal helped in ridding the state of Kansas of one of the most notorious charlatans, John R. Brinkley, the goat gland quack. Cahal wrote to me:

"As the depression-ridden decade of the thirties neared its end, there came a reassessment of problems and directions in many walks of life. People began to see a way out of their difficulties. They began to make plans and adjustments for a new period of growth and advancement. The profession of radiology was no exception.

"Meanwhile, the economics of medicine underwent a revolutionary change, which resulted from a vast increase in the utilization of hospital facilities. This trend

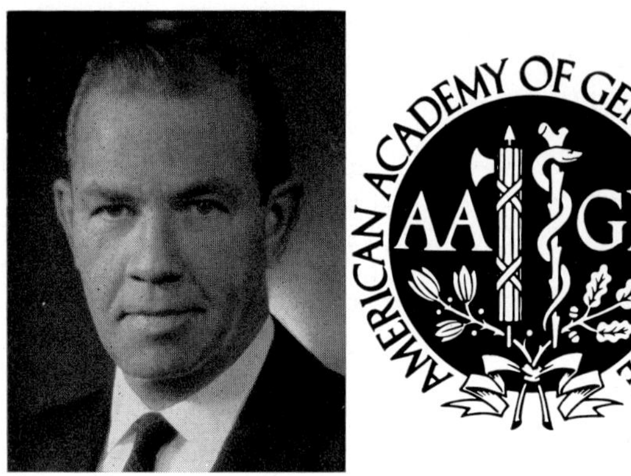

Mac Fullerton Cahal

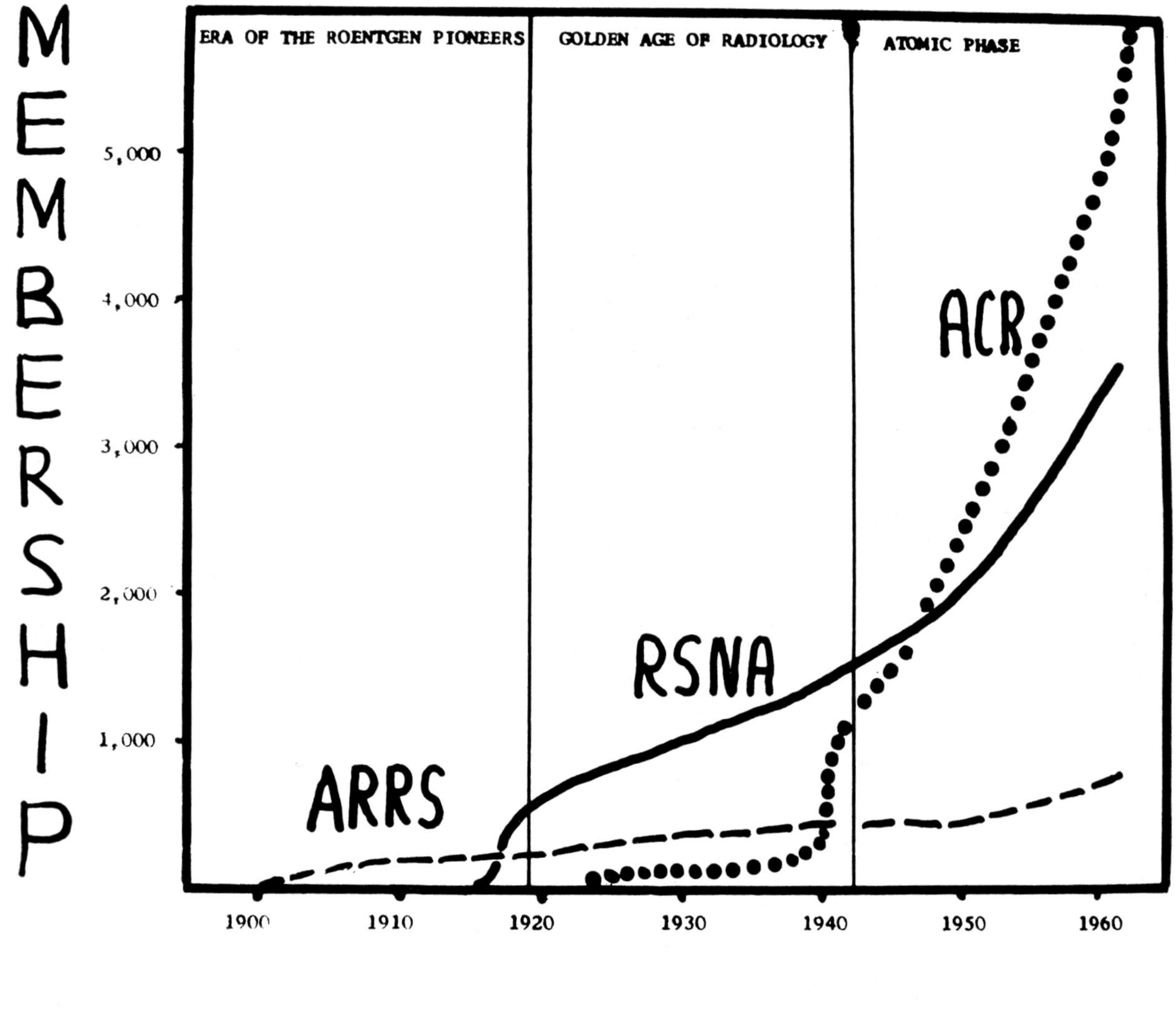

MEMBERSHIP

ERA OF THE ROENTGEN PIONEERS | GOLDEN AGE OF RADIOLOGY | ATOMIC PHASE

5,000
4,000
3,000
2,000
1,000

ACR
RSNA
ARRS

1900 1910 1920 1930 1940 1950 1960

has not yet been reversed. Patients and physicians alike became more and more dependent upon the hospital: Thereupon hospital radiology began to dominate the profession. The time of home-made automobiles had passed: big Detroit corporations owned the tools of production, and auto builders had to go to work for one of these corporations. The same thing was threatening in medicine, especially in radiology, where the equipment was becoming more and more expensive. The advent of hospital insurance further increased hospital utilization, compounded the problem, and raised new and collateral issues.

"So, in the winter of 1936 the Inter-Society Commitee was appointed. Its members had all been presidents of their respective state medical societies, and all three were serving in the AMA's House of Delegates. I was hired in February, 1937, started on the job in April, 1937, and immediately set up offices in the ICR headquarters, at Dr. Orndoff's office, 2561 North Clark Street in Chicago.

"One of my jobs was to create and improve communication channels with the rest of the profession. After launching the work of the committee, I went to Philadelphia to meet Dr. Ed Chamberlain, who was and is one of the most fascinating individuals I have ever met. Gene Pendergrass succeeded Chamberlain as chairman of the Chancellors. These two, and the three members of the Inter-Society Committee, Christie, Goin, and Skinner – each in his own way – influenced my personal philosophies and my character more than anyone else in the world, not excepting my own father.

"In 1940 came the Wagner "National Health Act." If passed, it would have imposed a system of socialized medicine, and turned radiology into a hospital, rather than a medical, service. This is when, in addition to my job as secretary to the Inter-Society Committee, I was appointed executive director of the ACR, so as to work closely with the AMA and the National Physicians Committee in marshalling public opposition to the Wagner-Murray-Dingell bills. We were successful in defeating them, but the fight is still on, and no let-up is in sight."

Mac Cahal has grown since his ACR days, and one of his addresses — the *Image* (of a physician) — has appeared in the *JAMA* of July 20, 1963. He is now the aggressive executive director of the AAGP, a good friend of the ACR. After all, the radiologist is the most generalist among specialists. Today organized medicine is unthinkable without its "lay" executives. The task of secretary of a medical society exceeds the capabilities of a part-time caretaker, even those of a semi-retired physician. Such a job demands an energetic and efficient full-time expert, who must be able to cover such varied fields as interprofessional communication, insurance intricacies, or legal advice.

In 1948, a trained lawyer, William Charles Stronach, became the executive director of the ACR. He has identified himself with the scope and the symbols of the ACR, with the sense of its struggles and with its spirit. In the face of periodical turn-over of elected officers, Stronach has come to represent — similarly to a trusted Civil Servant — a stable surface to stand on while elected officials like roaring waves roll on, over, and away.

Three radiologists from the Chicago area have recently devoted much time and effort in behalf of the ACR. Fay Squire, chief of radiology at the Presbyterian-St. Luke Hospital, is since 1955 secretary-treasurer of the ACR. His most cherished project is the creation of a *House of American Radiology*, to be located in the sprawling Medical Center in Chicago. For this purpose the ACR has purchased a piece of real estate, and funds are being saved for the start of a

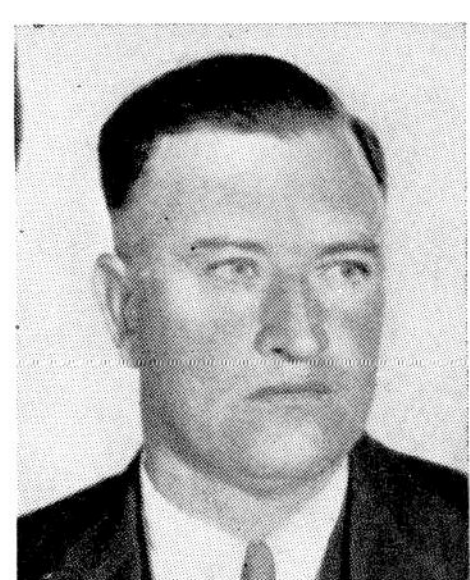

E. L. Jenkinson

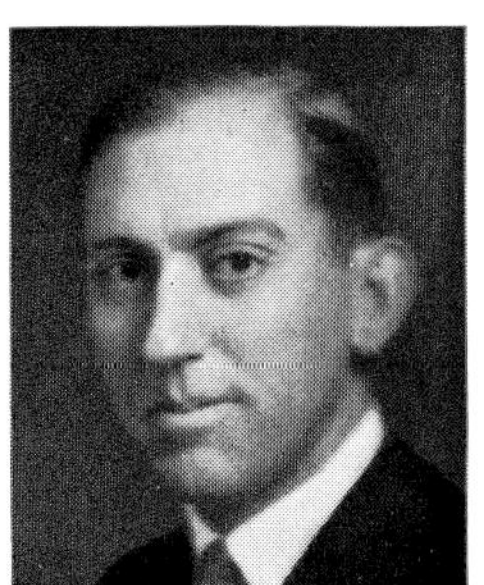

W. Ed. Chamberlain

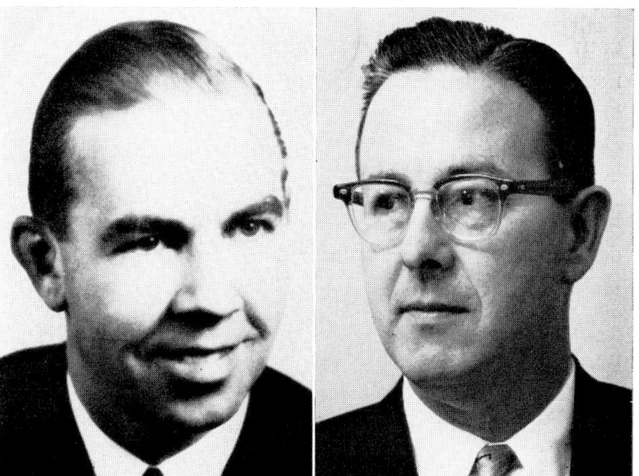

ACR's "lay" executives. Radiologists served turns as secretaries of the "old" ACR. The "new" ACR enjoyed in this respect the advantages of professional help. On the viewer's left is (then young) Mac Fullerton Cahal (who is now with the American Academy of General Practice in Kansas City). The other is William Charles Stronach, currently executive director of the ACR. They have contributed immeasurably to the development and present vigor of the organization.

building program. That *House* would house not only the offices of the ACR and of any other radiologic organization willing to move its headquarters to that location, but also the future *Museum of American Radiology,* presently in the planning stage.

Earl Edwin Barth, one of Jimmy Case's "boys," is currently the chairman of the Department of Radiology in Northwestern University. At one time or another he has occupied almost every significant position in ACR officialdom, for instance he preceded Squire as secretary-treasurer. During Barth's tenure as chairman of the ACR's Board of Chancellors, he started (in January, 1958) to send out a yellow-colored *Memo to the Membership.* With the December, 1958 mailing the name was changed to *Memor to the Membership Edition* (that particular issue carried also the sad news of the death of Warren Furey, clinical professor of radiology at Stritch School of Medicine — another Chicago radiologist who had served the ACR well and for a long time). The *Memo* contains mostly "confidential" items as opposed to the *ACR Monthly Newsletter,* or *Your Radiologist* (the latter is for non-radiologists).

The highest elected executive of the ACR is the chairman of the Board of Chancellors. The usual procedure is to let the prospective candidate work his way through the ranks, first in some committee, then — if he appears to be able to master more than a few parliamentary rules of order — he is "elected" to a more significant post, perhaps after a stage as councilor (the Board of Councilors is currently little more than a forum for the discussion of certain problems). Then the "kingmakers" pick him for the Board of Chancellors. If he works hard, does and says the right things, and stays in the good graces of the "kingmakers," his turn as chairman of the Board of Chancellors is assured. Thereafter, though, comes only the presidency of the ACR (which, in the current arrangement of things, is a figurehead position) and, perhaps, a gold medal.

Barth's *Memo* was continued by the subsequent chairmen of the Board of Chancellors, Arthur

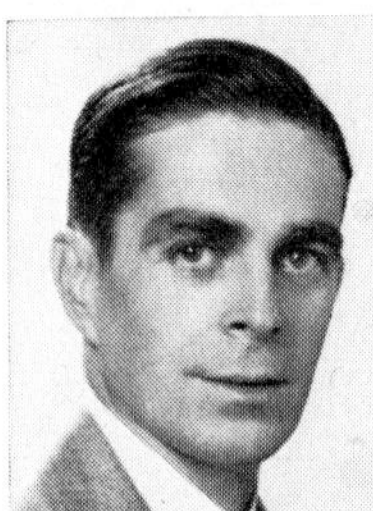

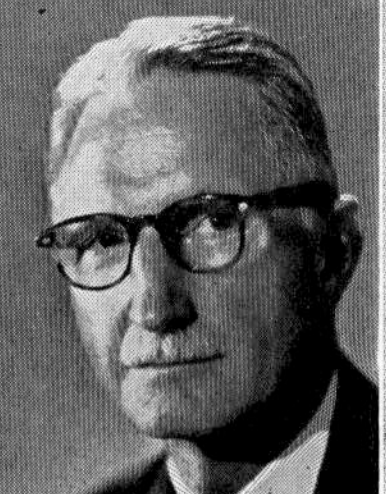

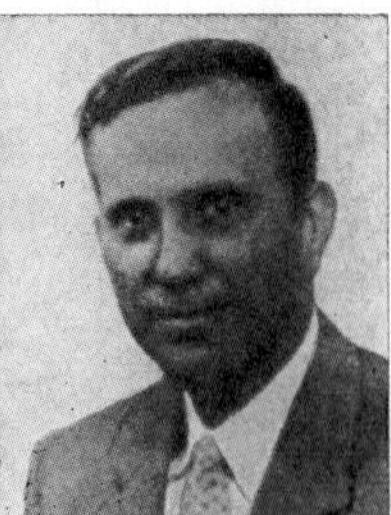

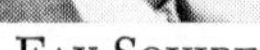

FAY SQUIRE EARL BARTH TY WACHOWSKI

Present of Tucson (Arizona), Theodor Wachowski of Aurora (Illinois), and David Carroll of Memphis (Tennessee). Ty Wachowski (a former track star at the University of Illinois), while not personally too interested in history as such, has actively supported the historic endeavors of the ACR. He went so far as to appoint a temporary (*ad-hoc*) committee to look into the possibility of creating a Museum of American Radiology and of preparing a History of American Radiology.

The first seal of the ACR contained a caduceus. Just such a twin-winged and twin-serpented staff was the

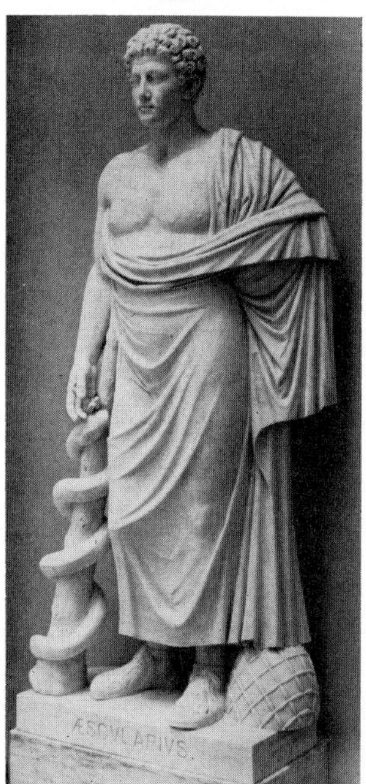

Courtesy: W. B. McDaniel, 2nd

ASKLEPIOS OF THE VATICAN. The original (by unknown artist) is in the Vatican. This is the photograph of a copy, which graces the stairway of the College of Physicians in Philadelphia. The latter's curator, Mr. W. B. McDaniel, 2nd, pointed out that this statue is also reproduced in Eugen Holländer's *Plastik und Medizin,* and that it is the only existing beardless statue of Aesculapius. Legend has it that the original (bearded) head of the statue was replaced, by order of Augustus Caesar, with a sculptured head of his physician, Antonius Musa. It is herein reproduced to show that the authentic Aesculapian (medical) symbol is the single-serpented wand.

symbol of Roman heralds, whose god (of communications) was heel-winged Mercury. The caduceus never became a true medical symbol although it was used in the insignia for the Medical Corps in both the British and the American armies – still the emblem of the *Journal of the Royal Army Medical Corps* has but a single snake. The recognized symbol of the physician is the single-serpented staff, shown in the antique statue of Asklepios, exhumed at Epidauros and preserved in the National Museum in Athens.

The club of Asklepios acquired its medical significance from the primitive method of treating Dracunculosis in the Middle-East. Dracunculosis is caused by female filaria which settle under the skin of (human) lower extremities, after which the filaria pierces the skin to eject its eggs. At this point the ancient healer would gently thread the (female) worm's tail into a slit made in a wooden stick: subsequent slow rotation of the stick permits the removal of the worm without tearing it. Nematodes in this family (such as *Dracunculus medinensis*) often reach a length of four feet, and are therefore popularly called snakes. When not removed they calcify and become visible on radiographic examination of the legs (*cf.*, the paper on experiences in Araby by M. Ghigo and M. Magrini in *Radiologia Medica* of October, 1959). The trade-mark of mythical Middle-Eastern medicine men – the snake on the stick – was later consolidated with the (quasi-corporate) image of a very competent Greek physician named Asklepios, deified after or perhaps because of his fatal encounter with a thunderbolt.

At the beginning of the Atomic Phase, the ACR replaced the caduceus in its seal with the (orthodox) single-serpented wand of Asklepios. Incidentally, a lone

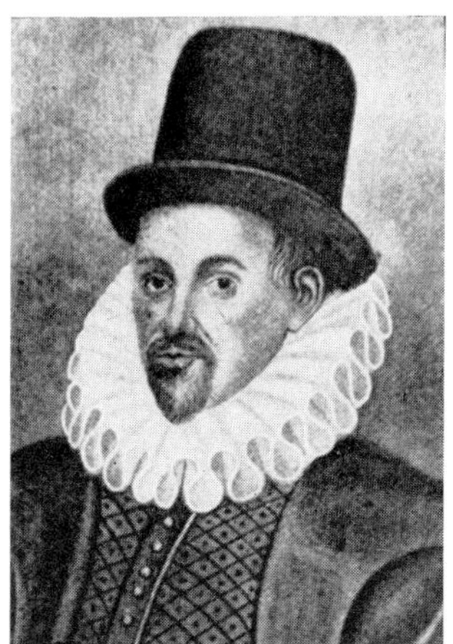

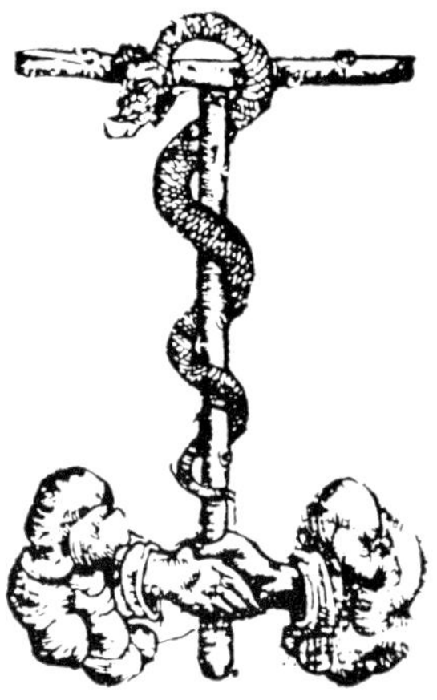

WILLIAM GILBERT. This physician and physicist placed the single-snaked crutch (seen on the right) on the frontispiece of *De Magnete* (1600), an opus for which he is regarded as the earliest recognizable forefather of Röntgen.

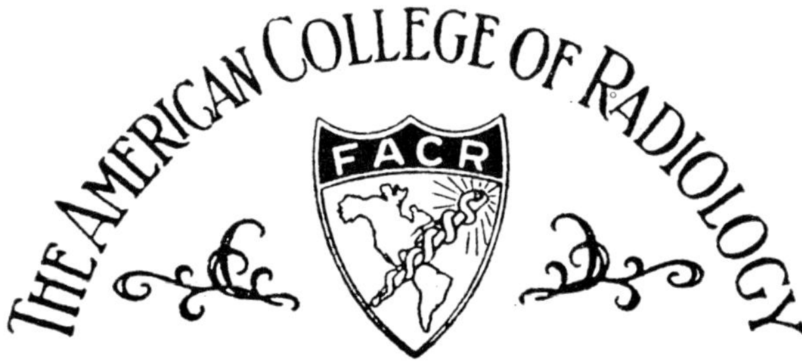

Founded by Radiologists of the United States, 1923

SIGN OF THE "NEW" ACR. At least one snake got lost in the re-shuffling process.

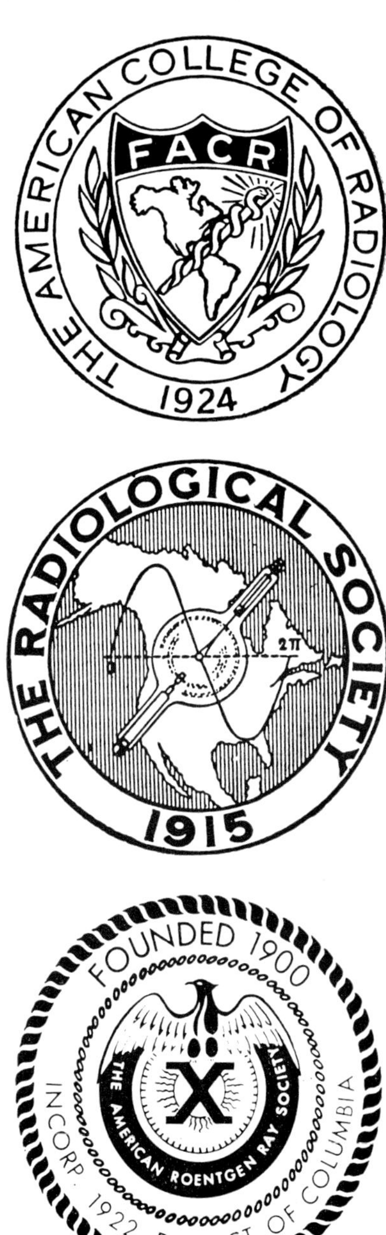

snake on a crutch appears on the frontispiece of *De Magnete* (1600), by the British physician and physicist William Gilbert (1540-1603), whom Glasser considers as the earliest recognizable scientific forefather of Roentgen.

In the complex of American Radiology, the ABR is the Membership Selection Committee for the ACR, as all those certified by the ABR are offered membership in the ACR. Many of them also join the RSNA, but comparatively few are later admitted into the ARRS and/or the ARS. The AMA maintains no membership records for its Section on Radiology. In the AMA Directory, members are listed with their declared specialty, but certification by any of the American Boards, and memberships in National Societies are included.

ATOMIC BEGINNINGS

The Atomic Phase came about so insidiously that, short of accepting an arbitrary dividing line, one is hard pressed to determine the precise date of its inception.

As early as 1913 two chemists, the Austrian Fritz Adolph Paneth (1887-1958) and the Hungarian born Georg de Hevesy used (natural) radioactive substances as indicators (the modern term is tracers) in analytic chemistry (*Nature* of May 1 and November 13, 1913). In 1923 de Hevesy employed radioactive ash assays in quantitative biochemical problems.

In 1933, the French physicists Irène Curie (1897-1956) and Frédéric Joliot (1900-1958) discovered induced (artificial) radioactivity (this event took place before they were married), while observing the emission of neutrons, protons and positrons produced when light metals were bombarded with alpha particles from a polonium source: the positron emission continued after removal of the source, thus indicating that a "new" substance had been formed. They reported their discovery to the Paris Academy of Sciences on January 15, 1934.

Because of his leftist leanings, Frédéric Joliot – better known as Frédéric Joliot-Curie (he appended the wife's name to his own) – had his portrait reproduced on numerous posters and postmarks originated in Iron Curtain countries. In the herein reproduced Roumanian stamp, his head is shown with an "atomized" peace dove.

Next, in 1934, the Italian physicist Enrico Fermi (1901-1954) – who was then at the Physical Institute of the University in Rome – devised a better method to produce radioactive isotopes (bombardment of neutrons resulting from the interaction of radon and beryllium powder), and among many other substances he prepared the first radioiodine (*Nature*, May 19, 1934). On November 9, 1935 (in *Nature*) de Hevesy, who was then at the Finsen Institute in Copenhagen, reported the use of neutron-generated P^{32} for the study of metabolism in rats.

A more abundant source of isotopes proved to be the cyclotron (1931), developed at the University of California in Berkeley by the American physicist Ernest Orlando Lawrence (1901-1958); in the *Physical Review* of October, 1934, he reported having accelerated *deutrons* (the modern term is deuterons) and thus produced his first radio-isotope – ${}_{12}Na^{24}$ "decaying" into ${}_{12}Mg^{24}$. Soon, various other radioactive isotopes were

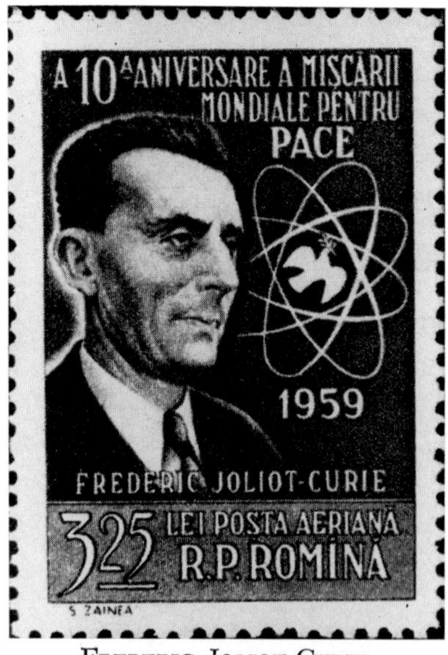

Frederic Joliot-Curie

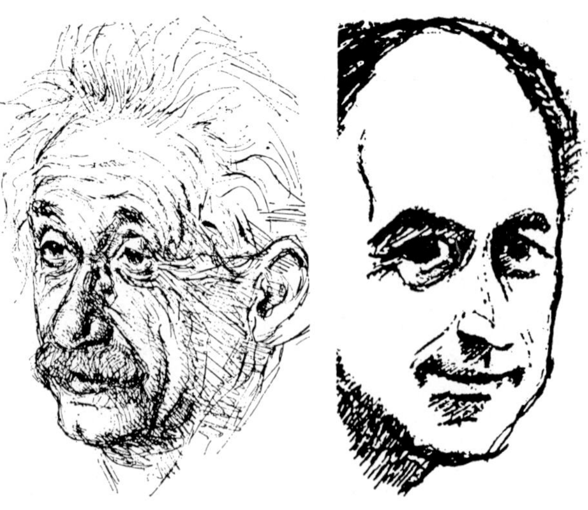

Albert Einstein and (Balding) Enrico Fermi

prepared and passed on to the Donner Laboratory of Biophysics and Medical Physics at Berkeley where, in December 1937, the physician John Hundale Lawrence (brother to the physicist) administered for the first time P^{32} to a patient with chronic lymphocytic leukemia (*cf., Archives of Internal Medicine* of June, 1956).

In 1938, at Massachusetts General Hospital, the endocrinologist Saul Hertz (1905-1955) performed the first thyroid studies with radioiodine – neutron produced at the Massachusetts Institute of Technology by the physicists Arthur Roberts and Robley Dunglison Evans. Their paper (in the May, 1938 issue of the *Proceedings of the Society of Experimental Biology and Medicine*) contains, among other things, also the now famous (*i.e.*, common) word "tagged."

THE ATOMIC PHASE

In 1905, Albert Einstein (1879-1955) proposed the Theory of Special Relativity. In 1915, he extended that principle to the General Theory of Relativity. One of the important predictions of his theory was that mass and energy are interchangeable and related by the now famous expression $E = mc^2$.

Einstein was a German-born Jew. He ranks with Galileo and Newton as a conceptual revisor of man's understanding of the universe. After having studied and taught in Berne and Prague, he became in 1914 director of the Kaiser Wilhelm Physical Institute in Berlin. At the time of Hitler's accession to power in 1933, Einstein was visiting professor at the California Institute of Technology. He never returned to Germany; at first he went to live for a few months in Belgium—his German citizenship was revoked and his possessions were confiscated in 1934. He then came to this country, and found a permanent faculty position with the Institute for Advanced Study, opened in 1933 at Princeton. Aside from being a genius at theoretical physics, Einstein was a mild philosopher, a devout zionist, and ardent pacifist.

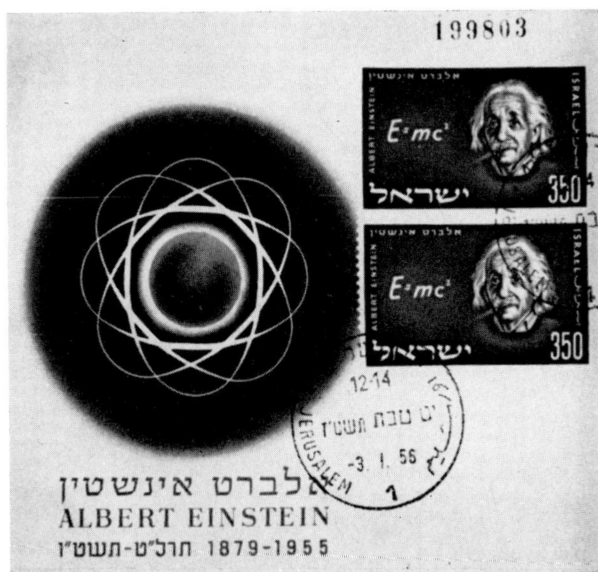

Courtesy: Stan Bohrer.

FIRST DAY COVER. This commemorative portrait stamp was issued on January 3, 1956, to honor the memory of Albert Einstein, one of the most brilliant theoretical physicists mankind ever had.

In 1938, the German physical chemist Otto Hahn achieved neutron-induced fission of uranium. Atomic fission liberates a frightening amount of energy, and the fear arose that a super-weapon based on nuclear fission might be under development in Germany. A group of scientists, including Niels Bohr, urged Einstein to "inform" Franklin Roosevelt of the feasibility of a super-bomb based on the fission of uranium, and of the need for producing such a bomb ahead of the Germans. Einstein's fear of Nazi supremacy must have been stronger than his pacifistic tendencies* because in September, 1939 Einstein put his name to a letter sent to Franklin Roosevelt. As an irony of sorts, the atomic explosion is one of the more spectacular demonstrations of the correctness of Einstein's $E=mc^2$.

At this point will be included a few details from the article *The First Pile,* published in the *Bulletin of the Atomic Scientists* of December, 1962 (that was the anniversary issue "honoring" the first two decades after the first chain reaction).

In the fall of 1938, Otto Hahn and Fritz Strassmann, working at the Kaiser Wilhelm Institute in Berlin, found barium in the residue material from an experiment in which they had bombarded uranium with neutrons from a radium beryllium source. Elements other than uranium had previously been found in similar experiments, but they differed from uranium by only one or two units of mass. This time the barium differed by 98 units of mass. Before publishing their work in *Die Naturwissenschaften,* Hahn and Strassmann communicated with Lise Meitner, an Austrian physicist who had fled the Reich and had gone to work with Niels Bohr in Copenhagen. Meitner reasoned that the uranium atom had been split, but even so some of the mass had disappeared, and she calculated (in accord-

*In retrospect Einstein may have developed a feeling of guilt for having signed that weighty letter; after World War II he became one of the more articulate members of the movement to "ban-the-bomb" and "ban-the-tests." He displayed quite often so-called leftist behavior, which alienated many of his USA fans. And yet, for a long time, USSR politicians (but not USSR scientists) regarded relativistic theory as something akin to heresy.

ance with Einstein's theory) the released energy to be about 200 mev for each atom fissioned.

Bohr then decided to come to the United States to discuss the matter with Einstein. Bohr arrived at Princeton on January 16, 1939. The news spread by word of mouth and reached Enrico Fermi, who was then at Columbia University in New York City. Italian-born physicist Fermi had been awarded the 1938 Nobel Prize for physics, and the Italian press had complained that during the festivities Fermi had not worn the Fascist uniform, nor had he given the Fascist salute after receiving the prize. Thereupon Fermi cancelled his return trip to Italy, and came instead to this country.

During Bohr's momentous visit to the USA in January, 1939 he attended also a conference on theoretical physics at George Washington University in Washington (D.C.). This is when and where Bohr and Fermi exchanged information, and discussed the problem of fission. Fermi mentioned the possibility that neutrons might be emitted in the process of fission. During the conversation the idea of a chain reaction was born.

On February 27, 1939 – at Columbia University – Canadian-born Walter Zinn and Hungarian-born Leo Szilard began to investigate the number of neutrons emitted by the fissioning uranium. Fermi and his associates worked separately on the same problem, and their results were published side by side in the *Physical Review* of April, 1939.

Further impetus to the work on a uranium reactor was given by the discovery of plutonium at the Radiation Laboratory in Berkeley, in March of 1940. This

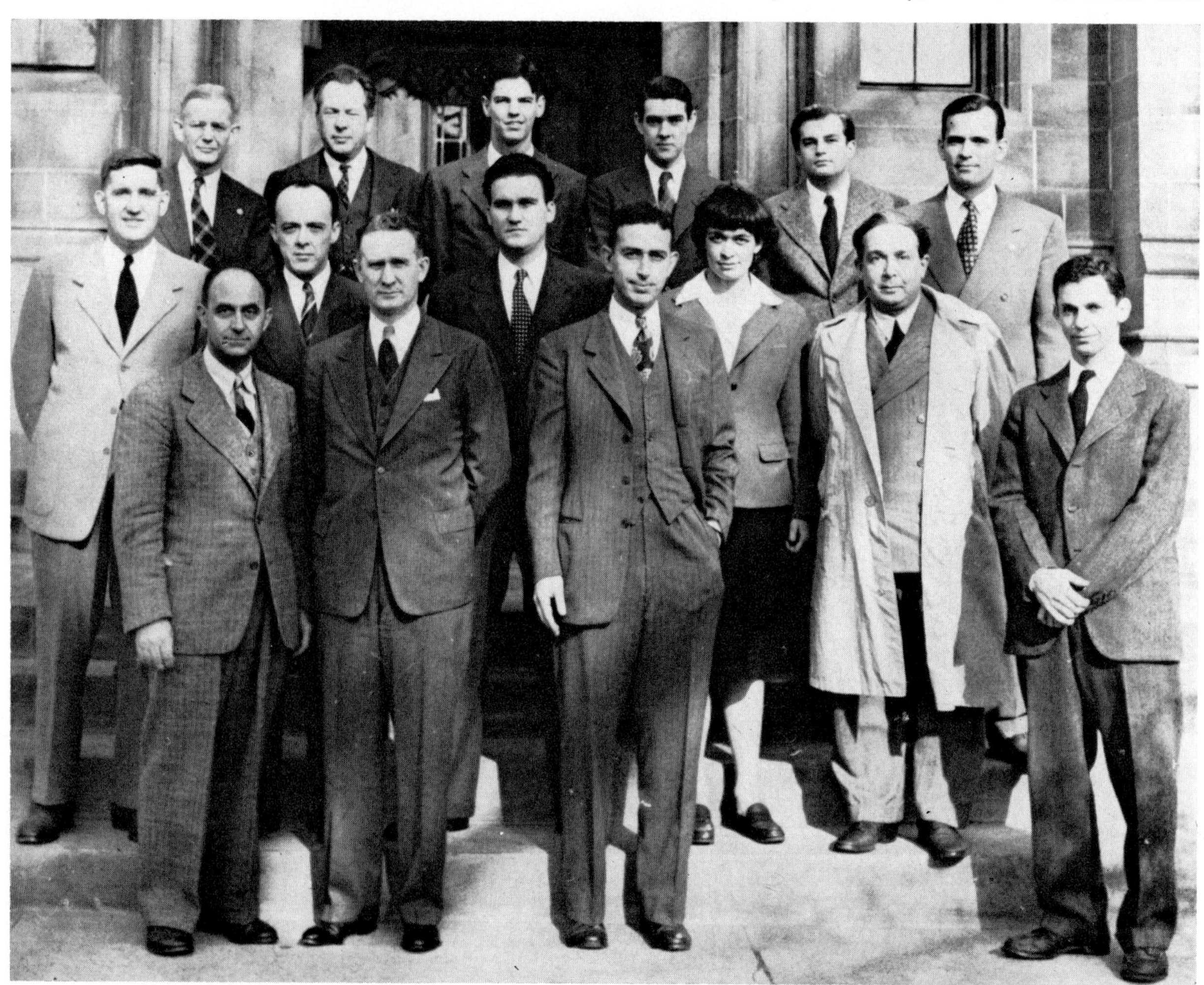

Courtesy: Argonne National Laboratory.

STAFF OF CP-1. This photograph was made on the steps of Eckhart Hall (University of Chicago) on December 2, 1946. Back row, left to right: Norman Hilberry, Samuel Allison, Thomas Brill, Robert Nobles, Warren Nyer, and Martin Wilkening. Middle row: Harold Agnew, William Sturm, Harold Lichtenberger, Leona W. Marshall, and Leo Szilard. Front row: Enrico Fermi, Walter Zinn, Albert Wattenberg, and Herbert Anderson.

element, unknown in nature, was formed by U-238 capturing a neutron, and then undergoing two emissions of beta particles. Plutonium, it was believed, would undergo fission as did the rare isotope of uranium U-235. Plutonium could be separated from uranium by conventional methods, and thence be used to make a bomb which would release that tremendous amount of energy. A bomb with U-235 was known to be feasible but at that time it was uncertain whether any means existed by which sufficient quantities of pure U-235 could be separated from U-238.

In July, 1941, experiments were started at Columbia University by Fermi, Zinn, and their associates to find a suitable moderating material for slowing down the neutrons (graphite was selected because of its easy availability). The key to the problem was the reproduction factor *k*. It had to be greater than one (more neutrons emitted by the splitting uranium atoms than were needed to "split" them), or else – with the inevitable losses – there could be no self-sustaining reaction.

Einstein's letter had the desired effect and the mighty power of the Federal Government was applied to the quest for nuclear knowledge.

Roosevelt named a Uranium Committee which in 1940 was reorganized as a subcommittee of the National Defense Research Committee, and on December 6, 1941 the project was enlarged to become a section of the Office of Scientific Research and Development (OSRD). On August 13, 1942 the Manhattan (Engineer) District was officially established in the Corps of Engineers of the US Army. In May, 1943 the Manhattan District took over all the work on the uranium project which until then had been under the OSRD. General Leslie R. Groves, in charge of the Manhattan District since September, 1942 acted as co-ordinator throughout the existence of the project. Early research in this field had been carried out by physicists at several universities, who later joined the Metallurgical Laboratory (another code name) at the University of Chicago under Arthur Holly Compton (1892-1962) to concentrate on the production of a chain reaction based on Uranium.[235]

The Atomic Phase started (officially!) on December 2, 1942 when Enrico Fermi (1901-1954) and his

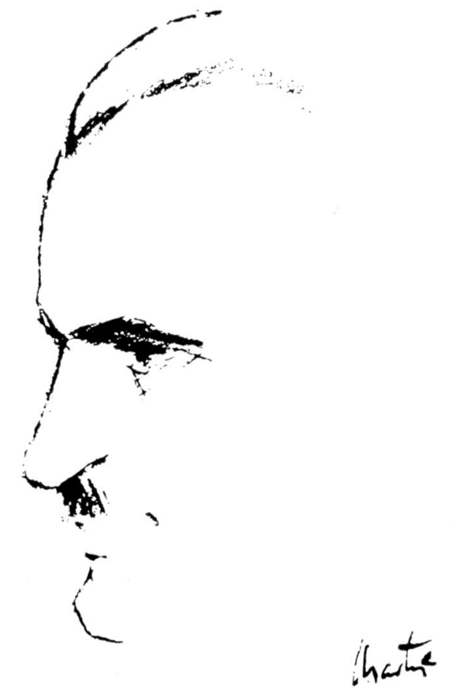

Courtesy: Bulletin of the Atomic Scientists.

ARTHUR HOLLY COMPTON. This drawing appeared as part of an obituary authored by Alexander Langsdorf, Jr., and published in September, 1962. The sketch is signed by Martyl.

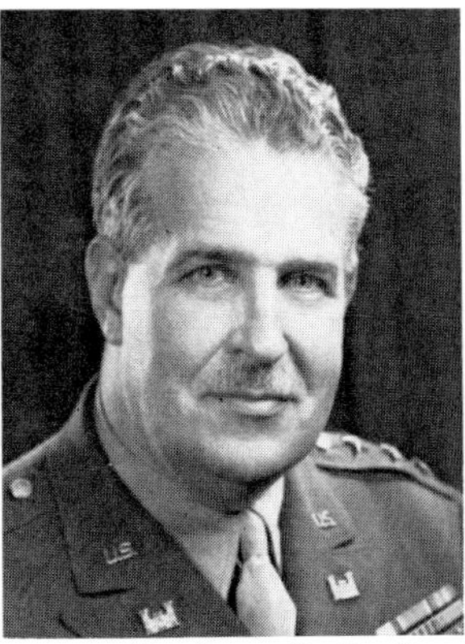

Courtesy: U. S. Army.

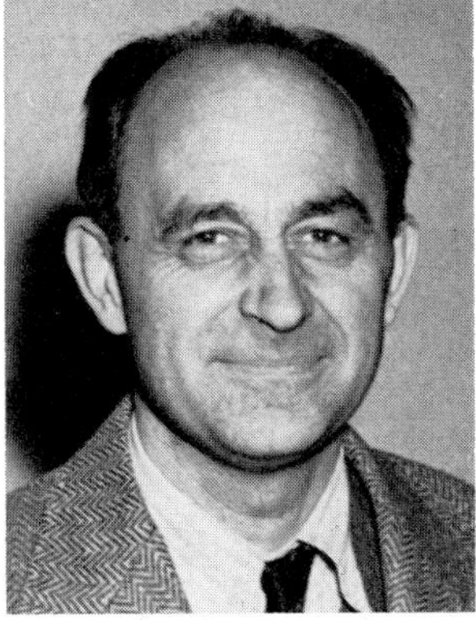

Courtesy: Argonne

GENERAL LESLIE R. GROVES. The dynamic military commander of the Manhattan Engineering District "got things done," but used to have scientists complain of his pet security regulation, the so-called compartmentalization. Groves insisted that one must know only what is necessary to get that particular job done, and no more. This is fine as long as one is moving on known territory. But when exploring the unknown, one never knows what (among things you are not supposed to know) could help you solve the problem at hand. Based on statements made in Groves' memoirs (*Now It Can be Told,* Harper & Brothers, 1962), regarding his views on development and delivery of the A-bomb, Groves has been called heartless, and something more profane than that. But Eugene Rabinovitch (one of his critics) justly remarked, "General Groves carried out his assignment . . . and his bombs ended the war. We have no right to reproach him (that)." The other is ENRICO FERMI. This photograph, taken on November 2, 1954, shows the face of the usually silent, but always smiling Italian-born nuclear physicist who was responsible for achieving the first chain reaction.

co-workers brought to criticality the first nuclear reactor, erected in the grandstands of Stagg Field (the stadium of the University of Chicago).

ARGONNE

The Metallurgical Laboratory was the birthplace of the reactor (a term used in preference to the barbarism pile). Its further development proved to be even more significant.

The history of the first decade of the Argonne National Laboratory was summarized by its 1957-1961 director, Norman Hilberry, in the *Argonne News* for September 5, 1951. The Metallurgical Laboratory had been organized at the University of Chicago in January of 1942 under a contract between the University and the OSRD. Two months later the Met Lab had about 150 persons on its payroll. During operation under the OSRD the Met Lab carried out the experimental program which culminated in the establishment of the first self-sustaining nuclear chain reaction together with the equally significant demonstration that the accompanying release of nuclear energy could be controlled positively and simply.

The first reactor – CP-1, means Chicago Pile One* – was moved early in 1943 from Stagg Field to a new

*There were 29 exponential piles before CP-1, according to Albert Wattenberg, the lanky lad in the foreground of the 1946 group photograph. He is now teaching physics at the University of Illinois in Urbana, pursues accelerator (synchrotron and the like) research into subatomic particles, and will co-edit Fermi's papers. Having been on the team of the first "pile," Wattenberg obligingly reviewed the "atomic" portions of this text, which were also critically reviewed by Theodore Fields, a health physicist from Chicago. Ted had been employed at the Met Lab beginning January 6, 1943, and he remembers that his first (backbreaking) assignment was to dismantle the graphite blocks from CP-1. The first day he found himself on top of a load of bricks, and needed help badly. He called out to a short guy who was standing around, and the guy helped him for 15 minutes until the assigned help returned. Only later did Ted find out that the short guy who had helped him was Enrico Fermi, not only a brilliant scientist, but first of all a warm, humble man.

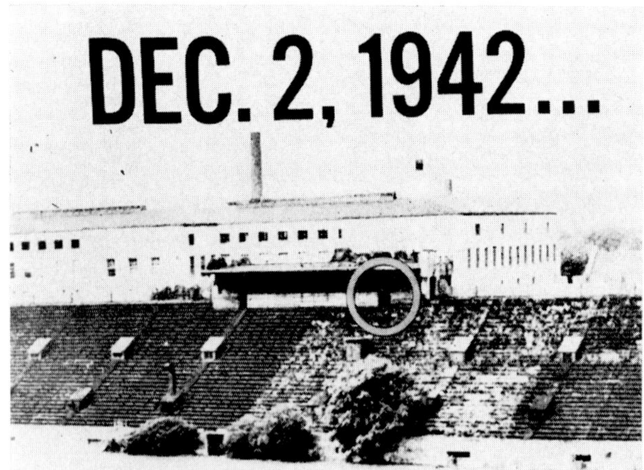

DATE AND PLACE OF FIRST ATOMIC CHAIN REACTION. Squash court under the West stands of Stagg Field on the campus of the University of Chicago.

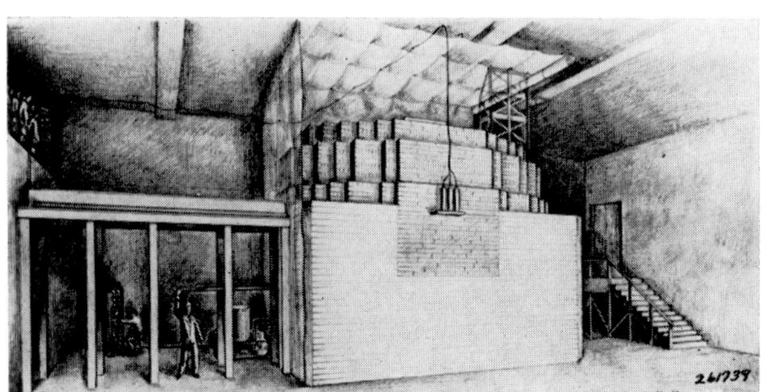

Courtesy: Pentagon Information Office.

FIRST ATOMIC REACTOR. Sketch drawn by Melvin A. Miller in 1946. Shows "zip" being pulled by George Weil.

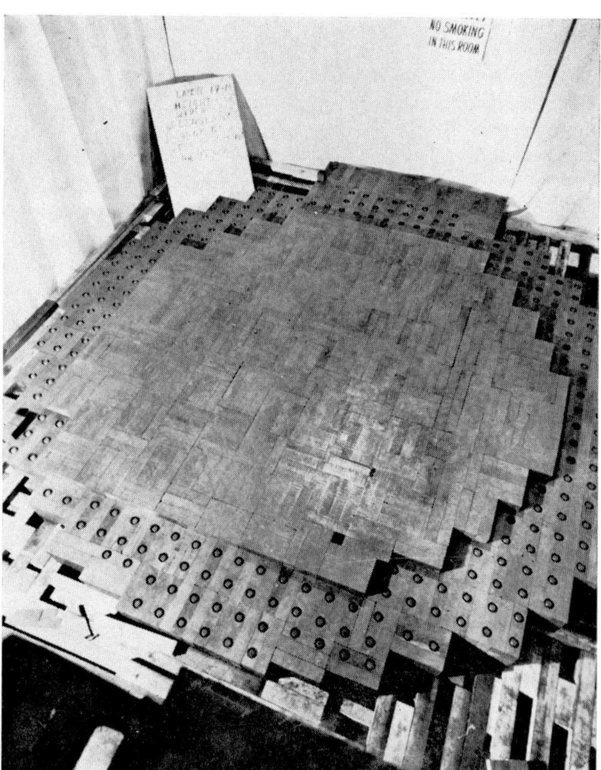

Courtesy: Argonne National Laboratory.

FIRST NUCLEAR REACTOR. Only extant photograph, made in November, 1942 at the 19th layer of graphite containing uranium metal and uranium oxide, which were spaced by layers of "dead" graphite. Layer 18, almost covered in the picture, contained uranium. Construction continued to the 57th layer, one layer beyond critical or operating dimensions. It resulted in a roughly spherical shape.

building in the Argonne Forest section of the Palos Park Forest Preserve. It offered additional isolation not obtainable in the city. This branch of the Met Lab was named the Argonne Laboratory because of its location and in 1946 this name was chosen for the laboratory as a whole.

At Oak Ridge (1943), the Met Lab in cooperation with DuPont designed its facilities including the reactor for Plutonium production. The Met Lab also carried out essential chemical studies on the new elements Neptunium and Plutonium which then existed only in submicroscopic quantities, and developed a tentative chemical separation process for the Hanford (Washington) production plant.

As new centers were developed at Oak Ridge, Los Alamos, and Hanford, the critical manpower needs were provided by the Met Lab. The first heavy water moderated nuclear reactor was designed, built and placed in operation at the Palos Park site of the Laboratory in the spring of 1944 and in a modified form was still serving in 1951. Both of the two pioneer Argonne research reactors, CP-2 (the reconstructed Stagg Field pile) and CP-3 (the first heavy water pile, later modified and designated CP-4,) were dismantled when the Palos Park site of the Laboratory was closed in

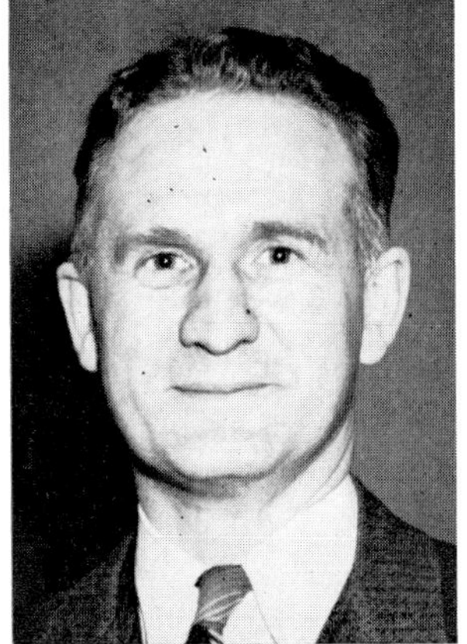

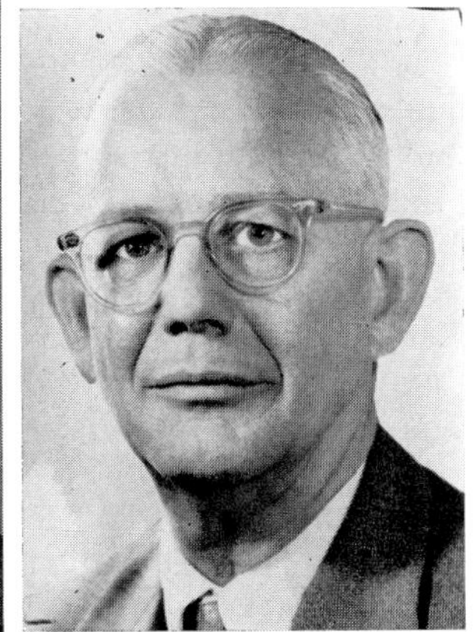

WALTER HENRY ZINN. First director of Argonne (from 1945 through 1956), is now building reactors with a private firm (General Nuclear Engineering Corporation), of which he is the president. On the right is NORMAN HILBERRY. His full name is Horace Van Norman Hilberry. He came to the Met Lab in 1942 (from New York University), rose in the ranks, and became director of Argonne in 1957. His main scientific interests are in cosmic rays, spectroscopy, and electrical discharges through gases.

DEC. 2 1942 START-UP OF FIRST SELF-SUSTAINING CHAIN REACTION
NEUTRON INTENSITY IN THE PILE AS RECORDED BY A GALVANOMETER

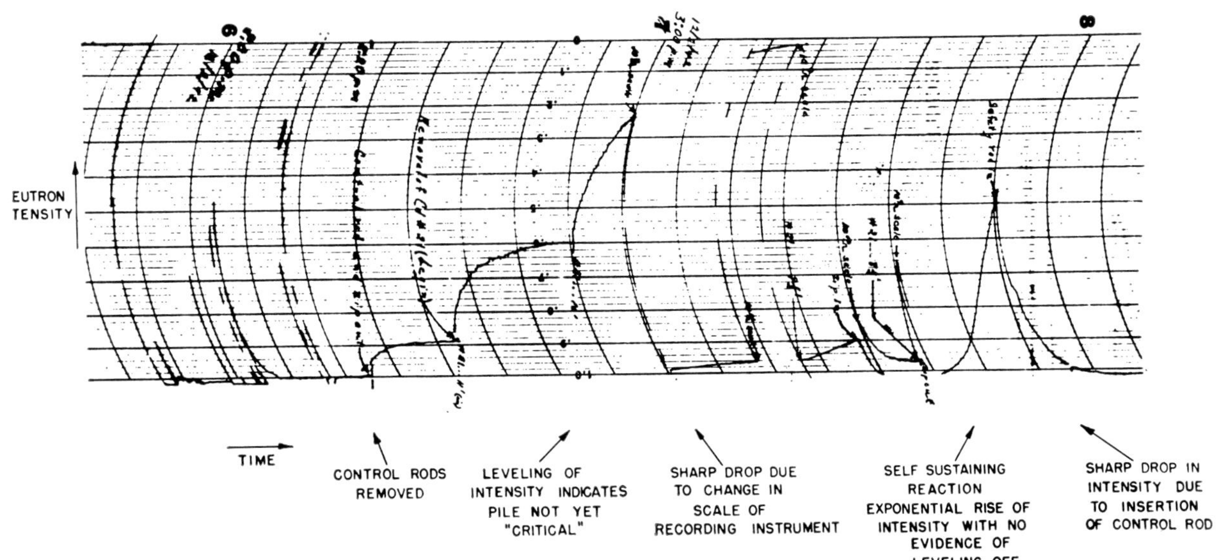

Courtesy: Argonne National Laboratory.

BIRTH CERTIFICATE OF THE ATOMIC PHASE. At about 3:25 p.m., on December 2, 1942, a final adjustment of the position of a control rod was made, and soon the number of neutrons liberated (created?) within the reactor exceeded the number of neutrons lost. After twenty-eight minutes of operation, a cadmium control rod called "zip" was pushed into the reactor, and the chain reaction ended.

1954. The present heavy water research reactor CP-5 began operation in February, 1954.

In September, 1944, the first Hanford reactor went into successful operation generating Plutonium and before the end of that year, the chemical separation plants began to deliver pure Plutonium. As the Hanford task was completed, Los Alamos requested an increase in their staff needed to expedite the program. Many members of the remaining staff of the Met Lab were transferred to New Mexico in the fall of 1944. With its major assignments completed and the staff seriously depleted, the Manhattan District began to wonder whether the Met Lab should not be disbanded and the contract with the University of Chicago terminated. On July 1, 1945 another group of scientific personnel was transferred from the Met Lab to the Clinton Laboratories.

By January 1, 1946 the technical staff at the Met Lab had dropped (from its high point of just over 600

May 17, 1955 E. FERMI ET AL 2,708,656
NEUTRONIC REACTOR
Filed Dec. 19, 1944 27 Sheets-Sheet 7

FIG.7.

Witnesses: Inventors: Enrico Fermi, Leo Szilard. By Attorney

Courtesy: Argonne National Laboratory.

U. S. Patent on "Neutronic Reactor." The inventors listed are Italian-born Enrico Fermi and Hungarian-born Leo Szilard. Work on the patent application was started six months before the actual CP-1 (Chicago Pile 1) went critical. As the Manhattan District reactor program grew, the patent application was expanded to include also the Oak Ridge and Hanford reactor prototypes. The growing file was guarded under a secret classification until December, 1944 when application was filed with the US Patent Office. The patent was finally issued in date of May 17, 1955. Patents on nuclear reactors had been granted (in the meantime) in some foreign countries, but in no case did the corresponding United States application have a disclosure adequate to meet the requirements of the US patent Office.

in the summer of 1944) to 200, and the total number of employees had decreased from 2000 to 1100. It was the low point in its history. Nevertheless, basic science projects continued unabated. The ground work for the Experimental Breeder Reactor was laid and the engineering studies which led to the techniques for use of liquid metals as cooling media were started. A new and more effective chemical process was developed for separating pure Plutonium.

A committee, appointed to offer suggestions for the future of Argonne, held its first meeting on December 2, 1945, the third anniversary of the start-up of the first reactor. In the spring of 1946 the committee offered a plan for organization of the Argonne National Laboratory. It included active participation of major universities and research institutions in the Middle West. The University of Chicago remained the operating contractor. The contract was signed and ratified in May of 1946, and Argonne National Laboratory began its official existence under the new plan on July 1, 1946 with Walter H. Zinn as Director.

A site was chosen in DuPage County within five miles of the Palos Park area where the experimental research reactors were then located. In August of 1946, the McMahon Act created the AEC to deal with all atomic developments. On January 1, 1948 the Argonne National Laboratory was requested and agreed to assume the responsibility of serving as the AEC's prin-

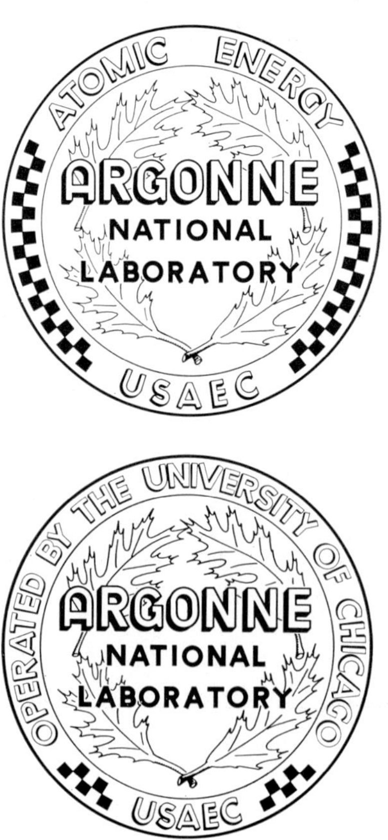

cipal reactor development center. In that same year ground for the first new buildings was broken and construction proceeded actively ever since.

In 1946, the Laboratory made a formal proposal to the Manhattan Engineer Division for a project to design and build a fast breeder reactor. This was the Experimental Breeder No. 1 (EBR-1). A major development was the use of liquid metals for transfer of heat energy to a standard working substance such as water. The question of an adequate construction site arose very early. By that time, the AEC had assumed responsibility and since other projects had similar demands, the National Reactor Testing Station (NRTS) was established near Idaho Falls. The EBR-1 was the first reactor built on that site. It was completed in the summer of 1951, and work on the loading of the reactor commenced. In August criticality was achieved. On December 20, 1951 the reactor was taken to full power, a turbine was activated, and four large electric bulbs were lighted by the electricity produced in the EBR-1. It was the first time in history when atomic energy was used for this purpose. The next day the reactor supplied all the power means in the building in which it was located. On July 17, 1955 Arco (Idaho) was lighted by power generated from steam heated in Borax-III, making it the first community to "go on atomic power."

True to its contract, Argonne continued to develop reactors, for instance they designed the BWR used in the first nuclear submarine. Most of their reactors have prosaic titles such as CP-5, their "work-horse." But they have also two which have received imaginative designations. There is Juggernaut, a low powered research reactor for physicistic purposes. The other is Janus, a 250-Kw research reactor with two faces (hence its name), one for low level irradiation of biological specimens, another capable of providing higher doses. Janus is the first nuclear reactor in this country employed entirely for biological research.*

A Liquid Metal Fuel Reactor (LMFR) utilizes as fuel molten bismuth in which highly enriched uranium is dissolved (about 500 to 100 ppm). In addition, up to 350 ppm each of zirconium and magnesium are included as corrosion and mass transfer inhibitors. This solution is circulated by pumps under relatively low pressure in a closed loop. In one section of the loop is a container with a graphite moderator; when the solution passess through the moderator, fission occurs and

*Scheduled for completion late in 1963 is their new Zero Gradient Synchrotron, planned in the 12.5 Bev range. They also have an electronic digital computer called GEORGE.

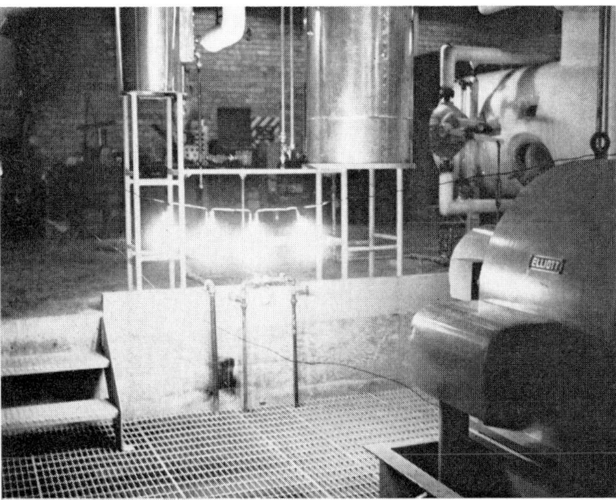

Courtesy: Argonne National Laboratory.

LIGHT FROM EBR-1. On December 20, 1951, the first four light bulbs were illuminated with electricity produced in the first Experimental Breeder Reactor located near Idaho Falls (Idaho). EBR means a reactor which "breeds" additional fissionable nuclear fuel (Plutonium) while operating.

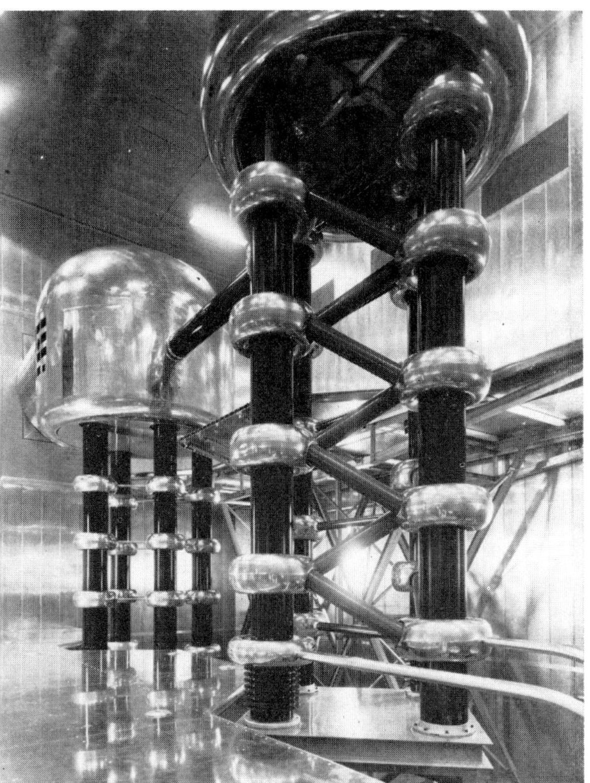

Courtesy: Argonne National Laboratory.

ACCELERATOR, SR. In 1932, Sir John Douglas Cockroft and Ernest Thomas Sinton Walton built the first transformer-rectifier voltage multiplier, in which capacitors were used to produce the high potential needed to accelerate protons or other particles. They used this technique to disintegrate lithium, for which they were (later) awarded the Nobel Prize in 1951. The Cockroft-Walton accelerator shown in this photograph serves to pre-accelerate protons which will then be "fed" through a linac into the ZGS.

heat is generated, with a resultant temperature rise in the solution. At another section of the loop, a heat exchanger removes this heat, which serves to produce steam that, in turn, is used to drive a conventional turbine generator (Dennis Puleston).

According to a recent AEC report (1962), the costs of producing electricity from atomic fuel have been progressively reduced. It cost about 50 mills per kwh at the Shippingport (Pa.) protohype reactor in 1958. It is now less than 10 mills per kwh at the full-scale plants in existence. The estimate for a large plant, to be built at Bodega Bay (California) is for 5.5 to 6 mills. The total nuclear electric generating capacity in the USA is today (middle of 1962) about 850,000 kw, close to 0.5% of the total installed capacity. The world's natural resources of fossile fuel (petroleum and natural gas) are undoubtedly limited, and more and more reliance will have to be placed (in the not so distant future) on energy from nuclear sources, which will affect the international petroleum politics and the time is nearing when a crash program might have to be initiated to solve the problem of obtaining (slowly released) energy not only from fission, but also from fusion reaction (which is why the research on plasma in particular, and on solid state physics in general, is of so much political interest).

In the biological field, Argonne National Laboratory has brought many important contributions. There is a joint project of the Radiological Physics Division, the Health Division, and the technically independent Argonne Cancer Research Hospital (Director: Leon Orris Jacobson), intended to determine the amount of radium body burden. This investigation was made possible by whole body radiation counting equipment (including the iron chamber) developed by their Senior Biophysicist, Argentinian–born Leonidas D. Marinelli. So far, the team has examined about 250 persons who had ingested radium, including the survivors of the famous radium dial painters of the 1920s.

Austin Moore Brues, director of the Biologic Division at Argonne, is interested especially in historic studies with radio-carcinogenesis. Cancer causation at macroscopic levels was intensely investigated by the radiozoologist Miriam Posner Finkel, who is also interested in the effects of low-level irradiation (since such projects require statistically significant numbers of animals, Argonne has recently increased its holdings to 100,000 mice); her husband Asher Finkel* has worked on several subjects, including recently the biology of Deuterium.

In May, 1958 the participating institutions of Argonne National Laboratory formed Associated Midwest Universities (AMU) and in March, 1959 they established an office at Argonne. The member institutions extended over an area covering roughly a triangle from Pittsburgh to Oklahoma to the Northern tip of Minnesota.

THE ATOMIC CITY

In the Summer of 1942, a combined crew from the Manhattan Engineer District and from the Stone & Webster Engineering Corp. (Boston) searched for the site of a new "installation." On September 19, 1942 they selected a 94-square-mile tract in the Anderson and Roane counties in Eastern Tennessee, at the foot of the Cumberland mountains.

The Federal Government purchased the land, evacuated the inhabitants (about 3,000), and the place soon became a maximum security area, fenced and

*Dr. Finkel, who is currently director of the Health Division at Argonne, courteously provided printed material for this compilation.

ARGONNE SCIENTISTS. Argentine-born physicist Leonidas D. Marinelli (with glasses), and Milwaukee-born biologist Austin Moore Brues.

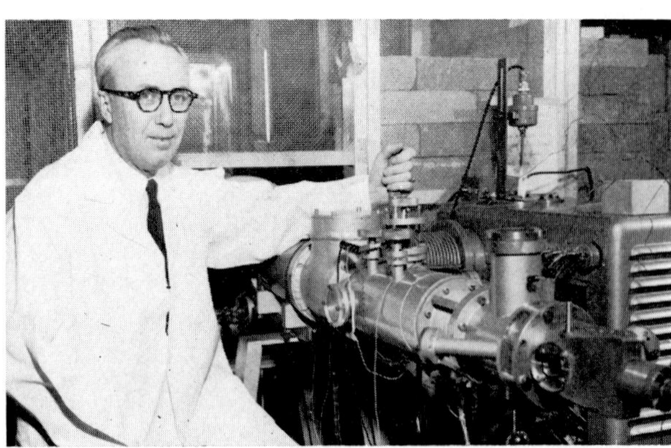

Courtesy: Argonne National Laboratory.

RADIO-BIO-PHYSICS IN ACTION. Leonidas Donato Marinelli operating a 250 kev Cockroft-Walton ion accelerator, used herein for production of neutrons. The vacuum setup is for removing gas from the continually pumped tube.

heavily guarded. In November, 1942 work started on the construction of headquarters for the Manhattan Engineer District. In the past that spot used to be called the Black Oak Ridge: they adopted as the name of their "installation" a shorter version, Oak Ridge.

On February 1, 1943 (only two months after Fermi's very first reactor had gone critical) ground was broken in Oak Ridge for the building of the X-10 pile, a Graphite Nuclear Reactor. The Oak Ridge Pile, the world's first production type of uranium chain-reactor, went critical on November 3, 1943. It produced gram quantities of plutonium, necessary for the development of a method of chemical separation of plutonium from uranium (the large plutonium-producing breeder reactors were later constructed at Hanford).

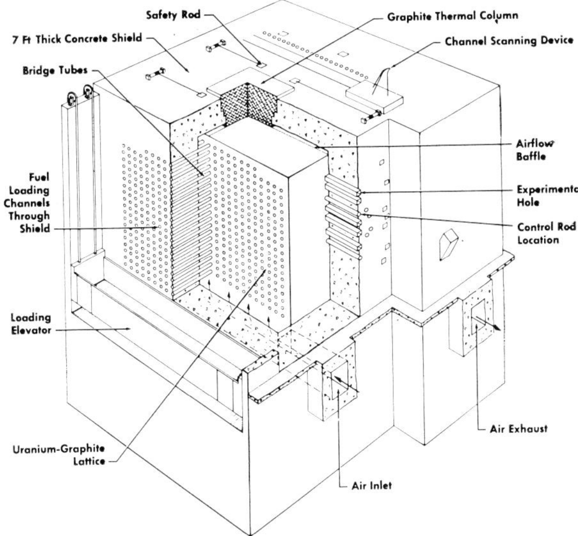

Courtesy: AEC.

GRAPHITE PILE. The word "pile" is an antiquated, obsolete, even frowned-upon, pseudo-synonym for nuclear reactor. But pile is what they called that first fifty-seven-layered graphite-uranium sandwich stacked up at Stagg Field in 1942. The name came from the vague similarity with Volta's electricity-producing pile. And since people who had been at Stagg Field designed the first large graphite-uranium reactor at Oak Ridge – it went critical at 5 a.m. on November 3, 1943 – they called it the X-10 (or Clinton) Pile. Its moderator is a 24-foot graphite (carbon) cube, in which holes are drilled for the fuel elements. It is air-cooled, which requires a tall discharge stack.

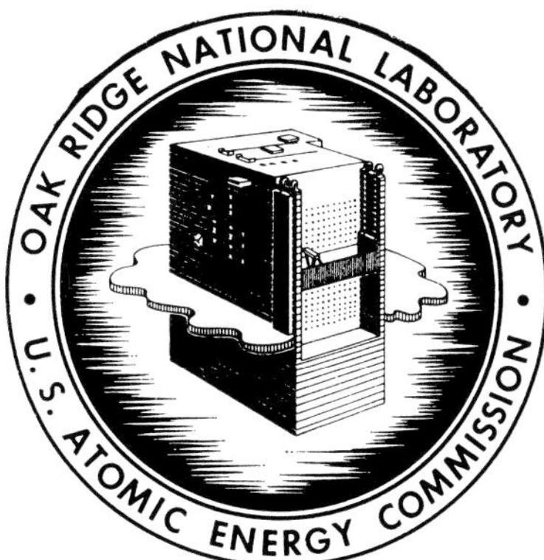

GRAPHITE REACTOR SEAL. Recent Oak Ridge mandala, featuring the face of the air-cooled graphite reactor.

Oak Ridge was built for the purpose of producing large quantities of "atomic fuel," the natural radioactive isotope U^{235}. This was the basic ingredient in one type of Atomic (fission) Bomb, and in the trigger for the Hydrogen (fusion) Bomb. In nature, uranium consists of about .7 of 1 per cent of U^{235} and of over 99 per cent of the stable isotope 238. The idea was to find an industrial method to "enrich" the uranium into a high(er) concentration of U^{235}.

On January 20, 1943 the Carbide and Carbon Chemical Company accepted a letter of intent for operation of a gaseous diffusion plant (for enriching uranium) and that building was started on September 10, 1943. They called it K-25. Later on the firm changed its own name to Union Carbide Nuclear Company. The gaseous diffusion process was developed by a group of scientists, with most of the credit going to Harold Clayton Urey. K-25 became operational on April 13, 1944 and reached full generating capacity in July, 1945.

On February 1, 1943 work began on the Y-12 electromagnetic U^{235} separation plant. It was built on the equipment ideated by Ernest Orlando Lawrence and was put into use on January 27, 1944. The electromagnetic plant was operated initially by the Tennessee Eastman Corporation, a subsidiary of the Eastman Kodak Company. They withdrew on May 5, 1947 when Union Carbide assumed also that operation.

Oak Ridge boomed and reached its peak in 1945 when it had 75,000 population. Employment crested at 82,000. Some of the people traveled seventy-five miles each day for work. The major secret that had to be preserved was the size of the Y-12 area (the elec-

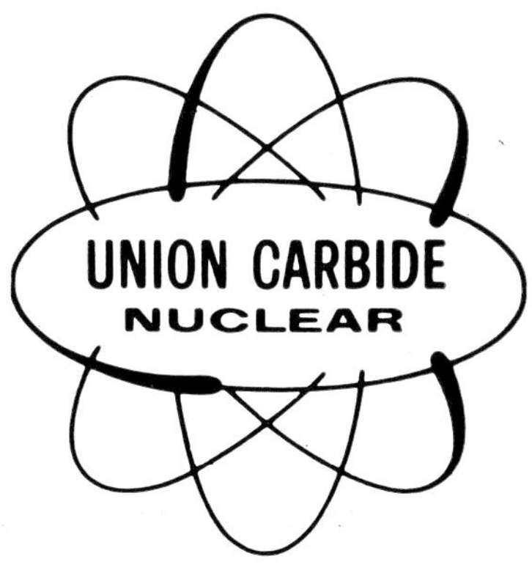

tromagnetic uranium enriching plant) which covered a surface in excess of 500 acres. Despite the large number of people who came and went, that secret was well kept from the outside: history has shown that there were, however, insiders who gave away most of the secrets.

LOS ALAMOS

The History of Project Y was written in 1946 by one of its physicists (David Hawkins) but most of it was only recently declassified, which is understandable: that is where the first atomic bomb was actually built.

The Los Alamos Project was one of a group of organizations, known collectively as the development of Substitute Materials Project (DSM), created early in 1943. While Project Y has been, of itself, small compared to other DSM projects, it occupied a crucial position.

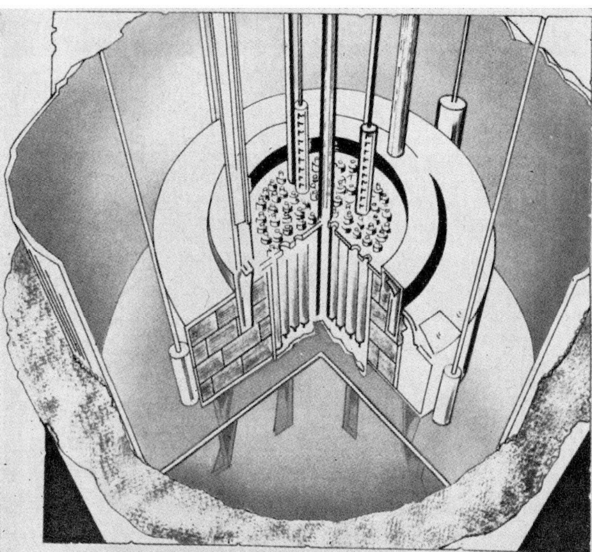

Courtesy: Bob Sulit's PORACC.

HEAVY WATER REACTOR. In 1944, heavy water became available in ton lots. Thereupon a "new" type of reactor was first built at Argonne. It consisted of a tank containing the heavy water as moderator, with uranium fuel rods dipped into it. Activity was controllable by pushing the rods deeper (which increases neutron flux), or retracting them. Most research reactors are of the tank type. The control-rod mechanism is usually on top of the surface plate. In a recent Oak Ridge design, that mechanism is beneath the reactor as the fuel rods have upper sleeves of neutron-absorbing cadmium. Many other refinements and variants are being developed (reactor technology). During operation there is heat production: by circulating the heavy water through a heat exchanger the reactor may supply power in the form of steam.

The first step toward a concerted program of bomb development was the appointment in June, 1942 of J. Robert Oppenheimer (from the University of California) as director of the work. Late in June a conference was called in Berkeley (California) to discuss the theory of the bomb and plan work for the future. A considerable part of the discussion was devoted to a new type of explosive reaction that had been considered by Edward Teller, a thermonuclear reaction in Deuterium (Teller is now known as the "father" of the fusion or H-bomb).

In October, 1942, it was decided to form a new establishment. The site of Project Y was selected in November, 1942. It was the Los Alamos Range School, located on an isolated mesa in the Pajarito plateau, by highway about forty miles north and west of Santa Fe (New Mexico). Its isolation and inaccessibility were regarded as very advantageous. Its subsequent growth to many times the original size was not foreseen. The main characteristic of the Los Alamos project was that a definite time schedule had been proposed: the bomb had to be ready for production by the time usable quantities of nuclear explosives became available.

The Los Alamos site, together with a large surrounding area, was established as a military reservation. The financial and procurement operations were handled by the University of California as prime contractor. The University received a letter of intent from the OSRD, superseded by a formal contract, signed with the Manhattan Engineer District on April 20, 1943.

Certain specialized equipment was brought to Los Alamos by the groups that were to use it. The largest single item was the cyclotron on loan from Harvard University. Two Van de Graaff electrostatic generators came from the University of Wisconsin. The Cockroft-Walton accelerator (D-D source) was from the University of Illinois. The Berkeley group brought chemical and cryogenic equipment. Thus work began at Los Alamos much earlier than would otherwise have been possible. Oppenheimer and a few members of the staff arrived in Santa Fe on March 15, 1943.

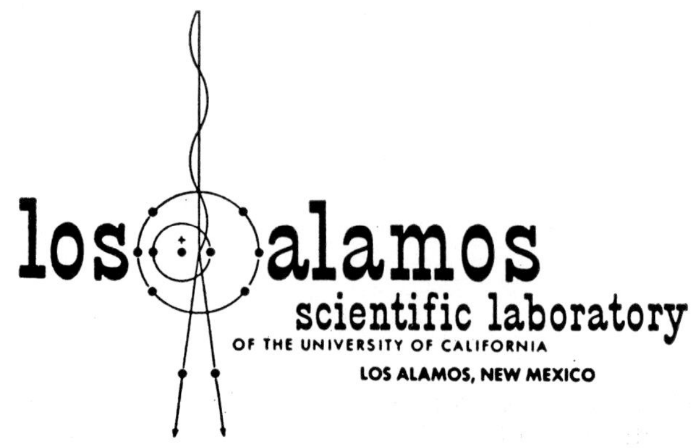

In December, 1943, the first representatives of the British atomic bomb project (known under the code name of Directorate of Tube Alloys) came to Los Alamos. Among these British envoys was the Danish physicist Niels Bohr, who had escaped from Denmark to England. Bohr was known under the pseudonym Nicholas Baker. Even in classified documents reference was made only to the name of Baker, never to Bohr. Early in 1944 Sir James Chadwick of the Cavendish Laboratory came to Los Alamos to head the British mission. The organizational problems encountered in the "wilderness" are difficult to imagine by outsiders. Incidentally, the Health Group was directed from the beginning by Louis Hempelmann, formerly with Barnes Hospital in St. Louis, now with the University of Rochester (New York). The really serious problem of the Health Group appeared in the spring of 1944 with the arrival at Los Alamos of the first quantities of plutonium, the toxicology of which was supposed to be about the same as that of radium, but definite differences are actually detectable.

At the time the Los Alamos Laboratory was established, it was not yet certain that the nuclear detonation could be produced. The first physical experiment completed at Los Alamos – in July, 1943 – was the observation of neutrons from the fissioning of Plutonium-239. The neutron number was measured from an almost invisible speck of plutonium found to be somewhat greater even than for Uranium-235. This result justified the decision already taken to construct the plutonium production pile at Hanford. Measurement of delayed neutrons also gave favorable results showing that such delays were negligible.

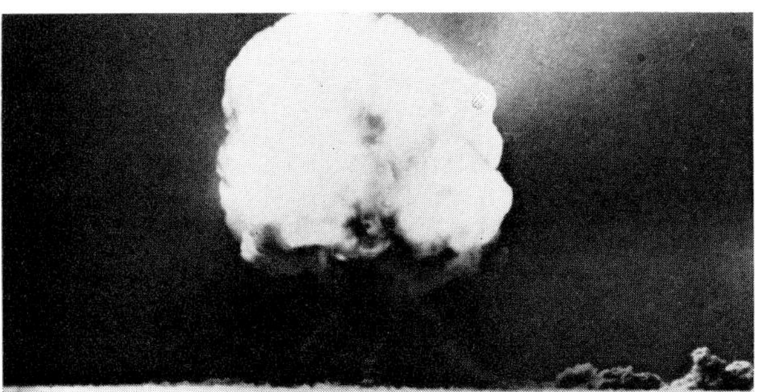

Courtesy: Los Alamos Scientific Laboratory.

First atomic explosion. Photograph of the Trinity test, taken fifteen seconds after detonation on July 16, 1945, shows the fireball rising high over desert air near San Antonio (New Mexico). Its yield was about 20 kilotons of TNT. In his memoirs, Groves recalls that on the day before Trinity, Fermi was offering to take wagers on whether or not the bomb would ignite the atmosphere – of course, Fermi said it would not! After the test, Vannevar Bush, James Conant, and Ernest Lawrence were upset for hours, and could talk of little else.

Actual development of the bomb started with nuclear studies and was gradually shifted to the assembly mechanism. The first major success was achieved with the Water Boiler, (a small tank type reactor with enriched fuel) which produced a divergent chain reaction, first accomplished on May 9, 1944. That series of experiments was continued until August, and determined nuclear quantities of interest, many of which had been predicted by the theorists with almost perfect accuracy.

An A-bomb is a run-away chain reaction in which the neutrons emitted by fission cause a logarithmically increasing number of fast fissions until all available "fuel" is used up. Take two hemispheres of pure U^{235} or plutonium (the "fuel"), each of which is subcritical when separated from the other. One of these hemispheres is embedded in a large mass of heavy material, called tamper, which forms the target end of a gun barrel. The other hemisphere serves as a projectile to be fired at the first hemisphere. Ordinary high explosives could be used to propel the second hemisphere down the gun barrel so that it would strike the first hemisphere at high velocity and weld itself to it in an overcritical assembly. Neutrons to initiate the fission reaction come from spontaneous fission, from cosmic radiation, or from some other neutron source. Another mechanism, later evolved, was the symmetric implosion technique (also discussed in several famous spy trials, and in standard textbooks, such as the well known primer by Ralph Lapp and Howard Andrews).

The method of detonating a nuclear bomb is to bring it into a supercritical configuration just at the time when it is to be detonated. The required speed of assembly depends upon the neutron background. As the parts of the bomb move together, the system should pass smoothly from its initial subcritical to its final supercritical state. But if it explodes before assembly has been completed, its efficiency is lessened. To decrease the probability of pre-detonation, and conse-

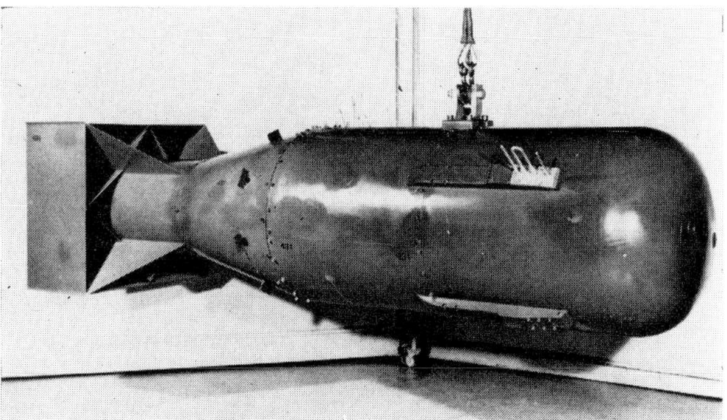

Courtesy: Los Alamos Scientific Laboratory.

First atomic bomb. Little Boy type, exploded over Hiroshima, was 28 inches in diameter, 120 inches long, weighed 9000 pounds, and yielded 20 kilotons of TNT. Fat man had a fusiform contour.

quent low efficiency, one must achieve either a higher speed of assembly or a lower neutron background.

During the first year at Los Alamos, assembly of the bomb was planned to be done with the Gun Method. The first guns were produced in the Naval Gun Factory in September, 1943 and were received at Los Alamos in March, 1944. Proof firing was begun in September with a 3″ Naval gun. In August, 1944 the entire Los Alamos Laboratory was reorganized and the plutonium gun assembly program was abandoned. Subsequent development of the Uranium 235 low velocity gun proceeded without meeting new basic difficulties, but the main effort of the laboratory was directed to the mounting difficulties of the implosion program. The proposal for the implosion assembly was to make use of the plastic slow tamper and active material under high-explosive impact. A subcritical sphere of these materials would be compressed into a supercritical sphere. This implosion mechanism was finally employed in the (experimental) Trinity explosion, and in the Nagasaki (Fat Man) bomb.

It is of interest to mention that all along, Edward Teller continued his theoretical, and to some extent practical, work on the fusion principle of nuclear explosion. At that time the name of the bomb thus conceived was the "Super."

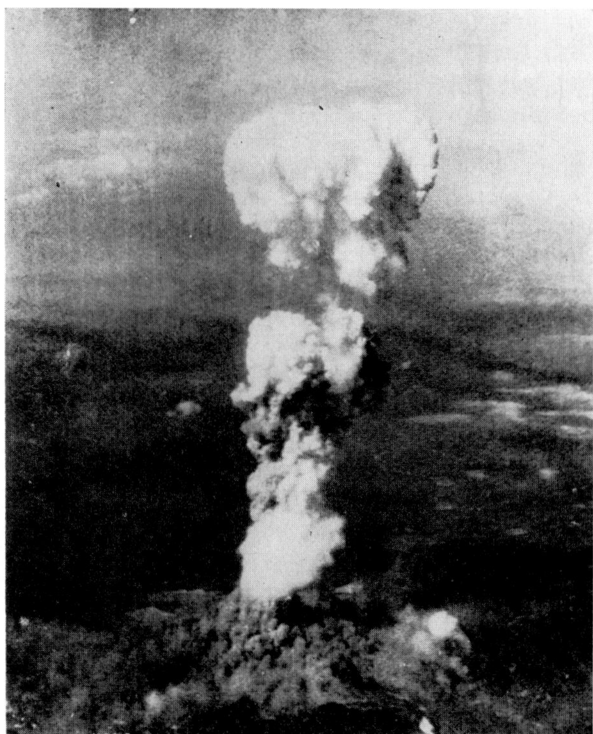

Courtesy: Los Alamos Scientific Laboratory.

First atomic bombing. Little Boy going off over Hiroshima (Japan) on August 6, 1945 sent smoke billowing 20,000 feet: its echo and the resulting fall-out can still be detected around the globe.

A rehearsal shot was performed on May 2, 1945 with 100 tons of HE (non-nuclear high explosives), stacked on the platform of a twenty foot tower. This was done at the site called Hornado del Muerto near Alamogordo Air Base. At the same location, at 5:29 A.M. on Monday, July 16, 1945, just before dawn was set off the first man-made nuclear explosion, called the Trinity test. It produced the intended blast, mushroom cloud, bluish glow, and excitement which has since become well known.

Immediately thereafter work started on preparing overseas delivery of the bomb, this being known under the code name Project Alberta.

The code name for an A-bomb using Uranium-235 gun assembly was Little Boy. On August 6, 1945 at 9:15 A.M. Little Boy was detonated over Hiroshima. On August 9, 1945 Fat Man (it was to have been dropped over Kokura but this was prevented by bad weather over the target) was exploded over Nagasaki at 11:50 A.M.

On October 16, 1945 the Los Alamos Laboratory received a certificate of appreciation from the Secretary of War. On that occasion, J. Robert Oppenheimer gave a short address in which he said, among other things: "The time will come when mankind will curse the name of Los Alamos and Hiroshima. The people of this world must unite, or they will perish." A few years later, Oppenheimer turned into what is called a security risk, but at that time he was already at the Institute for Advanced Studies.

The name Los Alamos Laboratories was in use until the present one, Los Alamos Scientific Laboratory of the University of California, was adopted in January, 1947.

During the war years, at Los Alamos, the only medical research done concerned the development of portable instruments to measure alpha radiation, and study designed to detect the minute quantities of Plutonium and Polonium excreted in the urine of laboratory per-

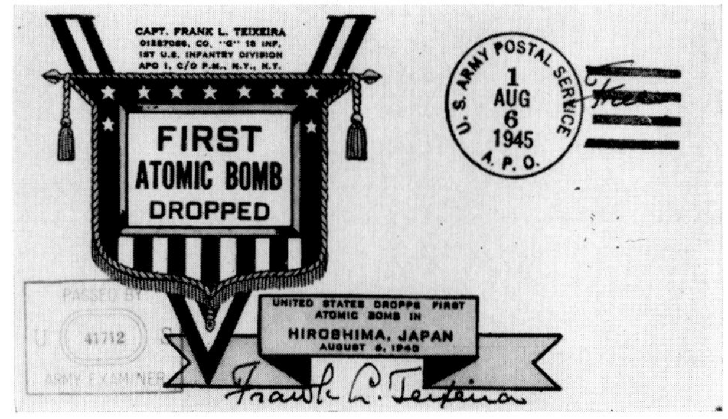

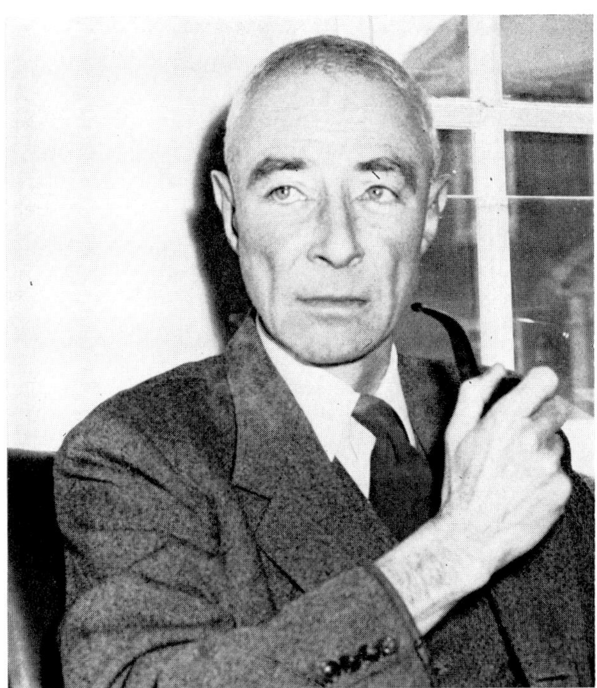

Courtesy: Alan W. Richards.

JULIUS ROBERT OPPENHEIMER. In 1943, Groves himself, against the advice of security officials, "hired" Oppenheimer as chief for Project Y. At that time Oppenheimer, one of Millikan's most gifted assistants, was a brilliant theoretical physicist (a theoretician's theoretician), but had no administrative experience, and his health was never too rugged. Nevertheless Oppenheimer did an excellent job, and the A-bomb went off! In 1954, after involved hearings, the AEC's five commissioners voted 4-1 to declare Oppenheimer a security risk, thus removing his "clearance," because of "fundamental defects in his character . . . close association with Communists . . . falsehoods, evasions, and misrepresentations." His staunchest foe was the then AEC chairman, Lewis Straus, which prompted a columnist's remark that nobody ever judges a Jew harsher than another Jew. Some of the hard feelings may have stemmed from Oppenheimer's aloofness toward and disdain for common mortals. I wrote to him several times, asking for a portrait and for a statement for this book, but never got an answer. Several months later, this photograph appeared in *Time Magazine* of April 12, 1963 (page 46) as the Kennedy Administration picked Oppenheimer to receive AEC's $50,000 Fermi Award (given in 1962 to Ernest Teller, another foe of Oppenheimer). Oppenheimer's scientific associates had asked the Government to do something about removing the moral stain which the Eisenhower Administration had placed on Oppenheimer, and the award was the result of that request. Said Oppenheimer *(Time)*: "Most of us look to the good opinion of our colleagues, and to the good will and conscience of our Government. I am no exception." Since then, a spokesman for the Johnson Administration emphasized that the award had no bearing on Oppenheimer's security clearance, which was not going to be reinstated.

sonnel.* On September 28-29, 1950 a meeting of medical and atomic laboratory directors took place at Los Alamos. Since then, somewhat more time and energy were spent on biologic studies of radiation, especially on RBE (relative biologic efficiency), for which the Cockroft-Walton has been used.

Los Alamos undoubtedly made history, but as yet it seems undetermined whether it should be regarded as a white or as a black page. *A quelque chose malheur est bon!* Maybe the question should be asked this way: had there not been the war-time urgency, and the "money-no-object" policy, how long would it have taken to reach the current level of "atomic" knowledge?

AEC

Deep secrecy still cloaked everything at AEC during the Trinity test. By contrast, the echo of the Little Boy detonated over Hiroshima — and some of its fallout — reverberated around the globe. Many of those who were working in the silent, secluded and smokeless facilities of Oak Ridge and at Hanford only then learned what they had helped to create.

After only one additional bomb — Fat Man, exploded over Nagasaki — a virtual but uneasy peace broke out. In 1946 the USA Congress enacted the McMahon (Atomic Energy) Act — this was recently recalled by a commemorative stamp, first issued in Brien McMahon's stamping grounds, Stamford (Connecticut).

*This information was offered by above mentioned Dr. Louis Hempelmann. The history of Project Y was procured through the kindness of Dr. Wright H. Langham, who is presently Group Leader of Biomedical Research at Los Alamos.

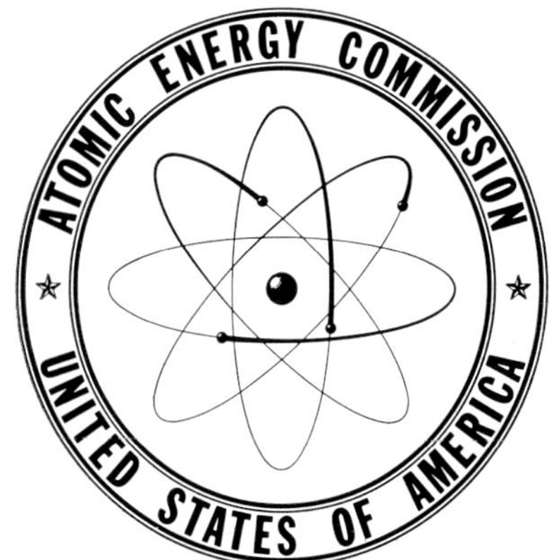

As of January 1, 1947 the Atomic Energy Commission (AEC) was formed and empowered with regulatory functions (also) over the distribution of radioactive isotopes, and/or other fission products. Since most of these were by-products of nuclear reactors, many radioisotopes were available in large quantities. The AEC adopted a seal with four concentric, eliptic orbits, slated to become world famous.

An inquiry was sent to the AEC and they answered by quoting several paragraphs from a letter written by the creator of the design for the AEC seal, A. W. Favale, who at the time was employed in the AEC's Graphics Section:

"In March of 1948, it was proposed that the AEC should have a seal. Through the Office of the Secretary, I (Favale) received a request to design and create a seal. I labored on this project for many months and came up with approximately ten designs. . . In January, 1949, a committee approved one of these designs which is the present (black and white) seal used by the AEC. In March of 1949, I completed the finished art work and the seal has been used since that date.

"To the best of my knowledge this design is an original created and conceived by me (Favale). No other model or drawing was used as a copy; because I did not want to create a symbol which would specifically indicate an atomic symbol, I consulted some of our scientists and at that time, to the best of their knowledge, they told me that the design presently shown in the seal did not mean anything. It is only symbolic of atomic energy showing the center of the nucleus with four electrons encircling it. . ."

AEC's archives provided additional information. A preliminary search of the principal registry of trade marks indicated that there were some forty-two marks containing one or more hypothetical electron orbits. These marks were then in use as trade-marks for such items as tooth powder, solvent reclamation powder, hanger brackets, alarms for vehicles, pressure responsive switches, computer-type machinery and newsletters. None of these were deemed to be the same as the then black and white seal of the AEC. A description of the official AEC seal in color was developed by the Heraldic Branch of the Office of the Quartermaster General, Department of the Army.*

PEACEFUL ATOMS

At the outset, the Met Lab supervised the work at the X-10 pile. On July 1, 1945, the Monsanto Chemical Company took over operation of X-10 which became a nuclear research center called Clin-

*This information was gracefully provided by Mr. Franklin Tobey, from the News Service Branch of the Division of Public Information of the AEC in Washington (D. C.). He mentioned also that after adoption of the AEC seal in 1949 it was determined that any subsequent design would be denied registration as a trade-mark under Sec. 1052, Title 15 U. S. Code. He specified that the description of the AEC seal was published in the *Federal Register* of March 19, 1957. No color combination the same as that incorporated in the official AEC seal has been found among trade and service marks.

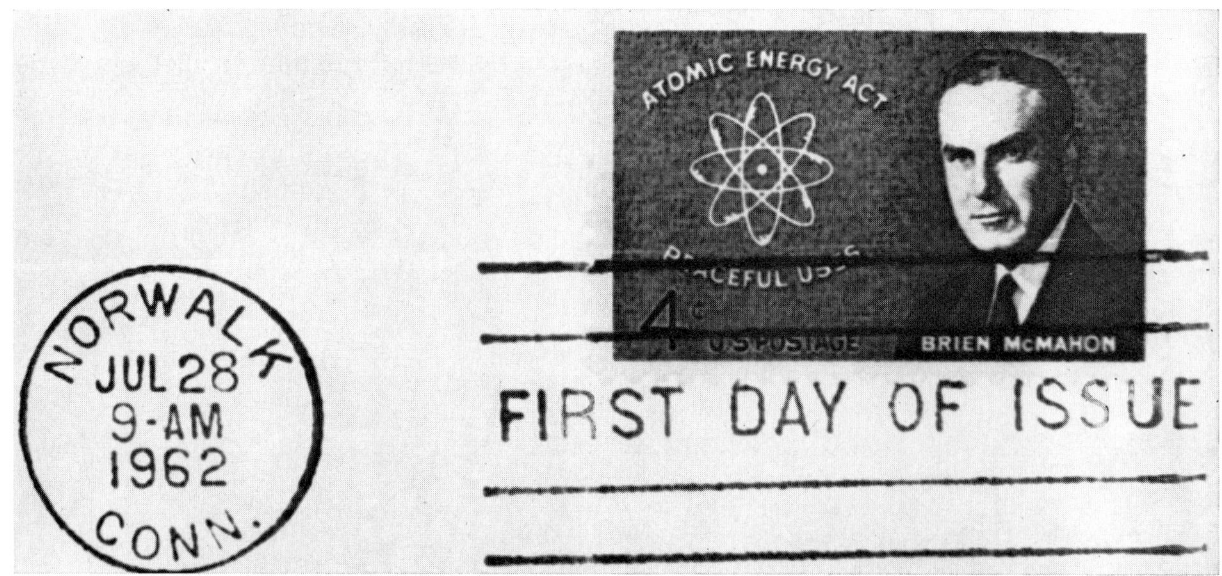

James O'Brien McMahon. His epic battle to put through the Atomic Energy Act is well documented and vividly narrated in Chapter 14 *(The Legislative Battle)* in the first volume of Hewlett and Anderson's History of the AEC.

ton Laboratories. In 1947, it was rechristened Clinton National Laboratories. On March 1, 1948, Monsanto was replaced by Union Carbide, and the name of the former X-10 facility was changed once more — this time for good — to Oak Ridge National Laboratory (ORNL).

The ORNL is today the world's largest supplier of artificial radioisotopes. Aside from the Graphite Reactor, which is still in full operation, several other reactors were built such as the *Low Intensity* (high neutron flux) *Test Reactor*, the *Bulk Shielding Facility* (known as the "Swimming Pool"), the *Pool Critical Assembly*, the *Tower Shielding Facility*, and especially the *Oak Ridge* (high flux) *Research Reactor*. Here was also constructed and tested the small (100-kw), completely automatic, swimming pool type of experimental reactor, exhibited at the Atoms for Peace Conference in Geneva (Switzerland) in 1955.

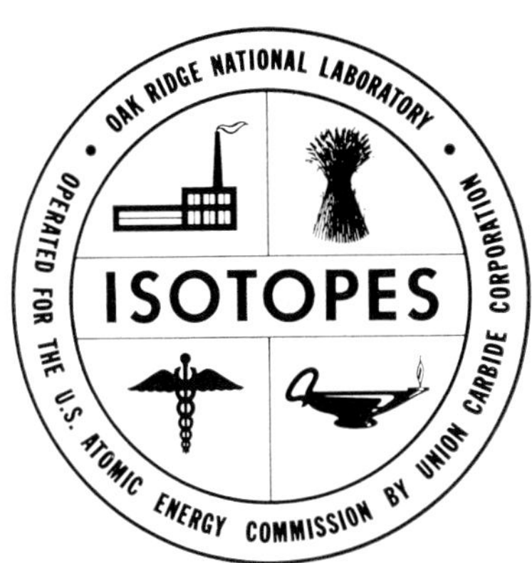

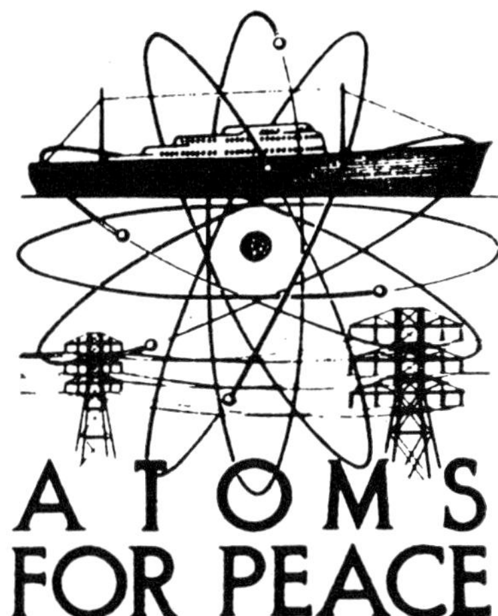

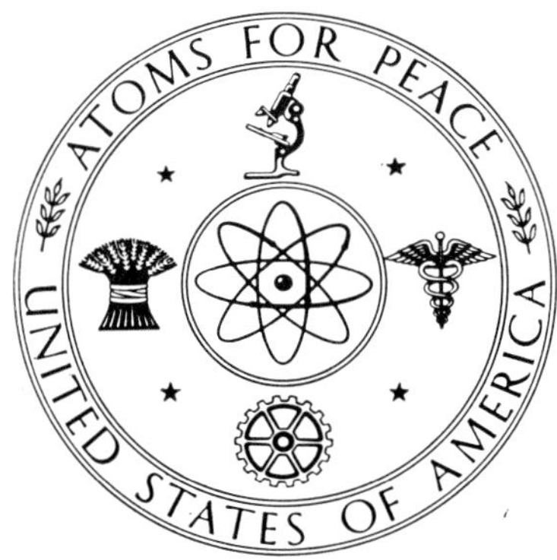

The Oak Ridge Institute for Nuclear Studies (ORINS) was incorporated on October 15, 1946. It consists of 38 member universities in the South and Southwest of the United States. The ORINS has both educational and research aims.

In addition to all that, Oak Ridge has also an ORACLE (Oak Ridge Automatic Computer and Logical Engine). It is a high speed, electronic, digital computer from the Princeton family of machines, associated with the name of the late John von Neu-

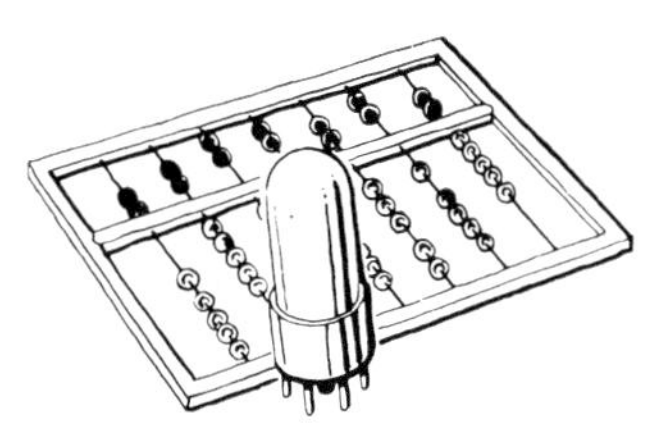

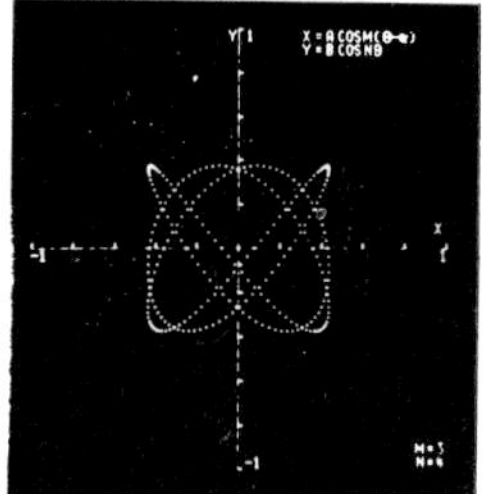

ORACLE ORBITIZED. The device of the Oak Ridge Automatic Computer and Logical Engine might well be an electronic tube superimposed on an abacus, but it is so sophisticated that it can draw "orbiting" curves

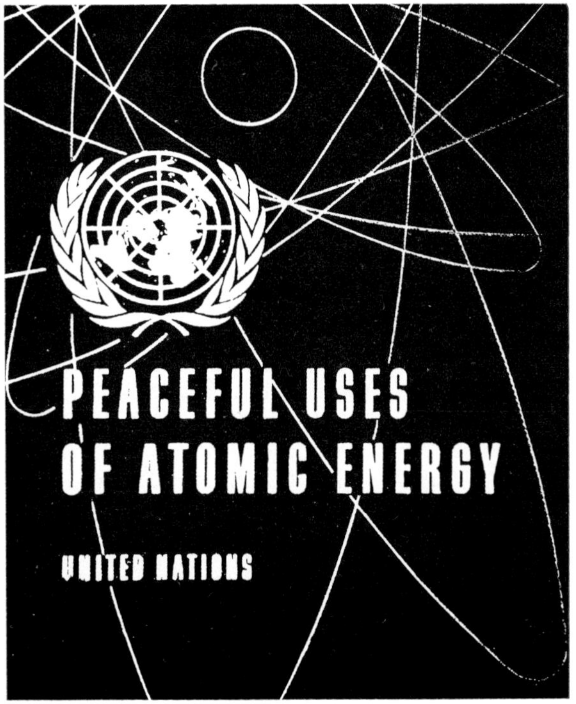

mann. This particular computer, built at the Argonne National Laboratory, was moved to the ORNL in September, 1953. It is now in successful operation, and does "most anything." It can even plot curves, some of which resemble those "fake" atomic orbits of Favale!

OLD BREMSSTRAHLUNG UNIVERSITY

During the period September, 1946 to June, 1947, training courses in Nuclear Technology were conducted at the ORNL. Those courses were the forerunner of the Oak Ridge School of Reactor Technology. It was soon discovered that the participants felt keenly the lack of a satisfactory designation for their site of learning. Of the great variety of suggestions, the name enthusiastically accepted by common consent was Clinch College of Nuclear Knowledge (derived from the Clinch river which flows through Oak Ridge).

In 1948 was held the first session of the School in Radio-Isotope Techniques. Right from the start the (now administrative) radiophysicist Paul Clarence Aebersold strongly recommended the formalization of their procedure for graduation. A poll of the trainees produced the admirable title of Old Bremsstrahlung University, to which they added a suitable seal, symbol, and degree. The seal contains the title Institute of Unclear Physics, retained from a typing error in a letter addressed to the then president of the ORINS (and of the University of North Carolina). The old-fashioned well symbolizes the un-Clinch-able thirst for knowledge. The degree is D.R.I.P, meaning Dabbler in Radio-Isotope Procedures.

As detailed in the Commencement Address, delivered by the Executive Dabbler'* they also have three honorary degrees: *causa laboris,* for the overworked staff of the Special Training Division; *cum grano salis* (with a grain of salt), for others whom they want to honor but whose level of attainment in the field of radioisotope technique they are inclined to question; and *pro tanto* (liberally translated, as far as it goes), to those who did not complete the entire course.

They were also blessed with the inevitable *alma mater* song from which we reproduce two verses:

Between guards and wire-fences,
Through the old red clay,
Where we now sink to our ankles,
There'll be grass some day.

Raise the background;
Drop the threshold;
Old Bremsstrahlung U.,
Hail to thee, our Alma Mater;
Hail, all hail, B. U.

The very first D.R.I.P. diploma was granted to Irvin Hummon. At the time of this writing 80 classes with over 4500 scientists from 55 countries have graduated from this course.

*The Executive Director of the ORINS, William Grosvenor Pollard.

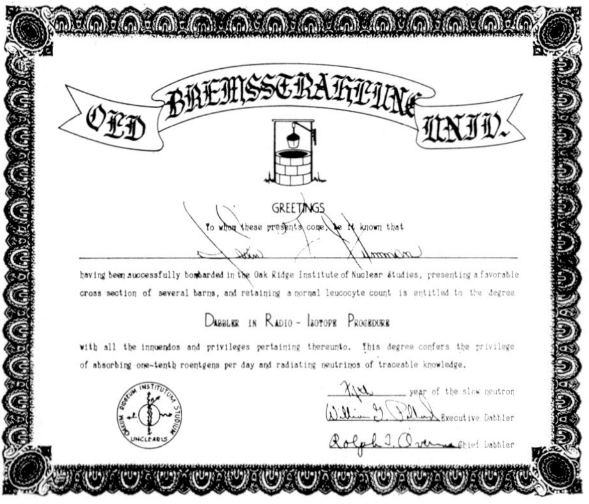

OLD BREMSSTRAHLUNG UNIV.

GREETINGS

To whom these presents come, be it known that

having been successfully bombarded in the Oak Ridge Institute of Nuclear Studies, presenting a favorable cross section of several barns, and retaining a normal leucocyte count is entitled to the degree

DABBLER IN RADIO-ISOTOPE PROCEDURE

with all the innuendos and privileges pertaining thereunto. This degree confers the privilege of absorbing one-tenth roentgens per day and radiating neutrinos of traceable knowledge.

OAKUM RIDGEUM INSTITUTUM STUDIUM UNCLEARIS

year of the slow neutron

Executive Dabbler

Chief Dabbler

FIRST DRIP DEGREE FROM BU. It was given to Irvin Franklin Hummon, director of the Department of Radiology in Cook County Hospital (Chicago).

MARSHALL BRUCER

In December, 1948 was formed the Medical Division at the ORINS, and from the very beginning, Marshall Brucer became its chairman. He built the Medical Division from an idea to the significant and widely recognized organization it is at present.

Chicago-born Marshall Herbert Brucer graduated from Rush Medical School in 1941 (at the time part of the University of Chicago), and then interned at the Mallory Institute of Pathology in Boston City Hospital. He went into the U. S. Army immediately after completing his internship, and served as Surgeon of the Airborne Command at Camp Mackall (North Carolina), and as a member of the Airborne Test Board. He "jump-tested" much of the equipment used. After his discharge Brucer joined the University of Texas Medical School in August, 1946 and worked his way up in the Department of Physiology until he resigned to come to the ORINS.

Brucer deserves beyond any doubt the title of "the" Atomic Physician. He acquired considerable technical knowledge, and designed several of the instrumentalities used in his investigations. Characteristic is the following quotation from a paper by Brucer, entitled *The Search for the Hole,* mimeographed in 1958:

"The science of radiation detection has progressed to the point where experts in electronics can needle the experts in interpretation. On the other hand, the experts in diagnosis decry the presumption of the oscillocographers. This is a portent of progress. It is a sign that medical science, though bloody and emasculated, is not yet dead. This study is the story of an argument – an argument on the interpretation of scans and the design of scanners. All the participants in this argument are members of committees – but they are not yet quite petrified. Occasionally, in spite of the anesthesia of committee membership (sometimes called "the sense of responsibility"), there is a quickening.

"The argument is presented here from the viewpoint of one side only. No attempt will be made to be "fair," to present "both sides of the question," to analyze dispassionately according to the gospel of 20th century decadence. I shall be emotional in this paper as my forefathers were emotional in 1850 when science was alive. I view with alarm the evil and somewhat stupid viewpoint of my opposition. When the article is finished, I shall return – like Pluto – to 20th century madness.

"The argument began when the Bell-Francis-Harris* crowd (may their mothers' milk turn sour) at the ORNL made a solid gold focused gamma-ray collimator. (The Division of Biology and Medicine restricts us to lead at 14 cents a pound). They attach this to a wondrous (but useless) spectrometer scanner. Their mechanism moves up and down and sideways. It wiggles as it makes marks on paper. It does everything – except find the hole. It couldn't find the hole.

"At the ORINS we have a standard scanning manikin. Her name is Anne Boleyn. In the neck of this manikin is a confusing array of mock-iodine activities. Some of this array represents hot areas, some warm,

*Persa Raymond Bell, J. E. Francis, Jr., and C. C. Harris are radiation physicists at ORNL.

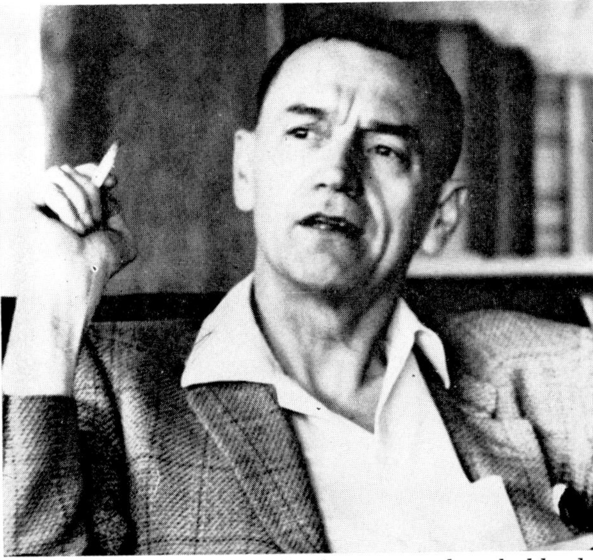

MARSHALL BRUCER. "Medical science, though bloody and emasculated, is not yet dead. Certain committee members are not yet quite petrified. Occasionally, in spite of the anesthesia of committee membership (sometimes called "the sense of responsibility"), there is a quickening!"

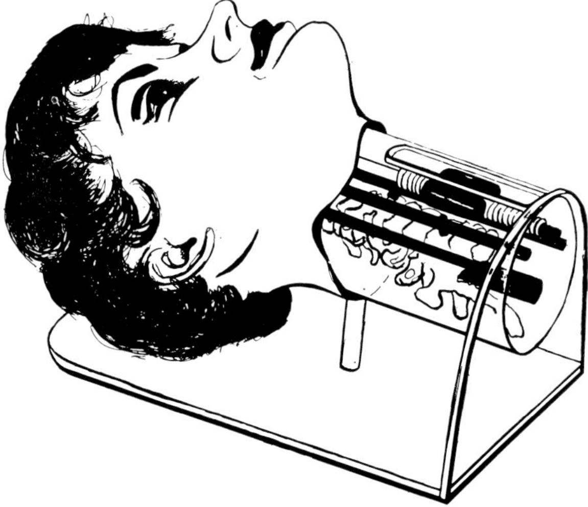

Courtesy: ORINS, Medical Division.

ANNE BOLEYN. They came with "gold" to find her "hole," but could not locate it!

some cold. (The head contains nothing in order to make physicists feel at home when they measure her.) The neck contains a removable mock-thyroid gland. The thyroid gland has two lobes, right and left. In the left lobe is a "hole." Both lobes (right cylinders roughly 3.5 cm. by 1 cm.) are filled with mock-iodine, which has spectrum similar to that of I^{131}; but the middle third of the left lobe is stuffed with a piece of rubber stopper about 0.9 cm. in diameter. When this was first made, the rubber stopper contained no activity. Every chemist in the world will testify that rubber is not an ion exchange resin superior to "Dowex 50." There *is* still a "hole" in the activity of the left lobe.

"The bully boys at ORNL tried to demonstrate the presence of the hole as the final test of the solid gold collimator, but they couldn't find the hole. Now this does not mean that a solid gold collimator is no good. It means that medical instrumentation is no longer a set of wires, tubes, and resistors neatly assembled. Three things are necessary in a scanner: the machine must have an inherent *resolution;* it must allow the technician to alter the factors of *definition* to allow the physician to make an *interpretation.* Each of these three is no good without the others. The solid gold collimator has the best of all possible resolutions (almost). At least it is good enough for today. The electronic gadgetry allows no variation in definition and hence no interpretation was possible. The bully boys said there was no hole, so we took the mock-thyroid and showed them where the hole was with our simpler and cheaper lead collimators."

In this particular instance, best results by Brucer and associates were obtained, not with the area scan, but with the profile (linear) scanner built on the concept created by Eric Pochin (of London).

In all of Brucer's activity at ORINS teamwork was the rule rather than the exception. This is evident from the medical reports on the Y-12 accident* of June 16, 1958, published in April, 1959 as the *Acute Radiation Syndrome* (ORINS-25). Another example is the comprehensive study of gallium-72 in *Radiology* of October, 1953 (proving that radiogallium is not safe for use in man). A set containing all of Brucer's reprints would fill a three-foot shelf. Many of them are only mimeographed, like the excellent *Radioisotope* (point, area, depth, linear, spectoral, and temporal) *Scanning* issued in January, 1958 as ORINS-20. Brucer caused two superb books to be printed:

ROENTGENS,
rads,
AND
RIDDLES

Edited by

MILTON FRIEDMAN, M.D.,
MARSHALL BRUCER, M.D.,
and
ELIZABETH ANDERSON

Oak Ridge
Institute of Nuclear Studies
Oak Ridge, Tennessee

U. S. ATOMIC ENERGY COMMISSION

A Symposium on Supervoltage Radiation Therapy

Held at the Medical Division, Oak Ridge Institute of Nuclear Studies

July 15, 16, 17, and 18, 1956

Radioisotopes in Medicine (ORO-125) appeared in 1955. It is the rich transcript of a course given by ORINS in September, 1953 (about that time Marshall Brucer was first told that his then few and odd neurologic symptoms were due to miltiple sclerosis). The material for the volume was quite extensive, and the editors (Gould Arthur Andrews, Brucer, and Betty Anderson) called it, in the beginning, the Two-Ton-Tillie. Aside from references after each article, it acquired an extensive final bibliography, with a table of contents for the bibliography itself. In the end, the nickname had to be changed to Ten-Ton-Tillie (817 pages).

The other book, *Roentgens, Rads, and Riddles,* published in 1959, is a transcript of the Symposium on Supervoltage Radiation Therapy, held at ORINS in July, 1956. The editors were Milton Friedman (the

---

*On another occasion Brucer spoke of radiation accidents which may occur despite (as he derisively specified) 100 percent effective safety protection. If and when such accidents occur, he suggested, in typical "paradoxical" Brucer fashion, to "push the panic button" and react accordingly:

"When in troubles,
When in doubt,
Run in circles,
Scream and shout!"

New York therapist*), Brucer and Elizabeth Anderson.

Gould Andrews is a combination internist-hematologist, who was instrumental in the decision to build the Cs^{137} total-body irradiation facility. Having gained experience with homologous marrow infusion ("blood graft") in patients with leukemia, he became a member of the team who cared for the injured in the criticality accident at Y-12. Even a temporary take of the bone marrow graft (which is the best that can be hoped for) may make the difference between death and survival after accidental irradiation in the mid-lethal range. Andrews wrote seventy-odd scientific papers, and numerous gems of human understanding in his exquisite letters to families of patients under his care.

Elizabeth Blagg Anderson is a former zoologist with an uncanny knowledge of English. She came to Oak Ridge in 1946 as a housewife (Betty's favorite job). Her husband, Edward H. Anderson, was one of the first three microbiologists hired for the Biology Division of the ORNL. After becoming a widow in 1952, she accepted the position of technical editor with the Medical Division of the ORINS.

*Orndoff recalls that in 1937, when the Michael Reese Hospital finally succeeded to sever its relationship with Max Cutler, their next therapist was to have been Milton Friedman, but Friedman decided to stay in the East. In his stead they appointed Erich Uhlmann who had come to Chicago for the ICR. Uhlmann was then the associate of Friedrich Dessauer (who had been helped by no other than Karl Frik to flee from Nazi Germany to Turkey).

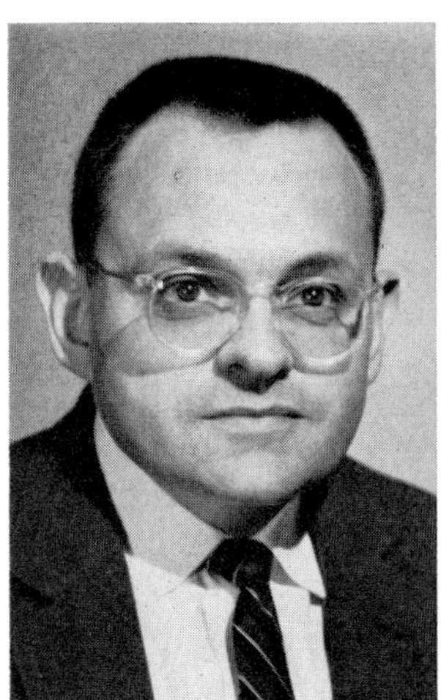

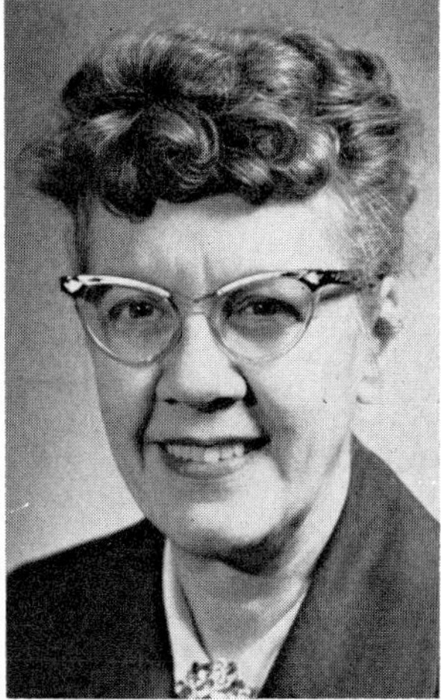

GOULD ARTHUR ANDREWS became director of the Medical Division at ORINS, after Marchall Brucer's resignation. ELIZABETH BLAGG ANDERSON. Technical editor of the Medical Division at ORINS, contributed considerably (often anonymously) to the quality of their publications. (Betty refused steadfastly to have her portrait published. Thereupon, unbeknownst to her, this picture was "stolen" on orders from Marshall Brucer, who is therefore entitled to this credit line.)

Betty Anderson's contribution may not be as apparent as it should. This is understandable because she follows a soft approach. One of her pet quotations is from Harry Shaw, "there is no such thing as good writing, there is only good re-writing." She likes to give credit to other people, for instance in her (often revised) ORINS Manual of Style she has inserted several Brucer gems as rules for *writing articles:* ". . . if you don't know what you are talking about, make it long!" and ". . . if you know what you are talking about, make a Midget Exhibit (*instead* of writing an article)."

Marshall Brucer was usually very outspoken, often to the point of offending those of his interlocutors who were unable to understand that it was all done in very good faith. In the Exhibit of Exhibiting, presented to the Society of Nuclear Medicine in June, 1957 at Oklahoma City (during Brucer's term of office as president of that society), he inserted the following sentences:

"It has been said that less than 1 per cent of scientists participate actually in scientific meetings. The other 99 per cent consider a scientific meeting a spectator sport. This 1 per cent has been called by George Meneely the performing dogs of science. As a part of institutional advertising, glib scientists go to many meetings; therefore, they become the best known, the big men in science, the performing dogs . . . (but) . . . most ideas of most scientists are worthless. A few ideas, however, may be worth reproducing. It should be possible for individual scientists to present these ideas

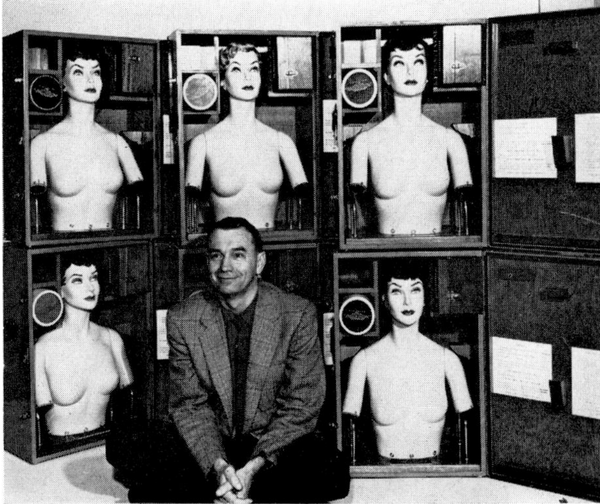

Courtesy: ORINS, Medical Division.

BRUCER'S CHORUS LINE. Lulu is now in Baltimore, Felicia in Tokyo, Maria in London, and Abigail in Egypt.

without presenting them first before a jury of performing dogs."

Another time, while reporting on a Seminar of Radiotherapy *(Management of Advanced Cancer)*, which consisted of independent papers followed by a few written questions, Brucer remarked: "The more I hear of such "seminars" the more I am convinced they are worthless. The general conclusion of this seminar was that cancer is a very dangerous disease."

The "performing dogs" did not relish his appraisal, and as a consequence Brucer received less official recognition than he deserved for his scientific stature and achievements. He was often invited to meetings outside the US, for instance in 1955 he was in Geneva, in 1957 in Tokyo and Manila, in 1960 in Tel-Aviv. Brucer devised phenomenal teaching techniques such as the production line of thyroid manikins — *les thyroid girls.*

The original manikins were all alike but their hairdresses were different, and there was of course a different sort of mock radioactivity buried in the "neck." Since those necks were so good-looking, many of the *girls* got "married."

Lulu is with Joseph B. Workman in Baltimore; Drusilla is with Raymond L. Libby in Los Angeles; Hortense is with Millard N. Croll in Philadelphia; Maria is with J. Eric Roberts in London; Abigail was on an AEC special project in Egypt; Bridgit is with Isadore Meschan in Winston-Salem; Grenadine is with Cuno Winkler in Bonn; Felicia is with Hirotake Kakehi in Tokyo; Nabby is with Joseph Sternberg in Montreal; Pandora is with E. Richard King in Bethesda, and lately Bonnie Boleyn (a fake sister of Anne) went to Baltimore to join Lulu for obviously "polygamic" purposes. The "unmarried" *girls* staid on to help in the ORINS teaching program at home. This group contains the very first such girl ever to be created, Abigail. The harem at ORINS boasts also of several subsequently sired sisters, namely Ibis, Chloe, Ophelia, Terry Toma (paired with Sara Coma), Jezebel, Katrina, Queenie, Rhoda and Euphemia.

Brucer's endeavors covered the entire field of Nuclear Medicine, for instance in 1960 he prepared a bibliography on human radiation counters. His last project at ORINS (with his radiotherapist, Barcelona-born Frank Victor Comas) was to study the effects of total body radiation in leukemia, using eight cesium-137 sources. The investigation proved, among other things, that in man the LD^{50} is way above the 600 rad (computed by extrapolation from animals) accepted by many authors.

Brucer weathered nonchalantly the inroads of demyelinization. When it exceeded the arbitrary limit which he himself had set, he quietly resigned

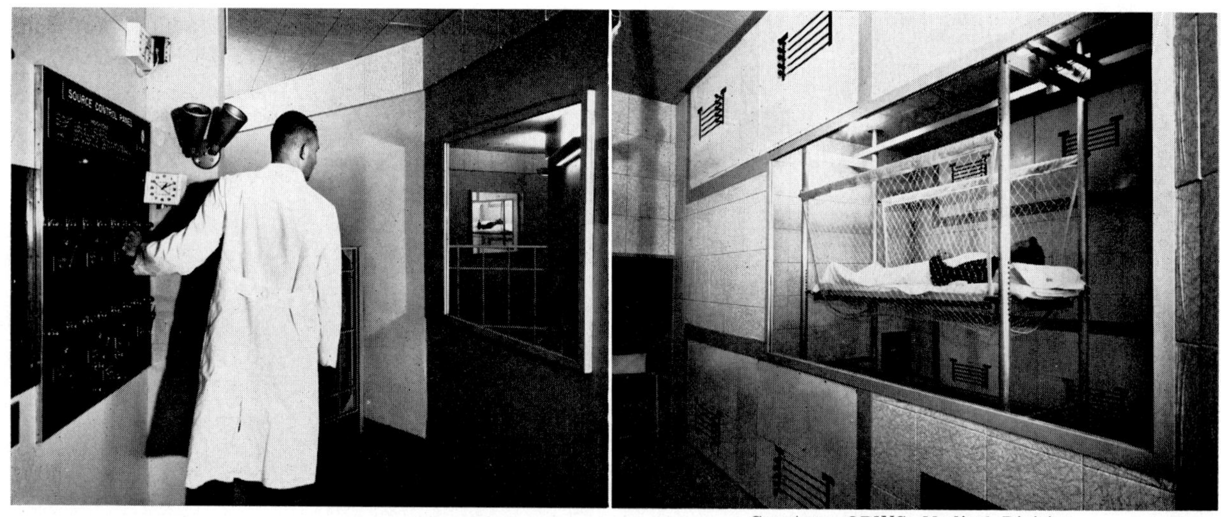

Courtesy: ORINS, Medical Division.

TOTAL-BODY IRRADIATOR. As described by Brucer in the *International Journal of Applied Radiation and Isotopes* (1961), the room design features a crooked corridor, but the operator can see the patient through a mirror. Patient is suspended in a rigid aluminum bed, with nylon curtains, and television receiver in line of sight. Eight sources of Cs-137, each of 500 curie strength, provide a maximum of 280 r/hr. With filters this can be cut down to 1.8 r/hr. Patients with leukemia were treated. Results have not been too promising, but they show that in man fatal total body irradiation with gamma-rays is beyond 1000 rem, possibly as high as 1500 rem, which is much higher than the LD-50 of 600 rem computed from experiments in mammals.

and left Oak Ridge on December 31, 1961. In his fourteen years at ORINS he had created the basis for, and may justly be regarded as one of the founders of, Nuclear Medicine.

Marshall Brucer had a penchant for lively controversy, so much so as to become at times astoundingly aggressive in the course of an otherwise trivial argument. Like Mencken, he was always willing to resort to strong invective, for which he was as strongly disliked by some as had been Mencken. And just like Mencken, Brucer enjoyed the search for the meaning of words, and for correct expressions: he contributed considerably to the acceptance of the terms brachytherapy (*American Journal of Roentgenology* of June 1958), and teletherapy. In the *Americal Journal of Roentgenology* of January, 1956 Brucer (& *al.*) described the automatically controlled pattern of a cesium source ("to end all rotational therapy"). Still, Brucer's name was probably more often mentioned in connection with cobalt-60 (rather than with cesium-137) irradiators.

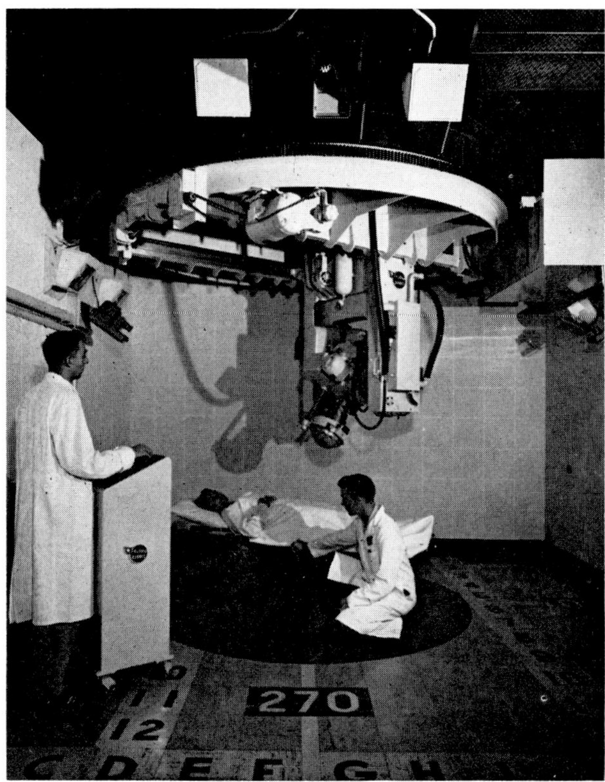

Courtesy: ORINS, Medical Division.

Cs-137 ROTO-THERAPY. This elaborate device, built by Barnes of Rockford (Illinois), permits (almost) all possible rotational patterns. It proved (if anything) that such complications are unnecessary (maybe not even desirable) in practice.

COBALT CREATORS

The radioactive cobalt-60 had first been produced in the cyclotron in 1941, when J. J. Livengood and G. T. Seaborg determined the half-lives of its two isomers (10.7 minutes and 5.3 years). Then, at the MIT, Martin Deutsch and his associates determined the energies of its gamma emissions, published in the *Physical Review* of November, 1945.

It is difficult (if not impossible) to determine who was the first to suggest that Co^{60} would be suitable for teletherapy. The earliest printed reference in this matter appeared in December, 1946 in the *British Journal of Radiology,* from the pen of Joseph Stanley Mitchell, professor of radiotherapeutics in the University of Cambridge. Here are a few excerpts from that 1946 article:

> "The most promising substitute for radium is now considered to be radio-cobalt, Co^{60}, of half-life 5.3 years . . . It is to be noted that the radiation from Co^{60} is eminently suitable for use in radiotherapy, being approximately monochromatic and of slightly higher mean energy (1.2 mev) than the mean energy of the usual filtered radiation from radium, which has the approximate value of 0.8 mev. . . There is no doubt as to the practicability of the manufacture of the necessary quantities of Co^{60} by means of the pile. The Canadian pile could easily produce several hundred curies of radiocobalt every six months, and a specific activity of the order of one curie per gm. should be obtained."

The suggestion to use Co^{60} as a teletherapy source of ionizing radiation was taken up in 1948 by Grimmett, who at the time was chief physicist of the M.D. Anderson Hospital and Tumor Institute in Houston.

Leonard George Grimmett (1903-1951) was born in London. He earned his way through King's College as a night musician (he was an accomplished pianist and later, in Houston, gave a few concerts of classical music). In 1932, he worked with Spear and then, still before World War II, Grimmett built a 10 gram radium beam unit with pneumatic transfer of the source (it was subsequently used by the Radiotherapeutic Research Unit of the British Medical Research Council). He was also an accomplished mechanic, and liked to build for himself shiny instruments, with nickel plating and crackle enamel. Thus he created a solid gold nozzle for a beam therapy unit. It is also said that he made a necklace of artificial rubies for his wife. After the war, during a brief spell as counsellor for the UNESCO in Paris, the always imperturbable Grimmett landed the Houston job by correspondence, and came to this country in 1947.

In 1956, during the ORINS Symposium of Teletherapy, Brucer declared: "Depending upon whether one is a Canadian, an American, Russian, or even an Englishman, Co^{60} production started (for teletherapy purposes) in one of these countries. I have selected 1951 as the first year in which Co^{60} was produced for teletherapy; however, as time goes on, the date of the first Co^{60} machine goes back further and further in history . . . I have in my files of newspaper clippings absolute proof of at least fifty "first" Co^{60} machines. All these people are liars, of course, because we have the first machine." This statement needs certain qualifications:

Grimmett originally envisioned a simple substitution of a radium-pack by a 10-curie radio-cobalt source. In the Spring of 1949 the Co^{60} project was discussed in the ORINS Medical Division by Brucer and Grimmett, and the plans were soon changed (on Brucer's suggestion) to a hectocurie and then to a kilocurie source. After a series of preliminary conferences, a joint meeting on Co^{60} sources and design problems was held on February 13, 1950, in Washington (D.C.) by the AEC Isotope Division and by the ORINS; at that meeting radiotherapists, physicists, and representatives of interested industry from the USA and Canada were present to discuss the problems and possibilities of Co^{60} teletherapy. In February, 1950, construction was started for a building to house the Co^{60} unit at Oak Ridge. In May 1950, the cobalt source was sent to be inserted into the high-flux nuclear reactor at Chalk

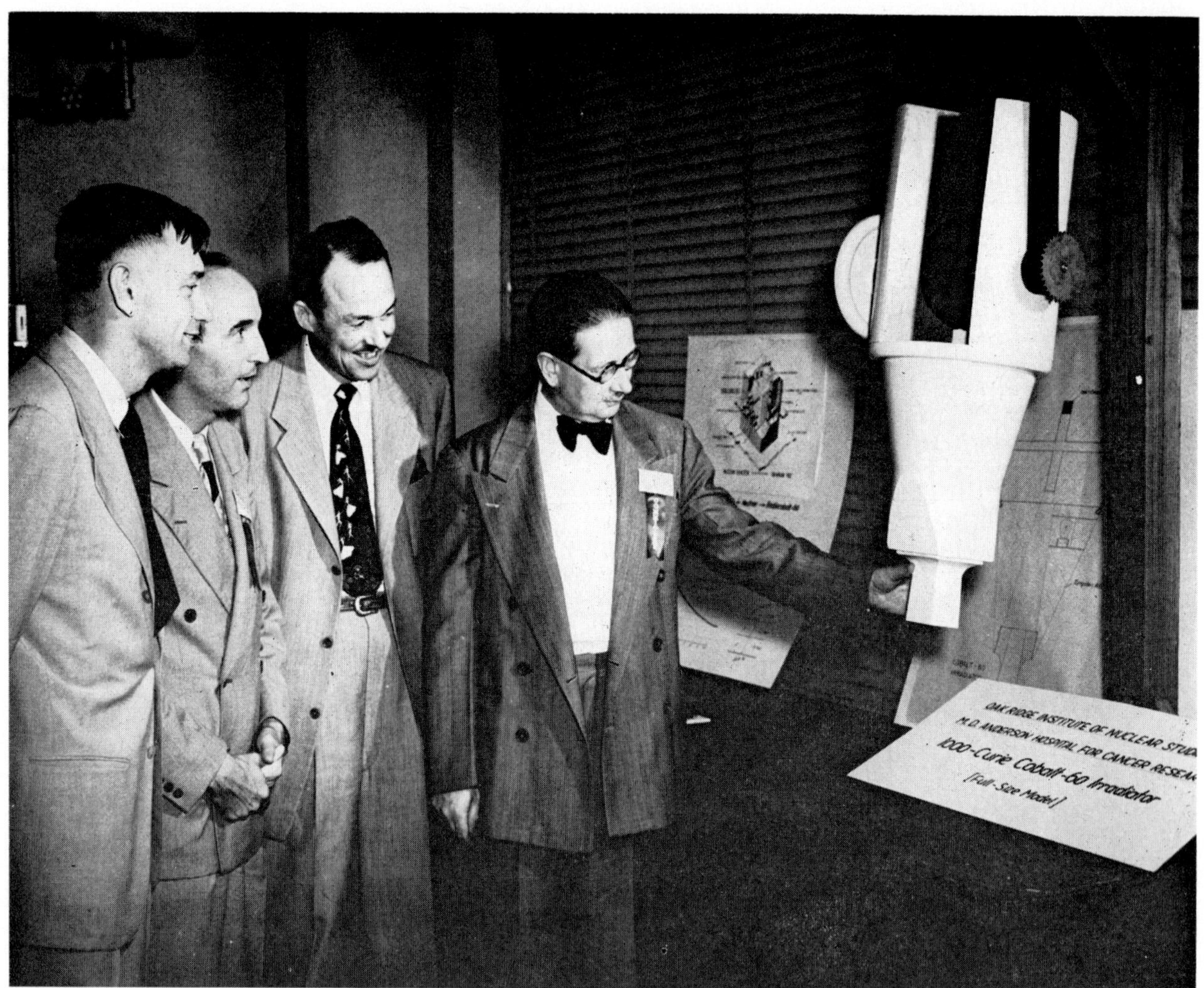

Courtesy: ORINS, Medical Division.

GRIMMETT'S Co-^{60} UNIT. This picture, made in May, 1951—days before Grimmett's sudden (coronary) death – appeared in the obituary in the *ORINS Newsletter* of June, 1951. It shows Leonard George Grimmett touching the nozzle of the mock-up. Looking on are (from the viewer's left) Marshall Brucer with Gilbert Hungerford Fletcher (radiotherapist), and Randolph Lee Clark, Jr. (surgeon) of M. D. Anderson Hospital in Houston.

River (Ontario, Canada); the insertion was performed on June 1, 1950. The contract between the M.D. Anderson Hospital (as future user of the unit) and the ORINS (as producer) was signed in July, 1950.

No attempt was ever made to conceal any of the ideas developed at ORINS (whether in connection with the Co^{60} project, or with any other topic of investigation). Indeed, Grimmett published the design for a thousand curie cobalt irradiator in October, 1950 in the *Texas Reports of Biology and Medicine*. This design is a dated, incontestable priority.

Many investigators started then to plan, and some even to work, along similar lines. At the (now defunct) Chicago Tumor Institute, the radiotherapist Max Cutler obtained a 200-curie Co^{60} source (from ORINS) and measured air doses as accurately as possible. At about that time the ORINS contracted with GE to have a container built (at Milwaukee); it was completed in November, 1951. The container was shipped to Oak Ridge and loaded at ORNL with the small (200-curie) source loaned by Cutler. Then, at ORINS, depth doses were determined and preliminary protection figures were computed and measured. In July, 1952 the neutron irradiation of the high intensity Co^{60} source which had been in the Chalk River reactor for about two years was completed, and the source was then shipped to Oak Ridge. The final study of stray radiation problems, treatment cones, and the production of isodose curves for clinical therapy completed the preliminary phases of this project in June, 1953. The unit was installed the same year at the M. D. Anderson Hospital and is still in operation.

I asked Marshall Brucer about Mitchell's priority, and this is what he answered in date of June 5, 1962:

"Grimmett is now dead, and so I cannot check up on it but my fifteen-year-old memory seems to say that Grimmett was still the originator. We lived together for two nights in a hotel room in Cincinnati. He spent most of the time telling me about how to make star sapphires which were apparently his real love. However, in between drinks (tea, not Ohio bourbon), he told me also about his troubles in making the "big" 10-gram radium unit, and his worse troubles in repairing it. When a big official from the Union Miniere du Haut Katanga (who had loaned the 10-gram radium source) came to visit the hospital, the pneumatic tube did not work properly, and the source got stuck in the middle. Grimmett pointed out that never again would he design anything but a completely "fail-safe" device. This is why we went into the internal rotating wheel in the first cobalt design.

"By telling me this story of his exposure to 10 grams of radium, Grimmett pointed out that ever since this design for the 10-gram unit, he had been thinking of something that would give a little bit more hope than the radium. One of the stories is that during a session while he was attempting to make a star sapphire in a bomb shelter during (I think) the V-1 bomb attacks on England, he thought of the idea of using this new "pile" production of something like Co^{60}. He had heard from some place that this might be done. My memory of this encounter seems to say that he gave this idea to Mayneord, who is in England a big shot both in political and in medical physics. Mayneord may have given it to Mitchell to write it up, for the *Recent Advances* are really part of the Mayneord document."

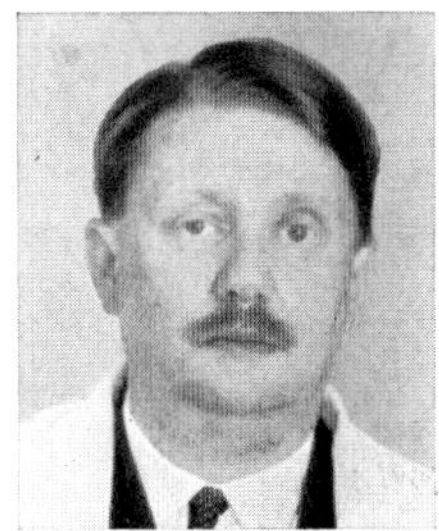

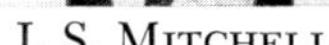
J. S. Mitchell

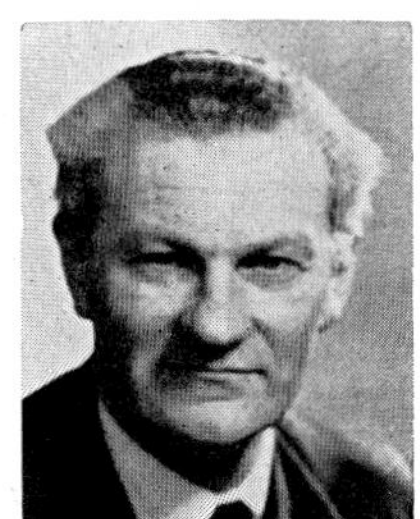
H. F. Freundlich

Be it as it may, Mitchell has undoubtedly the first published proposal for the use of Co-60 as a gamma source for teletherapy, and ought to get credit for it. Grimmett, just as undoubtedly, designed the first practical and usable container, but death and other adverse circumstances prevented him from being the first actually to put it to use.

With such a protracted time-table, it was inevitable that Co^{60} units were placed in operation before that first ORINS model. Grimmett never got a chance to see his creation: he died of coronary thrombosis in May of 1951.* In a photograph taken shortly before that, Grimmett is seen inspecting the mock-up of GE's container, while a young-looking, happy Brucer smiles approvingly.

The very first teletherapy unit ever to use artificial radioisotopes did not use Co^{60} as source. An $Iridium^{192}$ container was designed by the physicist Herbert Freundlich, and installed in J. S. Mitchell's department at Addenbrooke's Hospital in Cambridge (England). It has been in continuous clinical use since May, 1950. The disadvantage of its half-life being only seventy-four days was overcome by twin sources, one being "heated up" in the pile at Harwell, the other "used up" in the unit. An improved later model was provided with uranium metal shielding, and contained about 75 curies of Ir^{192}. The Cam-

*Biographic and other data on Grimmett were courteously supplied by Dr. Robert James Shalek, associate physicist of the M.D. Anderson Hospital, with details added by Dr. Brucer.

bridge unit is still the only one of its kind with an iridium source.

Rumor has it that somewhere in this country, in the year 1949 or 1950, a pit was dug in a basement floor, and a Co-60 source was tied to a string. The string was slipped over a pulley, and then — through a hole in the wall — the string was passed into the next (control) room. A lead screen with a rectangular window served as a collimator. The patient was positioned in front of the window in the lead screen, then the source was raised (by pulling on the string) until the source came to hang behind the window. It was held there for the treatment time desired, after which the source was lowered into the ground. That may have been the first "practical" application of cobalt teletherapy (of a sort), but the authors understandably refrained from communicating their experiences in print.

I searched at long length for any trace of that occurrence. I believed for a while that said basement was that of the Chicago Tumor Institute, but Brucer assured me that the 200-curie Co-60 source, for which Max Cutler had paid the cost, was decommissioned at Oak Ridge. Incidentally, Brucer recalls that the surgeon and radiotherapist Max Cutler got "sick" of hen fighting, fund grabbing, and all the other ordeals of the maladministration of certain cancer funds at the Chicago Tumor Institute, and took off for the Beverly Hills (California). The props of the Chicago Tumor Institute were passed on to the University of Chicago, but I found no trace of that historic 200-curie source.

CANADIAN COBALT CACHES

The first Co^{60} teletherapy unit was put into operation in 1951 in Canada. At the time the only installation capable of producing large quantities of radiocobalt was the heavy water reactor in Chalk River (Ontario). Two sources (each of approximately 1000 curies) were produced in 1951. One of these sources was delivered to the Saskatoon Cancer Clinic, and installed in a unit which had been manufactured, to the design of H. E. Johns, by the Acme Machine Shop in Saskatoon. The completed unit was installed in the Radiotherapy Department of Thomas Alastair Watson in the University Hospital in August of 1951. Thereafter, physicist Johns and his associates made extensive physical investigations in respect to output, isodose distribution and other factors. The photograph shows the unit shortly after installation. The male model is John McKay who, as the owner of Acme Machine & Electric Company was responsible for the construction and for many details of the unit. Subsequently the collimation system was modified but otherwise the machine is still the same and still in satisfactory operation as of the time of this writing. Later Picker manufactured machines based on this design.

In the meantime the other Co^{60} source from Chalk River had been delivered to the Development Division of Eldorado Mining & Refining Company where, under the direction of R. S. Errington and D. T. Green, another unit was built and installed at Victoria Hospital in London (Ontario) in October, 1951. The radiotherapist at Victoria Hospital was Ivan Smith. Shortly after installation, the first treatment with a Co^{60} teletherapy unit was given at Victoria Hospital on October 27, 1951. At University Hospital in Saskatoon, Watson treated his first patient with teleradio-cobalt on November 8, 1951.*

*These and other details were graciously offered by Prof. Thomas Watson, who teaches radiotherapy in the University of Saskatchewan in Saskatoon.

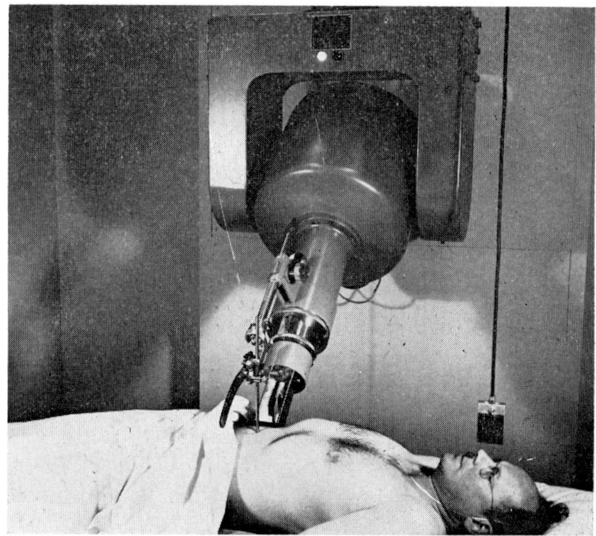

Courtesy: T. A. Watson.

FIRST COBALT TELETHERAPY UNIT. This model, designed by the physicist Harold Elford Johns, and built by John McKay at the Acme Machine Shop in Saskatoon (Saskatchewan), was installed in the Radiotherapy Department of Thomas Alastair Watson in the Saskatoon Cancer Clinic during the month of August, 1951. Then Johns proceeded to determine on it the first depth dose curves of Co-60. In the meantime the second Canadian 1000 curie source was built into an Eldorado unit at Victoria Hospital in London (Ontario). The first patient ever to receive cobalt teletherapy (from a conventional unit) was treated in London (Ontario) on October 27, 1951. Soon thereafter, on November 8, 1951, Saskatoon had its first patient treated.

A brief article on these two units appeared on December 15, 1951 in *Nature*. More detailed papers were published in the *Journal of the Canadian Association of Radiologists* of March, 1952 and in the *British Journal of Radiology* of June, 1952.

In the Saskatoon unit, the Co^{60} source was fastened to a motor-rotated wheel with which the source could be either "hidden" deep into the protective lead, or exposed at the end of a collimating tube so as to permit irradiation. In the Eldorado unit liquid mercury stored at the top part of the container, would flow by gravity to "turn off" the radiation; compressed air was employed to raise the mercury into the storage position, which "turned the radiation on." The Saskatoon head was suspended from a telescopic ceiling mount which was not only counter-balanced but could be moved along a track to cover a larger surface. The Eldorado unit was supported by a "gallows" mount connected to a pedestal. It had already such refinements as an adjustable aperture and light beam definition of treatment field.

The Eldorado Mining and Refining Company was formed in 1944. It marketed in the beginning radium and then Co^{60} sources for brachytherapy. In 1952, it began to manufacture the Eldorado unit for teletherapy. Their second machine was sold in New York City to the Fifth and Flower Hospital. The third Eldorado unit was installed in Chicago at Cook County Hospital's Radiation Center, directed at that time (1953) by Irvin Franklin Hummon, Jr. That was still a few months before assembly of the first unit at Oak Ridge. Actually, the very first Co^{60} teletherapy unit in the United States was a home-made device installed in Los Angeles.

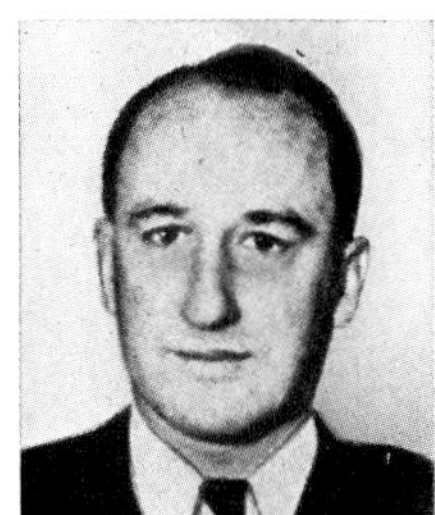

Thomas Watson

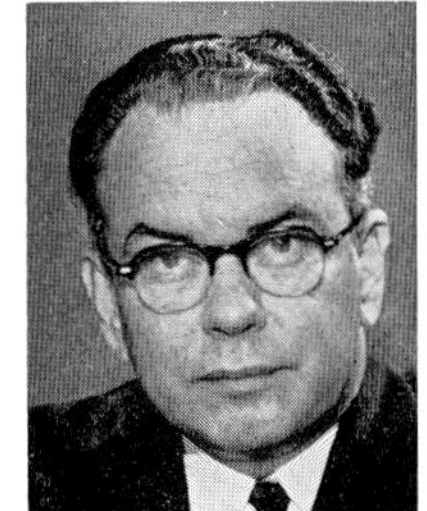

Ivan Smith

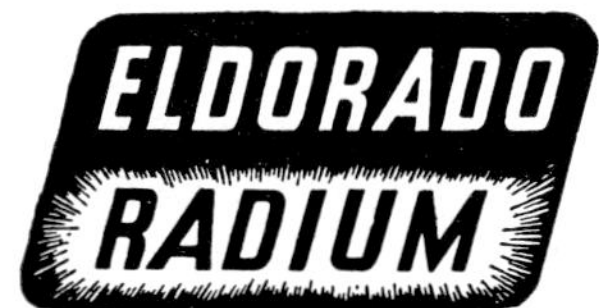

ELDORADO MINING & REFINING (1944) LIMITED

P. O. BOX 379

OTTAWA, CANADA

HOLLYWOOD HANDICRAFT

In 1951, Soiland's 4 gram radium bomb was still in operation at the Los Angeles Tumor Institute, and its mercury plug was working satisfactorily. But Soiland's ashes lay scattered in a Norwegian fjord, while the Atomic Phase had set in. The Tumor Institute needed something new, and Co^{60} seemed just the right thing.

In December, 1951 Brucer chaired a Symposium on New Developments in Teletherapy (at the meeting of the AAAS), published in *Nucleonics* of March 18, 1952. At that Symposium, James R. Mason (from AEC's Radioisotope Branch in Oak Ridge) acknowledged that only two large teletherapy sources of Co^{60} had been put into use, and both of these were in (the two previously mentioned) Canadian units. Approximately ten sources of 1000 to 1500 curies strength had been ordered by radiologists from the USA, and many pellets were being irradiated at Chalk River.

Here will be inserted a few explanatory excerpts from a letter by Marshall Brucer:

"Back in the late 1940s it took approximately two years for a reactor to produce even a small amount of Co^{60} in a Co^{59} pellet. But when I say a "small amount" I am thinking in terms of today. You remember the publicity in the early 1950s which pointed out that the first cobalt units had more radium equivalent than all

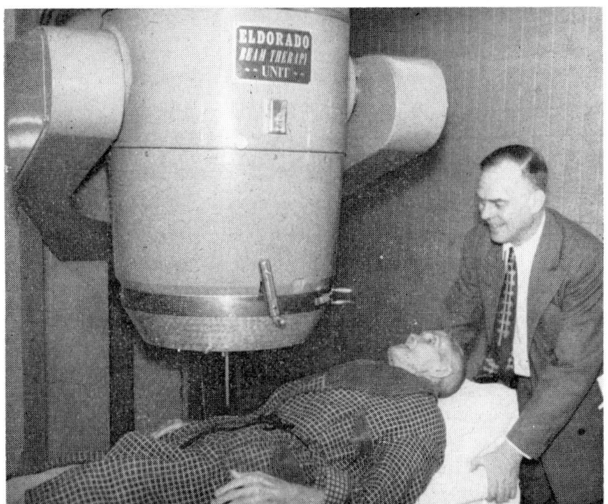

Cook County Cobalt unit. This unit was almost identical with the units installed by the Eldorado Mining and Manufacturing Company in Victoria Hospital in London (Ontario), and in the Fifth and Flower Hospital in New York City. It was the third such device made by Eldorado, and it is here shown in 1953, with Irwin Franklin Hummon (at the time director of the Radiation Center) positioning a patient. The source has since been replaced one time.

the radium available before World War II. Paul Aebersold, who was then director of the Isotopes Division of AEC in Oak Ridge, had been convinced by many people (Hummon included) that Co^{60} radiation was of great potential value in medicine. Aebersold decided, on his own responsibility, to begin producing Co^{60}. The Oak Ridge reactor had (at that time) a very low neutron flux, about 10^{11} barns, while the Canadian reactor at Chalk River had 10^{13} barns. Later the MPR was started at Los Alamos and that was for a long time the only Co^{60} producer in the USA.

"So Paul Aebersold got put into American reactors a fairly large number of one-centimeter right cylinders of Co^{59} and these were heated up to one, two, and even to (an unheard of) ten curies of radium equivalent. This was much better than (Grimmett's) ten – gram radium unit, and the source was (comparatively) small. By the time this material had been in the reactor long enough to make this amount of "million-volt radiation," we were already pointing out that there was no need to restrict ourselves to five or ten-gram radium equivalent units.* We began to think in hectocurie and in kilocurie figures. The Los Angeles Tumor Institute decided to use a 1000-curie source made from ten-curie pellets. This means the pellets had to be arranged along the surface of a large right cylinder. Their design had to be adapted to this peculiarity of the source which was very large, with tremendous penumbra and enormous shielding, but they wanted a Co^{60} unit "right away" and thus had to use what was available at the time."

*At this point in the letter, Brucer paraphrased Eric Roberts (the professor of physics at Middlesex), "if Co^{60} had been available in 1900, radium would never have been considered in medicine." And then Brucer added, "if $Cesium^{137}$ had been available in 1945, Co^{60} wouldn't have been looked at twice." I, for one, do not subscribe to the second statement.

Russell Hunton Neil (the physicist at the Los Angeles Tumor Institute) built a very ingenious, though bulky, container, and shipped it by truck to Oak Ridge. By then, Aebersold had grown willing to part with any number of the Co-60 pellets which were cluttering his irradiation facilities. So a clumsy source was built from juxtaposed pellets.

With Marshall Brucer's help that first composite source was inserted into Neil's container (shipping weight: 4,400 lbs) and returned to Los Angeles by truck (the picture of the container being readied for shipping at Oak Ridge appeared in that same issue of *Nucleonics* of March 18, 1952). For posterity we shall give the description of that first Hollywood source, printed in *Radiology* of September, 1953: it consisted of six stacks of eighteen pieces each (total: 108 pieces) forming a cylinder 4.33 cm tall and 3.5 cm in diameter; the cobalt pieces were in sealed stainless steel tubes with the outer end of each cone having a brass cover; therefore the 1080 curies of cobalt occupied 20.42 cc., weighing 181.74 gm; on February 25, 1952 the source had a specific activity of 5.94 curies per gram, the measured output on that date being 32 r per minute at 70 cm.

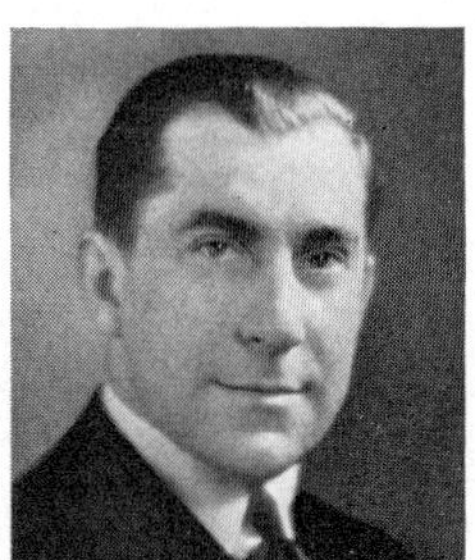
MAX CUTLER

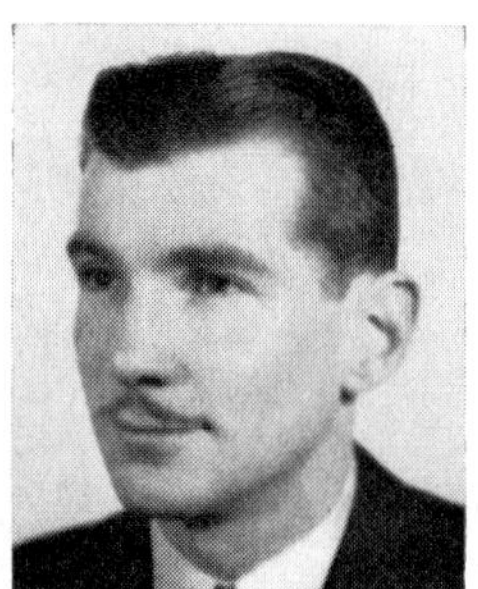
PAUL AEBERSOLD

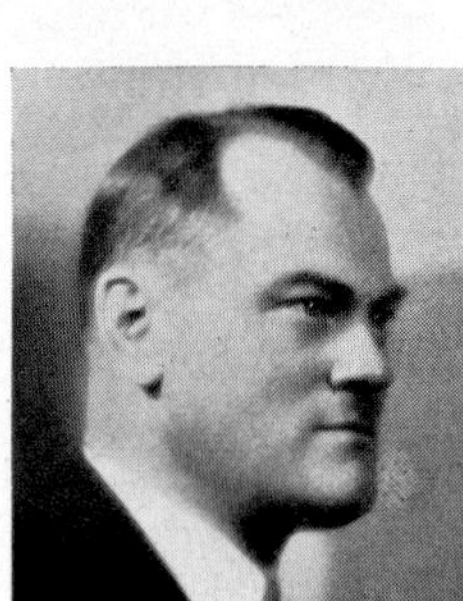
WM. E. COSTOLOW

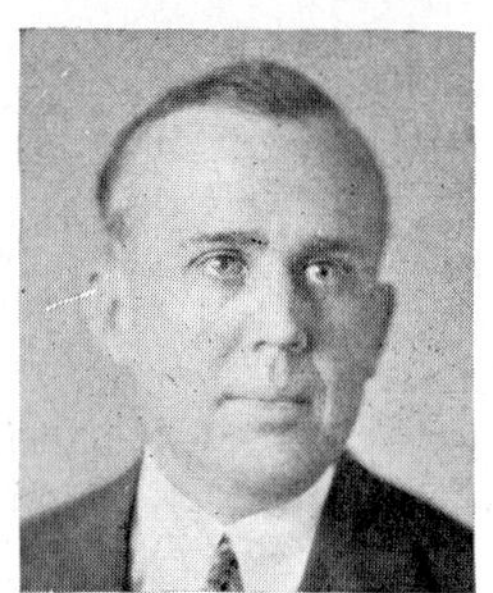
ORVILLE A. MELAND

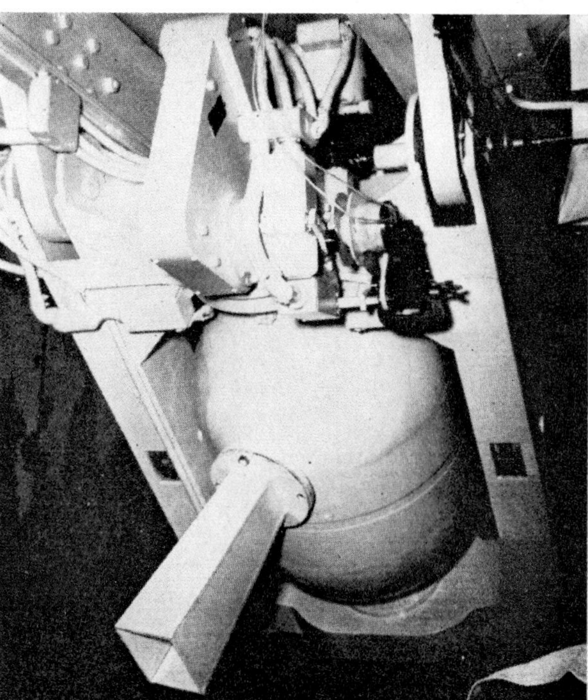
(Courtesy: RSNA)
LATI CO-60 APPLICATOR

At the Los Angeles Tumor Institute, the container was mounted in the basement room formerly occupied by the radium bomb, and the first patient (a young woman, 34 years of age, suffering from bronchogenic carcinoma) was treated by Costolow on April 23, 1952. By October, 1952 the number of patients treated with the new tool had risen to 104.

At the time of this writing I inquired about the fate of that first Co^{60} teletherapy unit installed for the Angelenos. William Evert Costolow (1892-1959) had passed away, Neil was working as a physicist for an oil company in Pasadena, and Soiland's former partner Orville Newton Meland replied melancholically that "the unit was in continuous use from that day until the first of this year (1962), at which time it had deteriorated to the extent that its output was much lower than is economically feasible. Everything decays!"*

DEVELOPMENT OF TELETHERAPY UNITS

In 1955, at the Atoms for Peace in Geneva, Brucer reported that there were about 120 Co^{60} machines in use around the world. In 1958, again at Geneva, Brucer and Simon* showed that only Atomic Energy of Canada (the young, "atomic" name adopted by the old Eldorado Mining) had produced 166 Co^{60} sources for teletherapy, while the USA had made 171 such sources. At least sixty units were then being used in Japan and at least 16 in the Soviet Union. Brucer and Simon computed a total of 300-350 cobalt therapy machines in operation around the globe.

Because of its skin-sparing feature, combined with a favorable depth dose pattern, Co^{60} teletherapy is today the "conventional" method for the irradiation of deep-seated malignancies. In 1959 a global Directory of Teletherapy Equipment was published by the International Atomic Energy Agency.

Not only Co^{60} but also $Cesium^{137}$ sources are used in teletherapy devices. The dead weight which results from the necessary shielding usually requires "power assist" but this is not always true of the smaller units.

In a small Co^{60} unit (for 10-150 curies) the Bryant Simons & Co. of London has built a pneumatic transfer

*Even the pristine philosophers of Stone Age times knew that mankind can only strive for, but can never achieve any significant degree of, permanency. This is why permanency had always been an attribute of divinity. Jahveh of the Hebrews inherited that concept of permanency and, by the same token, it was accepted in Christianity. Yet, from a strictly biologic viewpoint, life and lack of change are incompatible. From a religious viewpoint, the idea of permanency has resulted in many beautiful expressions, as this one by the Scottish clergyman Henry Francis Lyte (1793-1847):

Swift to its close ebbs out life's little day;
Earth's joys grow dim, its glories pass away;
Change and decay in all around I see;
O thou, who changest not, abide with me!

Since radioactive substances have a constant, immutable rate of decay, one might conclude that their essence is not very divine—could this be why so many people regard radioactivity as an evil?

*The first privately owned Co^{60} unit (306 curies) was installed by Norman Simon at his private office in New York City.

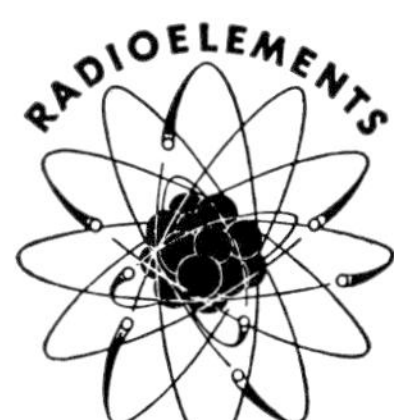

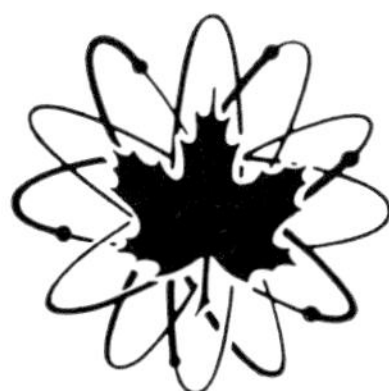

ATOMIC MAPLE. Soon after changing its name from Eldorado Mining and Manufacturing Co. to Atomic Energy of Canada, they replaced the boiling atoms with their (unofficial) national symbol, the maple leaf.

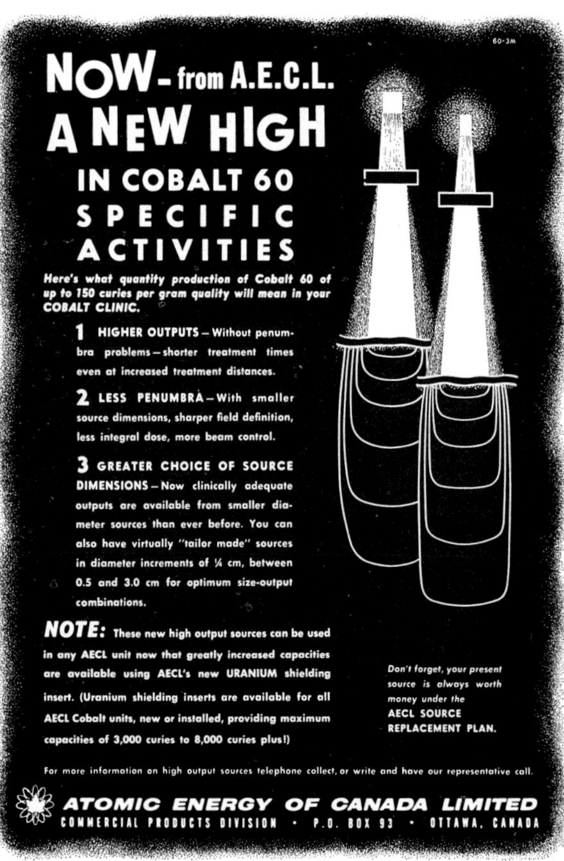

unit in which the source is stored in a lead safe in the wall, and pushed (with compressed air) into the applicator head only after the patient has been positioned.

Aside from varied strengths (the Elema-Schönander of Stockholm manufactures a Deka-Curie unit), these models differ also by whether they employ cobalt or cesium as a source, and by the mobility of the container.

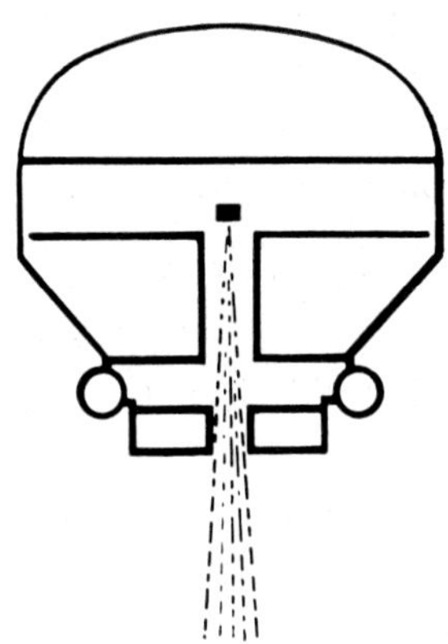

ELDORADO G. Schematic view of its head, which contains the "hot rods." A lingam-shaped representation of the latter appears on a recent ad, which depicts the rods with their depth doses.

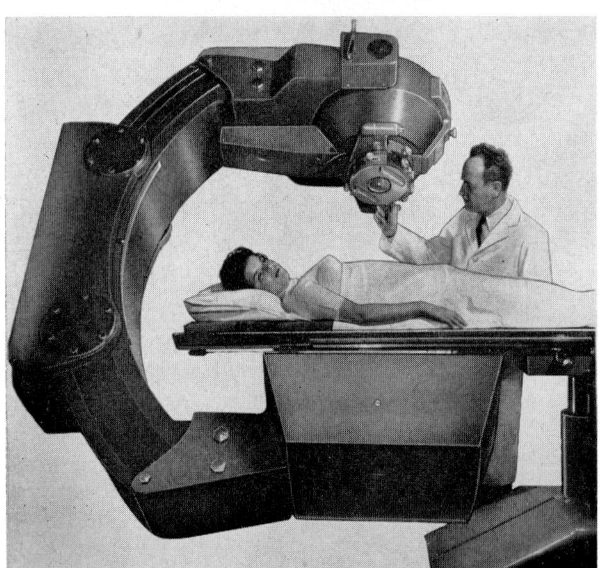

Courtesy: Atomic Energy of Canada, Ltd.

AECL's THERATRON. An early model (superseded by the Theratron 60) is shown with an impassible beauty between the beast's jaws, while the interested operator watches the outcome. The heavy lead block serves not only as a counterbalance for the head, it also attenuates the primary beam, which remains quite "hot", even after penetration through the target.

Atomic Energy of Canada had the Eldorado unit. With their chronologic priority they introduced also the Theratron, a rotational unit in which the source was mounted on one arm of a huge U; the other arm had a counter-balancing lead weight provided with a back pointer. The Eldorado and the Theratron be-

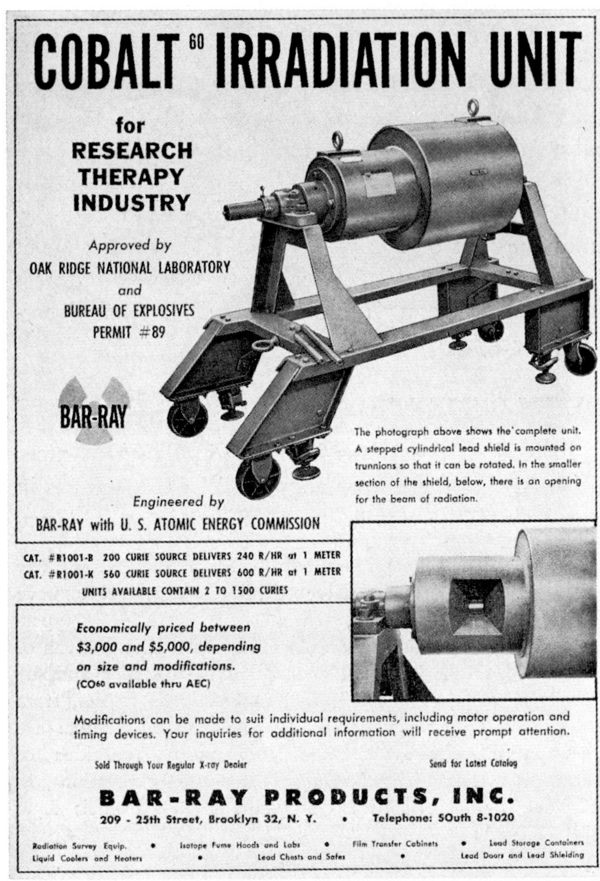

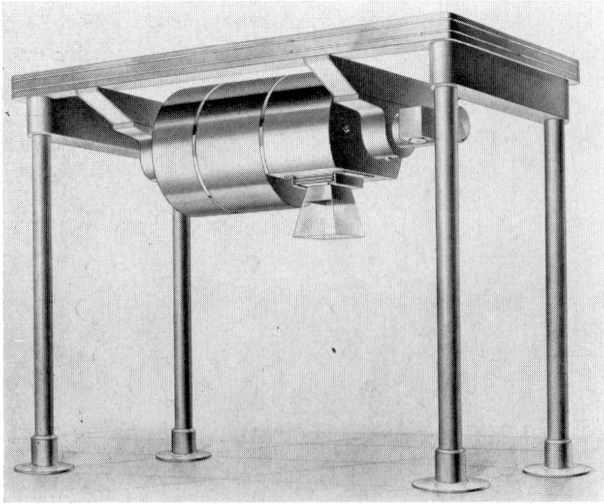

BAR-RAY'S MEMORIAL HOSPITAL UNIT

came the prototypes of most of the larger units subsequently built by other manufacturers.

The IAEA Directory (although compiled by K. C. Tsien before December, 1959) contains very valuable information. In it are listed forty-six models produced by eighteen firms in nine countries (Canada, France, Germany, Italy, Japan, Netherlands, Sweden, the United Kingdom, and the USA). Among Eastern countries it mentions only the Soviet Union, but Co^{60} irradiators are manufactured not only in Moscow, in Kiev, and in Leningrad, but also in Dresden, in Prague, in Budapest, and very recently also in Shanghai.

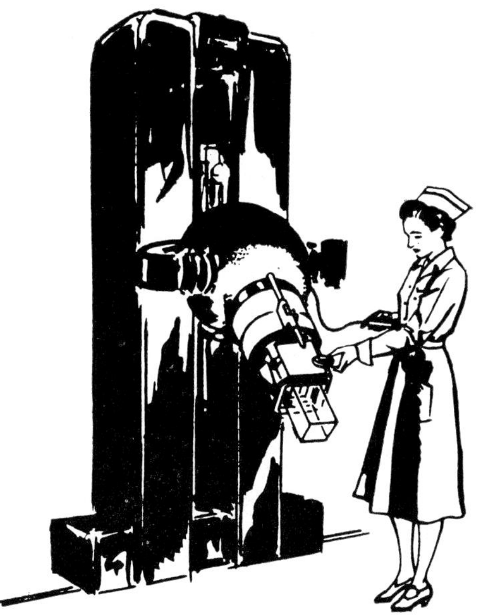

PICKER'S "SMALL" Co^{60} UNIT. It has a MacKay-Johns collimator, and can be loaded with sources of 1000-1500-curies.

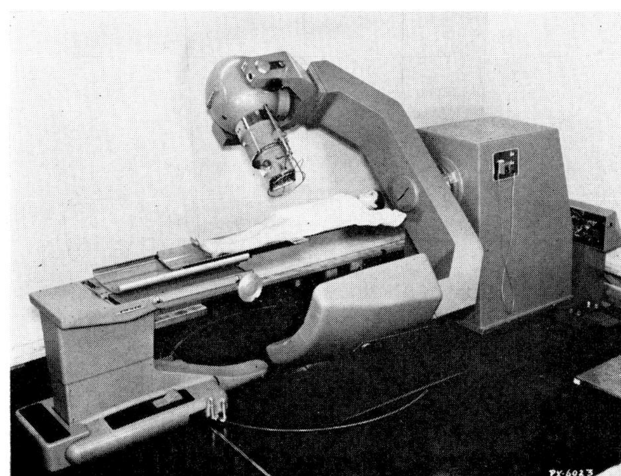

PICKER'S "GIANT" Co^{60} UNIT. The C-10,000 dwarfs its otherwise king-size female model.

An oddity, not listed in *Tsien's Directory*, is a model manufactured in 1953 (but presumably not after 1958) by Bar-Ray Products of Brooklyn. It consisted of a source encased in a cylindrical lead shield. The cylinder was mounted on trunnions so that it could be rotated. By such rotation, an opening in the cylinder would expose the source. Its low but massive frame was mounted on four heavy rollers. The ORINS had a slightly similar unit, painted in a dark, "screaming" red; one of their students thought of it as being a Red Menace.

In this country all major manufacturers produce Co^{60} units, most of which are either of the pedestal or of the heavy rotational type. Picker has recently issued the C-10,000 for moving-beam or fixed-beam teletherapy. It has a sensational 10,000 rhm output

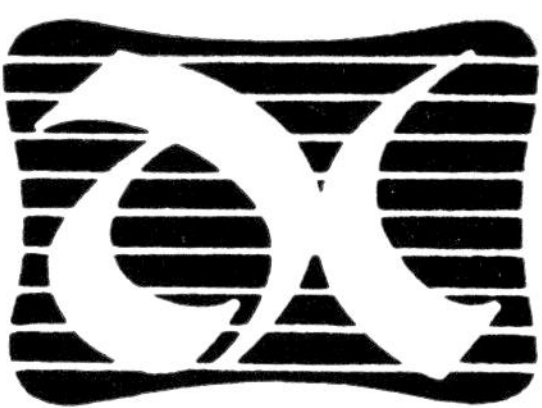

Courtesy: Dick X-Ray Co.

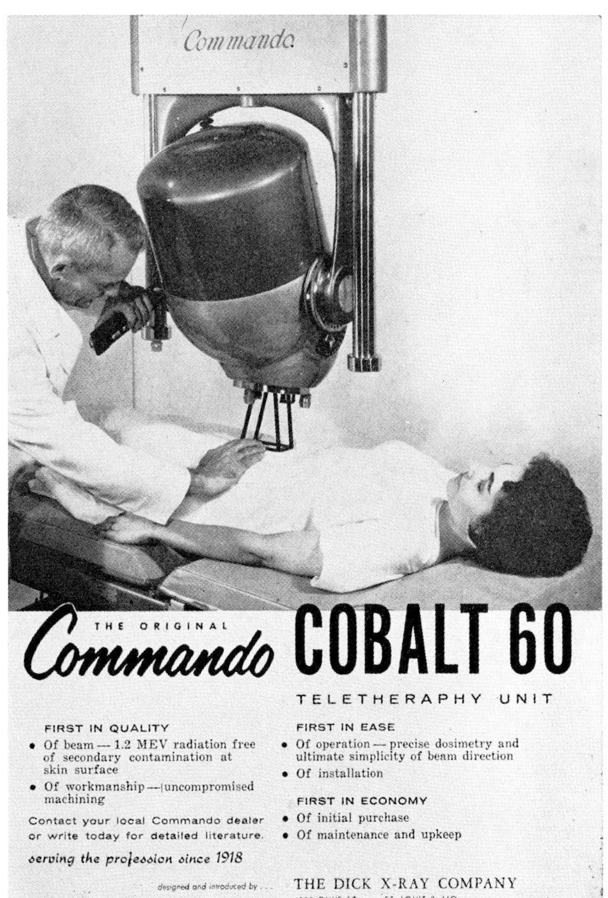

(almost double that of 2 mev x-ray units). Its arc during the moving cycle requires lowering the floor beneath the U. This unit of Picker's also has the distinction of being the most expensive anywhere on the market, except for custom-built installations. Indeed, when twin or triplet sources and other fancies are demanded, (as in the V. A. Research Hospital in Chicago), money must be no problem. Keleket, in combination with the Barnes Co. of Rockford (Illinois) — they had built Brucer's rotational cesium

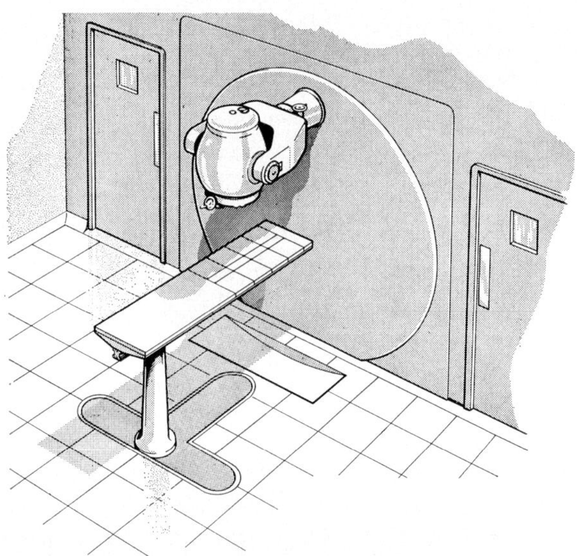

BRITISH MOVING FIELD Co^{60} UNIT. Mobaltron design.

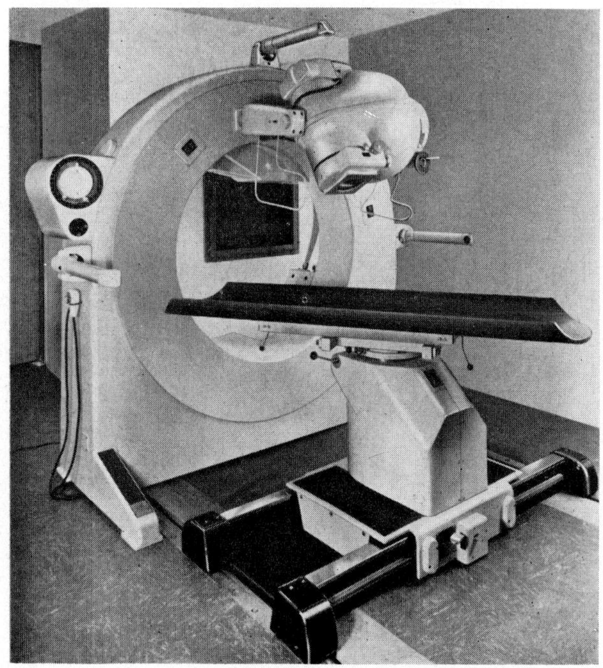

AEI ORBITRON.

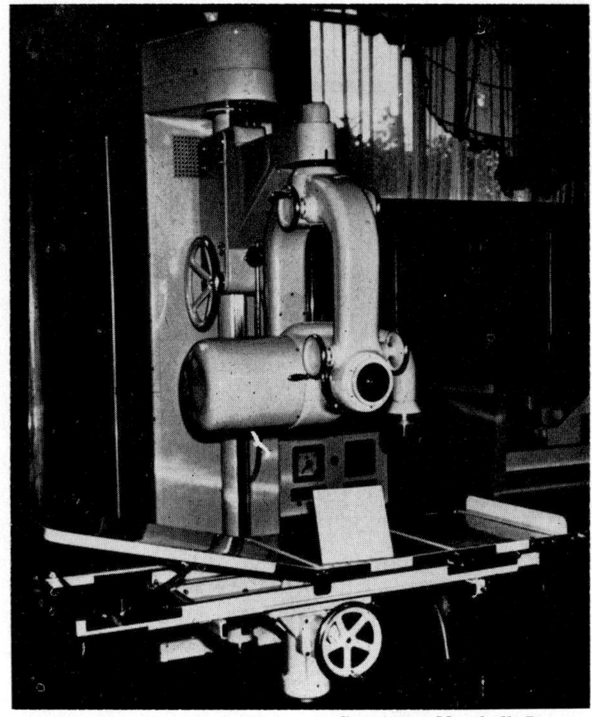

Courtesy: Marshall Brucer.

SOVIETIC Co^{60} UNIT I. It accepts deca-curie sources, and has an ingenious fail-safe feature: when tilted, the source "falls" back into the shielded position.

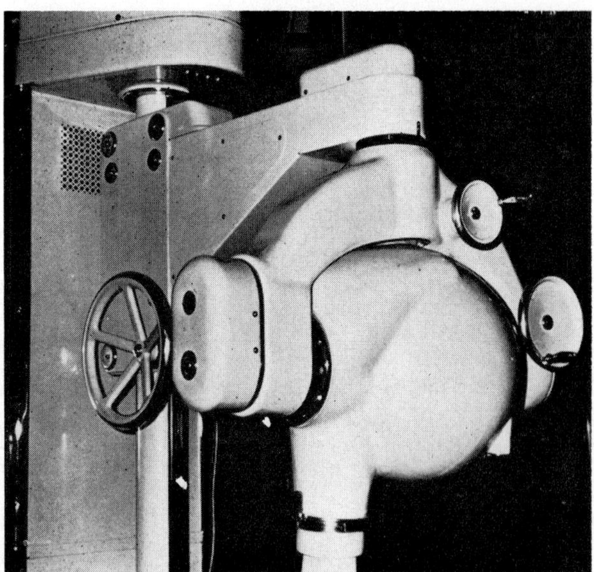

SOVIETIC Co^{60} UNIT II. Hecto-curie device, shown here from Marshall Brucer's collection at ORINS; in 1955, at Geneva, Sovietic therapists seemed to believe that hectocurie units were the largest sources necessary for adequate treatment; this is undoubtedly true, though treatment times can be shortened with bigger loads, meaning that one machine can be used to treat more people.

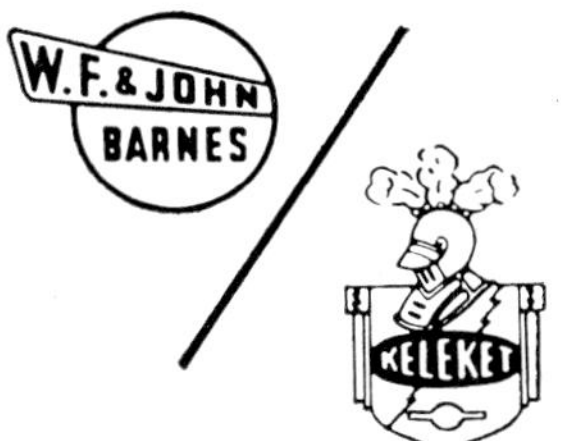

machine — came out with the Flexray (it is sometimes confused with Standard's 250 kvp conventional therapy unit called Flexaray). GE and Westinghouse likewise make Co^{60} units, and a few Cs^{137} heads are also available from the four larger American manufacturers. A small, mainly Ear, Nose, and Throat type of Co^{60} unit was offered for a while by the Dick X-Ray Company of St. Louis.

In 1923, Dick's total payroll numbered less than twenty-four persons, while in 1962 it exceeded 100. In 1933, they terminated the association with Keleket, and accepted thereafter a Westinghouse distributorship. In the past Dick had built some tubestands, and perhaps a few small transformers, but never major pieces of equipment. Manufacture of the Commando has since been turned over to Westinghouse.

The "heart of America" seal had been abandoned sometimes in the 1930s, and was not replaced until 1960, when they adopted the current monogram. It is a stylized and abbreviated cuneiform combination of the letters D and X (for Dick X-Ray), superimposed on a field of parallel lines symbolic or indicative of radiation.

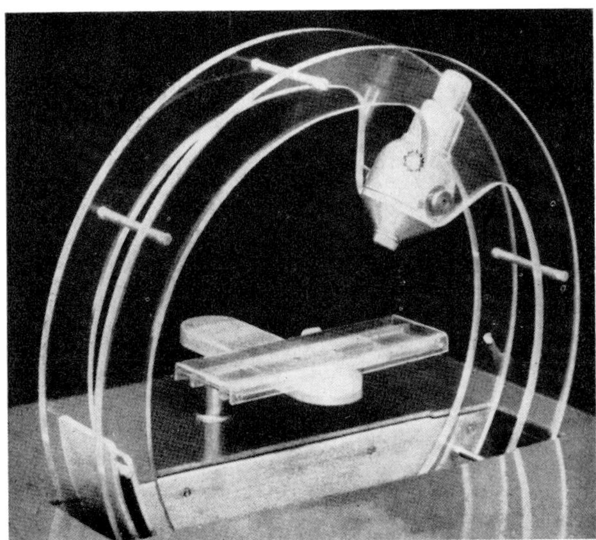

Courtesy: Smit-Röntgen.

DUTCH Co^{60} UNIT. Ingenious "satellite" arrangement, providing natural shielding of the source when "orbited" into the ground.

In Great Britain, elaborate teletherapy equipment is being manufactured by one of AEI's subsidiaries (the former Newton & Victor), by the locomotive manufacturer, the Hunslet Precision Engineering of Leeds (England) — they make the so-called isocen-

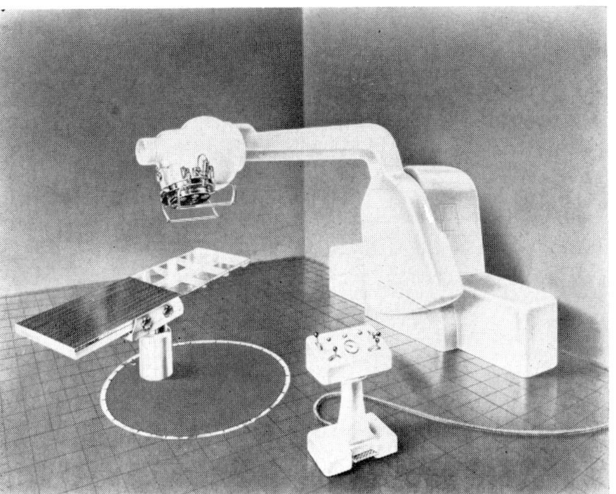

UNUSUAL BRITISH Co^{60} UNIT. Hunslet's 500 isocentric teletherapy device. It "points" at all times to the center of the circle drawn on the floor.

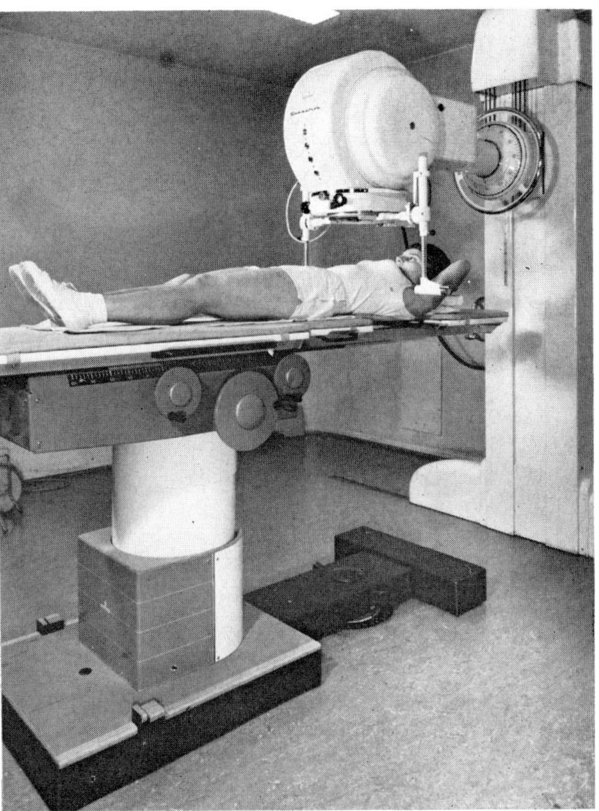

WEST GERMAN Co^{60} UNIT. SRW's stationery Gammatron 1, with elaborate table.

tric unit — and by Test Equipment (Models) in Sussex, successors to Nuclear Engineering of Greenwich. In France, Massiot Nucléaire (a Phillips subsidiary) makes both a stationary and a moving model. In Germany, SRW manufactures the Gammatron, which comes likewise in the two basic types. Smit-Röntgen of Leiden (Holland) has a diversified line in this field, including a rotational model which is half-sunk into the floor. In Japan at least three of the large firms manufacture teletherapy equipment, Shimadzu, Toshiba, and Hitachi.

In Italy, both Barazzetti and Gilardoni have developed (independently of each other) heads which contain both a Co^{60} and a Cs^{137} source. The two sources can be utilized (alternately) for irradiation.

Gravicert is the name of a 500 curie irradiator developed and built by Medicor in Budapest. The storage for the source is in the wall, and after the patient is positioned, the source is moved ("pulled") into the fixed container. At the end of the treatment period, the source returns by force of gravity into its storage space. This is the origin of the name, because *gravity* as*cert*ains that the source will return to its ultra-shielded location.

At the ARS meeting in Colorado Springs in May of 1961, K. C. Tsien reported on his continuing world survey of teletherapy units (published in the *American Journal of Roentgenology* of March, 1962). In mid-year 1961, he had computed the following figures of teletherapy units per countries: USA 386; Canada

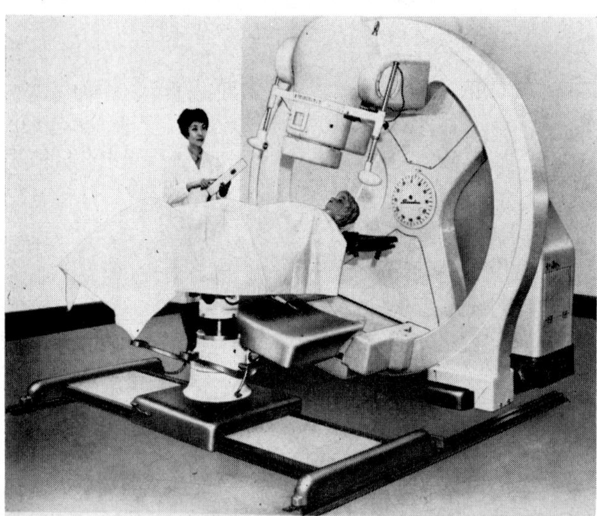

Japanese (Shimadzu)Co^{60} unit. 10,000 curie model with ringstand for rotational, and table on rails to add the pendular capabilities.

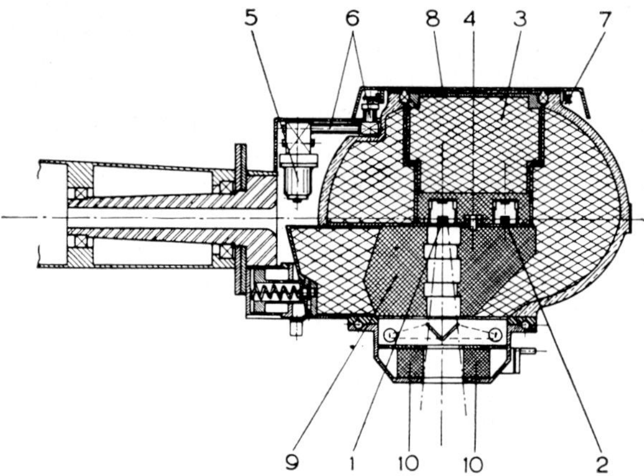

Italian twin-source head. This section of Gilardoni's Bisorgente shows the cobalt source (1), the cesium source (2), a drum (3) which rotates around the axle (4), the drum-actuating electrical motor (5) with its gearing (6, 7) and source-rotating platform (8), while the shut-off plug (9) is activated by compressed air; there is also a collimator (10). A similar unit is made by another Italian manufacturer, Barazzetti.

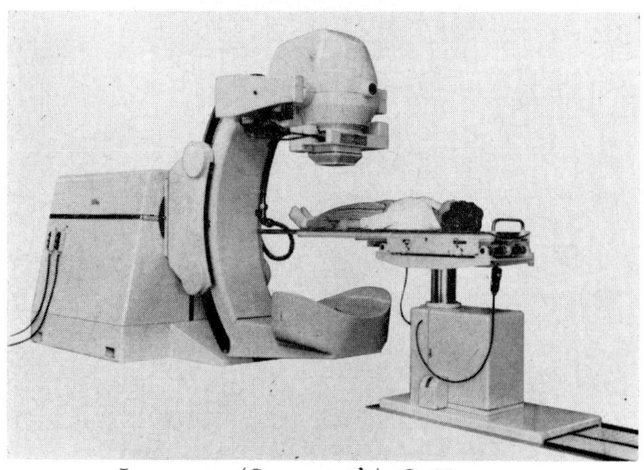

Japanese (Shibaura's) Co^{60} unit.

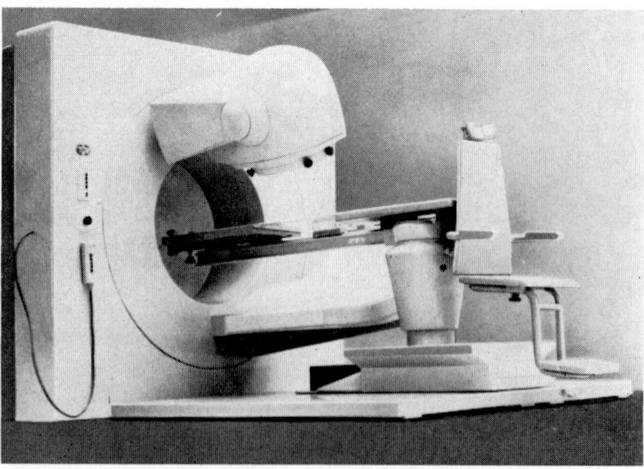

East German TCo 2000. Permits rotational as well as pendular irradiation, with a source of up to 2000 curies, giving 100 r/min at 65 cm distance.

36; Mexico 19; Argentina 11; Brazil 9; Japan 160; India 7; Philippines 4; USSR 180; Italy 83; Great Britain 47; France 45; others 20; estimated world total 1120.

In the (German) *MTA Radiologie* of October, 1963 Thomas Funke of Lorain (Ohio) reported his recent visit to the Picker plant in Cleveland. He inserted the statement, attributed to one of the Picker executives, that the Picker Company manufactures the containers for one third of the world's radiocobalt units, and for 90% of the world's radiocesium units. I checked these figures with Harvey Picker, and this is what he answered: "It is very difficult for us to be certain about the number of cobalt units we produce compared to other companies. Many other companies do not publish figures. This, of course, you know from our discussion about American competition. However, we can be reasonably sure that we produce over one-third of all Cobalt units produced in the world. Inasmuch as we are the only manufacturer of any size in the world producing cesium units, it is safe to say that we produce at least 90 percent of the world's production." His letter is dated December 4, 1963.

Current supplies of Co^{60} sources are in this country the ORNL; in Canada the reactor at Chalk River (Ontario); in England the Atomic Energy Research Establishment at Harwell (Berkshire) and the Radiochemical Centre at Amersham (Buckinghamshire); in Australia the (high flux) HIFAR in Sutherland (N.S.W.); and in the Soviet Union the Dubna and the Volga Laboratories (which sell their products through Soyuzreaktiv, a trust operated by their Ministry of Chemical Industries).

BROOKHAVEN

The history of Brookhaven can be gleaned from cursory remarks published by Dennis Puleston in May, 1959 in the *Journal of Metals*. The founding is well described in the final report of work by Columbia University, issued on January 15, 1948.

At the end of World War II, nuclear research centers functioned at Argonne, at Oak Ridge, at Los Alamos, and at the Radiation Laboratory in Berkeley, but there was no large center in the East. On January 14, 1946 George B. Pegram (dean of the Graduate School in Columbia University) wrote letters to various research institutions, calling a meeting to discuss the creation of a nuclear science laboratory in the vicinity of New York City. The discussion of the group at Columbia led to the formation of an Initiatory University Group (IUG) which met for the first time on March 26, 1946. They represented nine universities, Yale, Columbia, Princeton, Harvard, Johns Hopkins, Cornell, Rochester, Pennsylvania, and Massachusetts Institute of Technology (MIT). The Stone & Webster Engineers (Boston) were requested to survey two proposed locations. Delegates from above listed nine institutions formed the Associated Universities Inc. (AUI). On August 1, 1946 Philip M. Morse of the MIT was appointed director of the new laboratory.

Contrary to the requirements which prevailed at the time Oak Ridge and Los Alamos were being located, the site for Brookhaven was selected on the basis of easy accessibility. It was felt that it should be within one hour's drive from a railroad station of either the Pennsylvania or the New Haven: by traveling during the evening, a faculty member of any of the componet institutions should be able to spend one day at the

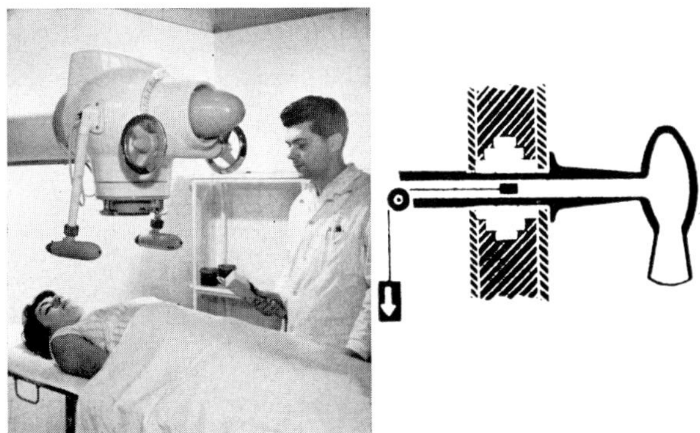

Hungarian Gravicert. Fail-safe is insured by gravity. This unit is manufactured by Medicor in Budapest.

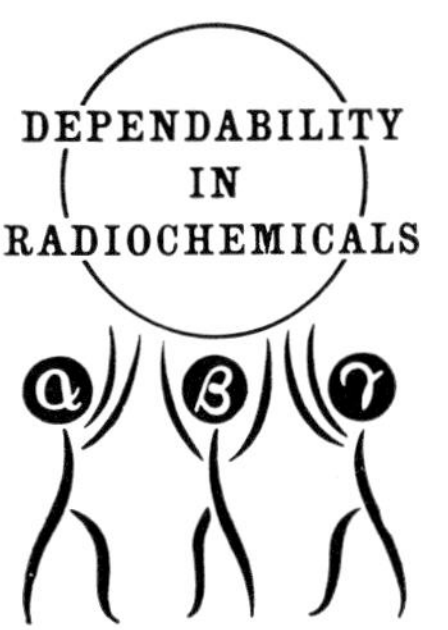

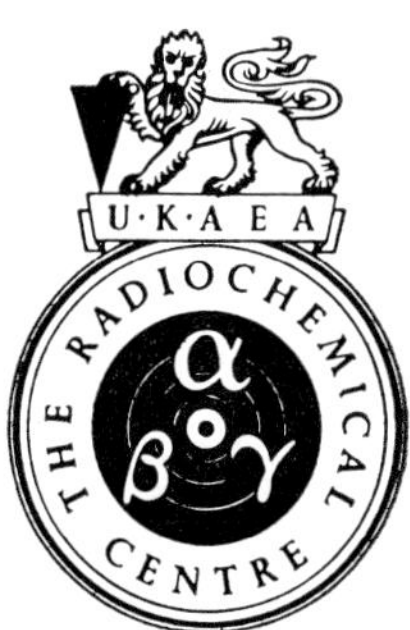

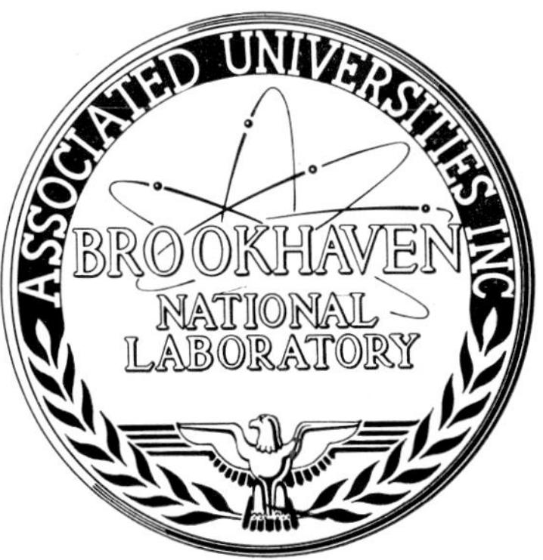

laboratory, and be back at his university the next day. Camp Upton, on Long Island, when it was taken over from the Army, was nothing more than a cluster of several hundred drab, barracks-type buildings and a small hospital, linked by muddy roads. The camp was set in over 6000 acres of parade grounds, scrub oak, and pine woods. It was located near the geographical center of Long Island, 70 miles due East of New York City. On January 7, 1947 a letter contract was made between the newly formed AEC and the AUI, and on January 13, 1947, the first AUI scientists moved to Upton. The existing barracks were converted into offices, laboratories, and dormitories, which saved almost one year in getting the research program under way.

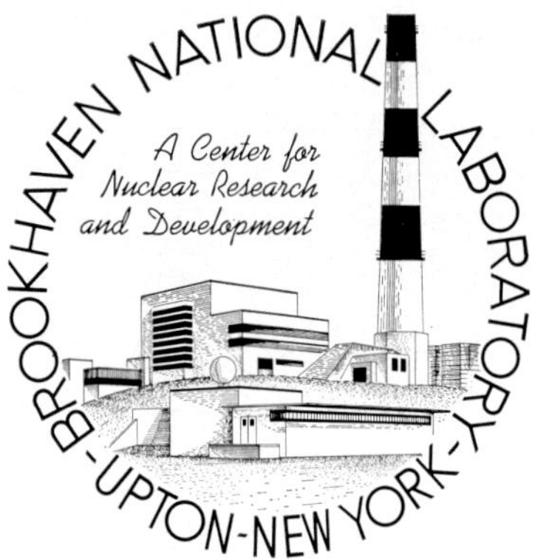

The first research reactor at Brookhaven was completed and brought to criticality in 1950. It consists of a twenty-five foot graphite cube separated into two halves by a 2.75 inch gap. Sixty thousand graphite blocks with a total weight of 700 tons make up the core, which is penetrated by 1368 round, parallel fuel channels, spaced eight inches between centers. The graphite serves to moderate, or slow down the neutrons so that the chain reaction can be maintained. Cooling is by forced air which is then exhausted through a 320 foot stack. The graphite cube and air-chambers are enclosed in a five foot thick shield of high-density concrete, reinforced with steel punching. The shield is penetrated by many horizontal experimental holes of various sizes for irradiation studies, and for the emission of beams of neutrons for use with equipment installed at the reactor faces. There are also conveyor systems for sending irradiation samples through the reactor at selected flux and time conditions. By means of pneumatic tubes, isotopes of short half-life can be shot directly from the heart of the reactor into awaiting experiments, in adjacent laboratories.

Until early in 1958, the reactor had operated at a fairly constant power level of 28 Mw. Then it was reloaded with highly enriched uranium and the central neutron flux was thus increased about six times.

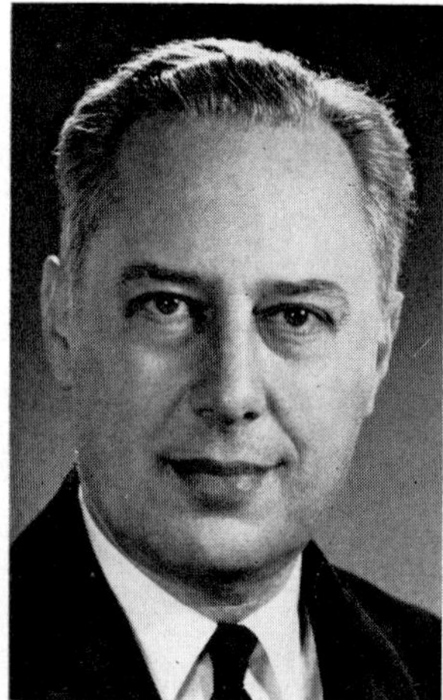

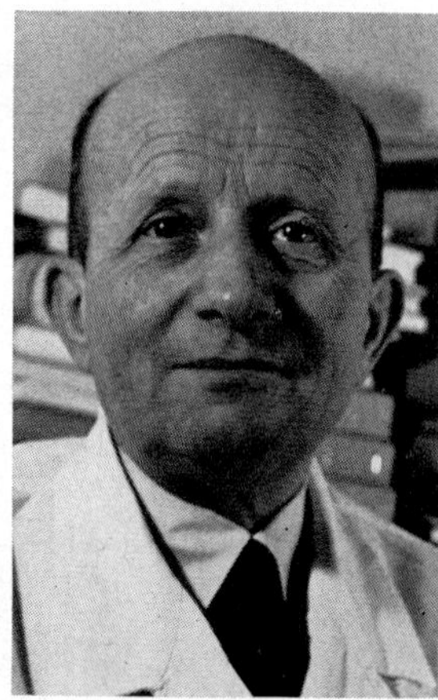

LEE EDWARD FARR. First chairman of the Medical Division of Brookhaven National Laboratory, and advocate of the use of an atomic reactor as a tool in medical research. His companion in this figure is HUGO WILHELM KNIPPING, a professor of internal medicine in Köln (Germany), who first became famous in 1924 with an eponymic respiratory test. Knipping believes in looking into any confines into which medicine advances, whence his interest in medical radioisotopes. He also believes, in true German magisterial tradition, that a physician must look beyond his immediate confines, whence his interest in artistic representations of medicine, and other "paramedical" subjects.

Lee Edward Farr* joined Brookhaven in 1948 and became the chairman of its Medical Division. On December 16, 1958, during the dedication exercises of the Medical Research Center at Brookhaven, Farr reminisced that their Medical Department was not organized until 1949. In that year it was started with a staff of two. From the beginning, the Brookhaven Graphite air-cooled reactor was envisaged as a tool to be used by all scientists in the laboratory. The Medical Department shared in this unique arrangement. Each basic department was given an opportunity to reserve to its own usage one or more ports of the 90-

*The information on Brookhaven herein provided was obtained from material graciously collected for this purpose by Dr. Farr. Incidentally, Farr (a Yale graduate of 1933, who dabbled first in pediatrics, then in internal medicine) has achieved international stature in the field of atomic medicine, and has published in 1961 in the Westdeutscher Verlag the polylingual *Nuklearmedizin in der Klinik,* in collaboration with Hugo Wilhelm Knipping, the professor of internal medicine at Koeln (Germany). My long time pen-pal Knipping is a clinician of world-wide repute, who has successfully endeavored in a variety of fields, from the study of respiratory physiology to the sanitary condition in India, and from investigations of cardiac insufficiency to the relationship between medicine and art (on the latter subject he has just published a volume in the Friedrich-Karl Schattauer Verlag in Stuttgart).

odd provided in the reactor. This had considerable impact on the philosophy of the Medical Department of Brookhaven, which since its inception has been concerned with the use of a nuclear reactor as an instrument of medical therapy.

The Medical Research Center at Brookhaven has now a 48-bed hospital, composed of four circular 12-bed nursing units. The Center has its own reactor, a 1-mw tank-type with light water-moderated and cooled fuel, and a forced air-cooled graphite reflector.*

In a statement on the *Role of a Nuclear Reactor in Medical Research and Therapy,* submitted on March 23, 1961 to the Subcommittee on Research and Development of the Joint Committee on Atomic Energy, Lee Farr discussed four aspects. Neutron flux can induce artificial radioactivity (used in activation analysis), and short-lived isotopes could be employed for biologic purposes without incurring the decay inherent in lengthy transportation. Most of all, Farr elaborated on the other two aspects, concerning therapy with "fast" neutrons, or through capture of thermal (slow) neutrons. He included a detailed history of their therapeutic usage.

The neutron was discovered in 1932 at Cambridge University by Chadwick while investigating cloud-chamber pictures of recoiled nitrogen atoms. In 1936 Ernest Lawrence and his associates used the Berkeley cyclotron for the study of biologic effects of fast neutrons. In the same year Gordon Lee Locher was the first to suggest in print that elements with high thermal neutron capture cross sections (such as boron) might have therapeutic uses by virtue of this property (assuming that prompt disintegration follows neutron capture), and that they might be introduced artificially into regions of the body to be irradiated. In September, 1938 Robert Stone first treated with fast neutrons a carcinoma of the upper alveolar ridge (using the Berkeley cyclotron); a total of 226 patients were subjected to neutron therapy, but bad sequelae *versus* the relatively few good results made them discontinue the procedure.

At this point will be inserted several paragraphs from a letter, dated January 22, 1964, which I received from Robert Stone:

"Last October Dr. Earl Miller spoke to me about sending you a list of the firsts that we were able to accomplish here at the University of California. I have been delaying answering you or him hoping to get some pictures. Since I have not yet found time to gather these together, I thought I would at least send the following information.

"Dr. Joseph Hamilton and myself were the first to use artificial radioisotopes in the treatment of patients. We treated our first patient for chronic lymphatic leukemia on March 23, 1936, with intravenous radiosodium. This is reported in the article by Hamilton and Stone in *Radiology* of February, 1937. I should say here that without the co-operation of Ernest O. Lawrence we would not have been able to procure radiosodium at that time in history.

"I was privileged to be the first person to use fast neutrons in the treatment of patients with cancer, again

*Among the biological research facilities at Brookhaven are a 10-acre field in which is centered a 2000-curie source of Co^{60}, a greenhouse where a smaller gamma source is located, and a thermal column atop the research reactor for the neutron irradiation of seeds and dormant buds. They own a digital computer, called MERLIN.

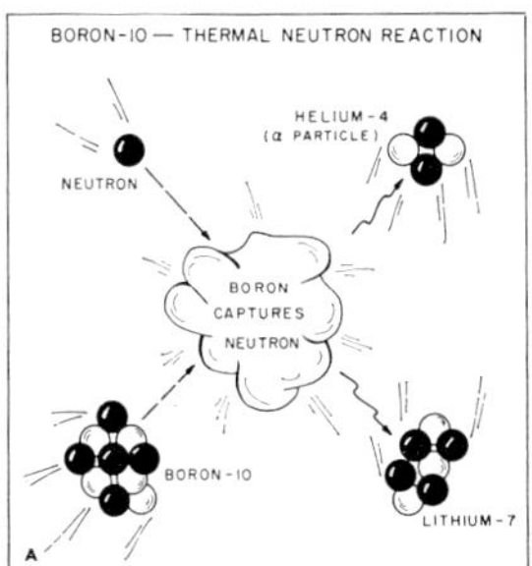

Courtesy: Brookhaven National Laboratory.

NEUTRON CAPTURE. Upon capture of a thermal (slow) neutron, the B^{10} atom disintegrates into an alpha particle and an energetic lithium particle with a large release of energy (2.4 mev); when that energy is absorbed in tissues it will show cytocidal effects.

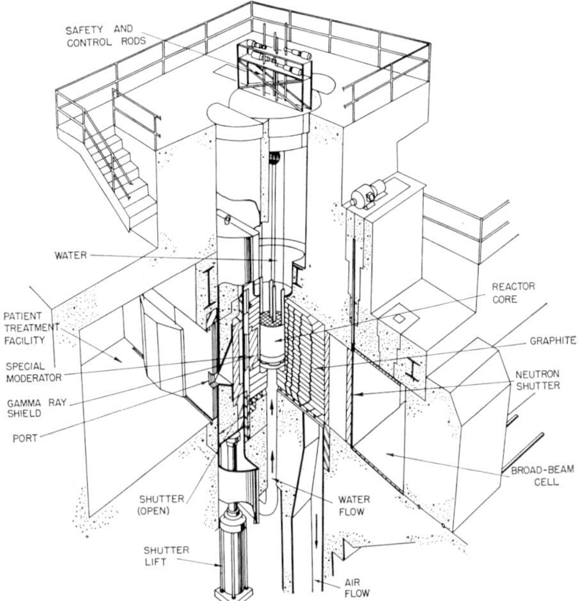

Courtesy: Brookhaven National Laboratory.

BROOKHAVEN MEDICAL RESEARCH REACTOR. Lee Farr believed that a reactor may function as a medical tool, and he tried his best to prove it.

because of the co-operation of the late professor Ernest Lawrence. In the initial studies I was aided by Dr. John H. Lawrence and by the biophysicist Paul Aebersold. That work was reported by Stone, Lawrence, and Aebersold in *Radiology* of September, 1940. Later in the study I was assisted by Dr. John C. Larkin until January, 1943 when the war effort took both of us away from San Francisco.

"After the war I was privileged to be provided with a synchrotron, which produced 70 mev x rays. We had it on the Campus in San Francisco, and it was for the sole use of biology and medicine. Our first treatments on this machine started in July, 1956, and are still continuing.

"Back in 1934 I was the first to use a radio-frequency transformer to produce one mev x rays for the treatment of patients. However, other people produced what were then called supervoltage radiations by different types of x-ray equipment. Some of those were in operation before ours. Dr. Mudd at Cal-Tech started clinical trials of 600 kv x rays in October, 1930 and by October 1933 was using 1000 kv x rays. The Memorial Hospital in New York had a machine that was operating at 700 kv in October, 1931. At Lincoln (Nebraska) a 650 kv machine went into operation in April of 1933. At the Detroit Harper Hospital a 500 kv machine went into operation in September, 1933. The Mercy Hospital at Chicago started to operate an 800 kv machine in October of 1933. The Tumor Institute of the Swedish Hospital in Seattle started in January of 1934 with 800 kv, and we started in May of 1934 with 1000 kv.

"I don't know whether there is any particular virtue in being the first to do something. The fact that one is first doing something different does indicate a spirit of adventure, and if firsts are quoted they might as well be put down in the correct order.

"The usual firsts to be quoted for the treatment of human diseases with artificial radioisotopes is John Lawrence with the treatment of a patient with leukemia

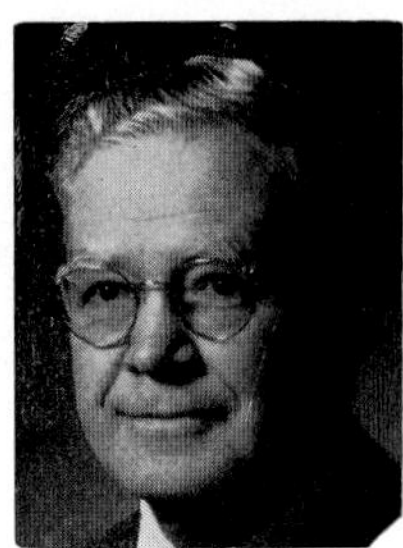

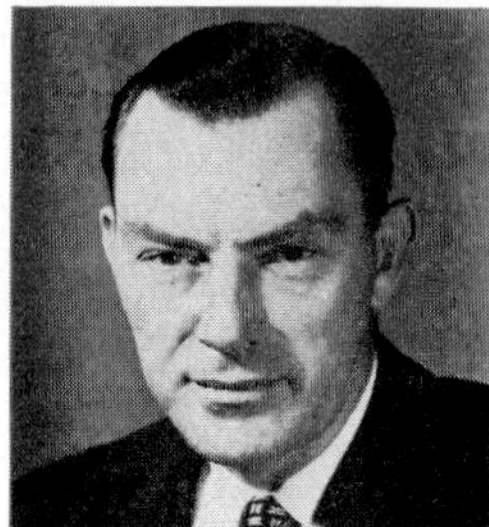

AT SAN FRANCISCO MEDICAL CENTER. Robert Spencer Stone (with glasses) is primarily a therapist, currently emeritus, but very active. His successor, Earl Roy Miller, is more interested in diagnostic problems, especially in cineradiography, but has given much of his time to the ACR.

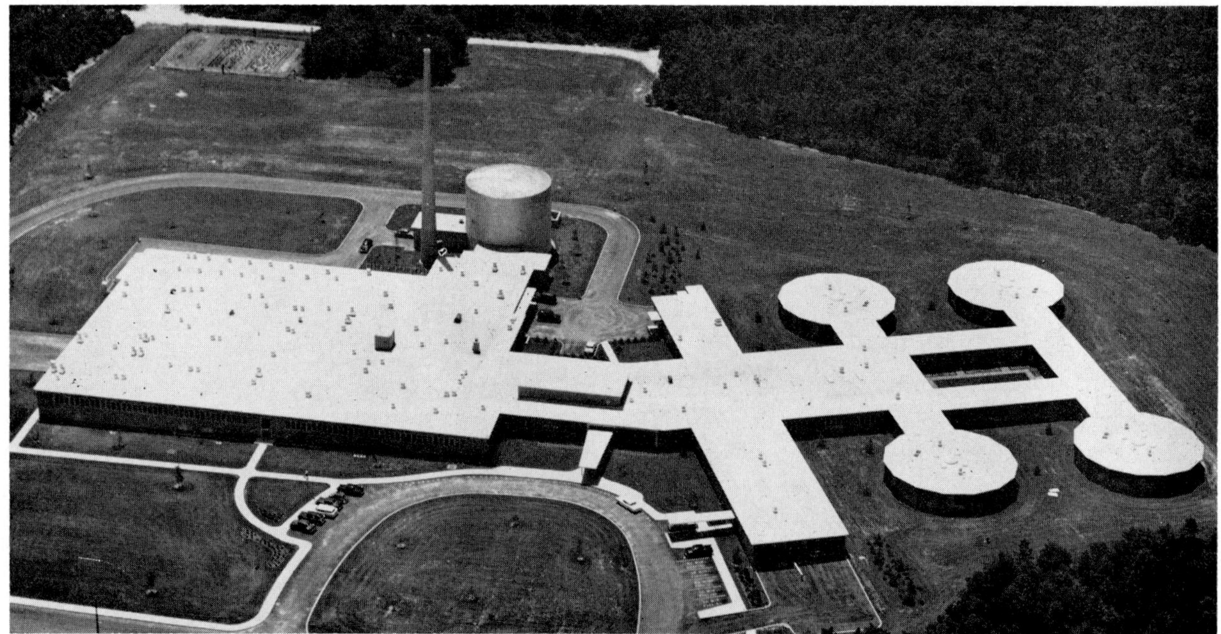

Courtesy: Brookhaven National Laboratory.

BROOKHAVEN'S MEDICAL RESEARCH CENTER. To the viewer's right are four cylindrical, 12-bed nursing units, next to the hospital service area. The rectangular area to the left contains the research laboratories. The medical research reactor is in the cylindrical tank-type building toward the rear, adjoining the stack, which is part of the air-cooling system for the graphite reflector.

of the lymphatic type, which he did for the first time on December 14, 1937. We gave up the work with radiosodium because radiophosphorus seemed so much more promising, more reasonable, and easier to handle. Since John Lawrence was the first to get interested in radiophosphorus in human treatments, Dr. Hamilton and I discontinued using the radiosodium, and left the field of treatment of leukemias to Dr. Lawrence with radiophosphorus. Signed: Dr. Robert S. Stone."

We shall briefly give a few additional details on early supervoltage therapy. Leonidas Marinelli had told me that in 1931, at the old Memorial Hospital in New York City had been installed a 700 kv transformer, which used a Lauritsen tube. The setup was illustrated in the *American Journal of Roentgenology* of March, 1933, and a similar Lauritsen tube had been used in the (above mentioned) Lincoln installation. Marinelli made several unsuccessful efforts to obtain a photograph of that tube from T. R. Folsom, a physicist who just then was searching the bottom of the Atlantic Ocean for the sunken submarine Thrasher. I wrote to Charles Lauritsen at Cal-Tech, and he replied he had no photographs, but could send me some of his early reprints, for instance the one in the *Physical Review* of December, 1928 in which he describes his 750 kv cold emission tube, which was operated from a four-cascade transformer. The room was 64x138 by 50 ft. high. The description of the installation, and the first therapeutic results were described by Mudd, Emery, Meland and Costolow in the *American Journal of Roentgenology* of April, 1934 and by Mudd and Emery in *Strahlentherapie* of October, 1935. I myself inquired with Folsom, at the Scripps Institute of Oceanography, and with Benedict Cassen (who co-signed a paper on the tube with Lauritsen in the *Physical Review* of September, 1930) but to no avail.

Incidentally, the turning point in making supervoltage palatable in radiotherapy was to a large extent the result of the excellent work done in Seattle by Franz Buschke and Simeon Cantril.

Returning now to the discussion of neutron therapy development, in 1940 Peter Kruger (who is now professor of physics in the University of Illinois at Urbana) reported *in vitro* experiments on the survival of transplants of animal tumors following irradiation involving the Boron-10 thermal capture reaction. The weak sources of termal neutrons available before 1950 precluded their application in human beings. As the Brookhaven Research Reactor was being completed, Farr and his team made arrangements with W. H. Sweet of the Neurosurgery Department of the Massachusetts General Hospital in Boston. Preliminary work conducted at Boston indicated that during the first hour after intravenous injection of boron in the form of borax, the concentration of boron was higher by factors of two or more in brain tumors than it was in the remainder of the brain. The first patient (with glioblastoma multiforme) was treated at the Brookhaven reactor on February 15, 1951. Definite tumoricidal effects were noted, but clinical results remained eqivocal.

Then the Medical Research Reactor was built, and it went critical on March 15, 1959. Patients are now being treated at this new facility.* Results in the patients under treatment will require follow-up for adequate evaluation. So far, animal experimentation (performed at Brookhaven since 1949) has proved that tumors can

*William Sweet is currently working in cooperation with the MIT. An operating room has been constructed directly below their research reactor's core. Only patients who have been operated upon (and had their tumor mass removed) are irradiated. Beneath the reactor the brain is exposed once more. The watery fluid which fills the space once occupied by the tumor is replaced with an air-filled balloon. The boron is then injected into trunk arteries leading to the brain, after which the patient is exposed to the neutron flux.

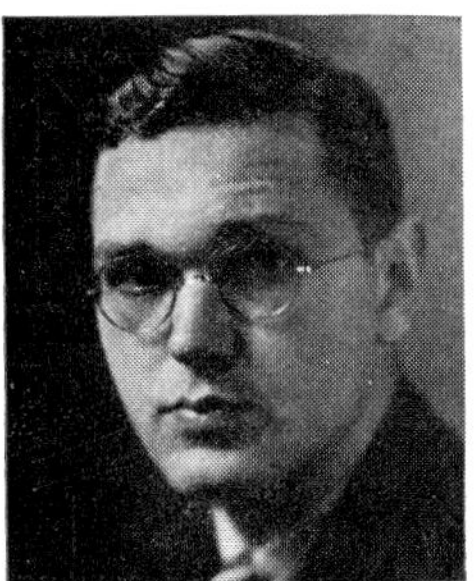
Simeon Cantril

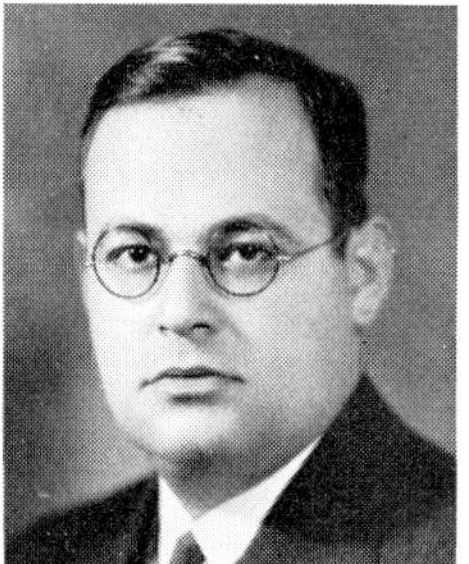
Franz Buschke

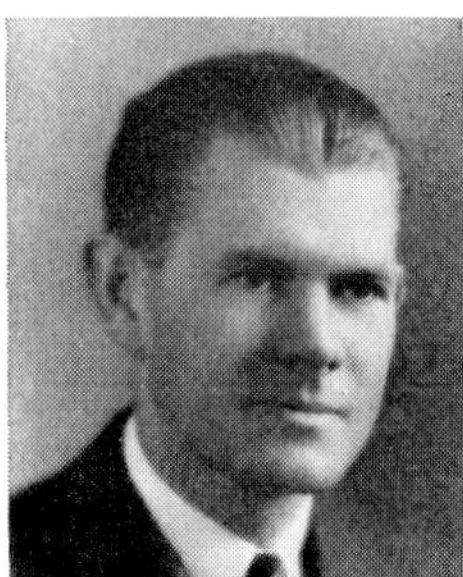
Clyde Emery

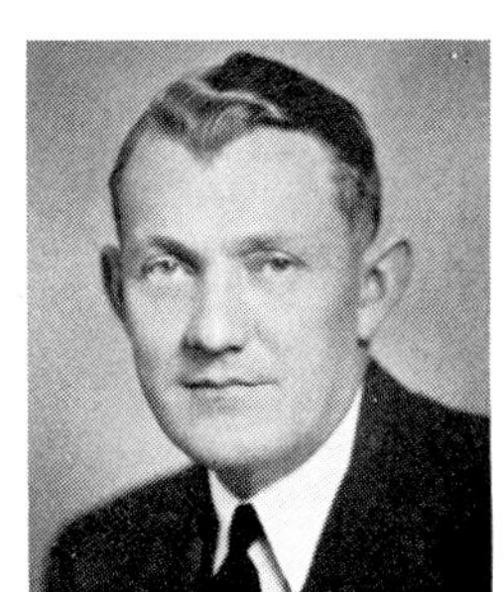
C. C. Lauritsen

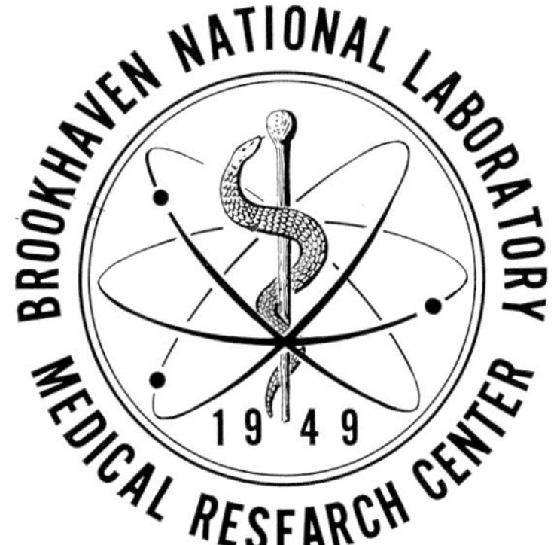

be completely destroyed by irradiation with boron-captured thermal neutrons. But animal experimentation cannot always be successfully extrapolated for the prediction of human response. This may have occurred to Brookhaven officials, or to Lee Farr himself, because at the time of my latest inquiry Farr* was no longer associated with Brookhaven. Only time will tell whether Farr's endeavor to use the reactor as a medical tool was the vain hope of a dreamer, or whether he was just too far ahead of his contemporaries.

AMF ATOMICS

In practice it is not so simple to obtain thermal neutrons directly out of a nuclear reactor if only because the gamma background must be kept low to protect the patient. Early schemes to produce "pure" thermal neutrons were based on the interposition of selective absorbers, but this caused *Bremsstrahlen.*

*Farr is now with M. D. Anderson Hospital.

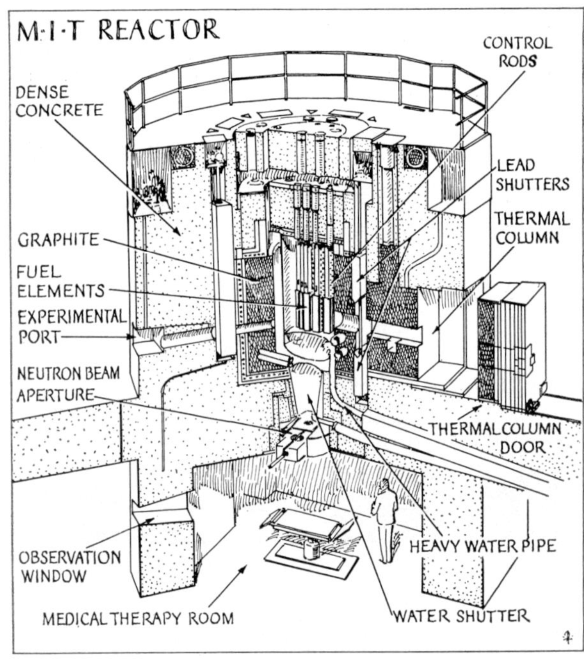

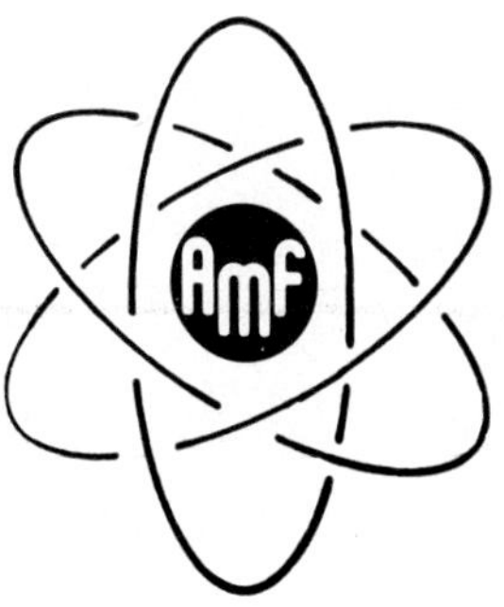

The Research Department of AMF Atomics in Greenwich (Connecticut) — a division of the American Machine & Foundry Company of New York City

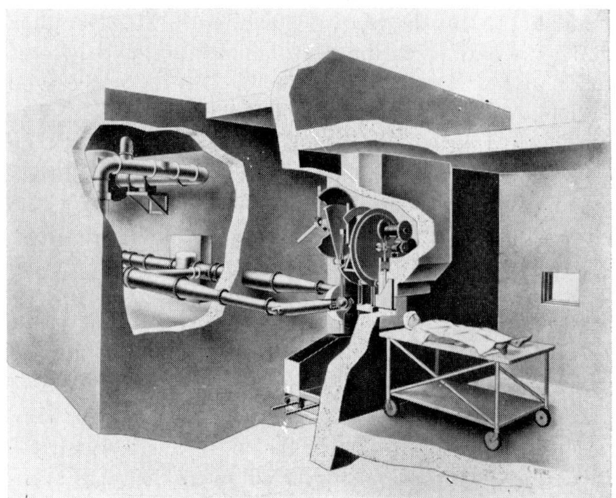

Courtesy: AMF Atomics.

AMF Atomics' SYFTOR. It is essentially a pulsing reactor with a moving shield between the heavy water and the target (diffusion-time discrimination). Adding at the proper moment a trigger amount of fissionable material will produce a pulse (surge) of neutrons. Most of them are fast, but they will be moderated by the heavy water, and will change to slow neutrons. By a gearing arrangement a shield with "holes" is rotated (orbited) in such a (synchroscreened) manner as to be in the "shield" position when gammas and fast neutrons arrive, in the "pass" position when thermal neutrons are "coming."

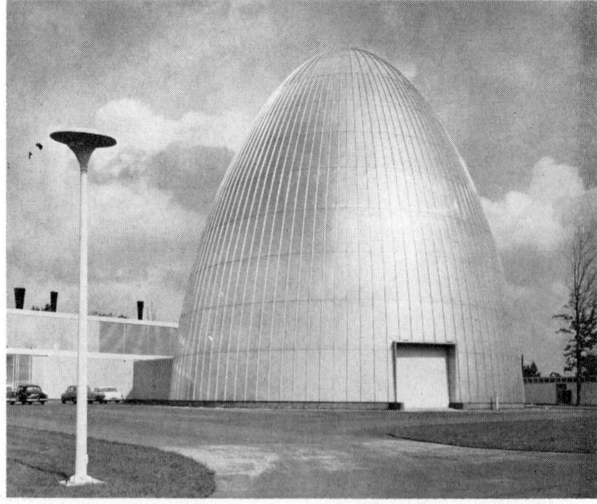

Courtesy: AMF Atomics.

IRL. The ovoid shape of this research reactor is located in Plainsboro (New Jersey). It is owned by Industrial Reactor Laboratories, a group of private industries, and was built by AMF Atomics.

— developed for this purpose the SYFTOR concept. The name is derived from *Sy*nchroscreened *F*ast Re*actor,* and alludes to the "sifting" of thermal neutrons out of the broad spectrum of reactor flux.

AMF entered the atomic business in 1942 when it began machining uranium for the Oak Ridge operations of the Manhattan District. AMF was knowledgeable in remote controlled machinery, and they started to develop remote handling devices for reactor refueling. After creating a special division — AMF Atomics — they built their first "civilian" (1 Mw) reactor in 1956 (at the Battelle Memorial Institute). In 1959 AMF constructed the 5 Mw facilities of the Industrial Reactor Laboratories (IRL) in Plainsboro (New Jersey): the IRL is a private venture of ten non-competing industries. In 1960 AMF built a score of reactors including the 10-30 Mw reactor for JAERI (Japanese Atomic Energy Research Institute) in Tokai-Mura; the 5-12 Mw reactor for the Oesterreichische Studiengesellschaft für Atomenergie in Seibersdorf (near Vienna); and the 1-5 mw pool for the Israeli Atomic Energy Commission in Rehovoth. They have also erected reactors in Turkey, Germany, Italy, Holland, and Portugal, and were considering one in Rawalpindi (Pakistan).

AMF Atomics also built Greece's first reactor, eponymized for Democritus. Its pool is set into the side of

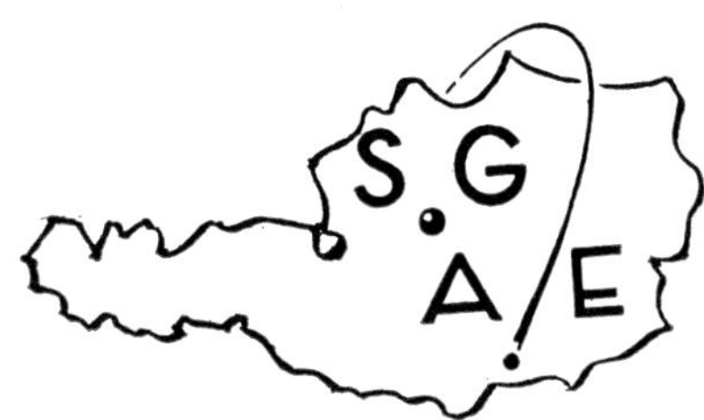

Austrian atomic seal. Mark of the Austrian Research Society for Atomic Energy, located in Seibersedorf, near Vienna.

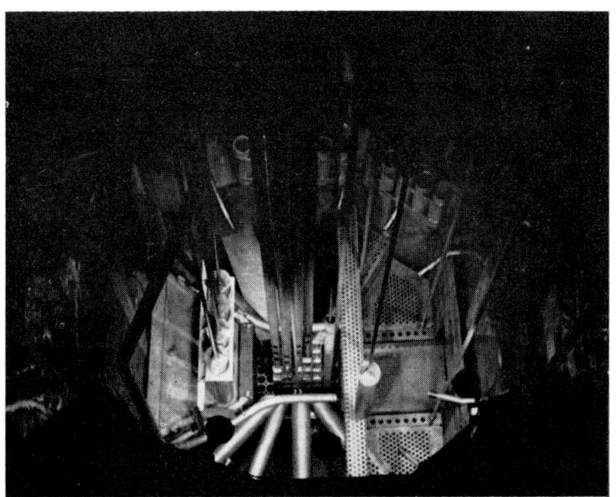

Courtesy: Oesterreichische Studiengesellschaft für Atomenergie.

Reactor core view. This photograph, by Christine Stanka, is "looking into" the innards of the Astra reactor, built by AMF Atomics in Seibersdorf.

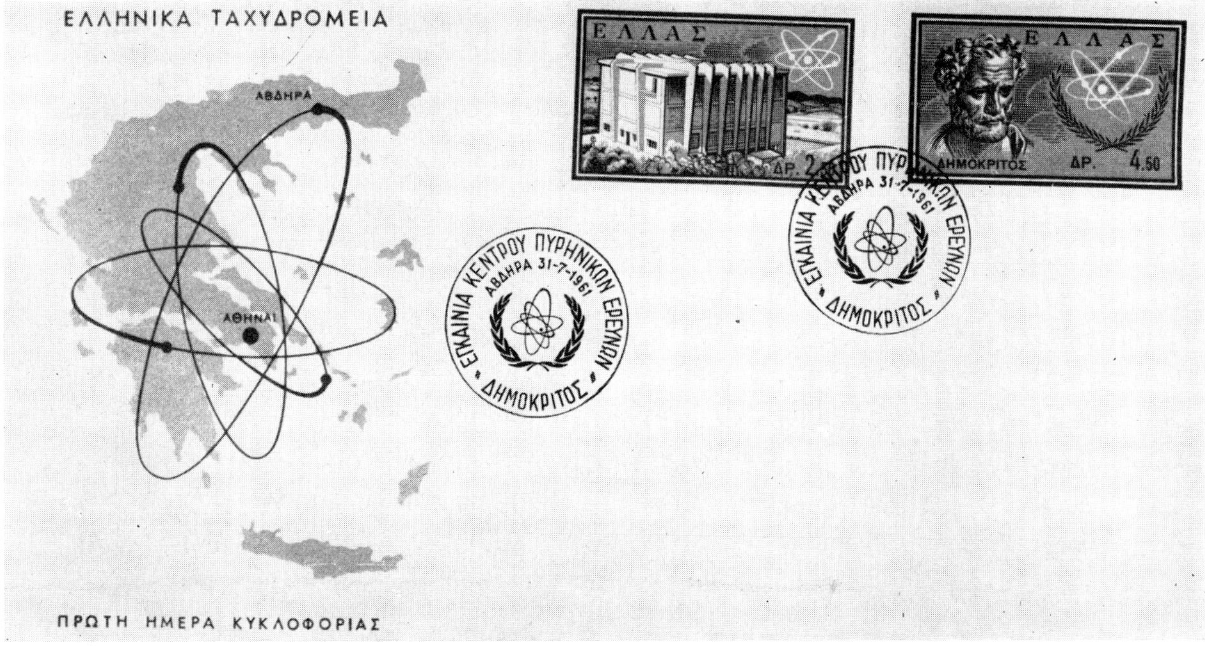

Courtesy: Stan Bohrer.

First day cover. Atomic stamps, issued on July 31, 1961, show the reactor building near Athens, and the head of Democritus.

Mount Himettus (near Athens); it achieved criticality on July 27, 1961.*

AMF Atomics has recently developed a light-water tank-type research reactor. They continue to manufacture a variety of atomic handling equipment, from simple manipulators to remote-controlled robot types* capable of recovery and neutralization of radioactive elements from crashed vehicles or otherwise accidented weapon systems components.

*Of major significance in the decision to build the Greek reactor was Queen Fredericka of Greece: for her unusual interest in, and knowledge of, matters nuclear she has been nicknamed the Atomic Queen.

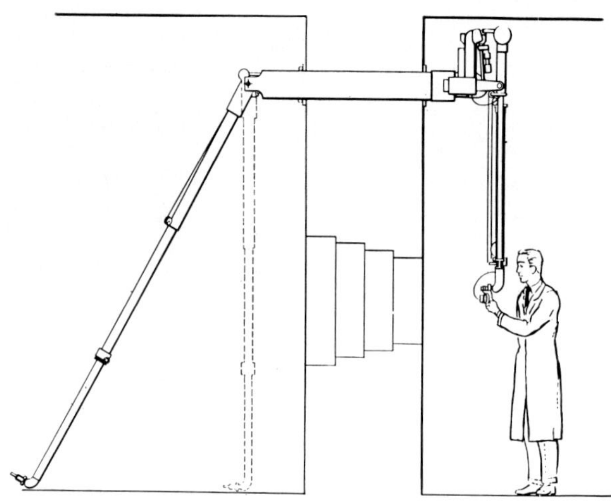

Courtesy: AMF Atomics.

MANIPULATOR. This AMF Extended Reach Manipulator is designed for extra reach – it has floor pick-up, in-cell storage, and other "modern" manipulator amenities, such as electric power assist and no loss of "close-to-the-window" handling capabilities.

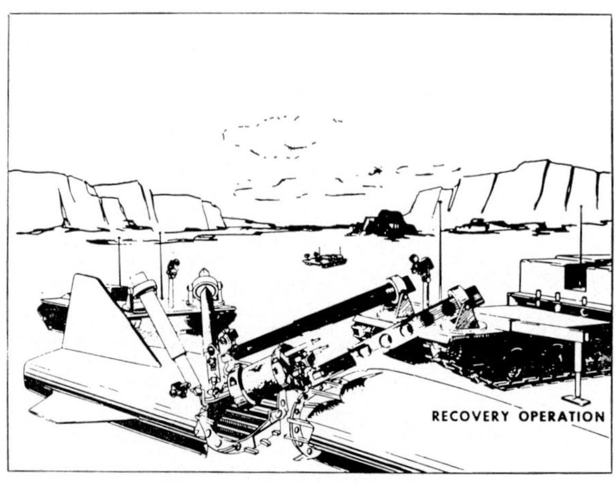

Courtesy: AMF Atomics.

REMOTE-CONTROLLED RADIO-ROBOT. This proposed mobile remote manipulator handling system may be operational at high but not at any level of radiation.

GENERAL ELECTRIC

Since 1946 GE operates for the AEC the plutonium producing Hanford Atomic Products Operation (HAPO) in Hanford (Washington), and the Knolls Atomic Power Laboratory (KAPL) in Schenectady (New York). GE's Atomic Products Division, headed by division manager Lyman Fink, consists of HAPO and of the Atomic Power Equipment Department (APED). The latter was established in 1955 at San Jose (California), with George White as manager. In the same year APED announced its dual-cycle, boiling water reactor design, which they regard as a major advance in reactor technology. In 1957 the APED dedicated its Vallecitos Atomic Lab.

In 1959 GE completed and placed in operation the 180 megawatt all-nuclear power plant for Commonwealth Edison at Dresden (Illinois), southwest of Chicago. I use the Dresden plant as a landmark when flying in that part of the country. It is located at the confluence of the Kankakee and Illinois rivers, and it is a beautiful site. This is particularly true when smoke from Chicago drifts into the area because of a Northeast wind, when one is trying to find his way, and when the sphere and smokestack finally pierce the haze, establishing an indubitable "fix" in space: that, indeed, is a most superlatively beautiful sight(ing)!

APED has built nuclear reactors from Moncloa (near Madrid) to Tokai-Mura (Japan), from Taiwan (Free China) to Caracas (Venezuela), and from Manila (The

*The cover of *Nuclear News* of March, 1962 carried the picture of the *Beetle,* a tank-shaped, robot-like vehicle built by GE for the USAF for just such manipulation of highly radioactive parts or structures. It had been ordered for a project which has since been dropped, but the strange looking contraption made headlines, and was pictured in newspapers and magazines.

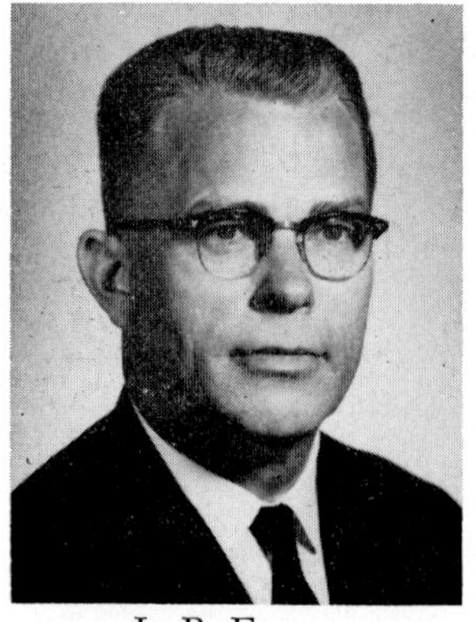

L. R. FINK

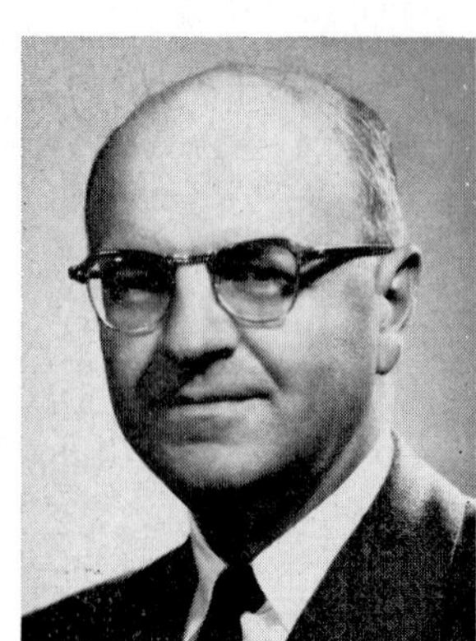

GEORGE WHITE

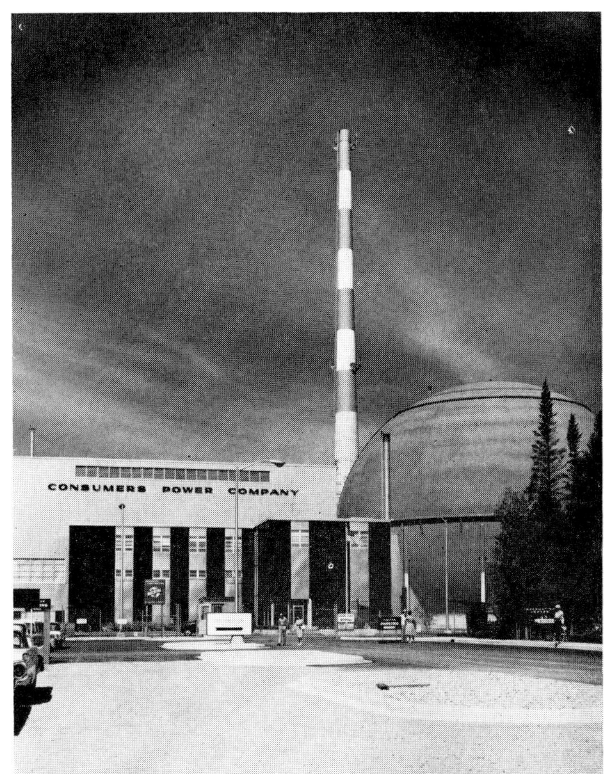

(Courtesy: General Electric)

BIG ROCK POINT. This is the 75 megawatt nuclear power plant, located near Charlevoix (Michigan). Full power production was achieved in March, 1963. A similar sphere and striped smokestag (for better visualization from the air) was built at the Dresden power plant.

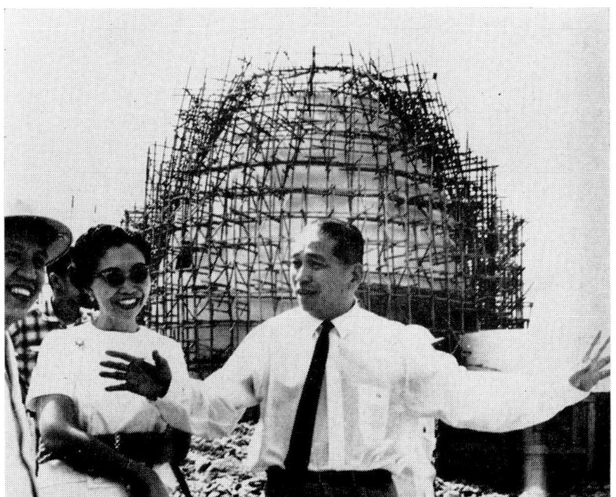

NUCLEAR REACTOR UNDER CONSTRUCTION NEAR MANILA. The figure in the foreground, with arms in abduction, is Paulino Garcia, a radiologist who was then directing the atomic energy program in the Philippines.

Philippines) to Garigliano (near Naples) and Kahl (near Frankfurt in Germany). GE has supplied 17 research, training and test reactors for university, government, and commercial research laboratories; nuclear fuel for 35 reactors; instrumentation for 40 reactors (including the first one scheduled for launching into space, the SNAP-10A).

REACTORS REPLETE

Nuclear reactors come in all sizes, even portable models are available for special purposes, demonstration or teaching. The SNAP (Systems for Nuclear Auxiliary Power), billed as the world's smallest nuclear reactor power plant, is being developed by Atomics International, a division of North American Aviation: it is aimed to deliver several kw of electricity from only a few hundred pounds of total power plant weight. A very tidy, almost house-broken, research reactor, dressed in stainless steel so that it can be placed right into the "living room," has been marketed — together with a well-orbited trademark — by Aerojet-General Nucleonics (AGN) in Southern California. Westinghouse built a number of reactors, and organized its own Astronuclear Laboratory. This listing is barely representative, there are several other firms in this field, for

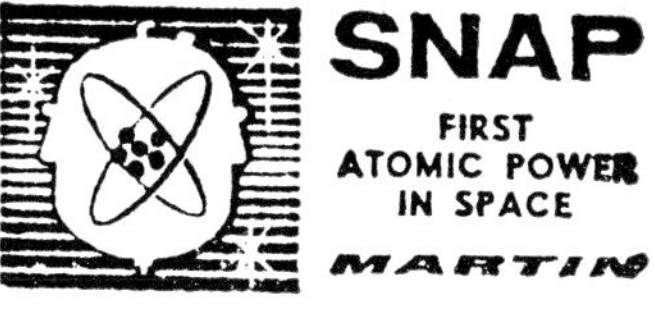

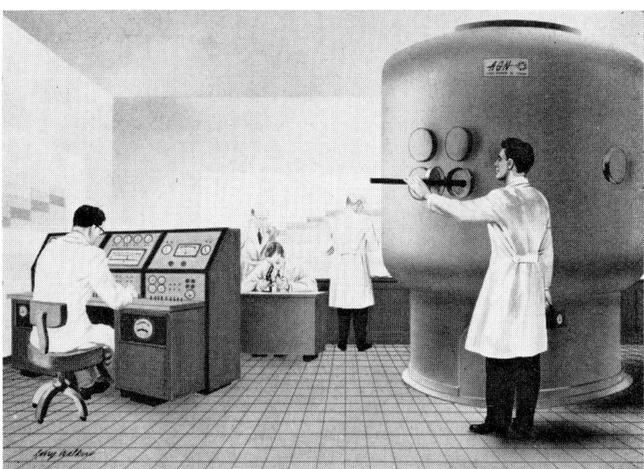

Courtesy: AGN.

AGN RESEARCH REACTOR. Aerojet-General Nucleonics' model 201 nuclear reactor in typical self-contained version with control console.

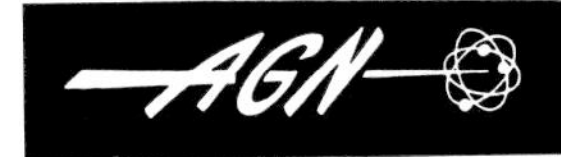

instance Babcock & Wilcox, and United Nuclear. And there is Allis-Chalmers, the builder of MIT's one megawatt thermal column and medical therapy facility with a water and boron-filled shutter arrangement.

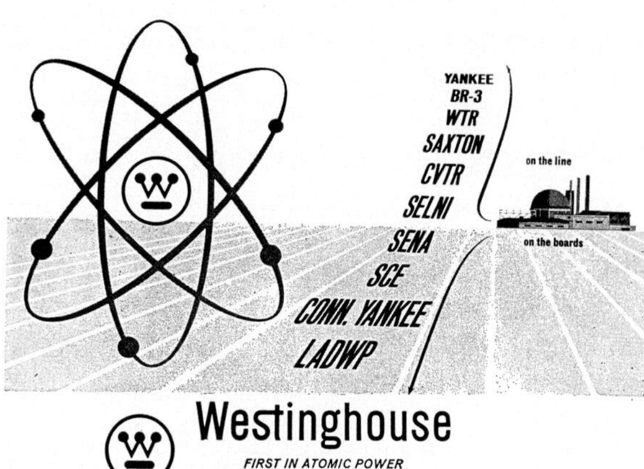

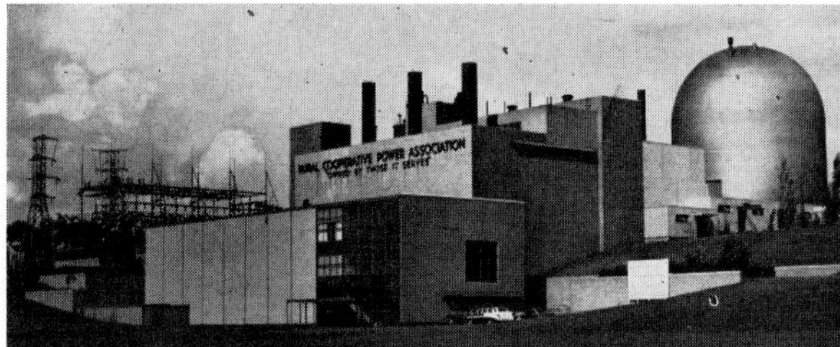

Courtesy: Allis-Chalmers.

RURAL REACTOR. This 58,200 kwt boiling-water power reactor is being built by Allis-Chalmers for the Rural Cooperative Power Association of Elk River (Minnesota), under the AEC Power Demonstration Program. It will be operated with the existing RCPA power plant, and will produce steam at the same temperature and pressure as that from existing boilers. The reactor and the conventional boilers are entirely compatible. This reactor is similar to the EBWR, but it has certain improvements, for instance spent fuel elements are transferred from the reactor vessel to the storage well entirely under water by raising the water level in the reactor vessel.

P.O. BOX 427 • OAK RIDGE, TENN.

GENERAL ATOMIC

John Victoreen once considered making hearing aids, but not of the smallest size, nor of the most inconspicuous shape: he was willing to settle for reasonable bulk and weight, provided the sound was of the highest possible fidelity.* A research reactor should be powerful, but it must not be expected to create power for power's sake; it has to be first of all inherently safe. Just such

*The problem is more complicated than that. Hearing losses vary in degree with certain wavelengths. The best hearing aid should provide sound at those levels at which the prospective wearer's audiometric test has shown preserved hearing. Any takers for the tip?

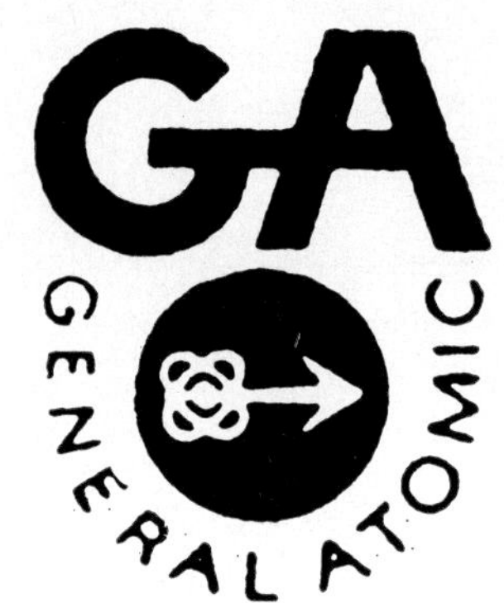

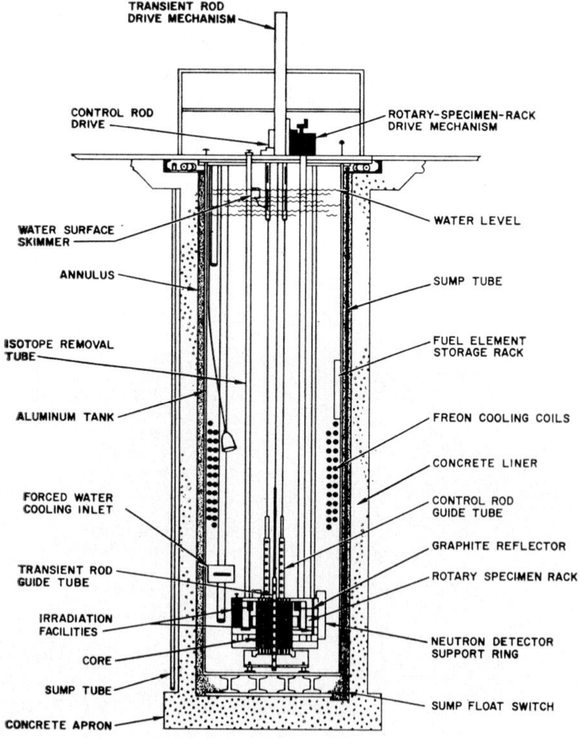

Courtesy: General Atomic.

GA's TRIGA MARK I. Tank arrangement for this U-ZrH fueled under-ground tank type of reactor with pulsing possibilities.

a development is TRIGA, a type of reactor designed, built, and marketed by General Atomic (GA) – a division of General Dynamics Corporation – in San Diego (California).

GA was founded in 1955 by the Vienna-born fission physicist and meson theorist Friedrich DeHoffmann (president of GA since 1959) — with the administrative assistance of John Jay Hopkins and Gordon Dean (from General Dynamics). DeHoffmann hired a group of physicists, established a laboratory in San Diego, and went to work. The TRIGA concept may be credited to three individuals, the theoretician Theodore Brewster Taylor, the solid state physicist Andrew Whetherbee McReynolds (both from GA) and Freeman John Dyson (from Princeton). They developed at San Diego a combined fuel-moderator element, using zirconium hydride as moderator. The uranium-zirconium hydride (U-ZrH) fuel rods are covered with aluminum, and contain an additive, to prolong core life. Its inherent safety is due to the physical property of the U-ZrH combination, which gives the reactor core a prompt negative temperature coefficient.

The acronym TRIGA derives from T(raining, R(esearch), I(sotopes), and G(eneral) A(tomic). The prototype TRIGA achieved criticality in May of 1958. That first model has been pulsed to instantaneous peak power levels of over 2 million Kw with no danger to observers, or the photographer. The prompt negative temperature coefficient of the U-ZrH combination suppresses automatically any power rise, even when the total available reactivity is rapidly inserted, and the reactor returns instantly to its usual operating level.

Since then over thirty TRIGA reactors have been installed in various places around the globe, from Urbana (Illinois) and Bandung (Indonesia) to Belo Horizonte (Brazil) and Ljubljana (Yugoslavia). And a TRIGA was installed as a purely medical reactor in the basement of the Veterans Administration Hospital in Omaha (Nebraska).

There is also a medical reactor group at GA in San Diego. It is directed by the hemato-radio-biologist William Frederick Bethard. They are currently carrying out neutron activation analyses of erythrocytes, leukocytes, and serum, and will also execute — on request — other specialized procedures in the field.

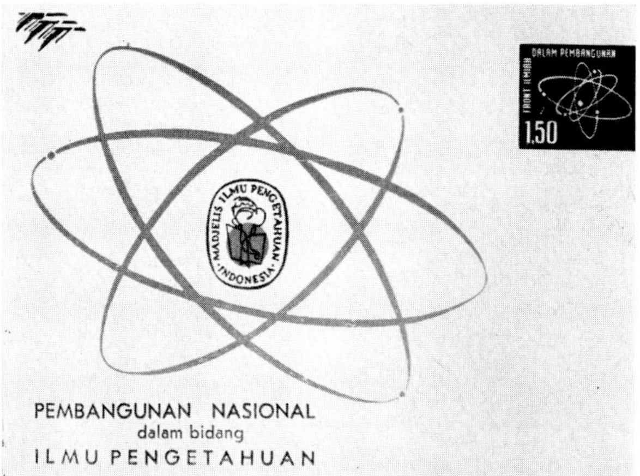

Courtesy: Stan Bohrer.

FIRST DAY COVER. Indonesian stamp, issued on September 24, 1962, to underline their nuclear program.

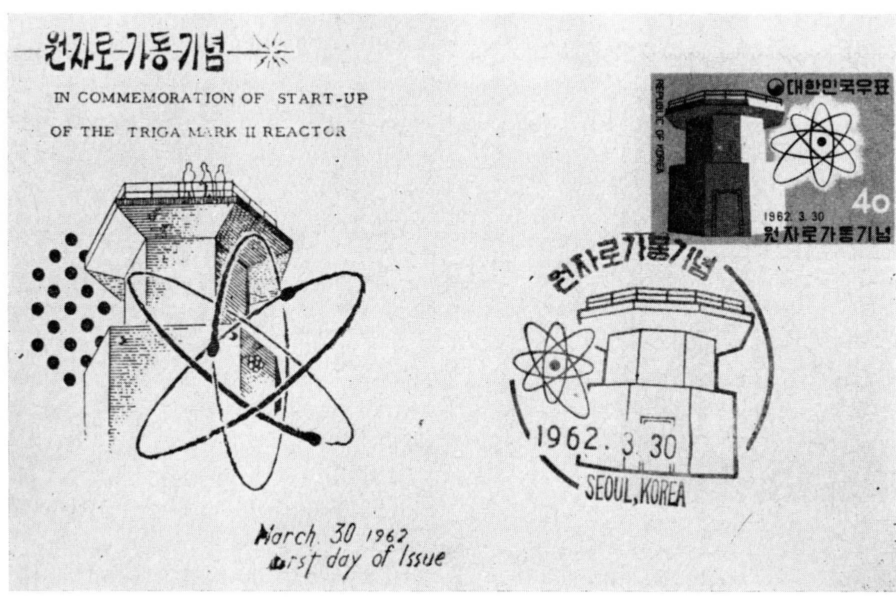

There are "pulsable" TRIGA models. One of these is the under-ground Mark I with a deep pool. The earth serves as shielding. The core is submerged in clear water (which provides additional protection). A central experimental tube extends through the reactor core at the point of maximum flux (for irradiation of small samples), and there is a rotary specimen rack. Extremely short-lived isotopes can be "propelled" from the reactor to the laboratory with the help of a pneumatic transfer system.

Similar facilities exist in the above-ground Mark II, which is routinely shielded by 7½ feet of concrete thickness. The Mark F is intended especially for pulsed operation (for which it has a thermal graphite column). It could become the forerunner of a model built for thermal neutron capture therapy, if and when that method were to become effective and established.

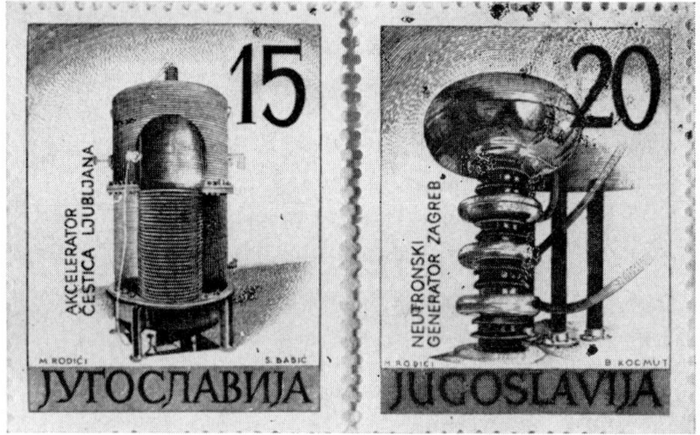

Courtesy: Stan Bohrer.

YUGOSLAVIAN STAMPS. First issued on August 23, 1960, they depict the accelerator at Ljubljana (where the Triga reactor was constructed), and a Cockroft-Walton, located at Zagreb. As we shall see, there is a reactor at Belgrad.

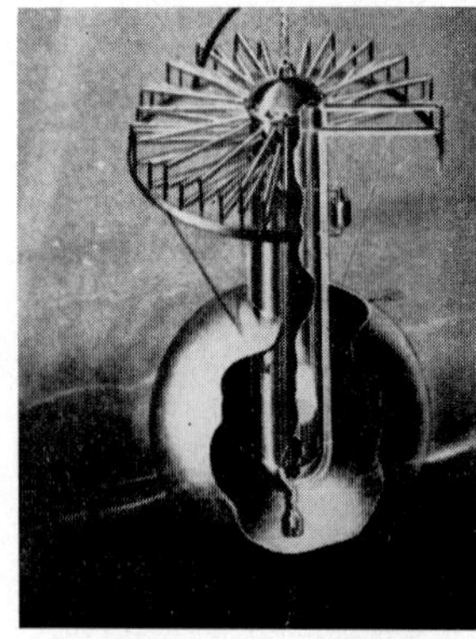

Courtesy: General Atomic.

ATOMIC PACKAGE POWER PLANT. Sketch of planned 50 kw undersea, self-sustaining power plant.

GA has many other nuclear programs and interests, including controlled thermonuclear experiments; beryllium oxide-moderated, high-temperature, gas-cooled reactors for both small-unit central station powers and for merchant ship propulsion; thermionic cells for (future) space vehicle propulsion; and its mother company (General Dynamics) built the nuclear submarines George Washington and Patrick Henry, first to fire "atomic" rockets from beneath the surface of the sea. There are also several subsidiaries trading under the generic name of General Atomic Europe (the first of these was in Zürich). At this point may be mentioned another atomic application to warfare. When a reactor must be very safe and very reliable, TRIGA-type U-ZrH fuel elements become quite important. They could be built into self-regulating, portable atomic power plants for underwater operation — a version of the 50-kw plant is on the drawing boards. By using a distant switching mechanism, such a powerplant may be turned on to provide a radio-signal on which a submarine could easily home in. Detection would be quite difficult because the signal would go on only when "remotely requested!" The currently fashionable method of sinking a strongly radioactive cache, and homing in on it with directional scintillation counters, is not fail-proof because such a radioactive marker beacon is fairly easy to detect.

These sketchy considerations of medical, para-medical, as well as extra-medical nuclear technologies have been inserted to emphasize the development of nuclear industries, which brings with it added radiation hazards (and inevitably some accidents). Such basic knowledge is also helpful for the understanding of the next section's expanded nuclear view(point?).

ATOMICS INTERNATIONALIZED

Formation of the International Atomic Energy Agency (IAEA) was approved during an international conference held in 1956 at the United Nations headquarters in New York City. The IAEA was actually created on July 29, 1957 and its first General Conference was held in Vienna (the permanent headquarters of the IAEA) in October, 1957. The main objective of the IAEA is "to accelerate and enlarge the contribution of atomic energy to peace, health, and prosperity throughout the world."

This atomic business has indeed become a world-wide proposition. Most of the so-called developed countries either have, or are planning to establish, not only research but also power (breeder) reactors,

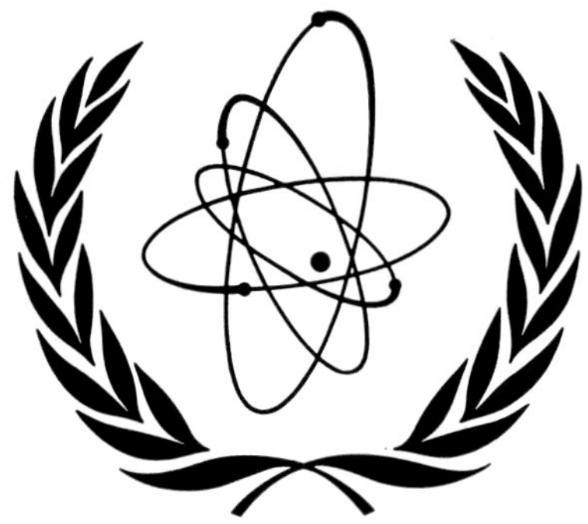

INTERNATIONAL ATOMIC ENERGY AGENCY
AGENCE INTERNATIONALE DE L'ENERGIE ATOMIQUE
МЕЖДУНАРОДНОЕ АГЕНТСТВО ПО АТОМНОЙ ЭНЕРГИИ
ORGANISMO INTERNACIONAL DE ENERGIA ATOMICA

which means plutonium, which in turn means (theoretical) bomb capabilities.

Reactor know-how inevitably leads to A-bomb capabilities. As emphasized in an excellent review in *Time* of March 9, 1962, the basic technology of nuclear weapons is well understood, the engineering problems have been simplified and the cost, so staggering in the early days, has been pared to the point where a bang can be bought for $500 million. Such advanced nations as Italy, Sweden, West Germany, and Japan could obviously do it. So, too, say U.S.A. scientists, could Austria, Belgium, The Netherlands, Switzerland, Norway, India, Brazil, Argentina, and Mexico. During the Manhattan Project, new instruments, materials, processes, even a new element (plutonium) had to be

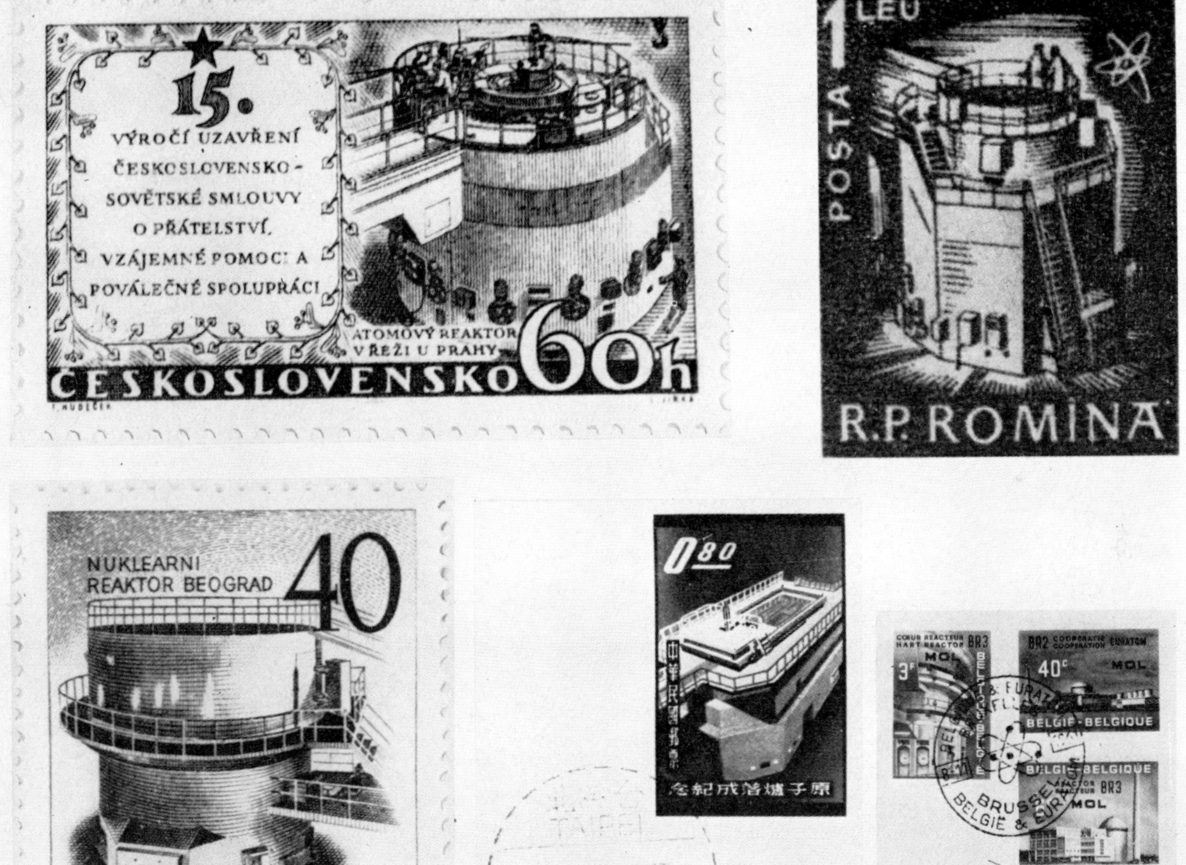

REACTOR PHILATELICS. These samples from Stanley Paul Bohrer's collection show Russian-built swimming-pool type reactors in Prague and Bucharest, and American-built research reactors in Brussels, Belgrad and Taipei. Power reactors seldom get this type of publicity.

created. New reference books had to be written in a new technical jargon. Uranium was a chemical curiosity, and the enriching processes had to be developed to get carload lots of it.

Today's candidates for the nuclear club need not repeat this painful pioneering; everything they need can be found in libraries. Only routine competence and a task force of 20 PhD.s and about 300 engineers could make something go boom.

It is still difficult to produce fissionable material, Uranium^{235} or Plutonium, but not as hard as previously. Nuclear "breeder" reactors cannot help making plutonium out of nonfissionable uranium while they are producing electricity. To separate the plutonium in "weapon-grade" purity is a difficult and dangerous job, done by remote control behind thick concrete shields, but there is little mystery about it.

Only a small amount of plutonium, about 10 lbs., is needed, as a detonator. Modern nuclear weapons (the Hydrogen or H-bomb) get most of their power from comparatively cheap fusion materials, such as Lithium and Deuterium (heavy hydrogen). The nation that makes or acquires a few plutonium detonators can upgrade them without much difficulty into city-busting H-bombs.

France exploded its first nuclear device in 1960, and is admittedly at work to perfect a fusion bomb. By the middle of 1963 they had four research centers devoted to nuclear science, 16 accelerators (including a 3.5 bev proton synchrotron), a plutonium production center,

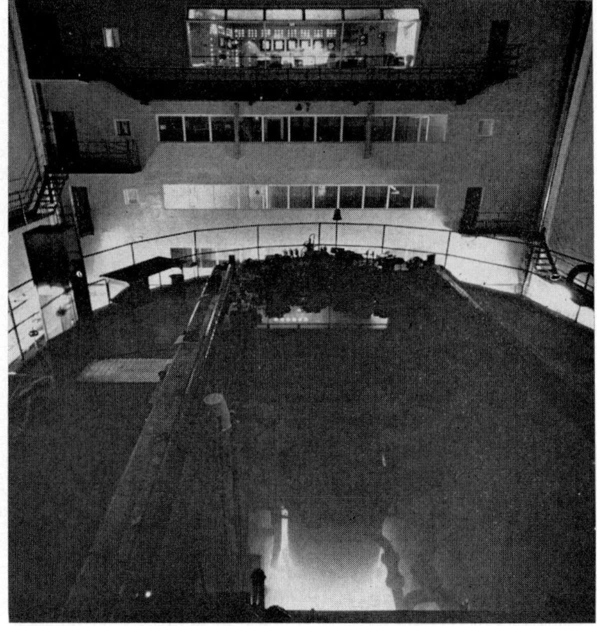

Courtesy: Allis-Chalmers.

SWEDISH REACTOR. Allis-Chalmers designed and built this 30 Mw high-flux research reactor in Studsvik for the Atomic Energy Company of Sweden. The reactor is cooled and moderated by ordinary (demineralized) water. The critical mass of U-235 is 3.00 kg. Construction started in 1957 and the reactor achieved criticality in May, 1960.

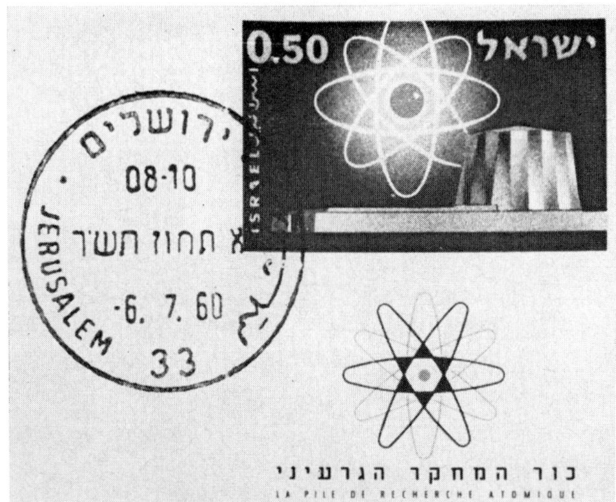

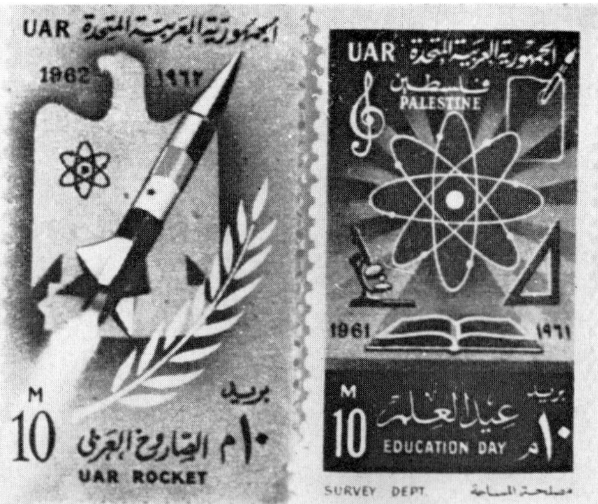

Courtesy: Stan Bohrer.

MIDDLE-EAST POTENTIALITIES. The stamp at left depicts the building for the reactor constructed in the Negev Desert (Israel) with French technical assistance. The two stamps at right indicate the joy of the United Arab Republics over the successful launching of a rocket, and at the same time their fervent desire of acquiring nuclear capabilities. Israel and the UAR are currently at odds. If they were to achieve some sort of agreement, with Jewish brains and Arab manpower they could build a state as influential as that of the Pharaohs at their time of glory.

17 reactors in operation (3 of them in power plants), 8 reactors under construction — in addition to a growing technical staff and the ambition of becoming a nucleo-military power.

Israel is completing a big power reactor in the Negev with French help and has the scientists to make the most of its plutonium output. Highly industrialized Sweden has a large corps of excellent physicists, big deposits of low-grade uranium ore and four reactors at work. At the moment, the Swedish program is purely for peaceful purposes.

India disclaims all desire to make nuclear weapons, but it has a first-class Nuclear Research Center near Bombay headed by famed physicist Homi Bhabha, and is working toward a large-scale nuclear power industry. Both Japan and West Germany have the heavy industry and abundant scientific skill, and could, if they chose, become strong nuclear powers in a few years.

Very little is known about the Chinese program, but they appeared to have started work about ten years ago. Chief of the project is the brilliant, French-trained physicist Chien San-chiang, director of Atomic Energy in the Red Chinese Academy of Sciences in Peiping. They have also other highly trained physicists. Joan Hinton, a woman physicist from the USA, who worked at Los Alamos during the bomb project, was reported

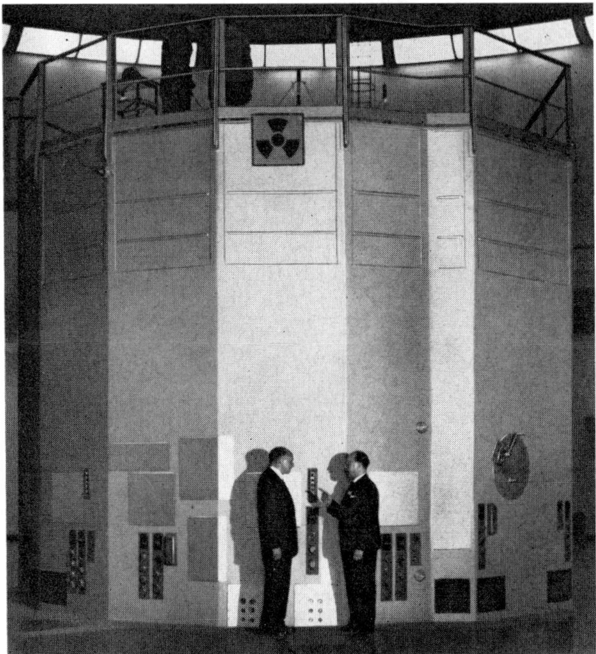

Courtesy: Allis-Chalmers.

ITALIAN REACTOR. The Ispra-1 heavy-water 5 Mw research reactor was designed and built by Allis-Chalmers for the Italian National Committee for Nuclear Energy, and is currently leased to Euratom. It first went critical on March 24, 1959.

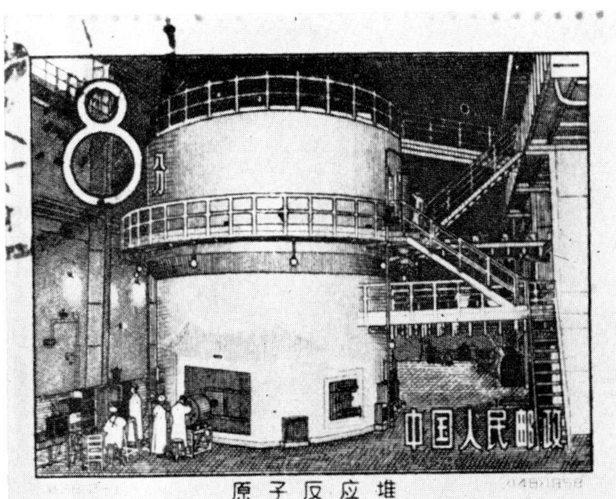

Courtesy: Stan Bohrer.

CHINESE RESEARCH REACTOR. Built on the outskirts of Peiping, this nuclear swimming pool was brought to criticality in 1958, for which a commemorative stamp was issued.

Los Angeles TIMES: September 4, 1962

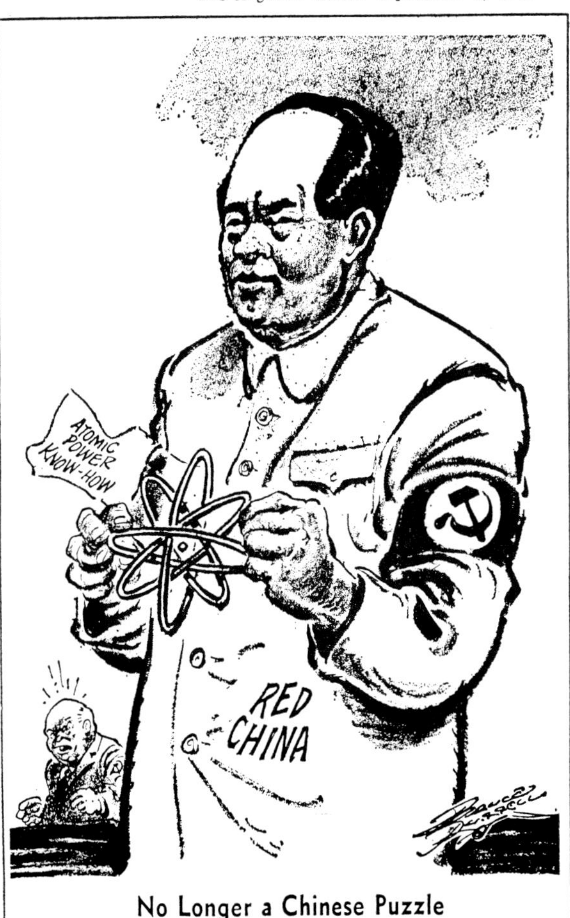

No Longer a Chinese Puzzle

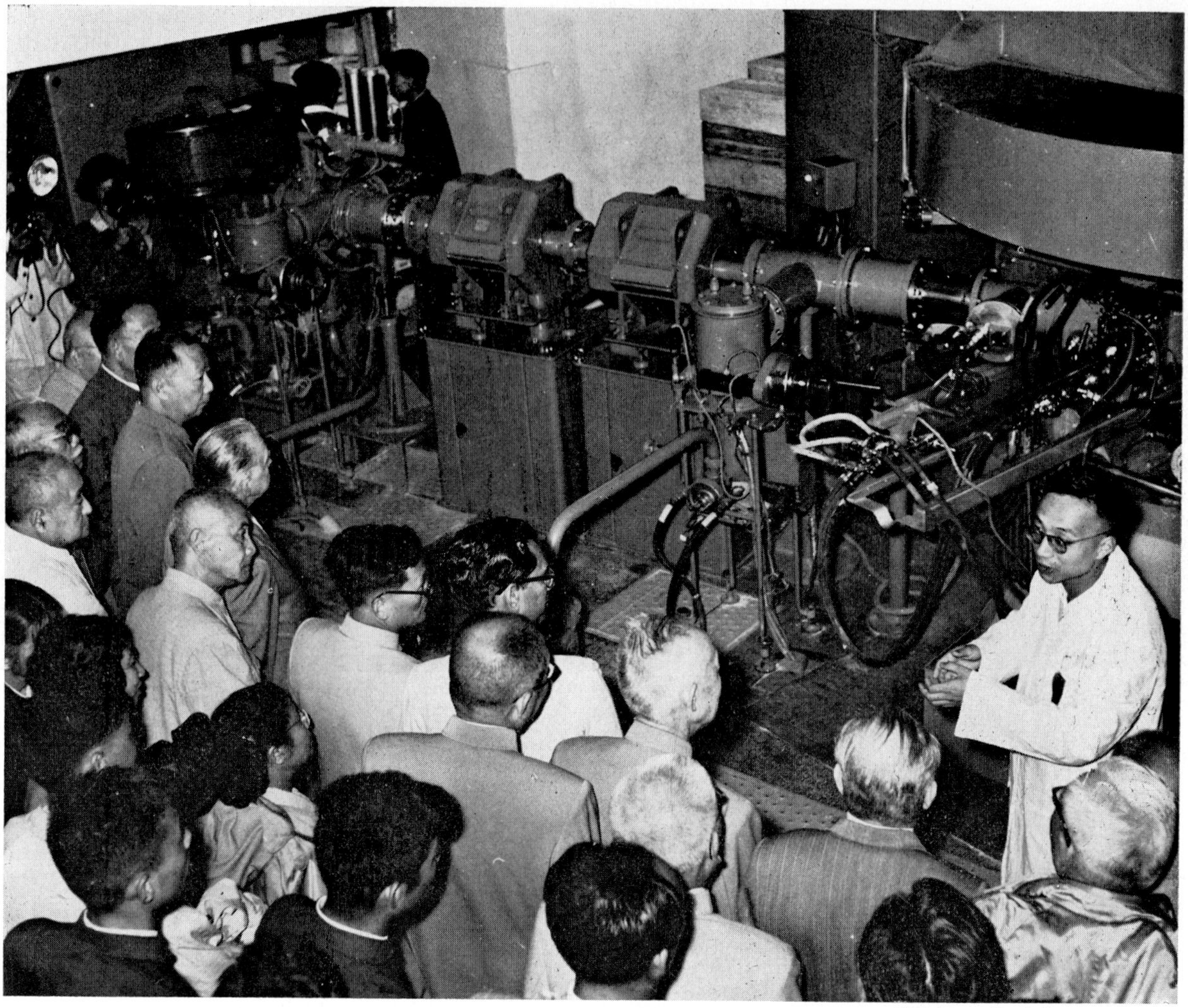

Courtesy: Sovfoto.

PEIPING CYCLOTRON. This cyclotron, and an adjacent 10 Mw research reactor, both of Soviet manufacture, were inaugurated on September 30, 1958.

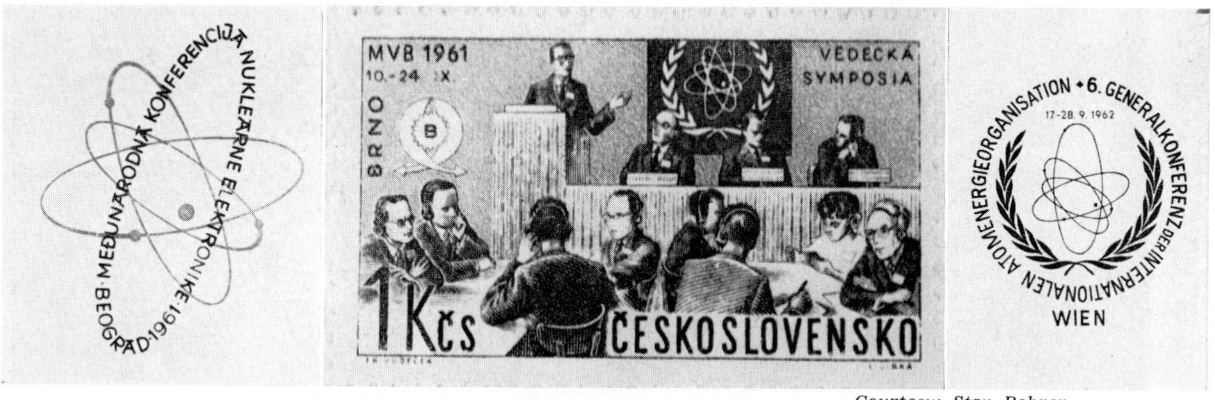

Courtesy: Stan Bohrer.

IAEA MEETINGS. Seals, stamps, and cancellations – all properly orbited – were issued in conjunction with several of the international conferences held under the auspices of the IAEA, such as those in Beograd (May, 1961), Brno (September, 1961), and Wien (September, 1962). Some "artistic" licenses are condoned in IAEA's tilted orbits, but not in its eccentric (?!) nucleus.

at a research center in Inner Mongolia. Italian-born physicist Bruno Pontecorvo, who defected from Britain to Russia, is believed to have worked for the Chinese. Most outside help came from the USSR in the form of scientists, technicians, and equipment. A Russian-built research reactor started working on the Chinese mainland in 1958, and it is believed that three other small reactors are now functioning. Rumors have it that a power reactor is also in operation.

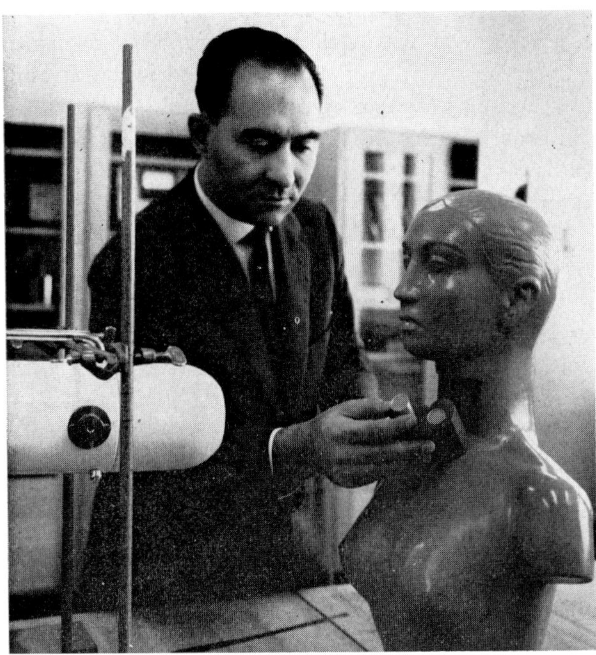

Courtesy: Paul Fent, IAEA.

IAEA MANIKIN. Godofredo Gómez-Crespo inspects the removable thyroid load of this austere dummy, built by, and located in, the laboratory of the International Atomic Energy Agency in Seibersdorf, in a building next to the previously mentioned Austrian Research Society for Atomic Energy.

A bit of history is always helpful for the understanding of a given situation. It all started with the Atoms-for-Peace proposal, issued in 1953 by President Dwight Eisenhower. That evolved a few years later into the IAEA, which was originally founded to provide assurance that the nations who were then in the nuclear club (USA, USSR, Great Britain), in spreading nuclear technology, would not be contributing to the spread of nuclear weapons. With 600 employees, and $7 million budget, the IAEA has become a very useful service organization, sponsors international conferences, and other means of imparting nonaggressive nuclear knowledge (such as training technicians). It is trying to develop standards of radiation safety, and waste disposal. From the beginning, the IAEA had been created (also) with the idea in mind that it would become the inspection agency to check on the entire world's nuclear installations. The members of the nuclear club (including the "sneaked-in outlaw" France, who exploded its own devices in the Sahara desert since 1961) have refused IAEA inspectors, even after an arrangement made in 1960 gave the IAEA inspection "rights" on thermal reactors below 100 megawatts (Mw). Recently, though, as a benevolent gesture, the USA invited IAEA inspectors to see four small research reactors in this country.

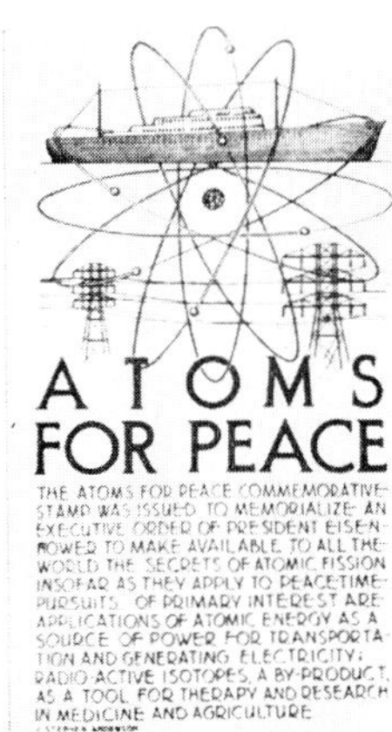

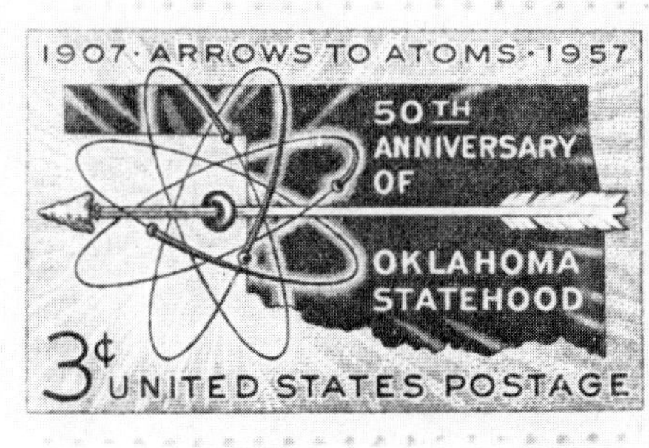

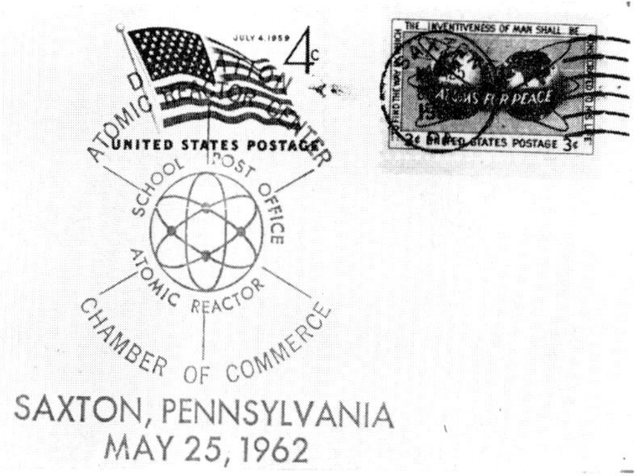

Courtesy: Stan Bohrer.

AMERICAN ORBITAL STAMPS. The *cachet* on the far left was used on the first day (July 28, 1955) of the twin-hemispheric (Atoms-for-Peace) stamp on the far right – the latter's inscription reads: ". . . to find the way by which the . . . inventiveness of man shall . . . be . . . consecrated to his life!" Use of the orbits in Oklahoma's anniversary stamp cannot be as easily justified as in the Saxton *cachet*.

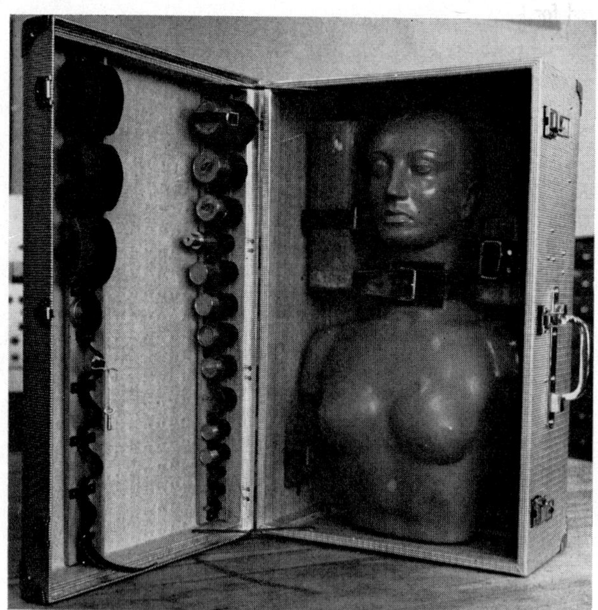

Courtesy: Paul Fent, IAEA.

MANIKIN'S TROUSSEAU. Although the IAEA placed all sorts of goodies in her bag (interchangeable glands and various standardized "loads"), and nature seems to have provided her with certain desirable appurtenances, her gaze must not be too appealing, because she never marries: when IAEA member states ask for scientific help in calibrating their machines, a scientific delegate of the IAEA accompanies the manikin on a standardizing visit to that member state. Both he and the manikin always get round-trip (*tour-retour*) tickets.

Outside the IAEA, bilateral agreements for providing nuclear materials and know-how have been signed between the USA and forty-four nations, and between the USSR and fourteen nations. In each case the USA as well as the USSR have retained the formal right to inspect nuclear installations in the countries with which they have signed agreements. This meant by-passing the IAEA, and it could result in the latter's "withering on the vine."

Recent "nucleo-diplomatic" difficulties arose from India's desire to have a power reactor. A contract is about to be signed with an American firm, the International General Electric, for the building of two synchronized 190 Mw reactors, which would mean a total of 380 Mw, and the capability of producing a sizable amount of weapon-grade plutonium. It seems that, sooner or later, the nuclear club will have to admit "new" members.

PRACTICAL NUCLEAR MEDICINE

Beginning in 1948, teaching facilities aimed at spreading the nuclear gospel were organized at various centers in the USA. There was the previously mentioned training facility at ORINS. Another one was at Cook County Hospital (CCH): at the then brand new Radiation Center, the combined team of Irwin Franklin Hummon, Jr. (physician), and Robert Stern Landauer, Sr. (physicist) started to initiate Midwestern physicians into the subtle and uncertain art of measuring thyroid uptakes of Iodine^{131}. At

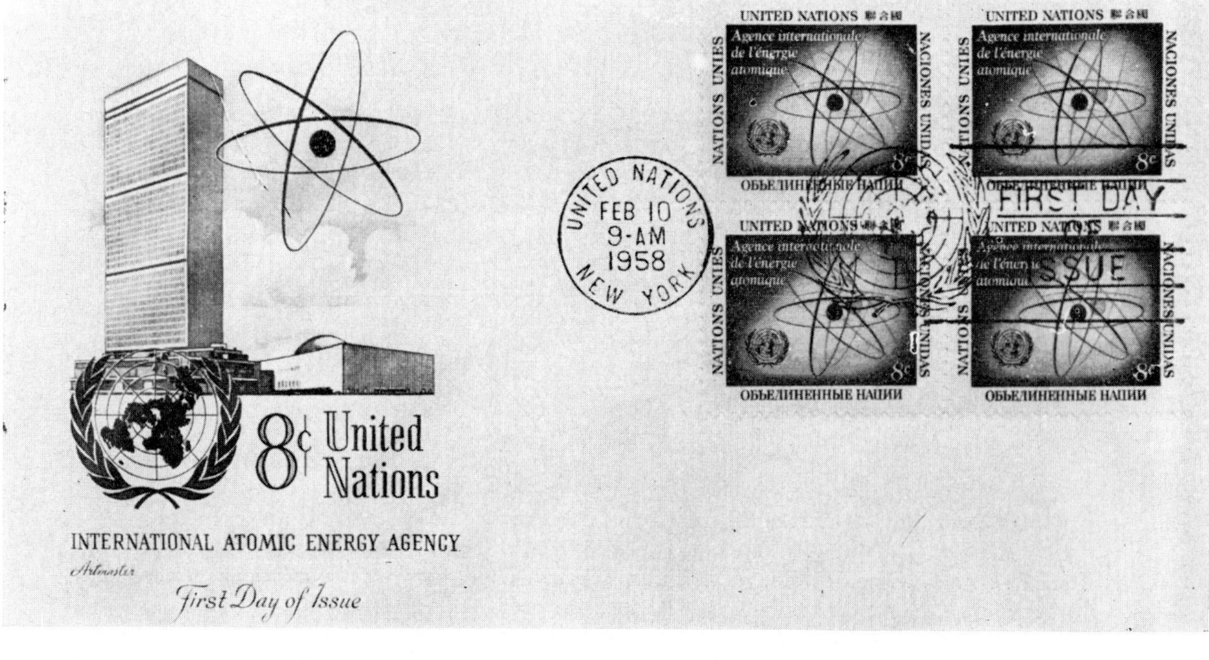

that same center were also accumulated significant series of therapeutic applications of the (now practically obsolete) radio-gold Au^{198}. $Phosphorus^{32}$ never quite became popular at CCH. Radioiodine (I^{131}) was used in the therapy of thyroid tumors, and in selected instances of heart failure and of hyperthyroidism. On the latter subject the recognized expert remains Frank Marion Magalotti (who since 1956 is director of CCH's Radiation Center as Hummon became chairman of the entire Department of Radiology in CCH).

On the East Coast Edith Quimby and Sergei Feitelberg at Columbia University (New York City) trained multiple groups of physicians.

On the West Coast of more than passing significance have been the achievements of a "nuclear medicist" who became a radiation casualty, the Czechoslovakian-born Bertram Vojtech Adelbert Low-Beer (1900-1955). At the time of his death he was teaching radiology in the University of California at San Francisco. He succumbed with a fulminating anaerobic septicemia, the terminal episode of a radiogenic myelocytic leukemia. His last article — a wonderful summary of the internal as well as external uses of P^{32} — was posthumously printed in the (previously mentioned) ORINS radioisotope course of 1953.*

OTHER USES OF CO-60

For the purpose of establishing the facts about the employment of Co-60 as a substitute for radium, I inquired with Isadore Meschan, professor of radiology in the Bowman Gray School of Medicine in Winston-Salem (North Carolina), and this is what he answered:

"After my Army service with the Western Reserve University Hospital unit, I returned to the School of Medicine at Western Reserve University in May of 1946, to serve first as a teaching fellow, then as an instructor in radiology. In July or August of 1946, Hymer Friedell was appointed as head of the Department of Radiology. As he had been associated with the Manhattan Project, he stimulated a number of us with an interest in radio-isotopes. The possible utilization of Co-60 as a radium substitute was suggested by him originally. I had had a fair amount of training with the utilization of radon needles and the like while I was in Australia, and was very anxious to work with Friedell on the use of Co-60. But in July of 1947, I left Western Reserve University to assume the chairmanship and professorship in radiology at the University of Arkansas School of Medicine. Friedell and I discussed the possibility of my pursuing this interest in Co-60 at the University of Arkansas, and this was done first by correspondence.

"The correspondence type of research met several snags and I then obtained permission from Friedell to pursue this interest on my own, and my first article on Co-60 with Raymond R. Edwards (a physicist from the University of Arkansas) and Paul Rosenbaum (at the time a physics student) appeared as the result of these efforts in the *American Journal of Roentgenology and Radium Therapy* of February, 1951.

"During that initial period Joseph Lewis Morton (now at St. Vincent's Hospital in Indianapolis), who was then teaching radiology at Ohio State University in Columbus, also became interested in Co-60 brachytherapy. Perhaps it was as a result of conversations with Friedell or with me; or perhaps he developed a spontaneous interest in this very obvious utilization. Morton's first exhibit on the subject *(Cobalt 60 for Cancer Therapy)* was presented – with George Callendine, Jr. – at the meeting of the ARRS in St. Louis in 1950. Whereas we removed the electron emission from Co-60 by encasing it in hyperchrome steel tubing, Morton and his

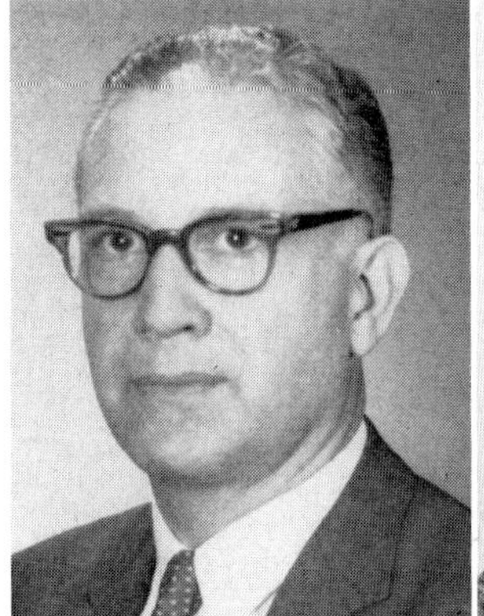

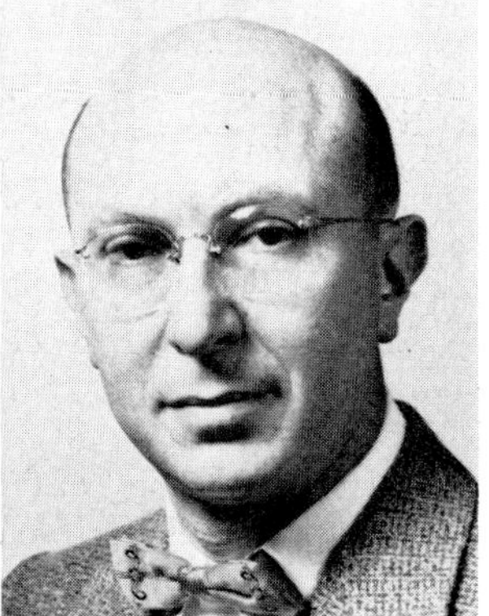

Co^{60} BRACHYTHERAPISTS. Joseph Morton (then of Columbus, Ohio, now in Indianapolis) and bow-tied Isadore Meschan (then in Little Rock, Arkansas, now in Winston-Salem) should get credit for developing this procedure, Morton especially for its use in nylon tubing, Meschan in stainless steel needle filters. It is difficult to determine who was the very first to have the idea: Meschan ascribes it to Hymer Friedell (formerly deputy-medical director of the Manhattan Project, now professor of radiology in Cleveland).

*His two middle names (Vojtech and Adelbert) were obtained from Low-Beer's "boss" and eulogist, professor Robert Stone. All other conceivable sources had been exhausted beforehand, including a distant Austrian-born cousin of Bertram, the Tulsa pathologist Leo Lowbeer (who volunteered the information that their leonine and bearish name was originally spelled Löw-Beer or Loew-Beer). The San Francisco Low-Beer was Bert for his friends: in his European days—he was already a recognized researcher—he used Adelbert as his first name (cf., *Strahlentherapie* of 1933).

associates used a nylon sheath, and emphasized the flexible, interstitial type of application. Among Morton's collaborators was William Myers a combination biophysicist and physician, particularly interested in the medical uses of radio-isotopes."

Meschan's name is actually much better known for his two popular works, *Normal Radiographic Anatomy* (of which there is a second edition), and *Roentgen Signs in Clinical Diagnosis* (1956), an excellent synopsis of the entire field, with many original ideas and observations presented without fanfare as if they were matters of fact (they were indeed taken for granted by several corps of residents in radiology).

At that point I wrote to Joseph Lewis Morton — who in 1959 had exchanged his academic position at Ohio State University in Columbus for the post of private radiologist in Indianapolis. Morton sent my letter to Callendine, who now lives in Worthington (Ohio). This is the copy of Callendine's reply to Morton, dated November 2, 1962:

"I have your letter dated October 22, 1962, along with the letter from Dr. Grigg to you which was dated October 20, 1962, concerning the historical development of Co-60 for use in therapy.

"I do not know who first thought of cobalt as a replacement for radium. I first came into the picture after you had more or less settled on this. I was always somewhat suspicious that Dr. Pool had probably reviewed the periodic table for a desirable radioisotope at the behest of either you or Dr. Myers.

"My recollection of the use of rigid needles is that we used both steel needles and aluminum needles prior to Dr. Meschan. We used these both in carcinoma of the cervix and in other types of malignancies including the roof of the mouth. After some experience with this technique we felt that the flexibility of positioning the sources in nylon tubing was much superior for most applications.

"I recall Dr. Meschan coming to Columbus to visit us at one time and that we reviewed our program with him.

"I believe that most of the exploration and evaluation of the different alloys were carried out by us. The alloy being used at the present time by all of the suppliers is the same Haynes Alloy 25 which we evaluated and decided was the most satisfactory. As I recall we discussed this alloy with first suppliers such as Abbott and Nuclear Consultants in St. Louis and later with Oak Ridge National Laboratories but for no good reason we apparently did not publish our explorations. I would have to go back and review some of the data books to determine exactly when this work was carried out.

"I hope this will help in your answer to Dr. Grigg. I think that in the establishment of historical priority the distinction between Dr. Myers' initial work with you in establishing feasibility studies and his subsequent association with the program should be made. Following the establishment of the feasibility facts, it is my recollection that Dr. Myers was not vitally interested in the practical problems of development to clinical usefulness, but became very actively interested in evaluating the possibilities of Gold 198 as an additional replacement material. My recollection is that the concept and development of the flexible interstitial method was hammered out in our group in the radiology department.

"I remember Dr. Henschke talking one time about a letter he received from a physician who had used woven flexible catheters with radium some years ago. This physician apparently wrote Dr. Henschke that he felt he was entitled first priority for developing the concept of the flexible method. I do not know the details of this but it apparently came to Dr. Henschke's attention subsequent to his referring to our work in an article which he had written."

I sent a copy of Callendine's letter back to Meschan, who replied that what he had said the first time is all he could recollect. I wrote to Hymer Friedell, who answered that he did not know who was the first who suggested the use of Co-60 as a radium substitute in either or both brachy- and teletherapy.

As in so many other instances of secondary priorities, the man who had the initial idea (even the one who applied it for the first time) is not as important as the name of the perfecter of the method, the one who transforms the idea into a workable tool of routine medical practice.

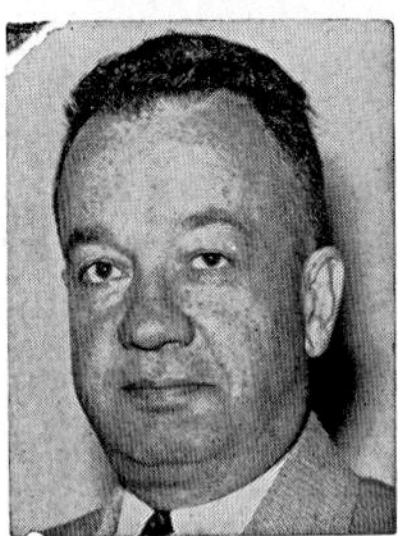
W. G. Myers

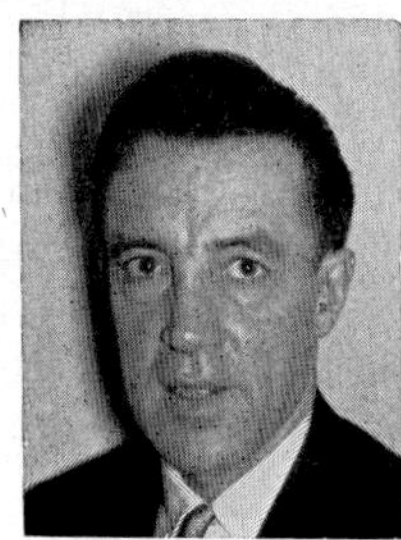
Ulrich Henschke

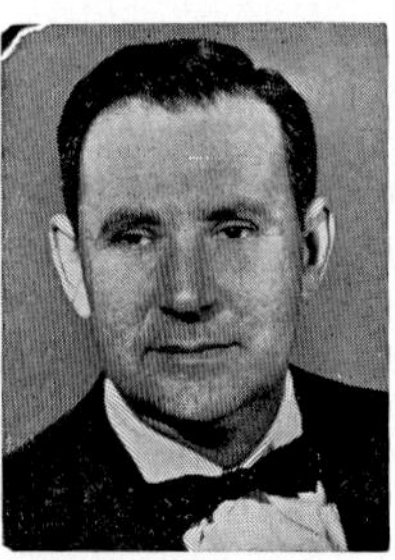
Hymer Friedell

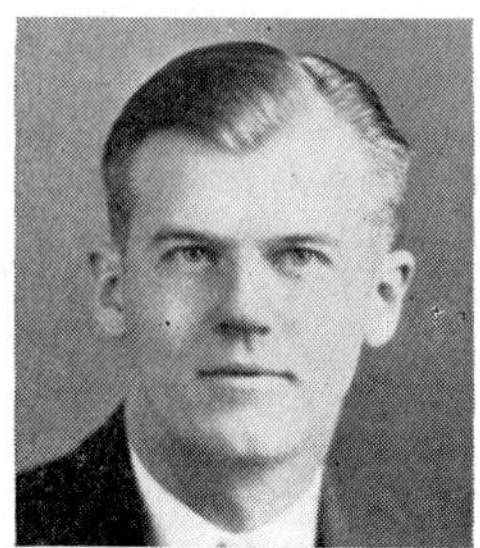
R. Van de Graaff

In summing up, the idea of using Co-60 in brachytherapy may or may not have been Hymer Friedell's. It was developed as a radon seeds substitute by Morton and his associates, as a radium needle substitute by Meschan and his associates.

OTHER NUCLEAR CONTRAPTIONS

The "electro-nuclear" appliances, classified under the generic term accelerators, may be circular or linear. The linear accelerators *(linacs)* are either electrostatic (the term accelerator is seldom used for this machine) or electronic (meaning that microwaves are employed as the accelerating vehicle).

The first electrostatic linear accelerator was conceived by Robert Jemison Van de Graaff in 1931, while he was working for the Massachusetts Institute of Technology (MIT). It is in principle a large metal dome, supported by an insulating cylinder. Negative electric charges are "sprayed" onto a high-speed motor-driven fabric belt, which whirls around within the cylinder, and transports the charges to the dome. By running wide belts at high speed (often as high as 60 miles per hour linear velocity), enormous charges can be accumulated and maintained on the dome. In 1932 – in an old dirigible hanger near Round Hill (Massachusetts), which served as his own shop – Van de Graaff built an improved version of his electrostatic generator. He succeeded in generating with it a beam of 5.4 mev, a record that stood until the end of World War II.

The idea of a linear accelerator was first suggested in Sweden by Ising, in 1924. In 1928, the Swiss engineer Rolf Wideroe (who is now the chief-engineer at Brown-Boveri) successfully applied the resonance principle in accelerating potassium ions to 50 kev, with an applied voltage of 25 kv. In 1931, in the Berkeley (California) Radiation Laboratory, Harold William Sloan and Ernest Orlando Lawrence developed a nonstatic accelerator wherein heavy ions were sent through tube segments. Each of these segments was alternately field-free, and then negatively charged. The ions "drifted" through the field-free segment toward the next (charged) segment which – like any respectable ideal – seemed always at least one step ahead (away). The procedure required accurate timing (a case of resonance to avoid out-of-phase situations): this is why increasingly longer segments were placed toward the end. With a 30-section accelerating tube, Sloan and Lawrence produced a 1.3 mev beam of charged mercury ions. For further improvements they needed a faster "vehicle," which did not become available until it was perfected in the radar developments of World War II.

This is where the Varian brothers came into the picture. During his varsity days, Russell Harrison Varian (1898-1959) had roomed with William Waalvord Hansen (1909-1949). That was in 1934 at Stanford. They had many arguments over what was the best way of producing million-volt x rays. Hansen thought that accelerating electrons by cycling them through a high frequency oscillating field ought to be a good way (which makes him one of the precursors of the beta-

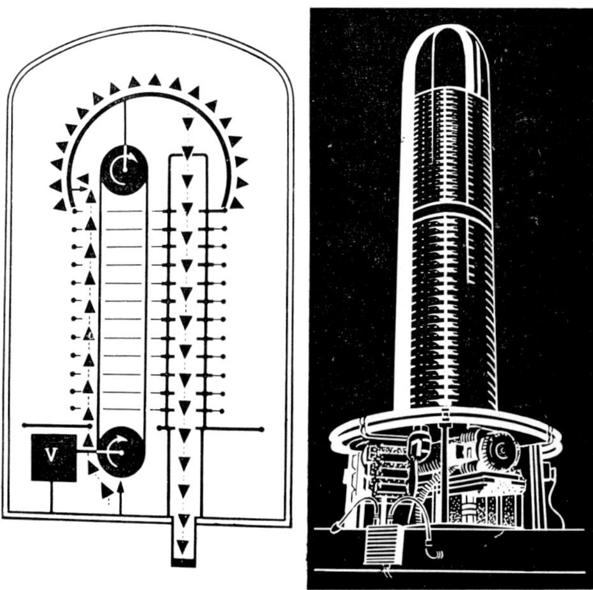

Courtesy: HVEC.

VAN DE GRAAFF ELECTROSTATIC LINAC. At left is the diagram of the belt, the dome, and the encasing cylinder. At right is the actual appearance after removal of the encasing cylinder.

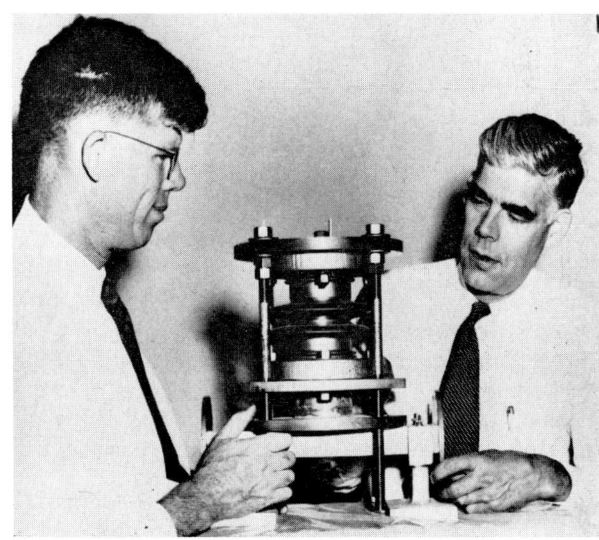

Courtesy: Varian Associates

THE VARIAN BROTHERS WITH A KLYSTRON. This photograph, taken around 1939, shows Russell Harrison Varian, with glasses, and Sigurd Varian, inspecting a twin cavity (oscillator type of) klystron.

tron). From this he came up with a special vacuum tube, a huge contraption, called the "oscillating sphere," sometimes nicknamed the "rhumbatron."

Russell's younger brother, Sigurd Furgus Varian (1901-1961) went for two years to the California Polytechnic, then took up stunt flying (in World War I "Jennies"), became in 1930 a commercial pilot (he was one of the first to fly scheduled Mexican and South American routes for Pan American Airways), later opened his own flying school, and finally decided to join his brother Russell, who had a sort of "electric" shop in their home town Halcyon (California). Sigurd had become concerned with the dangers of foreign offensive air power, and at the same time hoped to find something of value for instrument ("blind") flying. Both these "dreams" seemed possible if only one of Russell's ideas proved to be feasible. They spoke about it in 1937 to Hansen, who had stayed on in the Department of Physics (headed by David Locke Webster) at Stanford. Hansen was working on one of the rhumbatron's heirs, called the monotron.

A few weeks later the Varian brothers joined Stanford as non-salaried research associates: the departmental shops and stockpiles were to be placed at their disposal, and Stanford would contribute $100 toward materials and supplies. The Varian brothers had between them about $4000 on which they and their families lived for the next few years. It was agreed that if any financial return should result from their work, it would be divided equally in a three-way split between the Varians, Hansen, and Stanford University.

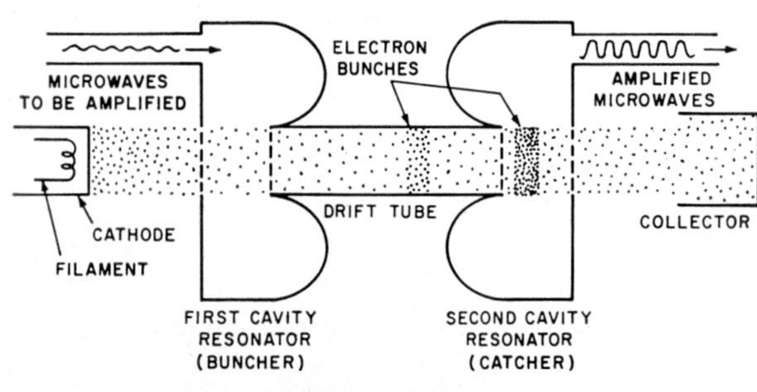

Courtesy: Varian Associates.

Diagram of oscillating klystron. Microwaves fed into the resonator cavity modulate the speed of the electrons emitted by the cathode (hot filament). Because of such modulation, the electrons travel through the drift tube in bunches corresponding to the frequency of the respective microwaves. As the electrons are "caught" in the second cavity, they give up their energy to the catcher, thus reproducing the microwave bunching pattern. With the exception of heat and similar losses, the potential applied between cathode and collector is added to, *i.e.*, amplifies, the initial energy of the microwaves.

Russell's idea was brilliant, but its actual implementation required mechanical skill, and much inventivity, because no "components" were available. Sigurd, an excellent "electro-mechanist," improvised the necessary instruments and parts. They both worked feverishly, and in a few months constructed the first, rudimentary model 'A' Klystron: it oscillated for the first time on the evening of August 19, 1937 in their laboratory at Stanford. This was not "announced" until January, 1939 and even then it remained a well-guarded secret because of its military importance. They had worked so hard that when they finally signed the contract, Sigurd collapsed; he was found to have active pulmonary tuberculosis, and spent the following six months in a tuberculosis sanitarium. Because the klystron became the heart (beam producer) in radar, the entire development was a hush-hush proposition, with an airplane instrument maker (the Sperry Gyroscope Company) opening up a special laboratory in Garden City (Long Island), manned by the brothers Varian, Hansen, and several associates from Stanford.

The klystron was used by the Allies in radar sets, which proved to be a significant factor in winning World War II, just as Sigurd had hoped it would. Today the klystron is ubiquitous in many fields, in tracking and guidance systems, and in communications (where it generates the microwaves for television, telephone, and other data transmissions). At the time of his death (he drowned after a crash-landing on the Pacific Coast of Mexico), Sigurd Varian had been retired because of ill health: he had willed to a local hospital in Puerto Vallarta (Mexico) $500,000 from his estate, valued at $3 million.

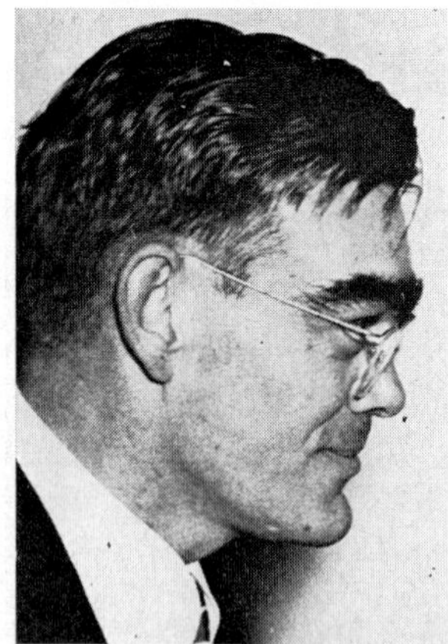

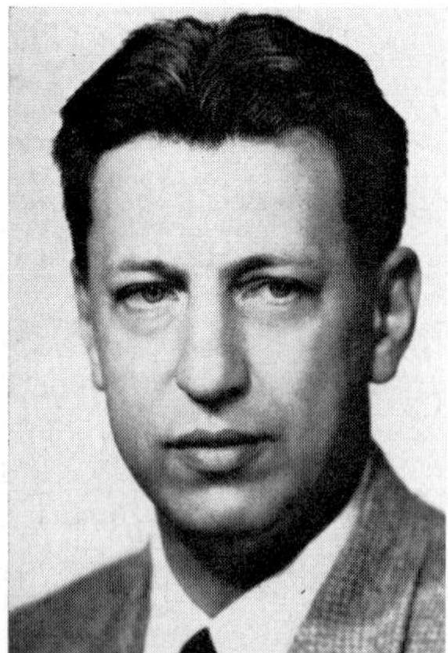

Courtesy: Varian Associates.

William Waalvord Hansen. At Stanford University, after years of search, Hansen finally built the first microwave, klystron-powered linac in 1949, and died the same year of pneumonia. On the viewers right is Edward Leonard Ginzton. The "linac specialist" and current president of Varian Associates.

In 1949, William Hansen and his associates at Stanford worked on the first high-frequency linear electron accelerator. They used one 10-megawatt S-band (2855 mc) klystron amplifier tube to produce an energy of 35 mev in a forty-foot long copper tube, which acted as a disc-loaded waveguide. It seemed as if the microwaves were returning the courtesies extended to them by the electrons in the klystron – in the linac the electrons were "riding" the microwaves fed into the copper tubing. A few months after this success, Hansen died of pneumonia, while working on the Mark III 1000 mev linac.

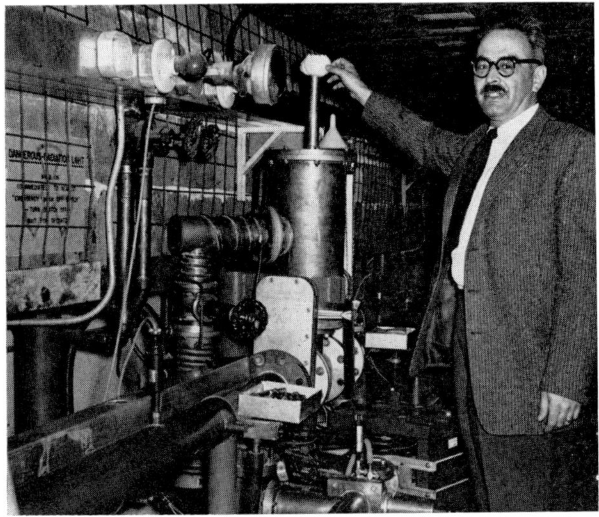

Courtesy: Varian Associates.

MARVIN CHODOROW. Director of Stanford's Microwave Laboratory, shown here at the side of one of their linacs.

The powerful klystrons needed to produce and amplify the microwaves for Hansen's electron linac had been developed for just that purpose by Russian-born Edward Leonard Ginzton (who was then director of Stanford's Microwave Laboratory), and by Buffalo-born Marvin Chodorow (who is now director of that lab).

VARIAN ASSOCIATES

The Varian brothers were opposite in many ways, yet they complemented one another in their strengths and weaknesses. Russ was a talented theoretical physicist, with unusual concepts and ideas, but all these would have remained speculations had it not been for Sig's initiative and tenacity in trying to transform them into working models.

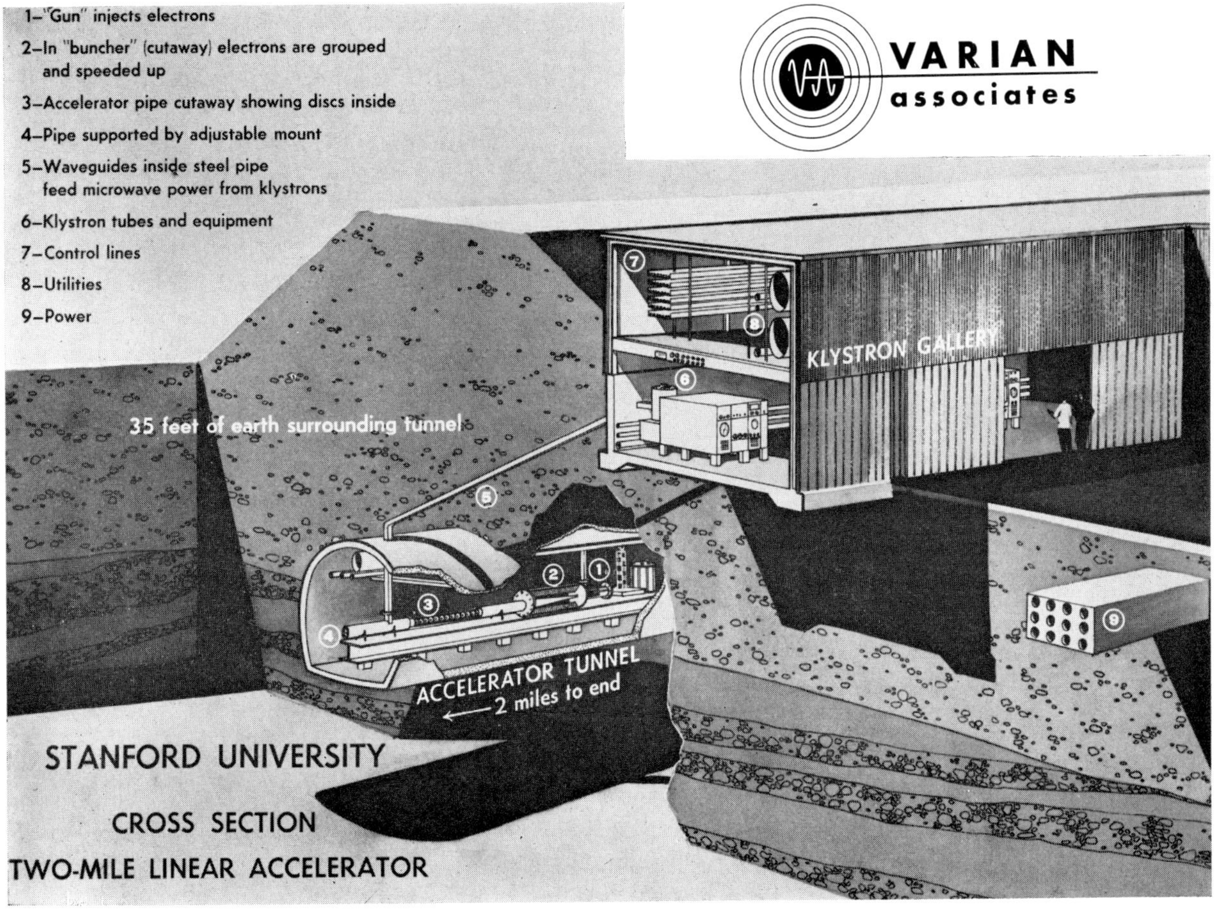

1–"Gun" injects electrons
2–In "buncher" (cutaway) electrons are grouped and speeded up
3–Accelerator pipe cutaway showing discs inside
4–Pipe supported by adjustable mount
5–Waveguides inside steel pipe feed microwave power from klystrons
6–Klystron tubes and equipment
7–Control lines
8–Utilities
9–Power

VARIAN associates

KLYSTRON GALLERY

35 feet of earth surrounding tunnel

ACCELERATOR TUNNEL
⟵2 miles to end

STANFORD UNIVERSITY
CROSS SECTION
TWO-MILE LINEAR ACCELERATOR

In 1947, in Garden City (California) Sigurd organized the meetings during which the company called Varian Associates was formed by six persons (the Varian brothers, Hansen,* Ginzton, and two other Stanford people).

Varian Associates had been formed with the intention to manufacture klystrons, and this they did. But they had also hoped to expand, and for that purpose a fundamental policy was established, and is still maintained: young people are encouraged to join, and grow up in the organization. It is set up as a company in which machinists, physicists, and engineers can participate in the management, as well as create and develop new ideas. Few incentives are as strong as that of developing one's own property, even when that property is only partly-owned.

Varian Associates grew into a bustling organization, with Ed Ginzton (born 1915) as chairman of the board, and Horace Myrl Stearns (born 1916) as president. More than half of their business is still derived from the manufacture of klystrons, but they have now a growing section of linacs (vernacular contraction from linear accelerators). Ginzton had been responsible for

*The headquarters of Varian Associates are now located on Hansen Way, named to honor the creator of the high-freq linac. Hansen Way is part of Stanford University's Industrial Park.

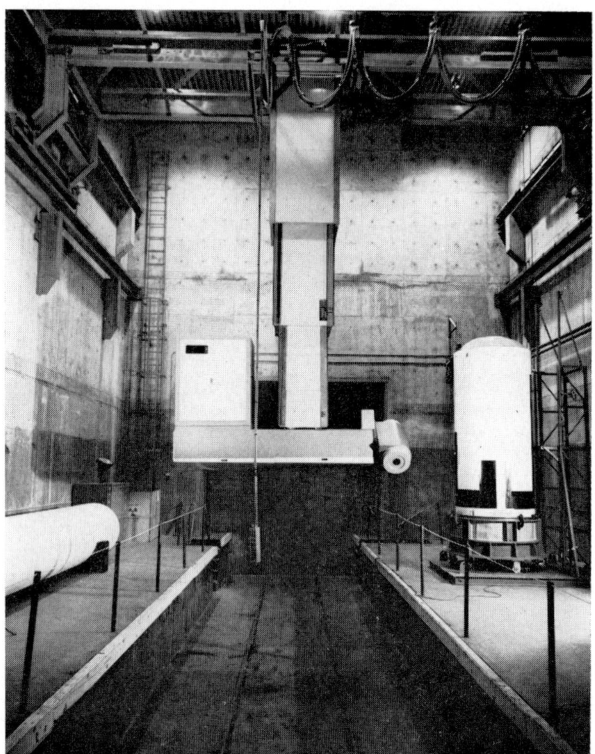

Courtesy: Varian Associates.

10 MEV RADIOGRAPHIC LINAC. It is shown with its telescopic hoist and bridge crane suspension, as used at the Naval Ammunition Depot in Concord (California). The white cylinder at right is a first stage Polaris motor. They had used their GE 2 mev Maxitron, then a Co-60 unit, but both were time-consuming, and necessitated about 100 exposures per motor, to detect cracks in the solid fuel. This linac (V7706), manufactured by Varian Associates, weighs about 8000 lbs., and has a rotating target (which prolongs target life). The Polaris motor rests on a motor-driven turntable for easy positioning. Vertical frame near motor is used to attach film holding devices.

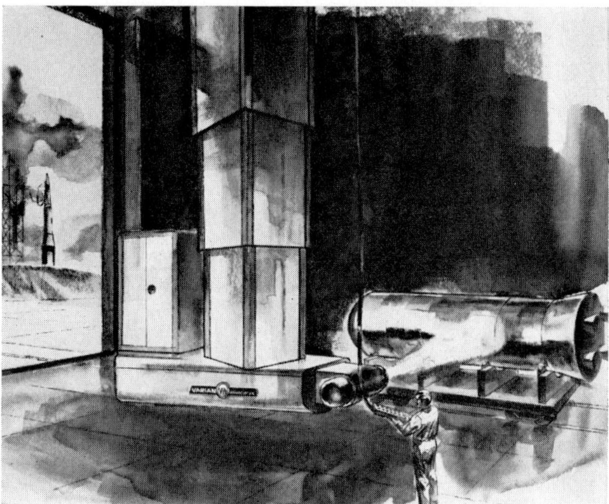

Courtesy: Varian Associates.

25 MEV RADIOGRAPHIC LINAC. Artist's conception of 25 mev model under construction at Varian for use by the USAF in radiographic inspection of Minuteman and other large, solid fuel, missiles.

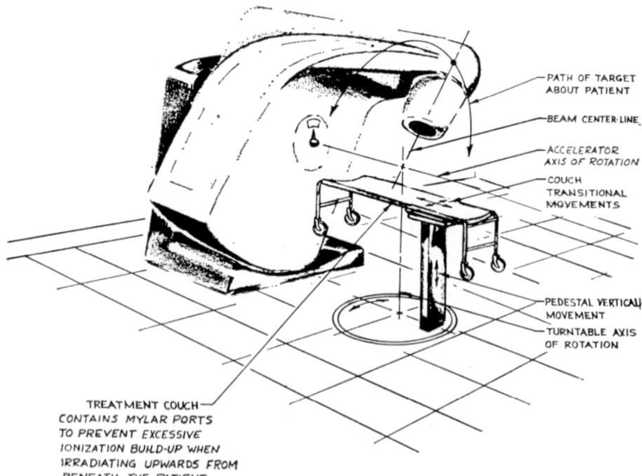

Courtesy: Varian Associates.

VARIAN MEDICAL RADIOTHERAPY LINAC. This 6 mev model was installed in 1962 in the Los Angeles Medical Center of the University of California.

the development and construction of all of Stanford's ten linacs, and directed the design of Project "M" – the Stanford two-mile linac – which has been approved by Congress, and will be operated together with the AEC. It is expected to be built in about six years, will cost $125 million, and its intense beam of electrons will have an energy of 20 bev at 600 kw. By increasing the numbers of klystrons, these figures could be raised to 40-45 bev and 2000 kw. Ginzton was retained as deputy-chief of project M.

Varian Associates delivered their first radiographic linear accelerator in 1961 to the Concord Naval Ammunition Depot, where it is used to inspect the solid fuel bonding within Polaris missiles. Medical linear accelerators are being installed in the Stanford and UCLA medical centers. Varian Associates with their USA, Canadian and European subsidiaries (they make, for instance, the VacLon pump and similar appliances in their Vacuum Products Division) had in 1961 sales totalling almost $60 million.

HVEC

In the commercial manufacture of both static and linear accelerators, an established reputation has the High-Voltage Engineering Corporation (HVEC) of Burlington (Massachussetts).

HVEC was founded in 1947. Its technical director is John George Trump, head of the High Voltage Research Laboratory at MIT. HVEC's current president is Denis Morrell Robinson, former chief of the British Radar Mission assigned during World War II to MIT's Radiation Laboratory. John Danforth is HVEC's chief-physicist, Van de Graaff their chief-scientist. In 1958 HVEC acquired controlling interest in Electronized Chemicals Corporation, a subsidiary which operates a radiation processing facility at headquarters. In 1958 HVEC sponsored the first bi-annual Accelerator Conference, which proved to be quite successful. In 1960 was formed High Voltage Engineering (Europe) N. V., in Amersfoort (Holland), for the manufacture of particle accelerators in Europe. Also in 1959 HVEC created a subsidiary in conjunction with the Goodrich Company, called Goodrich- High Voltage Astronautics, to pioneer in the development of ion-rocket engines and in other areas of space technology.

Reminiscent of multi-stage rockets, HVEC built in 1957 their first two-stage tandem Van de Graaff (Model EN) on the elegant charge-exchange principle for multiple acceleration stages. This increased its total energy to 12 mev. In 1961 they combined in a three-stage "tandem" a 5.5 mev negative ion injector, which boosted the final energy to 17.5 mev. In 1962 they

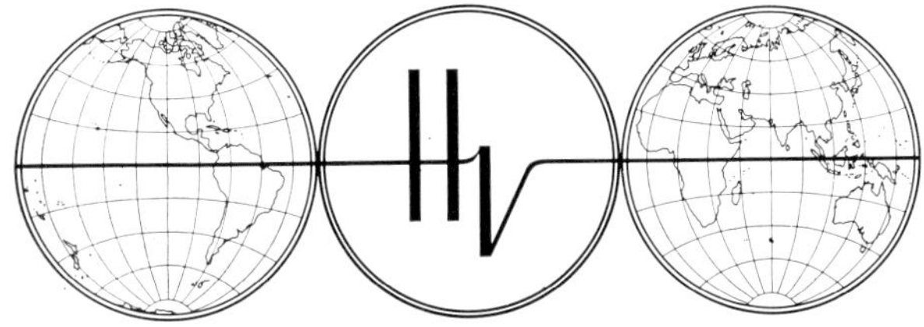

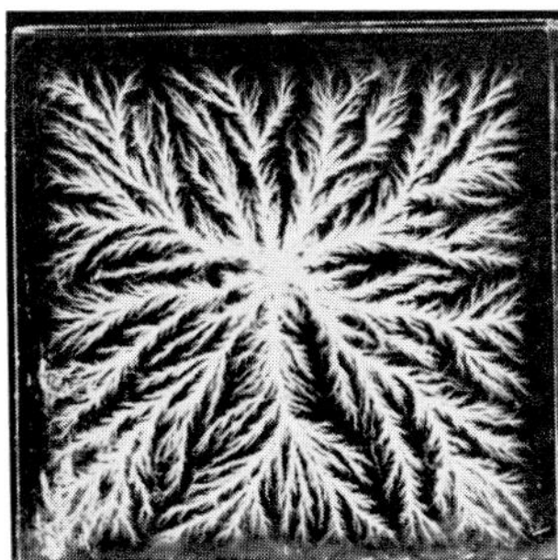

Courtesy: HVEC.

LICHTENBERG FIGURES. Unofficial HVBC insignia – the pattern is due to crystallization of lucite from electron discharge.

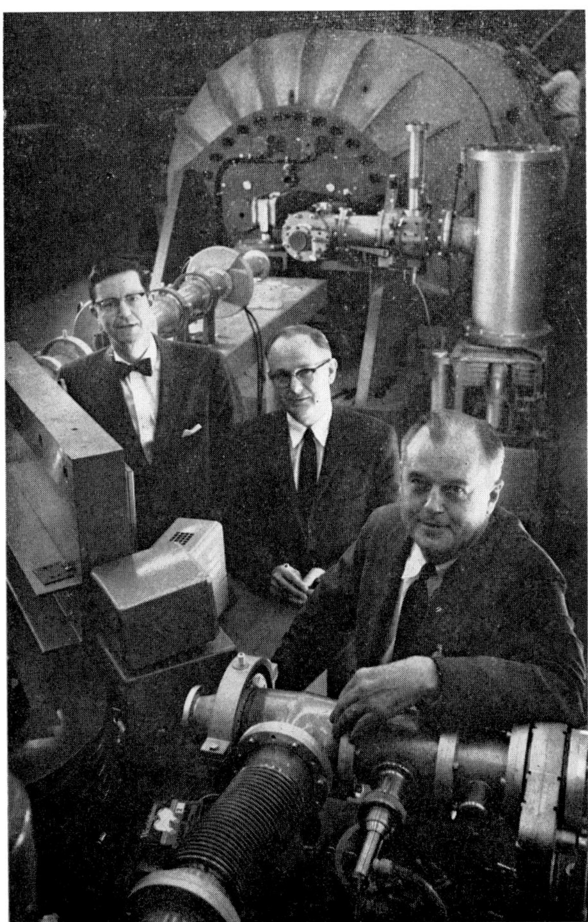

Courtesy: HVEC.

HVBC EXECUTIVES. Denis Morrell Robinson is in the background, John George Trump in the middle, and Robert Jemison Van de Graaff in the foreground.

reached 21.5 mev. An important use of the tandems is in the acceleration of heavy ions where by multiple charge stripping in the terminal, the final particle energy is several times the terminal potential. Tandem installations are in process at Yale, Minnesota and Rochester Universities.

At the Northeastern District meeting of the American Institute of Electrical Engineers, held in Boston on May 9, 1962, John Loring Danforth presented a paper from which a lengthy quotation is in order:

"The first 12-mev tandem was installed at the Chalk River Laboratories of the Atomic Energy of Canada, Ltd., in February, 1959. Since then, twenty-five additional tandems have been installed or are in the process of construction. In 1960 five were installed, two 12-mev tandems, two vertical tandems, two vertical tandems of a slightly larger size designed and built in the United Kingdom for English laboratories, and the one built in Russia. The capital cost of a 12-mev tandem Van de Graaff accelerator with accessories is approximately one million dollars, and the cost of the building, facilities, some experimental equipment and instrumentation is roughly the same. The larger models cost proportionally more."

The characteristic pattern formed by an escaping negative charge in a lucite block (Lichtenberg figures)

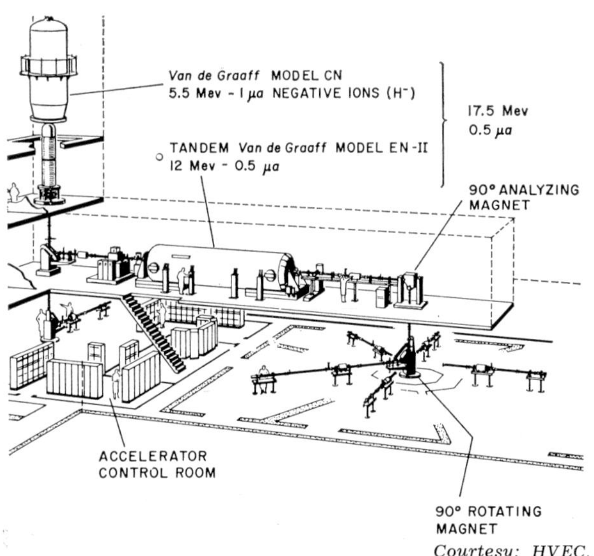

Courtesy: HVEC.

THREE-STAGE VAN DE GRAAFF. The vertical contraption is a 5.5-mev negative ion accelerator, the horizontal a 12-mev tandem, for a total energy of 17.5 mev. Of particular interest is the tandem's ability to accelerate heavy ions. It is the tool of the low-energy nuclear physicist in the investigation of proton-neutron relationship in nuclei formation.

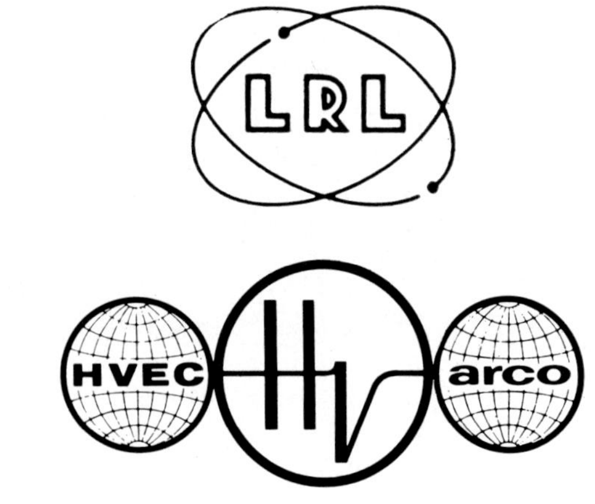

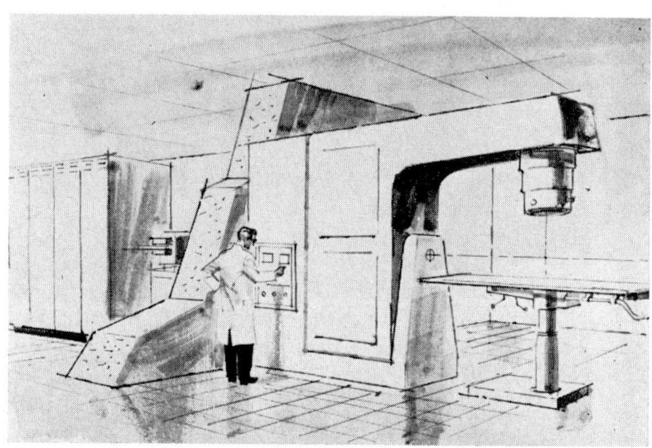

Courtesy: HVEC

6-45 MEV LINAC. HVBC and ARCO have installed both magnetron and klystron linacs. The herein illustrated variable energy machine can be used for therapy as well as for bio-physics research.

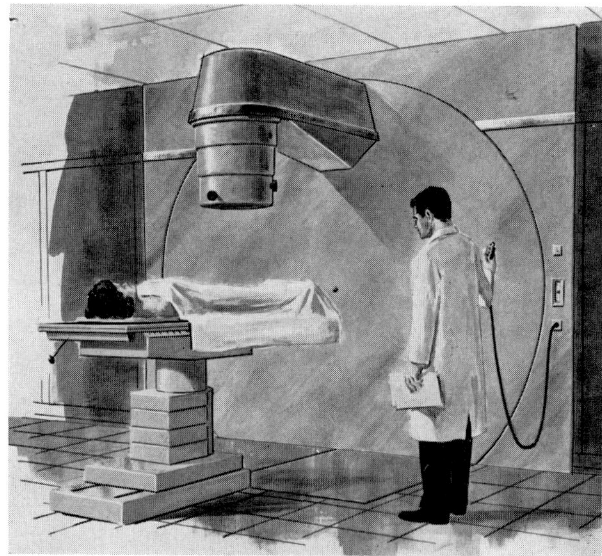

Courtesy: HVEC

LM-8: ELECTRONS OR X RAYS. 8-mev linac, in ultramodern rotational design, with isocentric capability, focal spot of five or less in diameter, delivers 300 r/min. at 100 cm, can be operated anywhere from 2 to 8 mev.

has been adopted by HVEC as unofficial insignia. It is obtained by placing a lucite block under a 2 mev electron beam, in which instance the electrons have sufficient energy to penetrate into the material. Lucite being an excellent insulator, some of the negative charge becomes trapped or stored within the volume of the block. The block is then removed from under the beam, and pricked lightly with a punch. This upsets the local electric field pattern of the stored charge. Following an erratic path of least resistance, the electrons flash out through the prick-point, causing the tree-like design in the block. This pattern is a crystallization of the lucite caused by the passing charge.

In October, 1953 engineers and physicists from the Lawrence Radiation Laboratory (LRL) of the University of California formed the Applied Radiation Corporation (ARCO) in Walnut Creek (California), and began building both magnetron and klystron microwave linacs.

The magnetron was developed in the United Kingdom in April, 1940 by J. T. Randall and H. A. H. Boot, who were working in the Physics Department of Birm-

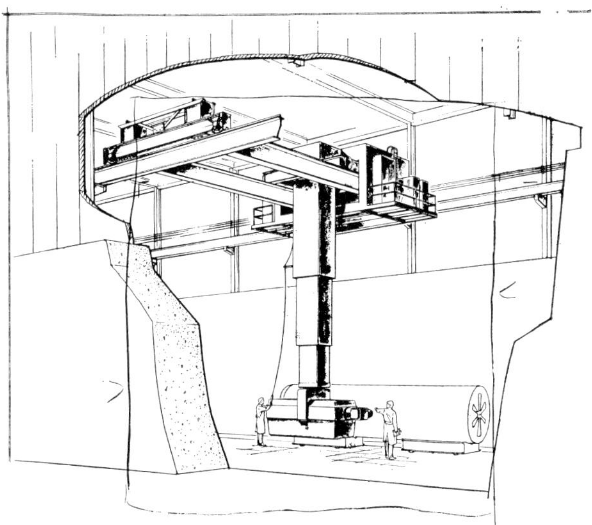

Courtesy: HVEC

RADIOGRAPHY OF SOLID ROCKET PROPELLANT. Standard industrial linacs are 3-15 mev models. A typical 8-mev linac produces 1000 r/min. at 100 cm with 1 mm focal spot; up to 6000 r/min. with 5 mm focal spot. Steel thicknesses up to 20 inches can be examined with a 15 mev linac which delivers 3000 r/min. with 1 mm focal spot. It is possible to build 25 mev linacs capable of delivering 25,000 r/min. at 100 cm.

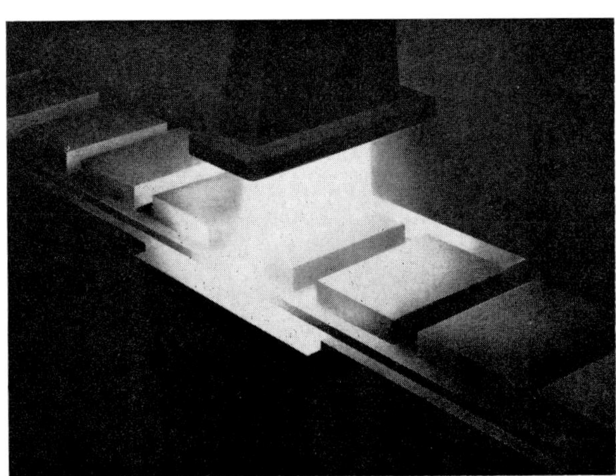

Courtesy: HVEC.

ELECTRON BEAM.

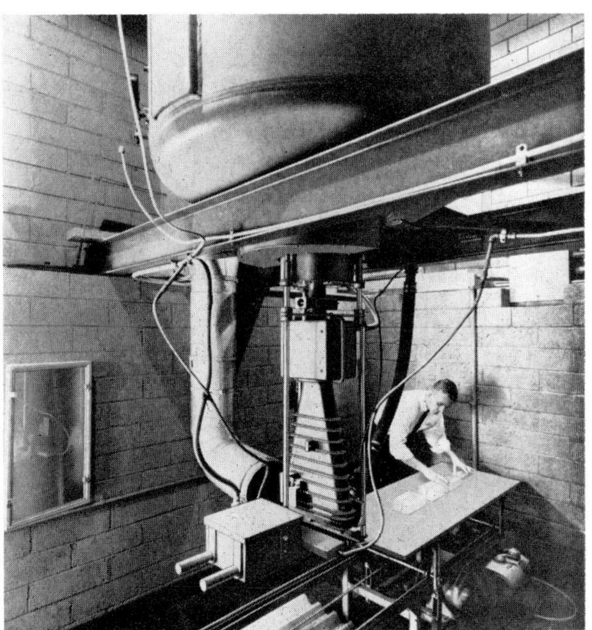

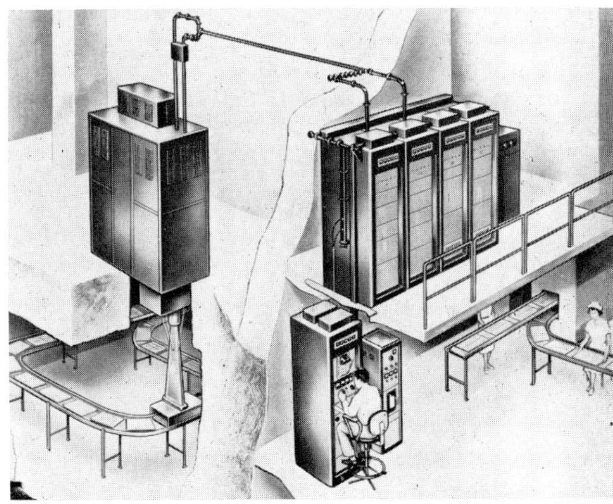

Courtesy: HVEC.

6 MEV HVEC LINAC AT ETHICON. After a research project in which a 2 mev Van de Graaff was used, an automated production line was installed with a 6 mev linac and a 3 mev Van de Graaff for continuous sterilization of packaged suture material.

ingham University under Sir Mark Oliphant. Randall and Boot simply married Hull's long-established split-anode magnetron with the resonant cavity of the klystron. The resultant cavity magnetron gave an output several hundred times that of any other oscillator. An early model, taken to the USA in the summer of 1940 by the Tizard mission (Denis Robinson was one of its members) came to be regarded as one of the most important items in reverse lend-lease. These details are from a letter by K. E. B. Jay, sent to me by Eric Walker, HVEC's x-ray specialist. Walker added that their recent linacs use the new Raytheon amplitron, a power tube which is driven by a magnetron.

To strengthen its hand, in 1960 the HVEC bought out the ARCO. Between the two of them they have manufactured some 180 single stage, Van de Graaff positive-ion accelerators (from 400 kev to 5.5 mev), and about 140 electron accelerators for therapy, radiography and electron processing. No doubt, it is becoming fashionable to use high energy electrons.

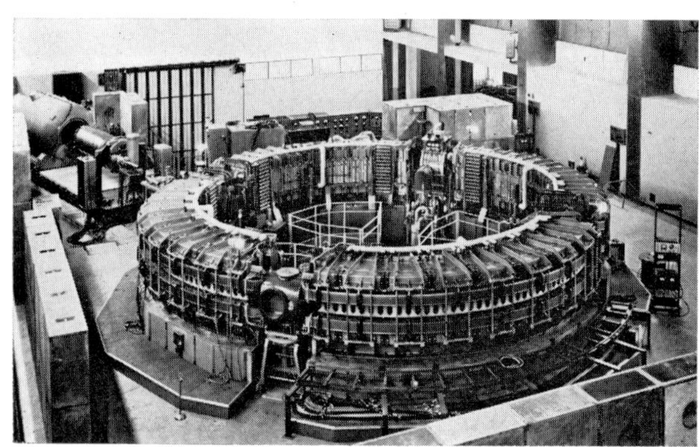

Courtesy: HVEC.

Synchrotron in Frascati (Italy). The contraption in the left upper corner is a 3 mev HVEC pulsed electron injector – the location is the Istituto Nazionale di Fisica Nucleare.

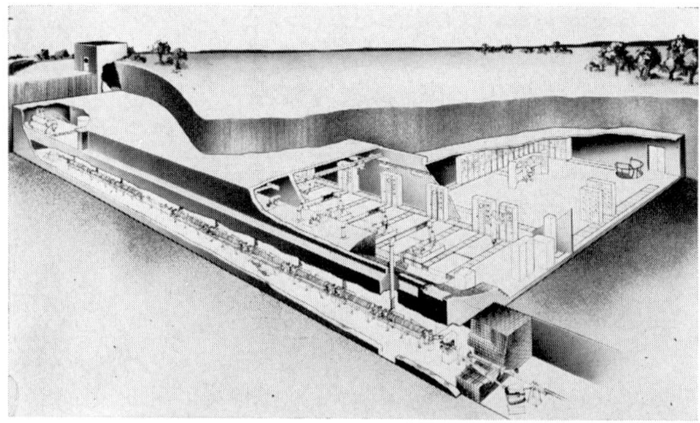

Courtesy: HVEC.

100 mev – 40 kw. Drawing of the National Bureau of Standards linac being built by HVEC in Gaithersburg (Maryland), where new laboratory of NBS is located.

Contrary to x rays, electrons have a "stopping point," beyond which they do not go, except for the *Bremsstrahlung* produced in the process. Rumor has it that at higher levels (30-40 mev), there is little or no significant therapeutic difference between an electron and an x-ray beam. Experience accumulated to this date is not sufficient for adequate appraisal, but it seems that there are certain areas in which electron therapy offers decided advantages, such as in oropharyngo-laryngeal malignancies, and in lymphomata.

In industry, linacs are used as a source of x rays (by interposing a target between the electron beam and the object under examination). Electron beams serve well in the sterilization of foods and drugs, even medical equipment can be so treated. At Johnson & Johnson's plant in Somerville (New Jersey) Ethicon sutures are sterilized with a Van de Graaff beam, and they have now purchased a larger linac.

Linear accelerators are very important in research, either as the main instrument or as a source of electrons for injection into other types of accelerators, as in the synchrotron of the Istituto Nazionale di Fisica Nucleare in Frascati (Italy). HVEC linacs are found in many places, at the Peter Bent Brigham Hospital in Boston, for the Medical Research Council at Hamersmith Hospital in London, and in Japan's Atomic Research Institute at Taka Iberazi Ken. And HVEC is currently completing a 100 mev linac for use by the National Bureau of Standards.

THE BETATRON

There are always several ways to skin a cat (with no allusion to the "electron peeler" of Lester Skaggs). That other way to accelerate electrons is the betatron, built by Donald William Kerst in 1940.

The betatron is a circular device in which electrons are accelerated by magnetic induction. It has a doughnut-shaped vacuum tube sandwiched between the poles of an electromagnet. Electrons injected into the tube receive a certain acceleration for each completed turn. At a cut-off, the accelerated electrons hit a target and emerge as x rays. The construction difficulty consisted in making the vacuum tube and in distributing the magnetic field, which must be smooth. That first betatron model worked fine the very first time it was "turned" on, on July 15, 1940. For its weight of 200 pounds, it had a beam with an energy of 2.3 mev.

In the *Dunlee Digest* of January-March, 1963 Zed Atlee wrote: "The betatron was conceived and developed by D. W. Kerst. (His) initial work on the betatron was done while he was in (my) employ. . . Original conception of the possibilities of such an accelerator goes to R. Wideroe, who published an article in 1928. Walton should share some of this honor, as he actually considered as early as 1927 a device employing electrostatic and magnetic focussing. The next milestone is marked by the efforts of M. Steenbeck, a German, who was issued a US Patent in 1937. From a communication from him it is evident that he did work as early as 1935. However, there is no evidence that he actually had a working device. Steenbeck gives credit to Slepian for having developed in 1922 the original concept of accelerating electrons in an electric field.

"It was this Steenbeck patent which started Kerst on his theoretical considerations. . . In February, 1938 Kerst, while in the employ of the General Electric X-Ray Corporation's Vacuum Tube Engineering Department, was given the above mentioned patent to study by the writer. Before leaving this position in August, 1938, he spent much time on the theoretical calculations involved in successful focussing of electrons, and evolved the basic design which he later built at the University of Illinois. In the beginning much speculation was done as to what of an orbit to employ. Kerst and the writer agreed that a circular orbit with the electrons admitted tangentially looked the most promising, at least from a vacuum tube construction standpoint. From this viewpoint the doughnut shaped vacuum tube evolved, which was built in 1939 for Kerst by J. Gosling, glass engineer of GE's Vacuum Tube Department.

"On April 12, 1938 Kerst wrote a short memorandum entitled "Electron Accelerator" which gave specifications for a 3 mev machine. He suggested a 5000 gauss field and 3 cm radius. In that memo he pointed out some possible stumbling blocks, mainly the problem of keeping the electrons in proper orbit.

"However, a few months later Kerst accepted a position at the University of Illinois. During 1939 and 1940 he worked on his first model, reporting success to the writer in a letter dated July 25, 1940. Based upon this work, a patent was granted Kerst in 1942."

Following are excerpts from a letter by Donald Kerst, dated November 21, 1962:

"I was introduced to old literature in betatrons partially by examination of a patent at GE where I went after obtaining my PhD at the University of Wisconsin in 1937, but most of the literature I found immediately after that by discussing it with my former major professor, Professor Breit.* A possibility of working on the problem did not occur at GE X-Ray, but when I joined the staff at the University of Illinois I was encouraged and had the necessary theoretical guidance and funds.

"It was possible to avoid the pitfalls encountered by others, whose publications I have read. I had hoped to get GE's interest renewed so that they could make the radiology and therapeutic betatrons at 20 or 30 mev, while at the same time I would construct a 100 mev machine for the Physics Laboratory at the University of Illinois. Things didn't work out quite this way. The 100 mev machine, which I had been designing, was constructed at GE for themselves, and the 20 megavolt prototype for industrial work came back to Illinois with me. The 20 mev machine worked right off. We just had the polarity of the injector backward, but this took only fifteen minutes to reverse.

"Immediately the Illinois staff and the government worked with Allis-Chalmers to try and get betatrons

*Russian-born Gregory Breit, a nuclear physicist who specialized in quantum electro-dynamics and in ionospheric studies, is now with the Sloane Physics Laboratory at Yale University.

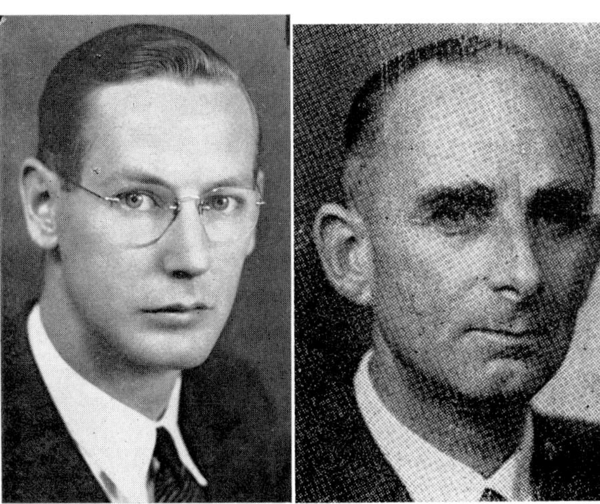

Courtesy: University of Illinois.

WILLIAM DONALD KERST. Photograph from the time when he developed the first betatron at the University of Illinois in Urbana in 1940. The other portrait is of ROLF WIDERÖE, the German-Swiss physicist who first conceived of the accelerating modality which is now called betatron.

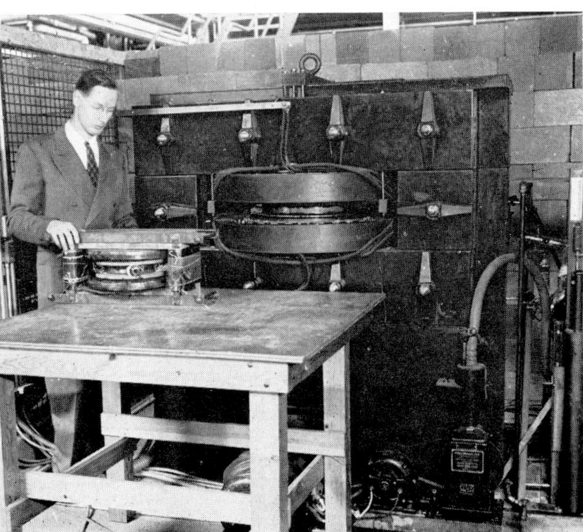

Courtesy: University of Illinois.

2.3 MEV & 24 MEV. Kerst with the prototype betatron in front of the 24 mev built at the GE Research Labs in Schenectady in 1941.

manufactured, which would be used in the war effort. Several were constructed during the war, and the very important sealed-off vacuum tube was developed by Professor Almy* of physics and Professor Hursh of Ceramics along with other members of the staff. Professor Gerald Almy and I were together throughout this work. His efforts in creating the sealed-off vacuum tube made the practical application of the betatron realistic.

"At the end of the war a patent situation developed since Allis-Chalmers, who knew how to make betatrons, received 20 inquiries. The arrangement that GE arrived at with Allis-Chalmers and with others who wanted betatrons was such that they did not inhibit the development of the field.

"Lester Skaggs came to the University of Illinois especially to work on the extraction of the electron beam (the "electron peeler"), which was accomplished in 1946. I am happy to see how far this application has gone.

"If you want to look at what I call history, why not read *Nature, 157*:90-95 (1946). In that historical account I have summarized the stages leading up to the development of the present betatron."

*Gerald Marks Almy is head of the Department of Physics in the University of Illinois in Urbana; his field of interest has also included spectroscopy and fluorescence of polyatomic molecules, and photonuclear disintegration.

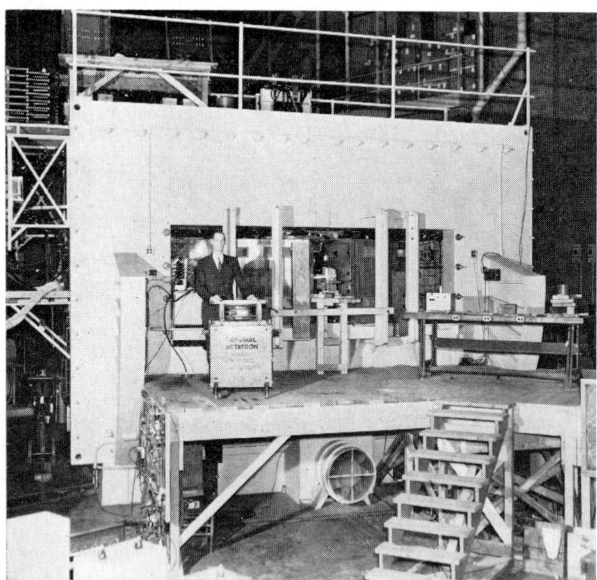

Courtesy: University of Illinois.

2.3 MEV & 340 MEV. Kerst with his primordial betatron in front of the herculean smasher in the Physics Research Lab in Urbana (Illinois). That platform has since been removed. The machine is operating just as well as it did on its first day – February 15, 1950.

BETATRONS BRED

In this country betatrons are built by the Allis-Chalmers (A-C) Manufacturing Company, with headquarters in Milwaukee.

In 1941, Kerst took a leave of absence from the University of Illinois, and went to GE's Research Laboratory in Schnectady (New York). With the machine shop facilities at his disposal, he built a 24 mev betatron which he brought back to Urbana to the University of Illinois. In exchange, GE received some of the patent rights on the betatron. In addition, Kerst designed the plans for a 100 mev betatron which he offered to GE, but they did not seem interested.*

Early in World War II the National Defense Council commissioned the University of Illinois to build a betatron for the production of high energy x rays needed in the examination of very heavy sections of war materials. By 1943 the University had designed and constructed such a machine, but it was still a laboratory

*These details come from Mr. Arthur Rudolph Wildhagen, associate director of Public Relations in the University of Illinois, who handled public relations of the Betatron development since its inception. The photographs herein reproduced are from a remembrancer album preserved in the Betatron building of the University of Illinois in Urbana. Arthur remembers having seen in the 1940s an article on GE's 100 mev betatron. They had built it as close as they could get to Kerst's original design. Still GE's 100 mev never operated fully satisfactorily. Later GE donated it to the University of Chicago: there (in Kerst's careful words) "a great deal of care (had to be supplied) to keep (it) performing properly." After "some" years it was scrapped (which is sometimes euphemistically called salvaged, although it means exactly the opposite as far as the structure's initial function is concerned).

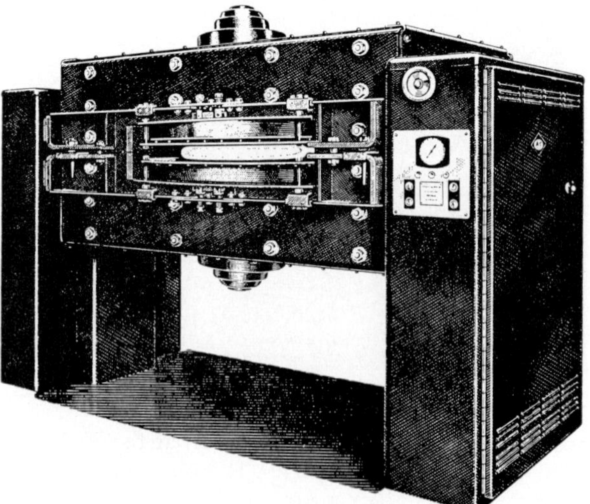

"OLD" *A-C* BETATRON. From a Picker advertisement of 1954.

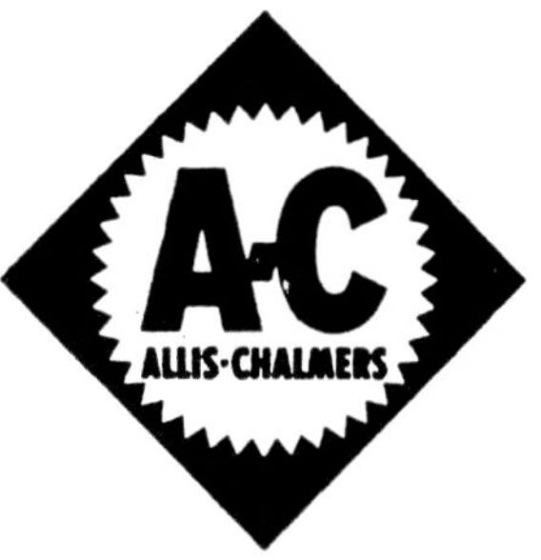

device, not a manufactured piece of equipment. Then Kerst went to join Project Y in Los Alamos, and he became the leader of the Water Boiler Group. That Water Boiler (a divergent chain reactor) was successfully operated in April, 1944. Then the University of Illinois betatron was transported to Los Alamos to be used in the study of implosion – the test implosion was detonated between two closely spaced bomb-proof buildings, one containing the high-voltage gamma source (the betatron), the other the vertical cloud chamber and recording equipment. By April, 1945 these test shots were giving significant data for the development of the assembly of the A-bomb. As he was busy at Los Alamos, Kerst asked A-C whether they would consider manufacturing betatrons on other government projects.

The beginnings of A-C in Milwaukee date from the year 1847 when the Reliance Works (supplier of flour mill stones) were started. Since then, through various acquisitions and mergers, A-C's production has come to cover all sorts of machinery, from tractors and locomotives to mining equipment and electric transformers. A-C engineers examined the betatron, and came to the conclusion that it was only a transformer, with the main difference that its secondary consisted of a vacuum tube. For this reason the new product was assigned to A-C's Transformer Section located in Pittsburgh.

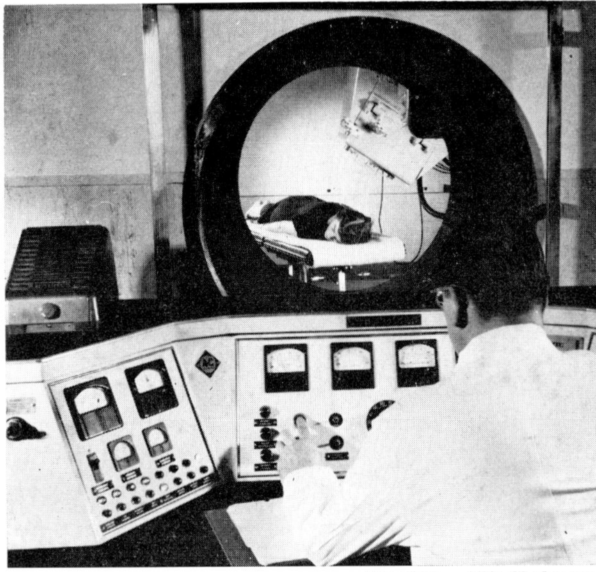

Courtesy: Allis-Chalmers.

BETATRON CONTROL BOOTH. Modern installation with patient "in focus".

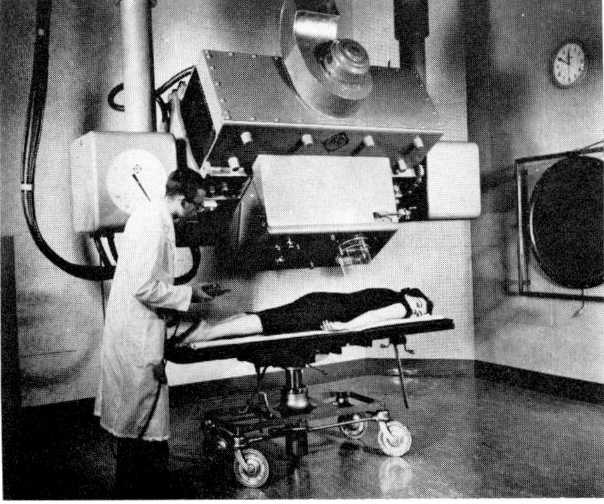

Courtesy: Allis-Chalmers.

"NEW" A-C BETATRON. Supported by two telescoping ceiling-mounts, it has power-assist positioning. Note observation window at viewer's right.

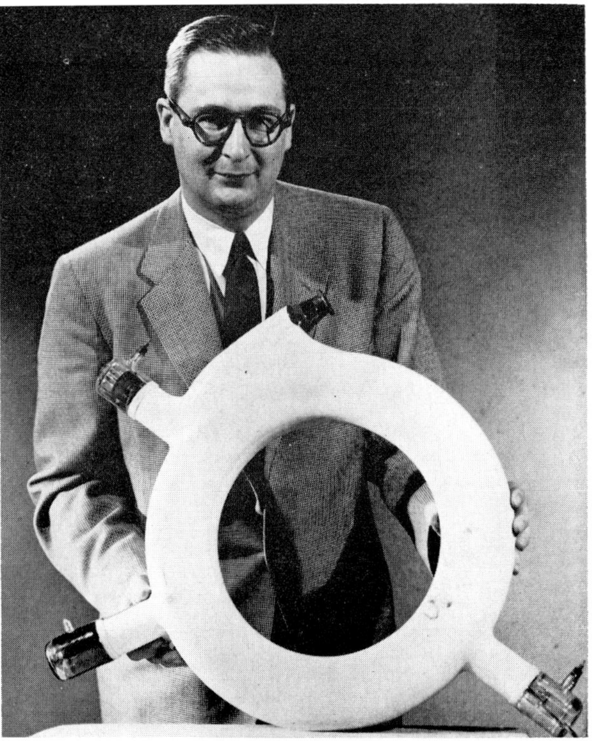

Courtesy: Allis-Chalmers.

ELECTRON BEAM DONUT. The "model" is Payson Gilbert Kirchhoff.

A-C helped to build the 80-mev betatron at the University of Illinois, which became operational in 1948, and was a pilot model for Kerst's crowning achievement, the design of the 340 mev betatron. The latter went into operation on February 15, 1950 – and it worked from the first moment the switch was turned on. The original 2.3 mev built by Kerst in 1940 is now preserved in the Smithsonian in Washington (D. C.). In 1957, Kerst went to work for General Atomic in San Diego, but he preferred the academic atmosphere, and is now in the Physics Research Laboratory of his *alma mater* in Madison (Wisconsin).

The betatron has three main parts – the power supply, the magnet, and the electronic control. The first contract between the National Defense Research Council and A-C, signed in 1944, covered the manufacture of the magnet. The first magnet built by A-C in Pittsburgh included an A-C patented welded pole structure which extended the life expectancy of the pole from one month to 20 years. This work was still supervised by the University of Illinois, which inserted a donut tube of their manufacture. The second contract with the National Defense Research Council in 1945 called for manufacture of the valve supply magnet as well as electronic controls. Late in 1945 Picatinny Arsenal insisted that A-C take a contract for a complete radiographic laboratory: A-C constructed the building, and installed the betatron ready for operation (with the University of Illinois as sub-contractor). In 1946, A-C hired one of the physicists of the University of Illinois and since then A-C assumes responsibility for the design, construction, installation, and service of both the betatron and everything connected with it.

In 1948, an A-C betatron was installed in the basement of the Research and Educational Hospitals of the University of Illinois in Chicago. In the same year it was used to treat the first of a long series of patients. The physical characteristics of that machine were studied and excellently presented in a book published in 1954 by their (former) physicist, John S. Laughlin. The medical aspect was handled by Ludwig (Lajos) Haas, an immigrant from Budapest (who had been famous in Europe as an expert in the interpretation of skull films). He was a typical scientist, quiet, modest, and dedicated. While on a Canadian vacation trip, he attempted to photograph a landscape, for which he stepped out of his car — evidently on the wrong side, because he was killed by an oncoming automobile.

Having learned that a Canadian group had a priority claim on the use of the betatron in human therapy, I endeavored to get the facts. Following are excerpts from a letter by Harold Johns, currently the head of the Physics Division in the Ontario Cancer

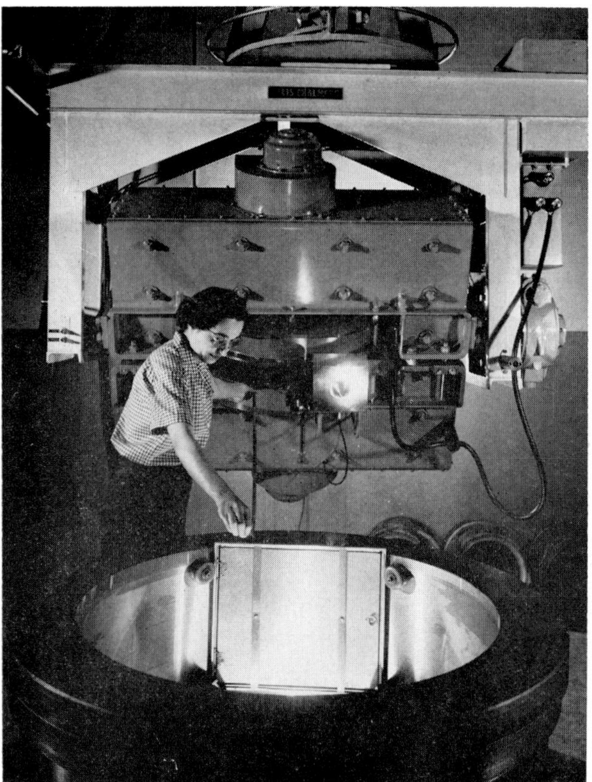

Courtesy: Allis-Chalmers.

INDUSTRIAL BETATRON RADIOGRAPHY. Inspecting trunnion and head assembly of a 10½ by 16 foot grinding cement clinker at Dragon Cement Co. in Siegried (Pennsylvania).

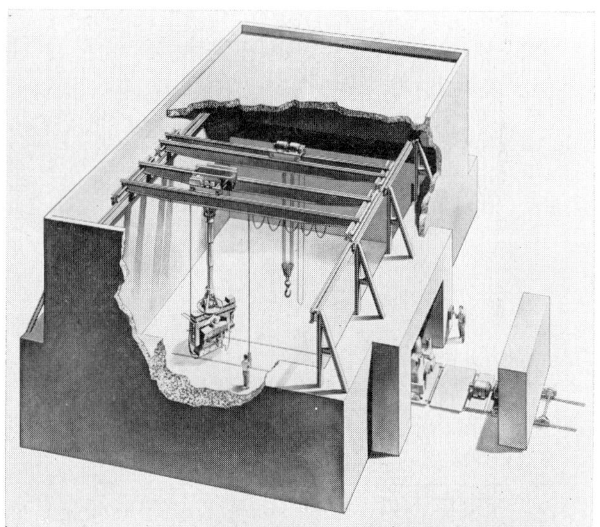

Courtesy: Allis-Chalmers.

TOOL MANUFACTURER'S X-RAY LAB. 24 mev suspended A-C betatron – with rails provided for "customer's convenience."

Institute in Toronto. His letter is dated June 18, 1963:

"I will try to give you my interpretation of history regarding these events. Certainly the first treatment of a patient with the betatron was carried out in Kerst's laboratory. The first patient was a graduate student of their department and all of the physicists and one or two of the radiobiologists tried to cure this poor devil of a brain tumor. All of this is writted up in the *American Journal of Roentgenology* in 1948.

"It was about one year later that we started treating patients on a routine basis in Saskatoon with a similar betatron. Our first publication dealing with this was in the same *Journal* in 1949. As far as I know, Kerst and his group never treated any more patients, and for about one year we were the only betatron running in this way. The second machine to be used in routine work was set up in Chicago by Dr. Laughlin. These three machines were all exact copies of the one made by Kerst.

"With regard to the Cobalt-60 unit the situation is again complicated. Our unit in Saskatoon was the first one to be installed. This machine was designed by myself in collaboration with Mr. J. A. McKay, our machinist in Saskatoon. We spent about three months carefully making measurements which have been described in the literature. While we were making these measurements, the Atomic Energy of Canada installed a machine in London (Ontario) for which they had a gala opening. They claim to have treated the first patients with Cobalt-60. I think it is perhaps true that they treated their first patient one day before we placed our machine in routine operation. I hope this answers your questions."

The first A-C betatron was supported by two columns. Their recent model is suspended from two telescoping ceiling-mounted tubes. In the beginning two separate vacuum tubes were necessary, one for the production of electrons, the other for x rays. Recent donut tubes have a built-in target, and the change-over from electrons to x rays or vice-versa can be

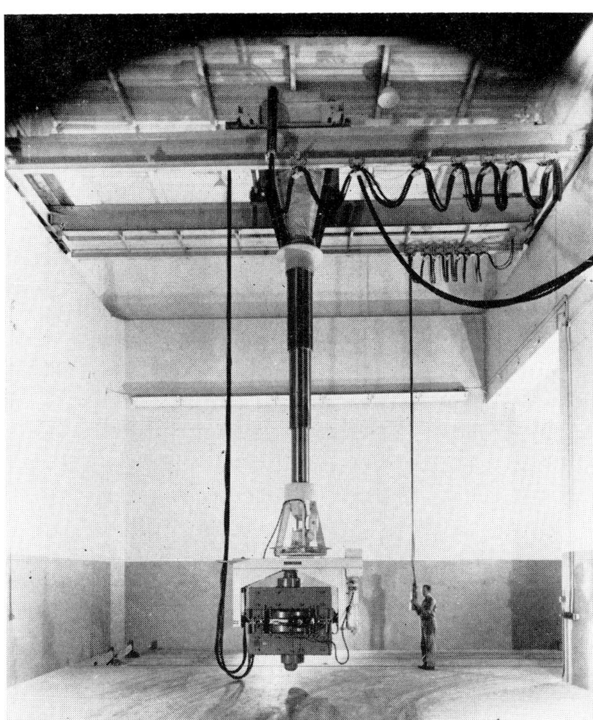

25 MEV RBI. Saddle-mount, telescoping tubes, and bridge crane suspension in A-C's own "x-ray lab" at West Allis works. See rails just behind operator.

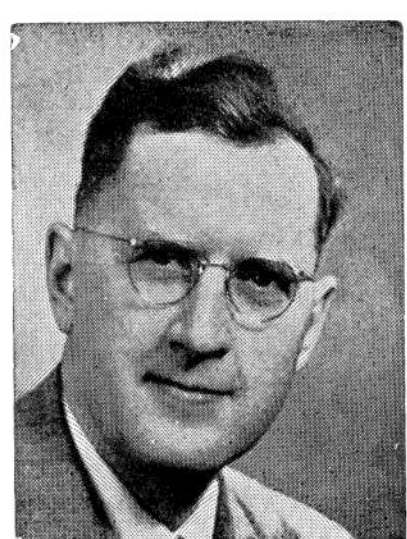

H. E. Johns

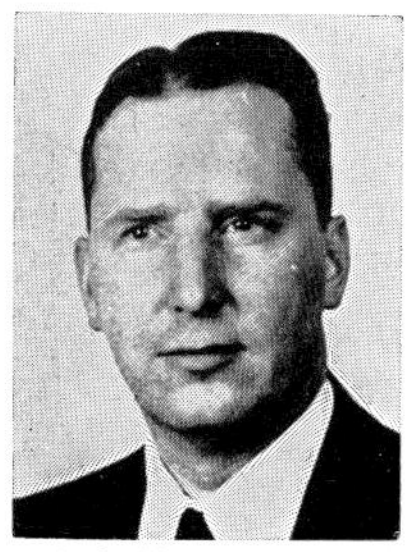

J. S. Laughlin

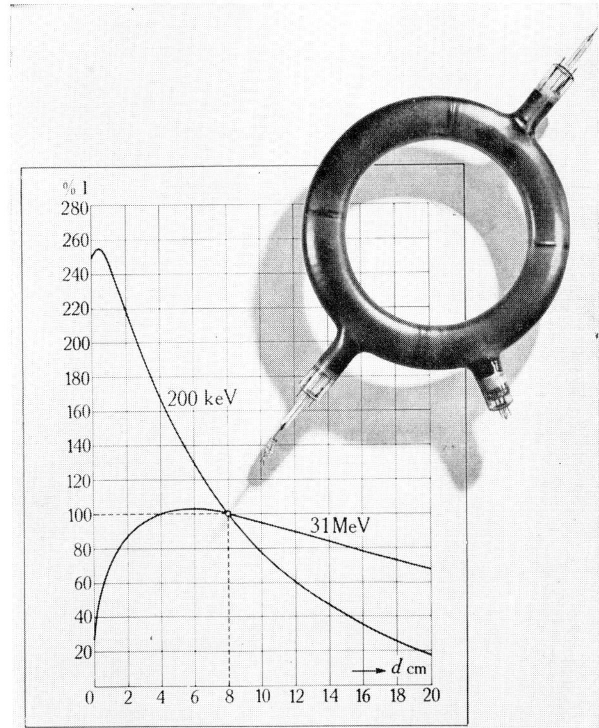

Courtesy: Brown-Boveri.

Betatron vs. conventional therapy. Comparison of depth dose curves seems to favor the betatron, but when patient survives a longer time than expected, one may wish he had used the 200 kvp rather than the 31 mev.

done by flicking a switch. The unit delivers at 22 mev with x rays 140 rhm (with electrons 300 rep at 90 cm).

Very valuable is the industrial utilization of the betatron. A good film of an eight inch thick section of steel would take nearly two days of exposure if one were to use a Co^{60} source of 50 curies (which, incidentally, is not too easy to handle); the same film requires only 20 minutes exposure with a 2 mev generator (because of its higher dose rate); it takes but 1½ minutes with a 25 mev betatron. Two hours of exposure of a film are needed for a ten section of steel when a 2 mev source is used; the betatron does it in four minutes.

One of the newest uses for a betatron (or for a linac) is to demonstrate in minimum time the integrity of missile propellants, *i.e.*, to make sure that no flaws, cracks, or voids exist in the solid fuel.

A-C makes two betatron models; 24 RCM is their medical version. The industrial betatron (22 RBI) can be suspended from a modified bridge crane with a stabilizing telescoping tube suspension system which permits inspection of the largest casting that can be brought into the "betatron laboratory" by railroad.*

*Information on A-C betatrons was graciously provided by Payson Gilbert Kirchhoff, who is a descendant of Sir John Leighton Charles Fischer (Bart.); Keeper of the Privy Seal and Promoter of the Virginia Colonies. I might have known more about A-C betatrons, for I was supposed to pick up Mr. Kirchhoff and fly him to a dinner at Lake Delavan (in the hope to extract more information)—but just about that time A-C decided to prohibit its valuable executives from flying in private planes. This order was even more surprising as it came soon after the A-C (one of the largest builders of farm equipment) played host to a Fly-In of Flying Farmers.

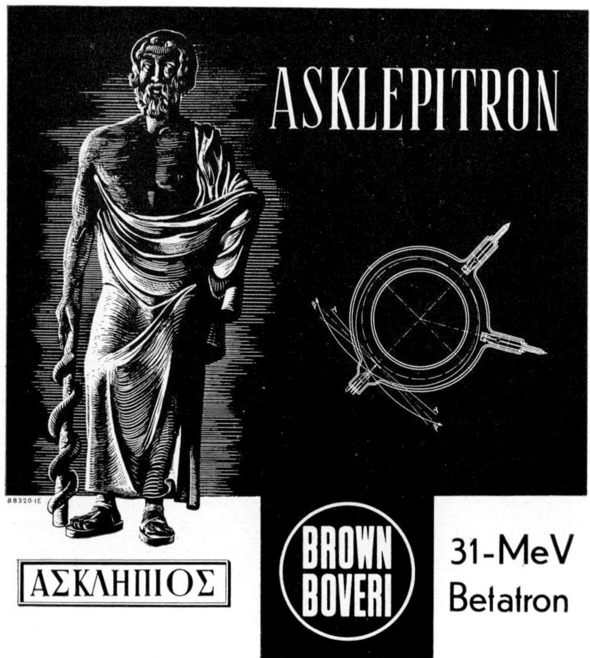

OTHER BETATRON MANUFACTURERS

In Europe the first betatron was constructed by SRW in 1944, but king-size models are built by Brown, Boveri & Co. (BB) of Baden (Switzerland).

BB (founded in 1891) operates at the present time 41 plants throughout the world, employs about 73,000 people, and does business in 83 countries. Its first medical betatron was installed in 1950 in the Department of Radiology of Hans Schinz in the Zürich *Kantonsspital.* They treated their first patient with betatron x rays in 1951, and installed an electron outlet in the winter of 1959.

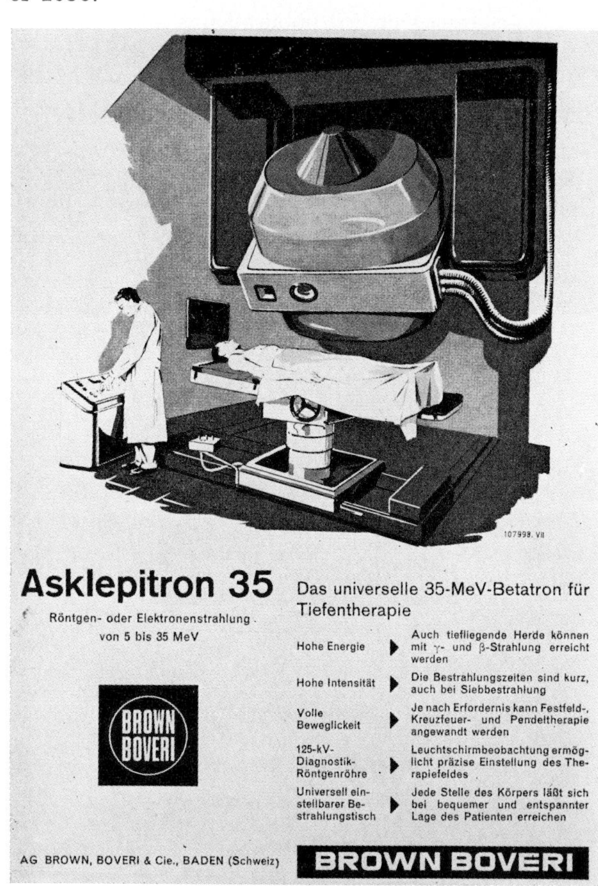

Courtesy: Brown-Boveri.

CEILING-SUSPENDED ASKLEPITRON. It has built-in 125 kvp rotating anode diagnostic tube, permitting precise preliminary positioning of the betatron beam, desirable with rotational and pendular treatment (albeit with such a depth dose rotational procedures are not too often necessary: on this I can get a good argument). Motor-driven table not only facilitates positioning, it can be transformed into a chair, and participates in motions for rotational and pendular procedures. This drawing was made from a photograph of the installation at the St. Ambrogio Clinic in Milano (Italy, where the accent is on crossfire gamma therapy. This ad appeared since 1959 in *Radiologia Clinica.*

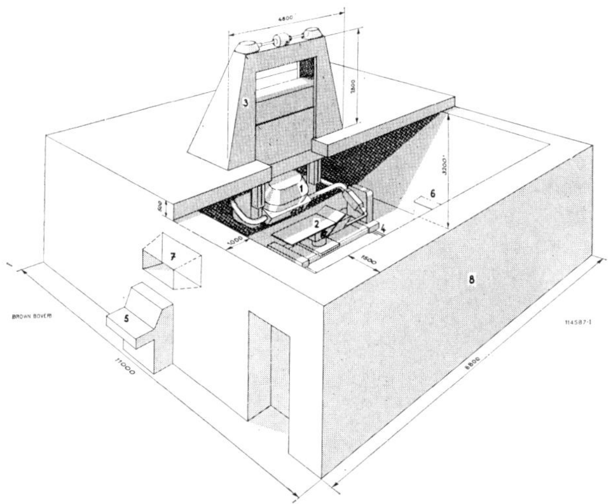

Courtesy: Brown-Boveri.

Asklepitron in concrete box. 1 – Betatron; 2 – table; 3 – crane; 4 – table rails; 5 – main control desk; 6 – controls for built-in diagnostic tube; 7 – protected viewing facility; barite concrete wall.

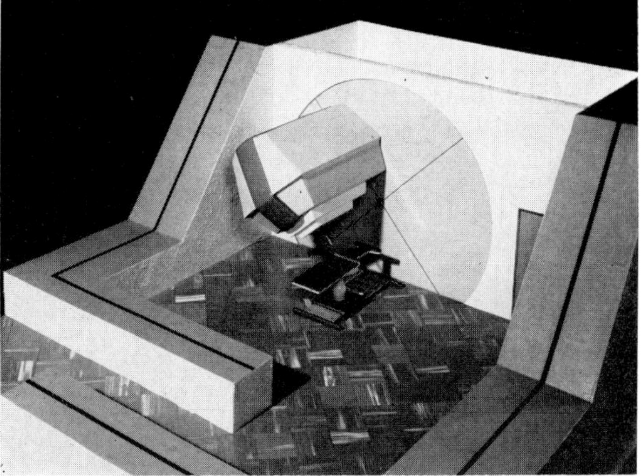

Courtesy: Siemens-Reiniger-Werke.

42 mev betatron. Model of a pendular installation.

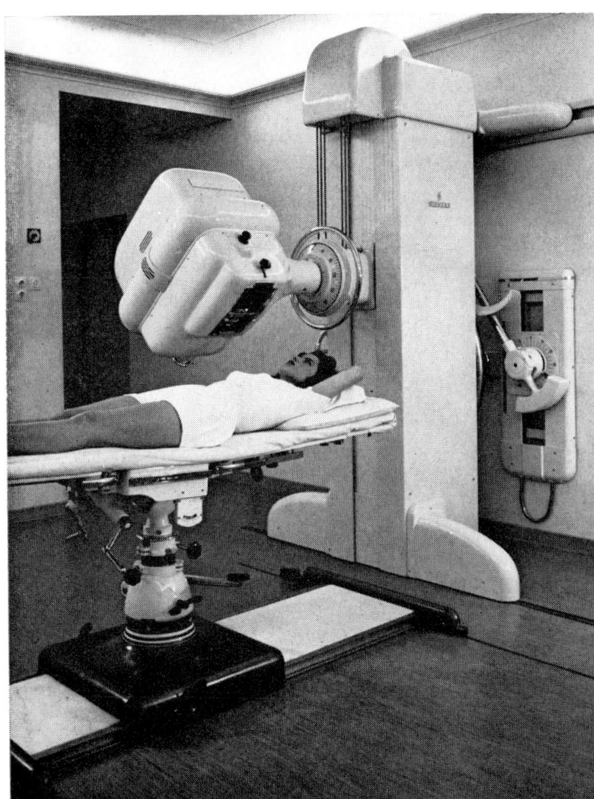

Courtesy: Siemens-Reiniger-Werke.

SRW 18 mev betatron. This machine is less bulky, and also otherwise quite comparable in size, weight, and maneuverability to a Co-60 irradiator. This is the installation at the University of Tübingen (Germany); it is set up for pendular gamma therapy.

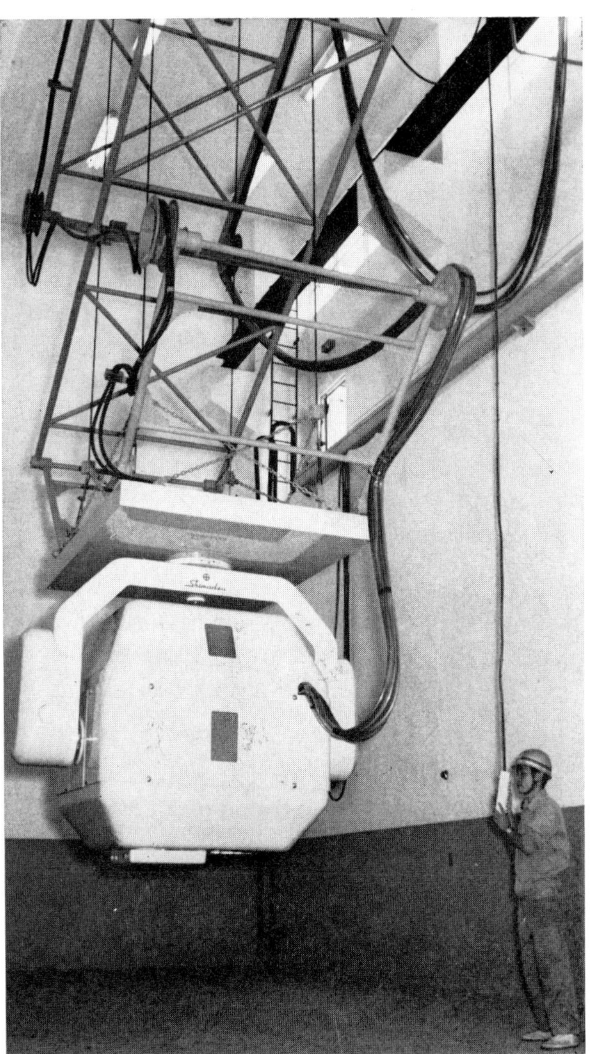

Japanese industrial betatron. Presumably 20 mev model, ceiling-mounted; this is an experimental unit, made by the Shimadzu Mfg. Company.

BB's earlier versions were rated at 31 mev. BB offers now the Asklepitron listed at 35 mev — its guaranteed output is 30 rhm for 31 mev x rays; for electrons it is 600 rep per minute at 100 cms. An interesting feature is the built-in 125 kvp x-ray source, which permits pre-evaluation of the field. An Asklepitron was recently installed at the Montefiore Hospital in New York City.

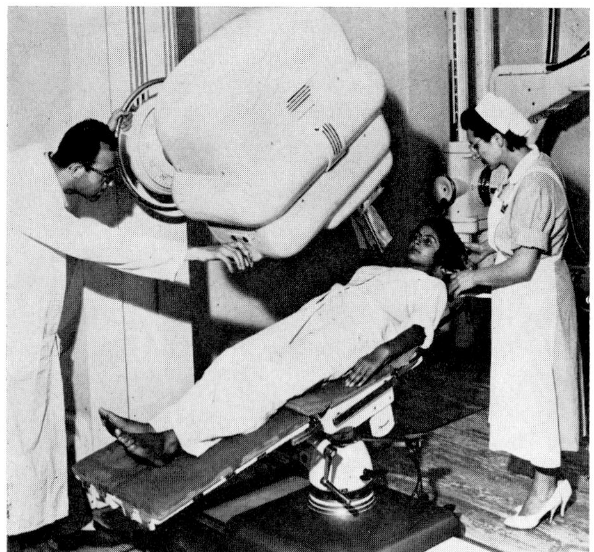

Courtesy: Siemens-Reiniger-Werke.

18 MEV ELECTRON BEAM. This installation is at the University of Rome (Italy), and was purchased from Gorla-Siama, a subsidiary of the SRW, which dominates the European medical betatron market.

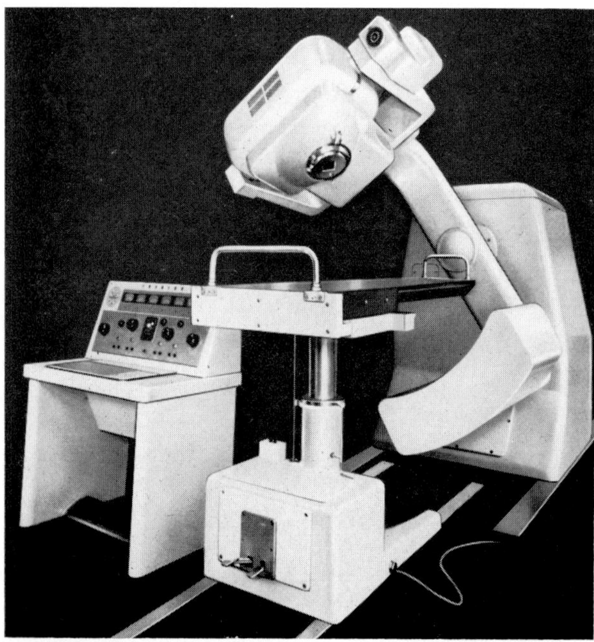

TOSHIBA ROTO-BETATRON. Another 15-mev model, which delivers 5 rad/min at one meter focal distance, weighs 900 kgr, and rotates 180° each way.

BB also furnishes crane-mounted betatrons for non-destructive testing. They sold for instance one such industrial model to the Tokyo Shibaura Electric Company, and another (tentatively) to the Soviet Union.

The European market for betatrons both medical and others is dominated by the Siemens-Reiniger-Werke of Erlangen (Germany). Their 15 mev *Elektronenschleuder* is light (900 kgr), and so small that it uses a casing of the same size as their Co^{60} unit (which may be why they called the latter gammatron).

A similarly manageable medical model was built in Japan by Toshiba. It comes mounted on a rotational device, and its output is 300 rhm, the weight 3080 lbs. At the time of this writing, an experimental, industrial ceiling-suspended betatron was built by another Japanese firm, Shimadzu (a friend of mine procured the photograph).

In England Metropolitan-Vickers built a few 20 mev betatrons. In the Soviet Union betatrons are constructed so far only for their own needs. They showed one with pendular capabilities at the International

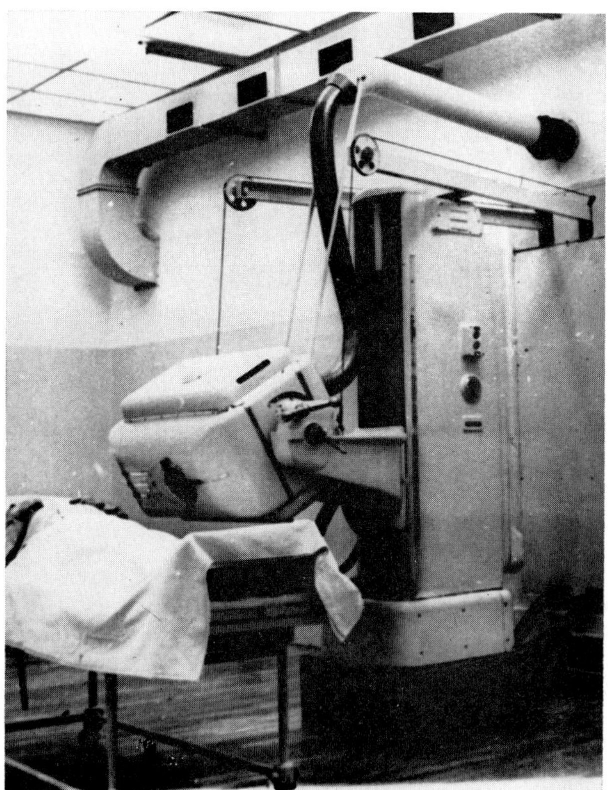

Courtesy: Chirana.

CHIRANA'S BETATRON. This is a 15 mev model, installed in the University Hospital in Hradec Kralove, a city in Bohemian territory.

Cancer Congress in Moscow in 1962. That model will eventually be exported through their usual outlets.

BIO-AIMED ACCELERATORS

At one time or another, all types of accelerators have also been used in biologic research.

Unicellular organisms as well as enzymes have been irradiated with the HILAC (Heavy Ions Linear Accelerator) both at Berkeley and at Yale; on the same subject (or rather object) the latter employed alternately their cyclotron. The cyclotron is a favorite in the study of cataract formation, for which it is used at Argonne; at the University of Chicago; and at ORNL. Very few people have access to the Synchrocyclotron; some of those who did aimed its powerful proton beam at the human pituitary. It seems that for biologic work in radiation, more people use Van de Graaff than other accelerators. For instance micro-organisms are irradiated in this manner at Brookhaven. But then even the "grand-daddy" of them all, the Cockroft-Walton, is still in operation here and there; it is employed for RBE studies both at Los Alamos and at Oak Ridge.

It is becoming fashionable to accelerate electrons for therapy in humans. The beam from a Van de Graaff — or from any other linac — exceeds many times the permissible dose rate, and must therefore be operated at a lower "injection" level for therapy.

Brookhaven has a variety of particle accelerators. With highly energetic and fast-moving particles directed at target atoms, their nuclear cyclotron produces beams of 11-mev protons, 20-mev deuterons, and 44-mev alpha particles.

The Brookhaven proton synchrotron has received the name Cosmotron because it produces energies (3-bev) as high as some of the primary cosmic rays from outer space. Protons are guided in a vacuum chamber by a doughnut-shaped system of electromagnets. By traveling in the same circular orbit through increases in the magnetic field, they are given an incremental 1000-volt boost in energy by a radiofrequency acceleration station. At the end of the 1 second acceleration period, having traveled some 150,000 miles, the protons are allowed to strike the target, which has been inserted in-

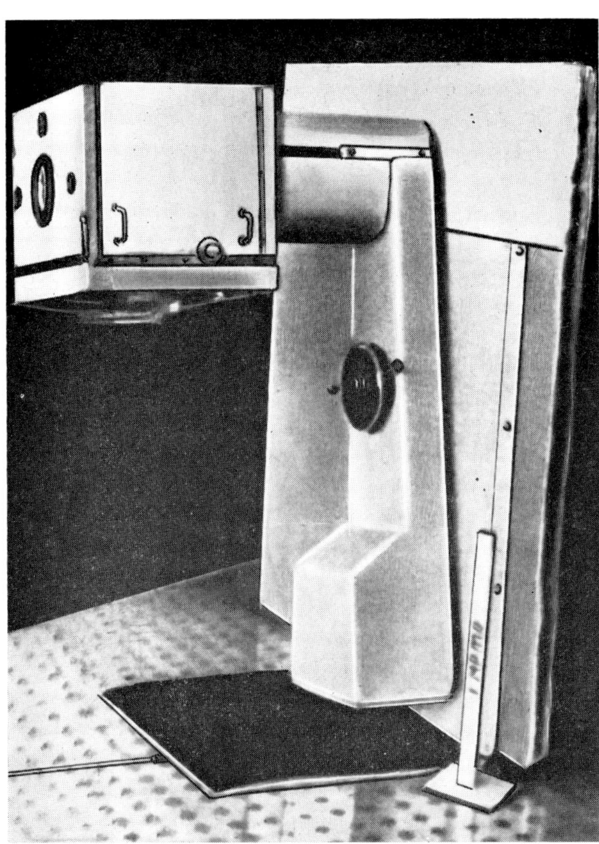

Courtesy: George Zedguenidze.

SOVIETIC BETATRON. This 15 mev model, with pendular capabilities was shown at the International Cancer Congress in Moscow in 1962. They make also a 35 mev betatron.

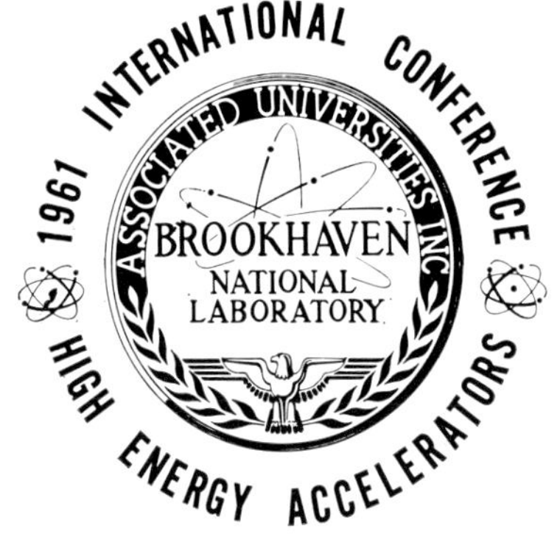

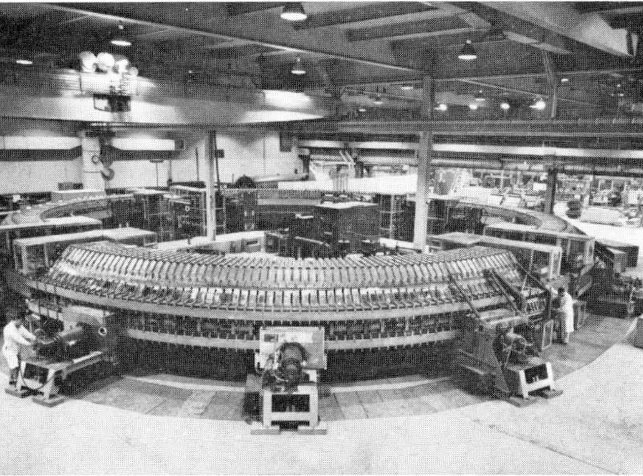

Courtesy: Brookhaven National Laboratory.

BROOKHAVEN'S COSMOTRON. 3 bev proton synchrotron, placed in operation in 1952, when it was the world's most powerful particle accelerator. A row of concrete blocks surround this structure to protect the operators.

side the vacuum chamber, but at a smaller radius. Nuclei of the target atoms are shattered into fragments, ranging in size from large chunks of the original nuclei to their component nucleons (neutrons and protons). In this way are studied many subnuclear particles such as the meson.

At the time when the first experimental beam was obtained from the Brookhaven Cosmotron in 1952, that was the world's most powerful particle accelerator. Very soon, the Bevatron of the University of California's Radiation Laboratory in Berkeley outpaced it, with protons of 6.2 bev energy. Then, in April 1957, the giant Synchrophasotron at Russia's Dubna Laboratory reached an energy of 10 bev. The steel requirements for the magnets for this latter machine reached the staggering figure of 36,000 tons. Man's quest for controlled nuclear interactions at higher and higher energies might well have ended there, for economic reasons alone. Then came a newly-developed concept. Known as the alternating gradient *synchrofocusing* principle, it made it economically feasible to build synchrotrons many times more powerful. Protons are focused in flight as they group themselves in a beam sufficiently narrow so that it can travel in a vacuum chamber of relatively small cross section.

The Alternating Gradient Synchrotron (AGS) built at Brookhaven, required only about 4,000 tons of steel to achieve 25 bev. Hydrogen gas is supplied to a cold cathode discharge as an ion source. The nuclei of the gas atoms in the discharge pass through a small aperture in the cathode to a Cockroft-Walton generator, which raises the protons to an energy of 750,000 ev. The second stage of acceleration is provided by a 50 mev linac, formed of 124 drift tubes totaling 110 foot length. At the end of the linac, the beam is guided into the main synchrotron ring, consisting of 240 magnet sections spaced in a circle one-half mile in circumference. At each of twelve locations around the ring, a radio-frequency acceleration station gives the beam an 8000 volt boost in energy. To reach the final energy of 25 bev, the protons must make about 260,000 circuits, or travel 130,000 miles. At their tremendous speed, the beam is bent magnetically to strike the target, or is deflected completely out of the vacuum chamber into an experimental area. Ejection increases the usefulness of the machine, because separate experiments can be installed along the beam path. However, an external beam presents a radiation problem that requires the erection of a heavy earthen dike as a backstop. Additional shielding is provided by the fact that the entire tunnel (housing the magnet ring) has been

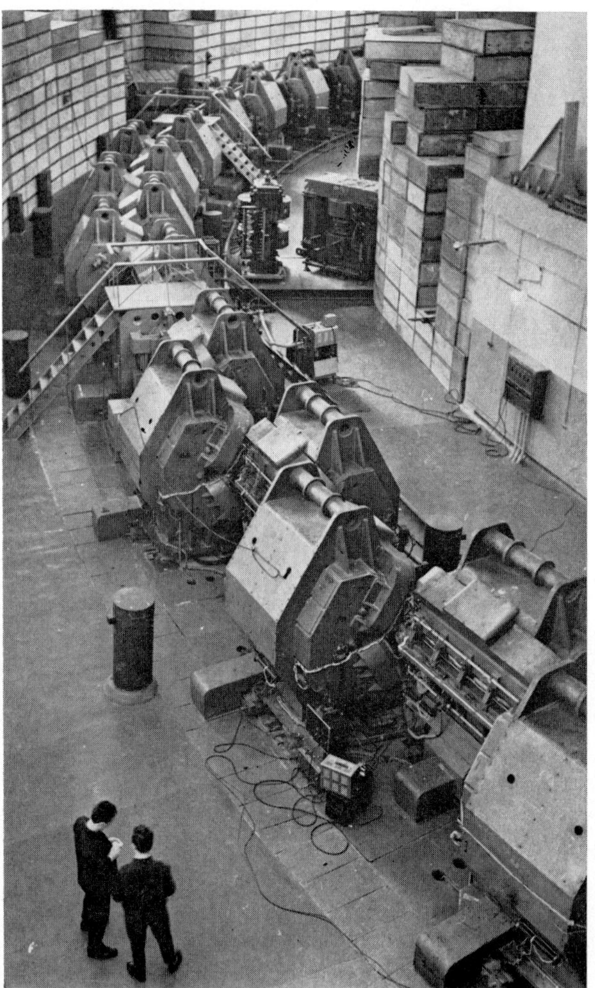

Courtesy: Sovfoto.

SOVIETIC ACCELERATOR. 7 bev model at the Institute of Theoretical and Experimental Physics of the Sovietic Academy of Sciences, placed in operation in April, 1962.

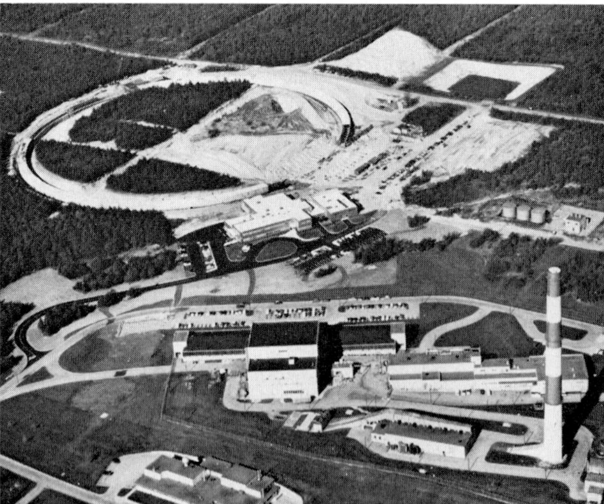

Courtesy: Brookhaven National Laboratory.

BROOKHAVEN'S AGS. Construction of circular 840 foot diameter tunnel to accommodate housing for magnet assembly. The Alternating Gradient Synchroton (AGS) required only 4000 tons of steel for 25 bev energy.

buried under a 10 foot bank of earth. In the main target building concrete shielding straddles the ring.

In 1930, the British physicist Paul Dirac (who had been one of Millikan's pupils) theorized that for every basic particle of matter there was an anti-particle. The first such anti-particle found was the anti-electron. Ever since, finding subnuclear particles and anti-particles remained a favored occupation of nuclear researchers. About thirty such anti-particles are now known (*i.e.,* supposed) to exist, including the recently found anti-Xi-Minus, discovered simultaneously at Brookhaven, and at a similar AGS, built at CERN (Centre Européen de Recherches Nucléaires) in Geneva (Switzerland). At the time of this writing, these two AGS are the most powerful accelerators in existence, but probably not for very long.

NUCLEAR TOWN

On July 21, 1961 (with the by-line of John Nicholson) the *Oak Ridger* (circulation: 8,307) carried a full page of symbols containing elliptical orbits. In the middle was the majestic seal of the city of Oak Ridge.*

From its 1945 peak of 75,000 the population of Oak Ridge had dwindled to 36,000 in 1947 when the (civilian) AEC took over. On March 19, 1949 the gates leading into the city were removed, making it an open community. In 1953 leasing of land for residential construction was permitted, and in 1954 two large housing projects were built after which schools and churches rose along the Turnpike, the city's main traffic artery. In the summer of 1955 Congress passed the

*Mrs. Betty Anderson called my attention to, and sent me the clipping of, this page from their daily newspaper.

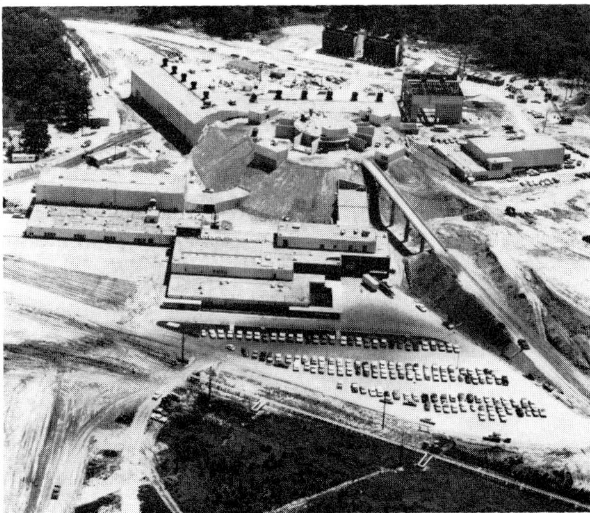

Courtesy: Argonne National Laboratory.

ARGONNE'S ZGS. This Zero Gradient Synchrotron is due for completion late in 1963 or early in 1964. Maximum energy anticipated is 12.5 bev protons. This photograph was made in June, 1962. A Cockroft-Walton feeds the protons into a linac which in turn sends them into the circular accelerating path. This research facility in the Midwest is needed to provide a place for corn-belt atomic scientists, who will no longer have to travel either East or West before they can "try out" some of their ideas. (P.S.: it is now in operation.)

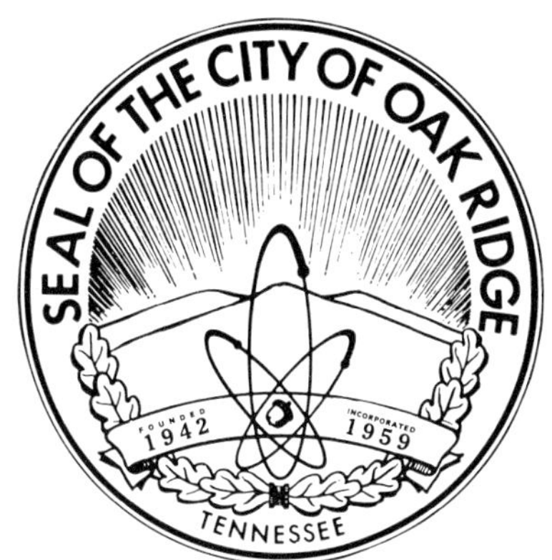

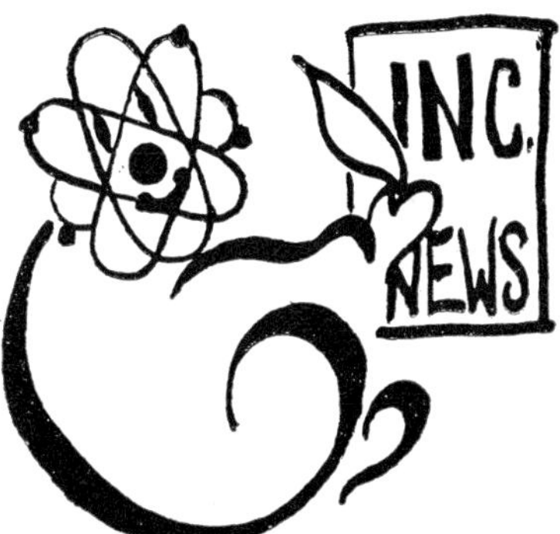

Courtesy: The Oak Ridger.

INCKY. Spearhead of the drive for incorporation of Oak Ridge (Tennessee) as a city.

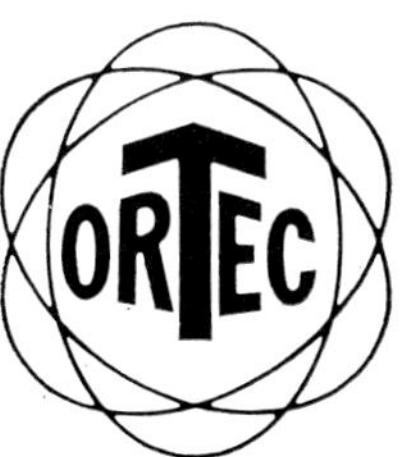

OAK RIDGE TECHNICAL ENTERPRISES CORP.

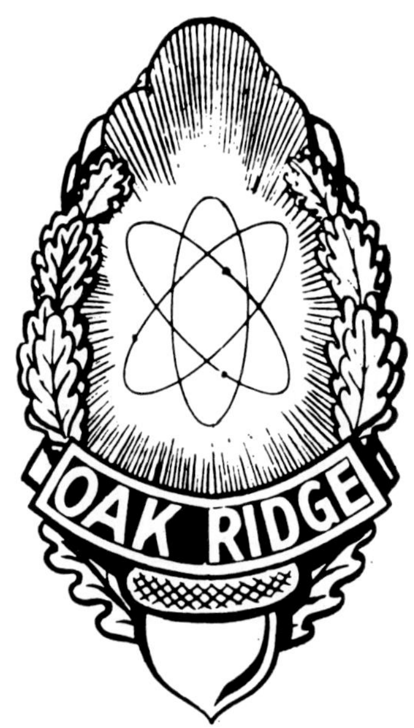

THE ACORN. Symbol of Oak Ridge High School.

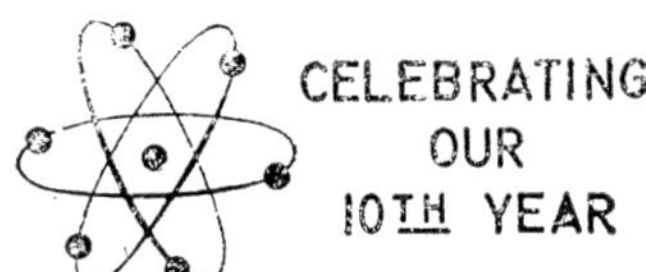

Atomic Energy Community Act, providing for the termination of federal ownership of Oak Ridge. After extensive preliminary planning – this is when Incky first showed his orbiting head – residents voted to establish municipal government under Tennessee law and city officials were elected. The seal of the town carries the orbits, and both the year when it was theoretically conceived (1942) and the year of incorporation (1959).

Today, with a population in excess of 27,000, Oak Ridge is again growing, if quietly. Instead of the old commissary there is a shopping center, and the makeshift dormitories have been replaced by hilly residential areas. And, to confirm the prediction of the *alma mater* song of Bremsstrahlung U., grass is growing in many spots where there used to be red clay. But there are still forbidden roads in Oak Ridge, where Federal ownership still extends to eighty of the total of ninety-four square miles in the area. Thus the nuclear town has preserved its peculiar atmosphere, and amidst acorns, asphalt, and automobiles linger on faded (ghost town) memories of bellicose secrecy, barracks, and barbed wire.

ORBITING ATOMS

Aside from modern representations of atomic orbits, Nicholson's story contained also a reference to the origin of the symbol. Favale was (almost) correct in stating that his orbits meant "nothing" in 1949. They had held quite a meaning in the past.

The New Zealand-born British physicist Ernest 1st Baron Rutherford of Nelson (1871-1937), who coined

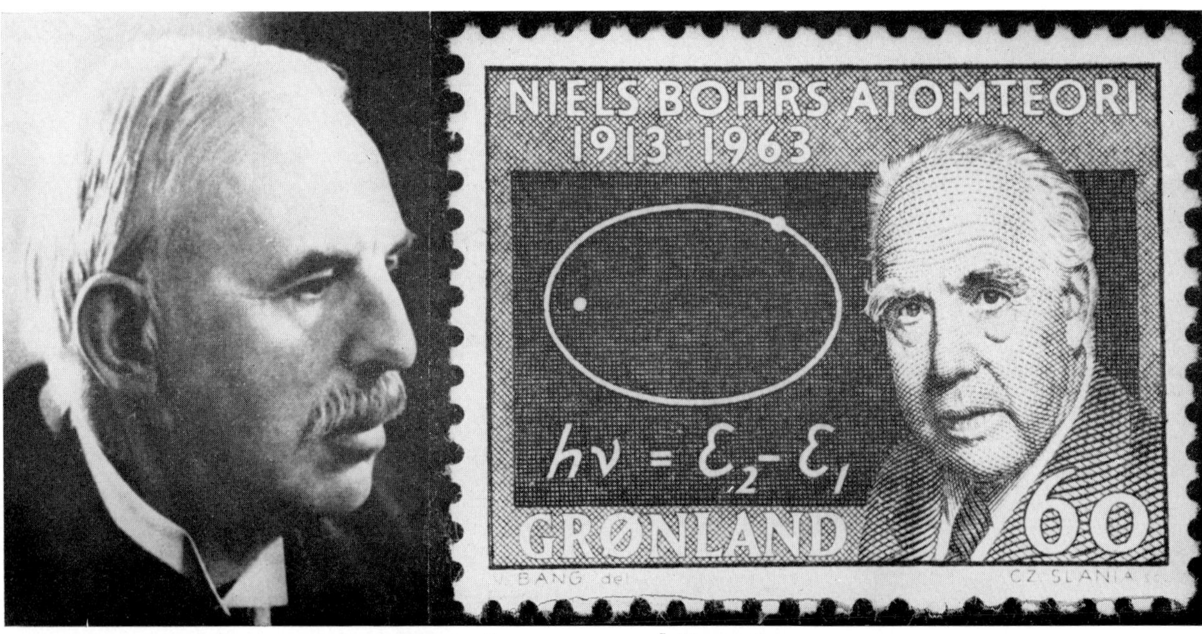

ERNEST RUTHERFORD and NIELS BOHR

the terms alpha, beta, and gamma rays, established in 1907 that alpha "rays" were really helium ions. That is when Rutherford postulated that the atom is a miniature solar system. To this his one-time associate, Niels Henrik David Bohr (1885-1962), the Danish physicist who was to give in 1945 a personal hand in the creation of the A-bomb at Los Alamos, added in 1913 the quantum theory. The result has been eponymized as the Rutherford-Bohr model.

The Rutherford-Bohr view of matter consisted of the theoretical model of an atom in which the center was occupied by a (heavy) proton, while the (light) electron circled in a (planetary type of) orbit. Louise Markel (librarian of the ORINS) played some of the old texts on nuclear physics against *Science Abstracts,* and located what may be the first diagrammatic representation of elliptical orbits — it appeared in the *Annalen der Physik* of September, 1916, its author being the German physicist Arnold Sommerfeld (1868-1951). I continued the search and "discovered" the most beautiful and elaborate combination of orbits in

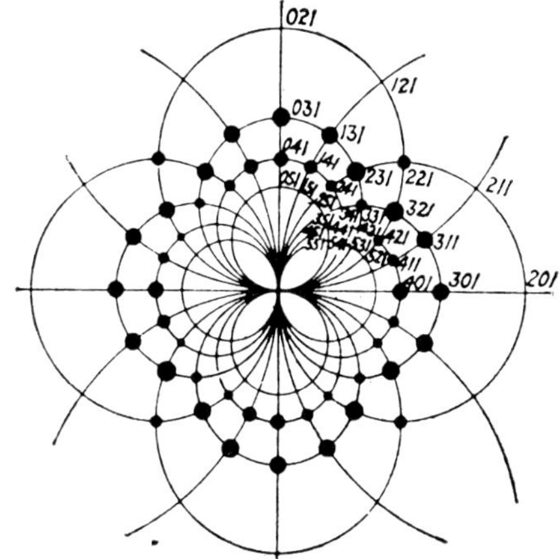

Courtesy: McGraw-Hill.

ANOTHER POLYORBIT. This stereographic projection of a Laue pattern of KCl is reproduced from the princeps edition of Clark's *Applied X-rays.*

APPLIED X-RAYS

BY

GEORGE L. CLARK, PH.D.

Assistant Professor of Applied Chemical Research, Massachusetts Institute of Technology

FIRST EDITION

McGRAW-HILL BOOK COMPANY, INC.
NEW YORK: 370 SEVENTH AVENUE
LONDON: 6 & 8 BOUVERIE ST., E. C. 4
1927

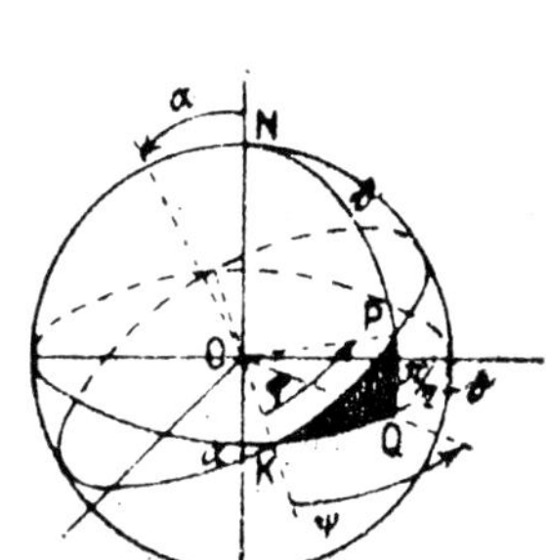

Courtesy: ORINS.

SOMMERFIELD'S ORBITS. From the *Annalen der Physik* (September, 1916) – these primordial elliptic pathways seem to be the first such (oval) pattern ever to appear in the literature – I am sure that earlier ones will yet be unveiled.

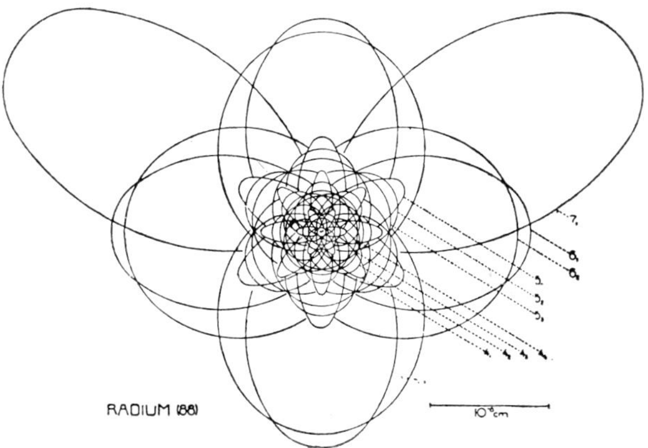

Courtesy: University of Chicago Press.

MILLIKAN'S ULTRA-ORBITED RADIUM. This was first printed in 1917 in *The Electron,* but the natural beauty of its multiple, interlacing orbits has yet to be surpassed.

the representation of the radium atom in *The Electron* (1917) of the American physicist Robert Andrews Millikan (1868-1954).

Another remarkable poly-orbit is the stereographic representation of a Laue pattern of KCL, reproduced

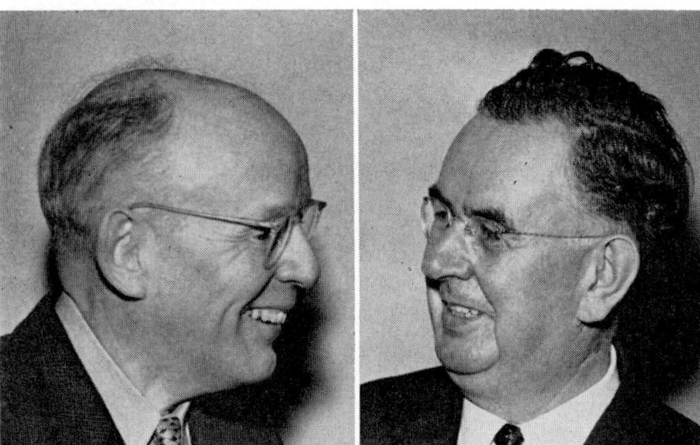

SMILING RADIO-PHYSICISTS. George Clark and hirsute Otto Glasser chatting in 1945 after the Symposium on Industrial Radiology held during the 50th anniversary of Röntgen's discovery observed at Marquette University in Milwaukee.

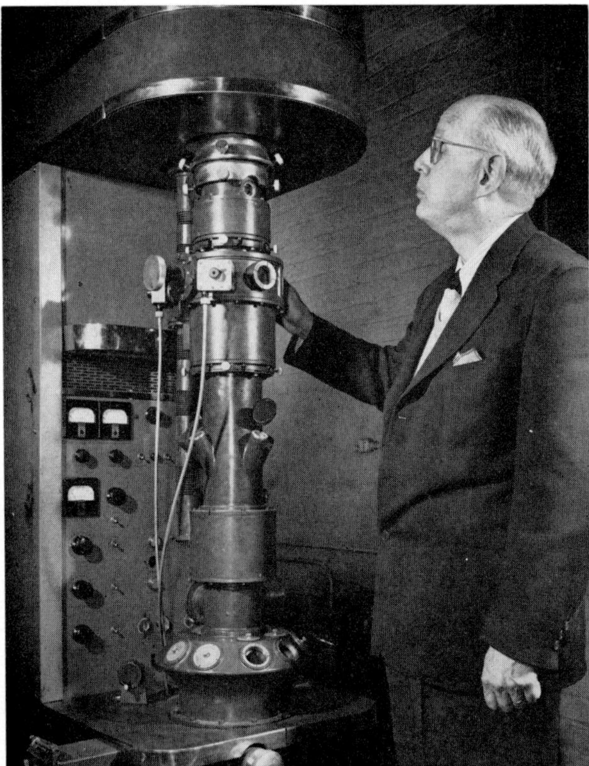

Courtesy: University of Illinois.

FIRST COMMERCIAL ELECTRON MICROSCOPE. In December, 1948 RCA built the first commercially-produced electron microscope, which was installed in the University of Illinois in Urbana. George Clark is "looking it over."

from the first edition of a classic, *Applied X-Rays,* first published in 1927 by the American all-time master crystallographer, George Lindenberg Clark. I have an autographed copy of the princeps edition.

The preface to that classic begins with the following sentence: "The primary motive underlying the preparation of this book is the presentation of x-rays as a new tool for industry." At the time less than fifteen radiostructures of crystals were known. Today – after the "alloy impetus" of World War II – the figure is up in the thousands. This boom is also shown by the fate of that book (published by McGraw-Hill): the second edition came out in 1932, the third in 1940, the fourth in 1955, and the next is overdue (it may yet be issued by Clark himself, fate willing!). Clark was born in Anderson (Indiana), and got his PhD at the University of Chicago (1918). He then became the associate of Duane (who may rightfully be regarded as the first American radio-physicist) at Harvard. Following three years at MIT, Clark went in 1927 to Urbana to teach analytical chemistry in the University of Illinois. In 1953, his title was changed to research professor of analytical chemistry, and in 1960 he turned emeritus. Clark published about 500 papers, and sponsored over 100 PhD theses in his chosen field – the structure of matter, as studied by x-ray crystallography. His works (some in manuscript) are to be deposited in the John Crerar Library.

In perusing old books, I found several representations of polyorbits, for instance the cardanic suspension, of which a more recent counterpart is Bernard Roswit's beam director for the angulation of x-ray tubes. The appearance of rotating fireworks is not dissimilar to orbits, but perhaps the closest to excentric ellipses are

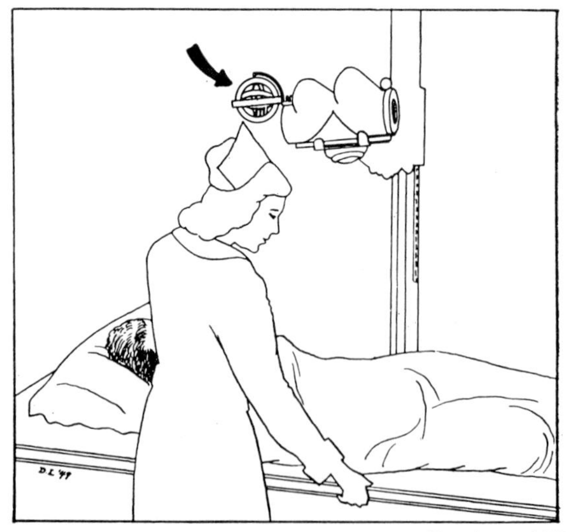

Courtesy: ARRS

ROSWIT'S "BEAMER". This illustration appeared in the *American Journal of Roentgenology* in January, 1951.

those on the plate of a star, from the *Original Theory or New Hypothesis of the Universe* (London, 1750) by Thomas Wright (1712-1786), who anticipated Herschel by 35 years in postulating a disc-shaped universe.

As a matter of fact, the polyorbital representation of the universe is very much older than that. A simple type of celestial globe, showing imaginary circles but not the stars or constellations, was painted on a mural (from about 50 A.D.), discovered in a villa at Boscoreale, near Pompeii. According to Derek J. Price, those early representations of the heavens evolved into the teaching armillary, undoubtedly influenced by Ptolemy's observing instrument, the armillary *astrolabon*. To these were later added the ecliptic with signs of the zodiac. This, then, combined with the age-old microcosmic representation of the macrocosm, spans the millenia between the antique Pompeian globe and the Rutherford-Bohr atom model.

It seemed desirable to check whether orbits had been used by the Manhattan Engineer District (MED) before Favale fastened them onto the AEC seal.

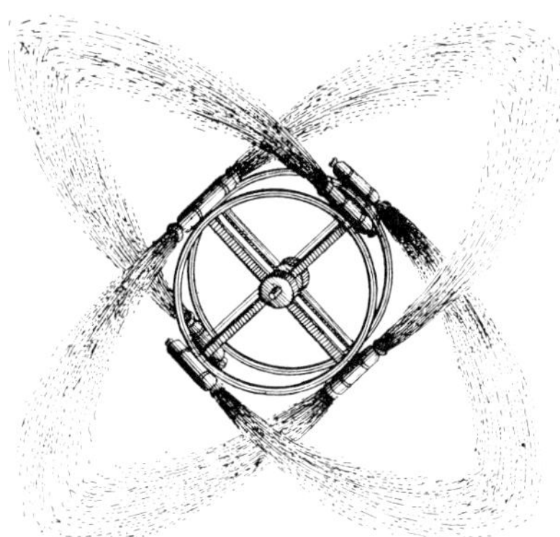

Courtesy: John Crerar Library.

MOVING STAR (1751). Firework display, shown in a French encyclopedia.

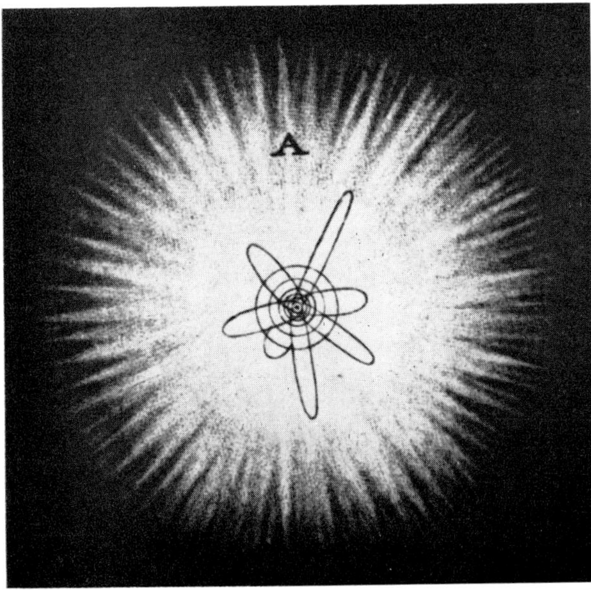

Courtesy: University of Illinois

ORBITING STAR. This is one of the 32 plates in copper and mezzotint from the very rare first edition of Wright's *Original Theory of the Universe* (1750).

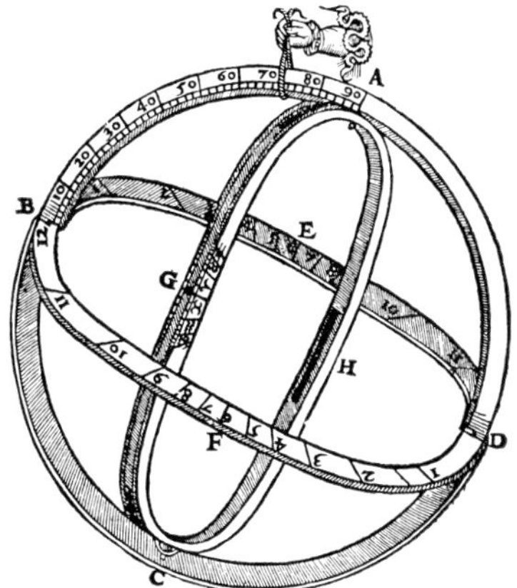

ANNULUS ASTRONOMICUS, a simplified version of the armillary or skeleton sphere, in which the rings represented celestial meridians and planetary orbits. It may be regarded as an ancestor of the "atomic" polyorbit. This particular picture of an "astrolabe" is herein reproduced through the courtesy of Dorothy Schullian, the expert in medieval medical history, who is currently directing the History of Science Collections at Cornell University in Ithaca (New York).

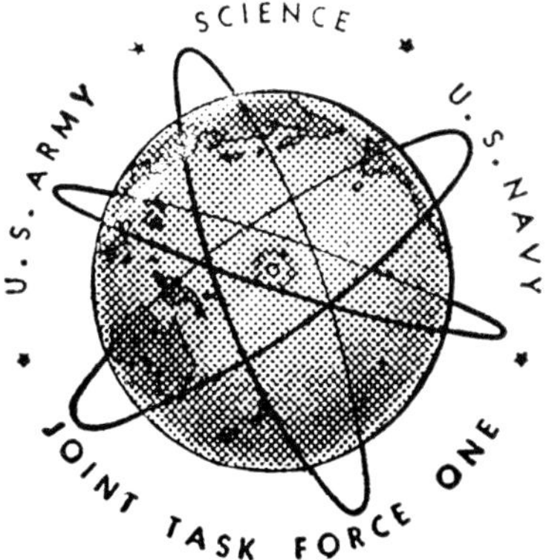

Courtesy: Stanley Paul Bohrer.

FIRST "FEDERAL" ORBITS. The earliest representation of atomic orbits on an imprint of the U. S. A. government appeared on the envelopes of Vice-Admiral W. H. P. Blandy, as he commanded the joint Army-Navy task force during the first postwar A-bomb tests on the Bikini Atoll (Marshall Islands). ABLE day was July 1, 1946 when first device was detonated in Operation Crossroads.

Wayne Range (the public communication officer of AEC's Oak Ridge operations) graciously came up with the glossy portrait of MED's patch as it had been worn on a sweater: a blue star, surrounded by a red circle, with a cloudshaped, white symbol on a blue background, and a similarly white lightning splitting a yellow ball. Wayne Range warned me to find the proper significance of these symbols, or expect some profane correspondence after publication. In the meantime I received from the Pentagon's Photo Branch a glossy of a similar (shoulder) patch, called the "atomic patch."

Marshall Brucer saved me by locating a clipping from the New York *Times* of October, 1945: it showed a wirephoto by the Associated Press with the "atomic insignia," explaining that the US Army was expected to issue this shoulder patch to about 3500 officers and enlisted men assigned to work on the A-bomb. The Army interpretation was that the blue field represents the universe, the small army service star signifies the command, the question mark indicates secrecy cloaking the project, and the tail of the question mark becomes lightning splitting an atom.

To all this Marshall Brucer added from his rich files the masthead of the *TEC* (Tennessee Eastman Corporation) *Bulletin* of 1946. That was a newspaper for the employees of the Clinton Engineer Works in Oak Ridge – carrying a not so hermetic seal, with the very words A-bomb and Manhattan Project.

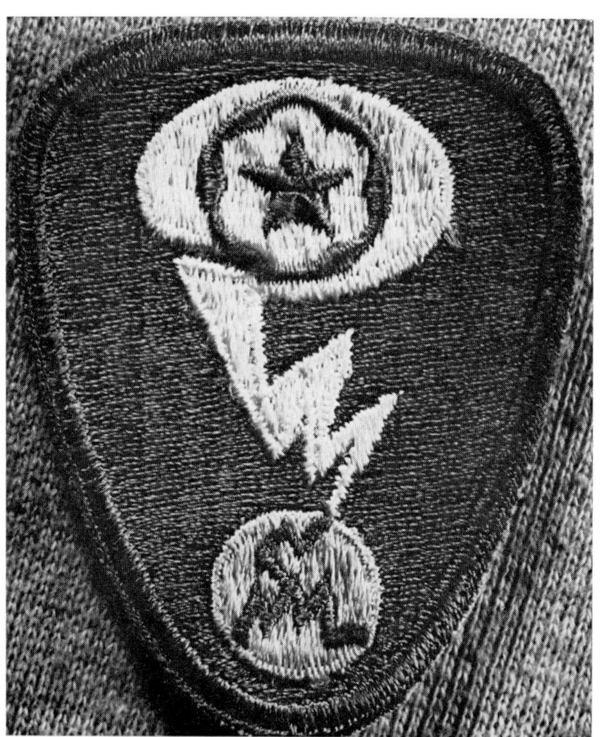

Courtesy: Wayne Range, AEC, Oak Ridge.

MED's "ATOMIC PATCH." This one adorned a sweater – the common variety was worn as a shoulder patch. In October, 1945 the U. S. Army distributed 3500 such patches to officers and enlisted men assigned to the A-bomb Project.

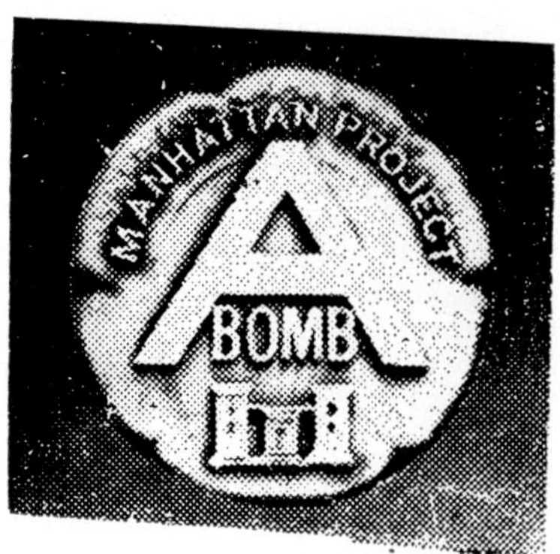

Courtesy: Tennessee Eastman Corporation

A-BOMB BUTTON. The Monday, October 22, 1945, issue of the *Y-12 Bulletin* (a newspaper for the employees of the Clinton Engineer Works of the Tennessee Eastman Corporation) carried the news that a certificate was going to be awarded to all those workers employed for more than six months between June 19, 1942 and August 6, 1945. Above button was awarded in bronze for six to eighteen months service, in silver for more than eighteen months service. The certificates were signed by Secretary of War Henry L. Stimson. This button was then reproduced on the masthead of the *TEC Bulletin,* and Marshall Brucer sent me a clipping from that publication. I wrote to Royal Tobey (sales manager of Eastman Kodak's X-ray Division), he in turn referred me to Jim Seat, current editor of the *TEC Bulletin,* and this is how we got the picture of the button.

MODERN ORBITING SYMBOLS

The orbits are used also by some commercial organizations which have only a vague relationship with the "atomic" business. Most prominently, though, the orbiting electrons, or reasonable facsim-

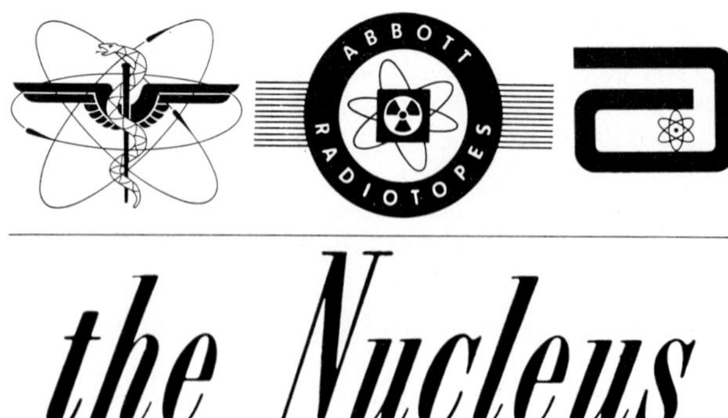

Copyright 1958, Nuclear-Chicago Corporation

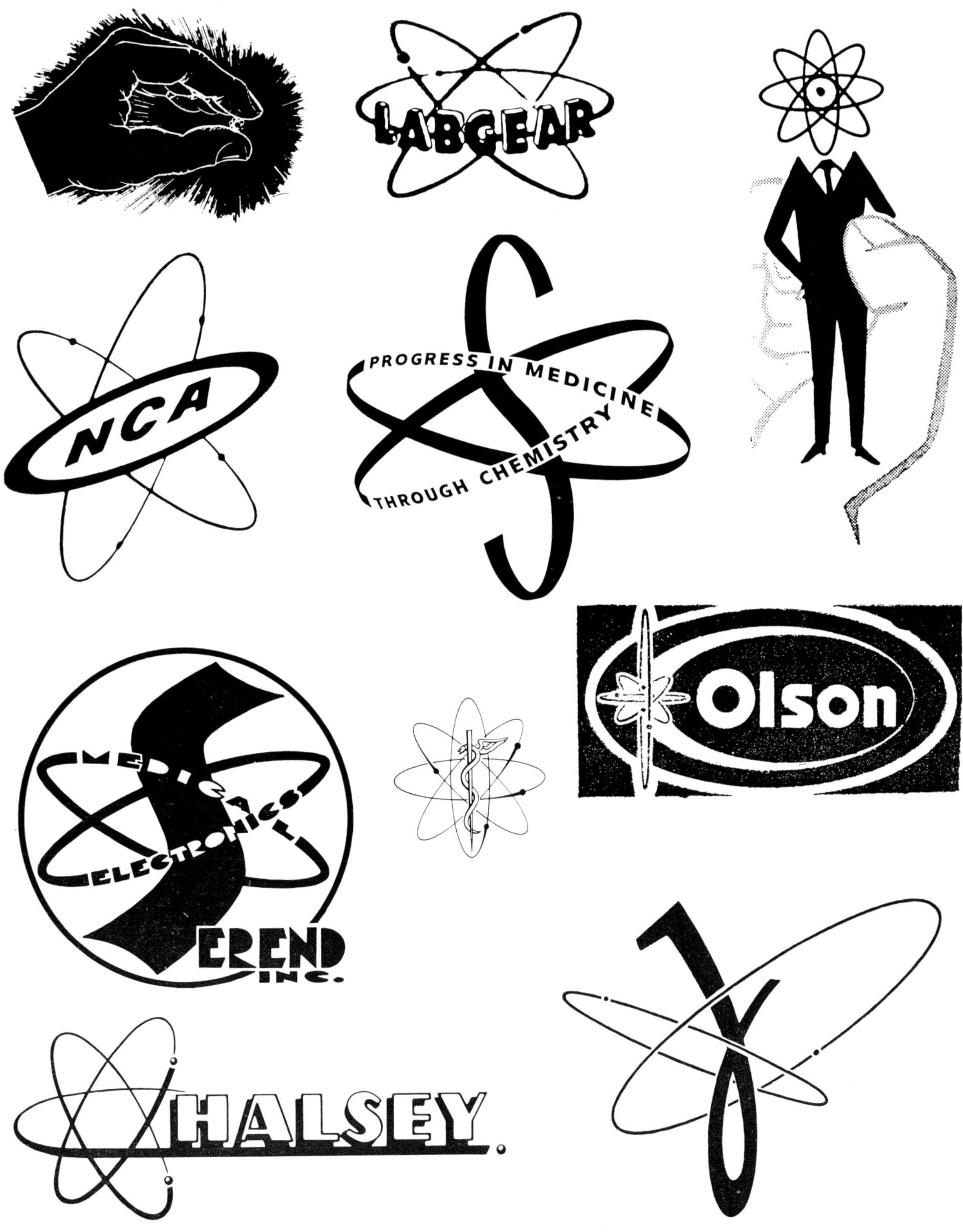

Atomic symbolism. Olson is a radio and television mail-order house. The single, winged snake belongs to Modern Medical Devices, a Brooklyn firm owned by a certified orthopod who sells a very ingenious black plastic envelope in which one x-ray film can be developed in daylight. Serend is also owned by a physician, Howard M. Edwards, who sells a miniaturized Japanese x-ray machine, so small that one would never suspect it could give the excellent service it does. The other S is from Strassenburgh Laboratories, a drug firm in Rochester (New York) – they sell, among other items, a sort of "strassionic" cough medicine. NCA is the Nucleonic Corporation of America, while the message is from the general manager of Martin-Nuclear. The hand holding the small atom is from Curtis Nuclear, the other hand indicates Atomic Personnal, Inc.

iles thereof, are displayed by specialized firms. Typical examples are found among the dispensers of "nuclear drugs."

Abbott Laboratories of North Chicago pioneered its Oak Ridge operations in 1948, built its own plant there in 1952. The manager of Abbott's Radioactive Pharmaceutical Division was Donalee Tabern (a former chemist known for his contribution to the development of Abbott's Nembutal and Pentothal), who became a co-founder of the Central Society of Nuclear Medicine. At least three Abbott seals contain orbits, including the miniaturized version fitted into their stylized capital initial. Abbott's wordmen proved to be up to their assignments and coined Radiotopes (from radio-isotopes), RISA (radio-iodinated serum albumin), and Radio-

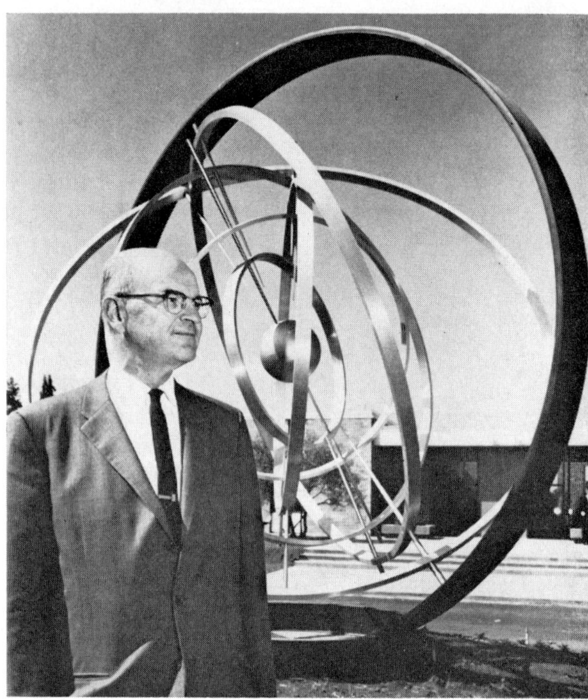

Courtesy: GE

GE ATOMICIZED "Orbits" of iron and anodized aluminum by sculptor John Slattery stand in front of GE's Atomic Power Equipment Department (APED) in San Jose (California). In front of the "orbits" is APED's general manager, George White.

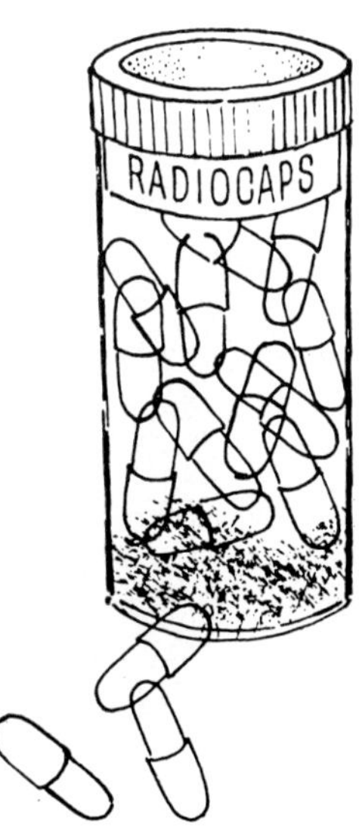

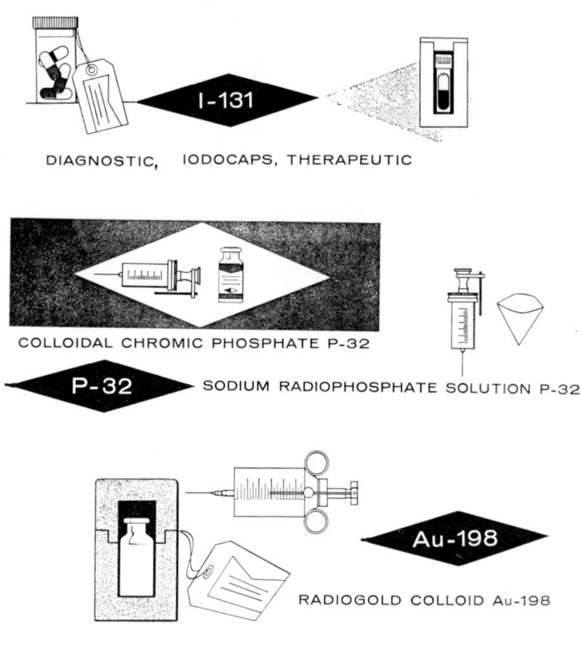

Volk RADIO—CHEMICAL COMPANY

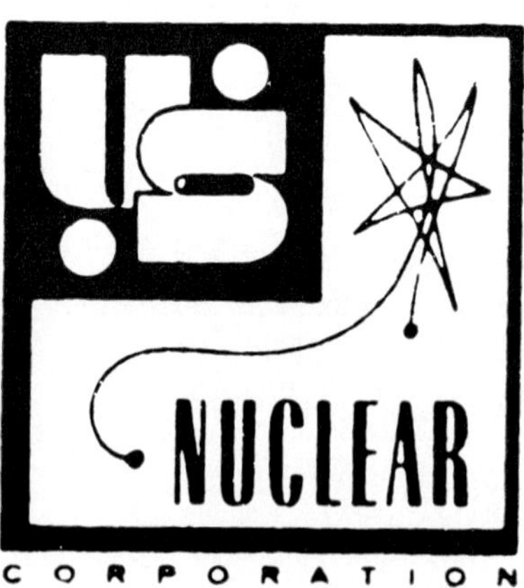

U. S. NUCLEAR CORPORATION was founded in 1959 in Burbank (California) as a distributor of radio-chemicals. They have since purchased Isotopes Specialties Company of Burbank, and Volk Radiochemical Company of Skokie (Illinois).

caps* (radio-active capsules). Isocaps is the same thing in the terminology of the radio-chemist Murray Volk's Radiochemical Laboratory of Skokie (Illinois). Their leaflets carry also the word iodocaps. Volk's favored is radio-medicines. The firm has built up a mail-order business of pre-calibrated radio-active material, especially for medical purposes, both diagnostic and therapeutic.

Radionuclides is the term found in the dictionary used by Nuclear-Chicago of Des Plaines (Illinois). This company was formed in Chicago in March, 1946. Its original name was Instrument Development Laboratories. It was founded by John L. Kuranz, Thomas E.

*To confuse the issue thoroughly, there are Radio Capsules which contain ultra-miniaturized telemetering devices: after being ingested, they will broadcast physiologic data to a receiver outside the body. Such capsules can be "radio-active," *i.e.,* battery-operated FM transmitters, or "radio-passive," *i.e.,* resonant circuits for re-transmission of pulses emitted by an external source. Incidentally, Herb Rich (from Curtis Nuclear Corporation) remarked that (atomically) radioactive capsules were first placed on the market by Reed-Curtis.

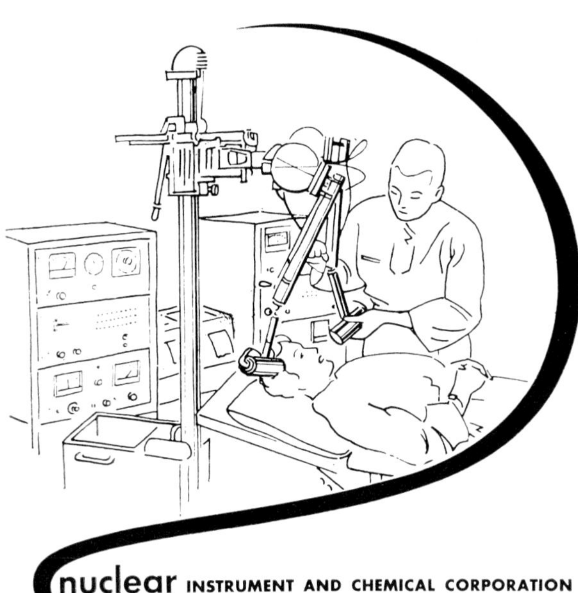

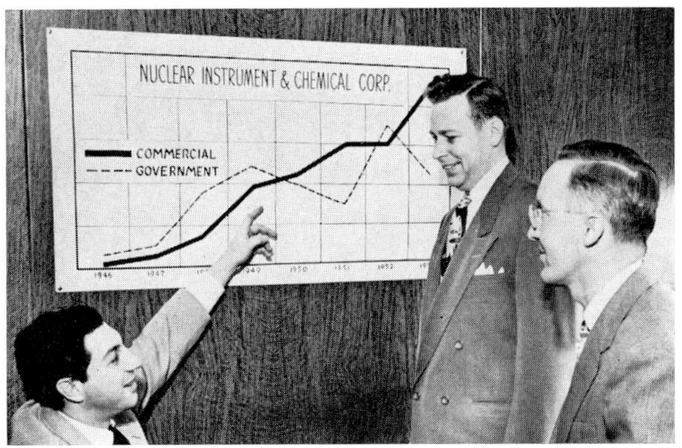

Courtesy: Nuclear Enterprises

FOUNDERS OF NUCLEAR-CHICAGO: James Schoke (pointing), Thomas Mitchell, and John Kuranz (with glasses). Only Kuranz has stayed with the company, and is now its vice-president and secretary. I met him at the Crystal Lake Airport: he flies his own twin engine plane, and so do I.

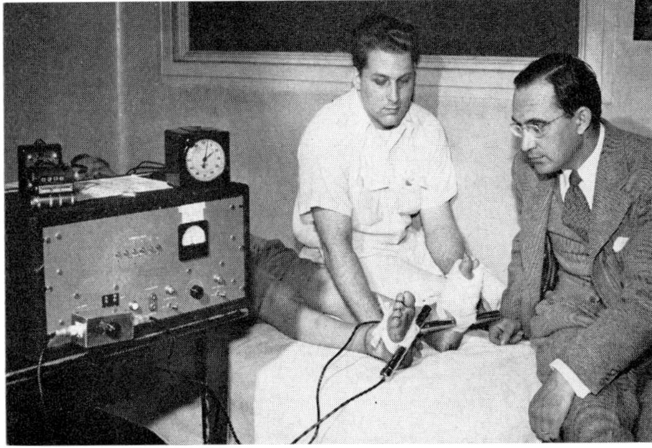

Courtesy: Nuclear-Chicago

COOK COUNTY HOSPITAL (1948). Fenton Schaffner and Morris Friedell (with glasses) use radiophosphorus and Geiger counter in studying a patient with arteriosclerosis. I know that scaler quite well, it is the same one on which I did my first uptakes, and it is still in good working order.

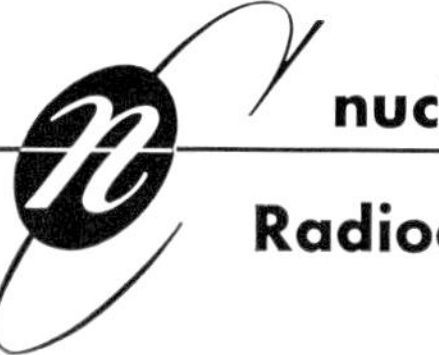

nuclear-chicago

Radiochemical Price List

Nuclear-Chicago liquid scintillation chemicals

PBD

PPO

POPOP

Liquifluor*

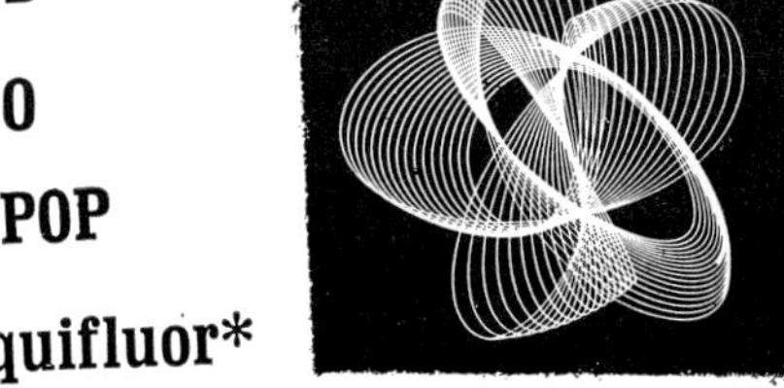

Scintillation Standards

Mitchell, and James A. Schoke, all of them formerly with Met-Lab's Instrument Division. Their first product was a binary scaler, which became almost the calling card of the company. Over the years they manufactured over 75 percent of all binary scalers ever made. The very first one, built in a one-room shop atop a delicatessen on 55th Street in Chicago, is still in daily use in a lab at the University of Wisconsin.

When it was incorporated in Illinois in 1947, it became the Nuclear Instrument and Chemical Corporation. The current name was adopted in 1954. In 1946,

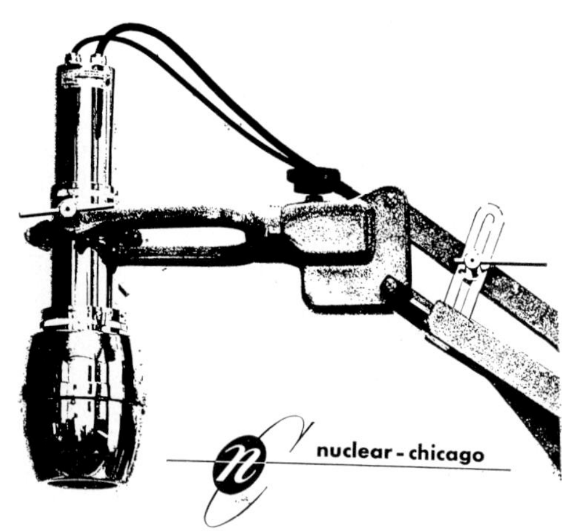

MEASUREMENT OF FAT DIGESTION AND ABSORPTION WITH RADIOIODINE LABELLED TRIOLEIN AND OLEIC ACID

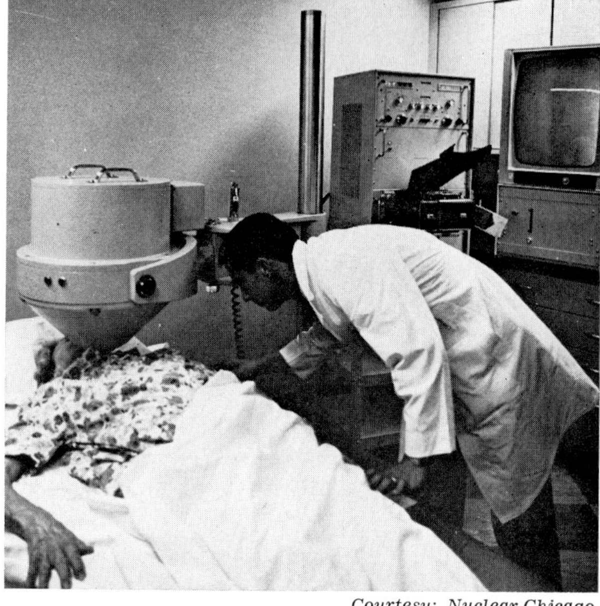

Courtesy: Nuclear-Chicago.

N-C's Anger Scintillation Camera. Latest, still partly experimental, scanning device uses 11″ circular crystal, 19 photomultiplier tubes, oscillographic tube, Polaroid camera and/or television viewing.

N-C's PHO/DOT Scanner (1963).

GEIGER - MUELLER TUBES

For All Radiation Detection Applications

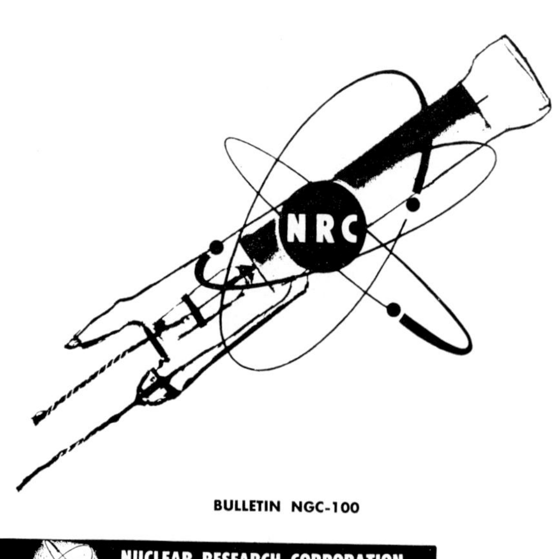

NUCLEAR RESEARCH CORPORATION
2563 GRAYS FERRY AVENUE · PHILADELPHIA 43, PA.

the company's net sales were $21,000 (the net worth $19,000 – by 1963 sales exceeded $13 million (the net worth reached $7 million). After the merger with Texas-Nuclear and with RIDL (Radiation Instrument Development Laboratory, a leading manufacturer of multichannel pulse height analyzers), and creation of Nuclear-Chicago Europa, N.V. (thus far a losing proposition), Nuclear-Chicago is now apparently the world's largest company in its field, has its own house organ *(the Nucleus)*, and markets everything from scintillation counters, scalers, and labelled (radioactive) compounds to subcritical (educational) reactors, isotope carriers, and nuclibadges. Among their "semantic" creations are the Mediac, a portable "thyroid" scintillation counter (adaptable also for blood volume and other measurements), and the Radiochromatogram (condensed from radio-active strip chromatogram) Scanner. As of late, Nuclear-Chicago employed about six hundred people in the five major plants and in the seventeen offices of the company. Nuclear's latest creation is the Anger Scintillation Camera, developed at the Lawrence Radiation Labora-

BENEDICT CASSEN. I have tried hard to obtain portraits of Curtis, Reed, and Libby. Cassen's cut is from Ben Orndoff's collection. I assume that difficulty was mainly due to the fact that Curtis and Reed had parted ways, and while the Curtis Nuclear Corporation exists as such, the C. W. Reed Co. is currently owned by Landwerk Electrometer.

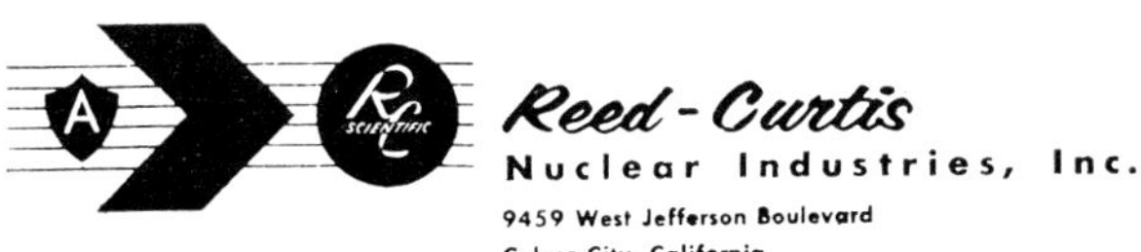

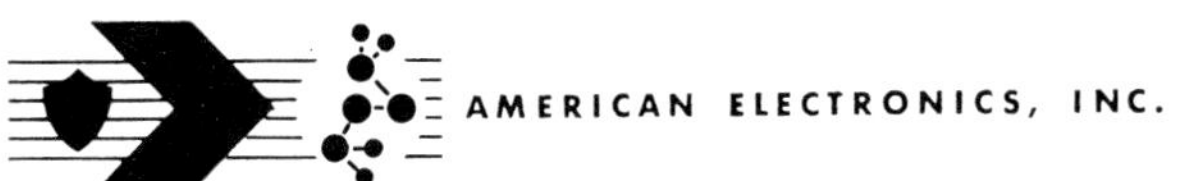

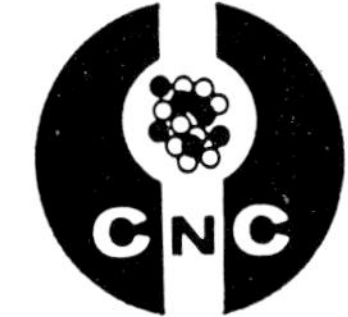

CURTIS NUCLEAR CORPORATION

"first in scanning"

THE ORIGINAL REED-CURTIS

Gardena, California

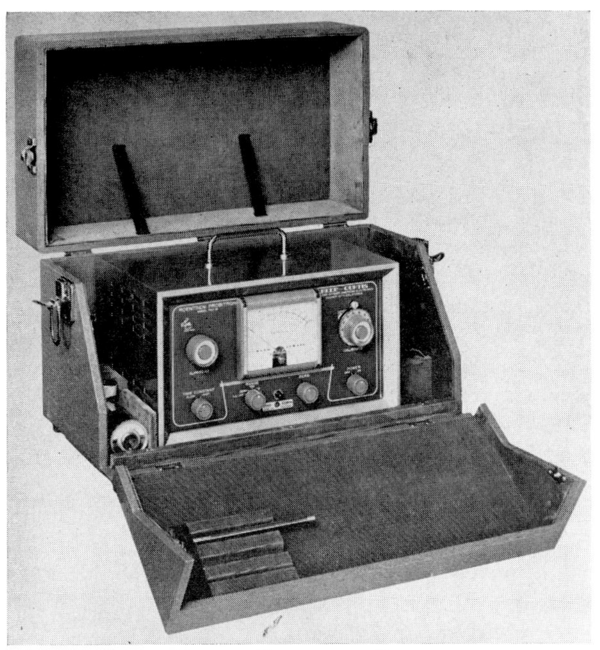

REED-CURTIS ROENTGEN-PROBITRON

Nationwide • SALES • INSTALLATION • MAINTENANCE

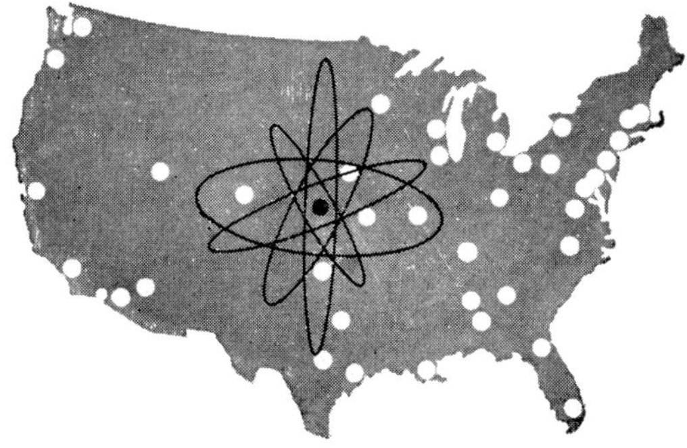

WESTINGHOUSE INSTRUMENTS FOR NUCLEAR MEDICINE... manufactured by the Reed-Curtis Nuclear Industries of American Electronics, Inc. Sold, installed, and serviced by Westinghouse X-ray representatives from coast to coast. Contact our local X-ray Office for a complete catalogue.

YOU CAN BE SURE... IF IT'S

1957 **Westinghouse** MEDICAL X-RAY

X-RAY DEPARTMENT · WESTINGHOUSE ELECTRIC CORPORATION
2519 WILKENS AVE., BALTIMORE 3, MARYLAND

tory of the University of California by Hal Oscar Anger. It has an 11" diameter round flat sodium iodide crystal, "viewed" by nineteen photomultiplier tubes, which feed their "overlapping" images into one cathode-ray tube screen. There it can be photographed (scintiphoto), or further fed into a television system. Completed pictures of the scanned area are obtained in one-half minute, instead of in half-an-hour. It also permits "stop motion" pictures of a radio-active substance flowing into and out of an organ, such as the kidney.

This brings up the problem of scanning. In 1958, Marshall Brucer remarked:

"It is considered somewhat quackish to talk of thyroid surgery without a neck scan. The true test of the usefulness of any gadget is that it changes somebody's mind about something. Because our therapeutic decisions have been influenced by scans, we feel that the scanner has passed through the gadget stage, and is now a diagnostic tool."

In the late 1940s the University of California at Los Angeles (UCLA) entered into a contract with the AEC for the study of "Peaceful Uses of Atomic Energy." Benedict Cassen, who was chief of the Medical Physics Section at UCLA, suggested that a scintillating material, optically coupled to a multiplier phototube, should make a good detector. Cassen's assistant, Larry Curtis, chose as the crystalline material calcium tungstate (developed by the Linde Company as part of a program to produce synthetic jewels), while the amplifier was built by Cliff Reed, then chief of UCLA's Electronics Section. This is how, after several trials and errors, was created the first scintillation detector. Early in 1949, Cassen, Curtis, Reed, and Raymond Libby devised an electro-mechanical device to move such a collimated

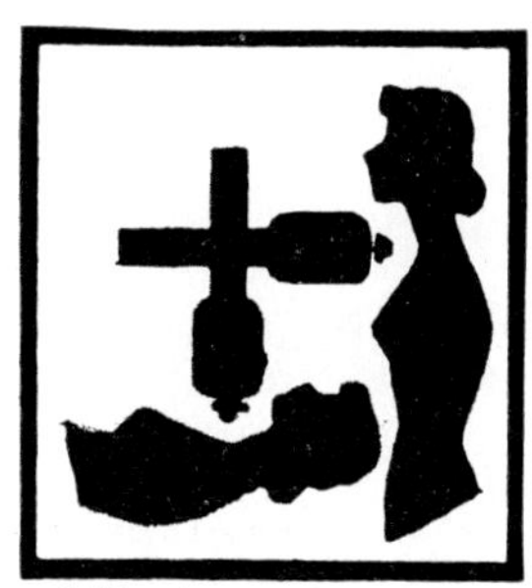

A flip of a switch provides vertical plane scanning.

TRI-D SCANNER

ATOMation inc.

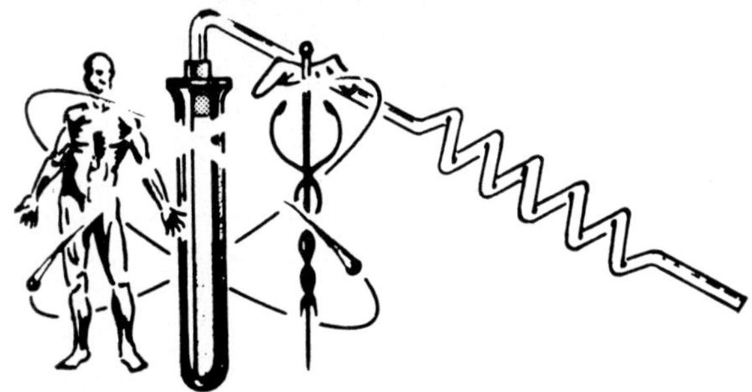

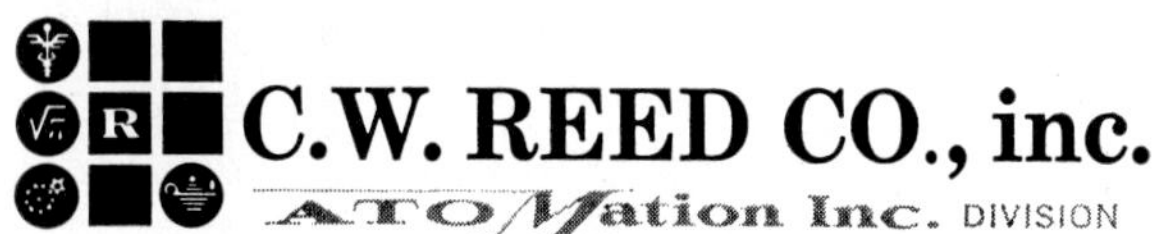

5959 S. Hoover Street, Los Angeles 44, California

Just off the board.......

UNIVERSAL

SCINTISCANNER

360°

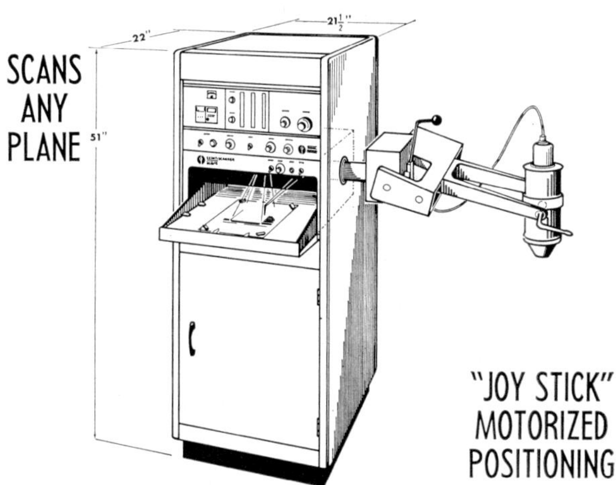

CNC's "ANY-PLANE" SCANNER. This is from an advertisement, which appeared in the *Journal of Nuclear Medicine* of July, 1961.

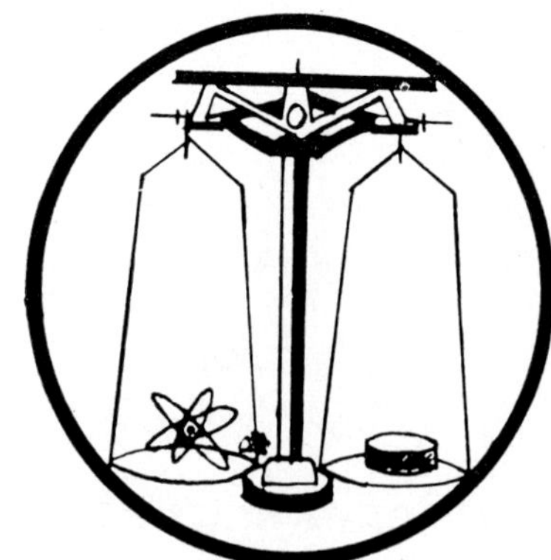

NUCLEAR MANDALA. This is the device of Bioassay, Inc., a laboratory for the radiochemical analysis of nuclides, located in Long Island City (New York).

scintillation detector back and forth across the area of radioactivity under investigation. The description of the very first scanner was published in *Nucleonics* of January, 1951. Then, with Cassen's approval, Curtis and Reed began building these scanners in a garage, and soon formed the R-C Scientific Instrument Company

Even before the scintillation crystal made the Geiger-Muller counter (almost) obsolete for thyroid applications, the Reed-Curtis Co. of Playa del Rey (California) had pioneered the Scintiscanner. Since then Curtis-Reed – Lawrence R. Curtis and Clifton W. Reed – went through several mergers and re-adjustments (at one time they had made arrangements with Westinghouse). The current name is Curtis Nuclear Corporation. Atomation Inc., a division of C. W. Reed Company, put out the read-o-matic computer scaler well

WHY THE PROBE IS MOVING- AND YOU'RE NOT CRANKING IT!
YES, BA'S NEW MOTOR DRIVEN REMOTE CONTROL VERTICAL DRIVE MAKES IT EASY- EVEN FOR US GIRLS TO OPERATE

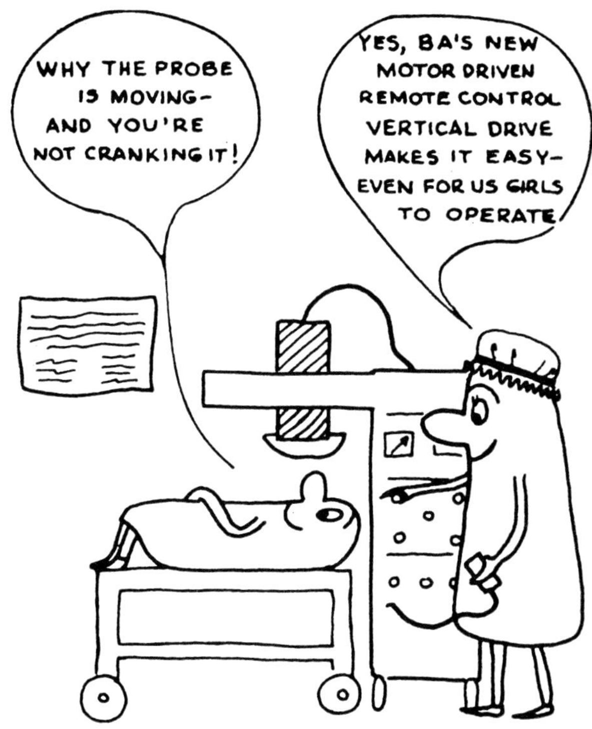

B-A's CS500 MEDICAL SCANNER. From *Scantastic*, Baird-Atomic's coloring book on scanners (1962).

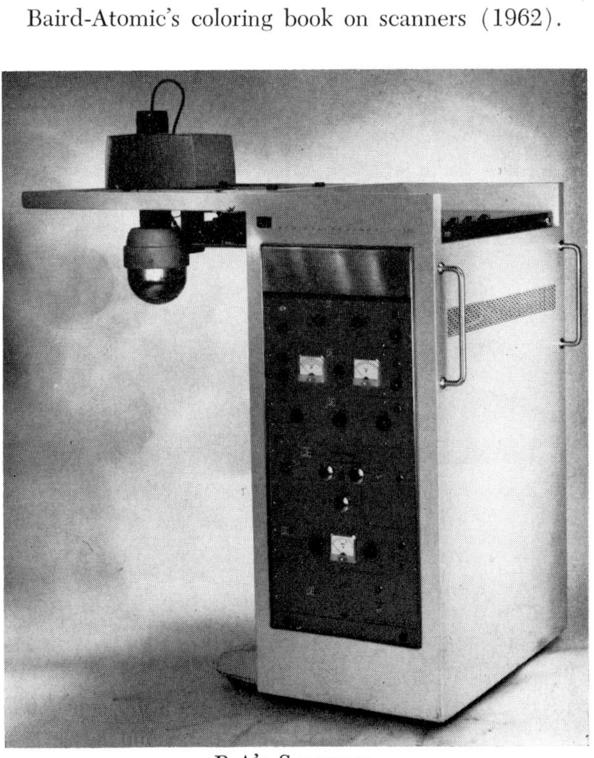

B-A's SCANNER.

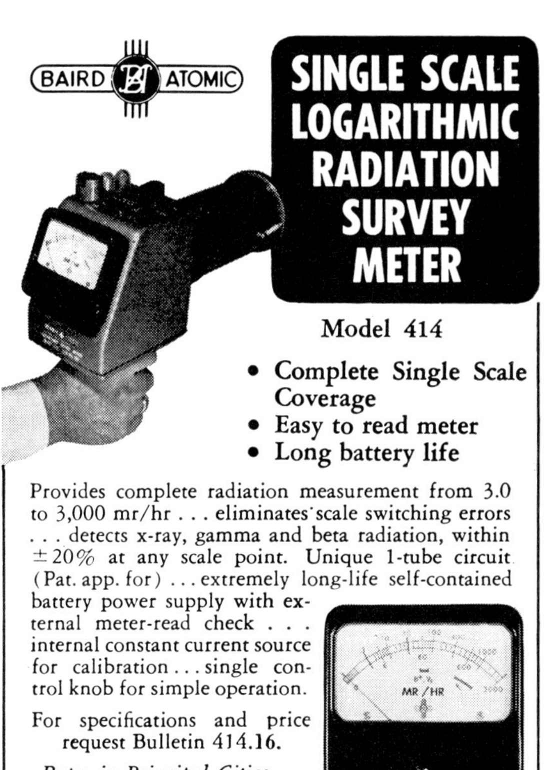

B-A CUTIE PIE. This is the code name used during wartime secrecy for the portable, battery-operated survey meter with long, cylindrical ionization chamber. This "early" B-A ad gives their first corporate name.

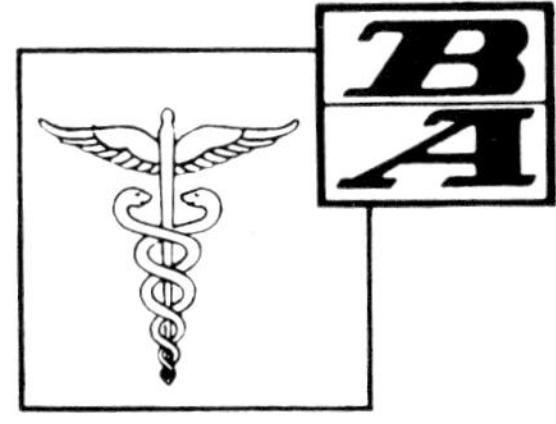

counting system, an automatized machine which calculates ratios, with associated paper tape printer; it is heir to the Automatic Spectra-Scaler built by Reed-Curtis, once the Nuclear Division of American Electronics. Reed's Radette (a scintillation counter similar to Nuclear-Chicago's Mediac) had been calibrated on one of Marshall Brucer's Oak Ridge girls (Jezebell, "married" in California). Atomation constructed the Tri-D Scanner, a dual detector system. Curtis's latest creation —which came out in 1961 — is the Universal Scintiscanner with "joy stick."

It is often difficult to keep track of the many short-lived "atomic" companies. Some are happy when they find someone willing to combine with them ("fusion"), the alternative being ("fission") complete volatilization.

Baird-Atomic in Cambridge (Massachusetts) makes the Positron Scanner (after G. I. Brownell and W. H. Sweet), a machine capable of twin tongue twisters, the coincidence positro-cephalogram and the asymmetro-gammagram. B-A's latest offering is a Medical Scanner, for the sake of which they have adorned their initials with an inter-twined snake symbol. B-A's subsidiary, Atomic Accessories of Valley Stream (New York) carries instead Saturn rings.

Saturn rings were also featured by the Radiation Instrument Development Laboratory of Northlake (Illinois). Atomium, Inc. of Billerica (Massachusetts) has a set of rings just for its "i".

Once upon a time the largest nuclear firm on the East Coast was "arrowed" Tracerlab in Boston. They prefer personalized prefixes, such as Tracermatic, its line of semi-automatized appurtenances. In 1958, Tracerlab marketed the first commercially produced total body scanner. Financial woes ended their marriage with Keleket. Both are now owned by LFE.

When Picker entered the nuclear field, they acquired only a conservative (written) seal, but the orbits appeared on the masthead of their (branched-out) house organ, the *Scintillator*. Tabern came to work for Picker, and they developed the Magnascanner: it permits both the conventional all-or-none "dot" stylus scanning, as well as the "extended range" photoscanning, with its multiple shades. Lately, Picker has purchased the plant, near Stamford (Connecticut), where its nuclear machinery was being produced.

The Scanograph, however, was not a scanner, just a portable scintillation detection unit constructed by the Nuclear Research and Development Company (NRD) in St. Louis. Also NRD creations were the Clinitron (another cousin to the Mediac), the Radimax (scintillation counter), the Radigraph (a scintillation counter system), and the Mediscanner. By that time they had changed their name to NRD Instrument

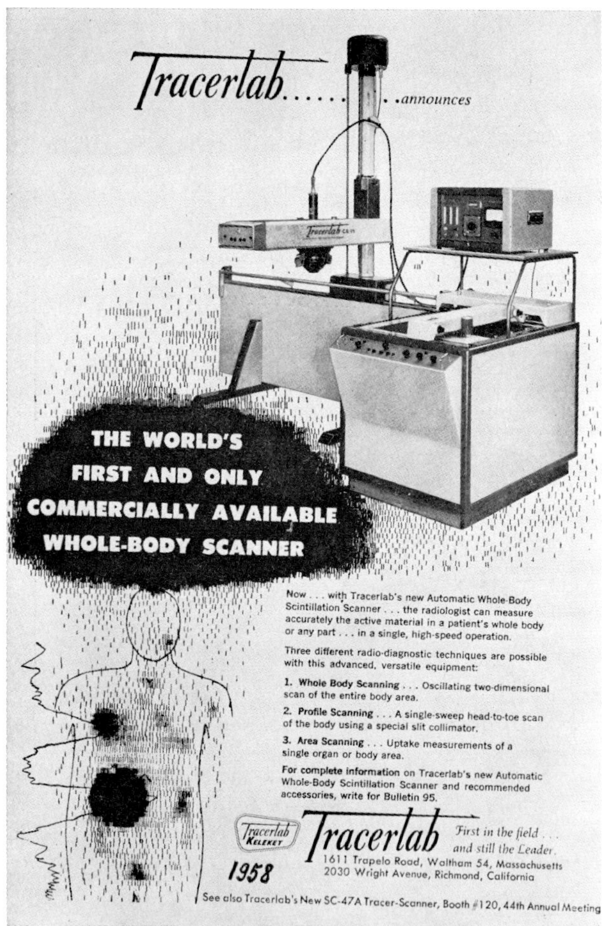

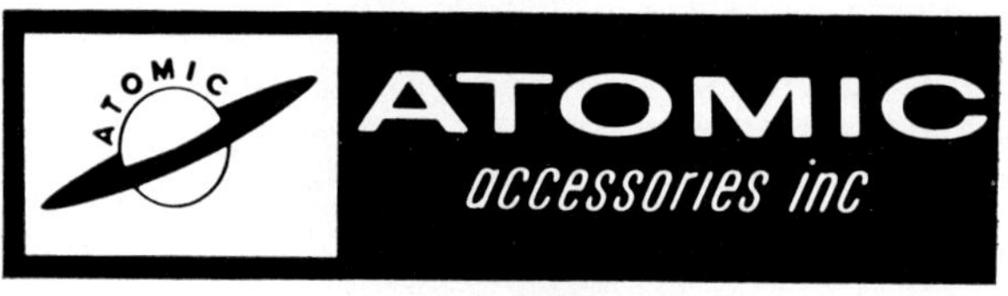

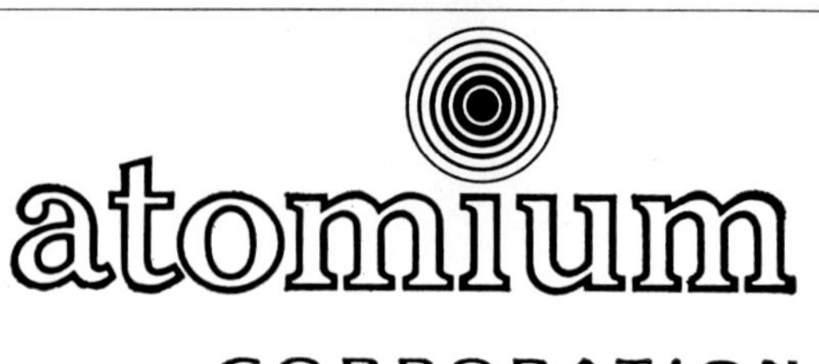

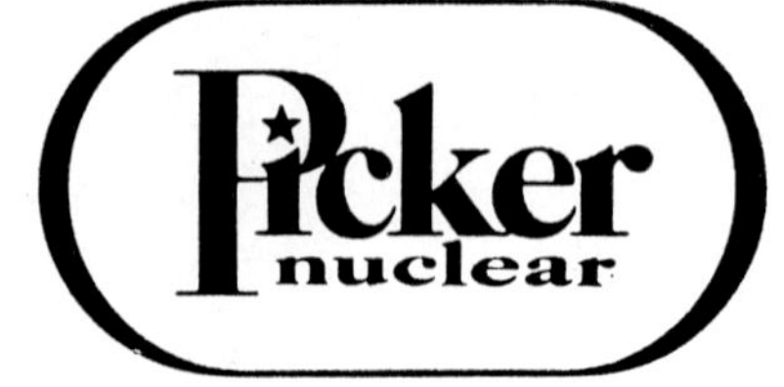

Company, and were a Division of the Nuclear Corporation of America (NUCOR). The latter sported for some time a stylized lower-case n, later turned to lop-sided orbits. NUCOR has discarded the old NRD sign, and has currently several affiliated sales organizations such as the Isotopes Specialties in Burbank (California), the X-Ray & Radium Ind. Ltd. in Toronto (Ontario), and the Nuclear Consultants in Long Island City (New York).

These must not be confused with the Nuclear Consultants Corporation of St. Louis — "originators" of Cobium-60, meaning Co-60 devices for brachytherapy, calibrated in milligrams of radium-equivalent. Their initials are NCC, not to be mistaken for NMC, the Nuclear Measurements Corporation of Indianapolis. The latter employs the tri-propelled radio-active danger signal in its insignia.

The danger signal is also used by other firms, for instance by the century-old pharmaceutical firm E. R. Squibb & Sons of New York City. Their "atomic" man is Paul Numerof, and their linguistic creation of the term Medotopes (presumably a condensation of medical isotopes). It has a large number of derivatives (all duly registered), *e.g.*, Rubratope, Cobatope, even the whimsical Robengatope (rose bengal), and the Albumotope Unimatic (RISA in a disposable syringe).

Three other firms will be singled out because their seals contain neither orbits nor other nuclear paraphernalia. The Atomic Instrument Company in Cambridge (Massachusetts) distributed its title around a cross pattern of parallel lines. The Radiation Counter Laboratories — located (not by coincidence) in the Nucleonic Park in Skokie (Illinois) — wrote their name into a triangle. The Landswerk Electrometer Company of Glendale (California), makers of various dosimeters, used the capital initials LEC.

PICKER
Scintillator

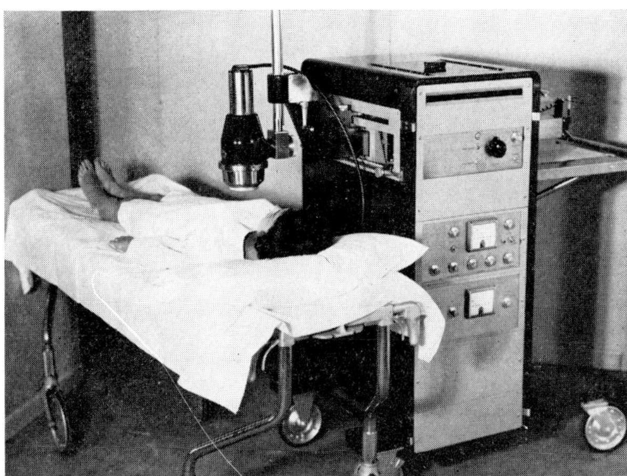

Courtesy: Picker.

PICKER MAGNASCANNER. Extended range photoscanner, one of several such models currently placed on the market by different manufacturers.

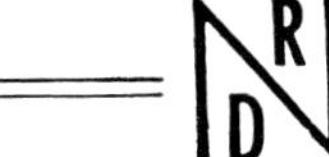

NUCLEAR RESEARCH and DEVELOPMENT, INC.

6425 Etzel Avenue
St. Louis 14, Missouri

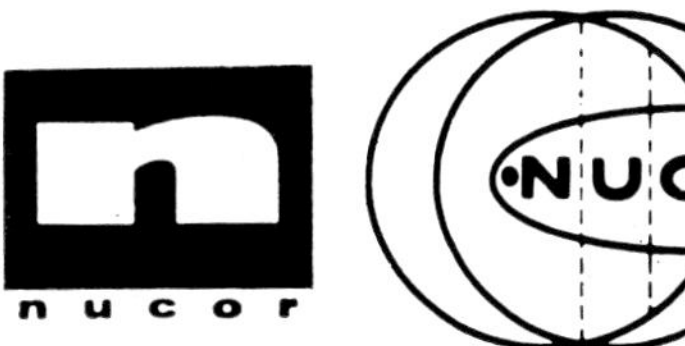

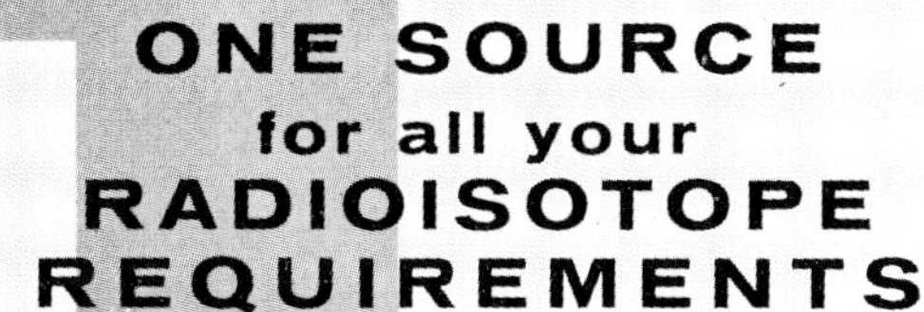

NRD Instruments

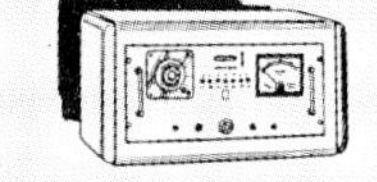

Radiopharmaceuticals

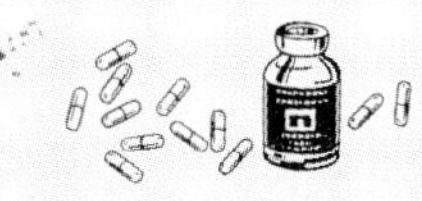

Consulting Service

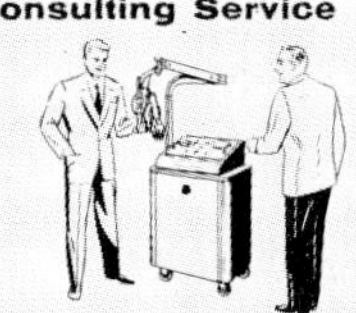

Now you can obtain all your radioisotope needs from one source. Only Nuclear Corporation of America offers these complete facilities:

NRD Instruments
Nucor Radiopharmaceuticals
Nuclear Consultants' Services

You can deal simply and easily with a single sales office for everything you need. Your requirements will be coordinated because we maintain a complete file for your laboratory.

The versatile line of NRD clinical instruments, proven by years of actual hospital use, will meet all of your needs.

A complete line of Nucor radiopharmaceuticals includes dosages shipped in precalibrated form ready to administer according to your specifications.

The physics consulting service offered by Nuclear Consultants is now being used by hundreds of hospitals. This program includes film badge service, health-physics control, instrument supervision and technician instruction.

For more details, including illustrated catalogs, consult the office nearest you.

nuclear corporation
of america, inc. 1957

SALES OFFICES:

Nuclear Consultants, Inc. 33-61 Crescent Long Island City, N. Y.
Nuclear Corp. of America 9842 Manchester St. Louis 19, Mo.
Nuclear Corp. of America 4754 W. Washington Blvd. Chicago, Ill.
Isotope Specialties Co. 703 S. Main St. Burbank, Calif.
Nuclear Corp. of America Box 7433, Sta. C Atlanta 9, Ga.
Export Dept. 431 Fifth Ave. New York 16, N. Y.
Canada — X-Ray & Radium Ind. Ltd. Toronto, Ontario and other major cities

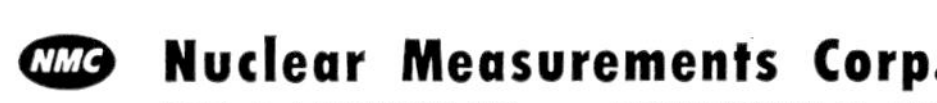

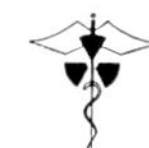

2458 N. ARLINGTON AVE. • INDIANAPOLIS 18, IND.

A number of firms have affiliated themselves with Nuclear Industries, Inc.,* which signs itself with the elegant lower case cursives *n* and *i.* Among these are Nichem of Bethesda (Maryland), "bottler" of isotopic labeled compounds; REAC (Radiation Equipment and Accessories Corporation of Lynbrook, New York), their maker of "atomic" instruments, such as the audio-visual warning device SCRAM; Tennelec of Oak Ridge (Tennessee), their "electronic" instrument maker; reactor Experiments (R/Ex) of San Francisco; Cosmic Radiation Labs of Bellport (Long Island); the arrowed Delta Instrument Corporation of Clifton (New Jersey), builders of the automated Thyrocomputer and the continuous monitoring (blood) Volumecomputer; the tri-

*NI is out of business. The component firms are continuing on their own.

PRICE LIST

MAY, 1958

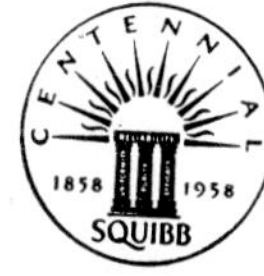

MEDOTOPES*

(RADIOACTIVE PHARMACEUTICALS)

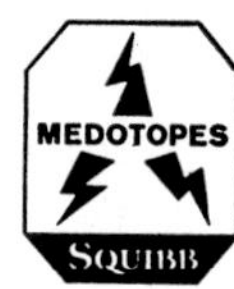

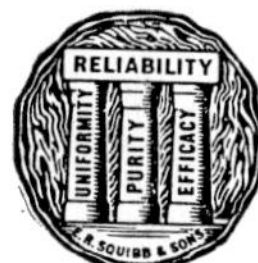

Supplied by

E. R. SQUIBB & SONS

DIVISION OF OLIN MATHIESON CHEMICAL CORPORATION

ATOMIC ENERGY COMMISSION BROAD COVERAGE LICENSE NUMBER 29-139-2

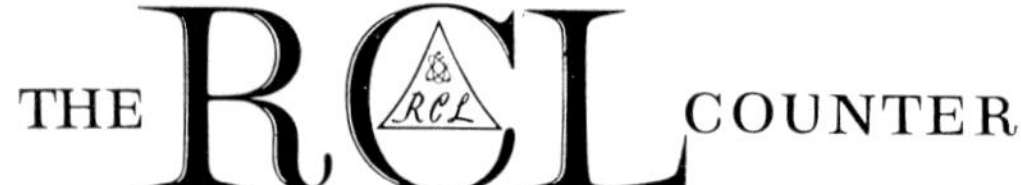

VOL. 7 PUBLISHED BY RADIATION COUNTER LABORATORIES, INC., NUCLEONIC PARK, SKOKIE, ILLINOIS, U.S.A. NO. 3

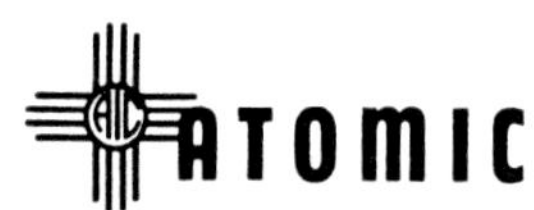

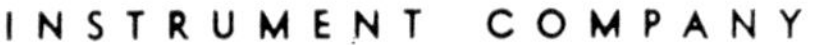

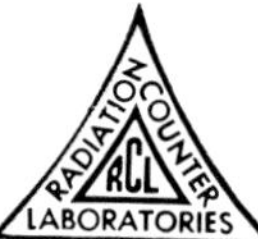

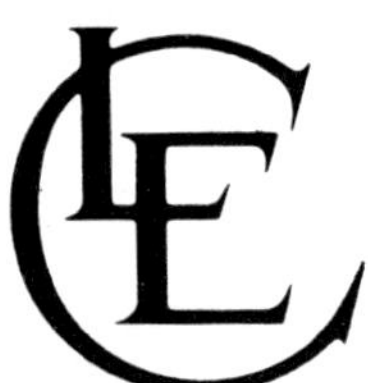

The Landsverk Electrometer Company

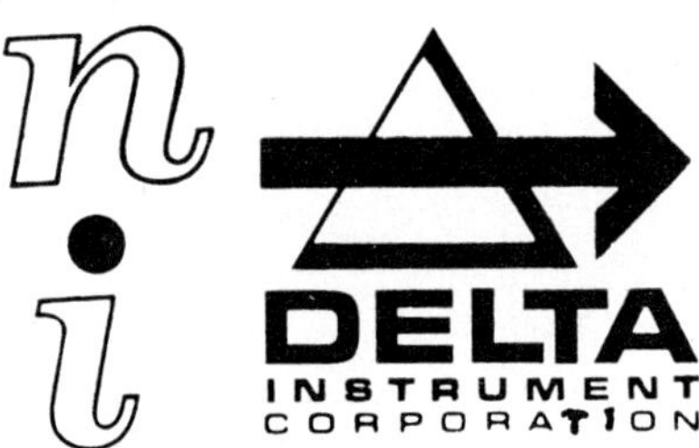

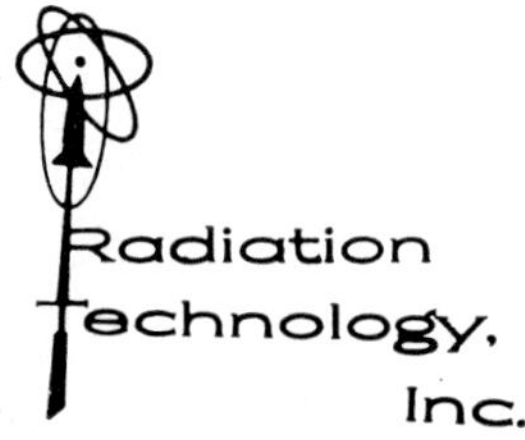

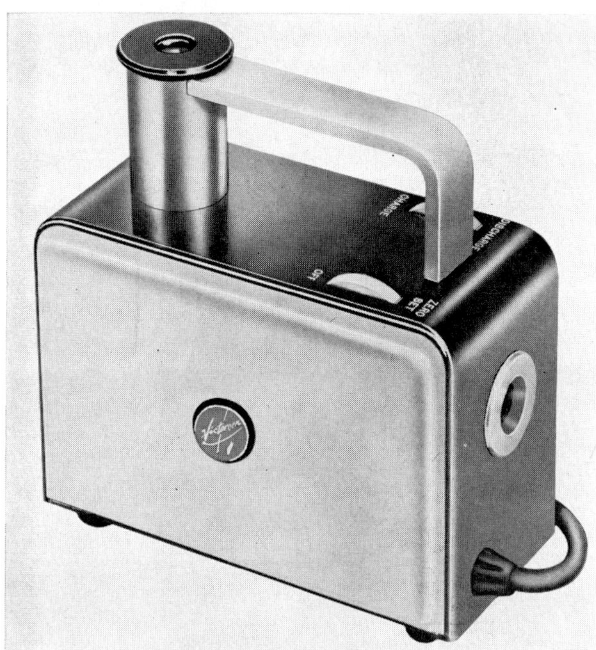

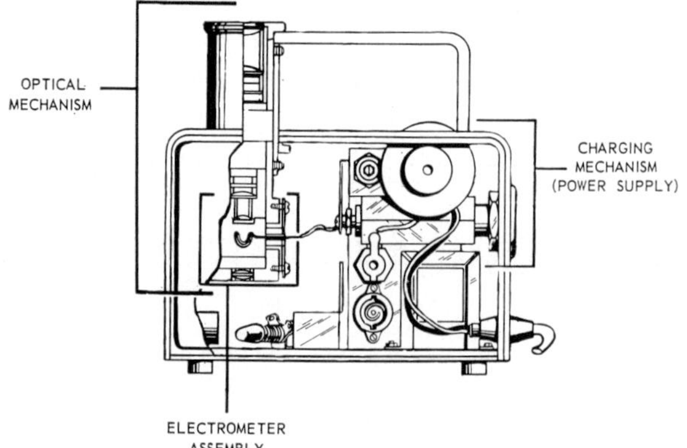

Courtesy: Victoreen.

CONDENSER-R-METER. Classic instrument, originally devised by Glasser and Fricke, seen here in its modern shape.

orbited Radiation Technology of Atlanta (Georgia); N.I.'s own headquarters were located in Valley Stream (New York).

The oldest (and one of the largest) maker(s) of radiacs is the Victoreen Instrument Company of Cleveland — one of their latest models in this category is the (transistorized) Thyac II. Of (more than) slight semantic significance are the names of some of their products, the Radector (a detector for both beta and gamma radiation); the Radgun (a sort of cutie pie with logarithmic response to measure both background and disaster levels); and the Minirad (a miniature gamma survey meter with four-decade logarithmic scale from .02 to 200 r/hr).*

VICTOREEN

Victoreen

WORLD'S FIRST NUCLEAR COMPANY

5806 HOUGH AVENUE • CLEVELAND 3, OHIO

Victoreen's Perscinticon was a portable thyroid and blood volume scintillation counter, similar to the type then popular in the industry. Among Victoreen's medical radio-measuring instruments can be listed the old reliable Condenser-r-Meter (for the calibration of therapy and other x-ray beams); the Iometer II (for continuous monitoring of the constancy of an x-ray beam); the Integron IV (for the measurement of cumulative doses on the skin); the Roentgen Ratemeter (for monitoring continuously the intensity of the x-ray beam directly in roentgens); and the Radocon, which is a cross between a dosimeter and a Roentgen Ratemeter (it serves to meter the prescribed dose at the skin over a wide energy range from 30 kev to 2 mev). The Victoreen Company has preserved its stylized tilted capital V, but it has also attached nuclear particles to its name, only their orbits are not quite complete.

*The Radector, the Radgun, and the Minirad are carried in Victoreen's catalog with Jordan's eponym. A search revealed advertisements of 1954 in which these products were being marketed by the Jordan Electronic Sales of Pasadena (California).

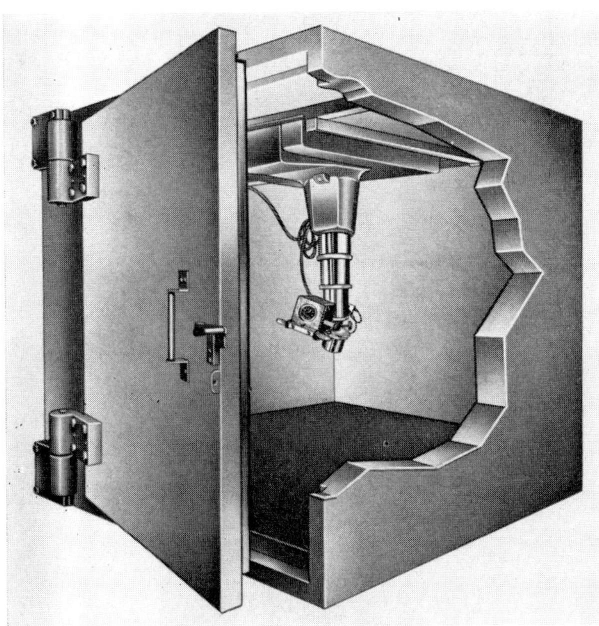

Courtesy: Metrix.

METRIX MX7 WHOLE BODY COUNTER (1962). Walk-in steel chamber with inside-ceiling-suspended detector for low-level gamma counting of humans and (other) large animals; sells for about $50 thousand; is manufactured by Metrix in Deerfield (Illinois), a company founded in 1960 by Stelios Regas, Max Chelf, and Ernest Carl Anderson.

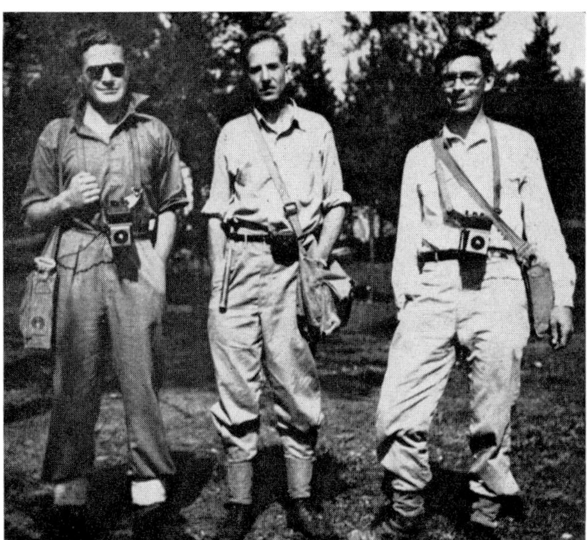

Courtesy: Nuclear Enterprises

FOUNDERS OF NUCLEAR ENTERPRISES, LTD.: R. W. Pringle (dark glasses), G. M. Brownell, and K. I. Roulston (glasses) in the Lake Athabaska area (July, 1949). Pringle and Roulston are carrying the first scintillation counters used in geophysical prospecting for uranium (instrument in side haversack, meter suspended in front).

Nuclear Enterprises, Ltd. of Winnipeg was organized in 1950 by three professors of the University of Manitoba, Robert William Pringle, a nuclear physicist, Keneth Irwin Roulston, an electronics specialist, and George McLeod Brownell, a geologist. They had developed the first scintillation counter for field use, and soon adapted it as an airborne instrument, which was flown exclusively by the USAEC for several years. With it were discovered some of the large uranium deposits in the USA, Africa, and France. The youngest of the three, Pringle, left his teaching position in 1955 to become the company's general manager. When they had to expand, in 1956, they made the unusual decision of setting up a British operation rather than an American one. Pringle was an Edinburgh graduate, and that is where he set up the plant and a sister organization, the Nuclear Enterprises (G.B.), Inc. The British branch – which makes the firm's big machinery, such as total-body counters – quadrupled in size, and, with about 200 employees as a work force, moved into a new plant at Sighthill (Scotland). At the Canadian operation they concentrated on chemical detectors. That department is headed by Boris Lionel Funt, who joined the company in 1954. They make all sorts of scintillation detectors,

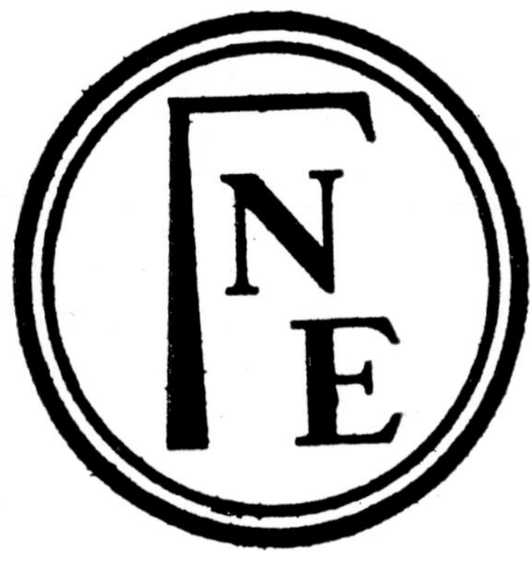

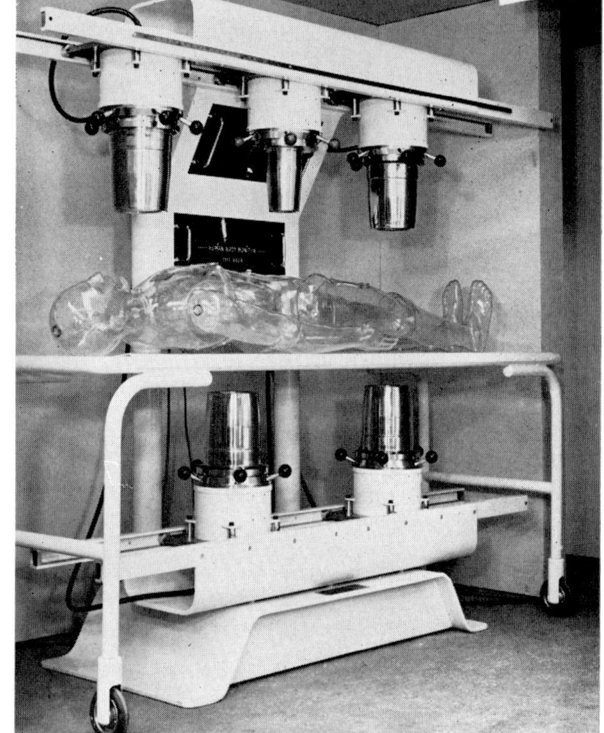
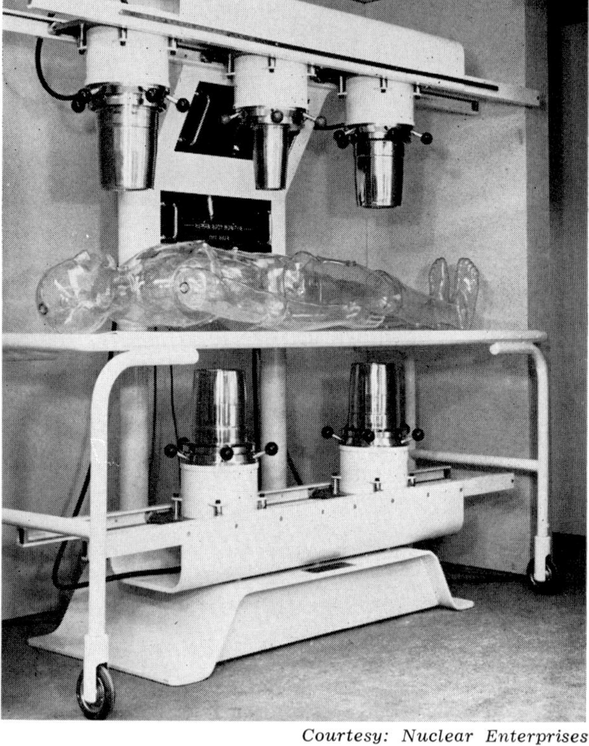
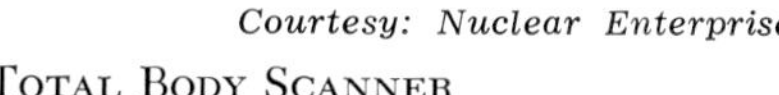

Courtesy: Nuclear Enterprises

TOTAL BODY SCANNER

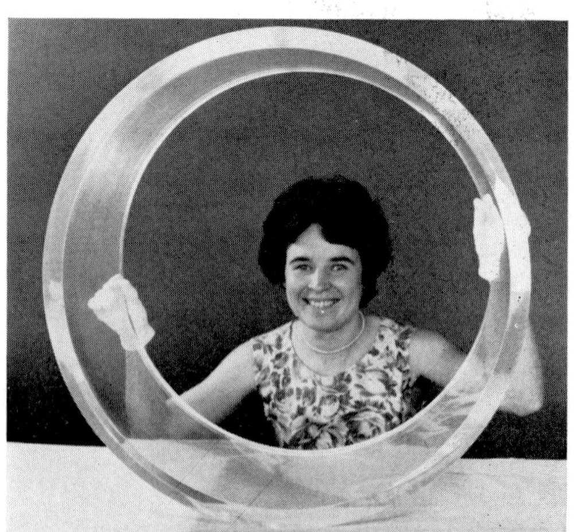

Courtesy: Nuclear Enterprises

NE 102 PLASTIC SCINTILLATOR. This annulus has 22″ interior diameter and is 12″ long.

not only plastic, liquids, and crystals, but also in film form (0.0003″ thick), in capillaries, and in fibre form. The mark of Nuclear Enterprises is the Greek capital letter gamma, sheltering the Roman initials N and E within a circular enclosure.

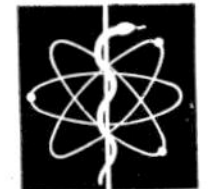
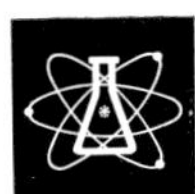
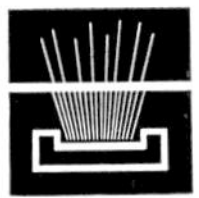
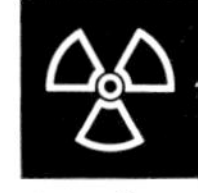
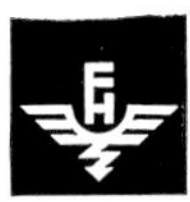

FRIESEKE & HOEPFNER SYMBOLS. This "atomic" manufacturer is located in Erlangen-Bruck (Germany). Their products cover the entire nuclear field.

ENCYCLOPEDIE CONSTAMMENT TENUE A JOUR

atome	**atome**
et	**et**
industrie	**droit**

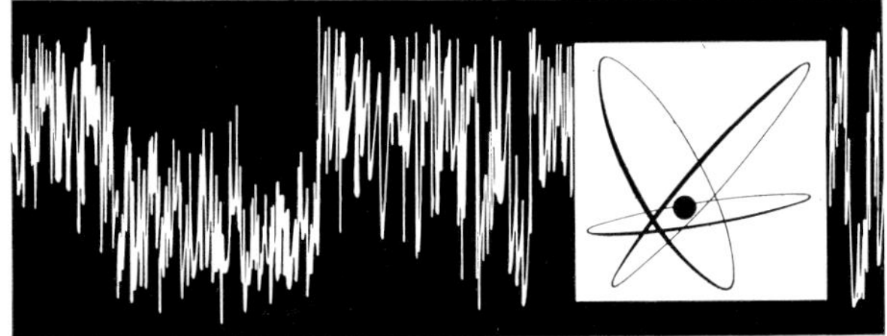

FRENCH LOOSE-LEAF ATOMIC ENCYCLOPEDIA. The two titles (atom and industry, and atom and law) are issued by the Librairie de Documentation in Paris.

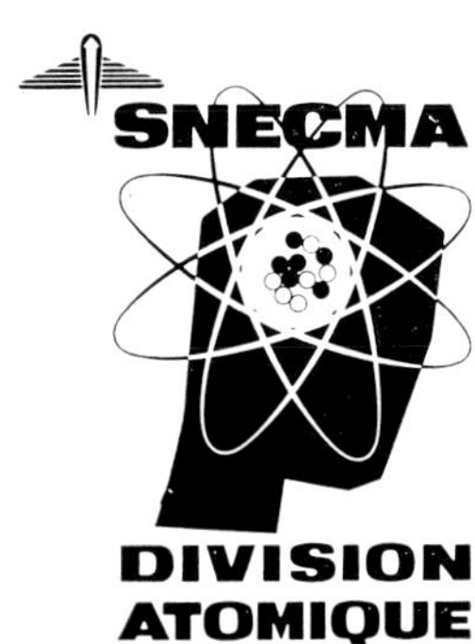

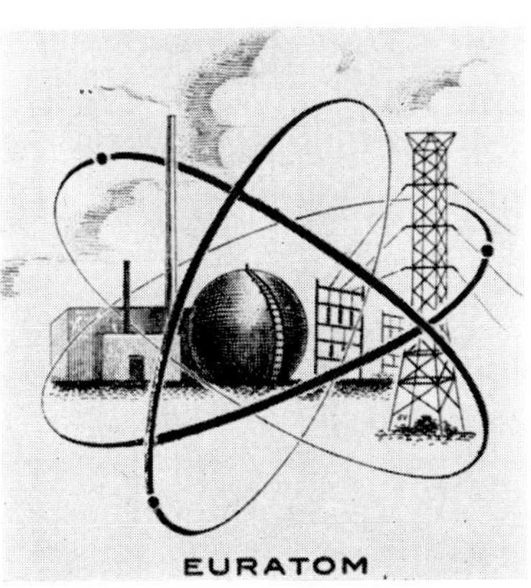

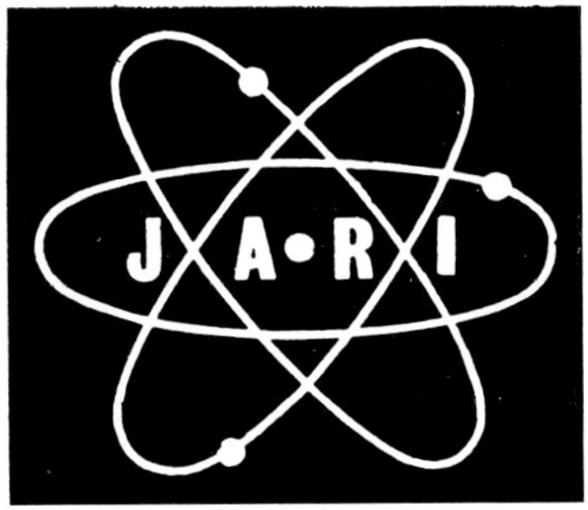

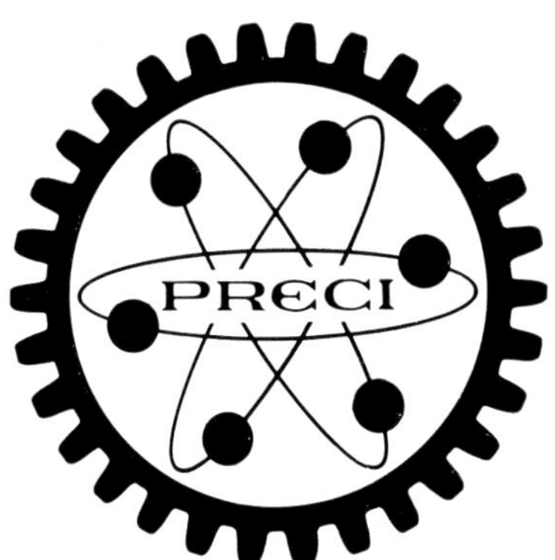

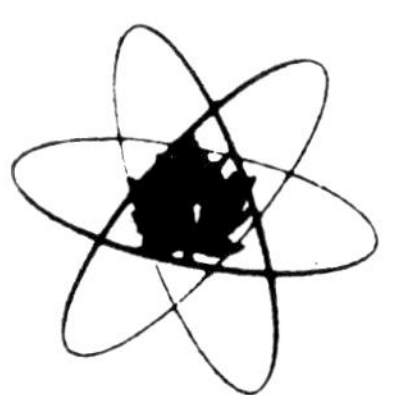

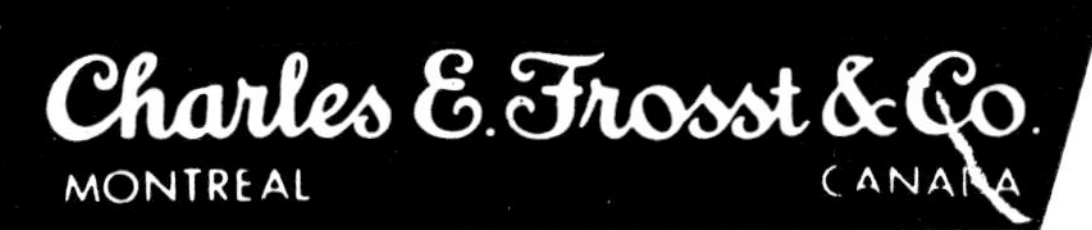

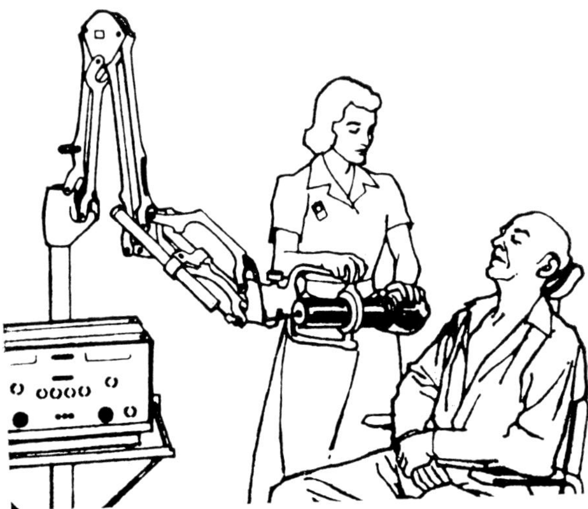

IODINE-131 UPTAKE MEASUREMENT. The sketch is from a Frosst advertising leaflet (they did not know its origin; it is a Nuclear-Chicago drawing).

So far, nowhere have the orbits been used as widely as in America. But it is not difficult to find examples of their utilization outside the United States. Beautiful designs are publicized by Frieseke and Hoepfner of Erlangen-Bruck (Germany), makers of all sorts of nuclear instrumentation, including a scanner, the Universal-Szintigraph FH 96. In France a loose-leaf atomic encyclopedia is issued by the Librairie de Documentation (Paris), and SNECMA, the airplane maker, has now its own atomic division. In England appears the *International Journal of Applied Radiation and Isotopes (JARI)*. And EURATOM, the European instru-

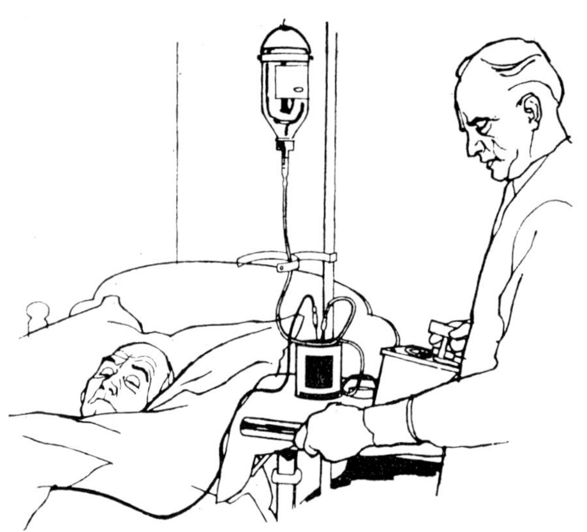

GOLD-198 INTRACAVITARY THERAPY. Sketch from Frosst leaflet, origin same as above.

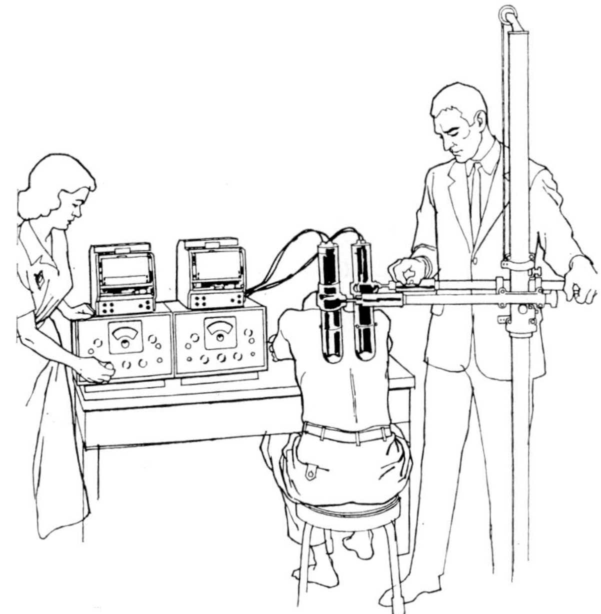

COMPARATIVE KIDNEY FUNCTION TEST. Sketch from Frosst leaflet.

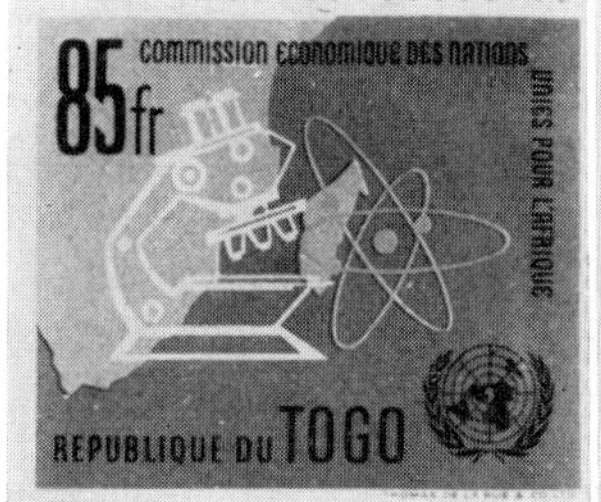

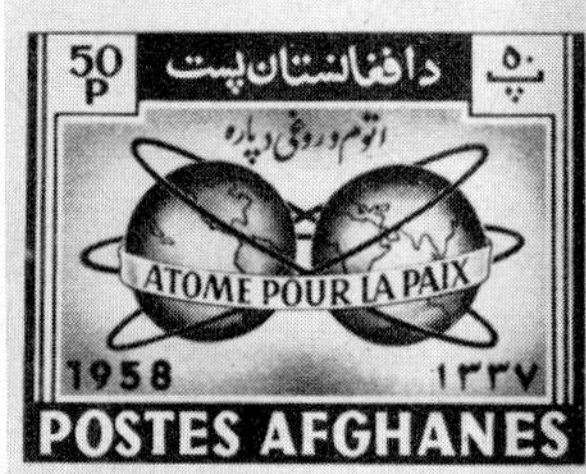

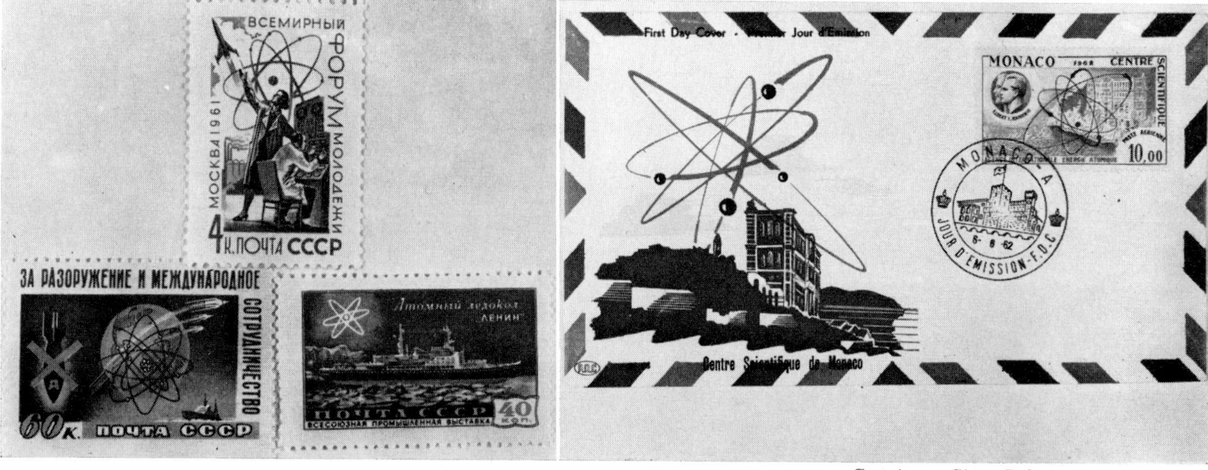

Courtesy: Stan Bohrer.

POLITICAL PHILATETICS. The orbits in the Sovietic stamps underline the fact that the successful sputniks could deliver atomic warheads. This is mitigated by the insistence on the word peace. The atomic ship shown on the two lower stamps is the nuclear-propelled icebreaker Lenin. Monaco's orbited first day (June 6, 1962) cover conveys the information that atomic instrumentalities and procedures are actively used in their recently opened Scientific Center.

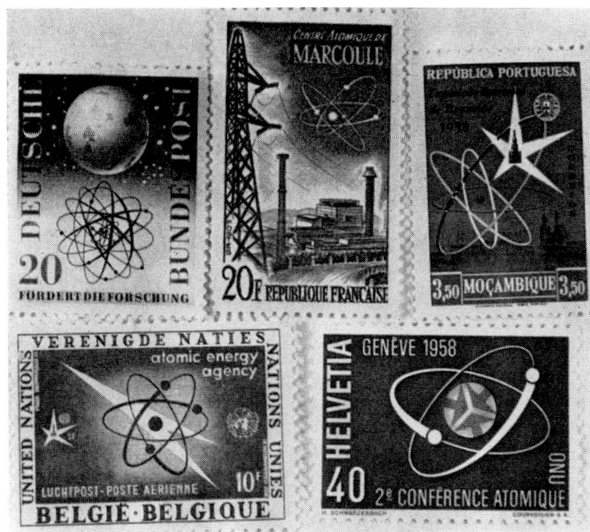

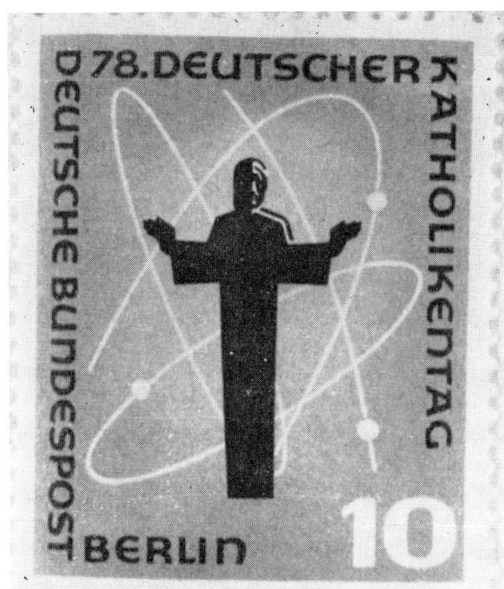

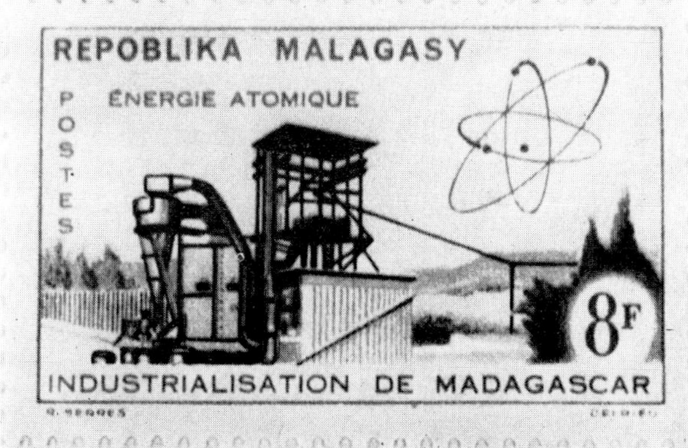

Courtesy: Stan Bohrer.

PHILATELICAL POLITICS. There must be a very sensible explanation for the use of orbits in each of these instances, but I could not find it.

ment for international atomic co-operation, is naturally very orbited. Neurosurgeons use the pneumotaxic x-ray localizer of Preci-Tools (Montreal) for intracranial orientation. The Canadian maple leaf replaces the imaginary nucleus in the orbits of Charles E. Frosst & Co. of Montreal.

And there are — as always — postal stamps, in this case with orbits extending from Moscow to Monaco, from Bonn to Geneva, from Berlin to Madagascar, and from Ankara to Afghanistan, as well as from Praha to Peiping.

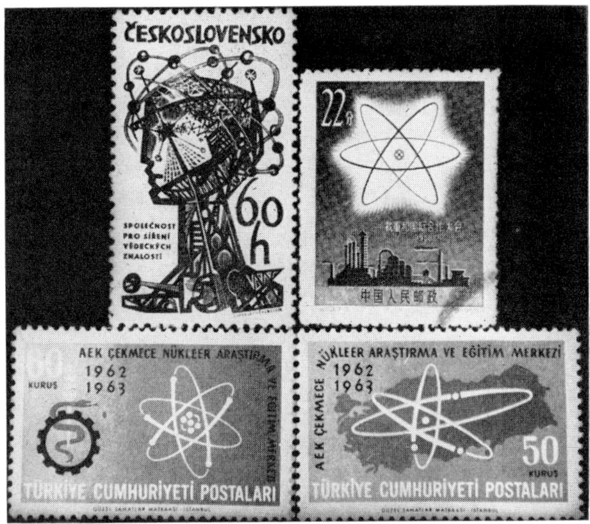

NUCLEAR VOCABULARY

Standardization of the nomenclature of radioisotopes procedures was advocated by Ervin Kaplan of Hines (Illinois) in the *Journal of Nuclear Medicine* of July, 1961. For *diagnostic* applications he suggested

HEALTH PHYSICS COMPUTATIONS

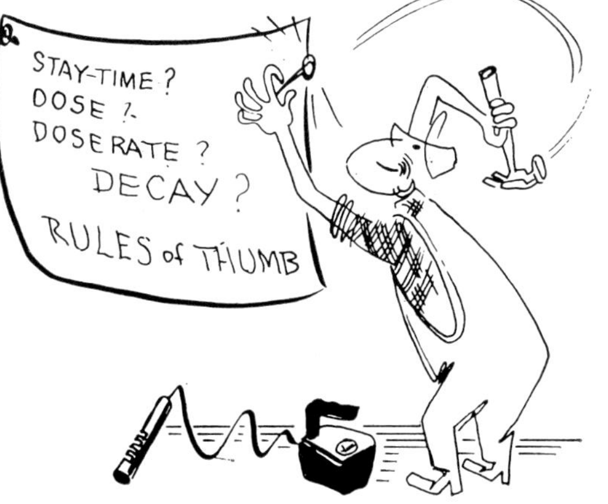

the use of five items: isotope, organism, function measure, method and author, *e.g.,* iodine 131 Hippuric Acid Cerebral Hemisphere Differential Circulation Volume (Oldendorf). For *therapeutic* procedures, he offered the following items: route of administration, isotope, therapy, disease or pathologic state, method, and author, *e.g.,* Interstitial Iridium 192 metallic pellet therapy for pelvic tumor by implant (Liegner).

RADIOLOGICAL SAFETY REQUIREMENTS

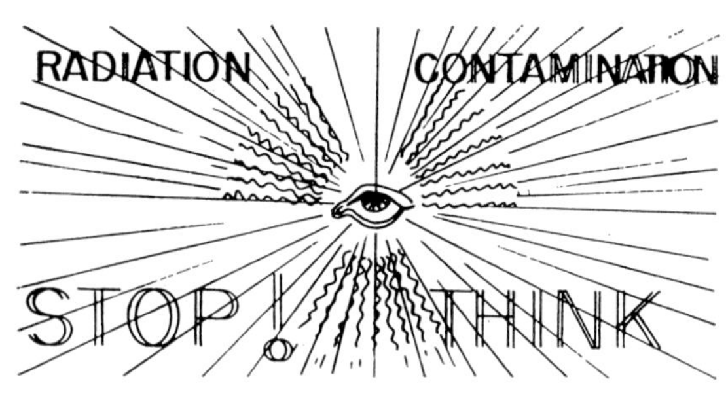

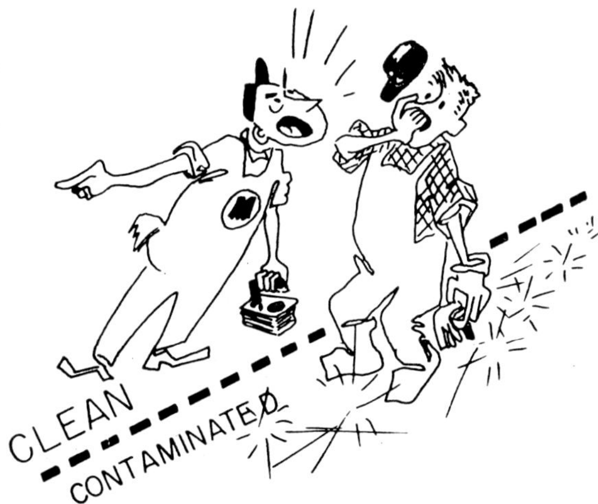

Courtesy: Bob Sulit's PORACC.

HEALTH PHYSICIST IN ACTION. One of the more desirable assets in a radiological team is an even-tempered contamination-(physic)ist.

HEALTH PHYSICS

OFFICIAL JOURNAL OF THE HEALTH PHYSICS SOCIETY

Volume I

KARL Z. MORGAN
Editor-in-Chief

W. S. SNYDER J. A. AUXIER
Editors

The nuclear upheaval brought with it expectations of groundbreaking diagnostic and therapeutic advances. Soon, though, it became clear that first of all one had to relearn a vast array of physicistic vocables. Introductory glossaries appeared in many of the texts devoted to the "new" specialty, as in the *Handbook of Radiology* edited by the radiologist (and radiophysicist) Russell Hedley Morgan, who teaches at Johns Hopkins, and by the physicist Kenneth Edwin Corrigan, director of radiological research in the Harper Hospital (Detroit). A word list is also included in the *Radiation Hygiene Handbook* (1959) edited by Hanson Blatz, director of New York City's Office of Radiation Control. This handbook is ostensibly intended for health physicists.

In the combined forms Radiological Health and Physicist the (always hard to define) health means the same thing as in Public Health: it implies preventive (safety) concepts, *i.e.,* radiation protection procedures. Not too long ago, radiologic safety officer was regarded as a better term than health physicist, but it did not prevail.

There are today in this country over one thousand recognized health physicists: they organized a Health Physics Society in June 1955 at Ohio State University, adopted a constitution and by-laws in June 1956 at the University of Michigan, had their first meeting in June 1957 at the University of Pittsburgh, and in June 1958 published the first issue of their official organ, *Health Physics,* edited by Karl Ziegler Morgan, director of Health Physics at Oak Ridge. Their seal is (naturally)

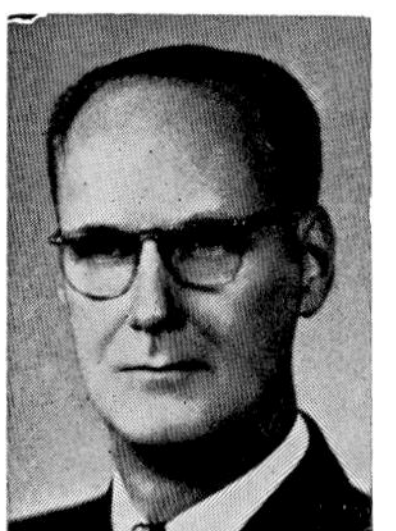

KENNETH CORRIGAN

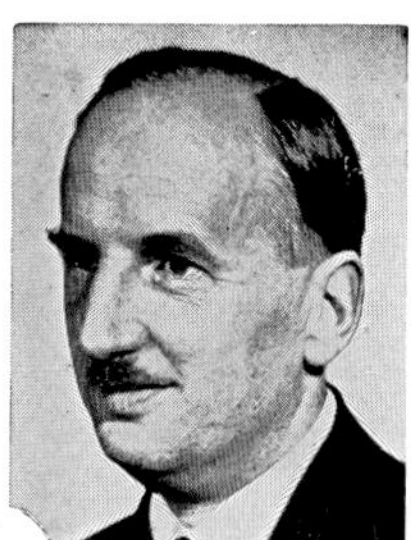

LLOYD KEMP

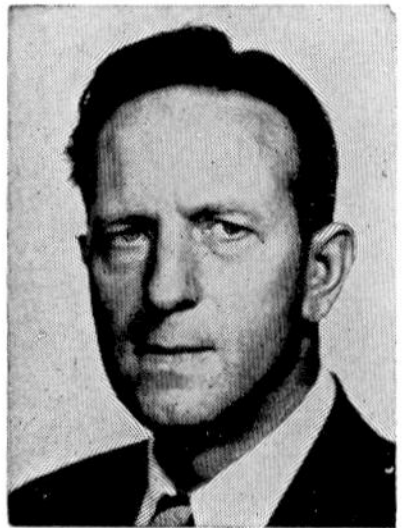

K. Z. MORGAN

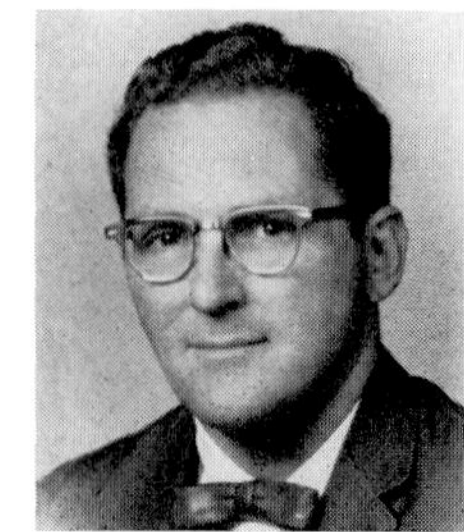

TED FIELDS

orbited, but they have not selected the one that I would have preferred.

Aside from revamping one's nuclear vocabulary, it became necessary, or at least desirable, to review related disciplines such as Kemp's *Radiological Mathematics:* to many this is not always as simple as its subtitle (Elementary mathematics applied to medical radiology) would imply.

ARS REVISITED

Late in the Golden Age of Radiology the American Radium Society was slowly dying. It had less than 100 members, and an obviously horizontal conformation. Among its members the actual (medical) radiologists had always been in minority. This is why the New York City onco-surgeon George Thomas Pack attempted to have the ARS name changed to American Cancer Society, or perhaps American Therapeutic Society. He failed, then the Atomic Phase came to be and the ARS revived.

The radioisotopes gave the ARS a symbolic "shot in the arm." It is true that radium is used less often than before, mainly because it is replaced by the cheaper Co^{60} in needles or in placques (without mentioning the packs).

While radon plants are being discontinued, and radium needles are used less and less for therapeutic purposes, there is an increasing demand for radium and beryllium sources, as a means of providing "neu-

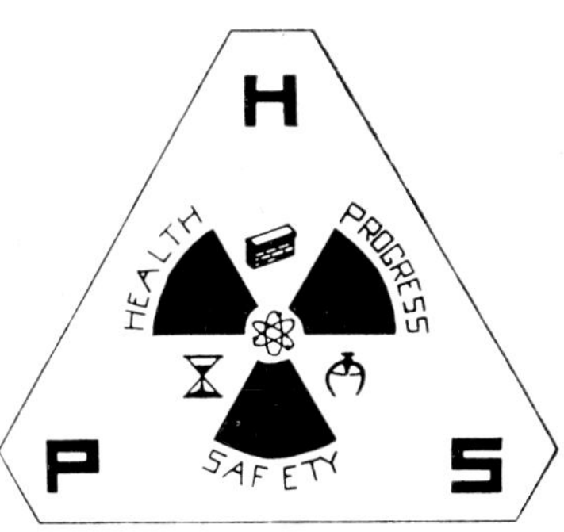

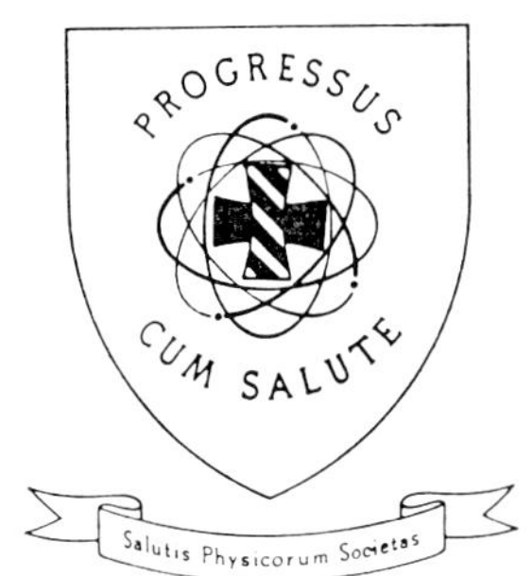

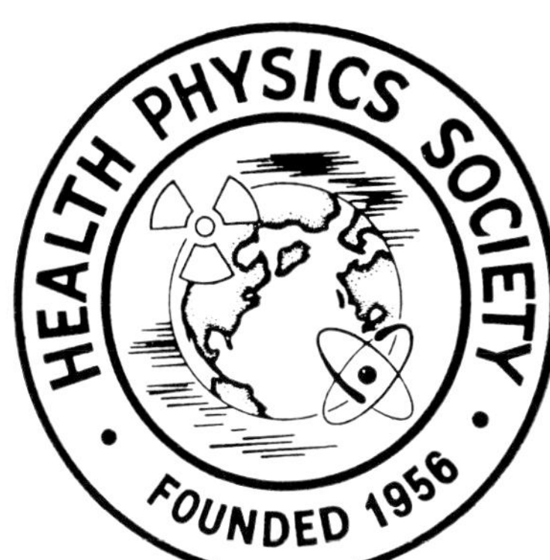

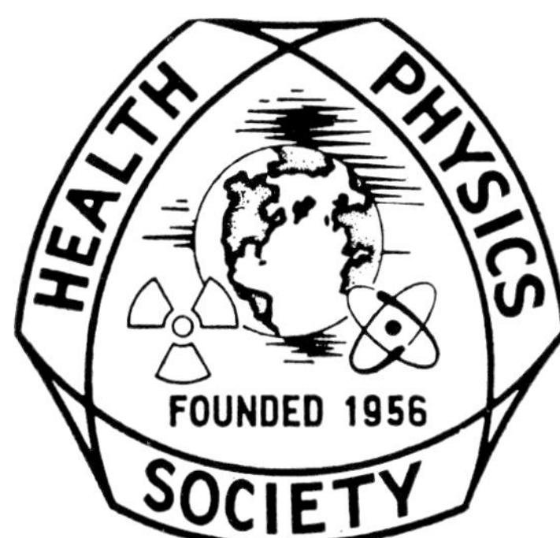

HPS INSIGNIA. The upper three were rejected in favor of the blunted triangle at the bottom suggested by the Health Physics Division of the ORNL in Oak Ridge. The "official" interpretation considers the globe as suggesting universality, the pinwheel meaning radiation, and the helium nucleus indicating the atomic age.

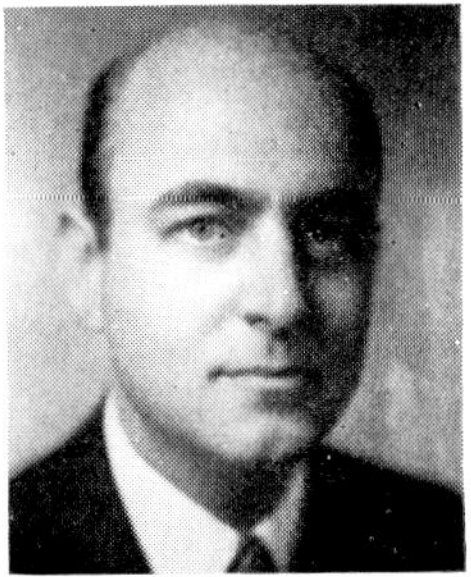

GEORGE PACK

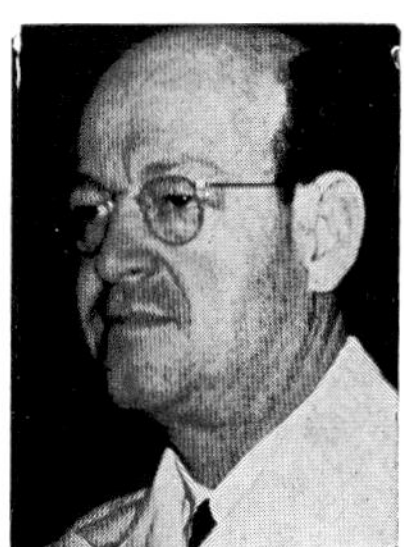

JESSHILL LOVE

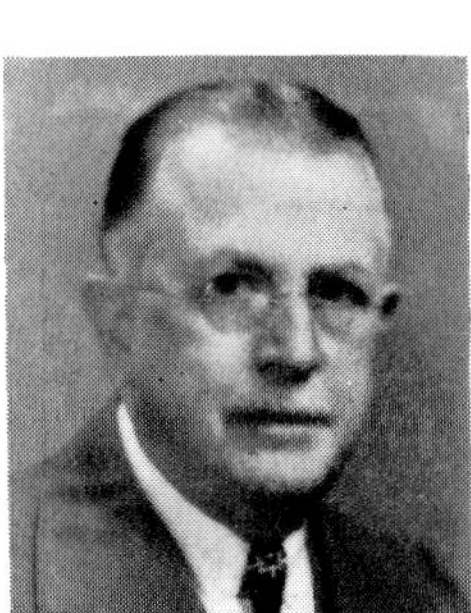

FRANK SIMPSON

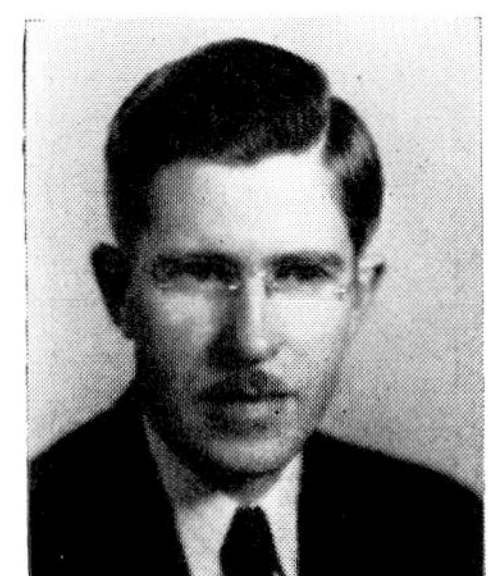

JAMES BREED

tron howitzers" for low cost radio-activation analysis (artificial neutron-induced radioactivity).

The era of the great radium therapists is past, but a few of the masters have survived the "cobalt revolution." One of the very first in this field had been Frank Edward Simpson of Chicago, remembered for a tract on *Radium Therapy* (391 pages), published in 1922 by Mosby. In 1933, Simpson took on an assistant, James Ernest Breed, who in 1938 took over Simpson's private Radium Institute. Today Breed continues to maintain a well equipped radium office in the Chicago Loop, with a daily turnover of 15-20 patients. He has several grams of radium (current price: $20/mgm.), distributed in various containers, and facilities for making special applicators. Many patients return again and again to the office for their daily or bi-weekly dose of "proximity irradiation." In certain instances the radium (or cobalt) source is simply attached to a long metallic rod, held by the attendant during the irradiation. I have heard residents from Northwestern call that rod the "sword," the procedure being nicknamed "fencing." Some of the younger radiotherapists from Chicago will display a quizzical smile when talking of Breed, but he remains undaunted.

Breed has some Co-60 at the office, but he prefers radium if only because it does not require periodic re-computation of dosages. He has published a few dozen papers on radium therapy, *e.g.*, one on carcinoma of the tongue (in *Radiology* of August, 1957), another on recurrent carcinoma of the cervix (in the *American Journal of Roentgenology* of March, 1962). Since biopsy may open channels for tumor spread, Breed – whose clinical experience allows him to recognize most malignancies before histologic confirmation – advocates preliminary irradiation prior to biopsy. He also stresses individualization of approach, and will adjust dosage in terms of patient and tumor response, rather than by virtue of a set number of roentgens. This, of course, is the art of medicine, which does not appeal to "modern" (mathematically-minded) colleagues, but Breed has a group of referring clinicians, who keep sending patients simply because of results achieved in past instances.

The revival of the ARS was accomplished by its change (for all practical purposes) into a society of radiotherapists. It is now bustling with young blood. The newcomers are not only enthusiastic, they crowd the meetings, and are willing to participate in all sorts of scientific endeavors. So far, these "Young Turks" have not taken over significant offices, but their accession is inevitable. Maybe at that time some of the out-dated procedures in public relations and in the keeping of archives of the ARS will be changed. At any rate, even as it stands today, the ARS seems to have a bright future.

RADIO- REVISITED

At the begining of the Atomic Phase it was thought that eventually radioisotopes would replace also diagnostic roentgen machines. So far this hope has not

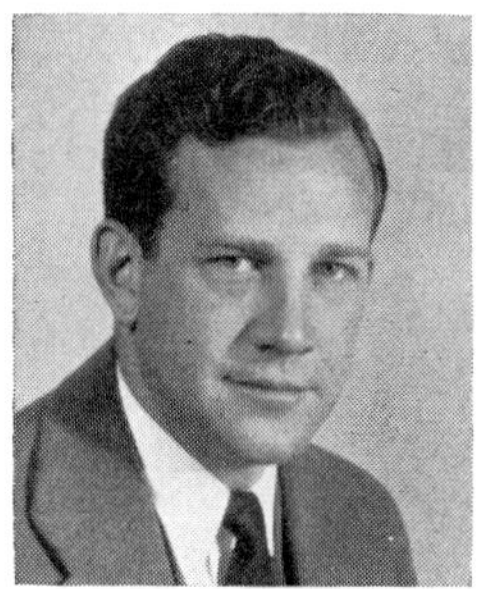

HAROLD JACOX

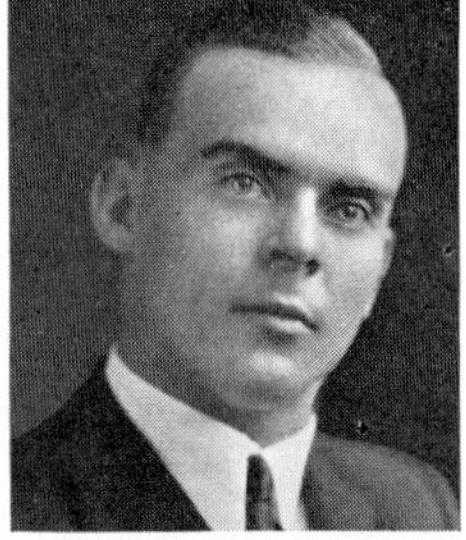

IRVIN HUMMON

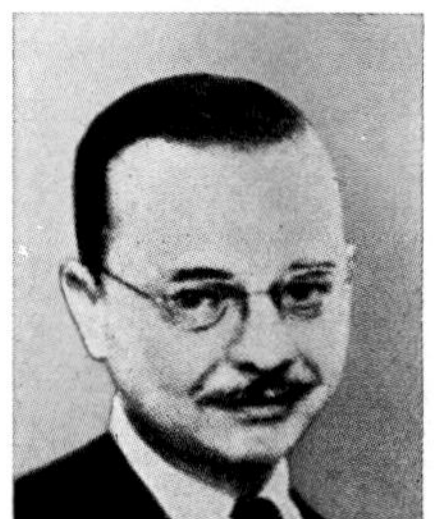

FERNANDO BLOEDORN

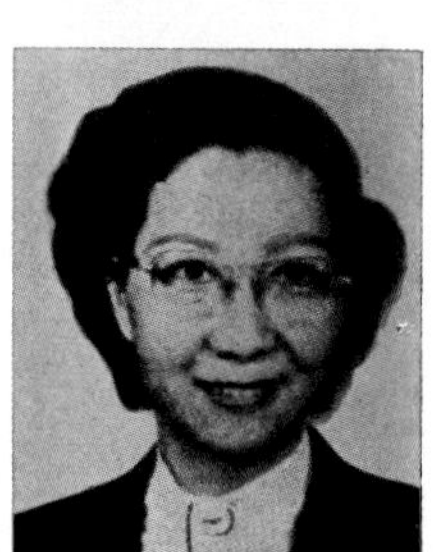

FLORENCE CHU

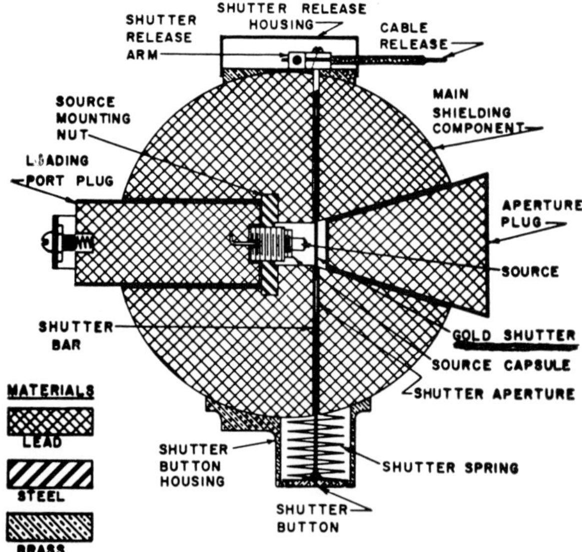

HEMI-SECTIONAL SKETCH OF PORTABLE ISOTOPIC X-RAY UNIT

Courtesy: Army Medical Research Laboratory, Fort Knox.

THULIUM-170 RADIOGRAPHIC UNIT. Gold, having a fairly high atomic number, is eminently suited for making shutters. And since this material is available in large (though decreasing) amounts at Fort Knox (Kentucky) – where this unit was built – the container has been provided with a gold shutter.

materialized, although very interesting results (especially under conditions which demand "portability") have been obtained among others by two radiobiologists, James Gus Kereiakes and Adolph Theodor Krebs, in the X-Ray Department of the (gilded) Army Medical Research Laboratory in Fort Knox (Kentucky): they used Thulium^{170} after having tried *X-Radiography* with *(Brehmsstrahlen* given off by) beta-emitting isotopes such as the combination Strontium^{90} — Yttrium^{90}.

In the *Dunlee Digest* of July-September, 1963 Zed Atlee mentioned — in a discussion of nucleonic x-ray sources — a peculiar "x-ray tube" in which the electron source was strontium-90. The electrons collided with a target of lead or platinum, after being focused by rings charged negatively by the source itself. The idea has a touch of genius, even if it may not (yet) be practical.

In the meantime the utilization of the prefix radio- boomed to new heights but with antique and long-accredited stand-bys.

To prove their airworthiness, some of these vocables were landed in the *Air Force Electronic Terminology* (1959) – where they have to live in competitive concubinage with a much longer list of terms which carry the same prefix radio-, but which have meanings related to communication, radar technology, and so on. Among radiologic terms therein contained were the following: radioactive (official abbreviation r/a), radioactivate ("to make radioactive"), radioluminescence ("produced by radiant energy, such as X-rays"), radiometallography, radiometer (radiometry), radiotransparent, radio-technology (ambivalent), and the inevitable radiology ("that branch of *physics* which deals with x-rays, radioactivity, and other high frequency radiation"). The Air Force editors had included this sampling of "foreign" terms merely to lessen the inherent confusion with their own *(radionic)* nomenclature. But they also mention the unique R/W which stands for radiological warfare. And there is the radiac, meaning any radiation monitoring or detection device.

Most of the above entries can be found in the unabridged Merriam-Webster (ed. 2., 1950) dictionary, which carried in addition a fairly large radio-collection including a few distinguished pieces of etymologic craftsmanship, such as radio-anaphylaxis (still with us!), radio(bio)chemistry, radiocinematograph, radiode (radium container, *i.e.,* applicator), radiodermatitis, radiodiagnosis, radiodontia* ("a de-

*The term radiodontia was coined before 1920 by Howard Riley Raper, D.D.S.; he was then in Indianapolis and had just invented his eponymized Dental Angle Meter which made dental projections mathematically reproducible, and thus created radiodontia itself. That definition from the 2nd edition of the Merriam-Webster is today inadequate, and was changed in their 3rd edition to "making and interpreting of radiographs of teeth. . ." The periodical *Radiodoncia* was started in 1940 in Buenos Aires by the Sociedad Odontologica Argentina de Radiologia.

Courtesy: Bob Sulit's PORACC.

RADIOLOGIC WARRIOR.

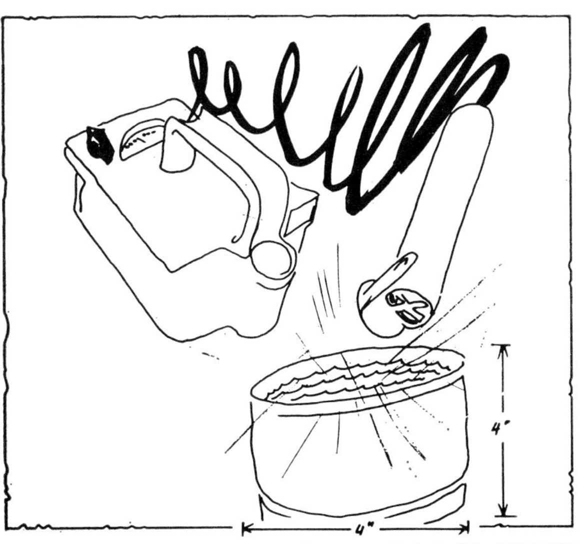

Courtesy: Bob Sulit's PORACC.

ROLLICKING RADIAC.

partment of dentistry concerned with making and interpreting radiographs of teeth and adjacent structures"), radio-element (including everything from radioactinium to radiozirconium), radiogenic ("produced by radioactivity" — this has also an alternate meaning, "eminently suitable for being broadcast by radio"), radionecrosis, radioneuritis, radiopelvimetry, radiophysics, radiopraxis ("the use of radiant energy . . . in medical practice"), radioscope (a device for detecting the presence of a radioactive substance), and radiostereoscopy (usual sense). It also brings radon (but not its long form—*rad*ioemanati*on*), and radioisotope (but not its abbreviated from — radiotope).

Two radio-experts are among the special editors named in the 3rd edition (1961) of Merriam-Webster's unabridged dictionary. They are Herman Eastman Seemann and George M. Corney, both of them physicists at Eastman Kodak and both of them listed in the Merriam-Webster as specialists in radiography. Indeed, they have inserted into the 3rd term radiographer (which was not in the 2nd), and equated it with x-ray technician. Several other radiowords (but not radioword) have found their way into the 3rd, for instance, radiohalo (halo in a mineral produced by radioactive emanation of some other included mineral), radiolysis (chemical decomposition by the action of radiation*), and radiotracer (radioactive tracer). Many "oldsters" have been preserved in the 3rd, *e.g.,* radiferous (containing radium). Radioscope acquired the second sense of fluoroscope. Radiosurgery is now defined as surgery with the radio knife (it used to be surgery with radium — in another dictionary). More important are the omissions from the 3rd, *i.e.,* radiopathology (Philip Rubin at the University of Rochester, in Eastman Kodak's hometown, authored in 1959 a syllabus on Clinical Radiopathology) and radio-epidemiology (title of a communication by AEC's C. W. Shilling at the International Symposium on Radiobiology in Rome in 1960). Both the 2nd and the 3rd carry the verb to radioactivate, but not the noun, although radioactivation by means of neutron bombardment (from the "primitive" radium howitzers to the sometimes very expensive neutron generators) is a favored tool in basic nuclear research.

The most important omission in the second edition of the Merriam-Webster is radiobiology but then, to antiphrase an old adage, "words are (not) like seashells on the shore: they show (also) where the mind ends, and not (only) how far it has been."

*This is usually employed in the sense of photolysis, but the article *Pulse Radiolysis* appeared in *Science* of August 9, 1963.

"IS IT SAFE, DOCTOR?"

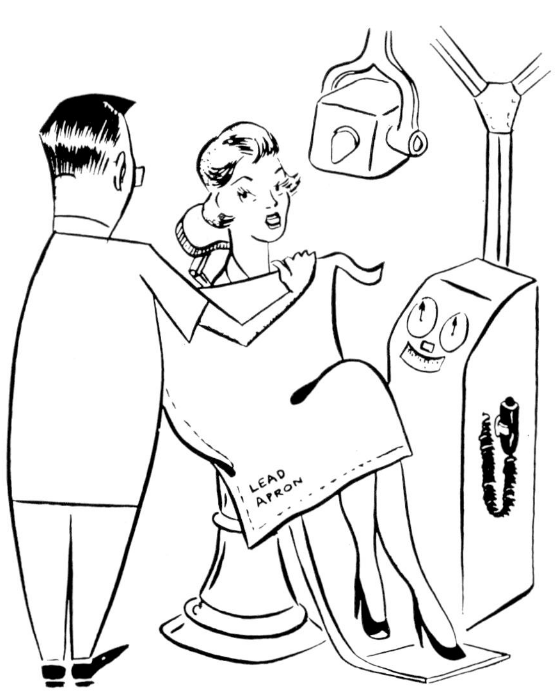

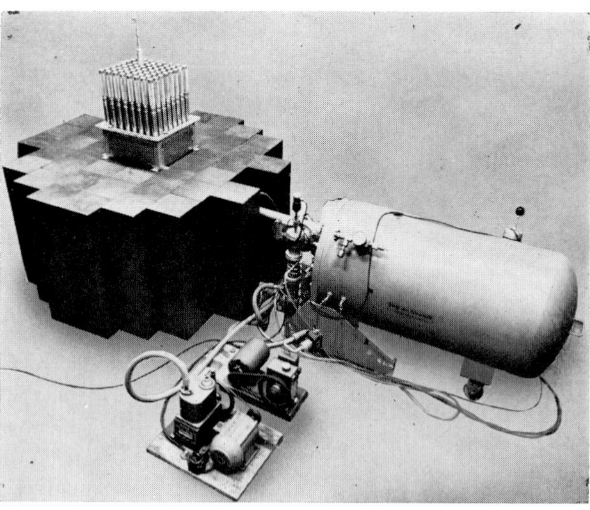

Courtesy: HVEC.

NEUTRON GENERATOR. The "modern" way of producing neutrons (for reactor research with subcritical assembly) is this 0.4 mev model AN-450 Van de Graaff, which emits pulsed or continuous neutron beams up to 10^{10} n/sec.

RADIO- IN DORLAND'S

The term radiology is defined (albeit with undue emphasis on light) in the scholarly Dorland* dictionary which, because of its fondness for French and Italian sources, carries a goodly number of radio-terms:

Radiability** (property of being readily penetrated by radiation), radiable ("capable of being examined by the roentgen ray") radioactor (apparatus for preparing radon), radiobe (bacteria-like condensations of sterilized bouillon exposed to radium), radiocancerogenesis, radiocardiography (angiocardiography), radiochemistry ("effects produced by radioactive rays"), radiochroism (capacity of a substance to absorb radiation), radiochromometer (penetrometer), radiocurable, radiocystitis, radiodiagnostics (art of radiodiagnosis), radiodiaphane ("instrument for performing transillumination by means of radium"), radioepidermitis, radioepithelitis, radiogen (any radioactive substance), radio-immunity (decreased radiosensitivity), radiokymography, radiolesion, radiolucency, radiometer, radiomutation (radiation-induced chromosomal change), radion (generic term for energized particles, *e.g.*, elec-tron), *radio-opaque* (as well as radiopaque, and the respective radiopacity), radioparent and radioparency (contracted radiotransparency), radiopathology (radiation effects), radiophobia, radiophylaxis (sensitizing effect of small doses of radiation), radioplastic (plastic models of organs reproduced by following roentgen measurements), radioreaction, radioresistance (decreased radiosensitivity), radioresponsive (favorable biologic response), radioslerometer (Villard's penetrometer), radiosensibility (synonymous with sensitivity in its biologic sense; figuratively, it might express a desirable quality in residents and other post-graduate medical students), radiothanatology (study of radiation effects on dead tissue), radiotomy (tomography), radiotoxemia, radiotrophic (influenced by radiation), radiumization (radium application), and radiumology (science — or art? — of radium therapy).

*Very few people have heard that Dorland (who was a gynecologist and obstetrician) had published with Hubeny a text on the *X-Ray in Embriology and Obstetrics* (1926), dedicated—in all seriousness—to their mothers!

**The slight discrepancy between radiable and radiability is not as pronounced as that between anxious and anxiety.

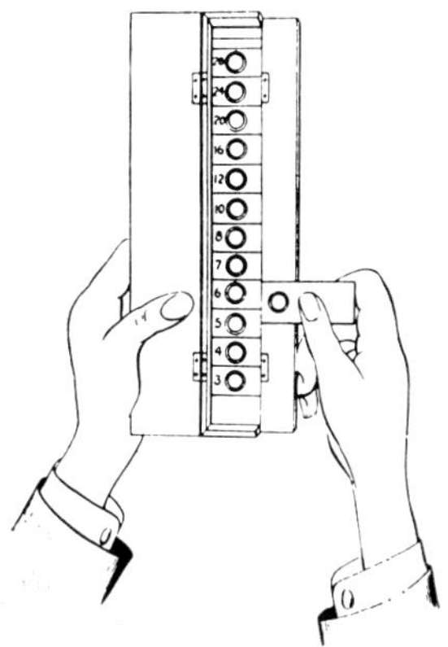

HOLZKNECHT'S RADIO-CHROMOMETER. It was also called penetrometer.

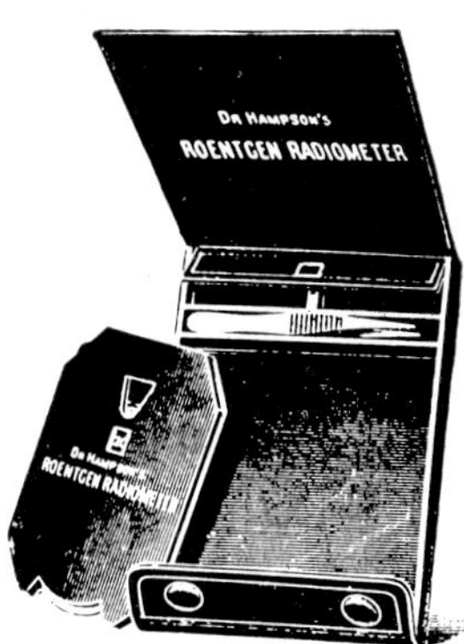

In 1811, the controversial Irish-born precursor of the germ theory and professor of Materia Medica in Baltimore, John Crawford (1746-1813), commented caustically:

". . . We are to consider the lax and indefinite use of words . . . (and) the quarrels that have obtained among physicians about mere words. . . Words thus to be guarded against are of two kinds. Some are names of things that are imaginary, such as are wholly to be rejected, and of such the medical nomenclature chiefly consists. There are other terms of considerable number in our science, that allude to what is real, though their signification is confused, and these latter must of necessity be continued in use; but their sense cleared up and freed as much as possible, from obscurity."

RADIOBIOLOGY

On February 7, 1959 the annual ACR Conference of Teachers of Radiology started with a panel on *Radiobiology in Medicine*. It was opened by Robert Spencer Stone, who defined radiobiology as "that field of science which is devoted to the effect of radiations upon living matter."

This is etymologically correct. The third edition of the unabridged Merriam-Webster calls radiobiology "a branch of biology dealing with the interaction of biological systems and radiant energy or radioactive material."

Conceived on just as wide a meaning was the listing of 4,600 biliographic references compiled before 1957 by the "naval" radiobiologist Friedrich Philipp Ellinger under the title *Medical Radiation Biology*: it contained even a chapter on photobiology, *i.e.*, on the biologic effects of visible light.

On December 6, 1960 (during the RSNA Convention in Cincinnati) Ellinger told me that Radiation Biology (a term which he likes better than the abbreviated Radiobiology) should be separated from Radiology, just as 100 years ago Pharmacology was separated from Internal Medicine. He doubted whether any of the existing societies would accept such a schism. I had no doubts, I knew they never would, and never should!

How did the term radiobiology originate?

In 1911 Oskar Hertwig (1849-1922), the German embryologist who studied the action of radium on animal cells, coined the word *Radiumkrankheit* (radium disease), and in 1913 in *Naturwissenschaften* (Berlin) he used the term *Radium-Biologie* which at the time had become quite fashionable in Germany. Also in 1913, Paul Lazarus published in Wiesbaden the first edition of his classic *Handbuch der Radium-Biologie;* he edited its second edition in München (1927), under the title *Handbuch der Gesamten Strahlenheilkunde.*

HANDBUCH
DER RADIUM-BIOLOGIE
UND THERAPIE

EINSCHLIESSLICH DER ANDEREN

RADIOAKTIVEN ELEMENTE.

UNTER MITWIRKUNG VON

PROF. DR. **E. F. BASHFORD**-LONDON, PROF. DR. **JEAN BECQUEREL**-PARIS, PROF. DR. **PAUL BECQUEREL**-PARIS, PROF. DR. **A. BICKEL**-BERLIN, GEH. RAT PROF. DR. **BRIEGER**-BERLIN, DR. **CAAN**-HEIDELBERG, WIRKL. GEH. RAT PROF. DR. **CZERNY**-HEIDELBERG, DR. **F. DAUTWITZ**-JOACHIMSTHAL, PROF. DR. **DEGRAIS**-PARIS, DOZENT DR. **FALTA**-WIEN, OBERARZT DR. **FÜRSTENBERG**-BERLIN, GEH. RAT PROF. DR. **GREEFF**-BERLIN, PROF. DR. **O. HAHN**-BERLIN, GEH. RAT PROF. DR. **O. HERTWIG**-BERLIN, PROF. DR. **C. KAISERLING**-BERLIN, GEH. RAT PROF. DR. **FR. KRAUS**-BERLIN, PROF. DR. **A. LABORDE**-PARIS, PROF. DR. **P. LAZARUS**-BERLIN, PROF. DR. **H. MACHE**-WIEN, DR. **L. MATOUT**-PARIS, PROF. DR. **ST. MEYER**-WIEN, PROF. DR. **C. NEUBERG**-BERLIN, HOFRAT PROF. DR. **v. NOORDEN**-WIEN, GEH. RAT PROF. DR. **PFEIFFER**-BRESLAU, OBERARZT DR. **PLESCH**-BERLIN, DOZENT DR. **PRAUSNITZ**-BRESLAU, PROF. DR. **E. SCHIFF**-WIEN, PROF. DR. **E. SOMMER**-ZÜRICH, PROF. DR. **STRASBURGER**-BRESLAU, DR. **SZILARD**-PARIS, PROF. DR. **WICKHAM**-PARIS.

HERAUSGEGEBEN VON

PROF. DR. PAUL LAZARUS

IN BERLIN.

MIT EINEM EINLEITENDEN VORWORT VON GEH. RAT PROF. DR. **FRIEDRICH KRAUS** IN BERLIN.

MIT 153 ABBILDUNGEN IM TEXT UND 2 TAFELN.

WIESBADEN.
VERLAG VON J. F. BERGMANN.
1913.

I had thought at first that the term radiobiology originated in Italy, as the periodical *Radiobiologia Generalis* was published in Bologna since 1932. In later years it lost the *generalis* but acquired a subtitle *(Archivio Internazionale)* and a staunch sponsor, the *Societá Internazionale di Radiobiologia.* That called for another change of name, to *Archivio Internazionale di Radiobiologia.* In October, 1937 Vallebona read a paper *(Le associazioni di agenti fisici diversi in radio-*

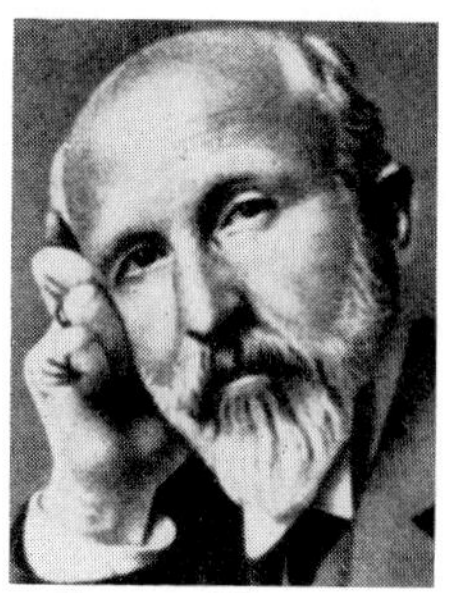
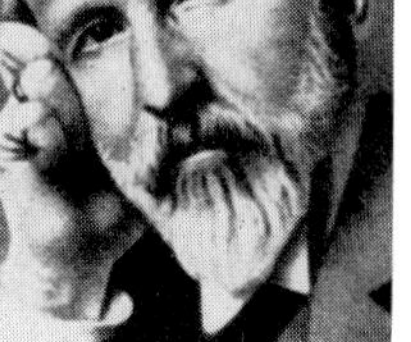

OSKAR HERTWIG

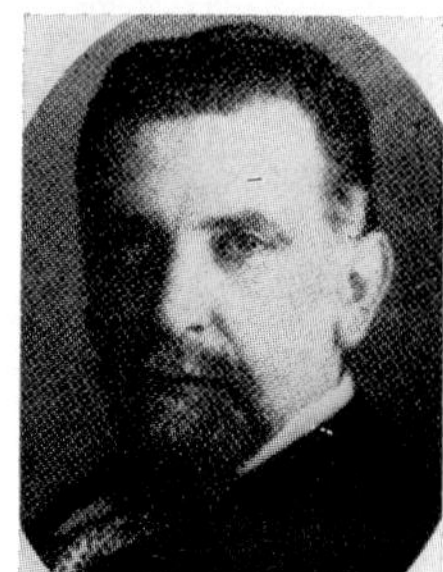

PAUL LAZARUS

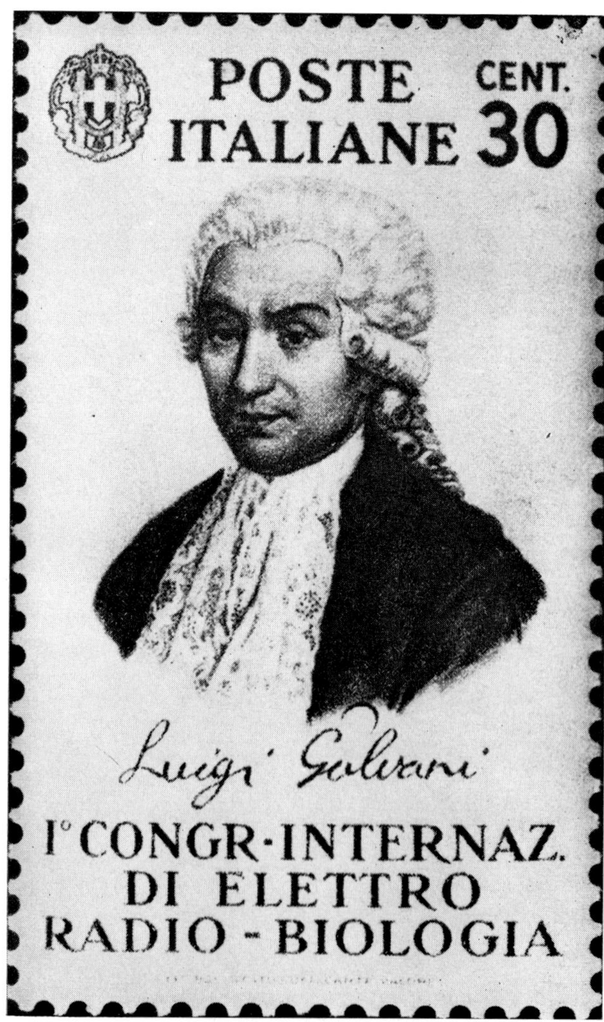

THIS STAMP WAS ISSUED IN 1934.

biologia) before the *Congresso dei Nuclei* (clubs) *Italiani di Radiobiologia* at its third annual meeting, held in Bologna: in that same town (re)appeared in 1946 the periodical *Radioterapia, Radiobiologia e Fisica Medica.*

The classic French text by Lacassagne and Gricouroff, *Action des Radiations sur les Tissus* (1941), which introduces the student to the basic notions of *radiothérapie,* begins with a definition of *radiobiologie.* In France, just as in Italy, the term radiobiology was used first by physicians, and carried therefore most of the all-encompassing sense mentioned by Stone and by Ellinger. It included evidently the so-called photobiology, and this is how St. Michael came to be the Patron-Saint of radiology.

The nomination was made by Vittorio Maragliano, G. B. Cardinale, and Alessandro Vallebona, from the Department of Radiology of the University of Genova (Italy), and was blessed in August of 1933 by local ecclesiastic authorities. Vittorio Consigliere, Bishop of Cerignola (Italy), remarked that there are several kinds of light (*luce,* in Italian); the light can be friendly and conducive to better vision, or light may be blinding. Although there is someone whose name is closely related to *luce* (the light), Lucifer – the angel of evil – he could not possibly have been selected as a patron-saint. The Archangel Michael seemed to be the better choice. The bishop offered also a witticism: in theology the light comes from the law; in radiology the law comes from the light.*

During the first half of the 20th Century, the term radiobiology was not commonly used in this country. It appeared, albeit sporadically, in the literature and in abstracts or quotations. There was for instance the article on irradiation of tissue implants in September of 1942 in *Growth:* its author, the very talented onco-histologist Leonid Doljanski (1900-1948) was himself a transplant from Berlin (*via* Berne) to the Hebrew University in Jerusalem; he was killed by accident during a political brawl.

Nor was the term radiobiology used in England prior to World War II. The question was submitted to the medical radiobiologist Frederick Gordon Spear, who had discussed the medical uses of the cyclotron in the 1945 Annual Report of the Smithsonian; he edited the first supplement of the *British Journal of Radiology* entitled *Certain Aspects of the Action of Radiation on Living Cells* (1947). In the *British Journal of Radiology* of February, 1962 appeared his presidential address (BIR) entitled *Questioning the Answers,* a quintessence of Spear's philosophic views on the relationships between radio(bio)logy and other disciplines. This is what Spear replied:

"I would say the term radiobiology was little (if at all) used in 1940 but was generally current in 1950. At

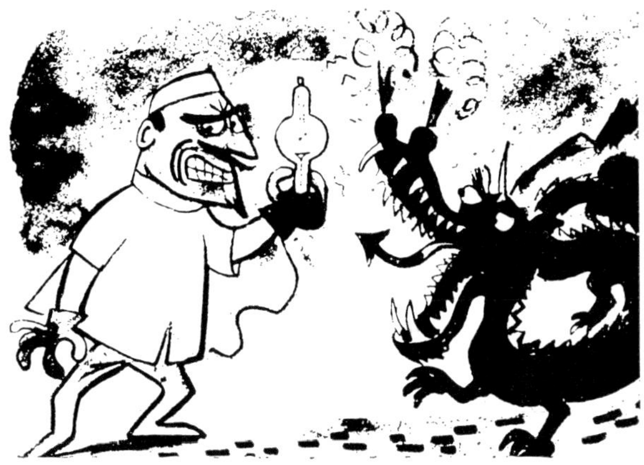

Courtesy: Dick Chamberlain.

St. Radio-Michael & the Dragon. In Christian art the dragon symbolizes Satan, who must be "trampled under the feet," as pictured in paintings of Christ and of the Virgin Mary. Many saints are represented fighting a dragon, such as (alphabetically) St. Cado, St. Clement (of Metz), St. Donatus, St. Florent (who killed the dragon which haunted the Loire), St. George, St. Keyne (of Cornwall), St. Margaret, St. Marthe (who slew the terrible dragon Tarasque at Aix-la-Chapelle), St. Maudet, St. Michael, St. Philip the Apostle (who killed a dragon at Hierapolis in Phrygia), St. Pol (who killed several dragons in Brittany), St. Romain (of Rouen), St. Samson (the archbishop of Dol), and Pope Sylvester. With that many exquisite witnesses, only hardboiled sinners can be so foolhardy as to dare to deny the existance of dragons. The most famous dragon-killer may have been St. George, but the undisputed patron of radiology is St. Michael.

*In *Paradise Lost* (6, 44), Milton wrote:

Go, Michael, of celestial armies prince
And thou, in military prowess next,
Gabriel; lead forth to battle these my sons
Invincible; lead forth my armed Saints. . .

Saint Michael is usually represented as a knight in armor, killing a dragon. On the saint's day (September 29), the so-called Michaelmas, it is customary in England to eat goose and pay the rent!

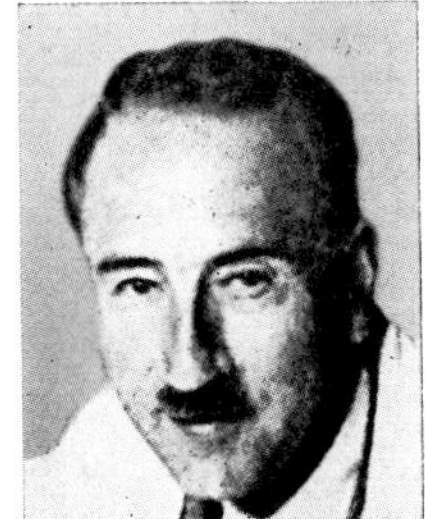

Antione Lacassagne

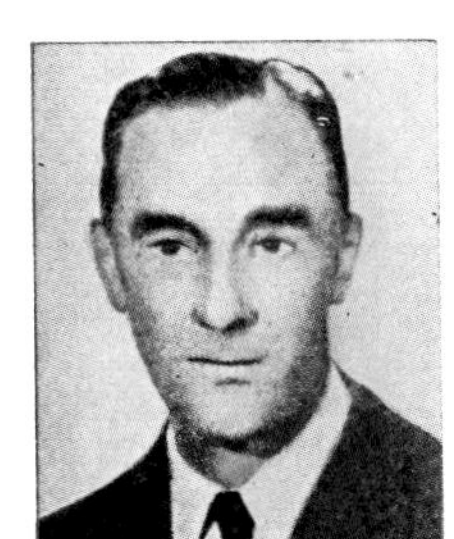

Georges Gricouroff

the 6th ICR in London in 1950 there was a separate Section of Radiobiology.

"I would date the introduction of the term (into English usage) around 1945. By that time the terms physical properties, chemical action, and biological effects of penetrating rays were being replaced as headings by radiophysics, radiochemistry, and radiobiology, and also by that time nearly 400 radioactive isotopes were known and their properties were being studied. It was not long before their chemical effects and biological actions were also being investigated and new fields of research were opened up, distinct from that in which conventional forms of 'external' radiation were still being used for radiological experiment.

"It was convenient to distinguish these two kinds of investigation and at the London (1950) ICR an attempt (initiated by C. B. Allsopp) was made to reserve the term radiochemistry for all those experiments which involved radioactive isotopes, and to use the term radiation chemistry for studies on the chemical actions of radiation in general. By analogy we therefore get radiophysics and radiation physics, radiobiology and radiation biology.

"This terminology is gradually coming into use but is by no means generally adopted yet. In any case the adjective radiobiological must, I think, be retained for use in either sense."

Having read Spear's answer I decided to have a look at pre-World War II ICR proceedings in the hope that some of the titles might contain the word radiobiology. To my surprise, the 2nd ICR (Stockholm, 1928) had a substantial Section on Radiobiology and Heliotherapy. I went back to the first London ICR of 1925 and they had only a Section on Radiotherapy. Why had Forssell created a new section?

I went through the content of the radiobiology section at the 2nd ICR and roughly half of the forty-odd papers presented were from Nemenov's Institute (Leningrad). In the Soviet Union, throughout the Golden Age of Radiology, Nemenov's Institute was the foremost center for both education and research.*

As we have seen, the first all-Russian Meeting of Roentgenologists took place in Moscow in 1916. The second, third, and fourth such meetings were held in Leningrad in 1924, 1925, and 1926.† At that fourth meeting, aside from two foreign guests (Hermann Holthusen from Hamburg and I. Seth Hirsch from New York City) they had an overabundance of papers on the experimental action of roentgen rays and radium on living tissue.

The best among these Sovietic contributions were offered the following year for presentation to the Stockholm ICR. Faced with such a plethora of papers for the Radiotherapy Section, Forssell and his Program Committee resorted to a (Scandinavian?) stratagem, and formed an additional section. I asked Elis Berven about it, and he replied that the term radiobiology was used in Sweden prior to that date, but I could not find any printed reference to prove this point. Orndoff believes that the term *radiobiologie* orginated in France, which seems quite likely but, again, I found no substantiating quotation. Under these circumstances it is my considerate opinion that either Forssell or one of his associates coined the term radiobiology – *ad usum Delphini* – for the benefit of international co-operation during the second ICR.

An account of the 2nd ICR was published in 1927 in the *British Journal of Radiology*, in the *American Journal of Roentgenology*, and in *Radiology*: that was

STRAHLENTHERAPIE.

Mitteilungen

aus dem Gebiete der Behandlung mit

Röntgenstrahlen, Licht und radioaktiven Substanzen.

Zugleich

Zentralorgan

für die

gesamte Lupusbehandlung und Lupusbekämpfung.

In Gemeinschaft mit

Dozent Dr. **Falta**, Wien; Primarius Dr. **Jungmann**, Wien; Dr. **S. Löwenthal**, Braunschweig; Oberarzt Dr. **Axel Reyn**, Kopenhagen; Dr. **H. E. Schmidt**, Berlin

herausgegeben von

Professor Dr. **C. J. Gauss**, Freiburg i. Br.; Priv.-Doz. Dr. **Hans Meyer**, Kiel.

Professor Dr. **R. Werner**, in Heidelberg.

Band I.

Urban & Schwarzenberg,

Berlin N. 24, Friedrichstr. 105 B. — **Wien I**, Maximilianstr. 4.

1912.

*Nemenov's assistant Sam Reinberg presented on September 24, 1921 to the Petersburg Society of Roentgenologists and Radiologists a case of congenital genuine dextrocardia (later published in the *Vestnik*).

†The fifth was held in Kiev in 1928, the sixth in Moscow in 1931, and the seventh in Saratov in 1958.

the first time when the term radiobiology appeared in print in the British and American literature (I must qualify this as being the earliest English reference in my files). The 1931 ICR in Paris had a Section on Radiobiology (the Heliotherapy was lost somewhere along the line), and so did the 1934 ICR in Zürich. There was also a significant Section on Radiobiology at the 1937 ICR in Chicago: on each of these occasions, the word radiobiology was printed in the respective programs, and appeared also in the specialty journals reporting the event.

The "approved" German term was *Röntgenbiologie* – in neighboring Copenhagen were printed in the mid-1930s several theses containing the term *røntgenbiologiske*. But it covered only x rays, thus one solution was to use this term in conjunction with Hertwig's *Radiumbiologie*. A better solution was to translate the word radiobiology, which is how *Strahlenbiologie* was born (it happens to be the title of a 1959 text by Hedi Fritz-Niggli of Zürich). At times, though, the term *radiobiologische* could be found also in German publications, for instance Halberstaedter used it in 1937 in the *Archiv für Experimentelle Zellforschung.*

At the beginning of World World II, the Berlin-Rome Axis had to be cultivated. Volume 65 of *Strahlentherapie* was therefore dedicated to the Italian Radiological Society, and carried portraits of Balli, Ponzio, Palmieri, and Perussia. Moreover, it had an article by Eugenio Milani of Rome, on the Italian contributions to *Radiobiologie.* That article had been translated from the Italian into German by Heinz Lossen. And on October 31, 1940 Lossen used in *Strahlentherapie* the term *Radiobiologie* and became effusive over the (excellent) 3 volumes of the *Trattato di Radiobiologia* (1937) of Ruggero Balli of Modena (edited by Mario Lenzi). Thereupon Milani returned the courtesy and published in 1943 (with Luigi Turano) the *Fondamenti di Radiobiologia e Röntgenterapia.* The axis has now receded into history (since 1958 appears in Milano the *Radiobiologica Latina),* and once again, the term *röntgenterapia* is no longer as popular in Italy as it had been just prior to and during World War II.

In this country the term radiobiology was more and more often encountered after 1940, for instance Stedman's Medical Dictionary, ed. 16 (1946), contains the following definition of radiobiology: "the branch of radiology which deals with the effects of radioactive substances on living cells." There existed a Sub-Committee of Radiobiology of the National Research Council, Division of Mathematical and Physical Sciences, Committee on Nuclear Science: in 1950 they issued a booklet (150 pages) by Harold Douglas Copp on research and training facilities for radiobiology in the USA and Canada. In the *Cumulative Index of Radiology* radiobiology was first listed in the third volume published in 1954.

It is of interest to note that when the two roots are reversed, the sense changes. The Spanish booktitle *Bioradiología humana* (Barcelona, 1953) by Manuel Taure Gómez could have been "translated" as radiologic anatomy. *Mutatis mutandis,* Hermann Rieder's *Bioröntgenographie* of 1909 was intended as a synonym for roentgen-kymography, and could have been "translated" as roentgen physiology.

The use of the term radiobiology is today as widespread as the fall-out. On August 15, 1960 the Third Australasian Conference of Radiobiology was held at Sydney University by the Australian Radiation Society. Even a stellar spread may be anticipated from Hermann J. Schaefer's article on the current problems in astroradiobiology published in *Aerospace Medicine* of May, 1951.

The question of what radiobiology means was submitted to several recognized authorities in the matter. All of them agreed on the generic (etymologic) meaning given by Stone, as well as by most of the recent dictionaries. Some of them believed that in practice the meaning of radiobiology is more restricted than its etymology implies. John Boland, a (formerly British) radiotherapist from Mount Sinai Hospital in New York City, would limit the coverage of radiobiology to ionizing radiations. Titus Evans disliked the term radiobiology, and preferred instead radiation biophysics.

Any and all statements to the contrary notwithstanding (and there were quite a few), in this country, radiobiology means today, — in its restricted sense — experimentation with ionizing radiation on subhuman subjects. In Europe the meaning of radiobiology includes also therapy on humans. The explanation for this geographic discrepancy is the fact that in Italy and France the term *radiobiologie* (respectively *radiobiologia*) was introduced and used by physicians (medical radiotherapists). In Great Britain and in this country, the term radiobiology was popularized by physicists and by other non-medical investigators. In recent years, though, with the preeminence of English literature on the subject, and the

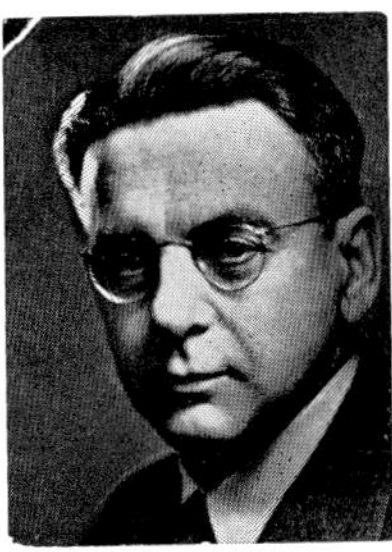
HERMAN SEEMANN

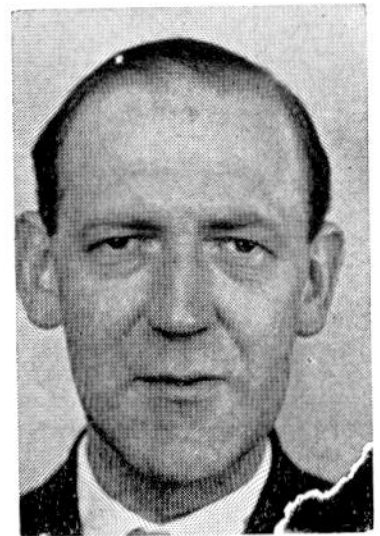
JOHN BOLAND

habit of abstractors to transliterate (instead of translating) the catchwords encountered in the articles abstracted, the Anglo-American meaning of radiobiology seems to hold a slight world-wide edge.

THE RADIATION SCARE(S)

Words are but tokens of the popular notion of things. As of late, the term radiation has come to evoke (especially in the minds of "common" people*), the potential somatic and hidden genetic hazards incurred when nuclear energy is "unleashed" upon living matter.

In 1959, Marshall Brucer described three peaks of radiation scare, which occurred among scientists in 1905, 1925, and 1955. Lagging behind each wave of professional hysteria was a peak of public radiation panic. Each time the professionals reassured themselves by strengthening their contempt for, and their knowledge of, the subject itself. In the public mind, the waves subsided mainly because of the inherent lassitude which people develop for any topic which is too often broached.

The *somatic* hazards of ionizing radiation became known in the very first weeks after Roentgen's discovery. Throughout that momentous year 1896 isolated occurrences, such as loss of hair, and then incurable skin ulcerations caused by overexposure to roentgen rays were well publicized, if poorly understood. After a few years, lasting radiation casualties, and then radiation fatalities, began to accumulate.

On April 4, 1936, a monument dedicated to the martyrs of radiology was unveiled in the garden of St. Georg Hospital in Hamburg. The main speaker at the dedication ceremonies, Antoine Béclère, was himself to become one of those martyrs. At the time of the unveiling there were 169 known instances of professionals who had died of, or whose death had been hastened by overexposure to, roentgen rays and/or radium. Their names were carved in the stone of the monument, and their biographies were printed in the *Ehrenbuch der Röntgenologen und Radiologen aller Nationen* (1937) which appeared as a supplement to *Strahlentherapie.*

By 1940, twenty-seven additional names had become known, and they were inscribed on two square stones added to the initial rectangular slab of the monument. By 1959, there were another 153 names, and two more stones were incorporated in the monument. In 1959, Hermann Holthusen, Hans Meyer, and Werner Molineus issued a second edition of the *Ehrenbuch,* again as a supplement to *Strahlentherapie.* It contains the names of 352 professionals whose death was directly or indirectly attributable to overexposure to radiation.

The eulogist's reputation was the only evidence required for inclusion of a new name on the list. From the "clinical" descriptions one can question whether several of those who have died in their 70s (a few in their 80s) with "anemic" conditions should have been included in the listing. Actually even malignancies of the skin, unless developed over teleangiectatic or otherwise damaged territory, are not necessarily caused by ionizing influences. Moreover, it is implied or at times outrightly stated that the pioneers disregarded the

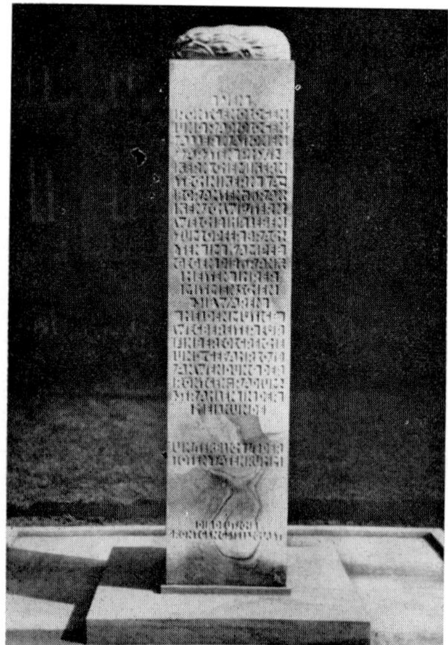

Courtesy: Hermann Holthusen.

MEMORIAL TO THE MARTYRS. This is how it looked when it was first erected in the garden of St. Georg's hospital in Hamburg. Today four stones with additional names have been installed around the central slab.

---

*In *A Man for All Seasons* (Robert Bolt's play based on the tribulations of Sir Thomas More) the Common Man says: "The sixteenth century is the Century of the Common Man—like all other centuries."

This Week MAGAZINE
February 22, 1958

The Truth About The X-ray Scare

Here is a report on the spreading fear which is keeping thousands of Americans from getting medical treatment they badly need — plus an authoritative guide to tell you when it's safe to have an X-ray taken

By A. E. HOTCHNER

danger and thus obtained knowledge for the benefit of oncoming generations. This is factually correct but, had they been truly aware of the dangers involved, one wonders how many would have continued to expose themselves to the invisible light. But they are dead *(De mortuis nil nisi bene)*, and several of them have contributed to the science or to the art of radiology. It is quite proper that their memory shall be honored.

As a token of courtesy to those who have sacrificed themselves — willingly or unwillingly — and were burned at the stake of radiation, we will list in chronologic order for each country the earliest recorded roentgen fatality.

In *Germany*, it was Friedrich Claussen (1864-1900) who opened a lay roentgen laboratory in February 1896 in Berlin, and exposed his hands to roentgen rays in at least one thousand public demonstrations before he succumbed to generalized carcinomatosis (after amputation of the right arm). In *Great Britain* the first such victim was Barry Blacken (?-1902), radiologist of St. Thomas's Hospital in London; in the *USA* it was C. M. Dally (1865-1904), Edison's glassblower; in *France* this "honor" goes to Jules Rhens (1871-1905) who suffered a dramatic burn while transporting inadequately shielded radium.* In *Belgium* M. Van Roost (1880-1924) had worked in an x-ray department only from 1900 to 1907, and his job had been to immobilize patients during exposures. The first recorded victim in *Italy* was Emilio Tiraboschi (?-1912), a radiologist in Bergamo. In *Switzerland* Henry Simon (?-1913) was a photographer who became the x-ray technician for the Cantonal Hospital in Geneva. In *Australia* J. F. Clendinnen (1860-1913) of Melbourne had been the first physician to use x rays in his practice.** In *Chilie*, Eckwall (?-1915) was a Swedish graduate in gymnastics and massage who became an x-ray

*Arthur Radiguet died also in 1905, after a prolonged suffering, but Rhens' tragedy was acute and thus more spectacular.

**He preceded in radiation death the internationally known Herschell Harris (?-1918), who was a radiologist in Sydney.

EHRENBUCH

der Röntgenologen und Radiologen

aller Nationen

Herausgegeben von

Hermann Holthusen, Hans Meyer

und Werner Molineus

Zweite, ergänzte und wesentlich erweiterte Auflage

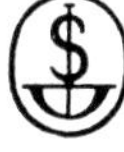

1959

VERLAG VON URBAN & SCHWARZENBERG

MÜNCHEN UND BERLIN

RUDIS-JICINSKY WITH CRYPTOSCOPE. The first secretary of the ARRS (shown "screening" a phthisic) was very interested in pulmonary tuberculosis. I have a photograph with Rudis-Jicinsky irradiating an experimentally tuberculized rabbit.

technician. In *Hungary,* Julius Schroeder (1866-1918) was a hospital radiologist in Györ. In *Spain,* Felipe Carriazo (1854-1919) was a private radiologist who also taught in the Medical School in Sevilla. In *Finland,* Anna Lönnbeck (1856-1920) was an x-ray technician. Both in *Denmark,* J. F. Fischer (1868-1922), and in *Japan,* Schichiro Hida (1873-1923), the first victims were radiologists. In the *Soviet Union,* Peter Baumgarten (1877-1925) was a private physician in the spa Pjatigorsk (Caucasus); in *Czechoslovakia* Rudolf Backer (1877-1925) was the radiologist of the hospital in Olomouc; in *Israel,* the Vienna-trained radiologist Josef Freud (1882-1925) was the first recorded victim. In *Austria,* it was the radiologist Alois Czepa (1886-1931) — only a thin partition separated his roentgen reading desk from the tubestand of a radiographic room in Childhospital in Vienna.* In *Portugal,* Carlos Leopoldo dos Santos (1864-1935) of Lisbon had worked with x rays since the year 1896. In *Yugoslavia,* B. Bressan ((?-1939) was a radiologist who died after suffering an amputation of the left arm in 1935.** In *Poland,* the first recorded radiation fatality was the radiologist Robert Bernhardt (1874-1950).

The genetic hazards of ionizing radiation were already recognized in the Era of the Roentgen Pioneers.

In the *Münchener Medizinische Wochenschrift* of October 27, 1903 Albers-Schönberg reported experimental evidence of somatic damage in testicles of rabbits exposed to roentgen rays. A few years later Ludwig Halberstaedter (1879-1949)* showed the existence of a similar effect upon ovaries of rabbits (*Berliner Klinische Wochenschrift* of January 16, 1906).

*Holzknecht died in the same year and also of radiation exposure.

**The *Ehrenbuch* mentions instead Zora Zec-Kuba (1895-1947) who died of aplastic anemia. She had worked as an x-ray technician for Laza Popovic.

The occurrence of genetic damage due to ionizing radiation was first shown by the (physician and) professor of anatomy in the University of Wisconsin, Charles Russell Bardeen (1871-1935), who found that undesirable congenital defects could be produced in the offspring by applying roentgen rays to spermatozoa in the toad (*Journal of Experimental Zoology* of February, 1907). The scientific proof of a causal relationship between exposure to roentgen rays and mutations in the fruitfly was published in *Science* of July 22, 1927 by the geneticist Hermann Joseph Müller who at the time, prior to his voyage to Moscow, was a zóólogist in the University of Texas.

At the banquet given at the Palace Hotel in San Francisco, during the mid-annual meeting of the RSNA in June, 1923, J. Wilson Shiels of San Francisco recited a poem of his own creation, entitled *Chief X-Ray Hawk Eye.* Quotation:

In the darkness of the screen room,
Where the tribe of cunning Ray-men
Stand protected from the tube-light,
So that many papoose Ray-men
May be given to their people.

*This therapist resided in Germany but then had to migrate to the Hebrew University in Jerusalem. He spent the last years of his life in New York City.

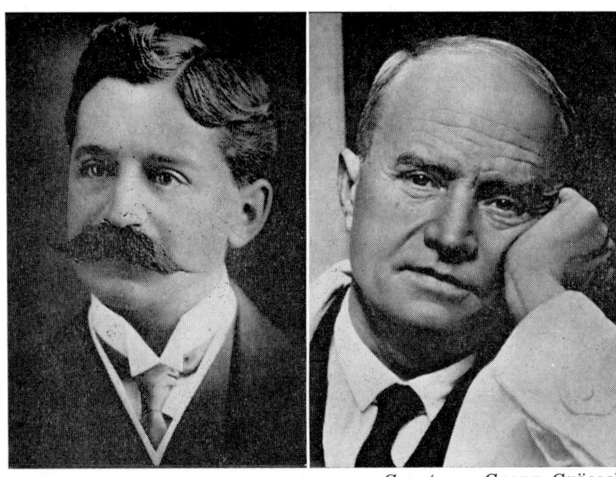

Courtesy: Georg Grössel

Harris & Popovic. Herschell Harris (of Melbourne) and Laza Popovic (of Belgrade) were not the first, but the best known radiation casualties in their respective countries.

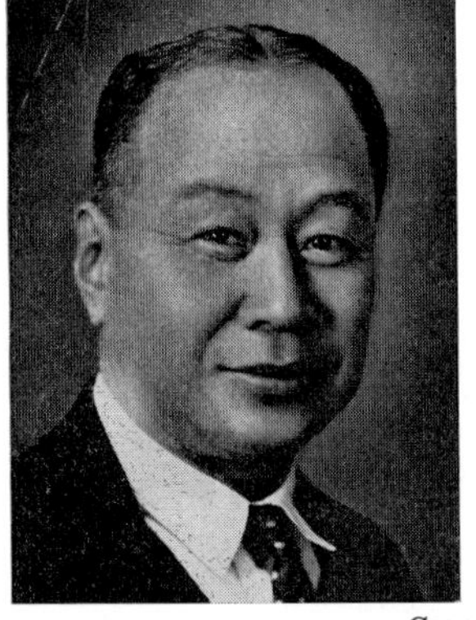

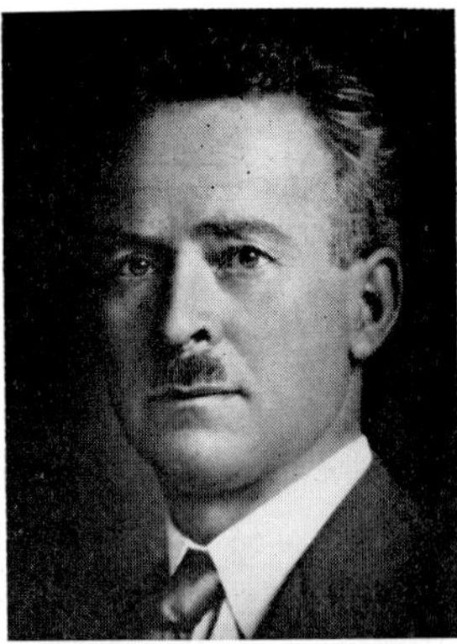

Courtesy: Georg Grössel and AGFA.

Koichi Fujinami studied in Vienna with Kienböck, returned to Japan, taught radiology in the University of Tokyo, wrote a scholarly radio-bibliography, and died as a radiation casualty, even if not the first in Japan. On the viewer's right is Joseph Freud. Born in Poland, MD Vienna (1909), became Holzknecht's pupil (1912), then assistant (1914), passed the examinations for the roentgen specialty (1919), went to Jerusalem as radiologist of the Hadassah Hospital (1921), and died there of (radiogenic) aplastic anemia.

The verses illustrate a misconception often used by laymen and ignorant physicians when making jokes about radiologists. A dose to the gonads of at least one thousand rads in one week would be needed for sterilization. The same thousand rads as total body radiation (or a correspondingly higher dose if fractionated) would have killed at least one half or more of those so exposed. Ben Orndoff told me that while he was a medical student, one of his teachers assigned him to experimental work, during which he held animals on a table, while the under-the-table x-ray tube was being energized, and that tube came very close to his gonads. After a few weeks of this work, he noticed a scrotal erythema, and soon his pubic hair fell off. He immediately discontinued those sessions of inadvertent "therapy," the erythema disappeared, the hair grew back, and he subsequently fathered five healthy children (who now have children of their own), and no mutations were observed in this "experimental" series.

Each of the three periods in radiologic history had its wave of radiation scare. The latest was by far the strongest.

After 1950, as bigger and better fission and fusion devices were detonated for "experimental" purposes, various groups pointed to the possible somatic and genetic damage resulting from fall-out, and demanded that such tests be discontinued. The composition of these groups varied widely, but political undertones were clearly audible in each and every instance. Some argued that even if somatic damage would be the immediate problem in case of a nuclear war,* as long as "peace" prevailed, there was no reason to incur genetic damage just because a few conservative politicos insisted that *Si vis pacem, para bellum* (if you want peace, you must prepare for war).

The *Bulletin of the Atomic Scientists* was founded in 1945 by Hyman Goldsmith and Eugene Rabinovitch (from the University of Illinois). It is well written, imaginatively illustrated,** and excellently edited. The basic theme in the *Bulletin* is that time is running out, and that the world is on the brink of nuclear war, as exemplified by their cover, based on a British suspense movie, in which a mad and dis-

Bulletin OF THE Atomic Scientists

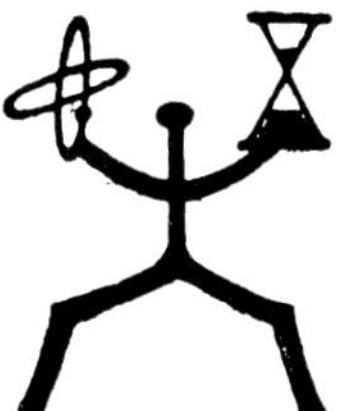

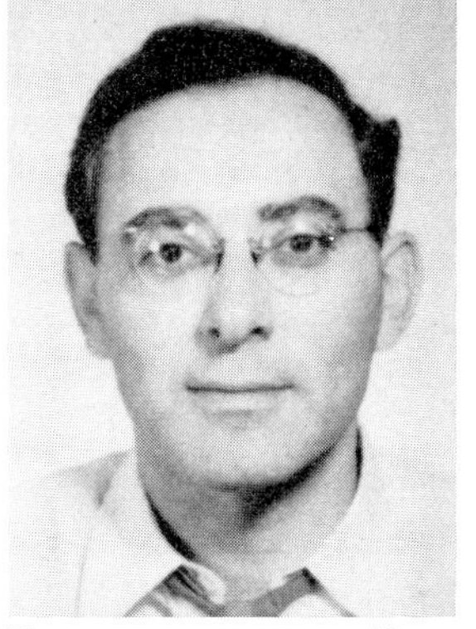

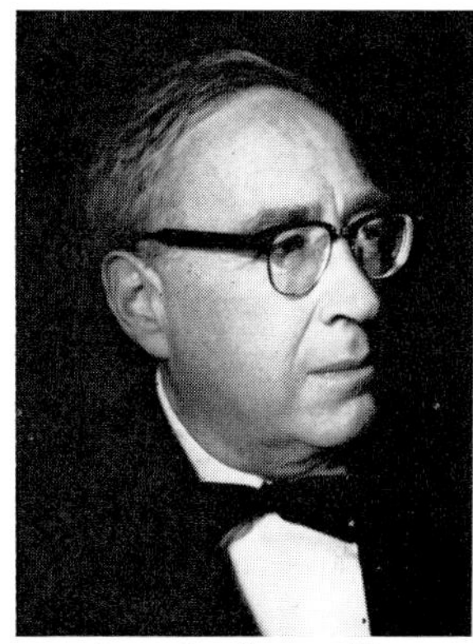

FOUNDERS OF THE BULLETIN. Austrian-born Hyman Goldsmith (1907-1949) taught physics at City College of New York, worked at the Met-Lab, and was head of the Information and Publications Division of Brookhaven National Lab when he drowned during a vacation in Vermont. At Brookhaven he collected full biographic files on most of the permanent personnel but left very little on himself. This shirt-sleeve shot is from Goldsmith's identification card, the only portrait of Goldsmith which J. E. H. Kuper (Brookhaven's health physicist) could locate. The other founder (and current editor) of the *Bulletin of the Atomic Scientists* is Russian-born photochemist and political writer Eugene Rabinovitch, who was formerly with the Met-Lab and is now with the University of Illinois. The formal portrait of Rabinovitch is herein reproduced from the artistic likeness executed by one of England's most exclusive photographers, Lotte Meitner-Graf (who graciously permitted its utilization).

*Most experts contend that the blast and heat caused by high yield nuclear weapons would exceed by far the damage inflicted through instant or delayed radioactivity.

**Many of its drawings are executed by Mr. Rainey Bennett. The editors of the *Bulletin* have graciously permitted the use of several of these sketches, one of which found its way onto the cover illustration.

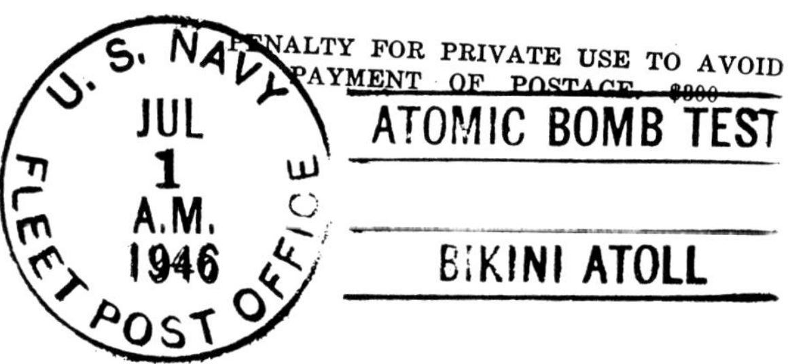

enchanted nuclear scientist threatened and almost succeeded to blow himself and London into smithereens; he was to have done it at noon. In 1960 and again in 1964 things seemingly improved. Each time the *Bulletin* turned its clock a few minutes back.

Most of the contributors of the *Bulletin,* all well qualified in their scientific pigeonhole, "know for a fact" that the holocaust of an atomic war would destroy both friend and foe. A very few went so far as to contend that anything is preferable to a nuclear conflict, even abdication of national sovereignty (in the vernacular this has come to be known as "better red than dead," with the quippy variant "better read than dead"). This obviously untenable position was never editorially subscribed, but its presentation has been tolerated. In recent years more emphasis is being placed on the need for achieving international understanding. But every so often, one or another distinguished *atomic scientist* will go into print with something as puerile as an (uninformed) eighth grader's political essay.

In the Atomic Phase science has become one of the main factors in — if not the very mainstay of — government. It is high time that scientists take over the government, not only in this country, everywhere in the world. To do so, however, one needs first of all political knowledge. "Certain" atomic scientists must understand that negotiations, *per se,* are meaningless. The improvement in the method of negotiations (more courtesies, better communications, added sincerity) will not solve the basic problem, just as symptomatic treatment never cures the basic disease. Everything, even nuclear testing, must be regarded as symptomatic of the general syndrome, not as the cause of (nor will its removal become the solution for) the problem. But there are signs — as the attitude of the Soviet Union during the Cuban crisis — which indicate that the problem is not insoluble. The time may not be too far when, once again, the USA and the Soviet Union will have to unite in the face of common peril.

Incidentally, the *Bulletin of the Atomic Scientists* was generally against nuclear testing, except — with some reservations — in the Fall of 1961.

To the outcry of "liberals" against testing, "conservative" physicists replied that — with the exception of a few isolated geographic locations where unique meteorologic coincidences had caused fleeting peaks — the total body radiation to the population coming from fall-out was a fraction of the (estimated) load coming from medical radiation sources.

This did not solve the dilemma "to test or not to test," but it distributed the overall pressure more evenly by coinvolving in the controversy physicians in general, and radiologists in particular.

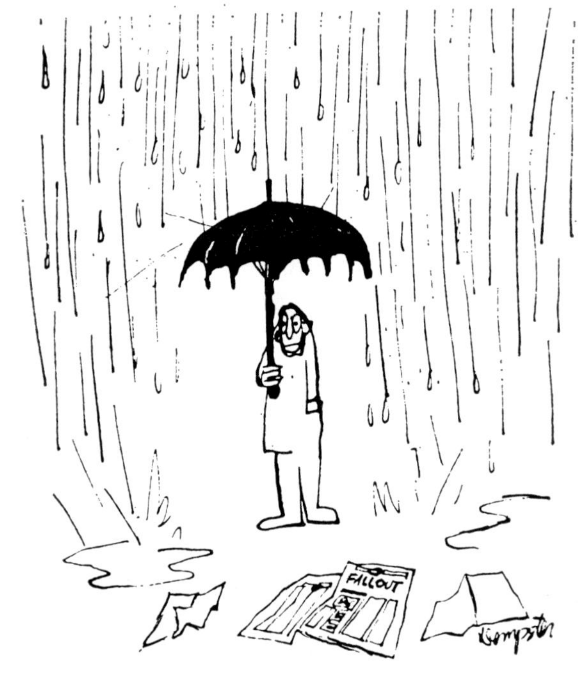

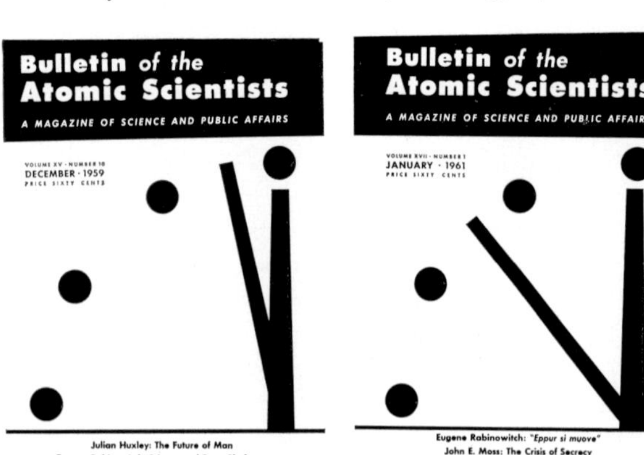

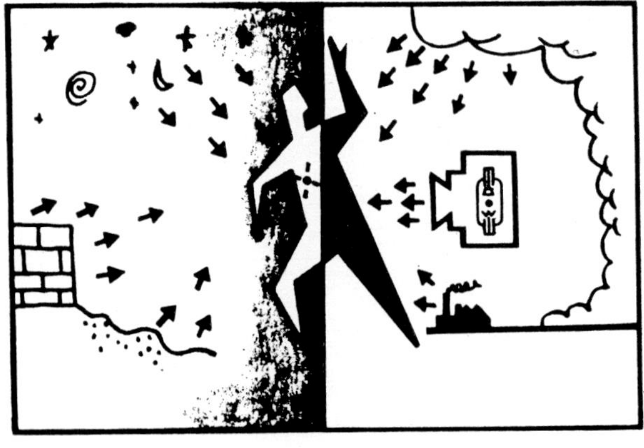

The "radio-geneticists" (most of whom never received a medical education) contend that genetic radiation hazards to humans are sufficiently proved by experimental results obtained in fast reproducing insects, and small mannals. This has led to often daring, and sometimes hysterical, extrapolations. Current concepts postulate that a single quantum of ionizing radiation causes cell damage which, in the gonads, may turn out to be a mutation. This is an (almost)* incontrovertible experimental evidence. But medicine is still an art, and we have not (yet) learned to predict biologic occurrences with any degree of accuracy. Therefore — on the advice of Voltaire's *Candide* — let us first look at the *clinical* facts.

Diagnostic radiology has been in existence since 1896, in current (often indiscriminate) use for most of the past four decades and yet, so far, there has been no demonstrable rise in obvious mutations. It has been stated (if you can believe such computations) that more dangerous than roentgen rays — mutation-wise — is the "civilized" habit of "overheating" the testicles by wearing pants: if the proselytes of Venus Castina find out about that, we may soon be fighting a drive which would have us change to kilts.

In the 1920s, Ira Kaplan, a radiologist from New York City, administered roentgen therapy to several hundred "apparently sterile" women, after all known medical procedures had failed to relieve their infertility. In every one of these patients, each ovary received 225 r (roentgen) in air, which is over 100 r tissue dose. Thereupon many of the irradiated women bore children, who grew up, married, and had children of their own. Since then, at periodic intervals, Kaplan exhibited photographs of their offspring (at the time of his latest publication there were about thirty grandchildren), and none had any demonstrable abnormal-

*There is a little-known mimeographed document K-1470, issued on May 2, 1961 by the Union Carbide Nuclear Company, and available from the Department of Commerce. Its author, Hugh F. Henry (a physicist at Oak Ridge), shows that a statistical average life-lengthening effect occurs at chronic life-time radiation exposure levels below about 2-5 rad/week. Also in animal experimentation, such as chronic internal exposure from injection of radioisotopes (plutonium, uranium, etc.) statistical life-lengthening effects occur at low level injections where higher doses shorten life. The title of that document: *Is All Nuclear Radiation Harmful?*

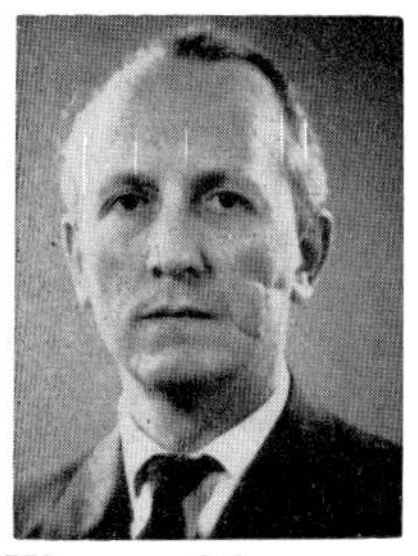

WERNER MOLINEUS

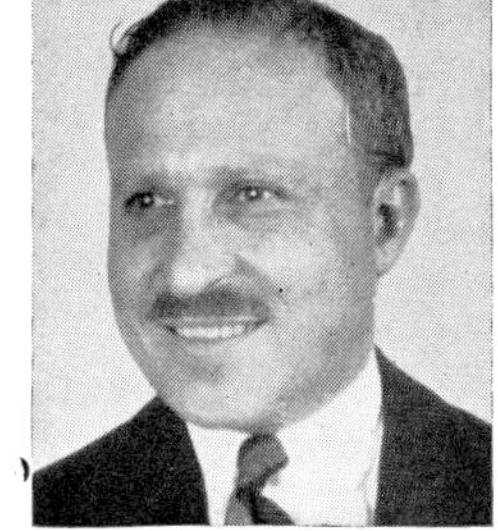

IRA KAPLAN

Why be concerned with radiation hazards

?

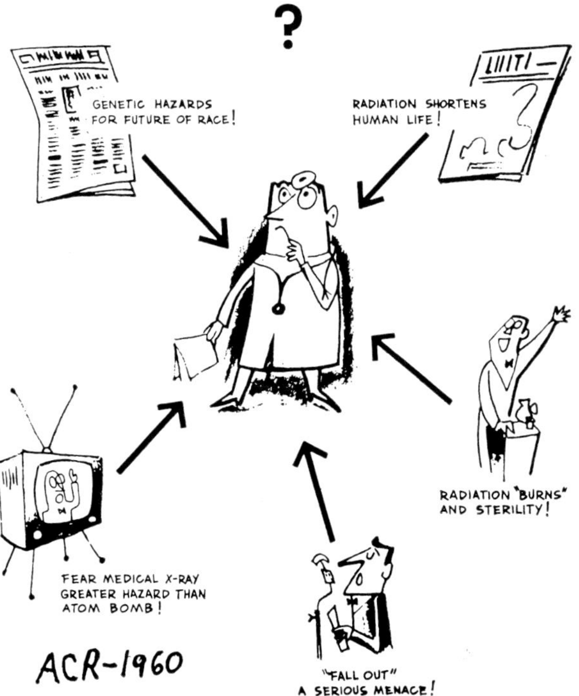

APPLICATIONS OF ATOMIC ENERGY

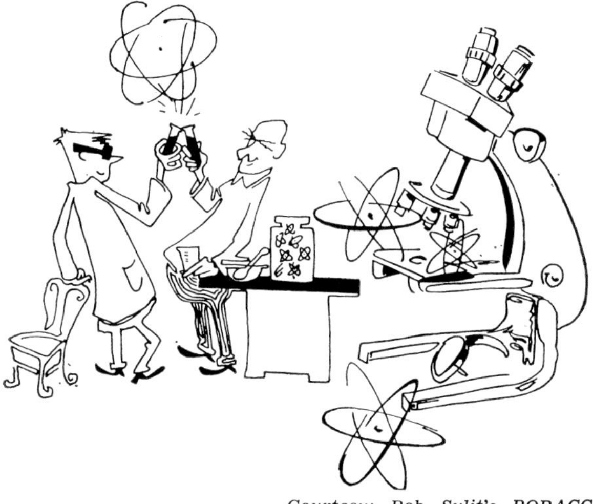

Courtesy: Bob Sulit's PORACC.

ISOTOPE INGESTION. A current fad is to provide captions for old movie scenes. One of these "mad scientists" says, "I hid my badge behind a lead brick. They will never know just how much we guzzled!"

ities. Modern geneticists want us to wait through the eighth generation before they grow willing to believe that there are no genetically damaged carriers among those descendants of irradiated ovaries. This may be theoretically valid, – but before it can be proved one way or another, all the staunch litigants will at best be memories. Roentgen therapy for dysmenorrhea (and infertility) is today hopelessly obsolete. But let us not forget that these thirty apparently healthy youngsters are with us either or both because and in spite of the ovarian irradiation inflicted upon their grandmothers.

The somatic damage inflicted by ionizing radiation in the high and medium dosage range is well known. We know very little about the somatic damage (if there is any at all) from chronic low-level exposure. Still, neither its promiscuous use, nor inadequate protective devices may ever be condoned. But there are faint indications that the pendulum of scientific opinion is about to swing back, and thus to reduce the overt anxiety over the genetic hazards of the invisible light.

Various explanations have been offered (aside from the genetic time-schedule) for the discrepancy in the experimentally demonstrable but clinically undetectable radiation-induced mutations. First of all, deaths due to lethal dominants occur too early to be of importance as human hazards. Lethal recessives do not manifest themselves unless and until mating takes place, and only then in certain proportions. As for the (allegedly few) "good" and (allegedly many) "bad" non-lethal mutations, said to be in the majority recessive, one might assume that imperceptible selection would take care of them, as it does take care of the presumably numberless "spontaneous" (cryptogenetic?) mutations, known to occur in the absence of measureable ionizing radiation. After all, there are populations living for millenia (on monazite beaches in India, on volcanic soil in the Andes) in the presence of a comparatively elevated "background" radiation. They are not impaired in any demonstrable way.

Several organizations are trying to find out more about these elusive hazards. The Industrial Medical Association has appointed its own Radiation Committee. A Johns Hopkins epidemiologist, Raymond Seltser, is examining the membership roster of the RSNA (the high-risk group) by comparison with the membership rosters of the (medium-risk) American College of Physicians and American Academy of Orthopedic Surgeons, and of the (low-risk) American Academy of Ophthal-

PRINCIPLES OF
RADIATION AND CONTAMINATION CONTROL

R. A. SULIT
E. J. LEAHY
A. L. BAIETTI

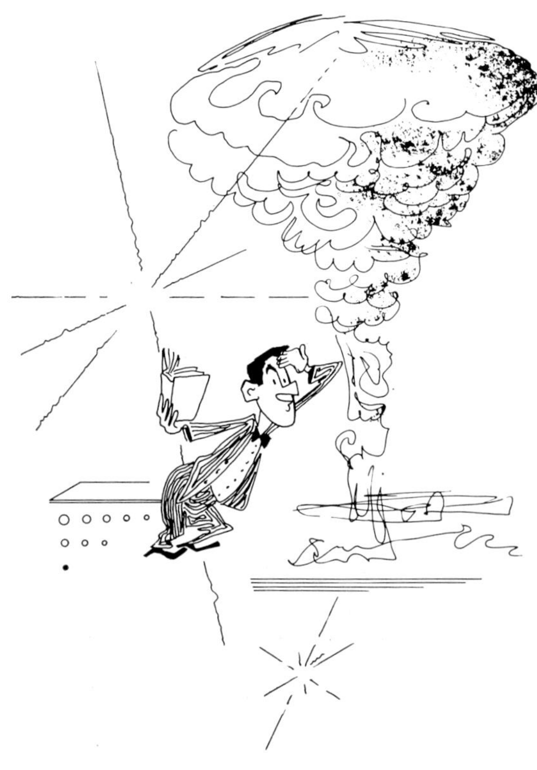

BUREAU OF SHIPS NAVY DEPARTMENT WASHINGTON 25, D. C.
prepared by
U. S. NAVAL RADIOLOGICAL DEFENSE LABORATORY
San Francisco 24, California

For sale by the Superintendent of Documents, U.S. Government Printing Office, Washington 25, D.C. - Price $2.00

PROTECTION PRIMER. This is the cover of one of three excellent volumes prepared by Bob Sulit and associates, with the avowed (?) purpose to serve as a do-it-yourself book if and when the big bang were to occur. Being printed by the Government, it is not copyrighted, so (with Bob Sulit's gracious acknowledgement) several of their delightful drawings have been "freeloaded."

mologists and Otolaryngologists. And the ACR is circulating a lengthy questionnaire among its members, with searching inquiries about the progeny.

There is little doubt that a few decades hence, some of today's more articulate "genetic radiation damage"-ists will be cited in the same humorous vein as the hazards to health which overcautious forebears ascribed to the 40-50 MPH speed of trains of one hundred years ago.

DOSIMETRY

The radiation scare became a welcome subject for the sensationalistic segment of the press. An aroused citizenry demanded thereupon that *something* be done about protecting them from radiation. Several conscientious science writers tried their best to soothe public anxiety. Somehow, the public as a whole was totally unaware of the fact that this commodity (radiation protection) had been on the books for over thirty years.

It is not possible to discuss protection without referring to dosimetry. We must be able to measure (or at least to estimate) the levels of radiation before we can decide what is to be considered dangerous, and how much so.

An abbreviated "History of Dosimetry" appeared, under the hermetic title *Therapeutic Limitations of Radioisotopes* in Urology, in the second number of the first volume of the ("throwaway") *Lederle Bulletin.* It was the talk given by Marshall Brucer before the mid-year meeting of the Chicago Urological Society (Edgewater Beach Hotel — January 27, 1957), under the sponsorship of the American Cyanamid Company, owner of Lederle Laboratory. Brucer's text (as most of his writing) is provocative, mainly because of his fresh approach to the problems, and partly because of the inherent Brucerian (mostly didactic) exaggerations. Following are excerpts from that address, based in part on a comparison between the amount of acetyl-salicylic acid in an aspirin tablet, and the quantity of radiation in a given unit.

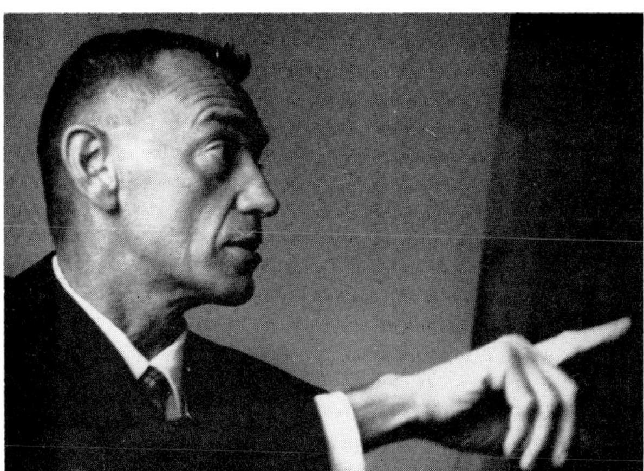

MARSHALL BRUCER (1963): "Let's have a protection-a-day plan!"

"A kind of constant used in biology is illustrated by some such figure as the maximum permissible concentration of Strontium-90 that is allowed in the body. But this is not a measured or a measurable figure. It is not an average taken from measurements. It is not a computed figure calculated from known physical laws. It is, however, the kind of figure that is used most in the field of medicine; and it is, properly speaking, a unit of radiation.

"The maximum permissible concentration figure is a kind of unit hitherto unknown in science. It is a biopolitical agreement. Biopoliticians have agreed that 0.1 microcuries of radiation from Strontium-90 is allowable in the body. Unfortunately for the progress of political science, the antithesis of its units is ever present. Whenever we make a biopolitical agreement, we also set up the potentiality of a biopolitical disagreement. This is what has happened and what is happening in the field of the biological units of radiation.

"After many years of argument, physicists agreed that when x rays from any direction, over any time interval, and at any energy, interacted within 1 cc. of dry air to the extent that one electrostatic unit of charge was formed, the unit of quantity of radiation called a roentgen (r) had by definition occurred. This unit was not a biopolitical agreement. It was a real physical measurement. It was arrived at with great difficulty and with a tremendous amount of labor, and it represents a unit similar to Avogadro's number. It has an error, but it can be measured with more than sufficient precision.

"In 1934, they made a minor change in the definition of the roentgen. In 1950, they made another minor change which, hidden within the meaning of the change, contained a major limitation. By this time it was known that, although the roentgen was a physical measurement of great precision, it had little to do with biological events. In 1953 in biopolitical convention the roentgen was finally discarded as a biological unit of radiation. The history of this upheaval in medical

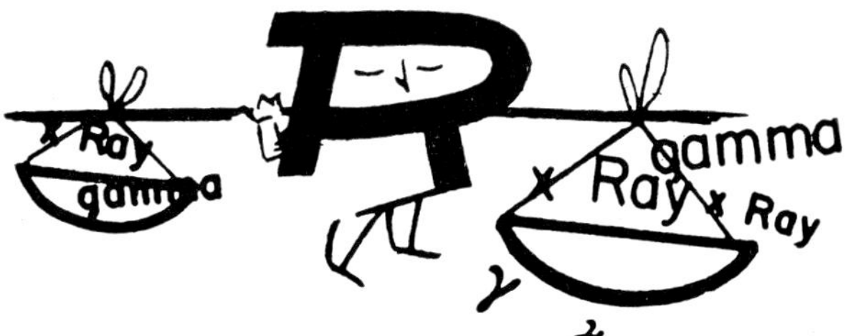

radiation physics is an interesting and instructive one.

"In 1895, Roentgen announced that discovery of a new kind of light. In 1897, Dorn made the first attempt to measure a quantity of x rays. In 1899, Rutherford improved Dorn's measurement, removed the obvious faults, and devised a concept of calorimetry that is in essence the concept we use today; but his methods, though suitable to the physics laboratory, were unsuitable in the clinic. Starting in 1900 Holzknecht, Kienböck, Sabouraud, and a host of others devised new ways of quantitating a dose of radiation that could be used in the clinic.

"As is always true in the history of medicine, when you have more than one method of measuring a substance, a co-ordination between these measures must be developed. The radiotherapeutic literature before 1910 is full of these co-ordination studies. One Sabouraud-Noiré dose was found to be equal to 5 Holzknecht units, and that was found to be equal to 10 Kienböck units.*

"It was suspected by some astute clinicians that where there are many units, probably none is any good, and so the problem was thrown back to the physicist.

"The physicist struggled with many devices for measuring radiation and finally, in 1908, Villard of France proposed a unit identical in essence to the unit we use today. Few people, however, believed him and it took twenty years of labor until, in 1928, the physicists meeting in biopolitical convention with a few radiotherapists agreed on the definition of the roentgen.

"While the first measurements of radiation from an x-ray tube were being thought over, a new source of radiation came into being and assumed a medical importance equal to that of the x-ray machine. This was radium. By 1910, it was admitted that nobody knew how much radium was how much, and so a unit for radium had to be devised. The unit that was agreed upon in biopolitical convention in Brussels in 1910 was

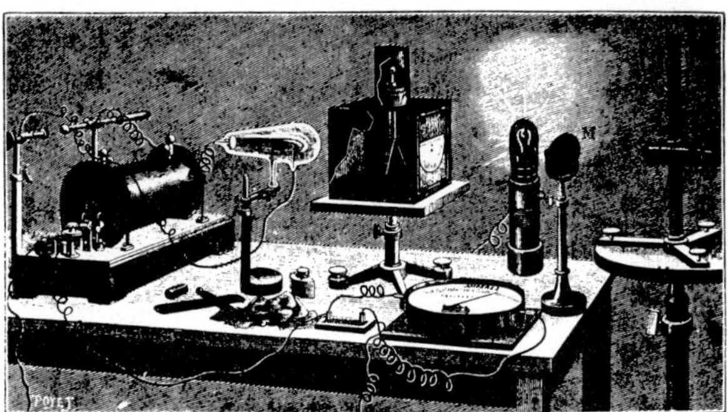

INITIAL IONOMETRY. Thus far most of the significant radiation dosimetry was based on ionization studies. In the first few weeks after the announcement of Röntgen's discovery, the Frenchman Benoist with his Roumanian associate Hurmuzescu began to study the ionizing effects of roentgen rays on a gold-leaf electroscope. Their observations were soon confirmed by Dufour in Lausanne (Switzerland), by J. J. Thomson in Cambridge (England), and by Righi in Torino (Italy). In this experimental arrangement of Benoist and Hurmuzescu, the electroscope can be observed with the mirror (M) and the telescope (L). The illustration is reproduced from the *Electrical Review* (London) of May 1, 1896.

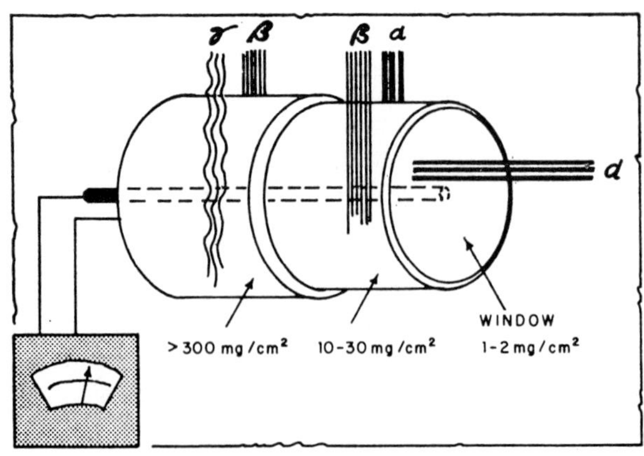

IONIZATION CHAMBER

---

*I thought it might be of interest to give a few physical details on the devices mentioned by Brucer as being employed at the beginning of the century.

In 1902, Holzknecht used the discoloration of irradiated alkaline salts as a measure of the amount of radiation. In 1904, Freund, and in 1906 Bordier and Galimard, employed for the same purpose the liberation of iodine from a solution of 2 percent iodoform in chloroform. These were soon superseded by Kienböck's quantimeter, with strips of silver bromide paper exposed on the skin of the patient under treatment, after which the strips were processed and their darkening compared with a standard. In 1907, Schwarz built a calomel radiometer, in which measurement of radiation was done by measuring the opacity produced by precipitation of calomel from a mixture of mercuric chloride and ammonium oxalate solutions. Most favored of all was the Sabouraud-Noiré and Bordier method wherein the dose of radiation was estimated from the color change of pastilles of compressed barium platinocyanide, placed on the patient's skin during the irradiation. In treatment the *full dose* of x-radiation was considered as that amount which caused a slight erythema to appear within 15-21 days, the skin having been exposed to the direct action of the rays without interposition of any filter, from a tube of medium hardness (about 6 Benoist). Four-fifths of this erythema or full dose (the latter term was preferred) would cause the hairs to fall out, a critical dose regarded as requisite for treatment of ringworm. Sabouraud's *Teinte B* corresponded to this full dose. Holzknecht moved the unexposed pastille under a celluloid band of graduated red-brown color until it appeared of the same tint as the exposed pastille: the scale divided the dose into five parts. Kienboeck divided his scale into ten equal parts, each of which he called X. Sabouraud's *Teinte B* equalled Holzknecht's 5 H, Kienboeck's 10 X, and Schwarz's 3.5 Kaloms.

the curie unit. It was an entirely different kind of unit from the roentgen, which has been under discussion so far. The curie unit was a unit of mass.

"But who could measure a unit of mass of radium when nobody had a very big mass of radium to play with in those days? Besides which, nobody was quite sure what radium was. Radium is one stop in a chain of decay of one element to another. What is radium today might not be radium tomorrow. Before the unit of mass of radium could be determined, the definition of what is meant by radium had to be achieved.

"It was simpler to change the unit of mass to a unit of rate of disintegration. It was easier to measure the rate of disintegration of radium than it was to weigh out a unit of mass of radium; and so physicists measured very carefully the rate of disintegration of what would be defined as 1 gram of radium. Unfortunately, when two people measure the same thing, there are bound to be at least two answers, and more people than two measured the rate of disintegration of radium. Therefore, the unit of radium was in peril.

"Whenever there is a disagreement in science and the disagreeing parties are equally respectable, the obvious thing to do is to appoint a commission; and so an International Commission was appointed to solve the problem of the rate of disintegration of radium. This International Commission, instead of measuring the rate of radiation, realized that this measurement only would have led to an additional argument about the accuracy of its measurement. Therefore they did something that is always much better than a measurement in the field of science – they decided on the unit by voice vote. The voice-vote method of determining a physical fact was born with the International Commission on Radiological Units and is now being followed uniformly throughout the field of science. We may not get the correct answers this way, but at least we have agreement.

"In 1930, the International Commission on Radiological Units met for the third time and decided that the curie was no longer a unit of mass of radium, but was 37 billion disintegrations per second of radium under very carefully defined conditions of packaging.

"But the International Commission was very specific about its definition of the radium unit. It noted that there were other kinds of radioactivity; and to keep its skirts clean it opposed fundamentally, absolutely, and without exception, the extension of the definition of the curie beyond the radium family.

"The definition of the curie was a biopolitical agreement, and it should be noted again that where there is a biopolitical agreement there can also be a biopolitical disagreement. In 1930, while the Commission was deliberating, the seed of dissolution of their agreement was being manufactured in California. The cyclotron was being invented. By 1932, the cyclotron was in operation and shortly thereafter not one, but hundreds of different kinds of artificially manufactured radioactive substances were being produced.

"But the curie was not a biological unit. It was purely a physical unit and its only claim to fame was its purity. While the commissions were arguing these units, biologists were using radiation and they were using it on people. Therefore other units had to be devised that were practical and usable by the practicing physician. About fifty other different kinds of units were proposed and were used by various physicians. One of the outstanding was the skin unit or rather the skin units.

"If radiation is applied to the skin under certain conditions and following certain very carefully specified procedures, something happens to the skin that even

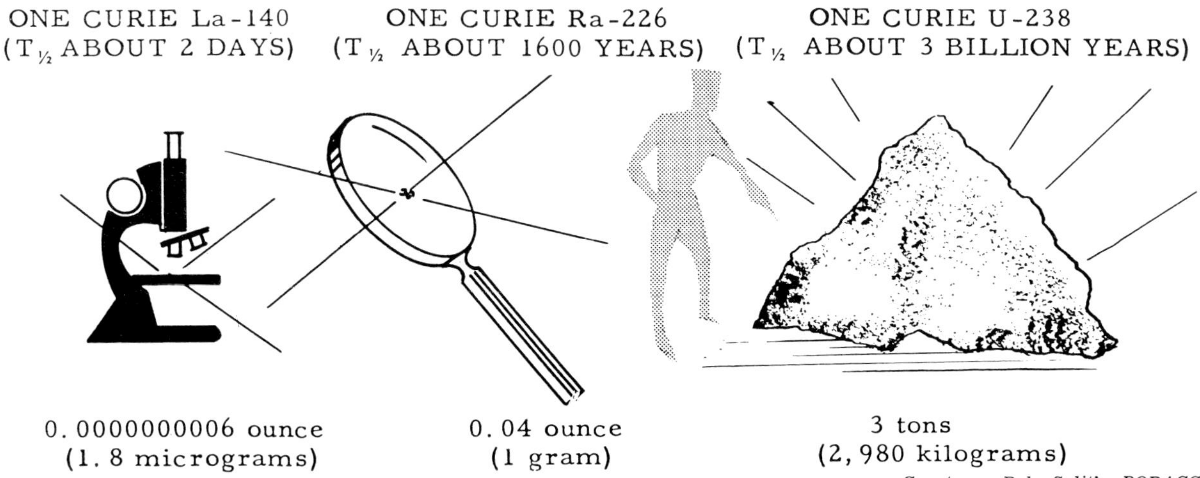

Courtesy: Bob Sulit's PORACC.

THE CURIE. A pound is a pound, no matter what its volume is. A curie is a curie, no matter what it weighs, provided 37 billion atomic disintegrations per second occur within it.

the physician can detect. By one definition that was used extensively, one skin unit of radiation would take the scalp hair off. Although this was hard on the patient, it was known fairly accurately that one skin unit was equal to four Hampson units, or 18 Kienböck units. It might not have been a good unit but at least it was a biological unit.

"(There was also) another kind of skin unit . . . called the erythema dose. The erythema dose was defined in many ways. A German method was to irradiate until a faint blush appeared on the skin. The French method was to apply the amount of radiation necessary to cause a second degree burn that healed without a scar. Again this was hard on the patient, but it was a biological unit.

"As would be expected, where there are many units one can find articles in the literature comparing the relative merits of the units. The skin unit was found to be approximately two-thirds of the erythema unit. Three German units were found to be equal to one French unit. The Buffalo erythema unit was found to be less than the New York erythema unit. There was a Chicago erythema unit, a Detroit erythema unit; and every city from civic pride alone had to have its own unit.

"All during the 1930s, the problems of radiation dosimetry, especially as used by the biologist, were difficult to understand. It was obvious to any astute physician that we did not know how much aspirin was in the aspirin tablet.

"By the end of World War II, a group of scientists in Boston began to get sensible about the problem. They devised the rhm unit. This was pronounced the "rum" unit, and it is to be expected that such a unit would come out of Boston since Boston was founded on the economy of rum. The rhm unit was defined as the number of roentgens per hour measured at a meter distance from the source of radiation. The important point about the rhm unit was that it was not a medical unit, nor a dosage unit, nor a protection unit. It was not even a political unit. It was purely and simply a statement of fact. So many roentgens, measurable with great accuracy, were measured by a detection device at a certain distance from a given source of radiation. This was such a sensible unit that it was forgotten by the medical profession almost as soon as it was devised.

"Along with the development of all of the physical units, many biological units were devised. There was the erythema dose of Seitz and Wintz. There was Jüngling's unit, which determined the amount of radiation that would stop the growth of bean sprouts. This was very useful for those physicians who felt that people were identical to bean sprouts. A unit was devised to measure the amount of radiation that would sterilize the eggs of the fruitfly or the amount that would cause the legs of a grasshopper to fall off. All these units were very useful for scientific papers and they were the kind of thing that medical students had to remember for the purpose of examination papers, but they confused the problem of dosimetry.

"In the 1840s, the American Government went through its period of "manifest destiny." The course of the empire was changed. One hundred years later the decade of "manifest destiny" in radiation occurred. The cyclotron was a success, and many of them were built. The chain reaction was a potentiality that became a probability and finally an actuality. From a little bit of radiation in 1939, the world was suddenly inundated by radiation in 1949. The neutron had been discovered and was now a biological hazard and also a biological hope. A neutron unit was invented. Because lots of beta radiation was available, a beta ray equivalent roentgen was invented; then an energy unit for beta rays (ev from mev to bev) was invented; a roentgen equivalent physical (REP) was invented; a roentgen equivalent man (REM) was invented. Each of these units was defined, redefined, and one unit followed another in rapid succession. The multiplicity of units caused confusion, but it was a confusion born from a newly realized understanding.

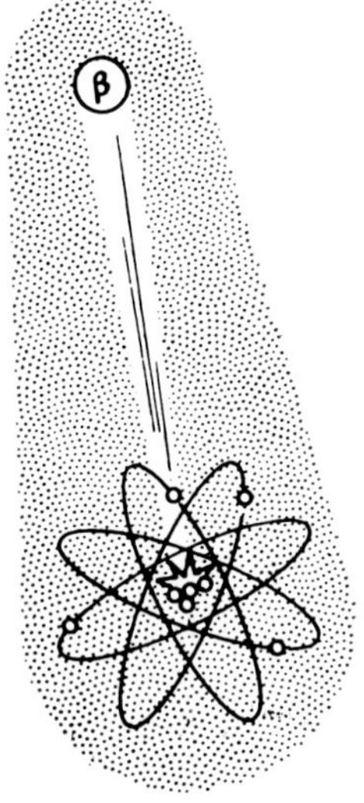

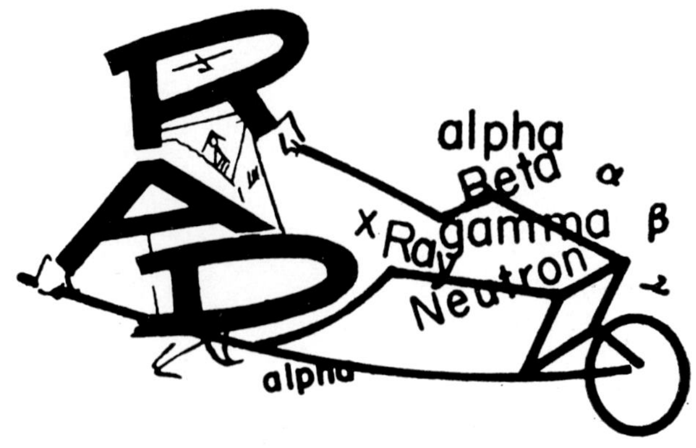

"Since the birth of radiation at the turn of the century, a few persons had been pointing out that the essential item for measurement was the number of ergs of energy absorbed by the tissue. With all the biopolitical agreements and disagreements, the definitions and the redefinitions, somebody finally made a measurement. A monumental piece of work was done by Spiers at the University of Leeds in England and published in 1945. Spiers had measured how many ergs of energy were absorbed in various kinds of tissue when one roentgen's worth of radiation was applied to the tissue. This work explained much of the confusion and set the stage for a new unit.

"By 1950, scientific politicians the world over recognized the need and that the time was right for a new unit. In 1953, the Commission met and ended a decade of confusion in a manner that only an international commission can accomplish. They passed a new unit. This time, however, they devised a unit that followed biological principles talked about for many years. They devised the "rad" and the rad was 100 ergs per gram of any kind of radiation absorbed in any kind of material. This was the first sensible biological unit that had been suggested within the field of radiation in fifty-seven years of radiation history.

"This does not mean that the roentgen has been discarded. The roentgen is still the fundamental physical unit of exposure. It is an absolute physical unit and hence it is very important. It is a unit that can be duplicated and measured with precision anywhere in the world today. It is a kind of unit that is similar to the units a pharmaceutical drug house* uses when it says there are five grains of aspirin in each tablet in the bottle.

"The roentgen is a calibration unit; but in spite of its usefulness to the physicist, it is worthless to the physician. Therefore the roentgen has been dropped, but only as a biological unit. The rad has been substituted, and probably this can be expected to be a sensible substitution with the next generation.

"The rad can be a biological unit. Unfortunately, up to a year ago it was impossible to measure the rad directly in tissue. It still cannot be measured directly in tissue, but it can almost be measured. We can, on an experimental basis, using chemical dosimetric techniques and very small, radiation-detection, glass-bead dosimeters, measure the absorption of radiation in animals. Within the next few years the rad promises to be a measurable unit, provided with a conversion table from roentgens. Therefore, after sixty years of very tedious work on the part of very many people, the stage is finally set for a physician to do radiation therapy.

"The rad, however, is in essence a biopolitical agreement. Therefore, it can be expected that a biopolitical disagreement will accompany it. The regulations that have been published for radiation exposure and for licensure to use radioisotopes are already speaking of "rem" units. They are speaking of relative biological effect. The modern radiobiologist has been raised in an era of confusion. It should be expected that this confusion will be perpetuated until the present generation dies."

*This pleonastic tautology eluded the red pencils of several editors, and was therefore preserved as a remembrancer (or hypermnemonic memento) for the recollection of future radio-stylists.

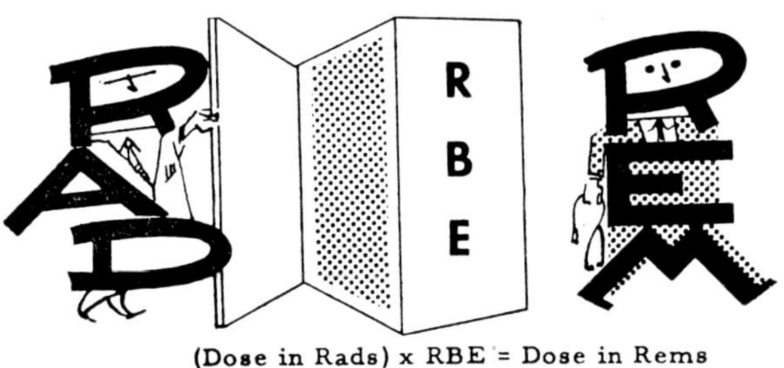

(Dose in Rads) x RBE = Dose in Rems

BRITISH PROTECTION

In the *British Journal of Radiology* of November, 1953, appeared several articles on the British X-Ray and Radium Protection Committee. First, F. G. Spear recalled that in April of 1899 a committee, appointed by the (British) Roentgen Society, collected evidence ("much of it confusing") on the harmful effects of x rays. Further discussions were promoted in 1915 and 1916, particularly on the question of protective devices for "X-ray operators," and a memo called the attention of the Admiralty and of the War Office to this aspect of military service. On March 29, 1921, a letter by Robert Knox in the London *Times* called again for the formation of a Protection Committee. Informal discussions started and it is now not quite clear when they were recognized as a formal body,

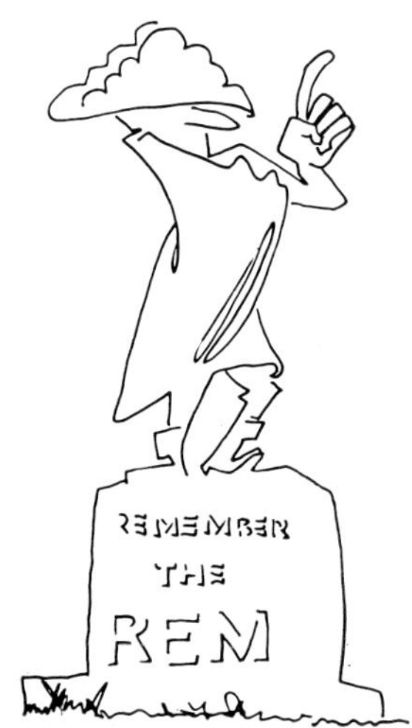

but that occurred about April, 1921. When so constituted, the Committee included Sir H. Rolleston (chairman), Stanley Melville and S. Russ (secretaries), Archibald Reid, R. Knox, G. Harrison Orton (the radiopathologist), J. C. Mottram, G. W. Kaye, S. Gilbert Scott, and Cuthbert Andrews. R. C. Lyster (from the Middlesex Hospital) had been prominent in promoting the committee, but he died in 1920 before its actual formation.

The Committee, which met in the BIR at 32 Welbeck St., published its first recommendations in July, 1921 (in the *Journal of the Roentgen Society*), with revisions in 1923, 1927, 1934, 1938, 1943, and 1948. The committee never had any statutory powers, but its recommendations carried great weight. Having no legal status, they modified their views from time to time to suit changing conditions. The (British) Medical Physical Laboratory — where George Kaye had his own Department — undertook the physical measurements requested by the committee, and inspected hundreds of hospitals, from the point of view of the committee's recommendations.

In the same issue of the *British Journal of Radiology,* there appeared reminiscences by S. Russ, and by C. Andrews, who recalled various details, for instance, in the beginning all they could say about protection against radiation was "let it be as little as possible."

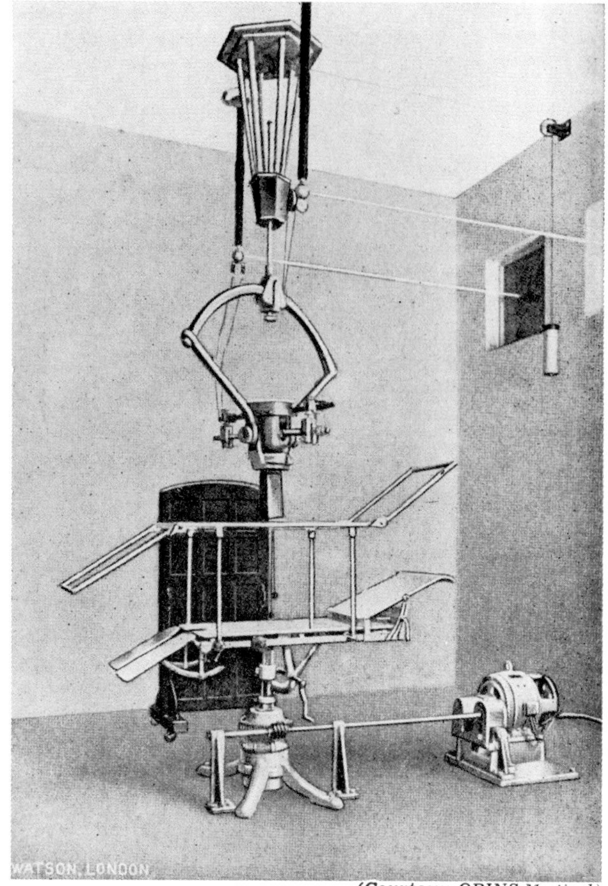

(Courtesy: ORINS-Medical)

KNOX'S ROTATING THERAPY COUCH

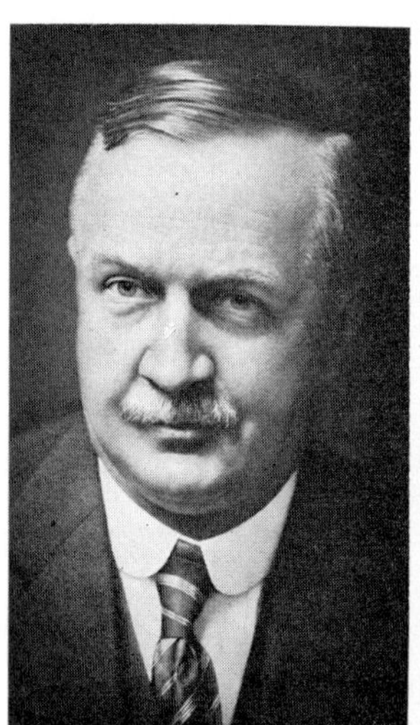

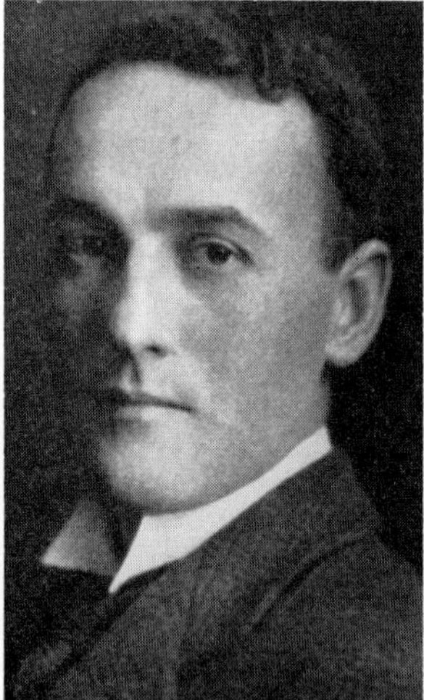

Courtesy: Georg Grössel - AGFA.

ROBERT KNOX. One of the best known among British roentgen pioneers, author of a classic textbook *(Radiography, X-Ray Therapeutics, and Radium Therapy),* and organizer of the BIR. But if only one achievement were to be recalled, it was the creation of the British X-Ray and Radium Protection Committee. A very young SIDNEY RUSS, the radium physicist, is shown on the viewer's right.

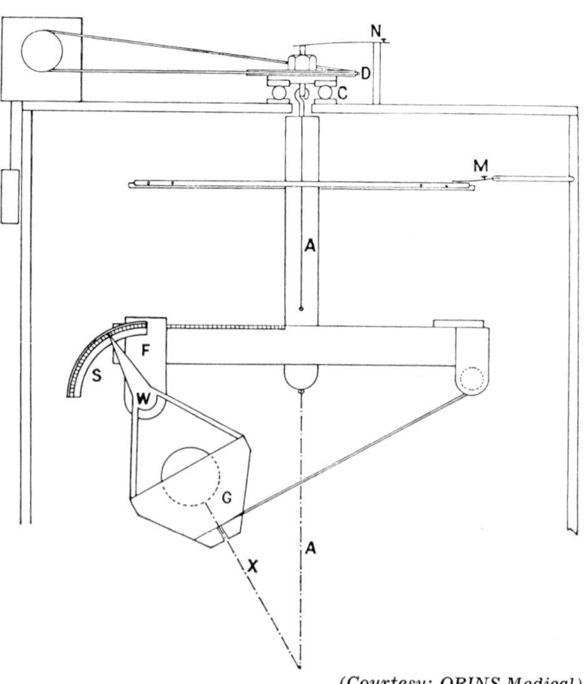

(Courtesy: ORINS-Medical)

KNOX ROTATING THERAPEUTIC TUBE STAND

At one time or another all committee members contributed to the expenses. The last article in that issue was by Sir Ernest Rock Carling, who had become chairman after Rolleston: he said *valle* to the Committee, which was disbanded in 1953. Its work was taken over by the British Ministry of Health and their Medical Research Council.

AMERICAN PROTECTION

During the annual meeting held in the Curtis Hotel in Minneapolis, on September 14, 1920 the ARRS formed the (American) Roentgen Ray Protection Committee. That was before the official recognition of the respective British Committee. The recommendations of that ARRS Committee were, however, issued only in September 1922, that is after those of the British Committee. Co-operation between these two bodies was quite close, and the recommendations were much the same. Later on, that particular committee of the ARRS was called Commission on Safety and Standards, with Pancoast as chairman, the members being Coolidge, Duane, Hickey, John T. Murphy, Bernard H. Nichols (of Cleveland), and Weatherwax. Their first report was published in the *American Journal of Roentgenology* of December, 1924.

The first Standardization Committee of the RSNA was formed in 1925, and its first report appeared in *Radiology* of March, 1926. Members of that committee were Ed Chamberlain, N. E. Dorsey, Arthur Erskine, Otto Glasser, F. L. Hunt, and the chairman, Eddy Ernst, Sr.

The Section on Radiophysics of the second ICR in Stockholm appointed an International Committee on the X-Ray Unit under the chairmanship of Manne Siegbahn, professor of physics at Upsala (Sweden); one of the secretaries was Edwin A. Owen who taught physics at Bangor (England), while the other secretary was Holthusen from Hamburg. The committee came up with what they called the "x-ray unit of intensity," better known as the roentgen. It was accepted on July 27, 1928. That second ICR in Stockholm was so very important also because of the creation of the International Protection Committee. It had been suggested by the British at the first ICR in London, and they had been assigned to prepare the necessary recommendations.

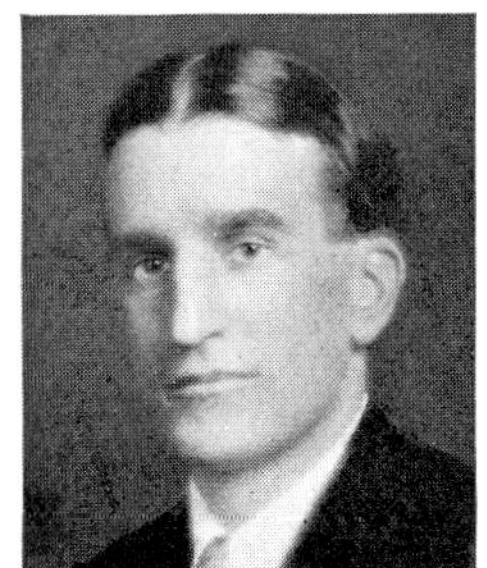

Lauriston Sale Taylor

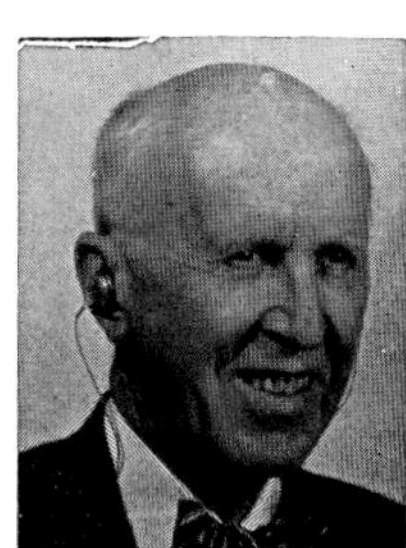

Bob Newell

In the very first issue of the first volume of *Health Physics* (1958) appeared the brief history of the (American) National Committee on Radiation Protection and Measurements (NCRP), by its permanent chairman, Lauriston Sale Taylor of the National Bureau of Standards (NBS).

The British Protection Committee had sent its suggestions to the more important national delegations and had asked them to appoint a respresentative to the ICR for the purpose of discussing protection problems. The NBS sent as an observer the (then 27 year old) Taylor. Serious difficulties arose in the course of the discussion, especially because the medical members of the

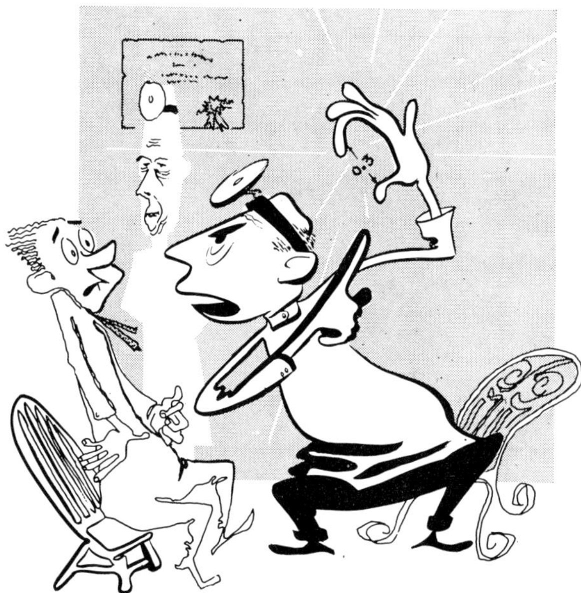

Courtesy: Bob Sulit's PORACC.

Permissible dose. During the Golden Age of Radiology it was known as the Tolerance Dose, having been conceived as an amount of radiation which can be tolerated without any injurious effects. Prior to 1934 a total radiation dose of 100 rem per year was regarded as quite innocuous. The ICRP recommendations, in effect from 1934 through 1950, limited it to 0.2 rem/day, which amounted to 60 rem/year. In the U. S. A., the accepted figures were lower, the ACXRP having advised no more than 0.1 rem/day, or 30 rem/year. In 1950 the ICRP revised it to 0.3 rem/week or 15 rem/year — and this is the figure on which the cartoon is based. Today it is 5 rem/year, but it may be lowered before this book is printed.

group expressed wide disagreement. The physicists then decided to act, and set up (in private talks held right there) an International X-Ray and Radium Protection Committee. The etymology of the title was "British" because they had organized it, and furnished the chairman (George Kaye) and one medical member (Stanley Melville). There were three other physicists on the Committee, Taylor, Rolf Sievert (Sweden), and Gustav Grossmann (Germany), and two physicians, the always argumentative Iser Solomon (France) and the then absent Ceresole (Italy).

On the recommendations of this international body, each country was to set up a national committee. The NBS sponsored the creation, early in 1929, of an Advisory Committee for X-Ray and Radium Protection; Taylor was the chairman, Pancoast and James Lloyd Weatherwax represented the ARRS, Newell and Failla the RSNA, Francis Carter Wood the AMA, and William David Coolidge (GE) and Wilbur Stanley Werner (Keleket) the manufacturers of x-ray equipment. The first palpable result of the Advisory Committee was publication of NBS Handbook 15 (May 16, 1931) on X-ray Protection. NBS Handbook 18 on Radium Protection appeared on May 17, 1934.

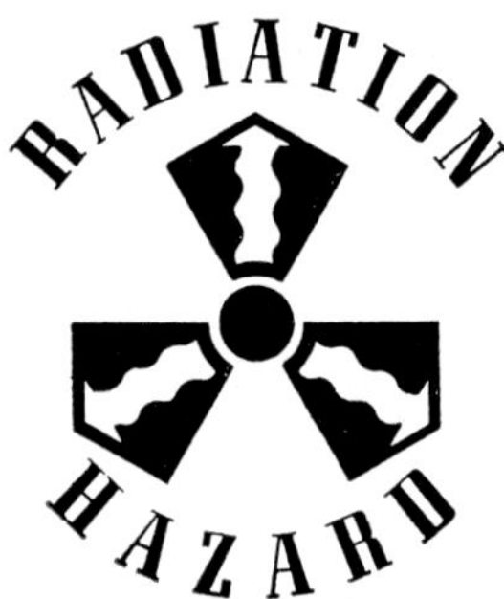

Courtesy: Marshall Brucer.

WARNING SIGN. Model used at ORINS around 1950.

The revised recommendations of the Handbook for X-ray Protection were issued in July, 1936, as NBS Handbook 20. This contained for the first time a permissible exposure level (then called tolerance dose) intended for occupational exposure: the figure recommended, 0.1 r/week, remained in force for twelve years (until 1948), and was used by the Manhattan Engineer District (MED).

In September of 1946, with the Atomic Phase in full swing, an informal meeting of the Advisory Committee was held to discuss the extensive revisions needed. Thereupon their representation was enlarged with the MED (Shields Warren and Karl Morgan) and the USPHS (H. L. Andrews and E. G. Williams). The expanded committee needed also a "new" name, which is when the one currently in use was selected: National Committee on Radiation Protection and Measurements (NCRP). It is just now in the process of receiving a federal charter. (It got it in 1964.)

The first post-war (re-organizational) meeting of the NCRP was held on December 4, 1946. The Committee burgeoned, and today it consists of eighteen subcommittees: with the main body they have a total of nineteen possible round-table combinations. The NCRP issued thirty-odd handbooks, many of which contain glossaries, needed to define the new terms successively introduced. Another important function of the NCRP is to keep lowering the level of maximum permissible exposure to ionizing radiation (they have been quite successful at that).

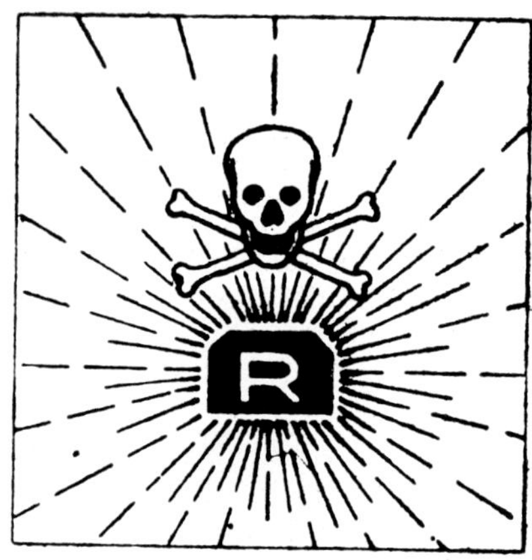

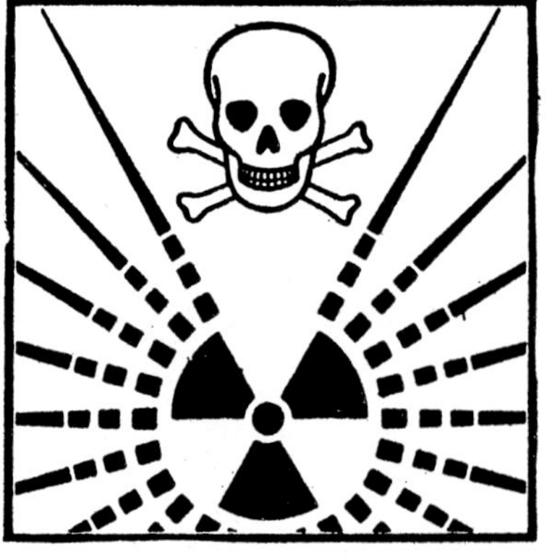

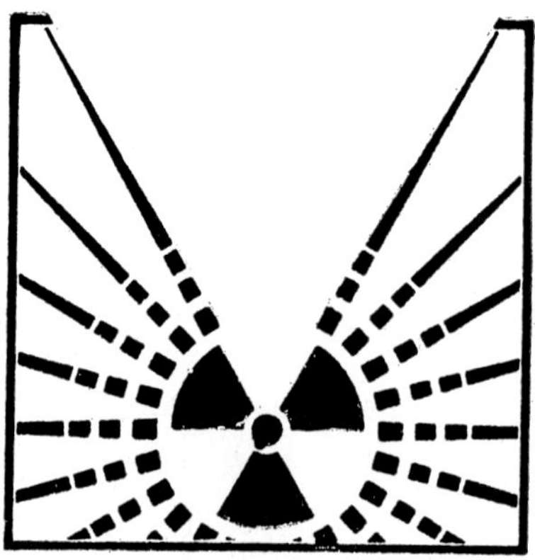

Courtesy: ILO

ILO ATOMIC DANGER SIGNS. The sign with the skull and the R is obsolete. At the 152nd session of the International Labor Organization (ILO) in Geneva in June of 1962, the other two signs have been approved. The trefoil with the skull (center) is for large sources, the trefoil without skull (right) is for lesser sources. Both signs, which are also approved by the IAEA, are used to label packages with radioactive material.

Prior to World War II, there occurred another international attempt to foster radiation protection: a *Handbook* on protective measures against dangers resulting from the use of radium, roentgen, and ultraviolet rays, written by Hermann Wintz (of Erlangen) and Walter Rump — the document was called CH-1054 — appeared in August, 1931 at Geneva. The effort proved to be just as ineffective as its sponsor, the League of Nations. A few years later, that international debating society became totally impotent. The League had been sterile since its very inception, but its deep-seated incapacitation became apparent only when it finally tried to enforce one of its decisions.

During World War II, all "international" co-operation ceased — not only in the field of radiation. In 1946, the international protection committee was reestablished. It, too, changed its name for the sake of the Atomic Phase, and became the International Commission on Radiological Protection (ICRP).

The ICRP meets during the ICR. For the time in-between, there is now the International Radiological Society. Its current president is Arthur Singleton. The secretary, Paul Flemming-Norgaard (and his office), remained in Copenhagen, where the IRS was founded during the 7th ICR.

ROENTGEN RADIACS

Radiac is a generic term and means radiation meter. Roentgen-radiac or x-radiac would be a device which measures x-rays.

The leading company in this field is the Victoreen of Cleveland. As previously mentioned, it furnishes the Gamma Dose Rate Meter, a Cutie-Pie, the Minometer II with the standard 200 mr pencil, and an improved version of the famous Condenser R-Meter. It also offers pocket dosimeters (indirect reading chambers), as well as direct reading chambers.

The Nuclear Consultants Corporation (NCC) of St. Louis makes the Townsend Roentgen Probe Model-RP-1, which measures gamma rays in body cavities using a unique tissue equivalent probe. This instrument was created because in the Atomic Phase people have come to favor the idea of measuring (whenever possible) the actual tissue dose instead of only computing it from tables. Atomic Accessories has the Roentgen Scinti-Probe and most companies have developed similar contraptions.

The Landswerk Electrometer Co. of Glendale (California) sells the Landswerk Roentgen Meter Model-L-64 for which they claim a wider sensitivity range and greater reading accuracy than available in any similar apparatus.

The radiation scare has also resulted in the development of gonad shields, lead mulages placed around the testicles (available in two sizes, for men and boys), imported by the Schick X-Ray Co. of Chicago. Bar-Ray

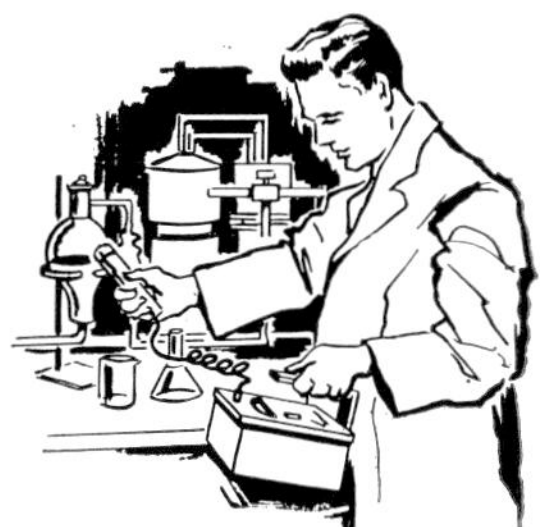

Courtesy: Victoreen.

LAB. RADIAC. The term has now a generic meaning — radiation detection and measuring device.

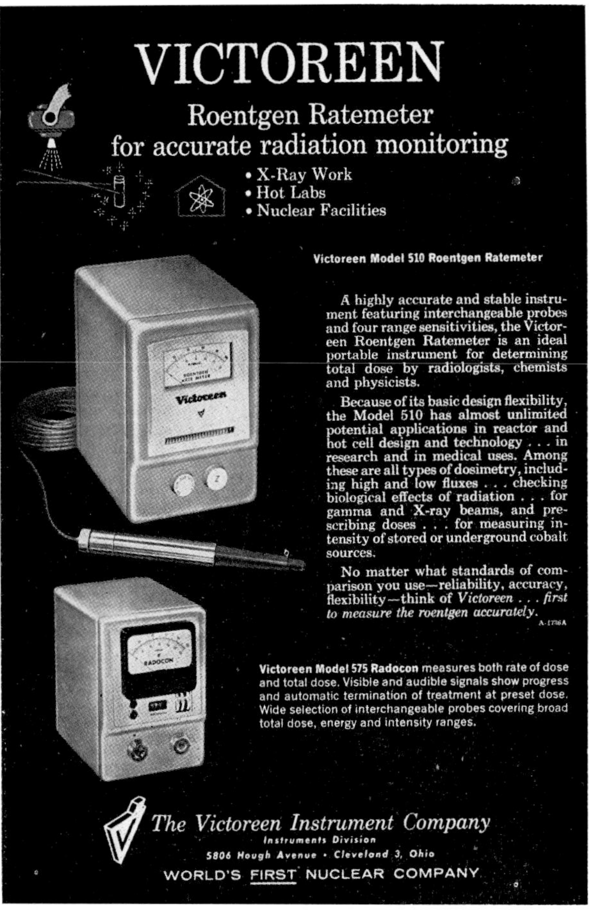

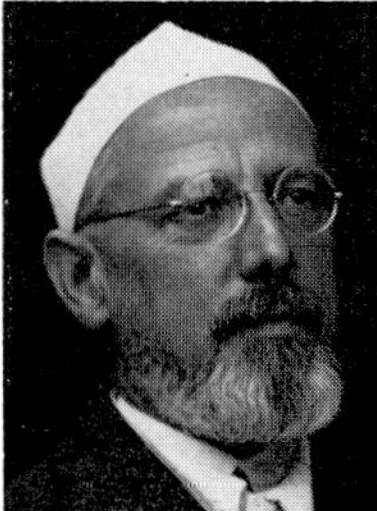

G. MAINGOT

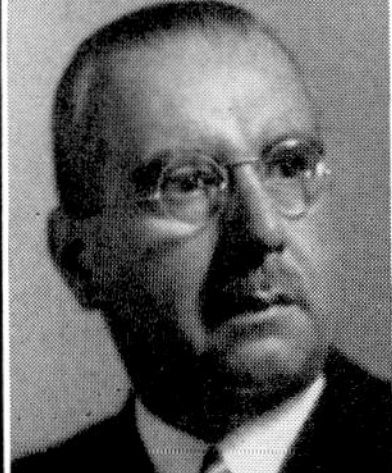

H. WINTZ

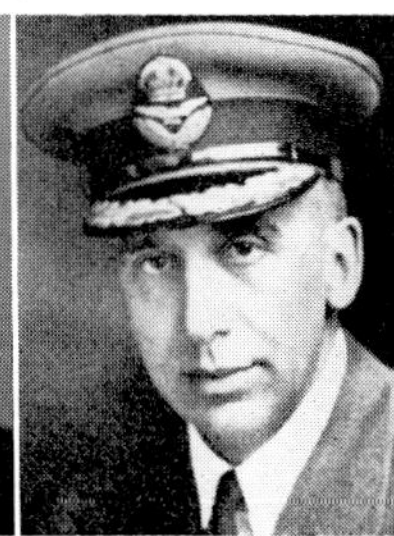

G. KAYE

Products of Brooklyn has an exclusive formulation of vinyl and lead, called Lead-X, from which it manufactures aprons and covers of various sizes, for various purposes.

Personal radiation monitors have been developed for physicists who are working in high radiation areas; they are called "chirpees" when sold to Civil Defense enthusiasts. Other "names" are sparrow, and REAC's Scram.

In this category may be mentioned another "atomic" development, the so called film badge, a small dental film placed behind filters of various quality and thickness; controlled development and densitrometric evaluation will then allow a fairly accurate computation of the dose to which the badge (and thus the individual wearing it) had been exposed during the time it was worn. R. S. Landauer, Jr. & Co. of Park Forest (Illinois) calls it the Laudauer Film Badge Service. Picker's version is named Guard-Ray while American Electronics of Los Angeles have christened theirs Dosifilm. Several other companies, including Tracerlab, offer similar services.

ATOMIC PHANTOMS

Atomic ghosts have real bones, but their lungs are molded in rigid foam, and their flesh is made of thermosetting isocyanate rubber. They are radio-equivalent (in general, and for human tissue). Furthermore, by adding bolus material, or by inserting an artificial tumor (material for one bronchogenic carcinoma costs about $30), one can duplicate almost any given therapeutic situation. Then, to complete the parallel with a voodoo doll, before assembly and clamping of the sections (of which the phantom is made), one may insert dosimeters into holes drilled into the very "heart" of the "tumor" itself. This is the basis of the RANDO system of *R*adiotherapy *AN*alog *D*osimetry, developed by Samuel W. Alderson of the Alderson Research Laboratories in Long Island City.

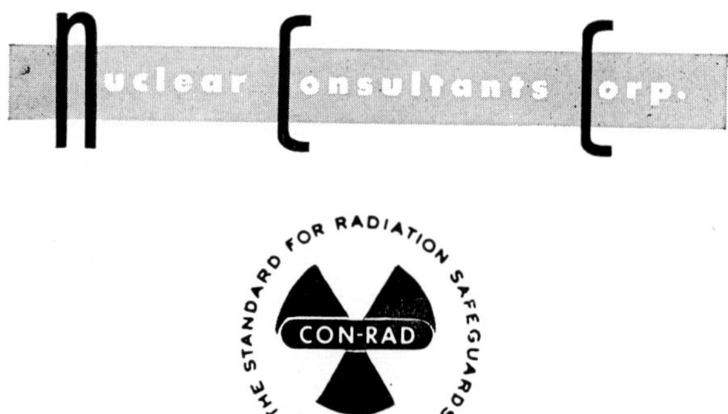

Both the REMAB (Radiation-Equivalent-Manequin-Absorption) and the REMCAL (Radiation-Equivalent-Manequin-Calibration) are useful in the study of actual dosages. In the orthovoltage range pre-calculation is never as accurate as pre-testing because of the "bone uncertainties." With super- or mega-voltage, bones are no longer a problem, but there appear "air errors," and those can be minimized with the manequin(s). Such a dark rubber ghost can also be helpful in re-creating radiation accidents, or in calibrating specialized research instruments.

PROTECTION PROBLEMS

In 1960, Marshall Brucer and Betty Anderson prepared several drafts of this subject,excerpts of which

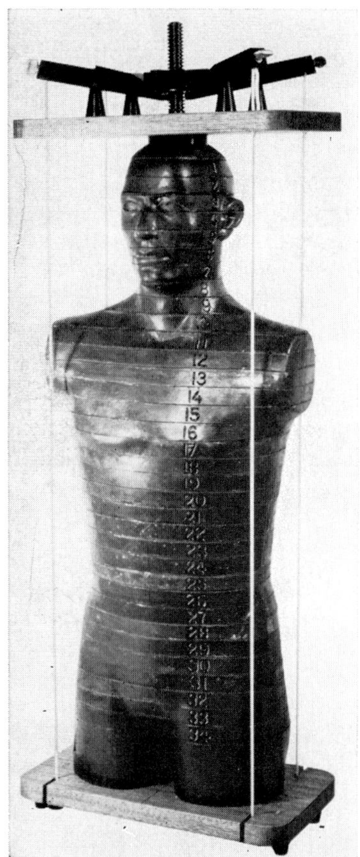

Courtesy: Alderson Research Laboratories.

ATOMIC PHANTOM. This is the average-man Rando phantom (5′8″ tall, 162 lbs. if completed with extremities), made of sections, which may be instrumented either by inserting ion chambers in the orifices provided, or by placing film sheets between adjacent sections. A special Rando data chart is provided to plot the actual readings. An average-woman was to have become available in early 1962. Phantom-patient matching is done by adding bolus material. For special instances one could conceivably obtain a custom-built (atomic) voodoo doll.

appeared under the title *Levels of Radiation* in the *AMA Journal* of January 7, 1961.

As a contractor to the AEC, the ORINS is exempt from its regulations. Nevertheless, since they teach students, the ORINS would like to follow all existing radiation protection rules and regulations. At one time they were about to establish the Radiation-Protection-

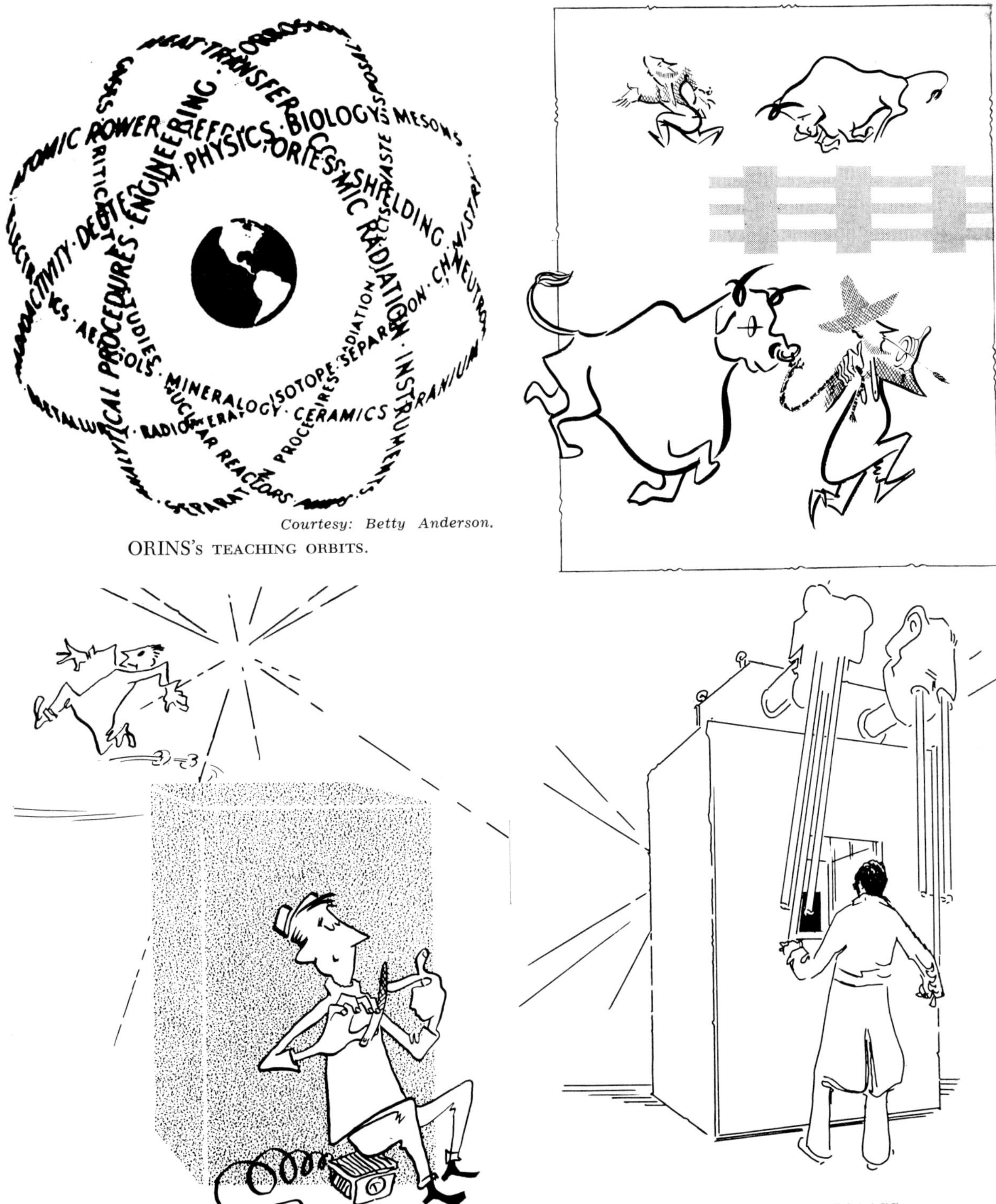

Courtesy: Betty Anderson.

ORINS's teaching orbits.

Courtesy: Bob Sulit's PORACC.

Protection is a matter of distance, shielding, and time of exposure, or a combination of these three factors.

Dose-of-the-Month-Club. After a very brief trial period they changed that to Radiation-Protection-Dose-of-the-Week-Club, in which each week a different set of rules promulgated by one or another organization would be followed. They soon found out that there were fewer weeks in the year than regulations.

As Brucer puts it, "Seventy-one national and international organizations have variable ideas on what radiation protection should be. Add to this the fifty highly individualized state governments in the United States that are rapidly developing uninterpretable regulations concerning unmeasurable quantities concerning an undefined risk and the problem becomes somewhat unmanageable."

A parallel may be established between the Pacific Ocean, a glass of water, and the various levels of radiation. If the event is properly arranged, a man can be drown with a glass of water, and it is also possible to work in and around the Pacific Ocean without drowning.

The same is true with radiation. Megacurie amounts of radioactive material – a disaster level of radiation – can be handled without getting hurt. Depending on the circumstances, one either domesticates a bull, or else keeps it fenced. It is always a matter of distance, degree of shielding, and duration of exposure. After all, one can look at megacurie sources through a very thick lead glass – the kind made by the Penberthy Instrument Company in Seattle. If necessary, those megacurie sources can be moved and otherwise worked upon with remote manipulatiors. In all those places warning signs must be displayed.

Kilocurie levels are used in teletherapy equipment; when properly shielded they cause no concern (leakage may at times become a problem). Curie levels are used in industrial radiography (leakage still one of the headaches), but so far not in medicine. The turning point is at the millicurie level, used for internal applications. Health physics computations, and protection measures are required with anything "stronger" than one millicurie. Below one millicurie the main problem is possible contamination which may raise the background to where measuring instruments become unusable. This is even more significant both in the microcurie (diagnostic), and at the millimicrocurie (low-level) categories.

De-contamination must consider the level of spilled radioactivity, which means the first thing is an adequate survey of the situation by a properly trained individual. Then, depending on the level found, remote manipulators (such as the Beetle) may be called for, or it is simply a vacuum-cleaning job. One of the latest methods uses ultrasonics — at REAC's Disontegrator, which can be operated by remote control, "wets" all the surfaces, forms bubbles (cavitation), and makes the cleaning solution more efficient.

RADIATION REVISITED

In the English language, the word radiation can be traced back to the beginning of the 17th century and perhaps beyond, but its frightening connotation is the by-product of the Atomic Phase.

Radiation came into international focus after the advent of fall-out, because science and politics do not mix so well. Today radiation is a powerful and destructive agent, as feared as any of the mysterious and evil divinities, created by the theurgic needs of primitive populaces. Many "modern" men would gladly give radiation "back to the Indians." Such regressive tendencies are but an expression of modern man's pathetic search for security in a world in which there is no security at all (except in the imagination of demagogues). After all, even a generation ago, if one became "sick of it all," he could retire to one of the obscure islands in the South Pacific and "get away from it all." Of course, combat proceedings during World War II would have taught him that there was no "escape" in the Pacific or anywhere else on the globe. Today, more than ever, one is a citizen of the world, and must think in global terms – especially with this fall-out!

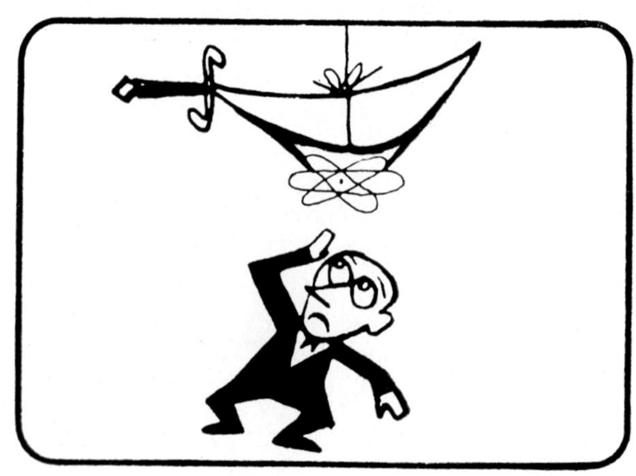

During the war, many radiobiologists, radiophysicists, and radiochemists — at Oak Ridge, Argonne, or Los Alamos — could discuss their findings only in secret conclaves. When the war was over, a first Symposium was held at Oberlin (Ohio) under the auspices of the National Research Council. They then decided to form a permanent association and the Radiation Research Society (RRS) had its first business meeting in New York on April 15, 1952. The first annual meeting was held at Ames (Iowa) on June 22-24, 1953 and Raymond E. Zirkle served as its first president.

The Radiation Research Society has two classes of membership. Full membership is reserved for those who have made contributions to the advancement of radiation physics, chemistry or biology by independent, original research or have performed special service considered equivalent. Associate membership is usually held by graduate students and by persons in lines of work relating to radiation but who are not professional, contributing scientists. At the beginning about 250 were members – the number now (1963) exceeds 900.

In February, 1954, appeared the first issue of *Radiation Research*, the official journal of the RRS, edited by the radiobiophysicist Titus Carr Evans from the State University in Iowa City. The RRS uses the term radiation in its broadest sense (ultraviolet, infrared, and invisible light, as well as ionizing wavelengths and energized particles), and is interested in all its aspects (physical, chemical, and biologic).

An International Congress of Radiation Research convened on August 11-15, 1958 in Burlington (Vermont). De Hevesy served as its honorary chairman. The *Proceedings* of that Congress were printed in 1959 as a supplement to *Radiation Research.**

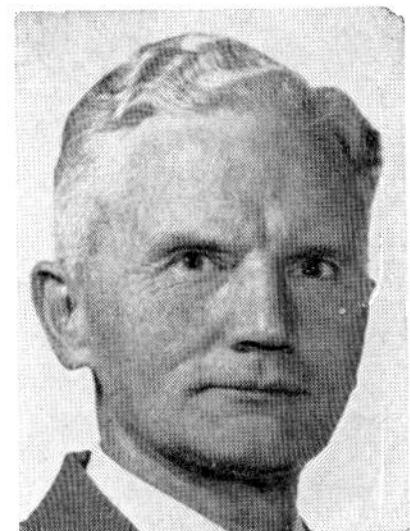

Carl Braestrup

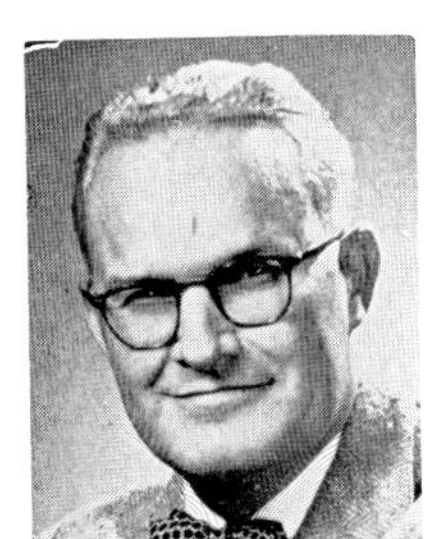

Harold Wyckoff

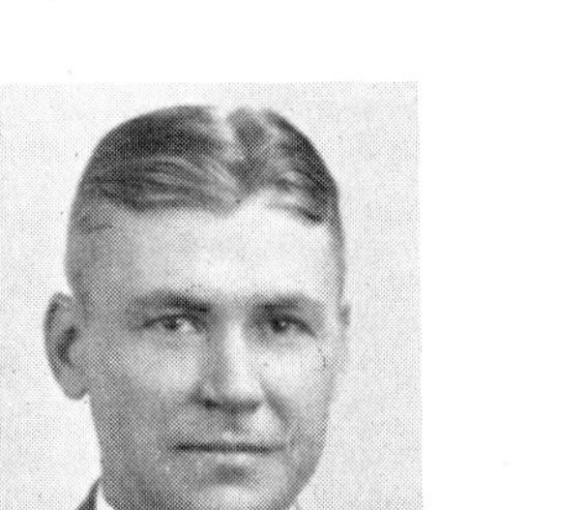

Raymond Zirkle

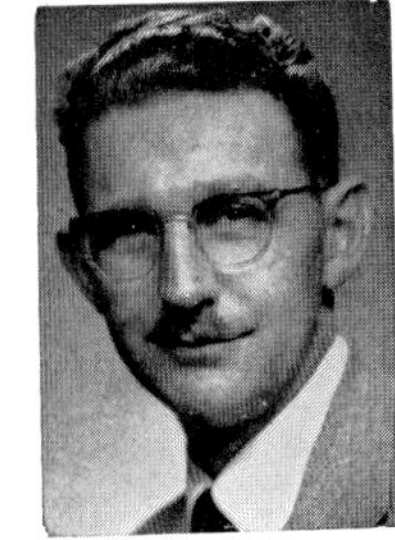

Warren Sinclair

FEDERAL RADIATION-OLOGY

The tremendous potentialities of radiation for both good and evil were also officially sanctioned by the creation of a special Subcommittee on Radiation (of the Joint Committee on Atomic Energy, 86th US Congress, 1st session). It took 966 pages to print the gist of its hearings, held on June 22-26, 1959.

And then, there is the Federal Radiation Council (FRC). It was established in 1959, by executive order, and later by statute, to serve as a co-ordinating body, and to advise the President with respect to radiation matters, directly or indirectly affecting health (including guidance for all federal agencies in the formulation of radiation standards and in the establishment and execution of programs of co-operation with the various states in the Union). Currently, the FRC consists of the heads of five federal agencies most directly concerned, the AEC and the Departments of Health, Education, and Welfare, Defense, Labor, and Commerce. Its first Secretary was Donald Roger Chadwick, a Medical Officer in the USPHS.

On May 13, 1960, appeared the FRC Report No. 1 entitled *Background Material for the Development of Radiation Standards.* This report introduced a new unit, the Radioactivity Concentration Guide (RCG), defined as that concentration of radioactivity in the environment which results in organ doses equal to those listed in the Radiation Protection Guide (RPG). Within this definition, the RCG can be established only for

*This information was courteously provided by D. D. Schottelius, a biophysicist from the State University of Iowa, and by the RRS's secretary-treasurer, E. L. Powers, a radiozöologist from the Argonne National Laboratory.

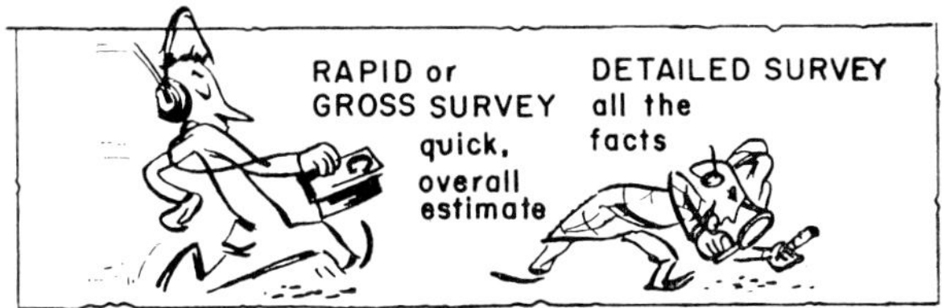

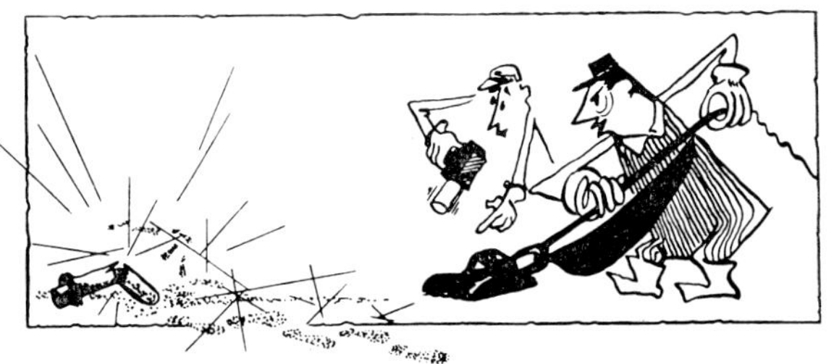

the circumstances under which use of its corresponding RPG is appropriate.

In August, 1959, the President directed the Secretary of Health, Education and Welfare to intensify activities in the field of radiation. The Secretary delegated that responsibility to the Division of Radiological Health of the PHS. The Division collects, collates, analyzes, and interprets data on environmental radiation levels, which are then published in the official *Radiological Health Data.*

It seems that the time is near when we shall have a Radiation-Protection-Dose-of-the-Day-Club!

X RAYS NUCLEARIZED

The Atomic Phase went "into effect" in 1942, but its influence on the design of x-ray equipment became significant only after 1950. Thence changes in built-in protection for both patient and operator became so pronounced that the State of New York decreed that x-ray equipment older than ten years (at the time the ordinance went into effect) was to be obsolete: even if the owner refused to junk it, that equipment could no longer be used on patients — lawfully, that is!

Until about 1950, transformers for diagnosis were usually rated at a maximum of 100 pkv, with from 25 to 500 ma. After 1950, the kilovoltage was raised to 115, then to 125, and (finally?) to 150 pkv.

High-kv has many advantages. For the same tube load, radiation intensity (behind the object) is about four times greater at 150 pkv than at 100 pkv. Consequently one may use a smaller focus, and get sharper detail, or a shorter exposure to offset motion. At higher kvp there is in addition comparatively lesser tissue absorption.

Above 100 pkv, one seldom needs 500 ma, except for high-speed exposures in children and/or in angiographic work. The usual combination is 125 pkv with 300 ma.

Throughout the 1950s the x-ray companies advertised increases in transformer ratings much like the horsepower race in postwar automobiles. Then the time came to attack the milliamperage. In 1957 Continental came out with the latest Panelmatic* which could go either to 1000 ma or to 125 kvp (but not to both at the same time) and provision for the energizing of any of three tubes. A Panelmatic model of 1960 was rated at 150 kvp and 300 ma; the maximum for that transformer (which has Selenium rectifiers) is 500 ma at about 100 pkv.

In 1961, Profexray's Jupiter J-950 was advertised at 900 ma and 150 kvp. These are maximum gain figures, qualified as follows:

900 ma at 90 kvp — up to 1/30 second
900 ma at 70 kvp — up to 1/5 second
600 ma at 130 kvp — up to 1/30 second
600 ma at 70 kvp — up to 1 second
300 ma at 150 kvp — up to 1 second

The Professional Equipment Company was originally a distributor of physical therapy machines, located on Ohio Street in Chicago. In 1937, they decided to go into the manufacture of small x-ray equipment, and brought out a portable unit rated at 80 pkv and 20 ma. In 1938, they offered it also in a mobile version, and a

*Engeln's Triplex may have been the first outfit wherein a single name was given to a combination of table, generator, and control. It is still being done, but on a limited scale. The name of the combination is often that of the table to which a figure is added, indicating the milliamperage of the transformer, as in GE's Maxiscope 200. Panelmatic is named for its upright (wall-mounted) control stand.

Profexray Rx

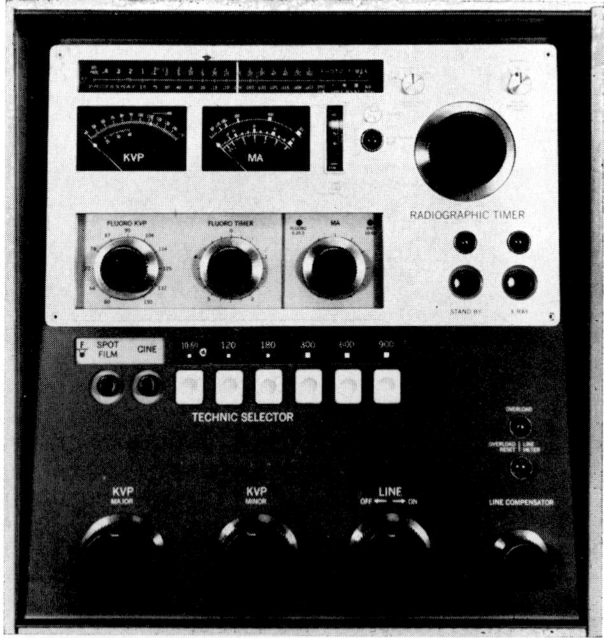

Courtesy: Profexray.

PROFEX-RAY'S J-950. Wall-mounted control stand, used in the latest Jupiter transformer series (up to 900 ma, up to 150 pkv, down to 1/360 sec.).

few years later they added a radimentary table to it. In 1946, they moved to 615 South Peoria Street, still in Chicago. They were then calling themselves Profex X-Ray. This is when they went into the 100 pkv – 100 ma units. In 1951 they expanded, and arranged their plant in Maywood, a suburb of Chicago. The firm had been founded by Leo M. Alexander (now retired), and Theodore H. Vatz (currently its president). Prior to the Jupiter series, Profexray's transformers were called "Rockets."

Keleket's Nova-Matic delivers 125 pkv at 500 ma, or 150 pkv at 300 ma. In the USA, early high kv units were put out by GE (in the Maxicon series, the KX-A gave 500 ma at 85 kvp, or 200 ma at 130 kvp) and by Picker (in the Pictronic series, the M-572 delivered 500 ma at 110 kvp, or 400 ma at 120 kvp, or 200 ma at 130 kvp).

Paul Hodges has insisted that the advantages of high-kv technique are of little consequence above 110 pkv. And since Hodges was once Mattern's technical adviser, Mattern manufactured the Medalist with 110 pkv at 300 ma (using a special tube made by Eureka); they also have the Master which goes to 125 pkv or 500 ma. Incidentally, the Mattern has become the Mattern X-Ray Division of Land-Air, Inc., an electronics firm

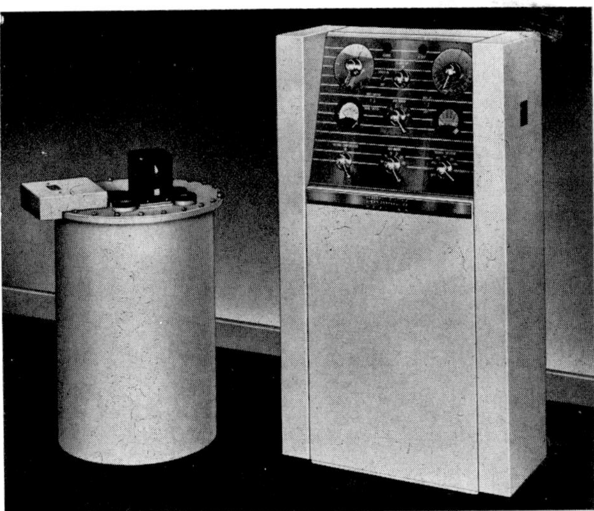

Courtesy: General Electric.

GE's KX-16. First gas-insulated transformer, a 100 ma full-wave rectified unit, introduced in 1950. Note the ¾-size control stand, with simple lines, accessible for servicing. These were superseded in 1963 by eye-level KXD 250, KXS 350, and KXR 600.

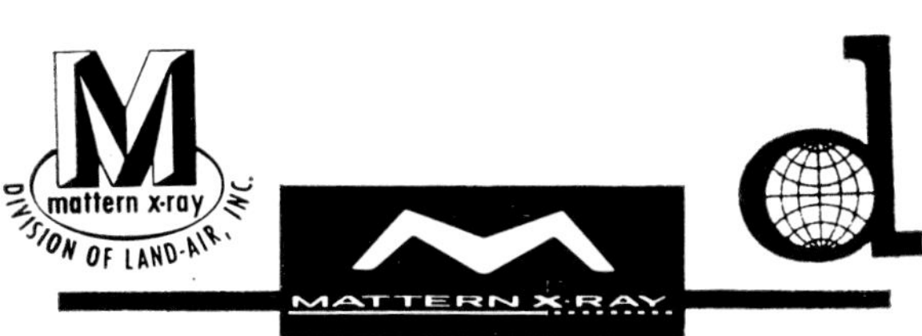

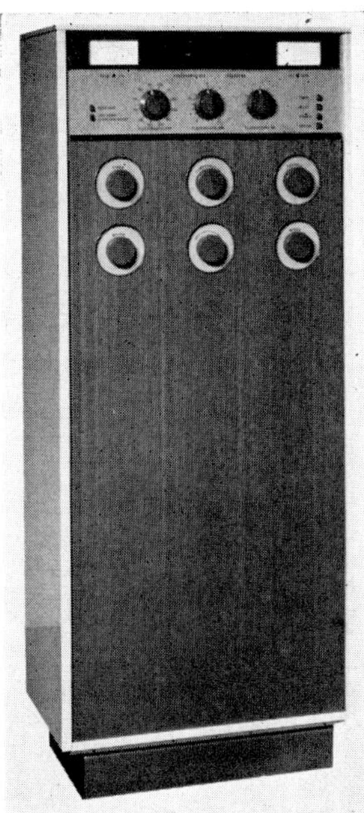

Courtesy: Keleket-Tracerlab.

KELEKET'S NOVA-MATIC. Classic wall-mounted control stand.

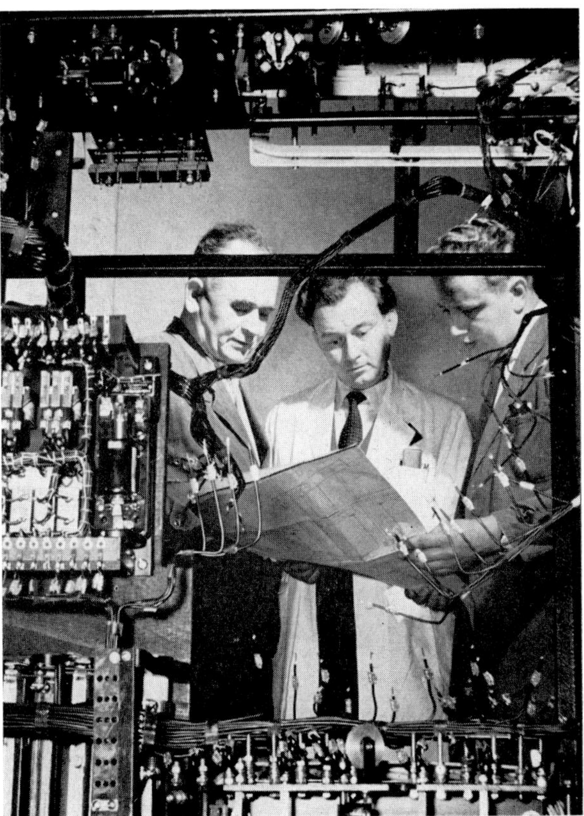

MODERN X-RAY MACHINERY can stun even the experts.

which is a subsidiary of California Eastern Aviation. They have therefore changed their seal to a more stylized pattern of the M. Lately another merger took place and they are now part of the Dynalectron Corporation. Then the Mattern operation was moved to a new x-ray plant built in Lake City (South Carolina). It is actually a new operation, because any such move is very traumatic — both GE and Keleket can testify to this effect.

The upright, wall-mounted, relatively slim control panel, which became popular at the end of the Golden Age of Radiology, is slowly being replaced by a shorter upright stand with slightly recessed (oblique) face, popularized by GE's Maxicon 100 ma and Picker's K-300 and K-500 generators. Printed circuitry is just coming into use. Even so, current equipment has more electronics in it than ever before. In the 1930s, it was still possible to "fix" certain things with a screwdriver, basic knowledge, a few wires and sufficient patience. This is hardly possible today except for changing fuses (of which there are also many more than in pre-war models).

GE's KX-19 had push-button Centraliner control merely meaning that there were seven buttons to preset the milliamperage. This has become a favored feature with many manufacturers. Some automation came into play. Picker has the "dial-the-part" anatomatic Century II and Westinghouse produces the Autoflex with milliampere-second timing. At one time or another, most manufacturers have offered certain automatic features. So far, complete automation has not become very popular in this country, if anywhere else. But cut-off circuits to prevent tube overload, and similarly useful electronic aids have caught on, and are now standard equipment.

A relatively recent feature (motivated by the radiation scare) is the limiting timer which cuts off the current after a total of five minutes of fluoroscopy. It must then be reset from the control, but Keleket has now an additional pedal-mounted switch for this purpose.

Both impulse and electronic timers are available. The 500 ma (and higher) generators come with a capability of 1/120 sec., the others go only to 1/60 or 1/30, but the Jupiter (Profexray) has 1/360 sec.

Since this section was written, GE placed on the market a whole series of taller (eye-level) control stands. Thereupon Mattern stretched the control stand of its latest offering, the Apollo, so named after the code name for the projected first American moon-flight. GE's latest transformer series goes up to 600 ma and 150 kvp, intended to compete with European 1000 ma triphasic transformers. The only triphasic x-ray machine ever marketed by an American firm was Picker's; that model is no longer in production, but Picker's European subsidiary builds triphasic transformers in Germany. In matters of x-ray technique, Europe has never been the Greece of American Rome (except for the fact that Röntgen was a German), but modern communications make cross-pollination an inherent feature of current technology. This is why GE's latest transformers have more automation, some are even fully automated. Solid state rectification has been used for years in electrical transformers, but after World War II it was adapted by European firms to replace the "expensive" kenotrons in x-ray transformers, and has since become very popular. Continental was the first American company to use solid state rectifiers throughout its com-

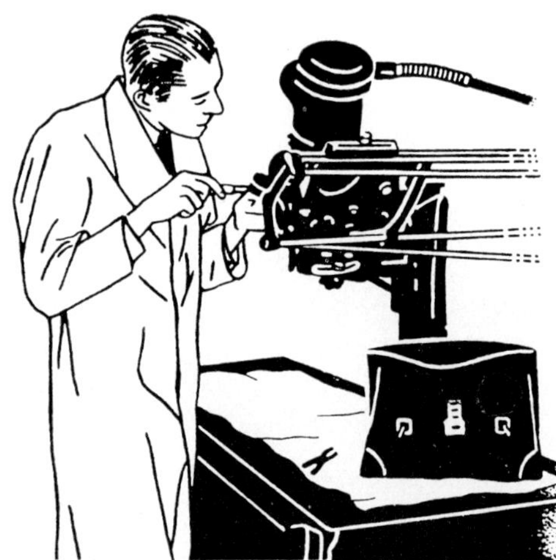

GE SERVICE. I have always preached that a machine — any machine — is only as good as the service available for that particular machine. Hence, availability of service is even more important than estimates of frequency of anticipated service calls. Incidentally, the serviceman usually comes prepared with little more than a pair of pliers and a screwdriver.

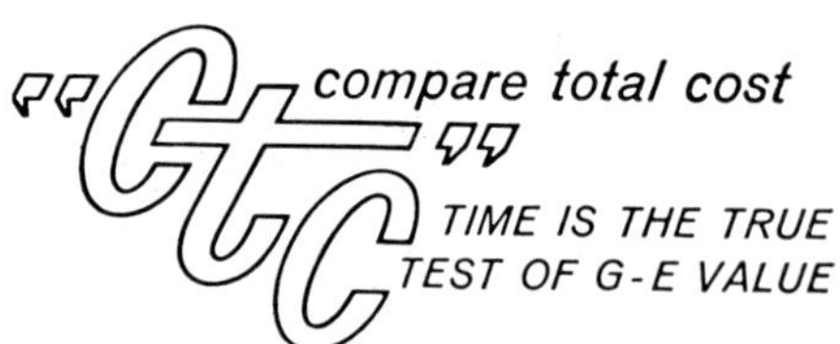

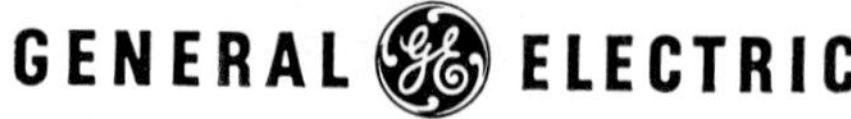

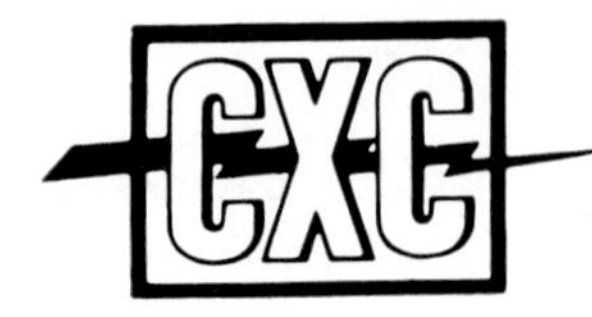

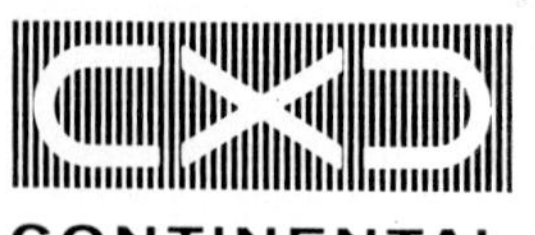

CONTINENTAL
1536 Clybourn Ave.
Chicago 10, Illinois

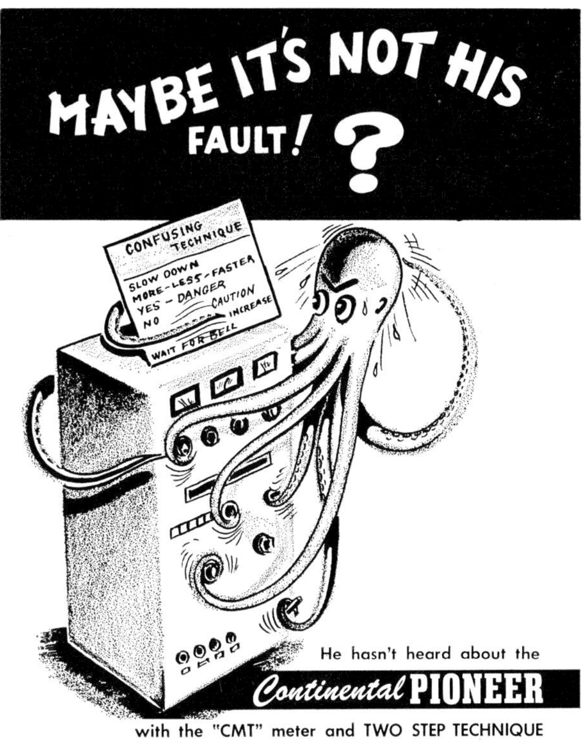

plete line of x-ray equipment — they adapted for this purpose their patented dual-bridge system; it was to replace their fully-rectified eight-valve transformer. When selenium rectifiers are being used, the kv drop depends on input kilovoltage, and may be as high as 10 percent at 150 kvp, which requires added compensatory circuits. In this respect silicon rectifiers are better (have much less kv drop), but they are more expensive. Keleket uses silicon rectifiers in some of its transformers, and GE employs solid state rectification in certain mobile units immersed in oil, where the desire to avoid excessive service justified the added initial cost. Some salesmen will extoll the virtues of a cheaper, stable, "so" dependable valve, but ultimately, solid state rectification will probably replace the kenotrons in most x-ray applications.

MOBILE UNITS

In 1954, Standard advertised the E-60, which had a capability of 60 ma at 89 pkv, as a mobile shockproof unit: this is no longer stressed today because nobody would dare to place on the market non-shock-proof equipment. In the meantime the kilovoltage race has had even more spectacular results in the "mobile" field than in conventional equipment. By 1956, most everybody had gone to 100 ma, like Mattern's Flexmobile which was rated to give 100 ma at 100 kvp full wave rectified, with rotating anode. The others had not yet reached 200 ma when Picker jumped in 1958 to the OR-300, not only fully rectified but also explosion-proof, and rated at 300 ma *or* 125 kvp. To date no cables are available for mobile units that would take more than 300 ma at 100 kvp.

Most manufacturers produce mobile units rated at 100 or 200 ma at 125 pkv, with 1/120 sec. timer, and with most other features of stationary generators. The mobile unit can then double as a second installation. When used in the operating room for cholangiography, it demands electrical factors almost as high as anywhere else in the body.

The most recent model in the group, GE's EP-300 has full automation; 12 kilovoltage settings (50 to 125 pkv), 6 milliamperage settings (3 to 300 ma), and 24 time settings (1/60 to 5 seconds) with automatic reset if the selected technique exceeds tube capacity. Moreover, x-ray value scale (XVS) calibration permits use of the simplified technique developed by Gerhart Schwarz* (*cf., Radiology* of November, 1959).

Such a "mobile automation" is in line with current advertising trends. Picker demands that "double-standard" radiography be discontinued ("portable" films were notoriously of poorer quality than "conventional" takes). Westinghouse in praising

*Gerhart is the son of the Austrian-born radiologist Gottwald Schwarz (who died in New York City in 1959).

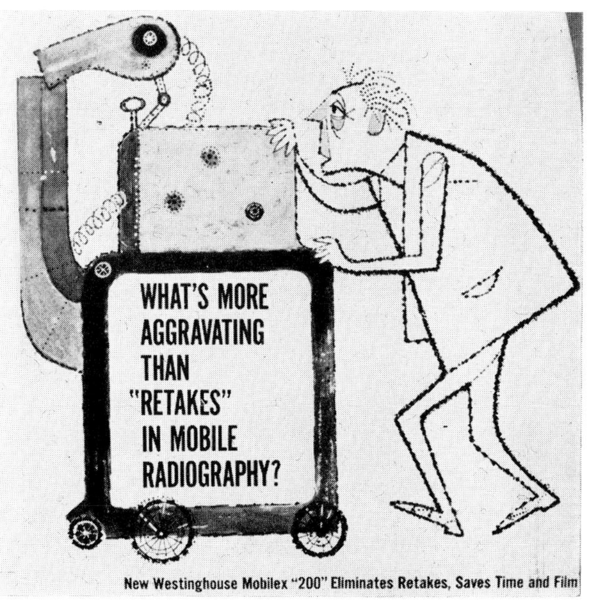

its own Mobilex, asks what could be worse than a re-take.

Truly portable units are no longer actively advertised in this country, perhaps because they are totally inadequate from a protection viewpoint. The only surviving next of kin in this class (10-30 ma at 60-75 pkv) is the dental unit. It consists of a grounded metallic casing, in which a small transformer with tube attached is submerged in oil. The whole thing is supported by a counter-balanced arm with several joints so as to make it easily adjustable to any height.

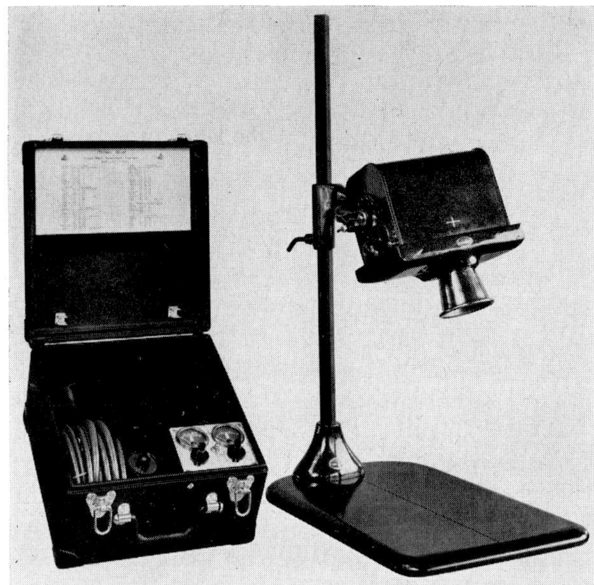

Courtesy: Picker.

PICKER PORTABLE. Pre-World War II model, at the time the only one in which a new tube could be installed without removing the oil.

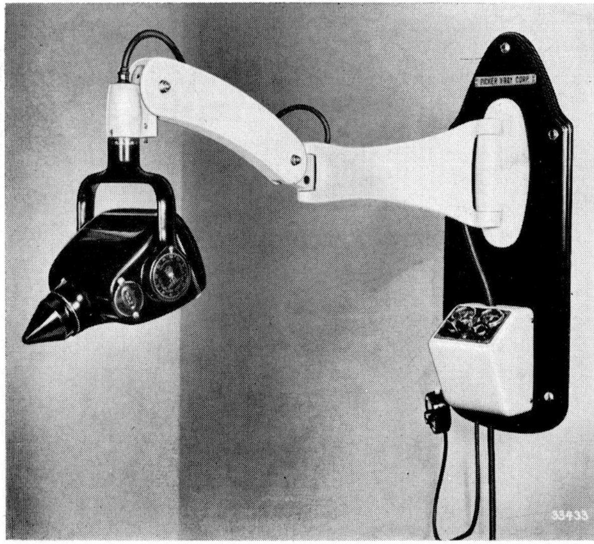

Courtesy: Picker.

PICKER DENTAL UNIT. Wall-mounted, flexible, and (relatively) inexpensive.

During the Golden Age fairly popular (among non-radiologists) was a mobile fluoroscope, which could also be used for radiography. It does not offer sufficient protection for either patient or operator, and is no longer "officially" built in this country, except perhaps on order, or for exportation. The one shown is the Continental Pacemaker 50 ma – 90 kvp.

MERTON MOSS

CONTINENTAL PACEMAKER 50-90
MOBILE RADIOGRAPHIC AND FLUOROSCOPIC UNIT
VERTICAL FLUOROSCOPIC POSITION
CATALOG NO. 749

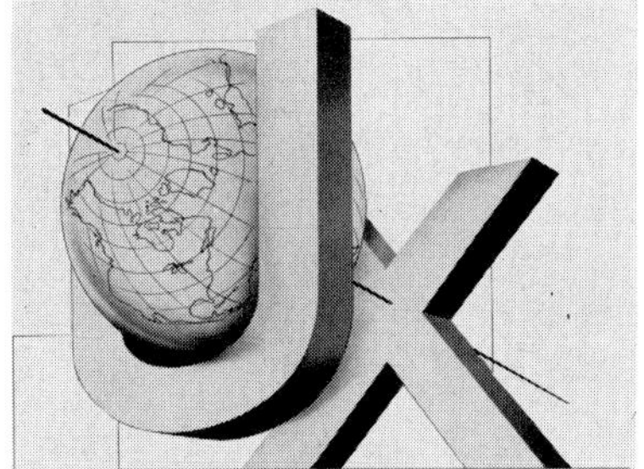

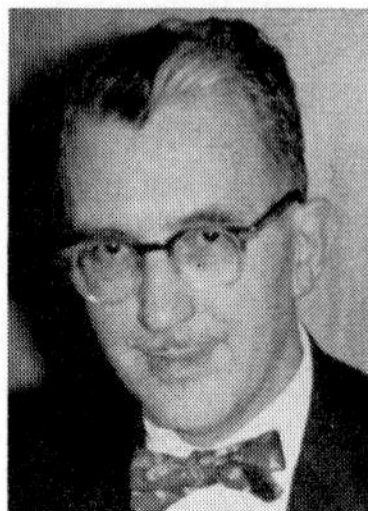

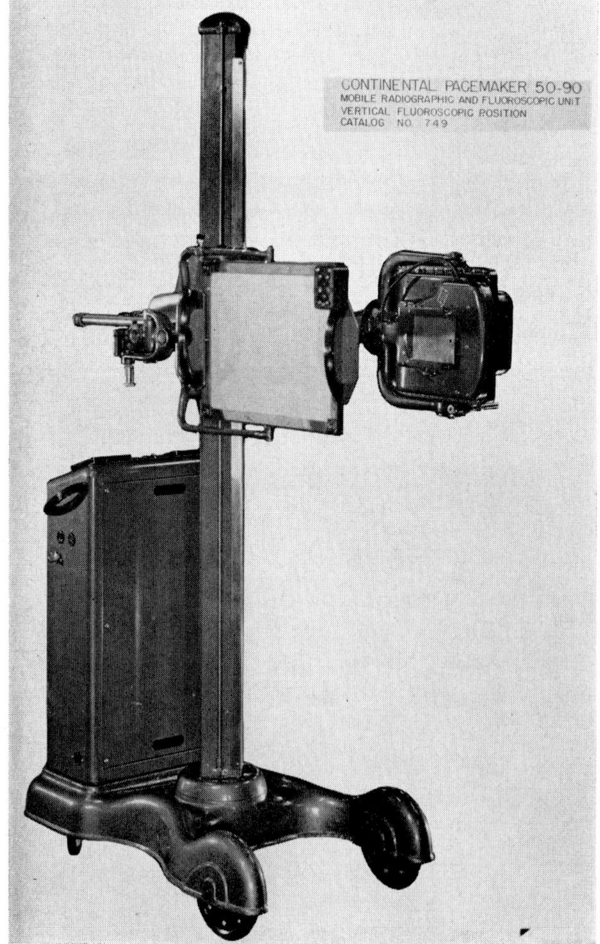

CONTINENTAL PACEMAKER

Merton Moss believes that the firm of which he is president, the Universal X-Ray Products, Inc. (Chicago). is one of the world's largest manufacturers of self-contained (monobloc) x-ray units. He uses for many of his models the suffix -master, for instance the Fieldmaster is a portable combination for the military, the Tilt-Scopemaster is a monobloc mounted on a hand-tilted table, the Mobilemaster is self-explanatory, and the largest in the series, the M. P. Master 200 is rated at 200 ma. Mert Moss, a soft-spoken (yet high-pressure) salesman-electrical engineer, has recently opened in Lincolnwood (a Chicago suburb) a Medical Merchandise Mart where several firms exhibit medical and dental (x-ray and other) equipment.

Another firm which specializes in monoblocs is the H. G. Fischer & Co., located since 1948 in its own plant in Franklin Park (a Chicago suburb). Just like Universal, they manufacture equipment for general medical, veterinary, osteopathic, and chiropractic practitioners (the R-B is built for the latter two groups).

The XRM (X-Ray Manufacturing Corporation of America) was organized in 1938 by Henry Abraham Hollmann (1881-1951) and Olav Olmholt (born in 1901), both of whom had been with Waite & Bartlett, then with Picker. They manufacture especially dental x-ray equipment, and are now a subsidiary of the S. S. White Dental Mfg. Co. XRM's latest offering is a mammograph.

Several other companies have become interested in making equipment for mammography, for instance Bucky International sells his own brand (made by Continental).

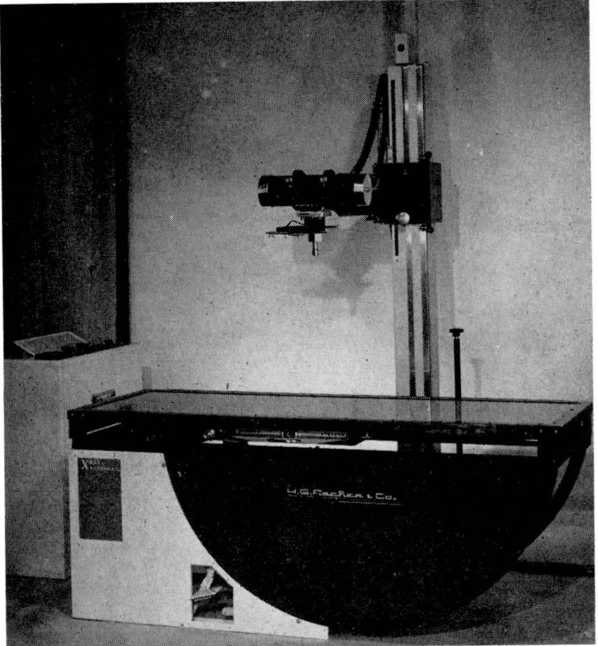

Courtesy: H. G. Fischer & Co.

FISCHER 35500G. Hand-tilted two-position radiographic table, with counterweighted Bucky, comes in two-tone finish.

H.G. FISCHER & CO.
FRANKLIN PARK, ILLINOIS

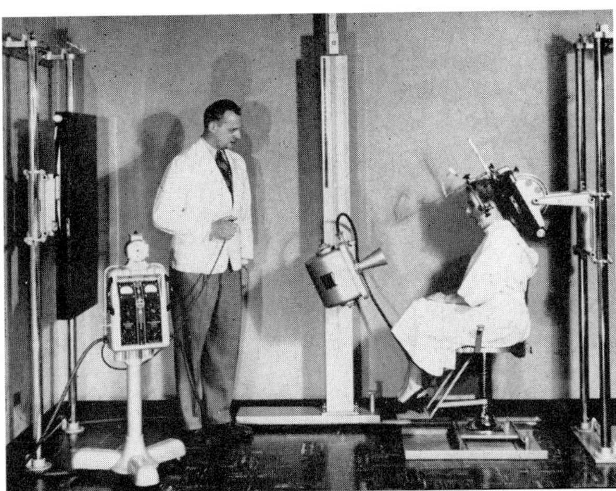

Courtesy: H. G. Fischer & Co.

FISCHER MODEL R-B. The "perfect alignment" unit with slotted wall-frame mounting board, floor-ceiling tubestand, turntable chair, and tilted Bucky (the 36″ Bucky, mounted on the wallstand behind the operator, can be attached to the tilting mechanism). Patient is held in position for open-mouth view of atlas-axis with the help of the Fischer-Thompson head clamp.

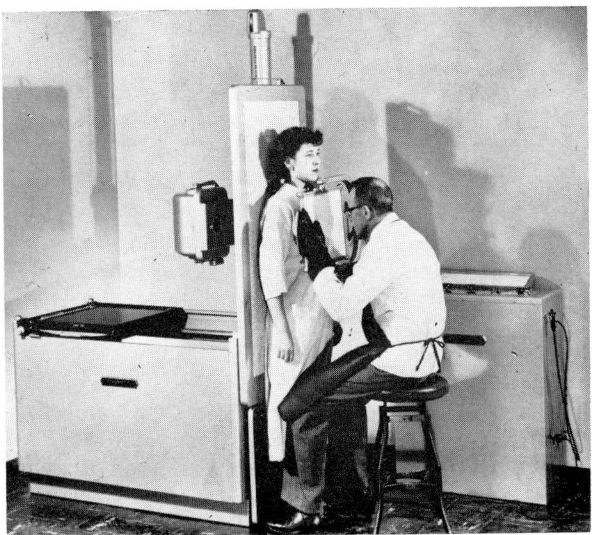

Courtesy: H. G. Fischer & Co.

FISCHER SPACESAVER. Pad and stirrups are available for the other end of the table. After such a close screening, the operator may feel the need for a bimanual pelvic examination.

But there is a new, almost revolutionary development which may change not only the portable and mobile categories, but in the long run also the stationary equipment. This development is the Fexitron.

At the Linnfield Research Institute in McMinnville (Oregon), experimental high dose rate tubes (field emission type — like Westinghouse's Micronex) were used for the investigation of high intensity radiation of biologic systems. Upon request, they built for the Army Medical Corps a prototype Model 880, which has

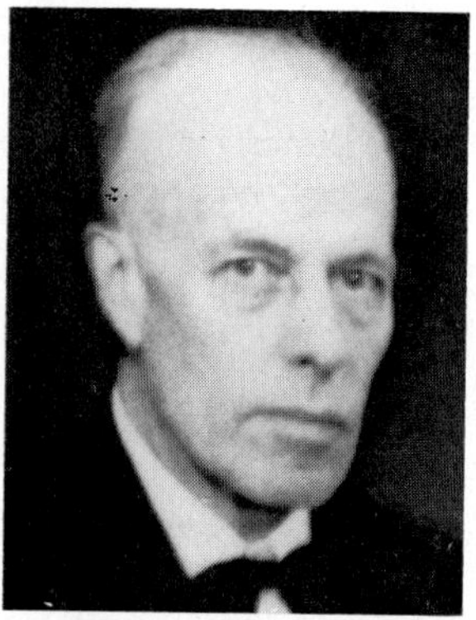

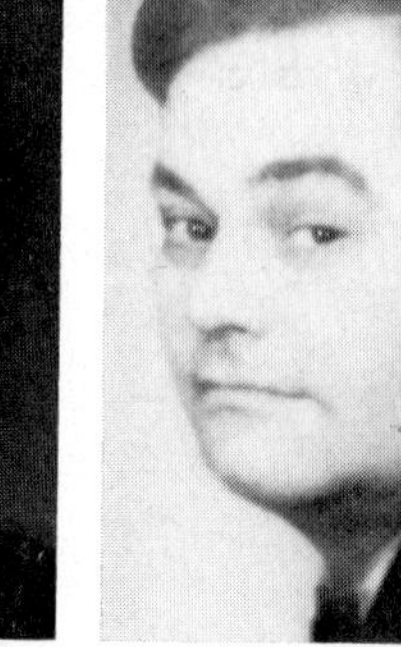

HENRY HOLLMANN OLAF OLMHOLT

These portraits and other data were graciously contributed by Henry Hollmann, Jr., who is now XRM's general manager.

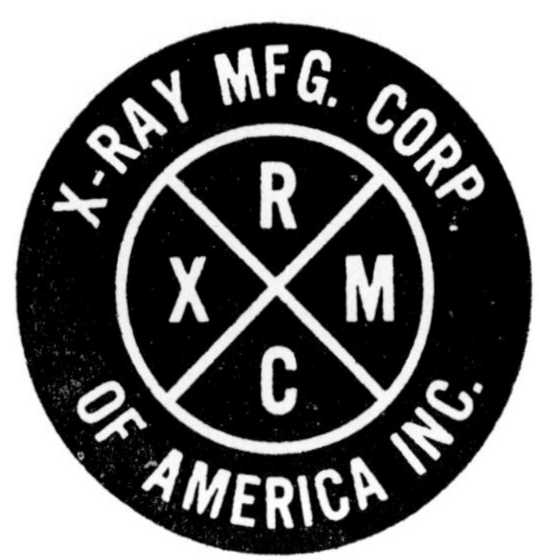

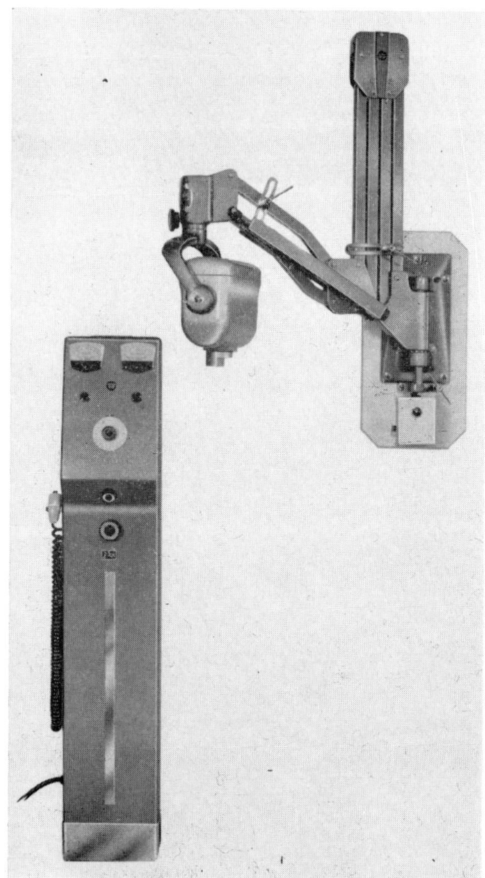

XRM's MAMMOGRAPH

a pulsed power source and a tube that does not require cooling equipment. The machinery is therefore miniaturized in a manner similar to a visual electronic flash. At increased tube current (2500 ma) with anode voltage continually variable from 70 to 120 pkv, the exposure time is 1/1000 sec., which eliminates motion blur. The unit uses a battery source, electrical storage capacitors and electronic switching. It can also be operated on standard 110 volts A. C., without special wiring. So far, the Field Emission Corporation has manufactured only a few units for the Army. Chest films exposed six feet with the Fexitron are quite satisfactory. In the near future they will offer the machine also for civilian use. It is of suit-case size — *and most important of all, total weight is below ninety lbs.*

Since this was written, there was placed on the market the Fexitron 845, a 40-pound rectangular instrument with removable tubehead, and x-ray source size reduced to 1.5 mm diameter. The same comes also in moble units. Details on its T-F emission x-ray tube were published by W. P. Dyke *et al.* in *Radiology* of February, 1961.

BRACKE-SEIB

A light-weight portable x-ray unit is being built for the US Army by Bracke-Seib in New Rochelle (New York).

Bracke-Seib started out in 1948 as the Eastern representatives for the Geo. W. Borg Company of Delavan

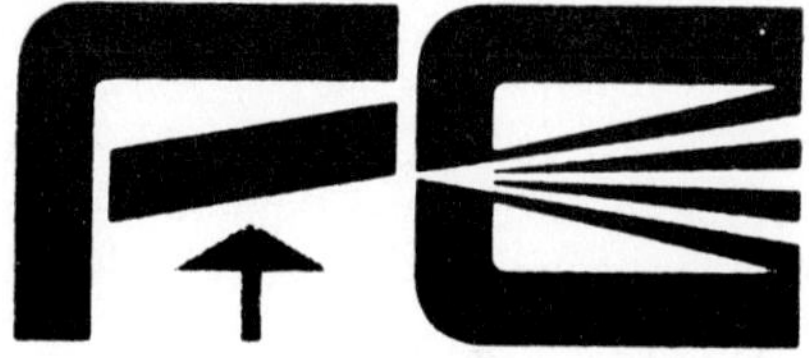

Field Emission Corporation

(Wisconsin). When Borg went out of business, Bracke-Seib – owned by Edward H. Bracke – decided to build custom-designed x-ray equipment and accessories.

The portable unit weighs sixty-two lbs., is operated from a 400 cycle battery, and 800 one-second exposures can be made before the battery must be recharged.

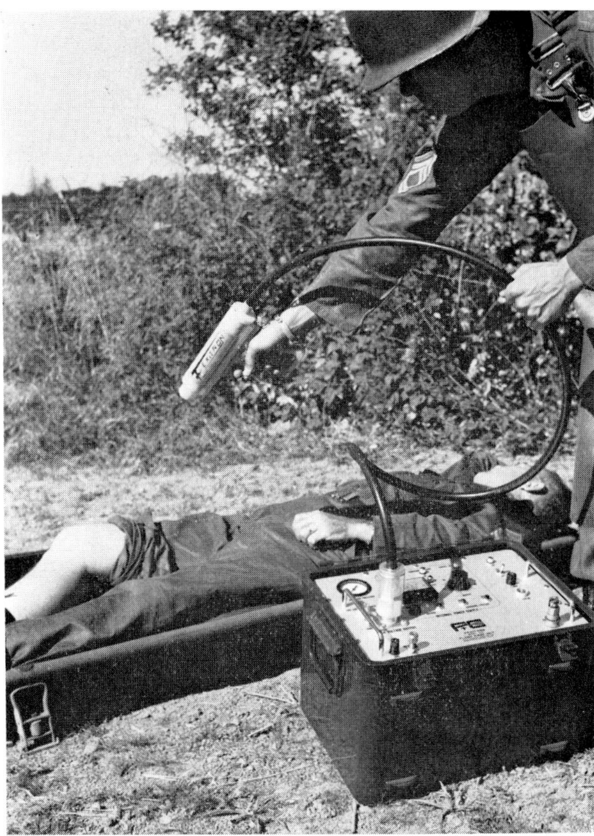

Courtesy: Field Emission Corporation.

FEXITRON 880. Field model, suitcase size, five pound tubehead, eighty pound total weight, battery or 110 volt AC power supply, 2500 ma, 70-120 kvp, one millisecond exposure; this is the prototype developed for the U. S. Army. Units for civil use are under development, the main stumbling block is a finer focus tube.

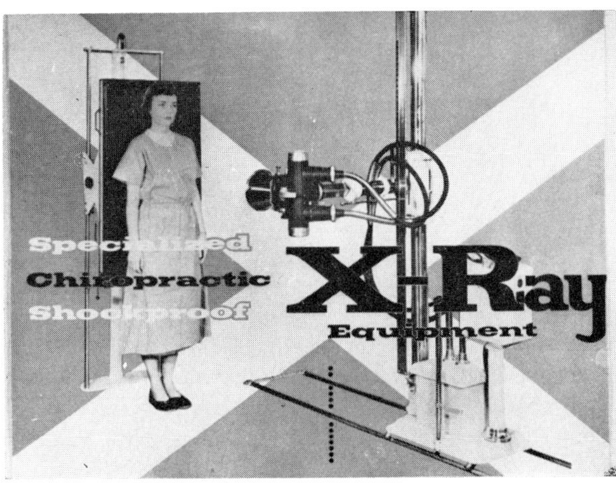

Among accessories manufactured by Bracke-Seib is the Wide Angle Cassette Holder – developed by Leon John Corbin, a radiologist at the VA Hospital in the Bronx.

TABLES AND TUBE MOUNTS

The (now hidden) pulley mounted on top of a heavy pipe with the other end of the pipe "rolling" back and forth along a floor rail, is still available as standard equipment. In most cases the Bi-Rail Tubestand, a rail on the floor and a rail on the ceiling with a pipe in between, is preferable. In Europe (especially in Germany), the counterbalanced ceiling mount had been employed for a long time. During the Atomic Phase, it also became popular in this country but usually in telescopic version. The telescopic suspension method is favored in the industry for moving very heavy parts (even betatrons). The ceiling mount frees access to the

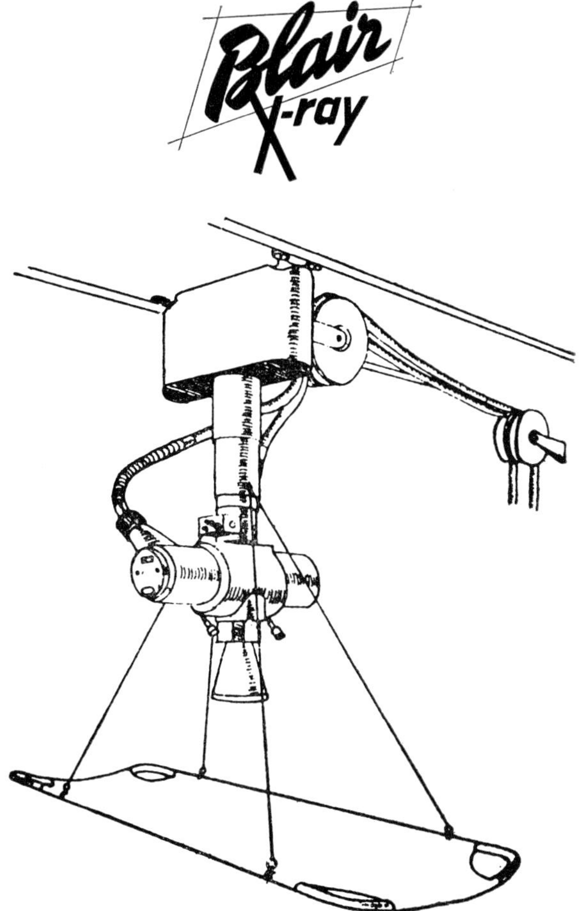

BLAIR'S CEILING TUBESTAND. The only one ever built with a litter lift.

table from all sides, and thus facilitates positioning. When (electrically) motorized, ceiling mounted tubes are quite easy to move.

Neither GE nor Picker use special names: they call them simply ceiling tube mount(s). So did Blair

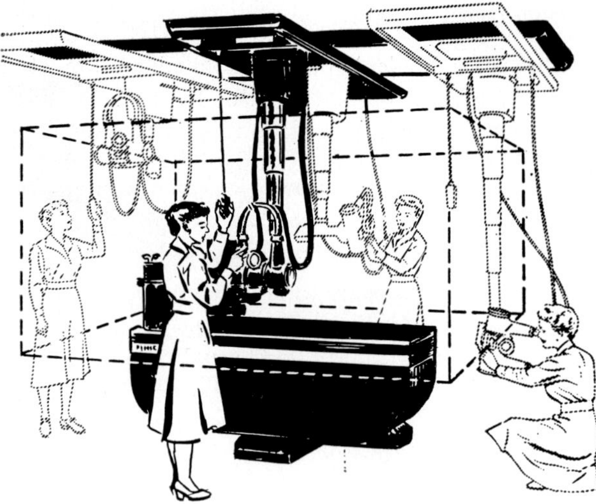

CEILING SUSPENSION. The advantages of the ceiling tube mount are demonstrated in this Picker advertisement.

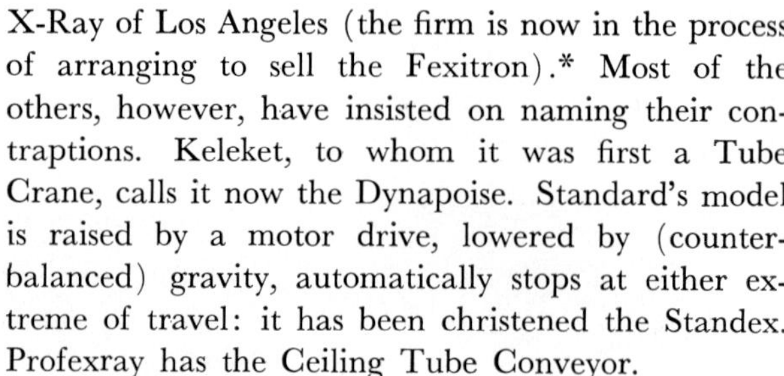

X-Ray of Los Angeles (the firm is now in the process of arranging to sell the Fexitron).* Most of the others, however, have insisted on naming their contraptions. Keleket, to whom it was first a Tube Crane, calls it now the Dynapoise. Standard's model is raised by a motor drive, lowered by (counterbalanced) gravity, automatically stops at either extreme of travel: it has been christened the Standex. Profexray has the Ceiling Tube Conveyor.

*Two brothers — Hugh H. Blair (president) and George R. Blair (secretary) — formed the firm which represented Philco Industrial Television in Los Angeles, and was recently selling Japanese x-ray equipment.

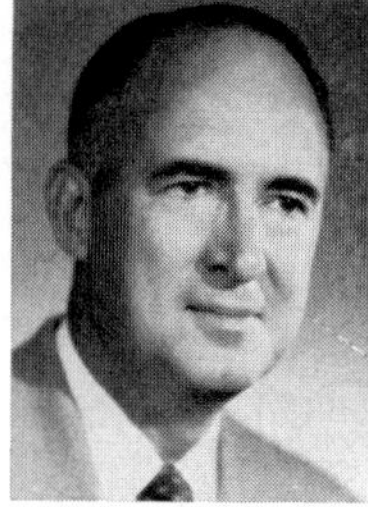

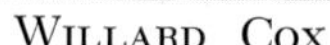

WILLARD COX

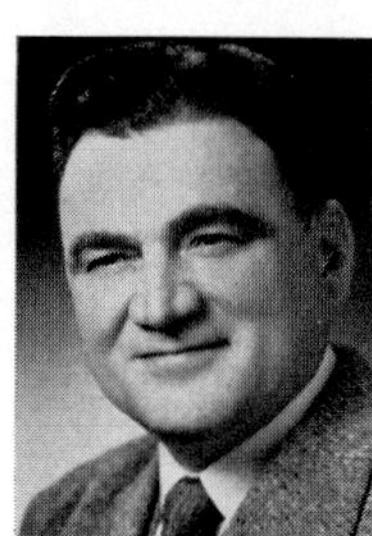

ART KIZAUR

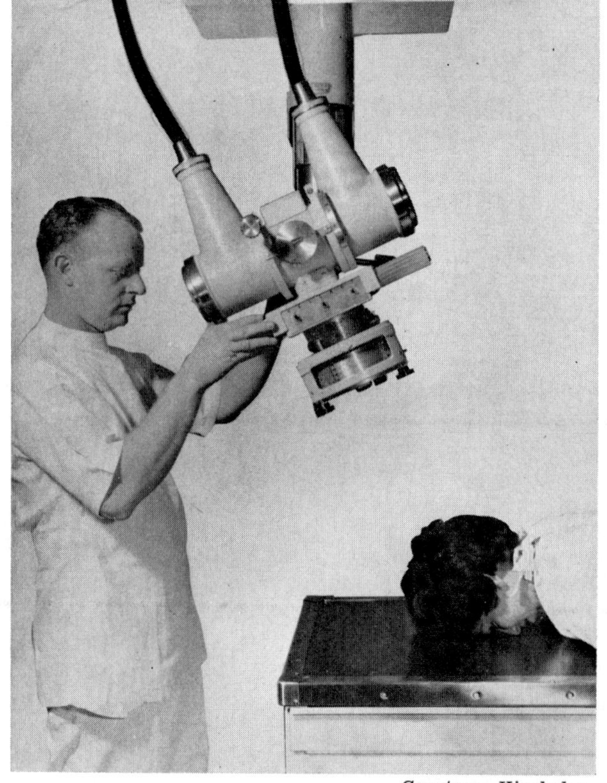

Courtesy: Kincheloe.

KELEKET'S DYNAPOISE. This was first called a Tube Crane, but Dynapoise (a telescopic model) is more euphonious.

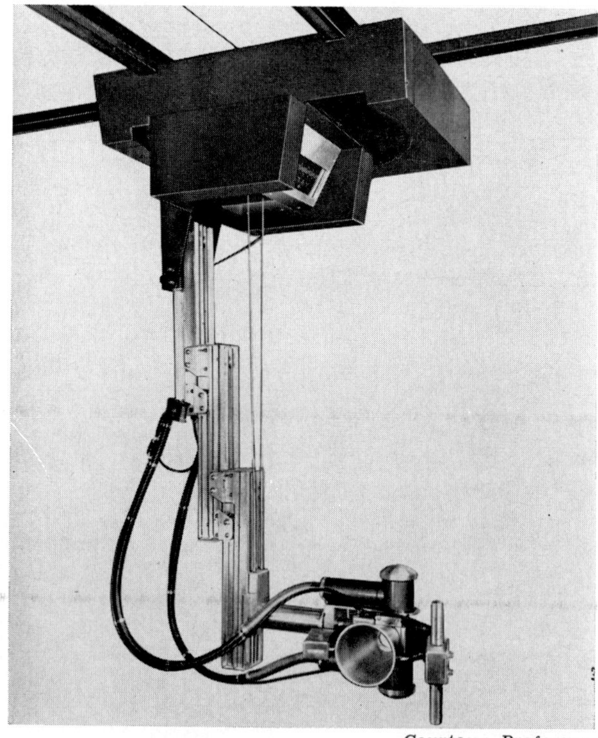

Courtesy: Profexray.

PROFEXRAY'S CEILING TUBE CONVEYOR. First model of hand-operated ceiling suspension; this is being sold in many foreign countries, including Japan, Australia, and Great Britain.

All the companies make a "lighter" table for General Practitioners, with a 50-100 ma, 100 pkv transformer, the latter sometimes encased with the tube in an under-the-table location for fluoroscopy. It can (usually) be raised for over-the-table radiography. These models are advertised in non-radiological journals. Any unit can be adapted for chiropractic necessities, which means simply adding a stand for their king-size cassettes. The one herein shown was manufactured by Mattern before its merger with Land-Air. The model may no longer be in production.

In the Golden Age, a table could be moved 90° from the vertical to the horizontal, and then some 15° into head-down Trendelenburg. In 1950 Keleket increased these 15° to 45° and called the respective table Super Tilt. GE put 30° on its Maxiscope but

GE's IMPERIAL was developed by GEXCO's former chief-engineer, the late Art Kizaur, and by Willard Cox (who left GE and is now a Standard dealer in Los Angeles). Their aim was to free the area around and underneath the table; to make the spotfilmer more readily accessible, and provide transverse movement of table top; to avoid suspending the fluoroscopic staging from underneath the table; and to raise the center of rotation above table top. All this was achieved by incorporating a ringstand in the table's supporting structure. At first only 60° of rotation had been planned, but it cost no more to include the full 360° orbital revolution.

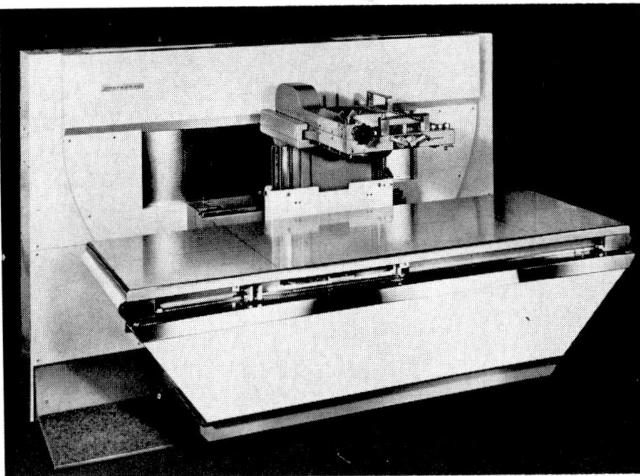

Courtesy: Profexray.

PROFEXRAY'S EMPEROR. Not only does it turn, it also rises.

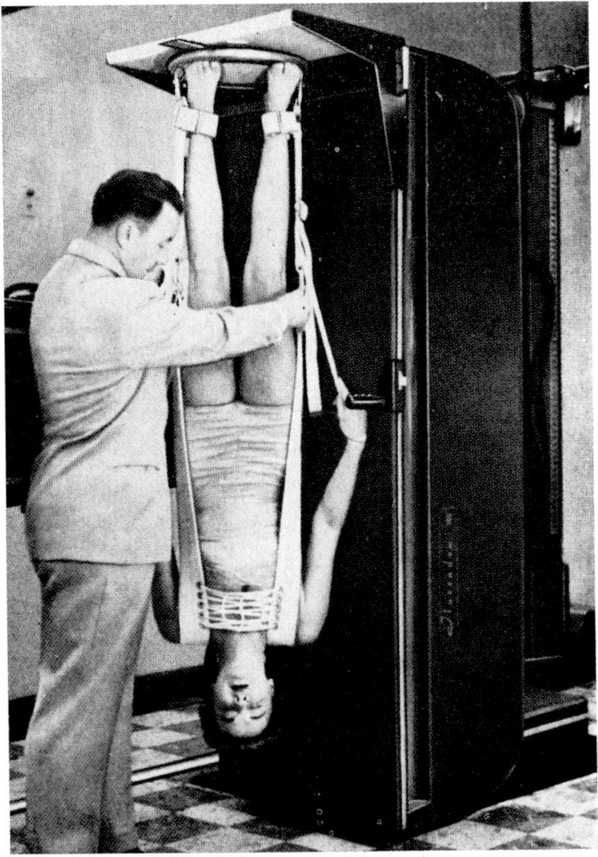

WESTINGHOUSE'S FLUORADEX. The caption to this advertisement read: "The new Westinghouse Trendelenburg Accessories provide maximum security and comfort." I believe it; do you?

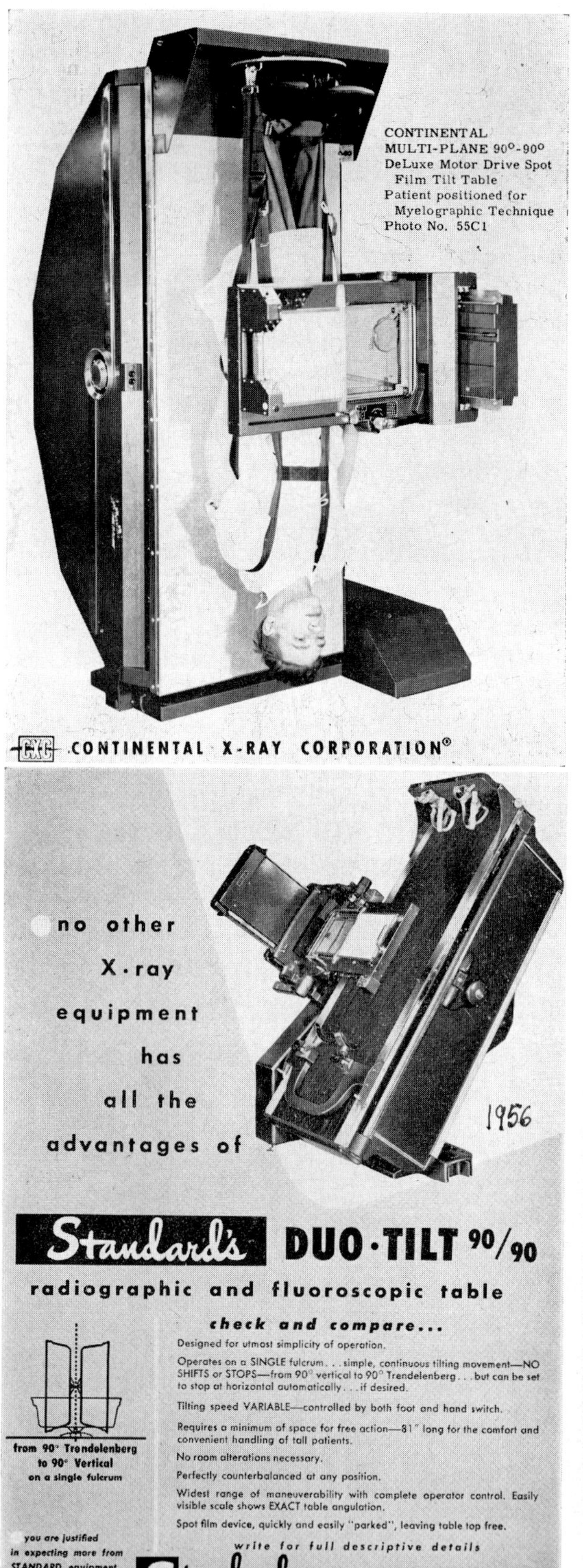

this was only a stopgap. In 1952 GE came out with the Imperial, based on a "new" concept whereby the table was fastened to a circular frame, being thus movable through 360°. Everything is centered, counterbalanced, and the patient does not have the sensation of being thrown off balance as he does when the center of rotation is (as usually) below the center of the table. In addition, the Imperial incorporated many luxury items such as longitudinal and lateral motion of the table top, slide-back parking of the spotfilm and all-around power-assist (for which GE had coined the euphemism Reflexomatic).

The success of the Imperial can be gauged from the fact that sooner or later all other manufacturers came out with similar tables. Profexray gave it adjustable height and called it the Emperor. Mattern named their version the Sovereign, and published a picture of a lady hanging by her heels just as GE had shown on the Imperial. Thereupon Westinghouse suspended its lady from heels tried to a Fluoradex 180, only Continental used a made model on their Multi-Plane.

One can recognize the 180° tiltable table by the fact that its pivot is centered to permit completion of the 15° Trendelenburg to its ultimate 90°. This is

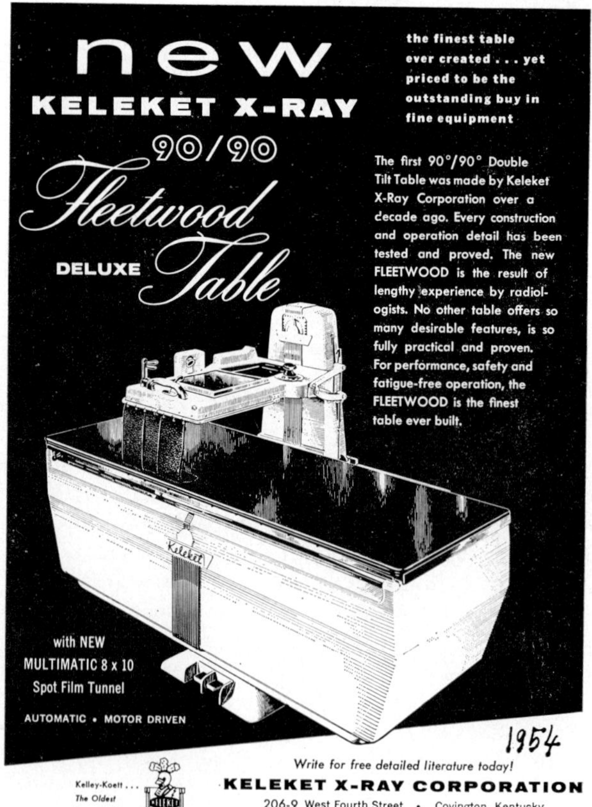

why Standard's model was called the Duo-Tilt 90/90, Keleket's Fleetwood 90/90, and Picker's Constellation 90/90. They all admit (in private) that there is only a limited need for such extremes: therefore all manufacturers continue to offer also the 90/15 models in improved versions (Standard's Ultima-105, GE's Monarch, Profexray's Emperor 15 with sliding table top). After all, with a shoulder support one can always place the patient the other way around and stand him on his head but how often is that desirable, let alone necessary?

Today, even the less expensive tables — for instance Picker's Centurion, Mattern's Medalist, GE's Regent and Aristocrat have been "cleaned up" and with a ceiling-suspended overhead tube, permit a cart to be wheeled close to the table for easy transfer of stretcher patients.

"Atomic" requirements have forced the enclosure of the tables. More recently on all tables metallic guards are interposed between the operator's lap and the under-the-table Bucky slit. The operator is supposed to wear an apron, and for added protection another lead rubber sheet is usually suspended from the screen. A recent table with all these protection refinements is Keleket's Nova-Matic: one of its unusual features is the ceiling counter-balanced screen carrier which comes in addition to the ceiling-suspended overhead tube, and to the various motorized motions of the table top.

A "new" feature by Westinghouse permits motorized angulation of the fluoroscopic tube (20° each way along the long axis of the table, totalling 40°), so as to allow "looking behind" certain anatomical structures. This feature has the beauteous name Panavision - so far it is available only on Westinghouse's most expensive table, the 180° Monterey. The latter has also motorized back-up as it stands up (into 90° vertical) which provides an additional 30″ of clear floor space.

There exists a futuristic development for encephalography. It is the Garcia-Oller Axioencephalographic Chair (it resembles what the Germans call a *Röhnrad*), which allows tilt along the tranverse axis into any of 360°. It is manufactured by the Stryker Orthopedic Frame Co. of Kalamazoo (Michigan), Stryker's also make a portable, radiolucent stretcher which can be placed directly on top of an x-ray table, to expose films without having to move injured patients onto the table.

When a permanent installation is desired in the operating room, there are surgical tables available with a slit for insertion of a cassette. This may be combined with a ceiling-mounted tube — of which there are explosion-proof versions approved by Underwriters Laboratories.

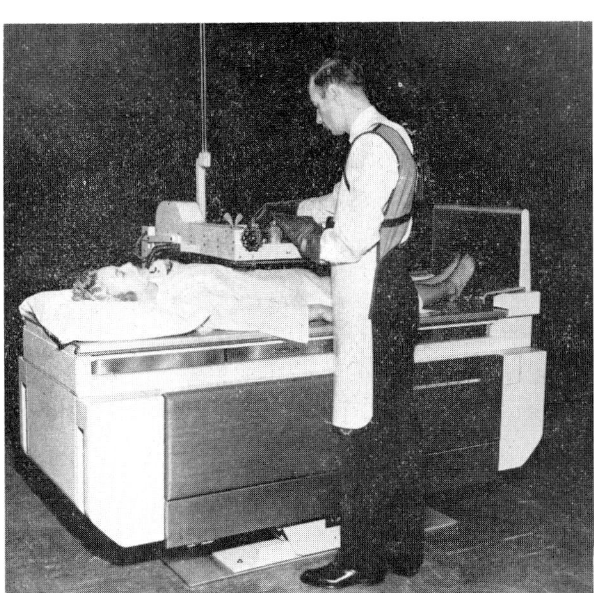

Courtesy: Keleket-Tracerlab.

KELEKET'S NOVA-MATIC 90/90. Note the side-guards for radiation protection, and the ceiling-suspended counterbalance; this table was being manufactured for Keleket by a Belgian firm, apparently with inadequate deliveries; since then Keleket has changed hands once more, is now a subsidiary of LFE (Laboratory for Electronics), and has become the American representative for the Italian firm Generay.

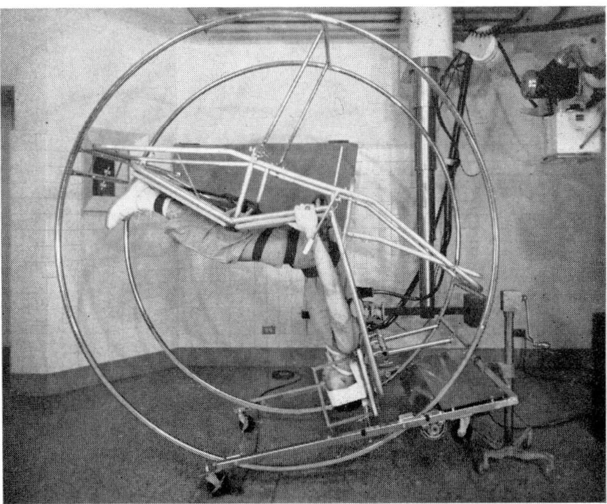

Courtesy: Stryker Orthopedic Frame Co.

STRYKER'S RADIO-CHAIR. García-Oller axio-encephalographic device.

SPECIAL TABLES

For over two decades, the Franklin X-Ray Company of Philadelphia is building specialized skull units. Upright as well as horizontal movable (Bucky-Potter) grid units were also available for a long time (such as Picker's wall-mounted Bucky Stand). Recently, these two features have been combined in a single unit, which in the Westinghouse edition is called the Chesapeake, while Continental calls its wall-mounted model the Verta-Vue. In both cases it is a multi-purpose unit adaptable for most radiographic procedures, including 72″ upright views of the chest, magnification technics, sinuses and skull studies, as well as lateral decubitus of the abdomen, and with a small attachment, even body section radiography.

For body section procedures there are available attachments (for use with most any table) such as the Laminographic auxiliary made by Picker, the Ordograph (with its exclusive hydraulic drive) manufactured by GE, or the mechanical model with motorized version made by Standard.

A table built especially for this procedure was the previously described Kieffer device, made by Keleket. Picker has constructed a special Tomograph, on the Grossmann principle used originally by Sanitas (Berlin). Neither transverse, nor helicoidal or other more complicated body section devices are manufactured in this country. And Liebel-Flarsheim has discontinued making the Kymograph.

Conversely spot-filming, which in this country was infrequently used during the Golden Age, is now very popular. Again, the semantic urge has created various denominations. GE refers to its models simply as 60-1, 60-2, and 60-3 (these are the semi- and automatic versions). Keleket has the Multimatic, Westinghouse a Nassau (with side loading), Picker has the Multifilmer, and the more elaborate and highly motorized Serialfilmer. Independent firms make the Scholz and Leishman spot film devices which can be installed on almost any table.

In the USA, Frank Scholz (of Boston) built the first commercially produced spotfilmer around 1930. In Los Angeles, Leroy Leishman (who had built a stereofluoroscope) formed in 1951 a company and began to produce automatized spotfilming devices. The firm was granted eleven basic design patents (no arms, no gears!), but financially the operation was not successful. In 1960 it changed from a partnership into a corporation, and in 1961 new management was brought in,

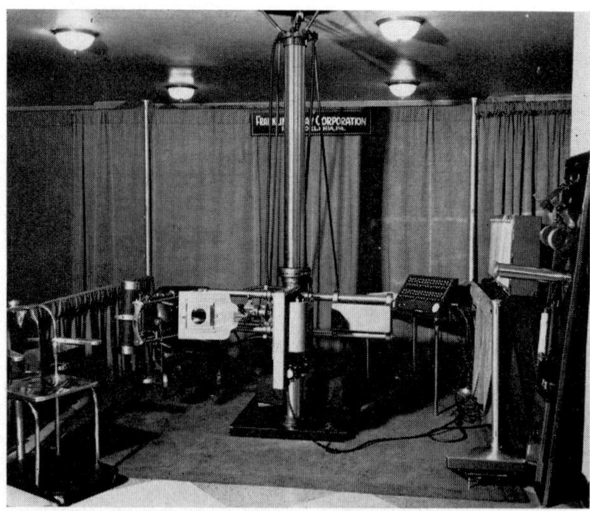

Courtesy: Charles W. Smith.

FRANKLIN HEAD UNIT. Exhibit at the ARRS meeting in Cincinnati (1949), where this unit was first shown. The Bucky head has been removed, and replaced with a Fairchild camera for angiography.

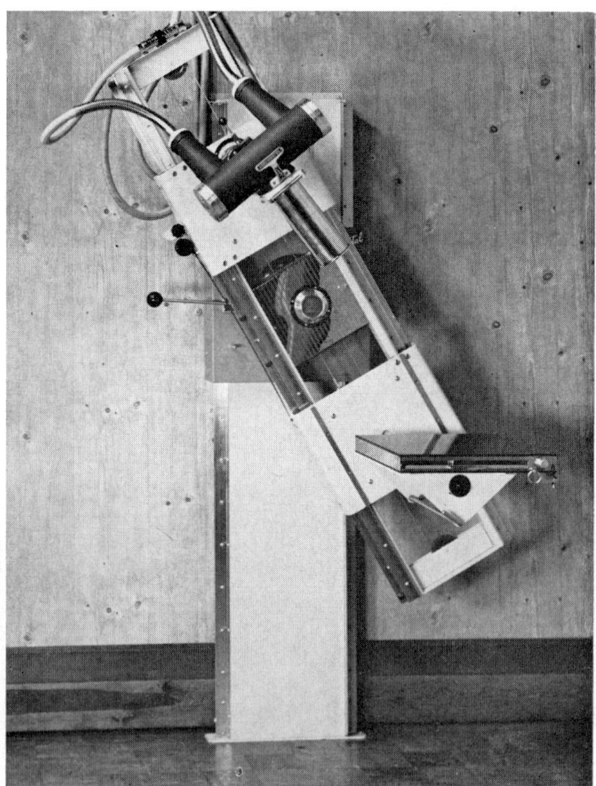

Courtesy: Continental X-ray Corporation.

CONTINENTAL'S VERTA-VUE. Bucky-tube positioning structure, useful for a variety of situations (skull and sinuses, vertical Bucky, horizontal Bucky, stretcher Bucky, magnification technics). A similar unit is being built by Westinghouse, but they were just out of glossy photographs of their model.

after which the Leishman company began making money. Its latest creation is the highly automatized Paragon, while the Fairmont is a manual, the Criterion a semi-automatic device. Both Scholz and Leishman refused to furnish portraits, and what I could find would not reproduce too well.

Most important in spot-filming is the availability of phototiming.

Phototiming is very useful in chest radiography – especially in photofluorography (in this country the latter is no longer used as a mass survey procedure because of its low yield, but it is still quite useful under selective situations, as in hospital admissions). Phototiming is even more desirable in spot-filming. The sensing device can be single or double, which varies from manufacturer to manufacturer. The electronic components are placed in the control stand (amid a few more fuses).

Following is a list of Westinghouse "firsts," compiled by their unofficial historian, Harry Jay DePriest. It is here reprinted between quotation marks, without subscribing to it nor rejecting any of the statements:

1. A tilting fluoroscopic table using shockproof tubes.
2. Constant potential therapy at 250 kvp.
3. Micronex super power radiographic unit for microsecond timing.
4. High voltage trigger tube.

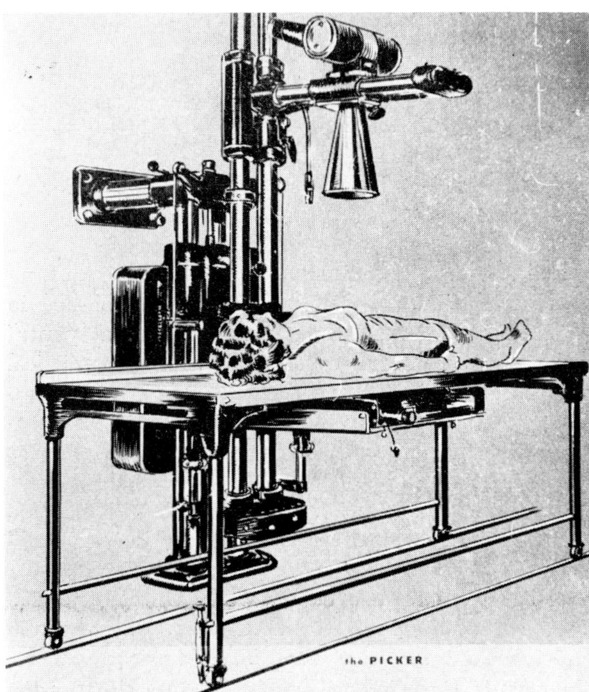

PICKER'S TOMOGRAPH. Built on the Grossmann principle.

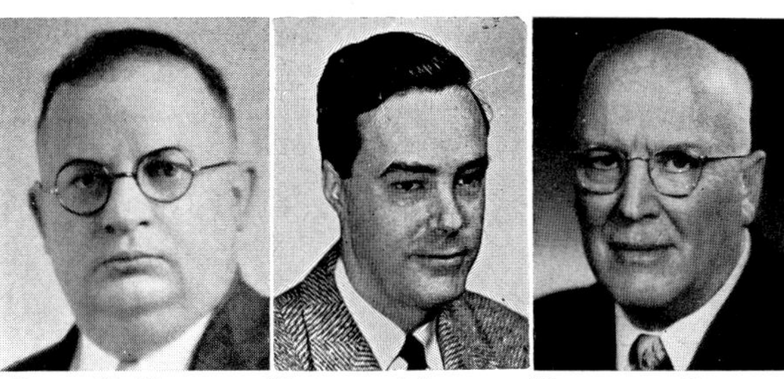

PAUL C. HODGES RUSSELL MORGAN HEINRICH FRANKE
(See also phototiming on page 145.)

5. Condenser discharge radiographic transformer.
6. First use of valve tube rectifiers.
7. First commercial phototimer using Morgan Hodges principle.
8. Fluorex image intensifier.
9. Cine with image intensification.
10. 180 degree tilt table.
11. Cyclex sequence programmer.
12. Motor-controlled fluoroscopic shutters.

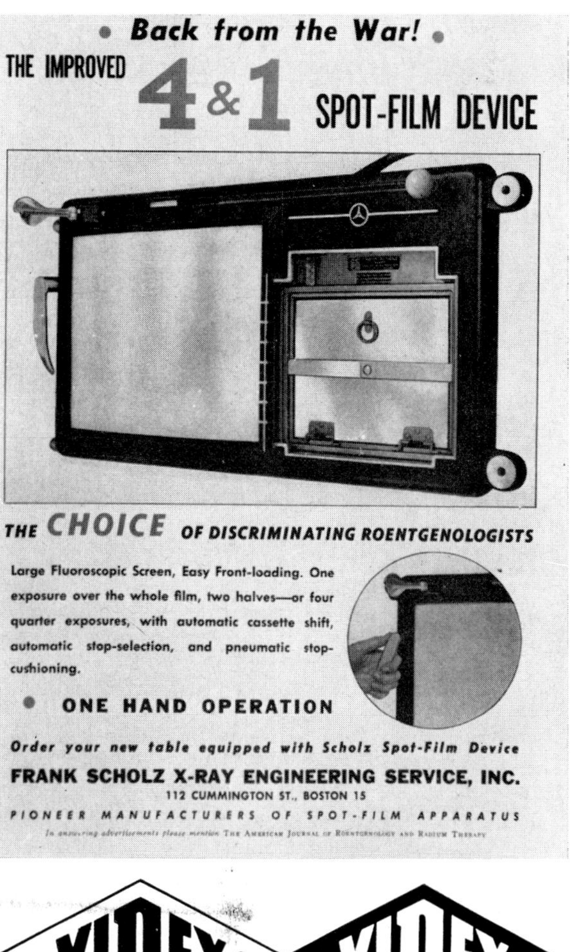

VIDEX® VIDEX®

13. Linear motion body-section device for use on all tilt or horizontal tables.
14. Operational radiation monitor for the first atomic submarine.
15. Tilt table on wheels.
16. Power assist for fluoroscopic carriages.
17. Electronic contactor permitting factor control for brightness stabilization.
18. Fluoroscope for first medical television program showing fluoroscopy.
19. First complete installation for tele-fluoroscopy (Greenbrier).
20. Monitoring equipment for first atomic power plant.
21. First completely-automatic tempering and replenishing system for darkrooms.
22. Transistorized thickness gauge for steel production.

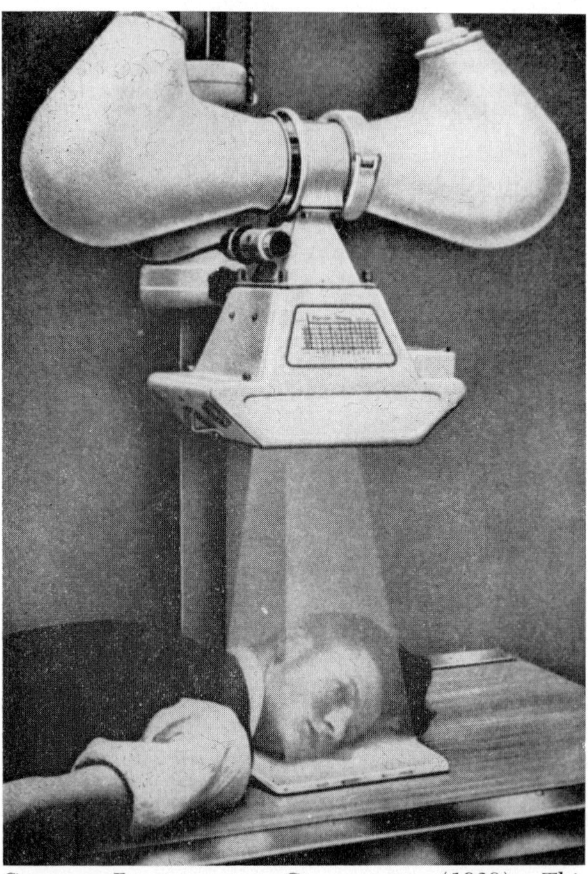

GERMAN RADIOGRAPHIC COLLIMATOR (1938). This Koch & Sterzel ad shows all the "refinements" currently hailed as the latest in collimator design. Similar adaptations to radiography of the old fluoroscopic shutter were then sold by most big German x-ray makers. In this country, production of such collimators began after World War II.

Also very useful in a spot-film device is a movable grid; in this country so far, only Picker has connected a vibrator to this grid to make it invisible on the film. Just such a "vibrant" spotfilm grid had been the subject of a 1923 patent by Waite (*cf.*, page 73).

In this connection the "atomic" desire for reducing radiation exposure has made the radiographic collimator a must. The first such collimator produced by the Howdon Videx Corporation of Mount Vernon (New York) was called an adjustable cone. The more expensive 1960 version is the Videx Fairfield 150, which has not only the slide rule for pre-calculating beam size, but also a light source to delineate the field covered. The latest model, just issued in 1963, is the 150 kvp Duocon-2, more compact, with semi-multiplane rolling diaphragms. The "lighter" Duocon-1 is for up to 125 kvp.

GE's version is called the Videx Palmer cone. The turret collimator is made by Dial-X Instruments. Picker uses the generic name radiographic collimator

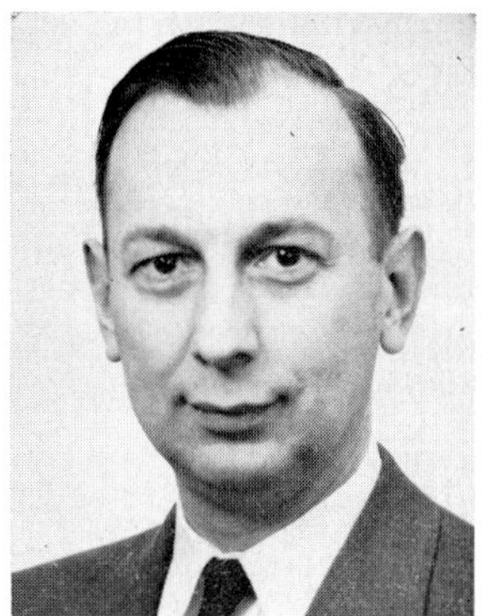

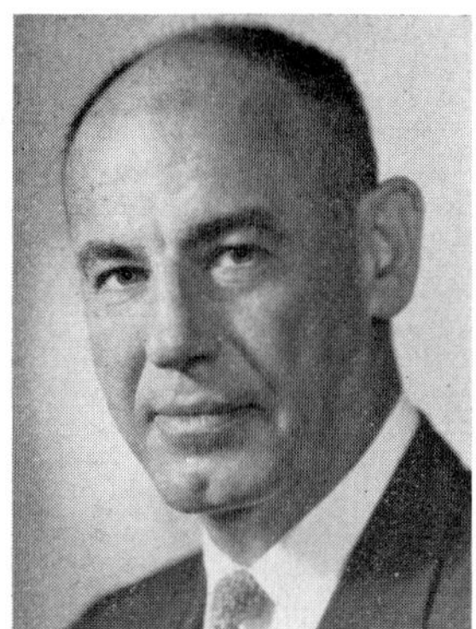

Courtesy: Westinghouse.

JOHN WESLEY COLTMAN. He built the first image intensifier tube in 1948 in the Westinghouse Research Laboratories in East Pittsburgh. It had been a project worked out by a team, and their pre-planned procedure was a case history presentation before the Industrial Research Institute in October, 1957 and published in *Research* in 1958. The only precursor was a "paper" patent (a theoretical description with no practical demonstration) issued to Irving Langmuir on November 3, 1937: we know today that it could not have provided any significant brightness gain. Coltman's achievement was the very first in the field. The first technical article on the second image intensifier (made by Philips in Holland) appeared in the *Philips Technical Review* in August, 1952 – and makes specific reference to Coltman's earlier work. On the viewer's right is RICHARD HALL CHAMBERLAIN, who was the first to use the then new 5280 image orthicon tube for direct television intensification of the fluoroscopic image.

as part of what they call the MDR (minimal dosage radiography), which stresses reduction in radiation by all methods available, from limiting the beam to processing the film.

IMAGE INTENSIFIERS

Whether by coincidence or otherwise, both the philosophic and the technical roots of image intensification were planted in Pennsylvania.

In the Carman Lecture of 1941, William Edward Chamberlain, who was then professor of radiology in Temple University in Philadelphia, discussed the need to brighten the fluoroscopic image. He de-

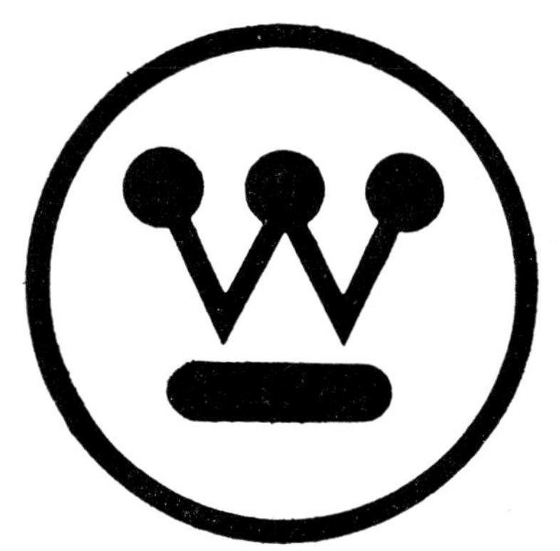

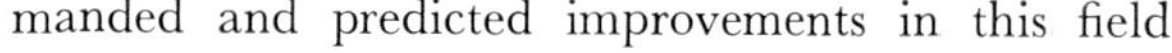

manded and predicted improvements in this field.

In the Carman Lecture of 1953, Richard Hall Chamberlain, (no kin to the previous one), who is now professor of radiology in the University of Pennsylvania, recounted the events which led to image intensification.

In *Radiology* of September, 1948 John Wesley Coltman, an electronics engineer from the Westinghouse Research Laboratories in East Pittsburgh, described a new vacuum tube. It contained a fluorescent (input) screen, in contact with a photo-electric surface (photo-cathode, input phosphorus): the quanta of light on the fluorescent screen were transformed into photoelectrons, (re-)emitted by the photocathode in an electron pattern similar to the original image. The potential across the tube (*i.e.*, between the two ends) accelerated these electrons, and focused them into a smaller (output) phosphorus. The end result was a gain in brightness over the initial image. The term amplifier tube is commonly used in electronics. Accordingly, Coltman named his method image amplification.

This vacuum tube became the heart of the Fluorex, which Westinghouse marketed for the first time in 1952. The earliest model had an input screen of 5″ diameter, rated at 200 times brightness gain. The im-

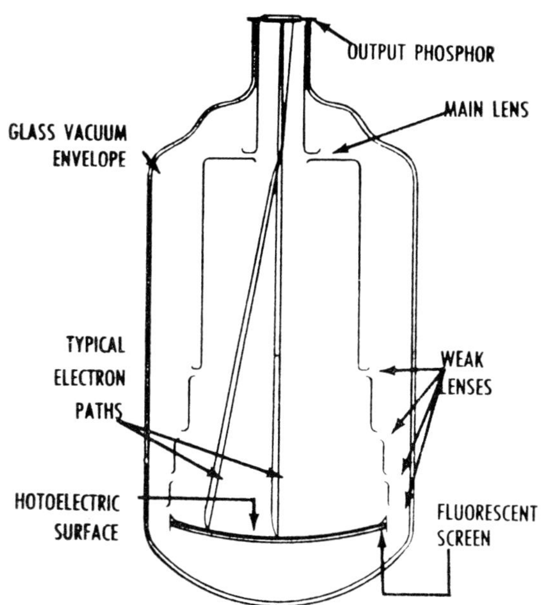

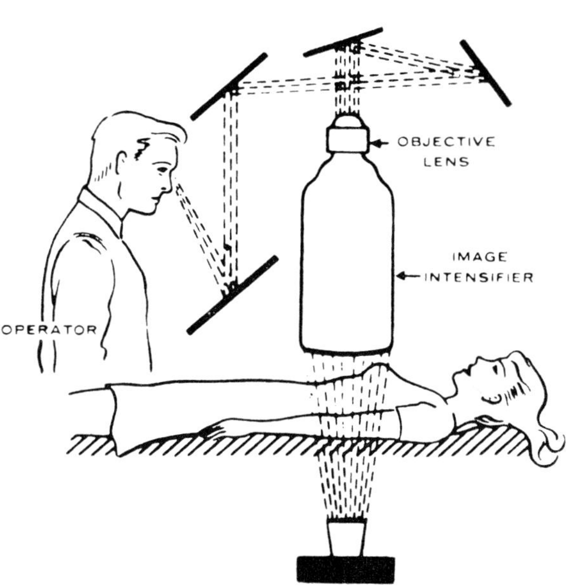

WESTINGHOUSE'S FLUOREX. Its first version had a brightness gain of about 200 times, but otherwise the radiologist was still looking toward the patient. The diagram at left shows the intensifier tube, the one at right is the optical (lens-mirrors) arrangement for magnifying the brighter but smaller image produced on the output phosphorus.

age on the output phosphorus was magnified by optical means and viewed through a mirror. Later models had a provision whereby the image could be split, and part of it was then recorded on a film strip in a movie camera.

In the winter of 1949, at the University of Pennsylvania, Dick Chamberlain and Sam Seal, working with engineers from the Radio Corporation of America (a kin to RCA-Victor), achieved the first successful television chain wherein the fluoroscopic image was picked up directly by the then newly developed 5,280 image Orthicon (television) tube.

This system permitted cinematographic recording, in addition to viewing by several monitors placed in distant locations. Television allows button-controlled contrast and theoretically a higher potential gain in brightness, up to 50,000 times, versus the maximum conceivable of 10,000 times for the electronic system. But with a television tube one is limited to a frame repetition rate of about 30 per second which places limitations on some of the functional studies. The number of images on the electronic system is limited only by fluorescent lag. Its disadvantage is the "limited" size of the input screen.

Amplification and intensification are synonymous in their wider meaning. In a restricted sense, though, to amplify implies to add something, and in this case nothing is "added" to the original fluoroscopic image (except for the sometimes inevitable electronic artefacts), there is only a change in brightness. Image intensification is a more appropriate term and it is the one currently accepted by the majority of users.

On seeing my historic exhibit at the 1963 ARRS meeting in Montreal, Russell Morgan remarked that in matters of screen intensification, the impact of Ed Chamberlain's Carman Lecture of 1941 cannot be overemphasized. Ed Chamberlain had referred to a 1937 patent of Irving Langmuir. Without that patent, Ed Chamberlain would not have raised the problem. In addition, Morgan mentioned an infrared image tube of World War II vintage as being another precursor of Coltman's first intensifier tube.

I wrote to Coltman, and this is what he answered: "Langmuir's was a "paper" patent in that no physical reduction to practice was ever attempted. In fact, it is now clear that his suggested arrangement could not have provided significant brightness gain. The IP25 infrared image tube, developed by RCA during the war

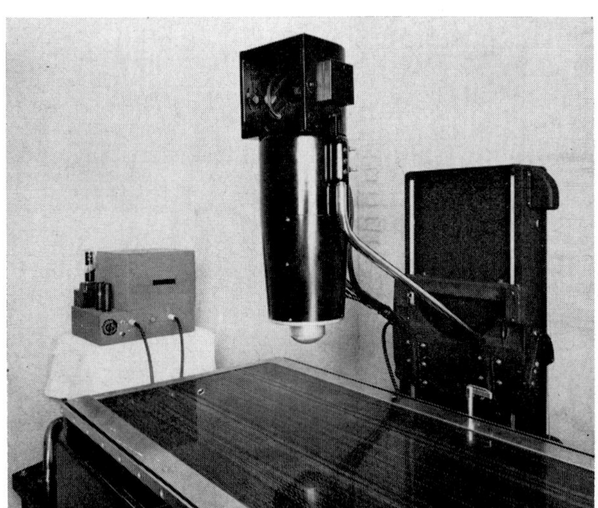

Courtesy: Westinghouse.

WESTINGHOUSE'S PRIMORDAL FLUOREX. This was the very first workable model. It was never produced commercially.

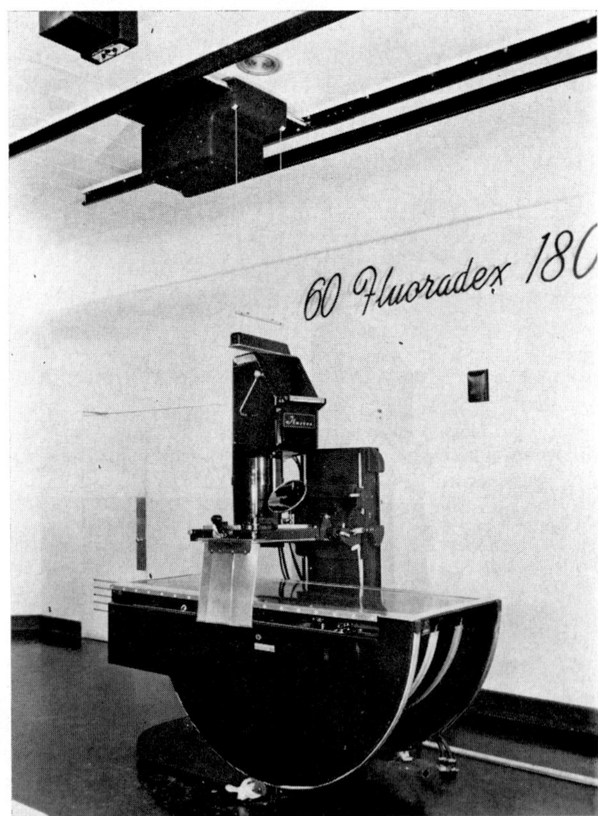

Courtesy: Westinghouse.

WESTINGHOUSE'S FIRST FLUOREX. First commercially available Fluorex image intensifier, mounted on the Duoflex table. Apparently, Philips brought out his commercial model a few months before Westinghouse's, but all electron-optical image intensifiers are based on, and their authors have referred to, Coltman's original publication in *Radiology* of 1948 as being the "pathfinding" item in this matter.

for use in the sniperscope and snooperscope, was described in the *RCA Review* of September, 1946. It influenced the design of the Fluorex, but there were between the IP25 and the Fluorex such differences in size, magnification, and especially the latter's high voltage, that design of the Fluorex was carried from first principles."

Russell Morgan informed me that in his laboratory at Johns Hopkins television equipment specifically designed for screen intensification was in use since early 1948. His system became the standard utilized in this country with orthicon intensification. The Bendix Corporation used Morgan's designs in the construction of television equipment which guided the first atomic submarine under the ice across the North Pole. And a medical variant was offered to the radiologic profession.

In 1955, the Friez Instrument Division of the Bendix Aviation Corporation (Baltimore) came out with the Lumicon, a complete television system. It was advertised both for diagnostic purposes and for monitoring of the patient's position during rotational radiation therapy. The Lumicon was overpriced, it did not sell, and its manufacture was soon discontinued.

In the beginning, the rest of the industry could utilize Westinghouse's Fluorex, or a similar tube made in Holland by Philips — while other manufacturers were feverishly at work to bring out their own versions. Improvements soon appeared, the size of the input screen went to 9″ and then to 11″, and the gain in brightness reached an advertised factor of 3000. It became fashionable to combine the electronic and the television methods into one system.

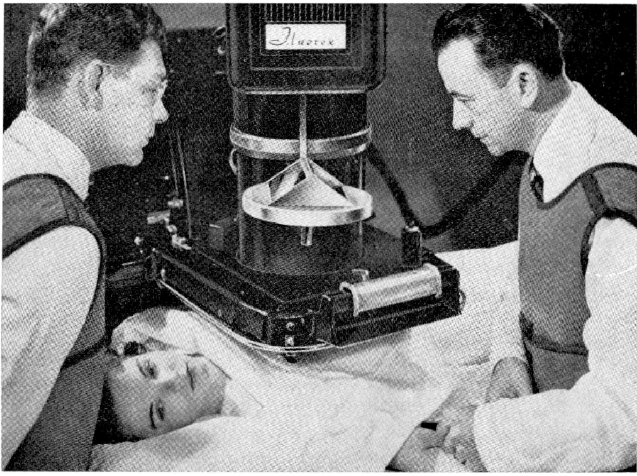

Intensified consultation. The need for prolonged accommodation being obviated by image intensification, one can easily demonstrate the findings to the referring clinician. The early models of Westinghouse's Fluorex had an optional prismatic mirror for simultaneous viewing by two observers.

As in Westinghouse's Televex,* the electronically intensified image is "split" optically, recorded on movie film, and at the same time fed into a television system, for further gain in brightness. This has the advantage of performing fluoroscopy with daylight, *i.e.*, central, retinal cone viewing, instead of the previous, darkroom, *i.e.*, peripheral, rod viewing. It permits monitoring in distant locations. And the television imagine can be recorded on magnetic tape which can be instantly reproduced.

The Ampex Professional Products of Red Wood City (California) brought out the VR-1000C console, which is their Videotape television recorder, adapted for radiographic purposes.

A relatively simple refinement, used by most manufacturers, is the so-called synchronization: the motor which turns the movie camera is placed in the same phase with the x-ray tube, so that the film advances during "idle" tube intervals. This can best be achieved through use of an x-ray tube "grid."

Both Picker and CE offered in the beginning the electronic type of image intensification - *e.g.*, Picker's Amplifilmer had initially a 5″ screen. Now both of them, as well as Keleket, have the combined electronic-television system, and use tubes with 9″ input phosphors. GE named its combination the Fluori-

*Westinghouse discontinued production of its Fluorex in 1959, and used Philips, Machlett, or SRW tubes. In 1964, Westinghouse resumed production of intensifier tubes at Elmira, starting with a 7-inch. Profexray (now a Litton subsidiary) set in 1963 the trend toward smaller sizes. All tubes eventually fade: replacement cost is $8,000 or more for the 9-inch — $3,000 or less for the 6-inch.

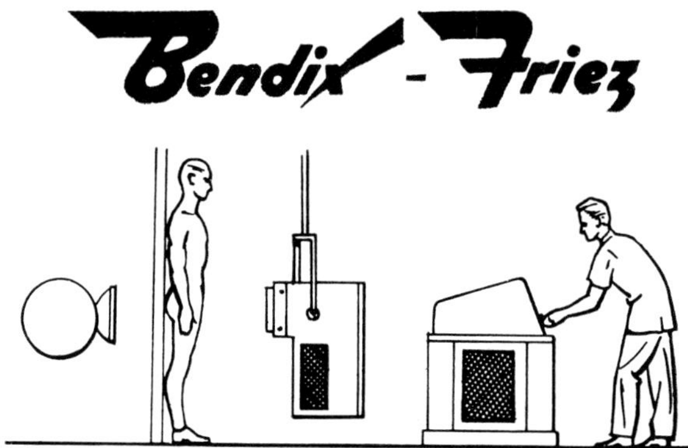

Bendix-Friez's Lumicon. It was the first (all-) television intensifier system, but apparently not very satisfactory and/or overpriced because its production was soon discontinued. Its most significant departure from the conventional was hardly noticed: with it the operator began to "look away" from the patient. This made remote controlled, push-button operation possible.

con, while Picker's version was called the Picker-Morgan Image Orthicon System. Television monitoring has led to Picker's Satellite and GE's Teletrol, remote control arrangements in which the radiologist sits behind a lead-glass wall, views the fluoroscopic image on a monitor, and directs the patient over a microphone. Various buttons are pushed to start and stop the tube or the movie camera or to move the screen or the patient up or down or sidewise. This being a highly competitive field, similar combinations have been advertised by both Keleket and Westinghouse.

At this point an attempt will be made to present an incurious view of current image intensification equipment. First of all is the matter of *size*. In the department of Paul Hodges at the University of Chicago all fluoroscopic examinations, whether of the heart or of the gastrointestinal tract, were performed on a five-by-eight inch screen, which was part of a special custom-built spotfilm device. It was quite adequate for routine work, therefore the currently available electron-optical image intensifiers, with input phosphors of eight or nine-inch diameter, are just as satisfactory for such routine procedures. Distance of the input phosphors from the patient's skin will determine whether all those inches of screen correspond with inches in the patient: this trivial detail is often forsaken by the preservation of a thick spotfilm device, with the intensifier mounted "on top" of the spotfilmer leading to the inevitable loss of *actually viewed inches* of patient. In cerebral angiography or angiocardiography, one would like to have the entire organ on the screen, and then eleven or twelve, or tomorrow's fifteen inches appear very desirable, so much so as to justify the bulk and other inconveniences of a larger machine like Marconi's special orthicon or Odelca's Cinelix.

The *brightness gain* advertised is the difference between input and output screen, and varies not only from tube to tube, but also in one and the same tube with voltage supply and with the age of the tube. Besides, the more gain in brightness the less detail, therefore tubes come in two or more ratings, usually with 1500 or 3000 gain. This is a theoretical figure if only because of the losses incurred during the optical magnification, "splitting," and attendant transfer of the image from the output phosphorus onto the observer's retina. And there is the highly important signal/noise ratio. A certain number of x-ray quanta* must hit the input phosphorus to form an image: below that minimal amount, no satisfactory result can be obtained – higher intensification would only intensify the noise (snow, static). But within these limitations, the radiologist who changes over to image intensification finds that new vistas open up, he really "sees" things, and no longer uses fluoroscopy solely to position the patient for spotfilms. While correcting the galley proofs, I learned that Thomson-Houston brought out a tube with 6000 brightness gain.

The addition of a *television* system is a great convenience because mirror (not to speak of telescope) viewing of the output phosphor in the upright position

*The quantum theory of fluoroscopic vision was proposed in an article by Ralph Sturm and Russell Morgan, which appeared in *Radiology* of November, 1949. Morgan is working on a modern revision of this concept, which has proved so useful.

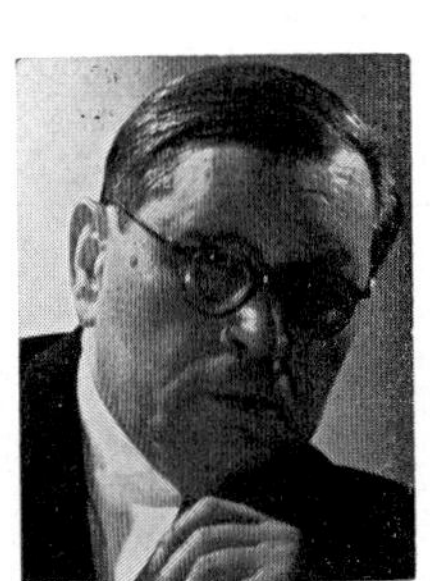
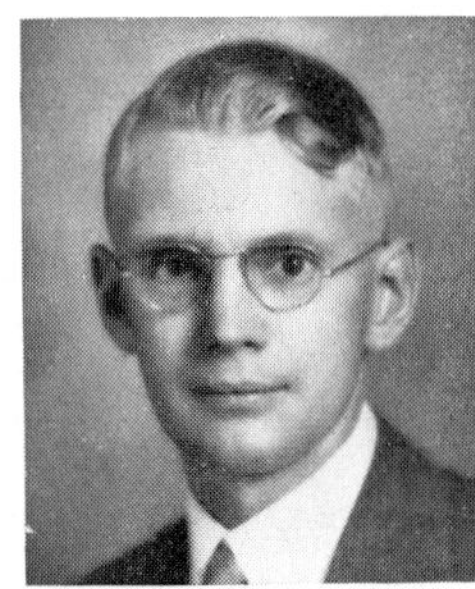

PIONEERS IN IMAGE INTENSIFICATION. On the left, with hand clasping tie, is the physician and technical wizard Robert Janker, known in Europe as the developer of fluorography. In his private *Strahlenklinik* in Bonn (Germany), Janker built in 1949 a television system for screen intensification with "fair" results. In 1952, using an electron-optical image intensifier tube provided by the German firm SRW, Janker obtained the world's first roentgen movie film with image intensification. On the viewer's right is George Christian Henny who, as Ed Chamberlain's radiophysicist, was in on the "prehistory" of image intensification. Henny stayed with it, and contributed considerably to its development.

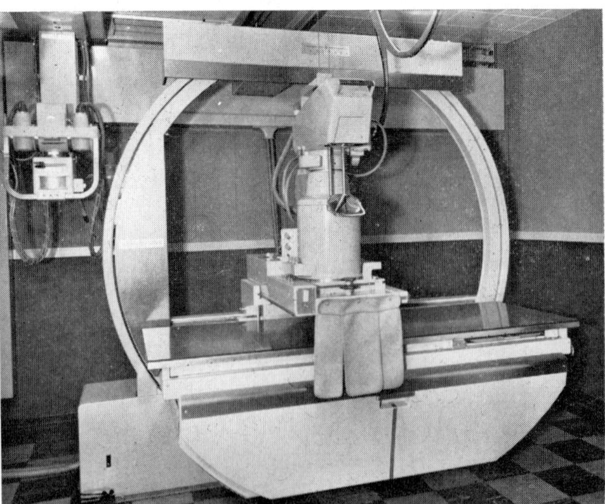

Courtesy: General Electric.

GE's FLUORICON. It is shown mounted on the Imperial table.

is cumbersome, to the point of producing torticollis. This can be mitigated by a more felicitous positioning of the mirror, but it does not compare with the ease of looking at a television monitor. The transition is of more than passing significance to the philosophy of radiology and deserves a bit of emphasis. Westinghouse's first Fluorex had mirror viewing, which was a serious departure from viewing of the screen. Still the radiologist was looking *toward* the patient; in recumbency the difference between it and conventional fluoroscopy (with the exception of brightness) was little more than trifling. Not so with Bendix-Friez's short-lived Lumicon, for that is when the radiologist began to *look away* from the patient. Soon television tubes were placed on top of electron-optical intensifiers, and more and more people became used to looking away from the patient. Remote control and remote monitoring have only finalized this situation. The exact consequences of such *looking away* cannot as yet be determined; historians are not supposed to be forecasters, and no prediction of gloom or glory will be offered, but I herewith ask an as yet unborn friend of mine (who will write the history of radiology fifty or one hundred years from now) to answer this question for me.

The decision whether to use an *orthicon* or a *vidicon* television tube depends on what one wishes to do with the installation. GE's Fluoricon utilizes the intensifier tube made by the (French) Thomson-Houston – with it you have no choice because they cannot mount the orthicon on it, it will take only the vidicon. The vidicon has the advantage of more lag, which means it does not flicker, and it is cheaper; but it has less gain, which is a handicap when intra-abdominal organs are examined. All tubes lose some gain with aging, and at a certain point the vidicon no longer picks up what one wants to see. The flicker of the orthicon can be palliated by using a green type of television monitor, which has sufficient lag to offset the flicker. And if one wants to take movies of the television image (kinescope), the more flicker, *i.e.*, the less lag the better!

This brings up the question whether everything should be recorded on *movie* film. The answer is yes, if one has unlimited time and money. It is not so difficult to process the film (Picker has now a very efficient, automatic device with and on rollers) and when only a few cases are done each day these can be viewed the same afternoon. Even storing these film strips and finding them is not so difficult – in the beginning! After a while rolls and reels begin to accumulate and things get tougher. Only when sorting material for a demonstration, or for educational purposes does one begin to

Courtesy: Picker

PICKER'S SATELLITE. There is complete duplication of controls at the machine and by remote, push-button mechanisms. The idea, however, is to do far-away fluoroscopy, by watching the television monitor above the control stand. Some radiologists combine the procedure, stay close to the patient while fluoroscoping, then actuate the cineradiography buttons by remote, television-monitored, control.

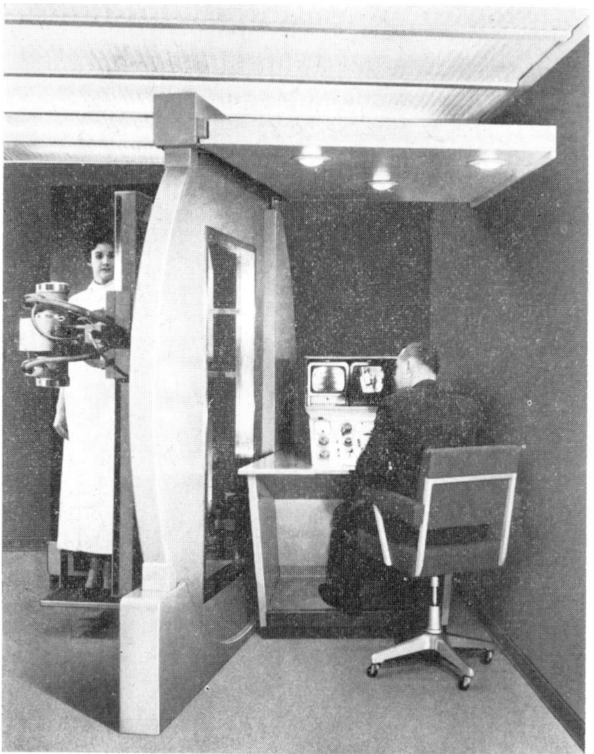

Courtesy: General Electric.

GE's TELETROL. Everything that has been said about Picker's Satellite is valid for the Teletrol, as well as for similar arrangements offered by Keleket and Westinghouse.

appreciate the job of a film editor in the movie industry. As I have said, this applies when not more than a few cases are done each morning. In a large institution, with forty or fifty daily fluoroscopies, continuous cineradiography during gastro-intestinal examinations is impractical (if at all possible). At the Children's Hospital of the University of Pittsburgh, Bert Girdany records every second of fluoroscopy on magnetic tape, transfers what is worth keeping on movie film, and reuses the tape. But one tape transcriber (aside from requiring the continuous services of a specialized engineer), costs about $50,000.

A side-issue is *sharpness*: most tubes have it — in the center. The difference between a good tube, and an excellent one is the quality of the peripheral image. In the USA electronic intensifying tubes are built by Machlett — under the Thomson-Houston license — but until recently their peripheral image was not the best. Picker's intensifying tubes are made in Chicago by Rauland, a subsidiary of Zenith Radio Corporation: they had difficulties with the gain in brightness, but the tube had less discrepancy between the center and the periphery. There is a continuous strive for improvement and, as of late, Picker tubes are as bright as Machlett's and Thomson-Houston's, and the latter two have less peripheral fall-off than before. Further changes are anticipated, recently the Thomson-Houston tube has acquired a magnification feature, whereby the central portion of the input phosphor is electronically projected onto the entire output phosphor, thus resulting in increase in size of the image, by sacrificing a part of the scrutinized anatomy.

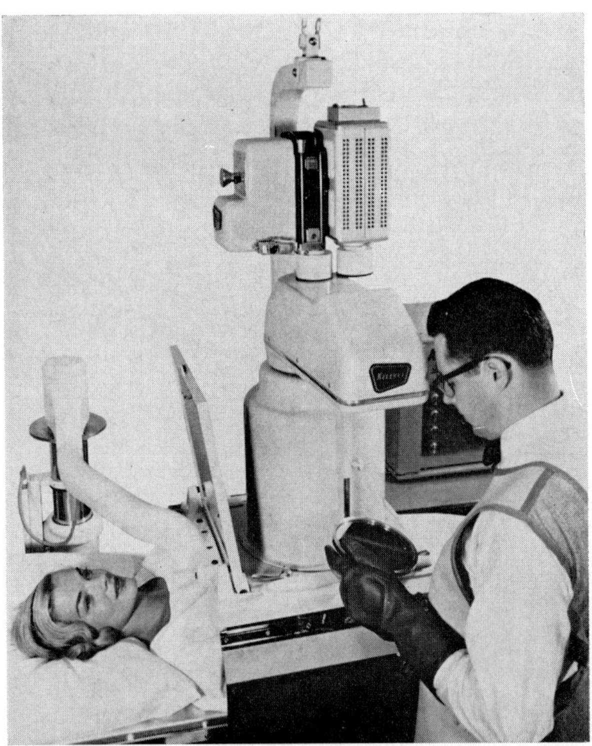

Courtesy: Tracerlab-Keleket.

KELEKET'S IMAGE INTENSIFIER. It is based on Machlett's Dynascope shown herein on the Nova-matic 90/90 table with ceiling-suspension. There is direct visual mirror-control, the image is split for recording on movie film, and for television pickup.

Regarding *radiation hazards*, image intensification reduces radiation exposure only during simple fluoroscopy. When cineradiography is performed, especially for intra-abdominal organs, the only way to reduce exposure to the operator is by going to one of those remote-controlled installations. As soon as the movie camera is turned on, the automatic brightness control (a sort of phototimer, indispensable for proper operation) jacks up the milliampherage to 5 or 10 or higher, while maintaining the 90 or more kvp required by the thickness of the part under examination. Julian Salik in Baltimore has a personal passion for peri-ampullary tumors — and believes he himself must position the patient; having a Picker Satellite, Salik stands next to the table during the fluoroscopy (thus establishing *rapport* with the patient, in a lighted room), then steps behind the lead glass wall, and watches the monitor while pushing the cineradiography button. Another solution for the high radiation dosage to the operator during cineradiography is to use a kinescope, in which the 16mm movie camera or a 70 mm still camera photographs the television image, thus obviating the need for increase in electrical factors. That means, however, to limit oneself to the 30 frames/second of the television scan — which is more than enough for gastro-intestinal examinations. It may not be enough for today's angiographic studies, and it certainly will be less than adequate for the vascular investigations of tomorrow.

Cineradiography demands additional tools, such as film processors. A special projector is needed, with instant reversal, slow-down, and single frame view-

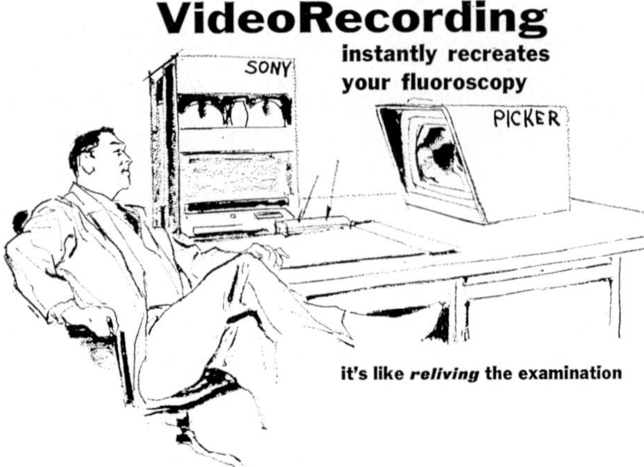

JAPANESE VIDEO-RECORDER sells for $12,000.

ing. An interesting name for a 35 mm projector of this kind is the X-Rayola (offered by Picker). There is a 16 mm model called the Weinberg-Watson modification of the Analyst II (offered by Eastman Kodak).

Most of these examinations are made with contrast media. It resulted in a demand for remotely controlled high-speed and high-power injectors. Picker, always a heaven for "x-ray gadgets," sells the Juan M. Taveras hydraulic injector.

There are some institutions and/or individual radiologists who cannot as yet afford the cost of image intensification. For angiographic work they can utilize devices which permit exposure of several large films. One such appliance is the Sanchez-Perez Universal Automatic Seriograph, manufactured by the Automatic Seriograph Corporation of College Park (Maryland), a subsidiary of Litton Industries.

The F-R Machine Works of Woodside (Long Island) came out in 1955 with a 12x12″ rollfilm cassette. It was incorporated in 1957 into a radiographic table — by then the rollfilm cassette had grown to a width of 17″ and was capable of taking fifty 14x17″ frames at a maximum rate of one frame per second. F-R bought the rights to the film changer from Fairchild. When F-R went out of the x-ray field, the film changer was sold to, and is now being produced by Franklin X-Ray Corporation in Philadelphia.

Very short-lived was the Cineray, which consisted of a trivial fluorescent screen, placed on a stand with a (modified) K-100 Kodak movie camera connected to a "synchronous" motor. With this simple contraption one could obtain satisfactory moving pictures of thin chests, but the dose rate loomed very high at a time when radiation protection was being (over-)emphasized. The American Teletronics of Anaheim (California) was created in 1959 to manufacture the Cineray: they went out of business in less than one year.

AMERICAN X-RAY INDUSTRY

There are today (early 1964) about 850 x-ray dealers in the USA and Canada, serving 8,500 radiologists and 20,000 additional physicians. There are ten manufacturers of x-ray equipment (tables, tube-supports, and transformers) with more or less nation-

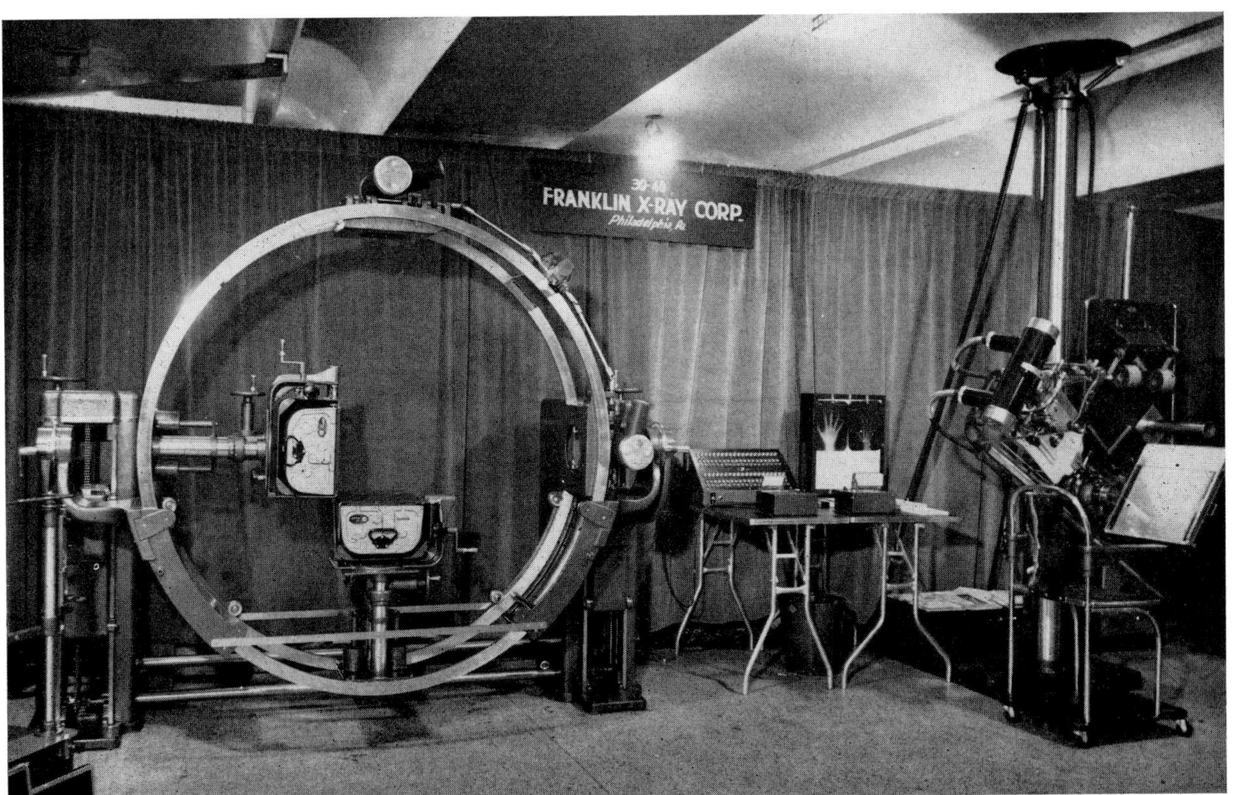

Courtesy: Charles W. Smith.

WAMPUS. Exhibit at the ARRS meeting in St. Louis (1950), showing the biplane angiographic unit devised by Ed Chamberlain of Philadelphia, using twin Fairchild rollfilm x-ray cameras.

wide sales.* Among these ten, the top three—in alphabetical order — are GE, Picker, and Westinghouse.

Ever since the "big merger" of 1916, Victor and then GE held an uncontested lead in the American x-ray industry. Shortly after World War II, GE lost that leading x-ray position, due to a number of circumstances, not the least important of which was that GE moved its x-ray operations from Chicago to Milwaukee. Picker was riding the publicity crest generated by its successful wartime production. Indeed, the Army Field Unit popularized the Picker label wherever the Armed Forces went, and they circled the globe. Then came the Fluorex, and Westinghouse could easily have become the leading x-ray manufacturer, not only in this country. But Westinghouse top management did not seem willing to make the necessary effort. There is a simple explanation: today, the entire investment in the American X-ray Industry (with the exception of accessories) is about $500 million, with $100 million yearly sales volume – "peanuts" when compared with $5 billion yearly liquor sales or even $1 billion toothpaste.

Thereupon Philips (in Holland) and Siemens (in Germany) produced their commercial models of image intensification a few months ahead of Westinghouse. As a matter of fact, Westinghouse never came close to leading the American x-ray industry, but Picker was unquestionably the first from about 1945 through 1960. Since then, with the advent of the Imperial table, with the Fluoricon, and now with the new transformers and eye-level control stands, GE has made a strong comeback. Today GE and Picker are almost tied for the first place. Also since 1960, Westinghouse is once again pushing hard for its share of the market.

No production or profit figures are available from either GE or Westinghouse. In the *Wall Street Journal* of August 4, 1958 appeared the information that CIT, a $2.5 billion sales finance company, purchased the until then closely-held stock of the Picker Company: the price was 341,063 shares of CIT common stock, valued at the time at $18 million. Picker had then 50 percent interest in a German x-ray manufacturer (Picker-Hartung) and has since purchased a nuclear instrument manufacturing plant in Connecticut. Picker has remained an autonomous organization (with Harvey Picker as chief-executive), and has in its Cleveland plant about 800 employees, one third of them in research.

Keleket was purchased by Tracerlab, a nuclear firm, whereupon the operations were moved from Covington (Kentucky) to Waltham (Massachusetts). Later on, in 1961, it passed into the hands of LFE (Labratory for Electronics). Now they are trying to reorganize their dealership and service outlets.

The other six are located in and around Chicago. The largest in this group are Standard and Profexray, with Continental a strong third. As mentioned, Fischer and Universal manufacture mainly monoblocs. And there is Mattern, first owned by Land-Air, then reorganized as part of the Dynalectron Corporation: they are currently in the process of moving out of Chicago.

In this context it is important to acknowledge the work done by the Radiologists-Manufacturers Committee of the RSNA, as detailed in Jesse Littleton's editorial in *Radiology* of October, 1962. Recently that committee completed a survey of radiologists in an attempt to find out what the profession thinks of the equipment available, and what improvements or deletions it would favor. It is a very laudable initiative,

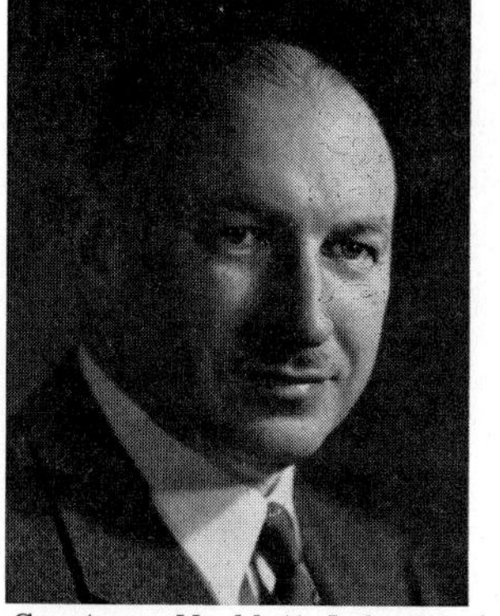
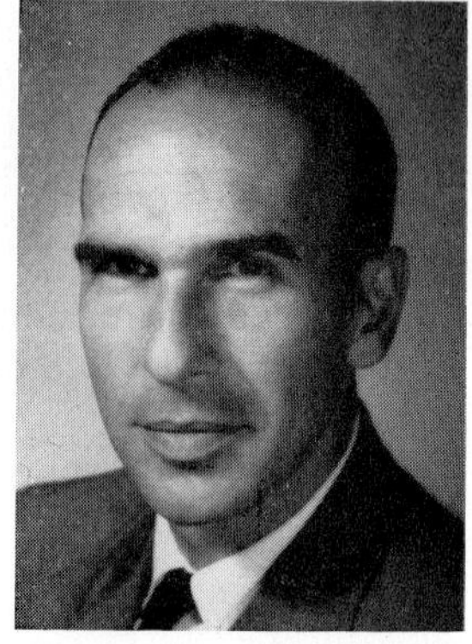

Courtesy: Machlett Laboratories.

W. E. STEVENSON. President of Machlett's after Ray Machlett's death. Stevenson retired in 1962. On the viewer's right is HARVEY PICKER, president of Picker X-Ray Corporation.

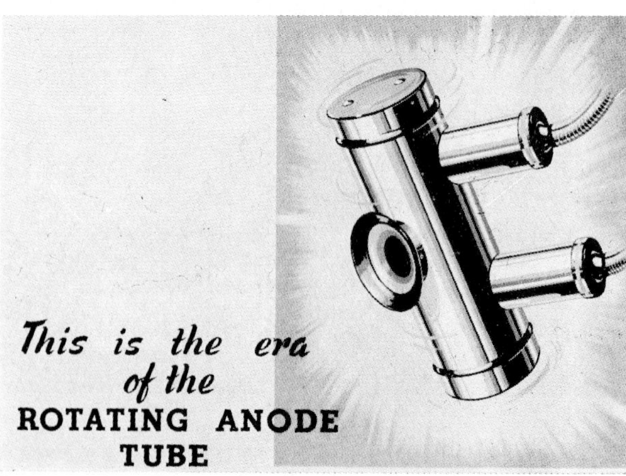

SELF-EXPLANATORY. From a Machlett advertisement of 1948 in the *British Journal of Radiology*.

*Smaller firms have been formed in several industrial centers. In 1955, in Toronto, Joseph Pritchard started his own company, which was incorporated in 1960 as the Pritchard X-Ray Mfg., Ltd. They make modern equipment, including a telescopic ceiling tube mount; a 90-15 and a 90-90 table; and various transformers up to 500 ma and 150 kvp. Pritchard is now trying to expand beyond his original territory, which is Eastern Canada.

and this type of communication channels between producer and consumer should lead to further progress and better understanding, and thus to a more desirable relationship between all parties concerned.

TUBES

A period of transition occurred at the start of the Atomic Phase, when both stationary and rotating anodes were fashionable. Today, in this country, only rotating anodes are being installed in new diagnostic x-ray equipment intended for use by radiologists - with the exception of truly portable, or special (such as dental or diffraction) apparatus.

Just as in other segments of the x-ray industry, it is difficult to pinpoint "firsts." The information obtained from the manufacturers was therefore reported herein, without necessarily underwriting its historical accuracy. I hasten to add that I have no reason to disbelieve any of the manufacturers' formal statements. It simply means that I have not had the time to check the technical literature for dates and priorities.

Since production of x-ray tubes has been discontinued in two plants (Westinghouse and Amperex*), there are today in this country four x-ray tube factories, Machlett (the one with the longest, though once interrupted, tradition); General Electric (the very oldest - GE made x-ray tubes in 1896 - but with a lengthy interruption); Eureka (which keeps up with what competition and the market demand, rather than as a trailblazer); and Dunlee (still budding, but aggressive, and already a strong contender for quality).

*Amperex was founded in 1926, and manufactured x-ray tubes from 1947 through 1958, x-ray housings from 1952 through 1958. Remembered are the "55" and the "3000" rotating anode tubes. In 1944 Amperex was purchased by the Philips organization, and today Amperex produces electron tubes and semiconductors.

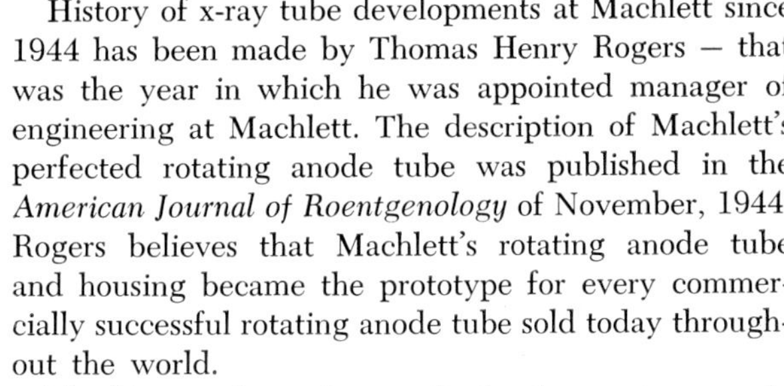

History of x-ray tube developments at Machlett since 1944 has been made by Thomas Henry Rogers — that was the year in which he was appointed manager of engineering at Machlett. The description of Machlett's perfected rotating anode tube was published in the *American Journal of Roentgenology* of November, 1944. Rogers believes that Machlett's rotating anode tube and housing became the prototype for every commercially successful rotating anode tube sold today throughout the world.

The history of rotating anode development was written up by Rogers in the Spring, 1947 issue of Machlett's *Cathode Press*. The model D Dynamax, introduced in 1939, achieved lubrication of its bearings by silver-coating — which proved to be extremely successful. In 1942 the heat-dissipating capacity was increased by 250 per cent by changing the design of the anode disc, as well as of the tube housing.

The race of transformer ratings made it imperative to increase tube loads. Still, tube ratings are (and always will be) below transformer capabilities. General Electric's HRT allowed loads up to 130 kvp at 500 ma. Even Eureka followed and came out with a 110 kvp job for a special, Mattern machine (the Medalist). Finally everybody had to go to 150 kvp. Machlett modified the Dynamax 150, and then also its Dynamax 50 so that both can take the 150 kvp. In addition, though, it was provided with a "grid."

In 1955, Charles Theodor Dotter (a former associate of Israel Steinberg, the pioneer angiocardiographer of New York City), professor of radiology in the University of Oregon in Portland, wanted to execute extremely fast film exposures of the heart during its "perfusion" with contrast media. At Machlett's, Tom Rogers built the Dynapulse for Dotter, which permitted millisecond exposures. It consists of a grid inserted between the anode and the cathode, aiming to stop the flow of electrons except at and for the time desired. The principle is the same as for any triode; as long as there is a nega-

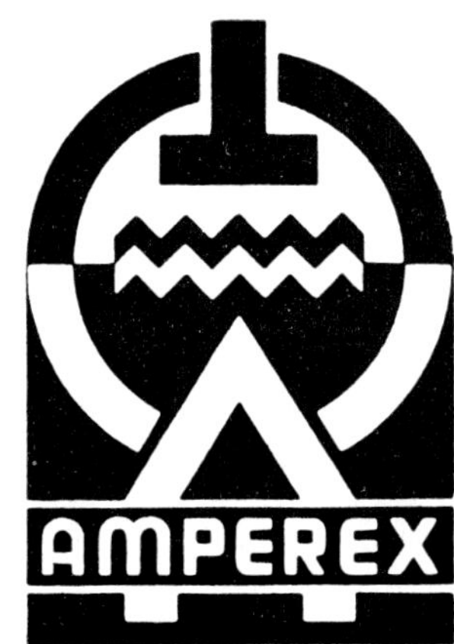

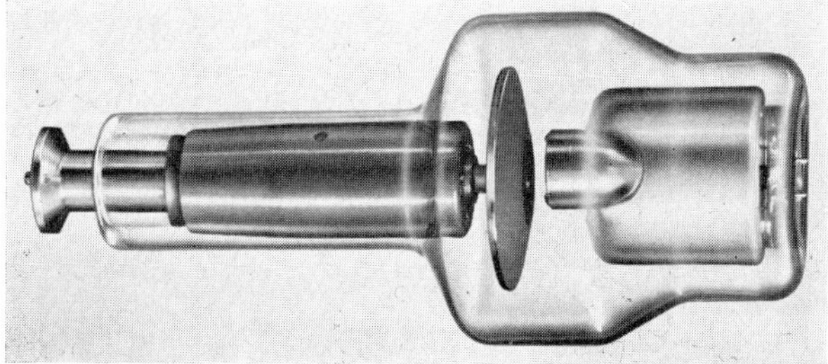

Courtesy: General Electric.

GE's HRT. Design of rotating anode tubes is now fairly standardized all over the world — with minor differences, and periodical raises in allowable tube loads.

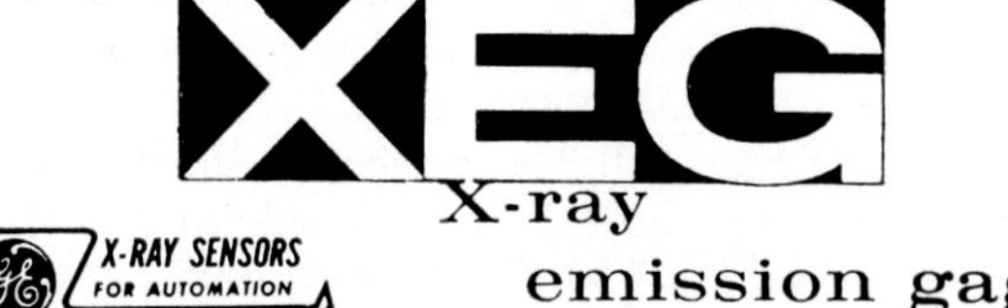

CONTINUOUS CHECKING. It consists of two main components, a vibration-resistant measuring head, and an electronic control cabinet — of course, in addition to the beryllium window x-ray source.

tive potential on the grid, no electrons will reach the anode! In 1959, Machlett's brought out the Dynapulse, a grid-controlled double-focus rotating anode x-ray tube; it had millisecond timing on its small (.5 mm square) focal spot, while the large (1.5 mm square) focal spot was of conventional design. This principle was then applied to cineradiography. Properly timed pulses keep the x-ray tube idle while the shutter of the movie camera is closed, and energize the x-ray tube when the shutter is open. This prolongs tube life, and saves unnecessary radiation exposure. Russell Wigh, professor of radiology in the University of Georgia, in Augusta, developed in 1959 a means whereby either Dynapulse or impulse timing could be combined with bi-plane film changers or conventional equipment.

In 1962 Machlett advertised the Stereo Dynamax, a rotating target having twin, grid-controlled focal spots which — together with an image intensifier — can be used for stereo-fluoroscopy or stereo-cineradiography.

Hasn't anybody thought of wiring bi-plane equipment for simultaneous viewing of both images (obtained from twin x-ray beams, placed at 90° angle from each other) on twin television monitors?

Since I wrote the previous paragraph, at St. Mary's Hospital in Rochester (Minnesota), Colin Holman of the Mayo Clinic produced electronic "subtraction" by superimposing on one television screen two television images of cerebral angiograms, one image in black-on-white, the other in white-on-black (photographic *Subtraktion* is, of course, the procedure proposed by Ziedses des Plantes). At the University of Melbourne (Australia), George Berci allowed orthopedists to view fractures in surgery on twin television monitors, each of which brought a "frozen" image at right angle with the other. Because of the electronic "freeze" feature, this was called the "stored telex-ray."

The development of beryllium window x-ray tubes was intimately connected with Machlett's, as described

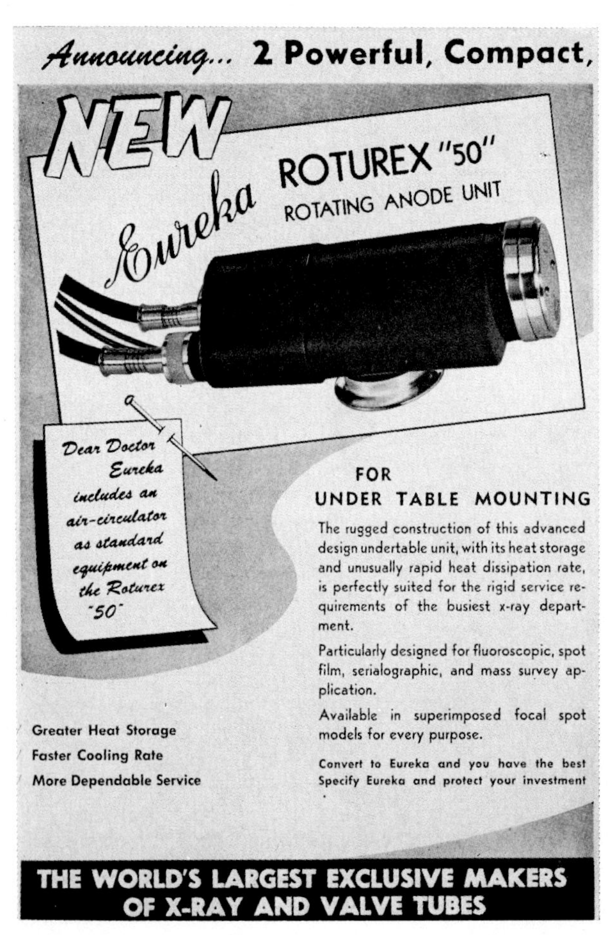

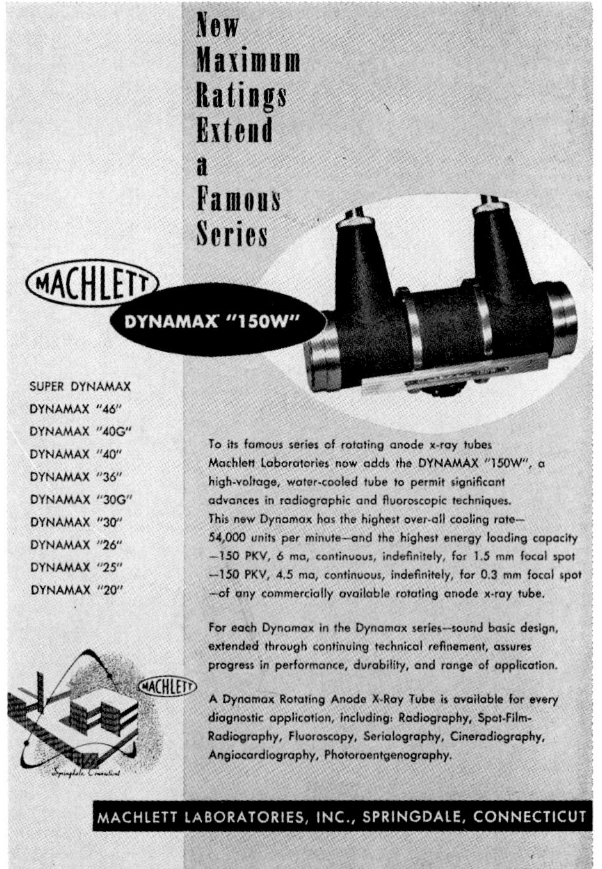

by Tom Rogers in *Radiology* of June, 1947. Beryllium sheets were used in the early 1930s, both in Germany and in this country, in an internal hood surrounding the target, to prevent the bombardment of the tube walls by secondary electrons. In this application the beryllium sheet did not have to be air-tight. In 1942, at Machlett's, a process was developed whereby beryllium could be made malleable, and with it the first commercially produced x-ray tube with vacuum-tight beryllium window was built and reported by Ray Machlett in the *Journal of Applied Physics* of June, 1942. During World War II these so-called diffraction tubes were used in various industrial applications. In the winter, 1945-46 issue of *Industrial Radiography* Tom Rogers reported the wide-angle 40° model AEG-50, a beryllium window x-ray tube capable of delivering at close range up to two million r/min. It made many applications practical, such as spotweld radiography, microradiography (for certain technics AEG-50 with molybdenum or copper targets were made available), thickness gauging (measurement of the attenuation of x-ray beam when passing through the material to be gauged for thickness), and radio-chemical analysis. It also resulted in the demonstration of radio-chemical effects, such as the color and other changes in irradiated gem stones (with the inherent danger of frauds), reported in 1947 by Frederick Pough and Thomas Rogers in the *American Mineralogist*. An improved version of the beryllium window tube, the OEG-60 — also with water-cooled grounded anode, but with 60° angle — came out in 1949. Its utilization made it possible to have one transformer and one tube for the production of x-ray beams from 3 to 50 kvp, covering thus both the Grenzstrahlen and the contact range.

Thomas Rogers, who is a member of the American Institute of Electrical Engineers (AIEE), presented at one of the latter's meetings (in January, 1952) the low drop, high voltage, high power valve, made with thoriated tungsten filament. It had been developed for industrial purposes, but was soon adopted by the x-ray industry, and by other tube makers. Some of the *princeps* publications can be found in the *Cathode Press* of summer, 1949, and in *Electrical Engineering* of January, 1953.

Two additional items from Machlett's history deserve special mention. One is the development of a production model of a sealed-off electron donut tube for betatrons — based on the electron peeler system, described by Lester Skaggs in *Radiology* of December, 1949. As reported by Rogers to the AIEE on January 18, 1954, the sealing-off of that tube was achieved by mounting a re-inforcing rim onto a beryllium disc of 0.5 mm thickness, which was then hard-soldered to the ceramic donut tube.

The first suggestion to use electron therapy was made

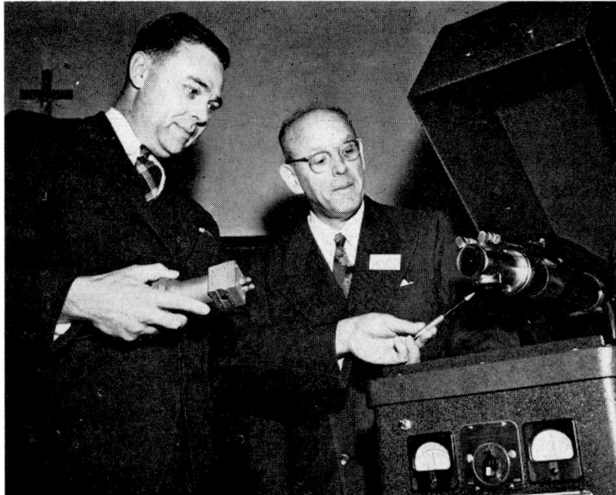

Courtesy: The Milwaukee Sentinel.

AEG-50 IN 1945. At the fiftieth anniversary of Röntgen's discovery, observed at Marquette University in Milwaukee, there was a Symposium on Industrial Radiography. Shown here are two of the panelists, Thomas Henry Rogers pointing to the AEG-50, while George Lindenberg Clark (the famous microradiographer) courteously watches.

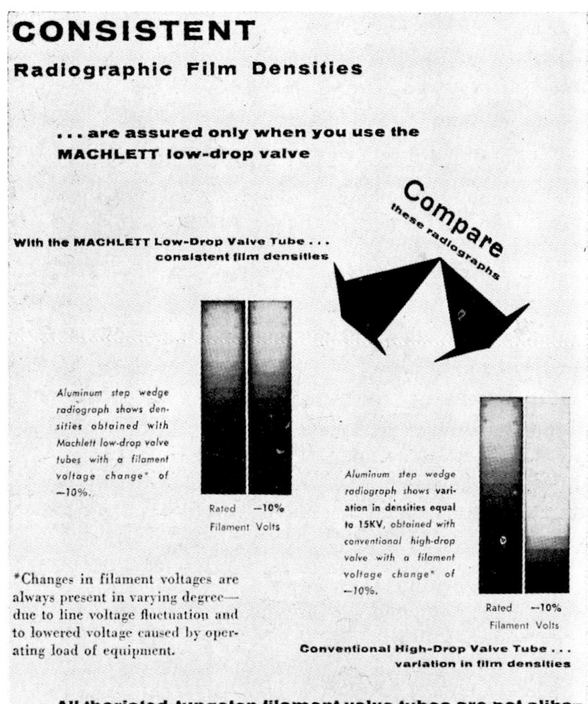

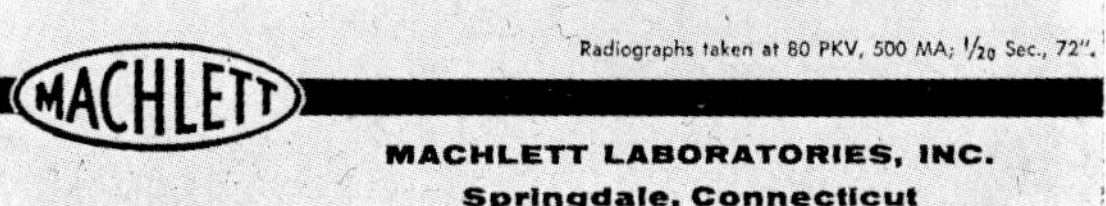

in 1934 in *Strahlentherapie* by A. Brasch and F. Lange. The first actual application of high energy electrons was reported by Ludwig Haas in the *American Journal of Roentgenology* of August, 1954: he had used the betatron at the Research and Educational Hospitals of the University of Illinois in Chicago. Today, electron therapy is being utilized in several centers in this country, by Hugh Hare in Boston, by Florence Chu in New York City, by Erich Uhlmann in Chicago.

The other item is Machlett's Dynascope, an image intensifier first built under a (French) Thomson-Houston patent. For this purpose Machlett constructed in 1955 a special photosensitive and display tube facility, because of the special requirements for such manufacture. Giant air-conditioners and peculiar housekeeping procedures are used to insure absolutely lint-free conditions. All structures are handled with Dacron gloves, or finger cots, beyond glass hoods, to avoid even breathing over these tubes. The Dynascope comes in two sizes, the ML-9411 (6″ screen), and ML-9421 (9″ screen), operated at 24-27 kvp. Machlett and (French) Thomson-Houston tubes are interchangeable in mechanical, electrical, and optical characteristics, and are cross licensed on new improvements.

Machlett Laboratories is no longer owned by the Machlett family. It is now a subsidiary of Raytheon. President of Machlett's, until recently, had been W. E. Stevenson, one of the old guard. In October, 1962, Thomas Henry Rogers became the general manager of Machlett's x-ray tube activities.

DUNLEE

The Dunlee Corporation was formed in 1946 by two chief-engineers. One of them was Dunmore W. Dunk, at the time Eureka's chief-engineer (he had been with GE X-ray in 1928). The other was Zed Jarvis Atlee, at the time chief-engineer of GE's vacuum-tube department (he had been at Schenectady since 1929). They were first located at 4558 West Congress Street in Chicago, and in 1959 built a new plant in Bellwood, a Western suburb of Chicago. Dunk died in a car accident in 1951, and Atlee is now Dunlee's president.

In the free-enterprise system, competition provides the "checks and balances" in business. In the late 1920s, the x-ray industry supported, both morally and financially, the re-entry of Machlett's into the manufacture of x-ray tubes. One generation later, after World War II, there was again need for an additional supplier of x-ray tubes of good quality, which is why Picker contributed financially to the creation of Dunlee.*

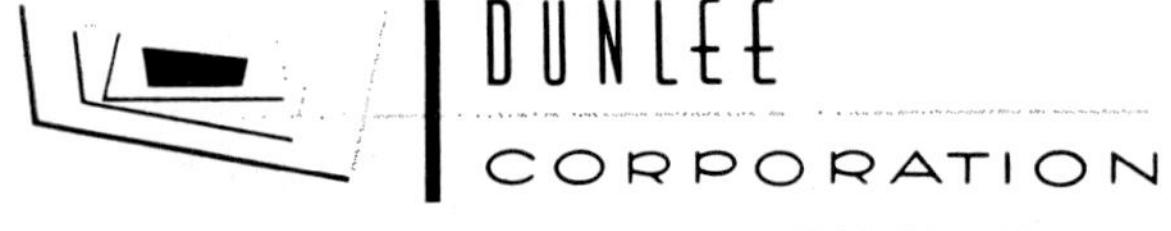

Zed Atlee is today this country's senior expert in x-ray tubes. With thirty-five years of uninterrupted activity in this field - from research, design, and manufacture to production, promotion, and marketing - he can speak authoritatively on any of these phases. Atlee is a forceful, aggressive, perhaps at times irascible personality. But even when, for publicity sake, he must stretch a point, he does it with dignity.

Following is a list of patented Dunlee "firsts," prepared by Atlee in January of 1963:

1. A Universal getter arrangement also providing end gradient shielding. U. S. Patent No. 2,502,070 filed January 19, 1949, issued March 28, 1950. Inventors, Atlee-Dunk.
2. Simplified electrostatic shield for thoriated tungsten filament valve. U. S. Patent No. 2,558,603 filed March 4, 1949, issued June 26, 1951. Inventor, Atlee.
3. Single focus tilted anode x-ray tube to prevent inverse runaway. U. S. Patent No. 2,671,867, filed November 24, 1950, issued March 9, 1954. Inventor, Atlee.
4. Tetrode x-ray tube. U. S. Patent No. 2,686,884,

*I perused Dun & Bradstreet's mammoth listing of million-dollar businesses in the USA, and found therein LFE, Nuclear-Chicago, Nuclear Corporation of America, Picker, Profexray, and Victoreen. There were no separate listings for the x-ray divisions of GE, Westinghouse, or Eastman Kodak.

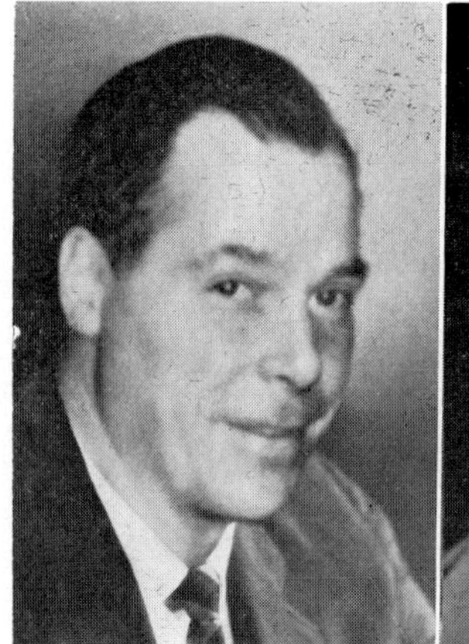
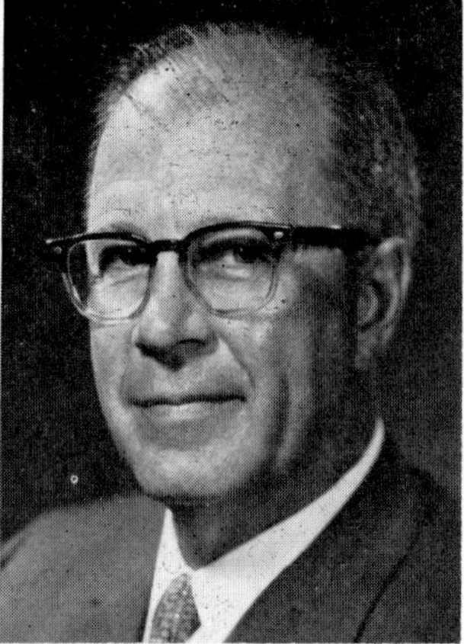

Courtesy: Dunlee.

DUNLEE'S FOUNDERS. Dunmore W. Dunk (on the left) and Zed Jarvis Atlee formed the company in 1946. Dunk died in a car accident in 1951, and Atlee is now Dunlee's president.

filed May 1, 1950, issued August 17, 1954. Inventor, Atlee.

5. Mechanical sealed Beryllium window, filed May 24, 1952, issued January 10, 1956. Inventor, Atlee.
6. Double focus double tilt x-ray tube, U. S. Patent No. 2,767,341, filed August 12, 1952, issued October 16, 1956. Inventor, Atlee.
7. 360° Beryllium window hooded anode x-ray tube, filed February 28, 1955, issued May 27, 1958, Inventor, Atlee.
8. Double focus double tilted target with 2 angles (skew bent), filed February 11, 1957, issued May 27, 1958. Inventor, Atlee.
9. Cerium target rotating anode tube for providing monochromation radiation, U. S. Patent No. 2,919,362, filed April 21, 1958, issued December 29, 1959. Inventor, Atlee.
10. Internal diaphragmed rotating anode x-ray tube, U. S. Patent No. 3,018,398, filed October 27, 1958, issued January 23, 1962. Inventor, Atlee.

GRIDS

Anti-scatter grids had to be adapted to the high kilovoltages demanded for the Atomic Phase. The largest American maker of grids, Liebel-Flarsheim of Cincinnati, now a subsidiary of the Ritter Co., increased the speed of its movable Bucky-Potter diaphragm, and gave it a new name: the Super-Speed Recipromatic. The grid ratio had to be raised from 6:1 to 8:1, then to 12:1, and even to 16:1.

At the latter figure, however, alignment became more difficult, and grid lines appeared on the films despite the motion. Today the 12:1 seems to be more often the favored.

Improvement in stationery grids has led to what they call the Microline types.

In 1959, Liebel-Flarsheim de-emphasized number of lines per inch, requesting its customers not to be misled by numbers. But in 1961 they introduced the Superfine model, and advertised it by emphasizing its 133 lines per inch.

L-F manufactures several other "x-ray items" (but no longer the Kymograph), including a mechanical timer, a 14x36″ grid-top cassette tunnel for osteopathic and chiropractic purposes, and the Young urologic table (replaced in 1963 with the Hydradjust, which is big enough to take an under-the-table image intensifier).

There are a few other manufacturers of grids in this country. Some of them - such as Stanley Ander-

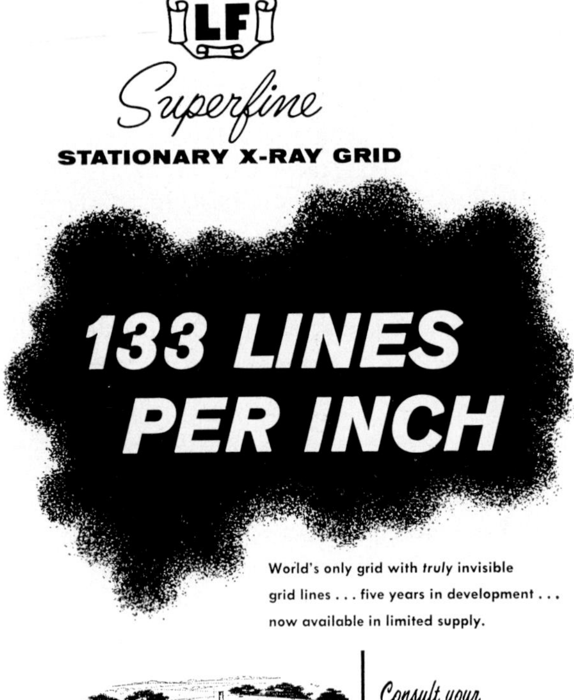

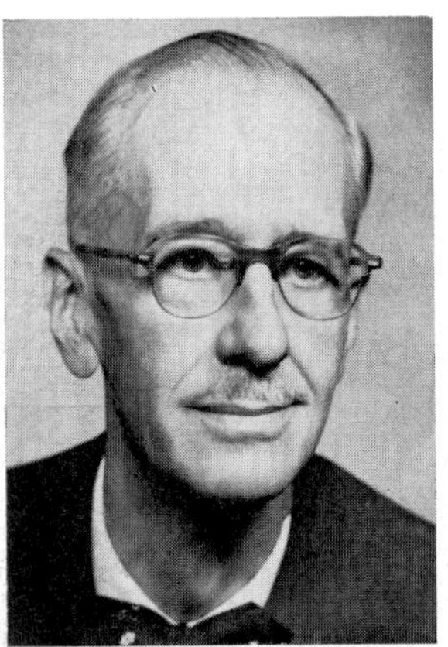

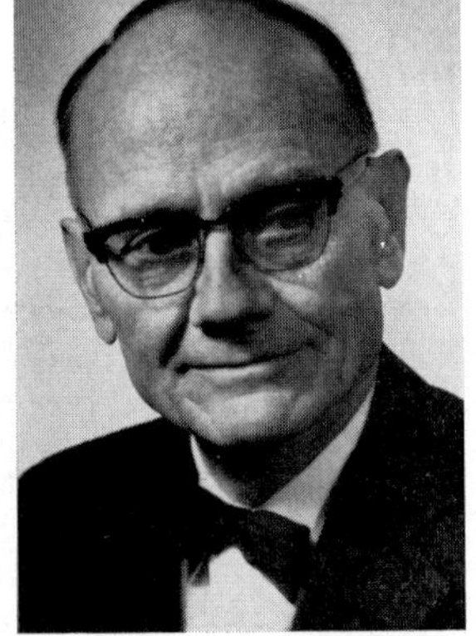

Courtesy: Liebel-Flarsheim.

JOHN FREEMAN OTTO. Long-time sales manager at Liebel-Flarsheim, stayed on as director of sales after L-F was purchased in 1957 by the Ritter Company of Rochester (New York). Otto was most compentent both on the technical and on the commercial aspects of his segment of the x-ray business. He died shortly after his retirement in October of 1962. On the viewer's right is WILLIAM JOSEPH HOGAN, president of Franklin X-Ray Corporation.

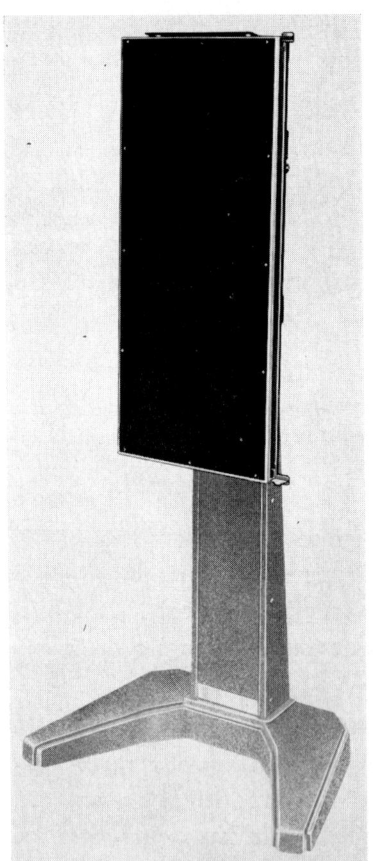

Courtesy: Liebel-Flarsheim.

L-F GRID-TOP CASSETTE. This is the 14x36″ model used when the entire spine must be exposed in a single view. Proper results require the use of a wedge filter to compensate for different densities at the various levels of the spine.

son's Monee Instrument Works in Monee (Illinois) - offer good quality, but limited rather than mass production.

SCREENS AND FILMS

If not spectacular, at least frequent, improvements are being announced in the production of fluorescent and re-inforcing screens.

This domain was "invaded" in 1946 by the Radelin Division of the (old) United States Radium Corporation of Morristown (New Jersey). In 1956, looking back over a decade, they claimed to have introduced the first PF (blue photoradiographic) screen free from significant lag, and developed the first FC (yellow, fluoroscopic) screen with finer detail. They also introduced such euphonious vocables as Rad-a-lert, the all-plastic fluoroscopic screen, and the Radelin aluminized TF reinforcing screen.

All manufacturers of screens, for instance Buck X-Ograph Company of St. Louis, have advertised their soil-proof intensifying screens produced from modern plastic material; they are more resistent both to discoloration and to abrasion because they have no varnished surface.

The X-Ray Division of the DuPont Company in Wilmington (Delaware) manufactures modernized models of the venerable Patterson screen but also a complete line of chemicals and of x-ray films. They have

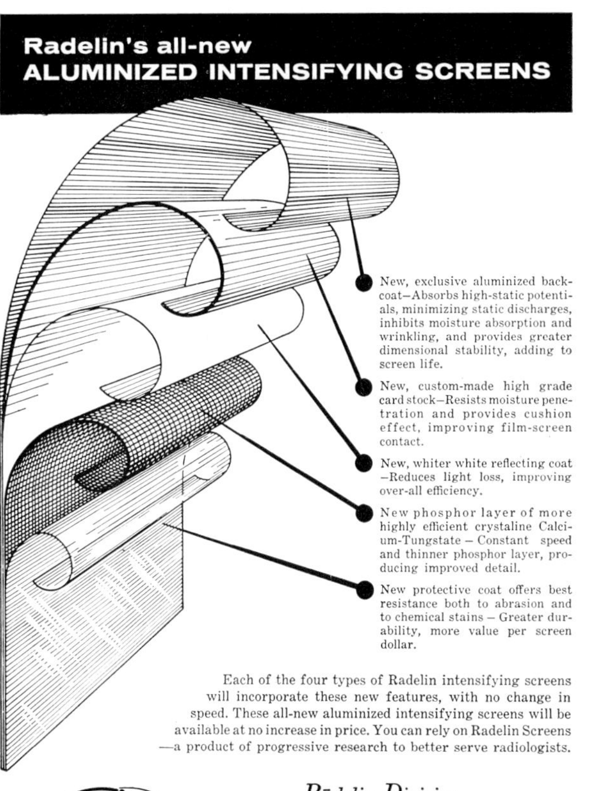

Buck SOIL-PROOF Screens

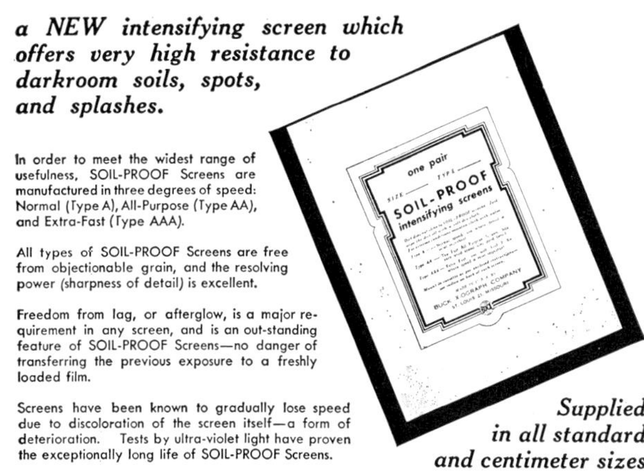

Supplied in all standard and centimeter sizes

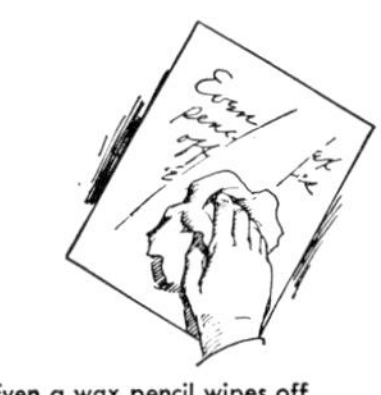

Even a wax pencil wipes off easily with a dry cloth.

The unusual resistance of SOIL-PROOF Screens to soils, spots, and splashes is due to the highly finished surface which contains no valleys, crevasses, or pores which collect and retain grimy materials. The surface of SOIL-PROOF Screens is a very tough water-proof plastic, strongly resistant to darkroom acids and alkalies.

To remove crystallized deposits of developer or fixer, dissolve the crystals with a wet swab; then wipe clean with a moist cloth. Don't try to remove the dry crystals, as in so doing you might scratch the screen surface.

for those who want the best rather than the cheapest.

BUCK X-OGRAPH COMPANY ST. LOUIS 36, MO.

★ *X-Ray accessories for those who demand quality* ★

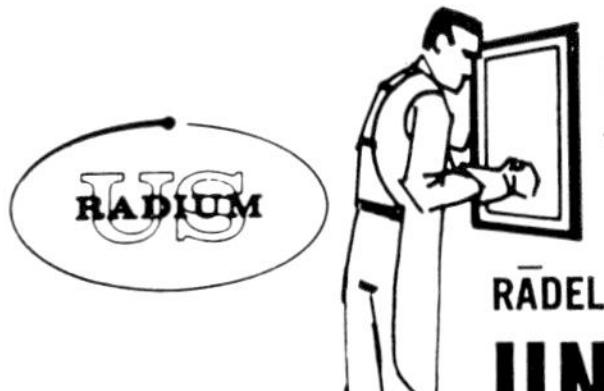

RĀD-A-LERT*—The new fluoroscopic screen for radiation control—and brighter too.

RĀDELIN DIVISION

UNITED STATES RADIUM CORPORATION

MORRISTOWN, N. J. | Offices: Chicago, Illinois and North Hollywood, Calif. Subsidiaries: Radelin Ltd., Port Credit, Ont., Canada and U.S. Radium Corp. (Europe), Geneva, Switzerland.

*PAT PENDING

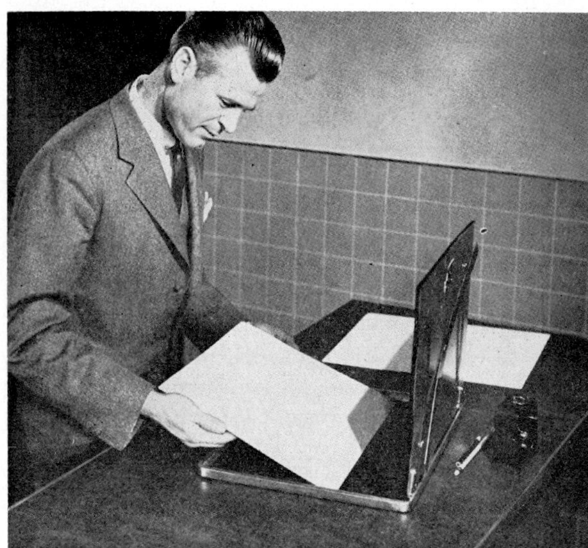

Du Pont "Patterson" Screens are

long-lasting...

Du Pont "Patterson" Screens have a hard, lacquer-type finish. It's carefully applied during the manufacture of these screens by skilled craftsmen proud of the exacting nature of their intricate work.

Inspect a new Du Pont "Patterson" Screen closely. Note its glossy surface. It even looks hard . . . and it is! Hard and tough. It's a surface scientifically made to resist wear of all kinds . . . the friction, digging, scratching of films placed in cassettes, as well as other abrasions.

This "built-in" characteristic of every Du Pont "Patterson" Screen explains why these screens consistently outwear all other intensifying screens. It's the reason why they do a better job over longer periods of time.

It is this quality of Du Pont "Patterson" Screen durability . . . plus the cleanability, perfection and uniformity of these screens . . . that explains why x-ray departments the world over prefer and insist upon intensifying screens bearing the famous name of "Patterson." Your dealer will gladly take your order.

A booklet, "Minutes That Matter," is your handy guide on the care of screens. A copy will be sent upon request. E. I. du Pont de Nemours & Co. (Inc.), Photo Products Department, Wilmington 98, Delaware.

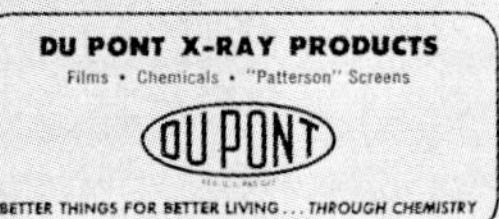

introduced a new base, called Mylar, of added tensile strength and impervious to water; on it the emulsion can get wet, but not the "film" itself!

Because paper is now frequently radioactive, and leaves "black dots" on developed films, Du Pont introduced NIF, non-interleaved films. This way of packaging has since been adopted also by other manufacturers.

Ansco's production of chemicals and films likewise covers the entire line and they, too, emphasize high speed screens and emulsions to minimize patient ex-

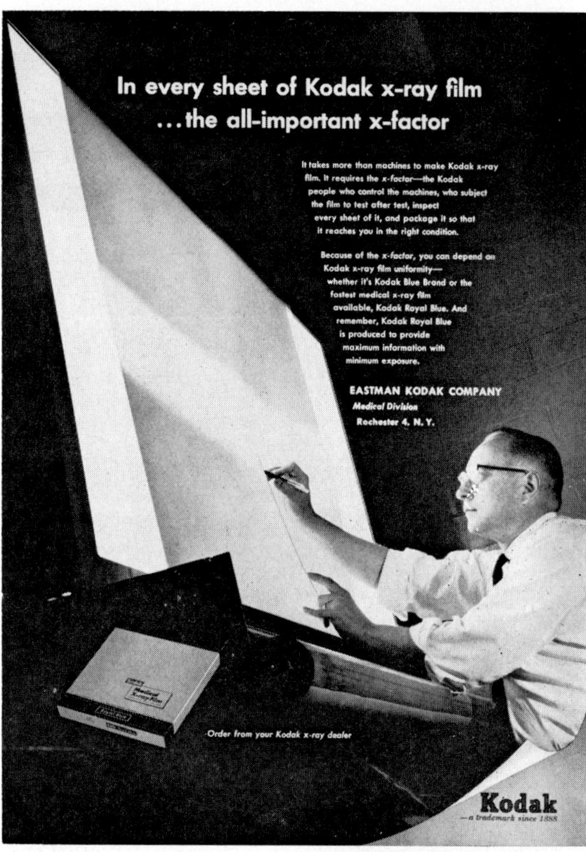

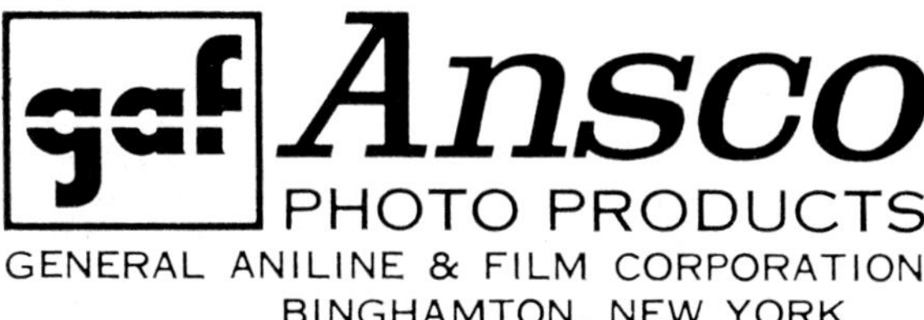

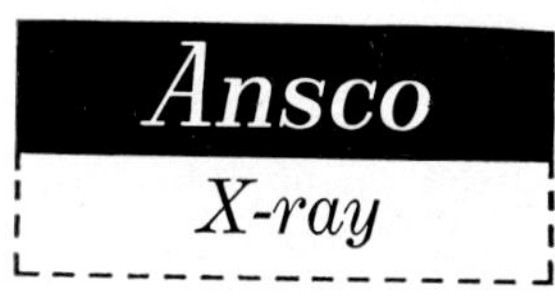

CONVENTION ISSUE

Ansco X-RAY NEWS

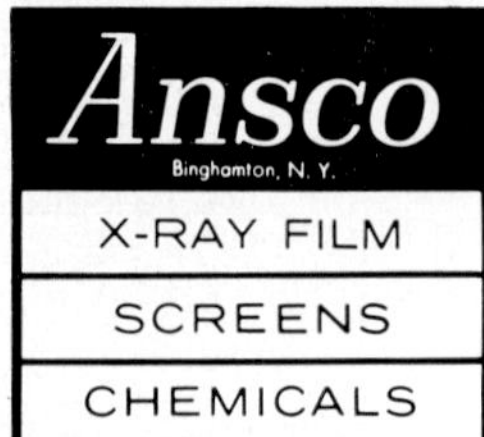

technical and commercial news for the radiological profession

ANSCO TO INTRODUCE NEW CHEMICALS FOR AUTOMATIC PROCESSING

posure (everybody is now so radiation conscious). Their semantic ventures include Bulkpak, a 300-sheet interleaved package, and Monopak, individually packaged sheets of non-screen x-ray film.

Incidentally, many people seem to have neglected the fact that excellent radiographs can be made without re-inforcing screens. Unusually sharp detail – desirable for textbook illustrations – can be had by combining (for extremities) non-screen film with movable Bucky-Potter technic.

Ansco (or perhaps only a part of Ansco) was once owned by the (German) Agfa, with a resultant change-of-hands during World War II. Now Ansco is (or, rather, would like to be) a division of General Aniline & Film Corporation. Recent ads stress this fact by using the terms GAF Ansco (just as it had been Agfa Ansco). But it seems that the legalization of their "concubinage" will require an Act of Congress and the payment of "damages" demanded by the former "husband" (Agfa).

Eastman Kodak's fast film is called Blue Brand.* The giant industrial complex called Eastman Kodak is today the world's largest all-around manufacturer of photographic equipment, both in and outside the x-ray industry.

AUTOMATIC PROCESSORS

In 1928, Glenn M. Dye, president of the Pako Corporation, introduced an automatic (mechanized) film processing machine for both roll and pack photographic film. It operated very satisfactorily, became quite popular, and filled a definite need in industrial photography. About 1938, Pako started research on the Filmachine, intended for the mechanical processing of x-ray films. The first prototype was built in 1942. World War II delayed the "civilian" applications of the Filmachine, but it was very successfully employed in this country by the Armed Forces and by a few private industries.*

Pako's first model 20 M Filmachine could process 120 films per hour, by using special hangers. Its mechanism

*Paul Chesley Hodges likes to point out that when properly exposed and processed, one cannot tell from the simple inspection of the film whether fine grain or coarse grain had been used in either or both the film and the re-inforcing screens.

*This information was taken from an historical paper written by the technical x-ray wizard Roy E. Wolcott from Champaign (Illinois). That paper appeared in November, 1945 in the *X-Ray Technician.*

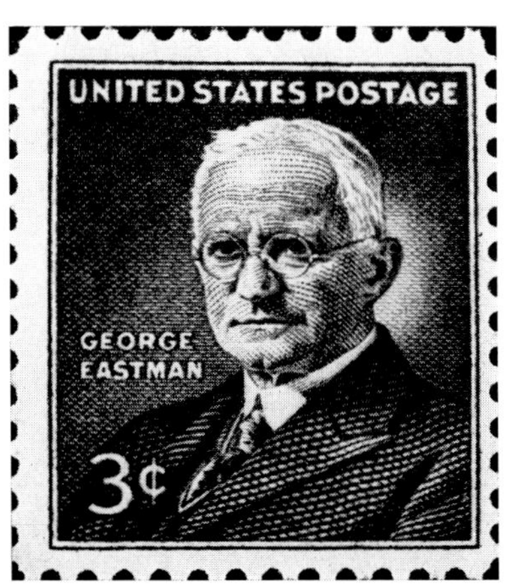

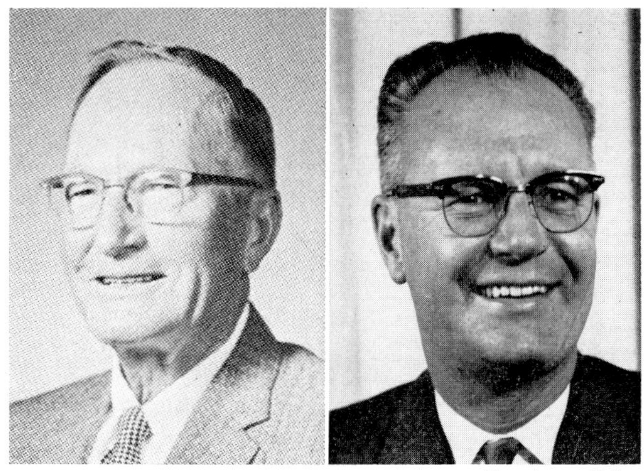

Courtesy: Pako.

THE DYES OF PAKO. Glen Morris Dye, "founder" of Pako, and his son, Harry Merwin Dye, currently chairman of the board at Pako's.

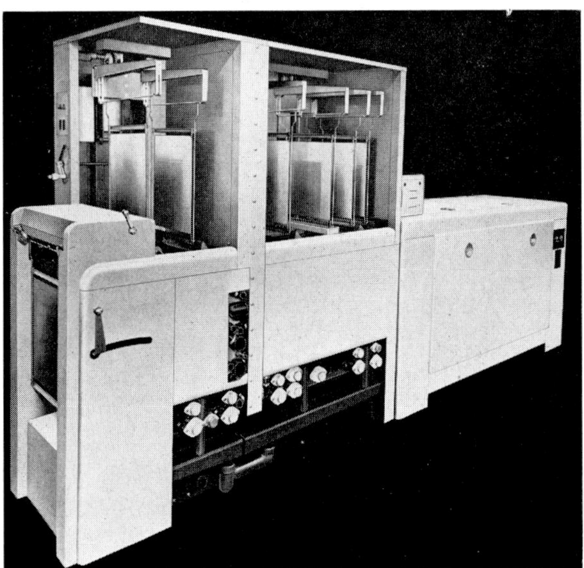

Courtesy: Pako.

PAKO X-RAY FILMACHINE. This was model 30, which handled up to 60 14x17″ per hour. Then came model 14, which delivered up to 120 14x17″ per hour, or handled films up to 17x28″ in size.

provided the successive dipping of the films in developer, washer, hypo, and then their advancement in the drying tunnel. Total cycle time for one film approached 40 minutes. Chemicals were rejuvenated by continuous circulation from separate tanks, with involved temperature and other controls.

The success of Pako's first model made it clear that automatic processors were here to stay. Indeed, soon several other manufacturers came into the picture.

Drying time was reduced in the Fax-Ray, manufactured by Oscar Fisher Co. of Newburg (New York) — more important, though, they used no hangers and of-

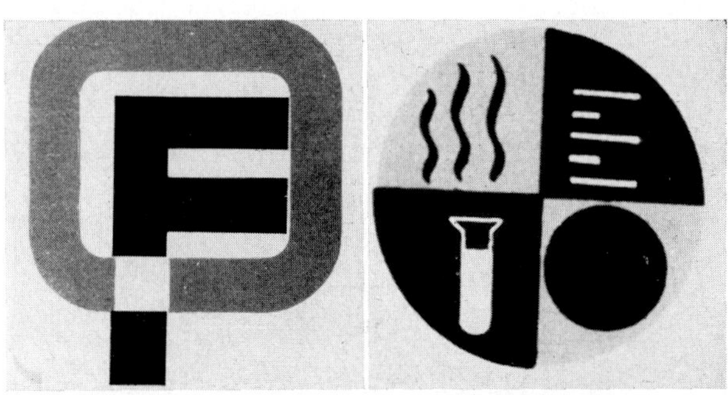

OSCAR FISCHER'S SEAL AND SIGN. This company, located in Newburgh (New York), manufactures an automatic processor called the Fax-Ray, and — among other things — installs and services the ("belted") automatic cassette conveyor made by the (Swedish) Elema-Schönander.

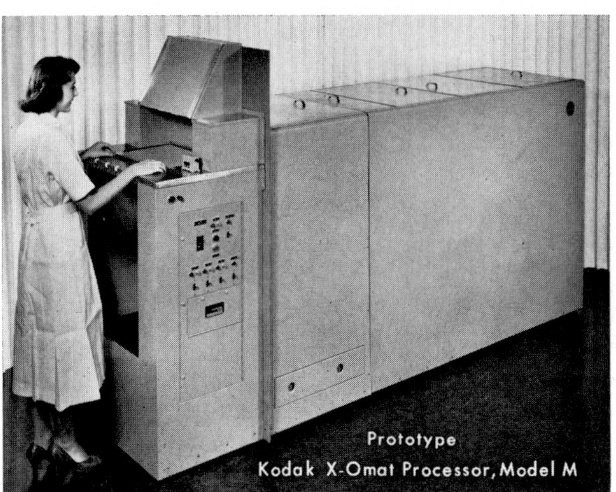

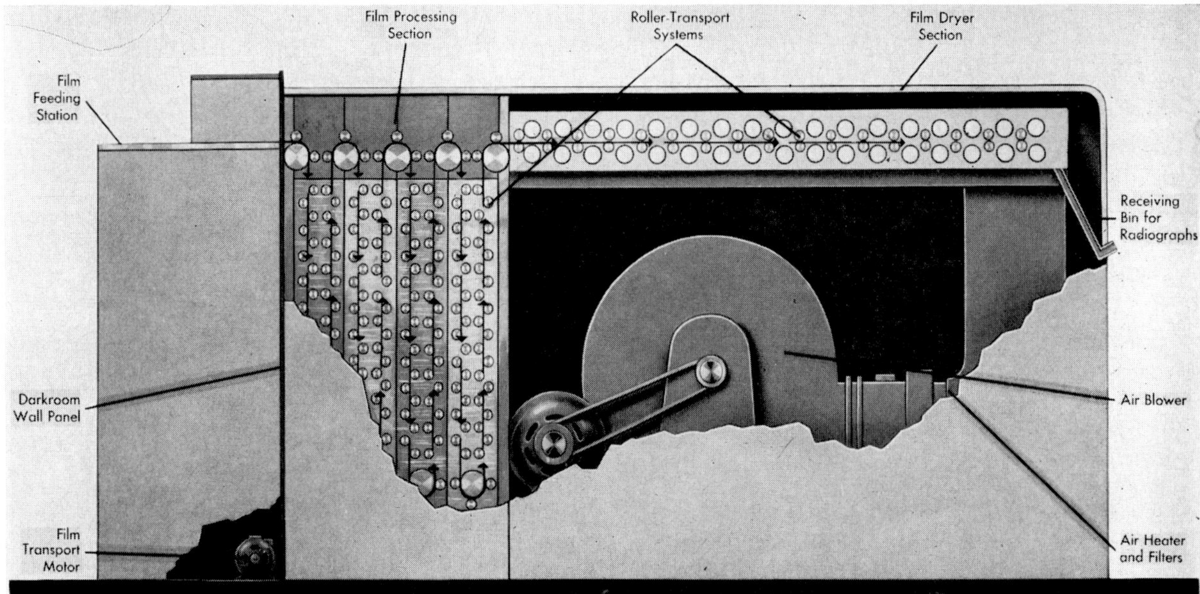

Courtesy: Eastman Kodak X-Omat Center.

CUTAWAY OF FIRST X-OMAT. As described by Harold Daniel Russell (Eastman Kodak Research Laboratories) in the January-February, 1959 issue of *Photographic Science and Engineering,* the six-minute rate of complete processing of Kodak Royal Blue and Blue Brand x-ray films is accomplished by (a) elevated temperature in all solutions, including the wash water, (b) use of hyperactive solutions, (c) optimum agitation by means of the wringer-roller transport system, and (d) drying of both sides of the film in a few seconds with heated jets of air while the film is being transported between rollers (to avoid water streaks). Eastman Kodak makes special solutions for automatic processors, including a hardening developer. They have, of course, also "compact" roller processors.

fered a loading magazine wherein up to a dozen films at a time were inserted, after which the machine fed itself and processed dry-to-dry in seven minutes. This was an improvement also over the B. F. Processor (and Isothermal dryer) manufactured by the Brown-Foreman Industries of Louisville (Kentucky), even though the latter allowed any type hangers, and processed at the rate of 200 films per hour.

Bar-Ray Products Corporation of Brooklyn sold the Hills Automatic Processing System, a "hanger" model, first shown at the ICR in Copenhagen in 1953 by Thomas Henry Hills, chief-radiologist of Guy's Hospital (London).

There was also the Rapi-dex, offered until 1960 by the Rapi-dex Company of Falls Church (Virginia), and since 1961 by the Capitol Research Industries of Alexandria (Virginia).

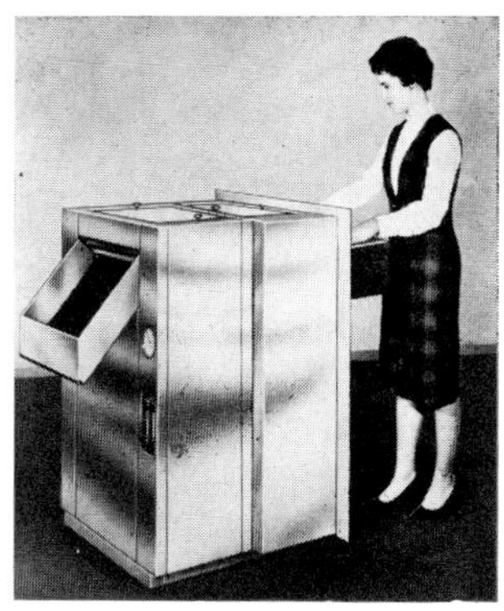

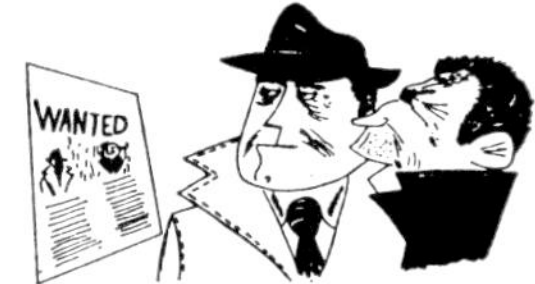

Private-eye Pakowett stops spots, streaks

Courtesy: Pako.

PAKOROL-XM. Pako's low-priced nylon roller x-ray film processor sells (now) for around $12 thousand. Pako is growing by leaps and bounds. On August 18, 1910, Glen Dye (then a young photographer from Lamar in Colorado) arrived in Minneapolis, and the same year formed the Photo Advertising Company. On their fiftieth anniversary they opened a new plant, located in Golden Valley (Minnesota). Pako makes all sorts of automatic processors, and markets many other photographic products, such as the wetting agent Pakowett.

The most significant improvement came in December, 1956 when the first model (M) of the Kodak-X-Omat was previewed. It had nylon rollers, and film sizes could be intermixed; its work rate depended on whether 5x7″ (1200 per hour), 8x10″ (600 per hour), or 14x17″ (240 per hour) were being processed.

Eastman Kodak's nylon rollers were an immediate success. Soon Pako had to bring out the Pakorol-X, with similar rollers and in other ways comparable to, but perhaps not quite as "solid" as, the X-Omat. Pre-cornered films (to save the need for, and the time of, cutting corners) were first brought out by Du Pont, then adopted by all other film manufacturers. This is just another proof of the wide acceptance of automated processing in general, of roller processors in particular. The recent trend is toward "compact" models, which would bring the blessings of automation also to medium-sized hospitals. This is all to the better. After switching to automation, there occurs a period of adaptation, during which technicians must sharpen their accuracy of exposure as they are prevented from "compensating" (or rather from thinking they do so) in the darkroom. In the long run, if the x-ray department is sufficiently busy, automatic film processing proves to be a time-saver (*i.e.*, also a money saver).

The overall quality of the production in teaching departments has been further improved by assigning an experienced resident to check all films as they come out of the processor, and order retakes while the patient is still on the floor. The success of the processor is attested by the fact that other manufacturers are joining the bandwagon: in 1962 Carr, and in 1963 Picker introduced their own models (Picker's is called the Pixamatic, and has an automatic loading mechanism, as has

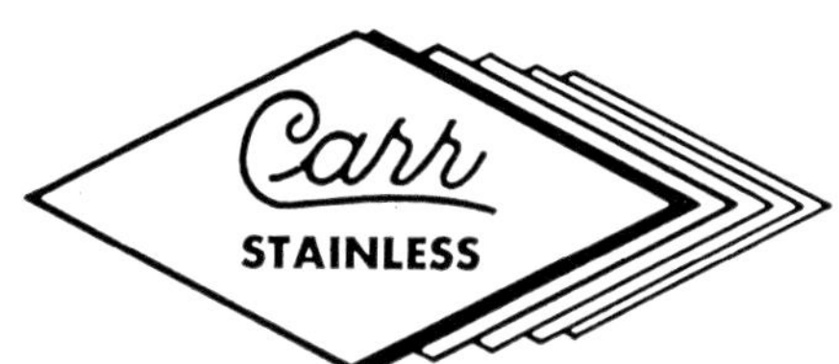

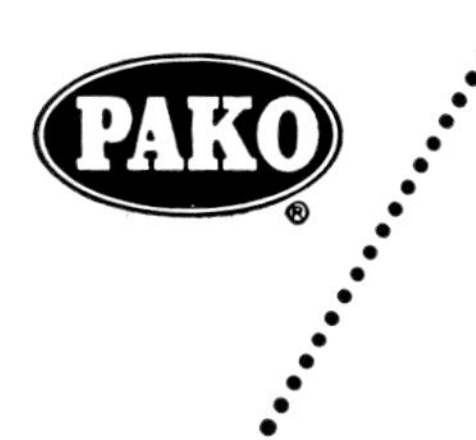

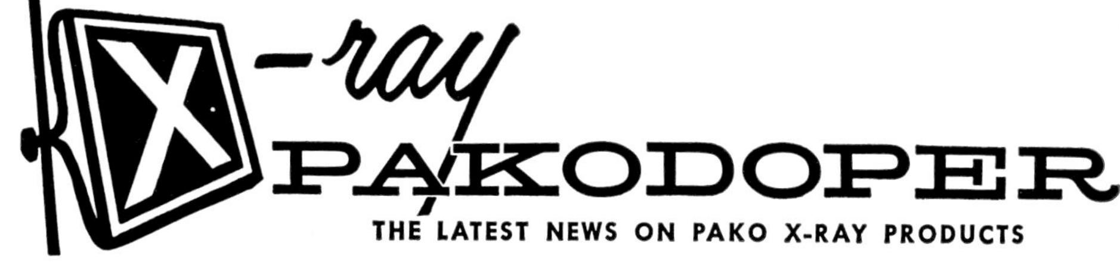

the new Pakorol). Now "hot" solutions are beginning to be used in non-automatic processors (Oscar Fisher's Fastanx), a long-known procedure which has recently found new friends (*cf.*, Robert Moreton in *Radiology* of March, 1963).

SOLUTIONS

The Atomic Phase had its impact even on processing chemicals, in part because of automation, but also because of the desire to reduce exposure times.

Roller type processors have apparently three common difficulties, developer deposits on the rollers, excessive foam, and improper hardening, with consequent softening, sticking, or edge frilling. Soon a softened film gets stuck, and the machine has to be stopped.

These difficulties can be obviated (to a large extent) by the use of special chemicals. The Philip A. Hunt Co. of Palisades Park (New Jersey) founded in 1909, sells the Graph-O-Mat developer and fixer, compounded especially for roller type processors. Of course, Eastman-Kodak offers its brand of chemicals, prepared for the same purpose.

"Hotter" developers — more concentrated solutions, perhaps less bromide, with anti-fog agent added — have been offered as a means of reducing radiation exposure in the conventional (tank type of) processing.

Picker sells the "heated" PIX, GE the Supermix, or MED (Medium Exposure Developer).

Changing solutions is messy and time-consuming, which explains the postwar growth of XSS (X-Ray Solutions Services), the advertising organ for several firms, among which the largest is Albert Acan (whose anti-foggant is called Raydene). But automation is now the catchword, so Acan sells a $6,000 roller processor made by Harper. This prompted Eastman to put on the market just as cheap a model — there will soon be a processor in every backyard.

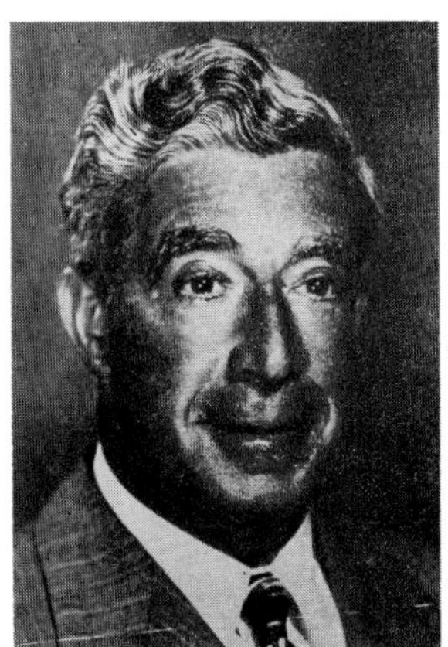

Courtesy: *The Philip A. Hunt Company.*

PHILIP ARTHUR HUNT. Born in New York City, was placed in an orphanage at age 6, earned his own living at thirteen, ten years later – in 1909 – founded the Hunt Company, which today claims to be the "largest exclusive manufacturer and supplier of photographic chemicals." The Graphidone activator chemical system (said to prevent the degradation of the developing agent) is one of the contributions to rapid processing chemistry coming from the Hunt Company's research. Hunt products are now being used in twenty or so countries. Philip Hunt died in a car accident.

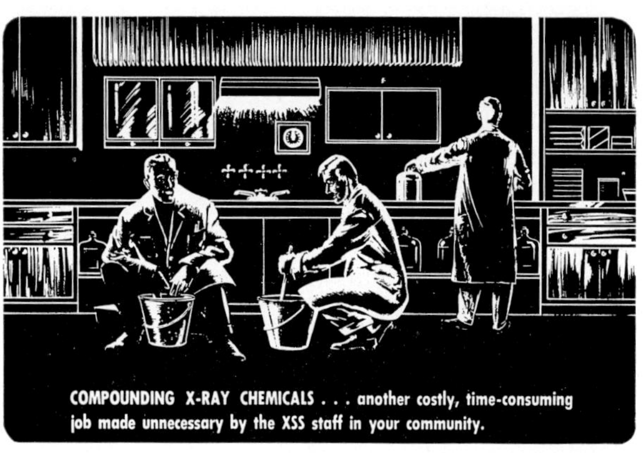

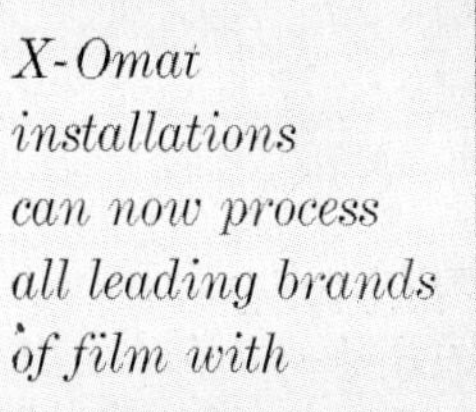

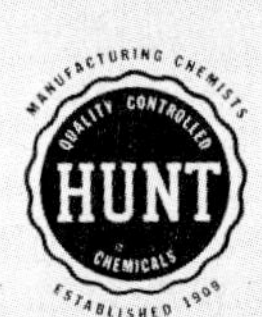

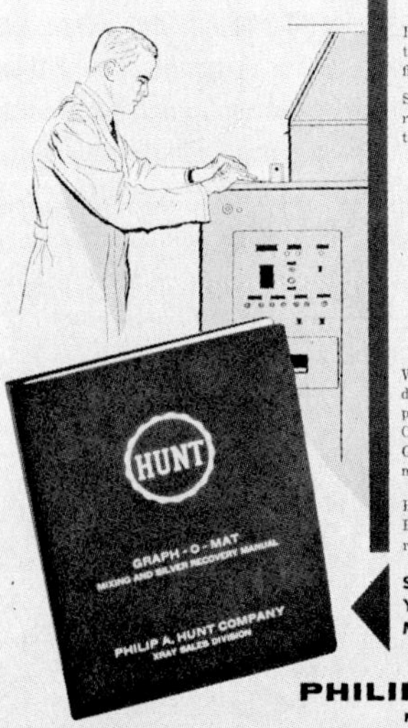

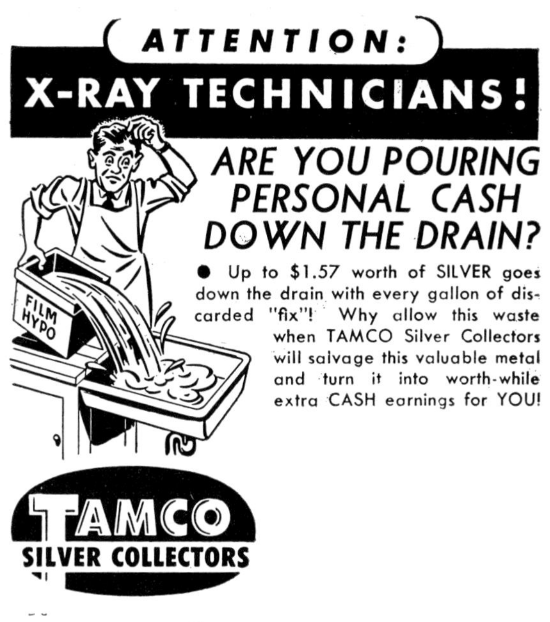

In your negotiations, be sure that you retain your silver rights! Remember—the silver earnings will be YOURS . . . .or theirs!

TAMCO
ULTRAMATIC

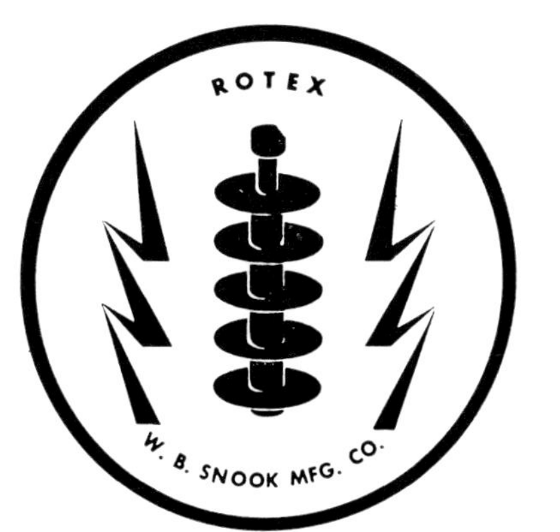

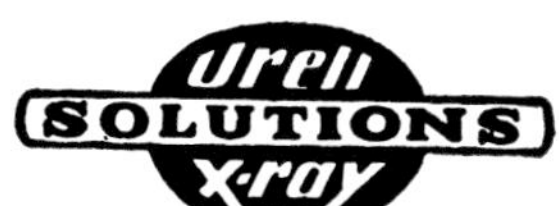

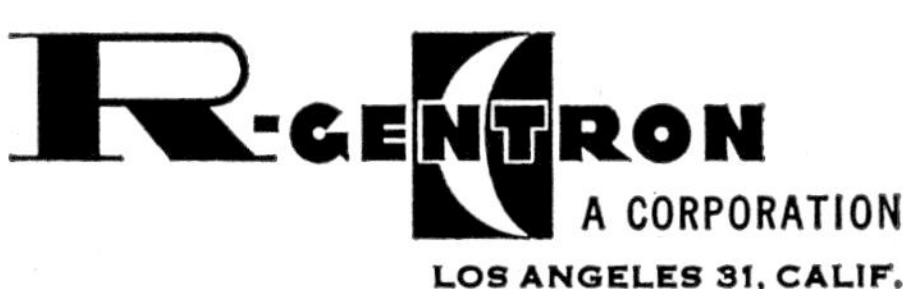

Advertised for a long time was the silver collector of the States Smelting & Refining Companies of Lima (Ohio). In 1954, their ads were asking, "Are you pouring personal cash down the drain?" Many must have heeded that warning, because in 1959 their trade-mark TAMCO Ultramatic showed dollar signs floating about a happy face.

The W. B. Snook Mfg. Co. of Palo Alto (California) has been formed by Walter Bonnard Snook for the marketing of an angiographic cassette changer (production now discontinued) and of various models of Rotex, for electrolytic recovery of silver from hypo. Both the changer and the Rotex had been developed with the active participation of Charles Duisenberg, a radiologist from Palo Alto. There is no kinship between Walter Snook and Homer Snook, and no connection between this Snook Mfg. Co. and the old Philadelphia firm by the same name.

On the West Coast, solution services are offered by Urell, Inc., of Los Angeles. Urell developed a silver-saving-system with a peculiar trade-mark, R-Gentron. The explanation for that trade-mark, offered by Howard Lewin (of both Urell and R-Gentron), is as follows:

"1. The Latin name for silver is Argentum.
2. The alchemical symbol for silver is the crescent moon.
3. 'Tron' as a suffix always (today) connotes electromechanical apparatuses.
4. To belabor the play on words, we feel that the name is rather suggestive of Konrad Roentgen's patronymic."

XERO-RADIOGRAPHY

The fact that certain insulators, for instance selenium, when x-irradiated, become relatively good conductors of electricity, is the basis of a new method of recording x-ray images. It is called xero-radiography from the Greek term *xeros* (dry), because dry pigments are used to "reveal" the image after x-ray exposure.

Xerography is a dry photographic process invented in 1937 by Chester F. Carlson, a patent attorney and physicist in New York City. Exclusive rights to Carlson's xerographic patents were acquired in 1944 by the Battelle Development Corporation in Columbus (Ohio). In 1947 the Harold Company of Rochester (New York) sponsored further developments of xerography as an office-copying procedure, and was granted a sublicense under the Battelle-Carlson patents. The first 100 units of the commercial version appeared on the market in 1950. The commercial aspects have been taken over by the Xerox Corporation, and the method has since been widely accepted in the libraries of industrial as well as scientific organizations.

As recounted by Robert C. McMaster in the Summer, 1951 issue of *Non-Destructive Testing*, x-ray applications of xerography were proposed in Carlson's early patents, and were recognized early in the research at Battelle. At that institute, William E. Bixby and Michael D. Phillips developed xero-radiography into a practicable procedure. The first step is the sensitization of the special plate. That plate consists of a thin layer of sensitive photo-insulator on a suitable conducting backing plate. Sensitization means deposition of a uniform layer of electrical charge on the outer surface of the plate, which is done by moving above its surface a fine wire maintained at a high potential. Next comes the exposure to x-radiation, which produces a change in the sensitive layer (relative conductivity) resulting in surface charge leaks to the backing plate. This leaking is proportional to the local exposure to x rays, thus an image can be formed when the absorption of an interposed object causes differences in the intensity of transmitted x rays. The latent electrostatic image may be revealed by any physical process capable of depositing a pigmented powder in proportion to the charge density, surface potential, or field strength. In practice this is done by exposing the plate to a cloud of charged powder particles, or cascading over the plate a two-component dry developer. The powder particles cling to the charged areas, thereby bringing out the latent image. The powder image can be viewed in this condition, but for storage it must be made "permanent," either by an adhesive transfer method (like the one used to record magnetic-particle images in non-destructive testing), or by the electrostatic image transfer (with subsequent "fixation" of the pigment to the paper, as by heating).

Xero-radiography gives peculiar images, with an unusual wealth of soft tissue detail. Indeed, they have been used in mammography (see *American Journal of Roentgenology* of August, 1960). The plates will respond to x rays in any range, even in the 20 and 30 mev level emitted by betatrons, and have applications in industrial radiography, described in the May-June, 1955 issue of *Non-Destructive Testing*. Since the non-sensitized xero-radiographic plates are insensitive to light or x radiation, storage in that condition may be of significance under disaster conditions. But there are as of today still very serious limitations in the medical application of xero-radiography. The marketing of xero-radiographic equip-

Courtesy: Xerox Corporation.

Xero-radiograph I. This skull and spine were exposed at 45″, 75 mas, and 95 kvp with no bucky diaphragm.

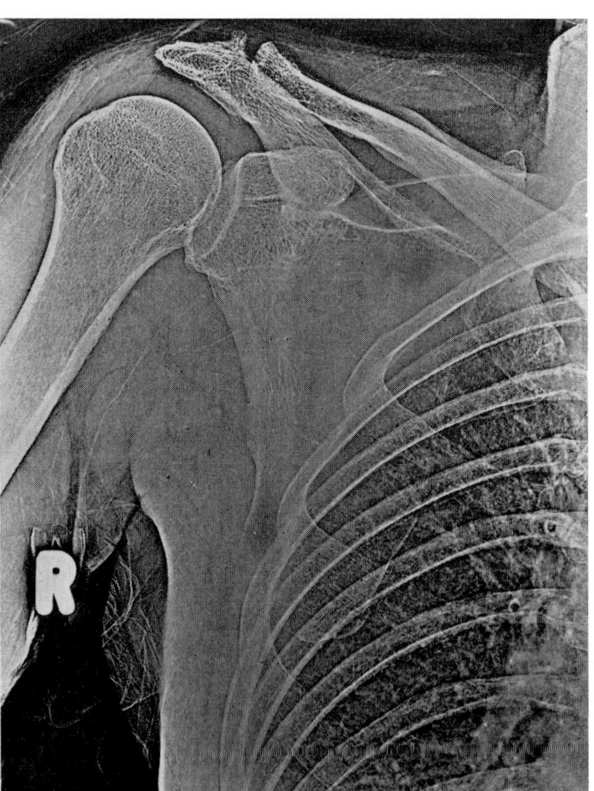

Courtesy: Xerox Corporation.

Xero-radiograph II. Exposure was made with 12:1 bucky diaphragm at 40″, 100 kvp and 75 mas. Note the excellent visualization of axillary hair and other soft tissue details – there was no retouching.

ment is in the hands of General Electric, under license to Xerox Corporation.

ONOMASTICON OF OPAQUE OFFERINGS

Future generations might find it difficult to assemble a list of contrast media used at the beginning of the Atomic Phase. The following compilation contains certain semantic peculiarities, as characteristic for the respective manufacturer as his trade-mark. These peculiarities also exemplify various adaptations

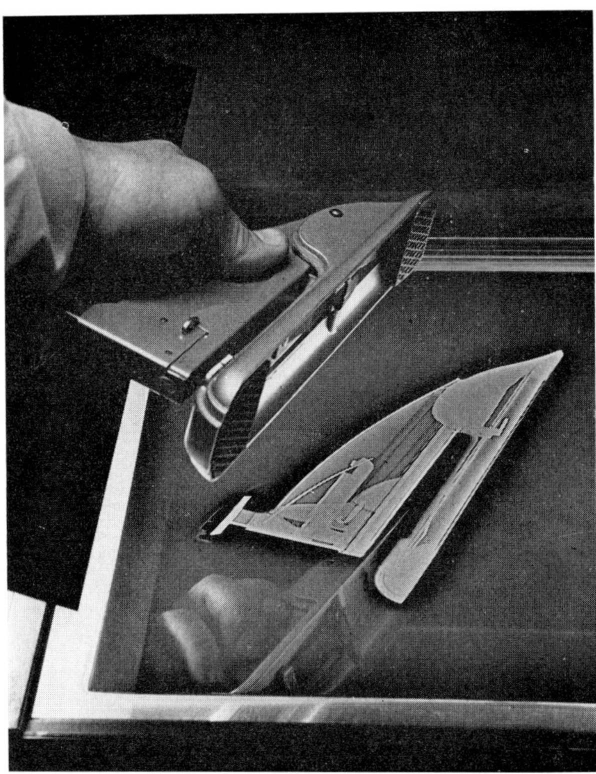

Courtesy: Xerox Corporation.

INDUSTRIAL XERO-RADIOGRAPH.

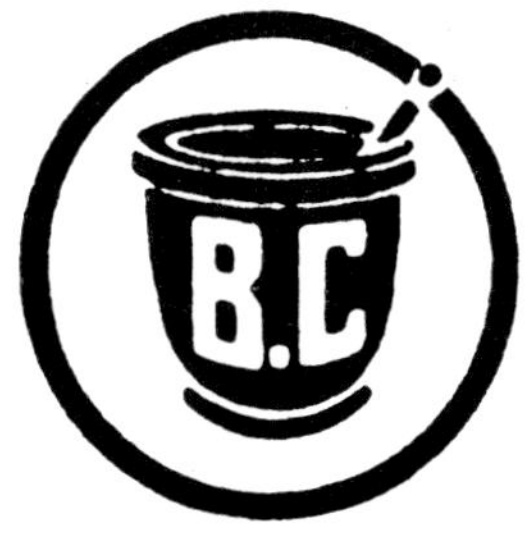

BELL-CRAIG, INC.

"Dependability Through the Years"

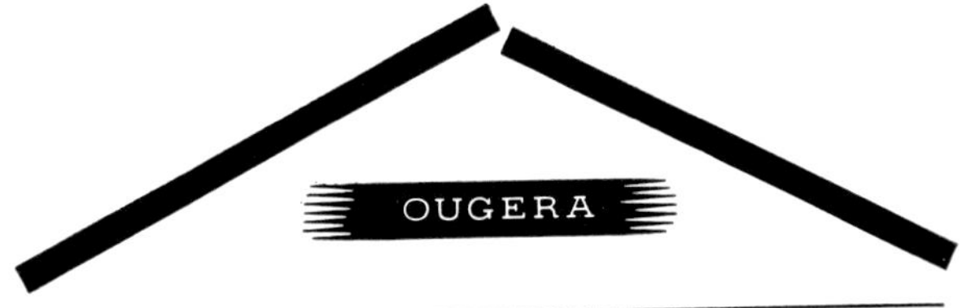

A HOUSE SERVING THE RADIOLOGIST

LIPIODOL® . . . . multi-purpose diagnostic
ETHIODOL® . . . . low viscosity contrast medium
VISCIODOL® . . . contrast medium for bronchography
ORABILEXT.M. . . . . . oral cholecystographic medium
COLO-BART.M. . . . . ready-to-eat gallbladder evacuant

HYTRAST®

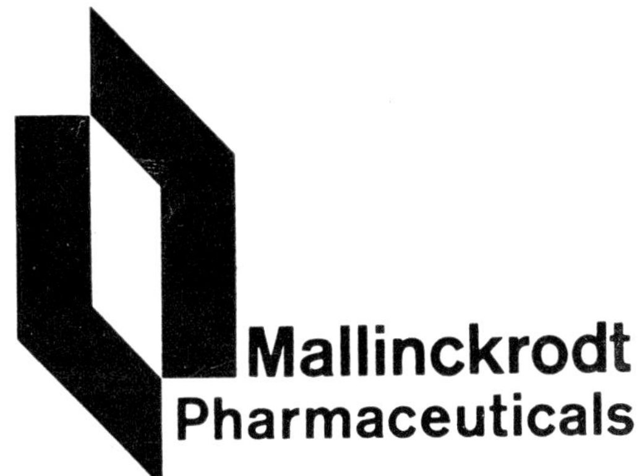

CONRAY®

(MEGLUMINE IOTHALAMATE 60%)
For intravenous urography

ANGIO-CONRAY®

(SODIUM IOTHALAMATE 80%)
For intravascular angiocardiography and aortography

of radiologic catchwords, and are therefore of etymologic consequence, which justifies their inclusion in this semantic treatise.

Bell-Craig of New York City compounds the Neo-Cholex, which is a fatty meal for cholecystography, and Medopaque-H, used in hystero-salpingography and in peroperative cholangiography.

E. Fougera & Co. of Hicksville (Long Island) is an American firm founded in the 19th century by a French immigrant. Many of their radiologic products are manufactured under license from André Guerbet. There is the Lipiodol Lafay, of which the newer version contains sulfanilamide and is called Visciodol. Fougera's newest bronchographic material is Hy-Trast. Their "uterine" lipiodol is named Ethiodol. A few years ago they introduced Orabilex, an oral cholescystographic substance which has recently been "removed" from the market.

Pantopaque is a heavy organic iodinated compound used in myelography. It was synthesized by the Eastman Kodak Research Laboratories, and is being marketed by the Lafayette Pharmacol. The latter's latest contrast material is a colloidal and otherwise "medicated" barium suspension, the Intropaque, prepared according to the formula recommended by Roscoe Miller

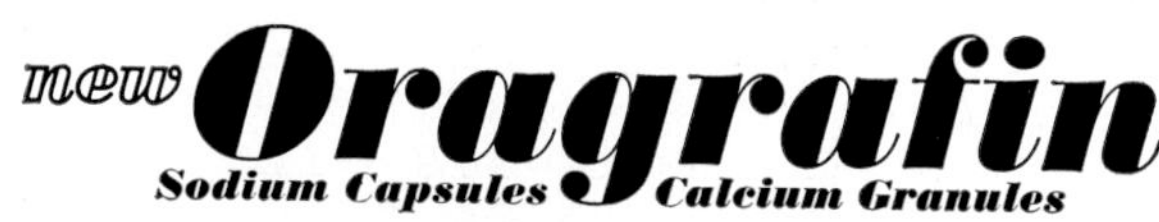

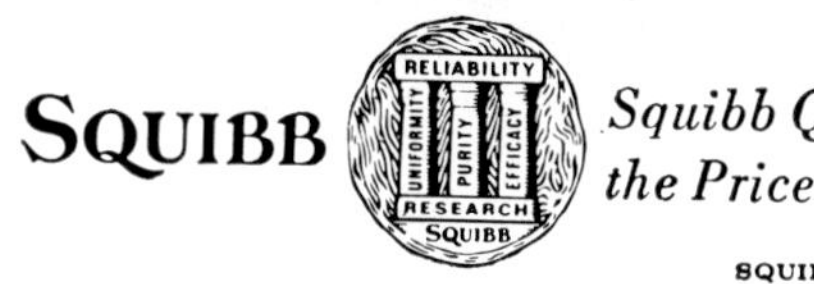

Squibb Quality – the Priceless Ingredient

SQUIBB DIVISION Olin

Now available

Thorotrast

(STABILIZED COLLOIDAL THORIUM DIOXIDE SOL.)

ROENTGENOLOGICAL CONTRAST MEDIA

A sterile, stabilized, highly dispersed solution of thorium dioxide. Thorotrast contains 24% to 26% thorium dioxide (by volume) suspended in 25% aqueous, repurified tapioca-dextrin 3219 plus 0.15% methylparaben as a preservative.

THOROTRAST IS HIGHLY RADIOPAQUE AND WILL PRODUCE SATISFACTORY OPACIFICATION OF THE CIRCULATORY VESSELS

Superior Diagnostic Value In . . .

THOROTRAST is relied upon in the performance of cerebral arteriography in patients who have arteriosclerosis or who are sensitive to iodine.

THOROTRAST is useful in locating and outlining cerebral abscesses and tumors; for the determination of cerebral arteriosclerosis and other atheromatous processes of the encephalo-arteries.

Arteriography with THOROTRAST discloses vascular abnormalities in suspect cases. THOROTRAST will visualize the location of a thrombus or embolism, as well as the development of collateral circulation. Arteriovenous aneurysm is readily demonstrated.

GREATER CONTRAST VALUE

SUPPLIED: in Sterile Vials, 12 cc., 25 cc., 100 cc.

Literature available upon request.

Testagar
& COMPANY, INC.
DETROIT 26, MICH.

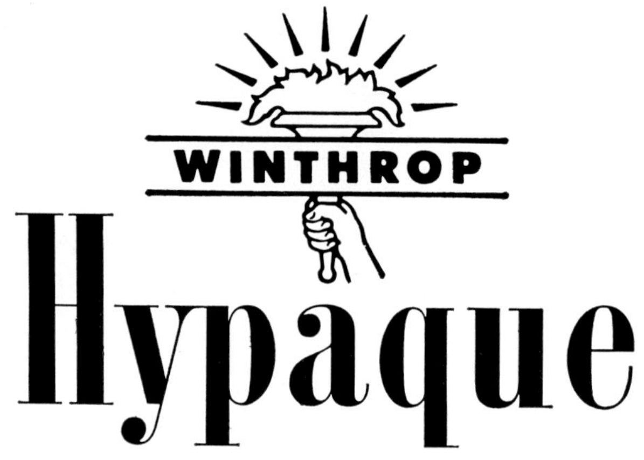

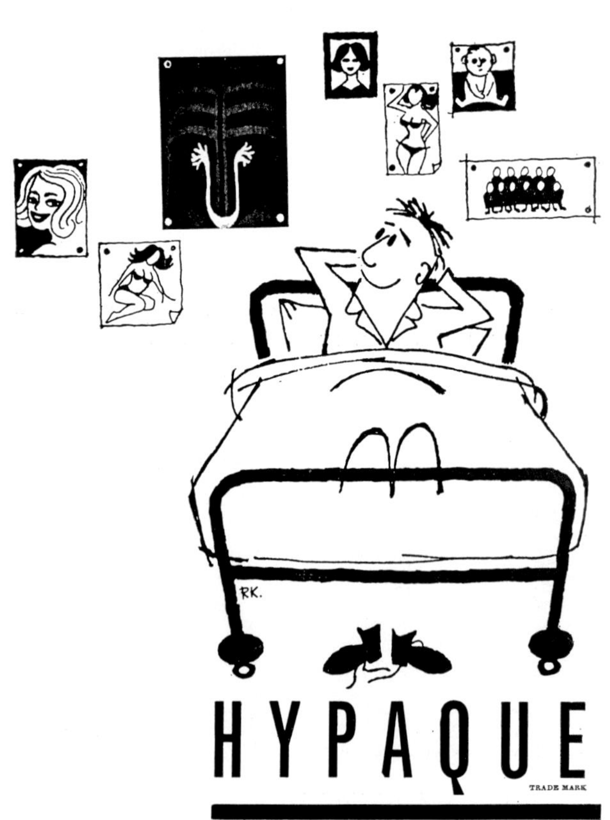

in the Department of Radiology of the University of Indiana.

Mallinckrodt Pharmaceuticals is a division of Mallinckrodt Chemical Works (founded in 1867) of St. Louis. The division was formed in 1913, and as a reminder of that date, they recently mailed to each radiologist a photoprint of the first issue of the *American Journal of Roentgenology,* originally printed as of November, 1913. In the beginning, Mallinckrodt Pharmaceuticals also sold photographic processing chemicals, but now they concentrate — in the radiologic field — on contrast media. Mallinckrodt's radio-etymon is *con* or *kon* (presumably from *con*trast). They had Miokon for intravenous urography, Pyelokon-R for retrograde examinations, Thixokon for uretrography, Urokon and Ditriokon for angiocardiography and other vascular opacifications. Their latest is Conray — with its winged derivate Angio-Conray. The firm is mindful of its tradition — their address is Second and Mallinckrodt Streets — and has therefore created and subsidized the Mallinckrodt Institute of Radiology, and is actively (*i.e.,* financially) supporting the ACR's attempts to create an American Museum of Radiology.

E. R. Squibb & Sons of New York City (now a division of OLIN) use *grafin* as the basic term. Renografin is for intravenous urography. Retrografin for retrogrades, and Cardiografin (a concentrated Renografin) and Renovist are used in angioroentgenography (their spelling). Cholografin is an intravenous cholangiographic medium. The intravenous Duografin, the (same-day) Oragrafin, opacifies in one shot both the renal and the biliary systems. Finally, Sinografin is used in sinuses, and for hysterosalpinography.

The Ortho Pharmaceutical of Raritan (New Jersey) makes the water-soluble Salpix for hystero-salpingography.

Schering of Bloomfield (New Jersey) had the cholecystographic medium Priodax, which it replaced with the (now also obsolete) Teridax. Their intravenous urographic substance is called Neo-Iopax.

Despite the adverse publicity given to the development of malignancies from delayed retention of radio-

BARIUM SULPHATE "M.C.W."
FOR X-RAY DIAGNOSIS

A soft, smooth, highly purified product, free from Soluble Barium Salts, Arsenic and other impurities, and is offered as a superior article in every respect for X-Ray Technique.

"M.C.W." PHOTOGRAPHIC CHEMICALS FOR X-RAY
including SODIUM SULPHITE ANHYDROUS PHOTO, SODIUM CARBONATE PURE PHOTO, PYROGALLIC ACID, HYDROQUINONE and other articles used in X-RAY photography.

SPECIFY "M. C. W." ORIGINAL PACKAGES

MALLINCKRODT CHEMICAL WORKS
ST. LOUIS NEW YORK
COMPLETE LIST ON REQUEST AJR 1919

visualization beyond the shadow of a doubt

Telepaque®
brand of iopanoic acid
well-tolerated medium for oral cholecystography and cholangiography

- gallbladder shadows with distinctly better contrast
- greater visualization of ducts
- no disturbance of gallbladder physiology
- convenient, economical administration

Supplied: Tablets of 500 mg., envelopes of 6 tablets, boxes of 5 and 25 envelopes; also bottles of 500.
Before administering consult Winthrop's literature for information about dosage, possible side effects and contraindications.

Winthrop LABORATORIES, NEW YORK 18, N.Y.

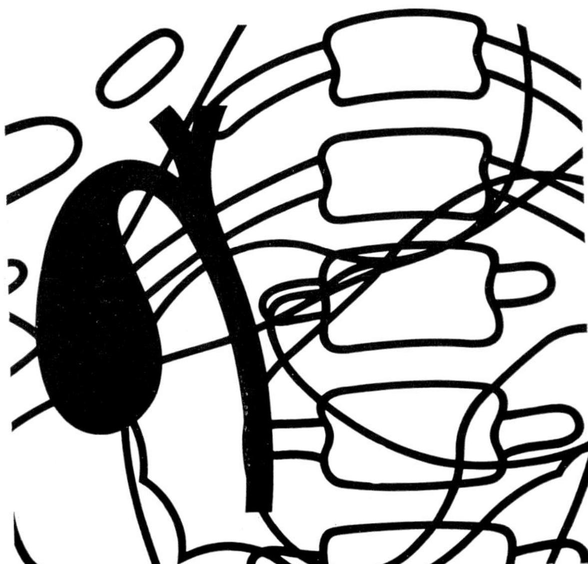

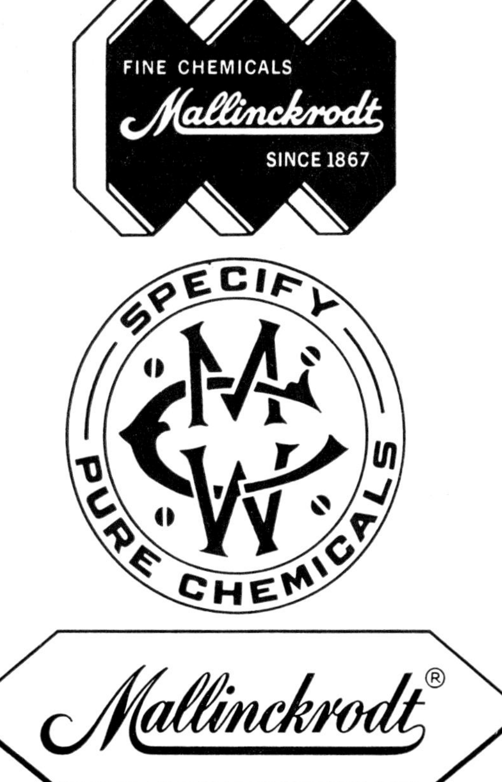

active Thorium, Thorotrast and Umbrathor (both containing Thorium dioxide) were advertised in 1957 by Testagar & Co. of Detroit. In 1964, the FDA ordered these substances removed from open commercial channels.

The Winthrop Laboratories of New York City sell Telepaque for per-oral cholecystography. They have replaced their Diodrast with Hypaque, which comes in various concentrations for various tasks, from intravenous urography to angio-cardiography. In this country Winthrop's ads carried for a while the portrait of Leonardo Da Vinci's Mona Liza as a comparison with the visualization obtained by using their contrast media. In Great Britain, a more lively, cartoon type of approach is used. Winthrop has also Skiodan, employed in urethro-cystography, and in the investigation of fistulae.

Barium sulfate can be purchased in its U. S. Pharmacopia version – in that way it has been packed by Mallinckrodt for almost half-a-century. A flavored brand, sold only by Buck, called Gastropaque, (allegedly) tastes very well. The "micronized" Barotrast, for use in double contrast examinations of the colon, is made by the Barnes-Hind Barium Products of Sunnyvale (California). A similar product is Picker's Micropaque (imported from England).

There exist special preparations, which have the consistency of peanut butter – such as McKesson's Rugar—intended for the delineation of folds. But that is something different from the current fad for "stabilized," "colloidal," "homogenized" barium suspensions. And when this fad began to cut into the sales of plain barium sulfate, even Mallinckrodt decided to join the fun, and announced its own Barosperse. A few years back, while still at the University of Chicago, Paul Hodges enlisted the aid of a biochemist (who specialized in colloids), and they decided that there was no advantage in using anything beyond plain barium sulfate. Maybe in a few years we will once more become convinced of the futility of trying to "micronize" the barium, but it would be more futile to plead that angle today.

The conventional barium suspension, even when stirred just before giving the enema, often separates, and the barium gravitates to the lower level, below the supernatant clear water. In the stomach this may be misinterpreted as retained secretions (don't accuse the patient of having eaten just before the examination, unless you have more evidence than that). Howard Steinbach and Joachim Burhenne (from the University of California in San Francisco) have studied the various micronized preparations (*cf.* the *American Journal of Roentgenology* of April, 1962). They favored Barotrast over Baraloid (Bell-Craig) and Baridol (Pacific-

Chemical). They finally measured several preparations with the Ba-test Areometer (sold by Svenska-Philips of Stockholm), and decided that liquid Micropaque (from the English firm Damancy & Co. of Ware) is just as "stable" as the Umbaryt C (from the German firm Rohn & Haas of Darmstadt.) Steinbach and Burhenne stressed the advantages of the disposable BE (Barium enema) Bag, made by Walker in Evanston (Illinois). Similar appliances are made by Travenol (a subsidiary of Baxter Laboratories in Morton Grove (Illinois) and by E-Z-EM of Long Island.

Excessive gas and other bowel contents cause shadows which may obscure most any roentgen examination in the abdomen. The classic method for removing these "shadows" is to give the (indestructible) castor oil, followed by cleansing enemata. The variety of alternate agents advertised for this purpose indicates that the perfect preparation procedure is still wanting.

The Lederle Laboratories of Pearl River (New York) has Neoloid, which is an emulsified castor oil preparation.

The Fleet Co. of Lynchburg (Virginia) offers several versions of its (retention) Fleet Enema.

Geigy Pharmaceuticals of Ardsley (New Jersey) sells the Dulcolax, which is an import from Germany.

Winthrop of New York City recommends the Lavema (a disposable retention enema container).

X-Prep is the name of the compound sold by the Gray Pharmaceutical Co. of New York City.

Most interesting is the brand name Roenten — a faintly sacrilegious combination derived from the title of its maker, the Brayten Pharmaceutical Company of Chattanooga (Tennessee).

CONTRAST CONQUERED

In 1953, Dwin R. Craig developed the first LogEtronic Contact Printer with automatic dodging and automatic exposure control for use in copying the "flat" negatives which are so common in aerial photography.

LogEtronics, Inc. was formed in Alexandria (Virginia) with Richard A. Johnson as president and Craig as technical Director. By 1959, their contact printers were selling in twenty countries and manufacture of LogEtronic equipment had begun both in England and France, with more than 300 units in operation around the globe.

Just as in fluoroscopic image intensification, it adds no details to the original negative. Existing details can be saved from a low contrast picture, and "brought out" through electronic modulation. This may be of value in microradiography, in press photography, in microscopic reproductions, and in conventional radiography, both medical and (especially) industrial.

Radiographic reproductions subjected to LogEtronics reveal more details, but they also have a peculiar, artificial appearance resembling the "plastic" pictures of two generations ago.

Another method of contrast enhancement was first described in June, 1957 in the *Journal of the Albert Einstein Medical Center* by J. F. Fisher (an engineer of the Philco Corporation of Philadelphia) and J. Gershon-Cohen (a radiologist at the Center).

The apparatus, called Exicon, is a television system which will enlarge selected areas from any x-ray film and by appropriate electronic controls can bring them in much better contrast on the (monochromatic) monitor.

In *Radiology* of March, 1958, the same authors described an Exicon which improved recognition of image

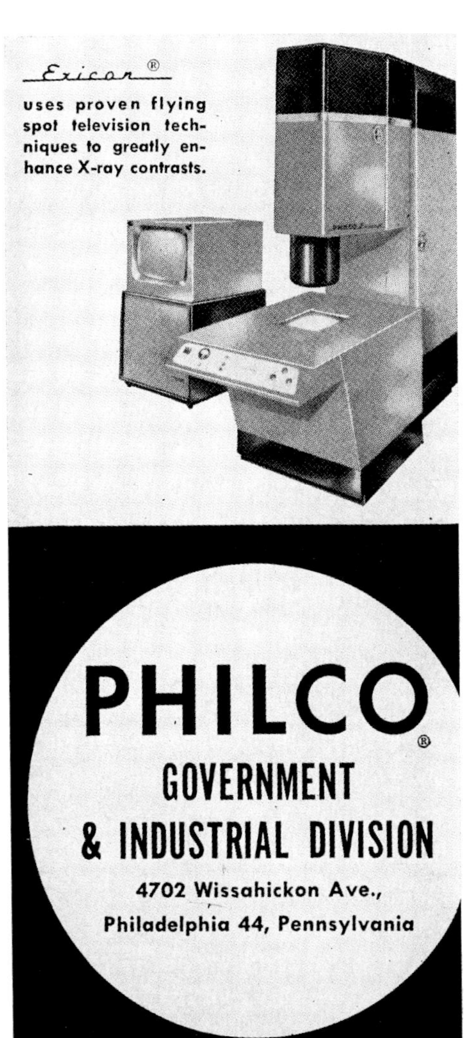

details by "translating" existing, even minute differences in contrast into television colors. And just as in color prints the polychromatic effect on the television screen permitted a certain depth perception.

MISCELLANEA

Several unrelated items will now be mentioned, mostly but not always because of their semantic connotation.

Disposable plastic enema tips are now available from several sources. The initial promotion of this item was made by Bell-Craig under the name of Cly-Tips – their latest "spiel" is that they can be furnished in decorator colors. Wolf X-Ray Products, which manufactures darkroom and related x-ray accessories, called their version N-ema Tips.

Wolf brought out the "Magic-Grip" consisting of a viewbox with tiny ball bearing rollers which hold the film in place without external support – the slogan says "flip it to grip it." This was extensively imitated, and a "poor man's version" was manufactured with a spring replacing the rollers; when the spring weakens, it "herniates" and goes "kaput."

Westinghouse manufactures a barium fountain, called the Bariumette. For the other orifice, there are various custom-built containers, which will hold (and continuously stir) 20-30 gallons of barium; by using disposable tips, enemata can be administered during an entire fluoroscopic morning without further manipulation, and with unquestionable uniformity of concentration, though without solving cross-contamination.

Television has found many applications in the medical field, for instance in microscopy. Recently, Motorola offered closed circuit television for viewing x-ray negatives (the usual films) over any of the monitors installed in the hospital. It is doubtful whether the detail (resolution) of the image is sufficient for diagnostic evaluation.

In 1947, Manoel de Abreu of Rio de Janeiro ideated and developed simultaneous tomography, which he then described in the *American Journal of Roentgenology* of November, 1948. A number of cuts are made with a single exposure. This requires proper spacing of the respective cassettes, and varied screen speed. Most screen and cassette manufacturers have offered the materials needed for this procedure, which may be called polytomography. Some of the names used are more whimsical than that. Halsey calls its cassettes the Multi-Sette (for 7 cuts) and the Multi-Sette, Jr. (for 3-5 cuts). Radelin prefers to call the method "plesiosectional tomography," for which it offers Plesiosettes (cassettes) and Plesio-Tomo screens.

There exists the Cordis Corporation in Miami (Florida), a firm organized in 1957 by a physician, Wm. P. Murphy, Jr. They manufacture instruments for use in conjunction with x-ray examinations of the cardiovascular system. They have an intercalative angiograph, a Cordis injector, a catheter pressure standard, heart pacers, and recently they added the Rotacor (designed by Manuel Viamonte, Jr., currently a radiologist in Miami), which is a power-driven cardle for rotation of the patient around his longitudinal axis. Such a de-

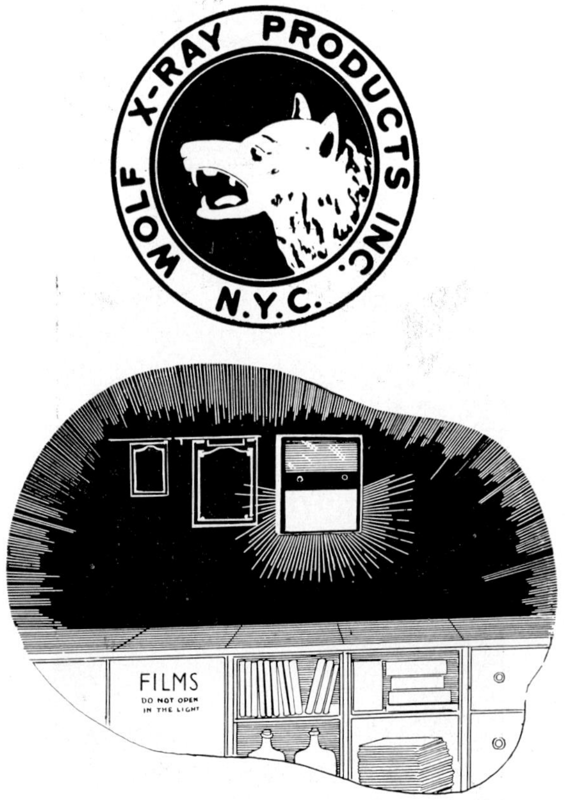

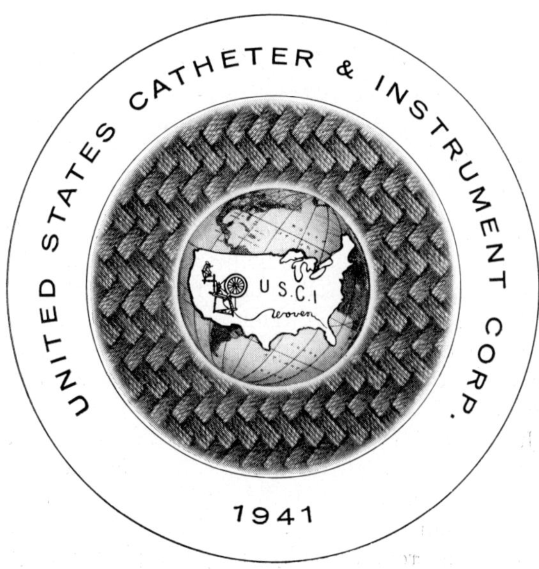

vice is not only valuable in cardiac examinations, it is quite useful in the fluoroscopy of elderly or otherwise invalid patients. This cradle is placed on top of, and fastened to, the x-ray table top.

Several firms manufacture catheters for use in the various natural and preternatural conduits of the human body. The seal of one of these firms is herein reproduced.

Very popular have become foam rubber positioning blocks which are almost completely radiolucent, warm to the touch, featherlight and also otherwise very comfortable. They are marketed by several of the companies for instance DuPont. Picker calls his brand Collo.

Picker has recently combined with Polaroid in offering the MD/RR (Minimal Dosage Rapid Radiography) in which the 3000-X Polaroid radiographic packet is used. It is a self-contained system for ten second processing of a positive image on paper. It comes as the Picker Portable Polaroid Processing Unit. The Ansco (day-light) Speed-X R processes (darkroom-loaded) single-coated "opaque base" film, viewed by reflected light. These units are useful in orthopedics, and in emergencies, but seldom achieve the detail of conventional radiography.

At this point it may be recalled that film badges have become almost an identification mark for those working in radiology (indeed, in many "atomic" installations, the badge serves both these purposes).

To conclude this section, a brand of Medical X-Ray Gloves made of lead-loaded Neoprene will be included: its manufacturer is Charco X-Ray Sales Corporation of Charleston (North Carolina), mentioned mostly because of its interesting trade-mark.

THERAPY EQUIPMENT

In this country, the design of currently available roentgen therapy equipment has changed very little in the last three decades — could this be the reason why they refer to it as apparatus?

Gustav Bucky, the developer of the first stationary grid, was also a pioneer in the development of Grenzs-Strahlen therapy, using very soft radiation (it is done today with very radiolucent Beryllium-window tubes). Bucky's son is the owner and operator of the International Medical Research Corporation (New York City), which sells the Bucky Combination Therapy Apparatus, formerly made by XRM, now by Continental.

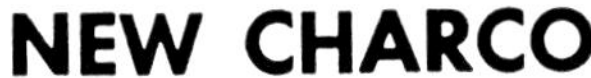

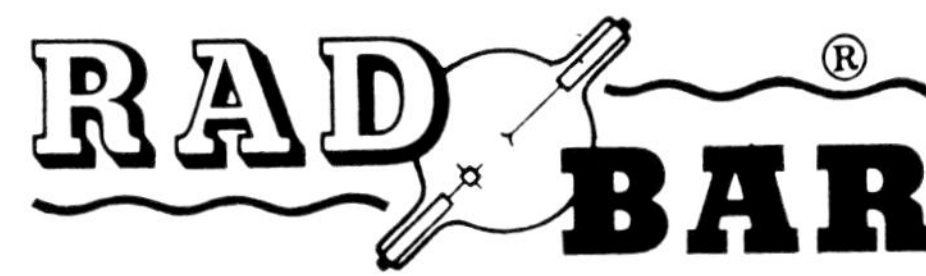

MEDICAL X-RAY GLOVES

Made of Lead – loaded Neoprene

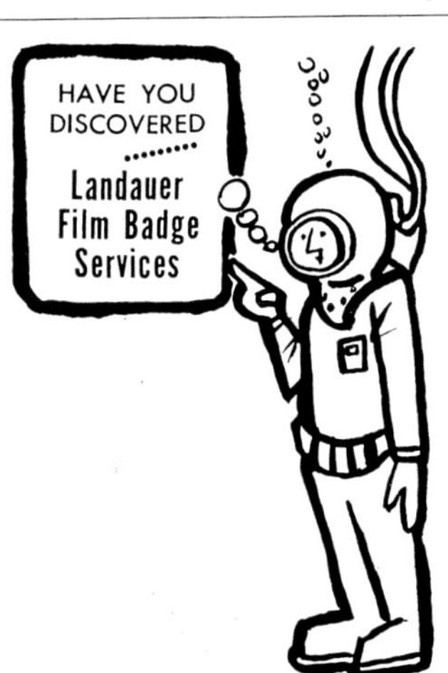

"America's Finest Film Badge Service"

BUCKY

The Pioneer Name in X-Ray announces

The BUCKY COMBINATION THERAPY APPARATUS for the RADIOLOGISTS

The one unit that fills the gap by providing all therapy modalities from a depth dosage of 140 KV down to 5 KV

INTERMEDIARY • SUPERFICIAL • CONTACT & GRENZ RAY THERAPY

Model G-3
Completely mobile, no installation needed

HIGH OUTPUT . . . . The unit can produce up to 20,000 r units per minute, and so it is ideal for:

1. Cavity therapy of all kinds. Special radiation cones are supplied for different applications.
2. Whole body radiation for the treatment of leukemia. The prescribed dosage can be given in one radiation at distances greater than 200 cm. focal-skin distance in approximately 1 minute.

SAFETY FEATURE Bucky provides positive radiation control. The safety protective automatic filter slide circuit affords the ultimate in patient protection. No radiation can be produced with this apparatus above 15 KV unless added filtration is provided. A special filter ring is provided for unfiltered radiation.

VERSATILE Unlimited field sizes for X-ray or Grenz ray therapy in one radiation can now be obtained due to high output.

EXACT DEPTH CONTROL is assured by stepless half-value layer control from 3.0 to .011 (mm. al).

ADAPTABLE Counterbalanced tube holder arm permits the positioning of the tube port in any position, without loosening or tightening any locks. No special wiring or current required since the units operate from standard house current of 110 volts on a 20 Ampere fuse.

DURABLE Long tube life guaranteed by overrating of tube voltage.

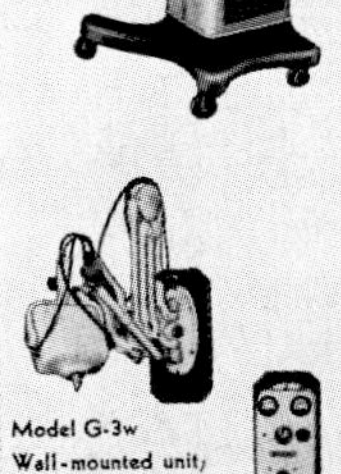

Model G-3w
Wall-mounted unit, tube holder arm and control unit installed according to your specifications. Takes up no floor space.

Write for comprehensive literature on this and time-tested BUCKY straight Grenz Ray and straight X-Ray machines.

MIR The International Medical Research Corp.
60 East 42nd Street • New York 17, N. Y.

Sales and factory-controlled Service in all major Cities and Countries

ORIGINATORS of the COMBINATION THERAPY UNIT AND GRENZ RAY THERAPY APPARATUS

It offers a depth potential from 5 through 140 kvp. This covers the gamut from *Grenzstrahlen* and contact to superficial, and well into the intermediate range.

Picker's Zephyr Minor goes up to 85 kvp, GE's Maximar-100 to 100 kvp, Standard's Ther-X to either 100 to 150 kvp. The latter comes also as a mobile unit (used at one time for irradiation of the parotid gland in cachectic oldsters).

In the 250 kvp constant potential or work-horse category are Standard's Flexray; a similar Keleket model; and Westinghouse's Coronado (which has selenium rectifiers, and replaces their demized Duoflex).

GE has the old Maximar-250 but also a newer Maxitron-250 and a newer yet Maxitron-300, none of which is a constant potential unit. A truly novel development was Picker's Vanguard, an application of the automatic "monitor" principle to roentgen therapy. They did not give the actual voltage (which was probably around 220 kvp), but the setting was in r per minute and HVL (half value layer). The machine turned itself off when the pre-set number of roentgens had been reached on the monitor placed at the radiation site. Later models utilized for support twin telescopic ceiling mounts.

The largest x-ray transformer in this category remains GE's Maxitron 2 mev. Over the years it proved to be a very dependable tool, though expensive and demanding as regards building requirements for the initial installation. Contrary to radio-isotopic teletherapy units, the Maxitron can be "unplugged" at

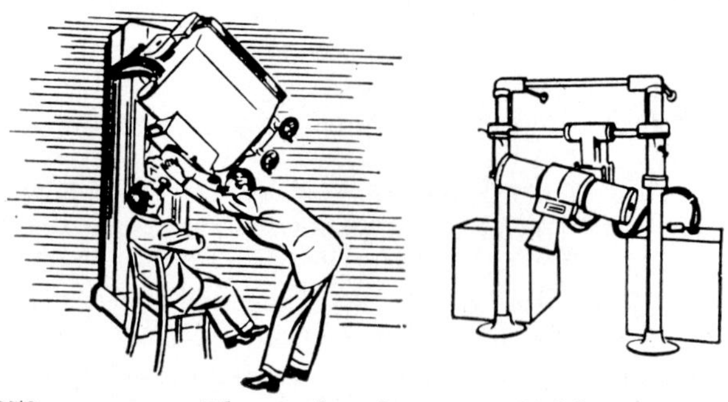

250 KVP UNITS. The single-column is a Keleket version of GE's Maximar 250, with about the same factors: it was issued in the late 1940's and did not survive the move from Kentucky to Boston. The twin-column is Standard's resilient Flexray, a work-horse whichever way you look at it.

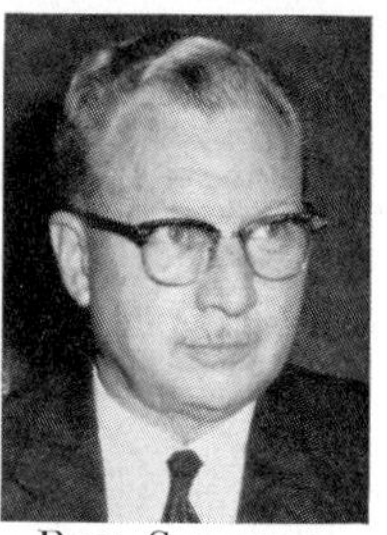

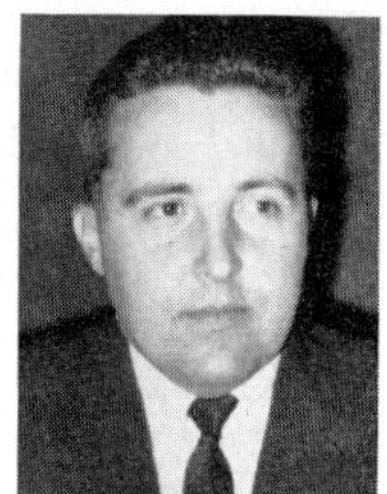

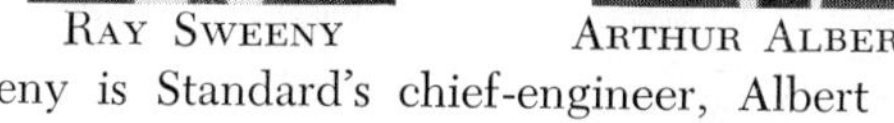

RAY SWEENY ARTHUR ALBERT, JR.

Sweeny is Standard's chief-engineer, Albert the vice-president in charge of sales.

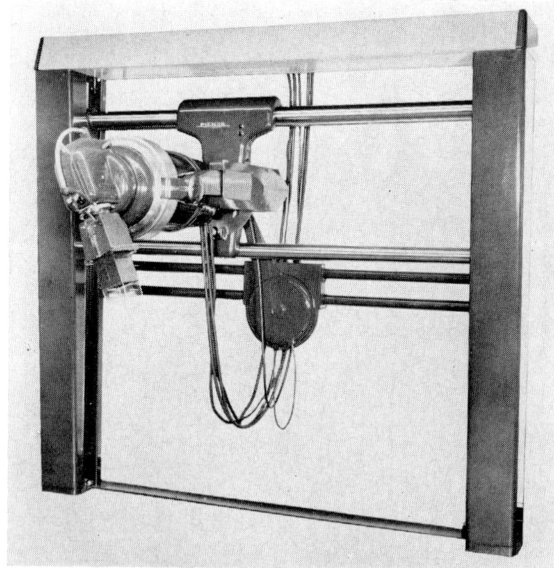

PICKER VANGUARD: turning itself off after reaching pre-set r-level.

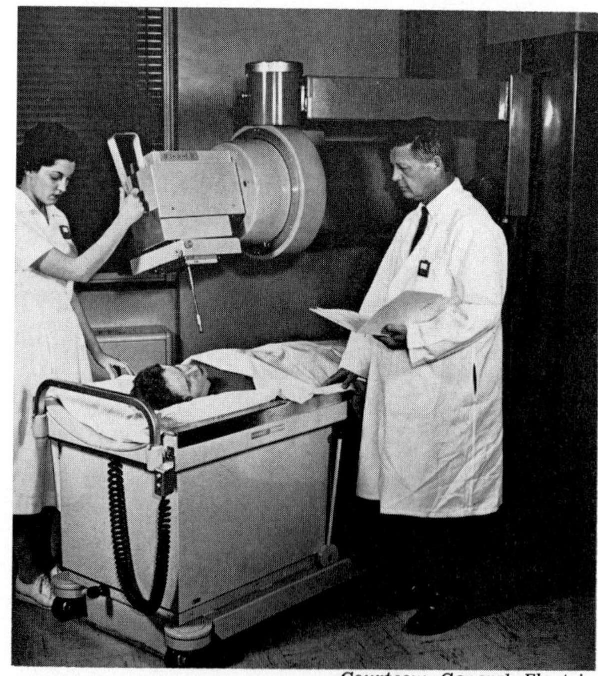

Courtesy: General Electric.

GE's MAXITRON 300. A relatively new (modern-looking) style, but the "innards" are similar to, and as reliable as, those of the Maximar 250.

any time, simply by flicking a switch!

But quite significant is the fact that "radiotherapeutic" advertisements of anti-emetic drugs display in the background very unconventional equipment. Tigan - a product of Roche Laboratories (division of Hoffmann-La Roche) - comes with what resembles a GE Maximar 400. Bonadoxin - a product of Roerig (division of Charles Pfizer) - sports a rotating cobalt unit. Copywriters are quite adept at re-creating the most acceptable public image: their choices would seem to indicate that - all the statements to the contrary notwithstanding - the 250 kvp unit is losing ground, and could hardly qualify as the current "work-horse" in radiotherapy.

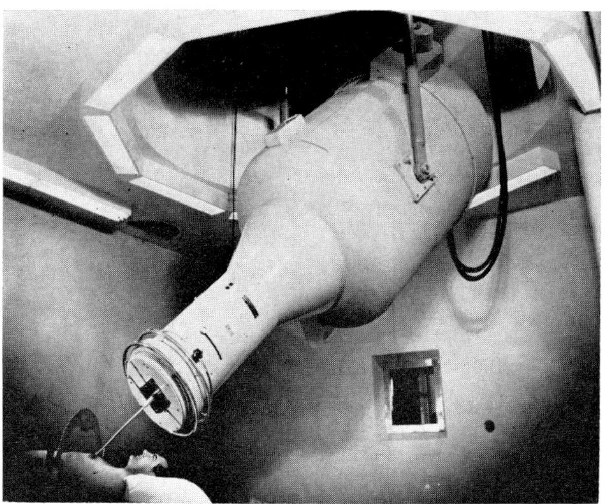

Courtesy: General Electric.

GE's MAXITRON 2000. This 2 mev unit was first introduced in 1944, it is quite dependable, and can be "unplugged" with the flick of a switch. Co-60 units do not have the latter but so many other advantages that they practically prevail in the range between 0.5 and 3 mev. Above that a small betatron may be the better buy.

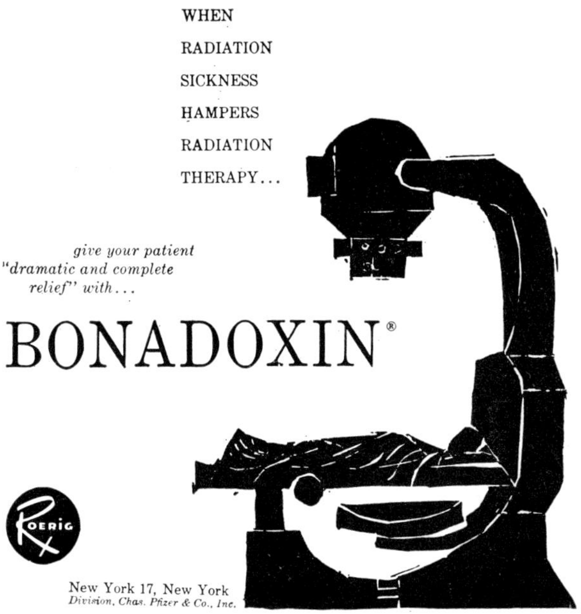

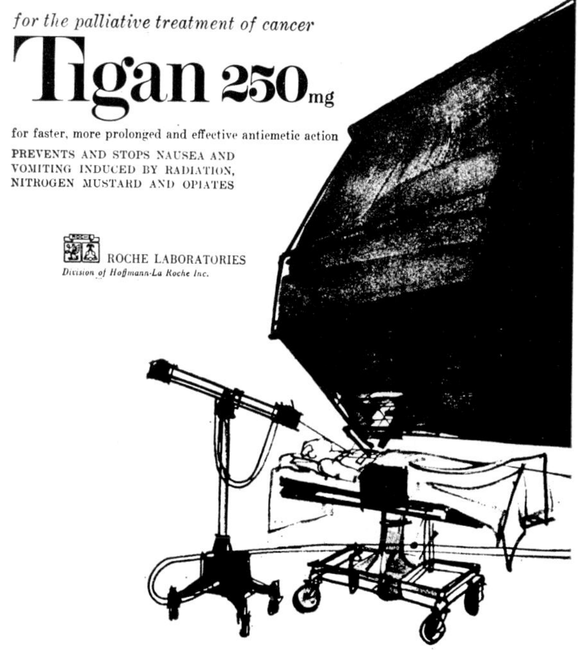

LEASING

Fusion devices (H-bombs) are being stock-piled as a deterrent to enemy attack. This is an expensive proposition, for which taxes have remained high. With the existing tax structure, leasing of all sorts of equipment became a way of preserving capital, while the lease is fully tax-deductible as an operating

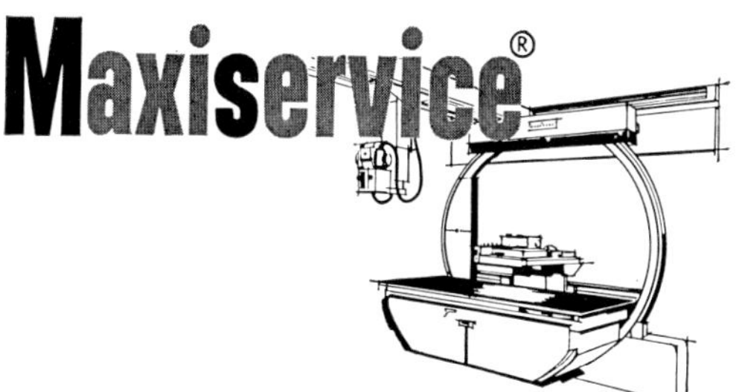

Now–lease the General Electric X-Ray equipment of your choice, including the Imperial II, through the exclusive Maxiservice plan

expense. However remote, leasing may thus be regarded as a product of the Atomic Phase.

GE's Maxiservice plan has been the first to provide such investment-free x-ray equipment. But that is the only "free" thing about it because the monthly rental is quite expensive. GE maintains the equipment in functional condition, except for damages due to carelessness or similar events.

Shortly after this innovation on the part of GE, Picker began to ask courteously of his potential clients: ". . . if you'd rather rent your x-ray apparatus . . .?" Standard's advertisements confirmed peremptorily: ". . . you can lease *our* equipment!"

Very recently GE is trying a new method which may be good news. It is their PMS (Planned Maintenance Service), contracted on a year-round basis. Only experience and time will tell if it is actuarially sound at the current premium level, or whether the premiums will have to be increased until they price themselves out of the market.

ODD ADS

Quite a bit of advertising copy had to be perused for this survey of the American x-ray manufacturing industry. In the process, several unusual or amusing, and a few impertinent advertisements were discovered.

In *Radiology* of November, 1945 Du Pont referred to a Patterson fluorescent screen, and fluted, "Too bad Roentgen never saw *this* screen. . ."

The 50th anniversary of the ARRS was marked in 1950 publication of "golden" issues of the *American Journal of Roentgenology*. On that occasion, several manufacturers committed historic *gaffes*. Standard, for instance, reproduced in its 1950 ad the picture of the Standard Interrupterless advertised in the first number of the *Journal of Roentgenology* of 1918 – implying that the *Journal of Roentgenology* was the same thing as the *American Journal of Roentgenology*. Actually, as we have seen, there were hard feelings at that time

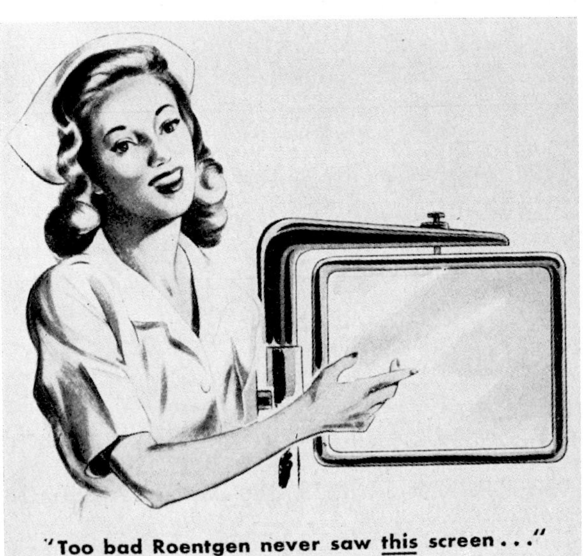

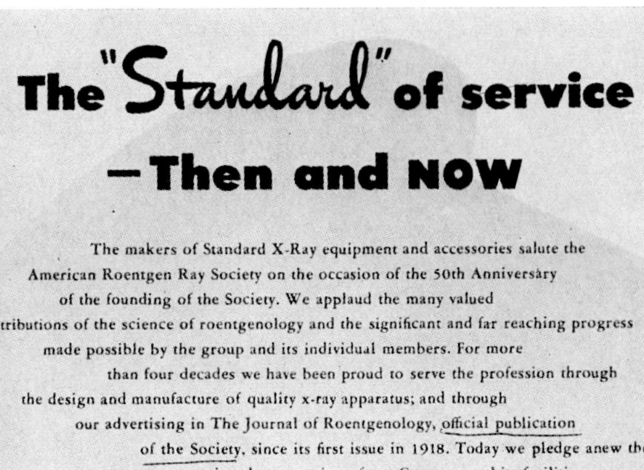

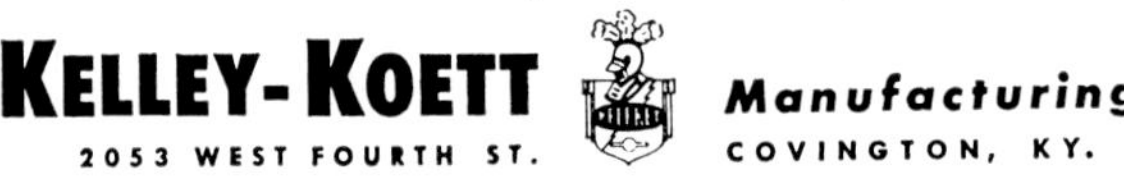

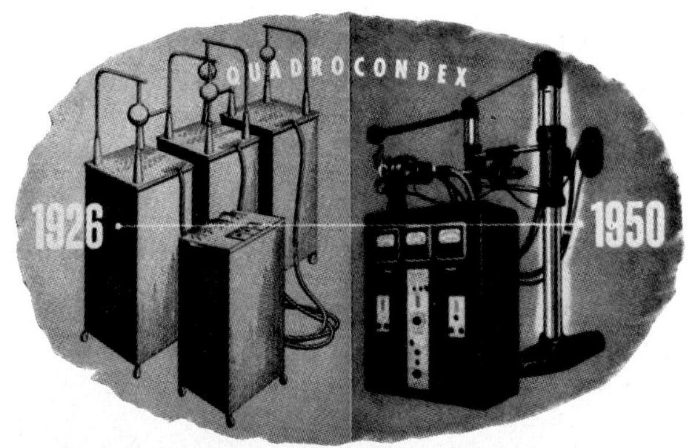

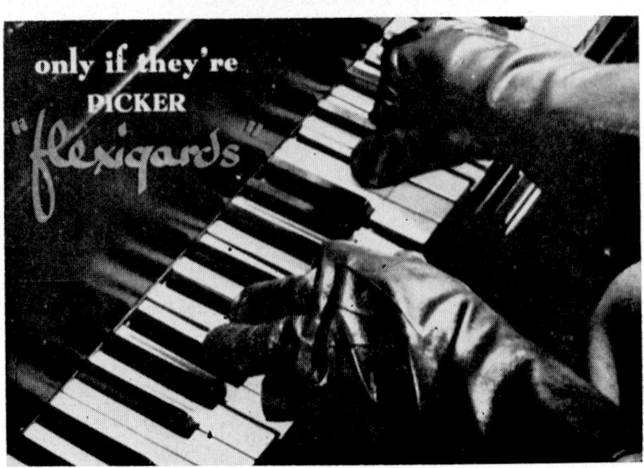

between the ARRS and the Western Roentgen Society precisely because the two names were confusing.

In the "golden" issues, Keleket billed itself as both "the oldest original name" and "the oldest name in x-ray", with the dates 1900-1950. Actually, Keleket was not founded until about 1903 or 1904. As a name in the x-ray business, GE is older than Keleket, on the strength of Edison's activities of 1896. Through Waite & Bartlett, Picker can also claim to be if not "older original" at least "older" than Keleket.

In those same issues of 1950 Westinghouse asserted that production of its Quadrocondex therapy generator is continuing since 1926 – but the x-ray division of Westinghouse was brought into being only in 1931. Quadrocondex and Duocondex had been Wappler denominations for equipment with condensers in the circuit of the transformer.

In January of 1954, in *Radiology,* Picker showed its Flexigard lead rubber gloves being no impediment to piano playing. Have you tried it?

In 1956, Ansco conducted a publicity campaign during which a pair of beautiful twin sisters were shown in various bust or full body postures; the caption insisted that monochorionic, monozygotic, and polyembryonic twins only *look* alike, while Ansco x-ray films *are* alike. Oddly enough, at that time, in my experience, Ansco x-ray films were everything but consistent from one box to the next.

The Heico Company of Strodsburg (Pennsylvania) had one of the corniest advertisements on record. It showed a lady dressed in a white gown (actually a cross between a night gown and a formal dress) with a nurse's cap, holding a developed x-ray film clamped in a hanger; this female figure was photo-mounted against a Saharan background, while the text (intended to promote their special dryer) said "switch on the Sirocco!"

But the most preposterous of them all was a GE release of September, 1958 in both *Radiology* and in the *American Journal of Roentgenology.* It started with the relatively innocuous question, "Just what did you have in mind, Dr. Roentgen?" The answer though, came close to what a radio-spiritist (or should he be called a roentgeno-spiritist) would certainly regard as utter sacrilege!

The following Victoreen advertisement is herein reproduced because it is informative and, in addition, carries a message of its own, over and above the intended publicity.

IT'S A FEMTO WORLD

The day of "medium-range" thinking has passed when we speak of an instrument's measuring capabilities – it's now an age of the "very small" and the "very large". Consider for a moment the task of creating new prefixes to accommodate this new way of thinking–the task which befell the International Union of Pure and Applied Physics when it met recently. Out of this meeting evolved some exotic new additions to our vocabulary.

Just what did you have in mind, Dr. Roentgen

Was it a diagnostic x-ray unit? Did it include automatic phototimed spot-film unit? Would design be function-mated to the needs of radiologists, whose specialty was born of your discovery?

If this is what you envisioned, Dr. Roentgen, you must have been looking forward to... THE GENERAL ELECTRIC REGENT

More alike than monozygotic twins

... Ansco High-Speed X-ray Films

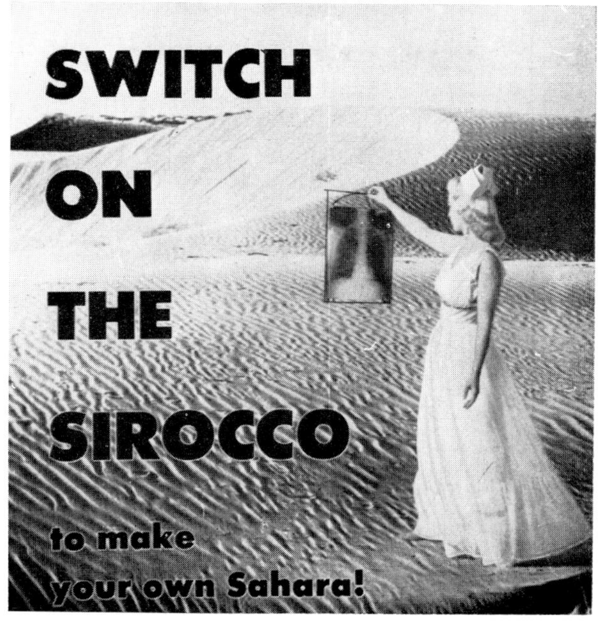

Deci-(10^{-1}), centi -(10^{-2}), milli- (10^{-3}) and micro-(10^{-6}) have long been in general use; nano-(10^{-9}) and pico-(10^{-12}) while still somewhat special are growing in popularity. FEMTO-(10^{-5}) and atto-(10^{-8}), new additions to the "very small" vocabulary are still earmarked "ultra-special". In the "very large" direction, the list reads as follows: kilo-(10^{3}), mega-(10^{6}), giga-(10^{9}) and tera-(10^{12}). While the scientific imagination is designing prefixes to describe future measurements, VICTOREEN scientists and engineers are designing the instruments which may ultimately make these measurements. The Model 475 Dynamic Capacitor Electrometer is one such instrument which was born out of many years of serious research and development into the femto world.

GLOBAL GLIMPSE

The Souvenir Number (1956) of the *Indian Journal of Radiology* contained an historic paper on the trends of radiodiagnosis in the Soviet Union, contributed by Y. N. Sokolov, editor of the *Vestnik Rentgenologii i Radiologii.* Sokolov introduced his contribution with a very pertinent remark: due to the intensive (intentional or otherwise) interchange of information between civilized countries, similar scientific discoveries have been announced at about the same time in several countries - and yet, the appearance of local or national peculiarities has been just as unavoidable. I found out how true that is when I attempted to survey the manner in which x-ray equipment is being manufactured in various parts of the world.

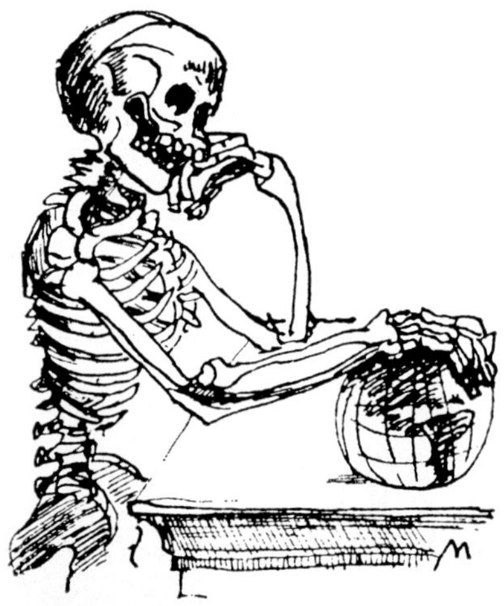

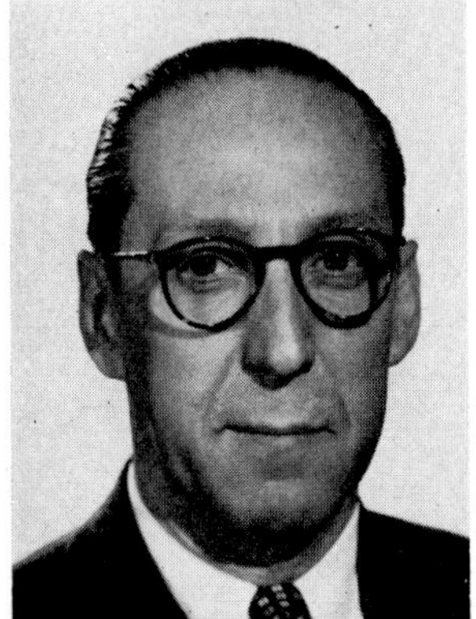

ARTHUR JAMES MINNS.

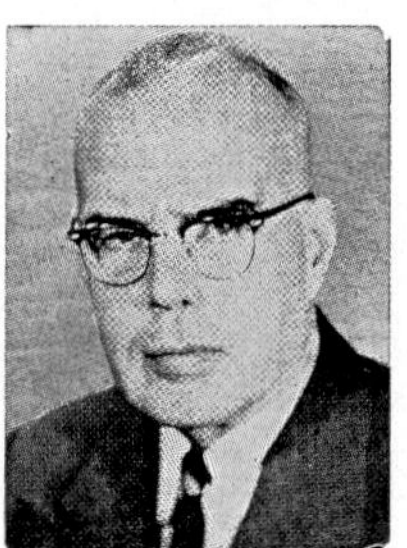

BRIAN DUNN

There is no single source of information for such a survey. The material was collected from advertisements published in many periodicals. In addition, credit goes to several knowledgeable technical executives, listed in the chronologic order in which they have contributed their "gems": A. M. Small, the managing director of the (Australian) Watson-Victor; Charles Pepin Donat, the manager for the Western Hemisphere of the (American) GE; Arthur James Minns, managing director of the (British) Watson and GE; Eric Frederick Walker, a globe-circling specialist in x-ray applications, formerly with Picker, then with Atomic Energy of Canada, now with High Voltage Engineering; Brian James Dunn, Sr., president of the (subsidiary) Picker International Corporation; Jiro Uyeno, managing director of the (Japanese) Sanyei Electric Trading Company; Arturo Gilardoni, founder of the (Italian) firm by the same name; and Giuseppe Barazetti, Jr., from the (Italian) firm which carries the name of his father.

No survey of radiologic equipment in the USA would be complete without considering the sale outlets of foreign firms. Some of them have created subsidiaries on American soil, and a few of these initially foreign subsidiaries have grown into large organizations, productive and respectable in their own rights.

PHILIPS

The Naamlooze Vennotschap (anonymous company) Philips Gloeilampenfabrieken of Eindhoven (Holland) was founded in May, 1891 by Gérard

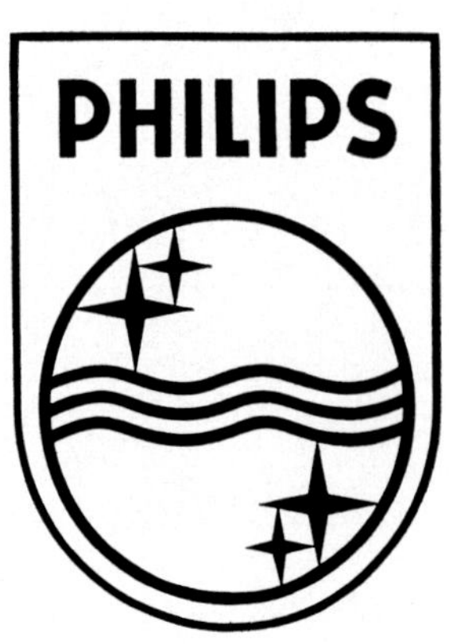

Philips (1858-1942) as a privately owned carbon filament electric lamp factory.

In 1894, the firm had financial difficulties, and was put up for sale. The price offered was too low, therefore the sale was never consummated. In 1895 Anton Frederik Philips (1874-1951) – Gérard's younger brother – joined the firm, and one of his first ideas was to offer Philips lamps for sale to the South African Republic, where electricity had been introduced in 1891. Anton Philips got his order, and from that moment on the firm prospered.

Today the Philips Company operates in more than one hundred countries, it has its own organization in fifty-six countries, and employs in excess of 214,000 people. It claims to be – with the exception of American companies – the largest electrical firm in the world. Since 1961 Frits Philips (Anton's son) is the firm's president.

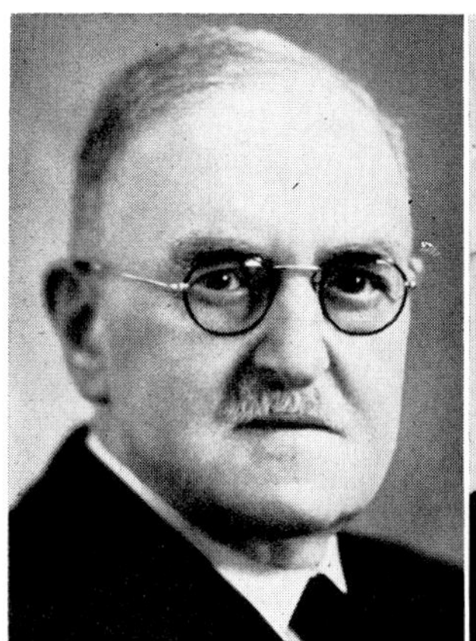

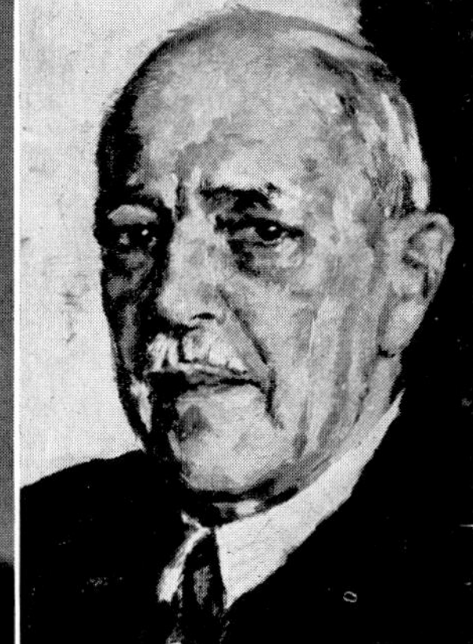

Courtesy: Philips-Eindhoven.

PHILIPS FOUNDERS. Gérard Philips, with glasses, and his brother, Anton Frederik Philips, created the lightbulb factory which grew into today's largest European manufacturer of electrical equipment.

NORTH AMERICAN PHILIPS COMPANY, INC.
750 S. FULTON AVENUE, MT. VERNON, N. Y.

Foremost in X-ray progress since 1896

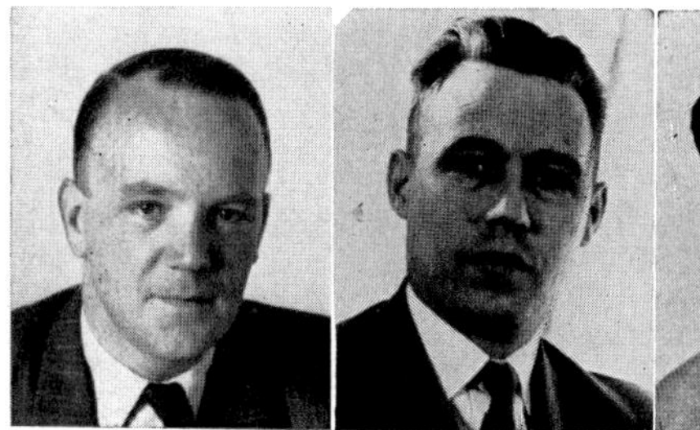

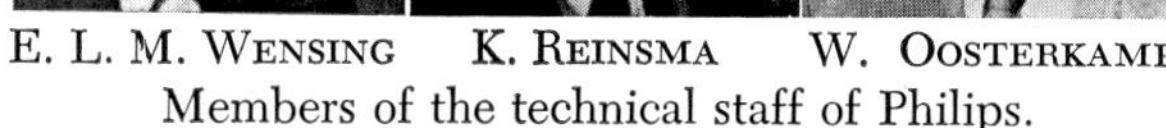

E. L. M. WENSING K. REINSMA W. OOSTERKAMP
Members of the technical staff of Philips.

Philips copywriters have used on occasion the ambiguous formula, "Foremost in x-ray products since 1896." In fact, Philips entered the x-ray business only when, prompted by World War I shortages, it began to manufacture gas x-ray tubes.

In 1923, Philips established an X-Ray Research Laboratory at Eindhoven. The first director of that Laboratory was the genial x-ray physicist Albert Bouwers, who graduated in 1924 in Utrecht (his thesis for the PhD degree was based on a study of the intensity of x rays). History was made in 1925 when Bouwers built the first x-ray tube in which the glass was welded" to a central "sleeve" of chrome-iron: that tube, the famous Metalix, was preserved as a trade-mark of Philips. In 1928 the Metalix became shock-proof. In 1929 Bouwers presented for the first time before the *Deutsche Röntgengesellschaft* his rotating anode tube, the Rotalix. It was not a new idea to distribute the heat load over a larger surface by rotating the anode, but that was the first time when the idea had been translated into an actual, workable model.

The Philips Company compiled upon request a list of their contributions to radiologic technology. Their list is herein reproduced but (as with similar lists by Picker or GE) this must not be construed as an implicit acknowledgment of these statements as being unquestioned priorities:

"Metalix" tube with protection against unwanted radiation (1925).
"Metalix" shock-proof and radiation-protected (1929).
"Metalix" portable x-ray unit – Junior – (1929).
"Rotalix" rotating anode tube (1929).

X-RAY RESEARCH AND DEVELOPMENT

A Selection of the Publications of the Philips X-Ray Research Laboratory from 1923-1933

Published by
N. V. PHILIPS' GLOEILAMPENFABRIEKEN
EINDHOVEN (HOLLAND).

200 kvp shock-proof and radiation-protected therapy unit (1930).

Condenser transformer with "Rotalix" for chest diagnosis (1930).

"Centralix" Dental X-Ray Unit, with both transformer and tube immersed under oil in a single grounded container (1932).

Mercury vapor high-tension x-ray valve, up to 200 kvp (1933).

Super D, high-power four-valve diagnostic unit with fully automatic optimal tube-load control (1933).

Radiation-protected, sealed-off, 400 kvp therapy tube (1934).

Contact therapy unit, also usable for cavities (1936).

Cascade high-tension generator for 2 mev (1937).

Neutron generator for 600 kvp (1938).

1 mev deep therapy unit with radiation-protected sealed-off tube (1939).

High capacity condenser discharge diagnostic x-ray unit (1939).

Thoriated tungsten filament high-vacuum x-ray valve (1942).

X-ray diffraction apparatus for crystal analysis with Geiger-Müller counter tubes (1942).

Installation for mass chest survey (1944).

Self-rectified, oil-immersed "Rotalix" rotating anode (1946).

Mirror camera for roentgen-photography (photographing the fluorescent screen) with automatic film transport (1947).

Electron microscope (1947).

"Compactix" universal therapy tank unit with electronic stabilization (control) of both ma and kvp (1948).

"Oralix" dental unit with .8 x .8 mm^2 focal spot (1948).

"Rotalix" with small (.3mm^2) focal spot for bone radiography and magnifying technics (1949).

The Philips empire comprises mostly firms which use the name Philips as part of their title.

Such is the case with Philips Ibérica (headquarters in Madrid, and branches even in the Canary Islands), with Philips Ethiopia in Addis Ababa, or with Philips Electrical Ireland in Dublin, Philips Iran in Teheran, Philips Liban in Beyrouth, Philips Electrical of Pakistan in Karachi, Philips Portuguesa in Lisbon, Philips Moyen Orient in Damascus, and Philips Rhodesian in Salisbury.

When desirable, the name of Philips was combined with that of the pre-existing company, as in Massiot-Philips (Paris), or Philips-Müller (first in Hamburg, then in Vienna). As convenience dictated, some of the firms purchased by Philips continued to be operated under their original names, for instance the Dansk Røntgen Teknik (Copenhagen), the O. Y. Dentaldepot (Helsinki), the Medisinsk Röntgen A/S (Oslo), or the Modern Pharmacal Products (Manila). In a few cases the purchase of certain firms by Philips was never publicized, as for Mullard of England or Smit-Röntgen of Holland. It is not uncommon to find in one and the same periodical (apparently) competitive advertisements of several Philips-owned subsidiaries, as if each of them were independent.

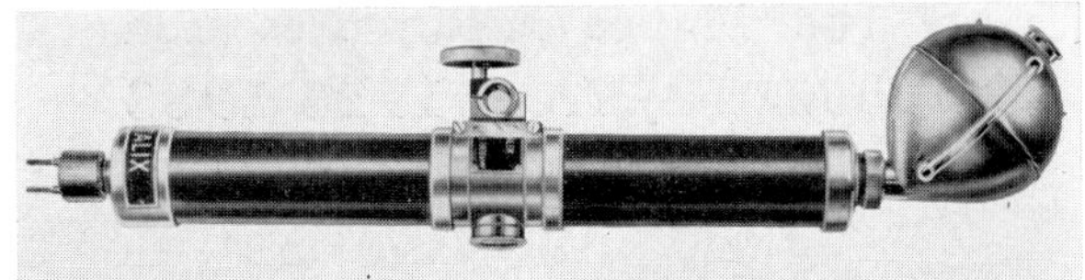

Courtesy: Philips-Eindhoven.

First Metalix (1925). The first Metalix tube (with glass sealed directly to the chromium iron cylinder) was shown to the British Institute of Radiology in December, 1923. It was placed in production around 1925.

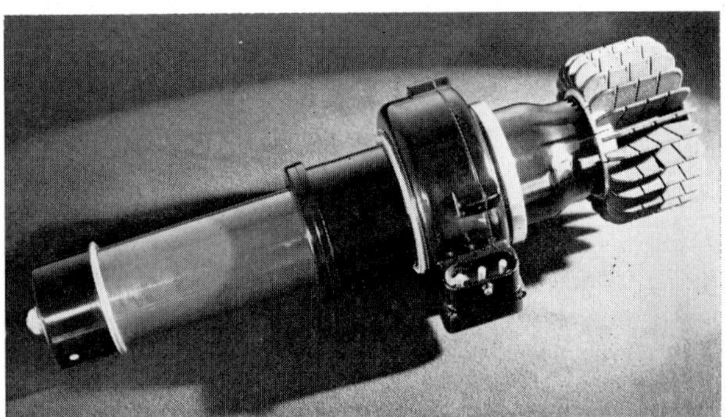

Courtesy: Philips-Eindhoven.

First Rotalix (1929). This is the first radiation-protected rotating anode tube created by Bouwers.

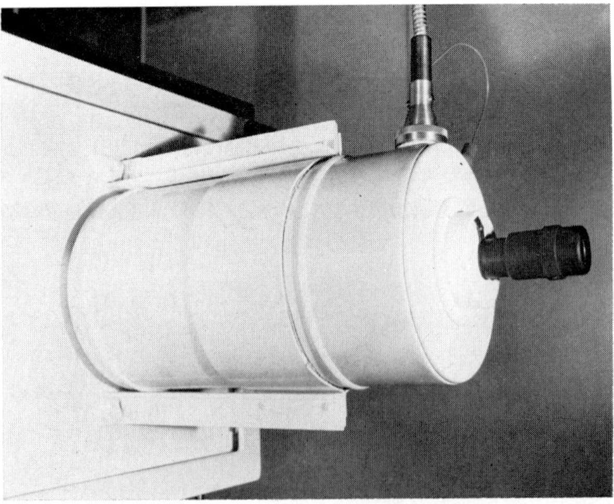

Courtesy: Philips-Eindhoven.

First Philips Image Intensifier (1953). Note the eye-piece, a very uncomfortable way of "looking" at the output phosphorus.

Philips apparatus is manufactured in many places around the globe. This means small items, and accessories. The bulk of larger Philips x-ray equipment is made in five locations: at Eindhoven, at Müller in Hamburg, at Massiot in Paris, at Philips Electrical Ltd. in London, and at Metalix in Milano.

It may be of interest to review briefly the development of the American subsidaries of Philips. The Philips Metalix Corporation was established in Mount Vernon (New York) in 1933, with the purpose of selling medical x-ray equipment manufactured at Eindhoven. Soon the subsidiary branched out to extra-medical territory, and began to import from Holland diffraction units in 1937, and in 1940 industrial x-ray transformers. In 1941 was developed at Mount Vernon the Norelco Crystal Analysis Unit (based on x-ray diffraction methods).

The North American Philips Company was created in 1942 with headquarters in New York City (the Germans had occupied Holland).

In 1944, North American Philips marketed the first commercial analytical x-ray instrument which did not require camera or films. It was called the Norelco Geiger-Counter X-Ray Spectrometer, known today as the Norelco Diffractometer. The first commercial x-ray spectrograph (Norelco) was marketed in 1948: its automatized version, the Autrometer, came out in 1955. The latter is nicknamed the "automatic chemist," because at the touch of a button it can identify and measure up to twenty-four elements in a specimen, and print the numerical results on a paper tape. There are also Norelco x-ray plating thickness gauges, based on spectrography (used for instance in steel mills, and in other types of manufacturing processes).

In the USA the medical part of Philips' x-ray business is currently handled by the North American Philips Company, located in Mount Vernon (New York), where they manufacture some parts. Most of the large equipment is imported from Eindhoven, Hamburg, and Paris. A few things are "farmed out," a practice which is relatively common in much of the American industry. I have seen Philips control stands put together (with printed circuits) by Continental in Chicago.

The simplest Philips x-ray table is the Examix, their most expensive is the Symmetrix 90/90, made by Massiot in Paris. In addition to the conventional x-ray transformers, Philips makes a condenser unit, called Maximus DLX, which delivers 300 ma at 150 kvp; or up to 1000 ma at 100 kvp. Philips has unique items such as the Pedestal Bucky Outfit. They make also the Contact Therapy CT-100 unit, and the constant potential 250 kvp rotational beam

Courtesy: Philips-Eindhoven.

HEART CATHETERIZATION. Note the mirror arrangement, a much easier way of "seeing" the output phosphorus. But people are already "looking away" from the patient, toward the television monitor.

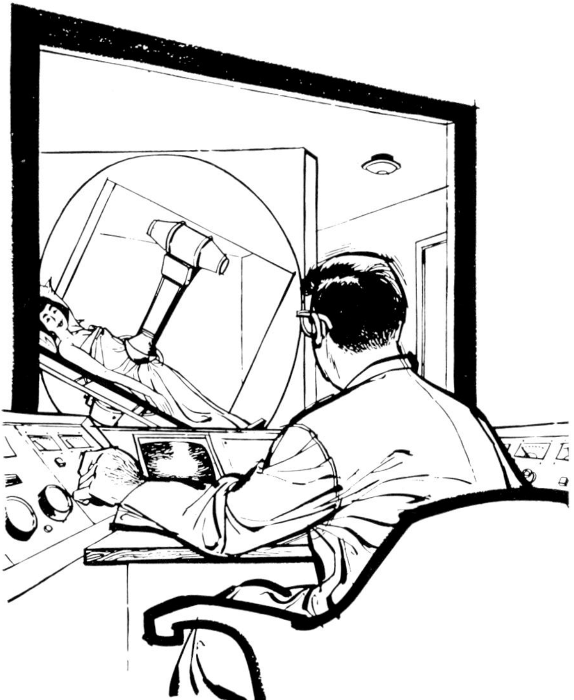

PHILIPS REMOTE-CONTROL VERSION. Shown for the first time at the 1962 ICR in Montreal, it is based on the ringstand (similar to GE's Imperial).

therapy unit TU-1 (which comes from Müller in Hamburg).

The Philips image intensifier appeared on the market in 1953, five years after Coltman's first announcement, but about the same time as Westinghouse's Fluorex. It had no special name. Its first version sported a 5″ input (phosphorus) with an awkward tubular (sometimes binocular) optical system. The brightness gain was wishfully advertised as being in the order of 1000. At carefully competitive intervals Philips improvements were announced, and they reached the 9″ size and 3000 times gain in brightness. They have also added the television technique, the split image with cineradiography, a synchronizing device (called cine pulse unit), and a ring stand for the "obligatory" remote control contraption. That same ring stand (structurally similar to the "skeleton" of GE's Imperial) was also used with their 11″ image intensifier (which has less gain in brightness than the 9″). Very useful is a small, mobile unit, the Surgex, which can be utilized in the emergency room or in surgery, to check the position of fractures at the time of casting or internal metallic fixation.

Although Philips equipment is comparable to the best available on the world market, it never reached in this country the sales popularity of any of the "big four" (Picker, GE, Keleket, and Westinghouse).

In the USA, the Philips subsidiaries are grouped in the Philips Electronic and Pharmaceutical Industries which include aside from those previously mentioned also the Philips Electronic Instruments, the (American) Philips Export Company, and several others such as the Anchor Serum Company of St. Joseph (Missouri), an outlet for the drugs manufactured or compounded by Philips Duphar of Amsterdam. Duphar has also an "atomic" subsidiary, the M. V. Philips-Roxane, an isotope bottling laboratory.

ODELCA

Another Dutch firm which has achieved worldwide fame is the (optical) creation of the previously mentioned Albert Bouwers.

Estonian-born Bernhard Voldemar Schmidt (1879-1935) had lost his right hand in early youth. After an optical apprenticeship in Sweden, he made a precarious living in Jena (Germany) by grinding lenses with his left hand. In 1926, he became associated with the Bergedorf Observatory near Hamburg, and in 1930 he devised a method for overcoming the aberration of spherical mirrors (a correcting plate at the center of curvature). That method was utilized in the famous Palomar-Schmidt telescope.

Helge Christensen is radiologist at the Roskilde Amtssygehus, a publicly owned hospital in Copenhagen. Just before World War II he wanted to acquire photofluorographic equipment for the hospital, but became disgusted with the inefficient optical components of existing machines. He came upon the idea to utilize

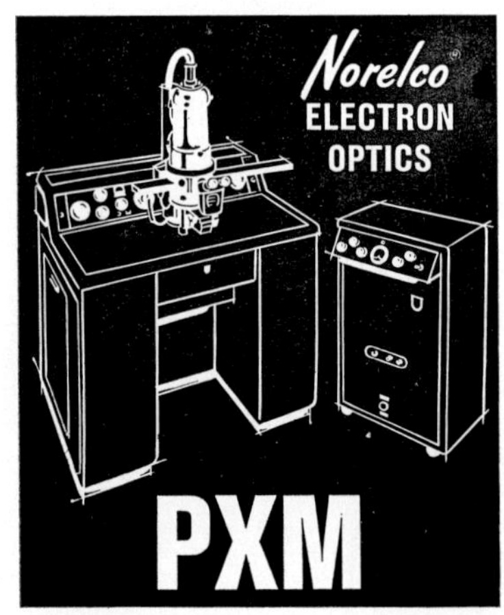

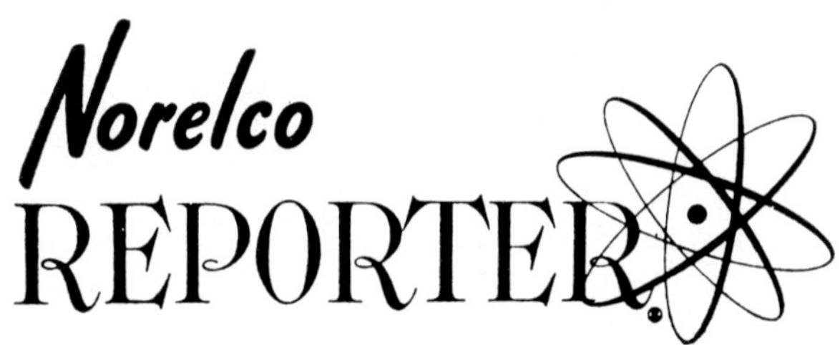

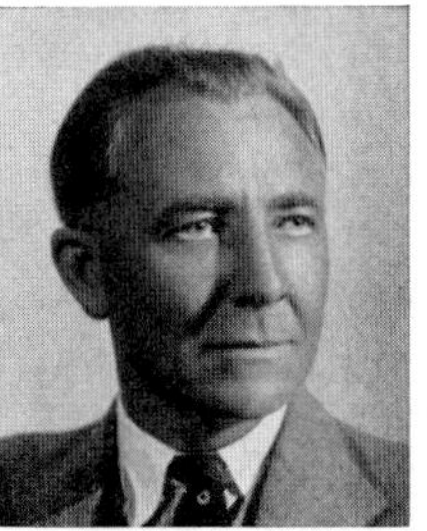
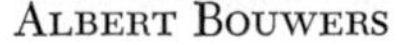
ALBERT BOUWERS

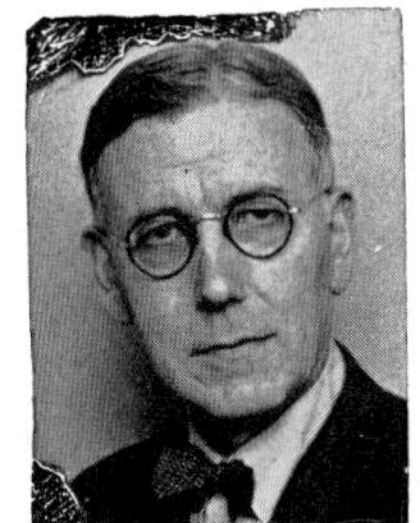
HELGE CHRISTENSEN

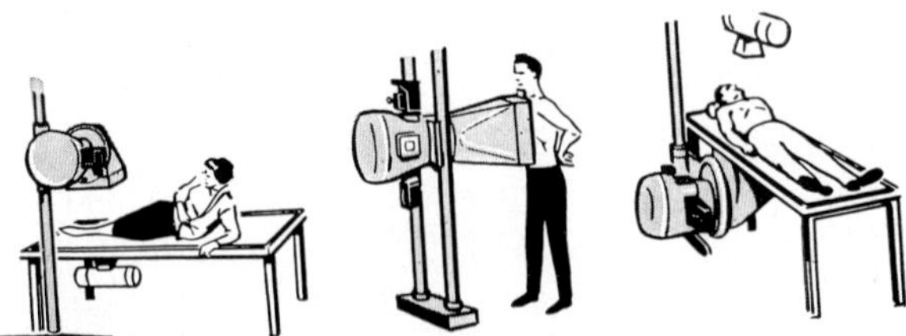
ODELCA. De Oude Delft's mirror camera comes in two sizes (70 or 100 mm) in-line or with angle-hood. It is a cheap substitute for conventional films, quite useful in admission examinations of the chest, rechecks of fractures, even tomo(fluoro)graphy.

the Schmidt principle in building a special camera, which he intended eventually to (but never did) use in television work. He consulted with several friends – including Heinrich Franke (from SRW) – but they all told him that such things had never been done before.*

*In his letter to me, Christensen remarked gleefully, "if they had heard of such things, it would have been superfluous for me to propose them." Most of Christensen's publications are in Danish, but he will soon come out with an English monograph on hip dysplasia in man and in the dog, with comparative anatomy being used to postulate the existence of hereditary factors in the appearance of aseptic necrosis.

GUARD AGAINST CONTAGION

from supine admissions with new X-ray camera

The Fairchild-Odelca, Angle-Hood, photofluorographic camera makes possible – for the first time – admission examinations of supine as well as ambulatory cases. Institutions will find it extremely effective in helping to minimize risk to personnel and other patients from unexamined carriers.

Highest quality photofluorography in ¼ the exposure time presently required

The Model X-70SA, Angle-Hood camera has the same outstanding features as the Fairchild-Odelca X-70S (In-Line): 75% less exposure time, excellent sharpness of detail, ability to stop motion, automatic safety devices. The versatility of the Model X-70SA permits conversion from upright to horizontal position . . . for a complete job of admission chest X-ray.

For complete information, contact your local X-ray equipment supplier, or write Fairchild Camera and Instrument Corp., Syosset, L.I., N.Y., Dept. 160-40T.

FAIRCHILD

X-RAY EQUIPMENT AND ACCESSORIES

1955

He set out with a mechanic, had the lens ground on calculations made by one of his friends from the Copenhagen Observatory, and built the first photofluorographic unit with mirror-camera (25x25mm rollfilm) which was used satisfactorily in his hospital for a total of 15 years. It is still in perfect working order, and is now preserved in the Danish Roentgen Museum.

In 1940, Bouwers decided – independently of Christensen, and of Schönander (Stockholm) – to apply the Schmidt principle in the building of a camera. He purchased two ordinary spectacle lenses, coated them, and

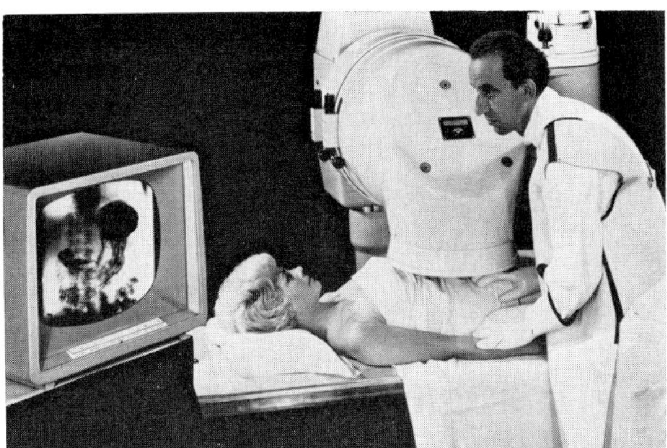

Courtesy: Odelca-Hicksville, Long Island.

CINELIX. Of all commercially available image intensifiers, the Cinelix has today the largest input screen. But this obtains only as long as the device is close to the patient. When mounted on top of a spotfilm device, screen size decreases proportionally. There are certain procedures in which a larger screen size is desirable – in those instances the unusual bulk of the Cinelix may have to be accepted and taken in stride. In this clever promotional picture the bulk is obscured by projection. The photographer had troubles with the male model (their sales manager) who wanted to remove the lead glove from his right hand. Then they forgot to put the "proper" image onto the television monitor – that lead glove is "invisible."

PRINCIPLE OF PHOTOFLUOROGRAPHY

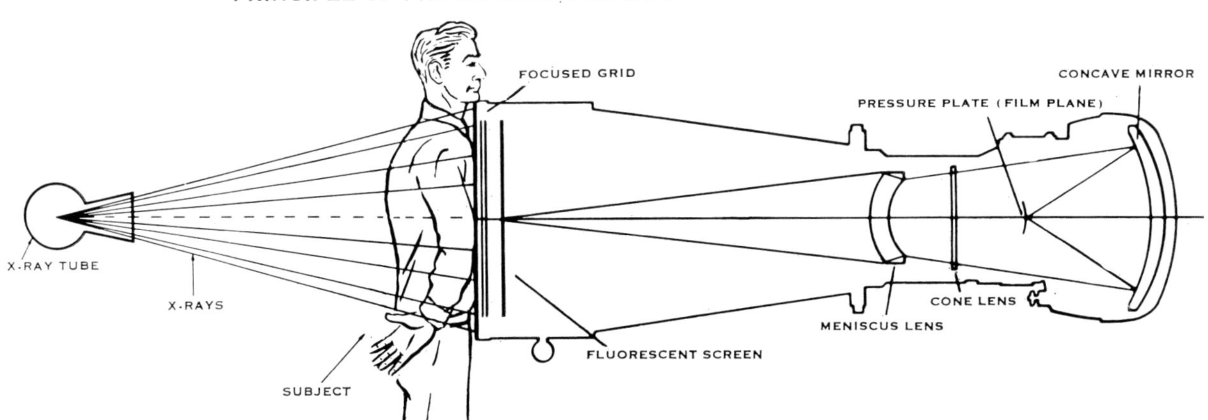

CINELIX 12½"

The electro-optical image intensifier with the largest screen (12½" diameter) in the world, now available in three models:

1 Cinelix 12½" for television-fluoroscopy

2 Cinelix 12½" for television-fluoroscopy and ciné-fluorography

3 Cinelix 12½" for ciné-fluorography and optical fluoroscopy

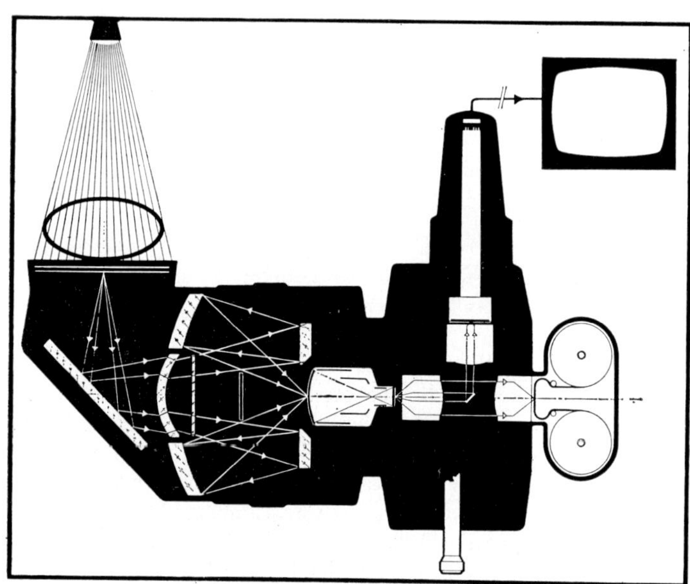

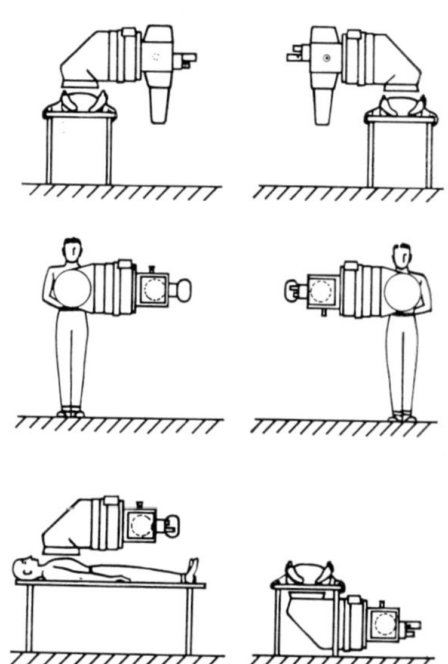

featuring:

- maximum diagnostic information both by television and ciné-fluorography
- substantial dosage reduction thanks to super-speed Bouwers' concentric mirror optics and unique light intensifying system
- possibility of enlarging x 2 the image electron-optically during TV-fluoroscopy and ciné-fluorography
- 35 mm ciné-fluorography up to 50 frames/sec by incorporated special "Old Delft" ciné-camera with 270° open sector
- facilities of adjusting contrast and brightness on the TV-monitor
- TV-fluoroscopy without adaptation
- 360° rotatability permitting examination of standing, recumbent or obliquely positioned patients.

For full information please apply to:

N.V. OPTISCHE INDUSTRIE "DE OUDE DELFT" DELFT-HOLLAND

1961

combined them with two spherical concave mirrors. The result was amazing: he had produced the fastest photographic lens achieved until that time, with an aperture of f/1. Then Bouwers left Philips, and purchased a small optical shop in Delft, which he called (beginning in 1941) N. V. Optische Industrie De Oude Delft.

In 1945, he brought out his first 70 mm photofluorographic mirror camera. Three years later appeared an improved model (with a reduction factor 6:1). This is the one which carried for the first time the name Odelca, from the initials of De *O*ude *Del*ft *C*amera.

The camera was constructed especially for mass chest surveys. It was later adapted also for various screening procedures, and evolved into a comparatively cheap way of checking alignment after casting of a fractured limb, and in similar situations. A few years later, the radiation scare, engendered during the Atomic Phase, made chest surveys less popular. The Fairchild Camera Company, which for a long time had been Odelca's representative in this country, went out of the x-ray business in 1960. Thereupon Odelca created its own outlet in Hicksville (Long Island). In the meantime, though, the inventiveness of Bouwers had centered upon a new application of the mirror camera, the Cinelix.

The Cinelix is a 12½″ optical image intensifier. Its mirror image is fed into an electronic intensifier tube: from there the brightened image is "split" between a visual check, a movie camera, and a television monitor. The Cinelix is the largest (also the bulkiest) image intensifier combination currently available.

Long before the Cinelix, Odelca mirror cameras were known and available from Japan to England, and from Italy to Australia. Today, De Oude Delft has 500 employees (as compared with 20 employees in 1941), and an established market also for its optical products other than those used in the x-ray field.

In fact, Bouwers returned to the "military" the courtesy which Coltman had received (in utilizing as a model RCA's infrared image tube): there is a Cinelix version utilized as a snooperscope!

SMIT-RONTGEN

In 1923, B. Th. Smit founded in Leiden (Holland) a private company under the name of Instrumentenfabriek Smit.

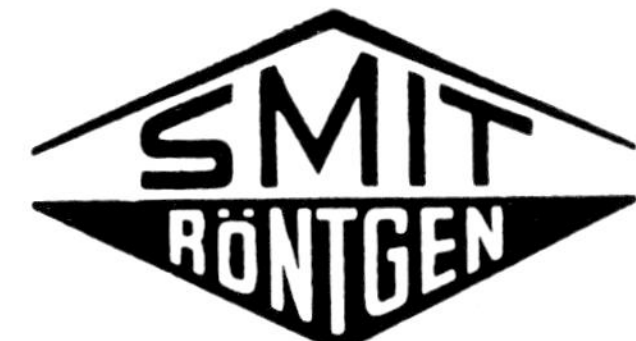

„Tandem Bona Causa Triumphat"

It was fairly successful in producing x-ray equipment (they had the US tables and the DS tubestands), and by 1930 their employees numbered 70. They reorganized after World War II by taking into a limited partnership a financier from Rotterdam, H. J. Bonda. The firm then became the Smit-Röntgen Apparaten Fabriek with 100 employees – by 1950, as they moved to a new location on Evertsenstraat the number had increased to 150 employees. In 1954 the company was incorporated as Smit-Röntgen N.V.

Smit-Röntgen makes various transformers, the Propensator (200 ma at 125 kvp, or 300 ma at 90 kvp); the

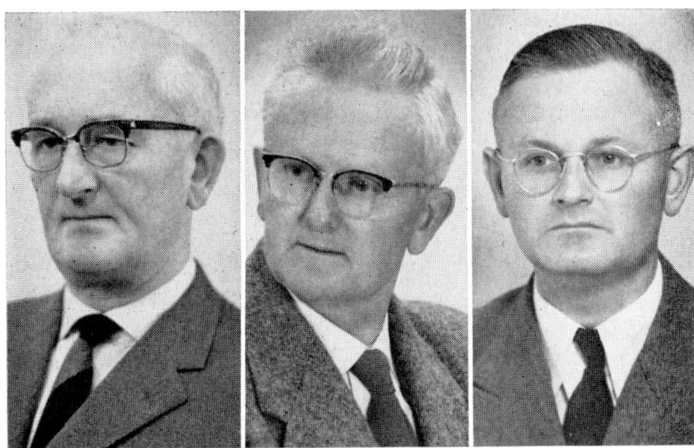

Courtesy: Bernhard Ziedses des Plantes

THE SMIT BROTHERS. On the viewer's left is the oldest, J. W. Smit (born 1899, the only one alive today). The others are B. Th. Smit (1900-1956) and P. A. Smit (1911-1958).

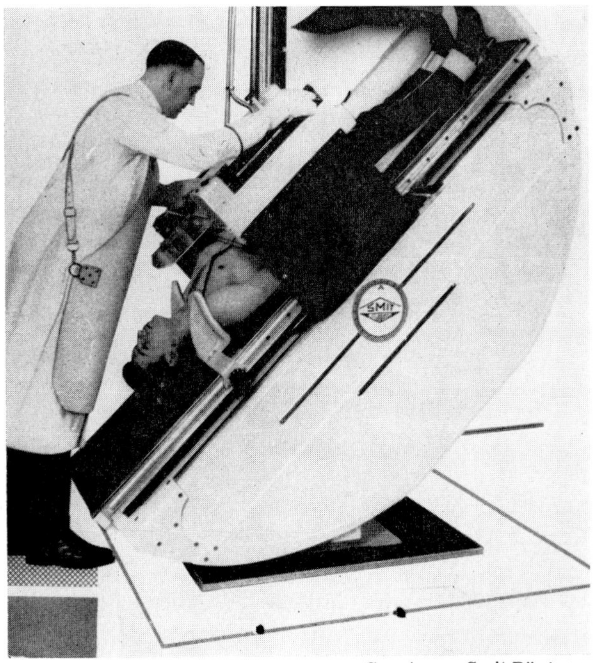

Courtesy: Smit-Röntgen.

SMIT-RÖNTGEN'S US-25. This is their best, 180° table.

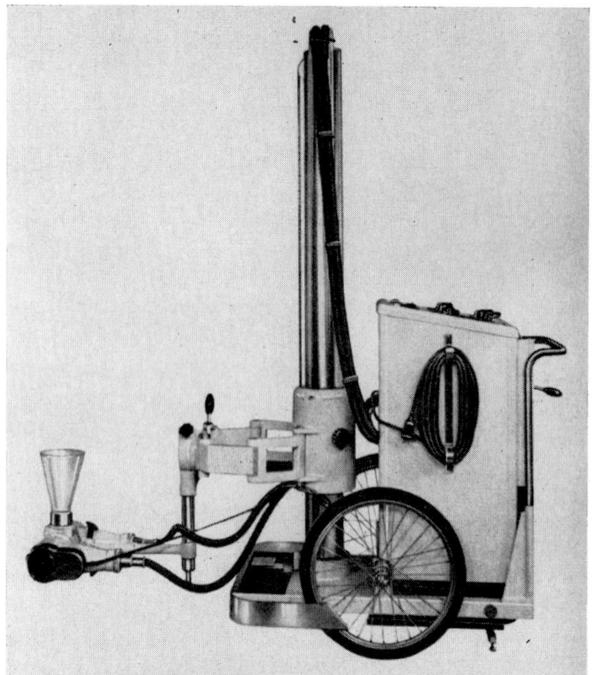

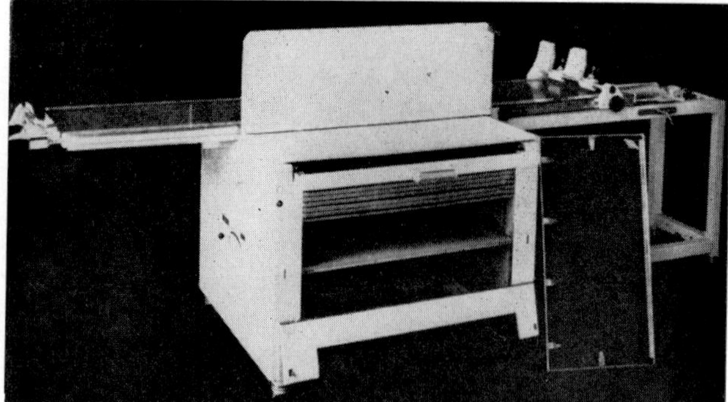

Courtesy: Smit-Röntgen.

SMIT-RÖNTGEN AORTA-ARTERIOGRAPH. Its sliding top is motor-actuated, and can be pre-set so that patient is moved after the second (or after any other) exposure. Ten cassettes (size 35.5x71 cm, for two square films of 35.5x35.5 cm each) are successively brought into position at the pull of a lever. Several wedge filters are provided for the correction of differences in subject thickness. This cassette-changer was designed by J. R. von Ronnen, who teaches radiology in the University of Leiden.

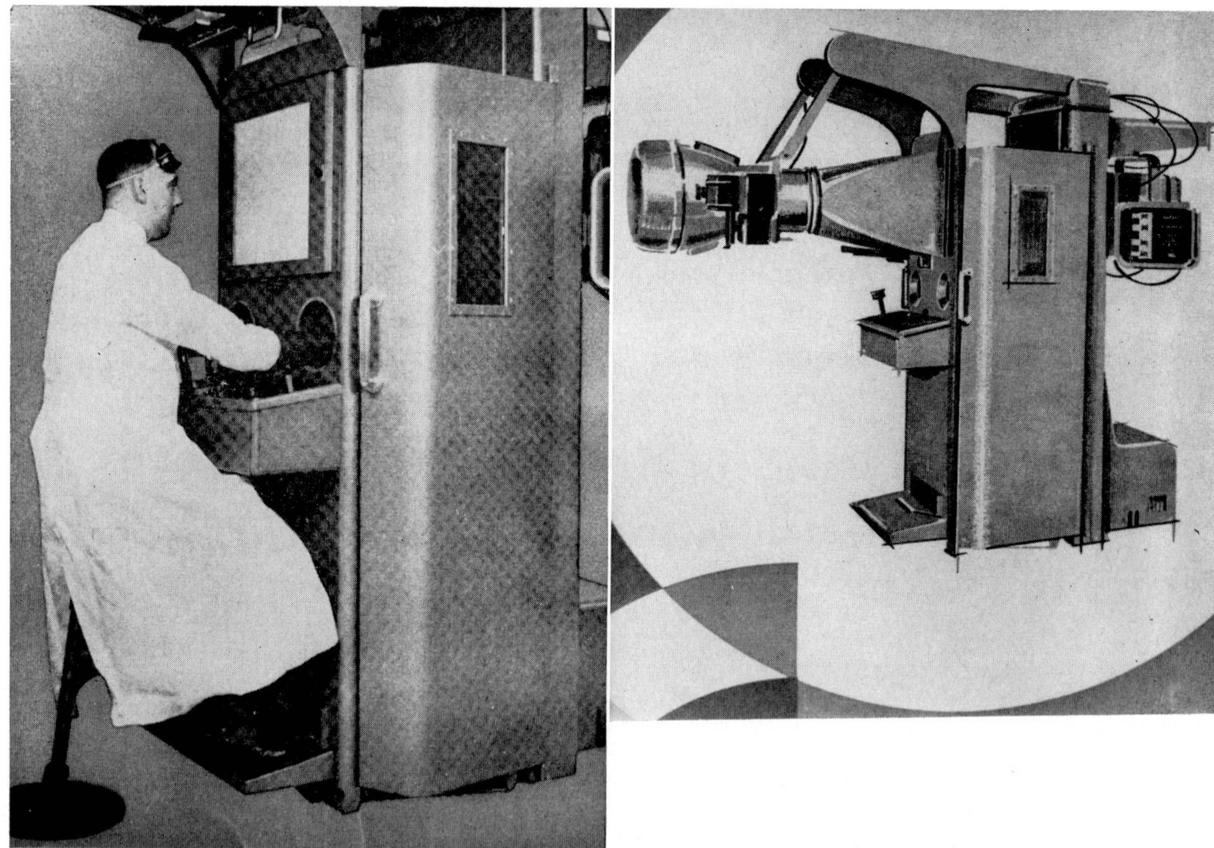

Courtesy: Smit-Röntgen.

PENETROMETER 160. Note the counterbalanced Odelca head, the heavy radiation protection, the lead-sleeved channels for reaching into the patient's compartment, and the convenient placement of the controls.

Provisor (400 ma at 125 kvp, or 500 ma at 110 kvp); and the triphasic Prominentor-6 (1000 ma at 100 kvp, or 100 ma at 150 kvp). Of their tables, the US-15 allows 15° Trendelenburg. The US-25 is center-pivoted, and goes therefore all the way to 90°. The SBC4 Serialograph is an automatic spotflim device. The Penetrator 160 is a fully enclosed (self-protected) photofluorographic stand: when its counterbalanced Odelca head is tilted out of the way, it becomes a just as heavily radiation-protected fluoroscope. The Mobilator (100 ma at 90 kvp) is a mobile unit with two bicycle type wheels in addition to the regular casters.

The Aorta-Arteriograph built after the specifications of Douwe Siurd Bartstra (a radiologist from Utrecht) had six ultra-long cassettes (35.5 x 140 cm). The model was lately re-issued in an improved version, following the suggestions of J. R. Von Ronnen, who is professor of radiology in the University of Leiden: it now has a sliding table top, and ten cassettes (35.5 x 71 cm), which admit two films each (of the 35.5 x 35.5 cm size, a standard size in Central Europe).

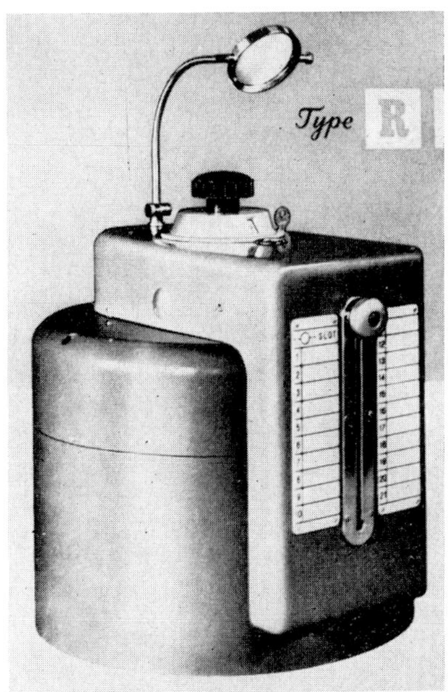

Courtesy: Smit-Röntgen.

SAFE FOR RADIO-ACTIVE MATERIALS. Note the mirror which allows one to "look into the well" without exposure to radiation. Inside the safe is a wheel with channels for storage of radium needles, and other brachytherapy devices.

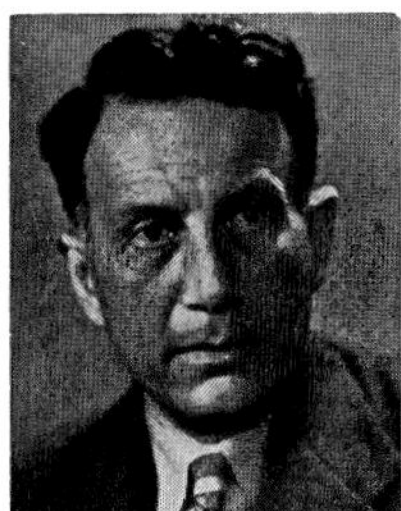
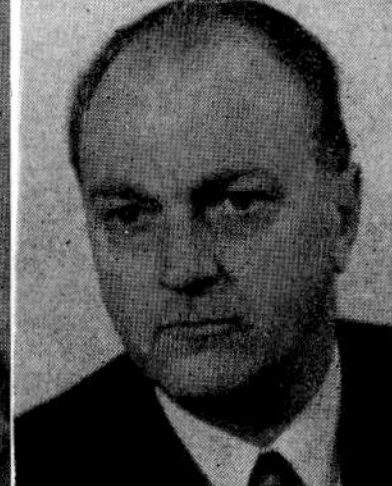
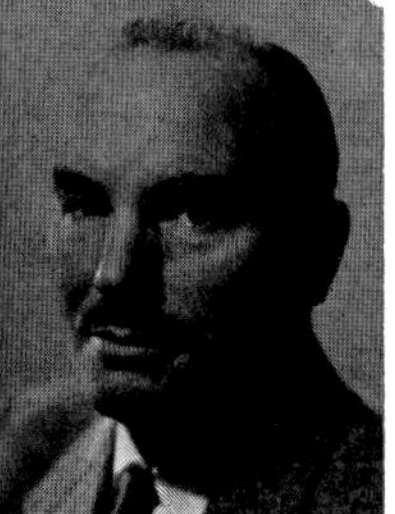

DOUWE BARTSTRA J. FEDDEMA J. R. VON RONNEN
Dutch radiologists with technical inclinations.

The ingenious safe RS-5 deserves special mention for storing radioactive needles. Twenty-one holes are provided in the "wall" of a rotating lead drum, which is "buried" inside a lead and steel block. On the upper aspect of the block is a knob with which the drum can be rotated so that one of those drum holes presents itself in line with and beneath a hole drilled in the block. To make life easier, there is a mirror so arranged that you can look into the hole without having to expose yourself, while an indicator on the face of the block shows which of the (numbered) holes in the drum has presented itself. The drum has its twenty-one holes placed in such a way as to leave another three "undrilled" spaces. The middle one of these three "undrilled" holes is aligned with the hole in the block when the safe is locked. There is at all times at least 100 mm lead between the radioactive sources and the outside. When loaded with one curie, the dose rate at the surface of the block does not exceed 6 mr/hour. Their clever rotating Co^{60} unit has been mentioned.

In this country Smit Röntgen is known mostly (only) for their Golden Grid (60 lines), and for the Jewel Grid (110 lines) - sold through the PTE (Physicians' Technical Equipment) Company of Milwaukee. Smit Röntgen is not a large firm, but it has always had imaginative engineering, products of good quality, and the company did its best to follow its motto - *Tandem bona causa triumphat,* which means in the end the good cause triumphs. Apparently the "bigger" cause is more likely to triumph: last year Smit Röntgen N. V. was purchased by Philips.

DAGRA

In the Netherlands, contrast media are made by the chemical and pharmaceutical firm Dagra N. V. of Amsterdam. They started to produce these media

DAGRA

during World War II, on demand, as drugs became scarce. Now they are selling them around the globe.

Their first preparation was an iodized oil for bronchography (Iodombrine), followed shortly by two cholecystographic media (Galisol for intravenous route and Galisol Peroral), replaced after the war (Bilombrine).

For urography they had di-iodo compounds (Pyelombrine M, Urombrine). Later they introduced the tri-iodo preparations for pyelography (Phelombrine M, Fortombrin M, and Plexombrine) as well as for intravenous cholecystography (Trilombrine, Felombrine), and for angiography (Angiombrine). A both shadowy and watery combination is used for hysterosalpingography (Hydrombrine 60) and for bronchography (Hydrombrine 160).*

*This information was gladly offered by Dr. W. van Rijn, their medical director.

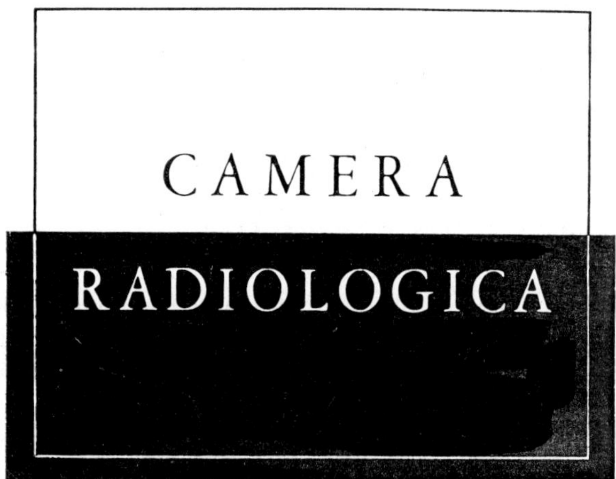

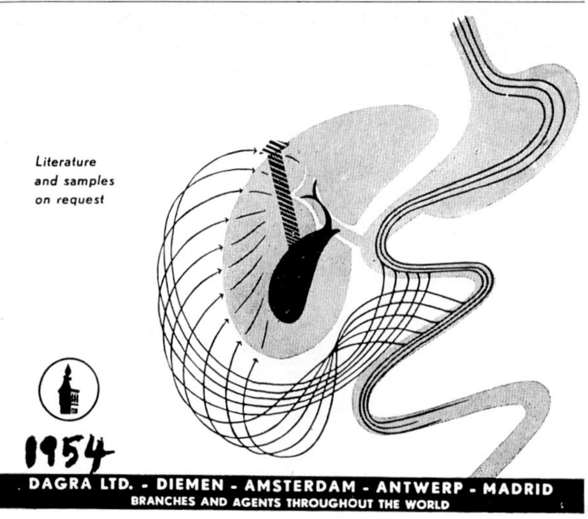

Dagra issues also a periodical, *Camera Radiologica,* which brings scientific articles in either English, French, or Italian. Topics are restricted to applications of (Dagra) contrast media.

SIEMENS

The German giant in the electro-medical field is the Siemens-Reiniger-Werke Aktiengesellschaft (SRW or SiReWA) of Erlangen.

SRW resulted from the merger of the electromedical section of Siemens & Halske (Berlin), Reiniger, Gebbert & Schall (Erlangen), Veifa-Werke* (Frankfurt/-Main), and Phönix Röhrenwerk (Rudolstadt/Thüringen). In 1925 they created a common sales outlet, the Siemens-Reininger-Veifa GmbH. The consolidation was finalized in 1932.

The name most prominently connected with the growth of SRW was that of Carl Friedrich von Siemens (1872-1941), the youngest son of the firm's founder, Werner von Siemens (1816-1892). Another SRW pillar was Max Anderlohr.

A dominant feature of SRW is that it produces (with its subsidiaries) every significant part that goes into an x-ray machine. And SRW manufactures every known type of x-ray equipment — if anybody else makes it *(Noblesse oblige!),* SRW will also make it. Because of cumulation with its component (ancestor) firms, the list of SRW "x-ray firsts" is quite lengthy.

*Veifa was created by Friedrich Dessauer, the roentgen-physicist who died last year of radio-carcinomatosis. He started Veifa in 1907 in the experimental shop which he had in his parents' home (Kurt Walther).

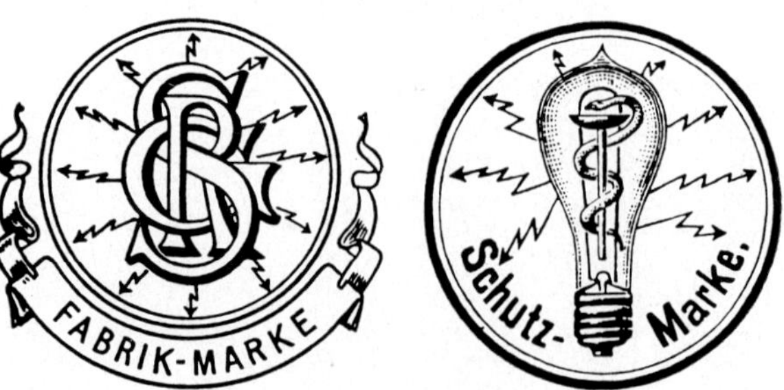

OLD INSIGNIA. These trade-marks were used by Reiniger, Gebbert & Schall. When the SiReWa was formed, it adopted a minor modification of the old SH symbol.

Roentgen tube with adjustable vacuum (*Deutsches Patent* – DP 91028 of 1896).

Roentgen outfit with Wehnelt electrolytic interrupter (DP 120340 of 1899).

Compression diaphragm after Albers-Schönberg (DP 156389 of 1902).

Orthodiagraph (DP 137349 of 1901).

Roentgen tube with tantalum electrodes (DP 156746 of 1903).

Roentgen tube with tungsten electrodes (DP 165138 of 1904 – practical realization was achieved only when methods of handling tungsten were developed).

Roentgen tube built into radiation-protective cover with shutters (1905 catalog).

Roentgen outfit with radiation-protective enclosure for the x-ray technician (1906 catalog).

Klinoskope; a metallic table for fluoroscopy in either upright or recumbent position, with provision for orthodiagraphy (1907 catalog).

Roentgen-cinematographic outfit after Groedel (DP 215648 of 1908).

Blitz roentgen outfit with exposures of 1/100 sec. (DP 250334 and 254117 of 1909).

Relatively fine grain reinforcing screen Sinegran (DP 229894 of 1910).

Scattered radiation diaphragms after Gustav Bucky (DP 284371 of 1913).

Transformer with four (six) hot-cathode-kenotrons for full-wave rectification (DP 202596 of 1915); the experimental model was shown to the Berlin Medical Society on January 26, 1916 but actual production did not start until after World War I.

Transformer with half-wave alternating current for energizing Siemens hot cathode roentgen tubes with separate adjustment of tube current, and introduction of kilovolt meter as a means of preevaluating penetration of beam (DP 296464 of 1916).

Complete shock-proofing through high-tension insulated conductors with a grounded cover - cables (DP 347029 of 1919); actual manufacture only in late 1920s.

First complete shock-proof and radiation-protected roentgen outfit with Siemens irradiation box (DP 417131 of 1919).

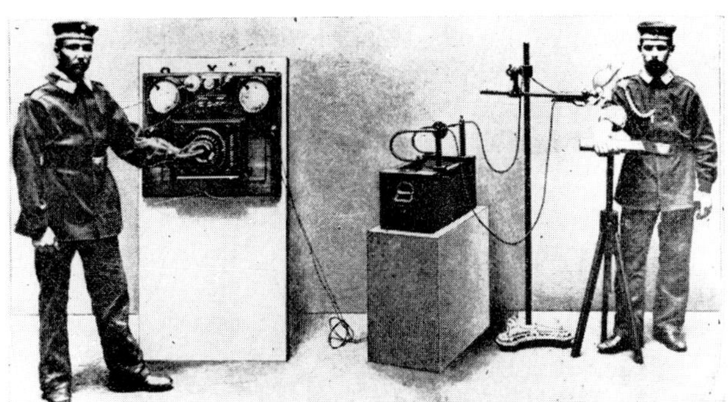

MILITARY MOBILE. "Portable" army unit, made in 1902 by Siemens & Halske.

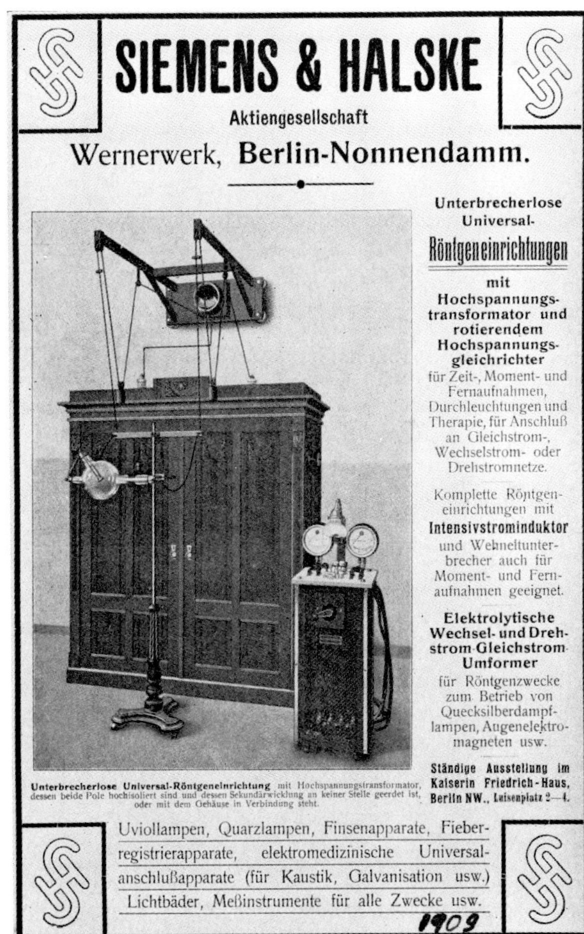

S & H AD OF 1909. A German-made "interrupterless" (which could be connected to AC, DC, or triphasic power supply) is shown. Also mentioned are coils, Wehnelt interruptors, ultraviolet and Finsen lights, as well as "all other" electro-medical instrumentalities.

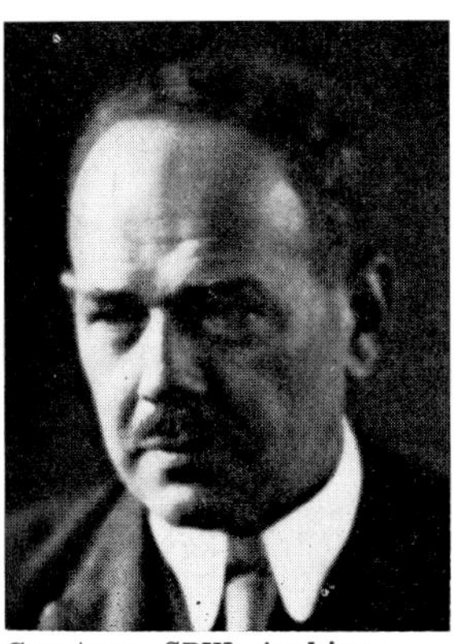

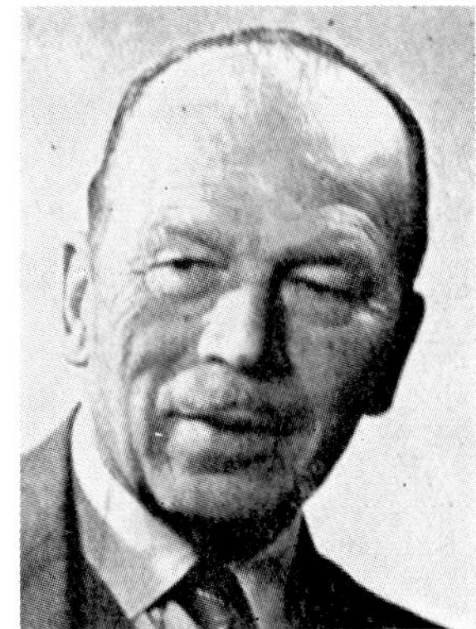

Courtesy: SRW Archives.

CARL FRIEDRICH VON SIEMENS. Youngest son of Werner von Siemens (founder of the original firm), Carl and smiling MAX ANDERLOHR "made" today's SRW.

Roentgen dosimeter with electronic amplifier tube for direct measurement of roentgen dose (1922).

Deep therapy generator Stabilivolt with constant potential, using condensers and hot-cathode kenotrons; at the same time introduction of hot-cathode rectification (DP 456512 of 1922).

Roentgen tube with double focus – Dofok-Röntgenröhre (DP 406067 of 1923).

Cassette changer after Berg – first spotfilm device (Registered model 845236 of 1923).

Four-valve rectification, Graetz design (1924).

Roentgen tube with internal radiation protection anode surrounded by shield with beryllium window (DP 473930 of 1925).

Deep therapy unit after Holfelder, completely shockproof and radiation-protected (1925 catalog).

Grenzstrahlen therapy unit after Gustaf Bucky (1926).

Condenser transformer for diagnosis with very short exposures (1927 catalog).

Roentgen tube with hollow anode for contact therapy (DP 567473 of 1928).

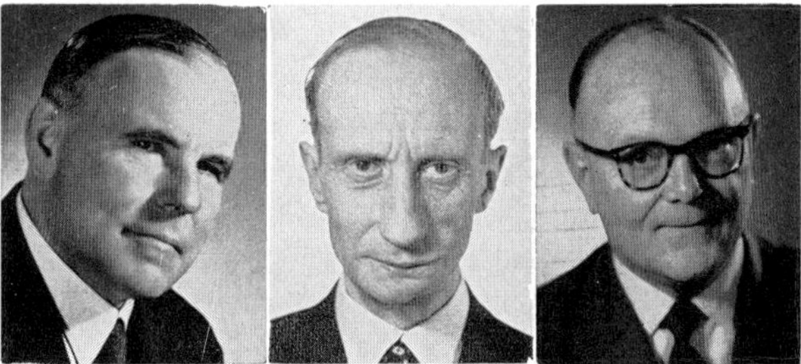

THEODOR SEHMER   VON BISSING   JOHANN PÄTZOLDT
Officials of Siemens-Reiniger.

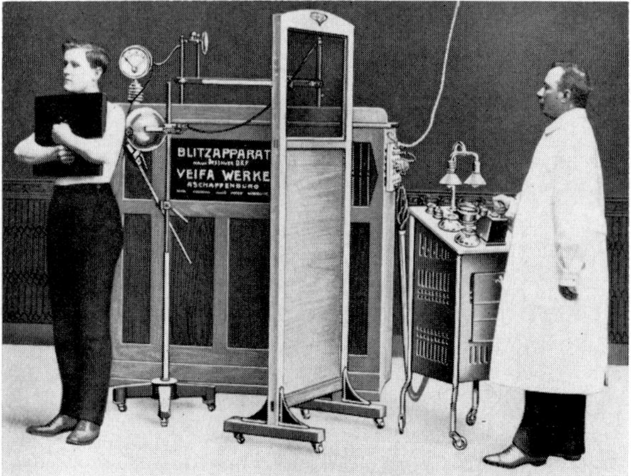

Courtesy: SRW Archives.

FRIEDRICH DESSAUER'S BLITZ (1909). One hundredth of one second exposures gave sharp detail even when the patient held the cassette. The machine was manufactured by the Veifa-Werke.

Triphasic generator, full-wave rectified, giving 2000 ma at 80 kvp (1928).

Grounded high-tension cables (1930).

Sinegran Rubra reinforcing screens with colored surface to minimize fluorescence (DP 660874 of 1930).

Long cone for better collimation of the beam after Frick (1930 catalog).

Transformer for 400-1000 kvp (1931).

Rotating anode Pantix with radiation cooling (1932).

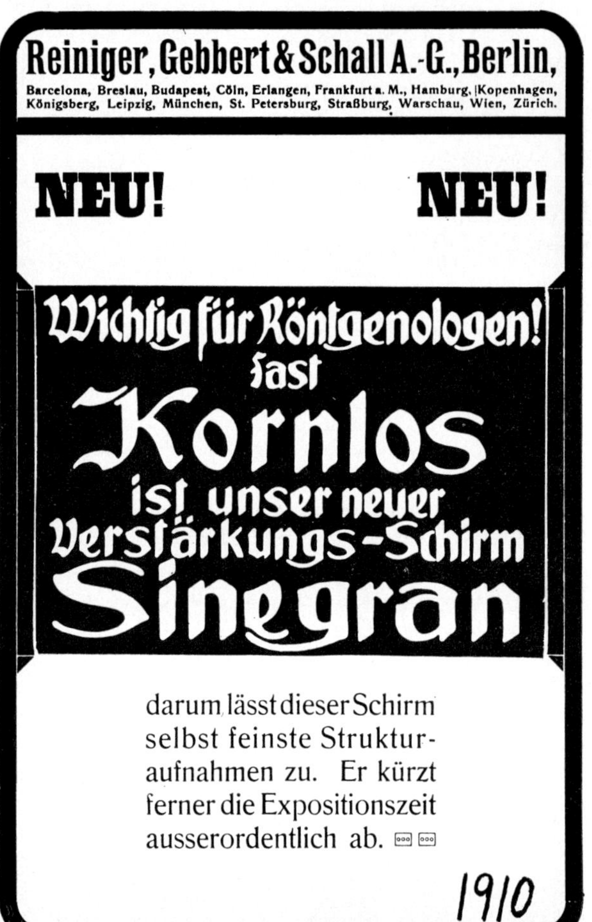

CORNUCOPIA. In copywriter's slang the barbarism which makes up the title of this caption – from the Latin *cornu copiae* (Amalthea's horn of plenty) – might indicate a copiously corny copy. The German copywriter of 1910 wanted to publicize the fact that the then new Sinegran re-inforcing screens had a very fine grain; he used the (already then ancient) trick of inserting the German word *fast* (meaning: almost) in the diminutive characters ahead of the needlessly capitalized *Kornlos* (meaning: grainless). Transliterations from foreign tongues are sometimes deceiving: the German word *Korn* means wheat, while the American corn is called *Mais* in Germany (and in France). Obviously, both this ad and the caption below it are *maisvoll* (full of corn)!

Introskop after Frick for body section radiography (1932 catalog).

Roentgenkugel, 22 cm metallic sphere containing transformer and tube under oil, giving 10 ma at 60 kvp (1933).

Beginning automation through pre-set milliamperage (1934).

Contact therapy unit after Chaoul (1934).

Explorator; fluoroscopic, spotfilm, and serial film device after Albrecht (1934).

Roentgen tube with pointed anode for cavity irradiation (1934).

Fully automated diagnostic control stand: one button each for kvp and mas, with circuit to prevent roentgen tube overload (1937).

Arrangement for indirect (screen) roentgen-cinematography after Janker (1937).

Rotating anode with grid-controlled exposure for serial and cinematographic ultilization (1937).

Planigraph for body section radiography on standing patient (1937 catalog).

Röntgenbombe; single container deep therapy unit giving 30 ma at 200 kvp (1938).

Transportable photofluorographic outfit for 24x24 mm rollfilm (1938).

63x63 mm photofluorographic apparatus (1940).

6 mev betatron for both electrons and x-radiation (1944).

Iontomat; phototimer built on principle of integral dosimeter with ionization chamber and cut-off circuits (1946).

Explorator Super; fluoroscopic, spotfilm, and serial film device with compressed air, fully automatized, push-button operation (1949).

Universal-Planigraph for body section radiography with patient in any position: 90/90° (1949).

Transversal-Planigraph for transverse body section radiography in either horizontal or vertical position (1949).

Rotational therapy unit with fluoroscopic control of the beam (1949).

Rotational and/or convergent therapy unit (1949).

Therapy unit with pendular motion after Kohler (1950).

Angiograph after Janker, serial films from screen image (1950).

Roentgen-cinematograph after Janker (1951).

Electron-optical image intensifier (1951).

Sireskop; table and spotfilm device with power-assist of all movements and electro-magnetic locks (1952).

Stabilipan; first therapy unit with selenium rectifiers; also fully automatic stabilization of both ma and kvp (1953).

Roentgen-cinematography based on image intensification (1953).

Roentgen-cinematograph after Janker with circular support (1953).

15 mev betatron for both electrons and x radiation (1953).

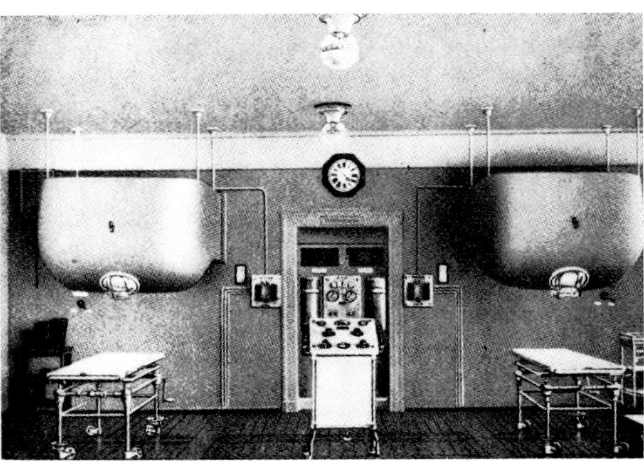

Courtesy: SRW Archives.

TWIN THERAPY UNITS (1921). Siemens & Halske installation with two ceiling-suspended tube containers, both shock- and radiation-protected.

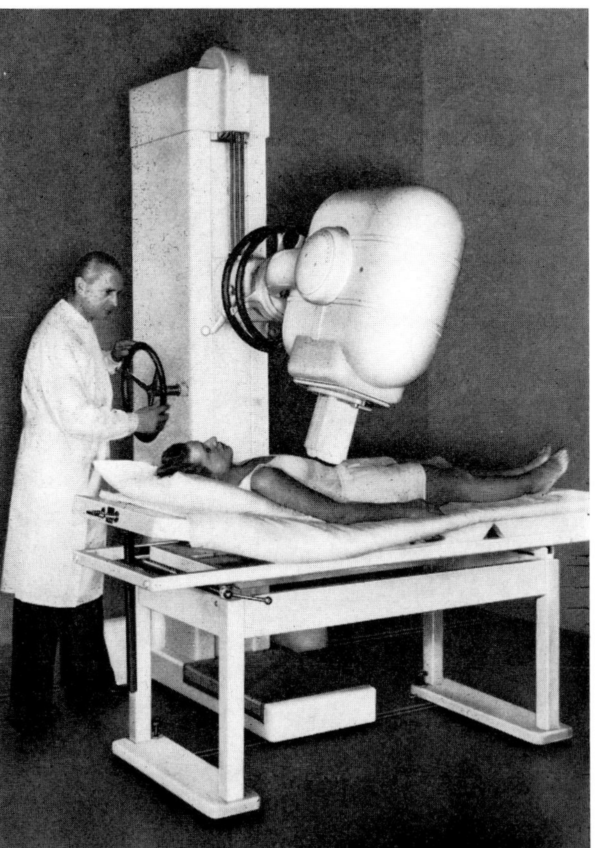

Courtesy: SRW Archives.

SRW RÖNTGENBOMB (1938). Comparable to GE's Maximar, it was a self-contained transformer-tube unit, capable of delivering 30 ma at 200 kvp.

Gamma meter with probe for actual measurements (also intracavitary) during radium and/or radiocobalt therapy (1953).

Gamatron; Co^{60} teletherapy unit (1955).

Improved transformer for diagnosis with selenium rectifier and added automation (1956).

Triomat; improved triphasic generator with photo-timing (1959).

Nanophos; rotating anode and transformer with selenium rectifiers in single, small casing, usable in mobile unit (1960).

42 mev betatron (1962).

Being a respectable organization, SRW has its own archives. This is why they were able to provide in such detail the list of accomplishments. Their archivist, Oefele, added pertinent remarks on the development of tubes, from which a few excerpts are given below.

The patent (DP 91028) obtained by Siemens & Halske for adjustable ionic roentgen tubes – dated March 24, 1896 – was presumably the first patent issued in the x-ray field. The construction of a gas tube with tungsten electrodes (DP 165138 of November 8, 1904) brought that tube to its maximum capability. Then came Coolidge's groundbreaking contribution, the hot cathode tube. Next were three significant steps, of which the first is the line focus, suggested by many precursors (including Rollins of Boston), but first built in 1918 by Reiniger, Gebbert & Schall (they followed the specifications of Goetze, a surgeon from Erlangen). The second improvement was the double-focus (Dofok) originated in the Phönix Röntgenröhrenwerk. The third was the rotating anode: the underlying idea had been expressed as early as 1896 by R. W. Wood* and in 1929 Bouwers had come up with a working model, but SRW made it practical by adding an adequate cooling system. It consists of a disc behind the anode, both being rotated on a thin stem: heat transfer occurs by radiation (at very high temperature). This particular cooling system is today universally used. SRW was also the first to introduce the grid into the rotating anode tube (1937) making it a triode. Finally in 1956 they came out with the Biangulix, a rotating anode with double focus, but each focus has its own angulation tilt with respect to the axis of the tube: this double angulation (called skewbent anode in Dunlee's

*Robert Williams Wood (1868-1955), professor of physics at John Hopkins in Baltimore, perfected also a method of color photography, and published science fiction, as well as an illustrated volume of non-sense verse, *How to tell the Birds from the Flowers* (1907).

Courtesy: SRW Archives.

SRW Universal Planigraph (1949). This ringstand (which preceded GE's Imperial) permitted body section radiography in any desirable (and in several from the patient's viewpoint undesirable) positions. It ushered in the modern "era of the ringstands."

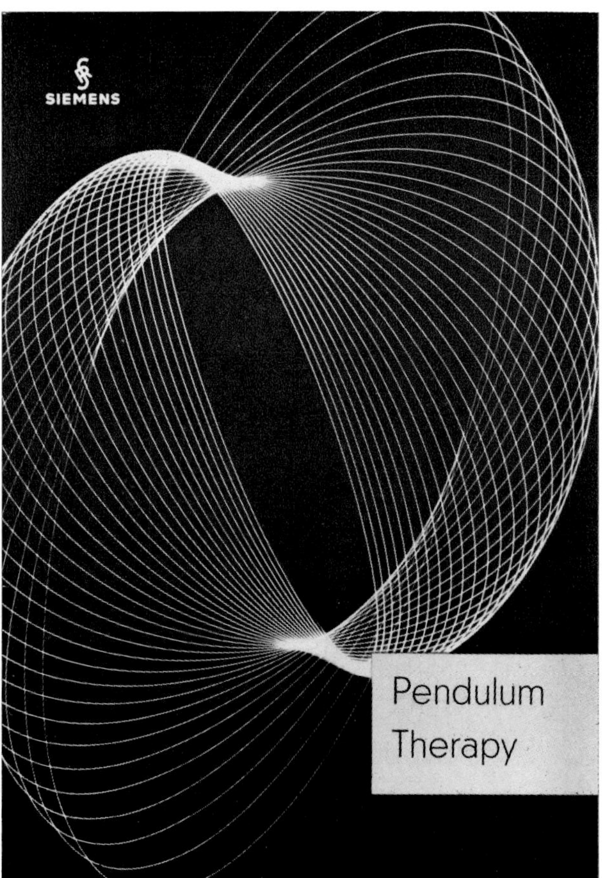

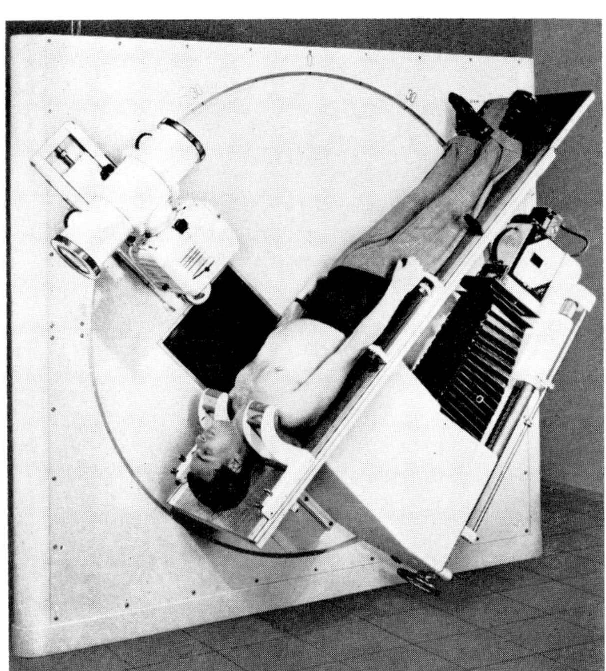

Courtesy: SRW Archives.

ROBERT JANKER'S ROENTGEN-CINEMATOGRAPH (1953). In GE's Imperial, which came out in 1951, the table's center of rotation coincides with the center of the ring-stand. Janker's patient is similarly centered (*was* is a better term, because this unit has been obsoleted by image intensification). Note the collimator, an accessory in common use (indicating light beam and all) since the 1930s. In this arrangement the camera "looks" at the fluorescent screen through a mirror. The angulation gives sufficient focus distance to the lens of the camera, and facilitates protection of sensitive photographic material from unwanted radiation.

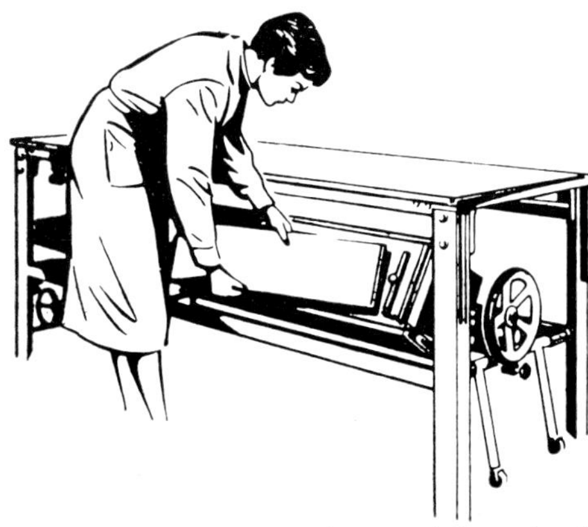

SRW CASSETTE CHANGER. This model is for lengthy cassettes, usable in angiography of the extremities.

book) is said to increase sharpness of details in the finished film.

All Atomic Phase refinements are available in SRW equipment. They have an all purpose table called Klinograph. Their better models, the Isoskop and Sireskop have both 90-90 motion and sidewise (lateral) displacement of the table top. In addition, the Sireskop comes with rotatory cradle attachment. Among their x-ray transformers, the Heliophos 4 delivers 300 ma at 125 kvp, or 500 ma at 90 kvp. The triphasic Tridoros 6 is rated at 300 ma at 150 kvp, 1000 ma at 100 kvp, or 600 ma at 125 kvp. They have several highload rotating anodes, for instance the twin-focus Biangulix, which will take 150 kvp. Their mobile 9″ image intensifier can easily be

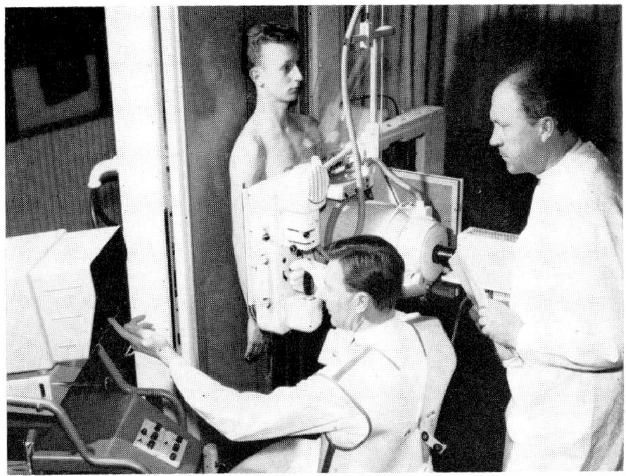

Courtesy: SRW Archives.

IMAGE INTENSIFICATION. The electron-optical intensifier is mounted on top of the automatized spotfilm device called Explorator. It has the expected television pick-up with monitor, and optional movie attachment. The radiologist is still seated next to the patient, but he is looking away from him. SiReWa has – of course – a very luxurious remote-control arrangement, intercom and all.

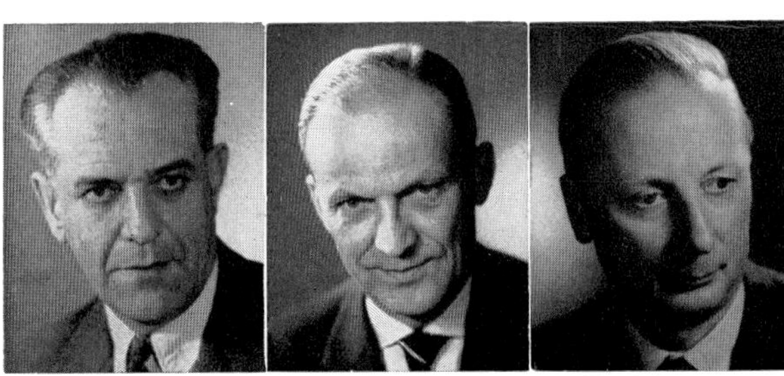

ALFRED SCHAAL W. GAJEWSKI F. MALSCH

SRW technicians: Schaal is an expert in matters of protection; Gajewski directs their photolab; and Malsch is a designer.

Bereits weit über **1000 Rotax-Apparate**

fest verkauft!

Dies ist für die **unübertroffene Güte** und **Leistungsfähigkeit** der Apparate das **beste Zeugnis.**

Jedes alte Röntgeninstrumentarium lässt sich durch Anbringung eines **Rotax-Unterbrechers modernisieren** und dadurch **zu Moment-** und **Fernaufnahmen** verwenden.

Der **Rotax** ist ein **Apparat der Praxis,** ist wegen seiner **Einfachheit** und **Leistungsfähigkeit** auf allen Gebieten der Röntgenarbeit und **Billigkeit allen anderen Konstruktionen vorzuziehen.**

Jeder Arzt kann sich davon in unserem Röntgenlaboratorium durch **eigene Anschauung überzeugen!**

— Die neueste Ausführung —
der Rotax-Röntgen-Instrumentarien

besteht in einer **fahrbaren Einrichtung** mit **Bleiwand** und **Bleiglas-Beobachtungsfenster** zum **absoluten Schutz gegen die Röntgenstrahlen** bei Durchleuchtungen, Aufnahmen und Therapie. Der Durchleuchtungsschirm ist hinter dem Bleiglas-Beobachtungsfenster bequem nach oben und unten verschiebbar. Schalter, Rheostaten, wie auch Rotax-Unterbrecher werden unter vollkommenem Schutz von demselben Standort aus ohne Platzänderung des Operateurs bedient.

Über 140 Zeugnisse von Röntgenologen u. Physikern.

Allmonatliche Röntgenkurse für Ärzte im eigenen Hörsaal!

Rotax Intensiv Induktor

Bleiglas

Bleiwand

„Rotax-Typ"
Die neueste Ausführung der Rotax-Röntgen-Instrumentarien.

Röntgenapparat ‚Motograph',

Hochspannungs-Transformator ohne Unterbrecher.

Der neueste und beste Apparat dieser Ausführung.

Referenz: Prof. Dr. Grunmach vom Königlichen Röntgen-Institut, welches mit dem Apparat zur grössten Zufriedenheit arbeitet.

Elektrizitätsgesellschaft „Sanitas"

Spezialfabrik für Röntgeneinrichtungen.

Friedrichstrasse 131d. **BERLIN N. 24,** Ecke Karlstrasse.

Düsseldorf, London, Brüssel, Paris, Mailand, Madrid, Oporto, Wien, Prag, St. Petersburg, Moskau, Odessa, Kiew, Warschau.

1910

wheeled into the operating room; it has television monitoring!

Among minor items may be mentioned a radiographic roentgen beam visual localizer; instead of the usual double-slot it has a multileaf collimator. Their floor-to-ceiling tubestand has electromagnetic locks. The SRW phototimer introduced in 1946 is called the Iontomat 6. They have a highly automatized control stand for the Triomat. Their therapy machines, for instance the convergent beam model, are offered with a special irradiation table on rails. The Dermopan with Beryllium window tube has a range from 10 to 50 kvp.

The international holdings of SRW will be discussed in the general context of the Global Glimpse.

E. G. SANITAS

At this point, a few lines will be dedicated to the memory of the firm Elektrizitäts-Gesellschaft Sanitas

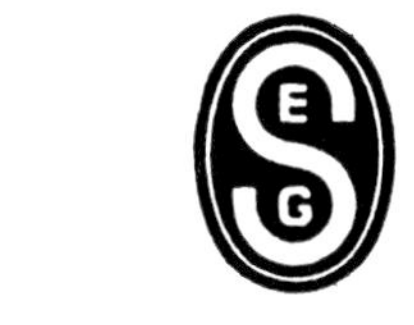

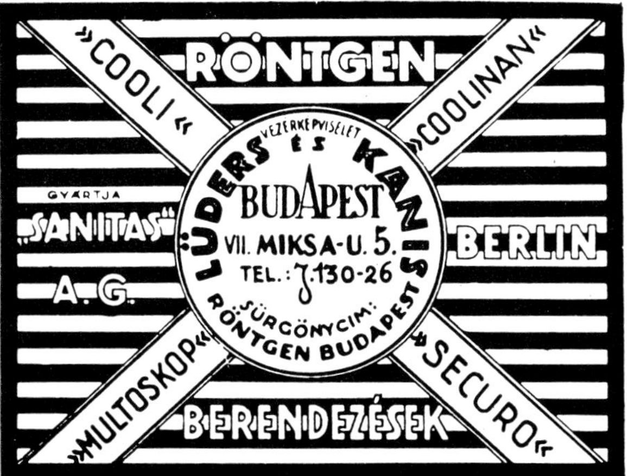

Courtesy: New York Academy of Medicine.

HUNGARIAN AD (1936). Sanitas was well represented in Central Europe and in South America, not quite as extensively in Asia.

(Berlin); it passed away early in 1960. Their time of glory did not extend much beyond the Golden Age of Radiology.

Among Sanitas "names" were the portable Coolifero, the medium-powered Coolinan with the table Sanitaskop, and the Supremos which was a combination suitable for both diagnosis and therapy. Their big generator Neograph pioneered push-button automatics.

Most of all, Sanitas will be remembered for having put on the market in 1933 the Tomograph, designed by Gustav Grossmann* - many subsequent single-plane contraptions issued by other manufacturers were copied from this initial model.

C. H. F. MUELLER

Within the Philips empire, the firm C. H. F. Mueller of Hamburg occupies a special position. It advertises as an independent organization, even in Sweden or France, where Philips has recognized factories and outlets. And Philips does not maintain separate sales offices in either Germany or Austria. This is presumably done to preserve Mueller's corporate image

*Of course, there were many precursors to the principle of body section radiography; among the best known were the Dutch Ziedzes des Plantes and the Italian Alessandro Vallebona. The very first, though, was Bocage in France.

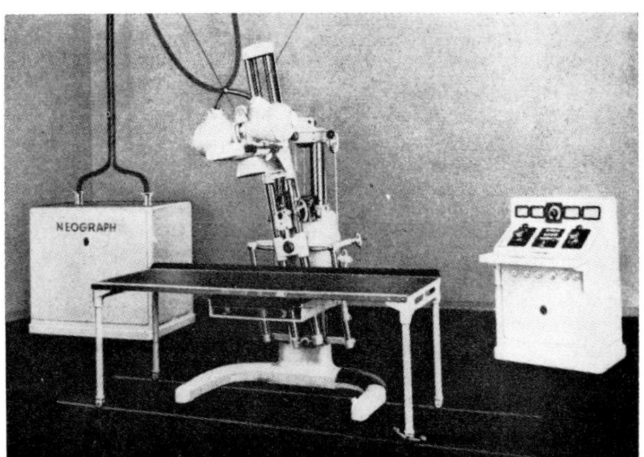

GROSSMANN'S TOMOGRAPH (1932). This is the very successful prototype (both technically and saleswise) of the often imitated classic, horizontal body section radiographic table.

←
SANITAS' ROTAX. Their most successful pre-World War I apparatus was undoubtedly the Rotax. Their "improved" model has been imitated and is still popular (with modern modifications) in the combined fluoroscop-photofluorograph encountered in European x-ray production lines. Sanitas held some of the Russian market well into the 1930's.

in the eyes of its Germanic consumers. There could hardly be another reason, as the Mueller company is owned by Philips. Very seldom have they used the denomination Philips Mueller in the titles of their products or subsidiaries.

Carl Heinrich Florenz Müller (1845-1912) was a glass-blower. His first shop dates in Hamburg from the year 1865. He kept in touch with the changing world, and when the time came he produced incandescent light bulbs; fluorescent tubes of the various types, Hittorf, Crookes, Geissler, Puluj, Lenard; and — after Röntgen's discovery — x-ray tubes. By 1897 his tubes had become well known around the globe, in 1901 a Mueller tube was awarded the Gold Medal of the (British) Roentgen Society. The Mueller Company made only tubes until after World War I. By the mid-1930s they had added a full line of transformers, tables, and other accessories, but that was only after Philips purchased controlling interests.

Mueller was primarily a tube manufacturer. Their current rotating anode is called Mueller-Duplo-Rotalix (Rotalix is a term coined by Philips): it has a twin-focus (.9 and 1.6 mm), and comes in several versions, including one with the top rating of 150 kvp. Mueller manufactures three image intensifiers, of 5″, 7″, and 9″ size.

Very popular is an image intensifier mounted on one arm of a U-shaped support. On the other arm is a single-tank transformer and tube. It is low-powered because not much of a load is needed to obtain a fluoroscopic image with the intensifier. On casters it can easily be wheeled into and out of the emergency or operating rooms. When equipped with an eyepiece or with a mirror system, it requires a lot of surgical draping. This is solved simply by adding a television pick-up, and everybody in the room can "look away" from the patient, and "see" it all on the monitor. Such a combination — which in Mueller's book is called BV-20 — will undoubtedly change things in orthopedics: once one gets used to it, nothing seems to be able to replace the ease with which bone fragments can be kept under control, and situations re-adjusted before they are recorded on celluloid. The surgical BV-20 comes also in a military model, the field unit BV-20T.

Image intensifiers are just as useful, perhaps even more so, in industrial fluoroscopy. Also there the television pick-up is an optional, at times indispensable, feature.

Incidentally — like all major manufacturers of x-ray equipment — Mueller has a line of small and medium-

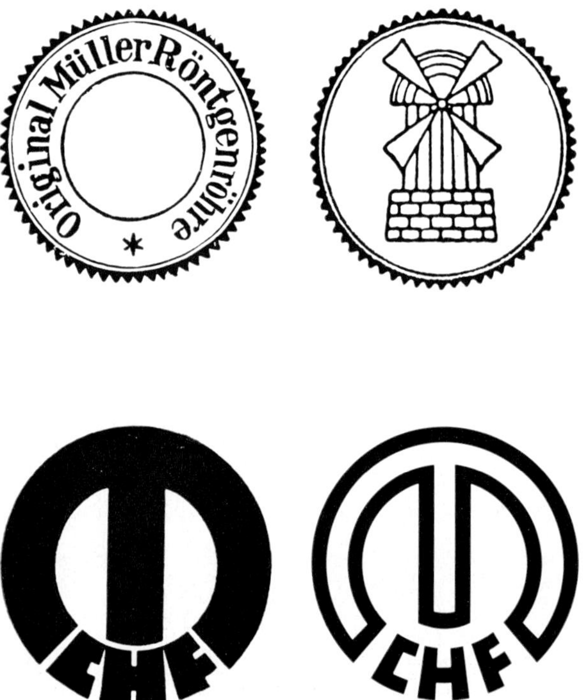

Courtesy: C. H. F. Mueller.

MUELLER TRADE-MARKS. The seal with the inscription was the very first ever used. It was replaced in 1910 with the windmill (in German MÜLLER means mill-operator). The stylized black-on-white CHFM was introduced in 1930. The change to the last shape was made in 1945, to indicate that something had been modified, while preserving the good, old name.

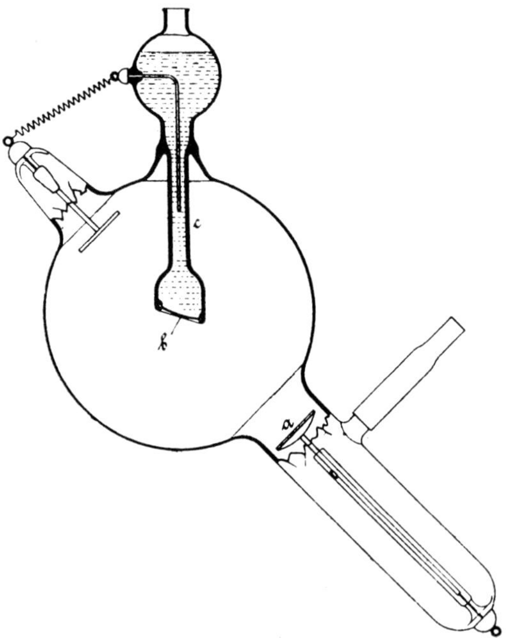

Courtesy: C. H. F. Mueller.

MUELLER TUBE OF 1899. Its German patent (113,430) was granted on May 21, 1899. The peculiarity was the water-cooled anticathode.

powered industrial x-ray units, from the Macrotank to the MG 150/300. The Mikro (91, 101, 111) is used in microradiography, and Mueller builds also a Spectrograph. As a Philips subsidiary, Mueller advertises and sells the (American) Norelco Autrometer.

Mueller transformers are called DA. There is the economical four-valve DA 301, which furnishes 300 ma at 90 kvp, or 150 ma at 125 kvp. Any of these can be combined with a phototimer – called Amplimat – for fully automatized exposures: only the kilovoltage has to be set, after which "the" button can be pushed. The condenser-transformer Maximus, sold also by Philips, is likewise a Mueller product.

Mueller tables are called UG*, for instance UG3 is

*The explanation for these symbols is as follows: BV means *Bildverstärker* (the German term for image intensifier), DA comes from *Diagnostikapparat,* and UG is an abbreviation of *Untersuchungsgerät* (examining machine, *i.e.,* table).

F E D
hart weich
A B
hard soft
+ C

Neuheit!

Welt-Record-Duplex-Röntgen-Röhre.

Von C. H. F. Müller, Hamburg.

(Patent Deutschland, England, America angemeldet.)

Courtesy: C. H. F. Mueller.

MUELLER DUPLEX OF 1900. The unusual thing about this tube was the fact that one of the anticathodes gave a soft, the other a hard(er) x-ray beam, for whatever good could come out of such a combination.

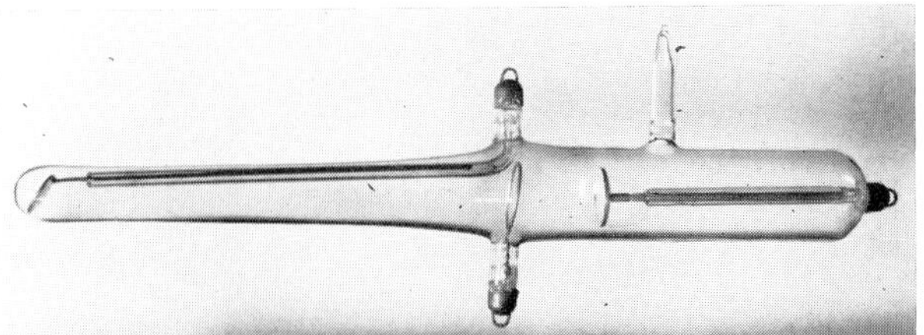

Courtesy: C. H. F. Mueller.

MUELLER THERAPY TUBE OF 1905. Just as 1897 had been a year of new designs in diagnostic x-ray tubes, so was 1905 a year of novelties in therapy tubes. The place where the x rays were generated was brought as close as possible to the treated territory. The electrons passed through the ring-shaped anode into the elongated "appendix" at the end of which they hit upon the anticathode.

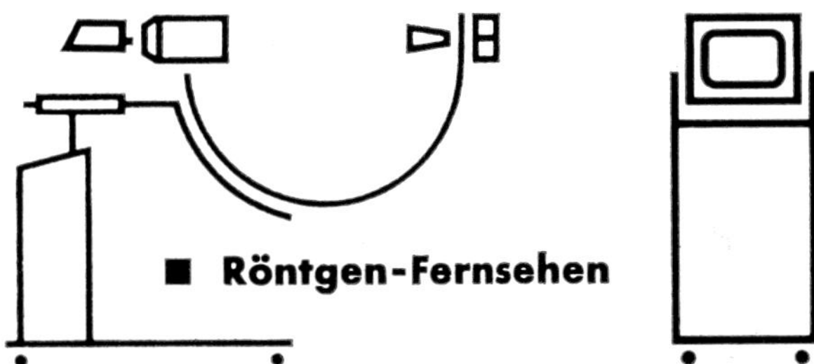

STYLIZED SURGICAL "SEE-ER." Sketch of Mueller's BV-20 shows control stand on casters, the Z-shaped support, the single-tank transformer and tube with cone attached, and on the other arm of the U an image intensifier with vidicon tube. The television monitor can be pushed around on its own casters. *Fernsehen* (seeing at distance) is the German term for television.

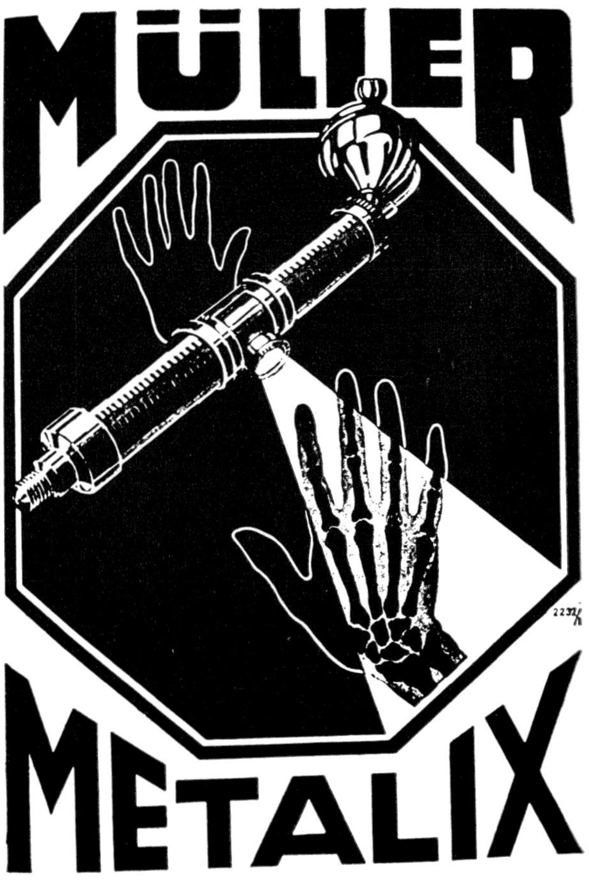

quite simple, and either hand- or motor-tilted, with one tube mounted on a floor-to-ceiling tubestand. In the USA ceiling suspension is just beginning to become popular. In Germany, ceiling suspension has been a stock item for decades, their luxurious tables are those which come with the column type of suspension (and the salesman can say, "see, nothing on the ceiling!"). UG4 is a table with motor-operated patient lift: it comes with the DK20, Mueller's highly automatized spotfilm device. The UG5 permits only 15° Trendelenburg.

Mueller's pièce de résistance in tables is the UGX, which allows rotation of the (cradled and fastened) patient in all three planes. The fore-runner of this table was the Omniskop built by E. Pohl in Kiel (Germany) in 1926, but even that could be mobilized only in two

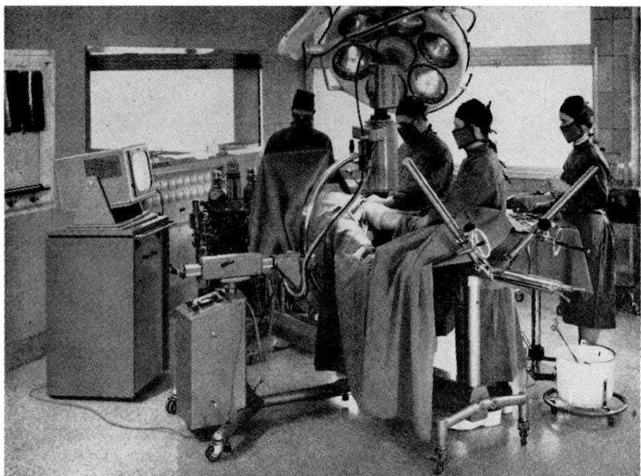

Courtesy: C. H. F. Mueller.

BV-20 IN-SITU. When television pick-up and monitoring is available, one can dispense with much of the sterilization (draping) problems connected with looking into the eyepiece or mirror of an image intensifier. Besides, everybody in attendance can see what is going on (an orthopedist friend of mine regards this as a very mixed blessing).

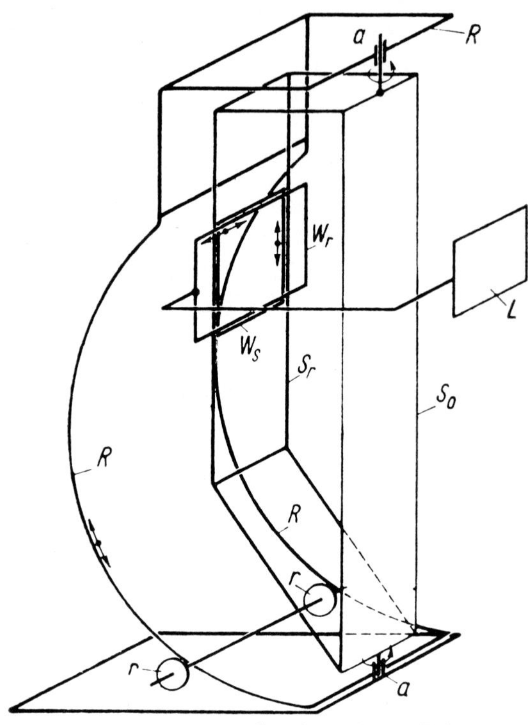

Courtesy: Georg Thieme Verlag.

POHL'S OMNISKOP (1926). The tube-screen carriage moved up and down, and side-wise. the patient could be reclined with the table, that is rotated about a transverse axis located in the center of the arc R. The patient could also be rotated around a longitudinal axis a-a, for which he was preferably cradled. This figure is from Rudolf Grashey's 1941 edition of Albers-Schönberg's *Röntgentechnik*.

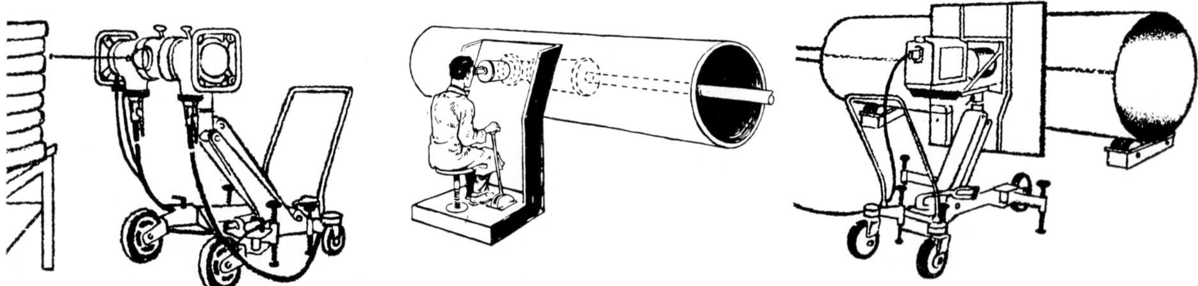

Courtesy: C. H. F. Mueller.

MUELLER INDUSTRIAL X-RAY EQUIPMENT. At left is the tubestand of an MG which comes in a constant potential 150 or 300 kvp. Image intensification is very useful in metalloscopy, because it allows softer radiation, and thus better contrast: with such intensification, one can see through 25 mm steel with the 150 kvp, through 60 mm steel with the 300 kvp. The sketch in the middle shows a stationary image intensifier, while the x-ray tube is held on a long shaft inside the pipe. On the right is the sketch of a mobile image intensifier with television pick-up, and distant monitoring.

planes. The UGX was first unveiled at the ICR in Copenhagen in 1953, together with the first commercial version of the Philips-Mueller image intensifier. Advertised as a machine for "functional" roentgen-diagnosis, is a combination of the UGX with a 28 cm image intensifier, coupled to the mirror lens of a 35 mm movie camera. Another special table is Mueller's UGF, which is simply a copy of the Koordinat (fixed tube and screen, with sliding table top), a Swedish idea (*cf.*, Elema-Schönander).

In the therapy line, Mueller advertises and sells Co-60 units made by Atomic Energy of Canada. Mueller's own RT-100 x-ray unit is rated from 10 to 100 kvp. The RT-250 comes in two versions, one with a simple column, the other with the famous TU-1 for either rotational, pendular, or convergent irradiating technics. The TU-1, designed after the ideas of the radiologist Werner Teschendorf, was first shown at the German Röntgenkongress in 1951. One wonders how "viable" these pendular and convergent (tangential) technics are in the era of cobalt teletherapy and particle accelerators? After all, it's only a skin-saver, no more, no less!

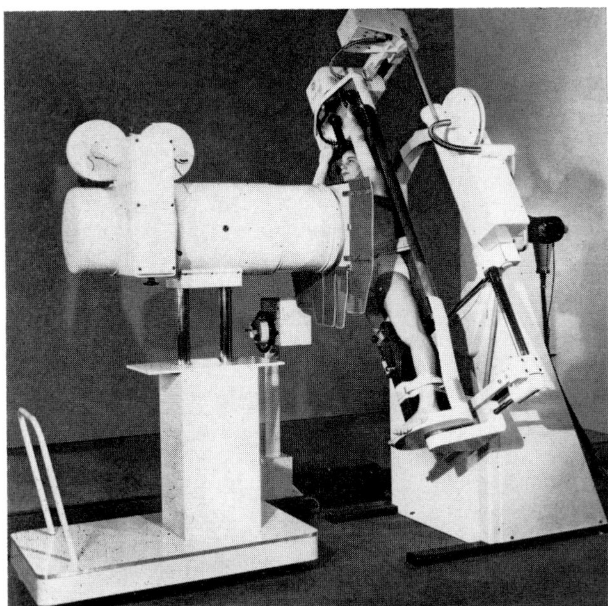

MUELLER'S UGX. In addition to the two planes of the Omniskop, the UGX has also a third plane of rotation, about an axis coincident with the x-ray beam. Patient is shown tilted along that axis to the patient's right. All these motions can be "inflicted" by remote control. The contraption in front of the "table" is an image intensifier with 28 cm input screen, "projected" through a mirror lens onto 35 mm movie film.

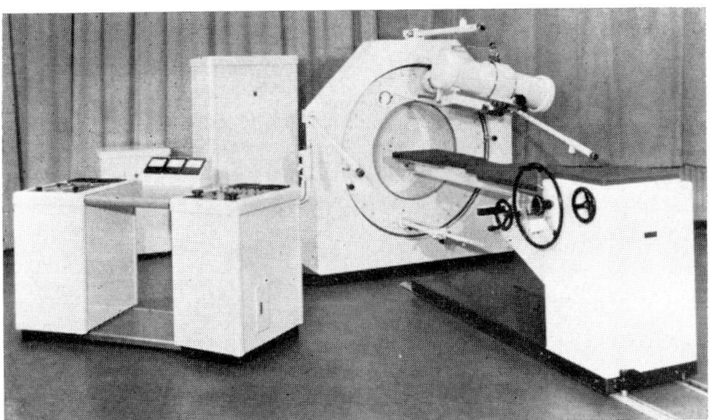

Courtesy: C. H. F. Mueller.

MUELLER'S TU-1. 250 kvp constant potential therapy unit mounted on special ringstand which, together with motor-driven irradiation table on rails, permits all sorts of treatment procedures (stationary, rotational, convergent, pendular, tangential).

SEIFERT

Richard Seifert & Co. of Hamburg is today the oldest privately-owned firm in the x-ray business. It was started by Friedrich Wilhelm Richard Seifert, Sr. (1862-1929) as an electro-technical shop on December 12, 1892 (in the wake of a protracted cholera epidemic).

Seifert, Sr. was a personal friend of C. H. F. Müller. Soon after Röntgen's discovery, an agreement was made whereby Seifert built all the electrical parts for the x-ray tubes made by Mueller. Their first co-operative

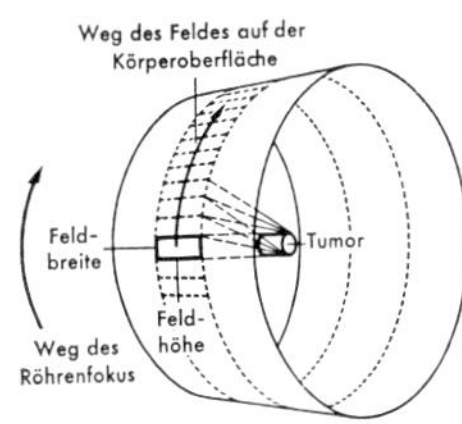

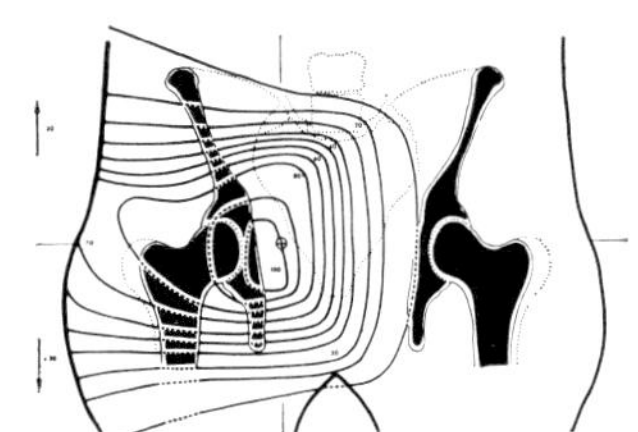

Courtesy: C. H. F. Mueller.

MOVING RADIATION TECHNICS. The dose-concentrating, *i.e.*, in the final analysis skin-saving, advantages of the convergent *vs.* simple rotational irradiation seem obvious.

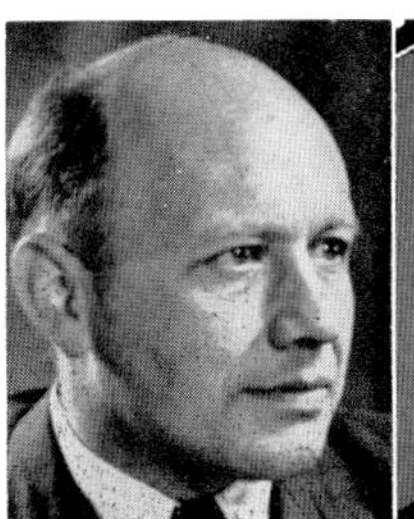

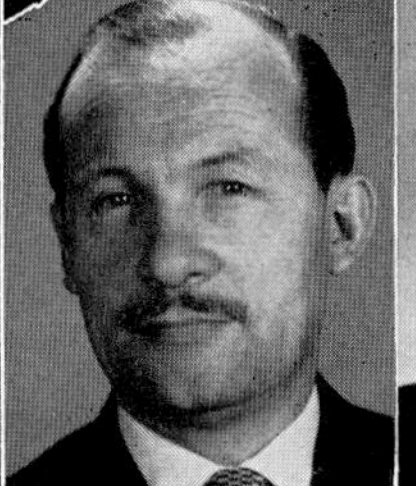

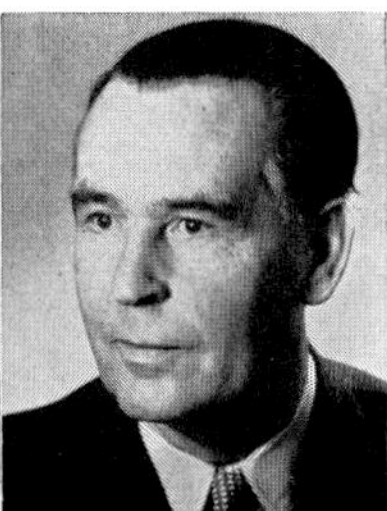

CURT NÄFCKE WILLI FLINDT I. INGWERTSEN

Officials of the C. H. F. Mueller Co.

venture in this field was the apparatus with which Voller produced in mid-January, 1896 his and Hamburg's first roentgen plate (of a healthy hand). It received world-wide attention, and was reproduced in the *Medical Record* (New York).

Later on a close friendship, and scientific collaboration, developed between Albers-Schönberg, Bernhard Walter, and Seifert, Sr. Most of the illustrations in the first edition(s) of Albers-Schönberg's *Röntgentechnik* (published by Lucas Gräfe & Sillem in Hamburg) were sketched by Seifert's draftsman. On Albers-Schönberg's request, Seifert built in 1903 an x-ray protection device, consisting of a lead-lined wooden box, with lead-glass window. It turned out to be one of the earliest, if not the first, model of what was to become a popular device only during the Golden Age of Radiology, the technician's booth.

After Müller's radiation death, his company was taken over by Liebermann, and Seifert, Sr. continued the previous agreement with him. Soon after World War I, though, Liebermann sold out to Philips, and this is when the gentlemen's agreement between the firms of Mueller and Seifert lapsed. Seifert hired one of Mueller's former glassblowers, and for a while produced his own ionic x-ray tubes.

In 1917 the founder's son – Heinrich Wilhelm Richard Seifert, Jr. – was taken on as an equal partner in the firm. After his father's death, and to this day, the son remained the firm's owner and manager.

Seifert, Jr., a Ph.D. in physics, made several significant contributions to the firm's well-being. He became interested in the industrial applications of x-ray procedures. In 1925 he began to switch pro-

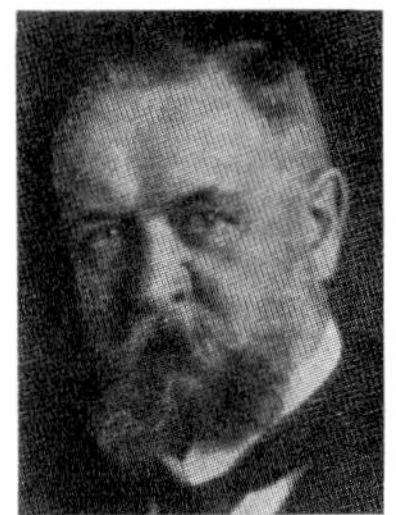

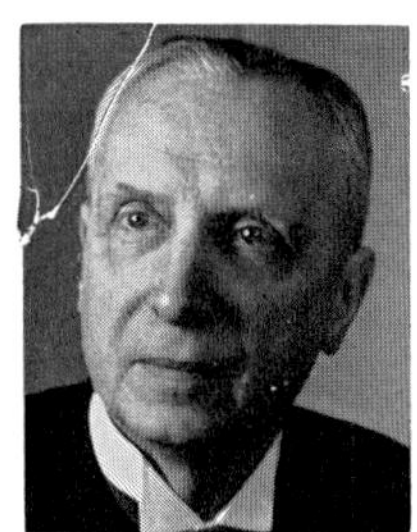

RICHARD SEIFERT, SR. (with beard) and his son, RICHARD SEIFERT, JR.

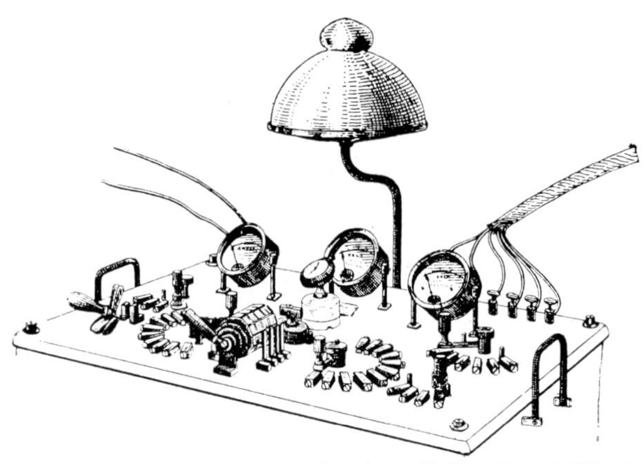

Courtesy: University of Illinois.

SEIFERT CONTROL STAND (1900). Reproduced from the first edition of Albers-Schömberg's *Röntgentechnik.*

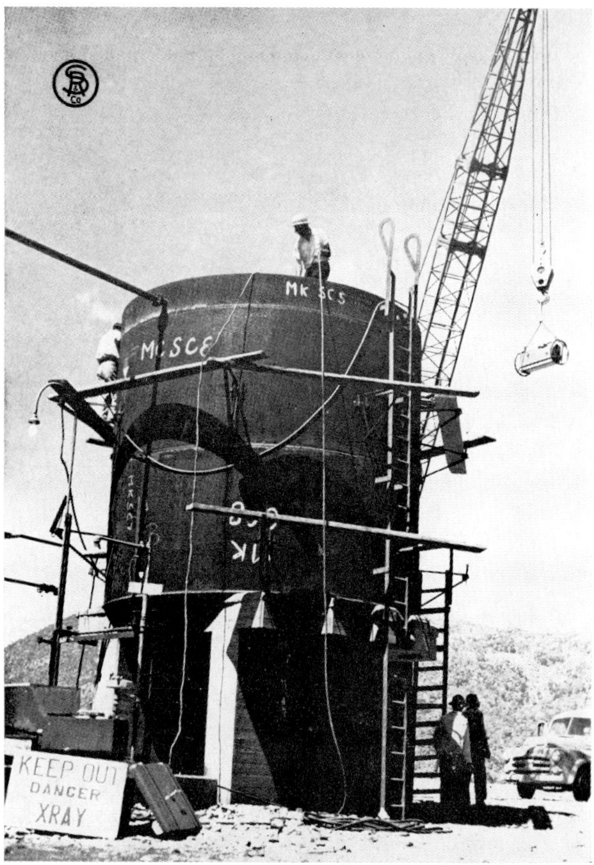

Courtesy: R. Seifert & Co.

SEIFERT'S ERESCO IN ACTION (1960). A 300 kvp single-tank Eresco x-ray unit is being hoisted for the checking of welds during construction of a large tank somewhere in the African tropics.

duction over to apparatus for non-destructive testing (as industrial x-ray machines are called).

The Allgemeine Elektrizitäts Gesellschaft (AEG) manufactured at that time x-ray tubes, and a friendly relationship developed between Seifert and AEG. In 1936, the latter made for Seifert an x-ray tube with small focus (.1 to .2 mm) which could take up to 150 watt loads. It was of little if any significance for medical purposes, but excellent for industrial applications.

Today Seifert produces only equipment for gross or detailed structural examinations. They have a constant potential transformer, called Isovolt, which comes in several sizes from 150 to 400 kvp. A single-tank unit (transformer and tube in a single, grounded casing), named Eresco, is available in five "degrees of penetrability" between 120 and 300 kvp. Seifert furnishes all necessary accessories, from darkroom to viewing equipment.

Several models of diffraction analysis units are offered, a recent one being the Iso-Debyeflex III A (named for the Dutch-Swiss physicist Peter Josef Wilhelm Debye, who is currently teaching chemistry at Cornell University in New York City).

The Seifert Company has kept up with the Atomic Phase. They offer image intensifiers adapted to their industrial machinery. In addition they are building containers for radioactive sources. Small, portable 50 or 100 curie Co-60 units are sometimes of distinct advantage in industrial radiography because of their independence from bulky electrical connections. The drawbacks are cost of source replacement, and heavy shielding, as well as other protection requirements.

SCHLEUSSNER

The world's oldest photo-chemical factory (one century plus !) is the Adox Fotowerke Dr. C. Schleussner GmbH in Frankfurt-am-Main.

Carl Schleussner (1830-1899), after getting his PhD in chemistry in 1857,* came to Frankfurt in 1860, and in the same year married Elise Rinn, daughter of a manufacturer of sealing-wax. Also in 1860, young Schleussner obtained a permit to install a "pharmaceutical laboratory" in the house of his in-laws, at nr. 18 on Römerberg.

On the 100th anniversary of that "pharmaceutical laboratory," the Research Section of the German Photographic Society held a festive session in the aula of the Goethe University in Frankfort, to honor the memory of Carl Schleussner. On that occasion John Eggert (of Zürich) retraced the changing concepts on what is the latent (dormant!) photographic image, and Robert Janker (of Bonn) discussed the methods and the medical importance of roentgen photography. The honor was rightly due because the founder of that "pharmaceutical laboratory" contributed considerably to the making of what is regarded as modern photography (and roentgen-photography).

At this point it may be of interest to recapitulate briefly the development of photography itself.

It all started with the ancient observation that certain colors fade when exposed to sunlight. Just how old this observation is can no longer be determined — it was found inscribed on Babylonian cuneiform tablets dating back to 3000 B.C. The alchemistic *Doctor universalis* Albertus Magnus Count of Bollstädt (1193-1280) is credited with the discovery that silver nitrate is light-sensitive.

In 1727, in Halle (Germany), Johann Heinrich Schulze used silver salts to make legible copies of written text. In 1822 — in Paris — Joseph Nicéphore Niepce (1765 — 1833) produced a picture (the first of its kind) by exposing a light-sensitive surface in a camera. In 1838, in London, William Henry Fox Talbot (1800-1877) made the first (silver chloride) paper prints, suggested the term "photogenic drawing," and deciphered Assyrian inscriptions, including that pristine reference to actinism. On March 14, 1839, before the

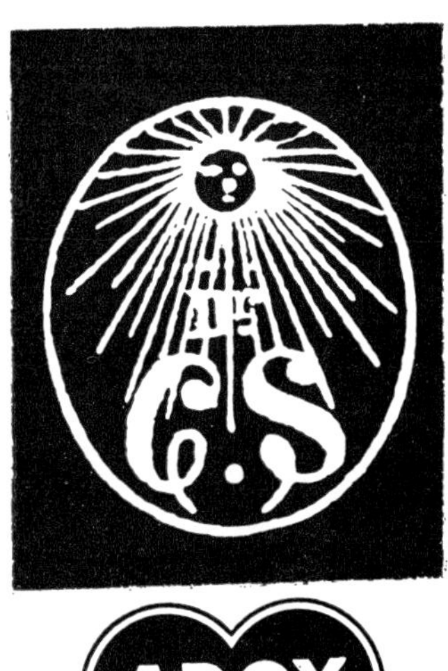

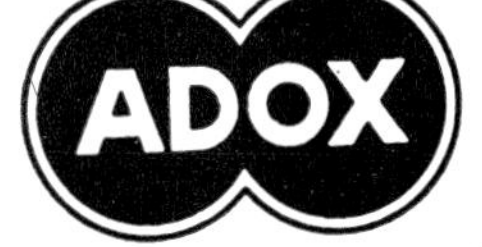

SCHLEUSSNER SEALS. The earliest (solar-bathed), and the latest.

Dr. Schleussner

*He studied for one year at Heidelberg with Robert Wilhelm Bunsen (1811-1899), whose eponym is recalled in the Bunsen burner, and in the Bunsen actinometer.

Royal Society, Sir John Frederick William Herschel (1792-1871) coined the term photography; he was also the first to employ the words positive and negative in the photographic sense, and to introduce the hypo (sulfites) as a fixer of the image. In 1850, the English sculptor Frederick Scott Archer (1813-1857) developed the *wet* collodion process, by which an emulsion could be coated on a glass plate. When traveling it meant carrying along a laboratory, with a tent-type darkroom, but many famous photographs have been produced with this *wet* process, including in this country the several thousand pictures exposed during the Civil War by Matthew Brady (1823-1896). In 1871, the English chemist Richard Lea Maddox came up with *dry* plates, meaning glass plates coated with an "emulsion" made by incorporating the photo-sensitive substance in gelatin.

Schleussner, upon starting in business, produced first the chemicals needed for the wet collodion process. When the dry process was developed, he turned to that new procedure. Schleussner's first dry gelatine plates were manufactured in 1879; he began exporting them to Austria and America in 1880; by 1881 his plates were universally acclaimed as a success.

In the 1890s, the yellow label *(Gelbetikett)* of Schleussner's dry plates had become famous the world over. Indeed, Röntgen used Schleussner plates to produce his very first roentgen-photographs. Carl Schleussner was then still at the helm of his enterprise, and there exists a letter - dated in Würzburg on May 13, 1896 - in which Röntgen thanks Carl Schleussner for a recent set of plates sent to him, and remarks that those plates had been faultless *(tadellos)*. In the same letter Röntgen goes on to inquire whether it would be possible to make plates

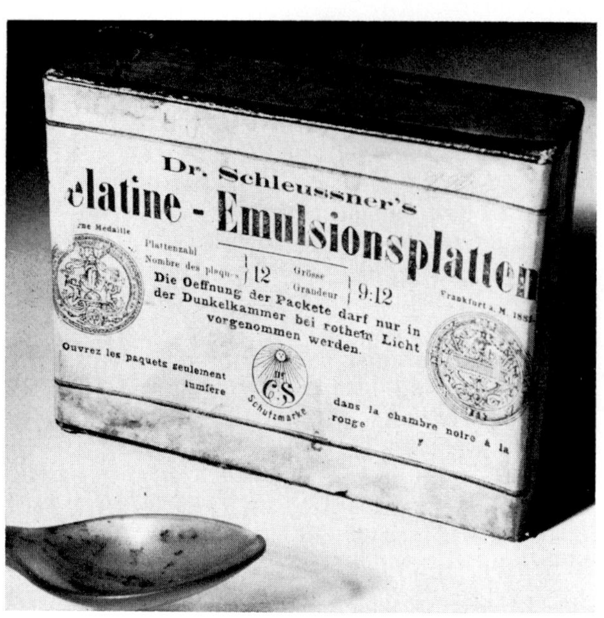

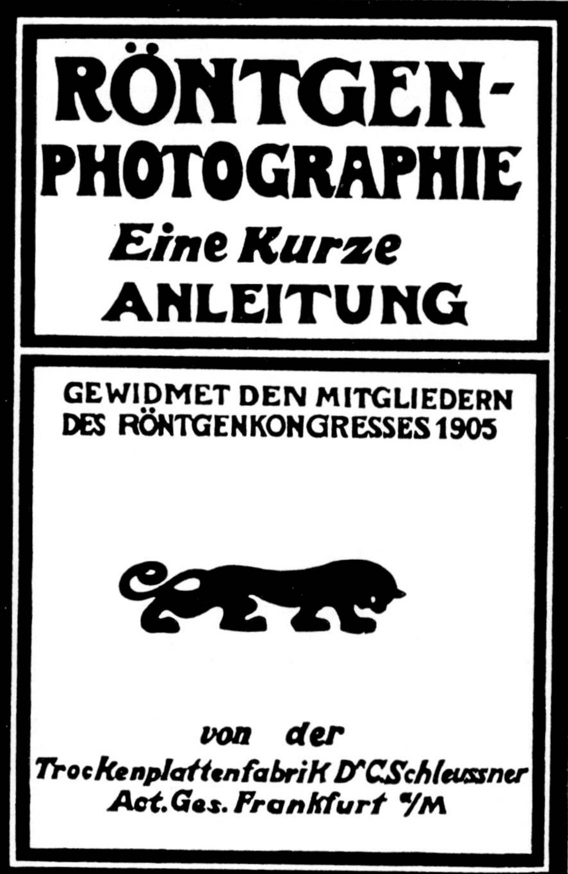

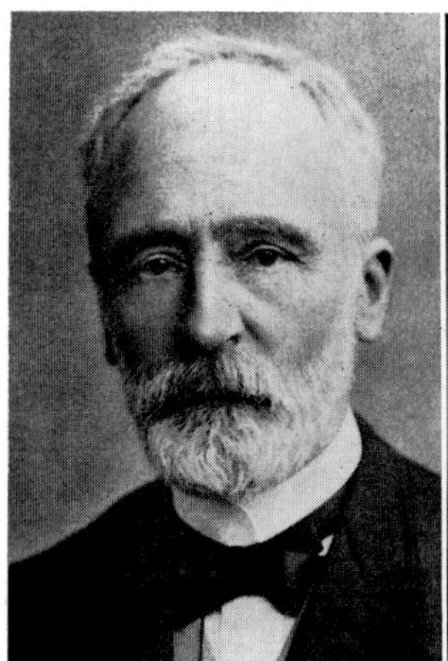
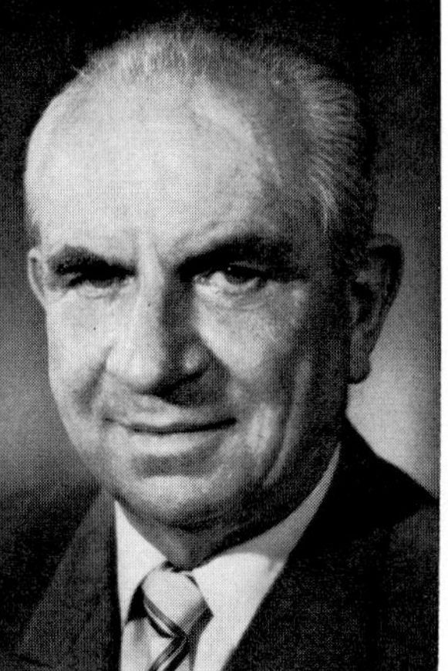

Courtesy: Adox.

SCHLEUSSNER STALWARTS. The bearded founder Carl Schleussner, whose signature constituted another of their seals, and his grandson Carl Adolf Schleussner, have been responsible for the firm's growth.

with a thicker (or more concentrated) silver salt coating, because he had found that "too many x-rays pass unused *(nutzlos)*" through what plates were then available.

Old Carl Schleussner did not stay around long enough to greet the 20th century. In 1900, appeared Immelmann's roentgen atlas: in the preface, Immelmann acknowledged that for the atlas he had used exclusively Schleussner plates. By 1905, Schleussner's roentgen plates dominated the world market. In that year, the first Röntgenkongress, Schleussner published (as a promotional booklet) Alban Kohler's *Anleitung zur Röntgen-Photographie.*

Old Carl not only created a solid photo-chemical business, he also sired a dynasty of photo-chemical businessmen to keep the fires lighted.

He was succeeded by his sons Friedrich and Carl Moritz Schleussner (1868-1943). Carl Moritz introduced the rollfilm in 1903; participated in the financially disastrous Deutsche Bioscop (also Bioskop and Bioscope) Gesellschaft (which produced the first artistic moving pictures); and authored a *Röntgenhandbuch* in 1909. By 1910 the Schleussner Company manufactured about 90% of all roentgen-photographic material exported from Germany.

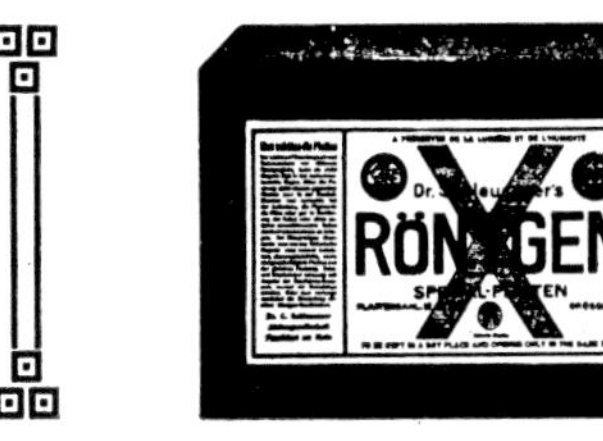

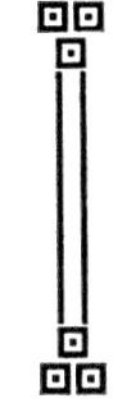

Röntgen-Spezialplatten

von vielen Autoritäten und von der Fachliteratur*)

ausdrücklich als die besten

aller vorhandenen Plattensorten für die Röntgenaufnahme bezeichnet.

Preisliste und Lieferung durch alle Handlungen photographischer Artikel oder direkt von der

Dr. C. Schleussner

Aktiengesellschaft

in Frankfurt am Main 27.

*) Professor Dr. Albers-Schönberg in Hamburg, Dr. Béla Alexander in Budapest, Dr. H. Gocht in Halle a. S., Professor Dr. A. Hoffa in Würzburg, Ingenieur Friedrich Dessauer-Aschaffenburg, Reiniger, Gebbert & Schall Aktiengesellschaft, Leitfaden des Röntgenverfahrens, Leipzig 1908, S. 324, Röntgen-Kalender, Leipzig 1908, S 93, Archiv für physik. Medizin u. medizin. Technik, Leipzig 1906, Bd. I, Heft 2/3, S. 200, Kompendium der Röntgenographie, Leipzig 1905, S. 252, 253 u. 269, Manuel Pratique de Radiologie Medicale, Bruxelles 1905, S. 41, Verhandlungen der Deutschen Röntgengesellschaft Hamburg 1908, S. 97, Deutsche Medizinische Wochenschrift, Berlin 1908, S. 1472, Orthoröntgenographie, München 1908, Zeitschrift für medizin. Elektrologie u. Röntgenkunde, Leipzig 1908, Bd. X, S. 11, Société de Radiologie Médicale de Paris, Bulletins et Mémoires, Tome I, Nr. 2, S. 43.

1910

Following the *Sturm* (stormy period) came the *Drang* (drive), during the "reign" of third generation Carl Adolf Schleussner (1895-1959). He took over in 1920, and soon changed the company into a family-owned joint-stock venture, with himself as president. In 1922 he patented the *Neo-Röntgenplatten,* sensitized to x rays more so than to light rays, which became the forerunner of material to be used without re-inforcing screens. A cache of *Neo-Röntgenplatten,* inadvertently stored for over thirty years, was found in the 1950s: the plates are in good shape, and very satisfactory roentgenograms can still be made with them. Some were shown (as a promotional feature) at the 1957 meeting of the Deutsche Röntgengesellschaft. In 1924, Schleussner began making x-ray paper, and in 1926 the double-coated Doneo x-ray film; in 1927 they built a factory at Neu-Isenburg, and came out with the double-coated Ixo-film; in 1931 they built a celluloid factory; in 1935 they observed their seventy-fifth anniversary; and in 1937 they put on the market the Ixotest for non-destructive testing, and the single-packaged Neotest.

On December 21, 1942 Allied incendiary bombs destroyed 90% of the Schleussner plant at Neu-Isenburg. It was rebuilt, but that demanded more "financial flexibility," for which a new corporate image and

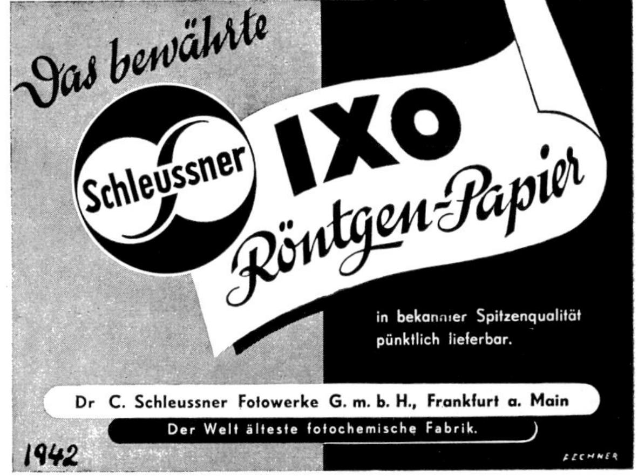

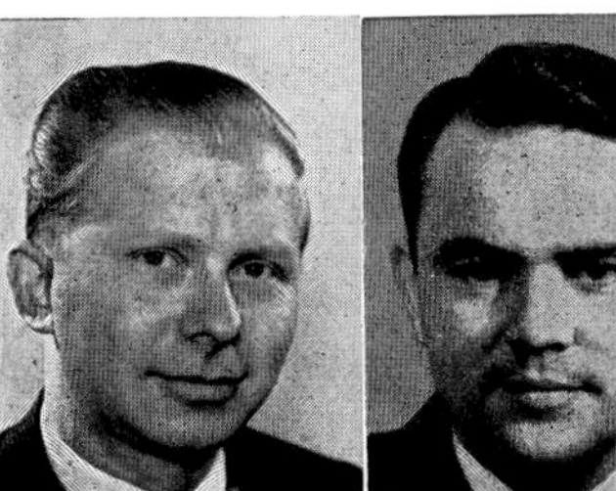

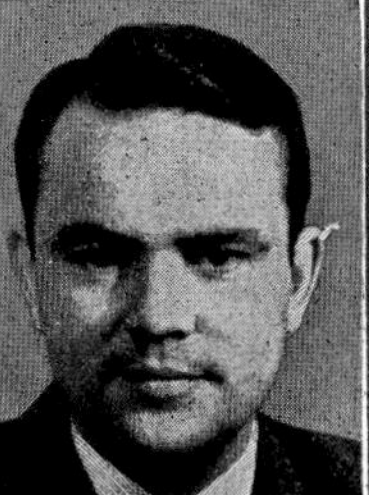

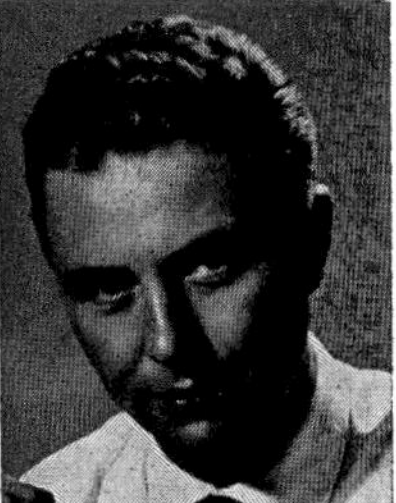

L. Ackermann H. Schleussner C. Schleussner

structure had to be created. That is why the new name Adox was adopted in 1947, but the Schleussner family retained controlling interests in the firm. Carl Adolf stayed on as "the boss" until 1952 when he became disabled by an accident which occurred in Brazil where he had gone to set up a new plant. Lately on deck was the fourth generation, Carlfried Schleussner and his younger brother Hans Schleussner, each of them with a PhD in chemistry, but with divergent ideas of diversification.

Current production includes Adox x-ray film (for use with intensifying screens), the single-packed non-screen Doneo, the Dozahn and Neodent (dental) films, as well as the attending line of darkroom chemicals. They make, of course, many photographic products outside the x-ray field, such as color film.

Adox also continued to support roentgen-historic endeavors, for instance they published Heinz Lossen's booklet on medical radiology in Frankfurt, and recently they issued in facsimile the civil office file on Röntgen, the original of which is preserved in the Bayerisches Hauptstaatsarchiv in Munchen under MK-17921.*

Late in 1962, DuPont bought Schleussner's photographic enterprise.

AGFA

A very fine European photochemical industry is the Actien-Gesellschaft für Anilinfabrikation (AGFA).

The firm started in 1867 as a dye factory located on the shore of the Rummelsburger Lake near Berlin. The current name was adopted in 1873, and use of the abbreviation Agfa as a trade-mark was introduced on April 15, 1897.

The firm became interested in photography only after hiring a chemist, named Momme Andresen, in 1887. He perfected chemicals for fine-grain developers, the Rodinal (1891), Methol, Amydol, and Glycin (1892). A photographic section was then created within the Agfa, with Andresen as section manager, and in 1893 they began to manufacture photo-sensitive surfaces. In 1908 a new plant was built in Wolfen, and Andresen became its director.

*This documentation was graciously provided by Dr. Lothar Ackermann, a radiologist from Frankfurt/Main who is scientific adviser at Adox.

Agfa

Next came the mergers. Photographic materials were being manufactured since 1857 by Eduard Liesegang in Düsseldorf, and by Friedrich Bayer & Co. in Elberfeld and subsequently in Leverkusen. Liesegang and Bayer merged in 1903. Further consolidation, which included the Agfa, took place in 1925 when the huge IG Farbenindustrie was formed: within it Agfa (whose headquarters were at the time in Berlin) no longer made dyes, but specialized exclusively in photographic equipment and materials.

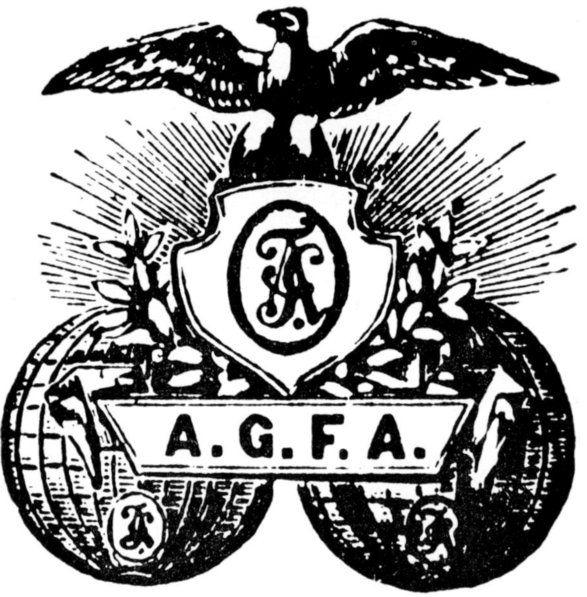

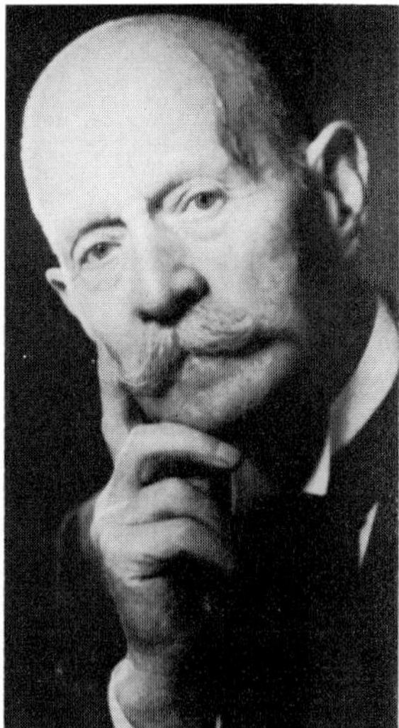

Courtesy: Agfa.

MOMME ANDRESEN. A dye chemist who developed Rodinal (a photographic developer based on paraphenylendiamin), Agfa's first photographic product. It is still being manufactured, and it still constitutes the basis of many liquid developers.

In the roentgen-photographic field, Agfa patented double-coating in 1896. It was intended to "catch" more x rays, as Röntgen had demanded, but double-coating of glass plates was very difficult; with the methods then available it was well-nigh impossible on film. Instead, Agfa successfully modified its emulsions, and raised their roentgen-sensitivity. The Agfa catalog of 1898 lists several sizes of single-coated roentgen plates and *Planfilme* (flat films!) up to 40x50 cm size, billed as requiring only one third to one fourth the roentgen exposure of regular dry plates.

In 1920, Agfa brought out dental film, and in 1922 double-coated x-ray film. In 1923, a special Röntgen-Abteilung was created within the Agfa. After the Cleveland fire of 1933, fire-resistant celluloid base was developed, and introduced in 1934. After the merger with IG Farben, oversea expansion was also intensified, and they purchased the American firm Ansco, which became Agfa-Ansco until the sudden scission at the time of World War II. Many photographic firsts were pioneered in the Agfa laboratories, to name only the Copyrapid system and Agfa-Color.

World War II destroyed the largest part of the Agfa installations, but on May 4, 1945 the first emulsion-machine was re-placed in operation in the photo-paper plant in Leverkusen. On April 18, 1952, Allied postwar control ceased, and two new companies were formed, the Agfa AG für Photofabrikation (Leverkusen) and the Agfa Camera-Werk AG (München), both owned by the Farbenfabriken Bayer AG (Leverkusen). Their regrowth was as phenomenal as all West German rebirth: in 1961 Agfa had 11,200 employees at its two plants (Leverkusen and München), is now the third largest European firm in the photographic (and roentgen-photographic) field, and sells its products in 133 countries around the globe.

In the re-building of postwar Agfa, a major role was played by Georg Grössel.

Georg Christian Grössel studied physics before he entered Holzknecht's Zentral-Röntgeninstitut as a technical associate in the late 1920s. From there Grössel went to Agfa and is still with them after thirty years. He worked at headquarters until World War II. Thereafter he became director of Agfa's Röntgen-Fachabteilung, located in Leverkusen. He is an expert in roentgen-photography, as well as in reproductions, in laboratory instrumentation, and in all-around photography. Grössel founded (and was for some time the editor of)

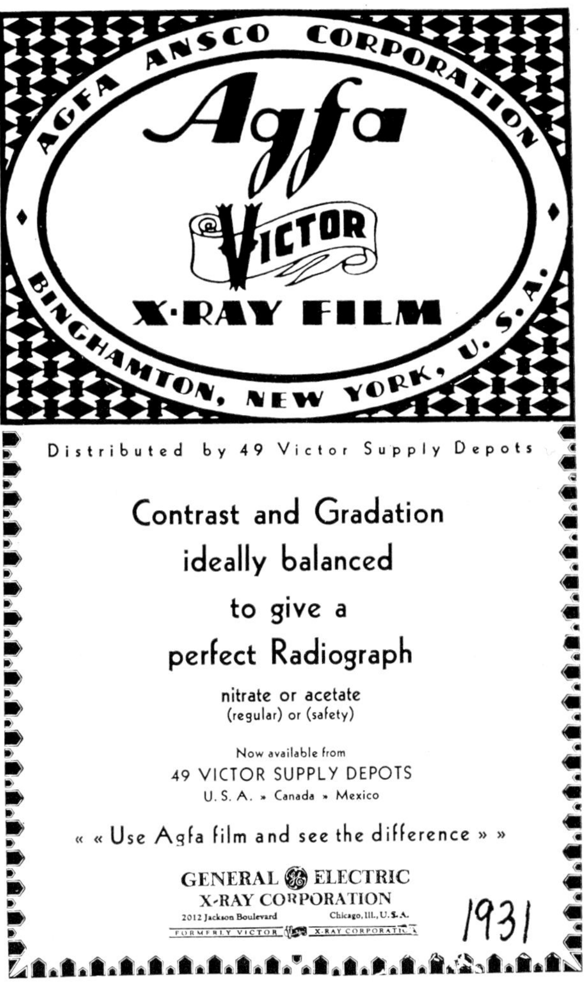

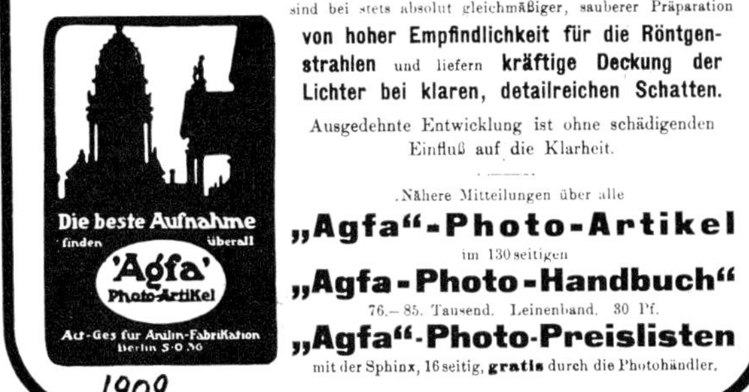

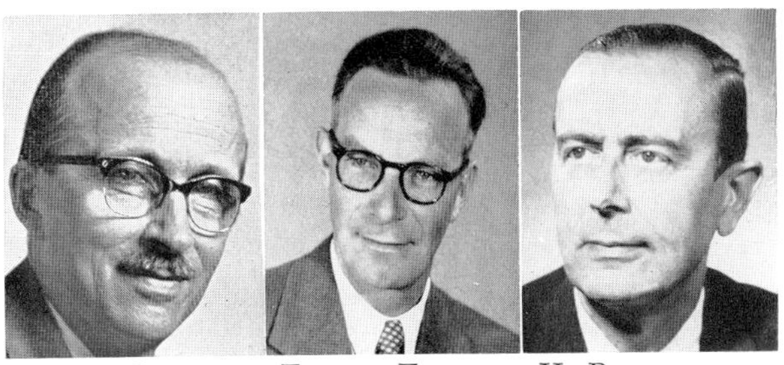

Georg Grössel Eduard Eylert H. Rindfleisch

Officials of the AGFA.

the postwar *Röntgen-Blätter,* published by the W. Girardet Verlag in Elberfeld. Grössel also revived Agfa's luxurious house organ, the *Röntgen-Hausmitteilungen.*

Agfa's roentgen products include the SSS-Roentgenfilm, used with re-inforcing screens, and the Sino-Roentgenfilm, a non-screen type adapted for medical use. For non-destructive testing of non-medical subjects (or rather objects), Agfa has the Texo-S-Roentgenfilm and the Texo-SH-Roentgenfilm, both of which require re-inforcing lead-screens. The Texo-I-Roentgenfilm is intended for high-energy radiations from betatron and radioactive isotopes. True to Agfa's long-time principle *alles aus einer Hand* (everything from a single - supplying - hand), they carry also roentgen paper, several other film types, and a variety of chemicals, including the *Röntgen-Machinen-Entwickler* developer for automatic processors.

In the historic field of roentgeniana, Agfa has printed in 1955 – on the fiftieth anniversary of the Deutsche Röntgen-Gesellschaft – a beautiful *Bilderbuch,* containing Röntgen's first communication, followed by portraits commemorating the first thirty-seven meetings of the German Roentgen Society. In 1959, for the ICR in München, Agfa printed another portrait catalog in which were reproduced the faces of up to four important figures from the radiologic past of each participating country.

In July of 1964, Agfa and Gevaert merged. The resulting firm is now called Gevaert-Agfa in Europe, while in the USA it is known as Agfa-Gevaert.

OTHER GERMAN FIRMS

Auer-Gesellschaft is a respectable German x-ray name: this (old) firm, still located in Berlin, makes fluoroscopic and intensifying screens, as well as cassettes, including *Simultan-Kessetten* for polytomography.

Cassettes, screens, as well as x-ray films are produced by the CAWO Photochemische Fabrik in Schrobenhausen/Obb.

A fairly complete line of x-ray tables and generators is offered by the Fritz Hofmann GmbH of München with the roentgen plant in Erlangen.

The firm was founded in 1922 by Fritz Hofmann (?-1947) in Erlangen. It employs currently about 300 people, and is owned by the founder's widow, Marie Hofmann.

They manufacture transformers with selenium rectifiers – from SR 230 (230 ma at 125 kvp) to the triphasic SR 700 D (maximum 700 ma or 125 kvp) – and electronic timer. Their table is called Metroskop, and

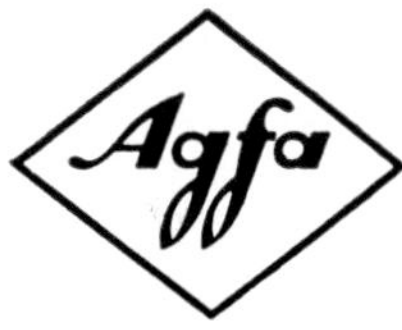

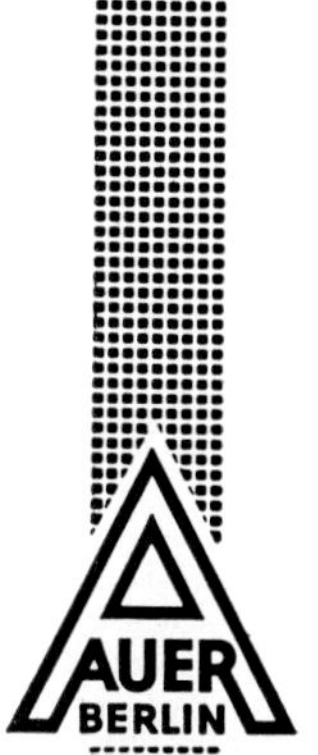

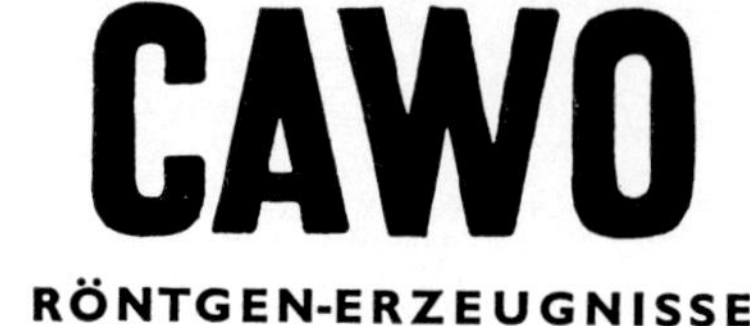

has 15° Trendelenburg; a newer model, Telemetroskop, permits 30° head-down position.

A peculiar device is the "Swing-diaphragm" (designed by Rudolf Raspe, a radiologist in Berlin), with which a view of the entire spine (from atlas to coccyx) can be obtained using a 30x90 or 20x96 cm cassette. It entails three exposures, starting from the bottom, with automatized interposition of a movable grid with adequate filtration so that the final product is properly penetrated over the entire distance. Utilization of this device would indicate that osteopathic (if not chiropractic) concepts have started to gain at least some acceptance on the Continent.

As far as opaque media are concerned, Endografin, Urografin and Gastrografin are produced in Germany by Schering, a firm which also prepared Biloptin and Solu-Biloptin for peroral cholecystography, and Biligrafin for intravenous cholangiography. The urographic and angiographic Opacoron is marketed by Cilag-Chemic of Alsbach.

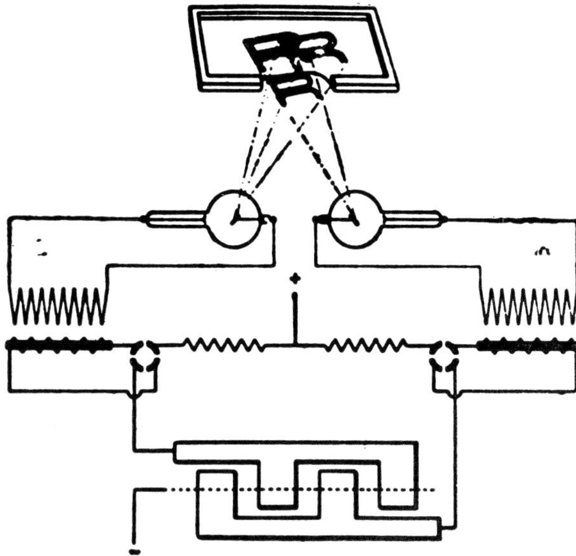

AEG STEREO-FLUOROSCOPE (1903). The interrupter energized the twin coil-tube arrangement in succession, to produce two distinct images, one for each eye. Even if separation were to have been achieved, one wonders what the fluorescent lag was in a screen of 1903 vintage.

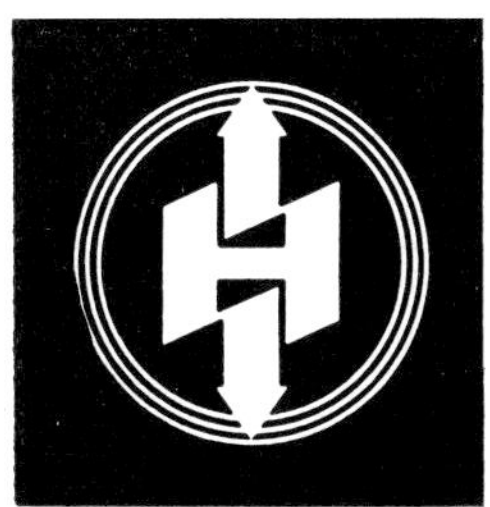

FRITZ HOFMANN GMBH

RÖNTGENWERK · ERLANGEN

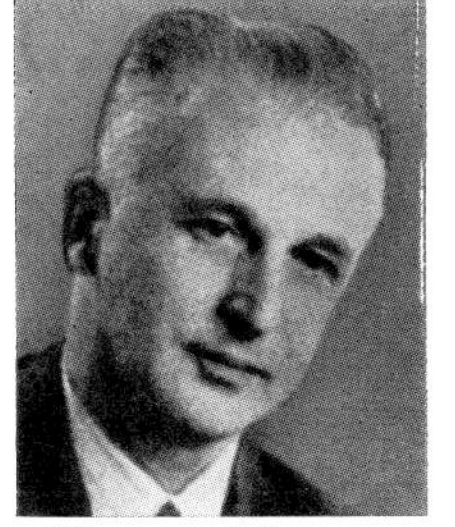
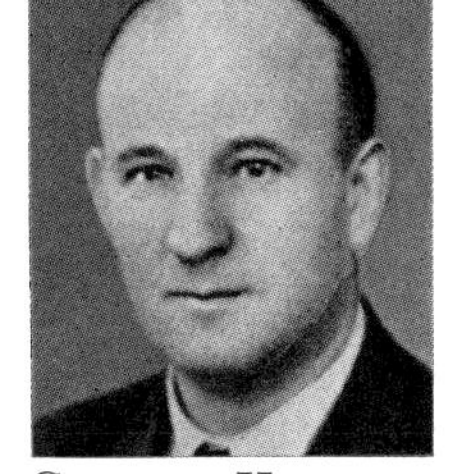

KONRAD MEYER GERHARD HUMMEL

Officials of AEG's x-ray tube factory.

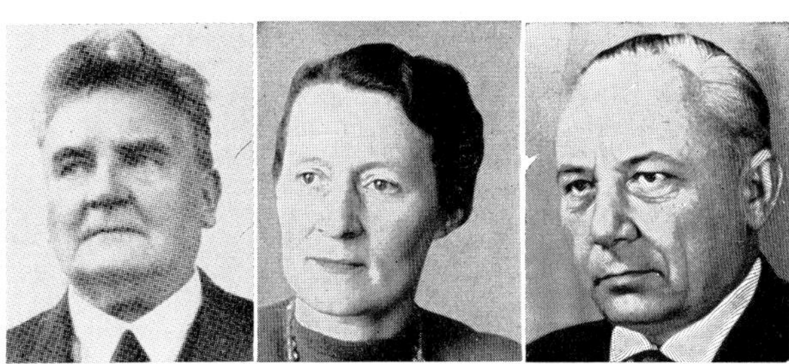

FRITZ HOFMANN MARIE HOFMANN KURT SCHWARZER

Officials of Fritz Hofmann Co.

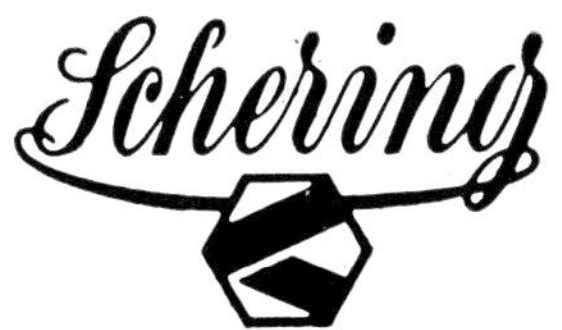

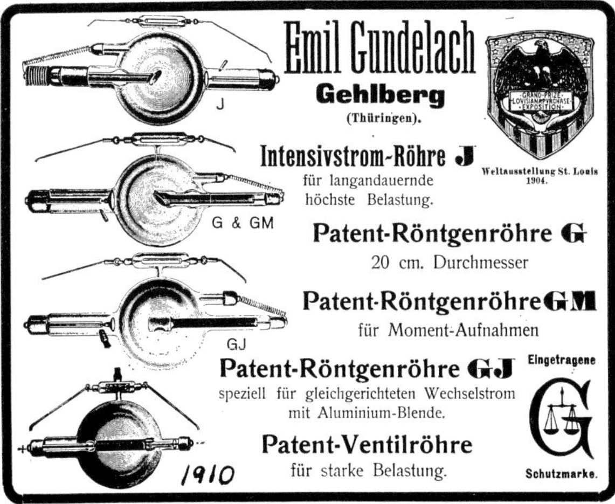

The Allgemeine Elektrizitäts-Gesellschaft (AEG) of Berlin has been involved in several x-ray ventures. One of their 1903 models was a special stereoscopic arrangement with two x-ray tubes having the anodes at pupillary distance: these tubes were alternately energized by a turbine interrupter, resulting in stereo-fluoroscopic visualization.

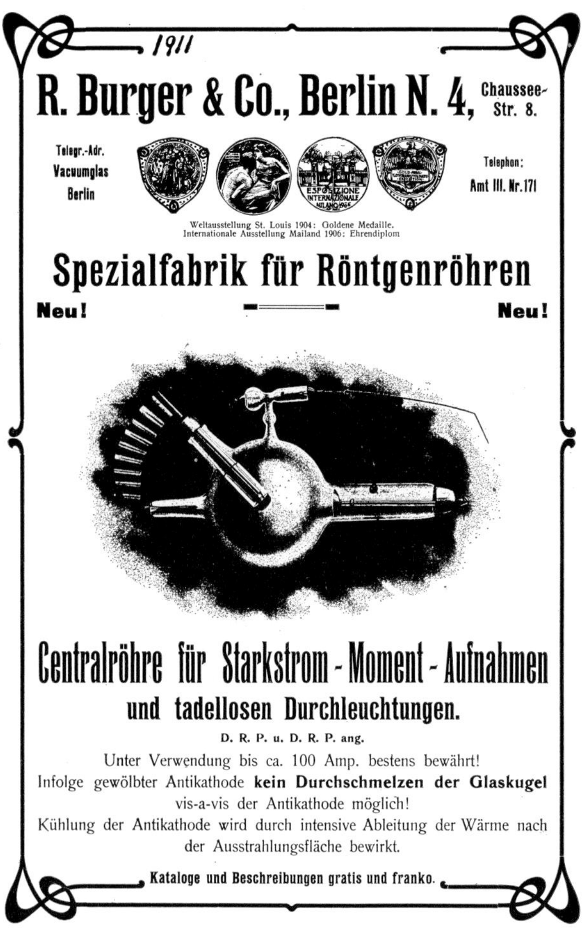

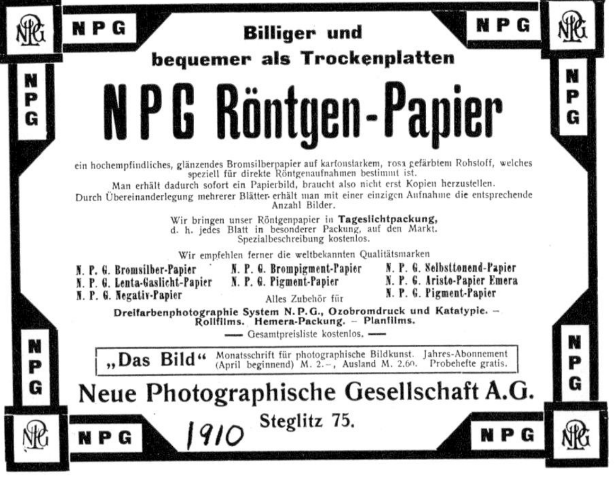

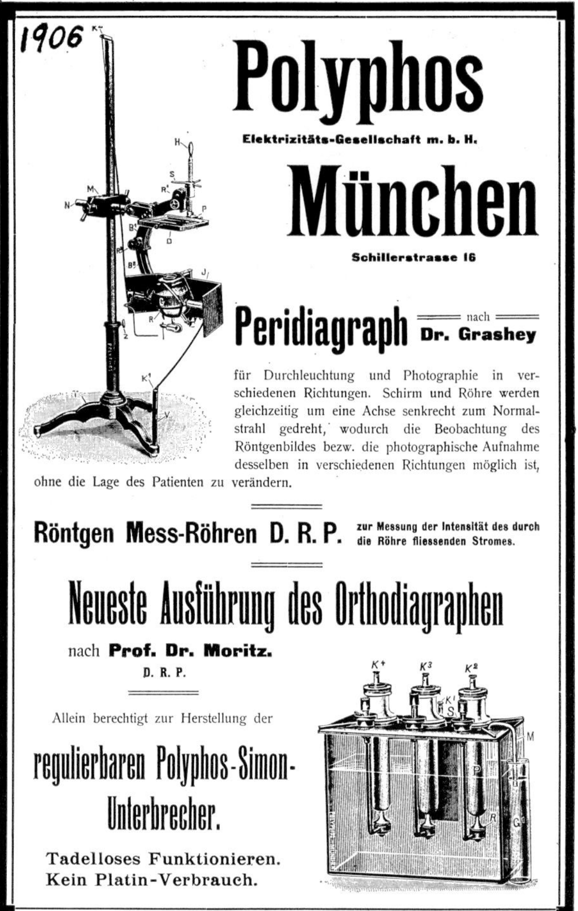

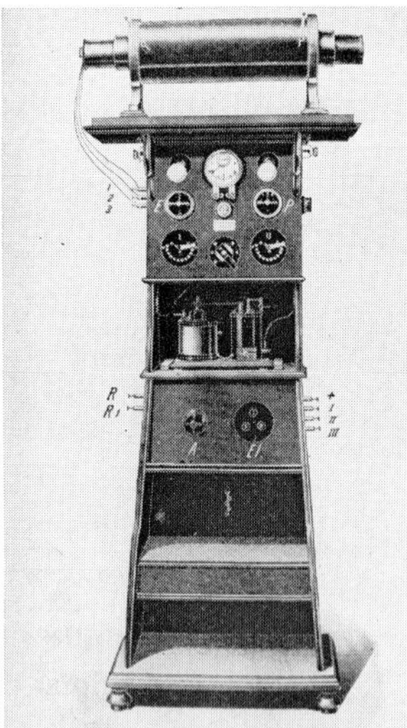

HIRSCHMANN COIL (1900). This arrangement was quite popular throughout the Era of the Roentgen Pioneers, most of whom were also electrologists. The coil was on top, the control surface at eye level, and the bottom of this wooden structure contained storage space for electrodes, x-ray tubes, and other accessories.

At this point will be mentioned a few German firms whose time of glory fell within the Era of the Roentgen Pioneers. None of them is currently in the x-ray business.

Prior to 1910, the best known German tube manufacturer was Emil Gundelach of Gehlberg (Thüringia): his trade-mark contained a balance framed by a capital G.

Very impressive were the advertisements of the tube factory R. Burger in Berlin (a relatively short-lived competitor of the firm Radiologie). Burger's device – a play on the German word *Burg* – was a tower resembling the insignia of the US Army Corps of Engineers.

The Neue Photographische Gesellschaft (NPG) in Steglitz, a suburb of Berlin, made an impressive assortment of photographic paper. They offered also the NPG Räntgen-Papier.

The Polyphos Elektrizitäts-Gesellschaft-mbH in München had a full line of x-ray apparatus, tubes, and accessories. They made Grashey's Peridiagraph (optional coupling of screen and tube carriers), Moritz's Orthodiagraph, and Rosenthal's precision x-ray tube (with anticathode of pure iridium). Polyphos marketed the opaque media Kontrastin, made of pure Zirconium Oxyde (described by C. Kaestle in the *Münchener Medizinische Wochenschrift* of December 12, 1909).

Another firm with a full line of both electro-medical and x-ray apparatus was that of W. A. Hirschmann in Berlin: they had a branch office in St. Petersburg (Russia) in 1909. Hirschmann's insignia was a snake wrapped around a lightning (medical electricity). The firm maintained a *Röntgenlaboratorium* at nr. 30 on Ziegelstrasse in Northern Berlin, and they accepted referred patients for either or both diagnosis and therapy. Hirschmann built one of the first vertical orthodiagraphs.

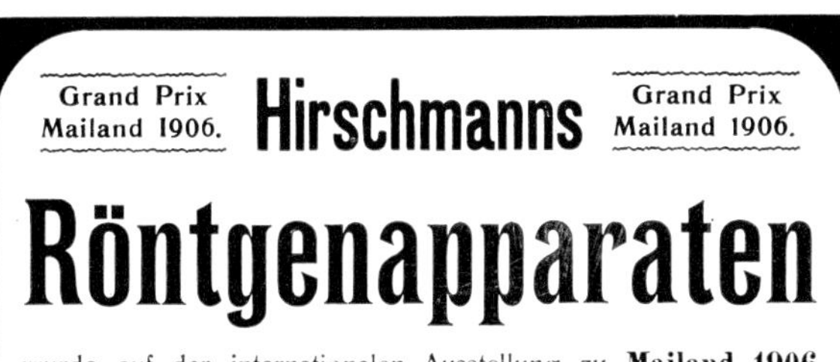

wurde auf der internationalen Ausstellung zu **Mailand 1906** der **Grand Prix** zuerkannt. Eine weitere Anerkennung der **soliden Konstruktion** und **gediegenen Ausstattung** dieser Röntgeneinrichtungen.

Den neuen Röntgenkatalog 16 bitte einzufordern.

Hilfsutensilien zur **Anfertigung** von **Röntgenaufnahmen**, zur **Durchleuchtung** und **Bestrahlung**, **Schutzvorrichtungen** gegen Röntgenstrahlen, **Schutzwände**, **Schutzhäuser**. **Sämtliche Hilfsutensilien** werden in meinen eigenen Röntgenlaboratorien auf ihre **Zweckmässigkeit** und **Brauchbarkeit hin erprobt**, so dass nur **praktisch verwertbare** und **handliche Apparate** zum Verkauf kommen.

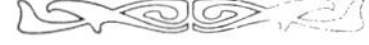

Den Herren Ärzten steht mein **Röntgenlaboratorium** zu **praktischen Übungen jederzeit zur Verfügung.** Seit 10 Jahren wurden in demselben ca. **25 Tausend Röntgenaufnahmen** und **Hunderte** von **Bestrahlungen** auf **ärztliche Verordnung** ausgeführt.

1908

W. A. Hirschmann

Hamburg Colonnaden 92. * **Berlin N. 24** Ziegelstr. 30. * St. Petersburg U.-Gogolja 4.

DEUTSCHE Picker G. M. B. H.

RÖNTGEN-NUCLEAR-ELEKTRO-MEDIZIN

KOCH & STERZEL

In October, 1904 two enthusiastic, enterprising, and energetic engineers, Franz Joseph Koch (1873-1943) and Kurt August Sterzel (1876-1960), founded a firm for the construction of electrophysical apparatus.

They had collaborated on several electro-medical patents, one of which was a workable rotary switch (1897) – it appeared, chronologically, after Lemp but before Snook. Koch & Sterzel (K & S) flourished, and their world-wide reputation as manufacturers of x-ray equipment became well established after World War I.

In *Röntgen-Blätter* of December, 1956 Kurt Bischoff (from the SRW) traced the history of triphasic machines. In 1916 K. Lasser (at the time an employee of Siemens & Halske) showed to the Berlin Medical Society the first triphasic generator (built for therapy). In the early 1920s Heinrich Chantraine expressed (and popularized) the desirability of low kilovoltage techniques as a means of obtaining better contrast in chest radiography. It required high milliamperage if one wanted to keep exposure time (and blurring around the heart) to a minimum. That is when the race for high-intensity generators started. K & S marketed its first triphasic transformer in 1924, and in 1927 they brought out the 2000 ma Titanos (Siemens' Gigantos 2000 ma reached the market only two years later, in 1929).*

*In Europe one can expect a lesser voltage drop on the triphasic (industrial) power supply—which is often 240 or 380 V rather than 220 V—than on biphasic (residential) current. Even today Europeans prefer triphasic generators. In this country Picker built at one time triphasic machines. Picker's German subsidiary, the Picker & Harting Vertrieb, in Espelkamp, manufactures the obligatory triphasic.

Among other K & S firsts may be mentioned the fact that in 1925 they pioneered the separation of kilovoltage control for fluoroscopy from that for radiography. In 1928, they announced the basic patent for automatic overload cut-off in the roentgen tube circuit. This *Röntgen-Automatik,* built into their generator Kostix (1934), employed a milliamper-second relay - it is today the standard method for automatization, employed the world over.

By 1943, the K & S plant employed about 3000 people. Over 600 patents had been taken out, and over 500 models had been deposited. There were in excess

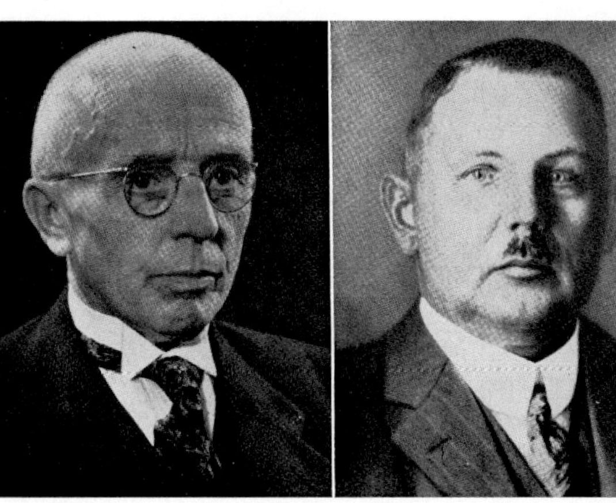

Courtesy: Koch & Sterzel.

Koch & Sterzel. Frank Joseph Koch, with glasses, and Kurt August Sterzel founded the company which was first located in Dresden, is now in Essen.

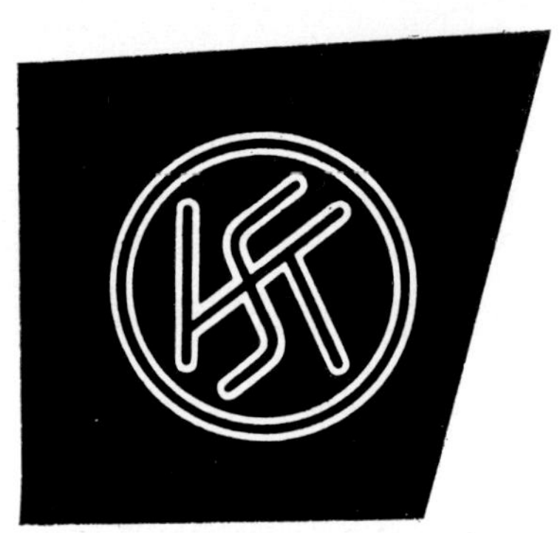

Koch & Sterzel, **Fabrik moderner Röntgen-Apparate.**
Inh.: Ing. **F. J. Koch,** Dipl. Ing. **K. Sterzel.**

Dresden-A., Zwickauerstraße 42.

Unterbrecherlose Röntgen-Einrichtung mit Hochspannungs-Transformator und automatischer Resonanz-Gleichrichtung,

Röntgen-Einrichtungen mit Intensivstrom-Induktor.

Die **80 Röntgen-Einrichtungen,** die wir in kurzer Zeit verkauften, sprechen für die Vorzüglichkeit u. Konkurrenzlosigkeit unserer Systeme. Man verlange Prospekte u. Referenzenlisten.

Bikathodenröhren D. R. P. ■ **Ventil-Röhren** D. R. P.
Universalblenden, Krypto-Radiometer mit Wehnelt-Skala
und alle sonstigen Nebenapparate.

Vertretungen und Alleinverkauf unserer Röntgen-Systeme:

für Berlin mit Norddeutschland .. .. .. ***Curt Westphal, Berlin NW. 6,*** *Karlstraße 26*
für Rheinland und Westfalen .. .. ***Teucher & Franz, Cöln a. Rhein,*** *Lütticherstr. 8*
für England und Kolonien .. .. ***W. Watson & Sons, London WC. 313,*** *High Holborn*
für Russland .. .. ***F. Schwabe, Moskau,*** *Schmiedebrücke.*

1908

K & S ad of 1907. The *unterbrecherlos* (interrupterless) rotary switch was similar to Snook's. Note among their representatives the Watson & Sons in London. Curt Wesphal (who was selling also Müller tubes) in Berlin, and Friedrich Schwabe in Moscow.

of 20,000 installations with the K & S trademark spread on the five continents, and they had built barely short of 1 million transformers.

During World War II the Dresden plant was bombed, and later the whole town remained behind the Iron Curtain. But K & S proved to be indomitable, ingenious, and industrious. They opened up a new plant in Essen, announced (since 1949) over 100 new patents, and in a comparatively short time issued an impressive new line of x-ray equipment.

Among their transformers, the automatized Kostix comes in various sizes, of which the largest furnishes 1000 ma at 50 kvp, or 300 ma at 150 kvp. Even their largest triphasic, the Titanos, has selenium rectifiers: it is built to service up to three tubes with 1000 ma at 100 kvp or 300 at 150 kvp. They are still building the

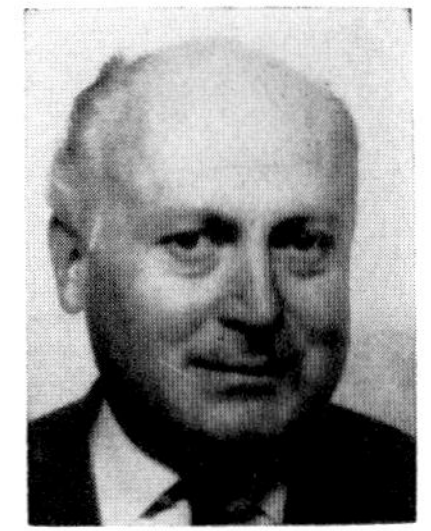

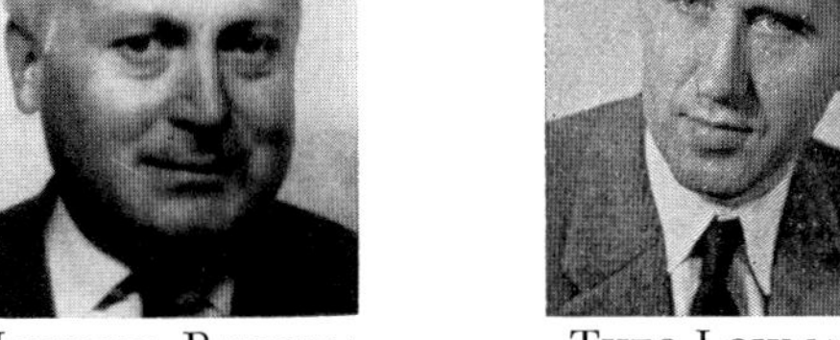

HERBERT PANDURA THEO LOHMANN
Chief-engineer and chief-designer at Koch & Sterzel.

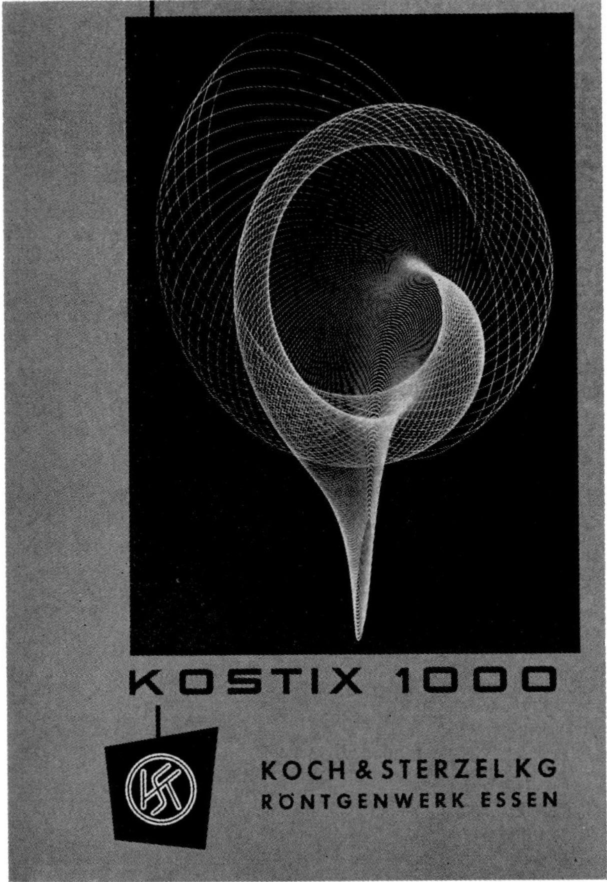

KOSTIX FUTURISTIC. This design appears on the cover of the advertising leaflet of K & S's Kostix 100 ma triphasic transformer, in an effort to emphasize the machinery's modern features.

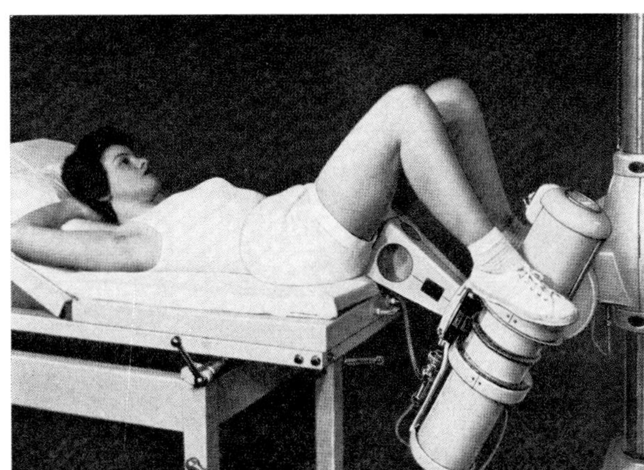

Courtesy: Koch & Sterzel.

K & S THERAPIX 250 KVP. Positioned for perineal (or sacral?) port.

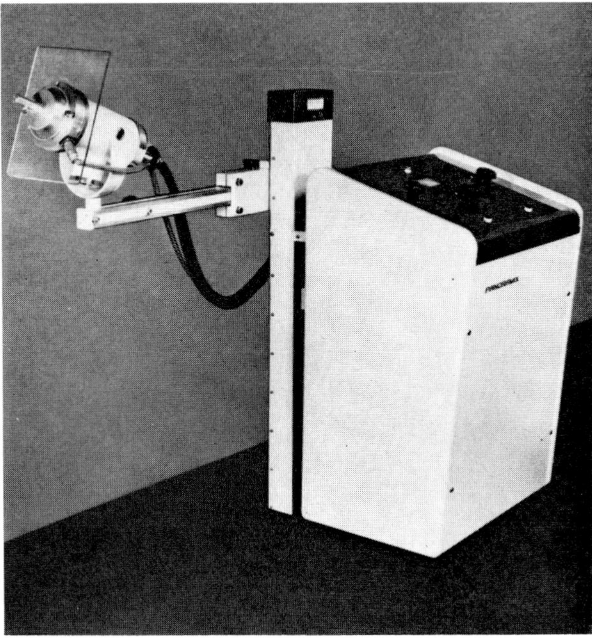

Courtesy: Koch & Sterzel.

K & S PANORAMIX. Intra-oral insertion of the x-ray tube manufactured by Comet (in Switzerland) produces a panoramic view of the teeth. Total dose is less than that from multiple exposures for each of 15 or 20 occlusal projections.

Ordix, a half-wave (non-rectified) transformer (230 ma at 70 kvp, or 100 ma at 125 kvp).

They have several smaller tables (Phoroskop, Viaskop, Mediskop), which come with 20-50 ma transformers and controls on the screen carrier. Their large table, the Ultraskop 2, has power-assist and other frills but only 30° Trendelenburg. Their fully automatized, push-button spotfilm device (Ultra-Zielgerat-DM) is one of the fastest in the industry. They purchase image intensifiers, and adapt them both to a mobile model ("surgical-orthopedic") and to stationary installations.

Photix is the K & S photofluorographic apparatus (which uses an Odelca), while their phototimer is called Luminix (it is ½" thick and of 17x17″ size, being interposed between patient and cassette).

K & S therapy machines come in the usual two sizes, the Therapix-C 100 and the constant potential Therapix 250. Custom-built rotational, convergent, and/or pendular arrangements are available for the latter.

Unusual is the proper term for a relatively recent dental development called the Panoramix. It consists of a special tube housing for a well grounded anode, so that the whole thing can be safely placed in the mouth.

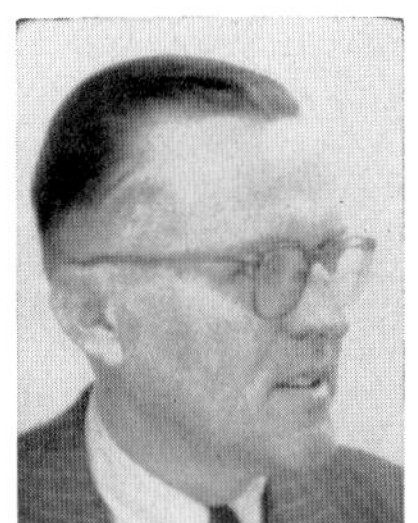
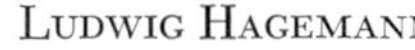
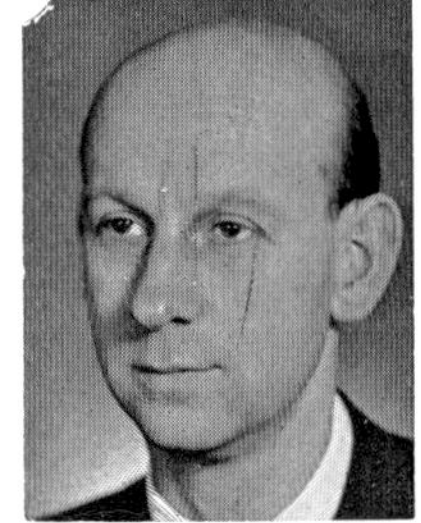

LUDWIG HAGEMANN KARL SCHMIDT

Koch & Sterzel officials.

A curved film is inserted between the lower teeth and the lips and cheek, and another curved film is exposed in a similar way for the upper teeth. The inherent magnification is an asset, rather than a liability, because distortion is not bothersome. And there is less total dose to the mandible and maxilla than there would accumulate from multiple small dental films. The tube is placed very near or right on the tongue; with the inverse square working the other way around, it may seem like a bit of plesiotherapy, but the tube is shielded at the point of possible contact with the tongue.

EAST GERMANY

The old Koch & Sterzel plant in Dresden was rebuilt, and manufactures a fairly complete line of x-ray equipment. The marketing is done by a central import-export outlet, located in Berlin, the Deutsche Import-Export Gesellschaft-mbH Feinmechanik-Optik.

The K & S plant is now called Transformatoren und Röntgenwerk (TUR), preceded by the initials VEB (*volks-eigener Betrieb,* meaning peoples-owned plant), or VEM (*volkseigner Maschinenbau,* meaning peoples-owned machine manufacture). In both cases it indicates that ownership has been taken over by the state.

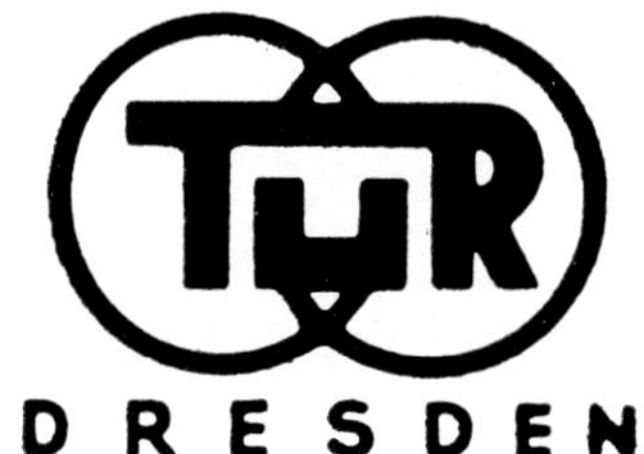

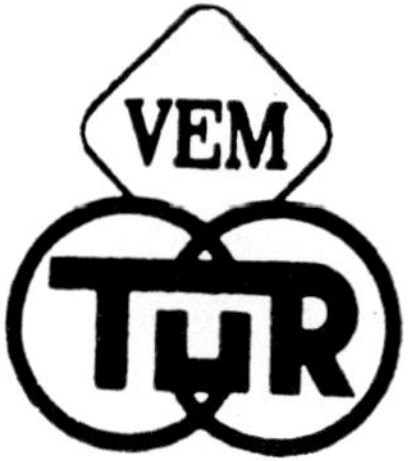

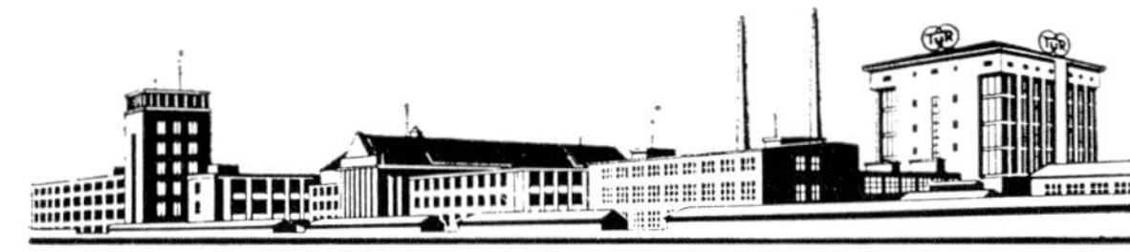

VEB TRANSFORMATOREN- UND RÖNTGENWERK DRESDEN

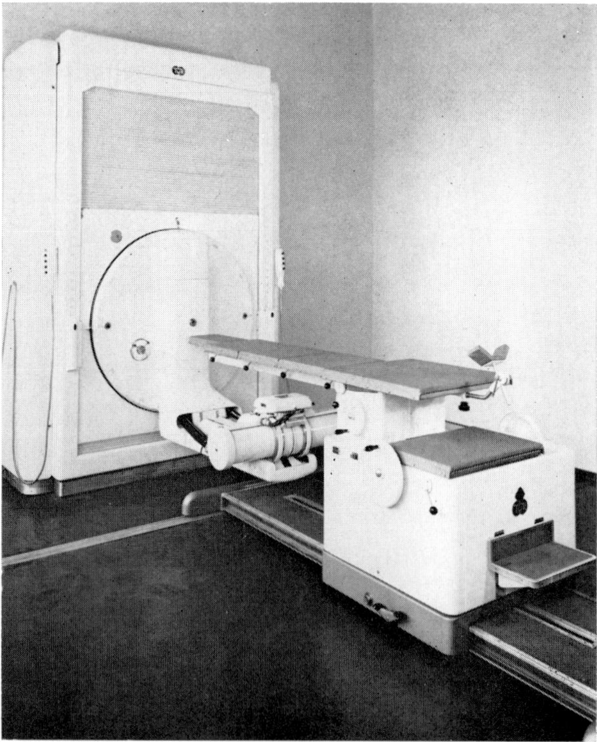

Courtesy: Feinmechanik-Optik.

TUR's TG2. 250 kvp constant potential therapy unit with rotational, pendular, and convergent capabilities.

TUR's largest transformer, the D 1000 is a fully automatized six-valve unit which delivers 1000 ma at 50 kvp, or 400 ma at 120 kvp. The mobile unit D 25-2 (which comes with the stand D 1-1) is rated for 130 ma at 125 kvp, or 300 ma at 45 kvp. The photo-fluorographic combination D 130 is very well shielded. TUR's best table is the DG 2: its automatized spotfilm device DZ 1 is quite heavy, and requires ceiling suspension. For therapy they manufacture the contact unit T 60, and a 250 kvp constant potential machine. The latter may be mounted on the ringstand TG 2, which looks like Mueller's TU-1, and does the same thing (from stationary to pendular, and from rotational to convergent). TUR makes also a diffraction unit, the M 60.

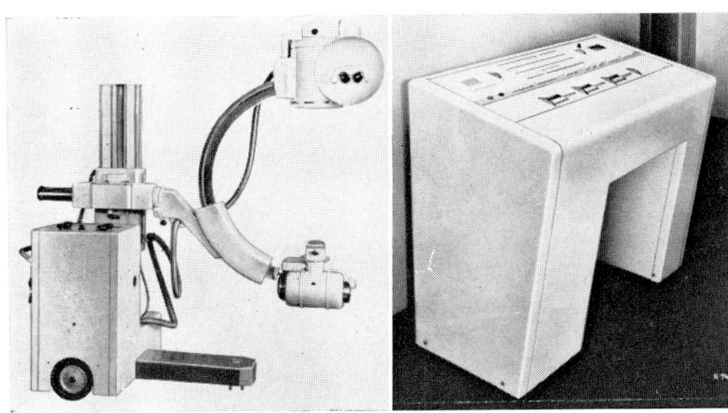

Courtesy: Feinmechanik-Optik.

TUR DIAGNOSTIC MACHINES. DO 15 is a surgical image intensifier, shown here as an optical system (not twin oculars). D 1001 is a triphasic six-valve transformer, with highly stylized desk-type control stand.

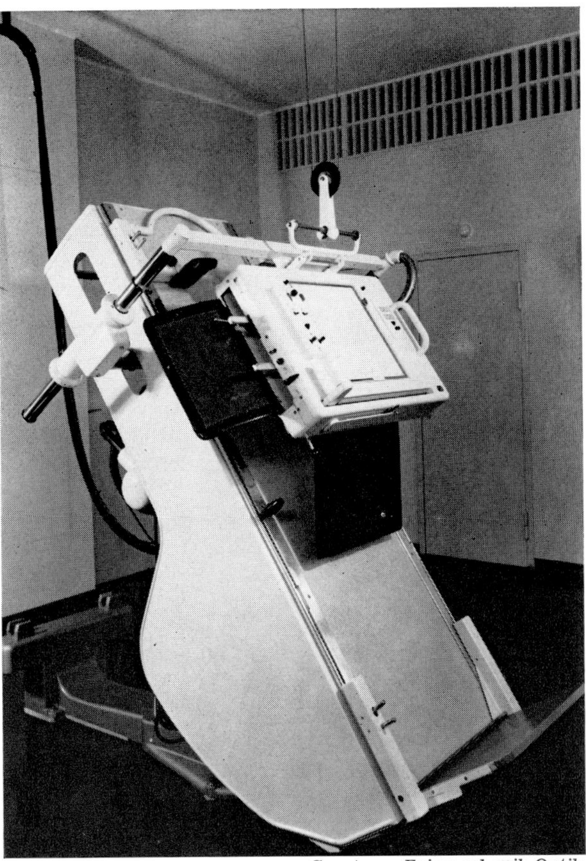

Courtesy: Feinmechanik-Optik.

TUR's DG 7. Latest roentgen table, with 30° Trendelenburg, and automatized spotfilm device – note front-loading needed for adequate utilization when image intensifier is attached.

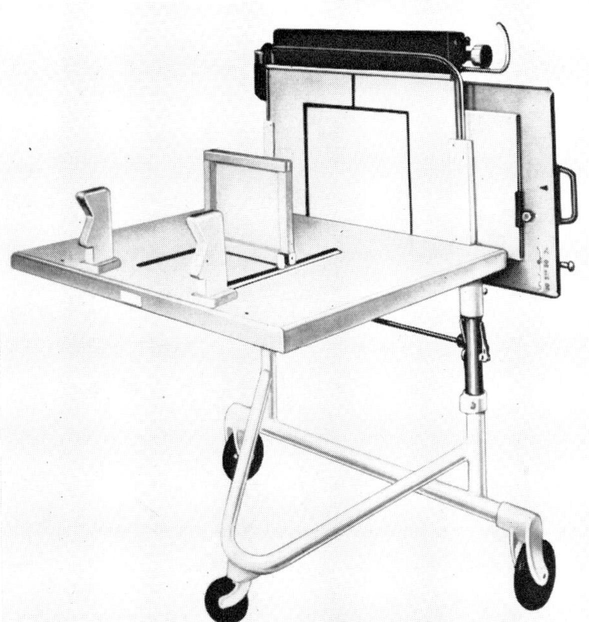

Courtesy: Feinmechanik-Optik.

PELVITRANS. Pelvigraph made by Gera.

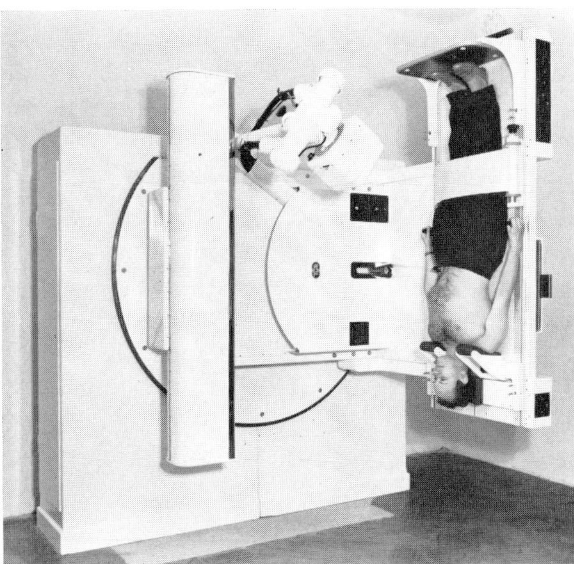

Courtesy: Feinmechanik-Optik.

DG 101. East German universal body section device, manufactured by Gera.

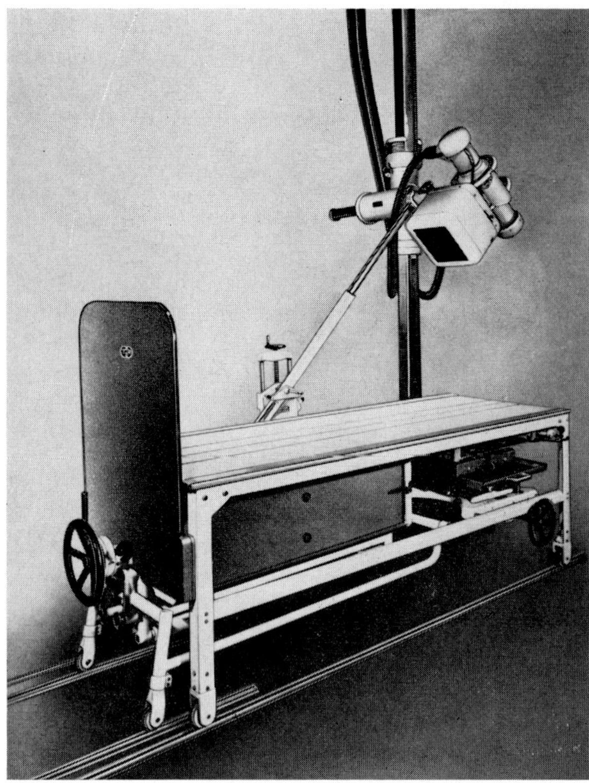

Courtesy: Feinmechanik-Optik.

DG102-1. East German Bucky table, with tomographic attachment, and multi-sectional capabilities — a stock item in Central Europe.

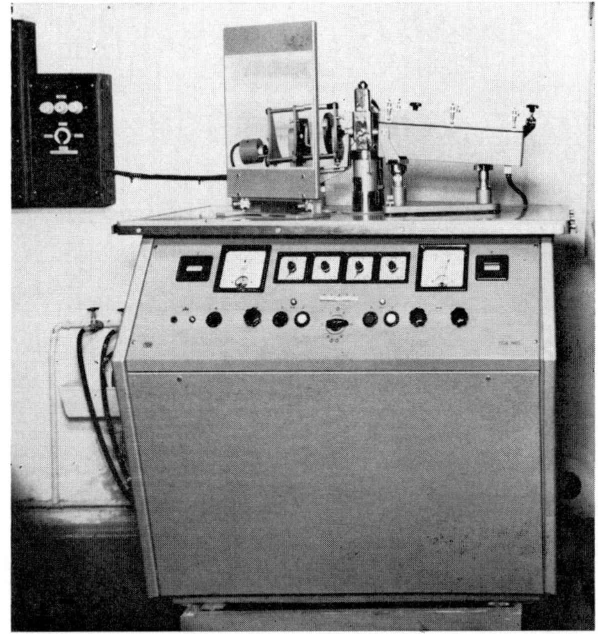

Courtesy: Feinmechanik-Optik.

TUR's M 61. X-ray equipment for *Feinstruktur* examination.

Several of the other German x-ray plants in the Eastern Zone have been re-opened. The Röntgenwerk Gera makes the dental units Perkeo and Piccolo, and several special tables, the Pelvitrans and a craniograph. Gera took over from TUR the manufacture of DG 101, a body section apparatus which looks very much like SRW's Universal Planigraph. A very interesting combination is the DG 102 (which was previously made

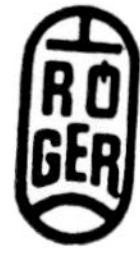

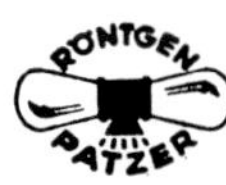

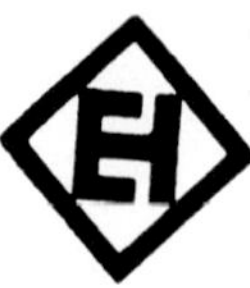

East German x-ray trade-marks. The first is that of the VEB Röntgenwerk Gera, next comes that of Ing. H. Patzer in Hermsdorf, last is that of Ing. Ernst Hüttmann in Dresden.

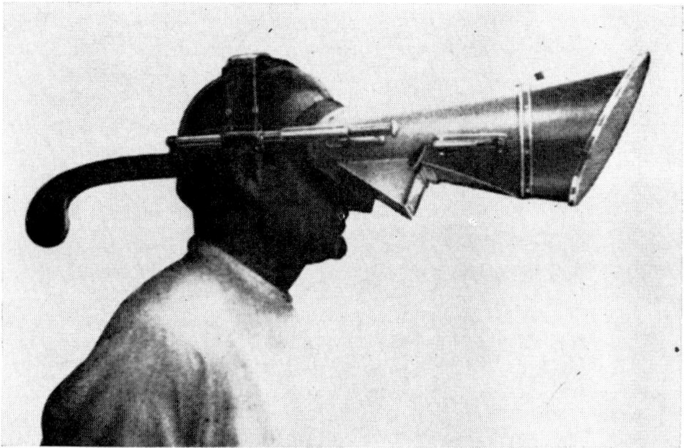

Head cryptoscope. The device weighs 2.3 kg (about 5 lbs.). It contains a roentgen beam field size indicator. It is a surgical cryptoscope, the fluoroscoping eye remaining in the dark, while the other eye is available for regular vision. This cryptoscope is currently manufactured by Patzer in Hermsdorf-Thüringen.

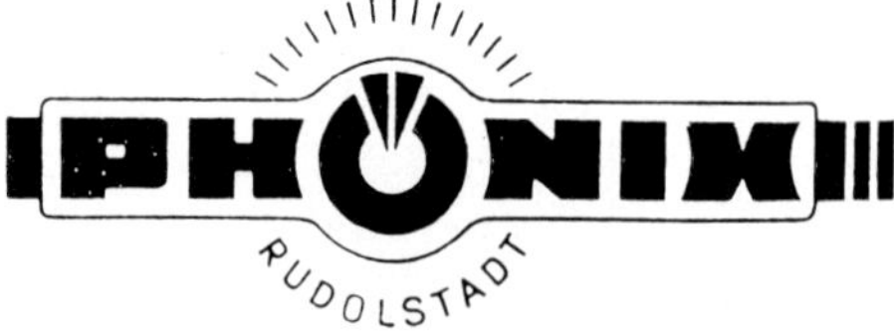

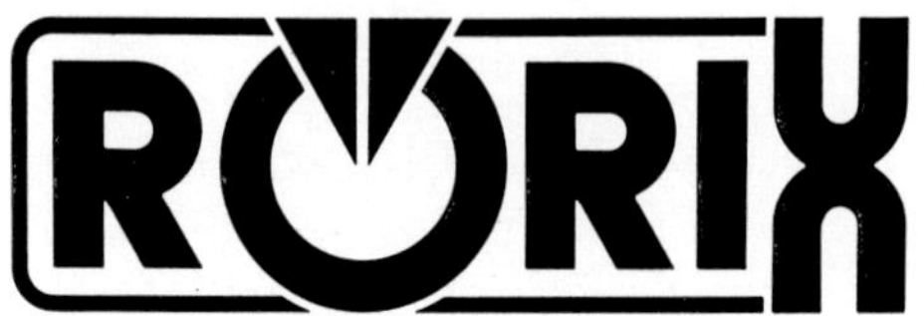

in the TUR plant), a table with a flat Bucky-Potter and a planigraphic attachment: it has space provided (beneath the Bucky) for polytomography, an attachment for radiographic magnification can be added, and a changer for one meter long cassettes used in peripheral angiography can be rolled under the table. That changer has, just like SRW's, four cassettes fastened to the four sides of a rotating drum.

The Chemische Werke Radebeul (the former Heyden) makes the intensifying screens for the "simultaneous" cassettes. All sorts of accessories are manufactured by Ernst Hüttman in Dresden, and by Patzer.

The Phönix Röntgenröhrenwerk in Rudolstadt (Thüringen) was founded on September 1, 1920. That is where in 1928 was developed the Dofok (double focus) tube, based on an idea of George Kucher*. Phönix was one of the firms which merged to form the Siemens-Reiniger-Werke.

The tube-factory Radiologie, located in Berlin, had been destroyed by Allied bombers. After the war, the Radiologie plant was re-opened in Gera (Eastern Germany), but soon liquidated (on May 31, 1951), and its production taken over by Phönix. On July 1, 1961 the name Phönix was changed to Rörix, to indicate that

*Kucher was an engineer born in New York City on February 15, 1883. He left Rudolstadt before the outbreak of World War II, and it was not possible to determine his whereabouts. Information on Kucher, and the illustrations of Rörix tubes were graciously provided by the Rörix Company's commercial director, Mr. Rudi Jacobi, and by their sales manager, Mr. Alfred Beck.

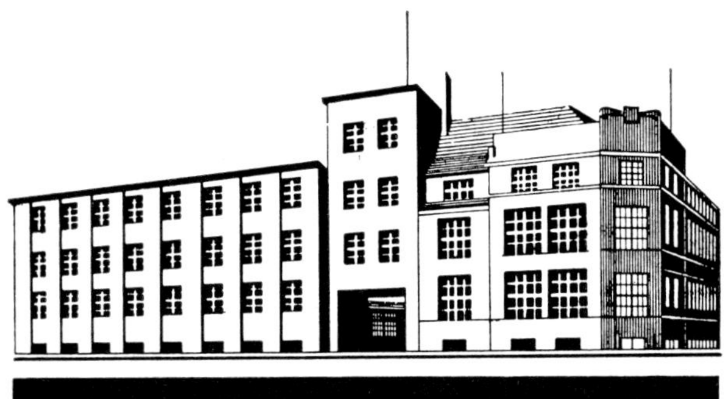

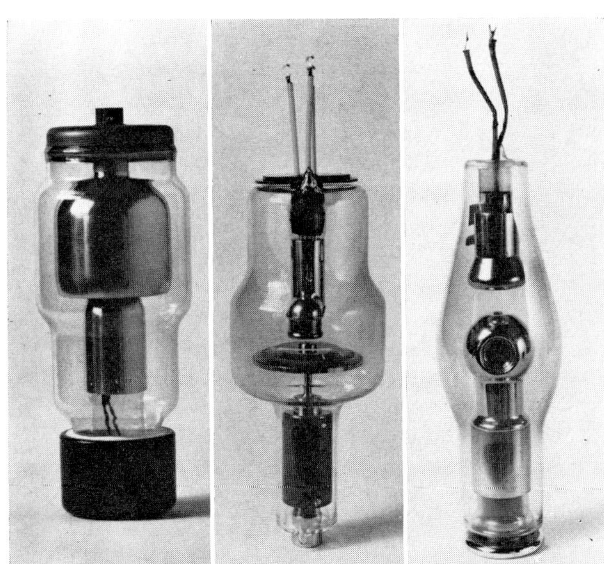

Courtesy: Rörix

RÖRIX TUBES. Shown are a kenotron with thoriated cathode, a 150 kvp rotating anode, and a 200 kvp therapy tube (with two wires connected to its filament), also used in *Grobstruktur* examinations.

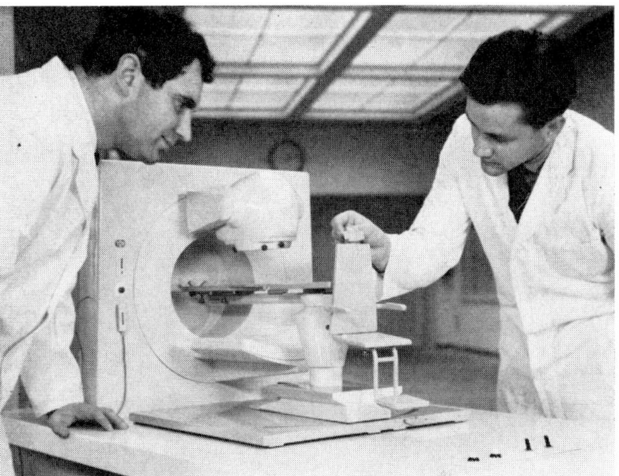

Courtesy: VEB TUR, Dresden

RADIO-ENGINEERS AT WORK. Magerstädt watches while Leukfeld replaces the headrest on the diminutive model of the TUR-TCo-2000 rotational cobalt irradiator.

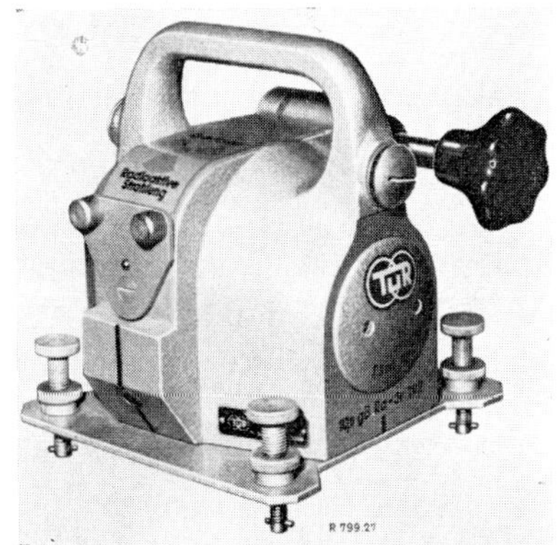

Courtesy: Feinmechanik-Optik

TUR's M IR-16. Radiographic container for up to 16 curies of Iridium-192, usable on steel thicknesses of 10-50 mm.

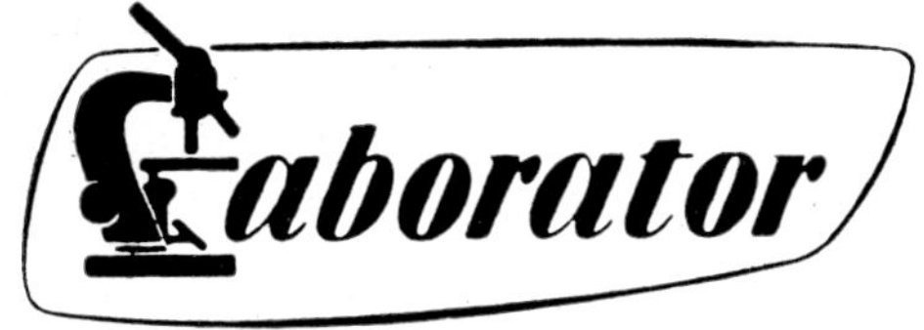

its production had expanded beyond x-ray tubes into power and other type of vacuum tubes. The insignia maintained a somewhat similarly stylized pattern, but now it resembles a power tube. Rörix production is of excellent quality (the same locale on Röntgenstrasse as before, and many of the old staff). It includes everything from 150 kvp rotating anodes and thoriated tungsten cathode kenotrons, to oil-immersed 250 kvp tubes for deep therapy and Grobstruktur and beryllium-windowed tubes for contact therapy and *Feinkstruktur* examinations.

East Germany is making a strenuous effort to carve a place for itself in this Atomic Phase. It is not easy: many of their physicians and other technical personnel have fled to the West. Life has always been so much harder East of the Iron Curtain. But Germans are Germans, and technical tradition counts. It would be unrealistic to underestimate East German echievements, apparent even in radiology. TUR builds several isotopic containers for non-destructive testing, one of which holds 16 curies Iridium-192. It is usable for thin welds, and other light metallic parts. Cobalt teletherapy units and linear accelerators are now in the works.

Then there is the Vakutronic in Dresden, where a full line of nuclear measuring equipment is being manufactured. That production makes up a section of a monumental East German catalog (8½x12″ size, 1728 pages) of various laboratory materials and instruments. The catalog is called *Laborator,* and has a microscop on its insignia. Among the countries currently called Sovietic Satellites, East Germany is undoubtedly the largest industrial manufacturer.

GREAT BRITAIN

Numerous mergers (amalgamations) and other "rearrangements" occurred in the British x-ray industry.

There existed for a long time the firm Schall & Son. Its founder, Schall, Sr., had been originally the third man of the famous German triumvirate of Reiniger, Gebbert & Schall. This is why even in the 1920s the advertisements of Schall & Son had to stress that they were selling British made apparatus.

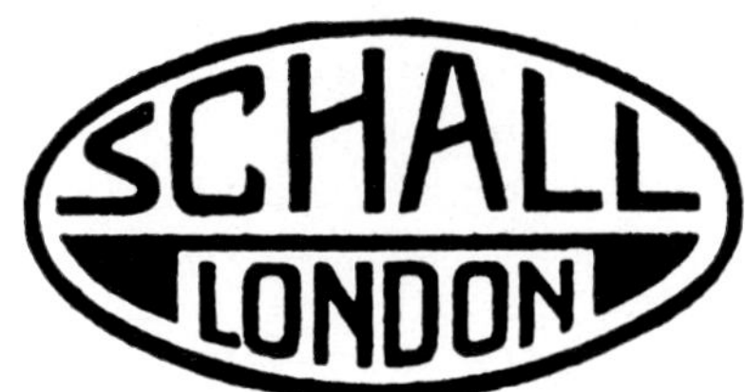

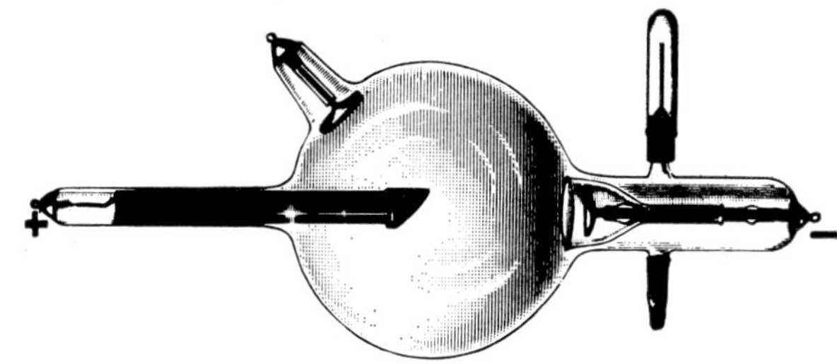

SCHALL TUBE (1903). This was captioned in the original ad as "heavy anode regulating tube."

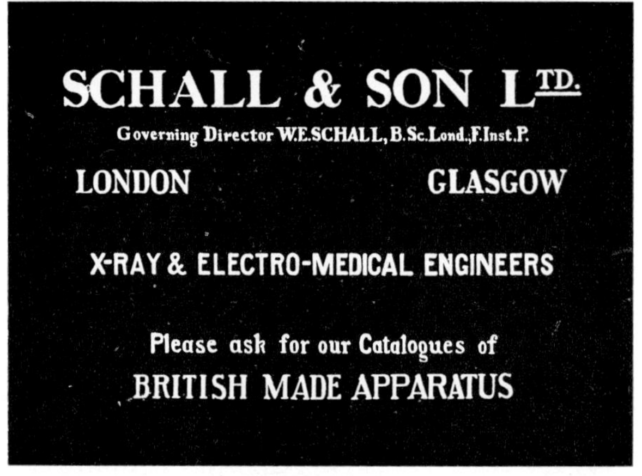

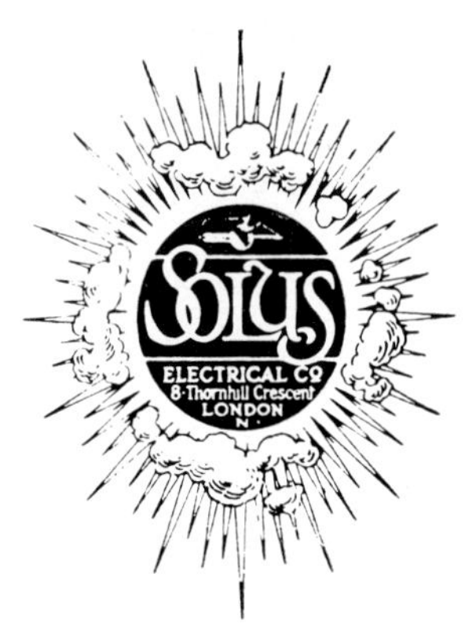

The "Son," William Edward Schall, Jr., is the author of a technical primer called *X-rays*, now in its 8th edition.

Another relatively old organization was the (sunny) Solus Electrical Company – in 1927 they were making tube stands for Metalix tubes. They also had a (mobile) 30ma Ward Trolley set. In 1946 Solus made a portable unit called the Supreme 85/15.

In 1947, the two merged into Solus-Schall, Ltd., and in 1948 they advertised the same portable unit modified for "chest radiology." In 1952, they began to place emphasis on accessories. They have become part of General Radiological, and as such a member of the Murphy group. The Solus-Schall factory is in Honeypot Lane, Stanmore (Middlesex); it manufactures industrial equipment.*

The fact that the sun or sun rays appear on several commercial seals of British radiologic maufacturers is possibly connected with the use of such a symbol in the crest of the British Institute of Radiology.

There existed in the early 1920s the General Radiological & Surgical Apparatus Company. Today the name is General Radiological (GR).

*This information was graciously obtained from Mr. C. E. Reiche of Sierex, Ltd. (London representative of the SRW), and from Mr. G. R. Woodall of Watson & Sons.

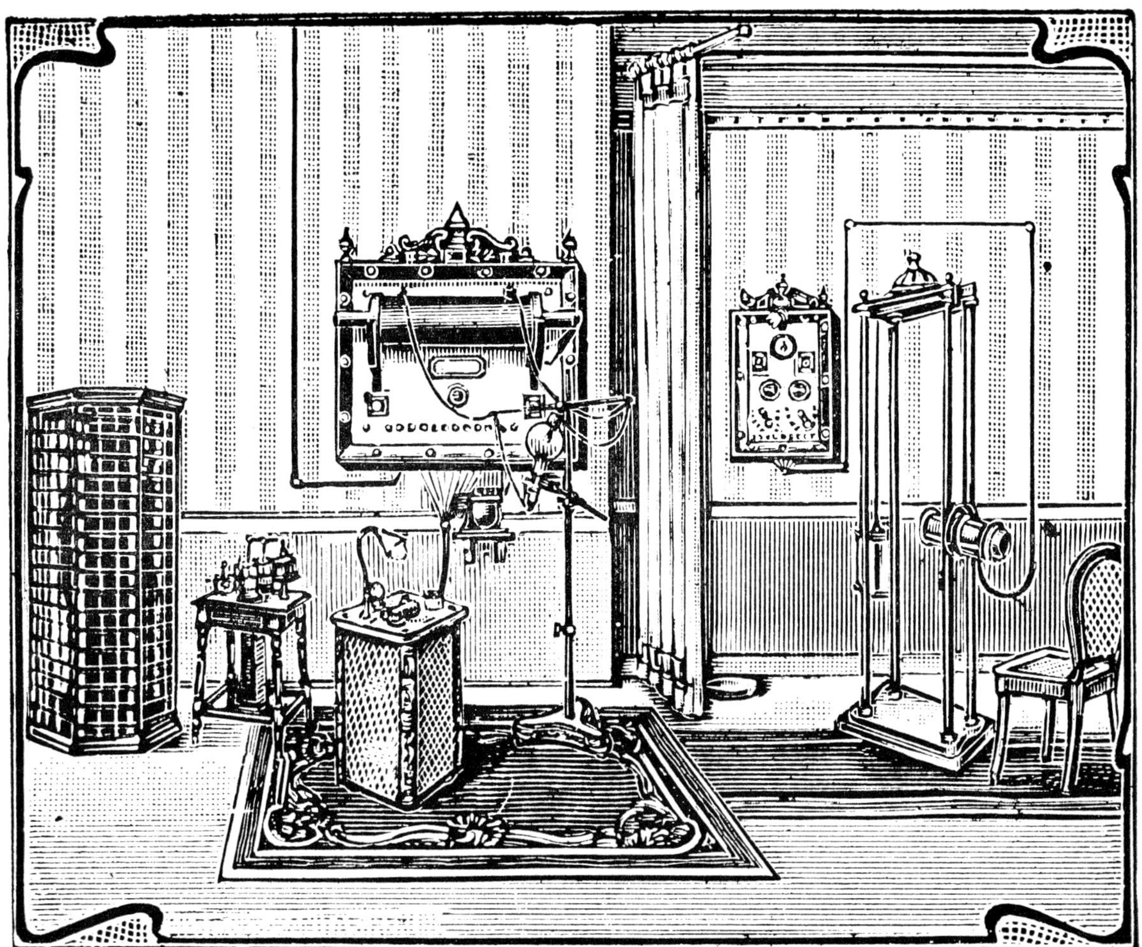

Sixty years ago (1903)! This is from an ad of the Sanitas Electrical Co., Ltd., 7a Soho Square, London, W., electro-manufacturers of repute. Note the solenoid or cage of autoconduction in left background: its terminals were connected to a source of high-frequency current (Apostoli's method), while inside the cage was an induction ring with Geissler tube for a rough estimate of current passed through the body of the patient (who was inside the cage). Their caption read: installation of x-ray and high-frequency apparatus, showing switch table from which everything is controlled, and apparatus for magneto therapy (sic!). The "magneto" was the "sparking" contraption to the viewer's right.

One of their famous machines was the Polydor with valve rectification: it had in 1927 the output of 250 ma at 150 kvp. At about that time they put on the market the Sectogrid, and a revolving Bucky-Potter diaphragm (the type which left a black spot in the middle of the film – at the center of rotation).

Like other British manufacturers, GR offers also "light" equipment, for instance the Cardioscope, a hand-tilted "couch" with tube-carrier independent of the screen carrier. But their main line is very much adapted to the Atomic Phase, including a 1000 ma or 150 kvp transformer with wall-mounted control stand, and a 90/90 Everest table (of 1959 vintage). GR also imports certain items (they were at one time representa-

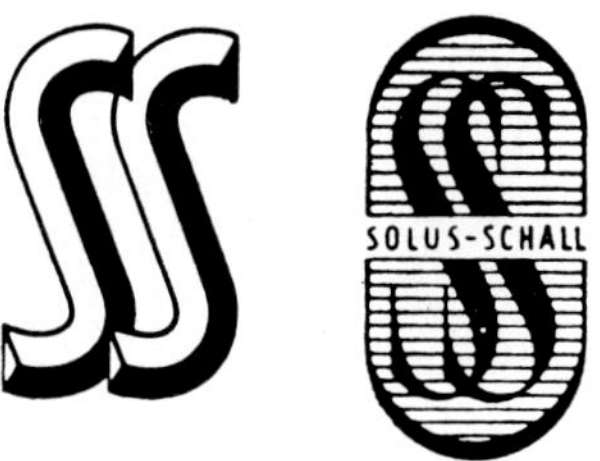

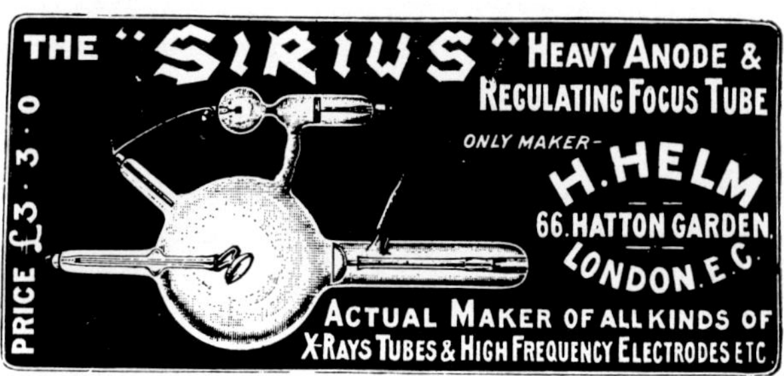

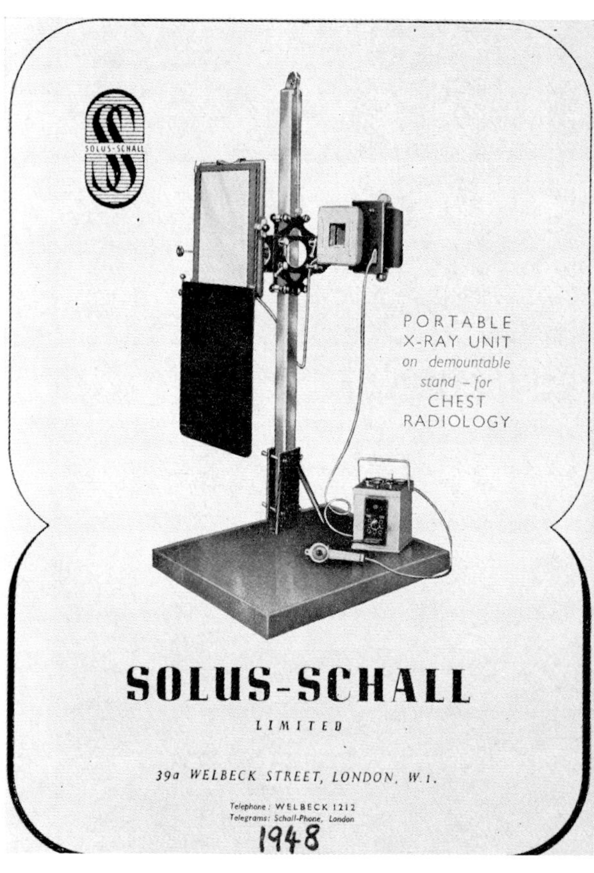

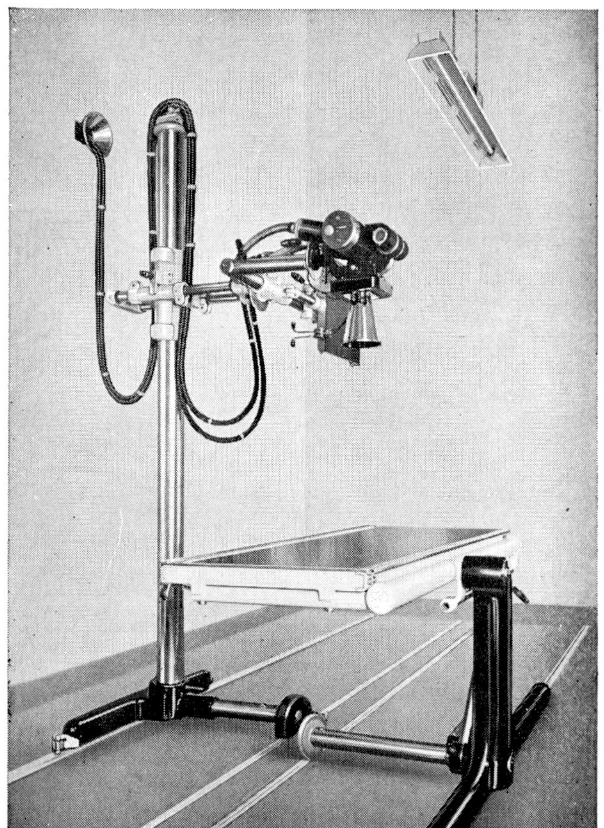

GR Cardioscope (1955). According to the ad, "the single pillar support permits undercouch screening over the whole length of the table making it ideally suitable for modern techniques involving the use of opaque media, such as intravenous pyelography." Any objections?

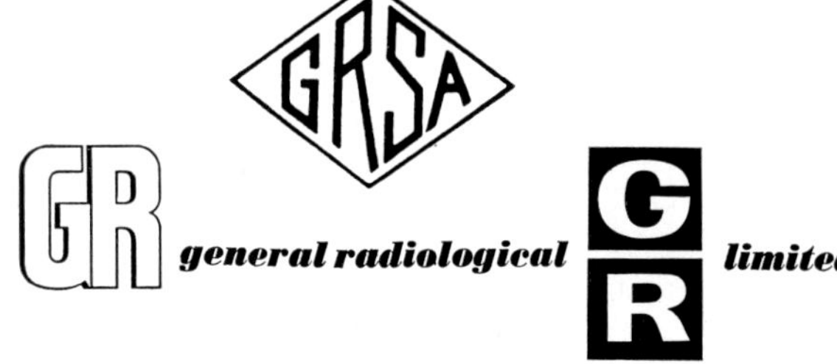

tives of Schönander), for instance they now advertise Profexray's Ceiling Tube Conveyor.*

At the time galley proofs were corrected, GR had started to build and sell their own motorized ceiling support, labeled TC-300. Another change was that GR had become a division of the (cinematographic) Rank Organization.

Mullard manufactures x-ray tubes (Guardian 125 and 150 kvp), tube housings and – since 1951 – also linacs. As previously stated, Mullard is now a subsidiary of Philips. Recently Mullard advertised – in combination with General Radiological – a 9″ electron-optical image intensifier.

Marconi Instruments, Ltd., originally a communications electronic manufacturer (since 1936), went gradually into the x-ray field, up to and including a 200 ma generator. In 1953 they produced a Universal (floor-to-ceiling) tubestand, in 1954 a Visual Diaphragm (light beam) Localizer, and in 1959 an overhead suspension mount (the latter two were for therapy equipment).

In 1954 Marconi decided – because of their electronic background – to get into image intensification.

*Another "foreign" ceiling tube support, advertised in British periodicals, is the one made by Picker, and sold by its London representation, the EXAL (Electronic & X-Ray Applications, Ltd.)

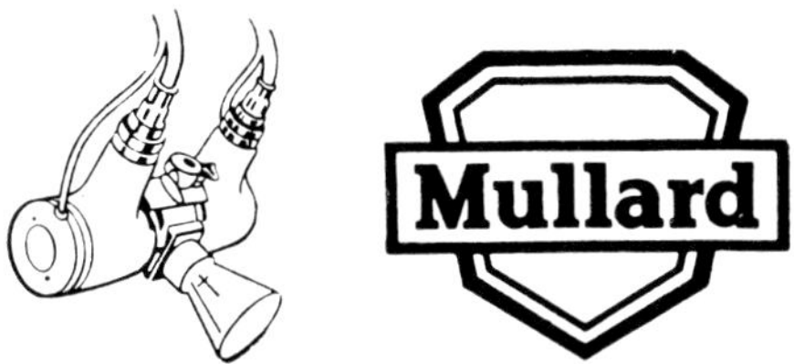

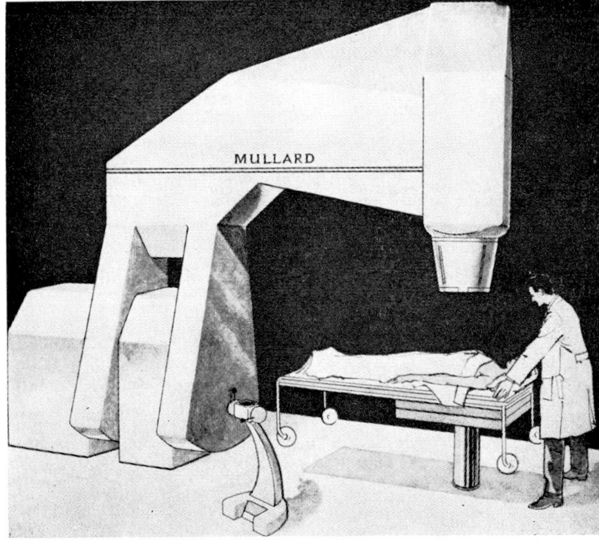

MULLARD LINAC (1961). 4.3 mev linear accelerator with high-frequency power source; output 350 r/min at 100 cm; light beam range finder; 270° gantry movement; single and double ended gantry available.

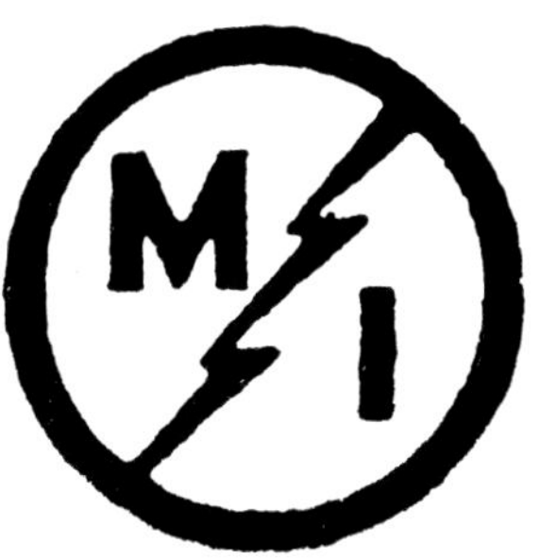

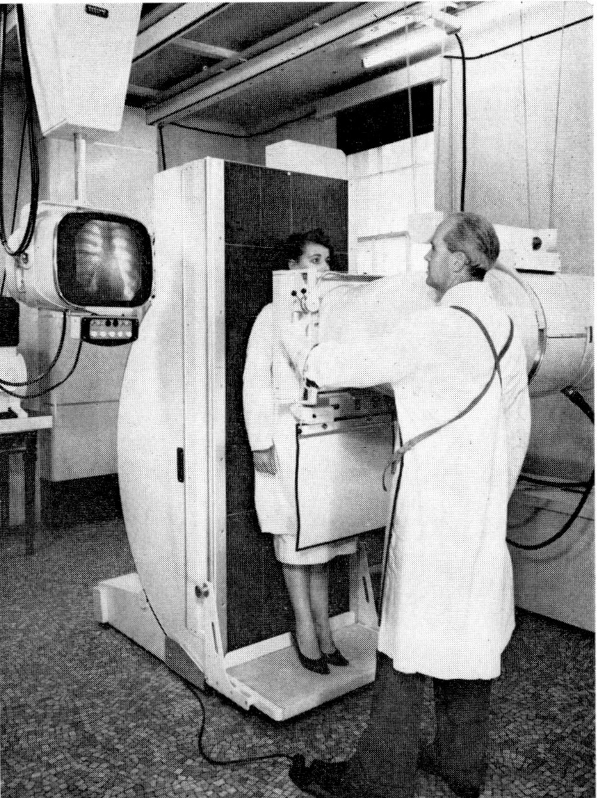

Courtesy: Marconi.

MARCONI IMAGE INTENSIFIER. It is mounted as close to the patient as possible to preserve the usefulness of its 12″ input screen. An Odelca mirror-lens brings the image within reach of a special 4½″ Orthicon tube, whence it appears on the ceiling-suspended television monitor and in any other desired monitoring area. In left background is visible part of the kinescope, a television-recorder.

In 1955 they made an initial arrangement with Odelca. In 1959 Marconi first showed at the München ICR its 12″ (Marconi) image intensifier. The image provided by the Odelca mirror arrangement is picked up (directly) by a very sensitive 4½″ Orthicon television tube, made by the English Electric Valve Company. The Marconi system uses a telescopic ceiling-suspended television monitor.

The Marconi intensifier differs from the Cinelix by having one-half inch smaller (12″) diameter of input screen, but this is much less than what can be lost by mounting the device on top of a spotfilmer — Marconi's intensifier was intended for direct mounting on the carrier, or else beneath the table (that removes the last vestige of the "old" way of positioning the patient on the table during fluoroscopy). The Marconi is just as bulky as the Cinelix (even though it does not have the electronic intensifier which in the Cinelix is interposed between the mirror image and the television pickup). For cine-recording, the Marconi provides a Kinescope, which is usually kept in the same room, although it could stay wherever a distant monitor were to be installed. In the USA the Marconi intensifying system is sold and serviced by Westinghouse.

Turning now to processing (and other "x-ray") chemicals, we shall mention the (abbreviated) X-Raysol 54, bottled by Johnsons of Handon, Ltd.

A well-known and well-advertised pharmaceutical manufacturer in this field is the May & Baker Company. They compound opaque media, for instance Diaginol, Arteriodone, and Vasiodone. Some may be imported.

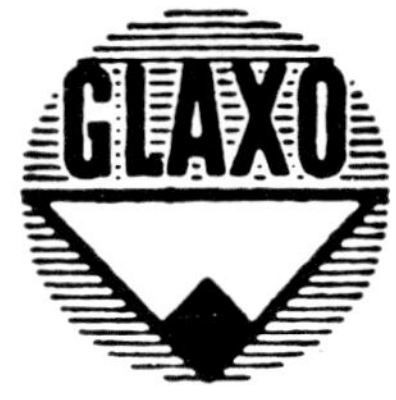

GLAXO LABORATORIES LIMITED
GREENFORD · MIDDLESEX · BYRon 3434

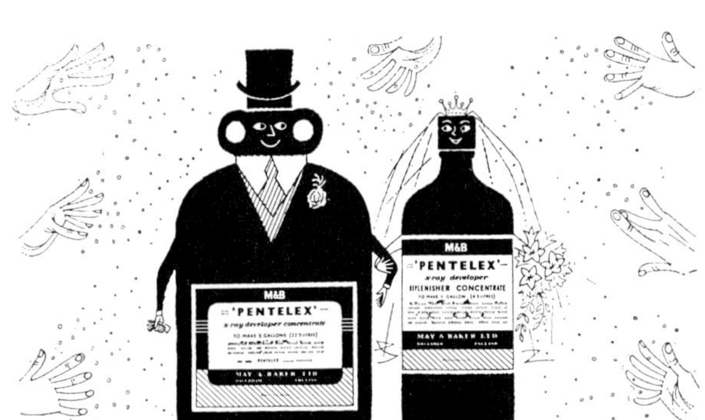

M & B's "Ideal pair." This May & Baker ad, which appeared in 1957 in *Acta Radiologica,* emphasizes that Pentelex and its replenisher are well suited for each other.

The NRD AUTOMATIC

X-RAY FILM PROCESSING UNIT

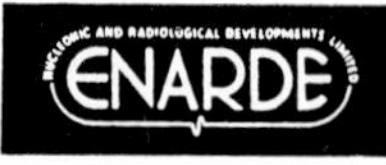

1954

Please write for full information to

NUCLEONIC & RADIOLOGICAL DEVELOPMENTS LTD.

22 MARSHGATE LANE, LONDON, E.15

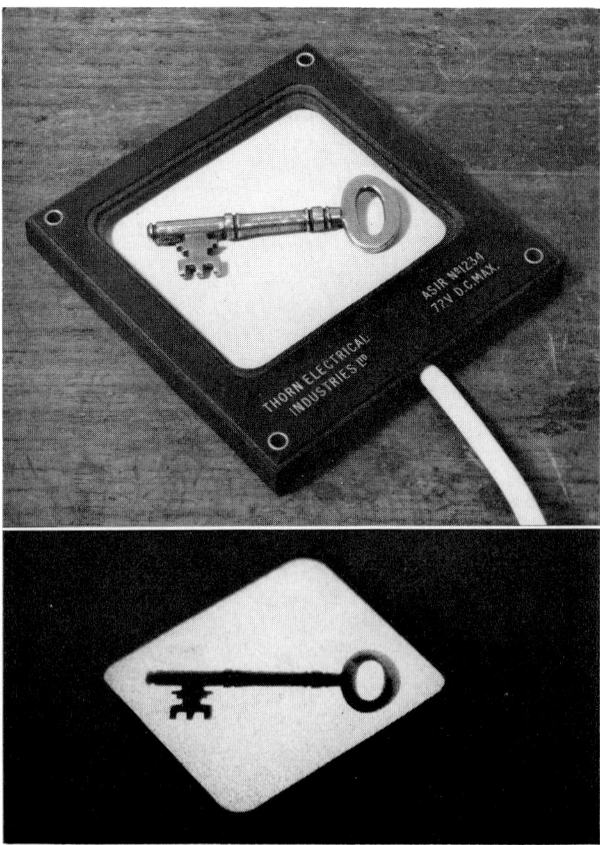

Thorn Image Retaining Panel

Their latest ads describe Biliodyl (for oral cholecysto-cholangiography) and Pulmidol (a soluble substance for for bronchography). For automation in processing, May & Baker have marketed "hot" solutions, the developers Pentelex and Exprol, and the hypo Perfix. In one of their advertisements, May & Baker gave the dates and places of installation of early automatic film processing machines in the British Isles. The first Fax-Ray Senior in the United Kingdom was installed in April, 1961 in East Glamorgan Hospital in Pontypridd — and uses Pentelex and Perfix. The first Procomat in the UK went into operation in May, 1961 at the General Infirmary in Leeds — and uses Pentelex and Perfix. And the Hills unit at Guy's Hospital (marketed in England by ENARDE) was redesigned in June, 1961 to reduce processing time from forty-five to eight minutes — for which they used Exprol and Perfix.

The Boots Pure Drug Company in Nottingham bottles opaque media. One of their brands is Pyelumbrine.

Perhaps the best known British maker of contrast materials is Glaxo Laboratories in Greenford (Middlesex), mainly because of the world-wide acceptance of Dionosil, the first soluble bronchographic substance. One of their advertising lines deserves to remain on record. In the early 1950s they played on the words "shadow of a doubt" to emphasize that the density of Pyelosil

October, 1919.

HARRY W. COX & CO., LTD.

beg to announce that they have effected an AMALGAMATION with the CAVENDISH ELECTRICAL CO., Ltd. The new combination will be known as:—

THE

COX-CAVENDISH

ELECTRICAL CO., LTD.

This step has been carried through with the loyal co-operation of the staffs of both the old Companies in order to give better service to the medical world.

The watch word will be "PROGRESS and SERVICE."

Apparatus can be inspected and purchases made at the Showrooms, 105, GT. PORTLAND STREET, W. 1, where a stock of small accessories for immediate delivery is held.

All communications by letter and telephone must be made with the Head Office situate at

TWYFORD ABBEY WORKS,
ACTON LANE, HARLESDEN, N.W. 10.

Telephone: 339 WILLESDEN.

NOTE:—The showrooms and offices at Wigmore Street are closed.

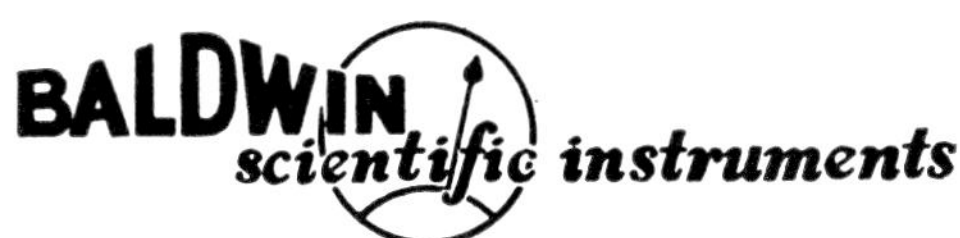

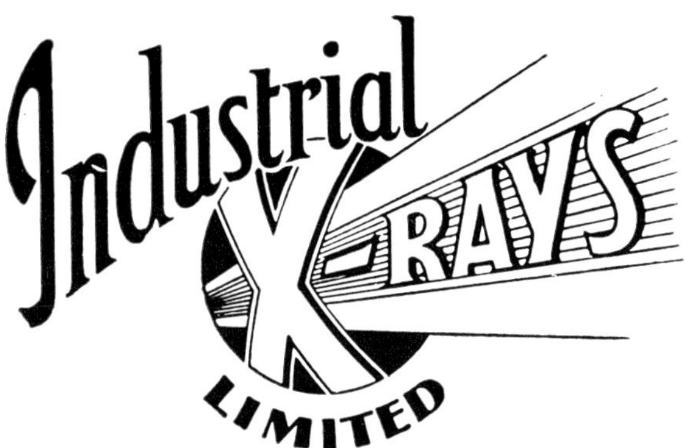

"Who's Who in X-Rays"

Every Medical Man and Hospital contemplating the purchase of X-Ray Equipment or Sundries should write at once for a copy of the above—a unique production profusely illustrating the various types of apparatus.

It will be sent gratis and post-free on request to the Publishers:

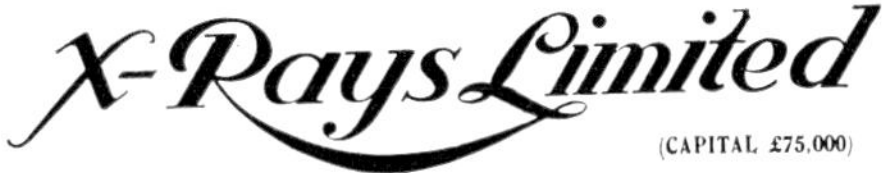

(CAPITAL £75,000)

Chairman of Directors:
SIR HENRY OUTRAM BAX-IRONSIDE, K.C.M.G.
(Director of Westminster Electric Supply Corporation, Ltd.)

Managing Director
J. W. MASON.

11 TORRINGTON PLACE, GOWER STREET,
LONDON, W.C.1

1928

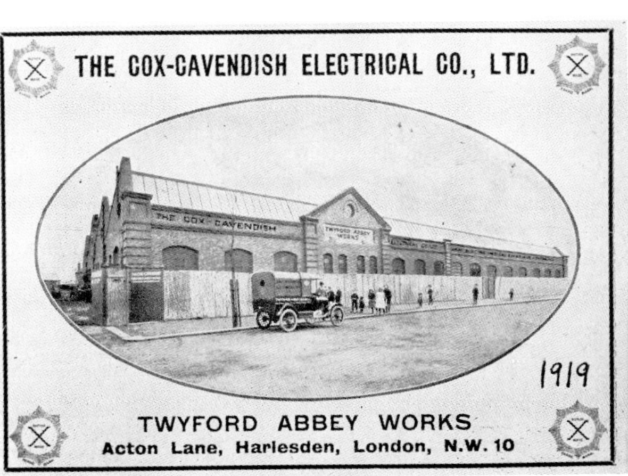

leaves no such questions. That was followed up with a series on the "subtleties of shadow" obtainable when using Glaxo media.

Thorn Electrical Industries in Enfield have placed on the market in 1963 the IRP (image retaining panel), a metal-ceramic surface coated with a special electroluminescent emulsion (phosphorus) to which a D.C. current can be applied. When electromagnetic radiation (of any wavelength) hits the energized panel, it will imprint its image, and that image (as that of the key, when the radiation is visible light) will stay on for half-an-hour or until the D.C. current is turned off, after which the panel can be re-used. X rays, infrared light, even radioactivity can be used as "light" source. To preserve the image, one simply lays a photographic emulsion on the panel for a contact print. The "phosphorus" employed is basically zinc cadmium sulphide. There are numerous potential applications of this novel apparatus, for instance in the orthopedic operating room. As of now, however, the "after-glow" can only be seen in a darkened room!

Dosimeters are produced by Baldwin Industrial Controls, a firm in Dartford (Kent). Among the manufacturers of protective equipment, W. S. Rothband & Co. is one of the older ones. Old-fashioned stainless steel tanks, and steel filing cabinets are made by Industrial X-Rays in Staffordshire, owners of a very interesting trade-mark. Cox's old firm, which merged into the Cox-Cavendish, is now no longer in the medical field, but makes industrial equipment.

Among firms which are no longer in the x-ray field (or no longer in existence) will be mentioned the Motterhead & Co. with its coils and transformers; the G. C. Aimer Co. with the "Welbec" Standard T. T. tube; X-Rays, Ltd. with accessories and with the spotfilmer Seriascope; and several quartz lamp manufacturers, such as the British Hanovia, who at one time were part of (or only in symbiosis with) radiology.

AEI

Associated Electrical Industries (AEI) is a group which resulted from the consolidation of several firms.

During the Golden Age of Radiology, GE had a wholly owned subsidiary in London, trading as the

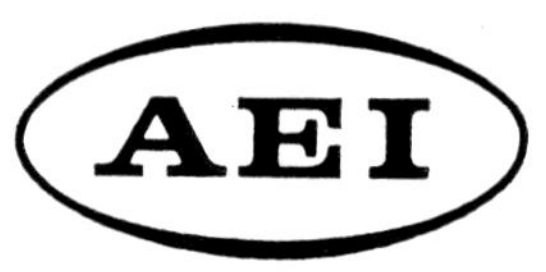

ORIGINAL HANOVIA
ALPINE
SUN

The New Successes of

Irritation Therapy
***with* Ultra-Violet Rays**

indicate a wide field of use for the Artificial "Alpine Sun" Quartz Lamp (Original Hanovia)

in the domain of

INTERNAL MEDICINE

Recent investigations show that in addition to general irradiation and the production of erythema on established lines of treatment, intense local irradiation of small areas producing third degree erythema (possibly to the point of Dermatitis bullosa) produces striking results.

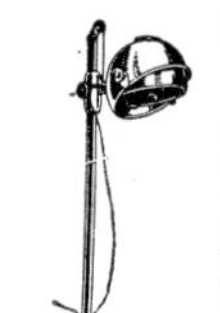

Prices from £15 for original Hanovia Artificial "ALPINE SUN." Available for direct and alternating currents.

Ask for Literature Set 8
mentioning your special branch of practice

1926

THE BRITISH HANOVIA QUARTZ LAMP CO. LTD.
SLOUGH - - - BUCKS.

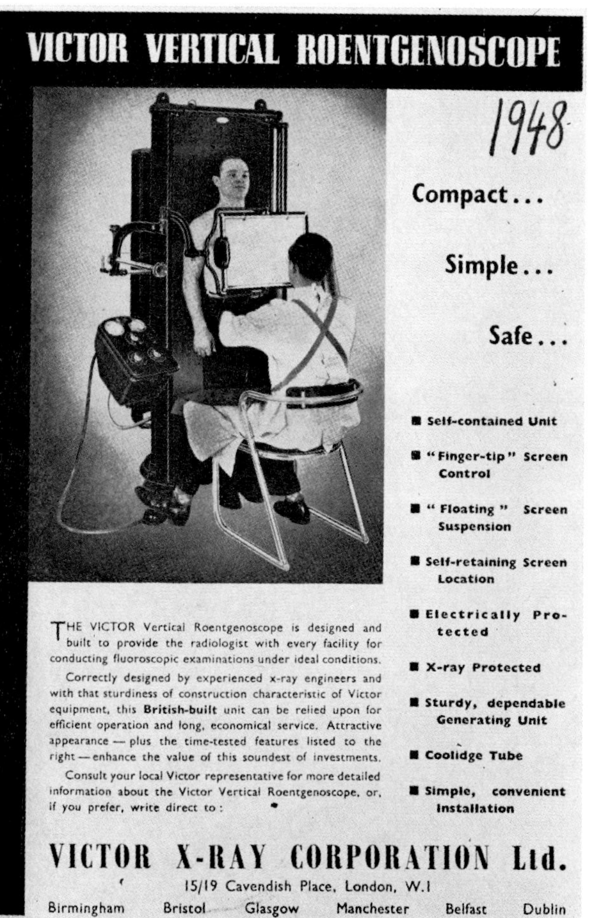

Victor X-Ray Corporation. As late as 1947, they were advertising their service organization and in 1948 the British-built Victor Vertical Roentgenoscope.

Another respectable firm was the Newton Wright Company — it descended directly from Sir Isaac Newton. In 1948, Victor and Newton Wright united to form the Newton Victor Company. During the war, Metropolitan-Vickers of Manchester had acquired interest in the Newton Wright Company, and when the Newton Victor merger came about, the "new" firm became a subsidiary of Metropolitan-Vickers, which in turn is part of the AEI. For adequate divisionalization, all x-ray activities of the AEI were combined in 1960 in AEI's Instrumentation Division.*

And so the Newton Victor Orbitron (a 2000 curie Co^{60} rotational teletherapy container) became the AEI Orbitron. The Victormeter (a dosimeter) has not been advertised after the merger. But Newton Victor's Resomax 300 — an x-ray therapy apparatus with resonant (no iron-core) transformer encased with the x-ray tube in a single container under oil is being manufactured. Several other items are also well introduced such as the AEI former Newton Wright Bucky Standard and the AEI Determinator (a lighted beam collimator for diagnosis). By far the most interesting piece of equipment is the Orthotron, made by Metropolitan-Vickers. That firm built in 1954 a 20 mev betatron, which was installed (and is still in operation) in the Christie Hospital in Manchester. The Orthotron is a travelling-wave

*These details have been obtained through the courtesy of Mr. Gordon Farqhar Gribbin, one of the directors of AEI.

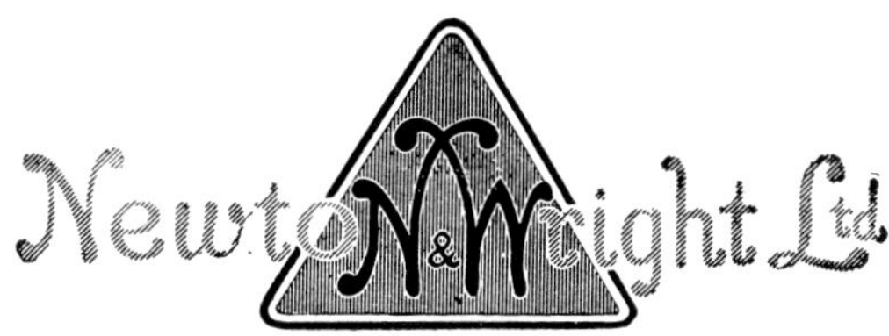

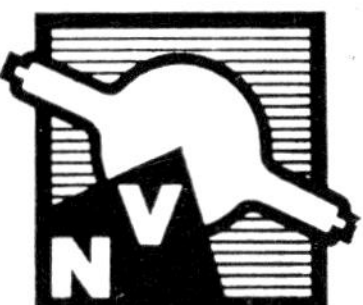
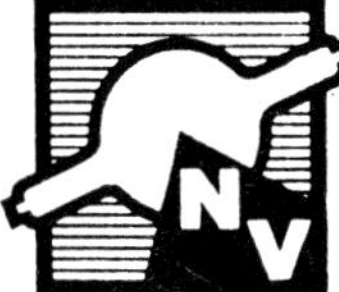
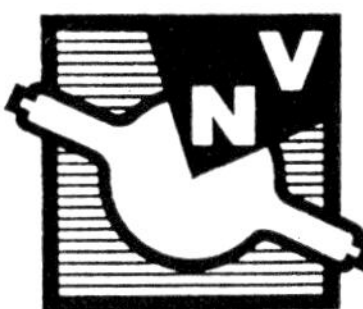

Newton-Victor's trade-mark. There must have existed a fourth seal, but I have never seen it.

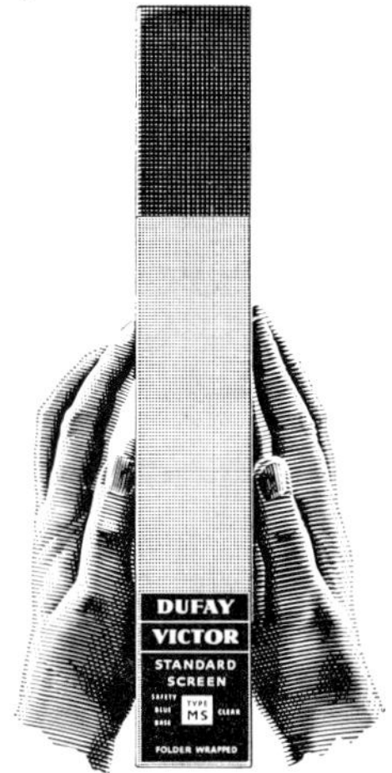

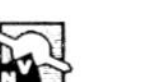

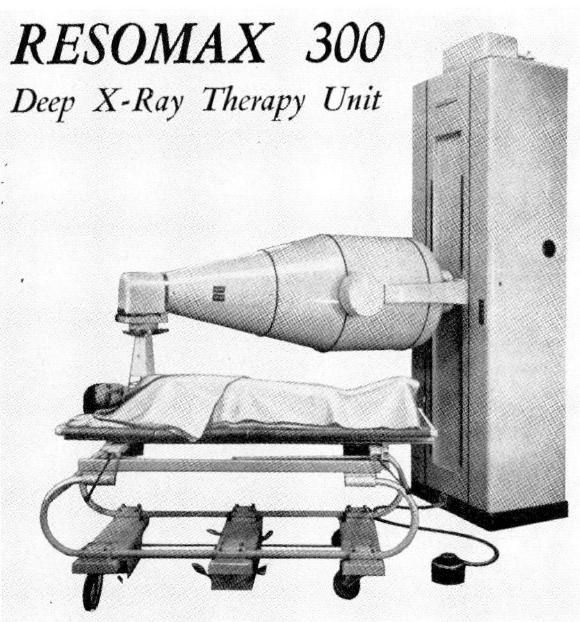

Courtesy: AEI.

Resomax 300. Having a hard time to live down the "foreign" origin of Victor, this 1955 ad begins by stressing that the machine is "all-British". Its resonant transformer has no iron-core: in its place comes the x-ray tube. The unit, which is now called AEI Resomax, performs quite well.

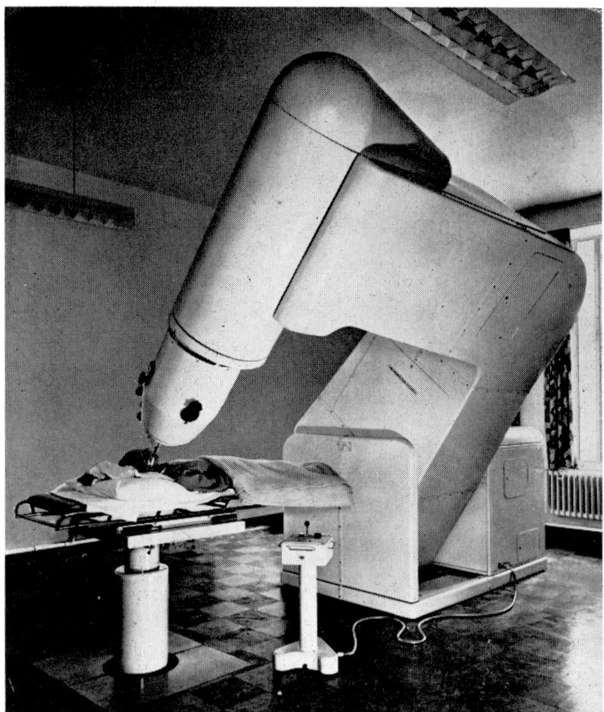

Courtesy: AEI.

METROPOLITAN-VICKERS ORTHOTRON is magnetron-driven. The 4-mev model in the illustration is installed at Mount Vernon Hospital (Middlesex). The maximum *live* voltage actually developed in any part of the equipment is below 50 kv.

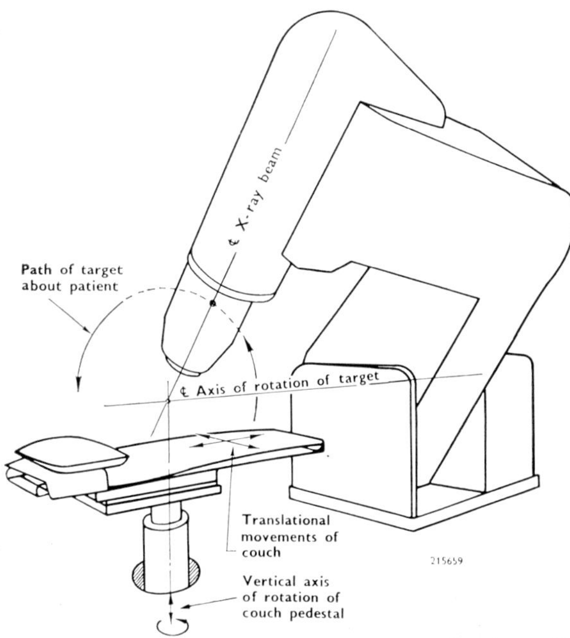

Courtesy: AEI.

METRO-VICKERS LINAC. The unit has isocentric mounting, so that the beam always passes through the axis of rotation of the target (gantry principle).

linac which was first constructed in an 8-mev version – installed in 1953 in the Hammersmith Hospital in London. Current models are in the 4-mev category: after filtration, they produce a uniform field of x-radiation 31.5 cm in diameter. At one meter from the target the output is about 200 r/min. This is high and the machine is therefore operated usually at a reduced pulse repetition rate, which prolongs the life of the magnetron, while still giving 100 r/min.

VICKERS RESEARCH

Advertisements of (another) Vickers 6 mev magnetron modulated linac began to appear in 1961. The manufacturer was listed as being the Vickers Research Ltd. in Sunninghill (Ascot, Berkshire). This company supplies also a linear accelerator with variable 12-35 mev energy, suitable for either electron and/or x-ray therapy. It comes with a three-meter accelerating tube, in which case maximum power is 500 watts at 35 mev. When five meters of accelerating tube are installed, the output goes to 2.5 kilowatts at 35 mev; it is then usable both for radiobiologic research, for isotope production, and for the sterilization of surgical and other materials.

There exists an "historic" connection between the names of Metropolitan-Vickers and Vickers Research.

The story goes back to 1828 when Naylor, Hutchinson, Vickers & Co. was founded. Its name was soon changed to Naylor, Vickers & Co.; George Naylor's junior partner was his son-in-law, who became the famous steel manufacturer Edward Vickers (1804-1897). The latter's name was retained in subsequent amalgamations from which resulted the Vickers' Sons & Co. A milestone was the formation in 1896 of the Vickers' Sons and Maxim. Another important merger occurred in 1927 – with the Elswick Engineering Works, founded in 1847 by the "father of modern artillery" William George Armstrong (1810-1900) – whence appeared the Vickers-Armstrong, Ltd. The acquisition of

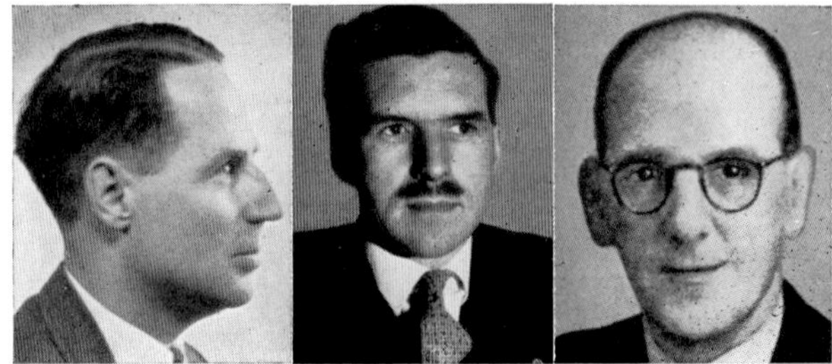

PHILIP MAY GODFREY SAXON R. W. ARMSTRONG

May is with Mullard; Saxon with Metropolitan-Vickers; Armstrong was with Newton Victor.

subsidiaries continued unabated, and the complex is known today as the Vickers Group.

In 1917, the Metropolitan-Carriage Wagon & Finance Company purchased the American shares which controlled the British Westinghouse (with plants in Manchester). In 1919, Vickers purchased Metropolitan-Carriage and all its "electric" stock, and formed another company, appropriately re-named Metropolitan-Vickers.

In January, 1926, a court ordered the Vickers Group to reduce its capital, and set up a commission to indicate the manner in which this ought to be done. The "recommendation" was for Vickers to dispose of all interests other than those directly connected with its main activities (steel, armament, shipbuilding). . . This is why in 1928 Vickers sold Metropolitan-Vickers. It entered into close co-operation with the (American) International General Electric Company. Then Metropolitan-Vickers acquired shares in the British Thomson-Houston, in the Edison & Swan, and in other "electric" companies in England. In December, 1928, the name of Metropolitan-Vickers was changed to Associated Electrical Industries (AEI), which is the holding company, while the name Metropolitan-Vickers was given to a new subsidiary (of the AEI) which carried on the business. The Vickers Group never acquired (officially, at least) any shares in the AEI. The new Metropolitan-Vickers did quite well, and expanded to where it is also making linacs.

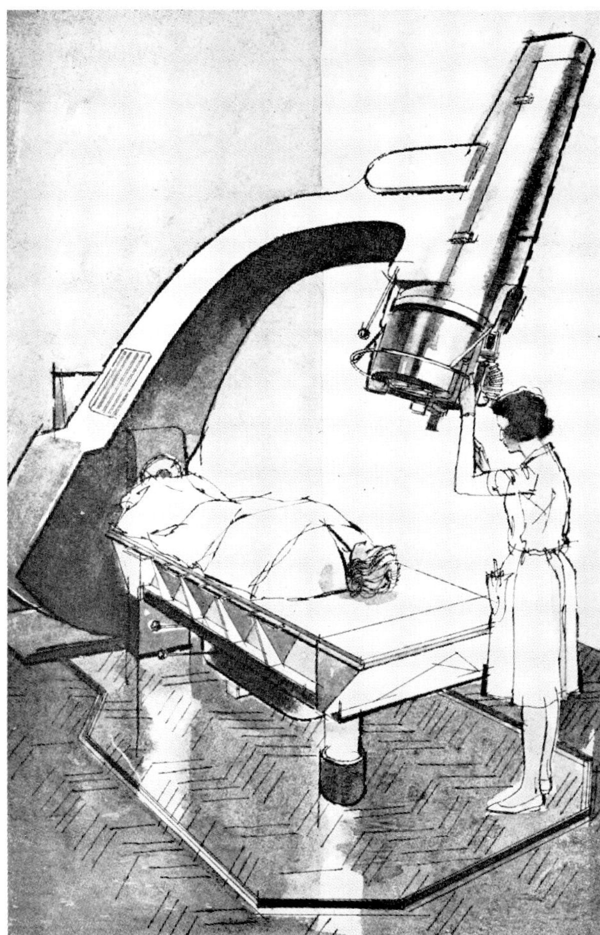

VICKERS RESEARCH 6-MEV LINAC. Sketch of linac installed in 1961 at Newcastle General Hospital (in Newcastle upon Tyne). Other units went to Guy's, the Westminster, and Royal Marsden. Its advantage is the miniaturization of the electrical components, which are thus housed either in the gantry or in the control unit (no separate apparatus room required). This linac has no connection with AEI (see text).

Vickers Research is a post-World War II "electronics-nuclear" diversification of the Vickers Group. Today Vickers' medical linacs are manufactured at the Vickers-Armstrong (Engineers) South Marston Works in Swindon (Wiltshire).

The Vickers linac has many interesting features. Its circuits are miniaturized, everything fits in the gantry; the only other machinery is the control desk, placed in another room in front of a lead-glass or liquid-filled observation "window." The gantry and pedestal unit is assembled and tested at the plant, and shipped as such. The best way of moving it into the treatment room is by making an aperture in the roof. That opening can later serve as a rooflight, or it may be filled in with precast concrete, should there be need for shielding.

Optional equipment offered with the unit is an oxygen chamber – resembling an oversized incubator – in which up to three atmospheres of pure oxygen pressure can be provided. Also optional is a servo-motor to accurately control the angular velocity of the gantry system. Other extras are wedge filter inter-locks, treatment record print-out, vacuum pump for bolus bags, and a 10° tilted couch.*

*Much of this information was graciously provided by Maurice Gordon Kelliher, the chief-physicist at Vickers Research Ltd.

Coolidge X-Ray Tubes

Important Announcement

The British Thomson-Houston Company Ltd. beg to announce that from 25th April, 1927, the main distributors of Coolidge Tubes in the United Kingdom and Irish Free State will be

Messrs. Watson & Sons (Electro-Medical) Limited
Sunic House, 43 Parker Street, Kingsway, London, W.C.2

The Victor X-Ray Corporation
Morley House, 314-22 Upper Regent Street, London, W.1

P4. *The British Thomson-Houston Co. Ltd.*

ILFORD

The history of Ilford, Ltd. goes back to 1879 when Alfred Harman started out as one of the earliest manufacturers of photographic dry plates. His first "factory" was in the basement of his own house on Cranbrook Road in Ilford.

His staff consisted of two men and three boys, with occasional assistance from his wife and housekeeper. Their output was distributed by Marion & Co. of Soho Square in London. In 1886, Harman organized his own firm as the Brittania Works Company. The demand for Ilford plates became such that he installed a separate factory on the Clyde Estate, within the area occupied by the present plate factory. The firm changed into a

JULY, 1908. *The Journal of the Röntgen Society.* vii.

NEW X-RAY PLATES

MADE ON A NEW PRINCIPLE.

For Particulars apply for Leaflet "R."

WRATTEN & WAINWRIGHT, LTD., CROYDON.

THE X RAYS.

In view of the demand likely to arise for Plates sensitive to these Rays, we have for some time past been conducting exhaustive experiments with every material likely to increase the sensibility of Plates to the

RÖNTGEN RAYS.

The net result has been that, instead of putting on the market a **SPECIAL PLATE AT A HIGH PRICE**, we can affirm with the utmost confidence that the very best and quickest results can be obtained on our **POPULAR PRICED**

A 1 PLATES,

which, with a Ruhmkorff Coil, giving a 3-in. spark, and using a Watson and Sons' or Newton's Focus Tube, will give a Radiograph of the Human Hand in from thirty seconds to one minute, showing full details of the bones.

These Plates, though only recently introduced, are meeting with such approval from professionals and amateurs that they may be said to be

THE PLATES OF THE SEASON.

FOR HAND CAMERA, SHUTTER, AND STUDIO WORK THESE PLATES ARE UNEQUALLED.

To be obtained of all Dealers of importance.

Any difficulty in procuring them should be notified to the Manufacturers:

R. W. THOMAS & CO., LIMITED,

THORNTON HEATH, NEAR LONDON.

Telegrams: "PEED, THORNTON HEATH." Telephone No. 9365. 1897

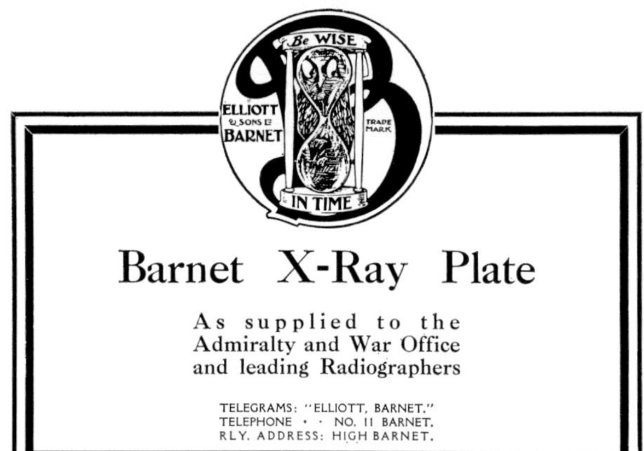

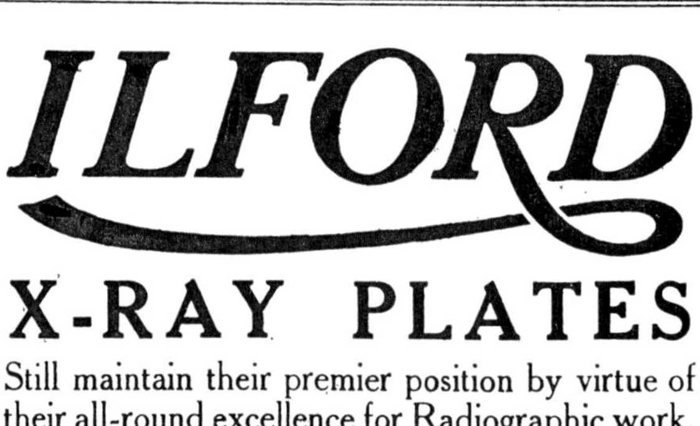

X-RAY PLATES

Still maintain their premier position by virtue of their all-round excellence for Radiographic work.

ILFORD X-RAY SCREEN PLATES are for use with intensifying Screens only, where exposures must be reduced to the minimum.

ILFORD X-RAY DENTAL FILMS are supplied in special moisture-proof packing. The perfect film for dental purposes.

The Ilford X-Ray Pamphlet sent post free.

ILFORD, Limited, Ilford, London, England.

Telephone: ILFORD 13 (3 lines). Telegrams: "PLATES" ILFORD

ILFORD REGISTERED TRADE MARK

1921

private limited liability company in 1891, and in 1898 to a public company. The name was changed to Ilford, Ltd. in 1900.

F. F. Renwick joined the company in 1899, and devoted his life to the application of science to photography. He died in 1943 after three decades as Ilford's director of research. Renwick became famous for his work on sensitometry. Together with Sir William Pope and others at Cambridge, he introduced British-made sensitizing dyes used in the first Ilford panchromatic plates in 1914 (that introduction was "accelerated" by the advent of World War I).

In 1919, was formed Selo. Ltd., jointly owned by Ilford, Thomas Illingworth & Co., Imperial Dry Plate Co., Rajar, Ltd., Paget Prize Plate Co., and Marion & Co.; in 1922 Selo began to manufacture roll films at Brentwood.

The consolidation process gained momentum. In 1919, Ilford acquired control of the Imperial Dry Plate Co., established in 1887, and with it of the General

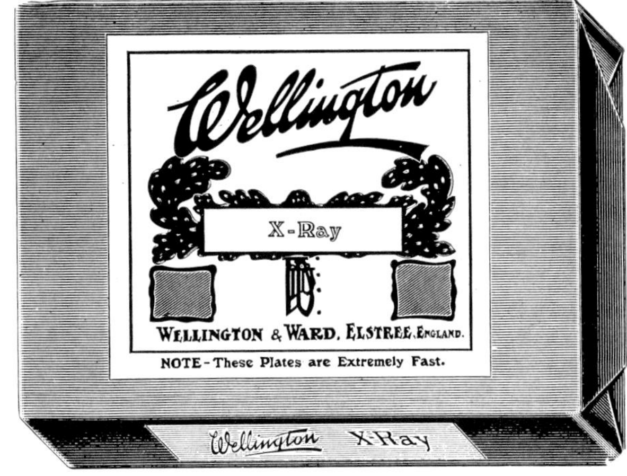

Wellington & Ward, Elstree, Herts.
London · Paris · Bombay · Calcutta, etc.

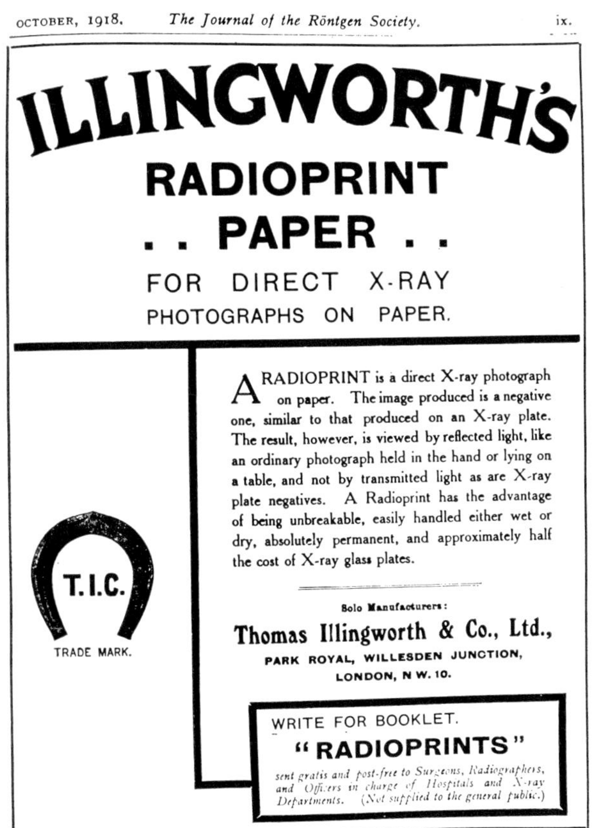

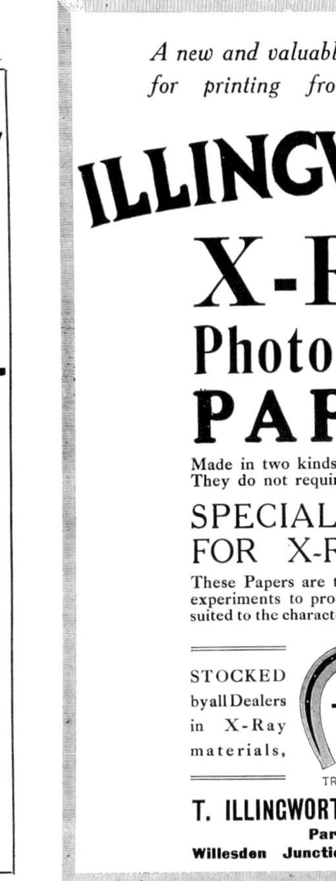

THE IMPERIAL DRY PLATE CO. LTD.

CRICKLEWOOD, LONDON, N.W.2

Dry Plate Co., controlled by Imperial since 1912. Thomas Illingworth & Co., founded in 1890, came under Ilford control around 1919. In 1928, Ilford absorbed the Amalgamated Photographic Manufacturers, Ltd. (formed in 1920 by Rajar, Paget Prize Plate, and Marion & Co.), of which the latter was the oldest, having been founded in 1860). Finally, Ilford purchased Wellington & Ward in 1929. In the beginning all these businesses maintained their identities but during 1930 they were reorganized and unified under the Ilford name.

In 1952, the film factory at Brentwood was provided with new high-capacity coating machines. By 1961, Ilford supplied more than 50 per cent of all x-ray film used in Great Britain. At the time Ilford, with 4500 employees, claimed to be the largest x-ray film manufacturer in Europe, but now the (Belgian) Gevaert is ahead of them. Until 1952, Ilford imported the film base from the USA: in that year Ilford completed building and installations of a British film-base producing plant, Bexford, Ltd., a joint venture of Ilford and B. X. Plastics, Ltd. In 1958, Ilford made a co-operative (color-film) arrangement with Imperial Chemical Industries, Ltd.

Ilford roentgen plates were well received during the Era of the Pioneers. Ilford plates were advertised in 1912 in the *American Quarterly of Roentgenology.* The importer was Meyrowitz of New York.

Currently Ilford has a complete line of films and screens, as well as of x-ray accessories and of chemicals, including those for automatic processors. Another Atomic Phase feature is the technique called "multiple radiography." It is the use of several layers of screens, each having a different intensification effect: with a single exposure one can thus obtain a "hard" and a "soft" film. In today's radiation-conscious era, such economy of exposure seems desirable not only in placentography. A similar multiple layer technique is used in Ilford's Polytomography — the female model for the advertisement of the former is particularly well built, presumably to show through how many bosomy layers one can penetrate. By way of history Ilford considers the introduction of Phenidone additive to developer

"NATURE."
GRANNY DEAR, PLEASE STOP WEL-WARD MAKING A BETTER BOAT THAN MINE — I WANT THE BEST BOAT
MY DEAR LITTLE SONNIE, YOUR NOISE IS CHILDISH, GIVE YOUR ATTENTION TO YOUR OWN BOAT-BUILDING IF YOU WANT TO MAKE THE BEST BOAT & WIN THE RACE & BEAT WEL-WARD. YOUR FOOLISH COMPLAINTS & TEARS WILL LESSEN YOUR CHANCE OF WINNING & ADD TO WEL-WARD'S REPUTATION
AND ALSO ADD TO THE REPUTATION OF THE
Wellington X-RAY PLATE
1920
GLUE

A Successful British Manufacture
ILFORD
DOUBLE D-C COATED
X-RAY FILMS
are of high speed and free from all trace of fog or veil
Prices and Terms on application
ILFORD, Limited
ILFORD, London, England.
ILFORD GASLIGHT PAPER
(Normal or Vigorous)
is perfect for X-ray prints.
No dark-room required
BUY BRITISH GOODS KEEP BRITAIN BUSY

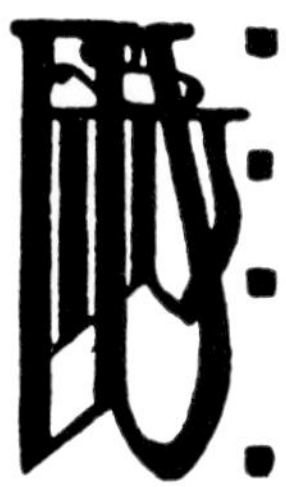

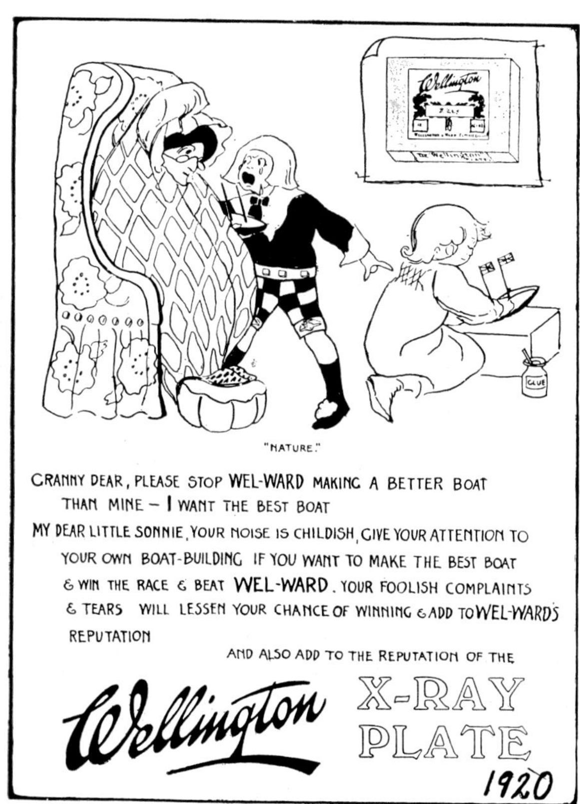

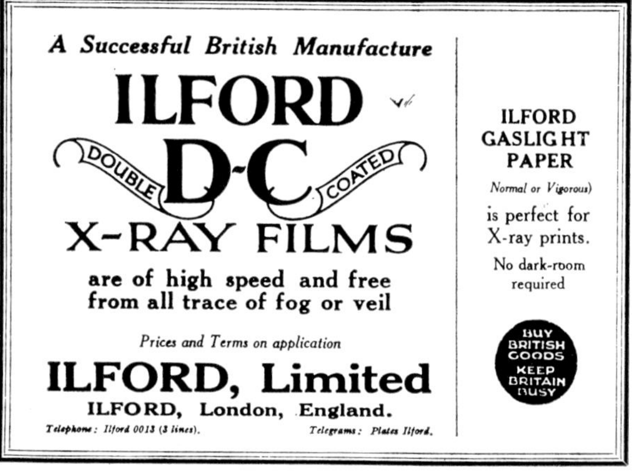

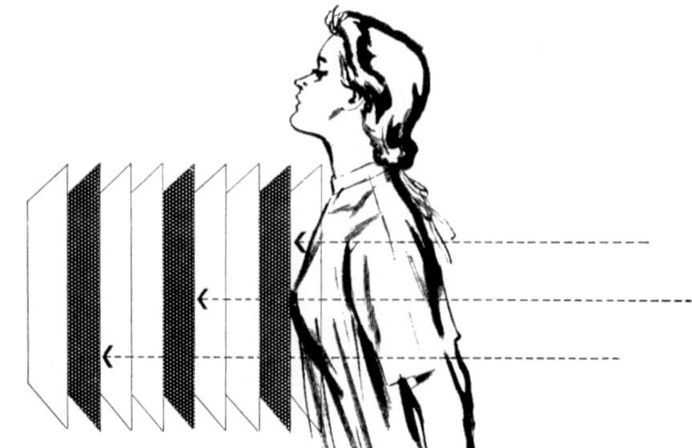

(Renwick) as one of the technical milestones in the field.

DEAN

Dean & Co. traces its beginnings to the end of the year 1896. As mentioned before, radiation contributed to the death of Alfred Ernest Dean. His son, Gerald Peter Dean, has recently gone into partial retirement, but is still chairman of their Board of Directors.

In looking back over the years, an impressive number of machines had been issued with the Dean insignia. A portable Field Service Unit was available in 1898. In the catalog for that year (Dean's first) there was also listed Dean's Exploring X-Ray Lamp (the advertisement read: "Perfectly insulated. Safe to handle. The only portable x-ray lamp extant."). In 1904 was issued the Harnack-Dean Precision Couch, having both overhead and under-the-table tubes, and a built-in sphere gap.

As the ICR convened in London in 1925, Dean had also the Empire Diascope, (an upright fluoroscope), and a therapy apparatus, for either constant or pulsating current, giving 10 ma at 200 kvp.

For the Atomic Phase, the company manufactures the Dean Gonad Shield, attached to a counterbalanced arm, supported by a heavy stand. As far back as 1952, the Dean Zenith Couch permitted 30° Trendelenburg – in 1959 it acquired a motor-driven footrest, and sliding table top. Their four-valve transformer had been offered for a long time in one of two models – 500 ma at 100 kvp, or 300 ma at 125 kvp. In 1961, the four-valve D-55 reached maximum ratings of either 1000 ma or 150 kvp. There exists also the Dean CD-40 Tubestand (with magnetic brakes) and the Dean Delineator (a lead leaf diaphragm with light beam to circumscribe the diagnositic field). In several advertising campaigns, the company stressed the ease with which Dean equipment can be serviced, and the ease with which Dean

A. E. DEAN & CO. (X-RAY APPARATUS) AED LONDON **LTD.**
G. P. DEAN
PROGRESS WAY · CROYDON · ENGLAND

ALFRED E. DEAN,

The Largest Maker in England

Of Apparatus in all Departments of

Electro - Therapeutics,

Including Radiography, High Frequency, Hydro-Electric and Light Baths, Finsen and other Light, Cautery, Electrolysis, X-Ray Tubes, etc.

INDUCTION COILS & STATIC MACHINES A SPECIALITY.

Contractor to the War Office, India Office, and Admiralty; British and Foreign Hospitals, etc.

Lists on Application.

82, HATTON GARDEN, LONDON.

8, Rue Victor Cousin, PARIS.
112, Sauchiehall St., GLASGOW.

1905

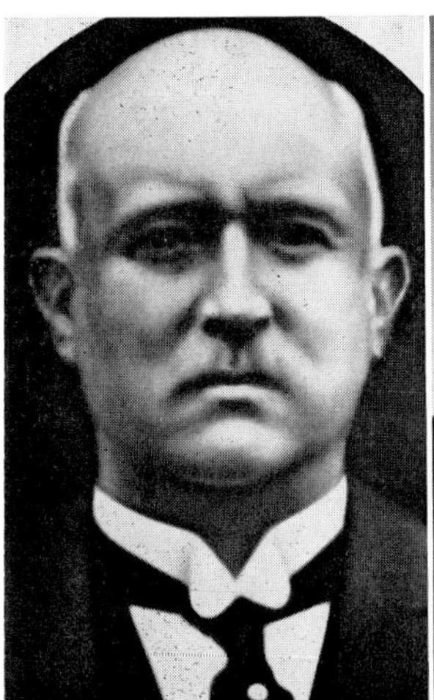

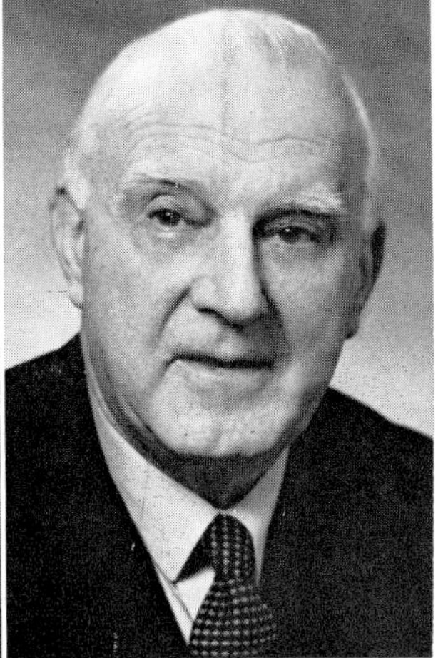

Courtesy: Dean & Co.

DEAN, FATHER & SON. Alfred Ernest Dean (with cut-out collar and stern, "fatherly" glance), and Gerald Peter Dean.

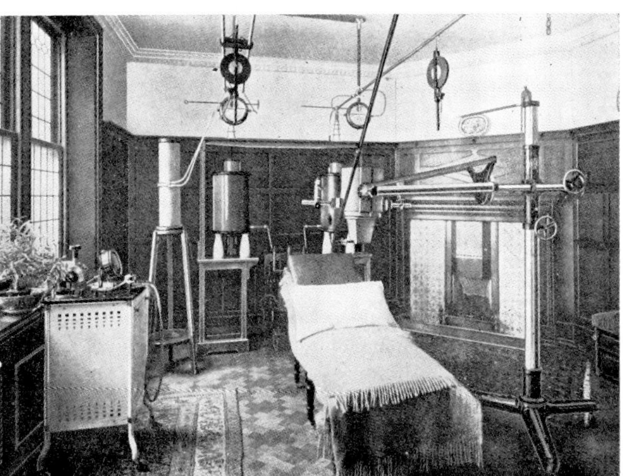

DEAN DEEP THERAPY UNIT. (1927). A sopha served as irradiation table. Note the fireplace in the background.

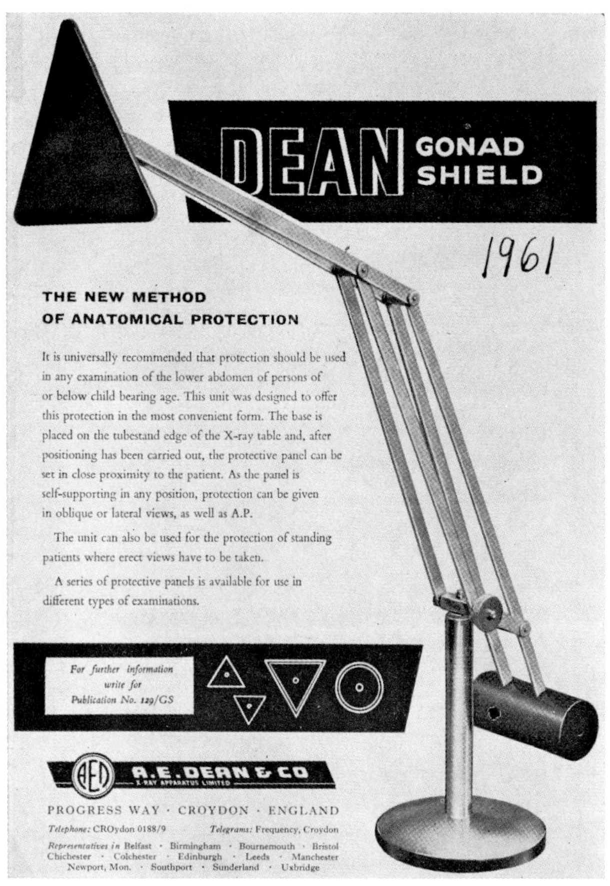

servicemen can be commandeered. Since World War II (after an air raid destroyed the offices they had at Baldwin's Garden in London), both the Dean plant and their offices are located in Surrey, on Progress Way.

WATSON

Watson & Sons can be regarded as the world's oldest manufacturer of electro-medical equipment. Their beginnings date back to William Watson (ultra-Sr.) and the microscope-making firm Watson & Sons, which was established in 1837. After Roentgen's discovery, Watson naturally participated in the endeavors of the pioneers. Herein reproduced is an advertisement which appeared in the *American X-Ray Journal* of 1898. A similar ad, except for the addition of the picture of a coil and a few modified wordings, was printed in 1901 just below the *manchette* (masthead) of the (British) *Archives of the Roentgen Rays.*

Toward the end of the Era of the Roentgen Pioneers, things were not too satisfactory for Watson. Thence a separate firm, called Watson & Sons (Electro-Medical), Ltd., was formed in 1915 with C. H. Watson as chairman of the Board, and Geoffrey Pearce as managing director. The "things" did not improve as fast as expected, and in 1918 the firm was purchased by the General Electric Company (GEC), Ltd. of England.

Watson & Sons had a tradition not only as an electromedical manufacturer, but also as an importer. They

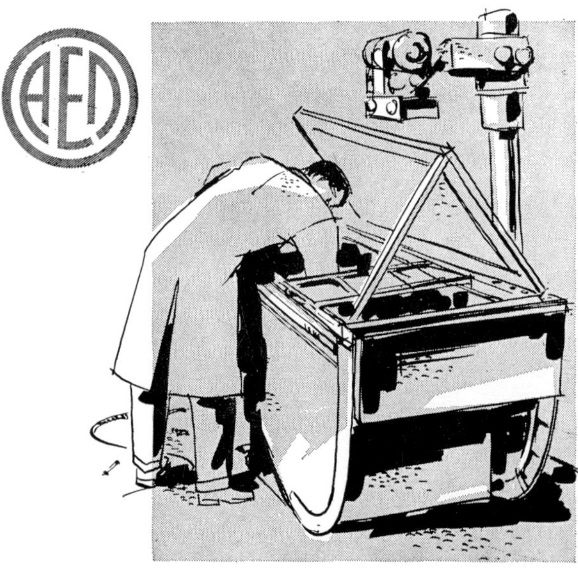

AFTER SALES — SERVICE. This is the main caption of a Dean ad of 1961. It also emphasizes the easy serviceability of a Bucky table when its top is hinged. Availability of service is a most important factor in the selection of any machine.

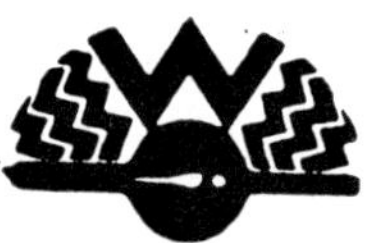

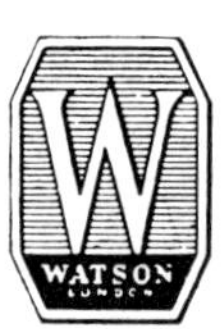

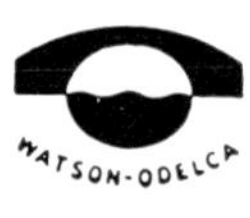

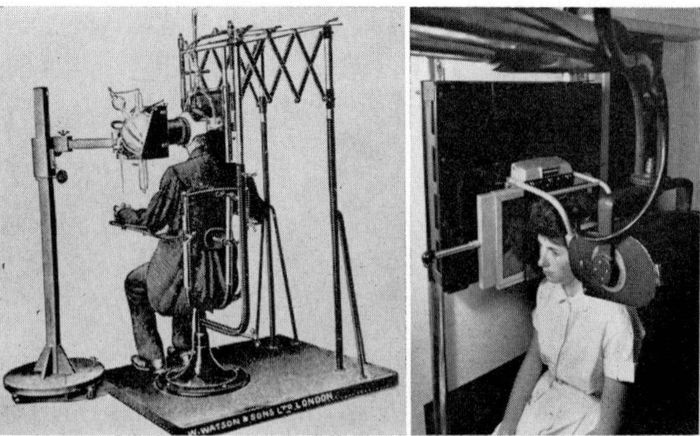

SPANNING FIVE DECADES. Watson chair for cranial radiography (1909) and Watson Cephalostat (1959), designed by Sydney Blackman. The Cephalostat is shown attached to a "Kingsway" dental pedestal.

were Koch & Sterzel's representatives for Great Britain and for the colonies throughout the Era of the Roentgen Pioneers. In the Golden Age of Radiology, Watson imported Mueller x-ray tubes; all sorts of radium applicators from the then Belgian Congo; and Iodeikon (the first cholecystographic substance produced in 1926 by

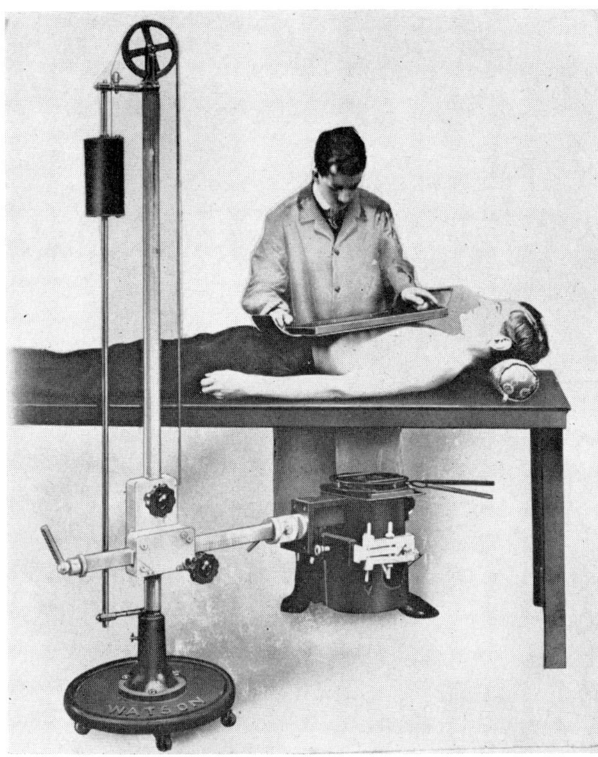

Courtesy: Watson.

WATSON ALL-PURPOSE TUBESTAND (1913). Note the guided counter-balance, and the hand-held fluoroscopic screen.

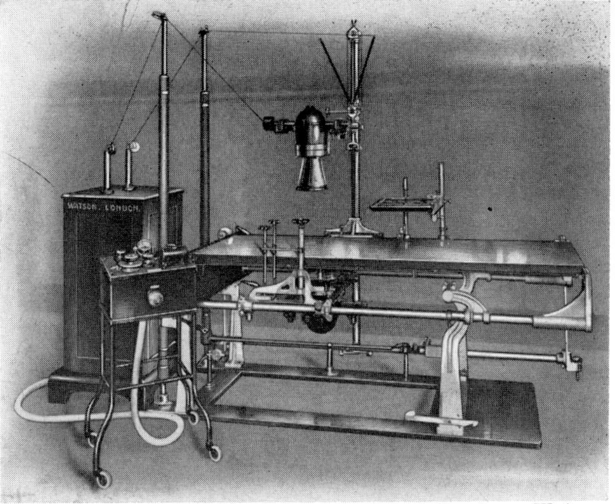

Courtesy: Watson.

WATSON UNIT (1923). Hand-tilted table, over- as well as -under-the-table Coolidge tubes, and self-rectified 30 ma transformer.

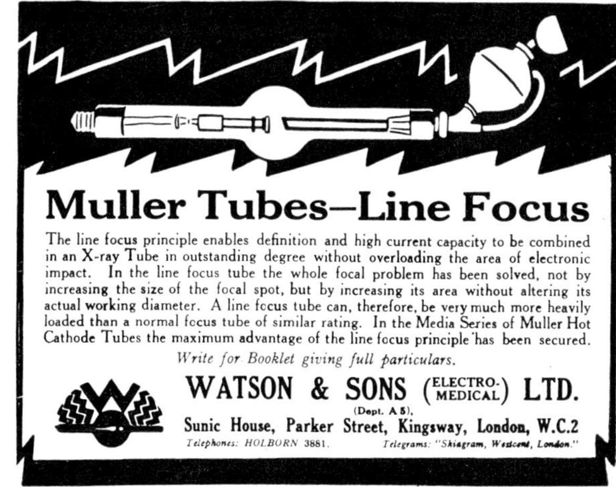

W. WATSON & SONS' BRITISH X-RAY APPARATUS

Is of Highest Possible Quality Throughout.

YIELDS FINEST RESULTS. EASY TO MANIPULATE.

Watson's Heavy Discharge Induction Coils—absolutely reliable. All sizes up to 24-inch spark.

Watson's Vacuum Tubes. The "*Penetrator*," as supplied to the United States Army Medical Dept., is unsurpassed for deep tissues, 35s. ($8.75); large size, 40s. ($10); the "*Reliable*" Tube, 25s. ($6.25)

Mr. Campbell Swinton's Adjustable Cathode Tube, for regulating penetrative power and vacuum, 35s. ($8.75)

Watson's Fluorescent Screens, from 15s. Accumulators, Primary Batteries, Rheostats, Etc.

Watson's Intensifying Screens reduce exposures 70 per cent. Size about 12x10 inches, 35s. ($8.75). Mahogany holder for same, and dry plates with inner frames and plate glass, 22s 6d. ($5.60).

Dr. Hedley's *Portable* combined *Localizer and Tube Holder.* No calculations necessary. The best bedside tube holder; accurate localizer; with instructions, 30s. ($7.50).

Watson's Hospital Outfit: Induction coil, 10-inch spark, £33 10s.; 12-volt Accumulator, £4 10s, 9d. Rheostat, 1s. 1d.; Tube Holder and Localizer, 30s.; two Penetrator Tubes, 4s.; Reliable Tube, 1-5s. Premier Fluorescent Screen, 5s. 5d. Complete in strong traveling case, 1s. 15d. Total, £53 2s. 9d.

Watson's Army Medical Outfit, for use in the *Field*, as supplied to British Army Surgeons. Self contained, always ready for use, not liable to injury. Full particulars on application

Complete catalogue (No. 7) of all that is latest and best in X-Ray Apparatus, mailed free on application.

W. WATSON & SONS, Established, 1837. **313 High Holborn, London, England.**

Opticians to British Foreign Governments. And 78 Swanston Street, Melbourne, Australia.

Awarded 38 Gold and Other Medals. Three Highest Awards, World's Columbian Exhibition, Chicago, 1893

When writing to advertisers mention The American X-Ray Journal.

Mallinckrodt) from St. Louis. For a long time Watson & Sons shared with the (British) Victor X-Ray Corporation the franchise for Coolidge hot cathode tubes in Great Britain.

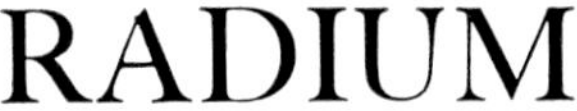

Sole Agents for the British Empire (excluding only Canada) of the

ANGLO-BELGIAN MINING CORPORATION

THE UNION MINIÈRE DU HAUT KATANGA (RADIUM SECTION) OPERATING IN THE BELGIAN CONGO

A PRACTICAL HANDBOOK

Radium: Its Production and Therapeutic Application

55 pages, 10 plates, numerous figures of applicators, etc.
POST FREE ON REQUEST

WATSON & SONS (ELECTRO-MEDICAL) LTD.

SUNIC HOUSE, PARKER STREET,

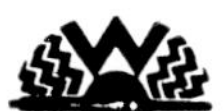

KINGSWAY, LONDON, W.C.2

Telephone: Regent 1227-8. Telegrams: "Skiagram, Westcent, London." Cables: "Skiagram, London."

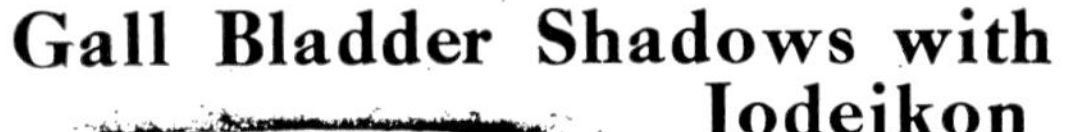

Iodeikon

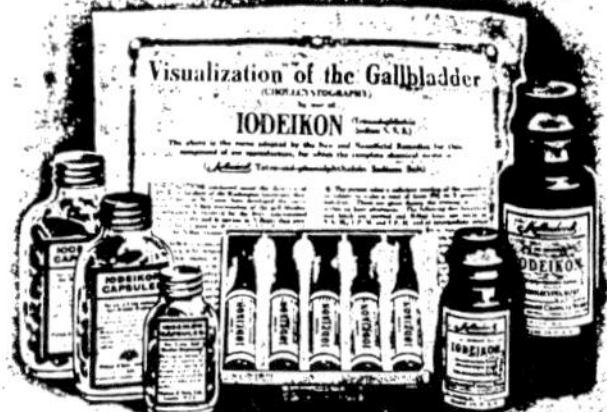

(Tetra-iod-phenol-phthalein Sodium)

The original product manufactured by the Mallinckrodt Chemical Works, St. Louis, U.S.A., in collaboration with Dr. E. A. Graham and his associates.
This product serves a similar purpose in X-Ray examinations of the gall bladder to that served by Barium Sulphate in X-Ray examinations of the stomach.
It is excreted by the liver, concentrated in the gall bladder, and is opaque to X-Rays. It is suitable for both oral and intravenous administration and is easily tolerated.
IODEIKON is supplied in powder form, loose and in single dose ampoules; also in Keratin-covered gelatin capsules.

Send for full particulars and prices to sole selling agents in Great Britain:

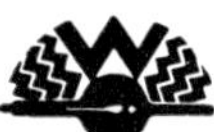

WATSON & SONS (Electro-Medical) LTD.
SUNIC HOUSE, PARKER ST., LONDON, W.C.2.
Telephone: Holborn 3881. Telegrams: "Skiagram, Westcent, London."

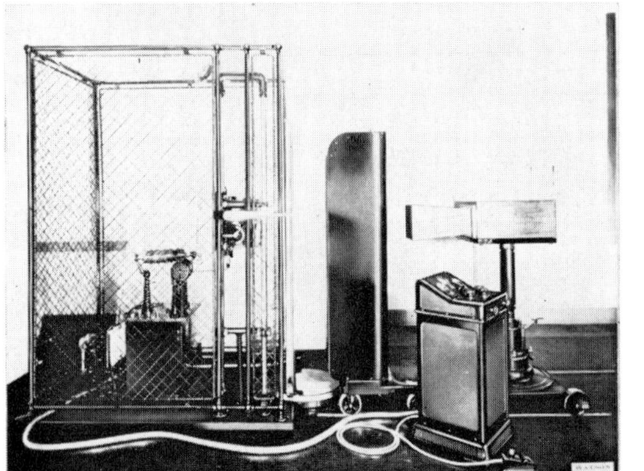

Courtesy: Watson.

REYNOLDS-WATSON CINE-RADIOGRAPH (1935). Decades later, Reynolds was to write a history of cine-radiography.

It may be of interest to mention that in 1935 Watson produced in co-operation with Russell Reynolds the first commercial (16 mm film) cine-radiography equipment. Despite the use of a non-shockproof, stationary x-ray tube and other "primitive" components the results were sufficiently impressive to demonstrate the immense possibilities of the method. Really satisfactory results had to await the development of image intensification.

With the coming of the Atomic Phase the name Sunic House had become hopelessly obsolete. From the old location on Parker Street in Kingsway (London), Wat-

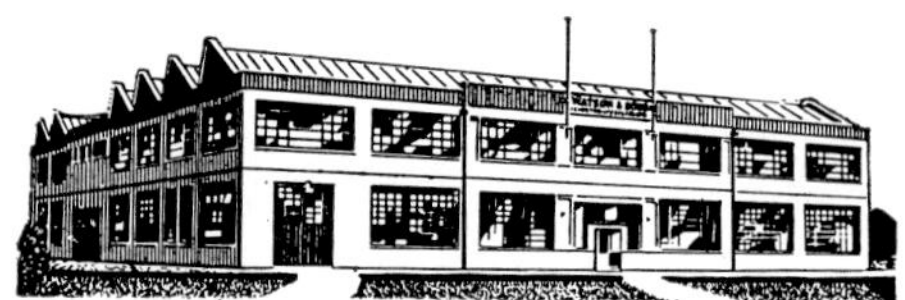

WATSON & SONS
(ELECTRO-MEDICAL) LIMITED

Associated with The General Electric Co. Ltd. of England

EAST LANE · NORTH WEMBLEY · MIDDLESEX, ENGLAND

Telephone: ARNold 6215 *Telegrams:* SKIAGRAM, WEMBLEY

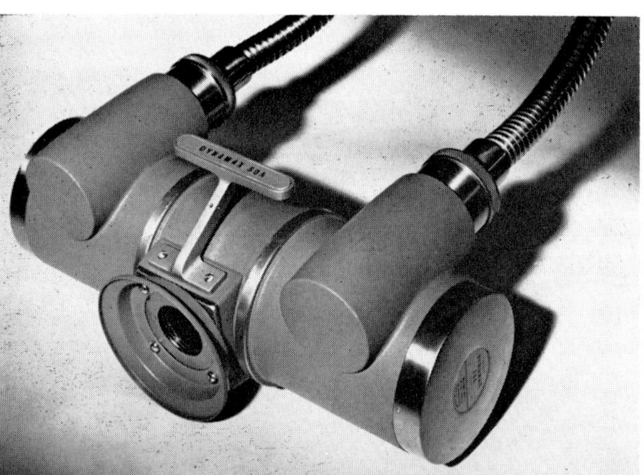

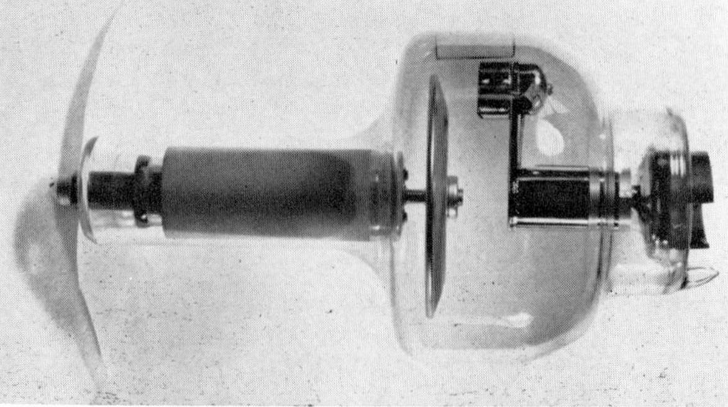

BRITISH-BUILT DYNAMAX. Housing for Dynamax 50A, and insert for Super-Dynamax 150, manufactured by British Machlett in Wembley.

son's moved to exurbia at Wembley in Middlesex, but preserved its traditional cable address, Skiagram. Today Watson & Sons (Electro-Medical) Ltd. is the largest manufacturer of x-ray equipment in England. Since 1948, at the same Wembley location, is the (British) Machlett X-Ray Tubes, Ltd., which makes all sorts of valves and x-ray tubes, including the latest 150 kvp rotating Dynamax "triodes." The British Machlett is owned by the same GEC (the GEC name is used on some occasions, as for heavy alloy "radiation-insulating" materials). The three firms are actually a single company, and the legal relationships are bridged simply by having one managing director – the (in also many other ways unique) Arthur James Minns, who combines deep-seated technical knowledge with an unusual talent for salesmanship.

JOHN SHAYLOR A. J. MINNS A. W. C. SEYMOUR

Shaylor is chief-engineer of the British Machlett; Seymour is home sales manager at Watson & Sons; and Minns is boss to both of them.

G.E.C. **heavy alloy**

supplied in densities 16.8, 17.0, 17.5, 18.0 g/cc (nominal)

for balance weights and screening purposes

PERCENTAGE TRANSMISSION

100 50 10 5 1 0·5 1·0

LEAD 16·8 g/cc 18·0 g/cc

0 1·0 2·0 3·0 3·75 INCHES

Broad beam absorption of Gamma-radiation from Cobalt-60. Density: 16·8 g/cc. and 18·0 g/cc.

This piece of G.E.C. Heavy Alloy, 13 in. diam. by 6 in. deep and weighing 660 lb., is probably the heaviest product ever made by powder metallurgy. Manufactured for the United Kingdom Atomic Energy Authority.

1961

THE GENERAL ELECTRIC CO., LTD. Component Sales Dept.
Osram Division, East Lane, Wembley, Middlesex. Tel: ARNold 4321

Watson's have an assortment of tables, beginning with the hand-tilted Beaver-III and Windsor, and the motor driven all-around "work-horse" T-252. The previous three models permit 100° tilt, while the Autonome V, with its 145°, reverses in 55° Trendelenburg, which suffices for almost all needs; as added features the Autonome has two-speed tilt, motorized longitudinal and lateral sliding table top, and no ceiling supports. The Supertilt (which goes to 180°) uses a special harness so that patient does not need a footrest, which at times can be of advantage. The CTS is Watson's telescopic ceiling tubestand. Their automatized serial (spotfilm) changers have no special names. Likewise, the tomographic attachment is simply called Layer

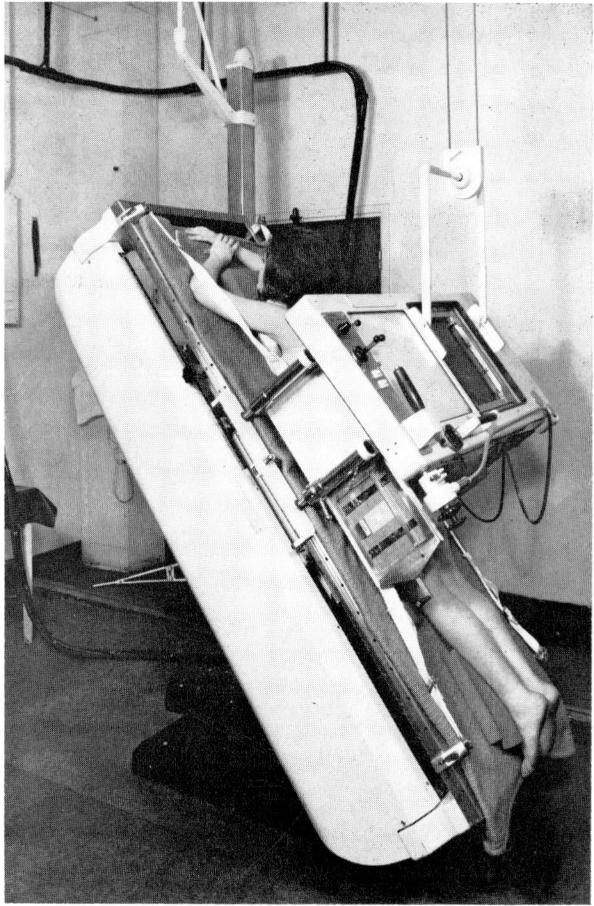

Courtesy: Watson.

WATSON SUPERTILT AT WESTMINSTER HOSPITAL (LONDON). The automatic spotfilmer is ceiling-supported the model is suspended in a shoulder-harness, the table can be tilted 180°, and an additional lateral setting is provided for horizontal-beam radiography.

Radiography; they have also an attachment for polytomography, one for under-the-table fluoroscopy, one for a five-drawer 14 x 17″ cassette changer, and one for x-ray magnification techniques. By arrangement with Odelca, Watson's offer the mirror arrangement for mass radiography, the Cinelix 12″ image intensifier, and use the latter in a special catheterization table (a close cousin of the Swedish Koordinat).

Watson's Universal Bucky Stand is fully adjustable as well as counter-balanced. In conjunction with a simple tubestand it will do (almost) as good a job as Continental's Verta-Vue. Watson's stand can be used for pelvimetry and for upright views of the paranasal

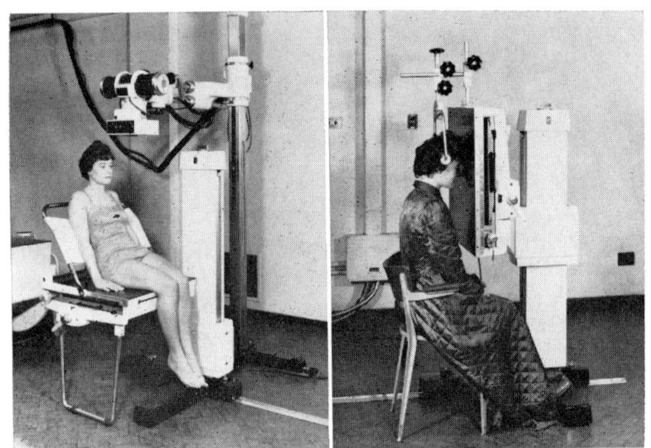

Courtesy: Watson.

WATSON BUCKY STAND. Provided with a backrest it serves well for pelvimetry, but might then be *hard* on the patient's nose during upright Waters' projection.

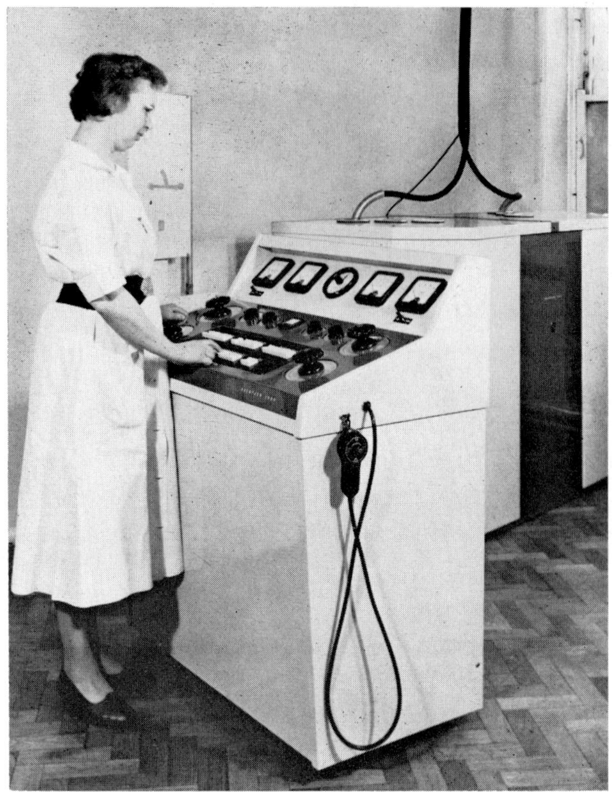

Courtesy: Watson.

WATSON ROENTGEN 1000. Installed at Chesterfield Royal Hospital, it has the desk-type control stand; a wall-mounted panel is optional. Roentgen 1000 is a six-valve job. As a valve-manufacturer, Watson has little incentive to switch to solid state rectification.

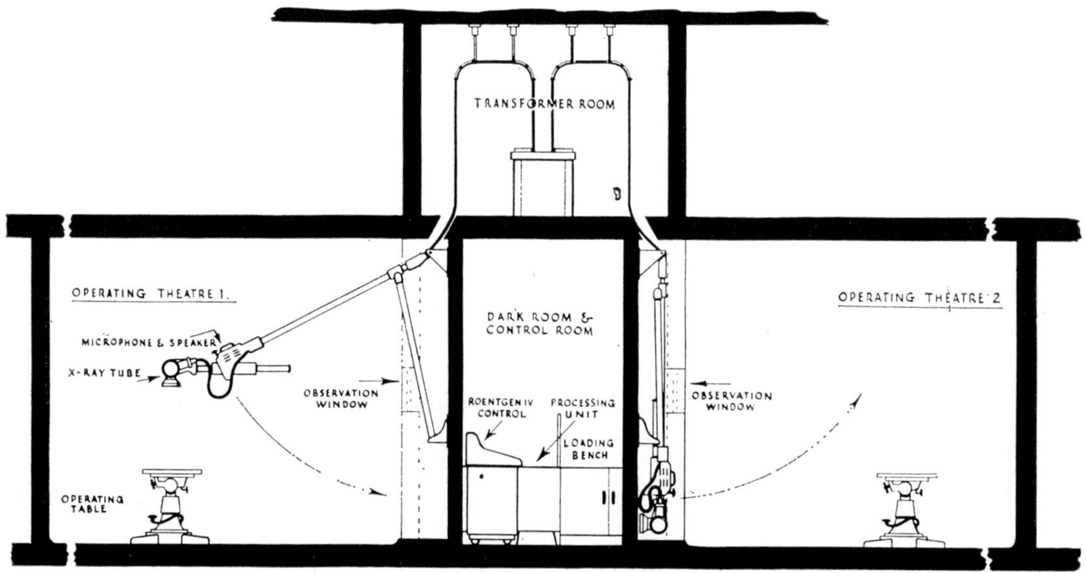

Courtesy: Watson.

RADIO-SURGICAL INSTALLATION AT ST. THOMAS' HOSPITAL (LONDON). The single transformer energizes both stations. There is a single control room which serves also for processing (Darkroom), since communication is by inter-phone.

sinuses (provided the head-clamp is attached after *cleansing* the Bucky's surface). Incidentally, Watson's have also a simple Bucky table with motorized 90° tilt.

Watson's generators carry Roentgen's eponym, and come in several sizes, from the Roentgen 100 (100 ma at 100 kvp) to the four-valve Roentgen V (500 ma at 100 kvp, or 250 ma at 150 kvp) and the triphasic six-valve Roentgen 1000, which can energize three double-focus rotating "triodes" (with 1000 ma at 100 kvp, or 500 ma at 150 kvp). At the other end of the line is the portable unit MX-2 (10 ma at 83 kvp, 20 ma at 76 kvp, or in fluoroscopy 3 ma at 88 kvp): its characteristic black control box has the dials elevated on a plane separated from the rheostats by a dihedral angle. Their largest mobile unit is the Mobilix 300 (its rotating anode can be energized to 300 ma at 102 kvp, or 200 ma at 125 kvp the cables are the limiting factor). Watson's have worked out a special stationary surgical solution, the Operating Theatre Tube Arm: in the resting position the arm is folded in a recess in the wall, while when needed it can be extended over the operating table. A single transformer can energize two such tubes in adjacent rooms: orders for exposure can be inter-communicated through a microphone-loudspeaker system incorporated in the arm.

Kingsway is the brand name of Watson's dental units. They build also three special gadgets, one of which is the ("linguo-plesio-therapeutic") Panagraph, similar to Koch & Sterzel's intra-oral tube. The second is the Rotagraph (after the model developed by Paatero of Helsinki), with which a tomographic (and yet panoramic) view of both the upper and the lower teeth can be obtained with a single or double exposure from a tube which rotates in an occipital semi-circle. The third contraption is the Cephalostat (which can be attached to a Bucky, to the MX-2, or to a Kingsway dental unit); it permits "arthrometric radiography" of the temporomandibular joints.*

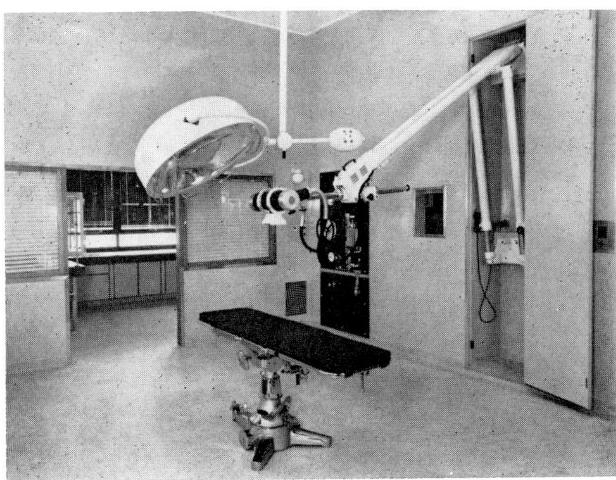

Courtesy: Watson.

WATSON SURGICAL TUBE ARM. When not in use, the arm folds away into a cupboard with flush doors. Communication with the adjacent control room is by means of microphone and speaker, incorporated in the bracket.

Watson's sell a lengthy list of darkroom and other x-ray accessories, but many of these are made by other firms, such as their Sirius fluoroscopic screens, manufactured by Levy-West. Lucidex grids and grid cassettes are Watson's own make and brand. The Cold Cathode Tube Illuminator is advertised as having a life expectancy of 10,000 hours. And Watson's sells the Co^{60} units of Atomic Energy of Canada.

CUTHBERT ANDREWS

If not the oldest in the business, the Grand Old Man among British x-ray manufacturers, Cuthbert Andrews, is certainly the most colorful. He started in the x-ray business in 1910 in a basement at 35 Hatton Garden (London) with an initial cash capital £100 allowed by Mueller of Hamburg. When imports of glass from Germany were cut off by the outbreak of World War I, Andrews persuaded one of the big British glass houses to make soda-glass bulbs for him.

From 1925 to 1933, Cuthbert Andrews manufactured also major x-ray apparatus, on the average one com-

*The Panagraph, Rotagraph, and Cephalostat were described in the *British Dental Journal* of November 15, 1960 by Sidney Blackman, the director of the Department of Radiology in the Royal Dental Hospital of London.

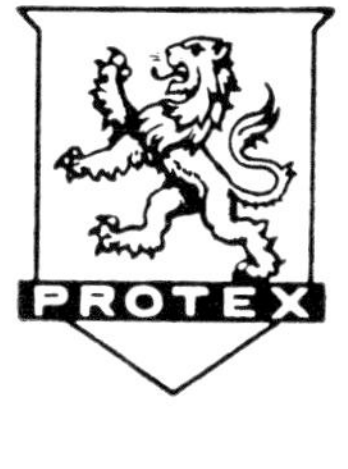

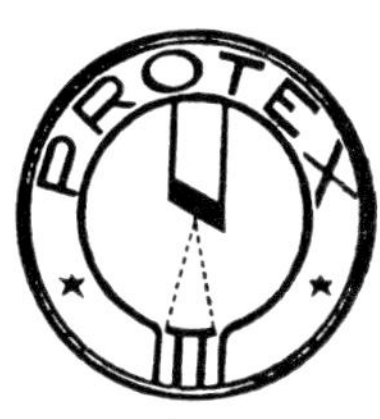

Trade-mark.

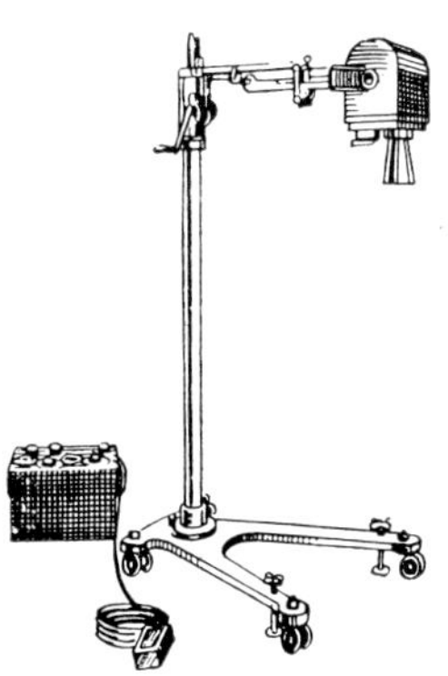

THE PORTEX PORTABLE UNIT

plete hospital installation per week. Slowly, these and other activities were given up, and in 1948 the tube-manufacturing was discontinued; in the course of thirty-eight years the firm had made over 30,000 tubes, of something like seventy-five different types and ratings. They still sell several gas tubes, made on order (of course, for demonstration and historic purposes only).

Cuthbert Andrews has issued catalogs which have become something of a collector's item: Blue (1934), Orange (1939), Red (1952), again Blue (1955), Ivory (1958), and the latest 50-year anniversary Golden (1960) edition. This catalogue, called *Everything X-Ray,* is written in a didactic, almost paternalistic style, with careful avoidance of inaccuracies, almost as impartial as a consumer's research paper. It is also rewarding for several historic details included. The catalogue describes mainly x-ray and darkroom accessories, and in addition a portable unit, the Portex. The trade-mark of Cuthbert Andrews is Protex, with the Imperial Lion. Significant perhaps is the fact that his office is now located in Bushey (Bissei in Domesday Book), in a building of which a part dates back to 1250. Incidentally, Cuthbert Andrews has been president of the BIR — and those who enjoy sentimental radio-reminiscences should read his *Inaugural Address.* In its own (not entirely accurate) way it is a little masterpiece.

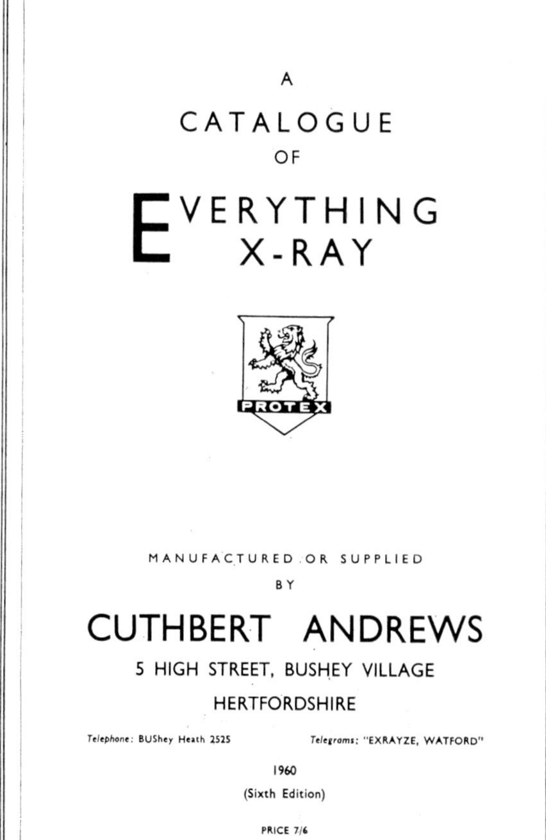
A CATALOGUE OF EVERYTHING X-RAY

PROTEX

MANUFACTURED OR SUPPLIED BY

CUTHBERT ANDREWS

5 HIGH STREET, BUSHEY VILLAGE

HERTFORDSHIRE

Telephone: BUShey Heath 2525 Telegrams: "EXRAYZE, WATFORD"

1960

(Sixth Edition)

PRICE 7/6

SWEDEN

Individual instances (including nostalgic distaff reminiscences) to the contrary notwithstanding, it seems that a cult for their own traditions, combined with courtesy and cool detachment toward strangers*, are age-old Scandinavian traits. During a casual acquaintance, the typical Swedish radiologist will seldom offer more than smiling aloofness to the foreign neophyte, especially if the latter proves to be inquisitive. It is not all *nordisk* disdain; much of it is pride coming from their solid, unquestionable achievements. Excellence is quite apparent also in x-ray equipment made in Sweden.

Among several traditionalistic aspects of Swedish x-ray apparatus is the preference for two separate units instead of a single, tilting table: they use an upright (Forssell Standard) fluoroscope, and for recumbent fluoroscopy a fixed, horizontal board (as the transliteration of their term sounds). Another Swedish peculiarity which stems from Forssell times is the morning

*The sense herein intended for the term strangers comes closest to a word used in the Italian (Parthenopeian) slang: *forestieri!*

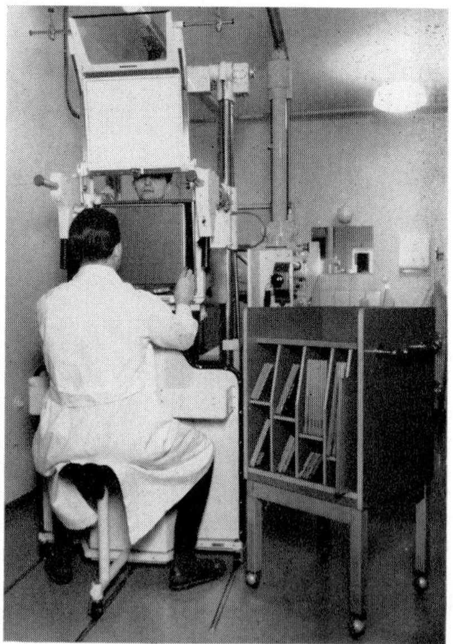

Courtesy: Elema-Schönander

FORSSELL FLUOROSCOPE. This is a 1963 model, with operator protected by a Forssell fluoroscopic console. Chest films are seldom routinely ordered in Sweden: accepted practice is to perform chest fluoroscopy and then "spotfilm" whatever seems worth recording.

conference between radiologists, clinicians, and/or surgeons: this is when the cases examined the day before are discussed by all parties concerned (clinical correlation).

As explained by Robert Thoraeus in *Acta Radiologica* of March-April, 1950 – in accordance with the Swedish system of periodical inspection of roentgen therapy installations – at the first inspection every new 200 kvp machine is subjected to a grueling two hours of continuous operation at the highest operating conditions used in practice (usually about 175 kvp and 15 ma). If an installation passes this test without a technical failure, a fairly reliable performance may be anticipated for the immediate future. The test also leaves sufficient time to examine the protective arrangements.

ELEMA — SCHONANDER

The oldest firm in the Swedish x-ray business was founded in 1890. It was taken over in 1902 by Bror Edvard Järnh (1879-1956), who renamed it Järnhs Elektriska AB (Aktiebolaget = stock company). This was the same Järnh who sponsored the creation of the first Swedish organization of radiologists. His son, Bertil Edvard Järnh, is currently one of the directors of the E-S.

AB Elema, created in 1917, was the Swedish representative of German x-ray manufacturers. Beginning in 1939 the two firms merged and became the Elema-Jährns AB. It was actually a tripartite combination with the KIFA (Kirurgiska Instrument Fabriks AB). Both the Jährns and the KIFA had plants in Solna, an industrial development in suburban Stockholm, with the Elema acting as the distributor. At the turn of the century, Jährns employed a dozen people: by 1952, the three firms had 625 personnel.

In 1921, Georg Schönander (1894-1958) founded a private x-ray firm, incorporated only in 1948. His plant was in Gröndal, and produced also x-ray tubes (including rotating anodes). Schönander originated many imaginative developments, such as the mirror optic for mass chest radiography (created independently of Helge

JÄRNHS

STOCKHOLM · SWEDEN

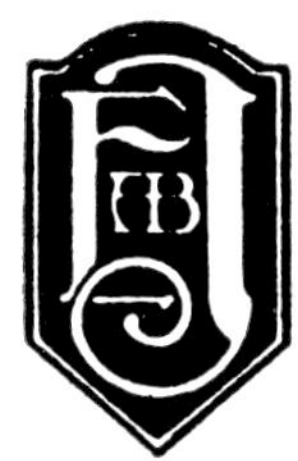

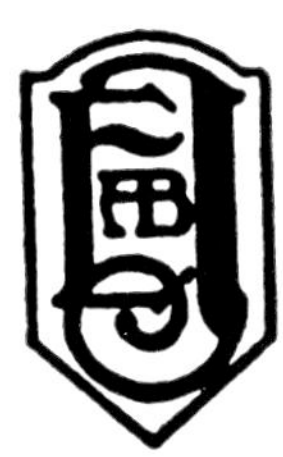

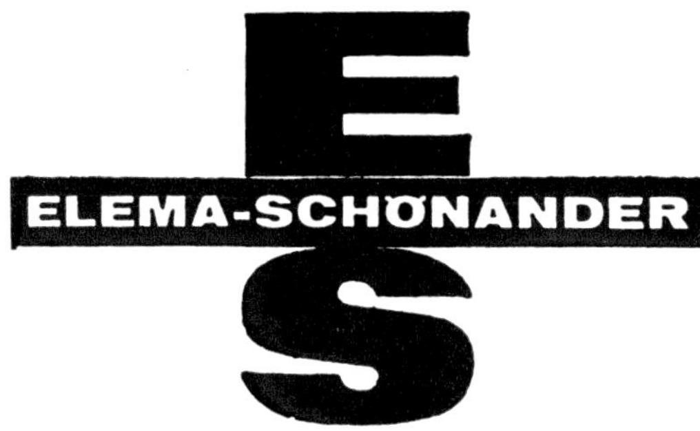

AKTIEBOLAGET

ELEMA

STOCKHOLM · SWEDEN

SCHÖNANDER

STOCKHOLM - SWEDEN

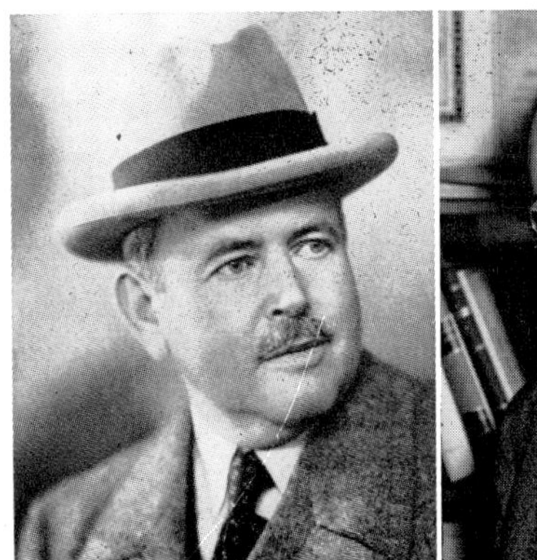

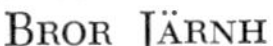

BROR JÄRNH

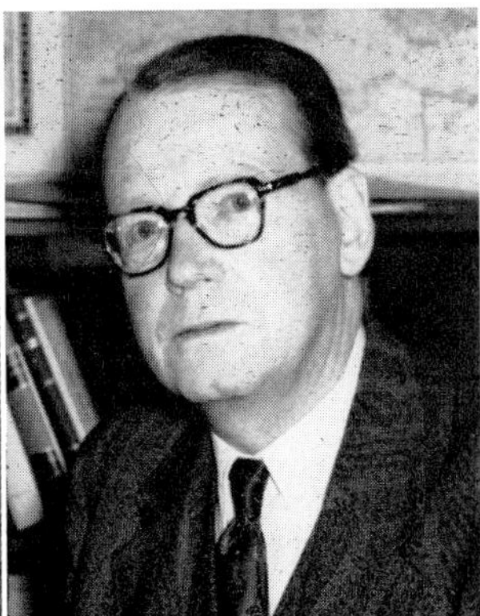

GEORG SCHÖNANDER

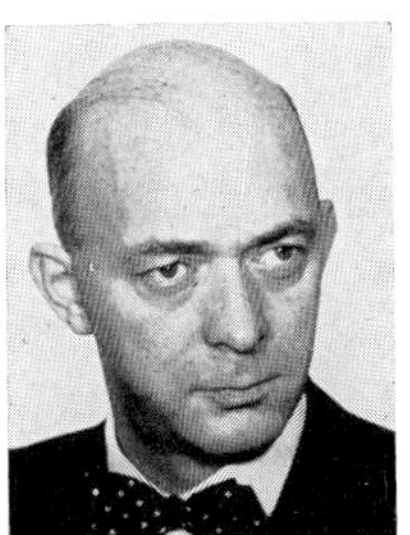

ERIC WASSER

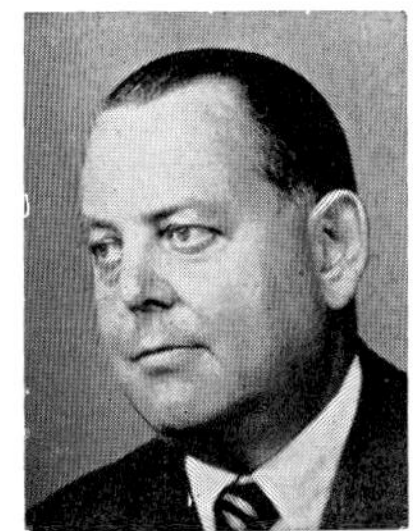

BERTIL JÄRNH

Directors at Elema-Schönander.

Christensen or Odelca). In 1947, he dared to put on the Swedish market a tilted table *(motordrivet universalbord)*. In 1950, he came out with the automatized DIK-1000: it delivered 1000 ma at 85 kvp, or 400 ma at 125 kvp *(högvoltsdiagnostik)*. But as the Atomic Phase advanced, Georg Schönander AB shared the fate which befell many private firms: after being "repossessed" by its bankers, and "absorbed" in 1955 by the Elema, its name re-appeared on the x-ray horizon in 1956 as the Elema-Schönander AB.

I had inquired with the senior Swedish radiotherapist, Elis Berven, and the following excerpts from his reply summarize the facts:

"Elema was a branch office of the German firm Siemens. The name comes from electro-medical apparatus. Elema's first director was called von der Burg; his successor was Weber, a typical German businessman.

"Kirurg-Instrument-Fabriks-Aktiebolaget (KIFA) was founded by Swedish surgeons, and produced surgical instruments.

"A young, energetic engineer, by the name of Schönander, appeared on the scene in 1921 as a (Swedish) representative for the (American) Victor X-Ray Corporation. He started a repair and service shop, soon expanded, and in 1934 built a factory, which was rebuilt in 1948 into a magnificent plant. In 1953, Schönander ran into financial difficulties, mainly because of serious illness.

"In 1946, all the supplies of the German firm Elema were confiscated by the Swedish Government, and sold to Elema's director, Weber, who had become a Swedish citizen. An arrangement was made between Järnh and Weber, whereby Järnh's sales organization was transferred to the Elema, while

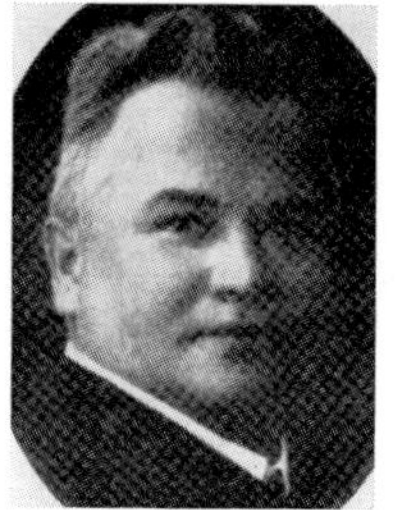

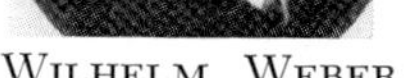

WILHELM WEBER

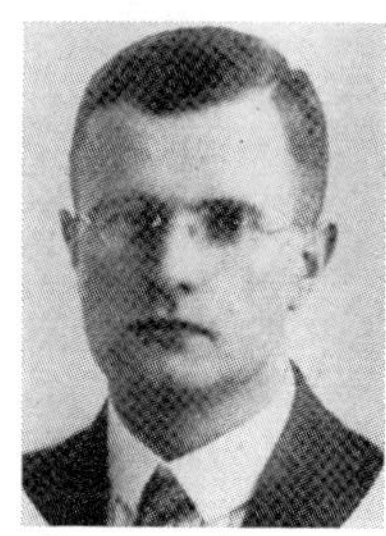

GUSTAV WEBER

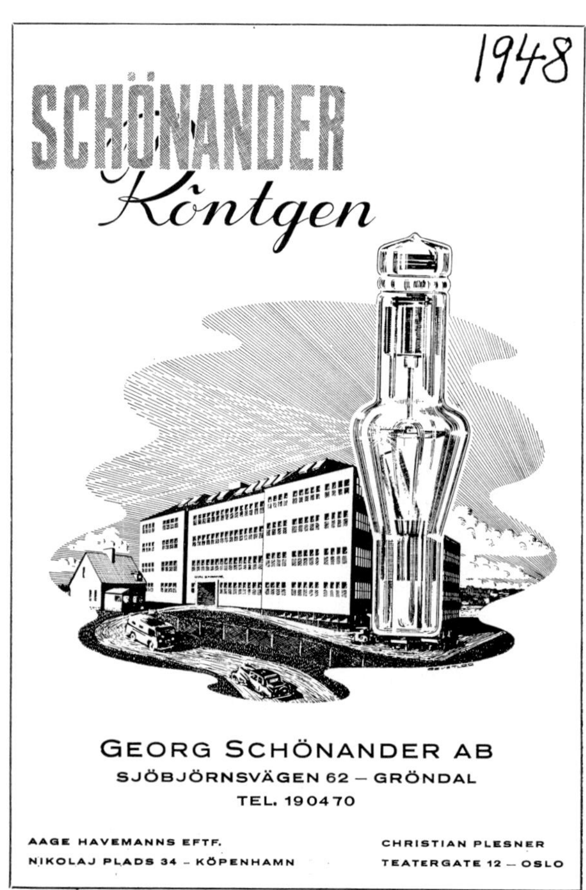

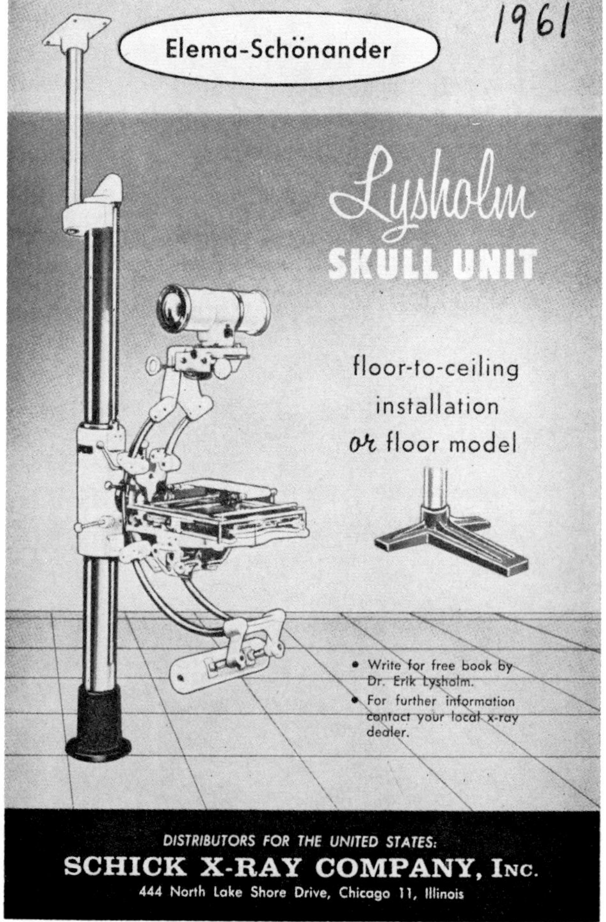

Järnh Elektriska AB continued to manufacture x-ray equipment. When Schönander died, his firm was first consolidated with Järnh's, then everything - KIFA included - became a single organization, Elema Schönander (E-S). The manufacturing division of E-S is under the direction of Järnh's son, while Weber is the commercial director."

Elema-Schönander (E-S) offers today a complete line of x-ray equipment. Most of it is manufactured at Solna. A few items (such as betatrons) are imported from SRW.

The E-S Pleromobil is a mobile installation with selenium rectifiers; the 303 CT model delivers either 300 ma at 90 kvp, or 75 ma at 150 kvp.

The automatized control stand of the Triplex Angiomatic 1003 2 CE is very impressive. The machine consists of twin triphasic transformers, with selenium rectifiers; there is provision for connecting five tubes, and two of them can be energized simultaneously.

The modern control stand for the selenium rectified Triplex Optimatic permits pulsed cineradiography with 1000 ma at 100 kvp.

In 1925, Erik Lysholm (whose eponym graces also their stationary grid) designed a "skull table" manufactured by Schönander. It was intended for the examination of paranasal sinuses and temporal bones. The design was modified in 1931 to include the entire skull,

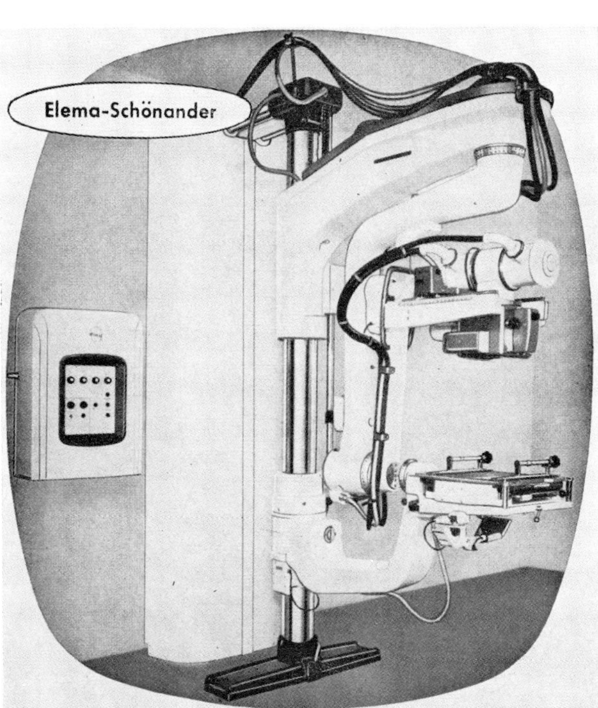

THE MIMER

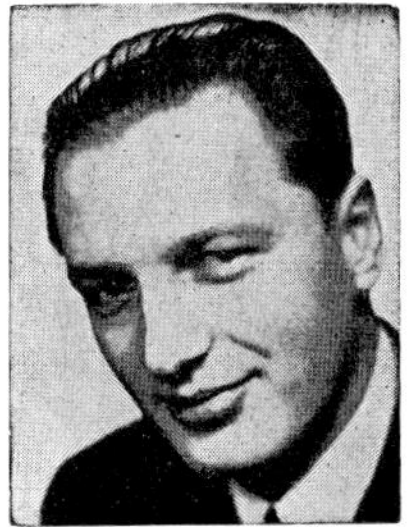

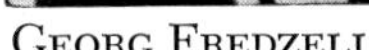
GEORG FREDZELL

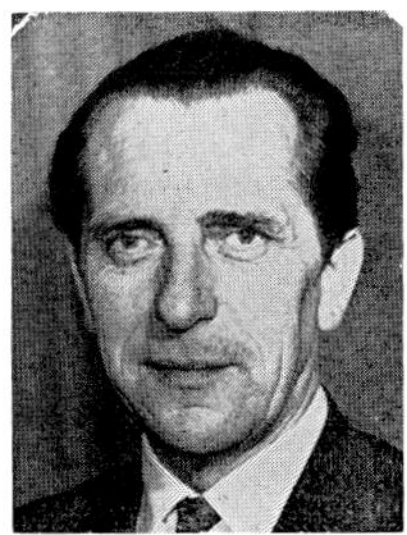
PAUL BUSCH

On technical staff of E-S

ANGIOGRAPHIC FILMCHANGERS

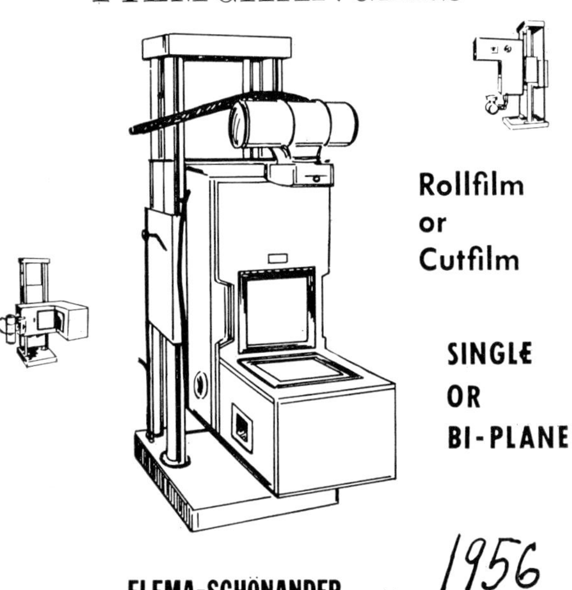

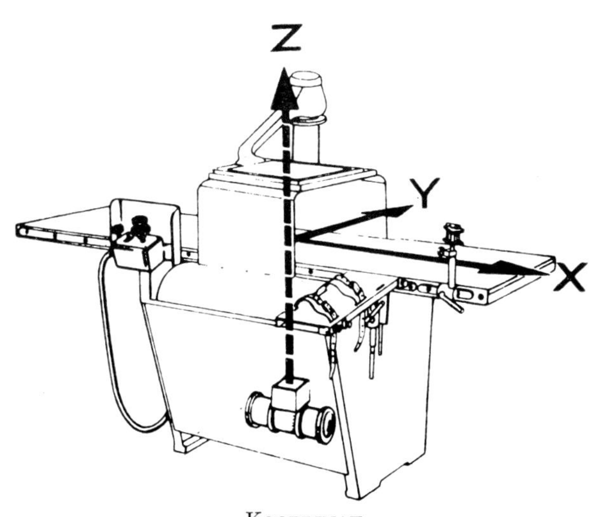

KOORDINAT

and then a more definitive model was built in 1935: it is still being sold (with minor modifications) by E-S as the CRT-4. The Lysholm craniograph is a short focal distance tube-Bucky combination with transparent table top (Plexiglass) and mirror appropriately placed to permit accurate centering and angulation of patient and beam.

Lysholm's design for a skull device became very popular, and was freely "adopted" by other ("foreign") manufacturers. After World War II the Italians added a tomographic attachment and increased the focal distance (such increase, according to expert Swedish opinion, is at best a mixed blessing). Nevertheless, such competition demanded a firm reply. Erik Lindgren (Lysholm's pupil and successor as chief-radiologist at Serafimerlassarettet) designed an improved skull stand, called the Mimer, issued in 1959, and described in *Acta Radiologica* of May, 1960. Its backbone is a heavy floor-to-ceiling column, which supports an arm for the Bucky and a cantilever with jointed arm for the x-ray tube; with this combination, the tube can be aimed at any point on the surface of a sphere with the radius of 80-90 cm. The Mimer permits 300° tomography, it can be used for arthrography, and for many routine radiographic situations, but it is mainly an ultra-elaborate tool for the craniographer, with or without contrast media.

The bi-plane 14″ wide rollfilm changer was still being advertised by Elema-Järnhs in 1954 when Schönander came out with the ingenious automatized twin AOT cut-film changer, which permitted six 10x12″ or 14x14″ exposures per second. It is now the E-S AOT: and the Triplex can energize twin tubes for the two-plane changer. With all that radiation around, a remotely controlled high-pressure intravenous injector becomes an invaluable commodity.*

For catheterization and other cardiac procedures E-S has the Koordinat table. The tube and the screen are fixed, while the motorized table top is sliding: after

*It seemed almost sacrilegious to find in the *Acta Radiologica* an ad placed by Medical Instruments of Portland (Oregon), describing the Shipps Automatic Injector for angiocardiography.

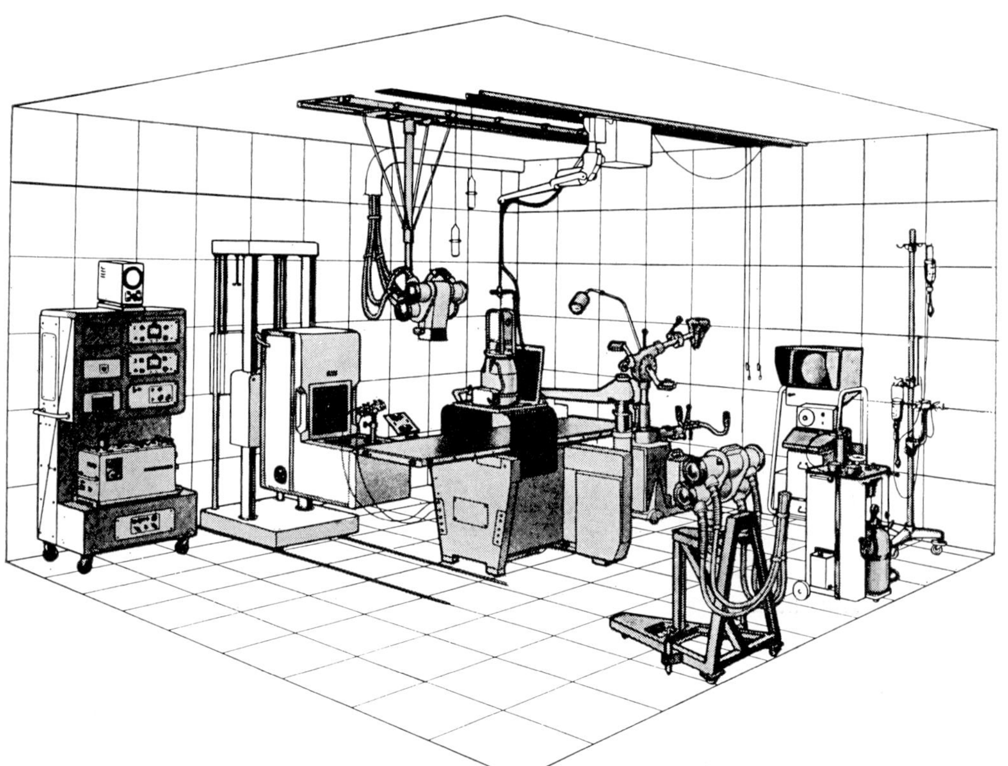

E-S Angiocardiographic room. In the center is a Koordinat table, with a ceiling-suspended 7″ image intensifier and movie camera (television monitor next to the wall). The film changer is on rails and can be slid underneath the margin of the Koordinat. The twin tubes on movable stand (in right foreground) are used for stereo-angiography with the film changer. The huge contraption next to the changer is an oscillograph and other physiologic detection and recording devices. The pressure-injector is located to the right of the twin stereographic pedestal.

fluoroscopy the (often anesthetized) patient can be slid over the adjacent AOT changer. A modernized version of the Koordinat has optional motor-tilt and image intensifier with television monitoring. The Atomic Phase is catching up with these changers. In a double AOT procedure, the patient gets very easily 40-50 rad, while cineradiography raises the patient to 4-5 rad (often to less than that).

E-S has an automatic processor, the Procomat, and a full line of darkroom accessories. Unique is their conveyor belt system for cassette transport, intended to minimize the carrying of cassettes from the radiographic rooms to the darkroom (automatic processor).*

For those (Swedish) morning conferences, E-S offers the Dekaskope: with it the radiographs can be prearranged on glass frames (10-15 frames are available per "magazine"). During the conference, one frame at a time can be slid in front of the illuminated surface. Another unusual feature is a plastic lens in metal frame (11x15″), which is used for the magnification of a large area.**

Today Elema-Schönander is controlled by the (German) Siemens-Reiniger-Werke.

*The chief-radiologist of Carle Clinic in Urbana (Illinois), Cesare Gianturco, has designed and built just such a mechanized cassette transport system in his Department. Only afterwards did he learn of the existence of the E-S transport unit. In Gianturco's system, magnetized strips attached to the backs of the cassettes actuate levers which then retain the respective cassette at the working place where it belongs (on the return trip from the darkroom). Lead veneer between conveyor and x-ray rooms prevents fogging from stray radiation while cassettes are in transit. Gianturco's main problem was actually architectural, as he had to avoid the (structural) pillars.

**Information on E-S was provided by Lennard Uppenberg from the E-S in Stockholm, and by Bela Schick, the E-S representative in Chicago.

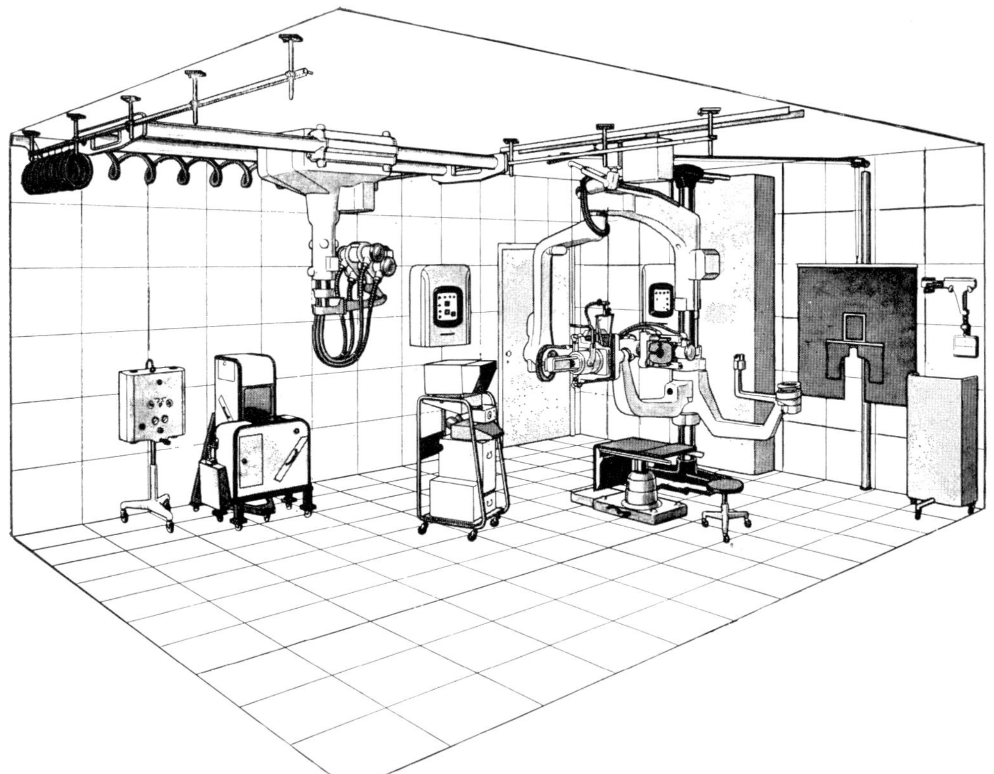

E-S Neuroradiologic room. The main piece of equipment is the Mimer in the right background, with an image intensifier and television monitor (in the middle of the room). Twin stereographic tubes are attached to the ceiling mount. The AOT two-plane film changer stands next to the wall in left background. Two interesting items of radiation-protection are the lead-screen on casters (in the right corner), and next to it a ceiling-suspended lead rubber apron, which can be moved to any desirable location in the room.

SVENSKA AB PHILIPS

The Svenska Aktiebolaget Philips is a Swedish subsidiary of the Dutch firm by the same name.

In Stockholm, Philips builds the Alternator, which is basically a viewbox with a rotating transparent belt. The regular Alternator has a belt corresponding to twenty viewing frames, for a maximum loading capacity of 360 small radiographs. The Super-Alternator carries the equivalent of thirty-one viewing frames. The viewing area can be "diaphragmed" with opaque surfaces located behind the opal plate. The motor-driven alternator belt is actuated either by a handswitch or by a footswitch. The latter comes in quite handy (footy?) during the loading phase. The idea behind the alternator goes back to Forssell's morning conference between radiologists and clinicians. Things work out much easier if all the films needed for a given morning conference have been pre-arranged by an aide, and are then demonstrated by flicking a switch, instead of having to handle bulky envelopes and/or sets of separate films. The cost of an alternator approaches nine thousand dollars. As a bonus feature to each alternator comes the Denoscope, a strong spotlight with a movable iris diaphragm. One of the most modern among Swedish hospitals, the Sahlgrenska in Gothenburg, has twenty-one alternators, and several more on order. Picker is now marketing a similar device.

Svenska Philips imports most of its equipment from Eindhoven and Hamburg, a few things from Paris. Mueller, for instance, makes a catheterization table which looks and acts just like the Koordinat. Actually, though, even Swedes have certain human frailties, and sooner or later develop a liking for French frills. Not too long ago Svenska Philips installed at the University Hospital in Lund a 90/90 Symmetrix table, with all the motorized, intensified, and televised conveniences available to Atomic Phase radiologists.* Somehow, progress always wins over tradition!

*This information was courteously provided by Karl Johann Fenz, director of the Svenska Philips. Fenz, who is a Dr. Ing. (Ph.D.) was formerly with Schönander.

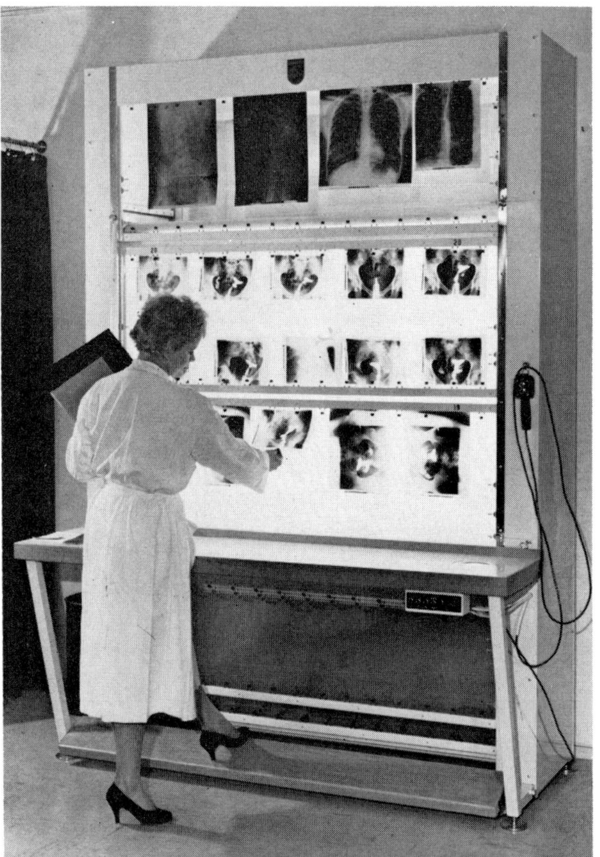

Courtesy: Svenska AB Philips.

PHILIPS ALTERNATOR. A viewbox with a motor-driven transparent belt on which up to 360 small radiographs can be pre-arranged for uninterrupted inspection (as during a conference). The belt can be moved forwards or backwards from the footswitch, from the handswitches located to the right just below table level, or from a remote control switch, seen hanging with its cables on the right column.

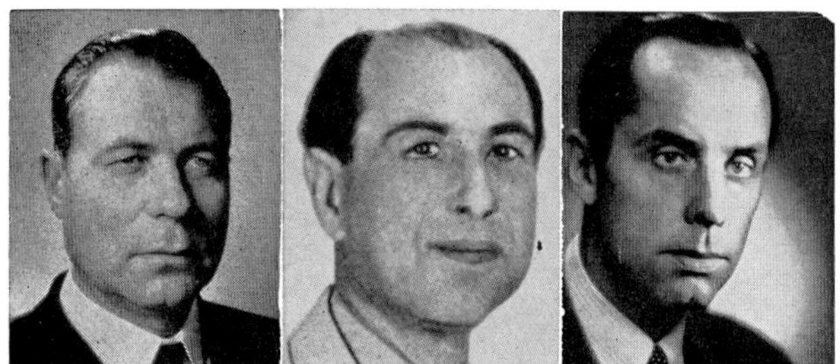

E. A. WESTERMARCK S. R. KJELLBERG EINAR WASTENSON

Wastenson is with Svenska Philips, Kjellberg is chief-radiologist at the Sahlgrenska, and Westermarck is with the Finnish firm which markets Paatero's Pantomograph.

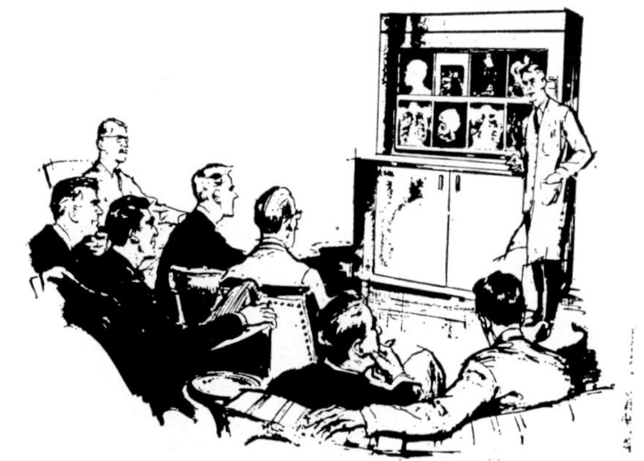

new PICKER *AutoViewer*

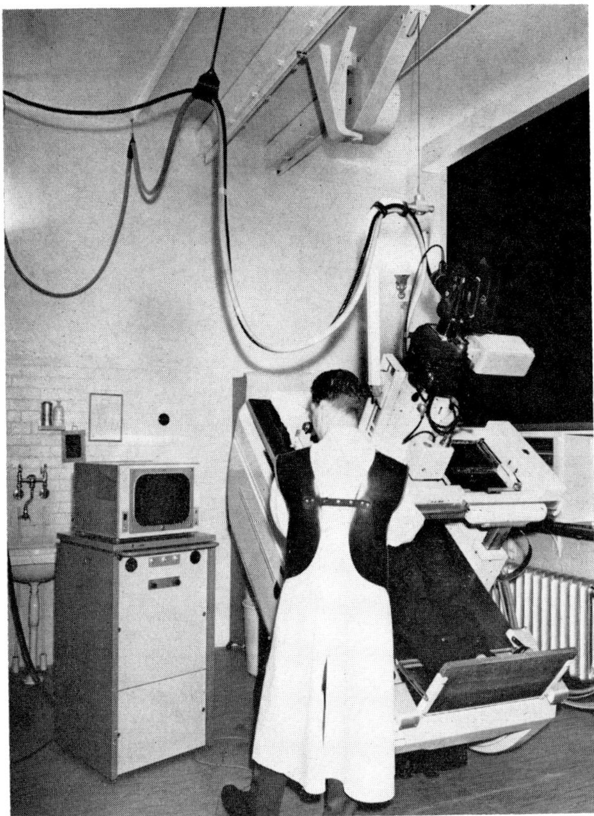

Courtesy: Svenska AB Philips.

SYMMETRIX AT LUND (SWEDEN). This 90/90 table is shown in the Department of Radiology of the University Hospital. It has also 9″ Philips image intensifier, movie camera, and television monitor.

DENMARK

The leading firm is Dansk Røntgen Teknik A/S in Copenhagen and Aarhus.

In 1898, Holger Larsen and Levring founded the firm Levring & Larsen, and began manufacturing electrical and optical appliances, as well as x-ray apparatus. In 1928, Dansk Røntgen-Teknik (DRT) separated from Levring & Larsen, the board of directors of DRT comprising Holger Larsen (who remained managing director until his death in 1963), Johan Kühl and P. M. Wilkens had been with Levring & Larsen since 1907.

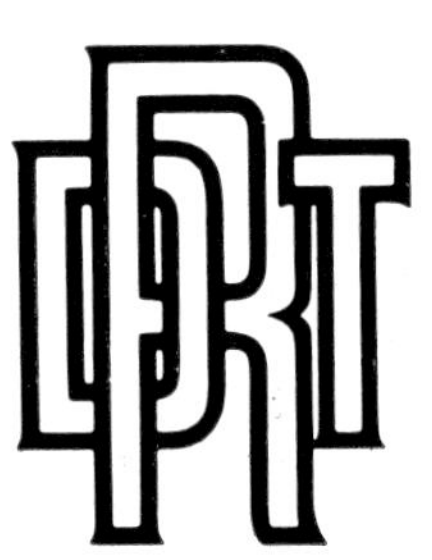

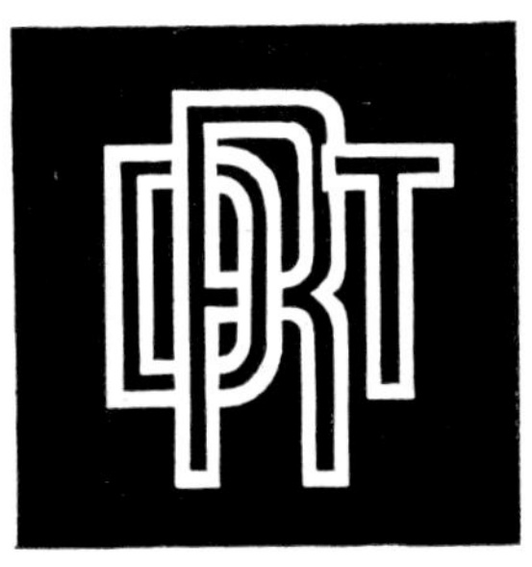

In 1936, J. Herholdt joined the board of directors, while Kühl and Wilkens became managing directors for the departments in Copenhagen and Aarhus. Early in 1959, Kühl sold his shares to the other members, left the firm, and died in August of the same year. In July, 1959 DRT was sold to Philips.*

---

*This information was provided by Mrs. Erika Knudsen from DRT. Some of it came from H. Pakkenberg, an historically minded engineer who had come to Levring & Larsen in 1920, went into the DRT in 1928, and was retired automatically in 1961 at the age of sixty-five. He is the author of several historical papers and booklets, dealing with radiology in Denmark, published by DRT.

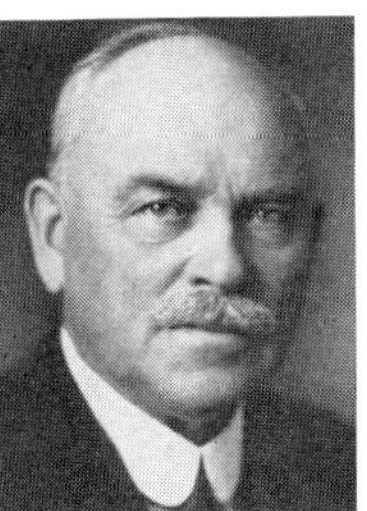

HOLGER LARSEN

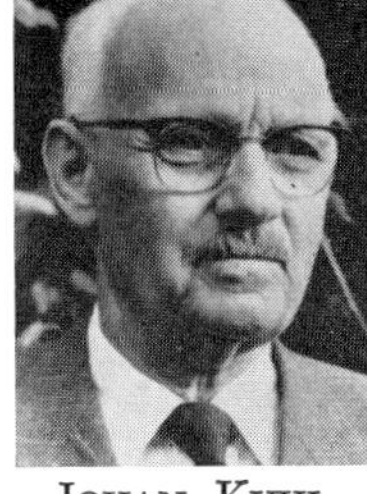

JOHAN KUHL

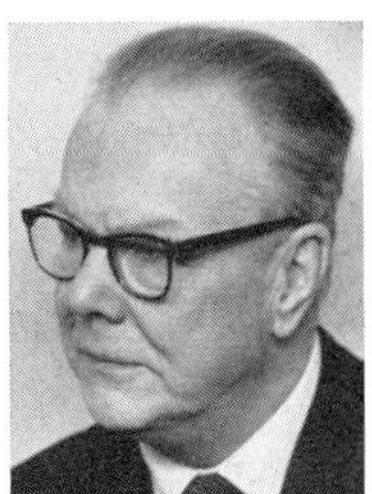

POUL WILKENS

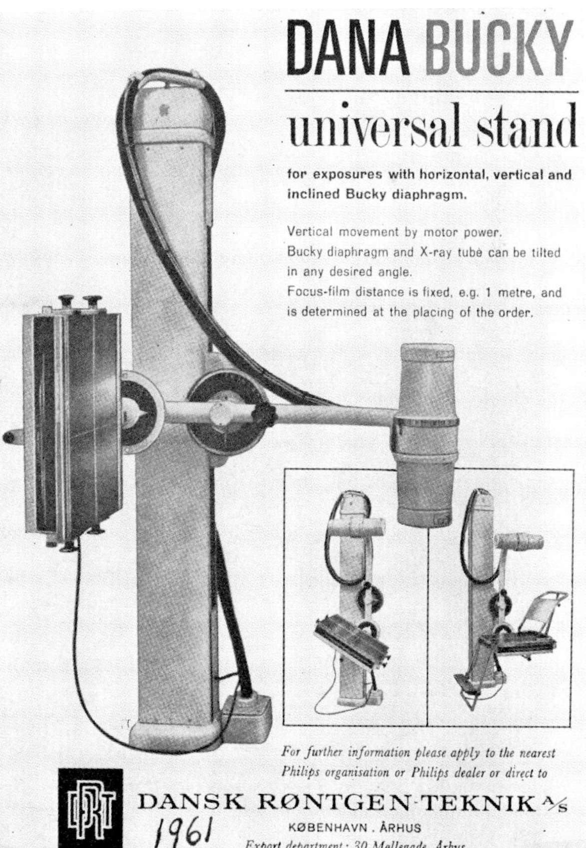

DRT manufactures mostly supportive equipment, the remainder is imported from Holland and Hamburg.

Danatom is a motor- (or hand-) operated 105° tilting table. It has a fixed floor-to-wall (not floor-to-ceiling) tubestand, while the table rolls on twin rails. Tomographic capabilities are built into the column, and there is space beneath the Bucky for simultaneous multisection radiography. Magnification attachment is also available.

The Dana Bucky Stand is similar to Continental's Verta-Vue, except that the Dana has a fixed tube-grid distance of 100 cm (about 3 feet).

DRT specializes in what they call "motor-driven clamp fitting." This means power-operated tubestands with remote controls. The system is used in the Dana Ceiling Suspension which comes in several models, the D-2 (motorized only for vertical motion, electromagnetic brakes for horizontal hand-motion), and the fully motorized EL-D. The previous two use four bands ("ribbons"), while for an operating room an elaborate wire suspension is utilized. Dana-Duplex is a simple telescopic ceiling suspension. The Dana Mobil (combined with the single-tank Philips Rotopractix) is unusual in that the tube can be lowered ("clamp-fitted") to a few inches above the floor, which is of advantage in veterinary radiography.

The very ingenious Dana Unit is a cross between the Danatom and the Dana Bucky Stand, with clamp-fitting thrown in for good measure.*

A very heavy, square, floor-and-wall supported column holds the Bucky, the independently movable tubestand, and in addition a board (called back rest).

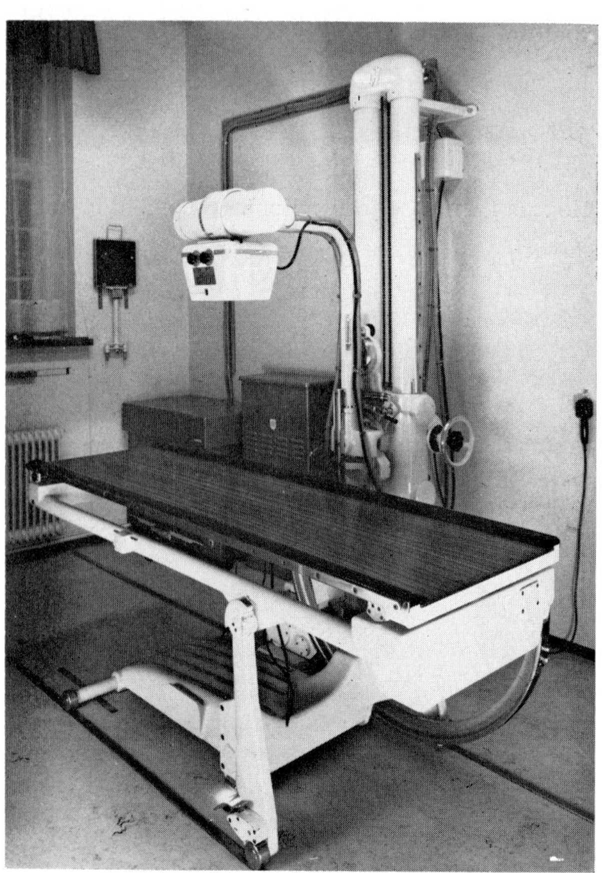

Courtesy: Dansk Rontgen Teknik.

Danatom. The name of this table derives its roots from Danish and tomography, optional attachments are available multi-layer even for magnification tomography. The table comes either hand- or motor-tilted (15° Trendelenburg). For upright exposures, with or without Bucky, the table slides back on the twin rails, it will go back sufficiently to allow a stretcher to be wheeled directly under the beam.

*In 1963 Liebel-Flarsheim introduced the Hydradjust, intended to replace the Hugh H. Young urologic table. The Hydradjust is supported by a square column, and looks somewhat like the Dana Unit. The Hydradjust's main feature is the possibility to place the image intensifier with television pickup underneath the table, that is as far away as feasible from the urologist's working space. Actually the Cinelix and the Marconi intensifiers, because of their large bulk, have occasionally been installed under the table. Liebel-Flarsheim were unaware of the existence of the Dana Unit at the time they designed the Hydradjust. At the University of Indiana, Campbell and Miller wrote the specifications for a urologic table with image intensifier and cineradiography mounted "below" (that table was built on a special order by Picker), and this is where Liebel-Flarsheim got the idea for the Hydradjust.

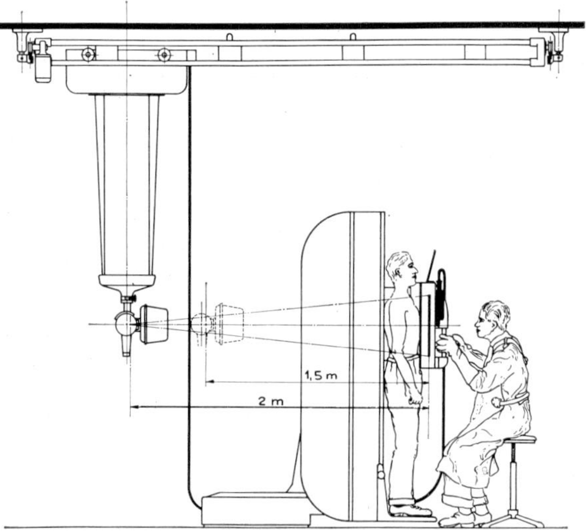

Courtesy: Dansk Rontgen Teknik.

Dana ceiling suspension. With "motor-driven clamp-fitting" one can fluoroscope at six or eight feet tube-screen distance, while handling the tube and diaphragm by remote control.

That board comes with an optional sliding top. All this has "clamp fitting" and constitutes a table which can be positioned by remote control. The arrangement is very useful whenever sterility must be maintained, as in urology, or in catheterization. Even oblique projections can be set by pushing "remote" buttons.

The Dana Automaskop is a viewbox with "clamp fitting." It has ten frames which take a total of 140 10x12″ films, and these frames can be moved by pushing buttons.

DRT products are marketed outside Denmark by the world-wide Philips organization. They have advertised Dana's ceiling suspensions, the Danatom, even the Danagraph (a darkroom identification printer), but so far little attention has been given to the Dana Unit, presumably because they did not want to hurt their other tables, the Symmetrix and Diagnost 60.

FINLAND

Yrjö Veli Paatero, who teaches dental radiology in the University of Helsinki, has been working since 1954 on a new way of making panoramic views of the teeth.

His solution is called Pantomography. In the orthopantomographic version the patient sits immobile, while the x-ray tube rotates behind his neck, and a curved, plastic cassette rotates simultaneously, in opposite direction, about the patient's mouth. During the motion, a narrow roentgen beam is directed through the neck

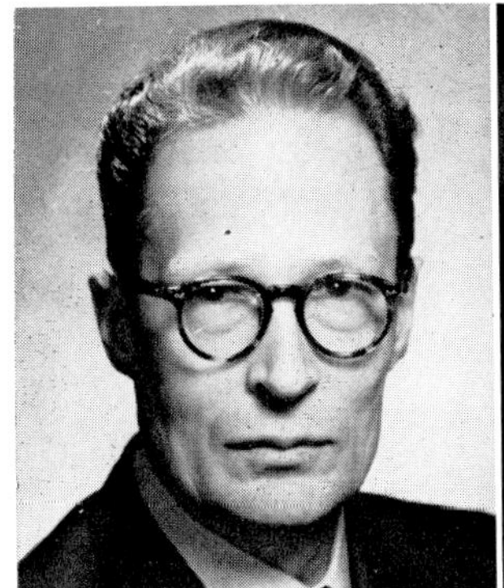

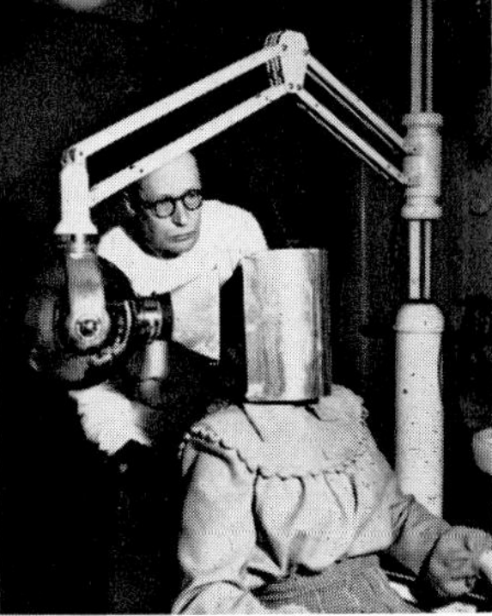

Initial Ortho-Pantomography. Yrjö Veli Paatero is professor of dental radiology in Helsinki. His first attempts to obtain panoramic views of the teeth by way of tomography were made in 1948, using a SRW Röntgenkugel and a curved cassette, fastened to the patient's face; then the patient was rotated with the dental chair.

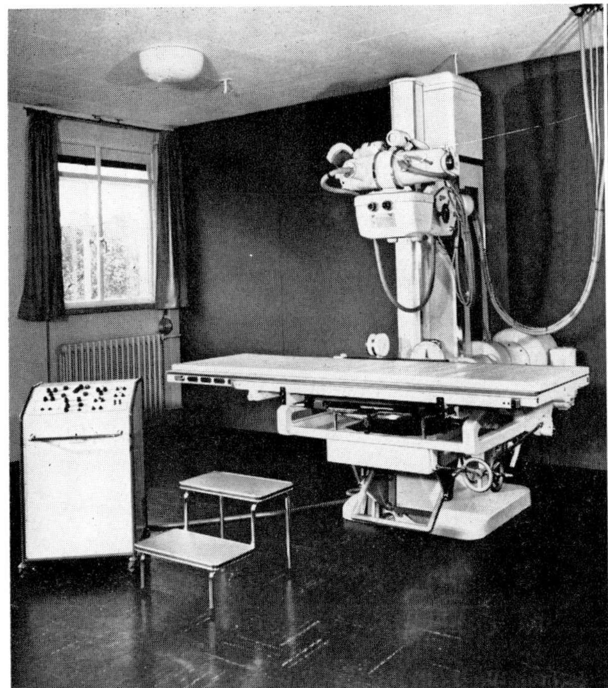

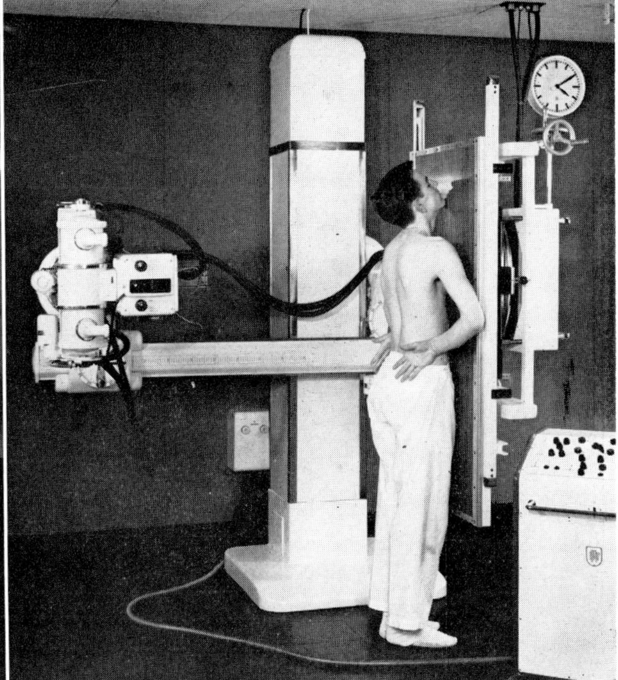

Courtesy: Dansk Rontgen Teknik.

Dana unit. Extremely versatile Bucky stand and sliding table top, useful in specialized procedures, from retrograde urography to heart catherization; it allows 15° Trendelenburg on its longitudinal axis, and from horizontal to 90° on its transverse axis. The whole thing can be operated by pushbuttons from the control stand.

onto the film. The beam turns successively about three rotational axes. One axis is for the incisor area, the other two for the mandibular rami region. In an earlier version, the patient was moved. Stereoscopic views can also be obtained, with a single exposure.

The first commercial Ortho-Pantomograph was built in 1959 by the Finnish manufacturer Lääkintäsähkö Oy, and distributed by Oy Sarjavalmiste AB of Helsinki.*

The ortho-pantomograph cannot replace the small occlusal dental films (with their fine detail obtained by actual contact with the part), but it offers an unusual survey view which resembles the drawings used on blanks for the recording of dental examinations.

*Their American representative is the Schick X-Ray Company of Chicago.

Similar devices are being built by the (British) Watson and by the (American) XRM. Watson & Sons have an arrangement with the Finnish holder of the patent. I inquired with XRM about their arrangements, and this is what they answered:

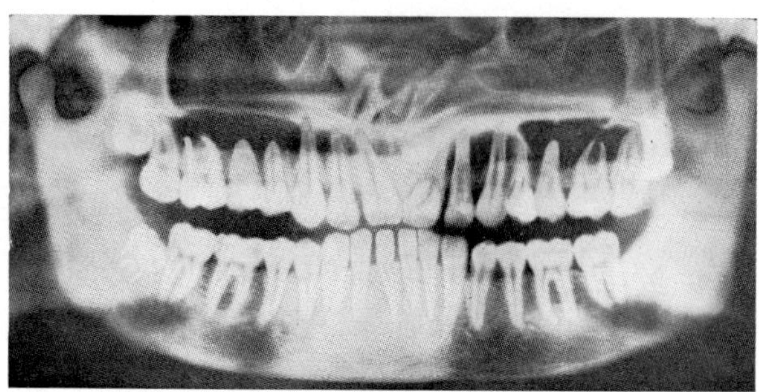

Courtesy: X-Ray Manufacturing Company of America.
ACTUAL ORTHOPANTOMOGRAM.

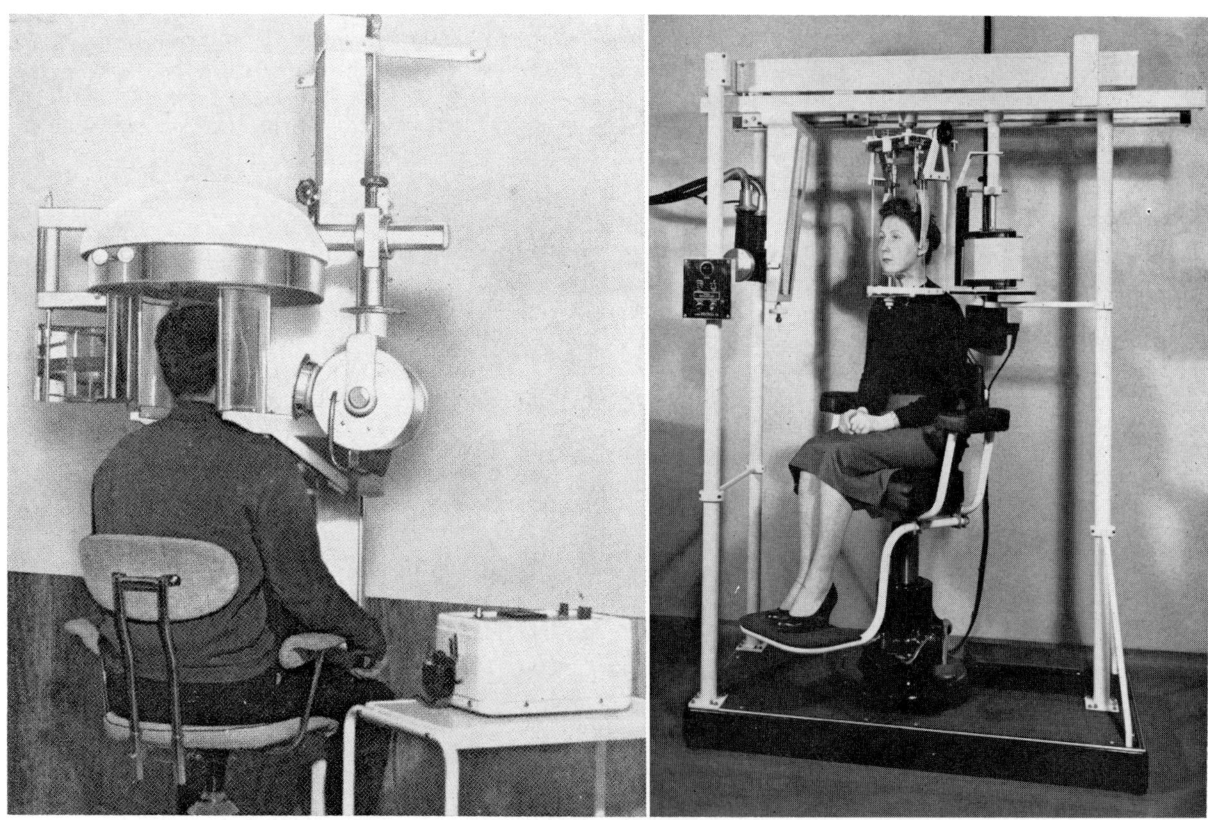

PRACTICAL PANTOMOGRAPHY. The male model holds still while tube and cassette revolve in opposite orbits in the Finnish version of the Orthopantomograph, manufactured by Lääkintäsähkö Oy. In the British Rotagraph, built by Watson, and shown here in Sydney Blackman's Department of Dental Radiology in the University of London, the tube is stationary, while the female model and the cassette rotate. So far the method has not become very popular because pantomographs have an inherent unsharpness (the Swedes call tomography in general an expensive way of getting poor x-ray films).

"The original motivation for the Panorex came from the need for a survey machine in the Air Force. Therefore the US Air Force and the National Bureau of Standards were given the assignment of developing the curved laminagraph principle, presently used in our Panorex. After this feature was developed, the manufacturers were invited to view the prototype, in 1955. The operation was unwieldy due to the need to carefully position the patient, but the system, in our opinion, showed merit. This is why the Automatic Chair Shift was developed and patented by XRM, and it is the basis for our Panorex."

XRM's PANOREX. Long Island version of the orthopantomograph, built by the X-Ray Mfg. Company of America.

BALTEAU

In 1919, Marcel Balteau (1891-1957) founded at nr. 91 on Rue de Serbie in Liège (Belgium) - *i.e.,* in uncontested Walloon territory - a small shop for the sale, installation, and repair of electrical motors. He employed 2 workers.

He must have offered something the customers liked, because the company expanded, and by 1930 was making high-tension transformers for power supply. Next came x-ray transformers and by 1935, Balteau was producing x-ray apparatus for both medical and industrial non-destructive testing. During the German occupation of Belgium (1940-1944), the firm was ordered to close down its x-ray section. In 1945 most of the plant was destroyed during an air raid. Reconstruction was started in 1946 with a work force of about thirty employees. Balteau's dramatic re-expansion coincided with the rebirth of Western Europe. After the founder's

Balteau

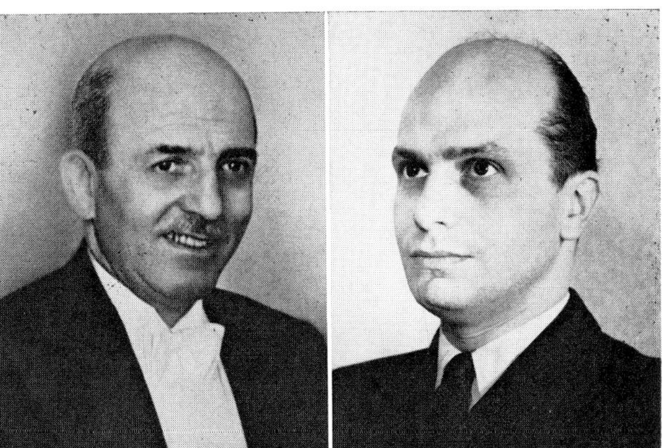

BALTEAU FATHER & SON. Marcel Balteau, with mustache, founded the firm. Pierre Balteau succeeded him as general manager, but died in a plane crash while returning from the U. S. A. where he had inspected the Stamford branch office. Currently at the helm of the company is another son, Georges Balteau.

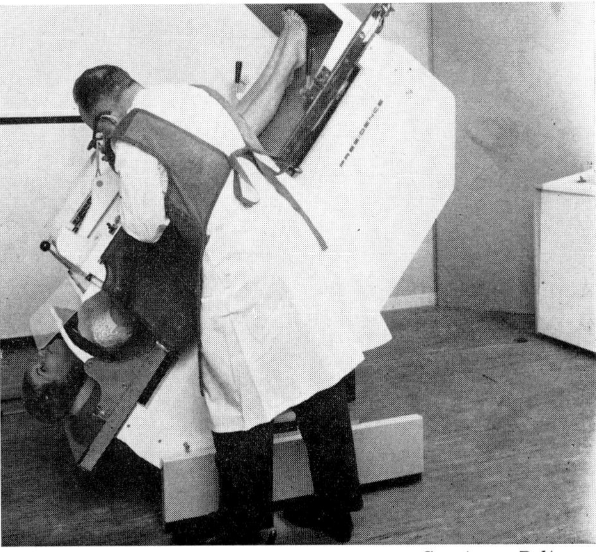

Courtesy: Balteau.

BALTEAU'S PRÉSIDENCE. Note the 180° travel, the automatized spotfilmer Polymat, and in right background the control desk of a Pilote.

death, his oldest son — Pierre Balteau — took over; four years later Pierre was killed in the same plane accident (crash landing of Boeing 707 at Bruxelles) in which died an entire USA Olympic ice-skating team. Thereupon the second son — Georges Balteau — became general manager of the firm. Today there are about 700 employees at Balteau's.

Balteau makes a fairly complete line of medical and industrial x-ray equipment. Single-tank construction (called Baltodyne) is utilized in a series of small machines, intended mainly for export, the Dynabloc, Minibloc, and Balybloc. Each has a fluoroscopic screen carrier mounted together with the Baltodyne and the control panel. The Balybloc has special provision for the protection of the operator. The Baltodyne comes also as a mobile unit (Toutix: 26 ma and 90 kvp). Congolix and Congostat are mobile units, but they have separate transformers, and higher ratings (80 ma and 95 kvp).

Balteau's big transformers are the Capitaine (which can energize 4 x-ray tubes at up to 700 ma or 120 kvp), the Pilote (for 2 x-ray tubes, up to 500 ma or 150 kvp), and the triphasic, selenium-rectified Commodore (for 8 x-ray tubes, up to 1000 ma or 150 kvp). An automatized exposure version of the Pilote is called Supermemorix.

Promotion is a table with 105° tilt, floor-to-ceiling tubestand, ceiling-counterbalanced screen-carrier, and fully automatic spotfilmer (called Automix). Présidence is Balteau's 180° table, with all the power-assisted frills; its automatic spotfilmer is the Polymat.

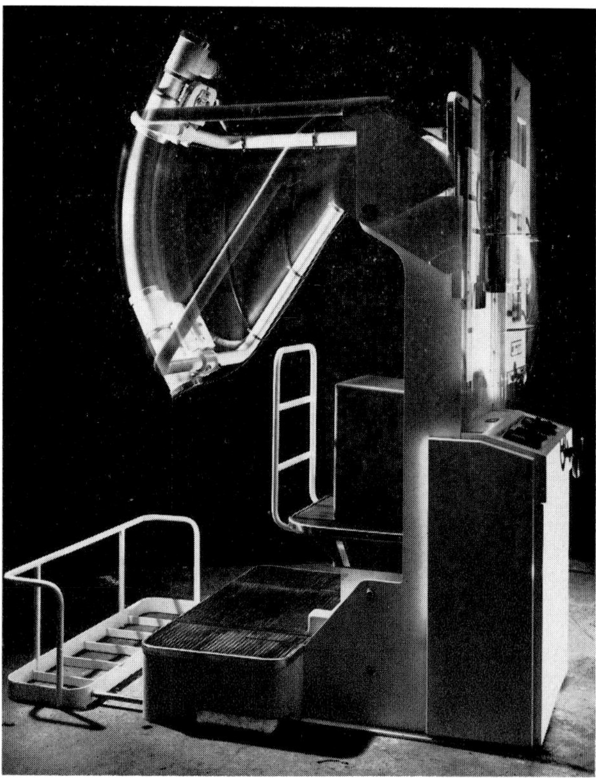

Courtesy: Balteau.

BALTOM-X (ALIAS BALTOMIX). Time-exposure, showing travel of the x-ray tube during tomographic exposure.

Balteau has several ceiling tube supports: the latest is called Zodiaque II, and consists of jointed arms, motor-operated by remote control. The Polarix is a Baltodyne bloc with image intensifier and television pick-up for "surgical" fluoroscopy.

In this country Balteau has a subsidiary in Stamford (Connecticut), mainly for the industrial line, which is well introduced in the airline maintenance business. For the USA medical audience Balteau has (so far) advertised only two body section devices (but not their single-axis Unitome): one was the conventional Baltom-X (in Belgium it is spelled Baltomix), the other was the transverse Cyclo-X, on which the patient is rotated.

GEVAERT

In 1890, Lieven Gevaert (1868-1935) founded at nr. 159 on Montignystraat in Antwerpen (Belgium) - *i.e.*, in incontested Flemish territory - a small shop, and began to make photographic paper.

In 1891, Gevaert hired a sixteen year old helper, Henri Kuypers (1875-1945), who was to become the firm's director general. In 1894, Gevaert built the first machine for continuously coating the paper with emulsion, and in the same year registered the firm as L. Gevaert & Co., with a capital of 20,000 fr. (about $400). Success came soon and the first branch office was opened in Paris in 1895; other branches followed in Milano and Moscow in 1906, in Berlin (Gevaert

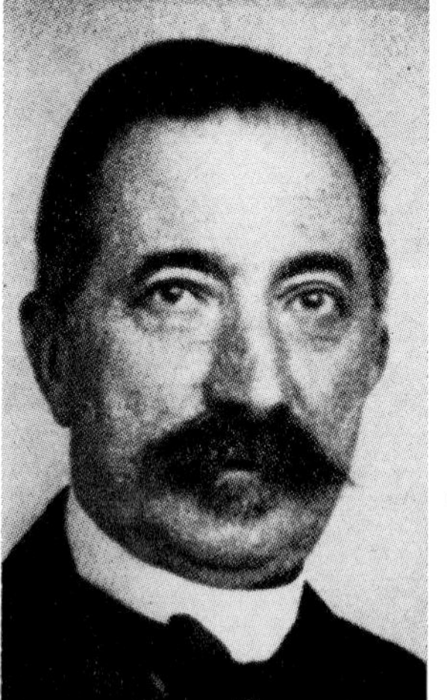

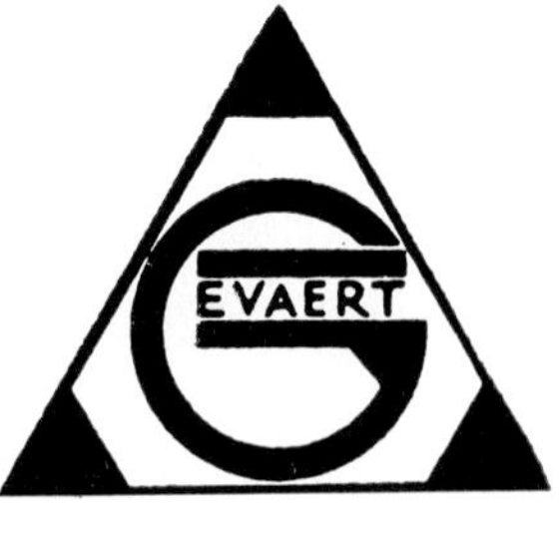

LIEVEN GEVAERT. Founder of the company which bears his name. The town where the factory is located — Mortsel — has erected a very impressive statue in his honor, with beautiful, tall pine trees in the background.

Werke mbH) in 1908, in London (Gevaert, Ltd.) in 1909, and in the USA (Gevaert Co. of America, Inc.) in 1920; the latter had even a small plant in Williamstown (New York).

The Gevaert headquarters are since 1897 in Mortsel, a suburb of Antwerpen. By 1905, their work force numbered about 150 people. In 1920, they were incorporated as NV Gevaert Photo-Producten. In 1929, Gevaert brought out the firm's first roentgen film (nonflammable). Today the total number of workers in their Belgian factories alone exceeds 8500.*

*Information was obtained from a 271 page book *(Lieven Gevaert; De mens en zijn werk)*, which is a collection of articles, published in 1954 in Leuven (Davidsfonds). This book was graciously offered for consultation by the director of research of Gevaert's X-ray Section, Philippe Lauwers. Lauwers (a physicist) is co-author (with the x-ray technician Ilse Lohstöter) in the monumental *Technik der Röntgendiagnostik* (Thieme, Stuttgart, 1961) by Hanno Poppe, radiologist in the Surgical Clinic of the University of Göttingen (Germany).

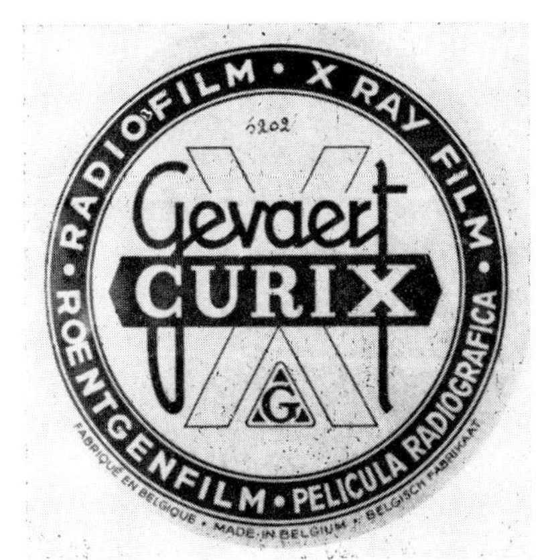

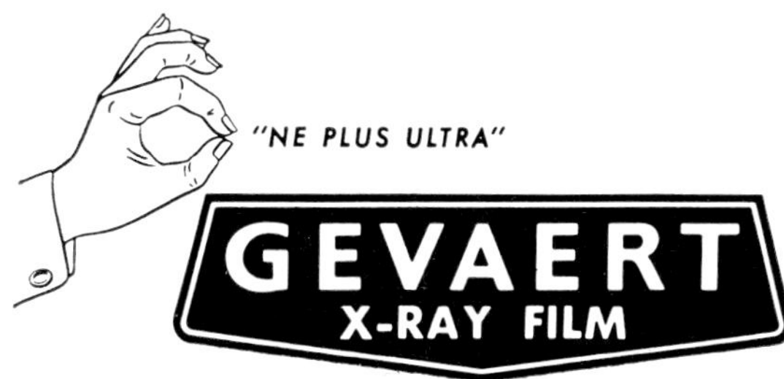

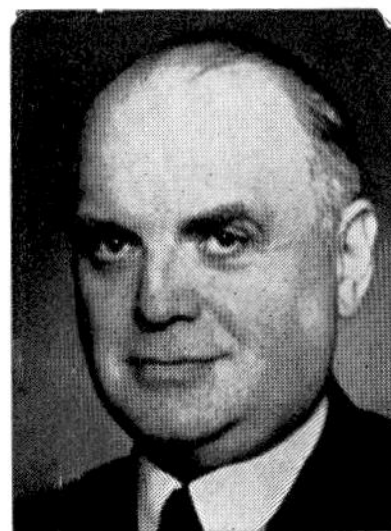

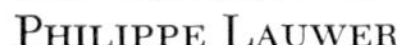

PHILIPPE LAUWERS

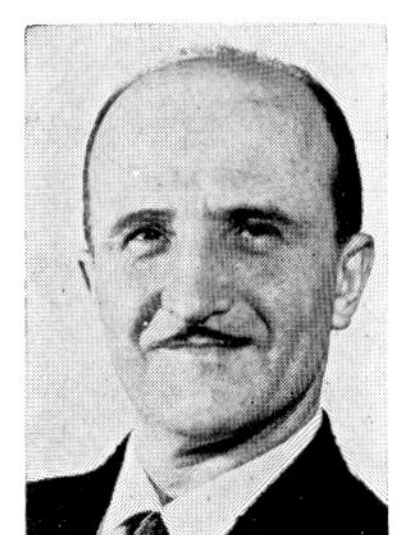

PHILIP STEINBERG

Gevaert manufactures a complete line of photographic x-ray products, from films to darkroom equipment and chemicals. Today, Gevaert is Europe's largest manufacturer of photographic materials including x-ray films — second only to Eastman Kodak.

The main brand names are Curix (high contrast film on blue base, for reinforcing screens), Curix Rapid (ultra-fast Atomic Age film), Osray (non-screen "bone and soft tissue" film), Dentus Rapid and Dentus Super Rapid (occlusal dental films), the photofluorographic Scopix (Scopix B for bluish screens and Scopix G for greenish screens), and the industrial Structurix (which comes in several grades and speeds.

Recently (1960) Gevaert brought out the Curix Matic automatic processor, and the G 120 A, a concentrated liquid developer for automatic machines.

Gevaert's representative in this country is the Low X-Ray Corporation of New York City: their advertising centered for quite some time on the Latin phrase *Ne plus ultra* (none better), which in Europe is usually spelled *Nec plus ultra.**

*Some of the seals herein reproduced were provided by Philip Steinberg, the manager of Low X-Ray Co.

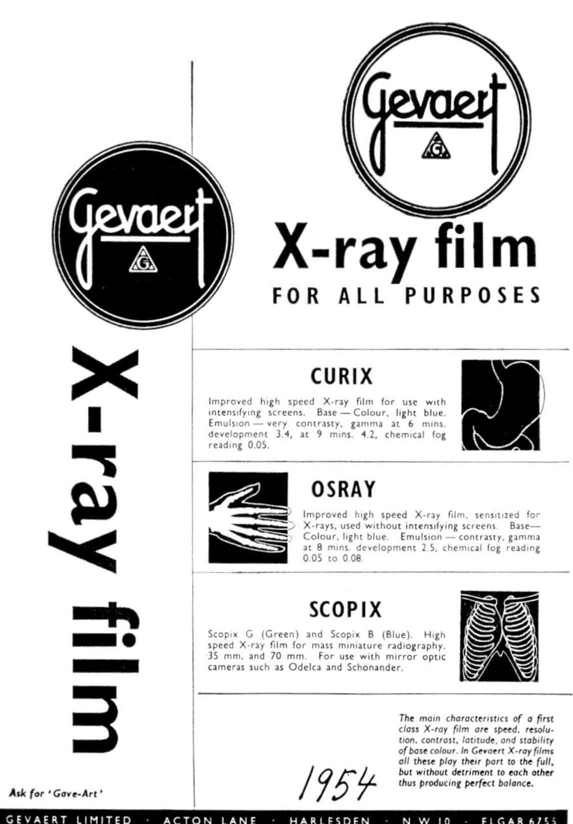

FRANCE

After World War II came several colonial repossessions, and somehow France and the Frenchmen continued to *cheminer* on the warpath all the way from 1939 through 1962. It revitalized their sagging fertility and, while before 1939 the French population was on the decrease, there are today many more Frenchmen than ever before (which is all to the better). Such a revitalization is one of the least

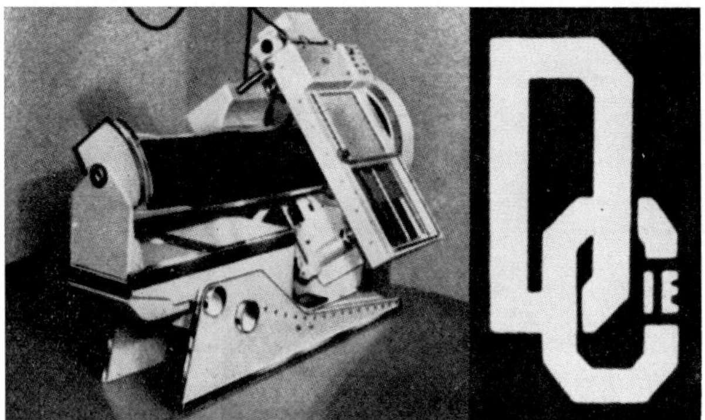

DUTERTRE'S ORIENTIX. Twin-axis 180° table with special feature allowing patient to rest in his "cradle" while the x-ray tube and screen (spotfilm) carrier rotate 180° about the patient.

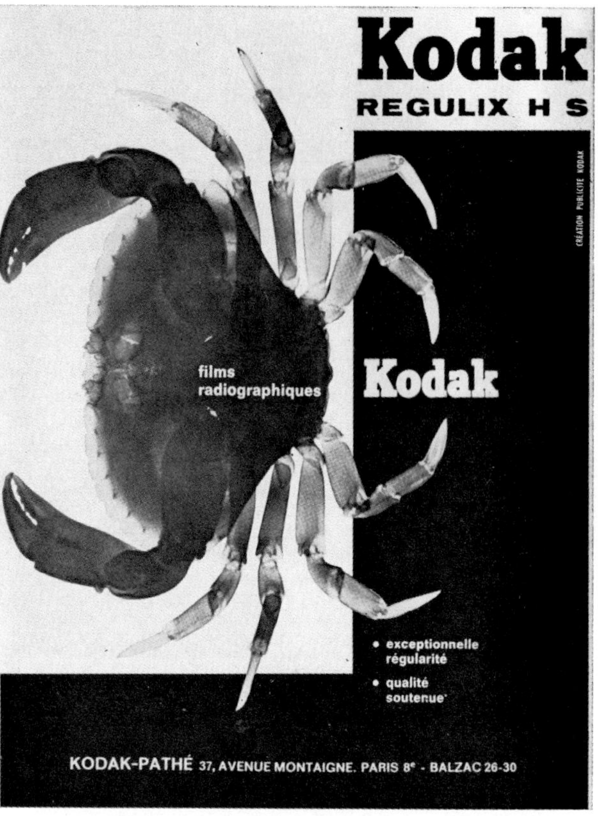

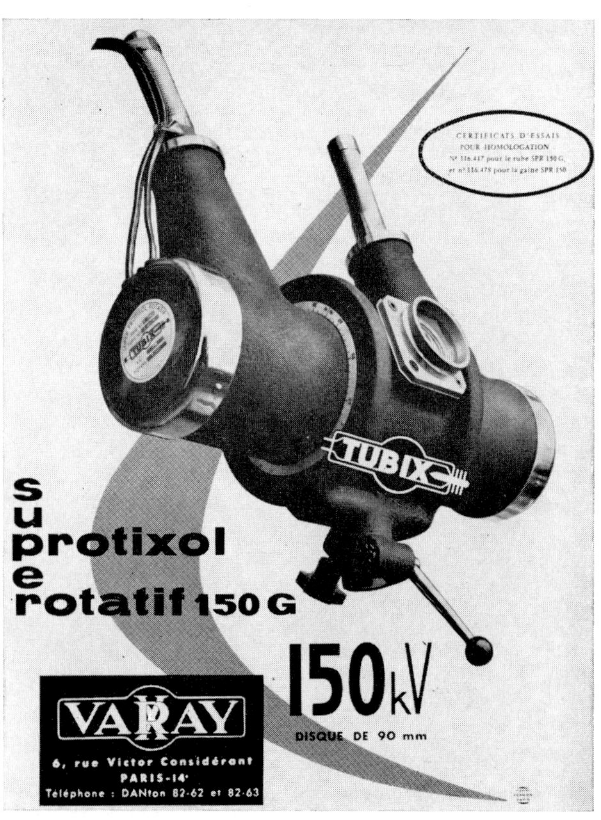

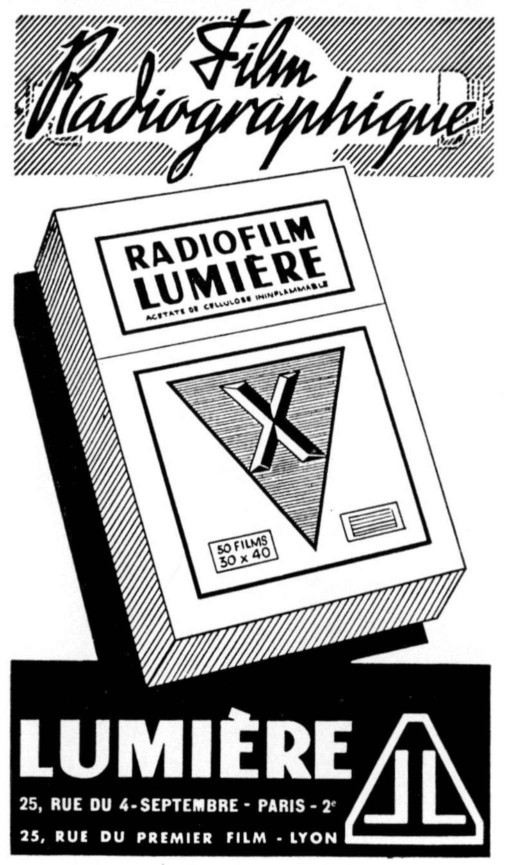

recognized consequences of non-nuclear warfare - the procedure can hardly be recommended, especially since an increase in population *per se* is regarded by some as a mixed blessing. Be it as it may, in the past decade France entered a period of economic prosperity, reflected also in the fact that some of the x-ray equipment currently made in France is among the world's most luxuriously styled.

This section will be introduced with remarks on miscellaneous French firms.

Dutertre & Co. in Arcueil (a southern suburb of Paris) manufactures several transformers, among which the Super Tetra X can deliver 800 ma at 90 kvp, 400 ma at 120 kvp, or 200 ma at 140 kvp. They have a telescopic tube support, the Pontix. The DCX is their more

Ancienne Maison ALVERGNIAT Frères
J. THURNEYSSEN
SUCCESSEUR DE V. CHABAUD
58, Rue Monsieur-le-Prince, (PARIS-VI)
Première Fabrique Française de Tubes à Rayons X
OSMO-RÉGULATEUR VILLARD — TUBES CHABAUD A ANODE DE PLATINE — SOUPAPES VILLARD
TUBES INTENSIFS A EAU — TUBES A ANODE DE TUNGSTÈNE 1919
RÉPARATIONS DE TUBES DE TOUS MODÈLES

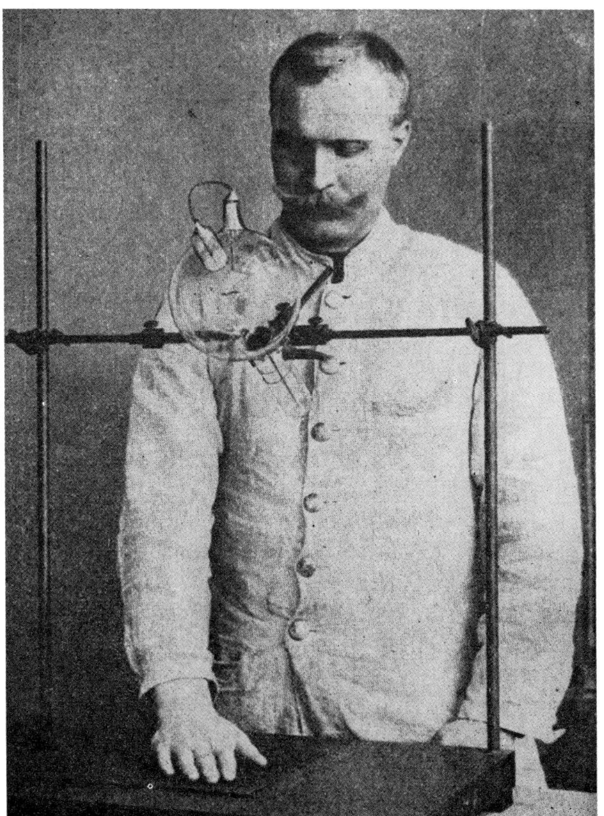

VICTOR CHABAUD. A "manual" type of stereo-radiography (about 1897).

Vous avez intérêt
à essayer la PLAQUE
RADIOX
"AS DE TRÈFLE"

Extrême Rapidité

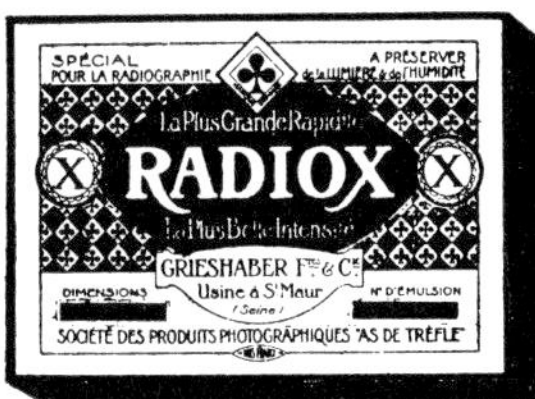

Grande Intensité

QUI CONSTITUE UN PROGRÈS
EN RADIOGRAPHIE
DÉMONSTRATION A DOMICILE 1921

Société des Produits Photographiques " **AS DE TRÈFLE** "
EN COMMANDITE PAR ACTIONS, CAPITAL: 2 MILLIONS
GRIESHABER FRÈRES et Cie
27, rue du 4-Septembre, PARIS

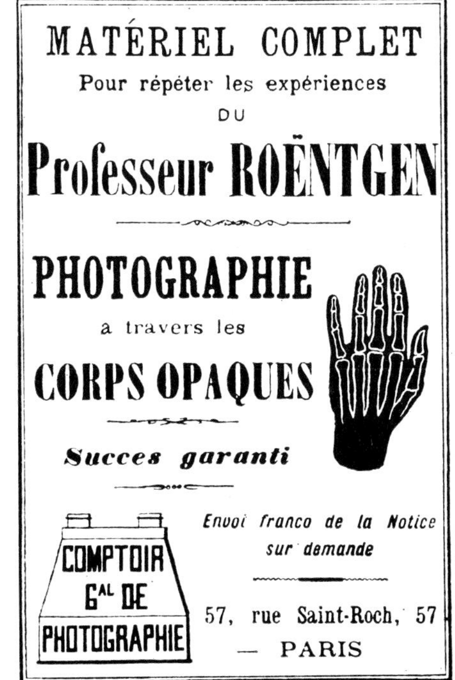

conventional table, the Super DCX is a deluxe model, while the most elaborate is called Orientix: it permits also rotation along the table's longitudinal axis, for which the patient must first be "cradled" so that he won't fall out during the "spin."

Varay in Paris makes accessories, as well as x-ray tubes. Their brand name is Tubix (they have one with 150 kvp rating).

The (SRW owned) Sinegran in Nantes manufactures screens with this brand name (in Germany Sinegran screens were available since before 1910). The French Sinegran screens are called Saphir (standard speed), Rubis (fine grain), and Diamant (high-speed). They offer, as a matter of course, also a set for simultaneous tomography.

Kodak-Pathé is the largest manufacturer of films in France. Because of their financial relationship with Eastman, Kodak-Pathé sells the X-omat in France (and in related or adjoining territories).

The venerable *radiofilm* Lumière is still being advertised and sold.

A French "contrast maker" of semantic significance is the SEPPS (Société d'Exploitation de Produits Pharn-

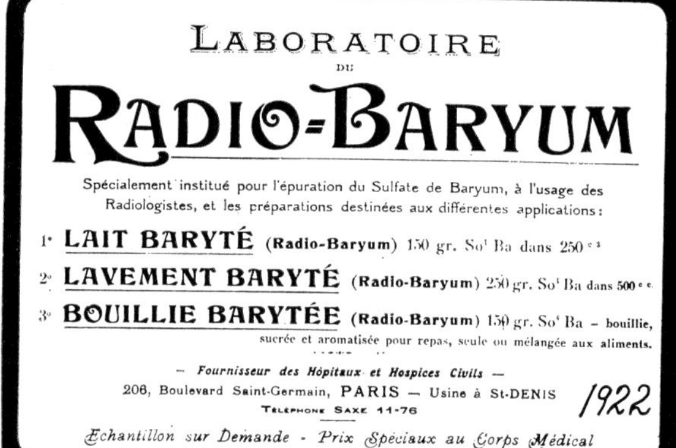

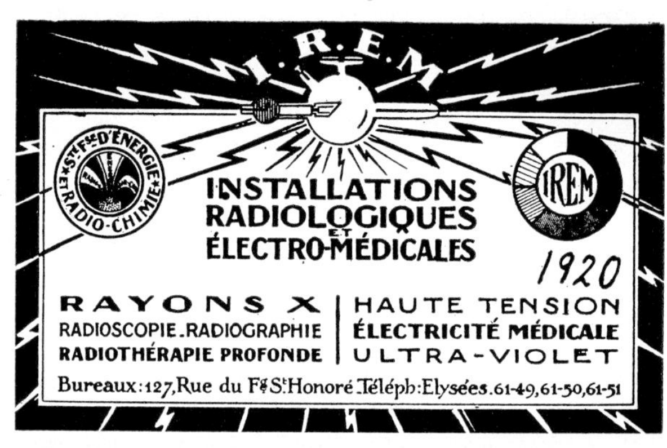

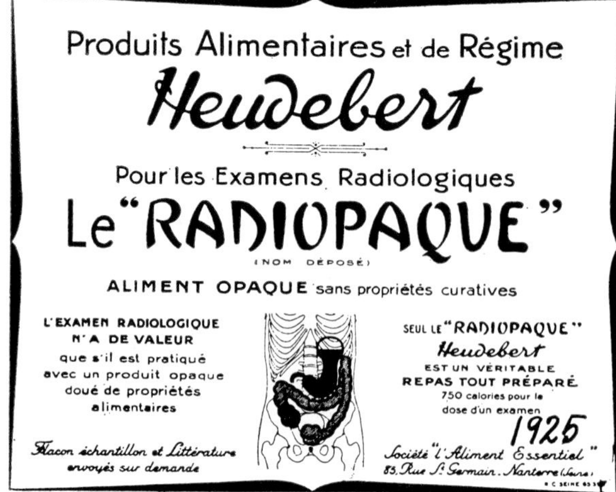

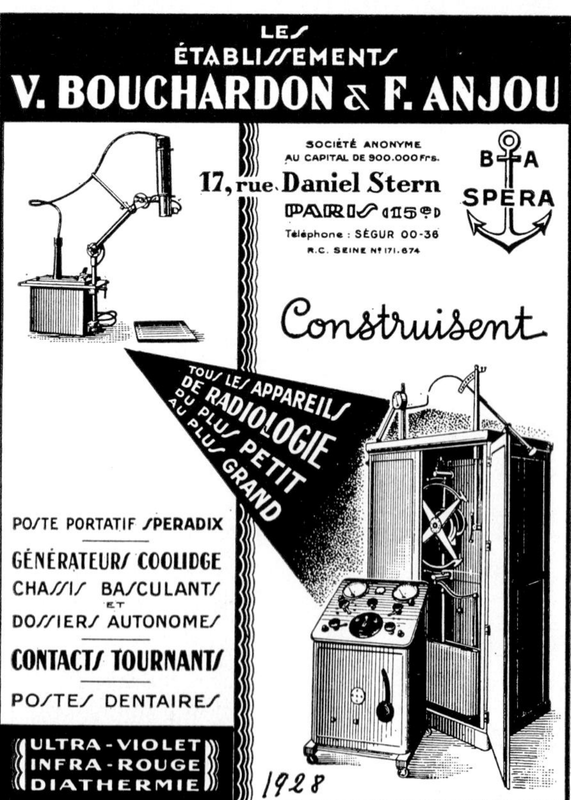

Produits Alimentaires et de Régime

aceutiques). Their nomenclature contains a single *genus,* Radioselectan, with several *species,* Radioselectan biliaire, R. vésiculaire, R. urinaire, etc.

Bladex is a cholecysto-stimulator (fatty meal) made by Biodica-Soudan.

It is not possible to pay tribute to all the significant names among French x-ray firms which are no longer in business, but a few will be remembered.

There was the "first" *(première)* French factory of x-ray tubes, founded by Victor Chabaud.

Radiox was the brand name of radiographic glass plates manufactured by the Grieshaber Brothers, who used an ace of spades as their trade-mark. A dragon was used as Crumière's trade-mark (he must have read Anatole France's *L'Ile des Pingouins*); their Draco-Radio was a medium contrast x-ray copy paper.

The Laboratoire du Radio-Baryum was marketing the usual barium suspensions, and in addition a condimented (seasoned) soup with barium (bouillie barytée). Heudebert topped this by bringing out the Radiopaque, which contained 750 calories per "barium meal."

The IREM (Installations Radiologiques et Electro-Médicales) was combined with the Société Française d'Énergie et de Radio-Chimie — so that they serviced all sorts of apparatus, and sold mesothorium and other radio-active materials to boot.

Then there was the Bouchardon & Anjou, which had a fairly complete line of x-ray equipment. Most of these firms capitulated at the time of the Great Depression.

ANDRE GUERBET & CIE

The largest maker of contrast media in France is the firm Laboratoires Andre Guerbet & Cie, located in Saint-Ouën, a "chemical" exurbia North of Paris.

Lipiodol Lafay (iodinated poppyseed oil) is still the first on their list, although no longer the one which makes the most sales. It was modified into Lipiodol F (fluide), which consists of the iodinated ethylic esters of the fatty acids in poppyseed oil. A variant is the Lipiodol Ultra-Fluide, used in sialography and fistulous instillations. Lipiodol Sulfanilamide is less likely to penetrate into alveoli during bronchography. Their latest bronchographic substance is the Propylix, which comes either in an oily or in a watery base.

Various hypertonic solutions are prepared for injection into vessels and canals, Acetiodone (up to 70%) is for intravenous urography, Diodone (up to 70%) for cholangiography, hysterosalpyngography, etc. Diodone comes also in a 35 per cent solution, which can be injected intramuscularly, or subcutaneously. The Diodone is even offered with Polyvidone (which is the Subtosan made by Rhône-Poulenc) for increase of viscosity, a quality desirable in hystero-salpyngography and urethrography. Intrabilix is a tri-iodinated intravenous cholecysto-cholangiographic substance. Methiodol is a myelographic medium. Vasurix is another vascu-

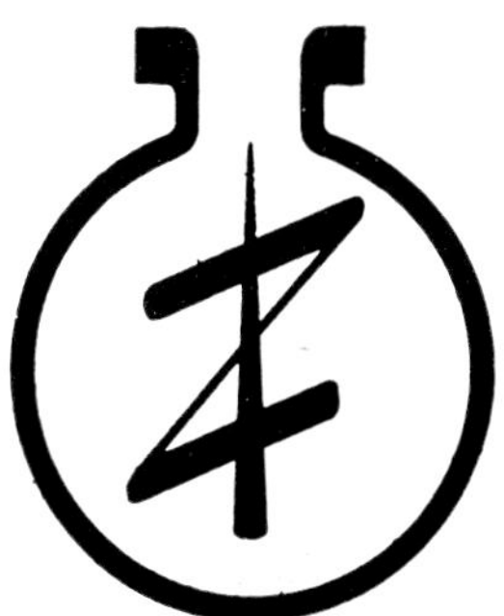

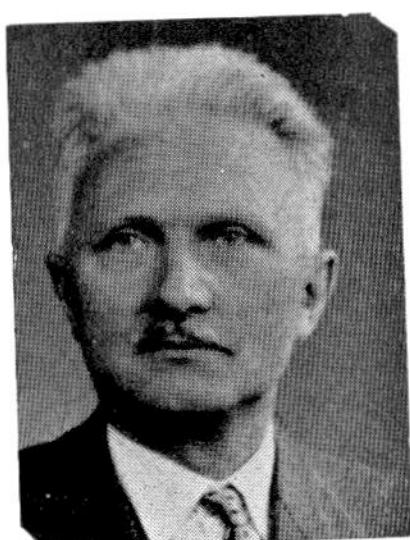

ANDRÉ GUERBET

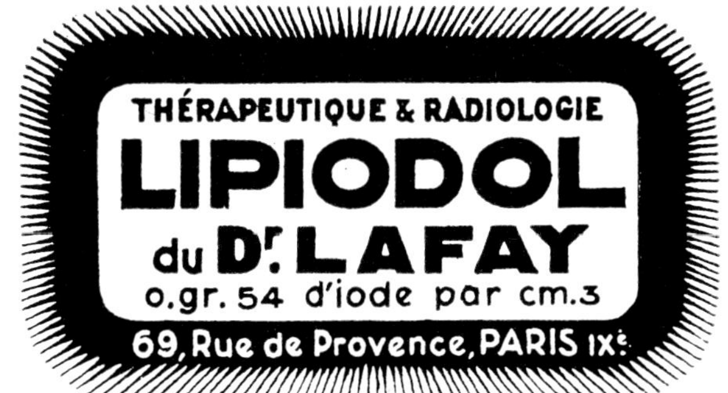

LIPIODOL GUERBET. André Guerbet's father was professor of pharmacy in the University of Paris. He was trying to develop an anti-syphilitic drug and came upon the idea to dissolve iodine in poppyseed oil. When he became ready to market the compound, the need arose to find someone under whose name it could be sold, because no university professor was allowed to maintain his position while being involved in a commercial venture (not officially, at least). This is how and why the eponym of another pharmacist (and friend of the family) was used: to this day it has retained the name of Lipiodol Lafay. The above ad dates from 1928, six years after Lipiodol was introduced as a contrast material by Sicard: he was looking for someone to work on this subject, but nobody wanted it. Then Forestier came along, accepted the topic, wrote the thesis, and both of them were thenceforth connected with the word Lipiodol. Lipiodol was also the pillar on which André Guerbet's business was first built. He was supposed to become an engineer (and was therefore studying at the famous *École Centrale*), but became sick, so it was decided that he should do something easy, which is why he went into pharmacy (this verbal information was obtained from one of André Guerbet's sons).

lar contrast solution (up to 50%), used mainly for arteriography,* and for urography.

Guerbet & Cie make a tri-iodinated peroral cholechystographic medium, the Orabilix (sold in this country by Fougera under the name Orabilex).

*In 1955, L. Sendra in Algiers built an injector and a changer (for 30x40 cm cassettes), utilized in what was called "enlarged angiocardio-pneumography" (cf., *Algérie Médicale* of February, 1955). It consists of a venous injection of contrast material (into the brachial, jugular, or crural vein) through a trocar so chosen as to admit in about two seconds 60-100 cc of concentrated contrast solution, followed by the same amount of physiologic saline.

MOYENS
DE
CONTRASTE
DES
LABORATOIRES
ANDRÉ GUERBET ET CIE
22, Rue du Landy - SAINT-OUEN (PARIS) - Seine

CHENAILLE

Chenaille, S.A. (Société anonyme = corporation) is a manufacturer of x-ray equipment located in Saint-Cloud, a former imperial (Napoleonic) residence, not far from Versailles. Chenaille's beginnings go back to the 19th Century.

In 1898, Drault, a mechanic, built an x-ray machine for Antoine Béclère. About 1903, Gaston Raulot-Lapointe* (an associate of Béclère) asked his brother Charles to go into the manufacture of x-ray equipment, and this is when the firm Drault & Raulot-Lapointe was formed. Their partnership lasted until 1930 when Drault retired.

In 1923, Manuel Chenaille founded an electro-medical firm, which in 1927 was incorporated as Établissements Chenaille. In March of 1936, the two firms merged and Chenaille & Raulot-Lapointe was incorporated. Shortly thereafter, Chenaille bought out the part held by Charles Raulot-Lapointe. Today Manuel Chenaille is associated with his two sons, Richard and Pierre.

It may be of interest to note that Drault and Raulot-Lapointe brought out in 1927 completely shockproof x-ray units. Today Chenaille has a fairly varied line of equipment.

They carry a number of single-tank units, which come as portables (Transportix with 20 ma at 90 kvp,

*He was a well-known radiologist, the first who recognized on fluoroscopy (in 1911) a smooth muscle tumor, subsequently removed in surgery.

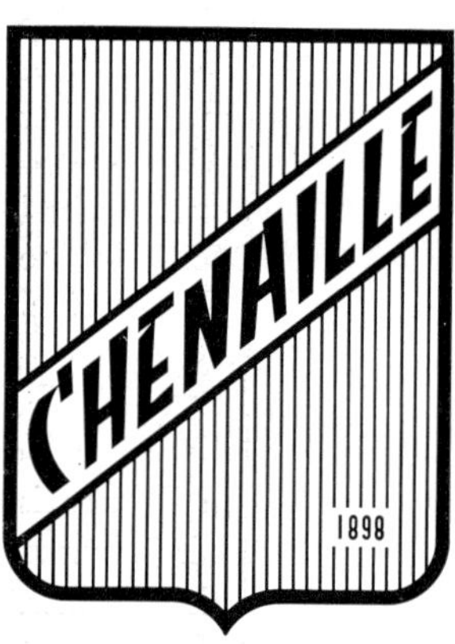

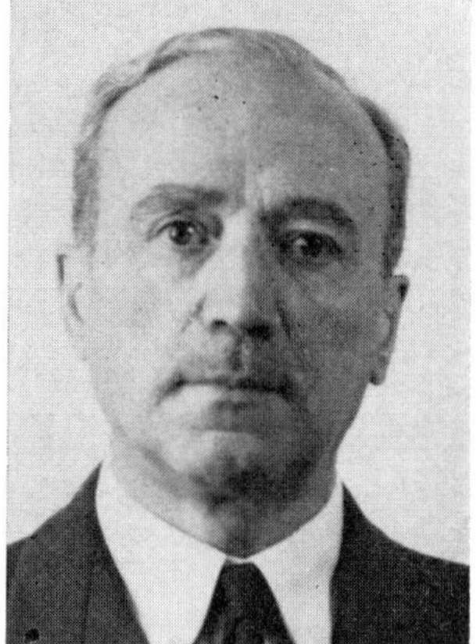

Courtesy: Chenaille.

MANUEL CHENAILLE. He founded his own firm in 1923. The date 1898 refers to the opening of a small shop by Drault (Béclère's mechanic), who shortly thereafter became associated with Charles Raulot-Lapointe. Drault retired in 1930, Chenaille bought the business in 1936, after which Raulot-Lapointe retired.

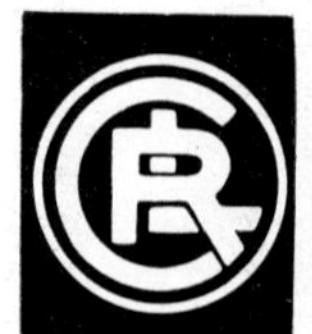

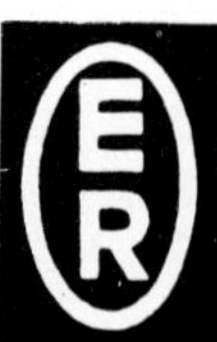

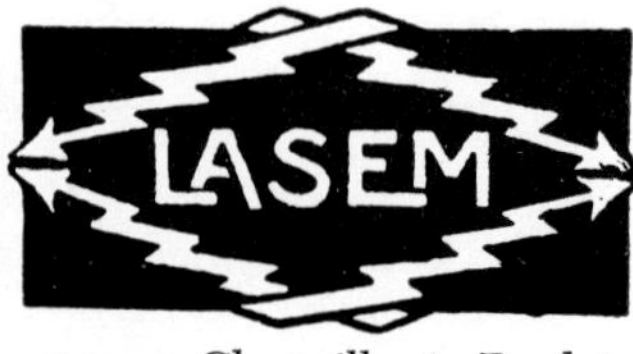

VARIOUS SEALS. The CRL means Chenaille & Raulot-Lapointe. ER comes from Electro-Radiologie (currently called Electro-Radiologie-Lasem), while Lasem is an old trade-mark from the 1920's.

or 40 ma at 85 kvp), or as "light fluoroscopes" (Verticalix), one of which is unusual in that it is supported by a wall-mounted column (Muralix). The newest is this category is the Scopirama C (better protected than the simple Scopirama).

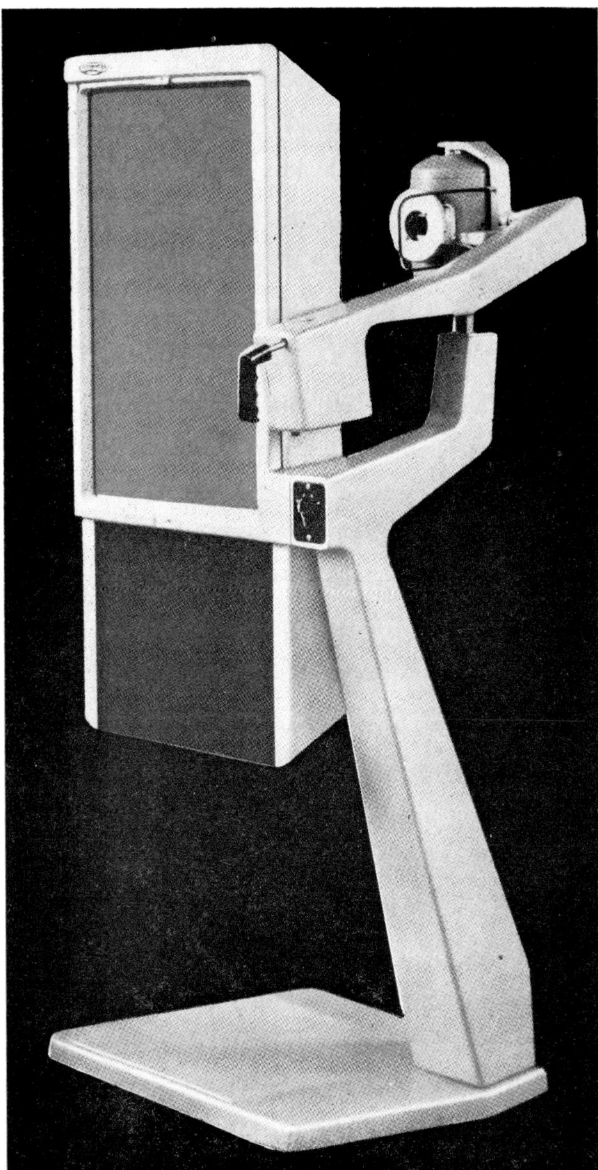

Courtesy: Chenaille.

CHENAILLE'S SCOPIRAMA. Very functional, and perhaps therefore seemingly futuristic, is the shape of this fluoroscopic unit, intended for general practitioners. The tube and the screen pivot on a support located midway between the two, on the connecting arm. The patient stands on the square footboard. He can be moved laterally so as to be brought into the beam. For height adjustments, the tube-screen arm is obliqued, whereby if the screen is raised, it also tilts a bit, and the tube is lowered, keeping it centered on the screen.

Chenaille offers two main table models, one hand-tilted (Simplix, Totalix), the other motor-operated (Raysix), with (unspecified, probably less than 15°) Trendelenburg, electromagnetic locks, floor-to-ceiling tubestand, and ceiling-counterbalanced spotfilm device Explorix.

A recent Chenaille first: in 1952, they began the evaluation of selenium rectifiers on radiotherapy transformers, and in 1953 they placed on the market a diagnostic generator with this feature. That was the first French-made apparatus using selenium rectifiers.

Chenaille makes a mobile unit (the Chirurgix, which replaced their previous Surgix) with selenium rectifiers; it comes in various models, up to 300 ma at 100 kvp, or 200 ma at 110 kvp. The stationery Selenix 500 delivers 500 ma at 106 kvp, or 100 ma at 140 kvp, while the Hexatronix (with six selenium rectifiers for triphasic current) goes to 1000 ma at 100 kvp, or 500 ma at 125 kvp. Also their therapy machine Sanix 200 is selenium-rectified (10 ma at 200 kvp).*

*This information was graciously provided by Jean Fischer, sales manager at Chenaille.

MASSIOT

I have seen a pre-print of their anniversary leaflet, called *65 Ans de Radioligie,* which has been the main source of information for the following summary.

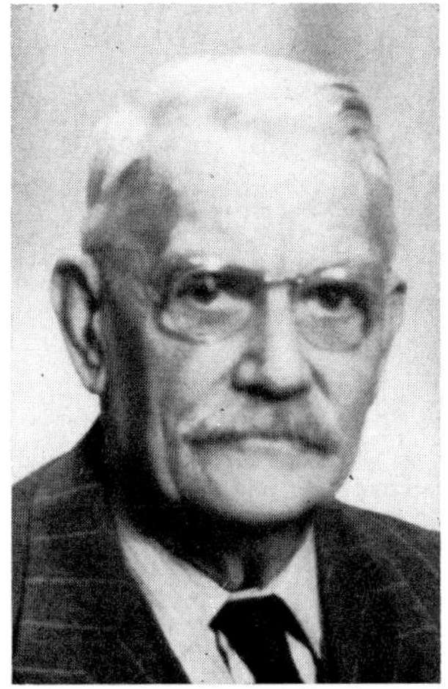

Courtesy: Massiot Philips.

GEORGES MASSIOT. While the ancestry of the firm of Massiot can be traced back to opticians of the 18th Century, it was really Georges Massiot who brought it to its highly respected place in the French x-ray industry.

The ancestors of Arthur Radiguet (1850-1905) had been opticians at least since 1782, date on which the shop (inherited by Radiguet) was founded. As mentioned in a previous chapter, Radiguet made, advertised, and sold x-ray equipment in the very year 1896. He also communicated some of his experiments with fluoroscopic screens to the *Académie des Sciences* in Paris. Among Radiguet's early contributions to radiology was a (kerosene immersed) copper interrupter for coils; a bibliography of radiologic literature of early days (compiled by a Dutch polyglote, van der Veldehuis, and later donated to the Physics Laboratory of Albert Weill in the Medical School in Paris); Bouchacourt's "lantern," a hand-held x-ray tube, precursor of today's portables; and Bouchacourt and Remond's endodiascopy x-ray tube with grounded anode, which could be inserted into various orifices (the inevitable necroses soon forced abandonment of this method). Radiguet had exposed himself to x radiation, and developed a severe dermatosis, especially on the hands. This was first treated with x rays, but breakdown of the skin made them discontinue such therapy after a few sessions. After several amputations, and five painful years, Radiguet died in December, 1905.

In 1898, a young engineer, Georges Massiot (1875-1962), came to work for Radiguet, became his son-in-law and finally his successor. Massiot built a foreign body localizer for Marie and Ribaut *(compas de repérage)*, and another type (the so-called *indicateur*) for Rémy. For Guilleminot, Massiot constructed the first orthodiagraph, and the first "bed" with a beam-centering device consisting of (under-the-bed) screen and mirror. In 1912, Massiot arranged a radiologic truck intended for the military, but reception was not too encouraging; indeed, in 1914 he was barely given permission to participate (at his own expense) in the planned military maneuvers; these maneuvers turned out to be much more serious than anticipated, and lasted until the armistice in 1918. But Massiot's *Voiture Radiologique* proved itself under stress.

After World War I, Georges Massiot returned to peaceful production. His first big showing came in May, 1925 when he exhibited in the (Military Hospital) Val-de-Grâce a new line of x-ray equipment, on the occasion of the Congrès de Médecine Militaire. Among his many achievements during the Golden Age of Radiology may be mentioned the integral ("absolute") protection device, built for Belot in 1927: the operator was completely separated from the patient, and the machinery was moved by a sort of remote control. In 1933, Massiot constructed another radiologic truck, this time for peaceful purposes; in 1941, on the demand of the French Red Cross, that truck was reequipped with a photofluorographic machine. To the ICR in Zurich (1934) Massiot presented for the first time his diagnostic tube Oleix, which was made both shock-proof and radiation-proof by being encased under oil, in a leaded housing. In 1936, the therapy tube

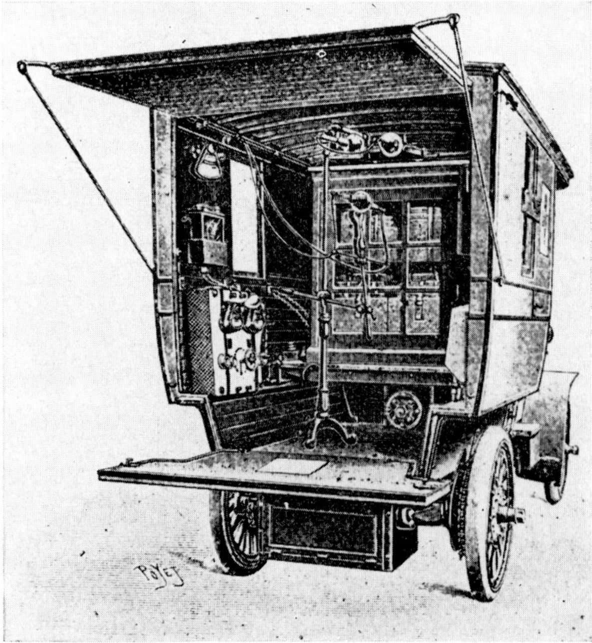

Massiot's Voiture radiologique. At first spurned, then anxiously adopted.

A l'occasion des

Congrès de Chirurgie et de Médecine

Première Quinzaine d'Octobre

Présentation de Nouveaux Modèles "RADIO"

Le "RADIOSTAT" Groupe radiodiagnostic idéal du PRATICIEN

Alimentation d'un Coolidge radiateur **30 milliampères**

Le "SCOPIGRAPH" Installation compacte et puissante du SPÉCIALISTE

Alimentation d'un Coolidge radiateur **100 milliampères**

Grand Contact Tournant CT 4 *bis*

(170.000 volts maximum)

Générateur Universel - Scopie - Graphie - Thérapie

GRILLES ANTIDIFFUSANTES R et M

Ces appareils sont exposés à la Faculté de Médecine au Stand de

G. MASSIOT

CONSTRUCTEUR

MAGASINS : 13 et 15, boulevard des Filles-du-Calvaire, PARIS (3e)

R. d. C. N° 8188. USINE A COURBEVOIE (SEINE) 1927

Oleix 200 kvp was constructed on similar principles. In 1934, Massiot built for Gérard and Sénechal a radiosurgical table with twin x-ray tubes, which gave two separate images of a given object on one screen: the angle was so arranged that the distance between the two images of the object was equal to the depth of that object. Massiot used twin tubes in 1939 for the stereoscopic fluoroscope of Bardon, which utilized a special binocular with synchronous obturator, so that each eye looked only at the image formed by the tube placed on its side.

In 1945, as the Atomic Phase arrived, Georges Massiot retired.*

His place was taken by his two sons, but one of them, Marcel Massiot, died in an accident in 1946. The other, Jean Massiot, became the firm's president, The next generation was already actively engaged in the business: Marcel's two sons were in the publicity department (Michel), and in isotopes (Gérard): Jean's two sons were in the technical direction (André) and in the manufacture of screens (Henri).

The house of Massiot tackled the Atomic Phase headon. In 1954, at the Radiologic Congress in Rome, was presented Massiot's image intensifier (Lynx). In October, 1954 the first radio-television apparatus was shown to the Medical Faculty in the University of Paris. In 1950, they started building two 4 mev linear accelerators, one of which was completed in 1955; the other was installed in 1961 at the Commissariat de l'Énergie Atomique in Saclay (France). They also branched out, and built Massiot-Fluor, a plant for the manufacture of screens, located in Ailly-le-Haut-Clocher. Another subsidiary, Massiot Nucléaire, constructed a rotating Co^{60} unit, the Mobaltron, and the Gammathèque, a storage container for the equivalent of 2000 mgm of radium.

And yet, despite these continuous successes, a change was in the offing. The European Common Market made it possible for all the German and Italian companies to compete for French customers. Besides, technical advances demanded considerable layout, just to stay in line with the competition. The need for strong financial backing became an actual necessity, and in 1959 conversations with the Metalix SA (the Paris representation of Philips) started. The merger was completed in July, 1960 and since then the company goes under the name Massiot-Philips, and is owned by the (Dutch) Philips. Jean Massiot is currently the president of Massiot-Philips, and Paul Botiaux (former director of Metalix SA) is vice-president of Massiot-Philips.

Even before the merger, Massiot offered a complete line of x-ray equipment, including their own reinforcing screens called Acrilix: Orion was of standard speed; Themis had high definition; and Phoebus was the high speed type.

The image intensifier is still called Lynx, but its heart is now a Philips intensifying tube.

Massiot-Philips has several "light" tables, such as the Celeroscope and Neo-Stator. Their best models are the

*He received in 1956, together with Maingot and Mario Ponzio, the Gold Medal of the Centre Antoine Béclère. Massiot is rightfully remembered as one of the pioneer *creators* in the development of modern radiologic equipment.

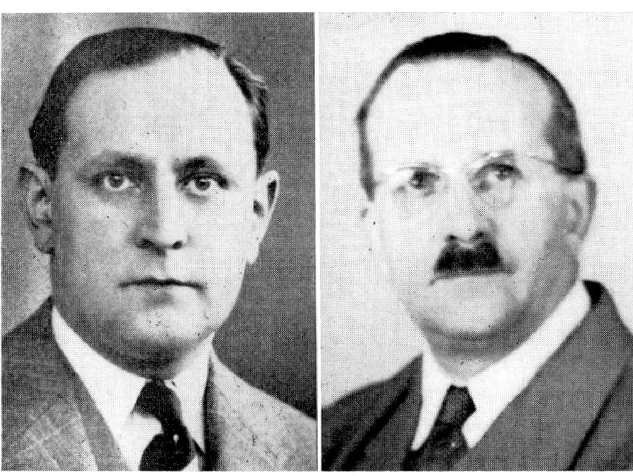

Courtesy: Massiot Philips.

Massiot 2nd generation. After the accidental death in 1946 of Marcel Massiot, Georges' other son, Jean Massiot (with spectacles and mustache) became and remained to this day the firm's president.

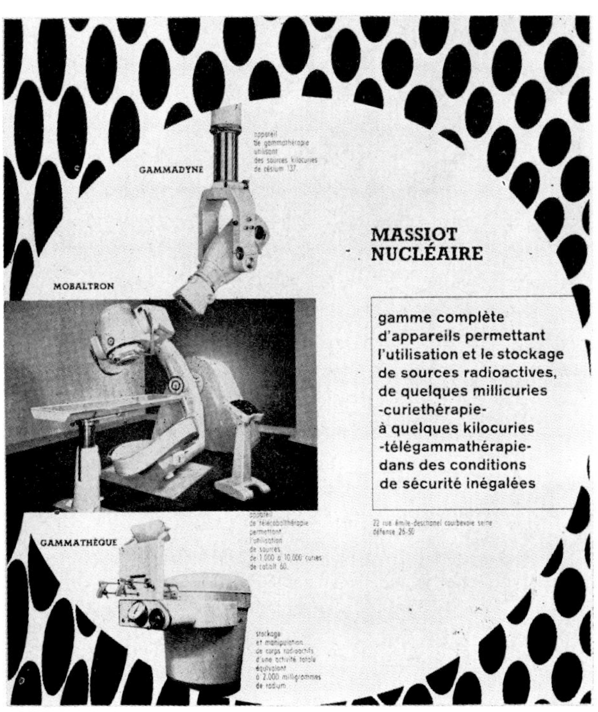

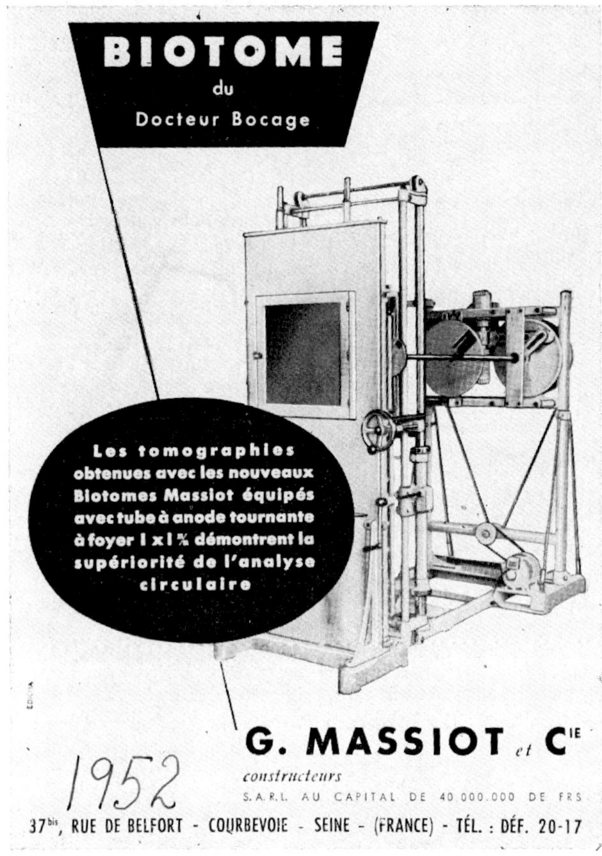

Symmetrix 90/90 (which outside France is advertised as a Philips table), and the Caducée. The latter comes also in a television-monitored, luxurious, remote-controlled version, the Tele-Caducée – eponymized for Edouard Cherigié, a radiologist from Paris – first shown in 1959 to the ICR in Munchen.

Outside France, the name Massiot became well known in the last decade mainly because of its association with the Polytome.

Massiot and body section radiography are old friends. Bocage was a French physician who practiced radiology while in the Army during World War I. After his return to civilian practice, in 1922, he devised the principle of body section radiography, including all the variants, which were later re-discovered by Grossmann (linear), Ziedses des Plantes (spiral, circular), and Vallebona (transverse). Kieffer in the USA built

am
pli
fica
teurs
lynx

MASSIOT PHILIPS
MATÉRIEL MÉDICAL
40 avenue hoche paris 8 carnot 08-24

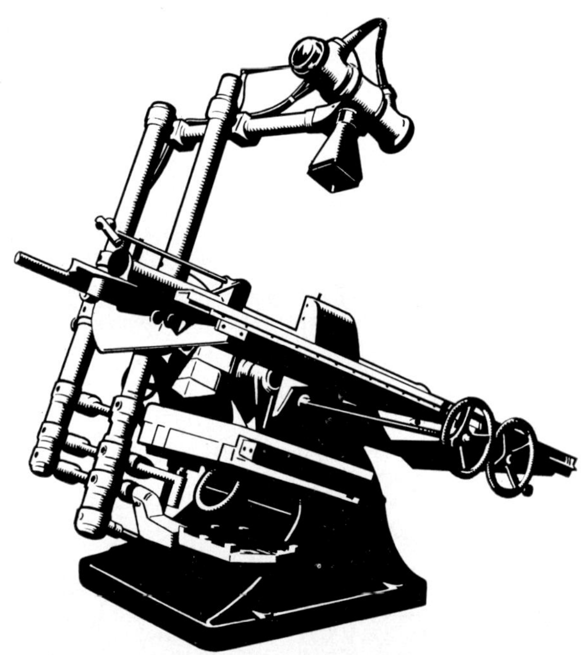

POLYTOME

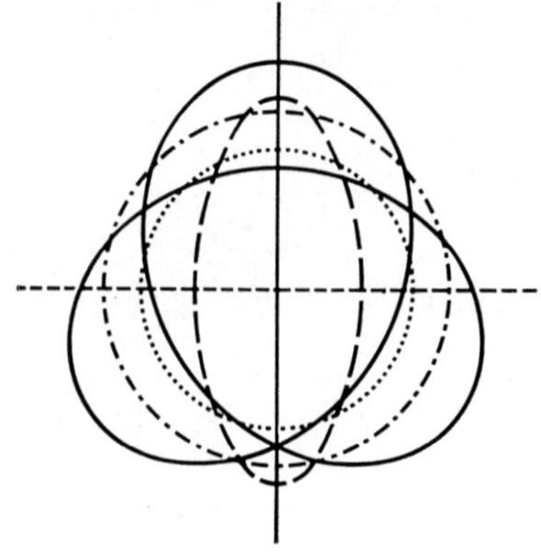

(independently) his own linear model. The first commercial tomograph was built and marketed in 1934 by Sanitas in Berlin (Grossmann's model). In 1937 Massiot constructed, from plans offered by Bocage himself, the Biotome which had a circular motion (still made and sold as late as 1952) and was quite satisfactory. Bocage himself did not stay in radiology, he became a dermato-venerologist.

The Polytome is the brainchild of an engineer (Raymond Sans), and of a mechanic (Jean Porcher). The latter is chief of the Radiologic Service Workshops of the Assistance Publique (Welfare Department) of Paris — and that is where the first model of the Polytome was built in 1949. The first commercial version of the Polytome was shown by Massiot in July, 1951 at the Belgian Radiologic Convention in Brussels. It was very successful, and so far over 100 such machines have been sold. The Polytome offers a choice of four obscuring motions (linear, circular, elliptical, and hypocycloidal): it may be a symbol of our age that the inscription of these four motions resembles the atomic orbits.

CGR

The Compagnie Générale de Radiologie (CGR), the largest French manufacturer of x-ray apparatus, was created in 1930, but its antecedent companies date from the 19th century.

In 1856, at nr. 4 on Rue de Savoie in Paris, Adolphe Gaiffe (1832-1887) opened a small, single-man optical and mechanical shop, which slowly branched out into the growing field of electricity and electro-medicine. His son, Georges Gaiffe (1857-1943), constructed since 1893 high-frequency apparatus for the famous "electrologist" Arsène d'Arsonval (1851-1940). After Roentgen's discovery, these high-frequency coils were also uesd for the production of x rays. In 1904, appeared the *meuble* (furniture) d'Arsonval-Gaiffe, which has also been immortalized in a painting: it could be used not only for high-frequency applications and for the production of x-rays but also as a source of high tension for wireless telegraphy. In the same year this furniture was bolted onto a (horse-drawn) carriage for use by the military. In the ensuing years, the Établissements George Gaiffe contributed many other items to the progress of radiology, for instance, Gaiffe's autonomous alcohol interrupter; the Blondel-Gaiffe interrupter (with gaseous dielectric) of which thousands were built; the radiologic credence-table with "shot-proof" *(increvable)* coils; Belot's tubestands provided with early protective shields; and the first French-made generator with a rotary switch. A typical feature of Gaiffe apparatus was

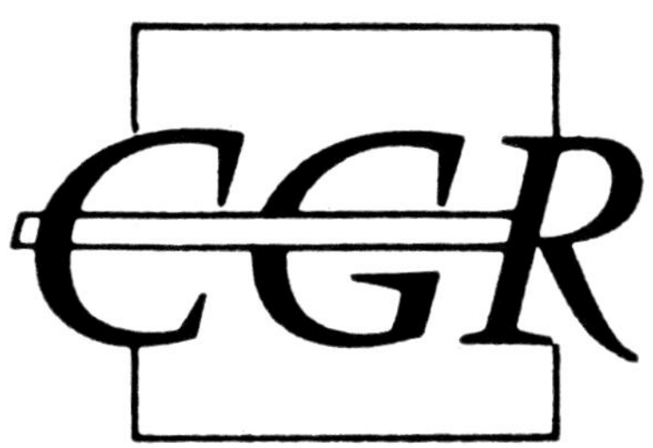

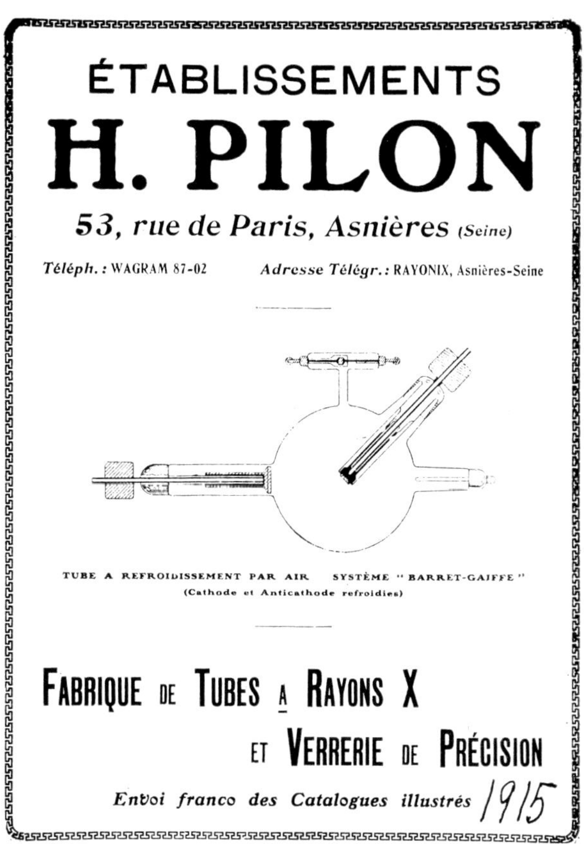

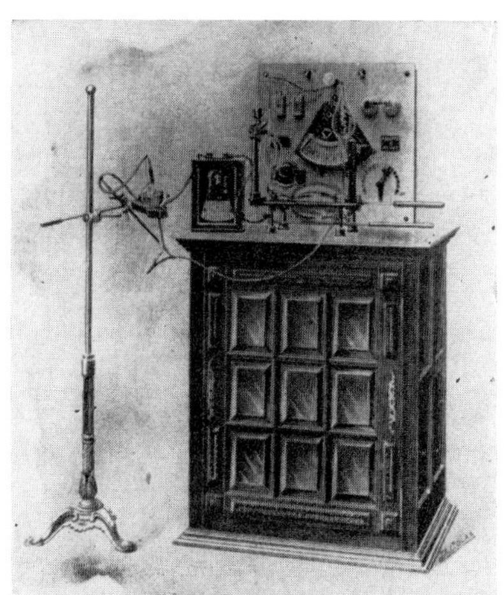

MEUBLE D'ARSONVAL-GAIFFE.

the large triangular measuring instrument on the panel. Georges Gallot (1864-1939), after having worked as a technician for d'Arsonval, was employed by Gaiffe, and became the company's sales manager. On January 1, 1914 Georges Gaiffe went into retirement. Gallot & Cie was created, and took over the physical and moral assets of Gaiffe's company. A few months later, at the beginning of hostilities in World War I, Gallot received from the War Ministry orders for radiologic automobiles, and delivered the first six of them within a few weeks. He built other "military" items, such as the portable *meuble* Ledoux-Lebard-Teilhard, and various foreign body localizers (Hirtz's Compass, Bergonié's Electro-Vibrator).

The Établissements H. Pilon, founded at Clichy in 1911 as an incandescent lamp factory, began to manufacture x-ray tubes in 1912. In the same year, with Belot's help, they brought out tubes with anti-cathodic mirrors made of tungsten, and Belot demonstrated these new tubes in December, 1912 before the Radiologic Society in Paris. In 1917, Pilon was incorporated, and in 1919 a merger led to the Société Gaiffe-Gallot & Pilon (GGP), with the advantage of being able to cover the construction of the major parts of x-ray apparatus, *i.e.*, transformer, table, as well as tubes. In the ensuing ten years GGP modernized many items, from the immersion of x-ray tubes into oil-filled protective housings to the creation of provincial branch offices (the first one in 1922), and from building a continuous current 500 kvp transformer for the "atomic" experiments of physicist Jean Baptiste Perrin (1870-1942) to the "innovation" of autonomous units for all sizes of pri-

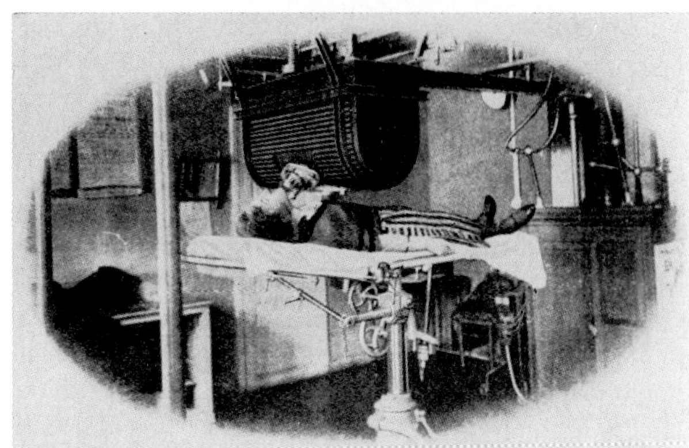

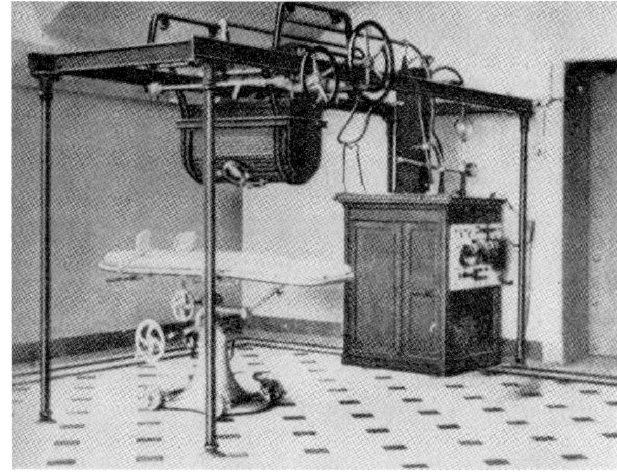

GGP THERAPY. *Bridge-supported oil-filled housing.*

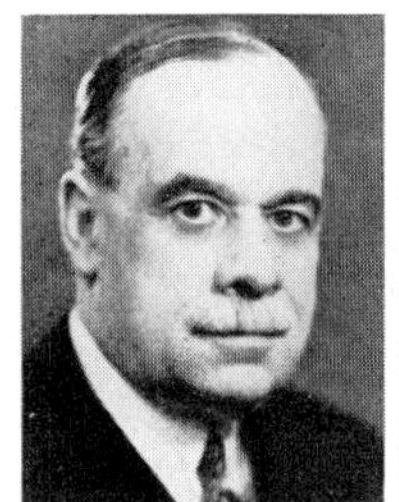

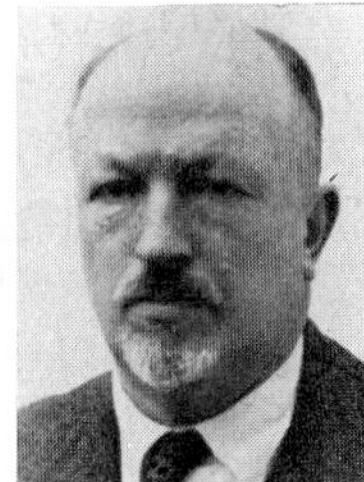

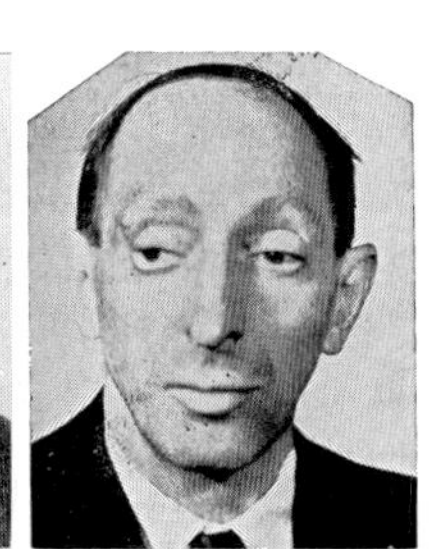

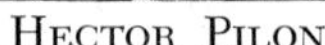

HECTOR PILON ISER SOLOMON EDOUARD CHÉRIGIÉ

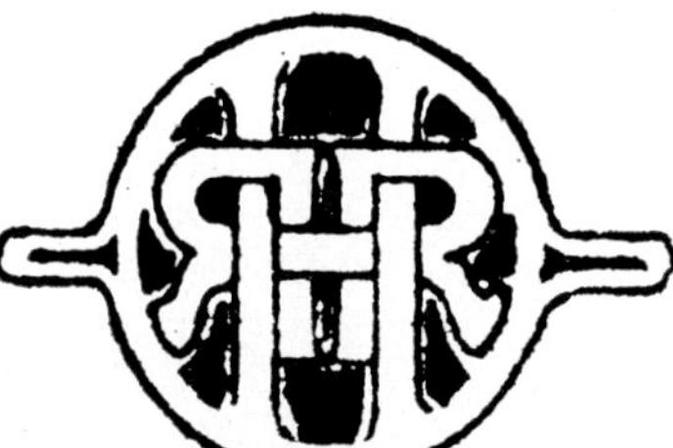

EARLY SEALS. Hector Pilon's trade-mark is easily recognized. The monogrammed RHR stands for Ropiquet, Hazart, and Roycourt. Hector Pilon's seal was maintained also after the merger into Gaiffe, Gallot & Pilon, indeed it can be found right after World War I in a highly stylized version surrounding a gas tube. All these early advertisements and seals have been culled from the commercial pages of the *Journal de Radiologie et d'Electrologie* published by the venerable Masson & Cie in Paris.

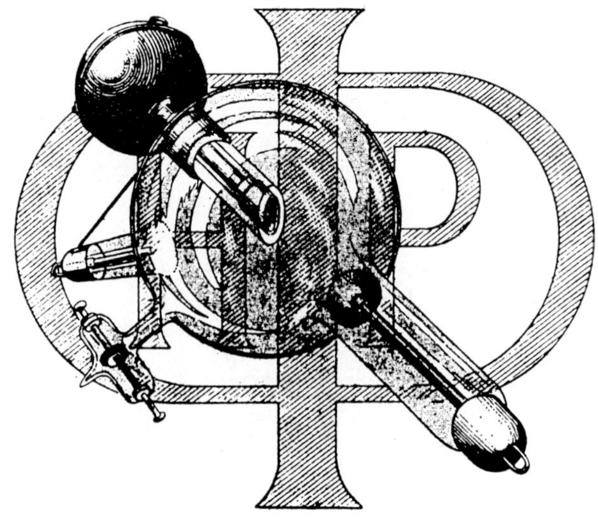

vate offices. GGP made also Henri Béclère's first Sélecteur (a spotfilm device); Nuytten's Tachygraph; a double oscillating Bucky-Potter diaphragm; and a device for hyper-stereo-radiography.

In 1891, Louis Bonnetti began building electrostatic influence machines for electrotherapy – since 1896 also for the production of x rays. His successor in 1901 was Eugène Roycourt who gave the enterprise an industrial character; he built in 1910 (for P. Villars and Abraham) an enormous static machine, with 20 discs of one meter each, which rotated at 1400 RPM, producing a potential of 500 kvp, capable of delivering 5 ma at 200 kvp continuously. Eugène died in 1912, and was succeeded by his son, Henri Roycourt.

At Amiens the pharmacist Claude Ropiquet was interested in electrical items since 1898, and built a mercury interrupter for (the primary of) a coil. Ropiquet had been in good relations with Eugène Roycourt since 1908. In 1919 a merger took place – with the help of a financier by the name of Hazart – and the Société Ropiquet, Hazart & Roycourt was born. In their first ten years, RHR created the Ionometer of Iser Solomon (about 1,500 of them were sold, and some are still in operation); France's first flat Bucky; and the tubestand for deep radium therapy at the Institut du Radium in Paris.

ROPIQUET, HAZART & ROYCOURT
Avenue d'Orléans, 71 — PARIS
USINE A AMIENS

Matériel ROPIQUET
pour le RADIODIAGNOSTIC et la
RADIOTHÉRAPIE PÉNÉTRANTE

BOBINES — INTERRUPTEURS — SUPPORTS D'AMPOULES
CHASSIS — TABLES pour Examens

IONOMÈTRE DU Dr SOLOMON
ÉLECTROTHÉRAPIE — HAUTE FREQUENCE
Machines ÉLECTROSTATIQUES ROYCOURT-BONETTI

In 1930, GGP and RHR merged, and thus the Compagnie Générale de Radiologie (CGR) was born. The CGR is a subsidiary of the Compagnie Francaise Thomson-Houston.

During the decade before World War II, they "homogenized" the existing organizations, but already in 1931, for the third ICR in Paris, the CGR showed the first French triphasic generator, the Tripharix 1000 ma; and a therapy transformer, the Janus, which could deliver 400 kvp of constant (or 600 kvp of pulsating) current. The self-protected twin-focus tube Roburix, and the oil-immersed tube-transformer combination called Securix appeared (the latter was used in the light fluoroscopic unit Clinix). After the advent of tomography, CGR built the (horizontal, linear) Oscillostrator, then the (vertical) Stratix. In 1938 the CGR made the first French rotating anode tube, the Movix. A 200 kvp 8 ma single therapy (transformer and tube in oil) bloc was supported by twin heavy columns. Finally they built a 600 kvp neutron generator for Joliot-Curie. World War II followed with its inevitable period of "hibernation."

Today the CGR, with about 1300 employees, is a strong organization, fully adjusted to the rigors of the Atomic Phase. In looking back over the *palmarès* (batting record), which combines also those of GGP and RHR, as well as CGR's own, a few dates ought to be mentioned:

First radiologic Belot bed (table) in 1907; Estenave's stereo-radiograph in 1908; Delherm's orthodiagraph in 1912; Belot's 100 mm therapy tube in 1912; first self-rectifying Coolidge tube in 1914; first oil-immersed, both shock-and radiation-proof 200 kvp therapy tube in 1919; a motor-driven tilting table in 1927; Simone

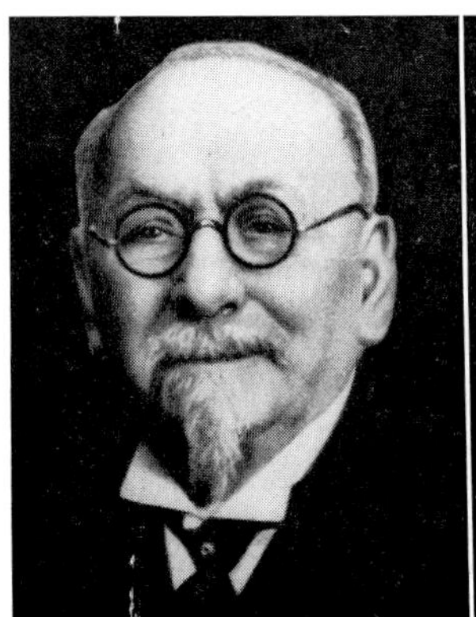
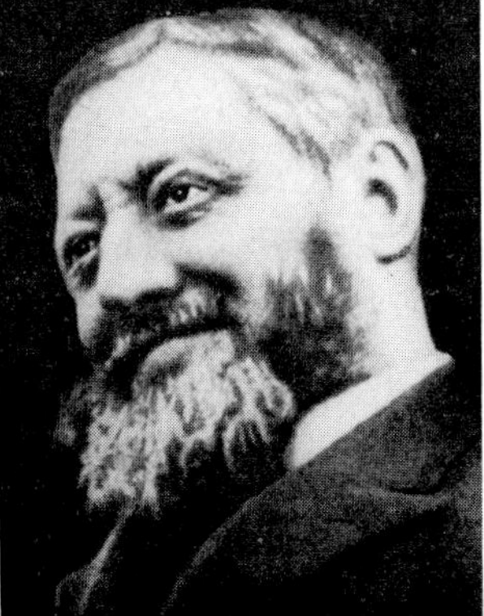

Georges Gaiffe & Georges Gallot.

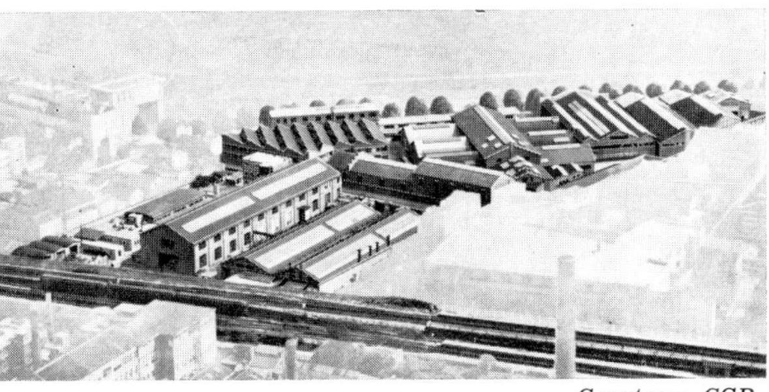

Courtesy: CGR.

Usines CGR. The plant, located at Issy-les-Moulineaux, used to be an airplane factory. It was purchased by CGR in 1949, and transfer of all equipment and machines to the new location was completed within less than one year.

Laborde's telecurietherapy apparatus in 1928; first water-cooled 100 kvp Coolidge tube in 1928; Dauvillier's rotating crystal spectrograph in 1929; first 300 kvp 3 ma Coolidge tube, and first 300 kvp pulsating current therapy generator in 1930; Delherm and Thoyer Rozat's kymograph in 1933; Super-Lumenix screen with zinc sulfate in 1937; Camerix for photo-fluorography in 1939; same, but with Odelca mirror camera, the Odelcamerix in 1953.*

From 1955 to the end of 1960, the general manager of CGR was Eugène Fournier, who had started with GGP in 1920. After his retirement, the top job went to Roger, who until then had been CGR's sales manager, as an illustration of the fact that (rightly or wrongly) Public Relations seems to be currently the most important aspect of any large industrial production. CGR carries a complete line of x-ray equipment. Since 1950, their plant is at Issy-les-Moulineaux (Southwest of Paris).

The race for bigger transformers demands corresponding increases in x-ray tube ratings. In fact, the various so-called automatic devices included in modern control stands are intented to protect the under-sized tube from the transformer's king-sized power. In 1947 CGR re-issued its pre-war rotating anode tube, the Movix (production had been interrupted during the war), and research started on a new model. It came out in 1957 as the Juvenix (always young and potent), followed in 1959 by the Juvenix-Record and Juvenix-Flash, with "thermically black" anodes, which rotate at 9000 RPM, and take up to 75 kw at 160 kvp. The Emitor, a cold emission valve, first built in 1959, can rectify (single-phase) tensions up to 175 kvp.

*This material was gathered from a beautifully printed brochure, issued by the CGR on the 100th anniversary of Gaiffe's opening of his first shop. That brochure has, in the guise of introduction, a sentence from the preface to the *Légende des Siècles* (1857): *On y trouvera quelque chose du passé, quelque chose du présent et comme un vague mirage de l'avenir* (one will find therein something from the past, something from the present, and a vague glimpse of the future). The volume lives up to its motto.

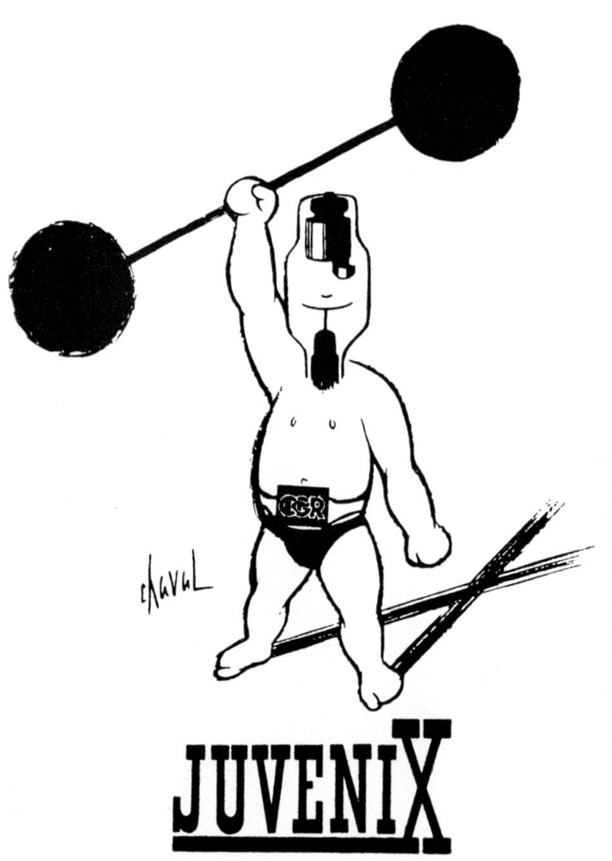

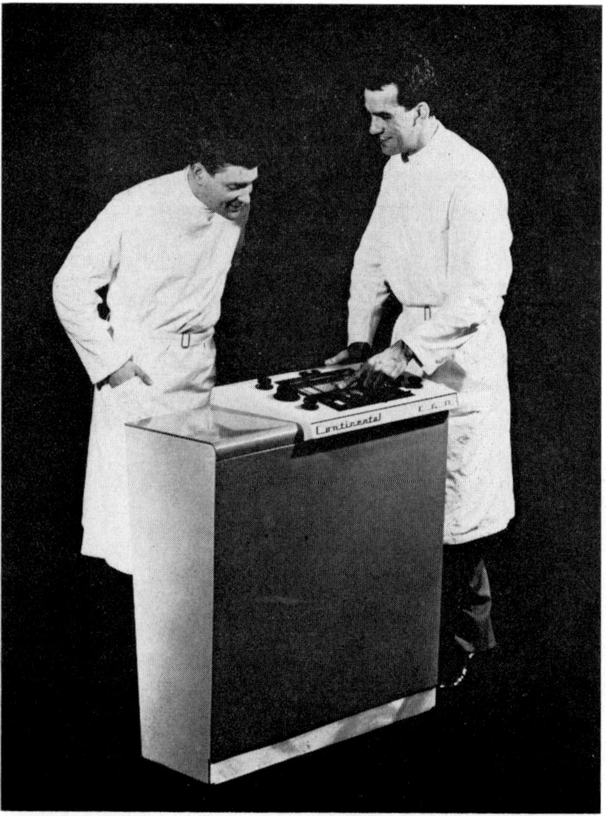

Courtesy: CGR.

CGR's CONTINENTAL. Highly automatized control stand of CGR's most potent triphasic transformer, rated at up to 1600 ma or 160 kvp. Like all other CGR equipment, it has simple, elegant lines, and comes in decorator colors.

Chenonceaux is the name of a four-valve transformer, first built in 1944; current versions go to 300 ma and 130 kvp. Langeais is the next largest with up to 500 ma and 130 kvp; Elysee has maximum ratings of 1200 ma or 160 kvp; finally, the triphasic Continental can deliver 1600 ma or 160 kvp.

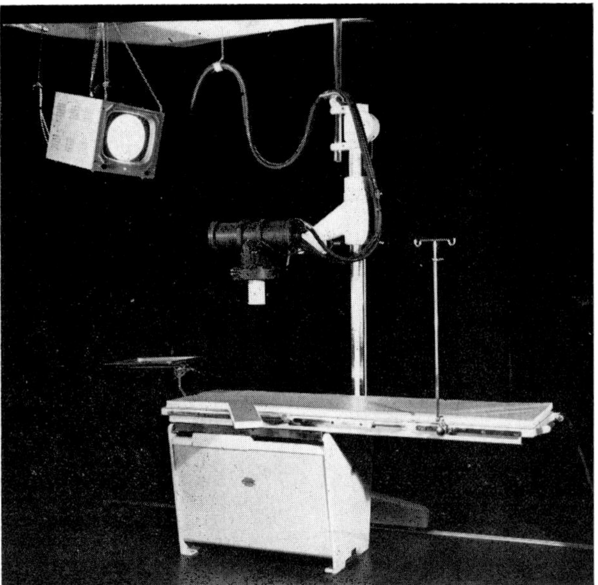

Courtesy: CGR.

CGR's NAVARRE. It has the "floating top" of the Koordinat, but the image intensifier tube is under-the-table. Note the television monitor suspended in properly tilted position.

CGR tables come in various editions, from the relatively simple Alsace, Ile-de-France, and Lorraine, to the 90/90 Champagne. Navarre has a sliding top, and is also in other respects similar to the Koordinat of Elema-Schonander. They use ceiling-floor tubestands, as well as ceiling-counterbalanced screen-carriers with automated spotfilm devices.

Among CGR's special tables is Dulac's Craniograph, the first such device with built-in tomographic motion. Princeps is vaguely reminiscent of Elema-Schonander's Mimer. Tomography is available also as a simple table attachment, connected to CGR's telescopic ceiling tubestand. They sell Vulpian's transverse body section device, the Pantomix. CGR has adapted the Odelca mirror camera to vertical (Stratodelca) as well as to horizontal (Tomodelca) layer radiography. Elbow Odelcas have also been used on Bucky tables (Gridiodelca), and

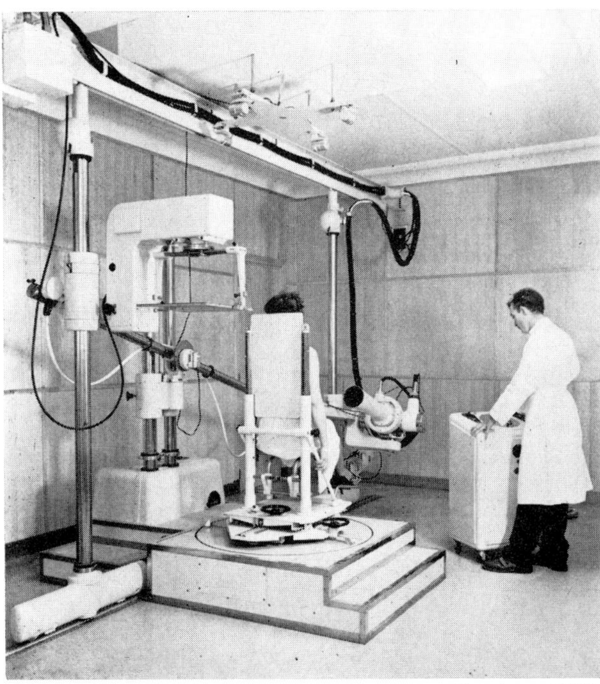

Courtesy: CGR.

CGR's PANTOMIX. Universal three-plane tomographic contraption, by Vulpian, is very impressive but never achieved a significant degree of popularity.

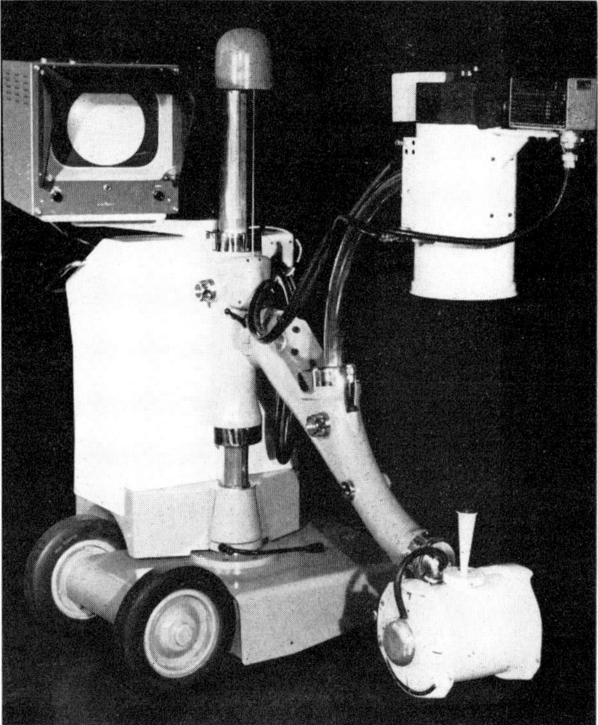

Courtesy: CGR.

CGR's TELECHIROSCOPE. It is designed to bring the blessings of radio-television to the operating room (*chir* is the root of *chirurgie*). The system has a Vidicon pickup tube, which is not as sensitive as the Orthicon, but the latest (French) Thomson-Houston image intensifying tubes have 6000 times brightness gain. One might object to the fixed location of the television monitor (atop the control desk). Bulky as a single unit is, it has the advantage of making away with a lot of cables.

for angiography (Angiodelca). The latter is a bi-plane unit, with twin Odelcas placed at right angles.

Magnilux is the CGR electron-optical image intensifier with the (currently standard) 6000 brightness gain, and with either a 16 or a 22 cm input phosphorus. The image from the output phosphorus is split between a 16 mm movie camera, and the Vidicon tube for connection to the television monitor and, if desired to a video tape recorder. When the Magnilux is combined with CGR's mobile unit Saphir (up to 200 ma), the result is called AC 80. When a television monitor is mounted on the same chassis, it becomes the (surgically convenient) Telechiroscop.

The Magnilux was also combined with the Craniograph for encephalography; and with the Navarre for angiocardiography. Magnilux on the Champagne, with the addition of remote control, of a monitoring stand atop the instrument panel, and of a lead glass divider, resulted in CGR's Explorateur Magister for *radio-diagnostic telecommandé* — including, of course, *radiotélévision* as well as *radiocinéma.*

The Bellatrix is a 5-90 kvp therapy tube head, the Intrix a contact device. A 250 kvp 12 ma radiotherapy machine is also available, in a fixed (Vega), as well as in a rotational (Antares) arrangement.

Courtesy: CGR.

CGR's MAGISTER I. It is basically the 90/90 Champagne table, with servo-motorized motions, shoulder-suspension, and under-the-table image intensifier.

Since 1955 they sell the CGR diffractometer, which is a goniometer with Geiger counter, and a monochromatic Guinier quartz blade, for radiocrystallography. They also build apparatus for radiometallography, and they make and sell (as a by-product of their own research toward attaining proper vacuum) a number of vacuum pumps.

CGR's house publications began with Gaiffe's monthly review, which appeared in twenty-three issues between March, 1910 and November, 1913. Gallot continued it since April, 1914, had to stop it during World War I, came out with it in November, 1917, but discontinued publication in 1918. Between 1922 and 1930 it appeared as the *Revue de la GGP,* and from 1930 to

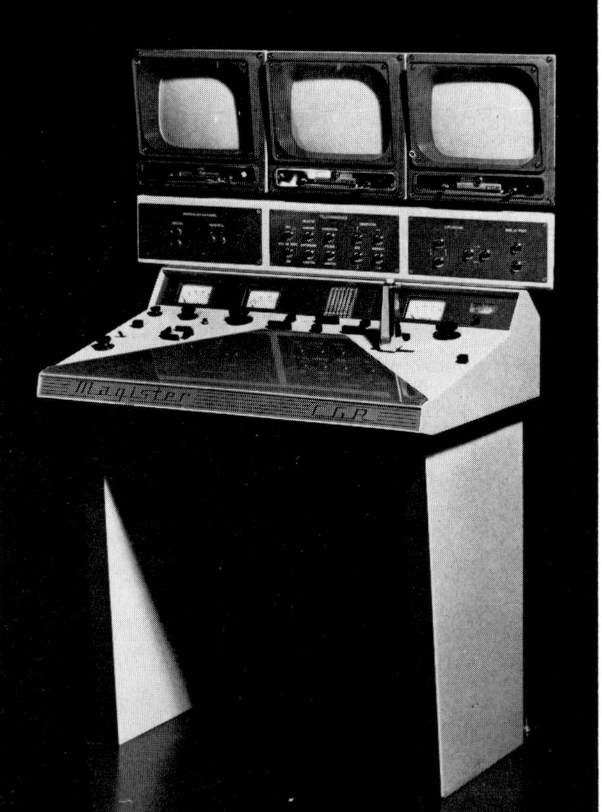

Courtesy: CGR.

CGR's MAGISTER II. The simple lines of this beautiful control desk resemble those of a Dior nightgown (of the evening dress variety). Note the push-buttons for remote control of the table. There is also a television monitor for visual control of the patient, thus obviating the need for an interconnecting "picture window". The desk, which comes in decorator colors, is almost as complicated as an airplane's cockpit — one can use dual instruction before operating it. And yet, this may very likely become the way of the future.

135 as the *Revue de la CGR.* After the hiatus of World War II, it re-appeared in 1952 as the *Rayonixar,* then returned to the name *Revue CGR* in 1954. It is lavishly published, but remains strictly promotional.

ITALY

The "oldest continuous name" among Italian manufacturers of x-ray equipment derives from Luigi Gorla, who began making electro-medical equipment in 1889.

Gorla's earliest (preserved) x-ray ad of 1896 is reproduced in the first chapter of this text. He founded the Luigi Gorla & Co. around the turn of the century. The firm was located at one time at nr. 20 on Lamarmora Street in Milano: this address is given in their 1913-14 catalog, in which are advertised Gundelach tubes. Gorla offered in the same catalog items manufactured in his own shop, for instance a peculiar seat, used for both fluoroscopy and radiography (price 500 Lire). He was also selling a portable, patented by U. Magini (an engineer), consisting of a hand-cranked electrical motor, a coil, and a gas tube mounted on a long wooden shaft; both the tube, and the *criptoscopio* could be stored in the box which contained the motor (price of this portable: 1500 Lire).

After World War I, Gorla no longer sold Gundelach tubes (Gundelach's Italian representative at the time was a certain Theodor Mohwinkel of Milano). In 1922,

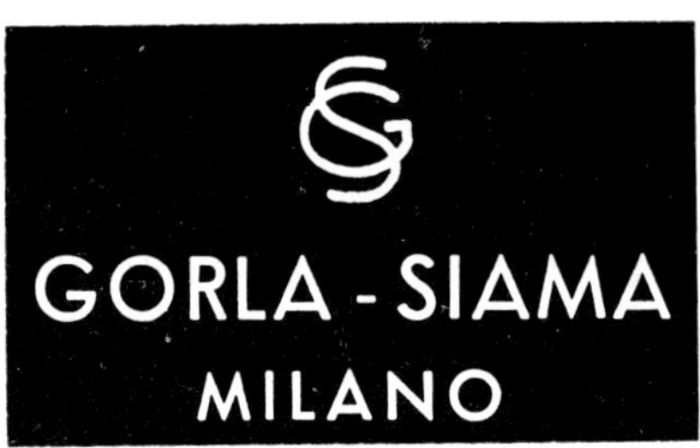

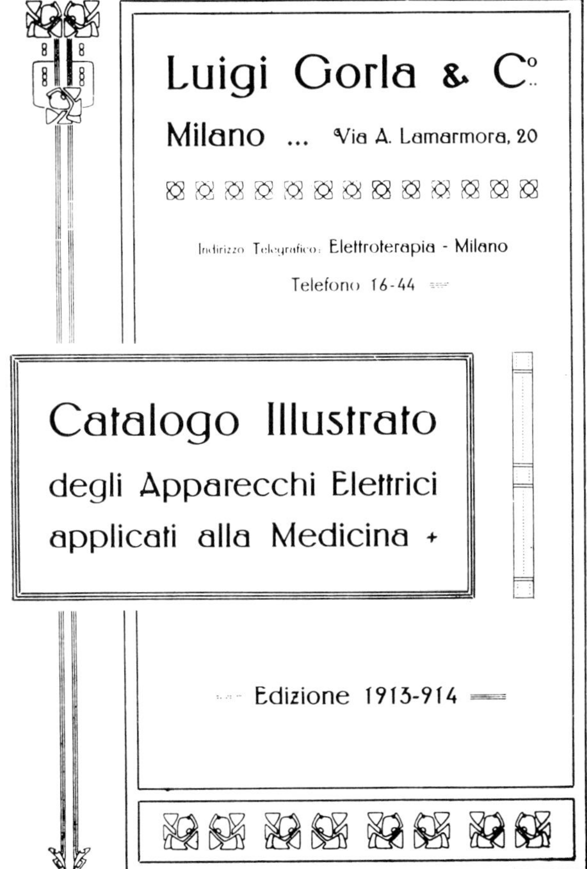

Luigi Gorla & C°

Milano ... Via A. Lamarmora, 20

Indirizzo Telegrafico: Elettroterapia - Milano

Telefono 16-44

Catalogo Illustrato

degli Apparecchi Elettrici

applicati alla Medicina

Edizione 1913-914

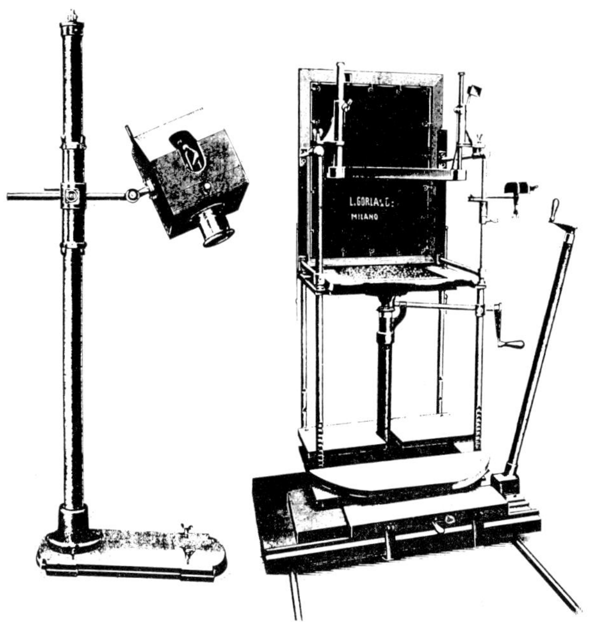

Courtesy: Gorla-Siama.

GORLA X-RAY EQUIPMENT (1913). The chair (price: 500 Lire) served for both fluoroscopy and radiography; note the frame provided for the fluorescent screen; the handcrank served to raise and lower the seat. The tube-stand (price: 450 Lire) came with the tube housing, movable diaphragm, and insulated compressor tube.

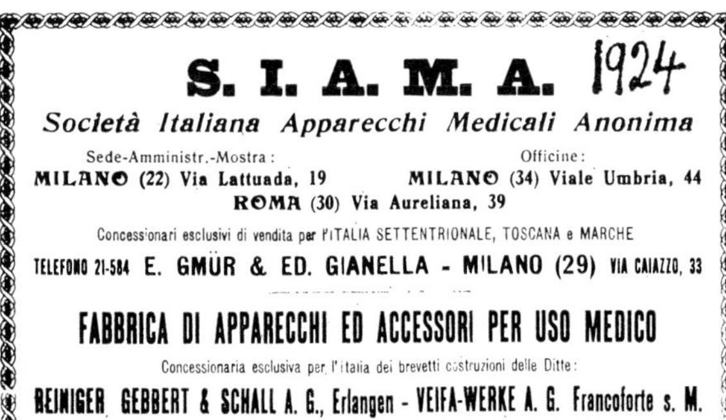

Gorla's firm was incorporated, thus acquiring the tail-piece SA (SA=*società anonima*). Business picked up, and in 1924 their biggest item was a combination therapy and diagnosis 250 kvp transformer eponymized for Scotti Brioschi. In the late 1920s the Big Depression supervened, and with it came the mergers.

SIAMA (Società Italiana Apparecchi Medicali Anonima) was a subsidiary of the German firms Reiniger, Gebbert & Schall, and Veifa. The electro-medical section of Siemens & Halske had its own representation in Milano. In 1929 – in Italy – SIAMA bought out Gorla, and in 1933 – in Germany – the above mentioned three firms merged into the SRW. In the meantime, Gorla-Siama had maintained its position, for instance in 1934 their two most advertised items were a portable, the Poliwatt, and a four-valve transformer called Neotetraval.

Today Gorla-Siama imports both SRW and Elema-Schönander equipment. In addition, in their Milano plant, Gorla-Siama manufactures certain apparatus, such as selenium-rectified transformers, up to the Selenix Gama 1000 (1000 ma at 50 kvp, or 125 ma at 150 kvp). Teleclinografo is one of their tables (15° Trendelenburg). They make a telescopic ceiling tube mount. The Monopan, a 6-60 kvp therapy apparatus, is advertised for what in Italy (and in France) is called *plesioterapia:* the term comes from the Greek vocable for striking (hitting), and implies that high local dosage of ionizing radiation acts similarly to a finger used on a percussion instrument (piano).

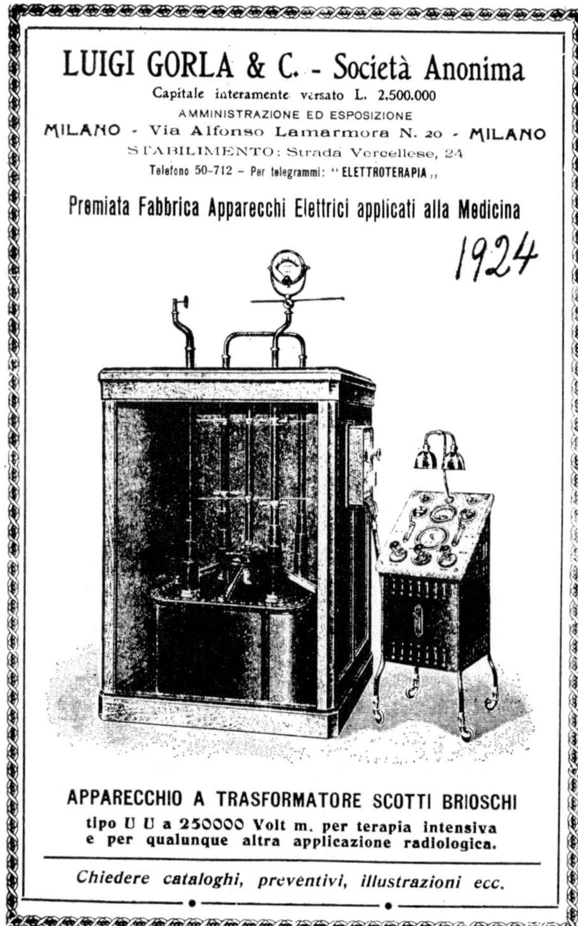

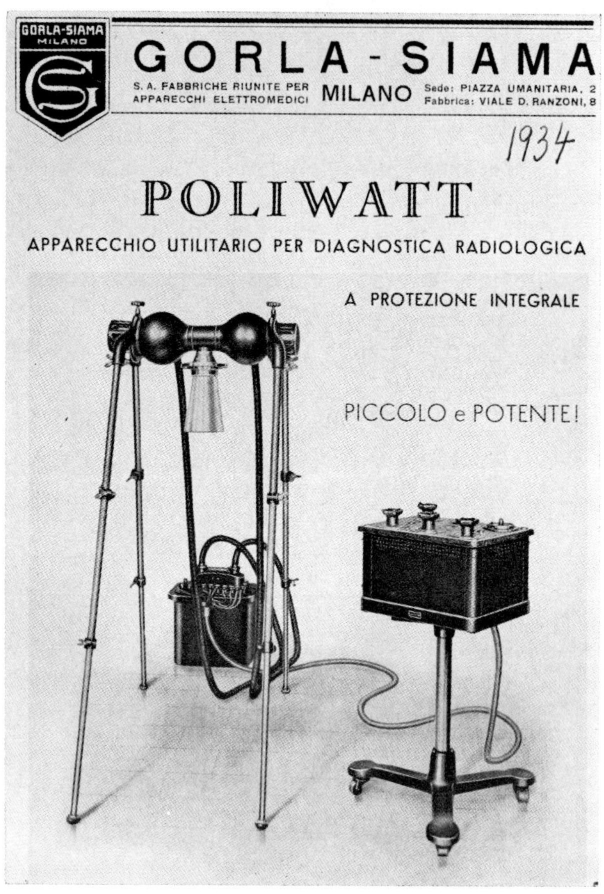

ITALIAN BYGONES

The casualty rate among Italian x-ray firms was comparable to, if not higher than, that found in other countries.

The second-oldest Italian manufacturer of electromedical equipment, A. Meschia in Milano, made the Ideal, a 100 ma transformer for diagnostic purposes, and all sorts of *trocoscopi, schermi* (screens) and

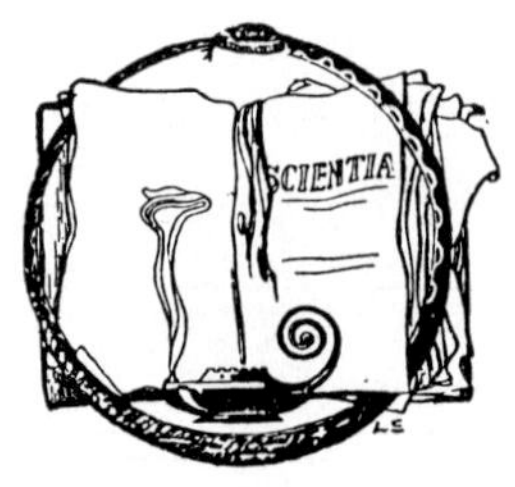

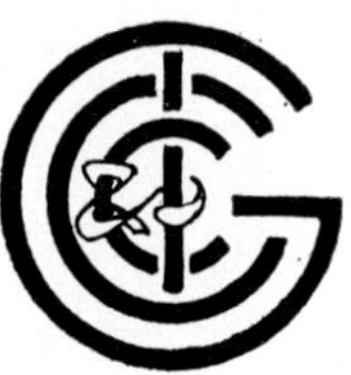

stativi murali (wallstands). Meschia also represented the now defunct tube factory Radiologie of Berlin.

The SA Giulio Cardolle of Torino had in 1923 the Beta transformer, with 250 kvp, giving 100 ma at 10 cm. spark for diagnosis, or 3 ma at 42 cm. spark for therapy. Their Alpha was a diagnostic transformer (with provision for up to 160 kvp therapy), Gamma a 300 kvp therapy machine, Omega a portable, Sigma (and dental Sigma) exclusively for use with Coolidge tubes. Cardolle's trade-mark was an open book showing their telegraphic address, the symbolic Scientia, illuminated by an Aladdin type of lamp.

In the 1930s, the Electromedical Section of Ing. Giampiero Clerici & Co. (with a rounded monogram framed by a capital G) manufactured in Milano a full line of x-ray equipment, from a portable (60 kvp at 30 ma) to DV6, a diagnostic triphasic (100 kvp at 600 ma), and TVC6, a triphasic for therapy with six valves and two condensers (10 ma at 250 kvp).

The Ampolla Itala in Rome and the Soffieria Monti in Milano made x-ray tubes. Müller of Hamburg and Philips were separately represented, the latter by a Metalix subsidiary. Among the importers, Enrico Gmür & Eduardo Gianella represented mostly German firms. The J. Iten & Co. — a printer gremlin mistreated the spelling in the ad — located likewise in Milano, brought in American apparatus; at one time they advertised Acme equipment.

Among obsolete names of Italian contrast media are Pielofanina, Colefanina, and Toriofanina, prepared by Carlo Erba SA, a Milanese drug firm which, contrary

APPARECCHI RADIOLOGICI

A. MESCHIA & C.

Un'antica marca
Una rinnovata organizzazione
Una moderna attrezzatura

Al servizio della Radiologia Italiana

1950

Sede e stabilimento:
MILANO - Piazza Napoli, 7
Telefono: 470.294

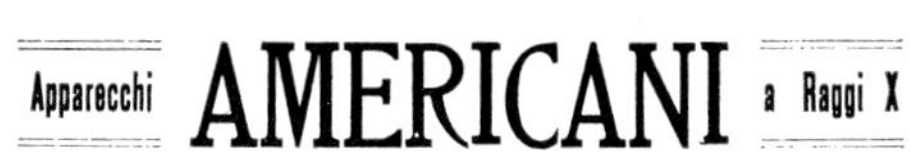

DIAGNOSTICA - TERAPIA

DIAFRAMMA POTTER BUCKY

CHASSIS IN ALLUMINIO

SCHERMI di RINFORZO PATTERSON

TUBI COOLIDGE

Ingegneri specializzati per l'impianto

I. JTEN & C.
Installazioni a Raggi X & Elettro-Medicali
MILANO
VIA TORINO, 47

1926

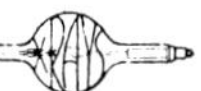

PIELOFANINA "ERBA"
per la pielografia endovenosa
Boccetta da gr. 20 di polvere
Fiale da cc. 50 di soluz. al 40%
» » » 20 » » » 70%
per la pielografia strumentale
Fiale da cc. 12 di soluz. al 20%

COLEFANINA "ERBA"
per la colecistografia orale
Metodo di somministrazione unica
Boccette da una dose
Metodo di somministrazione frazionata
Scatola per un esame

NOVIBARIUM "ERBA"
per la visualizzazione
delle pliche dello stomaco
Bario solfato con speciali doti di adesività e sospensività
Pacchi da Kg. 1

TORIOFANINA "ERBA"
per epato-splenografia endovenosa
Fiale da cc. 20
per la visualizzazione
delle pliche intestinali
Boccette da gr. 200

1935

CARLO ERBA S. A. - MILANO

to those previously mentioned in this section, is still very much in business.

RANGONI & PURICELLI

This is today the second-oldest Italian x-ray firm. Ugo Rangoni started his activities in 1910 as a Siemens representative. In 1914 he became a Gorla representative, and in 1920 he opened, on the side, a small shop in which he built x-ray accessories, including orthoscopes and trochoscopes. His seal was U.R.B. (Ugo Rangoni, Bologna).

In 1927, Edgardo Rangoni (Ugo's son) and Davide Puricelli (at the time Gorla's chief-engineer) created the Società Ugo Rangoni di Rangoni e Puricelli, with offices and plant in Bologna on Via Arienti 40, where it

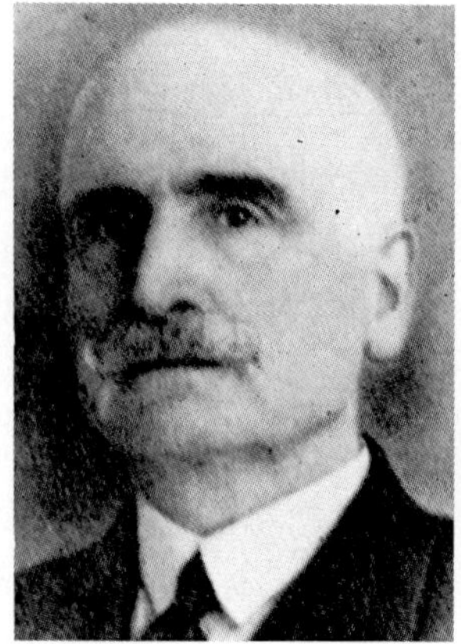

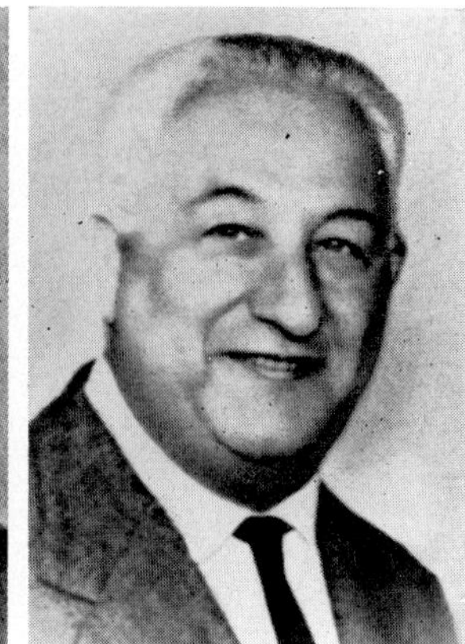

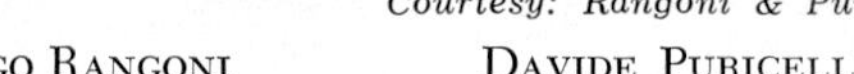

Courtesy: Rangoni & Puricelli.

UGO RANGONI DAVIDE PURICELLI

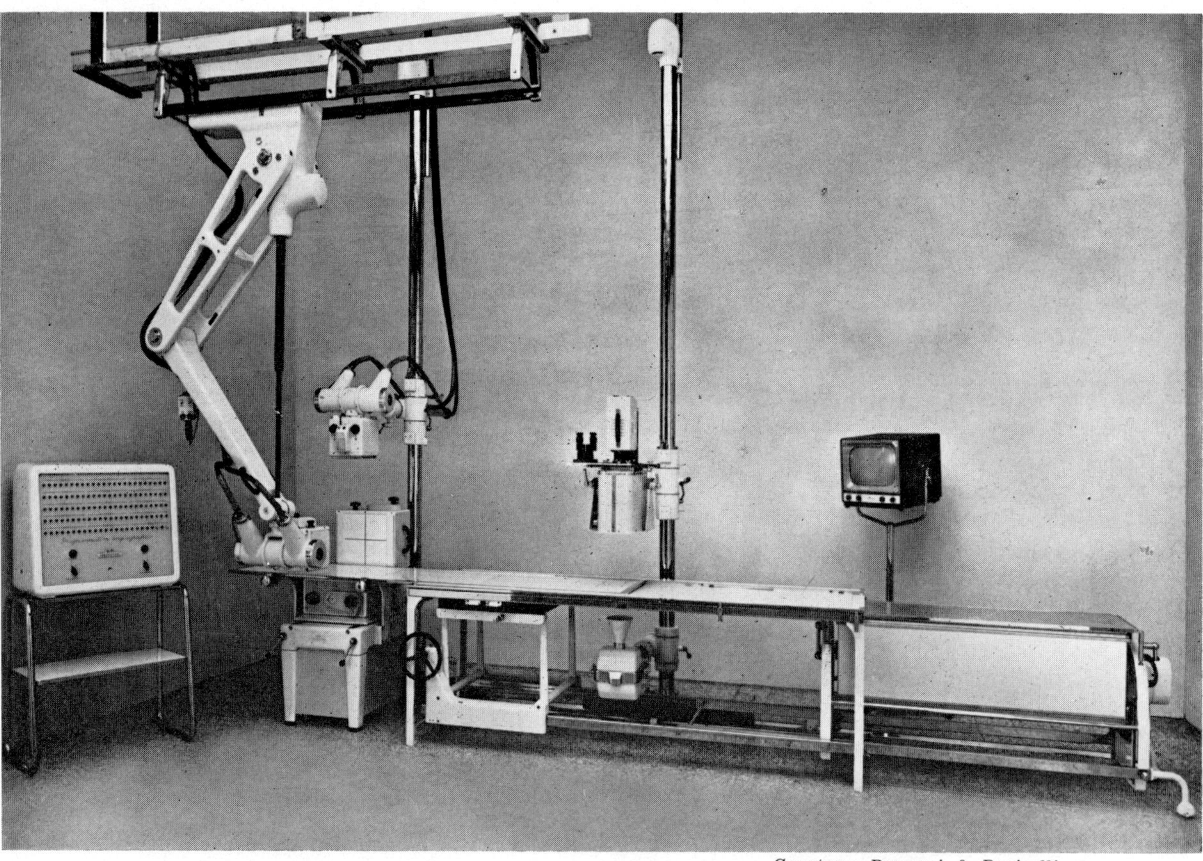

Courtesy: Rangoni & Puricelli.

R & P ANGIOGRAPHIC UNIT. The table has a sliding top, as well as provision for magnification radiography. Patient is first fluoroscoped (using image intensification and television monitoring), such as during insertion of needles or catheters. For peripheral angiography, table top with patient is moved over the long cassette changer (Angioskelograf). For heart or brain work, the table slides to the left, over the bi-plane Angioseriograf II. Note the twin tubes, one of which is supported by motorized jointed-arms (resembling Balteau's Zodiaque II). The contraption at the far left is an angio-programmer, to make the exposures at the precise pre-set moment.

was to remain until 1947. The firm was incorporated as Rangoni & Puricelli in 1935.

R & P's Righi Standard was a mechanical rectifier used for both diagnosis (500 ma at 65 kvp, or 200 ma at 110 kvp, or 100 ma at 115 kvp) and therapy (10 ma at 140 kvp). Duplex was a mobile unit, both shock and radiation-protected, with two tubes, alternately energized by a single auto-transformer — the apparatus was described by V. Putti in *Chirurgia degli Organi in Movimento* of June, 1938.

R & P's four-valve transformer is called Tetravalvo. Today's models are the Tetradyn S (500 ma at 110 kvp, maximum 130 kvp) and Supertetradyn, of which there are two versions, 1000 ma at 60 kvp (maximum 130 kvp) and 1000 ma at 100 kvp (maximum 150 kvp). They have also a triphasic with Selenium rectifiers called Triseledyn (700 ma at 60 kvp, maximum 140 kvp). They still manufacture upright fluoroscopes, for instance the Ortoscopio. Troco-radiostratigrafo is a combination horizontal Bucky table and tomograph. Their latest Duoscop has both a 90/15 and a 90/90 model.

Since 1955 R & P make all sorts of equipment for angiography. Their Securix table has a sliding top (like the Swedish Koordinat), which may be combined with a single-plane changer (Angiocraniografo), or with a biplane changer (they come with either cassettes or rollfilm). The changer can be placed at the end of the Securix table, to take advantage of the sliding top. An image intensifier, and a television monitor, have also been adapted to R & P equipment*

*This information was courteously supplied by Giacomo A. Garuzzi, one of the directors of R & P.

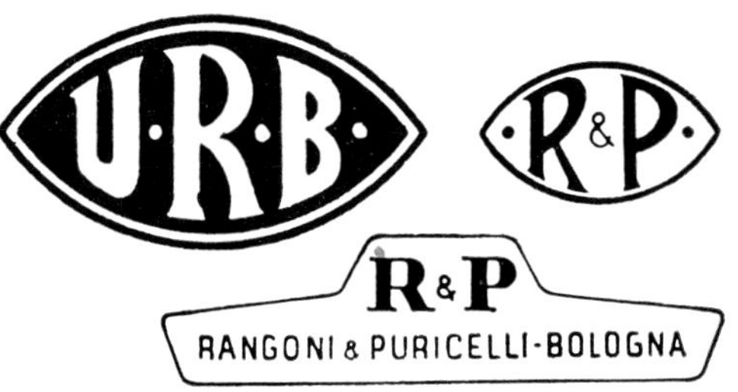

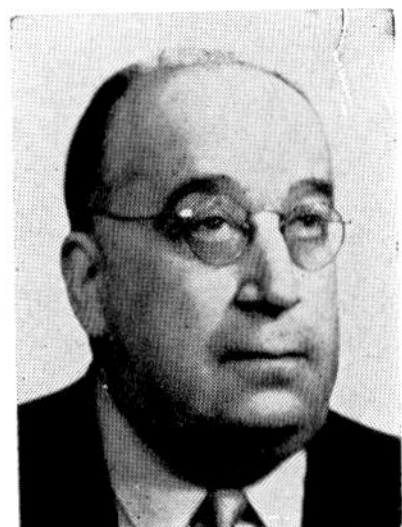
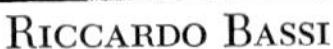
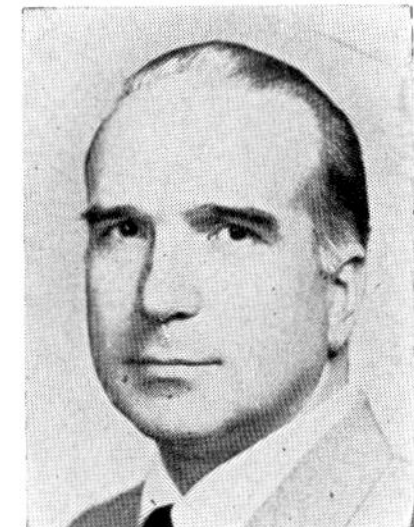

RICCARDO BASSI CARLO RANGONI

Officials of R & P

BARAZZETTI

This firm was founded in 1931 by Giuseppe Barazzetti, who started out as a constructor of Bucky-Potter diaphragms.

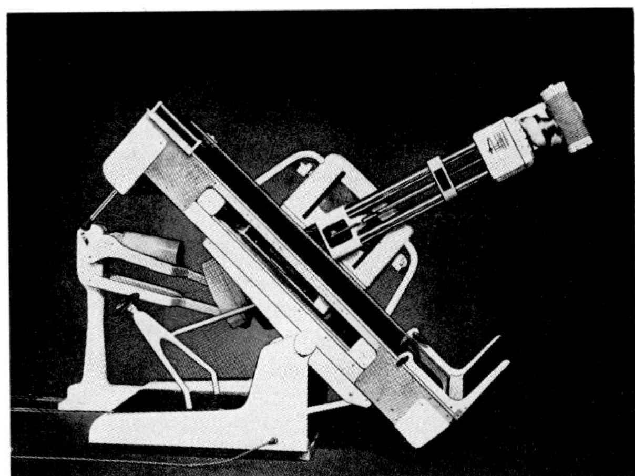

Courtesy: Picker.

BARAZZETTI'S GONIOTOMO. Two-plane tomographic unit, sold at one time also as the Picker Goniotome (Barazzetti didn't mind, as long as he got his money), as well as by the Exal (Picker's London representative). Actually, most Italian manufacturers lose money on x-ray tables, but make them to sell the other, more renumerative items, such as transformers or Bucky diaphragms.

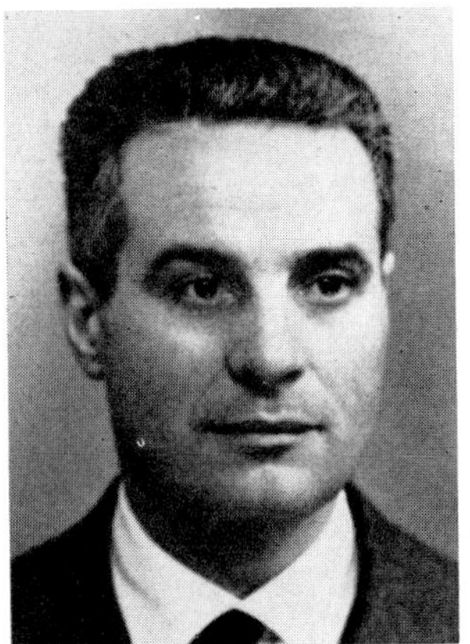
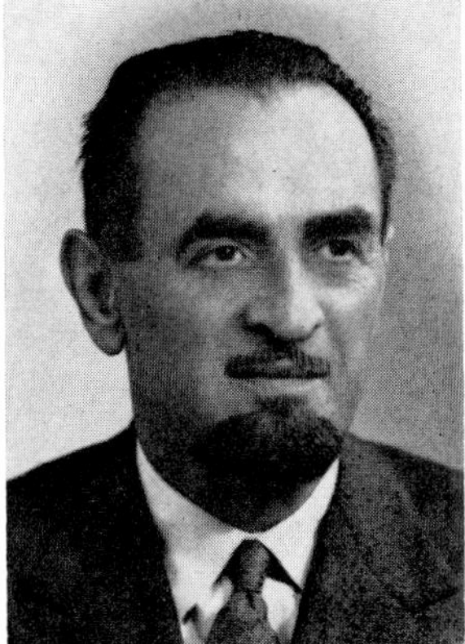

GIUSEPPE BARAZZETTI. He founded his firm in 1931, and in 1937 came to Chicago for the 5th ICR. Barazzetti was very successful in selling Bucky-Potter diaphragms (Philips bought from him over the years over 25 thousand Buckys). He opened a subsidiary in Brussels, and he still owns the Belgian Barazzetti (which makes slightly more than one half of the x-ray equipment purchased in Belgium), but the Italian firm of Barazzetti is now part of Generay. Man with goatee is ALFONSO FRONTINI. Another of the highly skilled, imaginative, and industrious Italian x-ray "artisans."

In 1934, he added a craniograph (patterned after Lysholm's) and a tomograph. Then he combined these two devices, and came out with the Craniotomo, which is still being manufactured. Neotomo is a horizontal, Goniotomo a horizontal and vertical, and Stratix a pluri-directional body section apparatus.

After World War II, Barazzetti expanded again, and began to build tilting tables. Giubileo is a 90/90 model with automatic spot film device Seriomat. The latest table is the Dirigon. Barazzetti's largest transformer is the Esatronic 1000/150, triphasic selenium-rectified, and highly automatized: it can energize five tubes, permits a maximum of 180 kvp, and exposures of three milliseconds.

The Barazzetti factory is located in Monza (a place where auto races are held). They produce a full line of teletherapy equipment, including the CesCoPan, which contains both a Cesium and a Cobalt source.

Barazzetti's latest contribution is a portable, battery-operated unit, which comes also as a mobile (surgical!) model. It is offered in this country by Keleket (Generay's representative): the unit is of the condenser type with 150 kvp maximum rating.

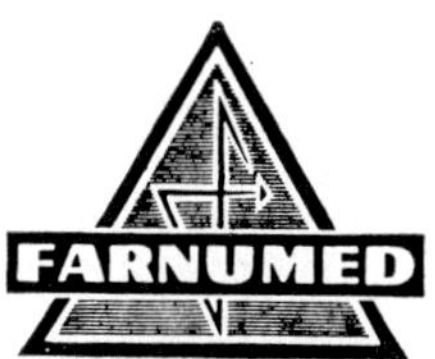

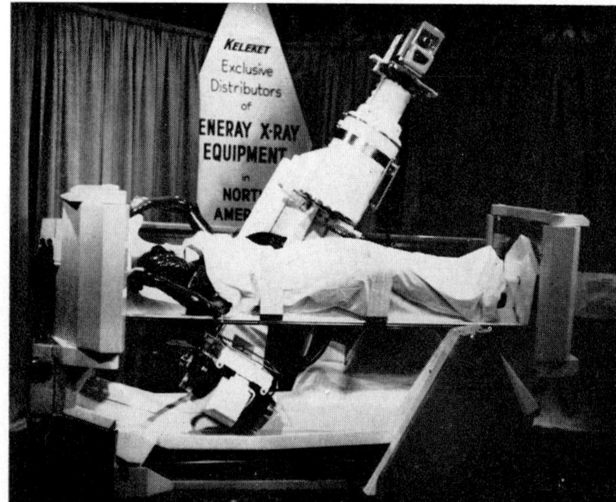

BARAZZETTI'S DIRIGON. After "joining" the Generay, Barazzetti had to prepare something spectacular for the 10th ICR in Montreal, and this was it: a remotely controlled twin-axis contraption, shown here with a mannequin. Keleket is currently Generay's representative in the U. S. A., since Keleket has some difficulties in delivering its own equipment (the Novamatic was "farmed out" to a Belgian manufacturer, with untoward results).

GENERAY

By the end of 1961, a financial organization from Milano - called La Centrale - bought out R & P, Barazzetti, and a firm from Milano called Farnumed - in addition to three x-ray tube factories, Columbus in Milano, Elsi in Palermo, and Fitra in Rome.

The explanation given was the same as in the case of Massiot of Paris. The Common European Market forced everybody in the x-ray business to compete with every other European x-ray manufacturer. To the manufacturer himself, a complete image intensifier-movie camera-television system with remote control and 90/90 table represents an investment of about $50,000, if only material and labor are considered. Besides, things can go wrong, work may have to be repeated or duplicated, and newer models must be designed and so on.

The Centrale permitted each firm to maintain its independence, but they were to pool their patents, dyes, and other manufacturing "secrets." The "merger" was finalized on February 1, 1962, and the resulting firm changed its name to Generay Generale Radiologica (of Milano).

FRONTINI

In 1930, Alfonso Frontini (who was born in 1900) purchased the assets of the J. Iten & Co. of Milano.

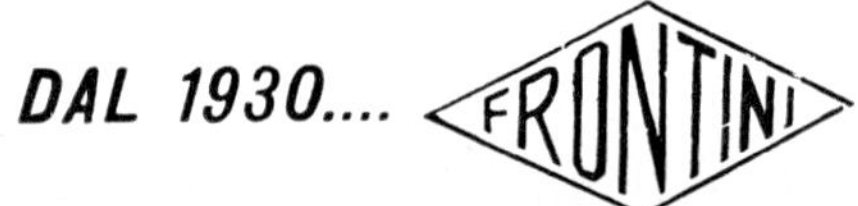

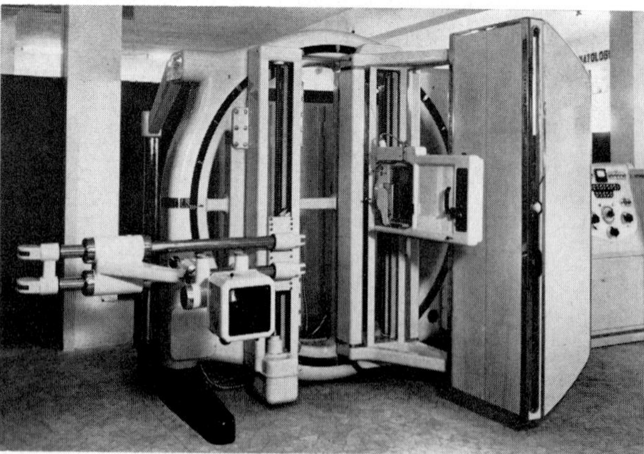

Courtesy:Frontini.

FRONTINI'S PANTOCLINO 180 (1956). Note the pedestal supported ringstand, as it was exhibited at the 33rd Milano Fair.

Of unusual design but very functional is Frontini's Pantoclino 180°, which is a 90-90 table mounted on a circular frame without ceiling support. Its transformer gives 125 kvp and 500 ma as offered especially for neuroradiology. The Pantoclino was first constructed in 1956.

OTHER ITALIAN FIRMS

Body section radiography has always been well thought of in Genova (where Alessandro Vallebona is professor of radiology): in that city is located the firm Zuder, makers of the Pluristrator, a device which permits several rotational and linear motions. The firm's

SG I
nuova
SAN GIORGIO
S.p.A.
GENOVA-SESTRI

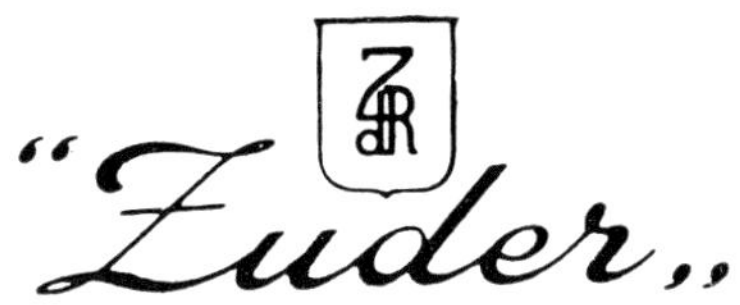

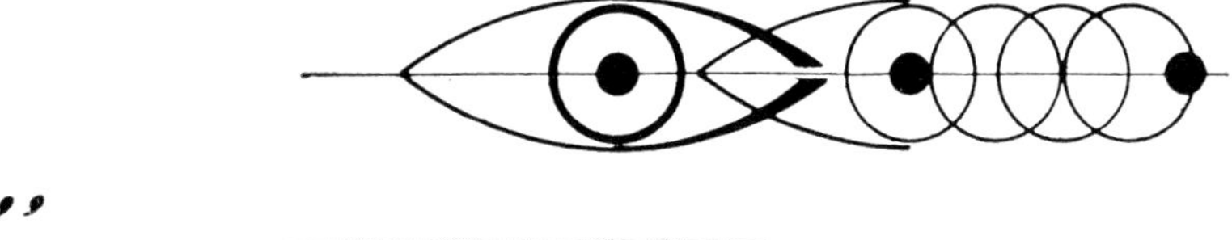

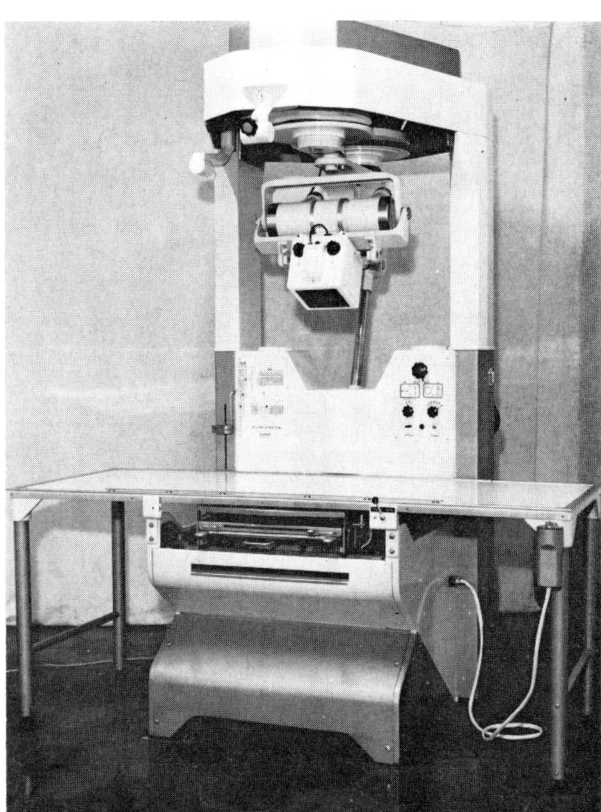

Courtesy: Zuder.

ZUDER'S PLURISTRATOR. This device can be used for circular (rotational) tomography, for unidirectional tomography (either transverse or longitudinal), for simultaneous multilayer technic, for routine (non-tomographic) radiography, even for magnification procedures.

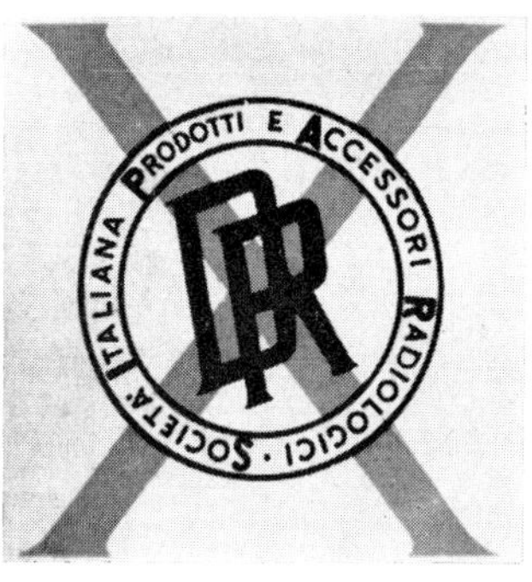

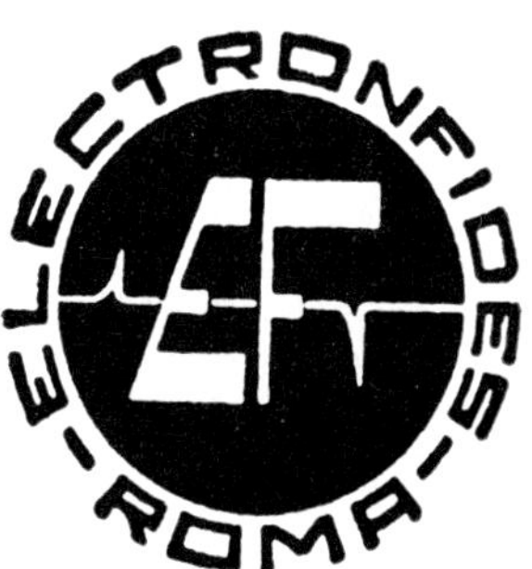

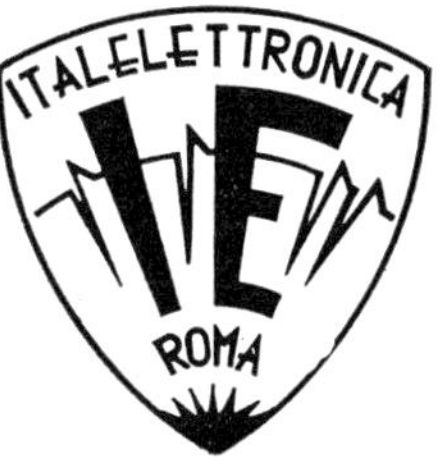

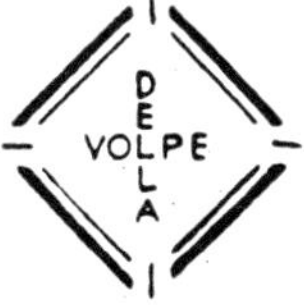

della Volpe

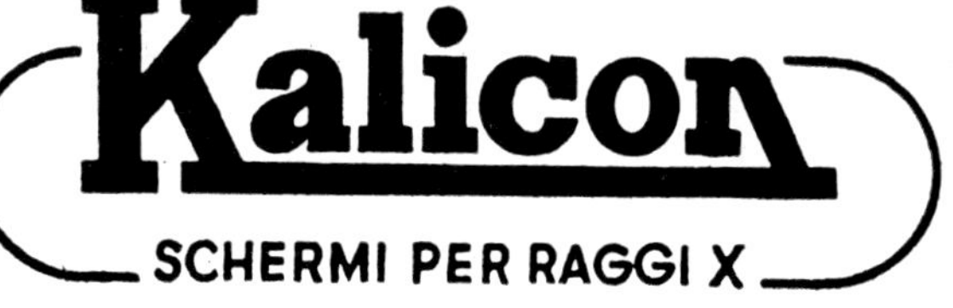

name comes from its two main cogs, G. Zurli and A. de Regibus.

Also in Genova (actually in a suburb, Sestri) is the plant of the Nuova (new) San Giorgio. Among other things, they make a horizontal table called Trocosimplex, a separate upright fluoroscope, the Ortosimplex, and energize both from a transformer called Mega-X 500.

In Milano (Italy's industrial center) is located the Società Italiana Prodotti Acessori Radiologici (SIPAR), which has an interesting trade-mark.

A tribute to the Atomic Phase is the Electronfides, an organization created in Rome, which provides all the services needed for radiation protection, including (dental) film badges.

In the early 1930s, the chemical laboratory of Lorenzo della Volpe (in Bologna) used the brand name Kalicon for its screens.* Today, Kalicon is the name of a factory in Rome, where fluoroscopic as well as reinforcing screens are manufactured. They offer the usual (fast, high definition, and standard) screens, and in addition bring in Ilford imports.

The big name in Italian photo-products is Ferrania (which is the name of the town in Savona where the factory is located). In the 1920s the firm M. Cappelli was selling *Lastre X,* while in the 1930s we find the

*The term is derived from the Hellenic *Kali* which means beautiful, for instance Venus Kalipigos (a statue less chaste than the one owned by the Medicis) was so called because of what the Greeks regarded as beautifully bulging glutei.

ferrania

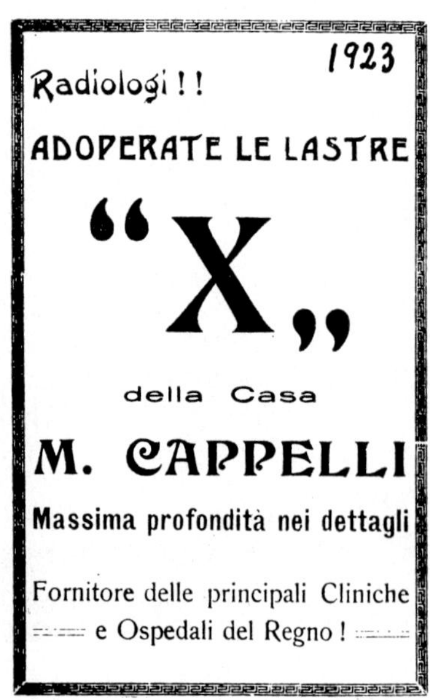

"FERRANIA,,

PELLICOLA PER RAGGI X

EMULSIONATA SULLE DUE FACCIE

PRODOTTO ITALIANO FABBRICATO

DALLA

FILM

1934

FABBRICHE RIUNITE PRODOTTI FOTOGRAFICI

CAPPELLI & FERRANIA

Capitale Lire 13.000.000 interamente versato

SEDE MILANO - PIAZZA FRANCESCO CRISPI 5

STABILIMENTO A FERRANIA (SAVONA)

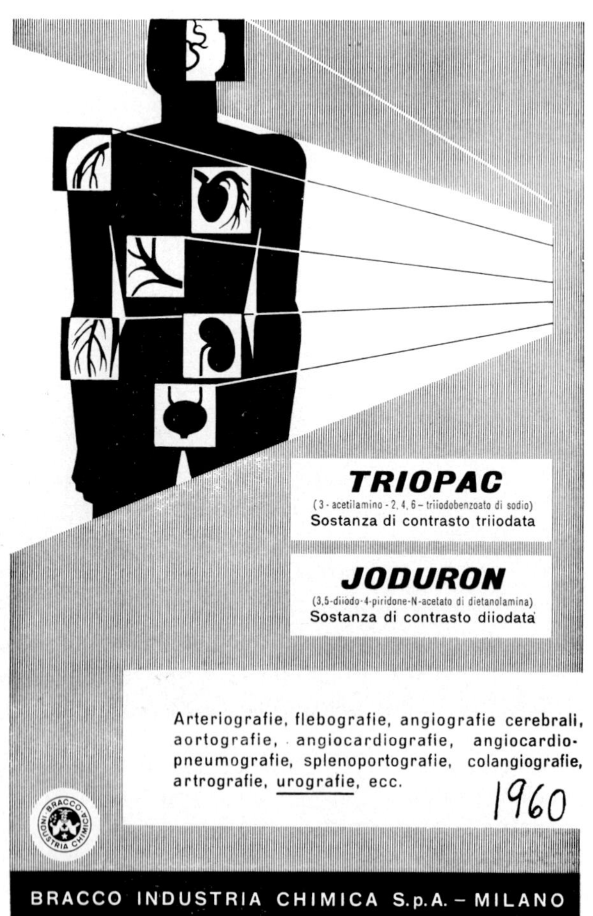

title Fabbriche Riunite Cappelli & Ferrania. Today they have a variety of x-ray films including the XS 320 (high speed), the N (normal speed), and the Simplex (envelope-packed non-screen films). A few years back they introduced the *Controtipo diretto,* a single-coated film for duplication of x-ray films without an intermediate; it can be processed in the regular x-ray solutions. Now Eastman Kodak makes a similar copy film.

Ferrania is part of the Fiat group, and has plants at Milan and Ferrania in Italy, and at Buenos Aires in Argentina. Regarding production of x-ray films, world's leading firms are in the order of volume, Eastman Kodak, Gevaert, Ilford, Agfa, and Ferrania. In Japan, Sakura and Fuji are big and growing (booming Japan, with 90 million population, consumes not much less than half of Western Europe), but so far they did not upset this order. Incidentally, Ferrania is selling the Pakorol in Italy. Last year, Ferrania was purchased by the Minnesota Mining and Manufacturing Company.

For "new" Italian contrast media, reference is made to the (oral cholecystographic) Jodobil and Cistobil and the (intravenous) Joduron and Triopac, made by the Bracco Industria Chimica in Milano.

GILARDONI

We have seen individual x-ray firms, very successful as long as they remained small. When they expanded, a point of diminishing returns (both figuratively and literally) was inevitably reached - and rapacious financiers repossessed the remains. An exception to this rule seems to be Gilardoni, an individual Italian x-ray firm, which at least so far kept on expanding.

Arturo Gilardoni graduated in 1939 from the Politecnico in Milano. He worked for two years in SRW's plant in Erlangen, was then employed as an engineer for Gorla-Siama. In 1945, he went in business for himself, and began to manufacture x-ray equipment. Gilardoni formed his company in 1947, and incorporated it in 1957. In 1958 he organized the APEL (Applicazioni Elettroniche), an x-ray tube factory. All these are located in his native Mandello Lario, on the shores of Lake Como — probably the most scenic location of any x-ray factory in the world.

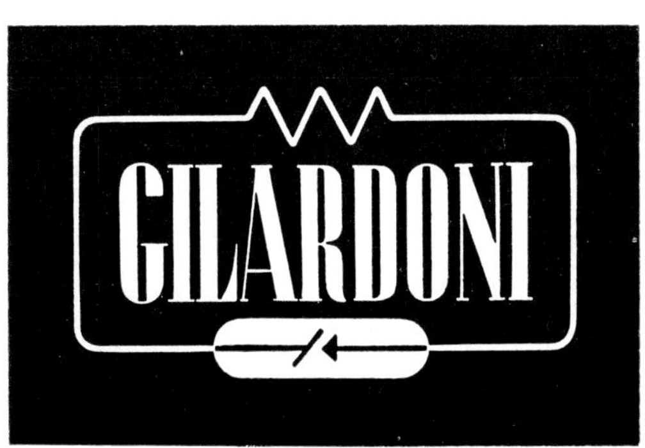

His production covers the entire x-ray field. The Gilardoni D2 is a monobloc, with peak load of 130 kvp. The Tetraselen is a selenium-rectified generator which delivers up to 1000 ma or 150 kvp. The Selenomatix is a triphasic, likewise selenium-rectified transformer: in addition to similar loads (as the Tetraselen) it offers an automatized ("anatomico-automatic") con-

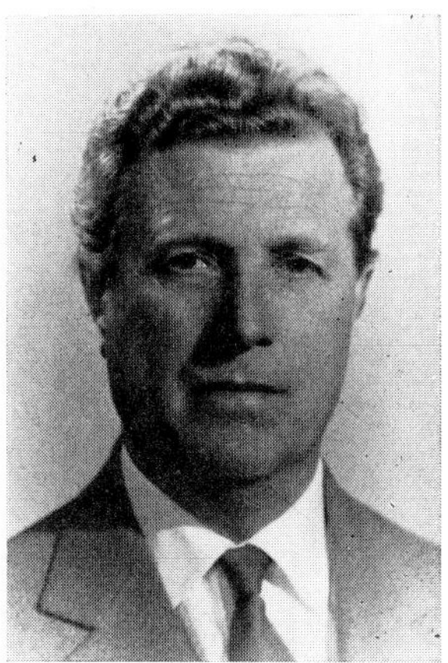

ARTURO GILARDONI. He may not be too popular with the competition, and many rumors have been circulated on his peculiarities, but his enterprises are (so far) very successful.

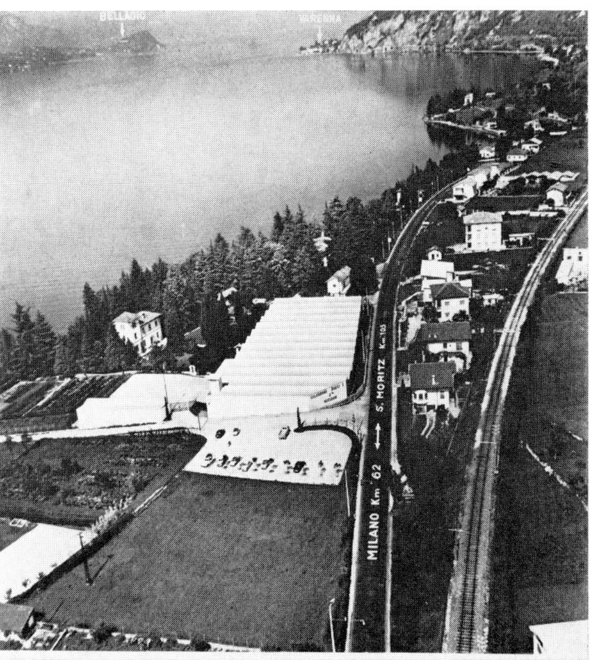

Courtesy: Gilardoni.

GILARDONI'S FACTORY. Lake Como makes quite a background for the main plant, seen as a "corrugated" white structure — it has actually a glass roof.

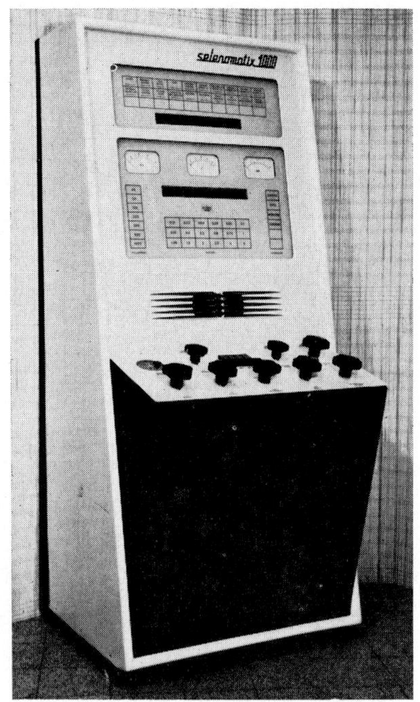

Courtesy: Gilardoni.

GILARDONI'S SELENOMATIX. "Anatomic-automated" control panel of Gilardoni's most potent triphasic transformer.

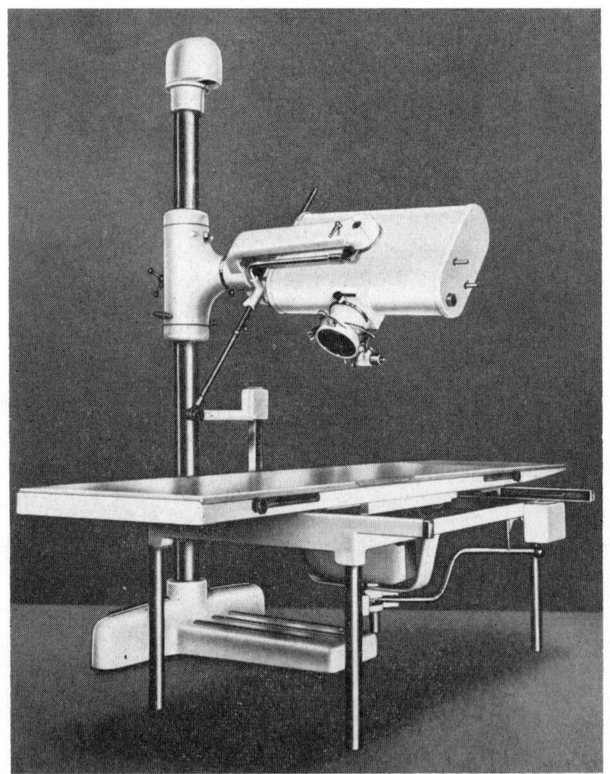

Courtesy: Gilardoni.

GILARDONI'S CINETERAPIX. Rotational attachment to his 250 kvp therapy unit makes the latter much more versatile regarding movable irradiation technics.

trol stand. Plinius is the name of a table with clean design and very functional lines — it has only 15° Trendelenburg, which may be why the firm is so successful (it does not go for unnecessary frills). Gilardoni's horizontal body section device is called Ascistrato.

The root *gil* is used in several names of Gilardoni equipment. The Odontogil is a dental model, the rotating Cobalt unit is called Gilatron 3000, the Cesium unit Cesagil 6000. Neodermo Be is a Beryllium window tube energized by a 5-80 kvp transformer, for coverage of the gamut from Grenzstrahlen to subcutaneous roentgen therapy. The T 250/12 (meaning 250 kvp and 12 ma) comes either as a stationary unit, or in a Cineterapix version with all sorts of "radiokynetic" capabilities.

Arturo Gilardoni is a member of the Society for Non-Destructive Testing of Evanston (Illinois). The Gilardoni plant turns out a variety of metallographic x-ray devices. The 250/12 comes in an industrial model, called MT 250/12, which is available as a mobile unit on casters. Scopix is an industrial fluoroscope, with adequate protection.

Arturo Gilardoni is not very well liked by the competition, but then the going is not too easy in the Italian x-ray industry, and he may have stepped on several unprotected feet. Whatever they may say about him, Gilardoni has succeeded where so many others have failed, and his company - at least at the time of this writing - appears to be prosperous, while some of his toughest competitors are now employees in the very houses in which they were the employers.

SWITZERLAND

Prior to World War II there existed the (now defunct) Swiss x-ray tube factory Radion - a firm "associated" with Phönix in Rüdolstadt (Thüringen). Today's Swiss x-ray tube factory is called Comet,

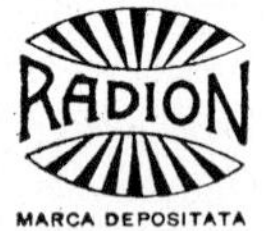

"RADION"

Soc. An. di Elettricità - Sede Zurigo

FABBRICA SPECIALE TUBI ROENTGEN

REPARTO RIPARAZIONI di Tubi per Raggi « X » di qualunque tipo e Marca

Filiale per l'Italia = MILANO (11)

Via Statuto No. 11 = Telefono 12.880

CASE CONSOCIATE

PHONIX - RADION. RUDOLSTADT / Thür.

VIENNA-BERLINO

Filiali: Frankfurt a. M. / Madrid / Praga

1925

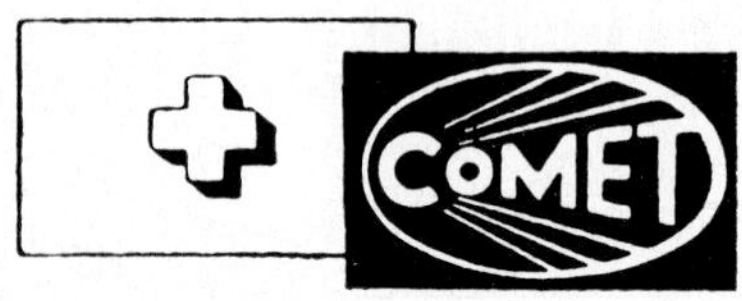

it is located in Berne, and its director is a patent attorney, named Beat Steck.

Comet was created in 1948, and in 1949 started to produce a stationary, 250 kvp therapy tube. In 1950 they approached Machlett, and obtained a license for the production of housings for rotating anode tubes. In 1954, an agreement was reached, whereby Comet would make also inserts for all types of rotating anodes manufactured by Machlett. This agreement was again expanded in 1961, at which time a tripartite arrangement was made to include the British Machlett.

Comet learned of the invention of a Swiss dentist (his name is Walter Ott) who had patented a method

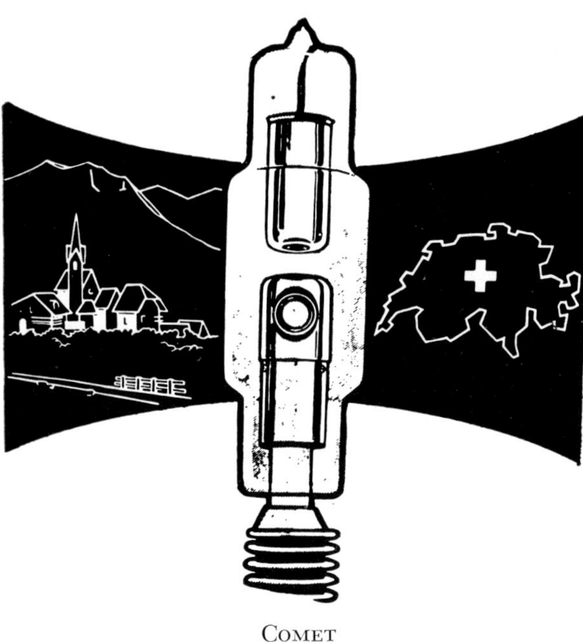

COMET

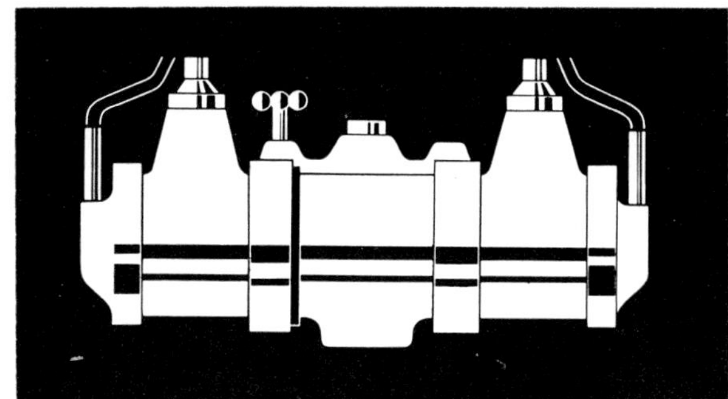

COMET'S TX-250 (1949). Comet's first product was a therapy tube for 250 kvp. Since 1954 they manufacture rotating anode tubes as a Machlett licensee.

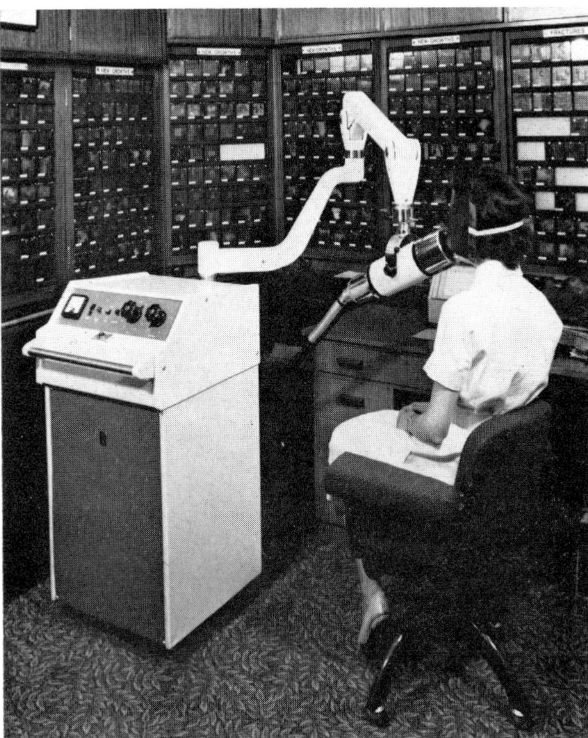

Courtesy: Watson & Sons.

WATSON'S PANAGRAPH. This is the British version of the pan-oral radiography, patented first by the (German) Koch & Sterzel, then – independently – by the (Swiss) dentist Walter Ott. In the background is the teaching collection of Sydney Blackman, a learned radiodontist in London.

of placing an x-ray tube in the patient's mouth so as to "get" all the teeth on a single x-ray film with one exposure. Comet started to develop such a tube, but when it reached the stage of production, they learned that Koch & Sterzel had a patent on it for several years. The inevitable altercations were finally resolved — in an amicable way — which is how the Panoramix was born. And since the British Machlett is in on all the (tripartite) developments, Watson has now on the market the Panagraph, which is very much the same thing.

Comet's advertising in Italian periodicals emphasizes that their tubes can be "over-loaded" without fear of damage. They have recently expanded into offering a full radiation protection service, including film badges.

In Burgdorf (Switzerland) Typon makes x-ray films. Their brands are called Typox, Typox-Rapid, and a fine-grain coating, the Progress.

Siegfried in Zofingen packs the Radiobaryt. Cilag-Chemie in Schaffhausen makes iodinated and other contrast media.

OTHER EUROPEAN COUNTRIES

Even before World War II, SRW had created several branch offices with manufacturing facilities, for instance the Siemens Electromedica Española in Madrid. Other Siemens licensees were located in Hungary and in Czechoslovakia. Today the successors to the two latter - Medicor in Budapest and Chirana in Prague - are state-owned. Both Medicor and Chirana manufacture a fairly complete line of x-ray equipment of good quality, and both of them export their wares not only behind the Iron Curtain, but also into neighboring Greece, into Egypt, and into several other countries, including South America.

MEDICOR

For a brief time after World War II, Hungarian x-ray equipment was sold under their (electrical) trade-mark Orion, as advertised in the *Indian Journal of Radiology.* In 1956 a new x-ray plant was erected in Budapest, and with it came a new trademark, the name Medicor, and later - in the guise of insignia - a winged-heel Mercury.

Medicor equipment has built-in protection for both operator and patient, as expected in the Atomic Phase. It actually goes back to a Hungarian Public Health edict, nr. 824 from the year 1939, which stipulated that during fluoroscopy the patient must be separated from the operator by a wall being the equivalent of at least one millimeter of lead. Such a lead cover was required not only on that part of the patient's body which faced the operator, but also on both sides of the patient. As a matter of fact, x-ray tables which incorporated this requirement had been available in Hungary for several years before 1939.

Nándor Ratkóczy, presently professor of roentgenology in the University of Budapest, had built a "pro-

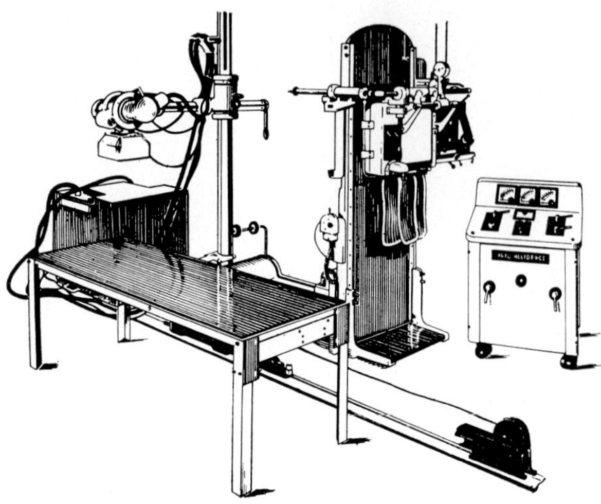

ORION'S AUTO-HELIOPHOS (1955). Kinship of this unit (made in Budapest) with SRW equipment is quite obvious, even in its designation.

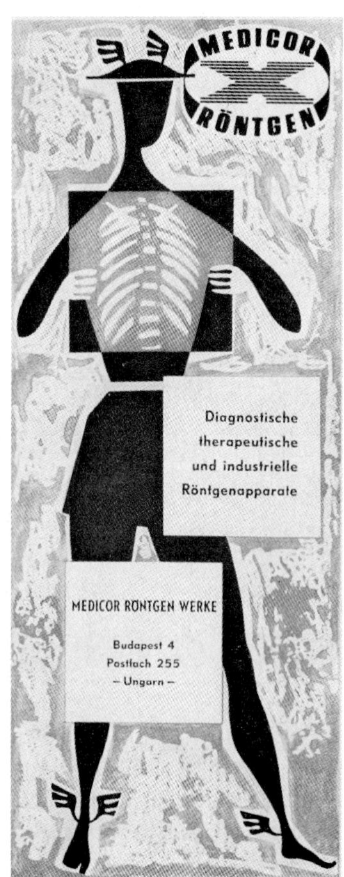

tective pulpit" in 1923 (before the one designed by Gösta Forssell): Ratkóczy's model was higher than the chairs available today, its protection reached almost to shoulder height. In 1927 Ratkóczy — in collaboration with László Huszár, the chief-engineer of Siemens' outlet in Budapest — constructed a complete enclosure for fluoroscopy, the Ratkóczy-cabin (or Ratkóczy-box). It provided absolute electrical as well as radiation protection (the latter by separating the patient from the operator), but it was restricted to upright fluoroscopy. Ratkóczy showed this box at the ICR in Paris in 1931 — Belot (who had a similar contraption built by Gaiffe, Gallot & Pilon) is said to have admitted that Ratkóczy's arrangement was more practical than his own brainchild.

In 1932, Zoltán von Hrabovszky, at the time chief-roentgenologist for the Hungarian Railroads, devised a special protective enclosure usable on a (horizontal) Bucky table for recumbent fluoroscopy. It was described as the Hraboskop in the first issue for 1933 of the *Magyar Röntgen Közlöny.* In 1935 — with Huszár's help and ideative cooperation — a Siemens Tele-Pantoskop table was modified to accept Hrabovszky's protective "sleeve" for use both in recumbent and in upright fluoroscopy. That improved Hraboskop embodied refinements which did not come into wider usage until after World War II, such as motor-driven footrest, automatized seriograph, stepping-ladder for operator, etc.*, all built in SRW's Budapest plant, the Magyar Siemens Reiniger Müvek.

*Hrabovszky designed also other x-ray accessories, for instance treatment chairs, one for the Chaoul method, another for gynocologic roentgen applications.

In the *Fortschritte auf dem Gebiete der Röntgenstrahlen* for February, 1925 Deszó Markó (then a young assistant radiologist in the Gróf Tisza Hospital in Budapest) proposed — as a protective procedure — to cover the "bulb" of the x-ray tube with a lead rubber sleeve. The "thing" was accepted and used by C. H. F. Müller, and contributed to the development of protective tube housings. In the first number for 1962 of *Magyar Radiológia,* the same Deszó Markó described the Gonaddefensor-tubus, an x-ray cone with a built-in triangular lead shield, used for pelvic radiography. In boys this lead triangle, when pointed upwards, projects its x-ray shadow protectively over the testicles. In females the same triangle, pointing downdards, protects the ovaries.

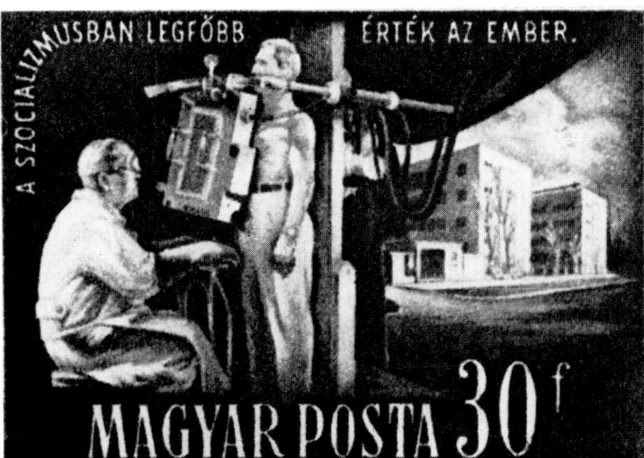

Courtesy: Stan Bohrer.

HUNGARIAN POSTAL STAMP (1951). Shown is a fluoroscopic examination with a tuberculosis sanatorium in right background. The apparatus is from the late 1930's — the operator sits behind a protective pulpit, has lead gloves, and wears goggles. The latter might be of transparent lead glass (if one may assume that the screen had no protective glass cover, which would be unlikely), or else the artist was unaware of the fact that adaptation goggles are removed during fluoroscopy.

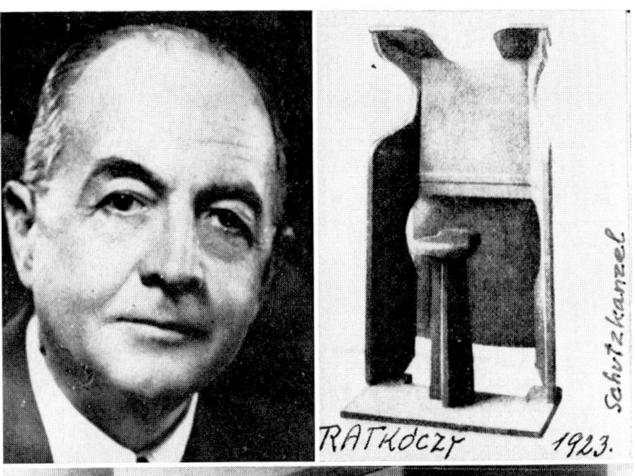

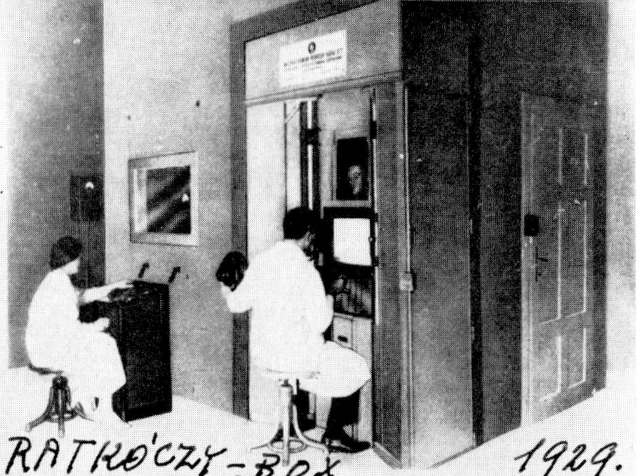

RATKÓCZY'S RADIO-PROTECTION. Recent likeness of Nándor Ratkóczy (who is teaching roentgenology in the University of Budapest) is shown with his protective pulpit (reproduced from *Klinische Wochenschrift* of 1924), and the fluoroscopic box (reproduced from *Röntgenpraxis of* 1931). The sign over the "box" reads Siemens-Reiniger-Veifa, topped by the monogram SH (Siemens-Halske). The inscriptions as well as the photographs are by courtesy of Ratkóczy himself.

Genoprot is a cassette-holder for chest radiography, devised in 1960 by Hrabovszky and Huszár, and sold by Medicor. Its special feature is a lead shield, which covers the patient's buttocks. The height of this shield is adjustable, and adjusting mechanism indicates the height at which the x-ray tube must be placed for proper centering of the primary beam. The lead shield prevents any significant amount of radiation from reaching the gonads.

One of Medicor's diagnostic outfits is based on the Diagnomax-125, a four-valve transformer (350 ma at 60 kvp, 220 ma at 125 kvp) with so-called "free automation," a feature developed in 1938 as the kilowatt-automation. When the factors set exceed the tube's capacity, the high tension switch is blocked, and a warning light appears; the respective circuits are pre-adjusted for the number of kilowatts the tube will take. The Diagnomax can be combined with the Uniscope (single-tube-table), with the Buckystrat (Bucky table with horizontal tomographic attachment), and/or with the Internoscope (twin-tube-table). In outward appearance, these combinations exhibit certain earmarks of filiation from the SRW line of apparatus.

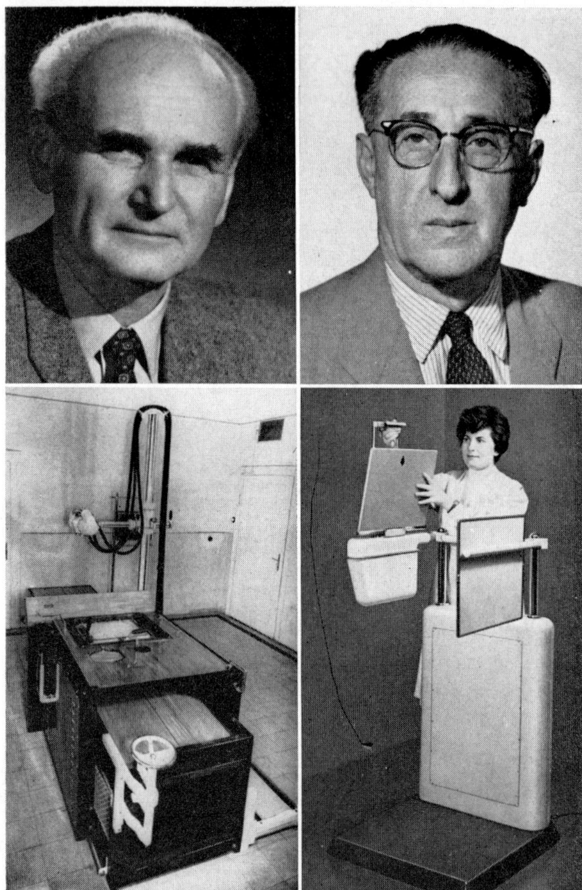

HRABOVSZKY & HUSZAR'S RADIO-PROTECTION. Zoltan von Hrabovszky and the bespectacled Lászlo Huszár have been associated on many technical ventures. The Hraboskop was a SRW table, herein reproduced from *Magyar Röntgen Közlöny* of 1933; it had been developed for urologic roentgen procedures, but was just as useful for fluoroscopy; until recently very few radio-people were aware of the magnitude of the secondary radiation emitted by the patient during any of the recumbent fluoroscopies. The lady shows the Genoprot, an arrangement intended to protect the genitals during chest radiography.

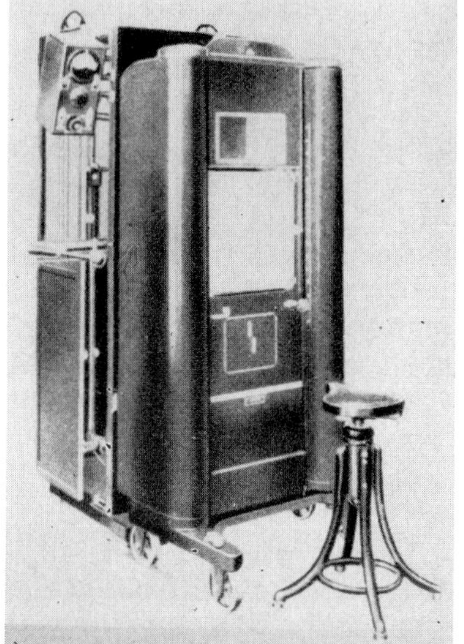

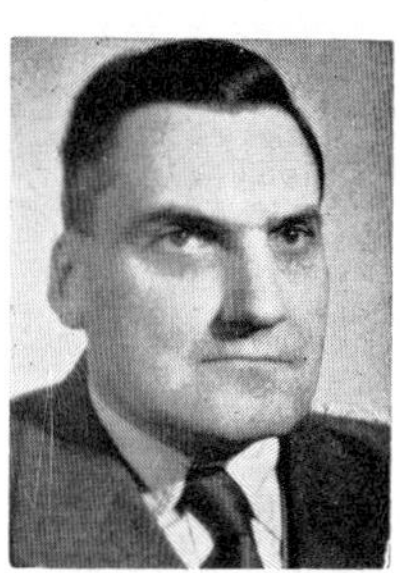

LASZLO BOZOKY

BELOT'S "PARAVENT" was custom-built by Gaiffe, Gallot & Pilon in 1927. Bozoky's portrait appears at this location fortuitously. He had no connection with either the Belot or the Ratkoczy box. Bozoky designed the Gravicert Co^{60} unit.

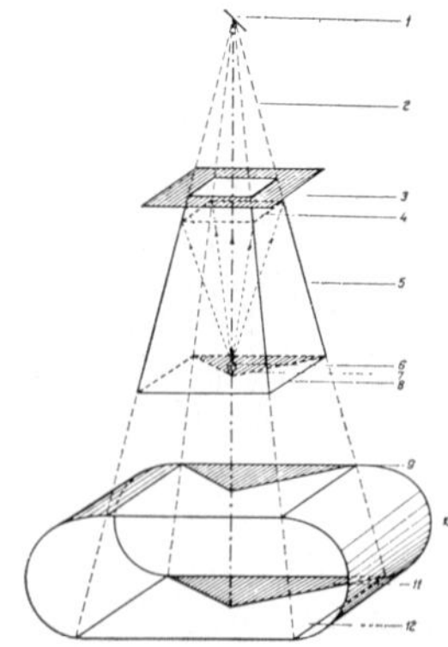

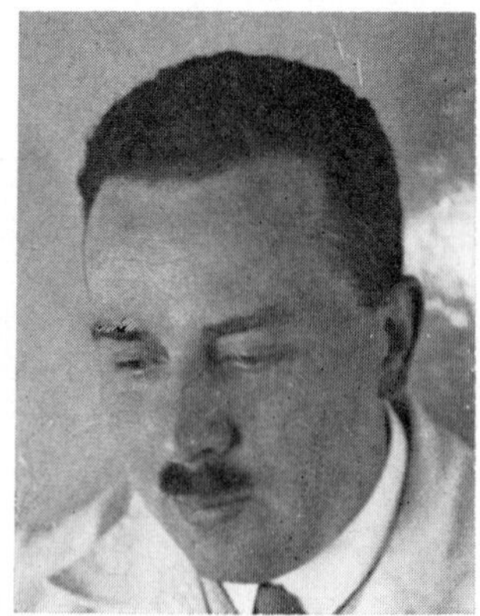

MARKÓ'S RADIO-PROTECTION. This photograph of Deszö Markó is from the time when he patented his protective lead-sleeve for x-ray tubes (1925). The sketch is of the lead triangle incorporated in a collimator (gonad-defense-tubus), herein reproduced from *Magyar Radiológia* of 1962.

Not so the Contrastor-150, a six-valve triphasic generator (1000 ma at 100 kvp, or 300 ma at 150 kvp), which has a control stand resembling elegant modern French design. It has double automation, (introduced in 1959) one part of which is the previously mentioned limiting tube circuit; the other, called "quick automation," has a selector panel with thirteen places for the various parts of the body. The Contrastor comes preferably paired with their best table, the UV-1, which has only 15° Trendelenburg, but motorized sliding table top, and a fully automatized spotfilm device, the Neo-Seriograph.

Medicor makes therapeutic x-ray apparatus, including the previously mentioned deca-curie cobalt irradiator Gravicert (designed by László Bozóky, chief-physicist of the Hungarian National Tumor Institute). Medicor sells the TH-250, a constant potential 250 kvp,

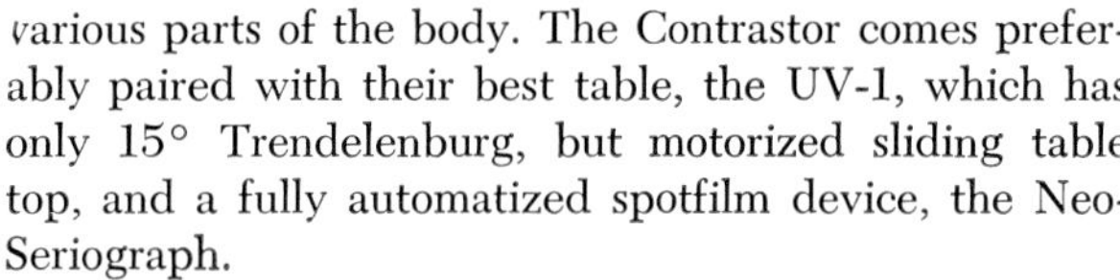

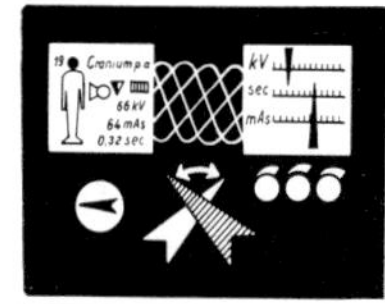
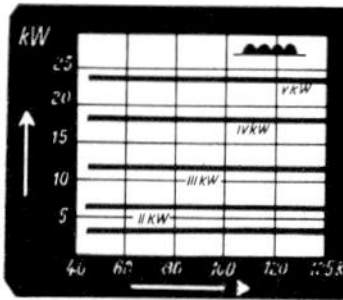
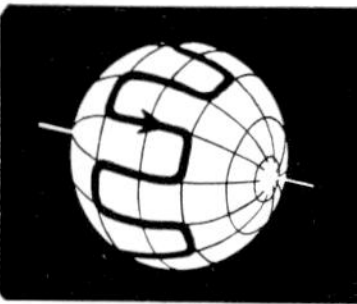

Courtesy: Medicor.

MEDICOR FIRSTS. At left is the dual automatic system, for alternative use of "free" or "rapid" automatic exposure control. In the middle is the kilowatt automatic system, a tube-overload cut-off system. The sphero-meandering pathway of the beam in the Spheroterix is shown at right. They also claim the Genoprot and Gravicert.

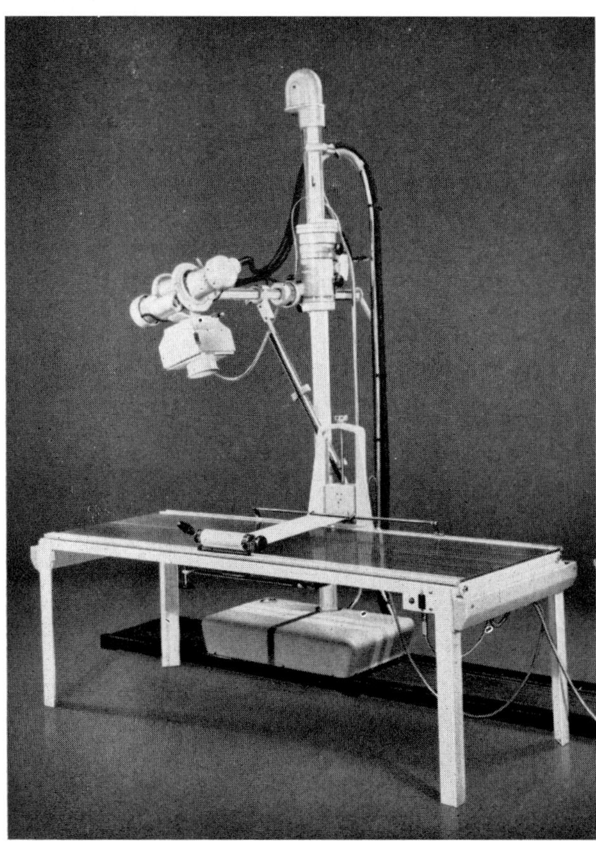

MEDICOR BUCKY TABLE.

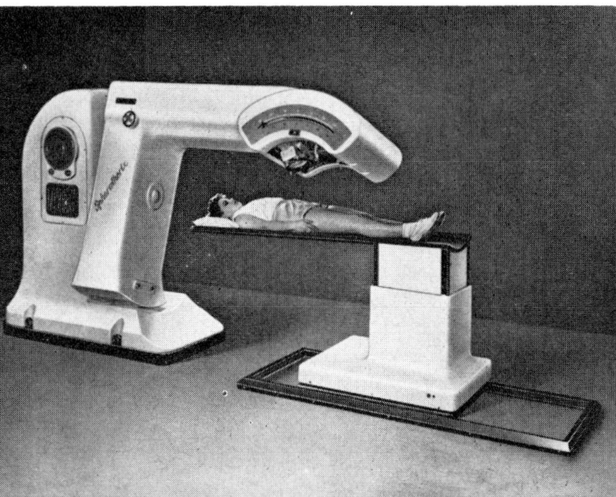

Courtesy: Medicor.

MEDICOR'S SPHEROTHERIX. This is a system developed by Huszár, and patented (Atomic Energy of Canada has purchased the American patent rights). The beam is directed toward a given point (always the same, regardless of the position of the head). Aside from the circular motion (on the gantry principle), the x-ray tube or any similar radiation source may execute a likewise motorized pendular motion along an arc which espouses the curvature of the tubehead. The sphero-meandering pathway of the beam, when both the circular and the pendular motions are "on," is shown in the preceding illustration. The basic principle is, of course, the intended skin-sparing effect.

15 ma therapy transformer, which delivers 90 r/min. at 50 cm focal distance. Their mobile 250 kvp monobloc industrial x-ray machine is called Stabil 250.

Medicor's *pièce de resistance* in the therapy field, is the Spheroterix, an apparatus designed and built by Huszár, who is currently Medicor's expert engineer. The Spheroterix cumulates all possible therapeutic tube motions, rotational, convergent, and pendular. By combining the rotational (equatorial) with the pendular (longitudinal) movement, the beam — although aimed at the center of an imaginary sphere — can be made to zig-zag a sphero-meandering pathway on the surface of that imaginary sphere. Such non-uniform coverage — similar to roentgen therapy through grid — is considered desirable on the (today still not quite orthodox) assumption that even when successful, roentgen therapy does not kill all viable tumor cells, but simply changes the ratio of tumor cells *versus* supportive stroma, thus favoring the development of an all-engulfing stromal scar. The well known failure of supralethal overdosage can then be explained very easily as the destruction of most stromal cell-seeds. Huszár's Spheroterix is built in the pure style of (Huszár's) gantry principle, which insures the dead aim at the center of the sphere, as well as the equatorial motion. In addition, an electrical motor in the head of Huszár's device moves the tube in a longitudinal plane. The controls permit separate utilization of any of these motions. Atomic Energy of Canada has purchased the rights to the USA patent for the Spheroterix (the basic design for the Spheroterix dated from 1951), but so far the Canadians have built it only as a rotational (equatorial) version.

Medicor has a house organ with an English edition, the *Medicor News,* printed on excellent paper. It includes some non-commercial contributions, for instance, a bird's eye view of the progress of radiologic technology by Irina Lagunova (of Moscow). Medicor has commercial literature in English because of avowed intent of selling its merchandise in Africa and Asia.

Incidentally, in 1960 was brought to criticality a Russian-built Hungarian experimental atomic reactor, located at Csillebérc, on the outskirts of Budapest.

CHIRANA

So far, the Hungarians must import x-ray tubes. The Czechs have excellent glassblowers (Bohemian glass has been famous for centuries), therefore Czechoslovakia has its own tube factory: they make a full line of x-ray tubes, including the ROD 30/40, a twin-focus rotating anode, for loads up to 30, respectively 50 kw, at up to 125 kvp. The ROS is another rotating anode, which takes 150 kvp of four-valve rectified current, or 130 kvp from triphasic generators. They make thoriated tungsten filament rectifying valves, and therapy tubes as well.

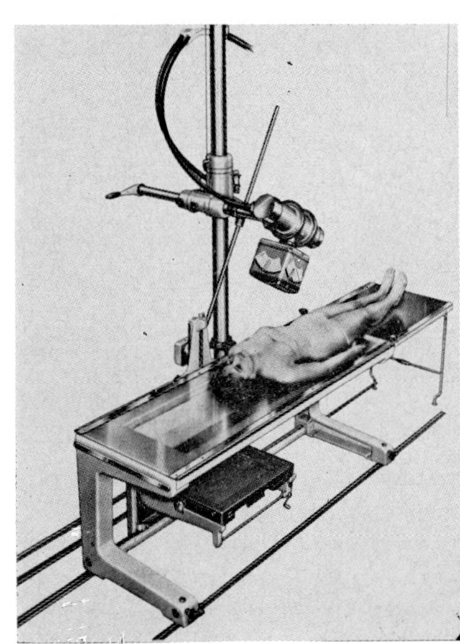

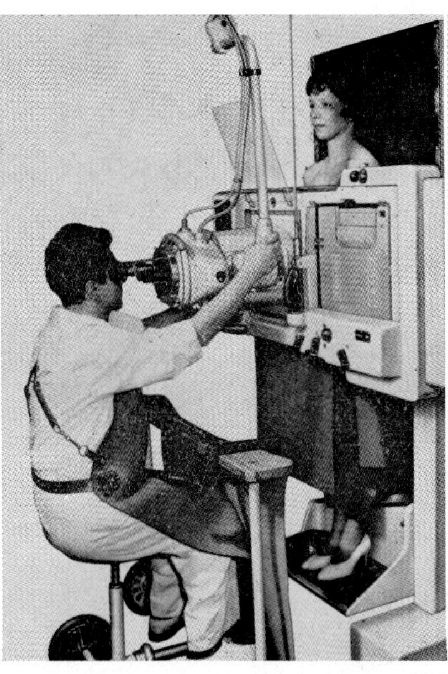

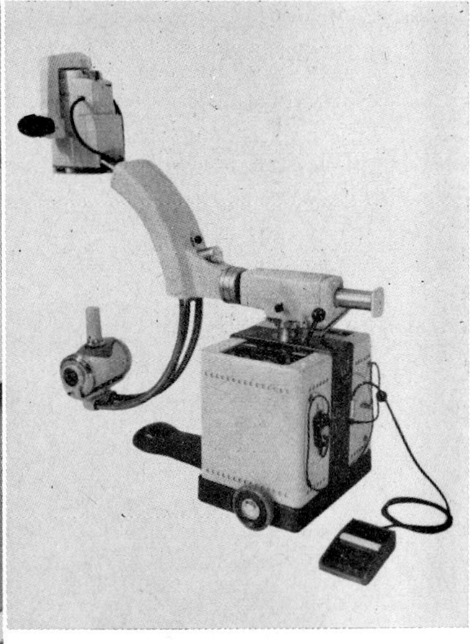

Courtesy: Chirana.

CHIRANA APPARATUS I. At left is the Planitom, a combination currently very popular in Central Europe: it has provision for single-axis tomography, for magnification radiography, for multiple-layer tomography, and for magnification (single- or multi-layer) tomography. Chirana's image intensifier ZOX 125A has a binocular system for viewing the output phosphorus; the table shown is the Motoskop. The third device is called Miniskop, again a very popular model of "surgical" image intensified fluoroscope.

The "people-owned" Chirana Národni Podnik in Prague produces a fairly complete line of x-ray equipment. Their design is now completely different from that of the SRW. Chirana places emphasis on function rather than on beauty. Their dental units are called Stomax and Minident. A truly portable (65 kvp with 4 ma in fluoroscopy, 15 ma in radiography) is called Chirax. Klinix and Internax are upright fluoroscopes (also capable of certain radiographic procedures), intended for general practitioners. Movex is a 100 ma, 90 kvp mobile unit. Chirana transformers include the Orthometa (200 ma, 100 kvp), Durometa (300 ma at 90 kvp, 100 ma at 125 kvp), Megameta (800 ma at 80 kvp, 400 ma at 125 kvp), and the Penetrix, a four-valve combination (800 ma at 110 kvp, 200 ma at 140 kvp). They make their own Bucky-Potter diaphragms, the S-3, and have a horizontal Bucky table with tomographic attachment. Urex is a urologic support with built-in tray and Bucky-Potter.

Both manually-operated and motorized tilting tables are offered.

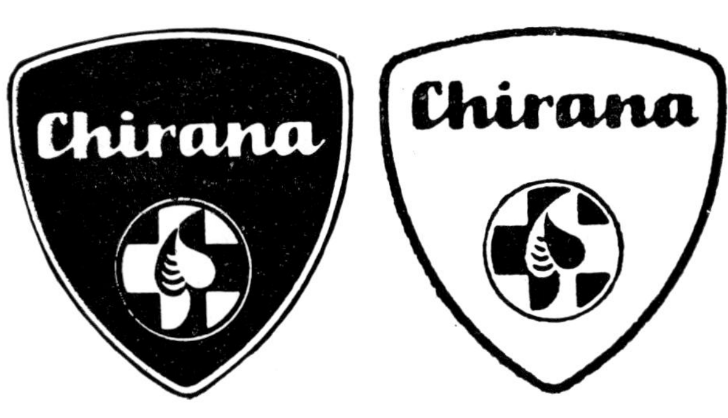

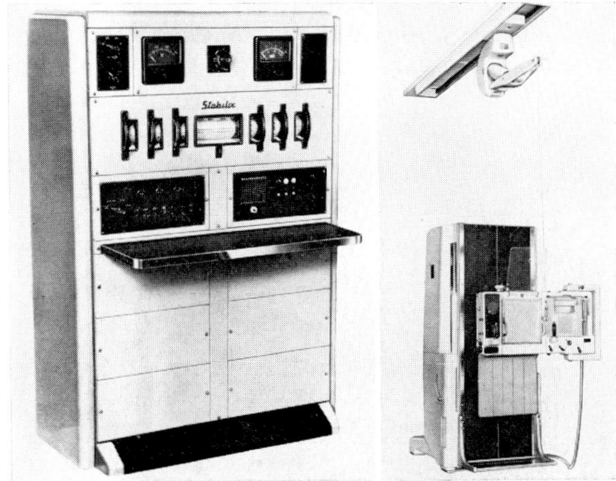

Courtesy: Chirana.

CHIRANA APPARATUS II. Control panel of the six valve, triphasic Stabilix 300 ma at 125 kvp, or 700 ma at 80 kvp, with electronic timer down to one millisecond. The table is a Motoskop 312 A, with ceiling-counterbalanced automated spotfilmer, and optional motorized footstand.

Most interesting, however, is the fact that Chirana is building 15 mev betatrons, similar to SRW's Elektronenschleuder. The first such betatron was installed in the Radiology Department of the University in Hradec Kralove. Chirana builds Co^{60} teletherapy equipment; the unit installed in the Radiology Department in Kosice, has television monitoring and voice-communication between operator and patient.

SOVIET UNION

In the USSR production of x-ray equipment is concentrated in the previously listed four factories, attached to major radiologic centers. They issue a

МЕДИЦИНСКИЕ
ИНСТРУМЕНТЫ,
ПРИБОРЫ,
АППАРАТЫ
и ОБОРУДОВАНИЕ

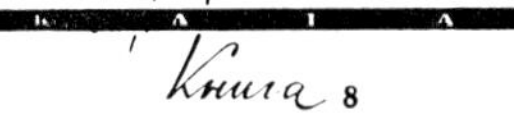

Разделы

13 — Рентгенология и радиология

14 — Физиотерапия

Всесоюзное Объединение
„СОЮЗХИМЭКСПОРТ"
СССР Москва

Courtesy: Medexport.

SOVIETIC RADIO-KATALOG. This is the eighth volume (434 pages) in a series of nine volumes (a general index is printed in a separate, tenth book) describing all sorts of medical instruments made and sold in the Soviet Union. Domestic buyers make their applications and receive the merchandise through channels: only when they have complaints or other difficulties are they supposed to communicate with the central Soyuz-med-instrument-torg. Foreign buyers make their purchases through the official Soyuz-khim-export. Volume eight, published in 1961, contains section 13 – roentgenology (prepared by an engineer, E. E. Troitsky) and radiology (prepared by the previously mentioned technical expert, V. V. Dmokhovsky), and section 14 – physiotherapy (prepared by a physician, A. N. Abrosov).

catalog, intended both for internal consumption and for export.

The stock x-ray item is RUD-110-150-2, meaning 110 kvp, 150 ma, and 2 tubes. It has a desk-type control stand, and a motor-driven 15° Trendelenburg tiltable table, with mechanical spotfilm device. There is also a separate horizontal table with tomographic attachment, permitting body section radiography both in recumbency and in upright position, the latter with the help of a wall-mounted cassette. A Bucky diaphragm is built into the tiltable table, while stationary grids are used for tomography and upright teleradiography.

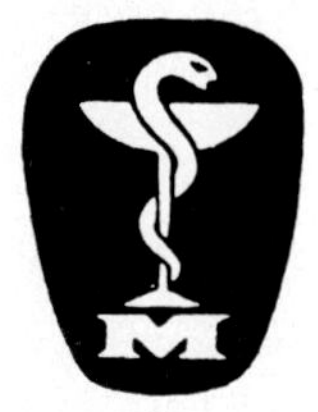

V/O "MEDEXPORT"
SSSR MOSKVA

A less elaborate version is called ARD-2-110-K4. It is a four-valve transformer with electronic timer, the shortest exposure being 1/25 sec. (the previous machine is provided with 1/50 sec.). It has a wall-mounted control panel, though the spotfilm device is less versatile.

The RUD-100-20-1 is a field unit, which can be transported in several wooden boxes. It is a monobloc unit giving 40 ma at 100 kvp, and has a stand for either vertical or horizontal radiography, with stationary grids.

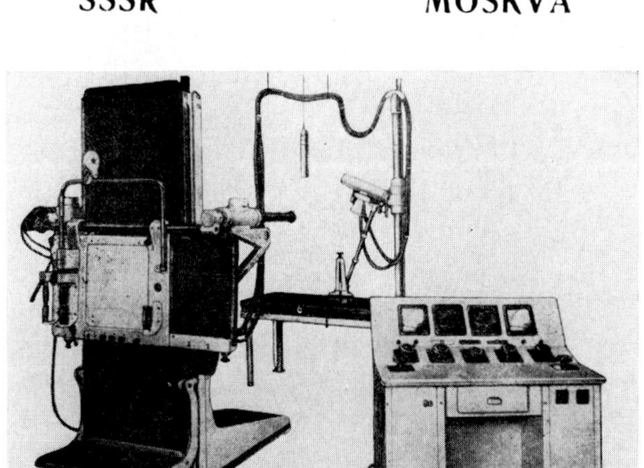

RUD-110-150-2. This is the best diagnostic equipment offered in the catalog (110 kvp at 150 ma).

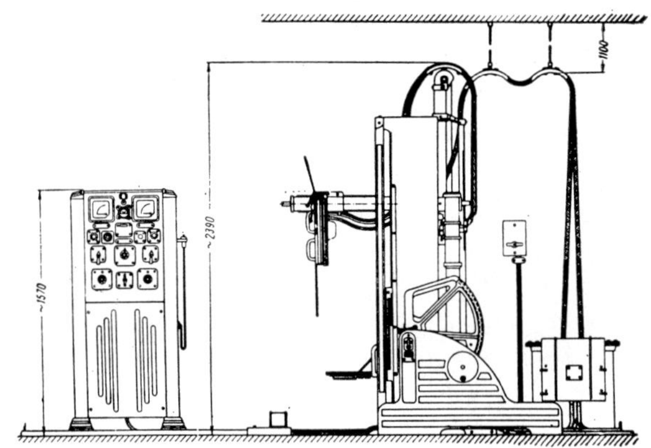

ARD-2-110-K4. This is the second-best stationary diagnostic unit offered in the Sovietic catalog; transformer has same ratings, the difference is in accessories and timer.

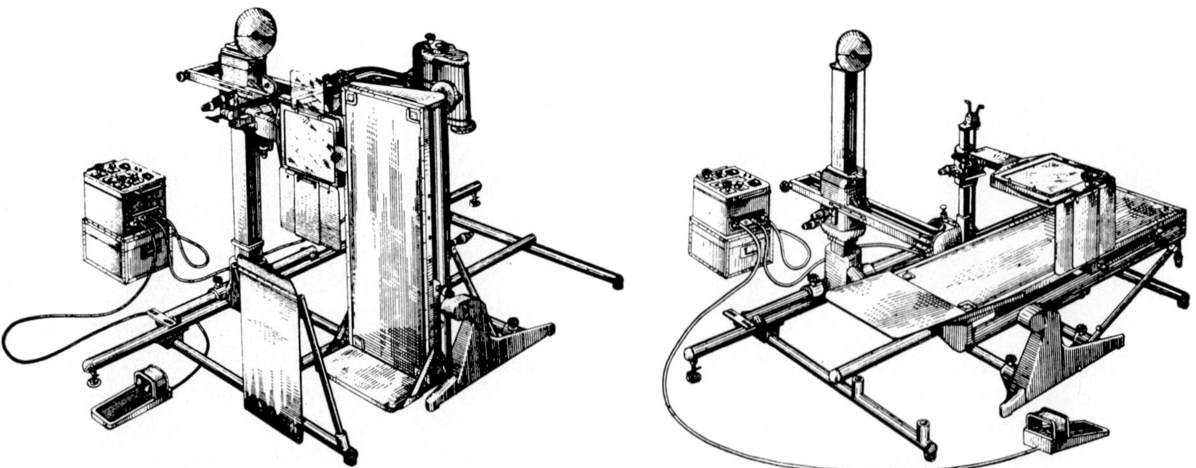

Field unit RUD-100-20-1. The figure 1 indicates a single tube. The transformer is rated at 40 ma and 100 kvp. An image intensifier is listed among optional accessories.

The catalog lists four other monobloc diagnostic machines, all of lesser magnitude than the field unit. One is a 20 ma, 90 kvp mobile apparatus. Another is also on casters, gives 12 ma at 75 kvp, and has a cryptoscope attached to it. The latter comes also with a hand-held cryptoscope, and the fourth in this series is a wall-mounted dental unit.

The catalog lists oil-, water-, and air-cooled line-focus (stationary anode) x-ray tubes, and several types with rotating anode. Of the latter, they offer for sale a 110 kvp, 10 kw model, and two types of twin-focus rotating anode with maximum load of 16 kw at 145 kvp.

They make a roentgen-urologic table, two types of fluorographic apparatus (one of these with mirror camera), and a ceiling counter-balanced roentgen-kymographic attachment. They have an electron-optical image intensifier (10 cm^2 input phosphorus and 1000 times brightness gain) with either binocular or monocular viewing; the latter permits adaptation of a "Kiev" movie camera instead of, but not simultaneously with, fluoroscopy. The image intensifier was built for use with the above mentioned field unit.

For pediatrics is listed a "respiratory-phase x-ray switch" with a pressure gauge for attachment to the

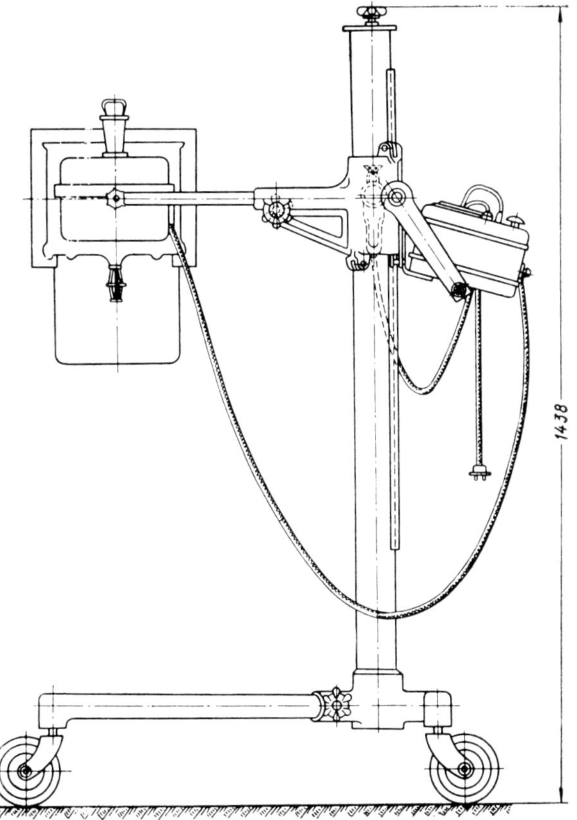

URPO-70-4.75 kvp, 12 ma single-tank fluoroscopic and radiographic unit on casters. The cryptoscope would permit fluoroscopy without darkening the room.

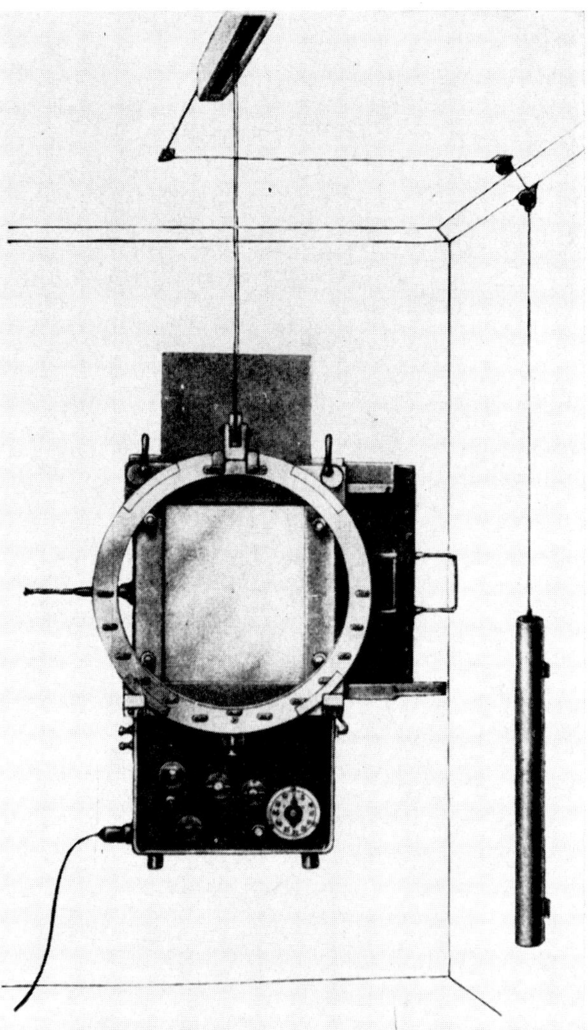

SOVIETIC ROENTGEN-KYMOGRAPH. It can be rotated in a horizontal plane through ± 90° in steps of 15°. The travel of the carriage can be set to 6, 12, and 36 mm, the exposures being varied in the ranges of .5-10 sec., 1-20 sec., and 3-60 sec., respectively.

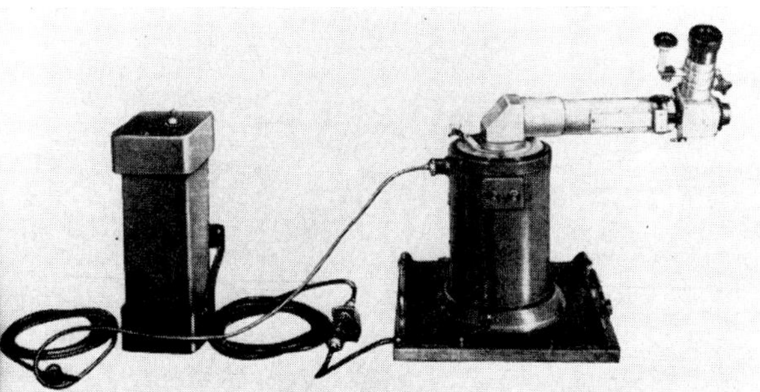

SOVIETIC IMAGE INTENSIFIER. Brightness gain is 1000; the device is primarily intended for fluoroscopy in upright position; it has no split-image provision, but a "Kiev" movie camera can be attached to the monocular for recording of the image on film.

chest, and a pneumatically operated on-off switch connected to the timer of the x-ray unit: this permits exposure at any desired stage of respiration. In the catalog, right after this item, are offered four models of spring-wound, hand-cocked Bucky diaphragm, and two models of mobile triphasic electric current generators with gasoline motors.

SOVIETIC "RESPIRATORY" SWITCH. A pneumatic mechanism actuates the exposure at any desired phase of respiration.

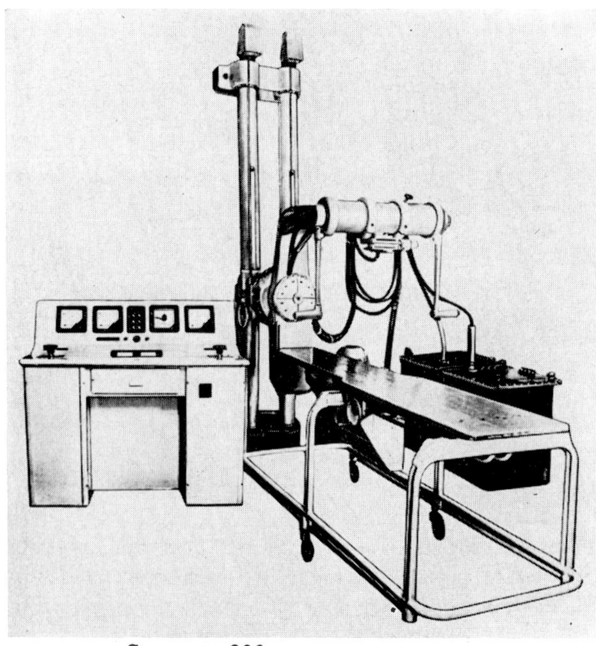

SOVIETIC 200 KVP THERAPY UNIT.

The RUT-200-20-3 is a therapy unit with 20 ma 200 kvp peak delivery. The 3 means three vacuum tubes (one x-ray tube and two kenotrons). It has a desk-type control stand, and oil-filled tubehead suspended from a single, pedestal supported column. The RUT-60-20-1 is a mobile therapy unit on casters, with beryllium-window tube, intended for contact levels (from 10 kvp).

The URDT-100-2 is an oil-filled monobloc which contains a transformer and two x-ray tubes mounted in parallel. Its maximum voltage is 100 kvp, with an aggregate current of 5 ma going through both tubes. Their catalog specifies that it is used "for superficial X-ray therapy (mainly, x-ray epilation)."

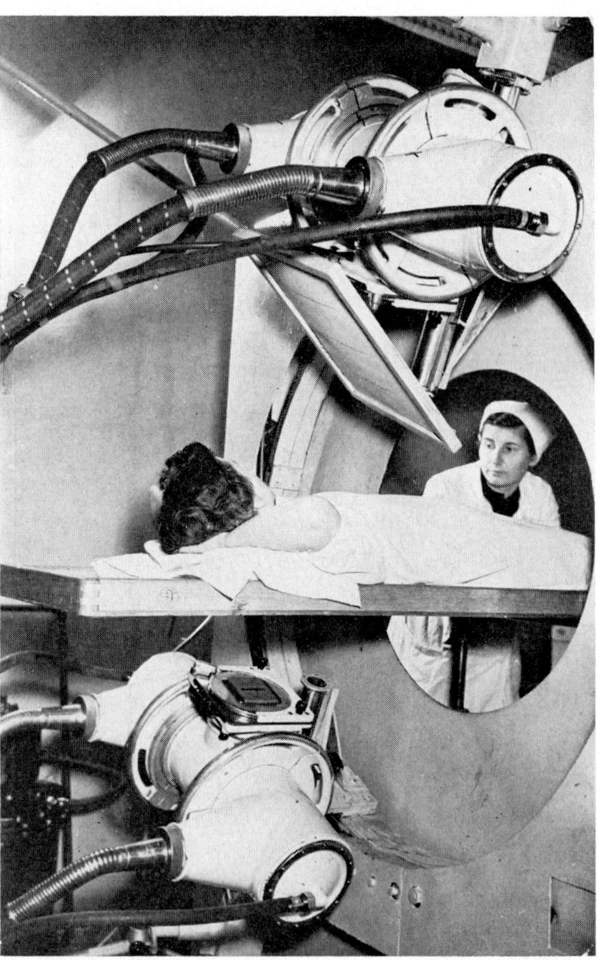

Courtesy: Sovfoto.

SOVIETIC TWIN-TUBE THERAPY UNIT (1956). The caption which came with the picture states that this apparatus was developed at the Molotov X-ray Institute in Moscow. Patient is being treated with "two continuously rotating tubes operating at different regimes."

The catalog is by no means exhaustive of the x-ray equipment available in the Soviet Union. First of all, in the past they have purchased selected units from foreign manufacturers. As the USSR does not recognize patent laws, they have utilized desirable improvements found in equipment made in other countries.

Then there is standard equipment which was not included in the catalog, for instance, the diagnostic unit URVv-110k-4-la, which is a variation of RUD-110-150-2, except that it has a single tube. Just like the other, its maximum is 150 ma, usable at 45 kvp, while at 110 kvp the maximum tube current is 60 ma.

Special equipment is being made on order in the Sovietic x-ray factories. Such a special order requires certain formalities (red tape) but if there is a recommended research project, the wish of the researcher will usually be accommodated. As an example, they have built elaborate rotational therapy devices, including one with two separate therapy tubes mounted on a rotating ringstand.

In the above mentioned catalog the sections devoted to "atomic" equipment are more impressive. There is an abundance of eponyms and code names as if they had been recently declassified.

An example of understatement is the fact that only a single, 400 curie stationary Cobalt unit is listed in the catalog. The Soviets make several models of large, rotating, 3000 curie (and over) teletherapy irradiators, for instance the Rokus.

Nor is included in the catalog their "Cobalt gun," a successor to the "radium gun" built in the late 1930s. The cobalt gun is an ingenious deca-curie unit in which the source is returned to the safe position simply by tilting the container.

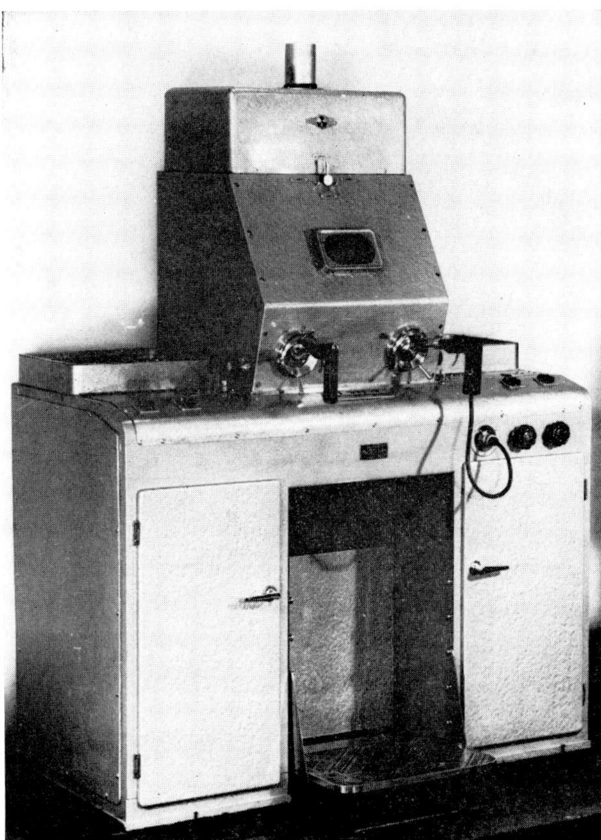

RADIOMANIPULATOR GRK-61. Note handles on face of unit for the remote manipulation of radioactive samples inside the hood.

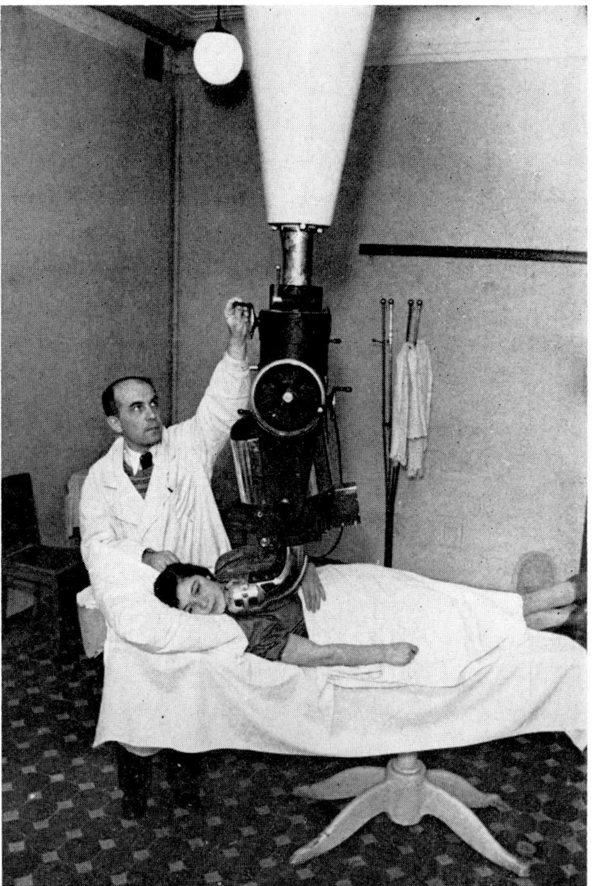

Courtesy: Sovfoto.

SOVIETIC RADIUM-GUN (1940). At the Central Oncological Institute in Moscow, M. Domschlak positions a patient with carcinoma of the sub-maxillary gland for treatment with the radium-gun. The pellet rolls from its lead-enclosure through the steel tube into treatment position (very close to the patient's skin). At the end of the treatment, the mid-section – containing the lead-enclosure and the steel tube – was tilted by means of the hand-crank, thus never-failing gravity returned the source to safe position.

Various sizes and intensities of radiocobalt-filled stainless steel filters (needles), and a lead-shielded boiler-sterilizer for these are shown in the catalog. Interestingly, the Russian term for radioactive (even for waste) storage receptacles is the transliterated English word container.

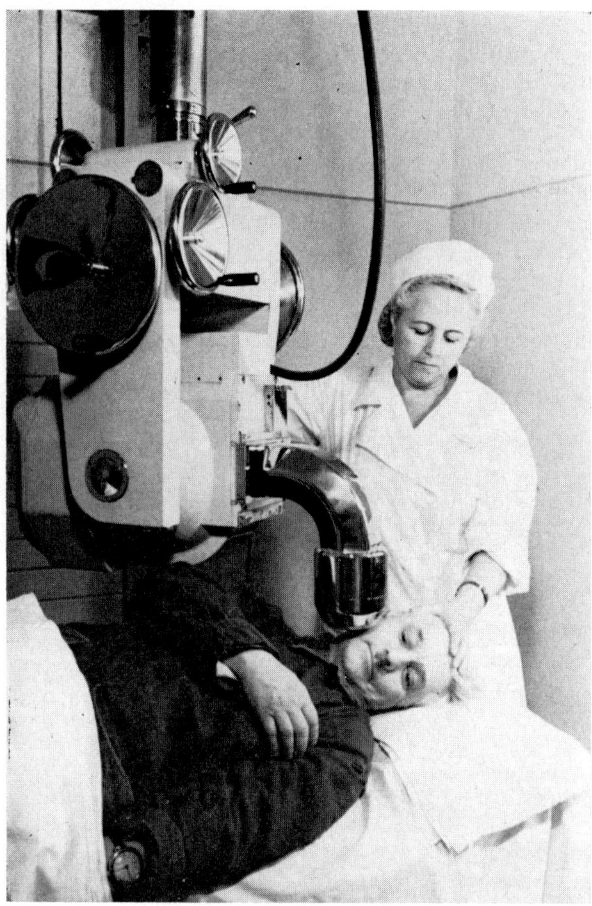

Courtesy: Sovfoto.

SOVIETIC COBALT-GUN (1955). In the Roentgenology-Radiology Department of the First Clinical Hospital in Minsk is used a deca-curie Co-60 irradiator, based on the tilting principle of the radium-gun. Hecto-curie units have been built on the same principle.

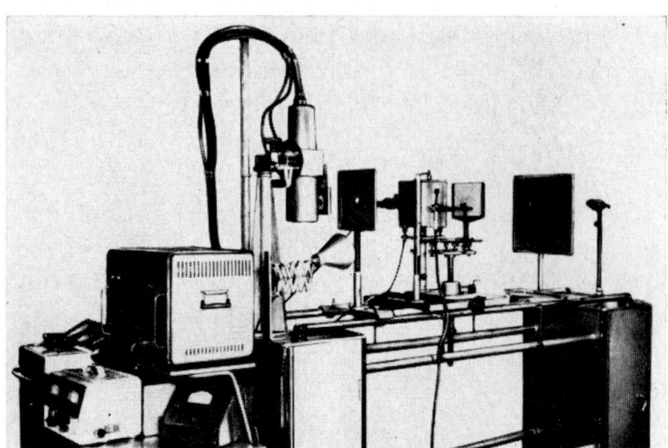

CALIBRATION STAND. Sovietic arrangement for calibration of dosimeters.

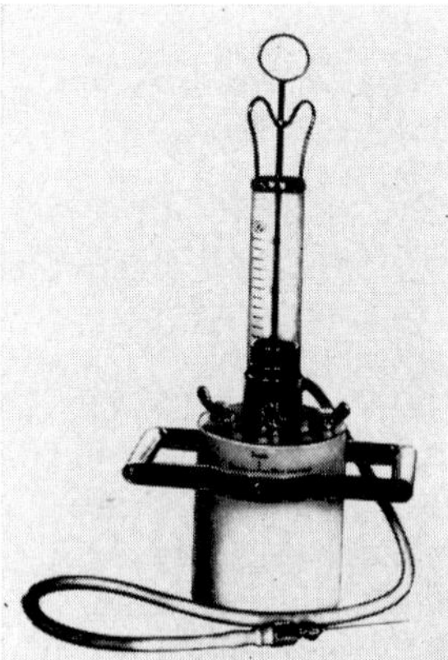

Courtesy: George Zedguenidze.

SOVIETIC GOLD UNIT. For intracavitary radiogold therapy.

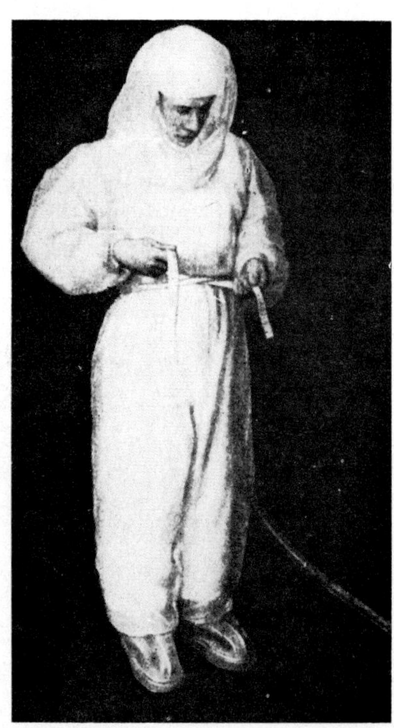

Courtesy: Sovfoto.

SOVIETIC PNEUMO-SUIT LG-4. 200-400 liters/minute of fresh air are pumped into the unit, both for respiration and ventilation, actually excess pressure is desirable to prevent entrance of contaminated air. It is intended as a protection against radioactive gas, and or aerosol, up to a concentration of 10 thousand times above the maximum permissable limit.

АТОМНАЯ ЭНЕРГИЯ–НА СЛУЖБЕ НАРОДУ
Здание первой в мире атомной
электростанции Академии Наук СССР
1955
ПОЧТА СССР
1

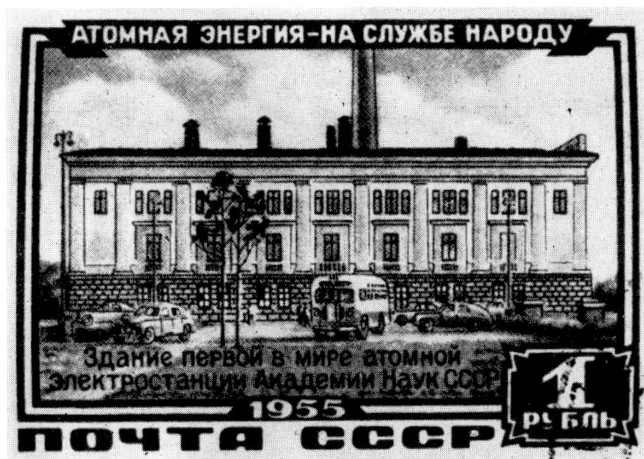

Atomic Electricity. The inscription on this stamp asserts that this is the picture of the world's first atomic "elektro-station," operated by the Sovietic Academy of Sciences.

No gynecologic radium applicators are listed, but there is in the catalog an item which seems old-fashioned in the Atomic Phase. It is a radon bath unit, type URV-1, and serves to prepare aqueous solutions of radon. As a safety measure, a "fume-hood" is provided for operating personnel.

Kaktus is the name of micro-roentgen-ratemeter (2-20,000 microR/sec.). Two battery-operated gamma-roentgen-ratemeters are listed, the Karagach-2 (50-100,000 microR/sec.), and the Loza (.02-500 R/sec.).

For radioactive isotopic measurements they have a Tyulpan ratemeter, Flox and Volna scalers, the Romashka scintillation (and well-) counter, the Kryzhovnik pulse-height analyzer, the Siren broad-band discriminator-amplifier, the Yablonya four-channel coincidence and anti-coincidence set, and the Eukalypt broad-band amplifier.

Thirty-five pages of Geiger tubes, gas flow counters, scintillation crystals, and photomultiplier tubes are included in that catalog.

Next are listed the Tiss universal radiation monitor, the Luch universal survey meter, the Svet-III scintillation meter, the Efir-II thermal neutron meter, portable survey meters for (uranium) prospectors, Sputnik-1 and Razvedchik-1 field survey meters, Malysh portable small size, fast and thermal neutron and alpha survey

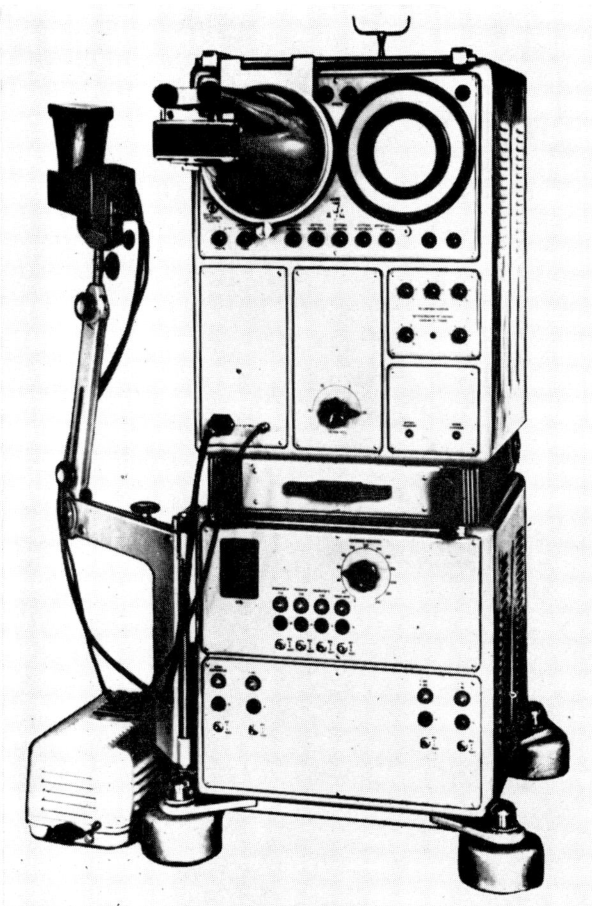

Ultra-sound in diagnosis. Sovietic model (1954); recently – in this country – the drug manufacturer Smith, Kline & French produced a similar unit.

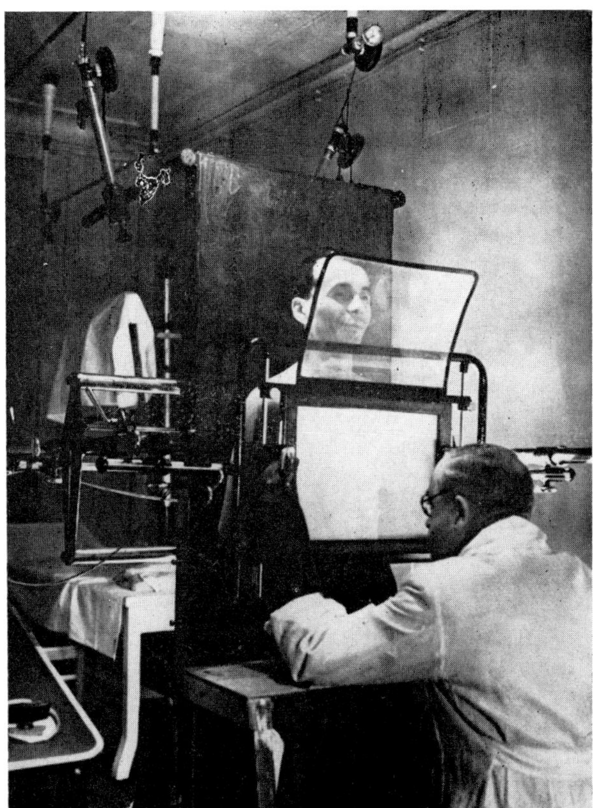

Sovietic fluoroscope (1930). Apparatus used in the medical department of a factory.

meter, as well as a variety of personnel radiation dosimeters, such as the Pioneer individual pocket indicator, and the Charnika neutron ratemeter.

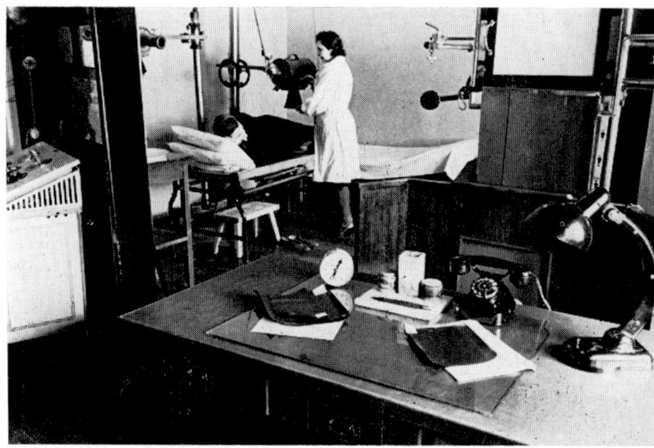

Courtesy: Sovfoto.

SOVIETIC X-RAY DEPARTMENT (1948). Located in the Central Institute of Balneology (Hydrotherapy) in Moscow.

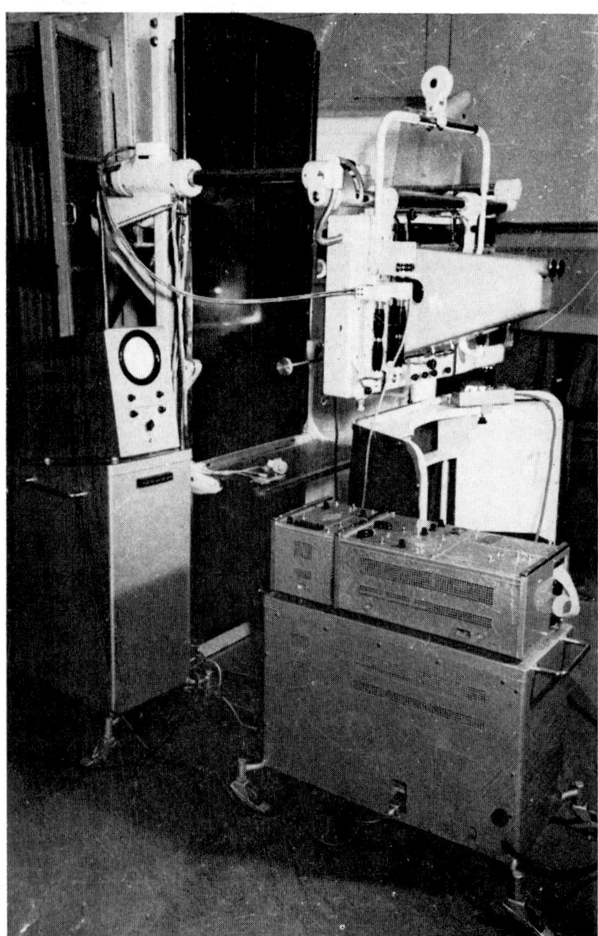

Courtesy: George Zedguenidze.

SCINTILLATION ELECTRO-KYMOGRAPH. Note the oscillograph and continuous recording of EKG.

The remainder of the catalog contains items of protective clothing, oscillographic and other electronic measuring equipment, electrotherapeutic apparatus (*e.g.*, ultrasound,* high-frequency, and radar therapy machines), ultra-violet and Sollux lamps of several denominations, hydrothermal therapy equipment, a variety of "aerosolizers" (for instance Mikulin's Hydroionizers), and finally a few outdated fancies, such as the "electro-mechanized percussion massage apparatus," or a "metal-screened cabin for the suppression of radio interference caused by high-frequency physiotherapy equipment."

In May of 1963, Manson Benedict, the MIT physicist, visited Sovietic nuclear installations, from Dubna with its 10 bev synchrotron, the most powerful currently in operation in the USSR, to the icebreaker Lenin, and from the Sm-2 high thermal flux reactor in Melekess to the Radium Institute in Leningrad. In June, 1963 Benedict gave the address of the retiring president of the American Nuclear Society. On that occasion, Benedict

*In the USA, ultrasonography is currently being promoted, manufactured, and sold by a corporate progeny of the (mail-advertising, but ethical) drug maker Smith, Kline & French of Philadelphia. Until now, they emphasized the "intracranial" applications of the method.

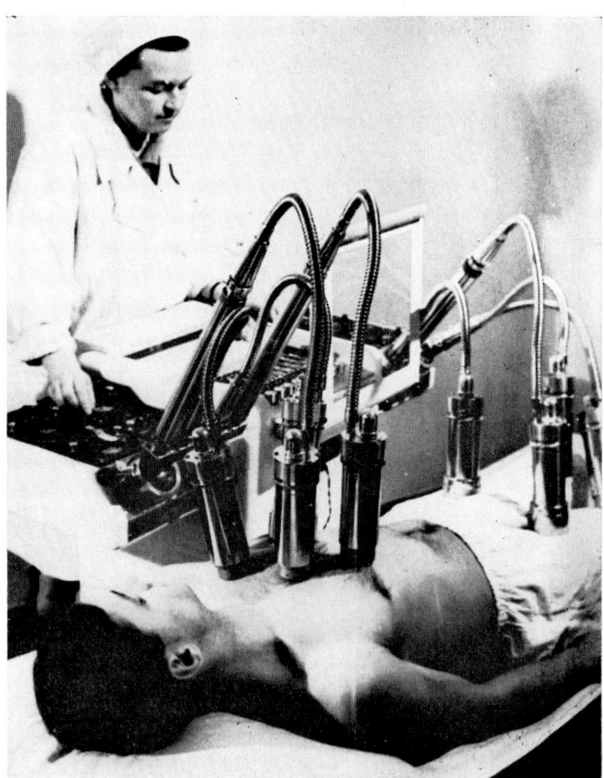

Courtesy: George Zedguenidze.

SOVIETIC CIRCULATION TIME DETERMINATOR (1956). Eight-channel scintillation counter used in the Chest Surgical Institute in Moscow.

compared the Sovietic and US nuclear capabilities. The US had ten civilian nuclear power stations in operation, compared with two Sovietic stations in operation. The total capacity of all stations built or authorized in the US was 3.5 million kilowatts, compared with one million in the USSR. Up to May 1, 1963 our stations had produced six billion kilowatt hours of electricity, compared with Benedict's estimate of 336 millions in the Soviet Union.

On the other side of the ledger are the 2 bev linear accelerator at Kharkov, which will have the world's highest energy of any linac for at least five years; the 70 bev proton accelerator under construction at Serpukhov, which will have the highest energy of any accelerator for some time to come. The SM-2 reactor has the highest thermal flux of any reactor in the world. Soviet research in nuclear physics and nuclear chemistry is on a par with US and Western European research. Scientific interchange between the US and the USSR would undoubtedly benefit both countries.

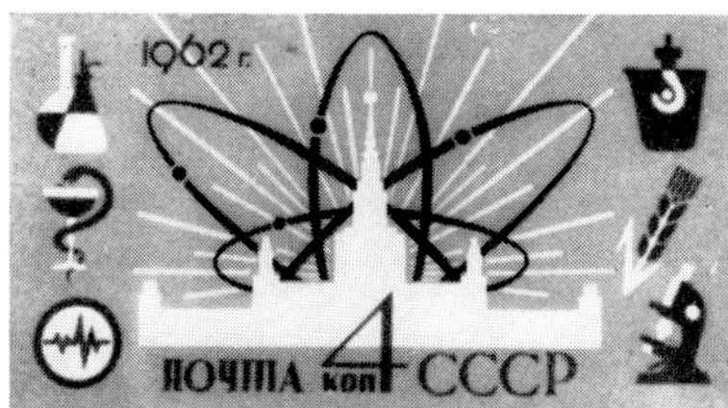

Courtesy: Stan Bohrer.

SOVIETIC ATOMICS. While differently arranged, the symbols are similar to those exhibited on the seal of the Oak Ridge National Laboratory.

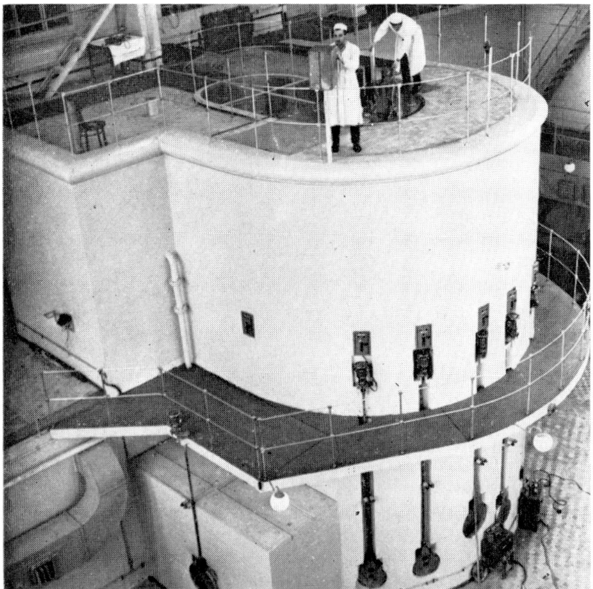

Courtesy: Sovfoto

SOVIETIC REACTOR. 2 mw experimental, heavy-water type, in the Institute of Physics of the Georgian SSR in Tiflis, from a photograph dated November, 1949.

X-ray technology in the Soviet Union has progressed steadily, if not spectacularly. From the primitive, barely finished tables of the 1920s they have advanced in the 1940s to clean-cut equipment, much of it still with exposed, overhead connections. Today most of their major radiologic centers have adequate machinery, especially for radioisotopic applications (reflecting their strive for nuclear warfare capabilities). There exists in the Soviet Union both the technical know-how and the skilled help needed for the duplication of practically all the refinements in x-ray apparatus developed anywhere else. However, at the beginning of the 1960s, there is as yet no sign that quantity production of luxurious x-ray equipment has been assigned any sort of priority among Sovietic goals.

AUSTRALIA

RADIOLOGY

NOVEMBER 1929

THE BOWKER DEVELOPING UNIT

(Patents applied for)

for x-ray film development

Advantages of the Bowker Developing Unit

1. NO DARK ROOM REQUIRED. May be operated anywhere, indoors or outdoors.
2. No necessity for special blinds, special curtains, bare floors, special doors, special room illuminations, special exhaust fans, etc.
3. No necessity to lock room during developing procedures. Outsiders may enter room without risk of fogging films.
4. Unit is ORNAMENTAL IN APPEARANCE and will not spoil appearance of room it is placed in. No unsightly tanks, view boxes, film cupboards, immersion heater, etc. are required, other than those included in the neatly constructed unit.
5. Whole unit may be mobile or portable in its smaller sizes.
6. NO MENACE TO HEALTH as operator does not work in the dark; ordinary floor coverings and room warming apparatus can be employed.
7. NO MORE SOLUTION THAN IS ACTUALLY REQUIRED FOR THE PHOTOGRAPHIC PURPOSES is used, thus greatly reducing the cost of chemicals.
8. RAPID DRYING OF FILMS.
9. GREATLY IMPROVED HANGERS, saving much time in handling, eliminating ugly marks on corners of films and eliminating bulging and abrasions.
10. In dental hangers. FILMS MOUNTED IN SERIES CAN BE VIEWED IMMEDIATELY AFTER FIXING WITHOUT THE NECESSITY OF SORTING AND FURTHER MOUNTING.

For further particulars apply to **JOHN BOWKER,**
V. C. A. Buildings,
Collins Place,
MELBOURNE, C. 1.
AUSTRALIA.

Intending agents please mark communications "Agency".

PIONEERING PROCESSOR. Only two were ever manufactured, but neither is in operation. The three Bowker brothers were then (but are not now) in the x-ray business. The unit was similar to a dental film processor (box with black sleeves). It did not catch on, one of the Bowker brothers went to work for WatVic, then returned to the photographic field proper.

In the land down-under they make (as yet) no x-ray tubes, no grids, no Bucky diaphragms, no mirror cameras, no angiographic changers, no image intensifiers, no automatic processors, no constant potential therapy equipment, and no linacs, nor any other type of particle accelerators.

Ultrays (Pty), Ltd. of Collingwood (Victoria) represents the (British) Watson & Sons and, in addition, builds a few tables. There is also the inevitable Philips subsidiary which, incidentally, makes some dental x-ray units.

The lion's share of the Australian x-ray market is in the hands of two "local" firms, Stanford and Watson-Victor.

STANFORD

At the time of World War I there existed a firm called Nightingale Laboratories, which manufactured as well as serviced Australian x-ray equipment. In 1919, one of their engineers, Joseph Henry Ford, left Nightingale's and with a partner, a fitter and turner called A. Stanley, founded the Stanford (Stanley and Ford) Works.

Stanford commenced operations at 316 Flinders Lane in Melbourne, constructing, maintaining, and repairing x-ray and electro-medical apparatus. Soon their slender finances ran low, and they accepted a third partner, Anthony Joseph Parer. Later his brother, Leandro Parer, bought Stanley's share in the partnership. Within a year the firm moved to a two-story shop at 214 Russell Street (Melbourne), and the name was changed to Stanford X-Ray and Radium Company. In June of 1921, Stanislaus Arthur Parer took over Anthony's share, and remained to this day Stanford's managing director (Leando is one of the directors). Premises were changed on several occasions until the factory and headquarters located in 1941 in Collingwood (Victoria), with branch offices covering most of Australia and Tasmania.

Aside from x-ray equipment, Stanford manufactures microscopes, projectors, laboratory and scientific apparatus. In the last fifteen years, they have installed over 250 complete major x-ray units, and over 500 mobile or minor units (dental apparatus not included).

In 1925, Stanford introduced the first valve-rectified x-ray generator in Australia, and in 1932 the first shock-

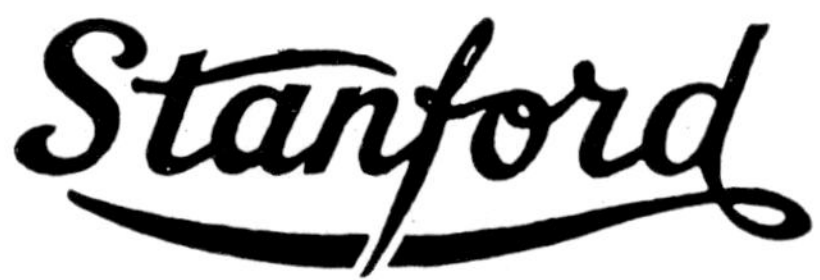

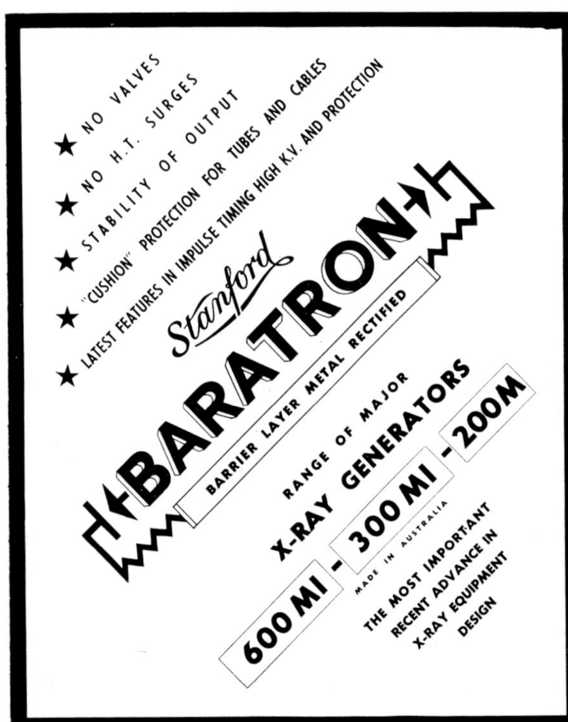

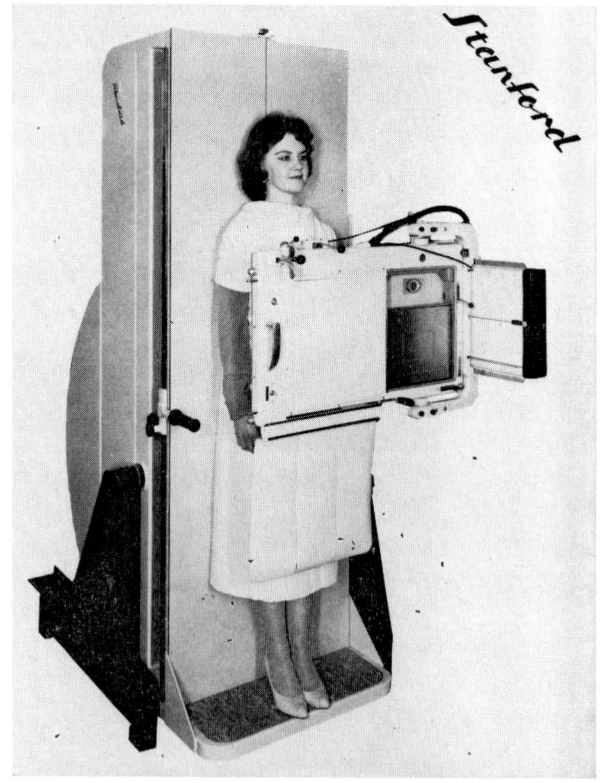

Courtesy: Stanford.

Stanford Universal Table. With Scholz spotfilm device.

proof mobile x-ray unit made in Australia. In 1936, they designed and produced the first Australian mobile laboratory for civilian chest x-ray surveys. At the beginning of World War II, Stanford's built the first Australian photofluorographic equipment using 35 mm film.

Stanford has currently a diversified line of x-ray equipment, from portables (15 ma at 75 kvp) to darkroom equipment.

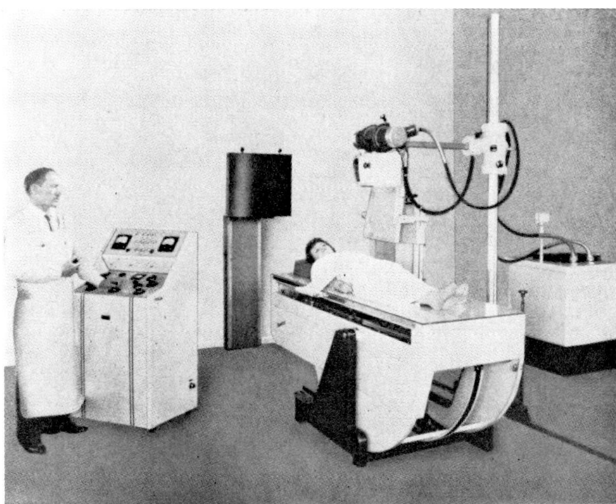

Courtesy: Stanford.

STANFORD INSTALLATION. Shown are the Baratron 600 ma (up to 140 kvp) transformer and control stand, with Universal tilt table. Note the monorail tubestand, and in center background the wall-mounted vertical Bucky stand.

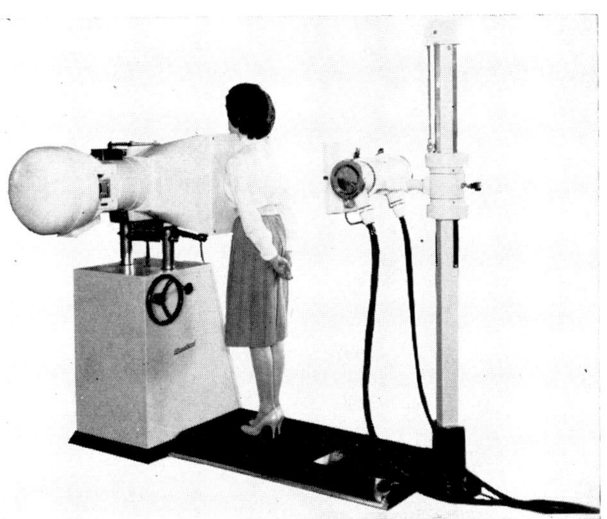

Courtesy: Stanford.

STANFORD ODELCA ARRANGEMENT. The Odelca elbow device is mounted on two columns neatly supported by a pyramidal base.

They make several mobile units, the largest of which has a valve-rectified (up to 250 ma or 125 kvp) generator, and rotating anode. In stationary units Stanford uses SRW-made selenium (barrier metal high tension) rectifiers. These consist of small elements of selenium-coated aluminum and other metals. Each unit is capable of rectifying 40 volts, and these units come packed in series in a tube. The tubes are then combined to obtain the maximum ma and kvp desired. There is no wear or tear, and breakdown of a single unit does not affect operation of the transformer. Another advantage is the "cushioning" effect against voltage surges. And much space is saved, while eliminating trouble-prone switch-gear.

Stanford uses the name Baratron for selenium-rectified generators, which come in three sizes, 200 ma, 300 ma, and 600 ma. The 300 ma can be operated at up to 130 kvp (for 100 ma), absolute maximum being 140 kvp.

Stanford's best table, called Universal, has a two-speed motor-driven 15° Trendelenburg tilt, and a Duplex semi-automatic spotfilm device. The table top is hinged to give free access to the Bucky diaphragm. They also manufacture a monorail ceiling-floor tubestand, with magnetic locks. The wall-mounted Bucky stand comes either non-tiltable, or tiltable with folding legs.

In the therapy field, Stanford makes a machine for superficial treatment. Its industrial version is called the 140-10 twin-valve.*

WATVIC

Like so many other important Australian enterprises, Watson & Sons was formed by immigrant Britishers, who had not done so well at home, but who turned out to be immensely successful in their chosen new location.

In 1888, Henry H. Baker (a grandson of William Watson) started business in Australia; his brother Frank Baker arrived six months later. They opened a factory in Richmond (Victoria), and called their business just like the London firm, W. Watson & Sons, Ltd. – yet, at no time was there any financial connection between the Australian and the British firms of Watson, except that the Australian Watson was and still is the representative for the British Watson's microscopes.

*This and other information on Australian x-ray conditions must be credited to the courtesy of F. W. Pierce, Stanford's director of marketing.

W. Watson & Sons' Ltd.

The Australian Watson prospered, and in the year 1896, when Röntgen's discovery came along, they began to supply x-ray apparatus to hospitals. Watson engineers always possessed "educated fingers" (this is an Australian saying), for instance they manufactured all sorts of scientific precision equipment, including specialized cameras for the Antarctic Expedition of 1908, later spectrographs, in 1918 even some instruments for the Australian Flying Corps. The "Watson House" in Sydney was built in 1925.

Watson-Victor is the name of a trading company (subsidiary of the Australian holding company W. Watson & Sons, which is the actual manufacturer of apparatus) formed in 1936 as the result of a reciprocal agreement between the (Australian) Watson and the (American) General Electric. Just as in London, the name Victor was selected as a company title because it suggested (without indicating outright) its connection with GE. By the terms of that agreement, Watson-Victor (WatVic) manufactured x-ray equipment under GE licenses until 1951, when this relationship ceased.

WatVic has tradition, and thus a feeling for history in general. A former chairman of the Board of Directors of the (Australian) Watson & Sons – J. P. Trainor – published in 1946 in Sidney the previously mentioned *Salute to the X-Ray Pioneers of Australia.* That booklet contains documentary information not available anywhere else.

Today WatVic has factories in Richmond, Collingwood, Turnstall, Finsbury (South Australia), and Glebe (New South Wales), and is the largest manufacturer of x-ray equipment in that part of the world - in 1961 their ordinary stock units received 12½ percent yearly dividends (which is "bloody

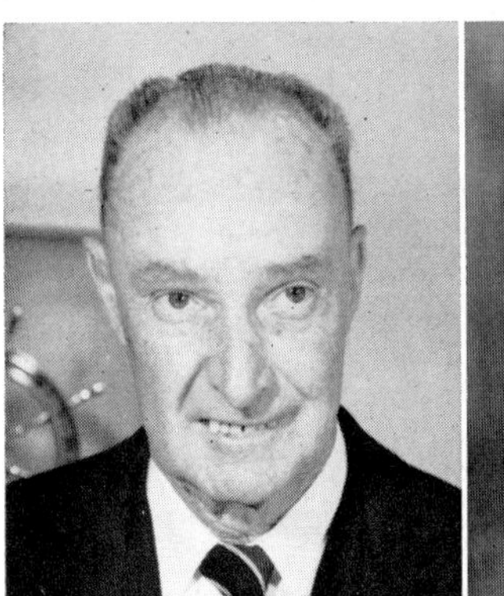

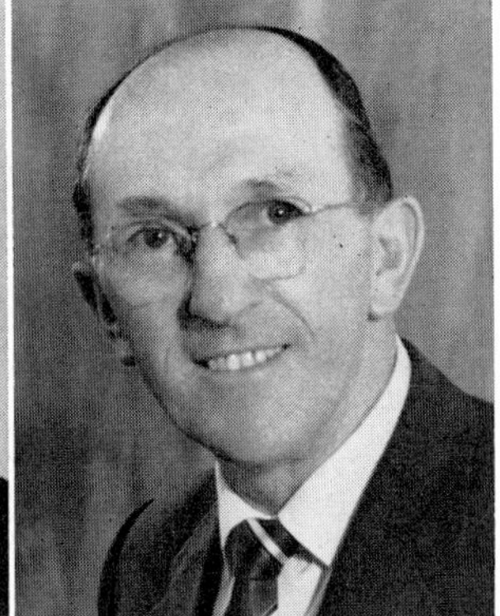

Courtesy: WatVic.

WATVIC BRASS. John Patrick Trainor and bespectacled Alexander Macleod Small.

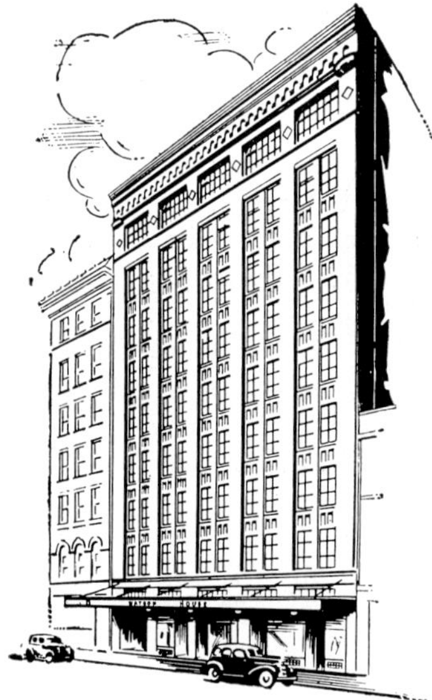

WATSON HOUSE. It is located on Bligh Street, in Sydney, and contains also a Research Laboratory, headquarters for the entire Watson Group, and exhibit rooms.

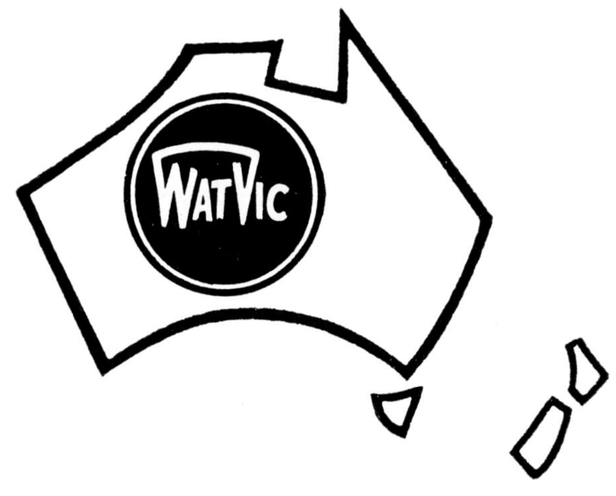

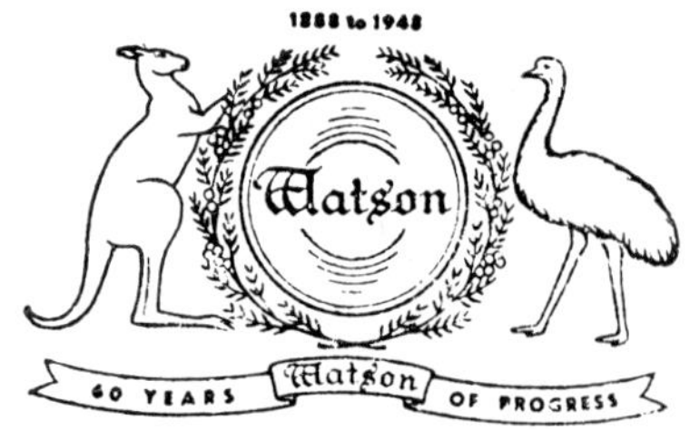

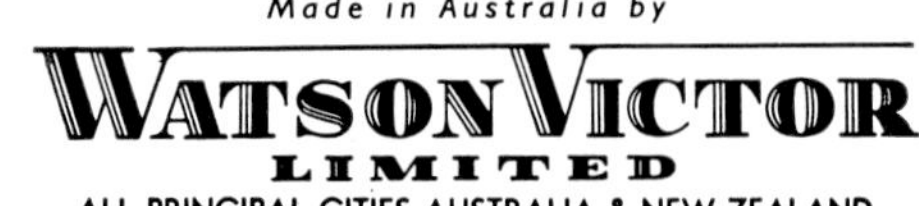

darn good"). Even though their relationship with GE has been terminated, some of WatVic's equipment is still reminiscent of GE styling.

Watson Victor's generators are called Konrad. They come in all sizes. Konrad 8 is a portable, Konrad 10 a dental unit. In the medium range is Konrad 300 ma at 120 kvp. There is a Konrad 600 ma (at 96 kvp), which

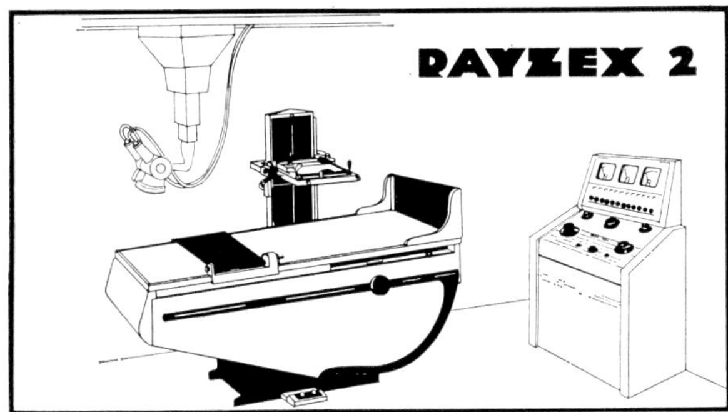

WatVic equipment. Rayzex is WatVic's name for tables (it is also WatVic's Cable Address), and this model — slightly reminiscent of GE equipment — has 25° Trendelenburg. The control stand is from a Konrad 600 ma old version (the new Konrad 600 has simpler controls).

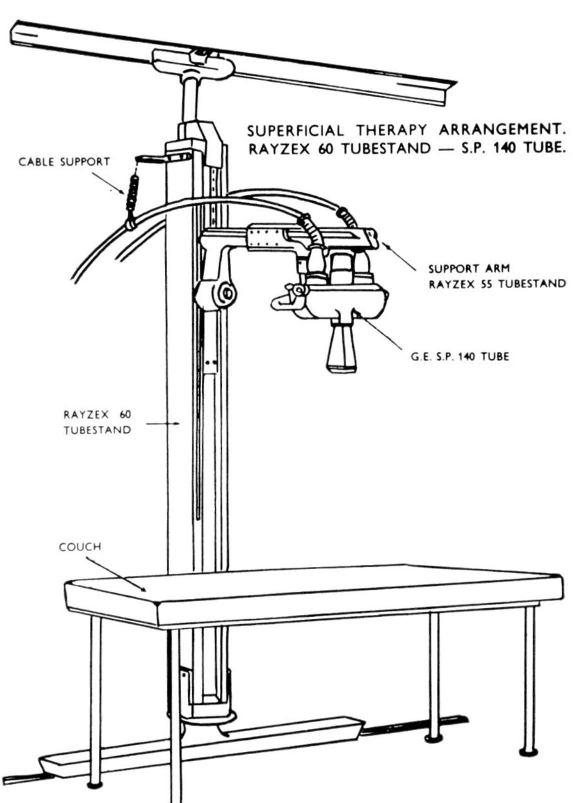

WatVic superficial therapy. Going up to 140 kvp, it permits whole body radiation of lymphomata with cutaneous localizations.

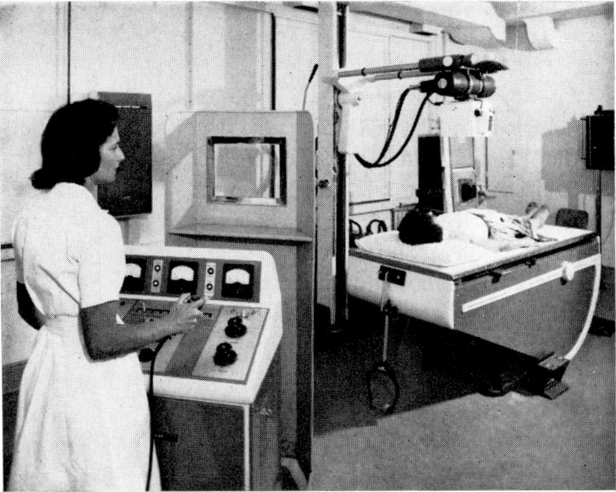

Rayzex at Western Suburbs Hospital in Sydney (Australia).

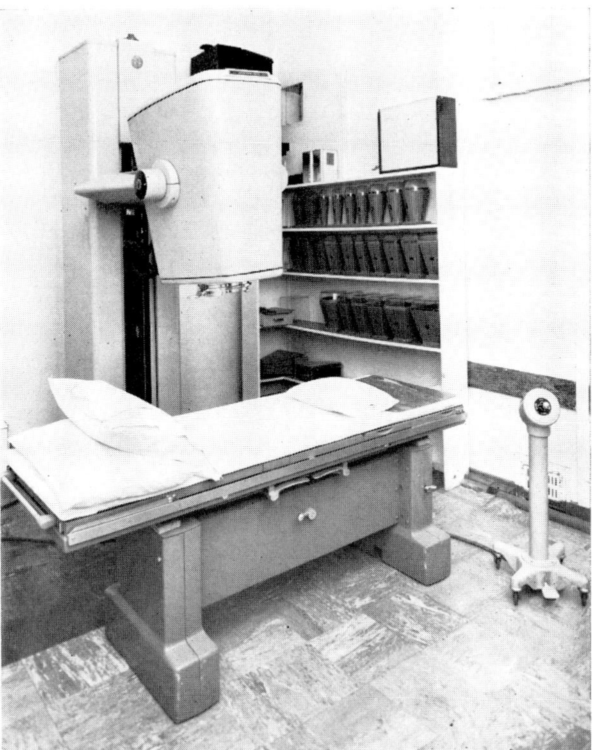

Courtesy: WatVic.

WatVic deep therapy. Rated at 250 kvp, 15 ma continuous, it is a single-tank unit similar to GE's Maximar. The x-ray tube is oil-cooled with a closed-circuit oil pump. The control unit is of the desk type with sloping panel. Safety interlocks are provided to switch the unit off unless proper filters are inserted, the safety doors are closed, and so on. The motors for the vertical and rotational movements of the tubehead are housed in the single support column.

can deliver at up to 130 kvp on some models up to 150 kvp. Konrad 600 has an electronic timer (from 1/100 sec.), and is so wired that it permits twelve exposures per second for high speed film changing technics.

Watson Victor's tables are called Rayzex. All have hinged tops for servicing of the (imported) Bucky-Potter diaphragm. Their most elaborate table, the Rayzex-2, has 25° motorized Trendelenburg tilt, and a telescopic ceiling tube mount is available. WatVic imports the (Bostonian) spotfilm device made by Scholz, and the (Italian) goniotome and craniotome made by Barazzetti.

Watson Victor offers a full line of darkroom equipment and accessories, including the sturdy Kontak cassettes.

Konrad ST140 is a therapy machine in the superficial range (5 ma at 30-140 kvp); its tubehead is best supported by a Rayzex-60 floor-to-ceiling tubestand. WatVic's deep therapy apparatus (15 ma at 250 kvp), with built-in Ionometer, resembles GE's Maximar, and has motorized vertical and rotational motion of the monobloc. Both of these come also in industrial versions.

JAPAN

Throughout most of Asia - everywhere else during a war - there is a relative penury of x-ray films, of processing material and facilities, even of the electrical power needed to energize radiographic equipment. Fluoroscopy requires less elaborate installations, and very little power, a hand-cranked device might conceivably furnish enough electrical current. This is why in Asia the stock-in-trade of x-ray sales is the small, preferably portable machine. The most generally usable combination seems to be a monobloc (transformer and x-ray tube immersed in a single, oil-filled housing), which can be mounted together with a fluoroscopic screen on a column, supported by a pedestal on casters. It can easily be rolled into a darkened room, or to the bedside of a patient - in the evening, with the lights out, one can get a great deal of information. Such a "castering column fluoroscope" is usually also quite satisfactory for bone radiography, even chest films can be made with it. Anything beyond that comes in the elective category and may (or must) be referred to better equipped centers. In a facetious way, one could state that a country is reaching a satisfactory sanitary situation only when the demand for larger x-ray equipment shows a significant increase.

In Tokyo, Osaka, and Kyoto there existed many "cottage industry" manufacturers of small x-ray equipment and accessories. Component parts would be machined in the workers' own homes, and brought for assembly to the respective factory. In Japan, as of late, the demand for larger x-ray installations is

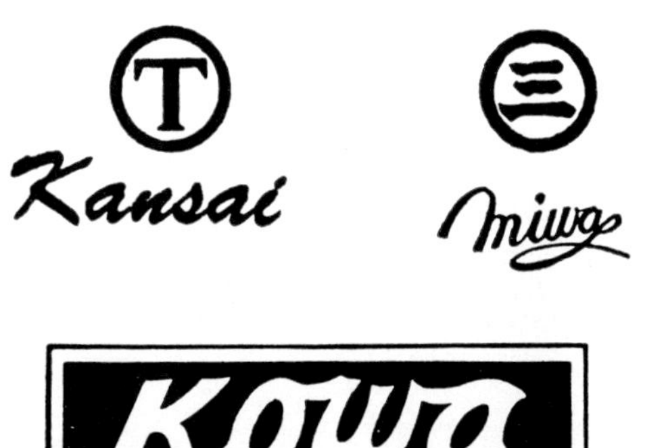

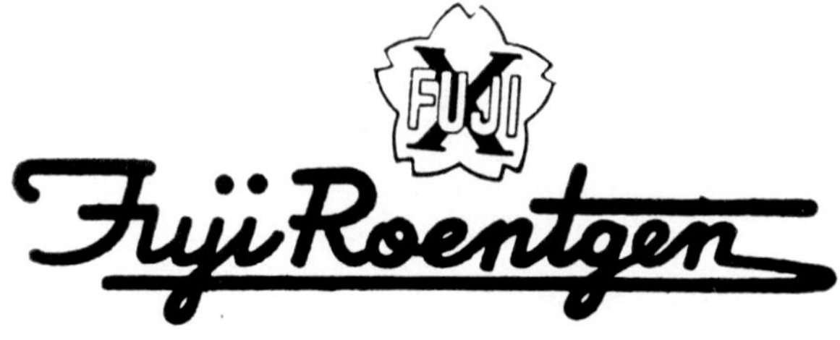

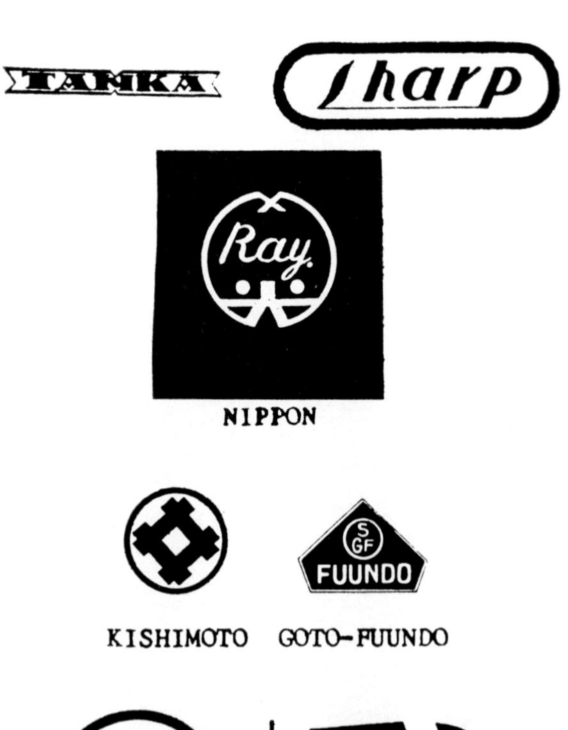

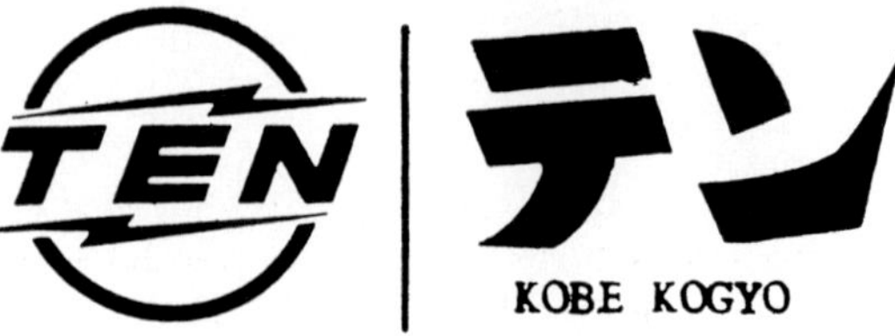

visibly increasing, therefore a number of small manufacturers have gone out of business, others are re-emphasizing the production of accessories, or have turned to making dental x-ray units.*

Tubestands, then horizontal Bucky tables, are the first items manufactured by a "new" firm. Next comes the big test, building a monobloc where the transformer and the tube must be immersed in the oil-filled casing (tropical heat and humidity can do things to those housings!). If that has been successful, the following step is a separate transformer and tube housing, and after that a tomograph, perhaps of the type in which the tube glides along a horizontal single or double rail, as made by Kansai (Osaka) or by Miwa (Tokyo). Thereafter, aside from branching into tilting tables, a few succeed to go into bigger transformers.

*Information for this section came in part from material collected by the Department of Commerce. Details were also obtained from Mr. Allan Chase, Commercial Attaché in Tokyo, and from other sources.

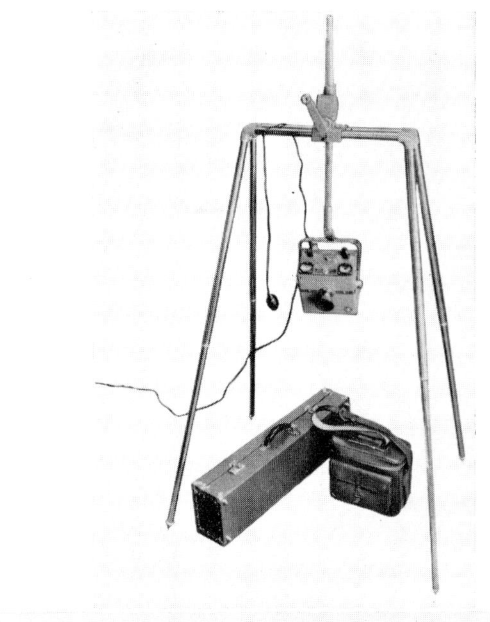

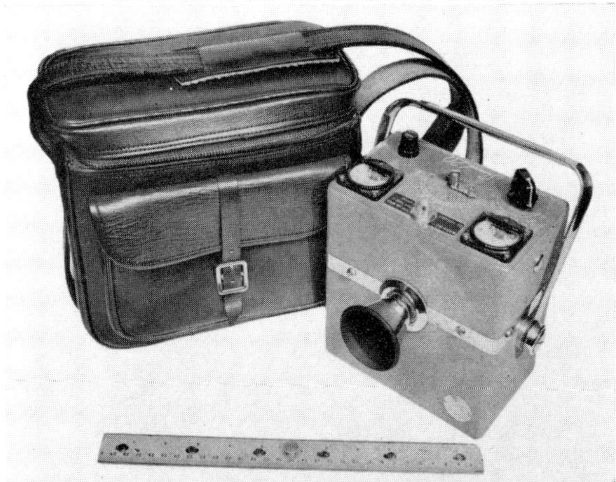

Courtesy: Serend.

ULTRA-PORTABLE. The 12-inch (30 cm) ruler shows the size of this 16 lb. unit (34 lbs. with stand and two cases). It has voltmeter and voltage regulator for the primary, its transformer is rated at 63 kvp and 15 ma, and the only other control (the first is the voltage adjuster) is the .2-5 second timer. The unit is sold in this country by Serend of Sterling (Illinois).

Among the companies created after World War II, Asia Roentgen in Tokyo stayed in the field of x-ray accessories. Kowa (Osaka) and Tanka Roentgen make portables, Fuji Rentogen made it to the 300 ma transformer size, and Acoma to the 500 ma. Hida Electric (Tokyo) is an older company, but it never went beyond portables. Sharp went out of business, but it had not been around for very long, while Dainippon Roentgen (Osaka) was dissolved after sixty years of existence. Mikasa (Tokyo) continues to hold on with portables, mobile, and Grenzstrahlen units. Nippon X-Ray (Tokyo) reached the 500 ma stage.

There are, of course, the representatives of the large Western companies, for instance SRW's is Fuji-Denki (formerly Goto Fuundo), Philips' is Matushita Electric Trading, Picker's is Kishimoto, etc.

Some companies have tackled from the beginning very difficult problems, for instance, Nippon Atomic Machines Mfg. (Osaka) makes betatrons, in the 6 mev and 15 mev group.

Five Japanese manufacturers of x-ray equipment are in the Al category. The Kobe Kogyo Company in Kobe makes x-ray tubes, and tube housings; lately the company has expanded into atomic equipment, cutie pies and all. Hitachi, with headquarters in Tokyo, is Japan's largest manufacturer of electrical equipment; although a relative newcomer in the x-ray field, Hitachi has now a complete line of radiologic machinery. A few more details will be offered on the other three important Japanese x-ray manufacturers, Toshiba, Shimadzu, and Sanyei.

According to Goro Goto, the unofficial historian of Japanese radiology, Shimadzu and Toshiba have

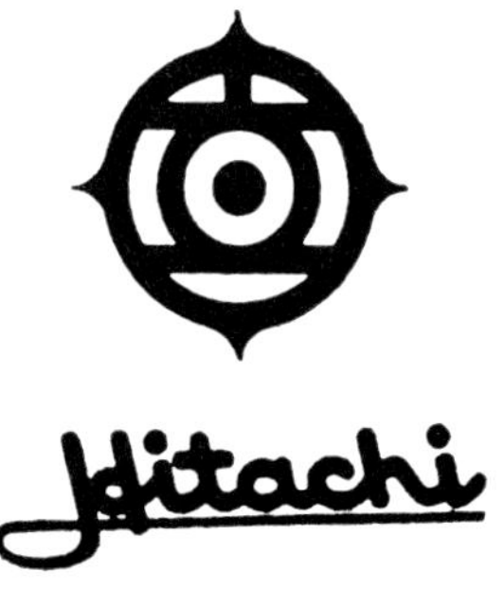

each about 35 percent of the Japanese x-ray market, Hitachi 10 percent, and all other manufacturers together about 20 percent.

TOSHIBA

The Tokyo Shibaura Electric Company (Toshiba), founded in 1875, is Japan's second-largest manufacturer of electrical equipment - with twenty plants, fifty-seven affiliated companies, about $120 million in assets, and over forty-two thousand employees.

Toshiba

Toshiba makes all sorts of radiologic equipment. It has its own tube factory, and among its subsidiaries there is one with the indicative name of Toshiba Nucleonics. Toshiba's production includes (almost) everything radiological, from grid-controlled 50 kw, 150 kvp Rotanodes to rotating Co-60 teletherapy units, and from reciprocating Bucky diaphragms to betatrons.

Toshiba's transformer KXO-15 500 ma at 90 kvp, or 30 ma at 150 kvp. The latter comes in two variants, KXO-15-1A, which has in addition an impulse timer, a synchronous timer, built-in-Bucky, and wall mounted control panel, while KXO-15-2A comes only with the synchronous timer.

Toshiba's better tables, the GMSE and FSE, have motorized sliding table tops and electromagnetic locks

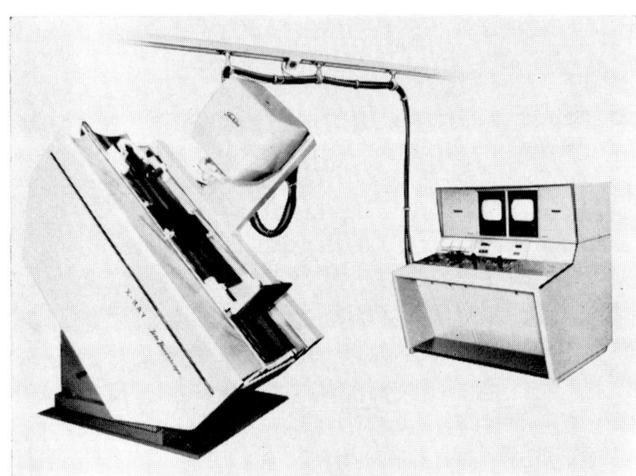

TOSHIBA X-RAY TELEVISION.

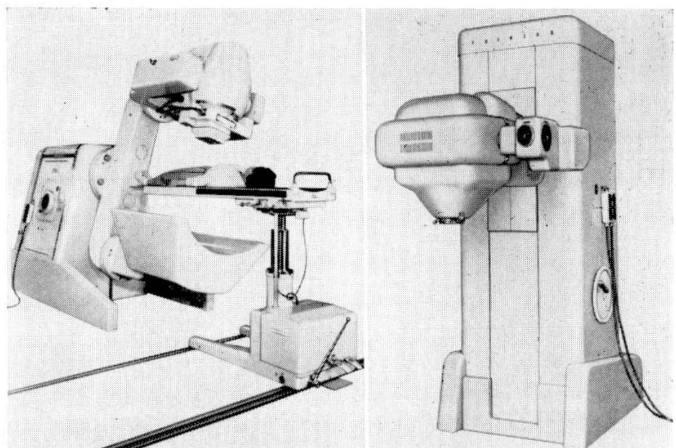

TOSHIBA THERAPY. RI-120-2 is a moving field Co-60 unit, while the upright machine is a 15 mev betatron.

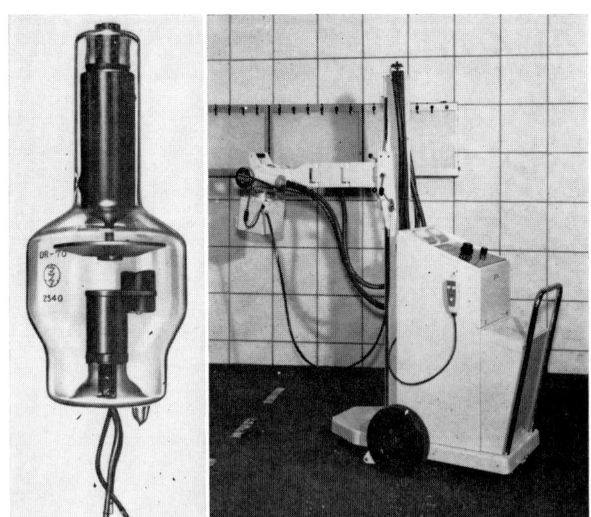

TOSHIBA MODELS. DR-70 is a rotating anode tube, while KED-M-3R is a condenser-type of mobile x-ray apparatus.

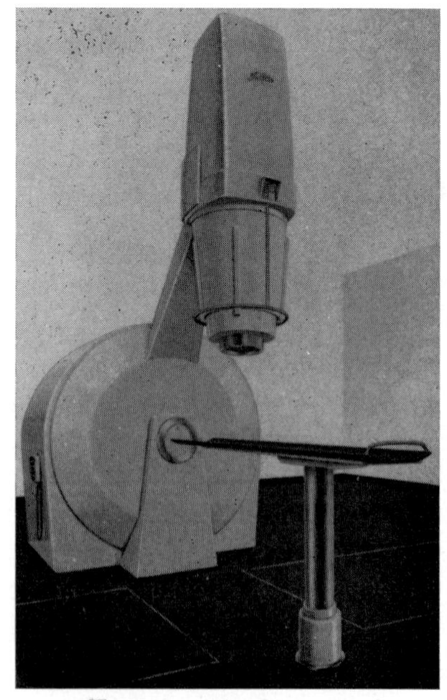

TOSHIBA MEDICAL LINAC.

The telescopic ceiling tube mount comes either remote-controlled (L), or in a manual type (M).

Toshiba offers a variety of upright fluoroscopes, mobile units in the 75-90 kvp range (monoblocs with fluoroscopic screen attached to a "castering column"), and several condenser units. One of the latter, the KCD-M-2 (30 ma at 60 kvp) comes likewise on a rolling column," and permits fluoroscopy both in upright and in recumbency.

Another peculiarity is the fact that Toshiba's catalog mentions for all these units the rating under prolonged usage. Any KXO can be operated continuously at 4 ma and 95 kvp. Their portable unit PK-40-1 is rated at 3 ma and 75 kvp for 20 minutes. The reason for this is the use as (make-shift) superficial therapy units. Such superficial therapy is being administered in the management of (potentially) infected wounds, with unquestionable if unorthodox results.*

*This procedure was extensively studied and relatively often utilized during World War II in the Soviet Union.

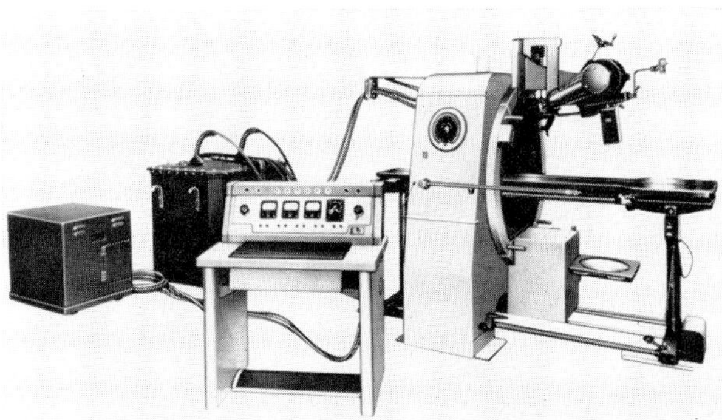

Toshiba KXC-18-3A. The ringstand as well as the other appurtenances and capabilities of this therapy unit closely parallel those of Mueller's Tu-1.

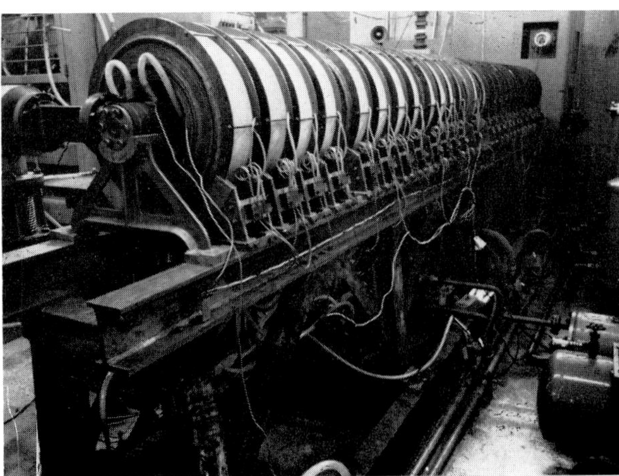

Toshiba 25 mev industrial linac.

Toshiba's dental unit is the TDX-IB. The Layergraph Type D is a horizontal tomograph with space provided for multi-layer cassettes. Several photofluorographic machines are available, the portable KCD-K-2, and the KCD-K-5RB for in-the-bus installation.

Toshiba's superficial therapy apparatus has the sign STX: STX-50-3 is a mobile 10-50 kvp unit carrying an end-type grounded-anode tube with beryllium window for contact dosage. KXC are deep therapy models: KXC-18-2 is a 25 ma, 200 kvp stationary unit, KXC-18-3A is the same thing mounted on a rotating device very similar to Mueller's TU-1. KXC-19-7 is a 250 kvp therapy unit with pendular capabilities.

SHIMADZU

Shimadzu Seisakusho is the oldest name among Japanese x-ray manufacturers. The firm was started in 1875 by Genzo Shimadzu as a small shop (located in Kyoto, center of classical Japanese culture): at first they manufactured scientific apparatus for use in schools. Continued prosperity made them branch out into electro-medical equipment, in 1896 they constructed the first Japanese x-ray apparatus, and succeeded in producing the first x-ray plates in Japan. Shimadzu contributed significantly to the development of radiology in Japan; among their pioneering achievements was the creation in 1927 of

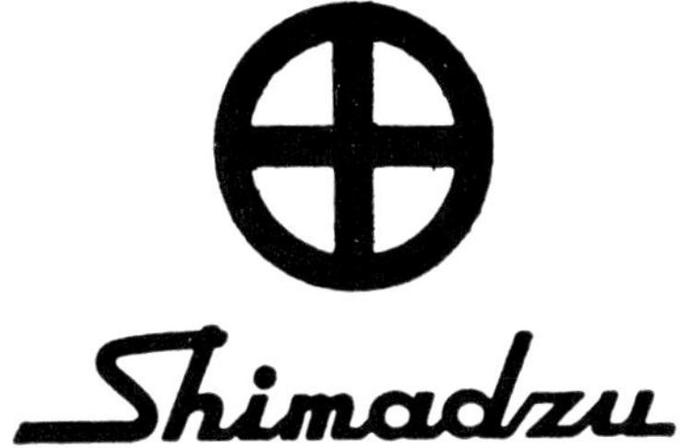

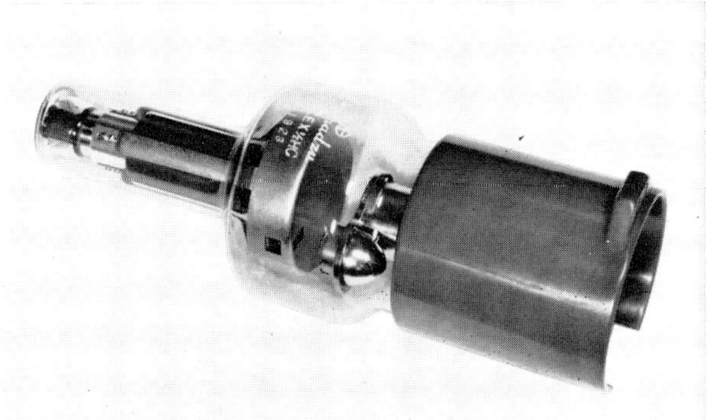

Shimadzu's O.F.R. less Circlex. The initials mean off-focus-radiation, and the whole thing amounts to inside-tube shielding which prevents the exit of anything but the useful beam.

a training school for x-ray technicians which, so far, has graduated over 1,100 trainees.

Shimadzu was incorporated in 1917. It reached its peak at the end of World War II with 12 plants and 18,000 employees. Today it has four plants, and 3,800 employees. The full name of the company is Shimadzu Seisakusho, Ltd., and its current president is Yosuke Suzuki, but they still have on their Board of Directors at least three members of the Shimadzu family.

Following an agreement in 1951, Shimadzu makes some equipment under a Westinghouse license. Shimadzu covers the entire field of radiology, both medical and industrial. They manufacture x-ray tubes and image intensifiers, fluorescent and reinforcing screens, Geiger counters and scintillation crystals, x-ray diffraction machines and betatrons (Shimadzu's cobalt irradiators have been on the market for several years). The company's capital is about $5 million.

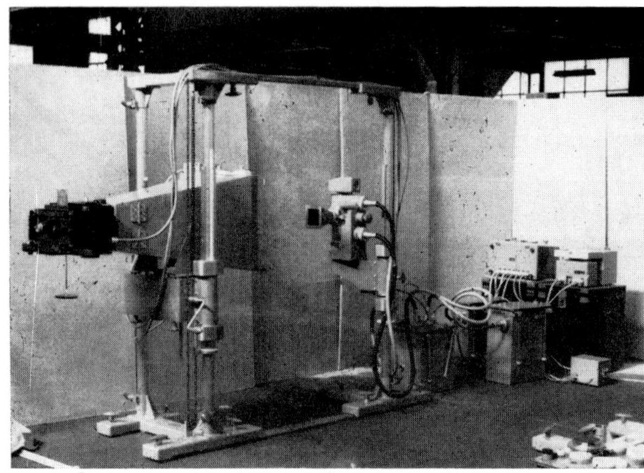

SHIMADZU'S PORTABLE CONDENSER PHOTOFLUOROGRAPH. It can be hooked up to residential power supply (because of its condensers), and has grid-controlled rotating anodes (to cut off the tail of the condenser discharge.)

Shimadzu equipment has very little resemblance to that made by Westinghouse (at least on the outside). Shimadzu still puts out inexpensive hand-cranked tables. BS-2SC is motor-driven and has a mechanical spotfilm device. The fully automated AS-2 permits 18° Trendelenburg tilt (13° when a rotating anode is used under the table); it has a multi-leaf shutter (M2-FR), and a pushbutton spotfilmer. In the de-luxe diagnostic combination YD125L-2, the AS-2 table is paired with a 500 ma, 125 kvp transformer, and wall mounted control panel. It has an electronic timer, electronic circuitry to protect the tube(s) from overload, and provision for an (optical) intercommunication system.

Shimadzu's rotating anodes are called Circlex. The Super Circlex type C has twin-focus, the largest of which (2x2 mm) can take a load of 40 kw at 150 kvp. The "OFR-less" Circlex suppresses "off-focus-radiation." Several models of triode Circlex are available: grid control is very useful in transformers with condensers (to cut off the undesirable tail-end of the condenser discharge). Indeed, grid-controlled rotating anodes are standard equipment on all photofluorographic machines, as the latter are often built with condenser-transformers to take advantage of weak sources of power supply. Mass chest surveys are still politically popular in the Orient — despite technological advances into the Atomic Phase, many people have retained the men-

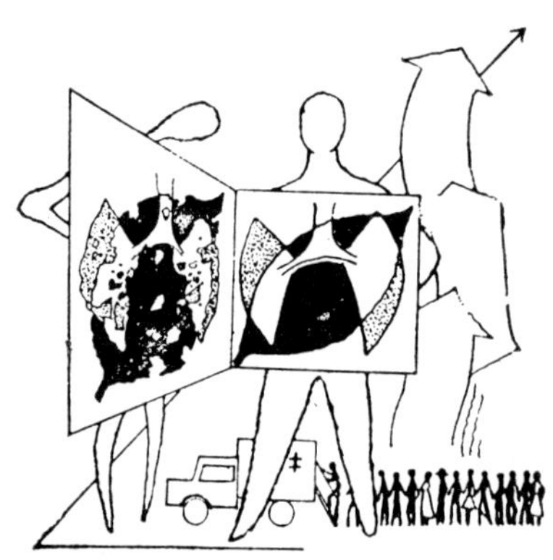

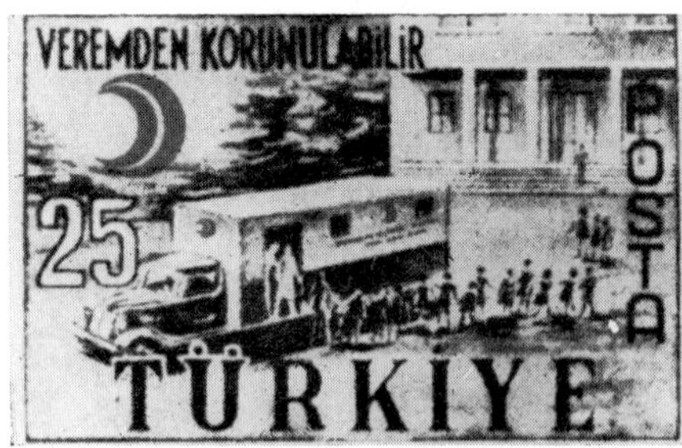

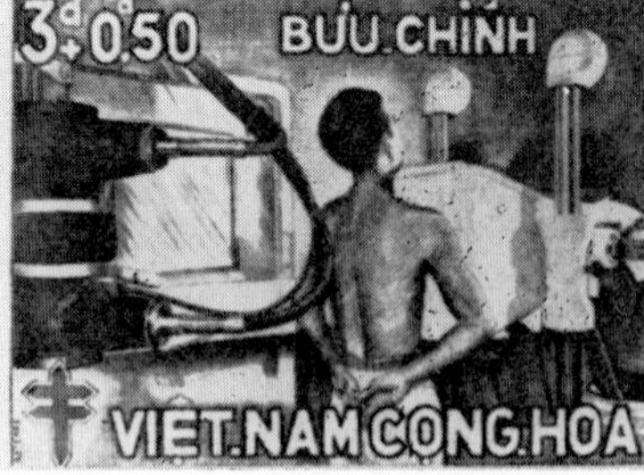

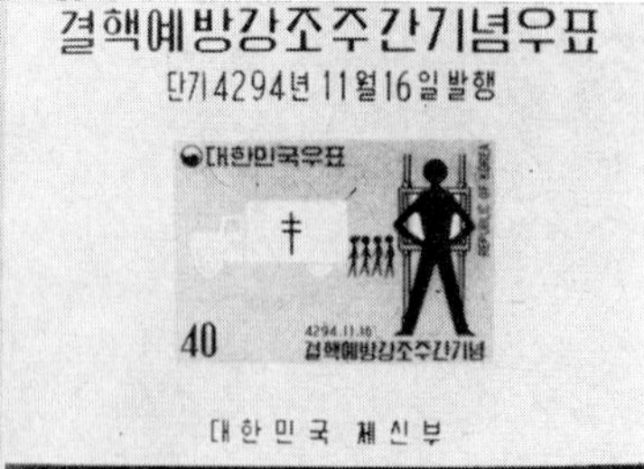

Courtesy: Stan Bohrer.

PHILATELIC PHOTOFLUOROGRAPHY. Since tuberculosis has been given the official stamp of "social disease," the "fight against" the "white plague" often acquires political overtones. This is demonstrated in three stamps showing children alighting from an "x-ray bus" (Turkey, 1957), a photofluorogram (Viet Nam, 1960), and both a bus and a schematic patient (Korea, 1961).

tality of the Golden Age of Radiology. The photofluorographic bus has become almost a symbol of sanitary improvement, but this is a side issue mentioned herein only to add that Shimadzu (like most other large Japanese x-ray manufacturers) makes several models of such survey equipment.

SHT250M-2 is Shimadzu's most elaborate deep therapy apparatus. It comes with a motor-operated treatment couch on rails, and with pendular motion of the tubehead. It delivers between 10 and 25 ma at from 80 to 250 kvp.

SANYEI

While it is not the largest, nor the oldest, the Sanyei Manufacturing Company is perhaps the most active of Japan's smaller x-ray firms. It was started in 1931 in Osaka (Japan's second-largest city) by Kikuji Uyeno and "two other" associates. In Japanese, *san* means (also) three and *yei* means prosperity, which is what the founders had wanted to presage for their ternary enterprise. The second part of the prediction came true, but not the first, because the "two others" dropped out before the company was incorporated in 1936. Today Sanyei represents the (American) Machlett, the (British) Watson & Sons, and the (Dutch) Odelca - and is

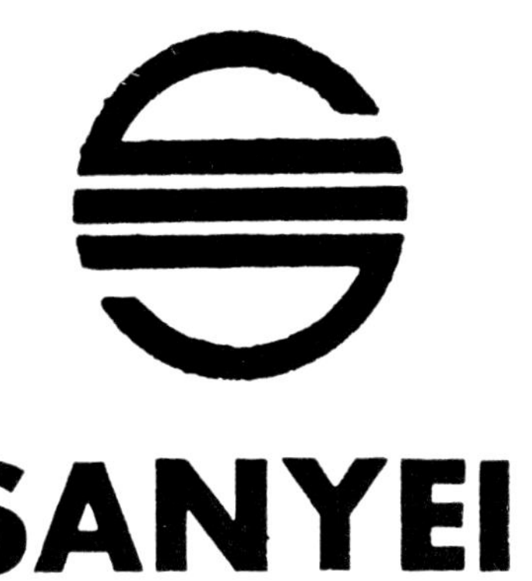

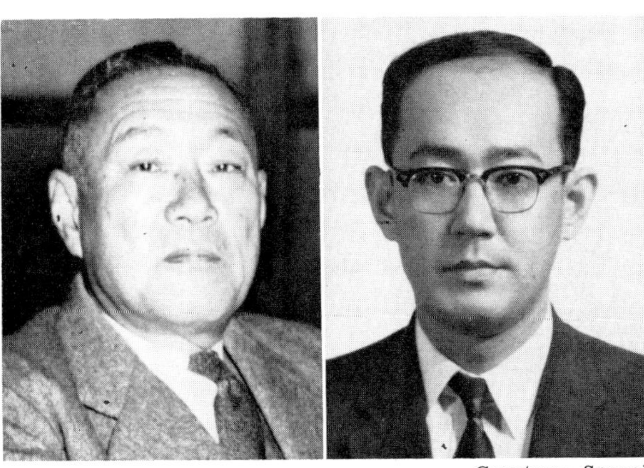

Courtesy: Sanyei.

SANYEI'S FATHER AND SON. One of Sanyei's founders (the most perseverent and optimistic of the three) was Kikuji Uyeno, who is currently its president. His son, the bespectacled Jiro Uyeno directs a trading subsidiary of the mother firm.

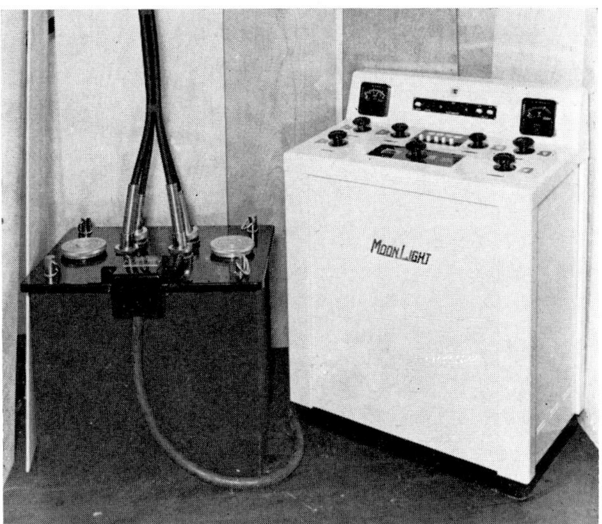

Courtesy: Sanyei.

SANYEI'S MOONLIGHT. Transformer rated 500 ma at 95 kvp, or 200 ma at 125 kvp, uses Machlett thoriated tungsten filament kenotrons, and its x-ray tubes are collimated with the "Light Beam."

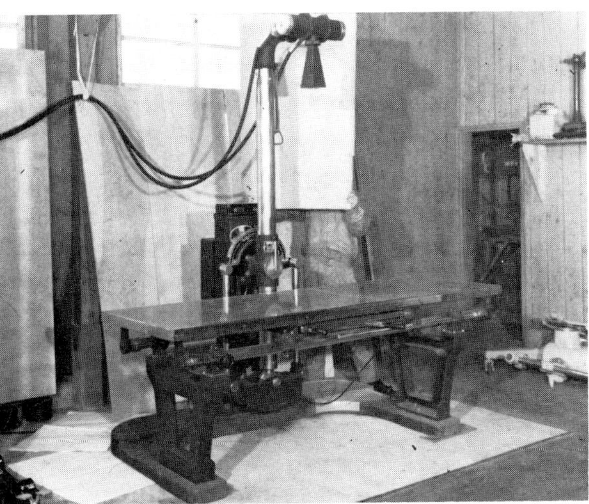

Courtesys: Sanyei.

SANYEI'S LAYERGRAPH. This reproduction has not been "cleaned up," its natural background shows up. White cloth is usually draped behind the "subject" to make the artist's life easier, in this instance an assistant held a white panel high up to "lighten up" things about the x-ray tube. The cluttered background fails to bring out the clean, orientally curved lines of the table.

therefore in a position to offer as good equipment as (most) anybody in the world. Besides, Sanyei builds its own tables, transformers up to 500 ma, portable and therapy equipment (they also manufacture varied electro-encephalographs, electrocardiographs, and multi-channel recorders).

Sanyei makes two hand-operated tables, the VH-1000 and the VH-2000. VH-3000 and VH-3500 are motor driven, have 15° Trendelenburg tilt, and semiautomatic spotfilming devices. Their transformer is called Moonlight and the multileaf collimator has the poetical name Light Beam. Sanyei's condenser units use (Machlett) triode rotating anodes, while the photofluorographic machines are built with Odelca mirror cameras. Among special devices, Sanyei has the portable PX-58, the (obligatory) mobile fluoroscopic unit mounted on the "castering column," and a Grenzstrahlen machine. An elegant horizontal tomographic unit (PT) is also available.

CHINA

On the island of Taiwan (Formosa) only repair facilities are available.

Many of the machines in operation on Formosa are of Japanese manufacture. The island had been occupied by the Japanese before and during World War II, and most of the physicians speak that language fluently in addition to Chinese.

Soon after introduction of embargo on the Chinese mainland, large quantities of surplus x-ray parts were left in storage in Hong Kong. An enterprising person bought them up, put them together, and made a few small x-ray units, which were soon sold to general practitioners. That industry was short-lived.

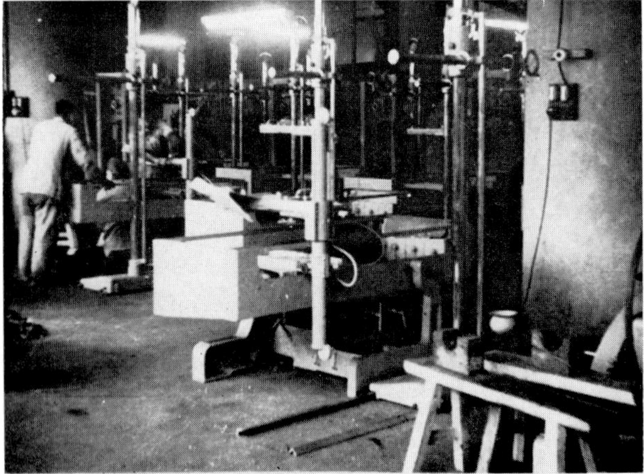

Chinese x-ray factory. View of the table room.

In the British colony of Hong Kong, most of the x-ray equipment is of one of three makes: (British) Watson, (Dutch) Philips, or (German) SRW. Only a few machines are of different manufacture, but almost all makes are represented, from the (Swedish) Elema and the (Australian) WatVic, to the (French) CGR and the (American) GE.* A few x-ray accessories, such as viewboxes, are manufactured in Hong Kong.

On the Chinese mainland, plagued by the political upheaval, the lack of above mentioned spare x-ray parts was keenly felt. Repair centers were set up in several places, one at Peiping, another at Tuncheng. An x-ray tube factory began operating in Shanghai sometime in 1954. By 1956, a visiting businessman was shown rotating anode tubes of Chinese manufacture. Tables and transformers had been built in China for many years. Even before 1956 (possibly as early as 1954) they started to put out complete installations.

*This information was courteously supplied by Hamdi Suao Rassim, the radiologist of Queen Mary Hospital in Hong Kong.

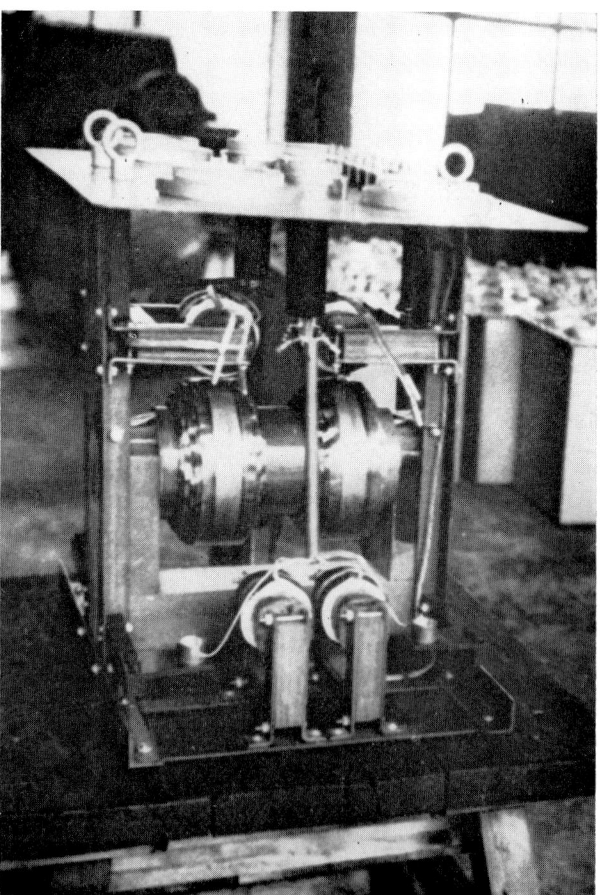

Chinese x-ray transformer. Innards seen before panels are applied.

The Chinese People's x-ray factory in Shanghai is called Wah Tung. One of their catalogs, printed about 1959, lists two complete x-ray outfits. The first is called 200-56, for its transformer which is rated at 200 ma for 70 kvp, or 100 ma for 90 kvp; the single rotating anode tube is supported by a column on rails, set alongside a motor-driven table, with under-the-table Bucky. The other installation, called 25-56 (25 ma) is a "castering column fluoroscope." The digits -56 presumably indicate the year 1956 in which these models had been designed.

The catalog depicts also two short-wave therapy units, electro-surgical apparatus, cassettes and re-inforcing screens, and a hand-held cryptoscope. The latter comes equipped with a radio-protective lead rubber skirt, suspended between the handle and the place where the patient is going to be located.

By Western standards, Chinese equipment is crude. Since it can be regarded as a beginning, one may anticipate the appearance of improved models. So far, however, judging from recent (September, 1963) reports, there has occurred no significant change in the quality of materials or workmanship.

But Russian-built reactors and cyclotrons are in operation on the Chinese mainland; Wah Tung has started building Co-60 teletherapy equipment; and having tested their first A-bomb, one wonders how soon will the Chinese have the H-bomb.

There seems to be very little Sovietic x-ray equipment on the Chinese mainland. Most of the new x-ray apparatus in China is imported from the (British) Watson and from Philips, somewhat less from Japanese manufacturers. The Chinese do not (or cannot) purchase significant quantities of x-ray equipment from East Germany, Hungary, or Czechoslovakia. From the very beginning there has been very little political or economic fraternization between Iron Curtain and Bamboo Curtain countries.

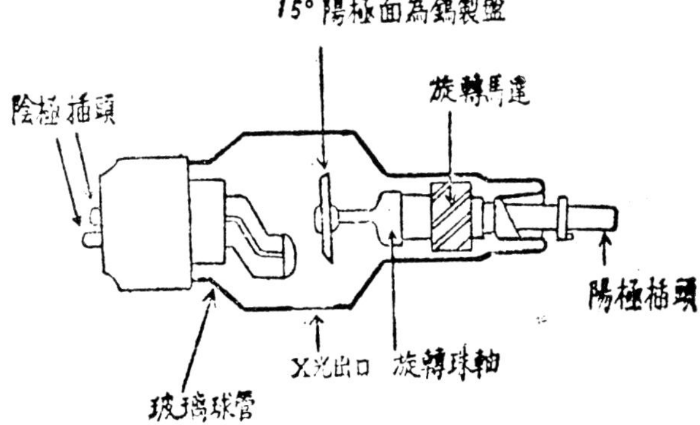

In the *Chinese Journal of Radiology* (Peiping) of December 29, 1958 appeared an article by Wang Shao-hsun entitled *Chinese Traditional and Western Medical Practices Combine, Create New Radiology.* Following are excerpts from the translation of that paper, graciously contributed by the Department of Commerce:

"In 1958, the Secretary of the Chinese Communist Party, who was also Deputy Minister of Health, in his

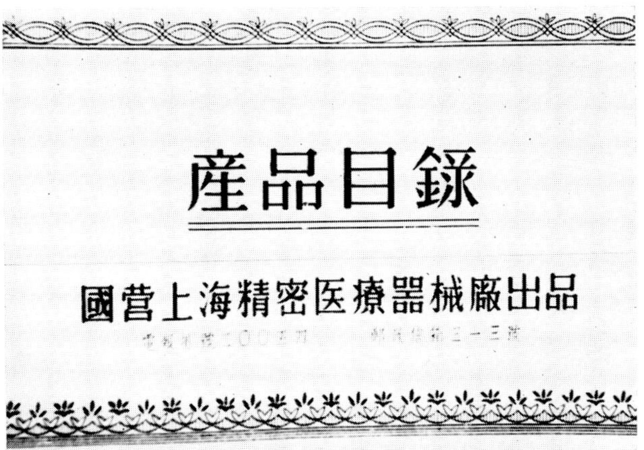

CHINESE X-RAY CATALOG. It contains also other "electric" machinery listings.

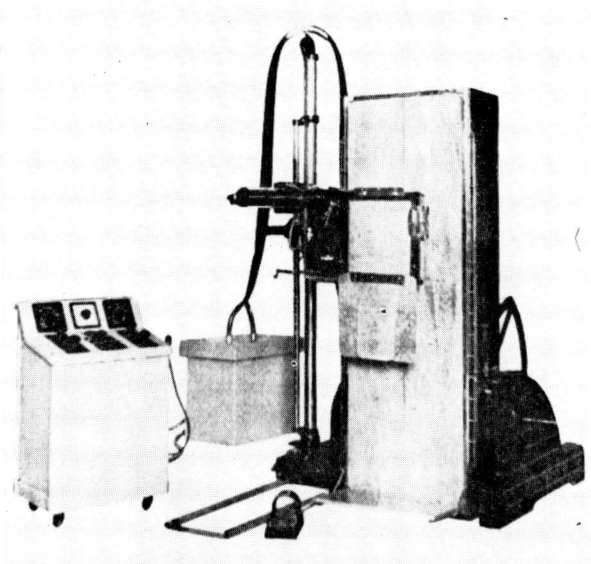

CHINESE DIAGNOSTIC UNIT. 200 ma, 70 kvp transformer, control stand, single tube, motor-driven table, and under-the-table Bucky.

presentation before the (Chinese) National Congress on the Exchange of Experiences for the Technical Revolution of Medical, Pharmaceutical, and Health Sciences, specified that "whether in the practice of preventive medicine or in the theoretical field, there are certain phases of traditional Chinese medical practice which cannot be surpassed by Western medicine. . . We must try to contribute medical science to the world . . . we must promote the combination of Chinese traditional medical practices with Western medicine to create a new Chinese medicine which will occupy the highest seat among all nations. . . (this) is also one of the most important items of the technical revolution."

"Generally speaking, there should be no question or difficulties in combining Chinese and Western medical practices in the field of internal medicine or surgery, because there is a tremendous amount of experiences in traditional Chinese medicine which is valuable for study and adaptation. However, the situation is somewhat different in the field of radiology. Radiology is a new medical science which was unknown in our (Chinese) traditional medical practice. Therefore, when promoting the movement to have "everyone study traditional Chinese medicine; every medical field must use both Chinese and Western medicine" there are several problems confronting the workers in the field of radiology: few of them study traditional Chinese medicine; those who do engage in such a study usually do not try hard to learn, conceiving that it has no value. But this is entirely wrong; traditional Chinese medicine has such a vast material and experiences that it could be applied by the dialectical method to any disease; combining Chinese traditional and Western medicine is useful also in radiology."

"Radiodiagnosis can be utilized to observe the effectiveness of Chinese traditional medical practices or

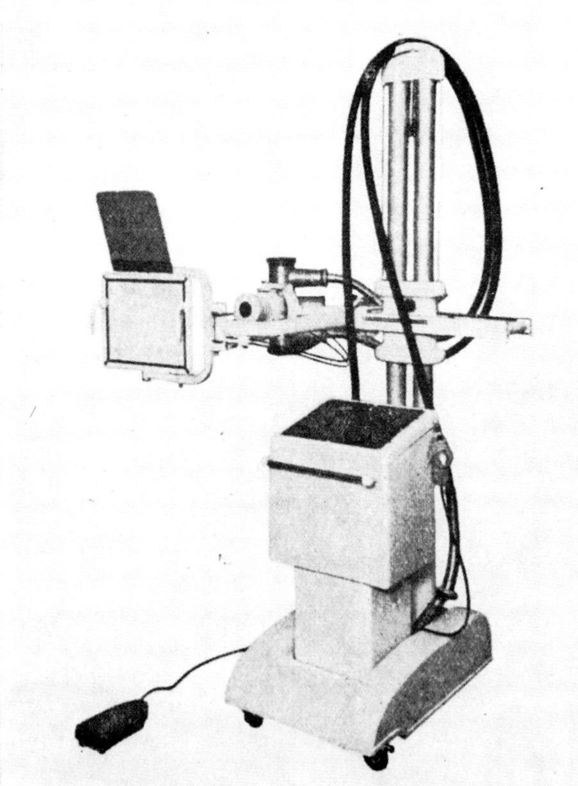

CHINESE CASTERING COLUMN FLUOROSCOPE. Low-powered 25 ma, 70 kvp monobloc transformer-tube under oil, usable also for simple radiographic procedures.

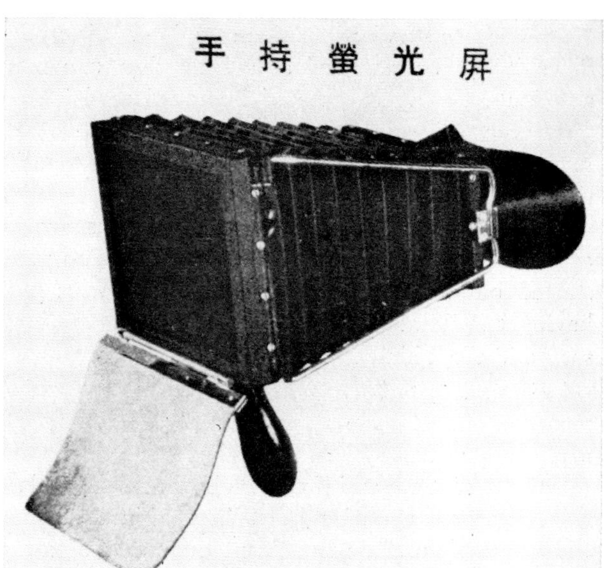

CHINESE CRYPTOSCOPE. Note the refinement added, a protective lead apron.

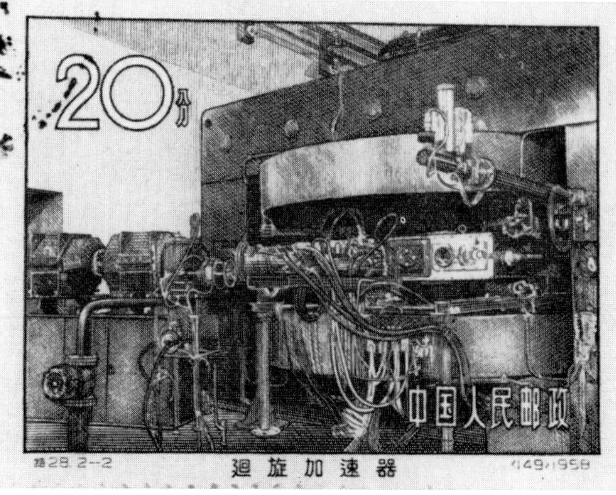

SOVIETIC CYCLOTRON IN PEIPING.

Chinese drugs . . . for example, when acupuncture or moxibustion therapy are used, functional changes of the gastrointestinal tract (such as peristalsis, motility, pyloric changes) may be studied by fluoroscopy . . . furthermore, radioisotopes could be employed to study patients treated by traditional Chinese medicine."

"Consider employing Chinese drugs as chemicals for making or processing x-ray films. All important chemicals for use with x-ray films are very expensive. Their supplies are usually short. If we spend some time studying such drugs we might be able to find some substitutes with a lower cost and more ample supply."

"In the field of radiotherapy . . . there is a very bright future . . . for the combination of traditional Chinese and Western medicine . . . it is well known that certain Chinese drugs increase blood circulation in certain parts of the body, as do acupuncture or moxibustion. They could thus be used to potentiate radiosensitivity which would increase effectiveness of radiotherapy when applied to those parts."

X 光學手冊

目 次

HANDBOOK OF ROENTGENOLOGY

1951

TABLE OF CONTENTS Page

Also in the *Chinese Journal of Radiology* of December 29, 1958 appeared an article on *The Usefulness of Acupuncture and Moxibustion in the Treatment of Radiation Reaction.* The latter would contribute to "defense medicine"* if traditional Chinese medicine could be used to cure acute radiation diseases. The effectiveness of treating radiation dermatitis by such Chinese drugs as crystallized egg white, egg yolk fat, and other yellow ointment has previously been alleged.

"Radiotherapy can be combined with traditional Chinese practices and drugs for the treatment of cancer. During the current national exhibit on medical, pharmaceutical, and public health practices in China, we

*This could best be translated by Medical Aspects of Civil Defense.

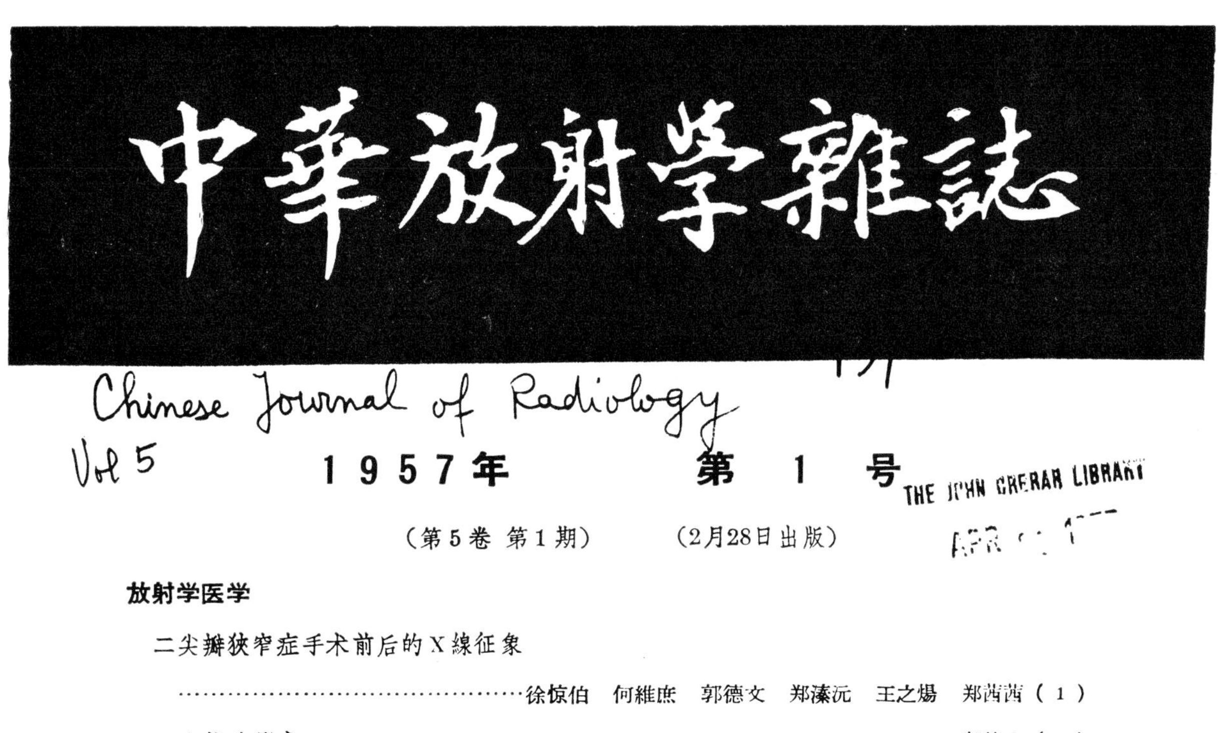

中華放射學雜誌

Chinese Journal of Radiology

Vol 5

1957年 第 1 号

(第5卷 第1期) (2月28日出版)

have seen many instances where cancer was not cured by Western medical methods, but was cured by traditional Chinese medical practices. It is very obvious that combining radiotherapy and traditional Chinese medical practices and drugs, the effectiveness of treating cancer could be greatly increased."

"This is just a rough outline of this subject. In order to combine traditional Chinese and Western medical practices, for the creation of a new radiological science, it is imperative to work under the (Communist) Party leadership, to emphasize political learning among the workers of radiology, and thus to study Chinese traditional medicine. In such a way we can promote traditional Chinese medicine to become the only new radiological science in the world for the well-being of the people."

However adventitious, this authoritative as well as articulate statement expresses the current (or, rather - it is hoped - only the currently desired) orientation of radiology on the Chinese mainland. To the Western mind, the statement is pure and simple scientific sacrilege. To make it utterly unpalatable also to what is presently called the Eastern mind, one might first have to adequately define the Chinese statement - in ideologic lingo - as a "leftist (radio-) deviation"!

Red China, less than two decades after its creation, is stronger than China had ever been. This was done with tremendous efforts, and by sacrificing the happiness and even the lives of many individuals. It would be foolish for any statesman to discount the potential shown by such an achievement. But from the lofty viewpoint of the historian, much of what the Red Chinese do and say today can be taken as the exuberant, sometimes ornery, or even destructive actions and words of teenagers, in the hope that maturity will make them understand the facts of life.

Ancient Chinese medicine survived millenia, which means that the patients must have been satisfied with at least some of its results. It is just as true that between 60 and 90 percent (depending on the type of practice) of those who consult a physician need no more than reassurance and placebos. Pierre Huard and Ming Wong's beautiful and historical *Médecine Chinoise* (Paris, 1959) indicates that the old Chinese used surgical procedures as well as many drugs. And yet, their most spectacular results were claimed with acupuncture or moxibustion, based on the "harmonization" of the two antithetic principles, the (female negative, dark, evil) Yin and the (masculine, positive, bright, beneficent) Yang. This dualism pervaded ancient Chinese thinking, from medicine to magic, and from philosophy to politics. In the physiology of acupuncture, it could be regarded as a symbolic representation of the sympathetic (Yang) and the even less predictable parasympathetic (Yin) systems. It is well known that acupuncture and moxibustion have achieved remarkable, if unpredictable, results in certain functional disturbances. "Modern" medical philosophers, much like schizophrenics, tend to disbelieve and reject as inexistent what they cannot comprehend. Some day the acupuncturist's fourteen mythical "vessels" may turn out to be as yet unknown reflex pathways of the neurovegetative complex. It would be scientifically (just as) sacrilegious to simply and haughtily reject the radio-acupuncturing proposal — except insofar as it implies the political subservience of medicine. One must never forget that mixing medicine and politics is like borrowing money from relatives: repayment of the debt, even with excessive interest, cannot remove all contingent obligations.

INDIA

We have seen the difficulties connected in Japan with the manufacture of small x-ray equipment. In India things are different, because there is as yet no local competition by organized large manufacturers. Moreover, beyond the stage of tubestands,

DEDICATED TO THE SERVICE OF THE COUNTRY

MADE IN INDIA

X-RAY MACHINES OF PROVED PERFORMANCE

PORTABLE 80 kV, 15 mA. STATIC 90 kV, 50 mA.
MOBILE 85 kV, 30 mA. STATIC 100 kV, 100 mA. (Complete with Tilting Table).

STATIC 100 kV, 200 mA. (Complete with Tilting Table)

In production for 12 years

RADON HOUSE

Factory: 89, Kalighat Road, Calcutta 26.
Office: 7, Sirdar Sankar Road, Calcutta 26.

1956

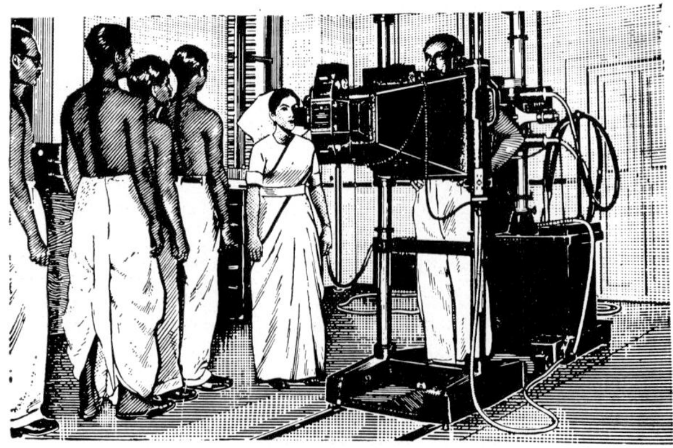

CHEST SURVEY. British Watson equipment in use in an Indian hospital.

tables and (small) transformers, the technical intricacies become insurmountable without special equipment and qualified technical assistance. A small Indian x-ray manufacturing firm exists since 1944 (at Bhowmik's) Radon House in Calcutta.

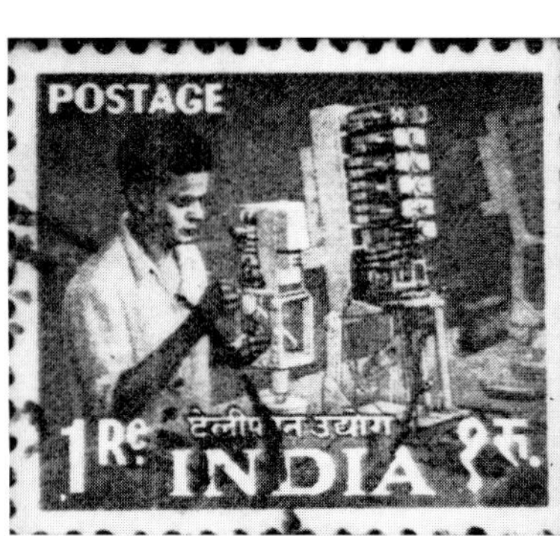

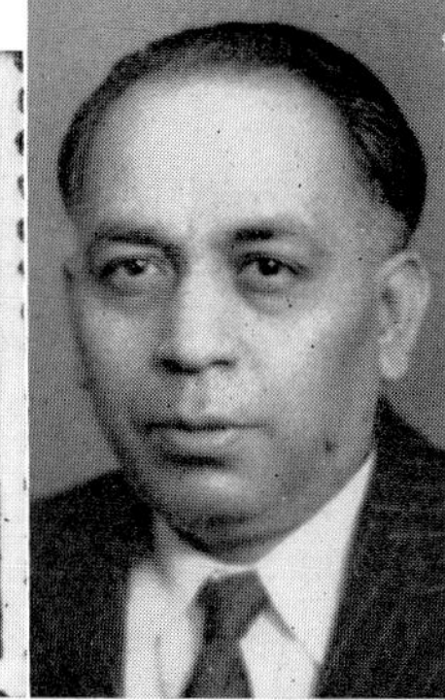

BIBHU BILAS BHOWMIK

With an MSc in applied physics (Calcutta) and an MSc in engineering (London), after five years in Europe (including France and Germany), Bhowmik returned to India to teach in the University of Calcutta, to create and operate the first Indian x-ray manufacturing plant, and to be a member of most of the Indian technical x-ray committees. Just like the stamp, he symbolizes the strive for the creation of "native" staffs and skills without which no industrialization program can ever be successful.

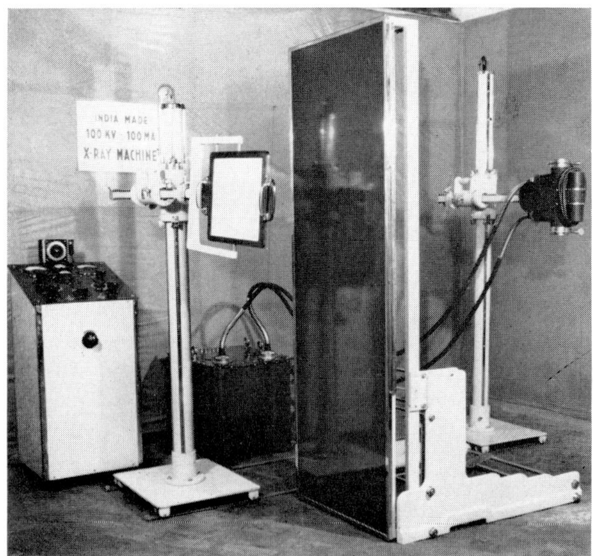

Courtesy: Bibhu Bhowmik

RADON HOUSE'S Indian-made 100 ma, 100 kvp transformer with two-position (up or down) table, and fluoroscopic screen supported by separate pedestal (1963).

Bhowmik makes a portable (15 ma at 80 kvp), and a mobile (30 ma at 85 kvp), both of which are available in the expected "castering column" fluoroscopic arrangement. Their largest installation is a 200 ma, 100 kvp with tilting table.

Siemens had always been very strong in India. They were represented (together with Elema-Schönander) by the East Asiatic Company. Now a new subsidiary has been created, the (Indian) Siemens Engineering & Manufacturing Co., and they are building an x-ray plant in Bombay.

Two other plants for the manufacturing of x-ray equipment are now in the planning stage, one by the (Indian) International General Electric Co. in Madras, the other by a Westinghouse licensee, the (Indian) Escorts, Ltd. of New Delhi.*

SOUTHEAST ASIA

The hiatus left by Siemens during World War II was filled by Watson, through its owner, the (British) General Electric Co.; by the (Australian) WatVic; by the (American) GE; and, after the end of the war, by Picker; and by Philips. Among the American firms, surprisingly active in Asia (by comparison with its local volume) seemed the H. G. Fisher Co. of Maywood (Illinois).

In Singapore WatVic, Siemens, and Philips are today the most popular makes. GE and Mueller are "also" used.**

In Malaya x-ray equipment is of Philips, GE, Watson, SRW, and Picker manufacture. No Japanese machines have as yet been introduced, but x-ray film is being purchased from Japan.***

As long as it remained a Dutch colony, Indonesia was Philips territory. Thereafter, because of the political situation, SRW and WatVic equipment began to be imported. The same situation obtained with French equipment in their former colonies.

---

*Information for this paragraph was provided by Dr. K. H. G. Krishnaswami, Dean of the Governmental General Hospital in Madras.

**This information was courteously supplied by Dr. Ben Cheng Tan, a radiotherapist in the General Hospital in Singapore.

***This information was obligingly offered by Dr. Manindra Nath Sen, radiologist in the General Hospital in Malacca.

AFRICA

British and French x-ray equipment prevail in the territories which were formerly under their mandate. As new nations appear on the mappamonde, they often show their independence by changing the suppliers of equipment (including x-ray machinery). Potential political allegiances play a role in the selection: this may be how and why (the Czechoslovakian) Chirana placed some of its wares in Egypt, and in Ghana. Equipment in missionary hospitals is usually determined by the donor. Since a great deal of money for the missions came from the United States, American x-ray equipment can be found almost everywhere.

As of today, no major x-ray installations are being manufactured anywhere in Africa. Even South Africa satisfies its needs through import - the major share of its market being divided about equally between WatVic and Philips.

I had seen a very interesting stamp, issued by Uganda, at the time when it changed its status from a British Protectorate into that of member of the British Commonwealth.

I inquired with the radiologist of Mulago Hospital in Kampala (Uganda), his name is John H. Roberts, as I wanted to know more about a technical x-ray stamp. This is the text of his letter:

"The present Mulago Hospital is completely new and was only officially opened during the Independence celebrations in October of 1962. The photograph for this stamp was taken in 1961 in what was called Nakasero Hospital. The diagramatic representation of part of the new hospital forms the background for the stamp.

"The equipment shown is made by Philips in Holland, as are most of the machines in the new department. The tube was an old 55 rotating anode with light beam diaphragm and the tube column of the type known as ACX. The table also is an ACX and is of the simple bucky type without fluoroscopy. The ACX is rated at 150 ma for 150 kvp. The Nakasero Hospital has been closed, and this particular unit (pictured on the stamp) has been moved up-country to a hospital at a place called Fort Portal.

"The "patient" shown on the stamp was one of the darkroom attendants, and the "radiographer" was a girl being trained as an Assistant Radiographer which is a local qualification. Since that time she has done very well at her studies, and has been accepted as a student for the full MSR diploma course at Exeter Hospital in England. She is now (February, 1963) about halfway through her course. On the stamp the apron worn by Miss Sanyi is shown in red: it was actually green. Incidentally, the ACX unit is now out of production, and has been superseded by the DSX (125 kvp at 200 ma)."

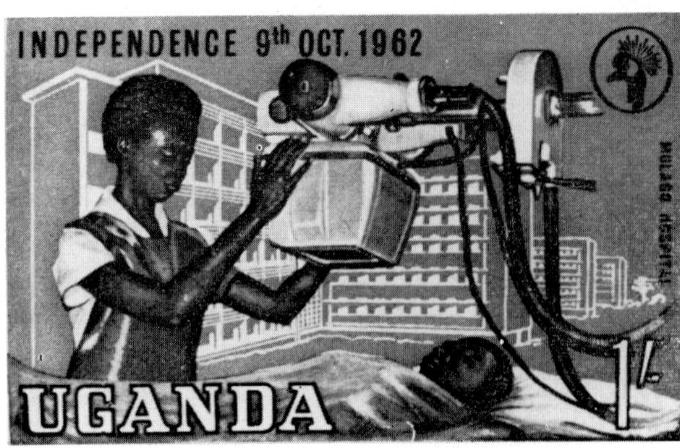

LATIN AMERICA

Prior to World War II, Central and South America were Siemens territory. After World War II, Philips gained entrance, but the conquest was far from being complete. The SRW manufacturing plant in São Paulo (Brazil) came under Philips control yet the operation was not too successful, and had to be discontinued. In the meantime American firms began to penetrate the South American market, especially Picker, and to some extent General Electric.

There are in Argentina several small makers of x-ray equipment. One of them is INAG of Buenos

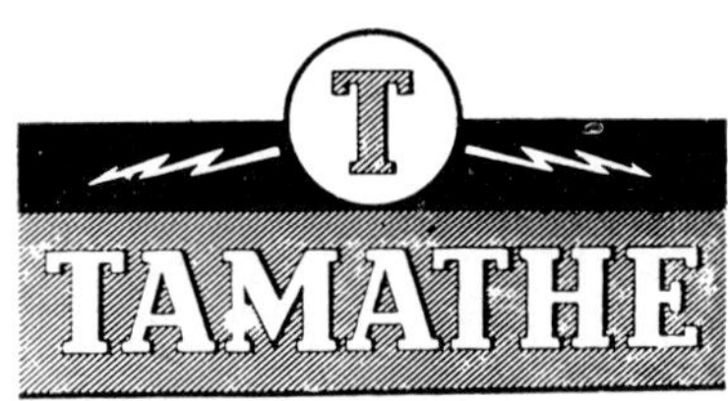

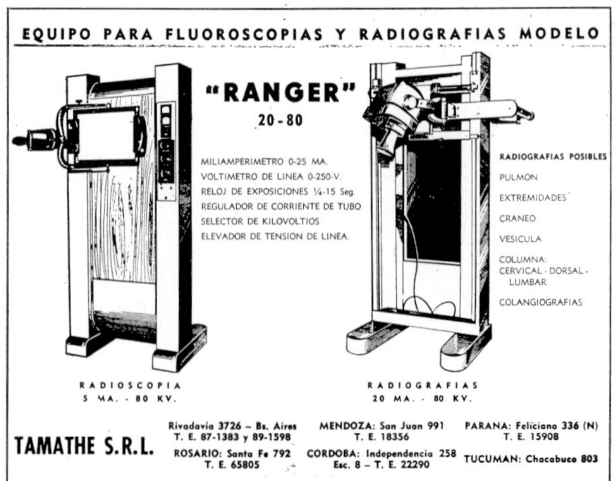

Aires, a former subsidiary and representative of SRW. During World War II, INAG was expropriated by the government and became *propriedad enemiga nacionalizada.* INAG continues to import certain equipment from SRW, for instance Telepantoskop tables. Since the early 1950s INAG advertises transformers of its own manufacture, the Sineval (no-valve) 50, 100, and 150 ma. By 1956 they had also a Tetraval (4-valve) 300 and 500 ma, with capabilities of up to 125 kvp. SRW has now, in addition, its own representative in Argentina.

In Buenos Aires are the headquarters of two other large South American importers of x-ray equipment. One of them is Tamathe, owned by a Yugoslavian immigrant, Juan Mathe. He does not have a definite representation, and his decisions to buy equipment here or there are determined by the balance of Argentinian foreign trade and the going rates of currency exchange. Tamathe has imported (German) Hofmann as well as Chirana machinery, occasionally even American equipment, for instance Continental's Ranger (an upright fluoroscope).

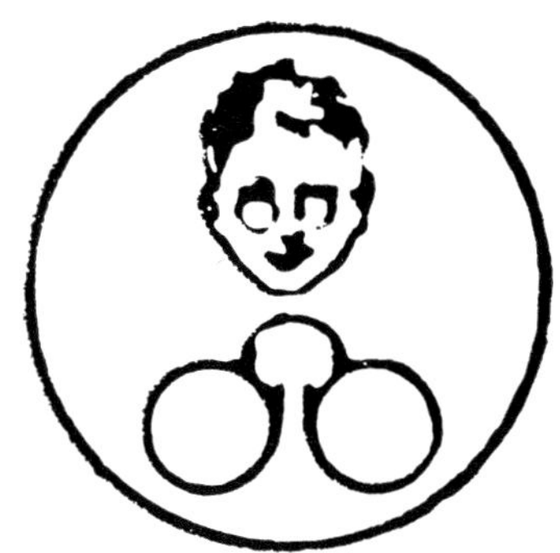

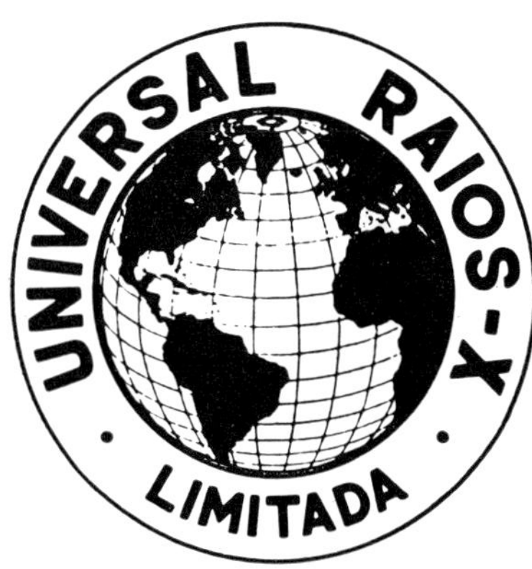

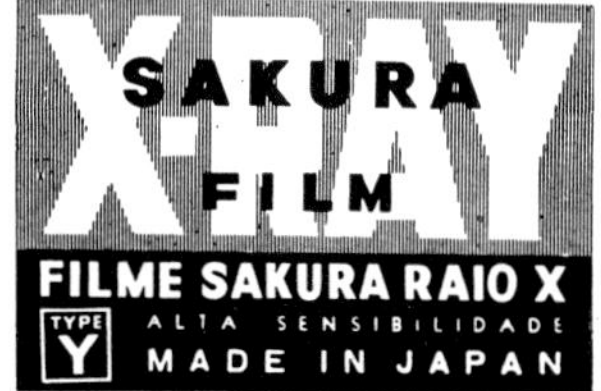

Lutz Ferrando - with a spectacled trade-mark - represented for many years the (German) Koch & Sterzel, but since World War II he has also imported (Dutch) Smit-Röntgen machines. German equipment is still the favorite in many places — according to Lidio Mosca, in Cordoba (Argentina) the majority of x-ray machines are either Siemens, Koch & Sterzel, or Müller.

But things have a way of changing. Today, Lutz Ferrando is the exclusive representative of the French CGR.

Small manufacturing plants of x-ray equipment have a high casualty rate. In 1961 Rayos X de America of Mexico City went out of business. The creation of local industry is recognized as a desirable feature: in the *Revista Brasileira de Radiologia* of January - March, 1959 appeared an article announcing the first complete installation made in Brazil (except for the Machlett tube and Bucky-Potter), a 100 ma, 100 kvp transformer with tilting table, named RX-58.

Casa Lohner (Rio de Janeiro) is the SRW representative in Brazil. The Brazilian market is today mostly a four-way split between Siemens, Philips, Picker and GE. This applies also to most other Latin American countries.

With regard to x-ray film sold in Central and South America, during and immediately after World War II, the (German) Agfa gave, and Eastman-Kodak and DuPont gained ground. Recently, though, there appeared the strong Agfa-Gevaert. Japanese firms have also started to export x-ray film to Latin America, for instance, Sakura.

THE BIGGEST

Only four firms can be considered as serious contenders for the unofficial title of world's biggest" manufacturer of x-ray equipment. Biggest would mean a combination of sales volume, number of sales outlets, and availability of service. X-ray equipment, like any other equipment, eventually goes out of order, and is therefore only as good as the service organization which stands behind it.

Prior to World War II the uncontested leader was Siemens, with more plants, more sales volume, and more service centers than anyone else in the business. Today, even though they gained a strong associate, the (Swedish) Elema-Schönander, it seems that Philips, with five major plants, is ahead. And yet, as far as production is concerned, the American firms must not be discounted. According to Eric Walker (of HVEC), during 1960 more than 50 percent of the world's production of radiological equipment was sold in the United States and Canada. Under these circumstances, even though American firms do not have the world-wide organization of either Siemens or Philips, production-wise they may very well be ahead. if only for the time being.

Between GE and Picker, the choice is difficult. GE was for many years ahead, but after World War II, Picker has significantly increased in volume, and has started a forceful international expansion.

Selection of any one of these "big four" as world leader is a matter of personal preference, because no figures have been made public. Together, these four firms make probably in excess of 80 percent (perhaps 85%) of the x-ray equipment manufactured today on this planet.

As I corrected the galley proofs, the question of who's the biggest in the x-ray world had not yet been settled. Most of those queried favored Philips.

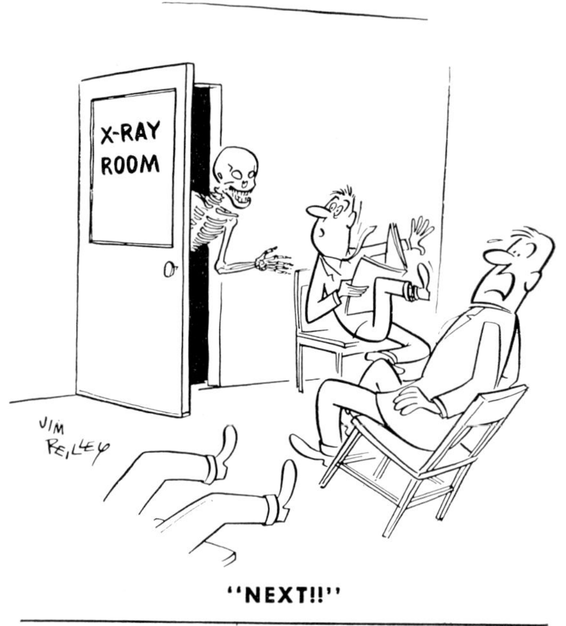

"NEXT!!"

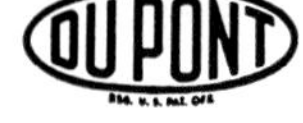

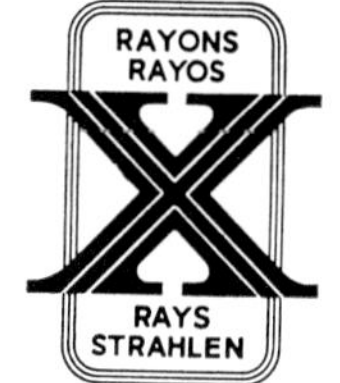

PHILIPS

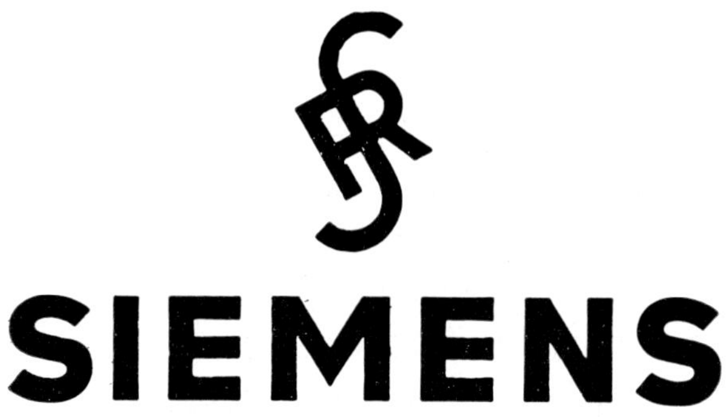

Progress Is Our Most Important Product

GENERAL ELECTRIC

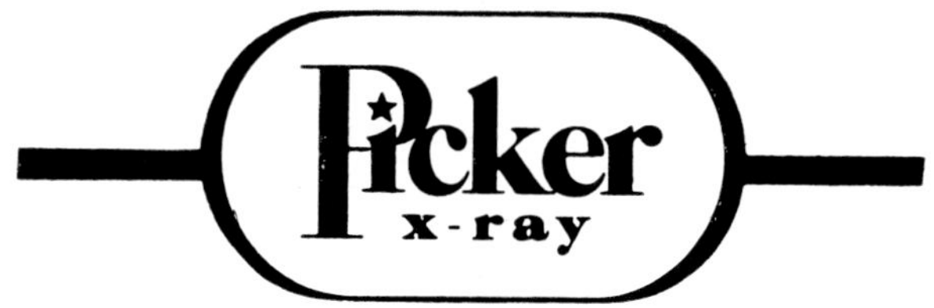

INTERMEZZO

At this point - after the glimpse at the globe - the time has come to return to radio-semantics proper. First, though, another section will be inserted. It is (considered) "politically unwise" to single out the Negroes among American radiologists, but such information is nowhere available in print. This is why I have tried to find out who was the first American Negro radiologist.

NEGROES IN AMERICAN RADIOLOGY

The earliest reference in this respect seemed to date back to 1900, when Heber Robarts surveyed the medical schools in this country. He sent out a questionnaire in which he asked about faculty interest in "x-ray science." Robarts listed G. W. Hubbard as teaching this subject at the (Negro) Meharry Medical College in Nashville.

Inquiry with their present dean (D. T. Rolfe) revealed that George Whipple Hubbard, who served as first president of Meharry from 1876 to 1921, happened to be a Caucasian.

The first Negro radiologist on the Meharry faculty was S. M. Utley, who taught from 1920 to 1930. Next came Charles E. Dillard, who is now in Cincinnati. His successor was Lawrence Disraeli Scott, who currently practices in Maywood (Illinois). Today Gadson Jack Tarleton, Jr., teaches radiology at Meharry.

Rolfe indicated that W. Montague Cobb, the professor of anatomy at Howard University in Washington (D.C.) and editor of the *Journal of the NMA* had collected considerable material on Negroes in medicine. Upon inquiry, Cobb courteously consulted his files, and replied that Peters was the first Negro radiologist certified by the American Board (in 1937).

Jesse Jerome Peters had been taught radiology by Leroy Sante beginning in December, 1920: on that date was completed the installation of the x-ray machine at St. Louis City Hospital No. 2 (the old Barnes Hospital, renovated in November, 1919 to house all Negro patients transferred from City Hospital No. 1). Later, Peters served as radiologist at the Veterans Administration Hospital in Tuskegee (Alabama) – where he saw the two patients with aneurysm of the left ventricle, reported in the *American Journal of Roentgenology* of March, 1941. Now, retired from the VA, Peters is radiologist at the Tuskegee Institute's Hospital, and teaches at the School of Veterinary Medicine in the same town. He remembered that while he served his radiologic apprenticeship in St. Louis, C. Bethany Powell was "taking his internship in x-ray at Bellevue Hospital in New York." Powell abandoned radiology, became the publisher of *Amsterdam News,* a Negro newspaper in New York City, and wound up in politics.

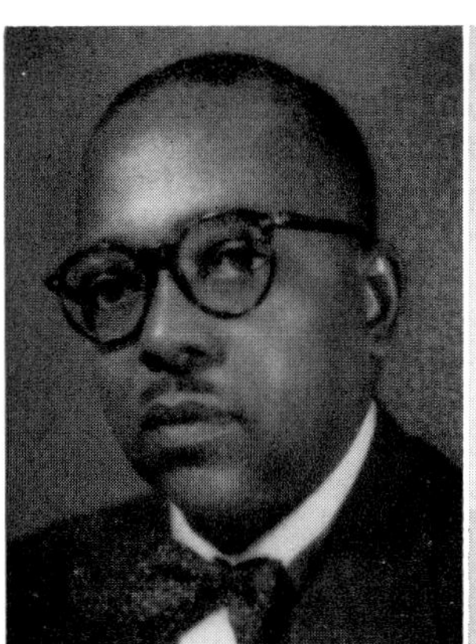

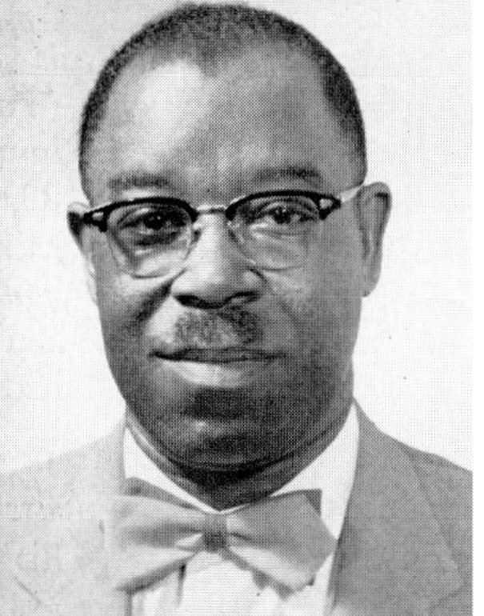

Jesse Jerome Peters & William Edward Allen, Jr.

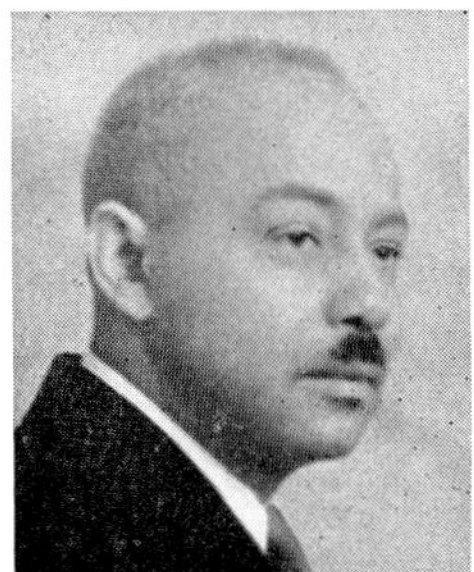

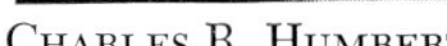

Charles R. Humbert

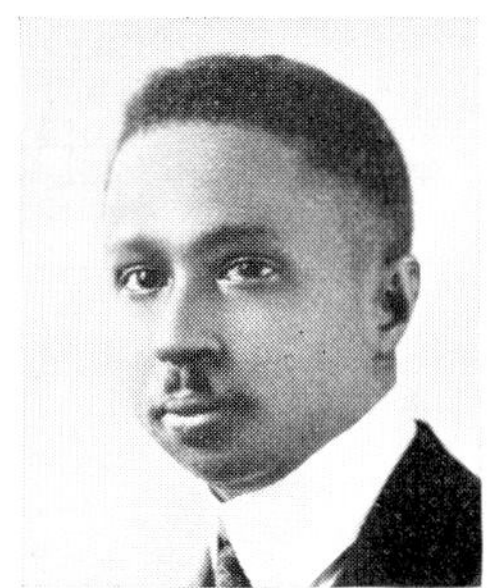

B. Price Hurst

Tarleton suggested that Allen in St. Louis might have more information. William Edward Allen, Jr., a Howard graduate, had his radiologic training in St. Louis City Hospital, was the first Negro certified in roentgenology in 1935 (in radiology in 1939), and in 1945 became the first Negro elevated to fellowship in the ACR. He is the chief-radiologist of the hospital named for Homer Gilliam Phillips (1880-1931). Phillips had been the hospital's most ardent Negro promoter, but was assassinated one year before hospital construction started. Allen, who is an expert in the interpretation of the "scout film" of the abdomen, has had several well received publications *e.g.,* the one on medical writing in the *Journal of the NMA* of January, 1948.

Allen provided the following data: the first two Negro radiologists in Philadelphia were Robert Henry and James Martin. B. Price Hurst was the first Negro radiologist to head a radiology department in a hospital, at Freedmen's in Washington (D.C.). Charles Humbert of Kansas City (Missouri) was also one of the very early Negro radiologists. Benjamin W. Anthony of Chicago was the first Negro to take a regular fellowship in radiology.

James Lemuel Martin, a 1906 medical graduate from Shaw in Raleigh (North Carolina), first went into general practice in Staunton (Virginia), from 1907 to 1917. He joined the Army and was wounded in France during World War I. After his return he gained some ex-

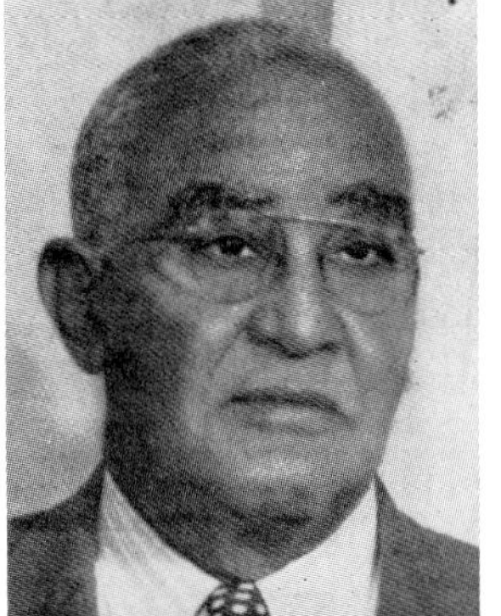

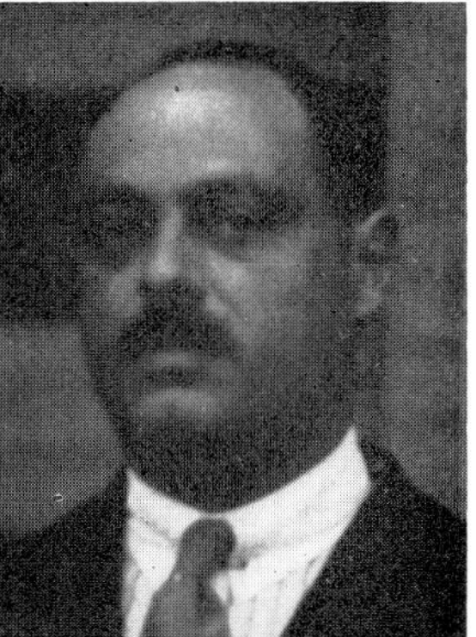

James Lemuel Martin & Marcus Wheatland.

This is the only portrait of himself which Martin gave to me. I cannot divulge the origin of Wheatland's picture (I hunted two years for it), but for authenticity I have the testimony of Ben Orndoff, who remembers him as a quiet, personable fellow, willing to joke about his own name (". . . without wheat this land could never be as great!").

perience in radiology at Freedmen's, was then accepted into the Graduate School of the University of Pennsylvania on April 20, 1921, and stayed on until 1936 as clinical assistant to George Pfahler – with whom he published (in the *American Journal of Roentgenology* of February, 1926) an experimental study on the combined effects of roentgen and of ultraviolet rays on carcinoma of the skin. From 1936 to 1944, Martin served as chief-radiologist at Freedmen's and as instructor in radiology at Howard. In 1944, he went into private practice in Philadelphia.

Robert Henry was the first Negro to practice radiology in Philadelphia, after having been trained at the Pennsylvania Hospital under David Ralph Bowen. In 1916, Henry founded the x-ray department at the Frederick Douglass Hospital, and was their chief-radiologist until it merged in 1940 with the Mercy Hospital (when Russell Farbeaux Minton became the radiologist of the combined Mercy-Douglass). At the NMA meeting in Detroit in 1960, Henry was the oldest living member of that organization.

The initial question was again submitted, this time to Henry: he specified that the very first American Negro to practice radiology as a specialty had been Marcus Wheatland of Providence (Rhode Island).

The secretary of the Rhode Island Medical Society summarized their records as follows: Marcus Fitzherbert Wheatland was born in 1868, graduated from Howard in 1895, and was licensed in the same year to practice medicine in Rhode Island. He became a member of their society in 1896, was a fellow of the AMA, and a member of the New England Roentgen Ray Society. Wheatland specialized in radiology. He died on August 16, 1934. No portrait of his, nor additional information could be obtained from any source, although both his *alma mater* (Howard University) and the NMA were queried. I finally found his portrait.

If one had to single out three foremost figures among contemporary Negro radiologists, the selection would be inherently biased by personal preferences. The following names are unquestionably outstanding: Allen, Lawlah, and Moseley.

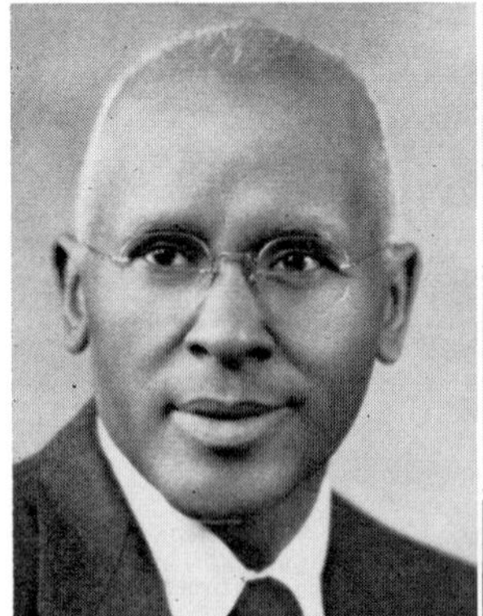
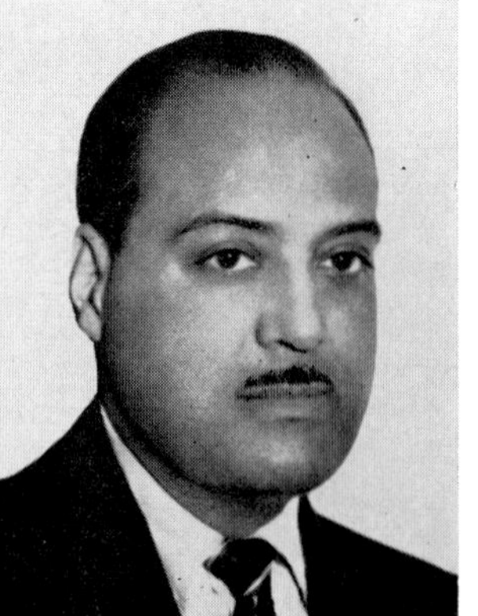

John Wesley Lawlah & John Edmund Moseley.

Allen is most of all an *organizer*. He also trained many residents in his department, and thus sponsored a number of young Negro radiologists. The first Negro to become a registered x-ray technician, Rose Peques Perkins, was a pupil in Allen's School for X-ray Technicians at St. Mary's Infirmary in St. Louis.

John Wesley Lawlah is primarily a *teacher*. Graduated in 1932 from Rush Medical College (Chicago), he served a fellowship at the University of Chicago under Paul Hodges. In the *American Journal of Roentgenology* of February, 1952 Lawlah described (with Pollack) the "gluteal bismuth ribs" found in a syphilitic patient from Provident Hospital. Before the paper appeared, Lawlah had moved to Freedmen's. Today Lawlah is professor of radiology at Howard and as such, most of his papers are signed by residents and associates, *e.g.*, the study of thoracic aortography in the *American Heart Journal* of January, 1957. As dean of the Medical School in Howard University, Lawlah has endeavored to improve the education of Negro physicians, both before and after graduation.

John Edmund Moseley, a graduate (1936) of the University of Chicago, had his radiologic training at Mt. Sinai in New York, and is now a radiologist at Sydenham Hospital in the latter city. Moseley is a radiologic *scientist*, who made original contributions, including a newly described disease entity (Sclerosing Osteogenic Sarcomatosis in *Radiology of January*, 1956), and a new sign (Thymic "Spinnaker Sail" in loculated pneumomediastinum in the newborn, *cf.*, *Radiology* of November, 1960). He has identified a series of cases of regional enteritis in children (in the *American Journal of Roentgenology* of September, 1960), and has recently published a book on the radiographic bone changes in blood diseases.

The only radiologic organization in America with exclusive Negro membership is the Radiologic Section of the NMA.* This section was first organized on August 8, 1949 in the Radkam Educational Building in Detroit, during the annual NMA meeting. The first secretary of the radiological section of the NMA was Darnell Mitchell of Detroit, the first president was Bill Allen.

At the time of this writing, all over the globe, but especially in the USA, the Negro is struggling to achieve integration, politically and otherwise. There can be no moral or scientific justification for segregation. In this context, though, I would like to de-

*NMA means National Medical Association, but it was selected so that its initials can also be read Negro Medical Association.

bunk a pseudo-scientific myth, the so-called equality between races. All the sacred pronounciations of anthropo-pundits to the contrary notwithstanding, the various races are not equal, certainly not in the (biologic) sense in which they are supposed to be. Each race is bound to follow its own biologic clock, which is a statistical average. Both extremes of "good" and "bad" (intelligent" or "cretin," or any other qualifications) and all points in-between are encountered in every race, only the proportions differ from race to race, at a specified moment in time. This is why individual evaluation of the person under scrutiny is the only sensible way of arriving at a proper judgment.

There is no race problem in American radiology. Because of current political pressures, many institutions are trying to "get a Negro," so as to show their willingness. Indeed, there are today more radiologic vacancies (from resident to chief of department) available to Negroes than there are qualified applicants.

In this country there are today — obviously — fewer Negro physicians, and among them fewer Negro radiologists, than there are - comparatively - among the white population. But the figures are slowly levelling off. The Negro lyrical (and phthisical) poet Paul Lawrence Dunbar (1872-1906) once wrote, "Slow moves the pageant of a climbing race." As long as the goal has not been reached, Negro destiny (both here and in Africa) is still ahead, still climbing. This may not be as undesirable as the situation of those who live in the past, and have no future for which to strive.

RADIO- NUCLEARIZED

In evaluating the popularity of the prefix radio- in the Atomic Phase, we find four periodicals which appeared with the title *Radiologia*. Two of these spelled it with a Spanish accent on the second í, as expected in Buenos Aires (1942), and in Panama City (1950). The third *Radiologia,* edited by Gheorghe Schmitzer, appeared in Bucharest (1956).

Schmitzer, whose main but not exclusive interest was in radiotherapy, is currently president of the Societatea

RADIOLOGIA

REVISTĂ A SOCIETĂȚII ȘTIINȚELOR MEDICALE

Redacția: București, str. Progresului nr. 8 – Telef. 41082

ANUL I IULIE 1 AUGUST 1956

Romȃna de Radiologie, and teaches radiology in the postgraduate program at the Coltea Hospital in Bucharest. The pre-World War II chief of radiology at that hospital had been Ermil Lazeanu, who came to Chicago for the fifth ICR in 1937, and contributed papers on cardio-radio-kymography. During the Golden Age of Radiology Amilcar Georgescu and Ion Jovin were among the better known radiologists in Bucharest. Oscar Meller, radiologist of the (Jewish) Caritas Hospital, was for many years secretary of the Roumanian Radiological Society. These were all representatives of the French (Bucharest) school of medical thought. Transylvania had been for several centuries part of the Austro-Hungarian empire, and therefore the Medical School in Cluj was under heavy German influence. The dignified teacher and wise clinician Dumitru Negru was professor of radiology in the University of Cluj (Roumania). With the advent of the Atomic Phase a younger generation of Roumanian radiologists is up-and-coming, after having accepted some of the Russian nomenclature: thus Ioan Bîrzu is now director of the Radiologic and Oncologic Department in the Cantacuzino Institute in Bucharest.

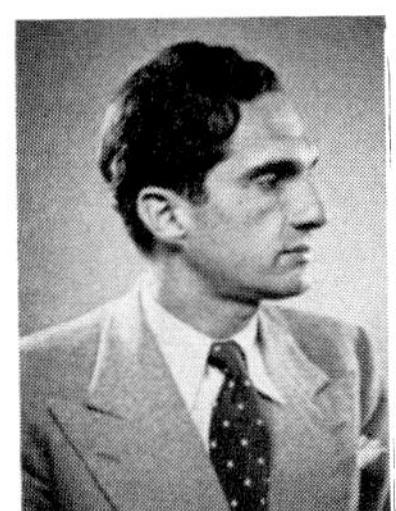

ION JOVIN

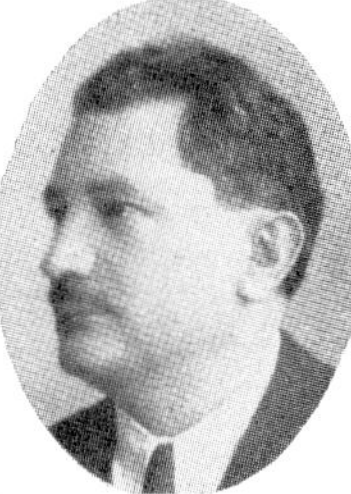

DUMITRU NEGRU

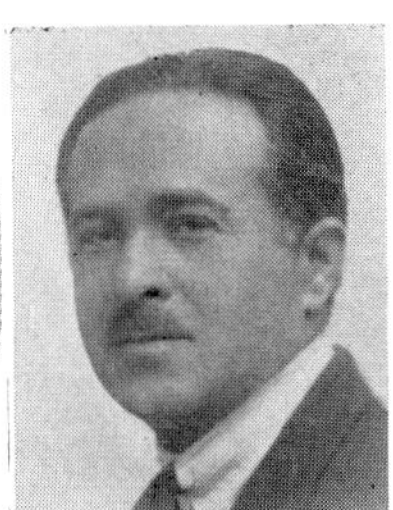

OSCAR MELLER

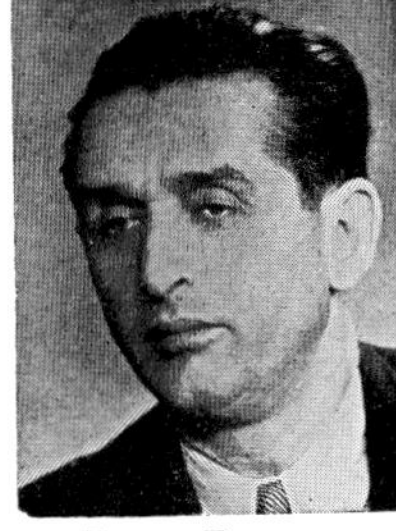

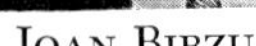

IOAN BIRZU

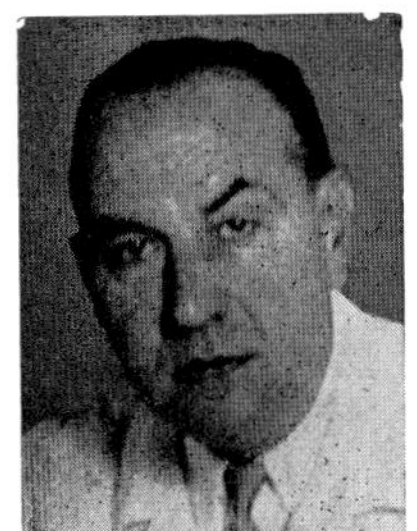

GHEORGHE SCHMITZER

ITALY

The fourth *Radiologia* is Eugenio Milani's pre-war Journal, re-issued in 1945 in Rome (Italy) by Sordello Attilj.

At this point a few Italian radiologists, past and present, and their favored professional preoccupations, will be mentioned.

Augusto Righi (1850-1920) was a physicist from Bologna who gave the paper on the nature of x rays at the first Italian Radiological Congress (1913). He was one of the real pioneers, and had a dozen papers on x rays, dated 1896. Another pioneer was Massimiliano Gortan (1873-1938), who died as a radiation casualty, had studied with Holzknecht, later founded (and was the first director of) the x-ray department in the Ospedale Maggiore in Trieste. One of Gortan's "pupils" was Aristide Busi (1874-1939), who delivered the *Corsi di Radiologia di Guerra* during World War I; he became in 1919 professor of electrotherapy and medical radi-

Radiologia

RASSEGNA INTERNAZIONALE TRIMESTRALE DI RADIOBIOLOGIA, RADIOTERAPIA, RADIODIAGNOSTICA, TERAPIA FISICA E FISICA APPLICATA ALLA MEDICINA

DIRETTA DA EUGENIO MILANI
DIRETTORE DELL' ISTITUTO DI RADIOLOGIA MEDICA DELL' UNIVERSITÀ DI ROMA

VOLUME V - No 1
GENNAIO - MARZO 1949
FASCICOLO 15

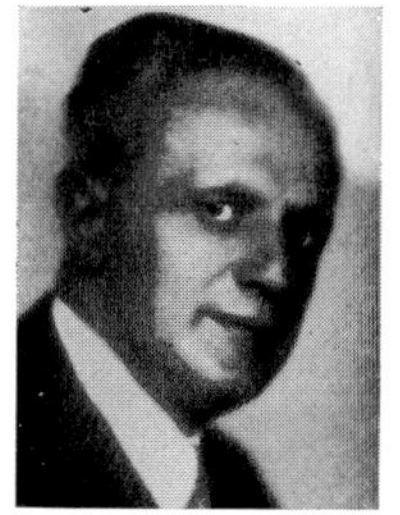

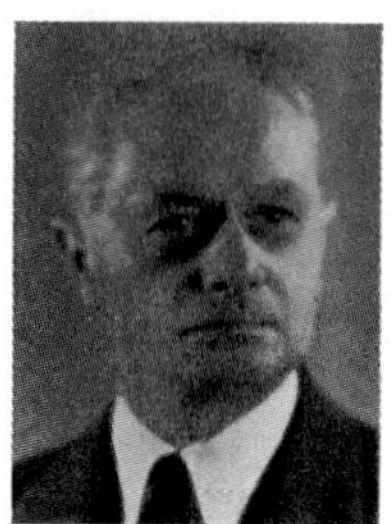

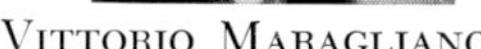

VITTORIO MARAGLIANO MARIO PONZIO

ANNO I. MARZO - APRILE 1933 N. 2

NVNTIVS RADIOLOGICVS

SCRIPTA AD REM PERTINENTIA RECENSET

DIRETTORE
ARISTIDE BVSI
ROMA

REDATTORI CAPO
PROF. A. SALOTTI — SIENA
PROF. L. TVRANO — ROMA

STABILIMENTO TIPOGRAFICO COMBATTENTI - SIENA

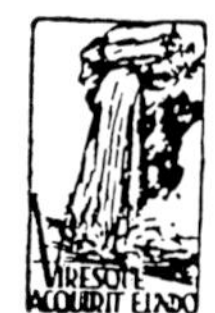

Istituto Bibliografico Italiano – Roma

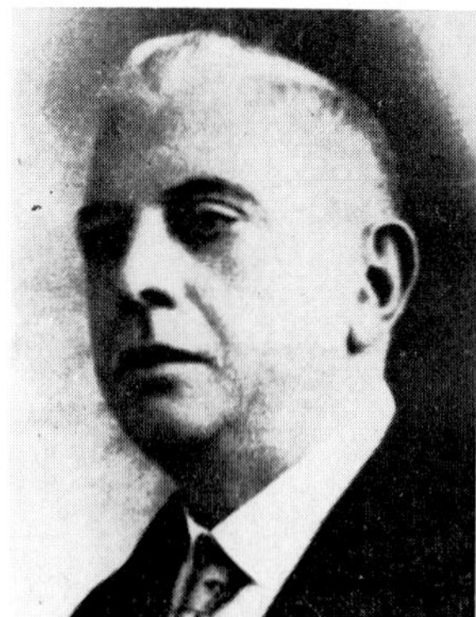

MASSIMILLANO GORTAN

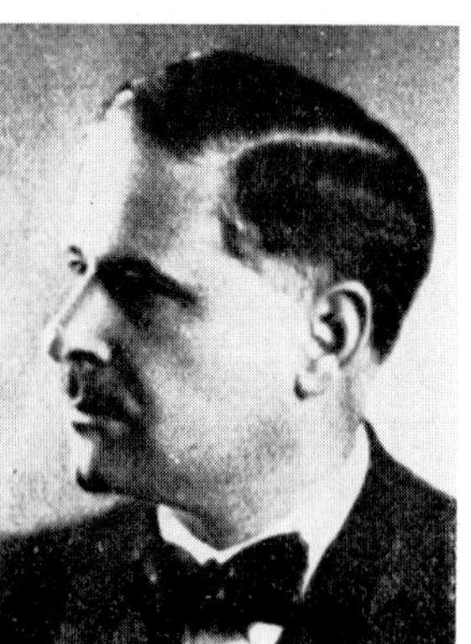

RUGGERO BALLI
Courtesy: Arduino Ratti.

ology in the University of Bologna (the name was "abbreviated" to medical radiology in 1924) until 1928 when he accepted the same position in the University of Rome. Four other Italian radiologists must be remembered, all of whom were born in the 1870s and lived well into the Golden Age; Pasquale Tandoja of Naples, Mario Bertolotti of Torino, Ruggero Balli of Pavia and Vittorio Maragliano of Genova.

Among Italian radiologic contributions may be mentioned the radioplastic heart model and the superteleroentgentherapy of Gian Giuseppe Palmieri of Bologna; the broken slit kymography (1929) and the new kymograph (1952) of Pietro Cignolini of Palermo; the polyanodic x-ray tube and the rotating cathode tubes of Mario Lenzi of Modena; the stabilizer of Enzo Pugno-Vanoni from Milano (he and Righi are the only nonmedical persons in this group); the axial transverse stratigraphy (1947) of Alessandro Vallebona of Genova; the lymphography of Franco Stoppani of Torino; and the study of intracranial calcifications of Fermo Mascherpa of Milano.

Two of the original founders of the Italian Radiological Society lived on well into the Atomic Phase. One of them was the society's perpetual secretary, Mario Ponzio (1885-1956), senior author of a Treatise of semeiotic radiology (1952), in three heavy volumes, and biographer of Italian roentgen martyrs: he died as a radiation casualty himself. The other was Felice Perussia (1885-1959), known as a radiobiologist, author (with Pugno-Vanoni) of a radiotherapeutic treatise, coiner of the term *plesioterapia*, and founder of *Radiologia Medica* (Perussia edited its first 45 volumes). He was succeeded in the job of editor by Arduino Ratti, formerly professor of radiology in Pavia, who also followed Perussia as chairman of the Department of Radiology in the University of Milano.*

There is a plethora of Italian radiologic journals, most of which are grouped in a Federazione Italiana della Stampa Radiologica. Aside from the previously mentioned *Radiologia*, and the respectable *Radiologia Medica*, there appeared the *Archivio di Radiologia* (Naples), directed by Carlo Guarini; *Radioterapia, Radiobiologia*

*The obituary of Perussia and other information on some of the famous names in Italian radiology were graciously provided by Professor Arduino Ratti.

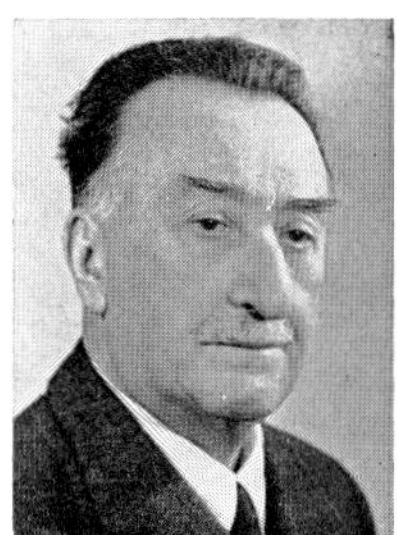
FELICE PERUSSIA

MARIO LENZI

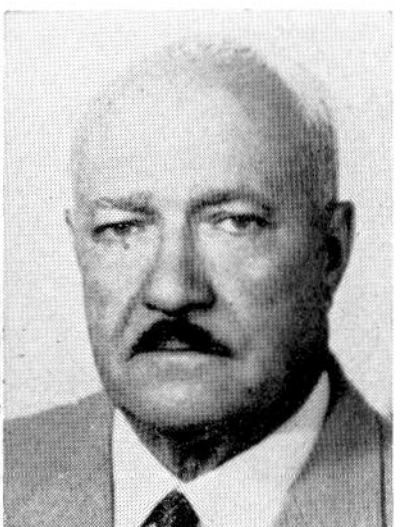
SORDELLO ATTILJ

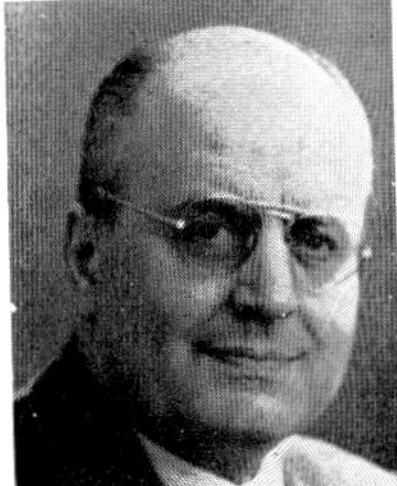
A. VALLEBONA

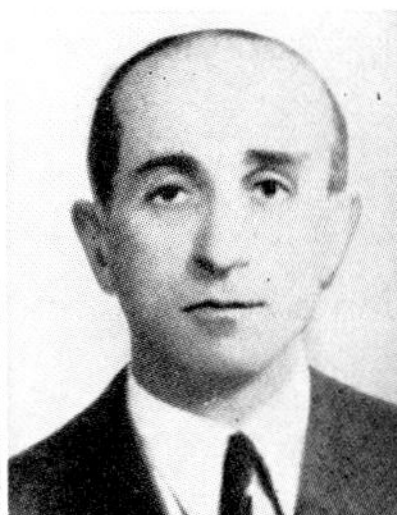
FRANCO FOSSATI

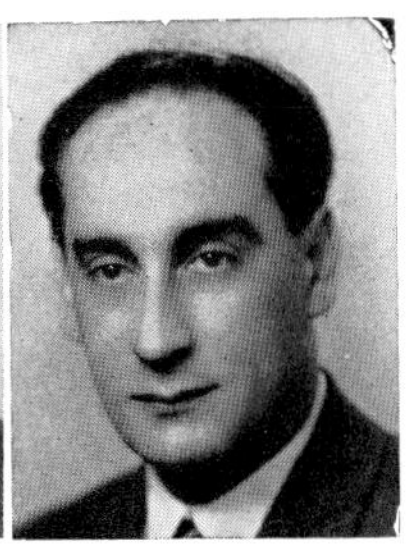
GIOV. SANQUIRICO

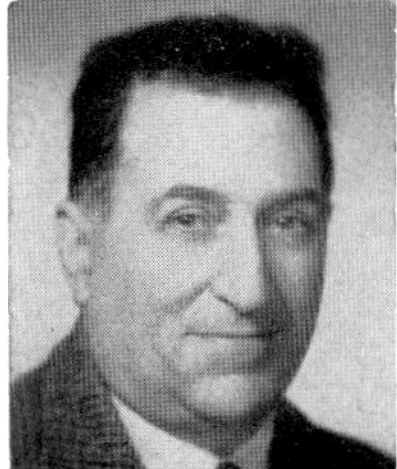
VINCENZO BOLLINI

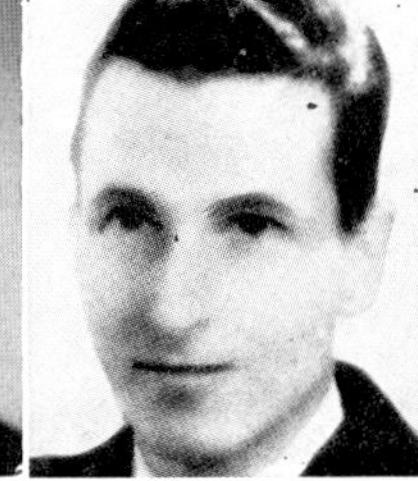
C.-HERNANDEZ

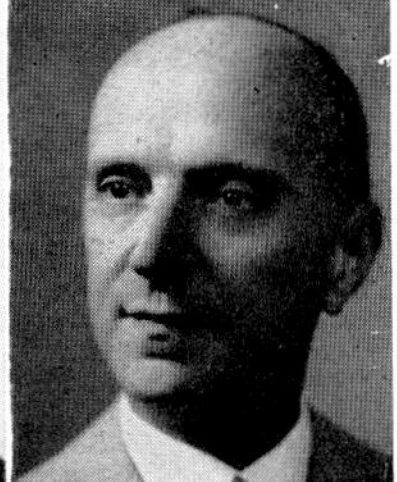
ENRICO BENASSI

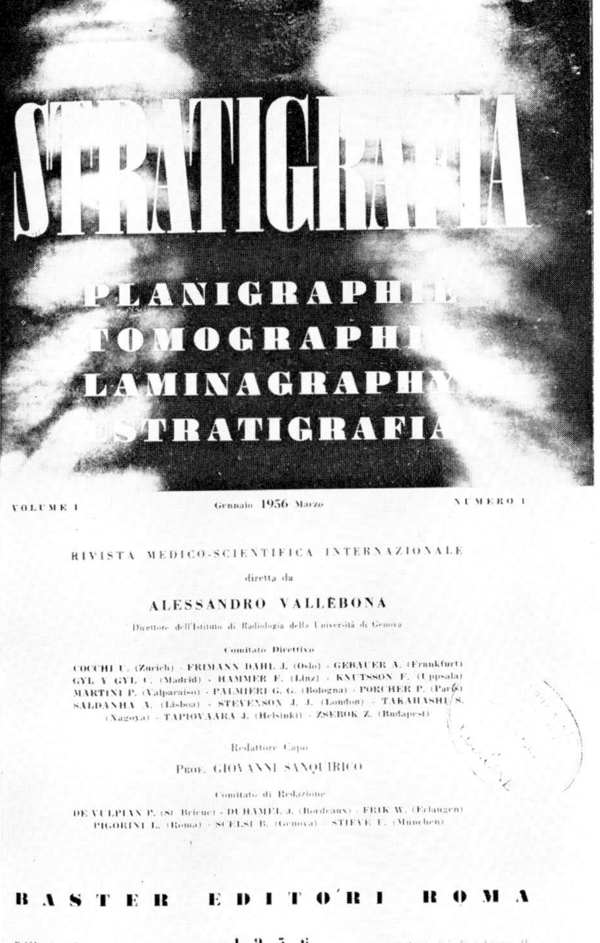
STRATIGRAFIA

PLANIGRAPH

TOMOGRAPH

LAMINAGRAPH

STRATIGRAFIA

VOLUME I — Gennaio 1956 Marzo — NUMERO I

RIVISTA MEDICO-SCIENTIFICA INTERNAZIONALE

diretta da

ALESSANDRO VALLEBONA

Direttore dell'Istituto di Radiologia della Università di Genova

Comitato Direttivo

COCCHI U. (Zurich) - FRIMANN DAHL J. (Oslo) - GEBAUER A. (Frankfurt) GYL Y GYL C. (Madrid) - HAMMER F. (Linz) - KNUTSSON F. (Uppsala) MARTINI P. (Valparaiso) - PALMIERI G. G. (Bologna) - PORCHER P. (Paris) SALDANHA A. (Lisboa) - STEVENSON J. J. (London) - TAKAHASHI S. (Nagoya) - TAPIOVAARA J. (Helsinki) - ZSEBOK Z. (Budapest)

Redattore Capo

PROF. GIOVANNI SANQUIRICO

Comitato di Redazione

DE VULPIAN P. (St Brieuc) - DUHAMEL J. (Bordeaux) - FRIK W. (Erlangen) PIGORINI L. (Roma) - SCELSI B. (Genova) - STIEVE F. (München)

BASTER EDITORI ROMA

Pubblicazione Trimestrale — 1956

e Fisica Medica, until recently edited by the regretted Palmieri; *Quaderni di Radiologia,* founded in 1930 by La Penna and reissued in 1951 in Padova by Pietro Perona; *Nuntius Radiologicus,* founded in 1933 by Busi (published in Florence, then in Siena, and now in Belluno) and currently directed by Luigi Turano of Roma; *Annali di Radiologia Diagnostica,* supervised by Armando Rossi of Parma; *Revista Italiana di Radiologia Clinica* edited by Adelchi Salotti of Florence; Vallebona's *Stratigrafia;* and Cignolini's *Radiologia Pratica.*

A bibliographic compilation of titles, called *Letteratura Radiologica Italiana,* is issued by the Italian Radiologic Society: the first 4 volumes (1895-1935) were prepared by Orlando Alberti; the 5th volume (1936-1940) is by Furio Cardillo; the 6th and 7th (1941-1950) are by Enzo Bollo who, like his predecessors, lives in Milano. Currently known as the unofficial historian and bibliographer of Italian radiology is Ettore de Bernardi (from Salerno) who is also the author of about seventy papers; some of these report his radiobiologic experimentations, others are on diagnostic topics, such as the roentgen evaluation of the painful abdomen, including possible relations between appendix and peptic ulcer.

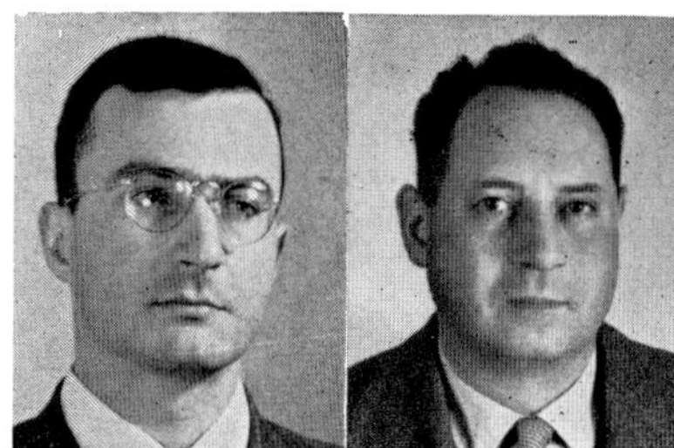
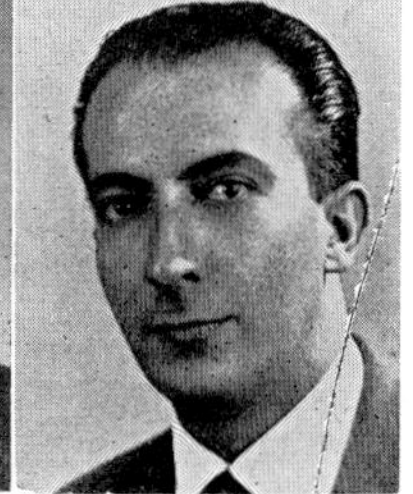
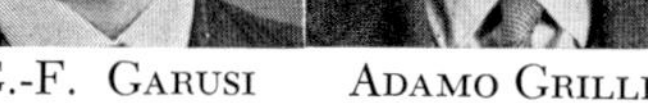

G.-F. Garusi   Adamo Grilli   N. Macarini

RADIAZIONI

DI

ALTA ENERGIA

Radiations de haute énergie

High energy radiations

Hoch - energie - strahlung

Radiaciones de alta energía

The latest Italian offering to the Atomic Phase is another journal (one more) called *Radiazioni di Alta Energia,* a private venture started in 1962 by Mainardo Tomiselli of Rome, in partnership with Rocco Rocco of Gorizia and Dino Catalano of Naples. The title on its cover is translated in French, English, German, and Spanish to show their interest in an international audience.

SPAIN

The Spanish Radiological Society was founded in 1943. Its official journal *Radiológica-Cancerológica* (edited by the venerable Carlos Gil y Gil) was first issued in 1946. In 1952 it changed its name to *Acta Ibérica Radiológica-Cancerológica* as it became also the official organ of the Portuguese Radiological Society.

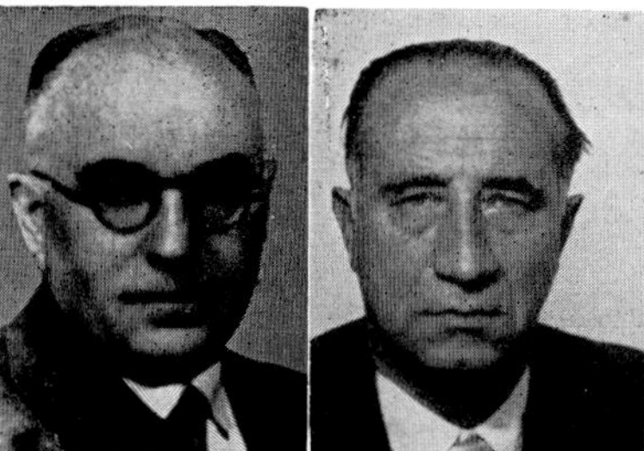
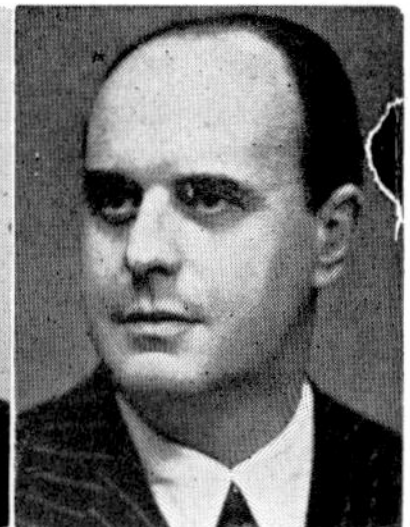

Carlos Gil y Gil   Celma-Hernandez   Arce-Alonso
Radiologists in Spain.

MIDDLE EAST

There are several internationally known radiologists who come from that part of the world. There is first of all Egyptian-born Henry Chaoul who lived most of his life in Berlin, where he was professor of radiology. Chaoul built the spotfilmer which was marketed under the name *Radioskop* in 1918 by Reiniger, Gebbert & Schall. And Chaoul is, of course, the originator of contact therapy. After World War II, he returned to Egypt, and settled in Alexandria. Last time I heard from him, he was back in München, being

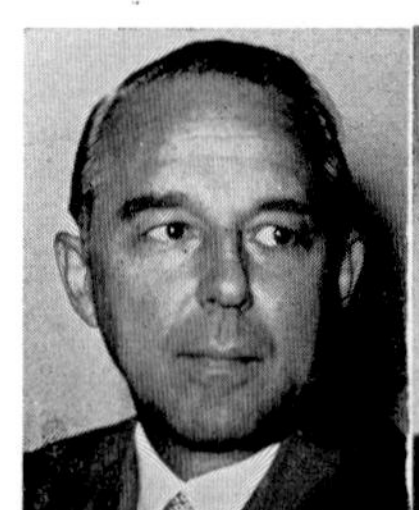
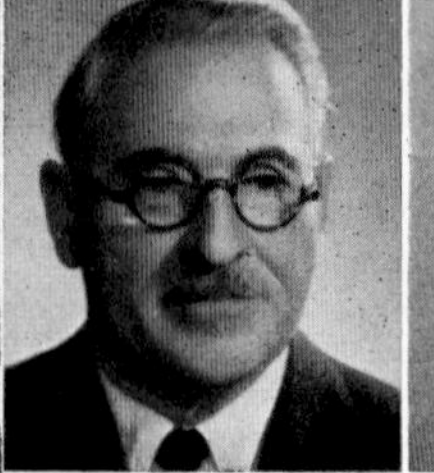
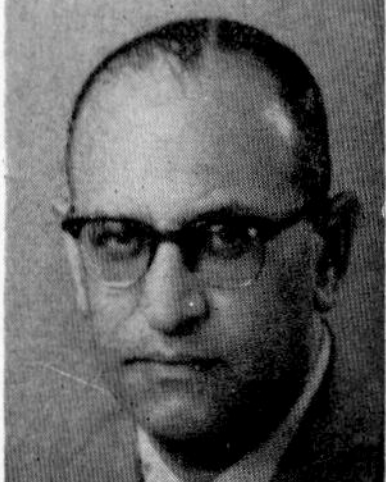
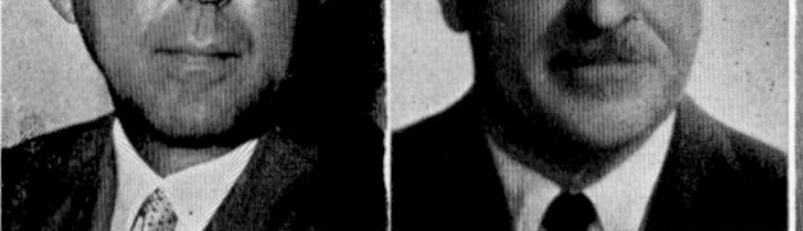

Kurt Greineder   Henry Chaoul   Erian Ghali

treated for radiation damage. In Beirut works Kurt Greineder, the expert in tomography. In Tel-Aviv is located the therapist Hans Salinger.

The Israel Radiological Society was formed in 1926 by Izhar Izkovitch, a radiologist from Haifa. He is still its president. There are about 120 radiologists in Israel, and all belong to that society. The chair of radiology in the Medical School of the Hebrew University was created in 1949. There are no radiological periodicals published in the Middle East. X-ray equipment in Israel is of high quality, and compares, on a *per capita* basis, with any metropolitan area in Europe or USA. More than half of the equipment is of Philips manufacture, about 30-40 percent is American (especially cobalt and therapy units). There are no x-ray equipment manufacturers in the Middle East, but viewboxes, cassettes, developing tanks and similar items are built, mainly on order, by Levant X-Ray, Ltd., the Picker representative in Tel-Aviv.*

Following are excerpts from a letter by one of the first two trained Egyptian radiologists, Nessim Abu-Saif:

"In 1925, x-ray work in Cairo was done by two "laboratories," manned by self-trained technicians, an Austrian Jew and a Swede. Mustafa Ragheb and I were resident surgeons at the Kasr-El-Aini University Hospital, when the Egyptian Ministry of Education selected us for radiologic training in England. We came back to Egypt three years later, in 1928, both with the following degrees: MRCS (Eng.), LRCP (Lond.), and DMRE (Camb.). We were both appointed lecturers in radiology at Kasr-El-Aini. Ragheb had charge of the administrative part, and did some diagnosis, I was more interested in radiotherapy. Six months later, Ragheb and I opened a private office on the side, for which we purchased Siemens apparatus. I did most of the teaching, and thus became the Egyptian delegate at the 1934 ICR in Switzerland. In 1937 Ragheb and I created an Egyptian Diploma of Radiology. In 1939 both Ragheb and I went to London, and became fellows of the newly created Faculty of Radiologists. Upon our return, Ragheb was made professor of radiology, and I became director of radiotherapy. Ragheb retired in 1954, at which time I succeeded in his position. Since then, other medical schools have been established in Egypt, another one in Cairo, a third in Alexandria, and a fourth in Assiut. The professors of radiology in these schools, and their assistants are all former pupils of mine."

To this I wish to add that Abu-Saif has currently the largest private practice of radiology in Egypt, both in diagnosis and therapy. He retired from the professorship about three years ago, but is still chairman of the examination committee for the Egyptian radiologic degree. In 1962 Abu-Saif succeeded in splitting the department of radiology at Kasr-El-Aini, and there are now separate chairs for diagnosis and for therapy. Both chairs are occupied by former students of his.

There are presently about 200 qualified radiologists in Egypt. The Egyptian Radiological Society was formed in 1949, in order to legally send a delegate to the ICR in London in 1950. Their first president was Ragheb, the first secretary was Ibrahim Abu-Sinna. Ragheb remained president until his death in 1960. The current president is Mahmoud El-Sayed, professor of radiology in Cairo University. The first professor of radiology at Kasr-El-Aini was an Irishman, Robert Augustin Gardner, assigned to that position sometime after 1930 – he was succeeded in 1939 by Ragheb.*

*This information was offered by the "dean" of Israeli radiologists, Dr. Izkovitch, and by Mr. Hans Herbert Aldor, the director of Levant X-Ray.

*This information was graciously provided by Erian Ghali, a radiologist in Cairo, a former pupil of Ragheb and Abu-Saif. Ghali has additional training in France.

הועד הארצי. חיפה
אגוד הרנטגנולוגים בישראל
ISRAEL RADIOLOGICAL SOCIETY
I.M.A.
CENTRAL COMMITTEE, HAIFA

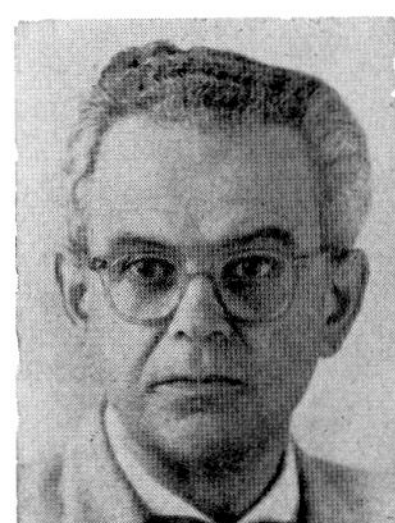
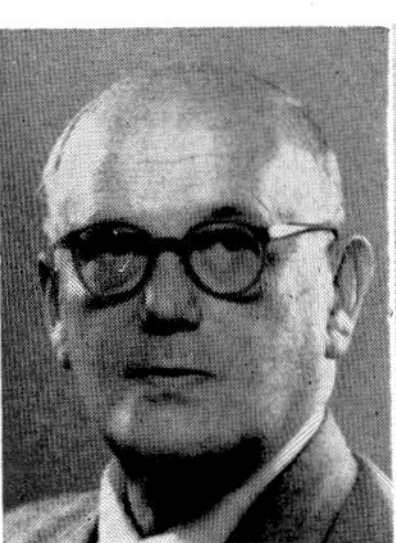
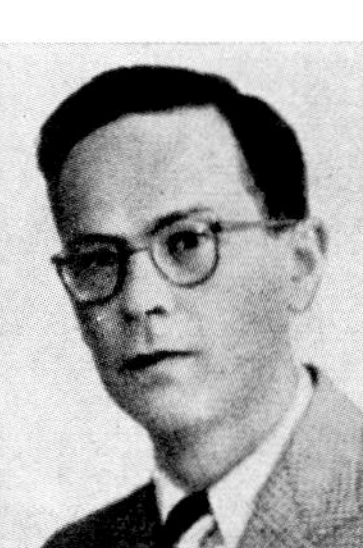
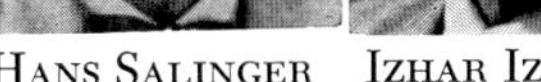
HANS SALINGER IZHAR IZKOVITCH HANS ALDOR

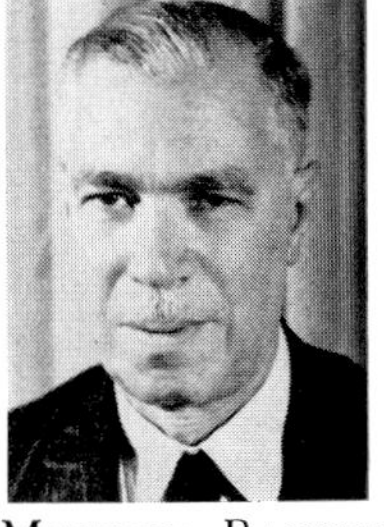
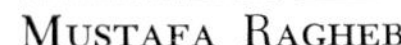
MUSTAFA RAGHEB

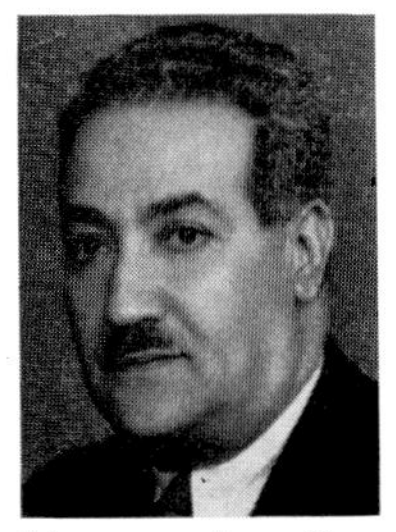
NESSIM ABU-SAIF

INDIA

The Indian Radiological Association was created in 1946.

Its first president was Maahadeo Dattatraya Joshi (owner of a private Radiological and Electrological Institute in Bombay), the Indian delegate to the 1950 ICR in London. The first secretary of the Association was Padamanur Rama Rau (1899-1956), who had been initiated into radiology in Holzknecht's department in Vienna; Rama Rau was for many years director of the Radiological Institute in Madras. Other founders of the Indian Radiological Association were the radiologists P. B. Mukerji of Calcutta, S. C. Sen of New Delhi, and K. P. Mody of Bombay. The official organ, the *Indian Journal of Radiology,* began to appear in 1947, its first editor being Kaikhuroo Peroshaw Mody (1885-1961). Mody was born in Bombay, where he attended Grant Medical College, after which he specialized in London and Vienna, and returned in 1913 to practice private radiology in Bombay (in 1936 he obtained the DMRE in London). After Mody's death, Narayanan Kutty Menon became editor of their Journal. The present honorary general secretary of the Indian Radiologic Association is Ved Prakash, a radiologist from New Delhi. Incidentally, the 8th Congress of the Indian Radiological Association was held in Madras on February 12-15, 1964.

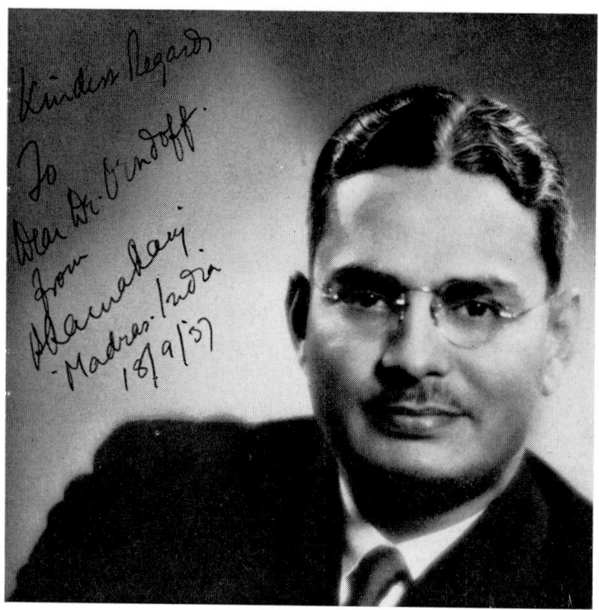

Courtesy: Ben Orndoff.

PADAMANUR RAMA RAU. First secretary of the Indian Radiological Association.

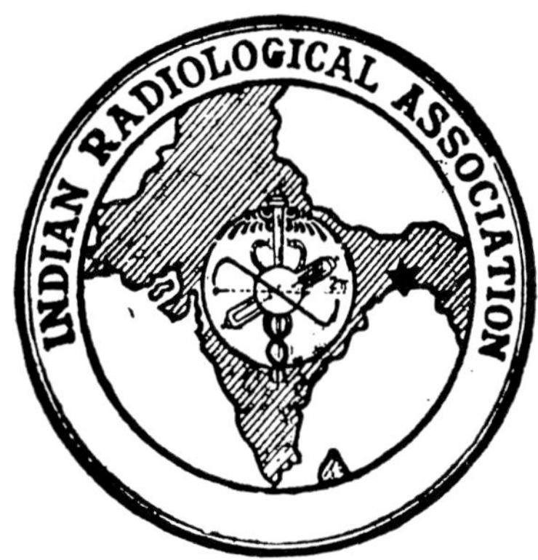

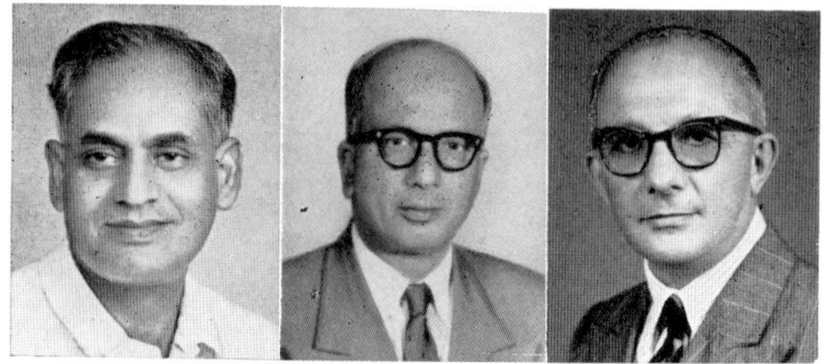

S. C. SEN VED PRAKASH R. F. SETHNA

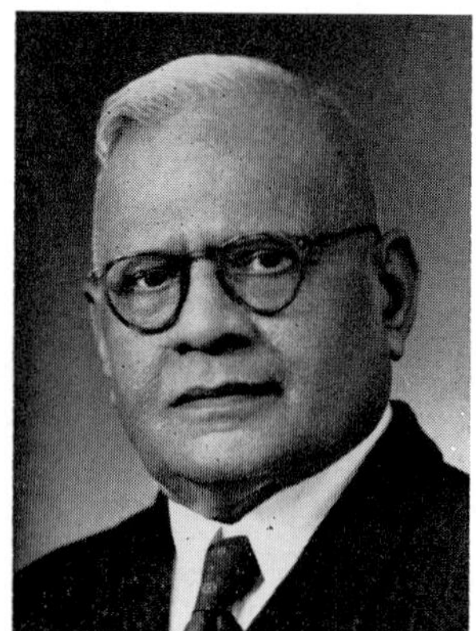

Courtesy: Ved Prakash.

MAAHADEO DATTATRAYA JOSHI. First president of the Indian Radiological Association.

PERKUMPULAN RADIOLOGI

Indonesia is a sprawling archipelago, covering about 3000 square miles. In May, 1952 - at the time when W. Z. Johannes founded the Indonesian

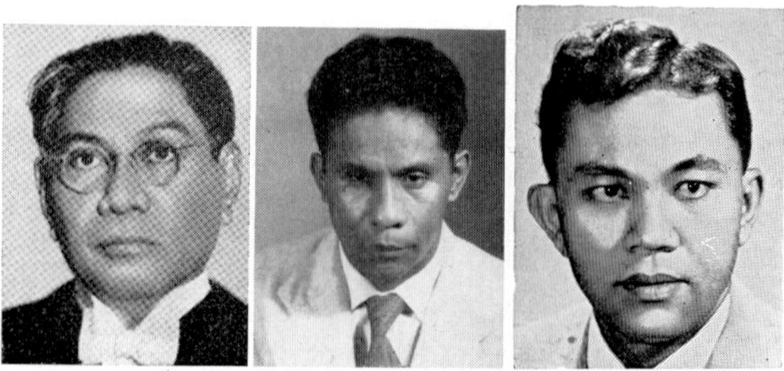

W. Z. JOHANNES G. A. SIWABESSY SJAHRIAR RASAD

Radiological Society at the University Hospital in Djakarta - Indonesia had less than ten fully qualified radiologists serving its population of 85 million.

Johannes was the professor of radiology in the University of Indonesia, and is regarded as the "father of radiology" in his country. At the founding of the Perkumpulan Radiologi Indonesia, Johannes became chairman of the society, his associate G. A. Siwabessy was elected vice-chairman, with Baginda Sjahriar Rasad as secretary. Siwabessy had been to England for training in radiotherapy, Rasad had studied both in Europe (at the Radiumhemmet, at the Curie Foundation, then in Great Britain with D. W. Smithers and Ralston Paterson), and in the USA (with Ross Golden), and is certificated by the American Board of Radiology.

In 1952, Johannes, while on a trip to Europe, died of the complications of a unusually severe Herpes Zoster. Although he had been a cripple for most of his professional life, he was respected as a gentleman, a scholar, and a teacher.

Thereupon Siwabessy became chairman of the Perkumpulan Radiologi, while Rasad stayed on as secretary. Rasad became professor of radiology in the University of Indonesia, and Siwabessy is the "boss" of the Indonesian Atomic Energy Institute.

One of the functions of the Indonesian Radiological Society is to certify radiologic specialists. The total number of radiologists has risen to about 20 (all trained by Johannes and Rasad), while the total population of the country hovers around 100 million. There is as yet much to be done, and they are hard at it.*

AUSTRALIA

The College of Radiologists of Australasia (CRA) was incorporated in 1959, but it was formed from the Australian and New Zealand Association of Radiologists (ANZAR), which was incorporated in 1935. The change from an association to a college allowed them to institute registrable diplomas for members and fellows. The term Australasia signifies the geographic area composed of Australia and New Zealand. The first president of the CRA was J. Stanley Verco, with Alan R. Colwell as its first secretary. Their seal is of the rubber stamp variety, and not suitable for reproduction. They are in the process of obtaining an official crest, but the design has not yet been approved.

The Radiographer was originally issued by members of the ANZAR. The official publication of the CRA was first issued in 1957 as the *Proceedings of the CRA*. The name was changed in 1959 to *Journal of the CRA*.

THE COLLEGE OF
RADIOLOGISTS OF AUSTRALASIA

135 MACQUARIE STREET,
SYDNEY, N.S.W.

Telephone: BU 3340 BU 3349 *Telegraphic address: Radiologist, Sydney*

PRESIDENT:
DR. E. W. CASEY

VICE-PRESIDENTS:
DR. R. KAYE SCOTT

HONORARY SECRETARY:
DR. ARTHUR B. SULLIVAN

HON. ASST. SECRETARIES:
DR. HAROLD J. HAM
DR. E. A. BOOTH

HONORARY TREASURER:
DR. E. A. BOOTH

EXECUTIVE COMMITTEE: Dr. E. W. Casey, Dr. R. Kaye Scott, Dr. Arthur B. Sullivan, Dr. Harold J. Ham, Dr. E. A. Booth, Dr. D. G. Maitland.

CHAIRMAN OF BOARD OF EXAMINERS: Dr. R. Kaye Scott.

CONJOINT BOARD: Dr. D. B. Pearce, Dr. B. L. Deans, Dr. E. W. Casey, Mr. D. J. Stevens.

FELLOWSHIP BOARD: Dr. Harold J. Ham (Convenor), Dr. E. R. Crisp, Dr. B. L. W. Clarke.

MEMBERS OF COUNCIL:
N.S.W.: Drs. E. A. Booth, H. J. Ham, K. E. Shellshear, D. G. Maitland, S. Wherrett, and A. B. Sullivan.
VICTORIA: Drs. E. W. Casey, R. Kaye Scott, Lloyd Dick, C. R. Laing and A. E. Piper.
QUEENSLAND: Drs. A. G. S. Cooper, H. Masel.
NEW ZEALAND: Drs. C. P. M. Feltham, E. R. Blakely.
S. AUSTRALIA: Drs. C. M. Gurner, B. S. Hanson.
W. AUSTRALIA: Dr. M. G. F. Donnan.
TASMANIA: Dr. K. J. Friend.

VOLUME I, No. I. JUNE, 1957.

PROCEEDINGS OF THE COLLEGE OF
RADIOLOGISTS OF AUSTRALASIA

Edited under the Direction of the Editorial Committee
For circulation to all Fellows and Members

EDITORIAL COMMITTEE:
E. W. Casey, E. A. Booth, H. J. Ham
D. G. Maitland, R. Kaye Scott, A. B. Sullivan

EDITORIAL STAFF:
Honorary Editor: W. Pook Honorary Assistant Editor: J. Bell

Honorary Associate Editors:
Radiodiagnosis: F. J. McEncroe
Radiotherapy: H. A. S. van den Brenk
Non-Medical: D. F. Robertson
New Zealand: B. M. de Lambert

JAPAN

Goro Goto, the expert in the history of Japanese radiology, prepared the following summary for publication in this text:

*These data were obligingly offered by Prof. Sjahriar Rasad.

*This information, and the illustrations reproduced herewith, were graciously provided through the courtesy of three Australian radiologists, who are secretaries of their respective organizations, B. S. Hanson (Adelaide), Craig Horn (Sydney), and J. K. Monk (Melbourne).

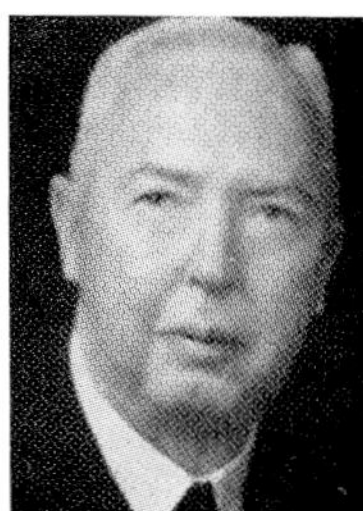

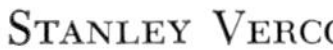

STANLEY VERCO

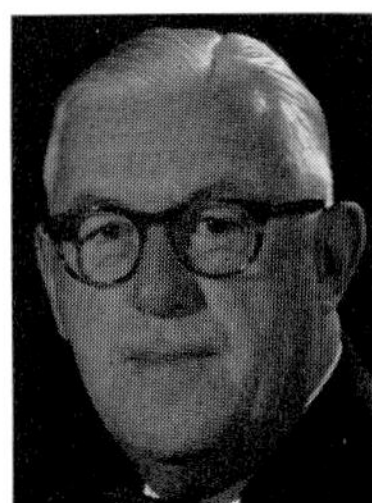

ALAN COLWELL

"Two circles of investigation and scientific discussion of roentgen problems were formed in 1913 in Japan. One of these was in Tokyo, and the initiative came from Gitoku Tashiro (1854-1938), Shichiro Hida (1871-1923), and Goichi Fujinami (1880-1942). The other was in Osaka, under the impulse of Masakiyo Ogata. Thereupon the first specialty periodical in this country in the field of radiology was issued in 1914 with the title *Irigakuryoho Zasshi* (Journal of Physico-medical Therapy), the editors being Keizo Dohi (1866-1931), Tashiro, Hida, Fujinami, Keichiro Manabe (1878-1941), and Ogata.

"The Nippon Rentogen Gakkai (Japanese Roentgen Association) was founded in April, 1923 with Tashiro as its first president. The secretaries were Hida, Fujinami, and Manabe. In the same year was started its official journal, the *Nippon Rentogen Gakkai Zasshi.*

"In 1933, some of the members separated, and formed another group. There being then the Golden Age of Radiology, they called themselves Nippon Hoshasen Igakkai (Japanese Radiologic-Medical Association), and issued their own periodical, the *Nippon Hoshasen Igakkai Zasshi.*

"By 1941 they became friendly again, the two groups were consolidated into the Nippon Igaku Hoshasen Gakkai (Nippon Societas Radiologica), and the two journals fused into the *Nippon Igaku Hoshasen Gakkai Zasshi* (Nippon Acta Radiologica), which has remained to this day Japan's most authoritative radiologic periodical."

The Journal of Radiology and Physical Therapy
University of Kanazawa.
(Editor, Dr. H. Hiramatsu)
Vol. 49 Nov. 1958

金沢医理学叢書

主幹 平松 博

第四十九巻

In Japan, Hiroshi Hiramatsu, professor of radiology in the University of Kanazawa, is since gogatsu, 1946 editor of the *Kanazawa Irigaku Sosho*: it publishes mostly original investigations from the entire field of radiology and electrology, performed under Hiramatsu's sponsorship by medical students working for their final thesis (also in many European universities, a final thesis is a pre-requisite for the medical degree).

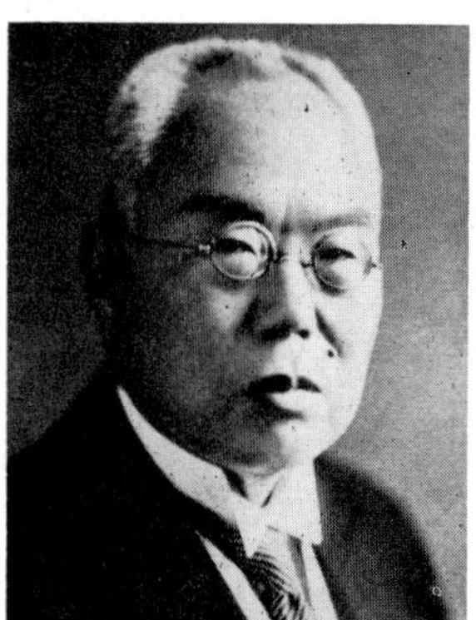

TASHIRO

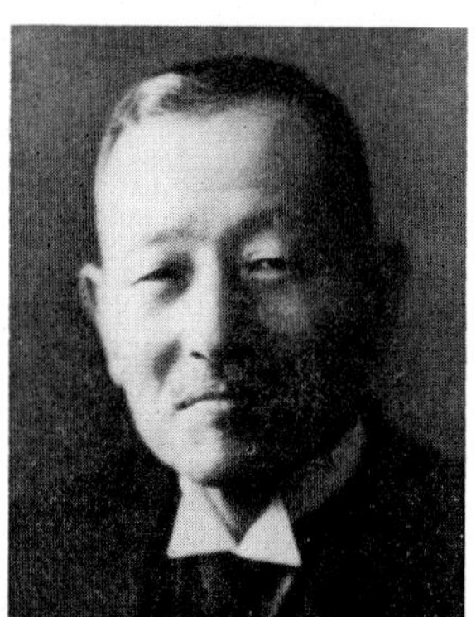

MANABE

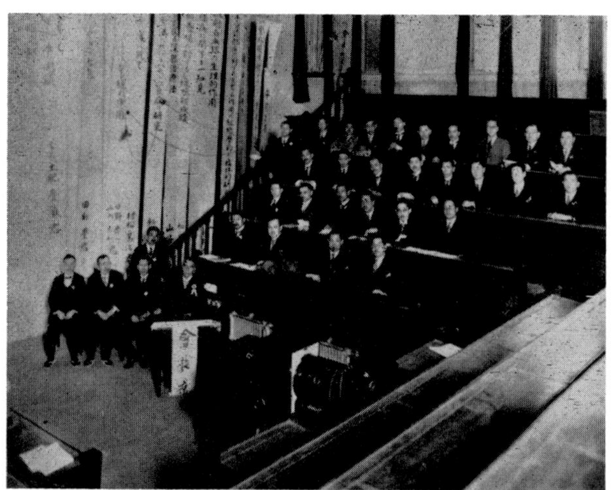

JAPANESE RADIOLOGICAL MEETING (1929)

HIDA

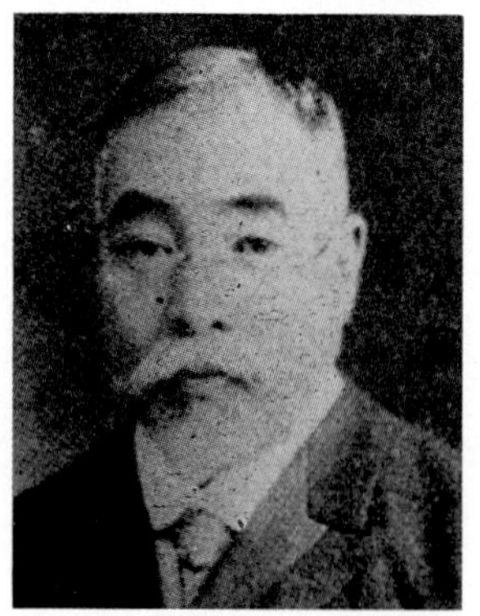

OGATA

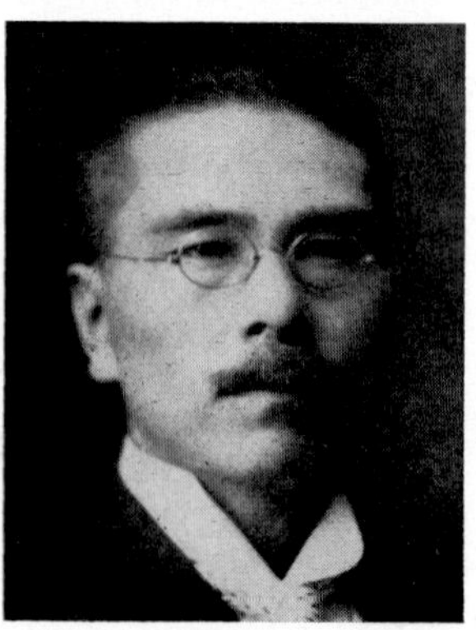

DOHI

The literal translation of *Kanazawa Irigaku Sosho* is *Kanazawa Medical Physics Series,* but on top of its cover is printed the English title *Journal of Radiology and Physical Therapy.*

During the Era of Roentgen Pioneers, Japan and the Japanese radiologists were in a period of Germanophilia, which persisted through the Golden Age of Radiology. From Fujinami's Roentgen Department at Keio University were issued the *Keio Roentgen Sosho* (series). The *Keiko* (fluorescence), the first periodical of x-ray technic was followed by *Nippon X-Sen Gishikai Kaiho* (Journal of the Japanese Association of X-Ray Technicians). After World War II, American influence inevitably increased the utilization of the term *hoshasen* (radiology), for instance in 1956 the Kanehara Book Company started the *Rinsho Hoshasen* (Clinical Radiology). A technical journal appeared, with the name *Nippon Hoshasen Gizitsu Zasshi* (Japanese Journal of Radiologic Technology). In 1960, some of Marshall Brucer's former trainees established the Nippon Hoshasen Eikyo Gakkai (Japanese Radiation Research Society) with its official periodical, the *Journal of Radiation Research.* The intelligent, industrious, and (usually) indomitable Japanese have rebuilt their country, and are now in the midst of a tremendous industrial and commercial boom. Their intellectual strength, capacity for hard work, and determination are some of the reasons why the country with the heliotherapeutic nickname (Land of the Rising Sun) and Japanese radiology have always been, and – within the foreseeable future – will remain, the most progressive in that part of the globe.

NUCLEAR RE-ADJUSTMENTS

Even in the USA the Atomic Phase did not come into full swing until after 1950. By then most of the true Roentgen Pioneers (those born before 1870) were either dead or, for all practical purposes, out of circulation. The officers of existing radiological societies (who had had their training during the Golden Age), faced a situation for which they were not quite prepared.

A new crop of physicists and their acolytes crowded the radiologic meetings, to the point where special sections had to be created for them. And if a Golden Age executive strayed into the "wrong" room, he felt

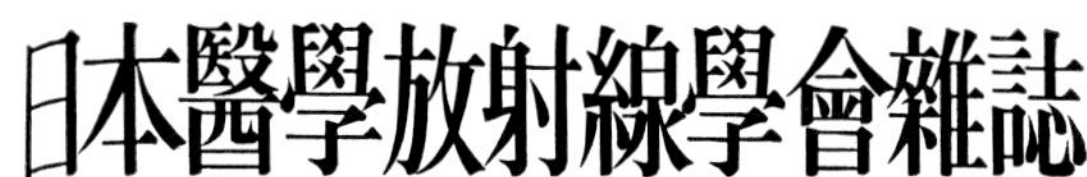

日本醫學放射線學會雜誌

NIPPON ACTA RADIOLOGICA

第十巻 第七號 Tomus X Fasc VII

昭和二十五年十一月二十五日發行 25. XI. 1950

目次 Contenta

原著 Originalia

社團法人 日本醫學放射線學會

NIPPON SOCIETAS RADIOLOGICA

日本醫放會誌
Nipp. Act. Radil.

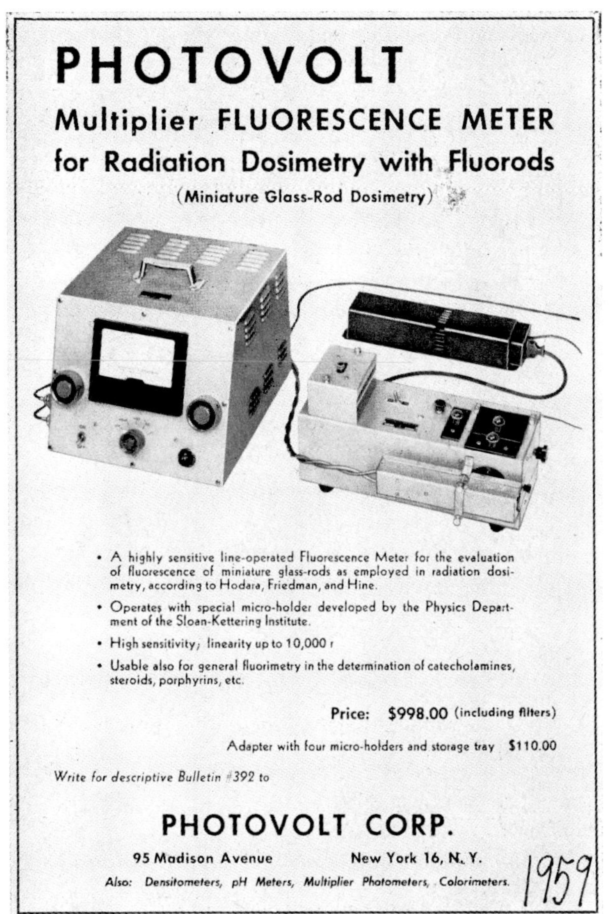

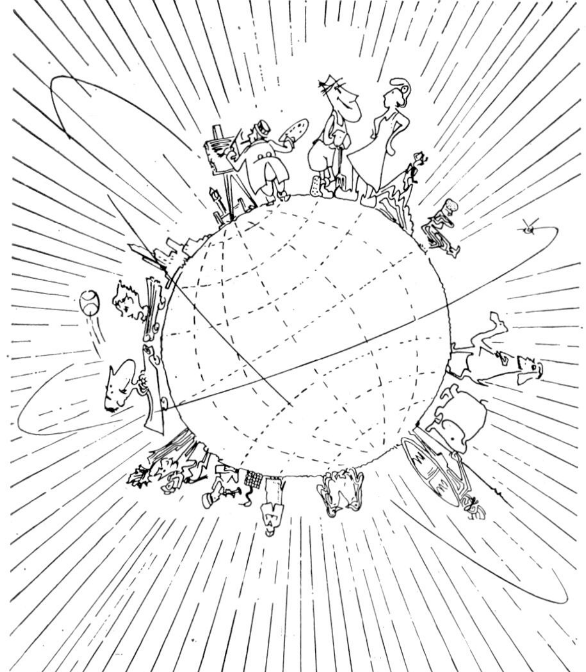

tempted to re-adjust his hearing aid because of such peculiar (radiologic?) words as chopper – which is a device for selecting electrons for injection into an accelerator during the preferred part of the cycle. In a crowd of isotopic buffs, he may be exposed to talk about radioactivation analysis – qualitative and/or quantitative investigations of artificially induced radioactivity, the "latest" method uses neutrons from a "pint-sized" 150 kvp linac. Or he would open his specialty journal, and find an article on gamma ray dosimetry, only to discover that it is no longer done with instruments familiar to him: they use instead radio-photoluminescent glass needles, a sort of detector proved quite useful in solid state dosimetry.

All these strange words, and the notions as well as the philosophy behind them, are (so far) no reason for alarm. Medicine is not (yet) a science, it is still ("only") an art. *Plus ça change, plus c'est la même chose!* No matter how significantly image inten-

HOWARD DOUB having edited *Radiology* continuously since 1941, is now, for all practical purposes, "the" radiologic editor.

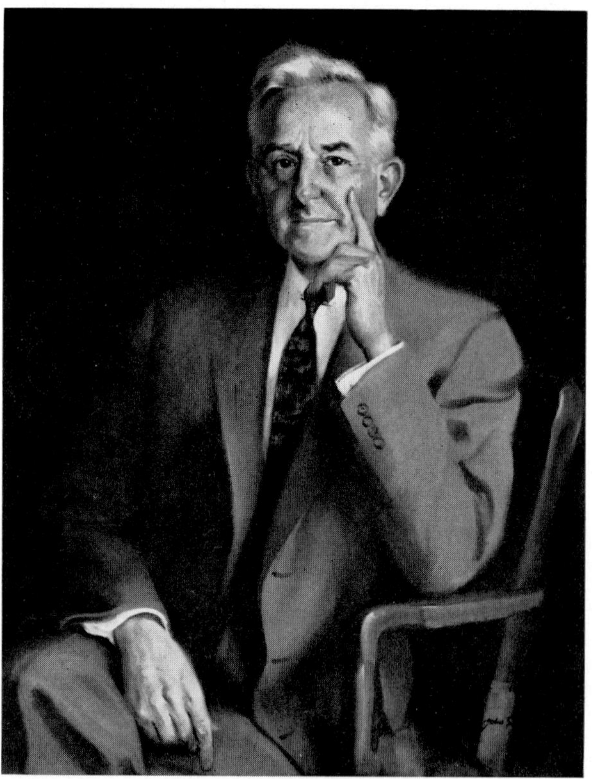

Courtesy: Kenneth Krabbenhoft

LAWRENCE REYNOLDS (1889-1961). Oil painting of the long-time editor of the *American Journal of Roentgenology*. Truly both a gentleman and a scholar, he donated his half-million dollar collection of historical medical books (including many incunabula) to his *alma mater*. The collection is now part of the Lawrence Reynolds Library at the Medical College in the University of Alabama in Birmingham.

sifiers and megavoltage sources might seem to have affected diagnosis and therapy, in the final analysis the "thing" always turns out to be a medical problem. The solution of medical problems requires the use of medical judgment which, so far, cannot (and may never) be replaced by physicistic computations or computers. Therefore, within the foreseeable future, medicine will be in need of, and will have a place for, radiologic clinicians.

But radionuclides kept on circling the globe, and appeared both as fall-out and in more useful shapes. Sooner or later this was bound to provoke wilful alterations in the names of many journals and societies in the field of radiology.

Detroit seems to be a favored spot for radiologic editorial offices, because at the time of this writing (and for over two decades) that is where both the ARRS and the RSNA edit their official journals. As a matter of fact, the Technicians' journal is likewise edited in Detroit.

During the lengthy tenure of the late Lawrence Reynolds as editor of the *American Journal of Roentgenology,* and during the continuing reign of Howard Doub as editor of *Radiology,* both journals have reached enviable positions in the world's specialty literature. In this context it is easy to overlook the contributions of so-called associates, such as Reynolds' secretary, Ruth Bigelow, or - in a different way - the significant help given in the publication of *Radiology* by the late Donald Childs, Sr.

The Yellow Journal's *Consolidated Indices* came out first (in 1939) - its sixth volume is currently being prepared for publication. The Gray Journal's *Cumulative Index* (started in 1943 by Marion Crowell and Florence Roper - the fifth volume will have appeared at the time this text reaches the bookstands) is so important because of the wide coverage inserted into *Radiology* by its *Abstracts of Current Literature.*

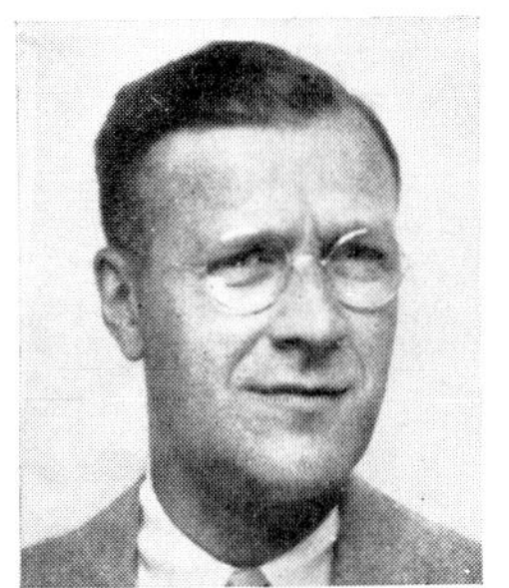

DONALD S. CHILDS, SR.

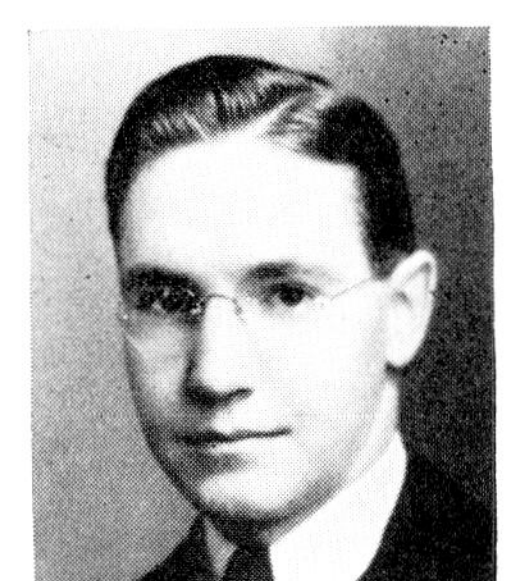

GEORGE WYATT

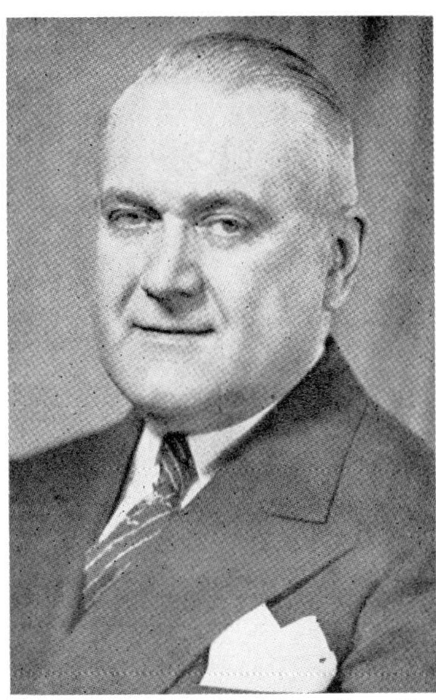

Courtesy: Kenneth Krabbenhoft

TRAIAN LEUCUTIA, current editor of the *American Journal of Roentgenology.*

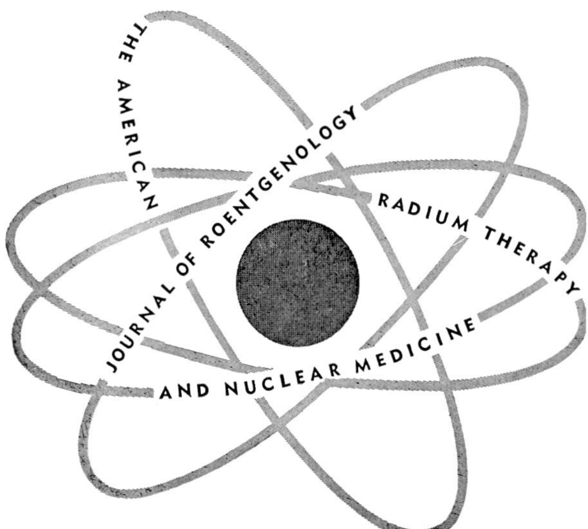

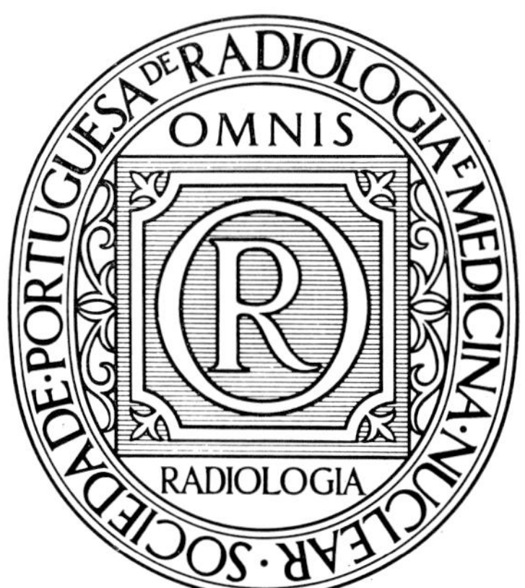

The original title of the Gray Journal, *Radiology*, was well adapted for all contingencies. Not so the Yellow Journal, which had to make its first re-adjustment in January of 1950, when George Marvin Wyatt's *Abstracts of Roentgen and Radium Literature* were replaced by Traian Leucutia's *Abstracts of Radiological Literature*. The second move came in January, 1952 (vol. 67) when the words *and Nuclear Medicine* were added to the title on the masthead — and this new label was orbited into the advertising section of the *British Journal of Radiology*.

At that time neither the Scandinavians, nor the Germans, or the Dutch (*Nederlandse Vereniging voor Electrologie en Röntgenologie)* had modified the names of their (Röntgen) associations. With the January, 1956 (vol. 84) issue, however, the (German) *Fortschritte auf dem Gebiete der Röntgenstrahlen* acquired the codicil *und Nuklearmedizin*.

It has been shown that in Romanic languages the coverage provided by the word radiology approximates ABR's former definition of diagnostic roentgenology. Therefore, when a nuclear change was called for, the official French radiological organ became (be-

AYRES DE SOUSA

ANGIOQUIMOGRAFIA

ENSAIO DA SUA APLICAÇÃO AO ESTUDO
DA HEMODINÂMICA

LIVRARIA PORTUGÁLIA
LISBOA — 1951

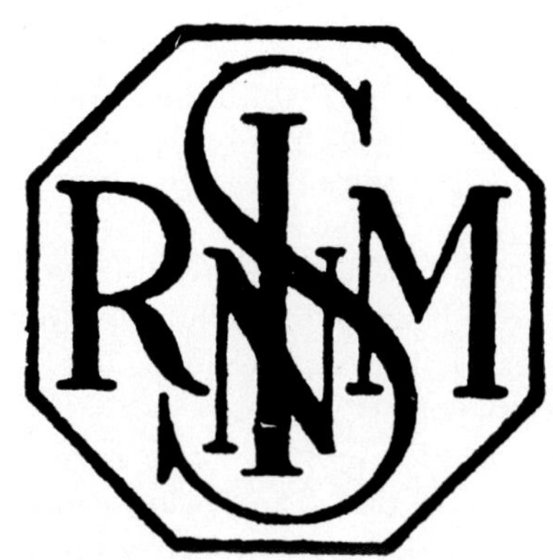

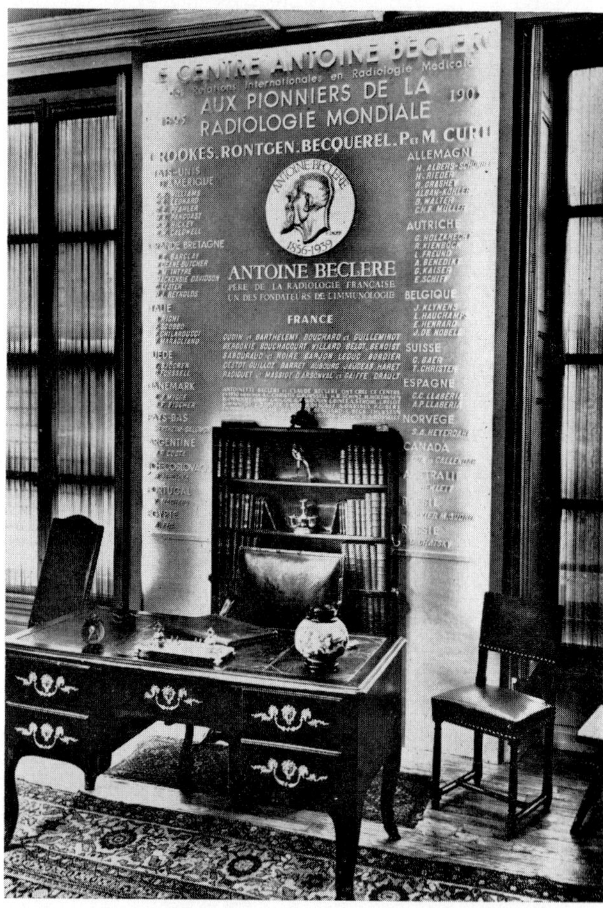

CENTRE ANTOINE BECLERE
des Relations Internationales en Radiologie Médicale
for International Relations in Medical Radiology
de Relaciones Internacionales en Radiologia Medica
für Internationale Beziehungen
in der Medizinischen Röntgenologie
7, RUE PERRONET - PARIS - 7° (France)
Tél. : LIT. 19-27 Adr. Tél. : CABRIRM-Paris
C. C. P. PARIS 8510-25

BULLETIN D'INFORMATION
pour les Sociétés Nationales de Radiologie

ginning with vol. 38, nr. ¾, March-April, 1957) the *Journal de Radiologie, d'Électrologie, et de Médecine Nucléaire.* Their professional organization, however, is still called Société Française d'Électroradiologie Médicale. By contrast, in Italy, Spain, and Portugal, nuclear appendages were attached to the respective titles.

The SIRM became the SIRMN, that is Società Italiana di Radiologic Medica e di Medicina Nucleare. The Madrid version is Sociedad Española di Radiología y Electrología Médicas y Medicina Nuclear, while in Lisbon appeared the Sociedade Portuguesa de Radiologia e Medicina Nuclear.

Portugal occupies a peculiar position of radiologic importance, out of proportion with its relatively small size.

It served as birthplace for some of the most important roentgen examinations with contrast materials, Egas Moniz (cerebral angiography), Reinaldo dos Santos (arthrography), and Lopo de Carvalho (angiopneumography) were all Portuguese. The big three's direct successor (a pupil of Moniz) is Ayres de Sousa, who developed his own, specialized procedure, called angiokymography. With his associates, de Sousa performed many other vascular studies, including microangiographic investigations into hemodynamics in general, of the skin in particular. Sousa is also an avid student of the history of radiology in Portugal.

The strange synonymy between the French *radiologie* and the German *Röntgenologie* was acknowledged by the Centre Antoine Béclère in Paris: as a

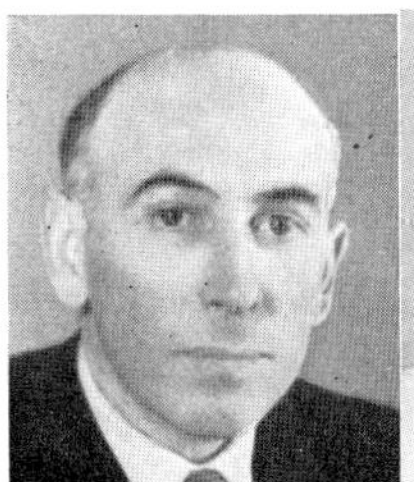
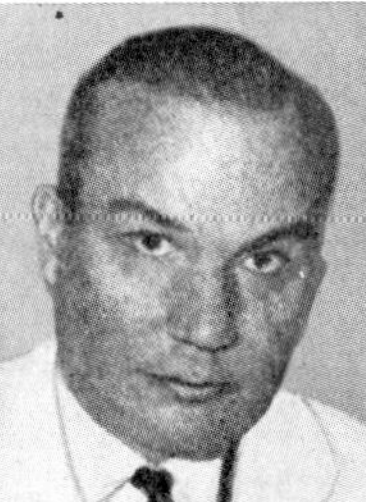
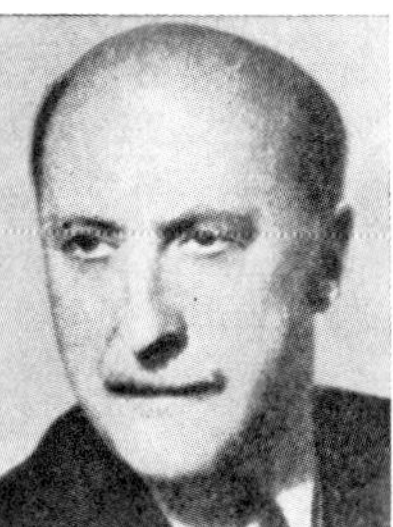

J. P. Betoulières Charles Proux F. Baclesse

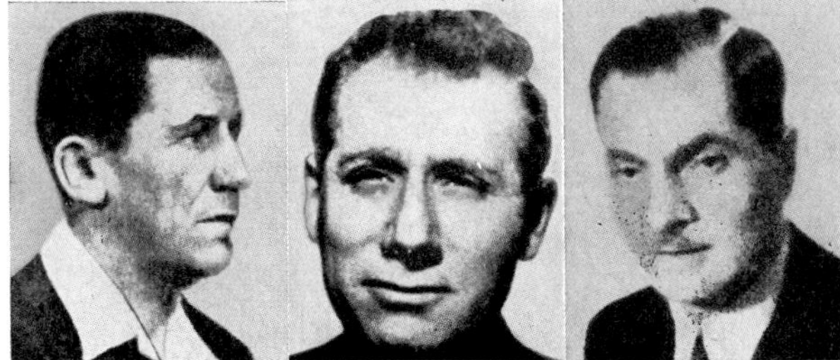

Pierre Porcher H. Fischgold G. Ledoux-Lebard

Contemporary French radiologists.

matter of fact when they had to translate into German the words "for international relations in medical radiology, they came up with *für internationale Beziehungen in de medizinischen Röntgenologie.*

A similar predicament existed for several decades in trilingual Switzerland, where the *Schweizerische Röntgengesellschaft* called itself in French *Société Suisse de Radiologie,* in Italian *Società Svizzera di Radiologia.*

In the *Bulletin du Centre Antoine Béclère* of March-April, 1962 Max Hopf (the current secretary-general of the Swiss Radiological Society) reviewed the history of radiology in Switzerland, a country in which Röntgen had studied and where he spent most of his vacation time. Around 1905 Albert Einstein had been a Swiss citizen: he prepared his first account of the Theory of Relativity while residing in Bern.

Turning now to famous Swiss radiologists, Theophil Christen (1873-1920), was a mathematics and physics teacher in Zurich and then in Bern, who contributed the concept of the half-value layer, so basic to therapeutic calculations. Special mention is deserved by the osteo-radiologist Emil Looser (1877-1936) of Winterthur; and Ed Stierlin (1878-1919) of Zurich, whose eponym is attached to the spasmodic emptying of the tuberculous cecum. The gynecologic radiumtherapist Max Steiger (1880-1924) of Bern became a radiation casualty, and so did the pioneer manufacturer of x-ray apparatus Friedrich Wilhelm Klingelfuss (1859-1932) of Basel.

The Swiss Radiological Society was founded on March 9, 1913 by Jules Curchod de Roll (1861-1937) of Geneva; Herman Hopf (1874-1930) of Berne, who became a roentgen martyr (his son is the current secretary, Max Hopf); and Hermann Suter (1878-1949) another radiation casualty.

The semantic ambiguity of the Swiss denominations became apparent in many ways, for instance in the titles of the expert medical roentgenphysicist* Adolf Liechti (1898-1946), who was at the same time professor of *Medizinische Radiologie* in the University of Bern, and director of the clinical *Röntgeninstitut,* which belonged to the same university.

On May 31, 1958 the Swiss decided to "uniformize" their "radiologic" nomenclature. They adopted the neo-German term *Radiologie,* but gave it the French

*Liechti's *Roentgenphysik* was brought out in a 2nd edition (Wien, 1935), revised by Walter Minder. This was the "correct" German term, as in Robert Fürstenau's *Leitfaden der Röntgenphysik* (Stuttgart, 1910), or Fritz Regler's *Grundzüge der Röntgenphysik* (Berlin, 1937). By contrast, Charles Weyl and Samuel Reid Warren called their volume, *Radiologic Physics* (Springfield, 1941).

Radiologia Clinica

Internationale Radiologische Rundschau
Röntgen, Radium, Licht - Forschung und Klinik
International Radiological Review
Roentgen, Radium, Light - Research and Clinic
Revue Internationale de Radiologie
Roentgen, Radium, Lumière - Recherches et Clinique
Rivista Radiologica Internazionale
Roentgen, Radium, Fototerapia - Indagine e Clinica

Organ der Schweizerischen Röntgengesellschaft – Organe de la Société Suisse de Radiologie
Organo della Società Svizzera di Radiologia

Radiologia Clinica

Internationale Radiologische Rundschau
Röntgen, Radium, Licht - Forschung und Klinik
International Radiological Review
Roentgen, Radium, Light - Research and Clinic
Revue Internationale de Radiologie
Roentgen, Radium, Lumière - Recherches et Clinique
Rivista Radiologica Internazionale
Roentgen, Radium, Fototerapia - Indagine e Clinica

Organ der Schweizerischen Gesellschaft für Radiologie und Nuklearmedizin
Organe de la Société Suisse de Radiologie et de Médecine Nucléaire
Organo della Società Svizzera di Radiologia e di Medicina Nucleare

meaning, which then (inevitably) demanded an atomic tailpiece. The full name was thus changed to Schweizerische Gesellschaft für Radiologie und Nuklearmedizin (used for the first time on the frontispiece of *Radio Clinica* of January, 1959) with transliterated French and Italian versions.

For many years *Radiologia Clinica* had been edited by Max Lüdin: after his death in 1960, editorship of the official Swiss organ went jointly to Adolf Zuppinger of Zürich and George Candardjis of Lausanne.

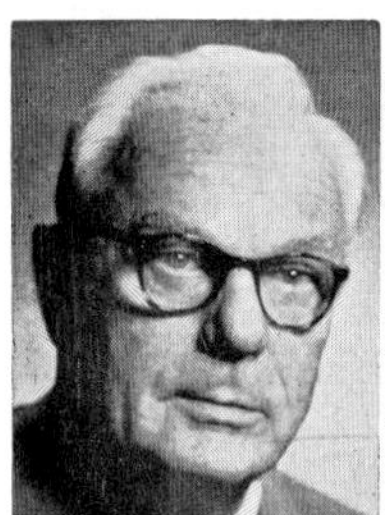
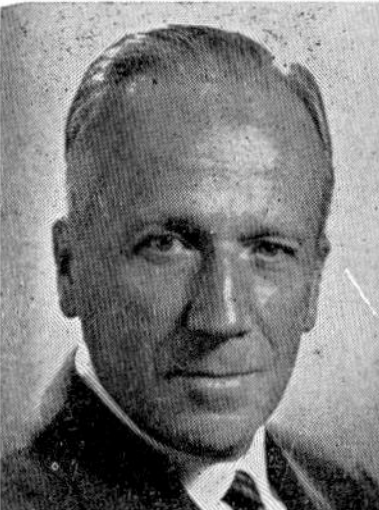
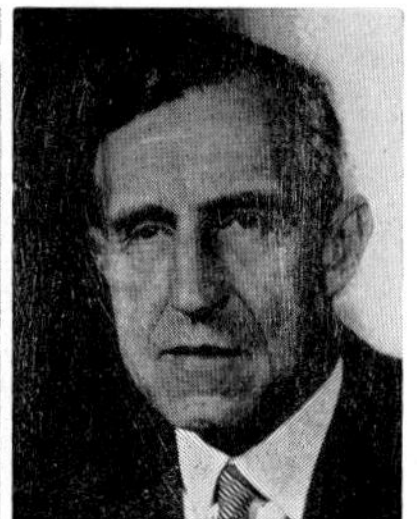

H. H. Weber   Erich Zdansky   Adolph Zuppinger
Contemporary Swiss radiologists.

SOCIETY OF NUCLEAR MEDICINE

Henry Leslie Jaffé, a Los Angeles radiologist, glibly recalled that on January 19, 1954 "twelve old men" met in a smoke-filled room in the Davenport Hotel in Spokane (Washington), and decided to form a Society of Nuclear Medicine (SNM).

Jaffé had not been in on the organizational meetings, it had been a strictly Northwestern society in the very beginning. One of the first officers, Norman Jeffries Holter – a physicist from Helena (Montana), who had been group leader in the atomic tests at Eniwetok in 1952 – was to recall the first SNM meeting in these words: ". . . we had a voluntary assessment of $10 to pay for rooms, booze, and food, and I was treasurer with an even $100 in the bag."

The SNM held its first annual meeting in Seattle in May of 1954 with Thomas Carlile (a local radiologist) presiding. The SNM expanded rapidly and at the sixth annual meeting (Chicago, June 17-20, 1959) it had over 1400 active members, and de Hevesy as an honorary fellow. The SNM had been created with local intentions in mind and shortly thereafter several other local associations were formed, such as the Central Society of Nuclear Medicine in Chicago, created by Irvin Hummon, Bob Landauer Sr., and Donalee Tabern. At the sixth meeting, the local societies merged into the SNM, and a sample issue of the projected *Journal of Nuclear Medicine* was distributed – it is regularly published since 1960.

Medical isotopology was built on radioiodine, and so was most of the equipment. Blood volume determinations seem destined to stay with us, and tracers are used on a large scale in physiologic research. But aside from Co^{60} in tele- as well as in brachytherapy, the use of isotopes in treatment has decreased. Not so in industry, or in agriculture and similar fields.

The possibility of using induced male sexual sterility as a method of controlling insect populations was well

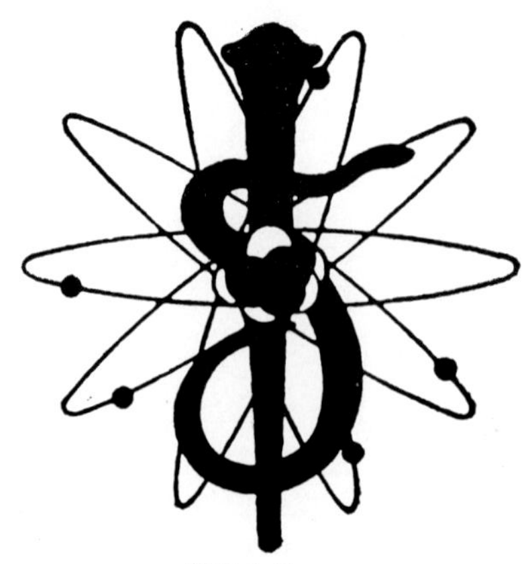

SNM Seal

illustrated in research that culminated in 1954 in the eradication of the screwworm fly from Curacao, a small island in the Netherland Antilles. It was based on the fact that the male screwworm is polygamous, the female monogamous. Male screwworms, after being sterilized by Co^{60} radiation, are released from airplanes flying low and slow over the screwworm infested territory. There is currently a large operation in progress in the Southwestern USA, and it is hoped that by the end of 1964, the screwworm will have been practically eradicated.

Cosmic radiation produces in the atmosphere a certain amount of radioactive carbon-14, which is incorporated into plants through photosynthesis. The addition of "new" C^{14} ceases at the time of death of the respective plant. The half-life of C^{14} has not been more precisely determined than 5568 ± 30 years. Still it appears to provide a satisfactory method for estimating the age of old wood up to about 15,000 years; the range might possibly be extended to as far back as 60,000 years.

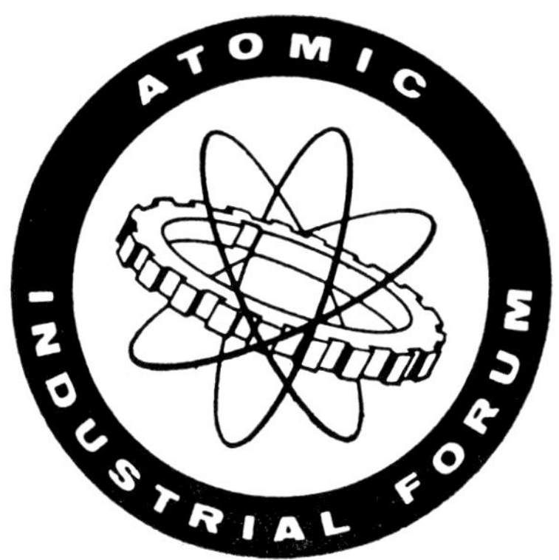

Nuclear knowledge is actively spreading in the populace, especially among the younger set. Recently the Boy Scouts have introduced an Atomic Energy Merit Badge. To qualify for the badge, the boys must demonstrate their grasp of the topic by answering certain questions, and performing certain practical tests. The badge itself is a model of the lithium atom (the three orbits) on a yellow background, enclosed in a green circle. To give you an idea of the test questions, two samples will be offered: (1) Given the names of Becquerel, Bohr, Curie, Einstein, Fermi, Hahn, Ernest Lawrence, Lisa Meitner, Roentgen, and Rutherford, you must explain, to the satisfaction of the merit-badge counselor, how a given person's discovery was related to another person's work in this group. The other sample herein offered is a *practical* one: (2) Make a cloud chamber, using simple material, then show the merit-badge counselor how the chamber can be used to see the tracks caused by radiation. How many members of the SNM would submit to such a test, and how many of them would pass it? As a matter of fact, the educational problem was one which the SNM evaluated with due seriousness.

To complete the new etymologic enterprise, tentative plans were made for the creation of an American College of Nuclear Medicine, and for the (hypothetic) American Board of Nuclear Medicine that would have to come with it. The ABR had issued "nuclear medallions" since 1956 (the actual mailing started in 1957). The ABR has since integrated in its standard examination procedures a reasonable number of questions on both the physical and the clinical aspects of radioisotopes, and in 1962 it discontinued separate examinations for the medallion. Whoever wishes now to be certified in therapeutic radiology must know "something" about isotopes.

A recent semantic addition is the term radioisotopology, used between quotation marks in the description of the Triga reactor at the VA Hospital in Omaha as it was published in *Radiology of* April, 1962.

RADIO-HISTORIC CENSORSHIP

In the 1962 edition of *A History of Historical Writing* (originally published in 1937, then reprinted in a Dover paperback), Barnes - whom some consider the most important living American historian - stated:

"... the whole row about (historic) relativism was a diversionary tempest-in-a-teapot designed in part to distract attention from the unwillingness of historians to face up to the real and vital threats to their profession. It was about like being distressed over a case of German measles or chicken-pox in the midst of an epidemic of typhus or bubonic plague...

"The breakdown of supernaturalism and the threats to the contemporary nationalistic, democratic, and capitalistic regime have created a mental confusion not unlike that which accompanied the downfall of (Rome's) classic civilization. The best exemplification of this trend in the historical field has been the immense popularity of Arnold J. Toynbee's *The Study of History*. Despite the fact that Toynbee is unquestionably the most learned living historian, his historical framework rested on theological aberrations, oddities, curios, and vestiges which should appal any reasonably well-informed college student.

"The historical procedure under Ingsoc (in the Orwellian nightmare of "Nineteen Eighty-four") involves the deliberate suppression and destruction of all existing documentation which conflicts with what passes for historical truth at any moment. Many readers will feel that we are still removed from any such situation as that... The truth is that we are already in just such a historical regimen. It is merely a matter of degree. Aside from a few despised "revisionistic" historical volumes, there has been no historical writing since 1939, even in the Free World, which has substantially challenged or departed from the basic policy of the country of the writer. It is well established that important documents dealing with the diplomacy of the second World War have been suppressed or destroyed. ... The documents finally published on such important wartime summit conferences as those at Yalta and Teheran were often badly distorted and some were suppressed."

This is also evident in the behavior of the executive committees of several of the current professional radio-organizations in this country. While the history of the ACR, RSNA, or ARRS is of no political consequence *per se,* the officials of the respective organizations will not accept for presentation at their meetings anything that does not conform with their views, meaning with what they believe should be told about the past of the respective organizations. But neither is the present spared. Marshall Brucer was chairman of the Program Committee of the Society of Nuclear Medicine (SNM) for the meeting in Montreal in 1963. As he did not intend to be present (for reasons of health) he decided to put on magnetic tape a few words to the membership, words that would then be "offered" to the audience present at the meeting. But the "committee" censored his proposed text, for reasons which were not publicly disclosed. I believe that what a former president of any society wants to tell the members of that society must not be suppressed. This is why I have reproduced the most incendiary paragraphs from that proposed speech, if only to prove my point which is that censorship in any form (but especially in professional organizations) is not only anachronistic, it is most of the time senseless. These are the words which Marshall Brucer was not allowed to say:

THE PARABLE OF THE THREE FISSIONS

"Once upon a time – in 1895 – a man invented a horseless carriage. It was very good for toting people around the countryside, and so it was immediately used by country doctors to take them out onto the highways and byways to deliver babies. This was a peaceful use of automotive energy, even though delivering babies increased the number of people who ultimately die of cancer, and we are fighting cancer.

"About twenty years later an American citizen, named Winston Churchill, found that war was boring because the soldiers didn't get any place. He pointed out that the horseless carriage could carry more than

LA BELLE PROVINCE DE QUÉBEC
AWAITS YOU
MON AMI!
MONTREAL
1963
Mark your Calendar Now!
10th Annual Meeting
The Society
of Nuclear Medicine
Queen Elizabeth Hotel
Montreal, Canada
June 26-29, 1963
ALOUETTE

one person. It could also carry shielding against the primitive weapons then in use. So he invented the tank, which was a horseless carriage with an iron pettycoat. It may not have seemed very new, but it was exceedingly practical.

"And it changed the face of the war so much that afterwards the USA created an Automatic Energy Committee, commonly called the AEC, for the regulation of these devices in peacetime. And a great president, who had been in on their military use, declared it an invention for all the people, and so he developed an "Autos for Peace Program." There were many practical things that could be done on this program, like water conversion, flame inversion, even political perversion. So an admiral was put in charge to ensure that the AEC would be for defense and not for offense.

"The first thing the AEC did was to buy 50,000 typewriters and to hire 50,000 monkeys to type 50,000 manuscripts each day. Each one of these manuscripts was then declassified. The result was a rain of white paper which covered the surface of the earth to exactly three inches. This was called a snow job, and it was a good thing.

"The old fashioned fossil fuel – used in these tanks – did not burn completely. Some of it spewed out at the back end, the deadly "blowout." There exists a branch of the American government, called the Department of Wealth, Spending, and Hellfire. That department is chuck full of highly resourceful scientists, and these scientists discovered that blowout is not good for mice. There were also a few intelligent scientists outside the department: one of them, called Paulus Lining, declared that blowout was carcinogenic, which meant it causes leukemia, which meant that henceforth most babies would be born with two heads, unless something was going to be done about it. So the department decided to get busy with the control of blowout, and started to make blowout less carcinogenic by publishing daily reports.

"Meanwhile – back at the ranch – a group of physicians and auto mechanics got together to discuss the wonderful things that could be done with blowout and its associated compounds. They formed a Society of Never-Never Medicine, SNM for short. At first the SNM went through growing pains, but as soon as those were over, SNM started to do things for its members. Then it debated on what to do next for its members. Then it began to debate on what members should be encouraged to debate on. Then it began to debate on the requirements of training debators on what to debate on. By then members of the SNM had joined another society, and there were not enough people left to debate on the training of debators to debate on the agenda for debate.

"All this time the AEC was growing, and it got so big that its typewriters formed a critical mass. Thereupon it fissioned into three parts: one portion wrote regulations for all people to follow; another portion inspected these regulations; the third portion investigated the first two portions.

"The Department of Wealth, Spending and Hellfire fissioned into one part which prohibited a number of things from going into human bodies; another part was searching frantically for more ways of spending money; the third part had the task of convincing the people to accept the work of the first two parts.

"The SNM fissioned into separate chapters of three members each, who voted gold stars to those who were still attending SNM conventions.

"This was a fairy tale, and most fairy tales are not true. But it might come true if the "debating for debating's sake" were to continue. If it does, I don't predict just "dire consequences," if it continues I simply predict doom."

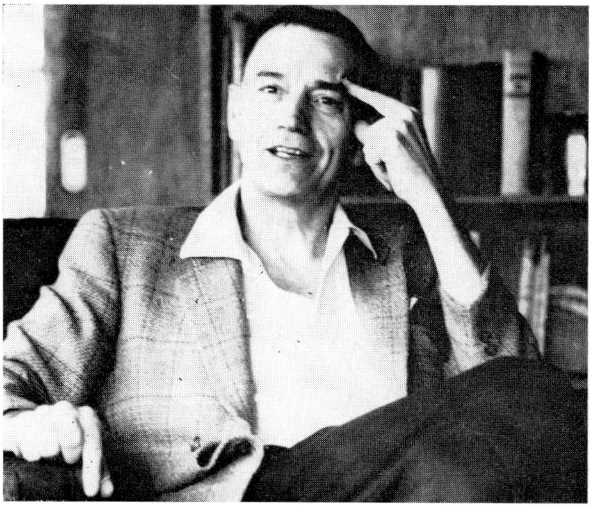

MARSHALL BRUCER.

RADIOLOGY IN LATIN AMERICA

The next best thing to a succinct survey of the development of radiology in Central and South America was James Thomas Case's address to the second Inter-American Congress of Radiology (IACR) in Havana (1946) - the address was published in *Radiology* of May, 1947. "South of the border," Case was in his lifetime the most respected, as well as the most popular *Yanqui* radiologist. At the sixth IACR in Lima (1958) Case was called the unofficial Ambassador of North American radiology. Contributions are currently being collected in Latin America - following the initiative of Arrieta Sanchez of Panama - to place a bust of Case in Case's radioshrine at the University of California.

Brief surveys of the development of radiology in various Latin American countries appeared in *Diseases of the Chest* of November-December, 1945. They had been prepared by the chairmen of local chapters of the American College of Chest Physicians, honoring the 50th anniversary of Röntgen's discovery.

The three stages of radio-historic development pursued peculiar time-tables in Latin America: due to local contingencies, in some places the Atomic Phase is still barely a few years old.

Roentgen pioneers appeared in most Latin-American countries in the very year 1896, but not too many authenticated first dates have been preserved.

In Lima (Peru), in October, 1896 the gynecologist Constantino T. Carvallo made roentgen plates of the hands of Nicolas de Pierola (first democratic president of Peru), and of Ricardo Palma (their great traditionalist writer).

At the time of Röntgen's first paper on x rays, Jaime R. Costa was teaching medical physics in the University of Buenos Aires. His Sala de Fisioterapia was in the Hospital Nacional de Clínicas: it is beyond any doubt that he produced roentgen plates before anybody else in South America, but there is no record of a definite date. In the *Anales del Circulo Médico Argentino* of January, 1900 Costa described his experiences and achievements in the article entitled *La practica de los rayos X.*

Edmundo Xavier was professor of medical physics in the University of Sao Paulo. He was probably the one who obtained the first roentgen plate in Brazil. Among his contemporaries were two Brazilian Roentgen Pioneers, Jorge Dodsworth and A. Alvin (who became a radiation fatality).

In other Latin-American countries exposure of the "first authenticated roentgen plates" occurred well after the turn of the century. This does not necessarily mean that roentgen plates have not been produced in that location at an earlier date, it simply means that no earlier records have been preserved.

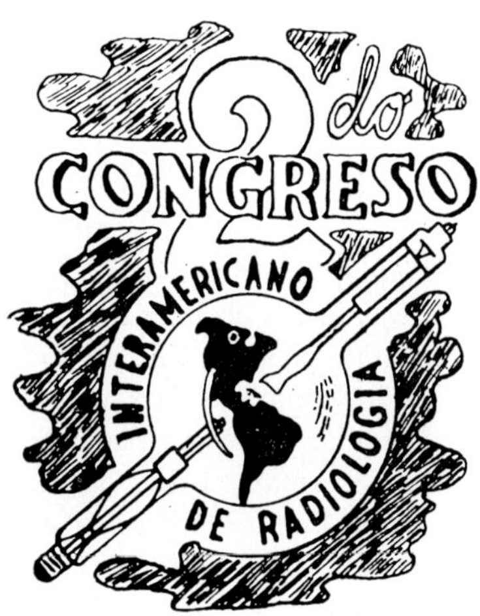

La Razon (a Buenos Aires newspaper) of June 22, 1897 related a strange incident. A suspicious box had been received at the customs house: it came from Buenos Aires and was addressed to Uruguay's president Borda. His life had been repeatedly threatened, indeed he was finally assasinated on August 25, 1897. The box appeared to be quite heavy, it was solidly built, and had an odor of phosphorus. On the suspicion that it might contain a bomb, an x-ray examination of the box was ordered. In the Laboratory of Physics of the University of Montevideo, Scoseria and Williman set up the necessary apparatus, and discovered by fluoroscopy that the box contained — of all things — an x-ray machine!

Zegers is presumed to have introduced x rays into Chile in 1897. Another early radiographer named Eckwall, a Swedish graduate in gymnastics and massage, worked as x-ray technician in the Hospital San Juan de Dios until he died in 1915 of numerous cancerous lesions of the hands.

In 1899 some demonstrations of x rays were made to the students of physics in the University of Mexico City. The first Mexican physician known to have regularly utilized roentgen rays in medical practice was a certain Joffre (in 1900); he was also the first to obtain series of chest films in Mexico in 1902 (those studies were published by one of Case's friends, Alfonso Pruneda, in an inaugural thesis on the symptoms and diagnosis of early pulmonary tuberculosis).

In Colombia the first roentgen equipment was purchased shortly after 1900 for the private offices of Isaac Rodriguez and of German Reyes in Bogotá. Later Julio Manrique had similar equipment installed in his office.

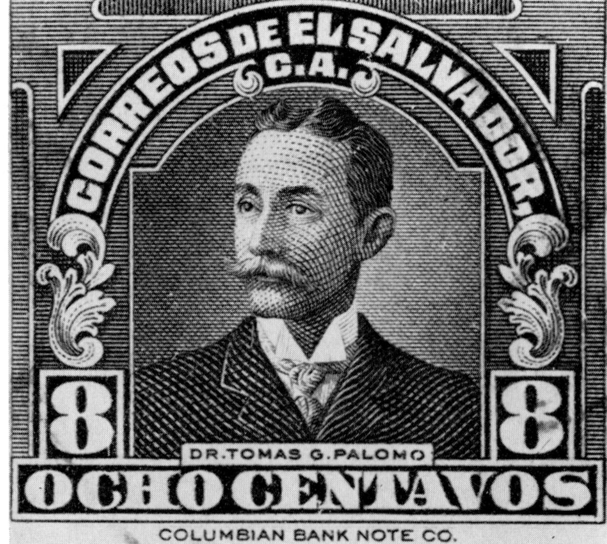

Courtesy: Stan Bohrer.

TOMAS PALOMO. For having introduced the first x-ray equipment into Salvador, his memory was honored in 1953 with this postal stamp.

In 1904 in Costa Rica, Jose Brunetti obtained American x-ray equipment and used it in his private medical office.

In Ecuador the first (small) x-ray equipment was introduced in 1906 in Quito in the private office of Pablo Arturo Suarez, who is remembered mostly as a hygienist. In the same year small apparatus was installed also in the private offices of Emilio G. Roca and Juan Federico Heinert in Guayaquil. The first large x-ray machine – a Gaiffe – was installed on May 24, 1908 in the department "Dario Moria" in the General Hospital in Guayaquil: it was operated by Juan E. Verdesoto Beltran, who is regarded as the first (medical) radiologist of Ecuador.

The Golden Age of Radiology was characterized in South America by the appearance of original investigators as well as by the creation of (mostly individual) teaching centers.

One of the two recognized Argentinian roentgen pioneers was Carlos Heuser (1878-1934), who published in the *Semana Medica* of July 24, 1902, a paper on the *radioscopia* of the abdominal organs. He is remembered mainly for having developed hysterosalpingography: his first article on the subject, entitled *Metrosalpingorradiografia* (in *Semana Medica* of December 23, 1926) contains the mention that in 1912 Dastugue had injected collargol into the uterine os, but had encountered complications, while Heuser used lipiodol since 1922, without any apparent difficulties. Heuser was awarded the gold medal of the RSNA in 1931 and – being one of Orndoff's personal friends – he came again to the USA in 1934 to participate in the American Congress of Radiology.

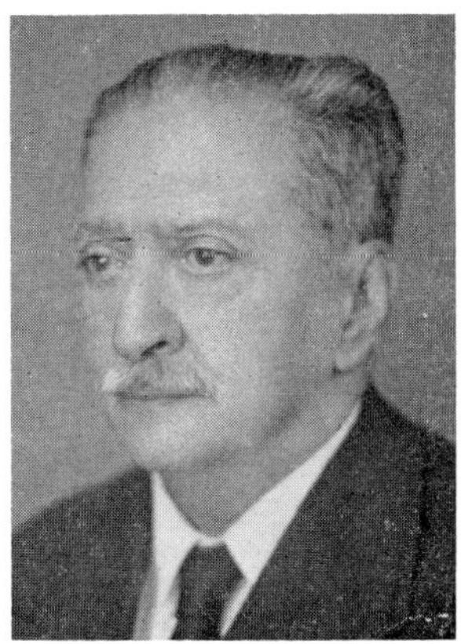

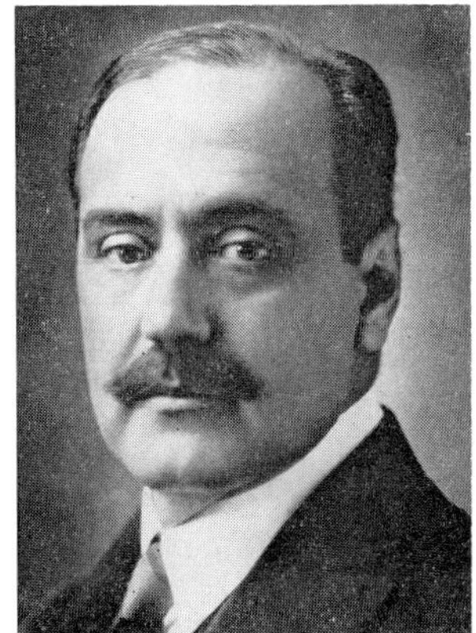

Courtesy: Georg Grössel - Agfa.
Courtesy: Mario Hinojosa Cardona.

JUAN VERDESOTO BELTRAN. Ecuador's first medical electro-radiologist wrote among other things on medical electricity in general, and in particular on its employment in radiology. He also investigated such varied subjects as "aortic aneurysm treated with Haret's electrolysis," "radio-diagnosis of dental abscess," and "scapulohumeral periarthritis." On the right, with black mustache is ALFREDO LANARI, first professor of radiology in the University of Buenos Aires.

Costa's Sala de Fisioterapía became the Instituto de Fisioterapía and when Costa died in 1909, he was succeeded by his associate Alfredo Lanari (1870-1930), who changed it into Instituto de Radiología y Fisioterapia. After Lanari's death, his position of professor of radiology in the University of Buenos Aires went to his younger brother Eduardo Lanari, and the name of the department was changed to Instituto Alfredo Lanari.

Humberto H. Carelli (1882-1962) had been the associate of Costa from 1901 to 1904 and then of Alfredo Lanari until 1911 when Carelli organized and became director of the (Municipal) Instituto de Radiología y Fisioterapía of Buenos Aires. He was the first radiologist in Buenos Aires who achieved high quality x-ray films in a consistent manner. In Argentina, Costa and Carelli were the first two who learned to irradiate successfully cutaneous epitheliomata. But Carelli became best known for his diagnostic acumen. He was a consummate master in the performance and interpretation of pneumoperitoneum for the detection of hydatid cysts, an infestation which is quite frequently encountered in South America. Carelli originated and first performed perirenal emphysema (*neumorriñon*) as a diagnostic procedure.

Jose P. Uslenghi, professor of radiology in La Plata, was first to inject Lipiodol into salivary canals, and published the first paper on that procedure in the first issue of the first Argentinian radiological journal.

Pablo Mirizzi in Cordoba was the first who suggested and performed per-operative cholangiography.*

Particular mention deserves Alberto M. Marque from the Children's Hospital in Buenos Aires, who collected 15,000 cases of bone pathology. Jimmy Case called it

*Instillation of contrast material through biliary fistulae had been done as early as 1918, but the first one who injected iodinated media directly into the common biliary duct at the time of surgery was Mirizzi, *cf., Bol. y trab. de la Soc. de cir. de Buenos Ayres* 16: 1133-1161 (October 5) 1932.

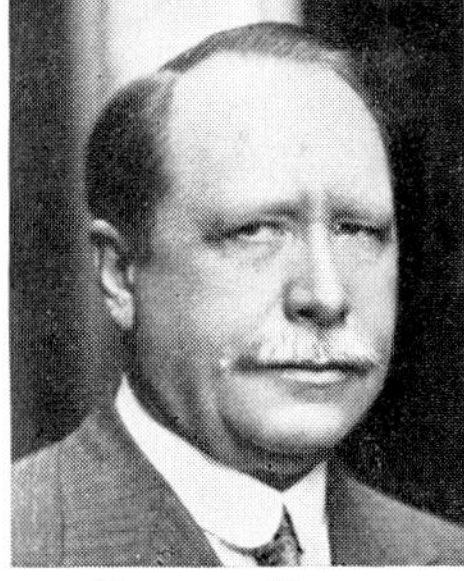

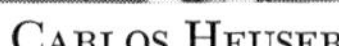

CARLOS HEUSER

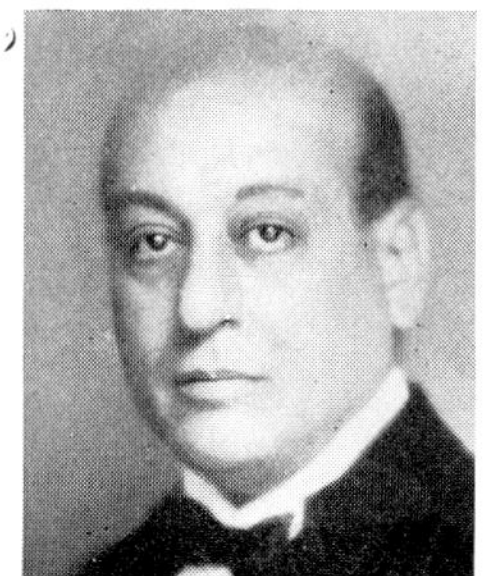

HUMBERTO CARELLI

the largest collection of radiographic material in South America.

The first x-ray department in Brazil was established by Henrique Carlos Gruschke in the service of Vieira de Carvallo in the Santa Casa de Misericordia (Sao Paulo) in 1899. Both Carvallo and Gruschke became radiation casualties, and after Gruschke's death his widow replaced him as director of the department.

Internationally famous was Manoel de Abreu (1892-1962), who obtained his MD degree in Rio de Janeiro in 1913, went for specialization to Paris, and returned to Brazil in 1922. His major achievement was the construction of a workable model of a photofluorographic machine in 1936. In Brazil this procedure is called *Abreugrafia,* there is even a Sociedade Brasileira de Abreugrafia in Sao Paulo. He made other significant technical contributions to chest radiology, for instance polytomography. Despite the many national and international honors received from both radiologic and phthisiologic organizations, de Abreu was a lonely, sensitive individual who wrote melancholy poems and philosophic essays on the eternity of life and related topics. He died of bronchogenic carcinoma.*

Two of the best known Brazilian teachers of radiology were—during the Golden Age — Roberto Duque Estrada in Rio de Janeiro and Raphael de Barros in Sao Paulo. The latter (an expert in osteo-radiology) is the founder of the Centro de Estudos (which carries his eponym) in the Hospital das Clinicas in Sao Paulo; he created also a school for x-ray technicians.

Another name of repute in Brazilian radiology is that of Barcello Ferreira and his pneumo-pericardium; the cardio-radiologist Eduardo Cotria conceived a device for evaluation of heart size, built for him by Casa Lohner; Abreu's former associate, Aguinaldo Lins, who is now in Pernambuco, continued the master's work on mediastinum in general, and on the vascular pedicle in particular; in the early 1940s Jose Jany (an engineer) and Moretsohn de Castro (a radiologist) developed a method of presensitization of the film for the production of cineradiography; and finally the well known radiotherapist, Mathias Octavio Roxo Nobre is still practicing in Sao Paulo.

In Uruguay Carlos Butler (1879-1943) was the first professor of radiology and director of the Instituto de Radiología in the Faculty of Medicine of Montevideo. He was succeeded by his former associate, Pedro A. Barcia (1888-1951). All present-day radiologists in Uruguary are directly or indirectly indebted for their education to one or both of these two pioneers.

In Cuba the "father of radiology" was Francisco Domínguez y Roldán (1864-1942), sometime health minister, who published a book on the thorax. One of his contemporaries, Emilio Alamilla, who taught Phys-

*A most beautiful eulogy, entitled *Manoel de Abreu, criador de métodos,* by Ayres de Sousa of Lisbon, appeared in the *Rev. brasileira de radiol.* of April, 1962.

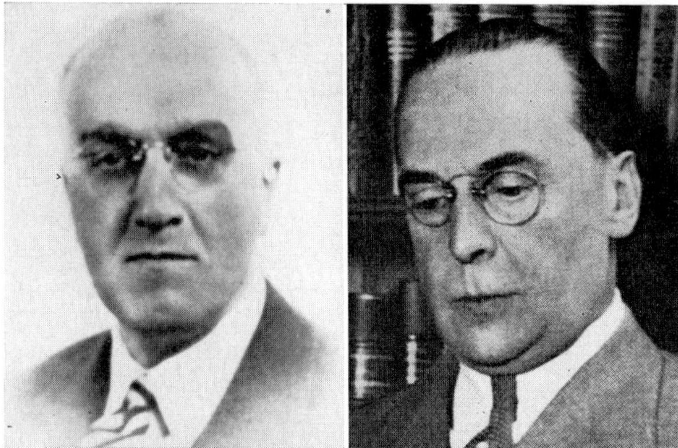

Pedro Alberto Barcia — Carlos Butler.

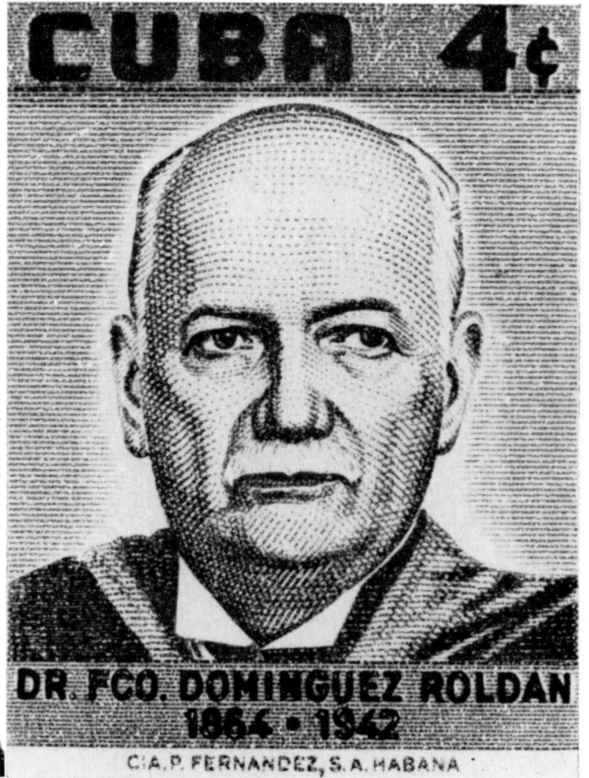

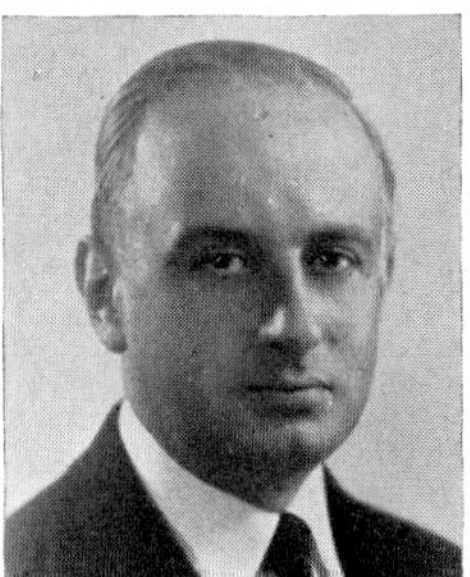

Nicolas Capizzano

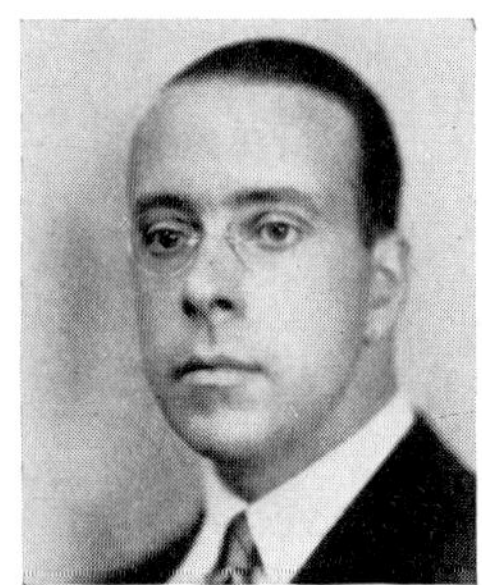

Jose Luis Molinari

ics in Habana since 1899, did much to establish medical radiology as a specialty in Cuba; he had the first deep therapy equipment on the island; Alamilla died in 1924 while on a visit to the USA. Francisco Cabrera Benitez was the author of *Radiodiagnostico y Fisiotherapía de la Tuberculosis* (1913). During the Cuban Golden Age of Radiology, the great teacher and original investigator was Pedro Leondro Fariñas y Mayo (1892-1951), who started to work in the specialty in 1912; he is remembered for his contributions to bronchography (including the detailed *broncografía al acecho, i.e.,* with spotfilms and replacement of oily with water-soluble contrast media), and to angiography, aortography and phlebography.

In Chile the first physician-radiologist was José Maria Anrique, the professor of physics in the School of Medicine in Santiago. His successor, José Ducci, may be regarded as the pioneer of radiologic teaching in his country: he established in the 1920s regular clinico-radiologico-pathologic conferences. To honor his memory, his former department was renamed the José Ducci Institute of Radiology in the Hospitál Clínico de San Vincente de Paul. Leonardo Guzmán, a therapist, founded the Institute of Radium in Santiago.

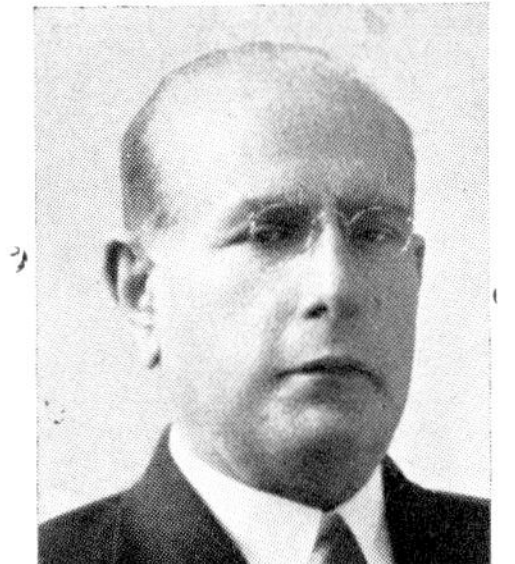

ESTEBAN CAMPODONICO

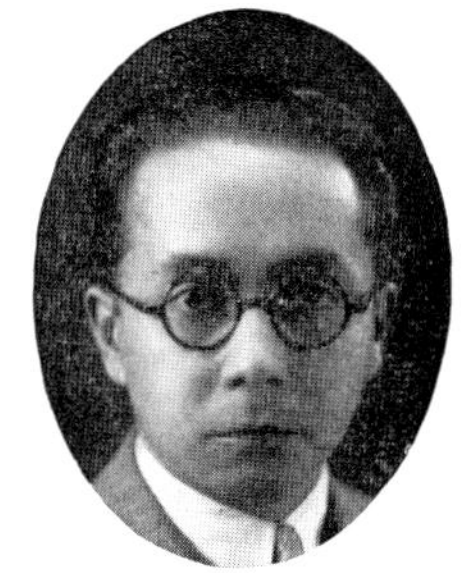

OSCAR SOTO

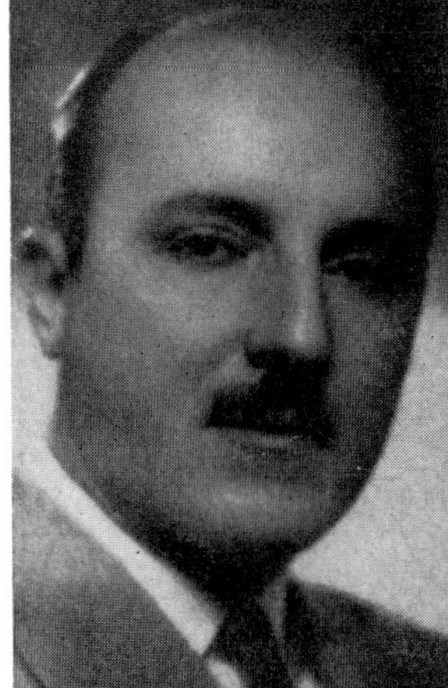

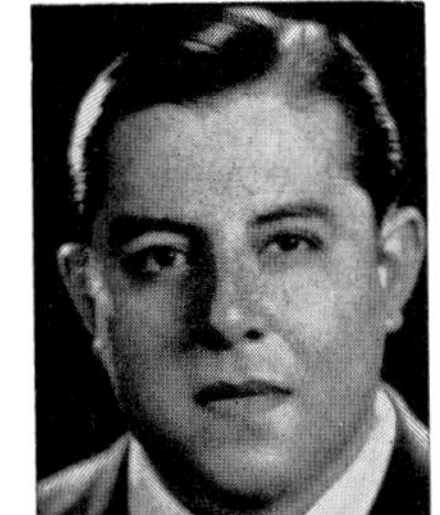

GERMAN ABAD-VALENZUELA

Courtesy: Mario Hinojosa Cardona.

JULIO MATA MARTINEZ. First professor of radiology in the University of Guayaquil, was particularly interested in angiocardiography on which he reported as the Relator Official to the 3rd IACR.

In Peru, after the more or less experimental exploits in the year 1896, the first roentgen equipment was installed in 1904 in the (female) Hospital de Santa Ana: the first radiologist to use it was I. Avendano, succeeded by E. Olivares. Better known was the "dean of Peruvian radiologists" J. L. Becerra from the (male) Hospital Dos de Mayo in Lima. The first recognized teaching in the specialty was organized by the Italian-born Esteban Campodonico (1866-1935), who was professor of radiology in the University of San Marcos. He was succeeded by Oscar Soto A., founder of the Instituto Nacional de Radiotherapia. In the history of Peruvian radiology, Campodonico and Soto occupy the same position as Butler and Barcía in Uruguay.

In Ecuador, aside from the previously mentioned pioneer Juan E. Verdesoto Beltran (1882-1954), well known is Arturo Terán Gostalle, the Argentinian-trained radiologist in the Hospital Militar in Quito. A very important figure was Julio Mata Martinez (1903-1950), the first (independent) professor of radiology in the University of Guayaquil; most of his publications appeared in the local periodical *Gaceta Medica,* and ranged in diagnostic radiology from cardiac catheterization to the syndrome of cord compression; Mata died in a commercial airplane accident over the Andes.

In Mexico the Swiss immigrant Gustavo Peter was one of the early radiotherapists. The Mexican "father of radiology" was Manuel Madrazo, who became a master of international relations in radiology (he was president of the eighth ICR in Mexico City in 1956). Among original investigators may be mentioned Carlos Gomez del Campo who opacified the aorta by direct puncture of the arch, a procedure so daring that it did not become popular.

In Venezuela the best known early radiologists were Rafael Gonzales Rincones and his brother Pedro Gonzales Rincones, established since 1917.

In Colombia, the pioneers were Isaac Rodriguez (1860-1928) and German Reyes (1864-1948). In 1919 a French radiologist, André J. Richard, went to Bogotá and when Richard left for the USA, he was replaced by the German radiologist Martin Weiser. Soon phy-

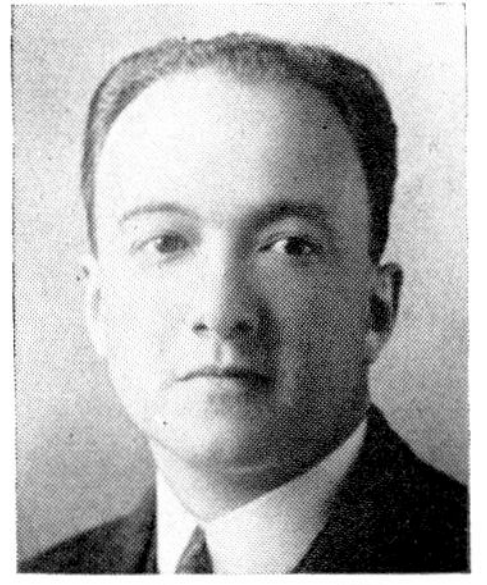

CARLOS TRUJILLO-VENEGAS

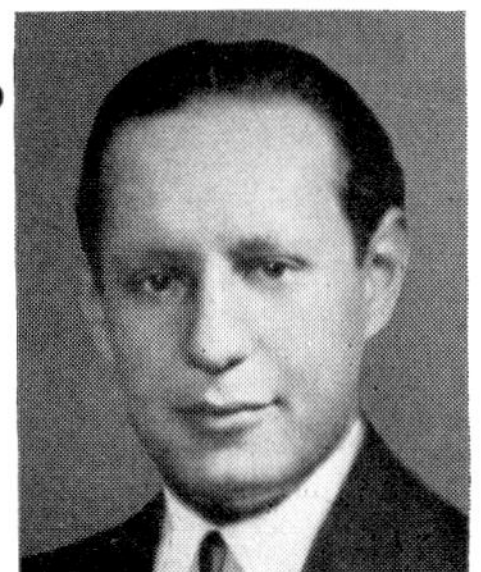

GONZALO ESGUERRA-GOMEZ

sicians graduated from Bogotá went for radiologic specialization to France, and then returned to practice in Colombia, as did Carlos Trujillo Venegas and Eduardo Ricaurte Medina. The pioneer in Medellin was Martiniano Echeverry, who became professor of radiology in the Universidad de Antioquia. Ruperto Irequi and Alfonso Flores were among early therapists who worked in the Instituto Nacional de Radium since its foundation in 1934. The director of that radium institute since 1942 was Roberto Restrepo, who died in 1954.

The best known name in Colombian radiology is that of Gonzalo Esguerra Gomez (brother of Alfonso Esguerra Gomez of Colombian paste fame), who gave the *Lección inaugural del Curso de Electro-Radiología* in the Facultad Nacional de Medicina in Bogotá on March 12, 1934. His part of the course was diagnosis, while electrology and therapy was being taught by Aquilino Soto. Gonzalo Esguerra Gomez has contributed numerous papers on varied diagnostic subjects, from roentgen findings in amebiasis and leprosy to familial pulmonary alveolar microlithiasis and pre-, per-, and post-operative cholangiography. Esguerra Gomez has his office in the Clínica de Marly, a private surgical-maternity hospital (formerly owned by his physician-father) on the outskirts of Bogotá; although French-trained, he has many friends in North America and has come several times to the USA.

RADIO- IN LATIN AMERICA

In Latin-American countries, the terms derived from the root radiology carry the same connotation as in previously mentioned Romanic languages. Carlos Heuser graduated in 1902 from the University of Buenos Aires with a thesis entitled *Radiología*.* The preamble to that thesis contained the following explanation: "I designate this work with the title 'Radiología' because I believe it to be more appropriate and more restricted to the different branches of this phase of science: radioscopy, radiography, endoscopy and radiotherapy."

Quite often, though, the South American *radiología* carries a diagnostic rather than the all-inclusive connotation.

*This information was elicited through the courtesy of Dr. Alejandro von der Becke, a biochemist in Buenos Aires.

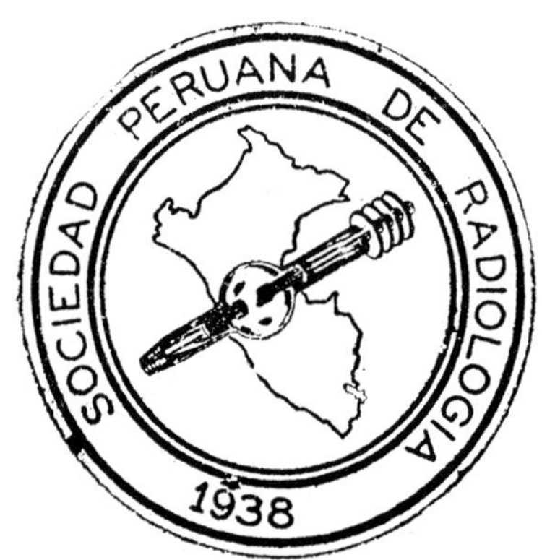

Revista Mexicana de Radiología

Organo oficial de la Sociedad Mexicana de Radiología A. C.

Registrada como artículo de segunda clase, en la Dirección General de Correos. Oficio Nº 30231 de fecha 24 de abril de 1952.

REDACCION Y ADMINISTRACION

Medellín No. 86. Tels.: 11-85-46 y 36-45-89 México 7, D. F.

Director: Dr. JORGE DESCHAMPS

Gerente: Dr. LUIS MARQUEZ

MANUAL DE RADIOLOGIA Y FISIOTERAPIA

LIDIO G. MOSCA

Premio Roentgen, 1951. Premio Decenal de Radiología, 1950. Miembro correspondiente de la Sociedad Austríaca de Radiología, 1950. Miembro correspondiente de la Sociedad Alemana de Radiología, 1952. Miembro titular extranjero de la Sociedad Francesa de Radiología, 1952. Miembro correspondiente del Sindicato de Médicos de Porto Alegre, 1952. Miembro titular del Colegio Internacional de Cirujanos, 1949. Miembro honorario de la Sociedad de Gastroenterología y Nutrición de Mendoza, 1954. Miembro honorario de la Sociedad Paraguaya de Radiología, 1953. Miembro honorario de la Sociedad Brasileña de Radiología, 1953. Miembro honorario de la Sociedad Radiológica Panameña, 1951.

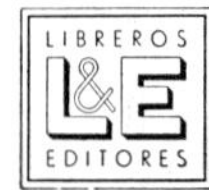

LOPEZ & ETCHEGOYEN, S. R. L.
JUNIN 863 - BUENOS AIRES
1956

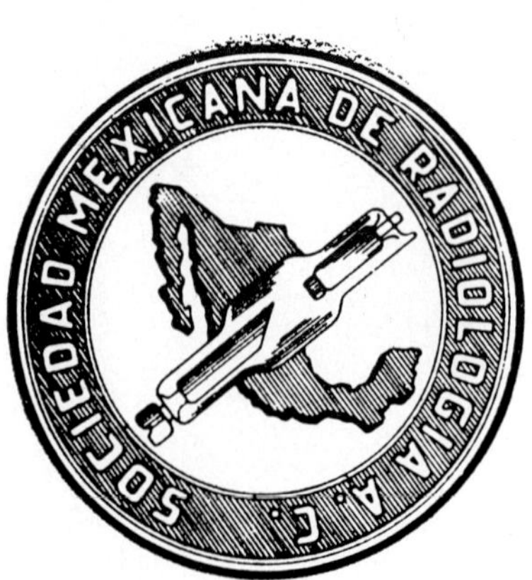

In 1951, appeared in Mexico City the *Manual de Radiología Clínica* by Juan José Quezada Ruiz. Lidio Mosca's *Manual de Radiología y Fisioterapía* (Buenos Aires, 1956) made it clearer yet that "electrologic" applications were not covered by the (South American) term radiology. And the leading article in the *Revista Brasileira de Gastroenterologia* of May-August, 1961 contains the word *farmacoradiologia,* meaning contrast examination of the gastrointestinal tract after anti-spasmodic and other medications.

Semantic analysis of the titles of radiological societies and journals in Latin America reveals a more or less uniform pattern.

The Sociedad Peruana de Radiología (founded in 1938, first president: Oscar Soto) has as its official organ the *Revista Peruana de Radiología* (started in 1946). The *Revista Mexicana de Radiología* was started one year later, in 1947, as the *Revista Mexicana de Radiología y Fiziotherapía,* because at that time its sponsoring society (founded in 1942) still carried the original name Sociedad Mexicana de Radiología y Fiziotherapía (among founding members of the Mexican Radiological Society were: Dionisio Perez Cosio, Guillerma Rodriguez Garza, Manuel Madrazo, Carlos Coqui, Juan José Quezada Ruiz, and Carlos Gomez de Campo). The physiotherapeutic tailpiece was deleted with the coming of the Atomic Phase.

The Sociedad Ecuatoriana de Radiología y Fisiotherapía was founded on December 29, 1950 upon suggestion of Efren Jurado Lopez. The first provisional president was Juan Verdesoto Beltran, with Mario Hinojosa Cardona as the first provisional secretary. The first definitive president was German Abad Valenzuela, with Remigio Torres as secretary. Their official organ, *Revista de Radiología y Fisioterapía,* was first published on November 18, 1954 in Guayaquil, under the editor-

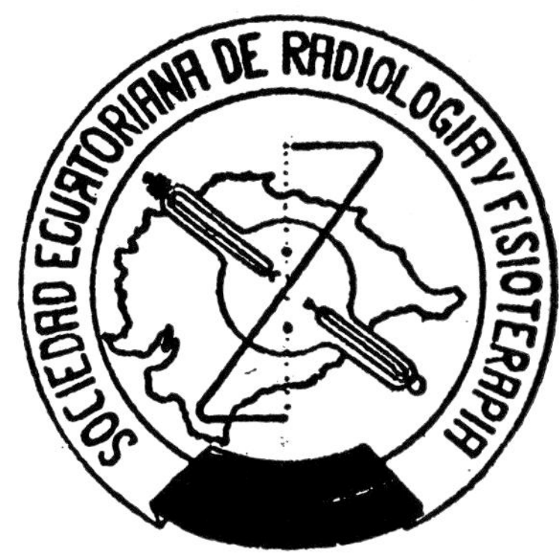

Revista de Radiología y Fisioterapia

Guayaquil-Ecuador

Publicación bimestral

Fundada el 18 de Noviembre de 1954

Vol. I - Noviembre - Diciembre 1954 - No. 1

Editorial

La seria responsabilidad que le corresponde asumir en los actuales momentos a la radiología ecuatoriana frente a la evolucion innovadora de esta rama del saber humano, hizo que se agruparan hace cinco años los radiólogos nacionales para fundar la Sociedad Ecuatoriana de Radiología y Fisioterapia

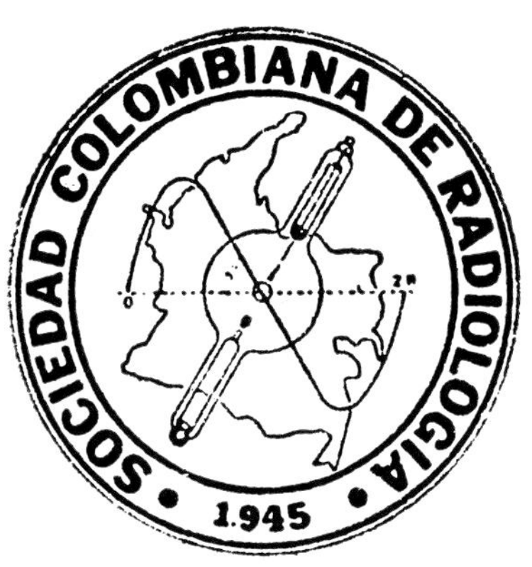

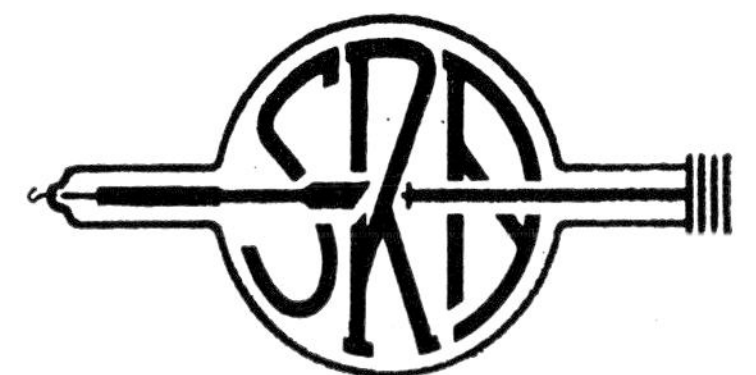

Sociedad de Radiologia del Atlantico

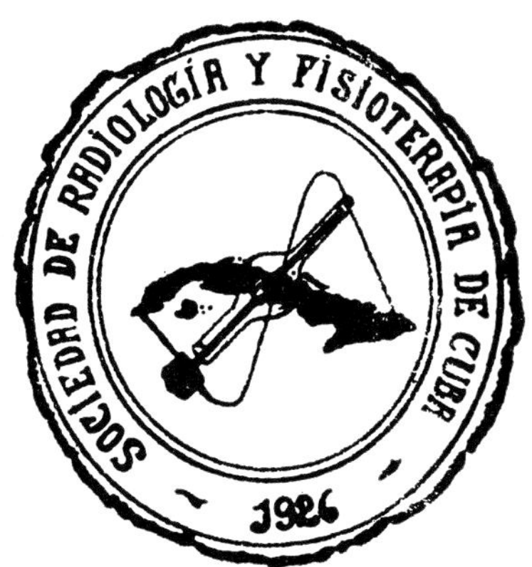

ship of Enrique Ortega Guzman (director of the Radium Institute).

The Sociedad Colombiana de Radioligía was founded in July of 1945, its first president being Gonzalo Esquerra Gomez with Francisco Convers as secretary. In Barranquilla (Columbia), Jorge Henao Echavarria founded in September of 1952 the Sociedad de Radiología del Caribe, and was its first president, the late C. Quintero-Hernandez being the first secretary. They used the name Sociedad de Radiología del Atlantico, which has recently become affiliated with their (national) Colombian Radiological Society.

The Sociedad Cubana de Radiología y Fisiotherapía, second oldest radiological society in Latin America, was founded in 1926 with Domínguez Roldán as its first president. Their official organ was the *Anales de Radiología,* started in 1929. *Radiología Oral,* published since 1948 by the Dental School in Habana, was about as short-lived as the *Anales.*

Latin American society denominations are usually all alike such as Sociedad Venezuelana (or Boliviana, or Chilena, or Paraguaya) de Radiología. The latter's president for 1961 was Quirno Codas Thompson, professor of radiology in Asuncion (Paraguay), a former associate of the late Pedro Barcía of Montevideo. An exception to the rule is the Sociedad de Radiología, Cancerología y Física Medica de Uruguay.

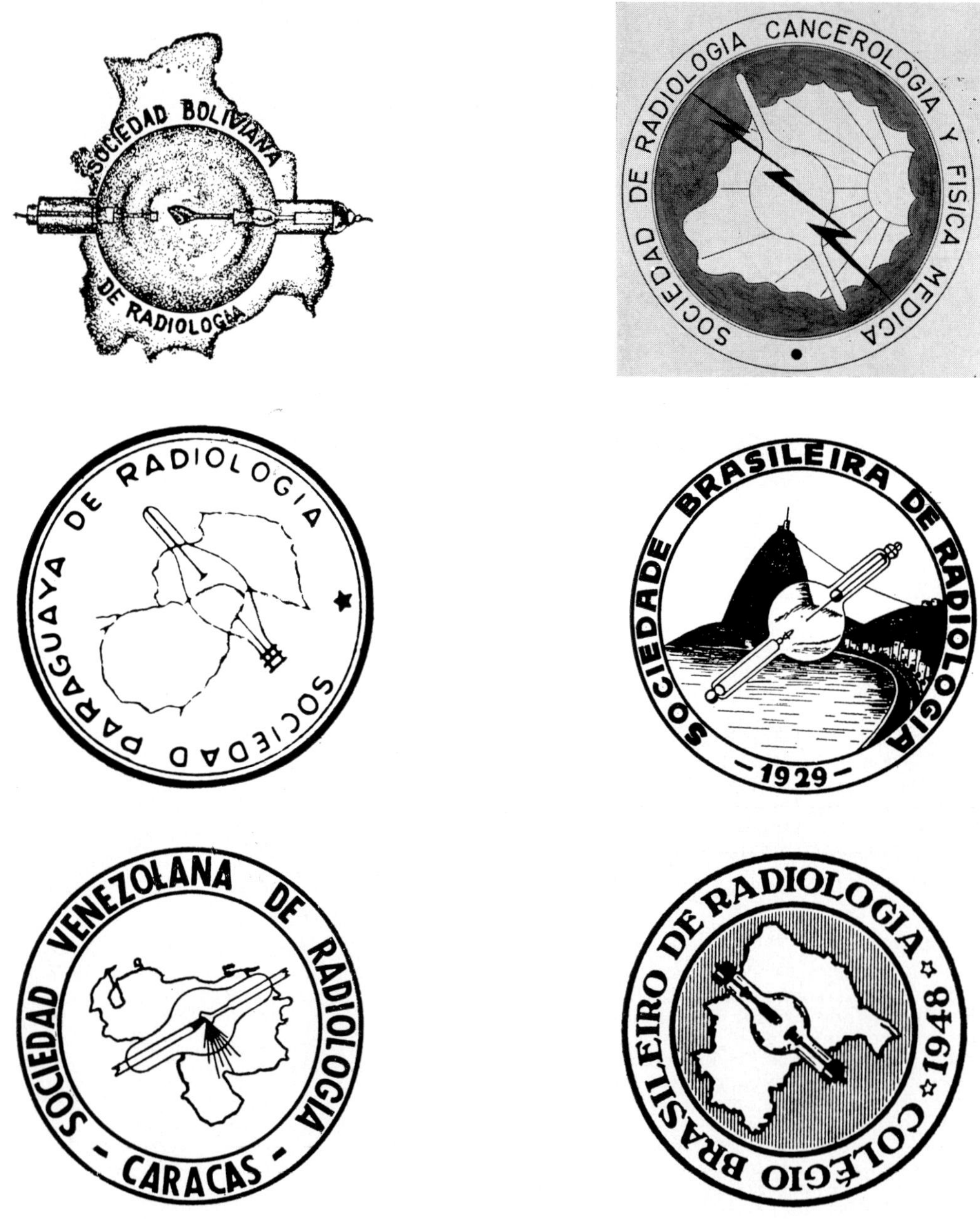

The Sociedad Brasileira de Radiologia was started in 1929 – its emblem is a roentgen tube superimposed upon the background of the harbor of Rio de Janeiro. The Colegio Brasileiro de Radiologia was founded on September 15, 1948 in Sao Paulo: the first president was Jose Maria Cabello Campos (professor of radiology in the University of Sao Paulo); the first secretary was Walter Bonfim Pontes (professor of radiology in nearby Sorocaba) who is also the editor of their official organ, the *Revista Brasileira de Radiologia*, published since 1958. There is further the Asociaçao Brasileira de Radiologia in Guanabara – their 1961 president was the radiotherapist Osolando Judice Machado. Similar regional groups have been formed in Minas Gerais, Ceara, and Pernambuco. Sao Paulo is more active (both scientifically and industrially) than Rio de Janeiro. In Sao Paulo are two other important organizations, the Sociedade Brasileira de Radioterapia, of which the current president is Roxo Nobre; and the Centro de Medicina Nuclear (with orbits in its emblem) directed by the Brasilian "atomic specialist" Tede Eston de Eston.

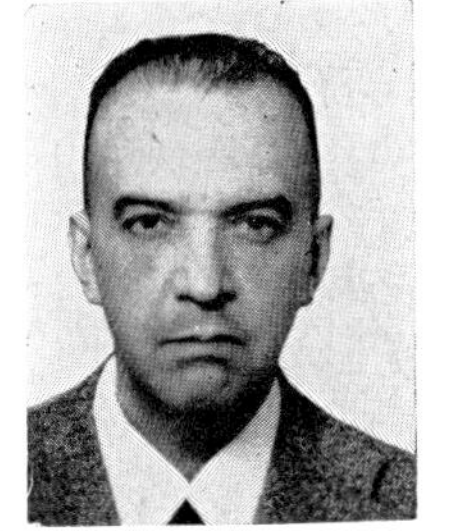
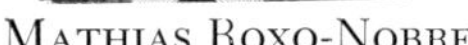

MATHIAS ROXO-NOBRE

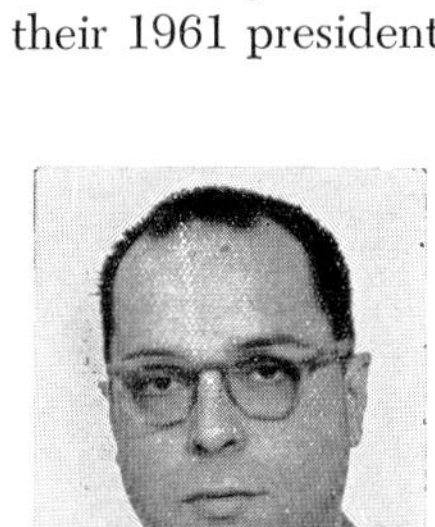
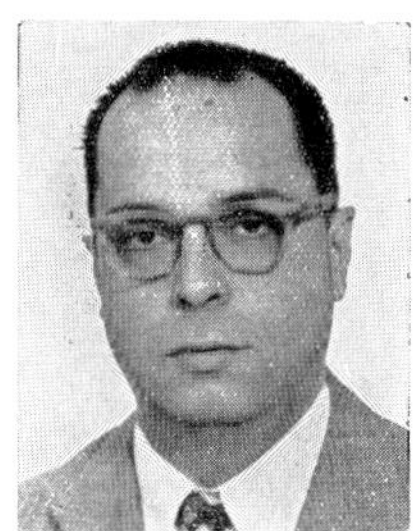

OSOLANDO MACHADO

Local radiologic groups are often started with less than ten members. The Sociedad Radiológica Panameña was founded in 1949 with Joaquin José Vallarino Zachrisson as its first president. The Society's permanent secretary is Luis Arrieta Sanchez, the editor of *Radiología,* its official organ, first issued in 1951. By 1955 the Panamenian Radiological Society had six members and, in order to have a bigger attendance, they were meeting together with five chest specialists. In 1961, the sponsorship of *Radiología* (Panamá) was enlarged, and it became the official organ of the Asociación de Radiólogos de Centro-America y Panamá (ARCAP).

The oldest Latin American radiological group is the Sociedad Argentina de Radiología. It was first organized in 1917, the founders being Alfredo Lanari, Carlos Heuser, Antonio DeNucci, Carlos Niseggi, Otilio Dast-

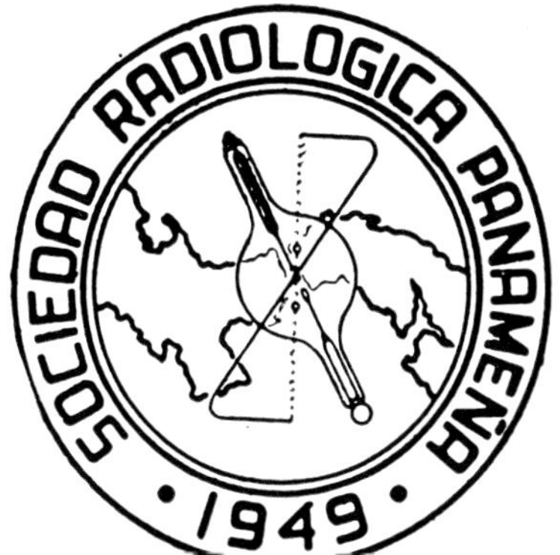

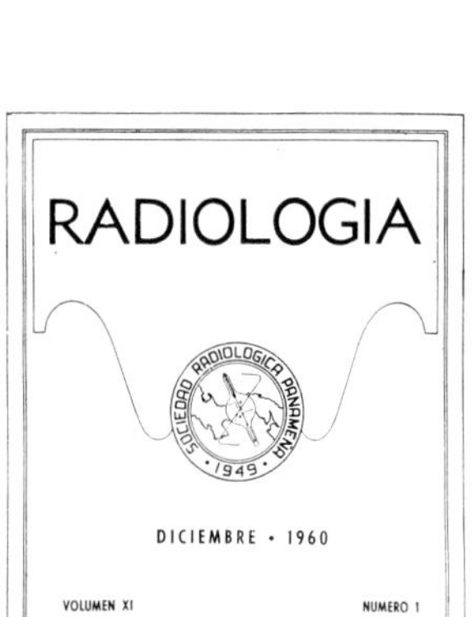

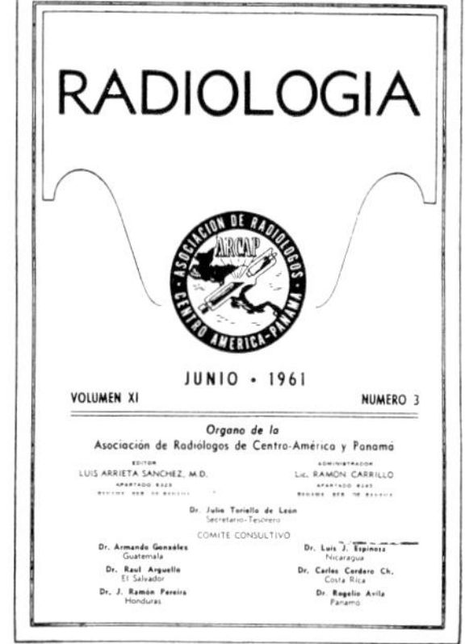

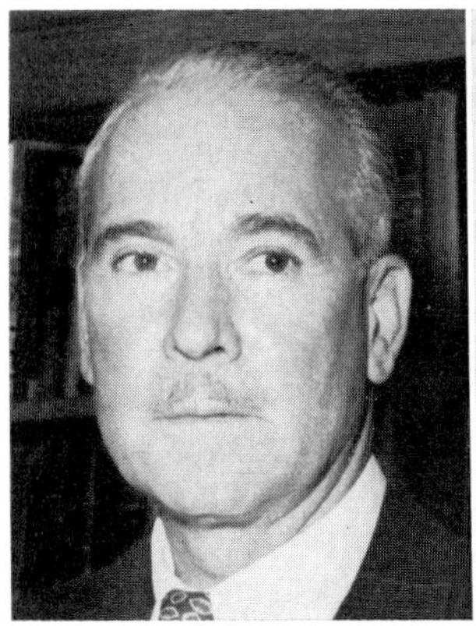
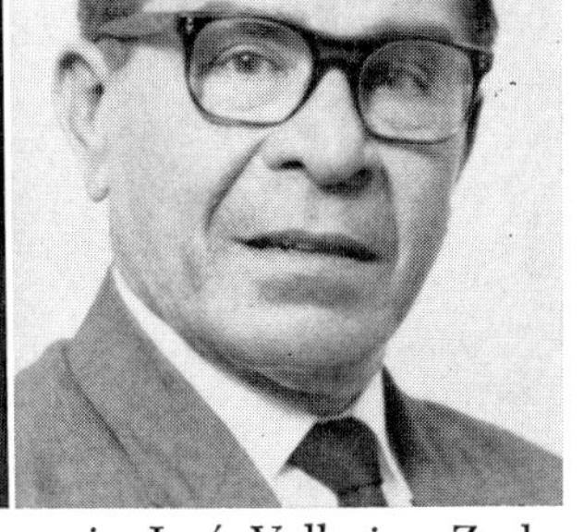

FOUNDERS OF THE SRP. Joaquin José Vallarino Zachrisson and bespectacled Luis Arrieta Sanchez, both of Panama City.

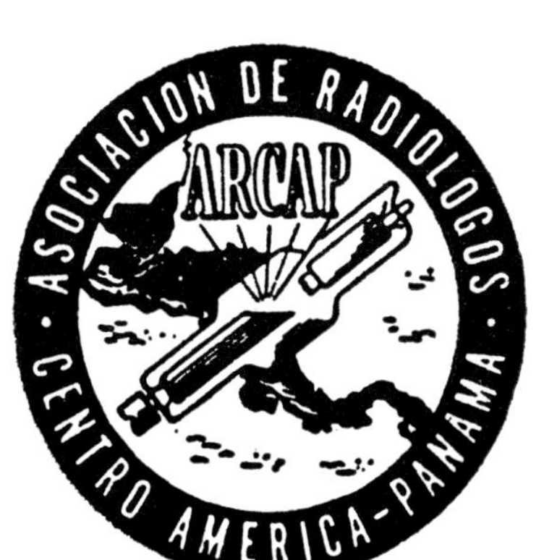

ugue,* Rafael Espindola, and Antonio Valdivesco. They published their transactions since 1923 in the *Revista de la Sociedad Argentina de Radiología y Electrología.* The electrologic appendix was lost during a subsequent re-organization.

There exists in Córdoba (Argentina) a regional group called Asociación Argentina de Radiología, which was founded in 1949; its first president was Di Rienzo, the first secretary Lidio Mosca. Córdoba is a metropolitan center with close to one million population. The coming of the Atomic Phase was acknowledged by creating a new organization, the Sociedad de Roentgenología y

*Dastugue was the one who performed in Argentina the first hysterosalpingogram with Collargol, but abandoned it because of undesirable complications. The very first hysterosalpingogram may have been done in 1910 by Rindfleisch, using thick bismuth suspension.

REVISTA

DE LA

SOCIEDAD ARGENTINA DE RADIO Y ELECTROLOGÍA

(CRÓNICA DE SESIONES)

Publicación de la Asociación Médica Argentina

TOMO I

BUENOS AIRES
DIRECCIÓN Y ADMINISTRACIÓN: SANTA FE, 1171

1925

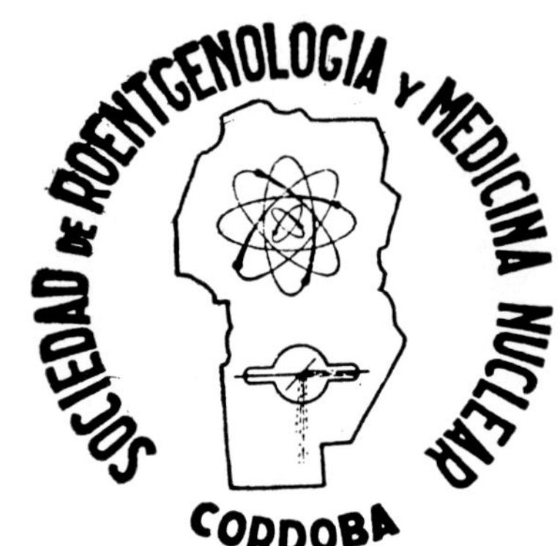

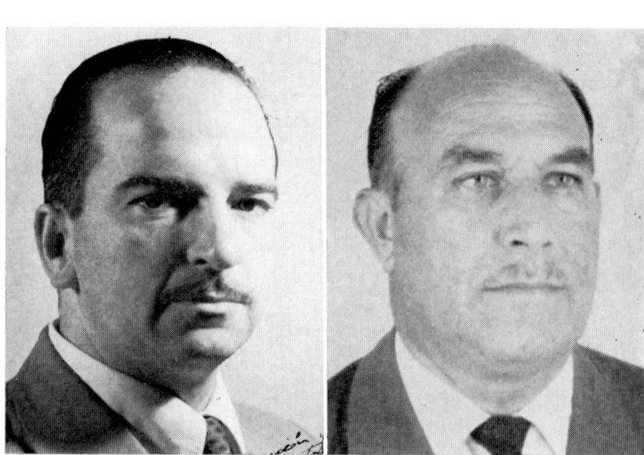

FOUNDERS OF THE SDRYMN. Raul Oscar Pereira Duarte and balding Carlos Anibal Oulton Clara, both of Córdoba (Argentina).

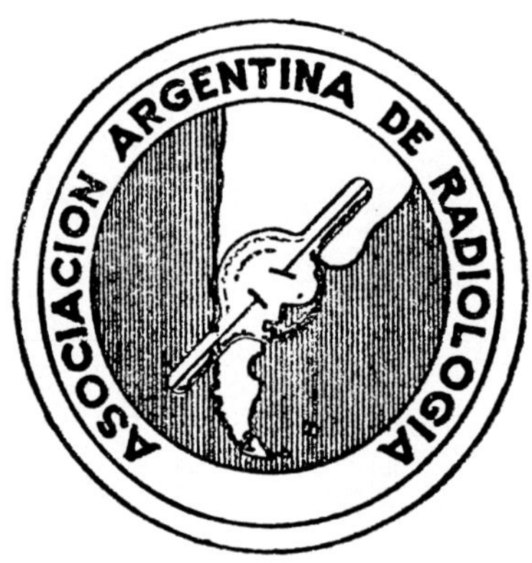

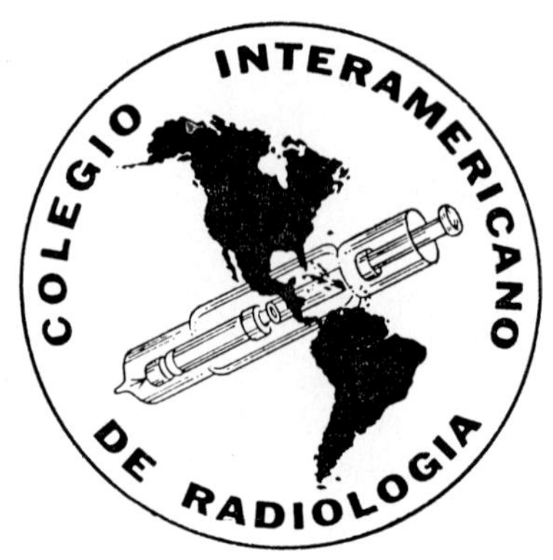

Medicina Nuclear de la Provincia de Córdoba, probably the only South American organization which uses the term *roentgenología.* This exception is explainable by the fact that many radiologists in Córdoba are German-trained, or of German extraction, such as Lidio Mosca, the chief radiologist in Córdoba Hospital (his mother came from Vienna, and he went back to that city for his medical and radiological studies).*

That roentgen-nuclear group in Córdoba was organized on November 30, 1959 with Raul Oscar Pereira Duarte as president and Carlos Anibal Oulton Clara (professor of radiology in the Universidad Catolica) as secretary: in 1961 they switched jobs, the secretary became president, and the president took the position of secretary.

The crowning achievement of radiologic organizations in Latin America is the Inter-American College of Radiology.

Its history was summarized by James Case in his presidential address to the fifth Inter-American Congress of Radiology (IACR) in Washington (D.C.) in

*My friend, Dr. Mosca, went out of his way to collect material for this presentation on Latin America. To illustrate the difficulties encountered, and to explain at the same time why certain significant information is not included in this section, I shall reproduce a passage from a letter by Dr. Mosca. It is in the original Spanish, only the names are deleted to protect the guilty: "Despues de haberle enviado ya variada documentacion en el dia de ayer, me llegan, por fin, algunos emblemas. Vd. no puede imaginarse el trabajo que costó conseguir dos emblemas. Primero escribí a colegas de ambos paises: nada. Despues a las embajadas de ambos paises en Buenos Aires: respuesta cortes pero evasiva. Por ultimo escribí a los Ministerios de Relaciones Exteriores de ambos paises. Asi consequi el emblema de . . . . Como . . . tampoco contesto, recurri a la representacion de Schering en . . . . Por fin, asi, llego." I have in my files carbon copies from over 150 letters sent to various Latin American colleagues, who never condescended to answer.

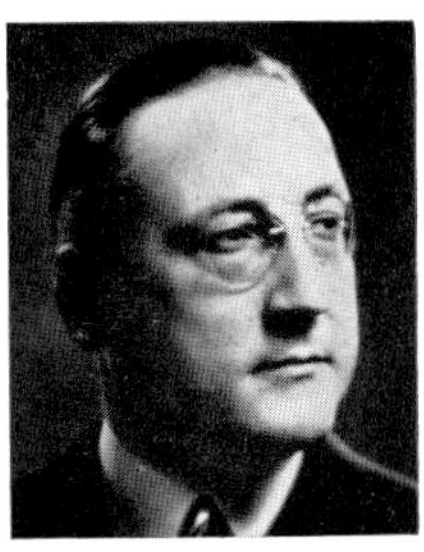

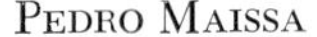

PEDRO MAISSA

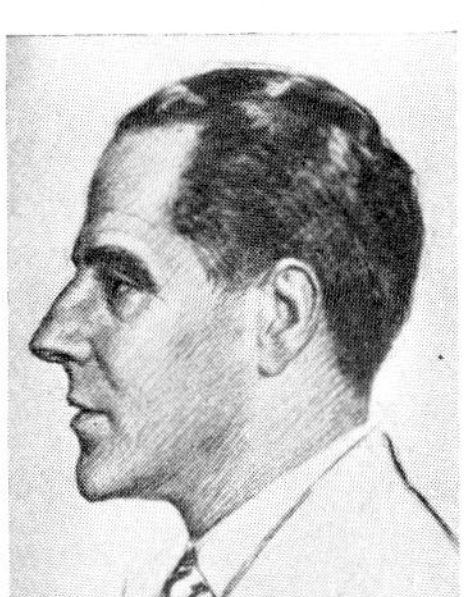

JOSE SARALEGUI

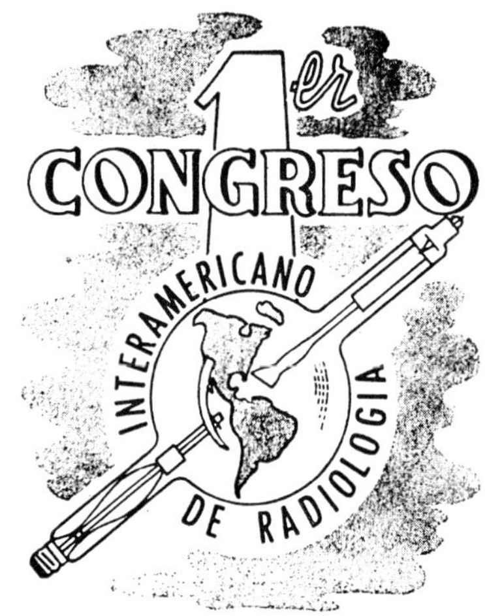

ACTA RADIOLOGICA INTERAMERICANA

ORGANO OFICIAL DEL COLEGIO INTERAMERICANO DE RADIOLOGIA

PUBLICACION TRIMESTRAL

Registro Nacional de la Propiedad Intelectual N° 414.010

Vol. VI — Octubre - Noviembre - Diciembre 1956 — N° 4

DIRECTOR:
Dr. PEDRO A. MAISSA. Bs. As., Argentina

•

UN ANIVERSARIO

Con el presente número, cumple ACTA RADIOLÓGICA INTERAMERICANA su quinto aniversario.

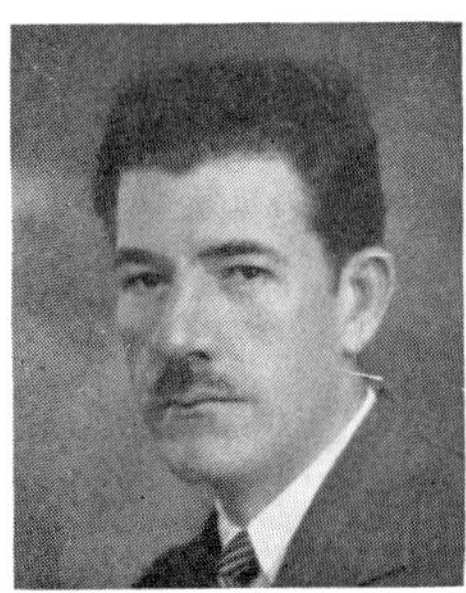

PEDRO FARINAS Y MAYO

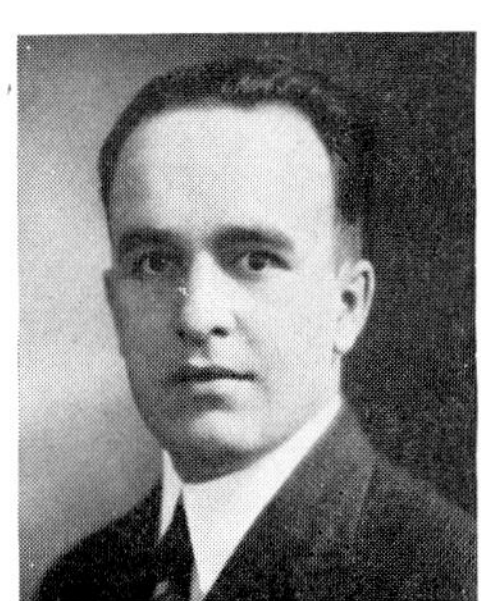

JUAN MANUEL VIAMONTE

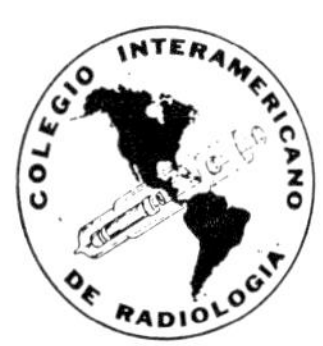

JUNE 1962
VOL. 1 • NO. 1

Radiologia Interamericana

ORGANO OFICIAL DEL COLEGIO INTERAMERICANO DE RADIOLOGIA

A Journal of Radiology and Nuclear Medicine

1955, published in *Radiology* of April, 1956. Since or before 1929 there had been attempts made to hold an all-American radiological meeting. Various names had been suggested such as Pan-American, but then it was finally organized as the American Congress of Radiology in Chicago in 1932. To that congress came 26 representatives from Latin America: seven from Argentina, five from Mexico, four from Cuba, two from Salvador, and one each from Brazil, Colombia, Ecuador, Guatemala, Panama, Peru, Puerto Rico, and Venezuela. They were relatively few when compared with the total of 978 radiologists and physicists registered. In 1937, during the ICR in Chicago, a group of forty radiologists from Latin America met several times to consider holding an inter-American congress of radiology. Among the promoters were prominent personalities such as

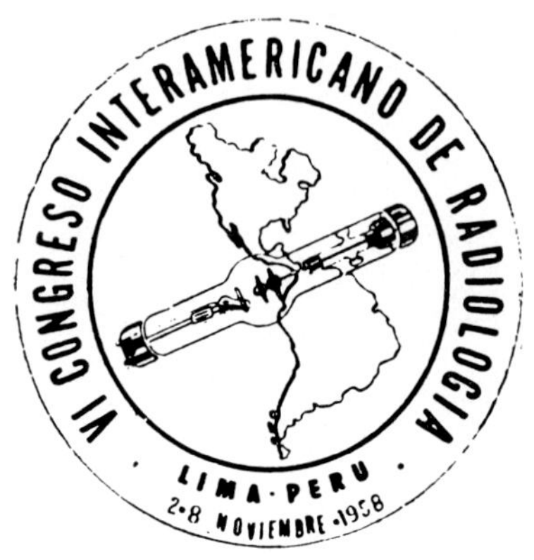

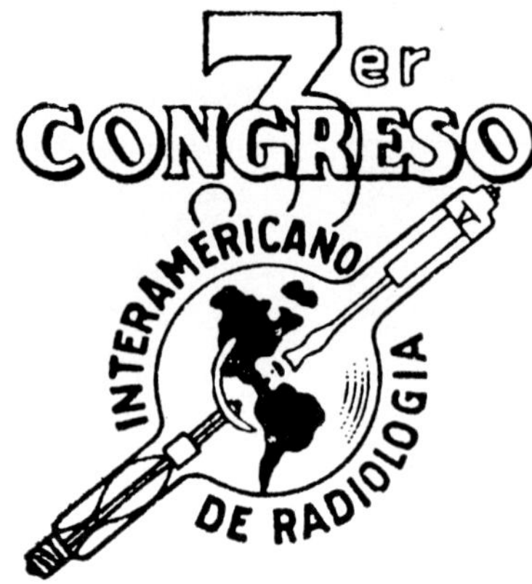

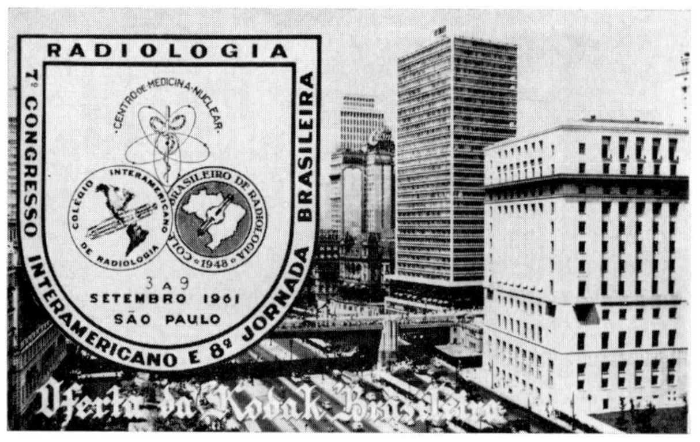

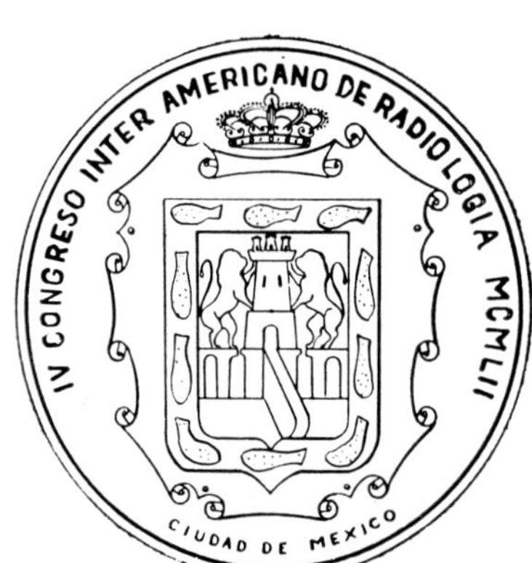

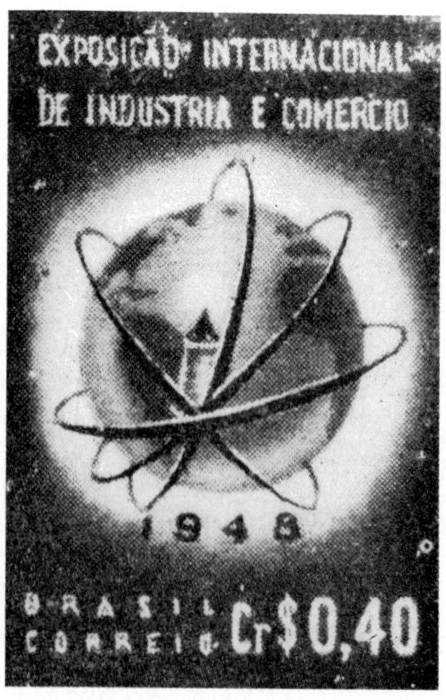

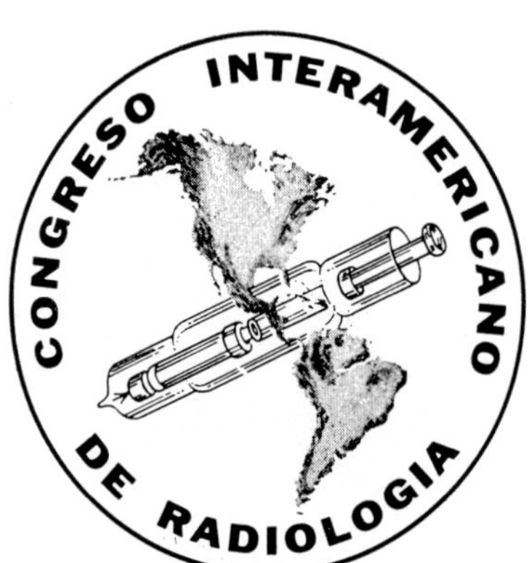

Fariñas y Mayo, Juan Manuel Viamonte (Habana), and José A. Saralegui of Buenos Aires.*

The first Inter-American Congress of Radiology (IACR) convened in Buenos Aires in 1943, under the presidency of José Francisco Merlo Gomez (1889-1948), an Argentinian radiologist with particular interest in neuroradiology. Mainly because of wartime, no radiologist from the USA was in attendance at that meeting. The first IACR bore an important outgrowth, the Colegio Inter-Americano de Radiología, with the same Merlo Gomez as its first president. In 1951, the Colegio began to publish its official organ, the *Acta Radiologica Interamericana,* edited by Pedro Abel Maissa, professor of radiology in Buenos Aires. It faded away about 1958, and was re-issued in June, 1962 under the new title *Radiologia Interamericana,* edited by Juan Angel del Regato, the radiotherapist from Colorado Springs. It has acquired the peculiar subtitle *Journal of Radiology and Nuclear Medicine,* in which the term radiology provides more than the (Latin American) diagnostic, though less than the (North American) all-inclusive coverage.

By 1963 it became clear that financial difficulties had forced the *Radiologia Interamericana* to discontinue publication. Once again the IACR had so-to-speak lost its voice!

The second IACR convened in 1946 (president: Pedro Fariñas y Mayo). The third was in Santiage de Chile in 1949 (president: Felix J. Daza B.). The fourth was called in Mexico City in 1952 (president: Manuel F. Madrazo). The fifth took place in Washington (D.C.) in 1955 (president: James Case). The sixth was in Lima in 1948 (president: Oscar Soto). Finally, the seventh IACR assembled in Sao Paulo in 1961 (president: Cabello Campos); on the occasion a gold medal was given to Walter Bonfim Pontes, its secretary-general. At that same meeting the presidency of the Colegio passed from Juan Manuel Viamonte (formerly of Habana, now in self-imposed exile in Miami) to Gonzalo Esguerra Gomez (Bogotá). The eighth IACR is scheduled for 1964 in Caracas (Venezuela).

*Saralegui was Carelli's successor in the Municipal Institute of Radiology of Buenos Aires. Saralegui introduced peroral cholecystography in Argentina, indeed at the American Congress of Radiology he received a gold medal for his scientific exhibits on this subject.

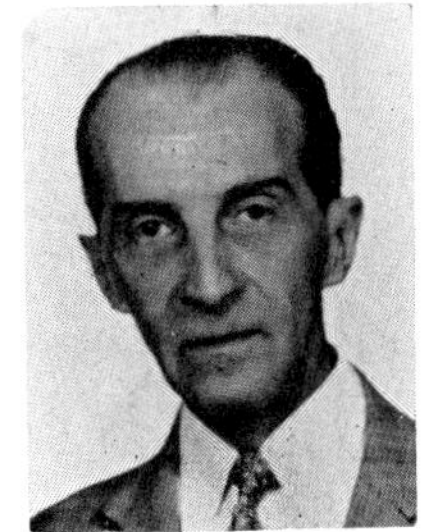

Jose Cabello-Campos

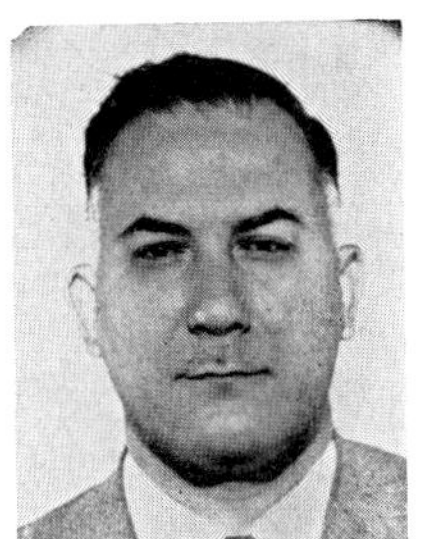

Bomfim Pontes

ATOMIC PHASE IN LATIN AMERICA

Latin American territories, barely in the early stages of the Golden Age of Radiology, were suddenly overwhelmed with nuclear requirements: this mixture of antiquated and ultra-modern is perhaps the most outstanding feature encountered today in Central and South American radiology.*

First of all there occurred in the past 20 years a dramatic increase in the number of qualified Latin American radiologists. There are now thousands of them in Argentina and Brazil, hundreds in most other South American countries and Mexico. In some places, the demand for trained personnel has been met by creating private teaching centers.

In Córdoba there exists the Escuela Privada de Radiología, directed by Sabino Di Rienzo, internationally known as a brilliant "broncho-radiologist" (he is also a sound therapist). In the past twelve years, his school has had 1,852 registered students: as an exemplifica-

*So far, however, there has been less than adequate interest in recording the history of Latin American radiology. This is unfortunate because *el medico que ignora la Historia de la facultad que profesa, no tiene disculpa en el tribunal literario de la justicia y de la razon; debe por lo mismo ser considerado como hijo bastardo de la medicina!*

ESCUELA PRIVADA DE RADIOLOGIA

DIRECTOR: Dr. S. DI RIENZO

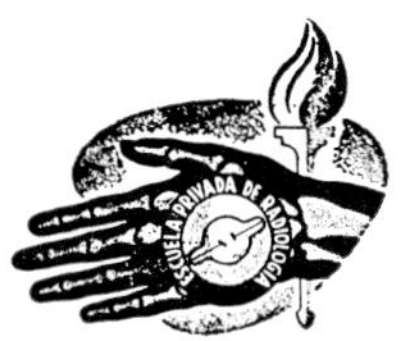

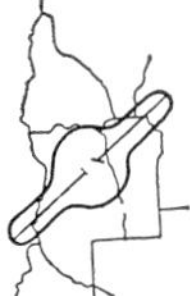

ESCUELA CUYANA DE RADIOLOGIA

(FILIAL DE LA ESCUELA PRIVADA DE RADIOLOGIA)

DIRECTOR: Dr. ALBERTO J. STORDEUR

tion, the course of cancerology held in 1960 from May 2 to October 22, consisted of 117 lectures. The school has its own emblem, and while its main object of teaching is radiology, it sponsors also certain artistic sidelines, from exhibits of paintings and sculpture to literary endeavors. Di Rienzo's school has a subsidiary, the Escuela Cuyana de Radiología.

There are now over 8000 qualified radiologists in Latin America. Such rise in numbers fostered competition and therefore an improvement in quality. As a result, there are now excellent radiologists in most Latin American countries. It is becoming increasingly difficult to select outstanding names without being biased. In fact, the names mentioned in the following paragraphs are unquestionably biased by the personal preferences of both Mosca and myself.

Lidio Gianfranco Mosca is the son of an Italian immigrant: the late Mosca, Sr. was born in Trieste, a territory known for generations as *terra irridente* (rebellious real estate). Lidio Mosca has a sensitive and cultured mind, is a gifted diagnostician, a pleasant speaker, and a talented writer. In the past few years he has been preoccupied with gallbladder and biliary duct problems, including the "syndrome of the stump of the incompletely amputated cystic duct," called in Spanish *muñon cistico*. But he has inherited his father's rebelliousness and therefore Lidio Mosca - who is also afflicted with a touch of socialism - is quite often "against" the powers-that-be.

At the time the manuscript reached the proof-reading stage Lidio Mosca notified me of his (first) arrest. Soon after he was transferred from a Córdoba jail to the Carcel de Caseros in Buenos Aires. I had to interrupt my work, and dictate frantic letters to important personages such as the Argentinian Minister of the Interior, the Interventor Federal de Córdoba, and the Argentinian Ambassador in Washington (D.C.), to ask them why they had "locked up" my pen pal. Thereupon, after forty-six days of "confinement," Lidio Mosca was released unharmed and a great deal wiser about the (un)-desirability of getting mixed up with certain politicians.

Lidio Mosca has delivered radiologic lectures in most, if not in all the important medical centers in South America. This is why I asked him to tell me who are his favorite Latin American radiologists. I

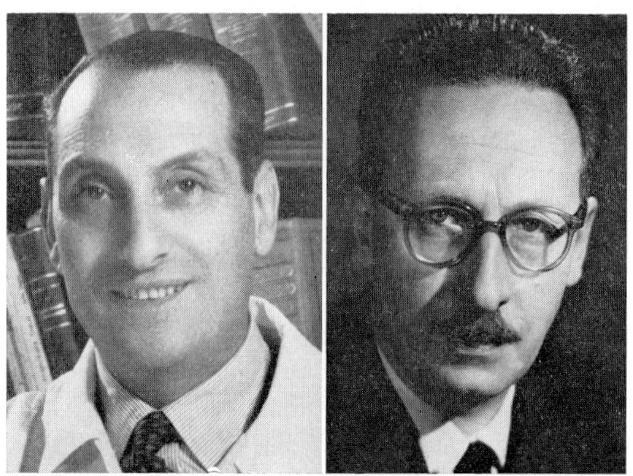

CORDOBA'S RADIOLOGIC INTELLIGENTSIA. Sabino di Rienzo and the bespectacled Lidio Gianfranco Mosca.

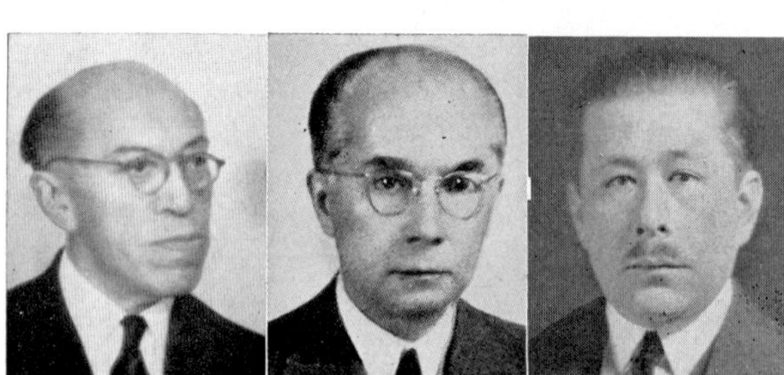

M. MELLA-VELOSO OSCAR SOTO A. PABLO A. SUAREZ

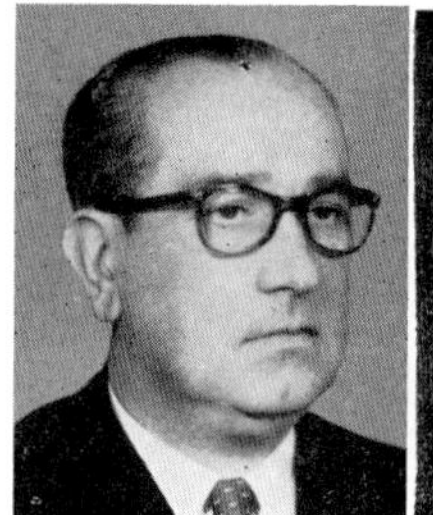

ADOLFO BURLANDO

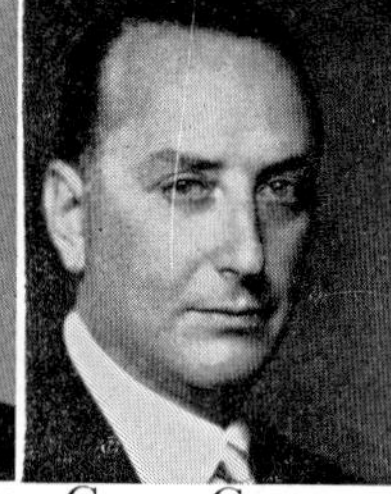

GUIDO GOTTA

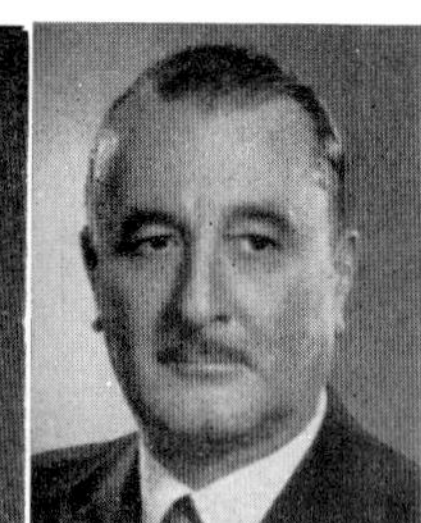

F. CIFARELLI

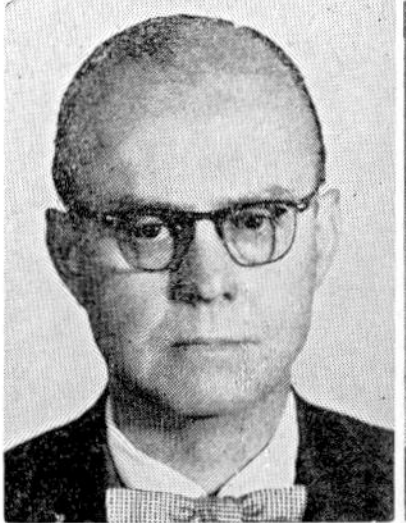

M. RIEBELING

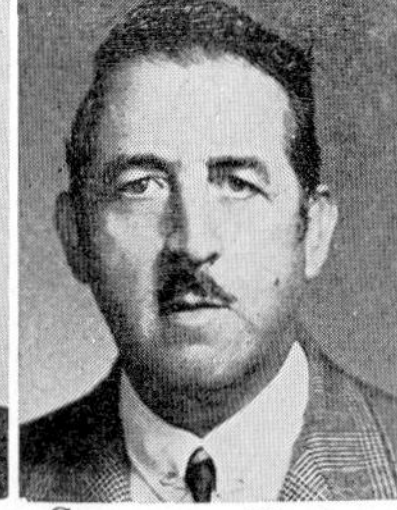

SANCHEZ-PEREZ

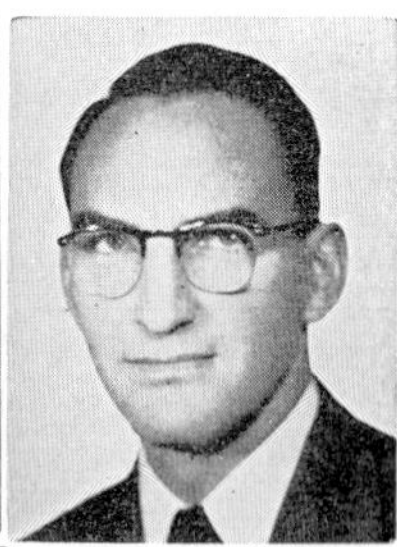

GUILLERMO SANTIN

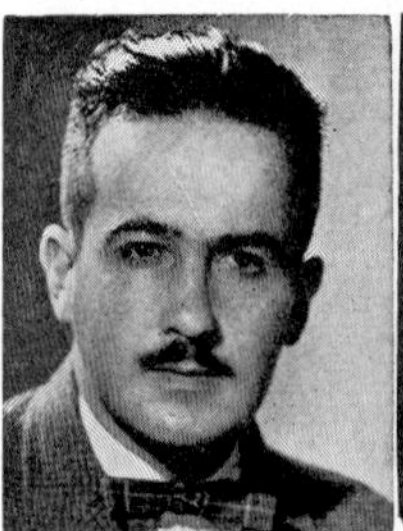

GAITÁN-YANGUAS

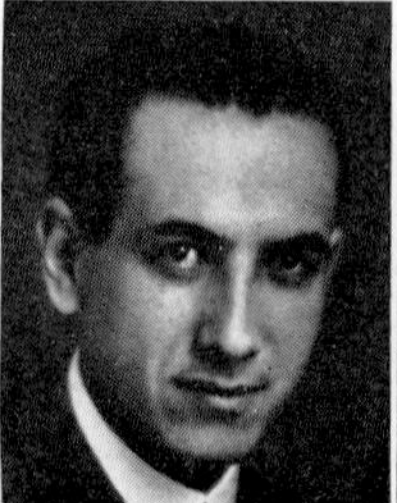

PEDRO GONZALEZ

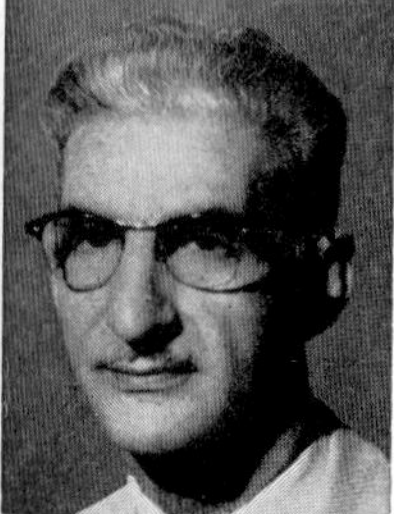

ENRICO BURLANDO

am convinced that his personal political preferences had no bearing on the names he selected. In his reply Mosca first inquired whether I want an assortment of "big names," meaning people whom they classify in the category *jarron* (literally flower vase). Such an individual is empty inside and yet decorative because with advancing age he usually acquires color, glaze, and polish - in addition to the rounded figure.

Actually many of these "flower vases" had given their measure of contribution in times past, but those things tend to be forgotten. And he who fails to keep up with the times will invariably be called a *jarron*, regardless of previous achievements. The corresponding term in some of the European countries is the equivalent of *constipated* which is not as picturesque (after all the Argentinian vase contained flowers), but carries similar (adopted) connotations.

To Mosca's list of names I added at least twice as many, chosen among the current radiologic intelligentsia (for some only the portraits are given).

In Argentina, a fine teacher and excellent diagnostician is Manuel Malenchini,* director of the Escuela Nacional y Municipal de Radiología. Another well known radiologist from Buenos Aires is Oscar Francisco Noguera.

*In 1963 Malenchini investigated a backache which was bothering him, and found an osteolytic lesion, whereupon he took his own life.

In Brazil, Camillo Segreto seems to be a talented radiologic organizer.

In Colombia, Alberto Torres Focke is professor of radiodiagnosis in the Universidad Nacional in Bogotá. Jorges Henao Echavarria from Baranquilla has first described in Latin America the roentgen findings of Cooley's anemia. Julio Manrique is currently director of the Colombian National Institute of Cancerology.

In Cuba, Eduardo Rivero (son of a roentgen pioneer) became known for his investigations of and improvements in pediatric bronchography. After the death of Farinas, his associate Clemente Rodriguez Remus built and installed the most elaborate and luxurious radiodiagnostic office found on any Caribbean island.

In Ecuador, Mario Hinojosa Cardona of Guayaquil has studied the thymus with the help of artificial pneumomediastinum, and has articles on roentgen investigations of the pancreas, on the post-bulbar ulcer, and on bone lesions due to malnutrition. Jorge Illingworth is a military radiologist.

In El Salvador, Amadeo Rivera y Solsona has studied the post-operative stomach and severe cases of scorbut.

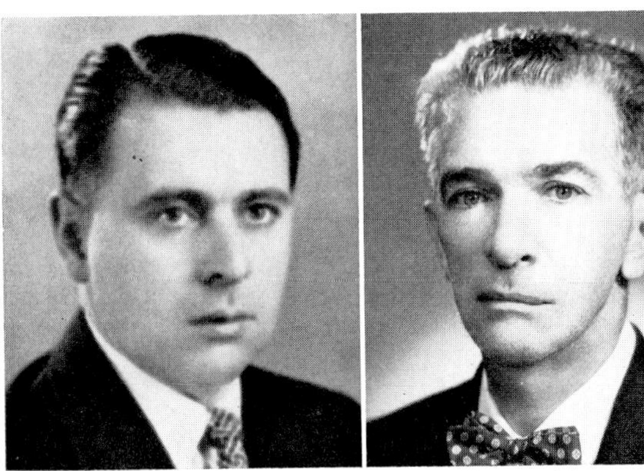

ALBERTO TORRES FOCKE — JORGE HENAO ECHAVARRIA.

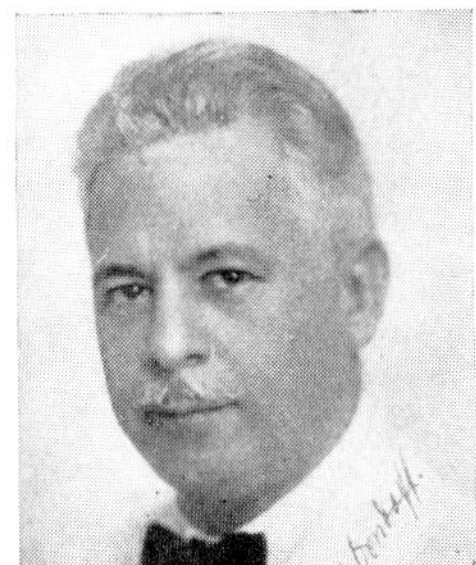

FILIBERTO RIVERO

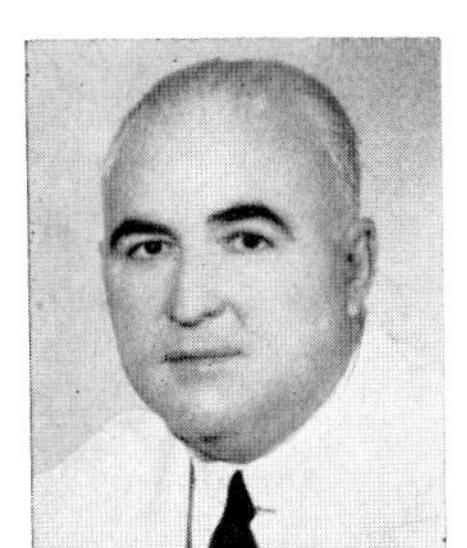

C. RODRIGUEZ REMUS

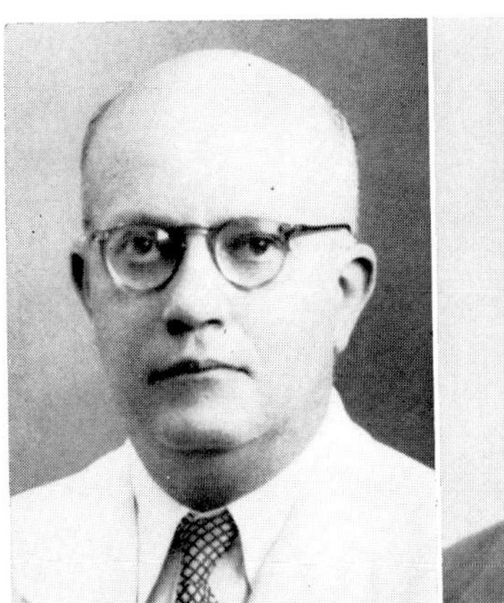

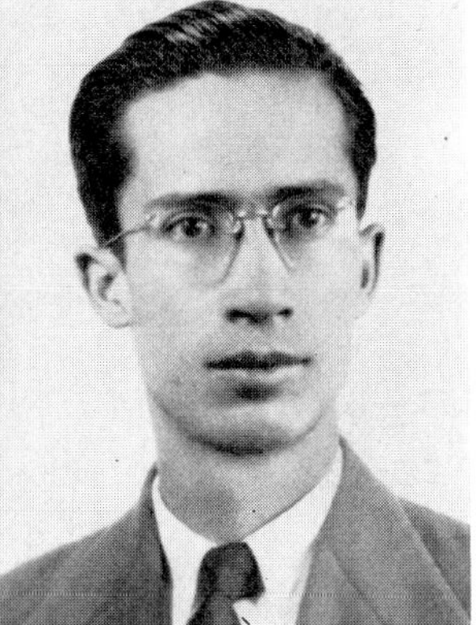

JORGE ILLINGWORTH — MARIO HINOJOSA CARDONA.

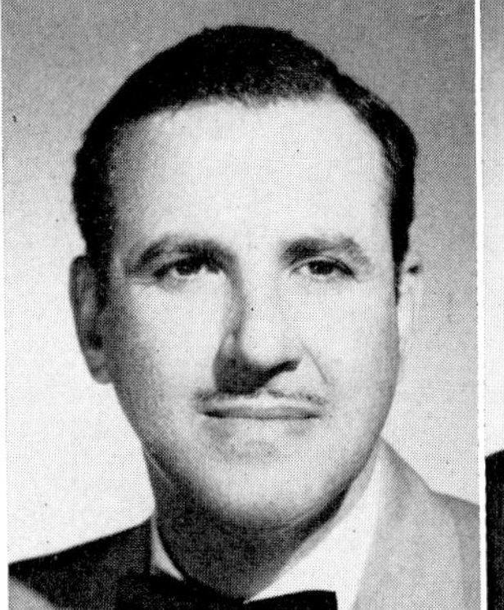

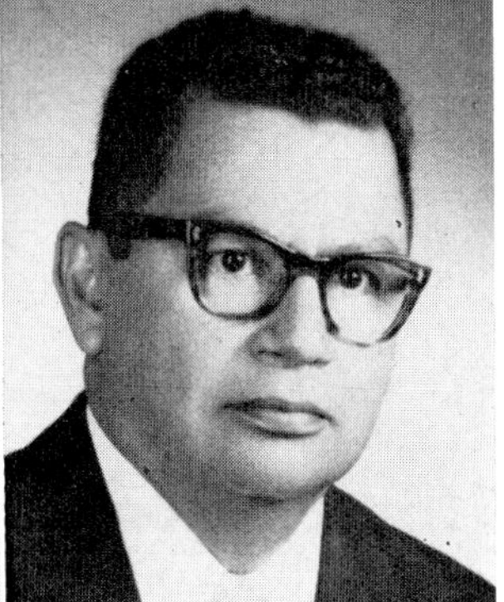

AMEDEO RIERA Y SOLSONA — JUAN RAMON PEREIRA.

In Honduras, J. Ramon Pereira is one of the active organizers of the ARCAP, and official of the Sociedad Hondurena de Radiologia.

In Mexico, Jose Manuel Falomir has done valuable work in spleno-portography. Jose Noriega is a therapist with much experience in cobalt teletherapy as well as in megavoltage. Narno Dorbecker is the best known Mexican cardioradiologist.

In Panama, Luis Arrieta Sanchez is a radiologic editorialist; one of his latest scientific endeavors was the administration of cholecystographic medium by enema.

In Peru, Julio Bedoya Paredes, who is professor of radiotherapy in the University of San Marcos, has many publications on radio-isotopes. Jorge de la Flor Valle (also from Lima) has done considerable work in the roentgen diagnosis of malignancies in various locations. Vicente Ubillus Arteaga, a remarkable diagnostician, is the chief radiologist of the Hospital San Juan de Dios in Callao.

In Uruguay, Alfonso Frangella, professor of radiology in the University of Montevideo, has compiled an excellent text on clinical radiotherapy, the first such title in South America. One of his associates, Helmut Kasdorf, is the author of an exquisite monograph on *linfopatías tumorales*. Another of Frangella's associates, the diagnostician Leandro Zubiaurre, was interested especially in gastrointestinal problems such as the cine-

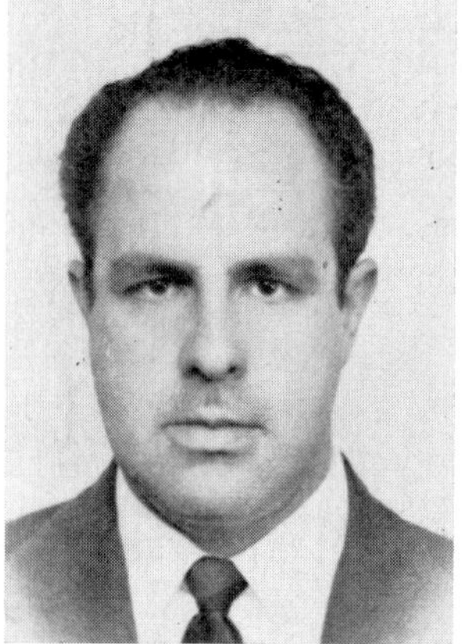

JOSÉ MANUEL FALOMIR.

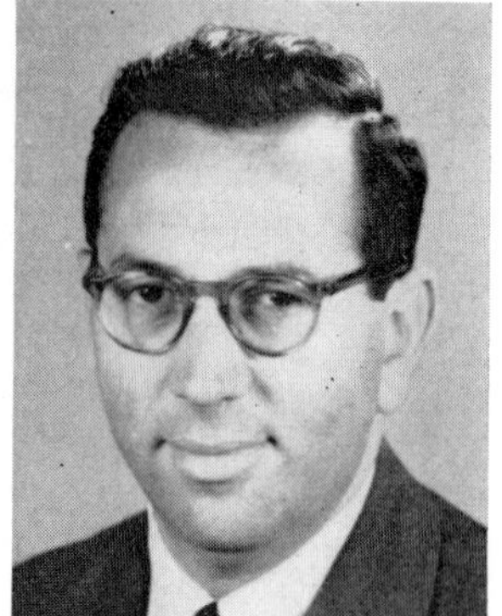

HELMUT KASDORF.

ALFONSO C. FRANGELLA

Jefe de Radioterapia del Instituto de Radiología de la Facultad de Medicina de Montevideo

•

LA RADIOTERAPIA EN CLÍNICA

Elementos de Física y Biología de las Radiaciones de RÖNTGEN y BECQUEREL-CURIE

Utilización terapéutica en catorce Especialidades Médicas (indicaciones, contraindicaciones y dosis)

•

MONTEVIDEO
"IMPRESORA URUGUAYA" S. A.
1942

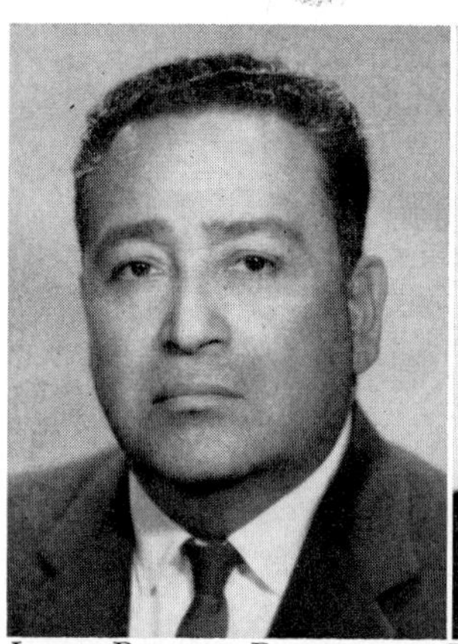

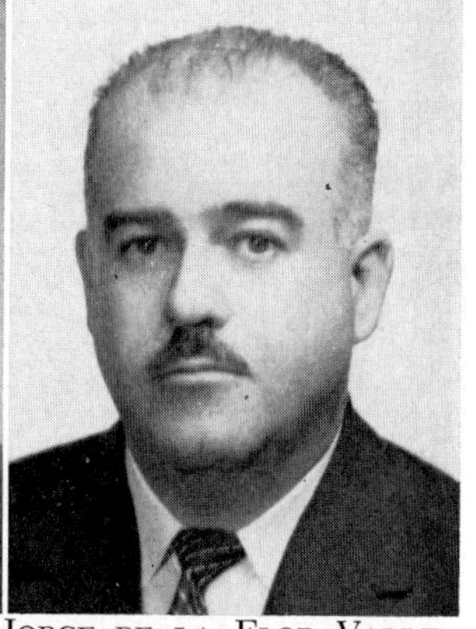

JULIO BEDOYA PAREDES — JORGE DE LA FLOR VALLE.

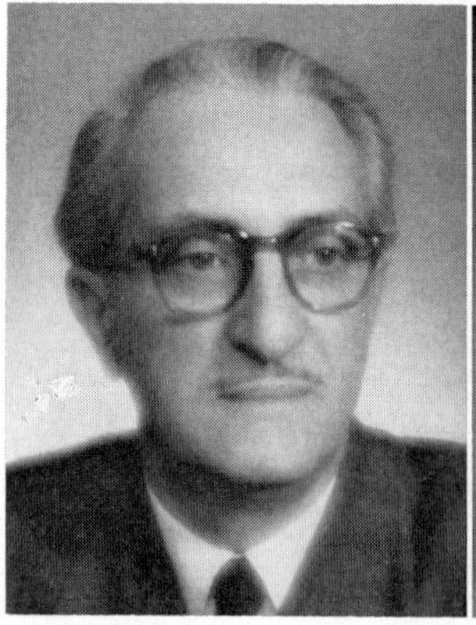

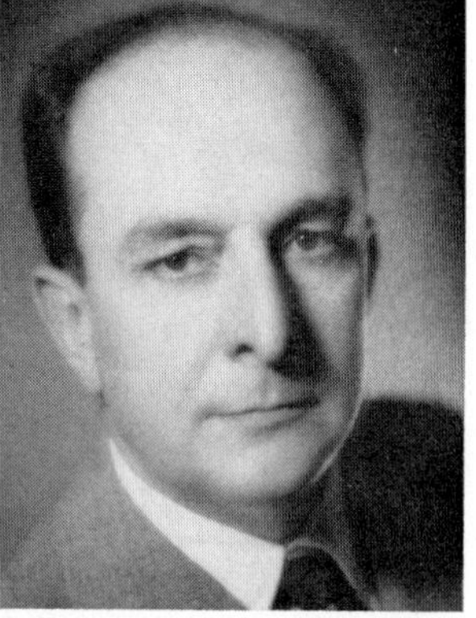

ALFONSO FRANGELLA — FREDERICO GARCIA CAPURRO.

radiography of the operated stomach or the examination of the lower abdominal quadrants. Federico García Capurro (former Cultural Attaché in Washington, and former Uruguayan Minister of Health) is mostly a diagnostician, although he has recently published a booklet on practical radiotherapy (1961); his main contributions are books on ecchinococcosis and the clinico-radiologico-therapeutic *Patología Digestiva,* first issued in 1942; he has published over 200 papers on varied subjects from bronchography to intestinal tuberculosis and from Hodgkin's disease to abdominal tumors; García Capurro founded in 1937 the Clinica Electro Radiologica (Montevideo). Well known are two Uruguayan radiotherapists, the brothers Raul Alfredo Leborgne and Felix Leborgne; the latter is the author of an important text on carcinoma of the larynx, based on tomographic studies of that organ; the former is one of the pioneers of mammography.

NEIGHBORLY ANIMADVERSIONS

A number of Latin American radiologists nurture a certain amount of resentment toward their North American colleagues. In *Radiología* (Panamá) of March, 1962 was started a new section (called *Crítica Bibliografica*) in which Mosca and Arrieta Sanchez joined forces to lambast the *radiologistas norte-americanos* for the latter's frequent failure to quote Latin American authors. The complaint is factually correct, but is it justified?

In the particular instances cited, the North American authors were undoubtedly at fault: they had described as "new" (*i.e.*, as their own) certain roentgen signs which appeared in South American articles printed two or three decades earlier. From a purist viewpoint such an omission is inexcusable — unless the respective contribution had not been recognized in the universal literature. The problem is simply one of communication: in the final analysis, how much can anyone be expected to read?

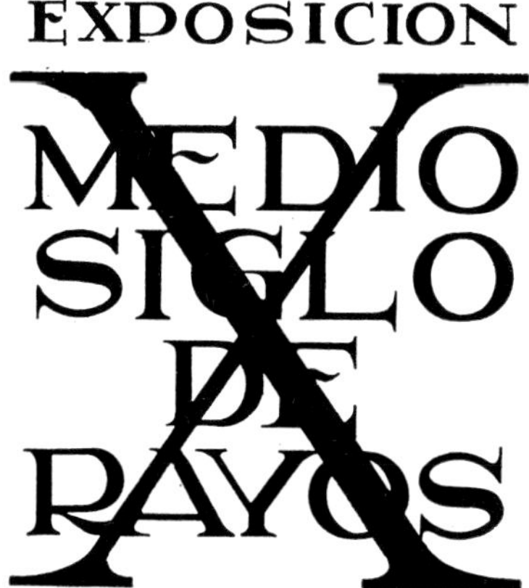

Courtesy: Alfonso Frangella.

EXHIBIT POSTER (1945). Half-century anniversary of Röntgen's discovery, celebrated in Montevideo. The preoccupation with radiologic history is just another proof of the level of intellectual maturity reached by Uruguayan radiologists. In the original, the X is in red, so it does not obscure the rest of the text.

According to UNESCO estimates, the world's 50 thousand medical journals publish 1¼ million original articles every year. At the NLM (National Library of Medicine) was placed in operation a bibliographic computer, called MEDLARS (Medical Literature Analysis and Retrieval System). The first issue of *Index Medicus* prepared with the MEDLARS was published in January, 1964: it had 15 thousand entries (of listed articles), and came out in five days instead of the previously needed twenty-two. Under the old system about 140 thousand articles were indexed every year. With the MEDLARS, this figure will be raised to 250

MINISTERIO DE SALUD PUBLICA

FACULTAD DE MEDICINA

LA EVOLUCIÓN DE LA RADIOLOGÍA EN SUS PRIMEROS CINCUENTA AÑOS

FOLLETO PREPARADO POR EL "INSTITUTO DE RADIOLOGÍA"

Montevideo, 1945

thousand – by 1969. Even then, it will mean one indexed article or monograph out of every five or six published. And that is currently the world's best system, and the world's least incomplete library.

In the *Bulletin of the Atomic Scientists* of November, 1963, John Maddox, the science editor of the *Manchester Guardian,* wrote: "Though it is fashionable to worry about the preservation of the increasing volume of scientific literature, comparatively little attention has been paid to the more fundamental issue of whether, in its present form, the scientific literature is worth preserving at all?"

In an open letter published in *Radiología* (Panamá) of March, 1960 Arrieta Sanchez took to task the editor of *Acta Radiologica.* Castellanos had sent an article for publication in these Scandinavian *Acta,* and the article contained a reference to a paper published in the *Archivos de la Sociedad de Estudios Clinicos de la Habana.* The editor of *Acta Radiologica* wrote back to Castellanos declaring that he could not take into consideration references to Spanish periodicals of little circulation. This sounded silly (and it gave Arrieta Sanchez a good case in point), but there was more to it than meets the eye. A Nobel Prize seemed to be at stake.

Agustin Castellanos y Gonzalez is a Cuban pediatrician of part-Chinese ancestry, who is now in self-imposed exile in Miami. In his princeps paper on the visualization of the heart and great vessels by intravenous injection of opaque media, which appeared in above mentioned *Archivos* (dated September-October, 1937), he mentioned that the cases therein reported had been presented before the respective society on October 22, 1937. There is always a delay between the date imprinted and the actual publication (and this delay is often greater in publications of Romanic language), but no serious people ever doubted that said presentation had been made at the time and place indicated. The associates of Castellanos on that first series were the radiologist Raul Pereiras and an intern, Argelio García Lopez. Those who might question the date ought to be told that Castellanos offered a monograph of 180 pages entitled *La Angiocardiografía en el Nino,* to the 7th Congress of the Association Médica Pan-Americana in January of 1938.

At a meeting in Atlantic City (New Jersey) on May 2, 1938 George Porter Robb and Israel Steinberg presented their *Practical Method of Visualization of Chambers of the Heart and Pulmonary Circulation* with reports of 215 injections made in 123 patients. That paper was printed in the *Journal of Clinical Investigation* of July, 1938. I corresponded with Steinberg who assured me that the first time Robb and he heard of

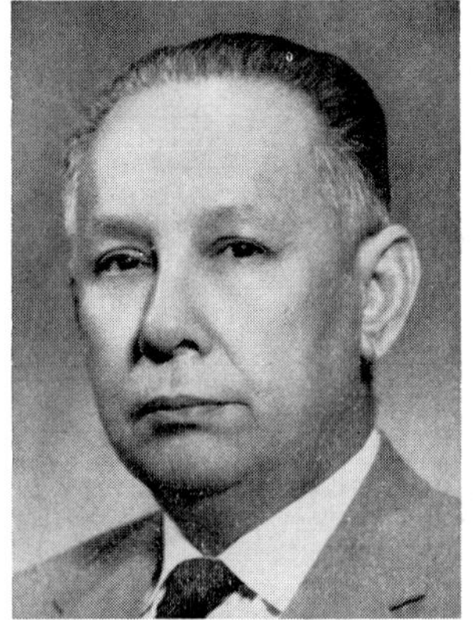

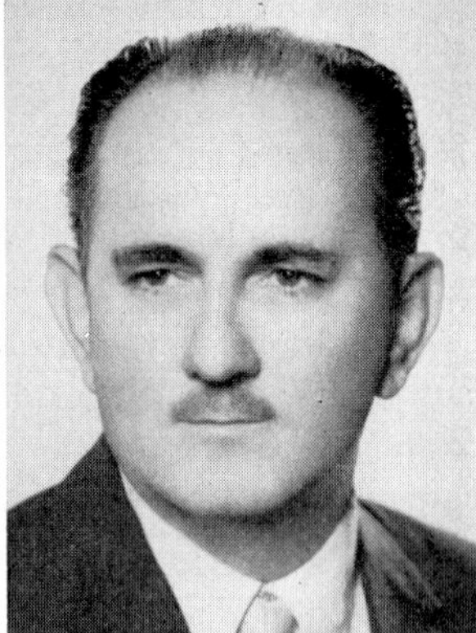

AGUSTIN CASTELLANOS Y GONZALEZ. His Spanish nickname is *El Chino Castillano,* attributed to his part-Chinese ancestry. It never carried any pejorative implication. Man with mustache is radiologist RAUL PEREIRAS.

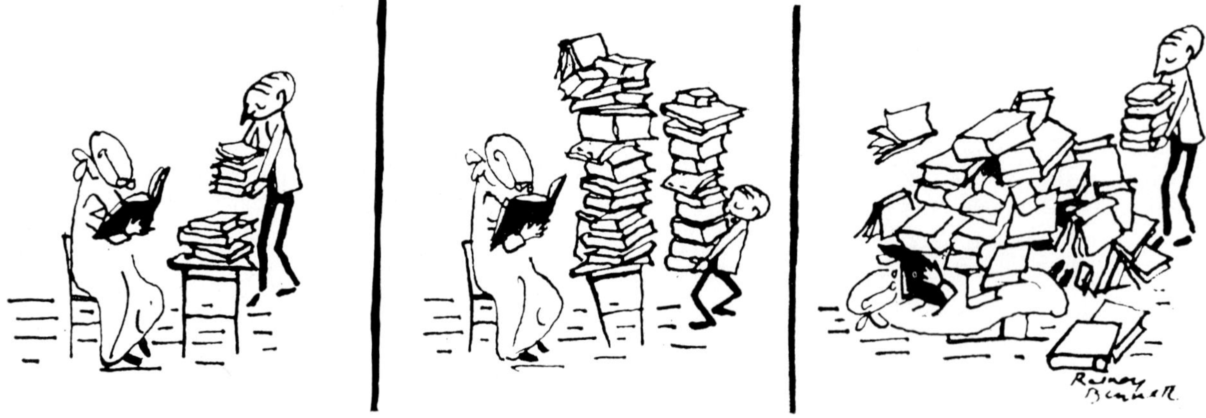

Courtesy: Bulletin of the Atomic Scientists.

CAN ANY ONE SCIENTIST READ ENOUGH? This excellent cartoon (by Rainey Bennett) accompanied the article *Information Crisis in Biology,* authored by the geneticist Bentley Glass, and published in October, 1962.

Castellanos was when they read a short account in the New York *Times* stating that Castellanos had presented a paper before a Pediatric Congress in Cuba; that was shortly before the meeting in Atlantic City.

Since there was a printed priority in favor of Castellanos, Robb (who had had the injection idea long before his actual presentation) obtained appropriate testimony. Arthur Christian DeGraff (professor of therapeutics in New York University), who had been familiar with their work, declared that Robb and Steinberg started experimentation in rabbits in the fall of 1935, and obtained their first visualization of the right chambers of the heart in man on January 30, 1937. Castellanos retorted by showing clinical charts of patients who had been injected in 1935 and 1936. Then Robb produced an affidavit from Magnus Ingvald Smedal, a radiologist who had been a resident at Boston City Hospital and had fluoroscoped Robb in 1933: the latter had volunteered to be the subject of an experiment, and was given intravenously 20 cc Uroselectan, but the heart chambers were not visualized. In reply, Castellanos dug out the information that in the very year 1931 he had injected a child with opaque media, for the same purpose, and with just as little success as Robb had in 1933.

As these claims and counterclaims were receding faster than a middle-aged hairline, the fact remained that in the English and German literature Robb and particularly Steinberg (who wrote numerous papers with his associates, especially with Charles Dotter) had been given priority. Once these things are picked up by textbooks it becomes very difficult to make a change. Whenever a new generation of physicians appears on the literary horizon they consult for historic background the textbooks of the previous generation. This is why erroneous credits, once established, will keep coming back like Scottish ghosts.

As a matter of fact there is only a limited priority that either Castellanos or Robb could claim. Werner Forssmann* published his original article on catheterization of the heart in *Klinische Wochenschrift* of November 5, 1929; it contained the idea that a (ureteral) catheter may be inserted through an incision in the cubital vein and advanced all the way into the right heart. In *Presse Médicale* of July 4, 1931 the Portuguese investigators Egas Moniz, Lopo de Carvalho, and Almeida Lima reported their experiences with angio-pneumography, meaning visualization of the pulmonary vessels after injection of sodium iodide through a catheter in-

*Since then, cardiographers have grown much bolder. They do not hesitate to catheterize a newborn's heart through the vessels of the umbilical chord, provided there is a clinical indication for such a procedure.

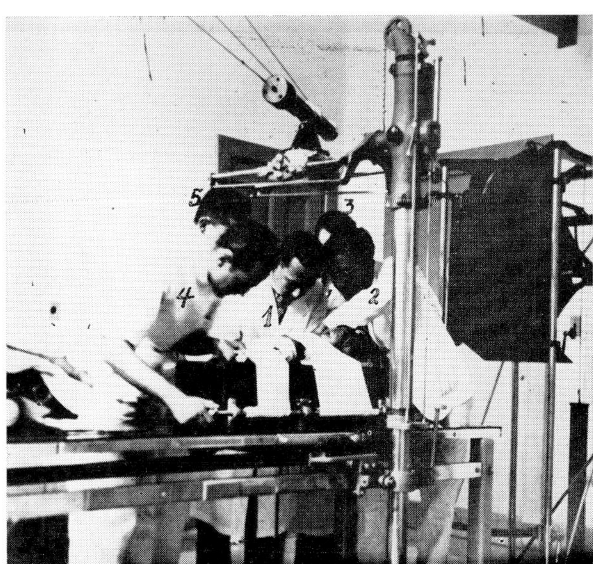

Courtesy: Agustin Castellanos.

FIRST PEDIATRIC ANGIOCARDIOGRAM (1937). The numbers identify those present: (1) Agustin Castellanos; (2) Argelio Garcia Lopez; (3) Angel Pausa, a medical student; (4) Enrique Galan. Garcia and Galan are physicians, (5) could no longer be recognized.

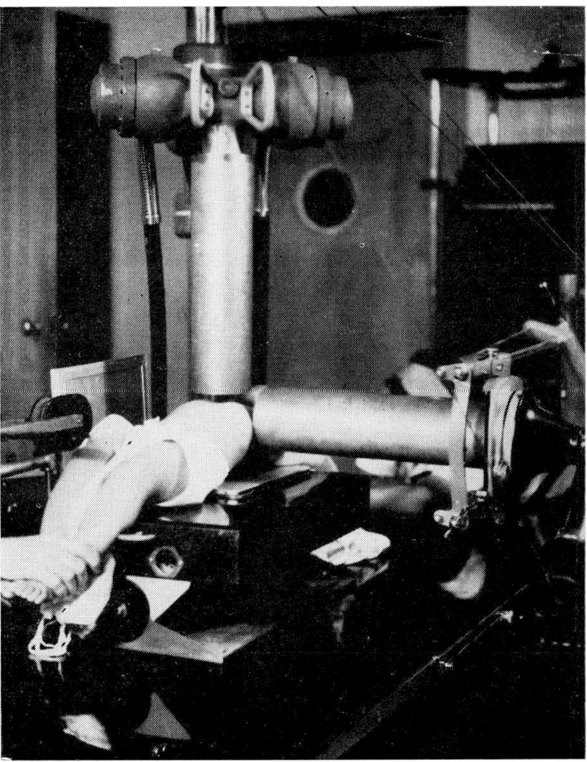

Courtesy: Agustin Castellanos.

BI-PLANE ANGIOCARDIOGRAPHY (ABOUT 1939). Castellanos is rightfully recognized not only as an angiocardiographic pioneer, but also as the developer of angiocardiography into a clinical tool. He still is one of the master diagnosticians in this field.

serted in the manner specified by Forssmann. The Portuguese had thus (inevitably) opacified, at one time or another, also the left heart chambers. They stated, though, that injection of a large amount of contrast material directly into the vein under pressure would not seem advisable because of the "unavoidable" extravasation and consequent bleeding. This we know was a fallacy, and the merit of Castellanos and Pereiras – respectively of Robb and Steinberg – was to show that large amounts of organic iodinated media could be injected with impunity, and will result in visualization of heart chambers and of great vessels. Such a priority would actually be of minor importance, and hardly worth fighting for.

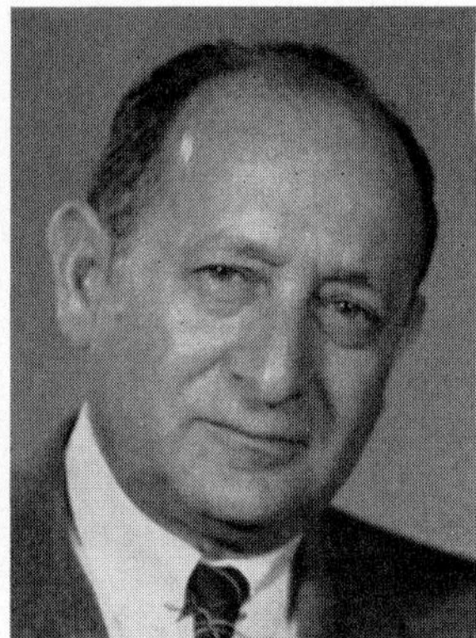

George Porter Robb and Isreal Steinberg.

But Castellanos and Pereiras on one side, Robb and Steinberg on the other, have done much more than that, each team on different categories of patients. Robb and Steinberg investigated adults, and were not primarily interested in congenital heart disease. Castellanos and Pereiras examined only infants, and particularly patients with congenital heart disease. They became consummate masters of angiocardiography and developed the technics as we know them today, which is the great merit of the two teams.

The original features of Robb and Steinberg's method were high concentrations of radiopaque solution (first 70% skiodan, then diodrast), oversized needle lumen, inspiration during injection to draw the opaque material into the vena cava and heart, and ether and cyanide circulation time measurements to syncronize opacification and filming.

Castellanos coined many of the terms used today, such as levogram and dextrogram, the title of his first communication being *Angiocardiografia radio-opaca.* He also developed cavography and retrograde (or counter-current) aortography, published in 1938 in the *Revista de la Sociedad Cubana de Cardiología.* Castellanos became professor of pediatrics in Habana, and in 1951 created a Fundación Agustin Castellanos. With the political upheaval in Cuba, Castellanos came to the USA; he told me that in revenge his personal library was destroyed. Reprints of his earliest publications, photographs of their bi-plane film changer, and the original film of the first angio-cardiogram are now preserved in the Army Medical Museum in Washington (D.C.).

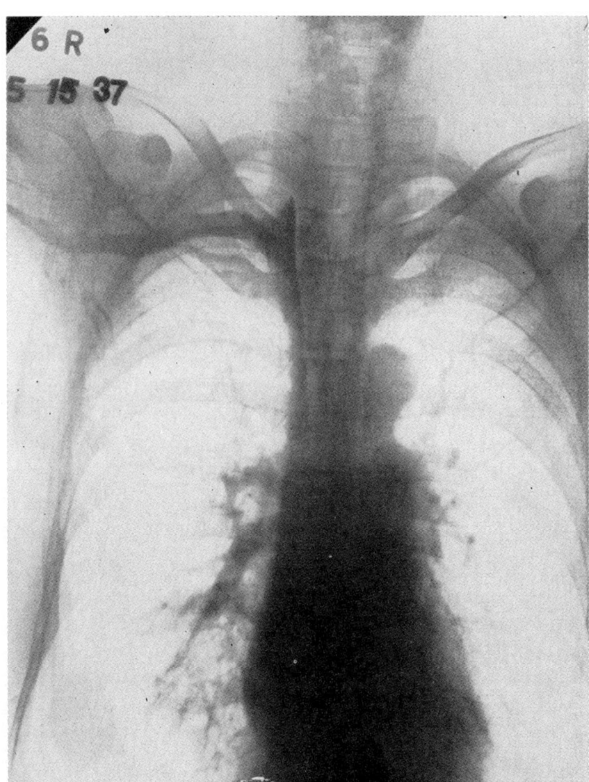

Courtesy: George Robb.

Robb-Steinberg angiocardiogram (1937). The patient was William Lee, age forty-eight, who had recovered from a middle lobe pneumonia. The film shows good visualization of the axillary and right innominate veins, the superior vena cava, the right atrium and ventricle, and the pulmonary arterial tree.

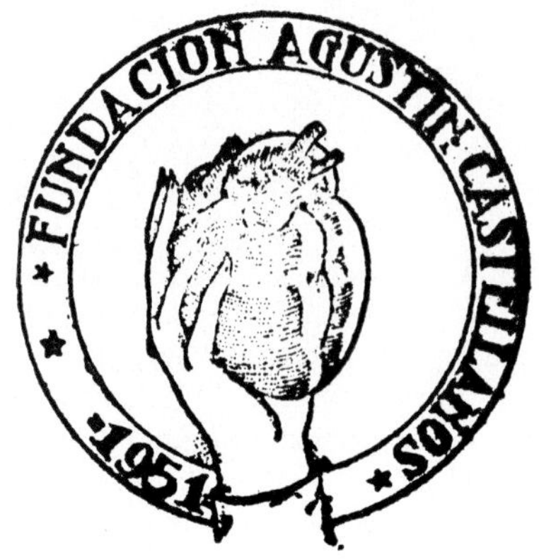

Werner Forssmann received a Nobel prize for having developed catheterization. Thereupon in 1959 Arrieta Sanchez, and in 1960 Carlos Coqui (of Mexico), demanded unsuccessfully that Castellanos and Pereiras be given the Nobel prize for their development of angiocardiography. The paper by Castellanos, intended for *Acta Radiologica,* was to have referred to his chronologic priority, and this might have seemed embarrassing to the Swedish editor - few people like to be told that what they know (or think they know) especially in matters of scientific priority is not so.

There is also the inability of most North Americans to distinguish between given and family names of Latin Americans. In Central and South America (as well as in Spain and Portugal) a person usually retains both the father's and the mother's family names. The child takes on the first half of the father's (double) family name, to which is added the first half of the mother's (double) family name. I have a very good friend (a Cuban-born radiologist), the son of José Maria Iglesias y Tourón and of Ernestina (no middle name) de La Torre Izquierdo: his name is Ignacio Iglesias de La Torre. The men are usually given a middle name, and my friend has been named for the pioneering jesuit, so his full name is Ignacio Loyola Iglesias de La Torre. To confuse the issue, some Latin Americans (actually intending to be helpful) delete the second half of their family name, and appear like a North American with one first, one middle, and one last name - Ignacio Loyola Iglesias (or Ignacio L. Iglesias). This complicates things because other Latin Americans delete their middle names, and use only the first given name, followed by both family names - Ignacio Iglesias de La Torre. It then takes more than superficial knowledge to decide which is what, even natives make mistakes on this count. Several solutions have been offered. One may use in European fashion a single first, and a single last name - Ignacio Iglesias. Or else the maternal family additive may be reduced to a single letter - Ignacio Iglesias de La T. Another way is to interpose between the family names a hyphen, such as Ignacio Iglesias-de La Torre. Finally, as in Spain, one may instead interpose the particle *y* (which means and), and come up with Ignacio Loyola Iglesias y de La Torre. Since my friend's father was born in Spain, the latter is the way Ignacio writes his name when he uses the long form, albeit he prefers the short Ignacio Iglesias. One must learn about these things because Latin American authors - just like everybody else - are unhappy when their middle and last names are confused, or when they are incorrectly indexed in alphabetic listings.

Many Cuban physicians have chosen to come to live in the USA, even if it entailed the loss of their properties in Cuba, and the difficulties inherent when one attempts to establish himself in another country. Among these physicians there were quite a few radiologists, several of them very well known, for instance the previously mentioned Manuel Viamonte, Sr., who for the past four years was the president of the IACR, and currently resides in Florida. His son, Manuel Viamonte, Jr., is associate professor of radiology in Miami University, has original publications in lymphography and other contrast procedures, and has designed a "rotating cradle" usable in angiocardiography and geriatric fluoroscopy, made and sold by Cordis Corporation.

The issues between Latin and North American radiologists can actually be reduced to a single one. It is a problem of recognition. Latin American radiologists want to be recognized as peers.

An old Spanish proverb says: *Quanto sabes no diras, quanto vées no juzgarás, si quieren vivir en paz* (if you like to live in peace, don't tell all you know, and don't judge everything you see). But I am going to side with Antonio de Solis (1610-1686) who insisted that *La*

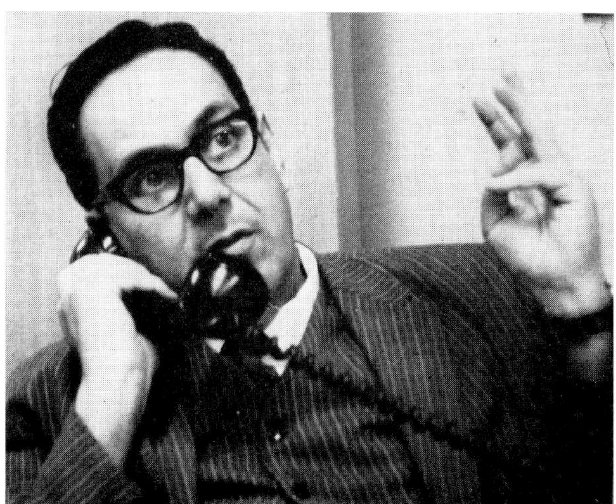

Ignacio Loyola Iglesias y de La Torre

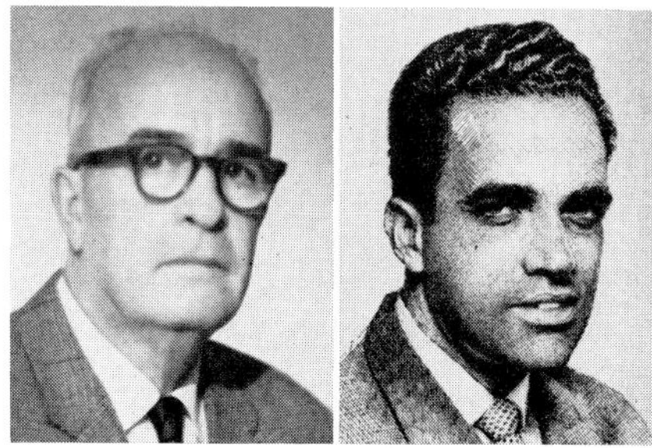

Juan Manuel Viamonte, Sr. & Jr.

verdad es el alma de la historia (the truth is the soul of history).

I have read the *Revista Brasileira de Radiologia* ever since its first issue came out, and I have been very pleased to notice the constant improvements in its material, and in the form of presentation.

There have appeared and are currently appearing many excellent single papers in Central and South American radiologic journals. On the whole, though, Latin American radiologic publications are not quite up to the average quality level found in the world literature. This can be explained in many ways, first of all by the lack of proper records going back over a span of more than a few years. Not many authors will admit that adequate documentation is a must before a good paper can be prepared. As Charles Dotter wrote in *Radiología* (Panamá) of December, 1956, "The personal honesty of a scientist cannot serve as a substitute for basic knowledge of the scientific (*i.e.*, statistical) method. The danger of an inaccurate conclusion is not measured in terms of good intentions, although they may excuse it." So far, few Latin American authors utilize adequate statistical computations (not to speak of double-blind procedures) in their papers, and all too often rely on empty statements such as "in more instances," "occasionally," or "almost always."

Then there is the Latin verbiage, so commonly encountered in many Romanic languages. A typical experience for the historian is to find an obituary containing two or three printed pages of strong adjectives and grandiloquent lament concerning the severe loss incurred by the scientific community. The dead man's life and labors are then declared to be so well known that only a bare rudiment of facts and figures need be included in the eulogy. This, of course, is only a subterfuge for the necrologist who does not want to take time out to inquire into, and/or to look up, the deceased's biography and bibliography. Such an obituary is a disgrace not only to the one who signs it but also to the editor who accepts it for publication.

There are today many outstanding Latin American radiologists who have contributed original studies and ideas, recorded in valuable papers. But they are not yet the majority. A Russian proverb contends that the future belongs to him who knows how to wait (obviously, similar statements have been made by numerous authors, from Longfellow to Disraeli). It was Calderon's idea to give time a break *(dar tiempo al tiempo fué siempre la accion mas cuerda)*. It is not a coincidence that the Spanish verb for waiting - *esperar* - comes from the same root as the Spanish word for hoping. And *esperar* has also another meaning, that of (great) expectations. It is indeed true that Latin American radiology is now standing on the threshold of a bright future, as bright as they decide to make it. The ultimate forecast is quite excellent - until then, to use a Rio de Janero colloquialism, they will have to *dar em jeito!**

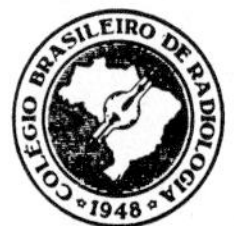

revista
brasileira
de
radiologia

órgão oficial do colégio brasileiro de radiologia
e da sociedade brasileira de radiologia

EDITORIAL

A crise da Radiologia

THE OPERATOR

It is almost anticlimactic to consider at this point the names by which roentgen operators had been called since pioneer days.

One of the first designations was *cathographer*, suggested by the editorialist of the *Electrical Engineer* of April 8, 1896. Forms based on the root electro-, such

*This is a slang expression, typical of what the Argentines call el *portugues brasilero*. You ask for tickets, and everything is sold out, but then the cashier says, *vo a dar em jeito* (maybe we can find some other way).

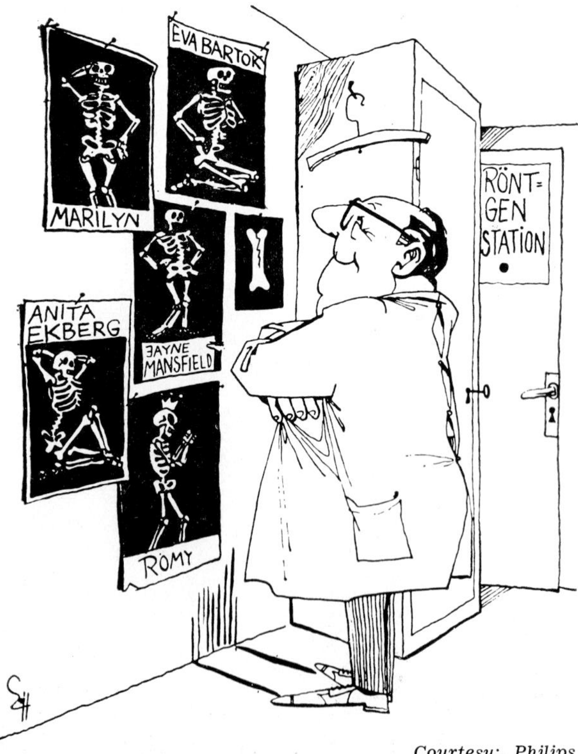

Courtesy: Philips.

THE "RADIOLOGIC OPERATOR."

as *electrologist,* appeared also quite early. The quaint term *electro-medicist* was printed in the *American X-Ray Journal* of March, 1898 with Kolle's by-line. The Romanic *electro-radiologist* came into use only after 1910.

Lewis Gregory Cole was for some time *skiagrapher* to the Roosevelt Hospital in New York City. Frederick Henry Baetjer (1874-1933) functioned as *assistant actinographer* at Johns Hopkins. Alexander Howard Pirie (1875-1944) was called a *lecturer in x-rays* in McGill University. Pancoast was a *lecturer in skiagraphy* in the University of Pennsylvania until 1912 when he became *professor of roentgenology.* An exception was Francis Henry Williams (1852-1936) who – for the sake of principle – remained to the end of his assignment, the *physician-in-charge* of the X-ray Department of Boston City Hospital.

In England one of the first titles used was *radiographer,* in fact Edward Warren Hine Shenton (1872-1955) – famous for his hip-line (could he therefore be called a "hipster"?) – started out as radiographer to Guy's Hospital. At that time, the term radiographer was reserved for physicians, because in the *Edinburgh Medical Journal* of June, 1912 Archibald M'Kendrick differentiated between (lay) *x-ray photographers* and (medical) radiographers. The term *radiologist* became popular in Great Britain before the end of World War I: Francis Hernaman-Johnson in the *British Journal of Radiology* of November, 1919 and Barclay in the *British Medical Journal* of September 11, 1920 worried about the place of the radiologist in medicine. Barclay wanted to lift it out of the cellar, both figuratively and literally!*

*The request to raise the x-ray department above the basement floor was often voiced, for instance in the *American Quarterly of Roentgenology* of March, 1910 by Rollin Howard Stevens (1868-1946) of Detroit.

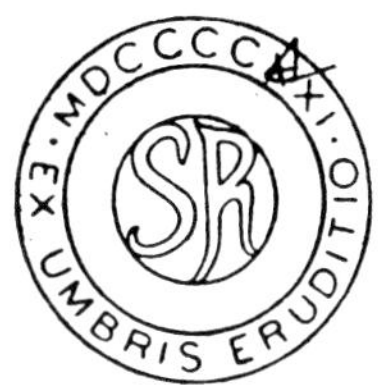

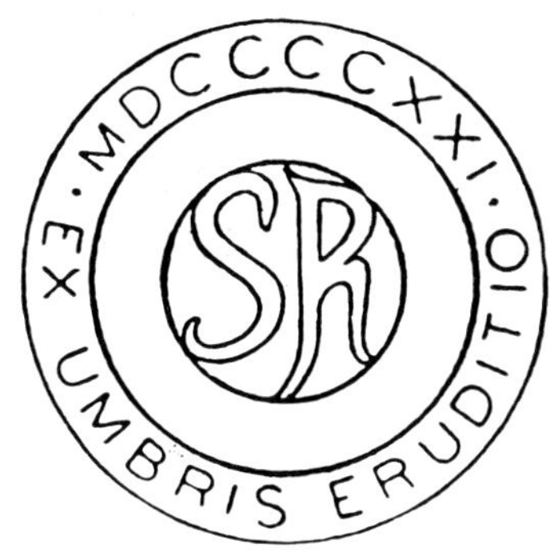

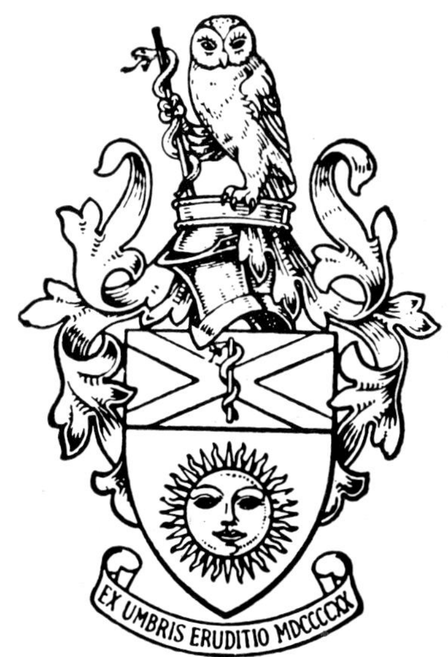

Society of Radiographers. Old round seal, and new coat-of-arms.

RADIOGRAPHY

Founded 1935

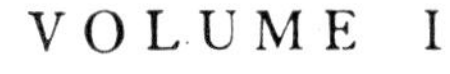
VOLUME I

JANUARY TO DECEMBER, 1935

PUBLISHED MONTHLY BY

THE SOCIETY OF RADIOGRAPHERS

32 Welbeck Street, London, W.1

In this country the term radiographer was suggested as early as February 19, 1896 in the *Electrical Review.* In the *American Quarterly of Roentgenology* of July, 1911 George Henry Stover (1871-1911) of Denver, who was to die a radiation death, formulated the "radiographer's property right in the radiogram." This problem was akin to the thorny question of who is entitled to see and show the films (only the attending physician!), discussed in *Hospital Management* of November, 1930 by George Milton Landau (1891-1956). He was to become chief-radiologist of Cook County Hospital in Chicago. The term radiographer (in the sense of radiologist) was used as late as June, 1924 in the *International Journal of Orthodontia*: the "correct" modern word is *radiodontist.*

In England the term radiographer is now used exclusively to indicate what in this country is called an x-ray technician. The (British) Society of Radiographers was founded in 1920. In 1927 they became affiliated with the BIR. They started their own journal, *Radiography,* in 1935: its first editor was the famous radiophysicist George Kaye. Incidentally, *Radiographer* is also the title of a publication of the Australasian Institute of Radiology, started in 1948 in Sydney.

X-RAY TECHNICIANS

In this country, the all-time *master x-ray technician* was beyond any doubt Eddy Clarence Jerman (1865-1936). He is also remembered as the founder of the American Society of X-ray Technicians (ASXT).

In the office of his father (who was a physician), Ed Jerman found a faradic battery, operated by a fluid cell and magnet. This is when his curiosity for electrical phenomena was first aroused, and this interest stayed with him for the rest of his life. In 1892 he became associated with the manufacturing of the Pattee static machine. On March 15, 1896 he produced his first roentgen plate. Since 1917 he was with the Victor X-Ray Corporation, assigned to the development of an educational program for x-ray technicians.

Jerman used to teach physicians and technicians in private x-ray offices, for a set daily fee and expenses. This is how he came to the attention of Samms, the president of Victor.

On October 25, 1920 a group of thirteen technicians (from nine USA states, and one province of Canada) met with Jerman at the Victor X-ray Co. in Chicago to organize a society.

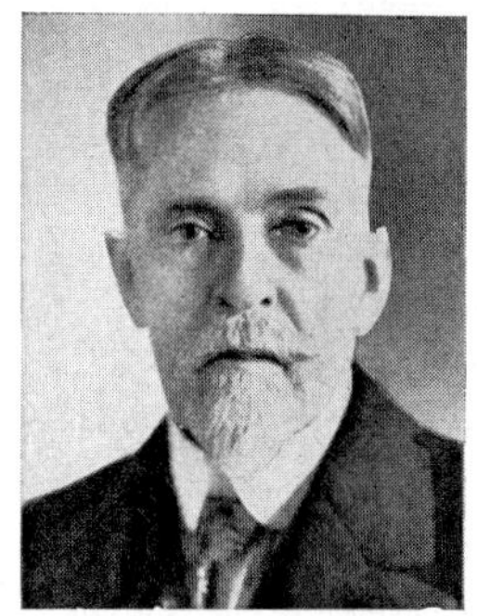
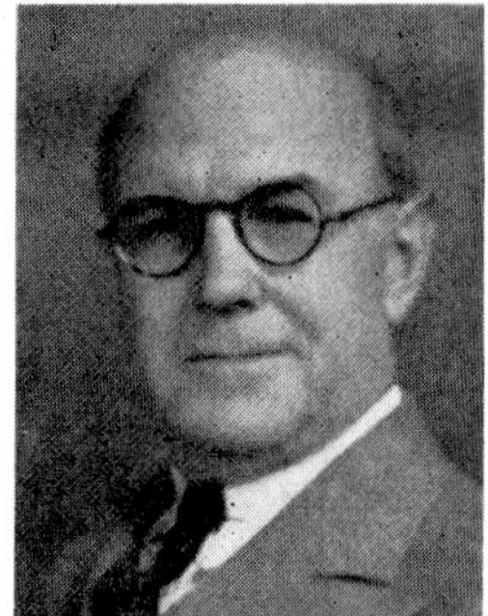

Courtesy: Radiologic Technology

Ed Jerman (with white goatee) and Tommy W. Lough, who was president of the Society in 1934 when he changed its name from Society of Radiographers to ASXT.

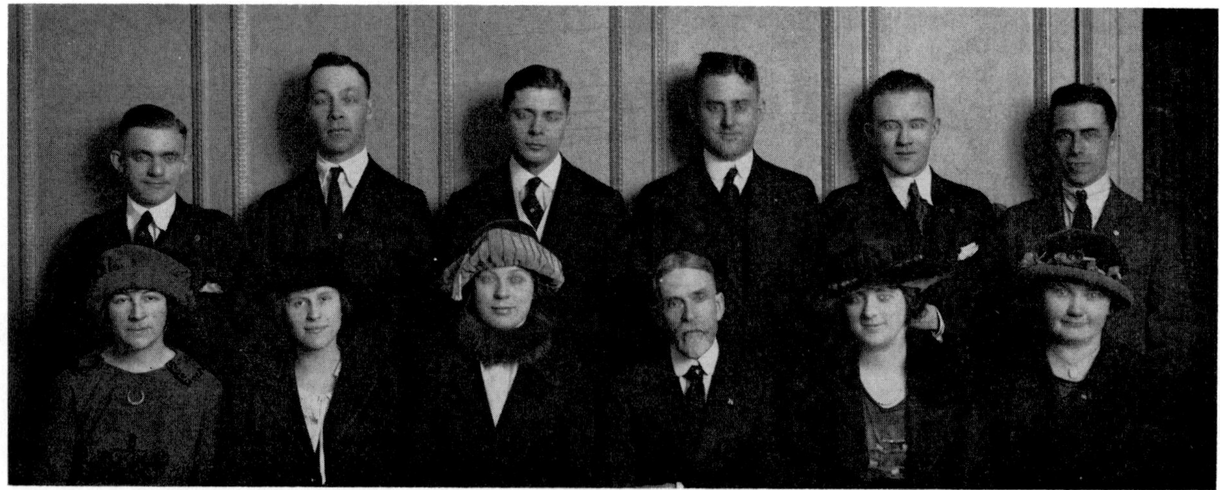

(Courtesy: Margaret Hoing)

Founders of the ASRT. From the left, standing: Glenn Files, C. W. Reed, H. A. Newman, W. H. Thompson, H. O. Mahoney, and C. J. Bodle; sitting: S. Christofferson, Freda Copple, Jessie Gordon, Ed. Jerman, Marie McDonald and Ruth Thoroman.

The following technicians were in attendance: P. J. Blegan, Webster (South Dakota); C. J. Bodle, Winnipeg (Manitoba); Alma G. Carbon, Minneapolis; Mrs. S. Christofferson, Portland (Oregon); Freda Copple, Kansas City (Missouri); Glenn W. Files, Chicago; Jessie Gordon, St. Joseph (Missouri); H. O. Mahoney, Duluth (Minnesota); Marie K. McDonald, Des Moines (Iowa); Herbert H. Newman, Tampa (Florida); Carl W. Reed, Minneapolis; Ruth Thoroman, Newton (Iowa); W. H. Thompson, Mobile (Alabama); and E. C. Jerman.

Incidentally, Glenn Files became well known for his work on GE's reciprocating Bucky grid (Files built one model with 100:1 ratio, from which the 16:1 was developed).

The day after that first informal meeting (on October 26, 1920) at the Morrison Hotel in Chicago, they organized themselves as the American Association of Radiological Technicians (AART), with Jerman as president and Freda Copple as secretary.

This information is taken from the *History of the ASXT* written by Margaret Hoing, a registered nurse who was trained by, and is still the x-ray technician of, Benjamin Orndoff.

In 1920 the RSNA appointed a committee of three radiologists — E. W. Rowe of Lincoln (Nebraska), Orndoff of Chicago, and Byron Darling of New York City — to determine whether or not there was a need for controlling the education of x-ray technicians. The committee suggested the establishment of a registry for the purpose of certifying x-ray technicians. The ARRS accepted an invitation to participate, and the two committees working jointly created the American Registry of X-Ray Technicians on November 18, 1922.

Sister Mary Beatrice of Oklahoma City was the first to take the Registry examination. She received a letter from the Board dated December 26, 1922, which notified her of the success. The certificate was dated in 1923.

The second meeting of the AART was again a Victor-Jerman affair. Many objections were raised, on various (commercially competitive) grounds, whereupon the meetings were discontinued. The organization was re-established in 1926 at the LaSalle Hotel (Chicago): current meetings are consecutively numbered by considering the 1926 reunion as number one.

Jerman became one of the first examiners on the Registry Board, and conducted the examination of the first one thousand American and Canadian technicians to be registered. In 1928, he issued his classic *Modern X-Ray Technic.* In 1929, he received an honorary D.Sc. Nevertheless, in 1933 he had to sever all connections with the Registry Board because of rumors that he might be using his position with the Registry to the advantage of GE. Like most of the pioneers, Jerman died with the marks of radiation imprinted on his skin.

The original name of the Registry — American Registry of Radiological Technicians - was easily confused with the AART. At the 1930 meeting of the AART —at the Sherman Hotel in Chicago — perhaps with reference to the British, the name was changed to American Society of Radiographers. This was all the more surprising because they had just begun in 1929 to publish their official organ, called

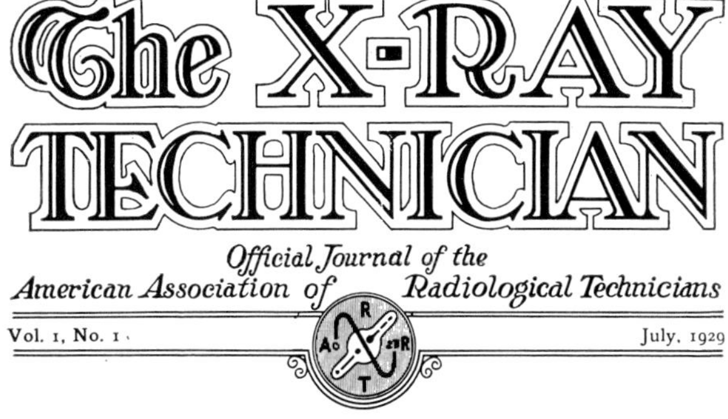

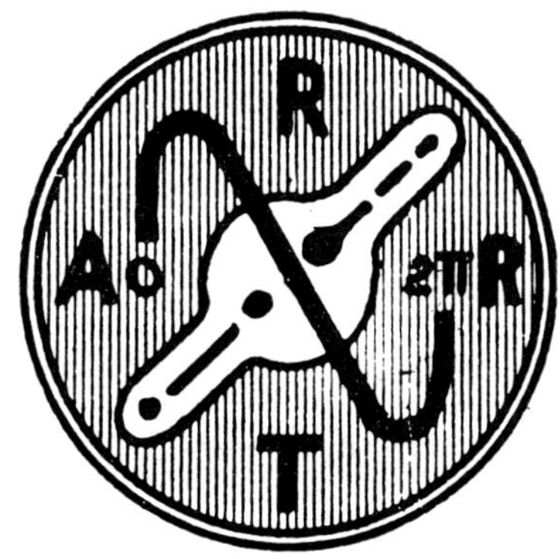

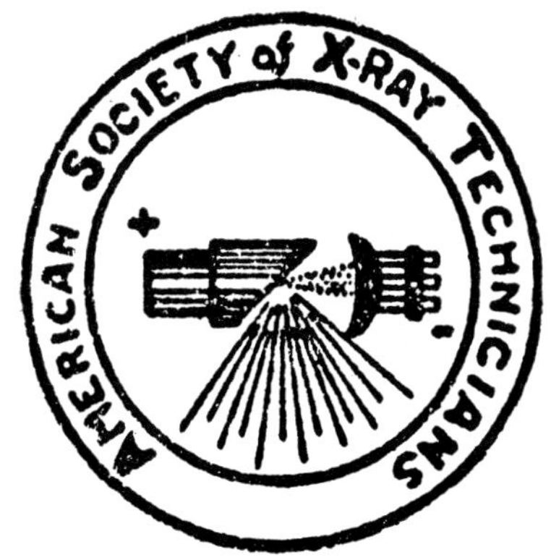

the *X-Ray Technician* (carrying the seal of the Registry), its first editor being Emma C. Grierson. Finally, at the Milwaukee meeting of the Society, in 1934, they adopted the current name, American Society of X-Ray Technicians (ASXT).

Most of the state and local societies of x-ray technicians, affiliated with the ASXT, changed their names accordingly. Several of their newsletters have delightful titles, for instance, the *Hawaiian Rays*, Arizona's *Desert Rays*, Kansas City's *Random Rays*, and Twin City's *Scattered Rays*. Arkansas has the *Ark-Sparks;* California, the *Technigram;* Colorado, the *Cassette Gazette;* Dallas, the *Grid Lines;* Oklahoma, the *Cathode Chronicle;* Pennsylvania, the *Keystone Target Practice;* and Montana, the *Live Wire*.

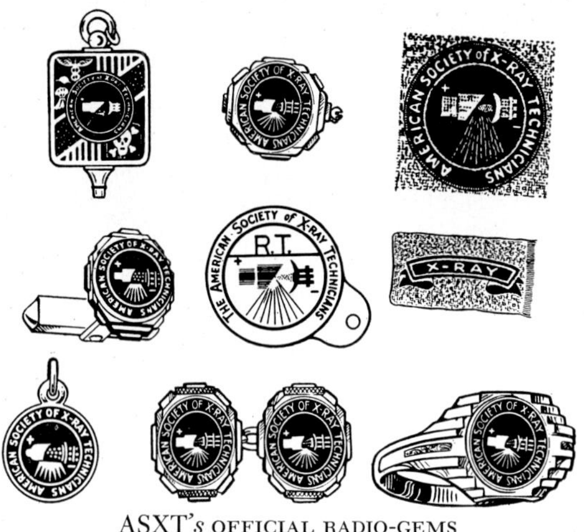

ASXT's OFFICIAL RADIO-GEMS

The development of the American Registry (and American Board of Examiners) of X-Ray Technicians was summarized by its longtime secretary, Alfred B. Greene, in a memorable article, *Quo fata vocant* (freely translated as Whither fate calls), which appeared in the *X-Ray Technician* of September, 1954.

In 1927, five years after the Registry came into being, a total of 470 technicians had been certified; of these, 362 were in good standing. Interest was at a low ebb, and it was questioned whether the Registry would continue or quietly fade away. The ARRS had already withdrawn its support. At this point an inquiry was sent to a long list of radiologists to determine how they felt. The response was startling: of 322 replies received, 302 favored continuance of the Registry, 17 were opposed, and 3 were non-commital.

Another seven years of uncertainty followed. In 1933, an attempt at formal training was finally recognized,

RADIOLOGICAL TECHNICIANS having proper qualifications and complying with the requirements of the Registry Board may be registered in

The American Registry of Radiological Technicians

The value of such registration in helping to maintain or improve the standards of this vocation is apparent. It has many other advantages to the Radiologist as well as to the Technician.

PERSONNEL OF THE REGISTRY BOARD

The Registry is under control of the following Radiologists:

President—DR. EDWARD W. ROWE Lincoln, Nebraska
For the *Radiological Society of North America*

Vice-President—DR. BYRON C. DARLING New York City
For the *Radiological Society of North America*

Secretary—DR. E. S. BLAINE Chicago, Illinois
Appointed by the *American Roentgen Ray Society*

Examiner—MR. ED. C. JERMAN Chicago, Illinois
Appointed by the *American Association of Radiological Technicians*

All communications should be sent to J. R. BRUCE, *Executive Secretary*
GUARDIAN LIFE BUILDING, SAINT PAUL, MINNESOTA, or care of
THE AMERICAN JOURNAL OF ROENTGENOLOGY & RADIUM THERAPY
67-69 EAST 59TH STREET, NEW YORK, N. Y.

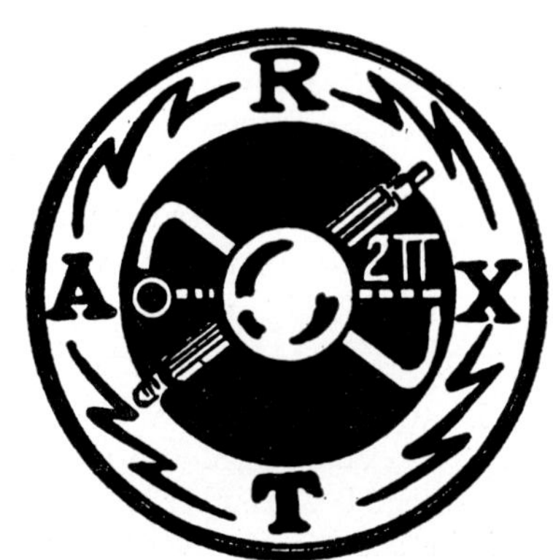

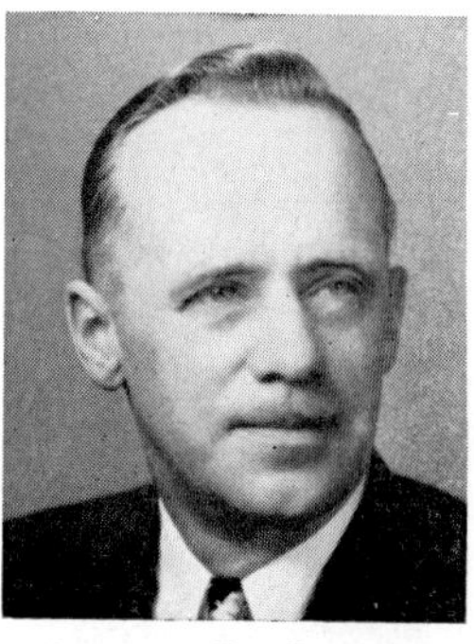

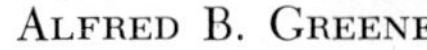
ALFRED B. GREENE

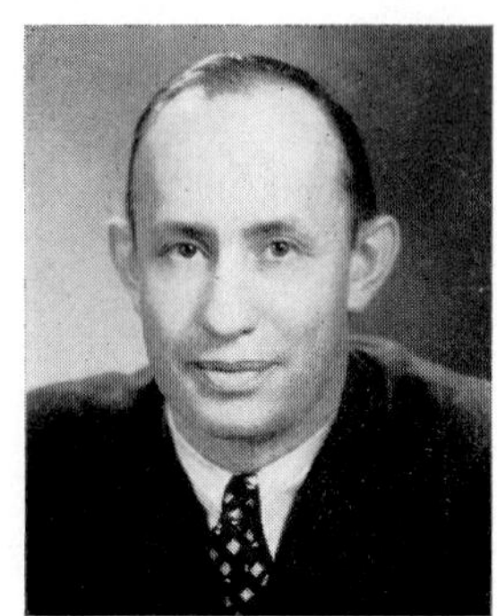

DAVID SHIELDS

and the Registry began its list of accredited training schools with three radiologists as instructors: Robert Arens at Michael Reese in Chicago; Bertram Cushway at Evangelical, St. Bernard's, and Englewood, also in Chicago; and Ernst Pohle at the University of Wisconsin in Madison. In 1934, there were 1,165 certified technicians, but almost 19 per cent had defected. By 1943, the total number had gone up to 4,558 certified technicians, with losses down to 14 per cent. During the next five years, until 1948, total registrations jumped to over 7,000 with almost 6,000 in good standing. In 1954, the total number of x-ray technicians registered in the United States exceeded 15,000. At that time they estimated a total of 39,000 x-ray technicians in the field (13,000 reported employed in hospitals, and of these only 3,800 certified).

The creation of the ARXT was sponsored by the RSNA, which continued such sponsorship until 1942, when it passed to the ACR. This was about the time when increase in the number of members of the ACR made the College the representative voice of American radiology.

Following are excerpts from notes prepared by David Shields on March 20, 1963:

"Jerman was the examiner for the Technicians' Registry through 1931. Whether his commercial connections were or were not detrimental to the Registry and to the Society remains a good question, but I had a personal experience in this respect. I had considered registration as early as 1925, but made no move, especially not after February 22, 1927 when Glenn Files told me that if I were to apply, he would blackball my application. This was the outcome of his failure in producing better pediatric films on a temporarily set up Victor-Snook against our old unit. Files declared his films were better, but I did not think so, and was supported by my radiologist, Dr. C. C. McCoy. Thereupon Files lost the sale, and this he never forgave me, especially because I had advocated the competitive equipment test. I joined the Registry only in 1939, following the assignment of a Cleveland radiologist, Dr. John D. Osmond, Sr., as a Trustee of the Registry.

"The September, 1962 roster of the Registry contains about 32 thousand names, ten thousand of whom are members of the Society. Affiliated with the Society are 58 societies (48 of them state societies). Large cities have non-affiliated societies, and even affiliated societies are permitted to accept non-registered x-ray technicians as associate members. A very conservative estimate of the total number of x-ray technicians in the USA exceeds fifty thousand, not including about five thousand students in the 700 approved (two year) schools of x-ray technology. Nor does this figure include those employed in osteopathic or similar services or those listed by the (apocryphal = not recognized by the ACR or AMA) Registry of American Radiography Technologists."

Examination and registration of x-ray technicians, which is today taken for granted, has contributed immensely to the development of radiology in this country. The significance of this fact could hardly be overestimated.

In ASXT's *News Letter* of April, 1961 appeared the information that at the mid-year meeting held in Minne-

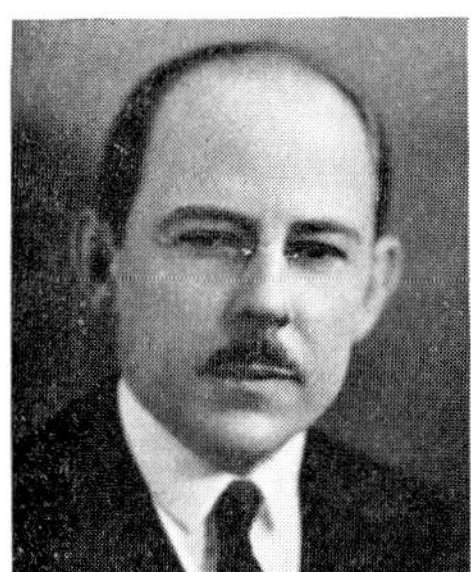
ROBERT ARENS

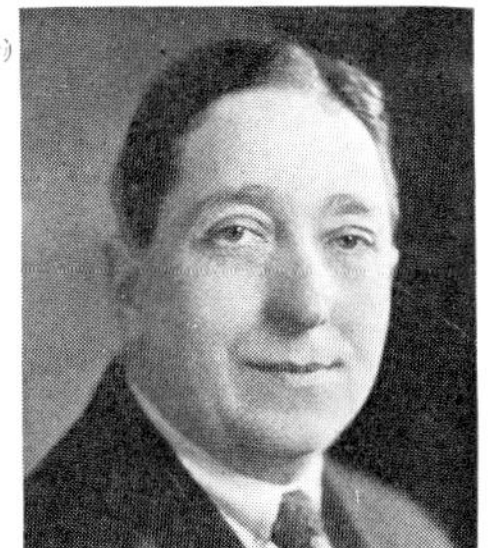
BERTRAM CUSHWAY

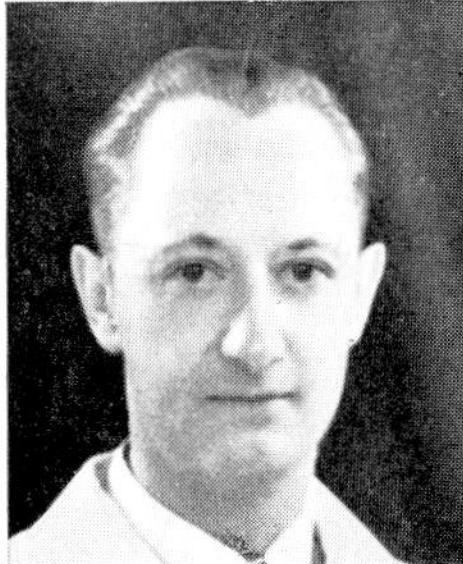
ERNST A. POHLE

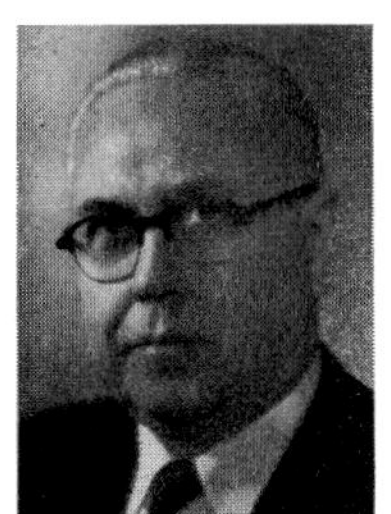
JOHN H. COONES

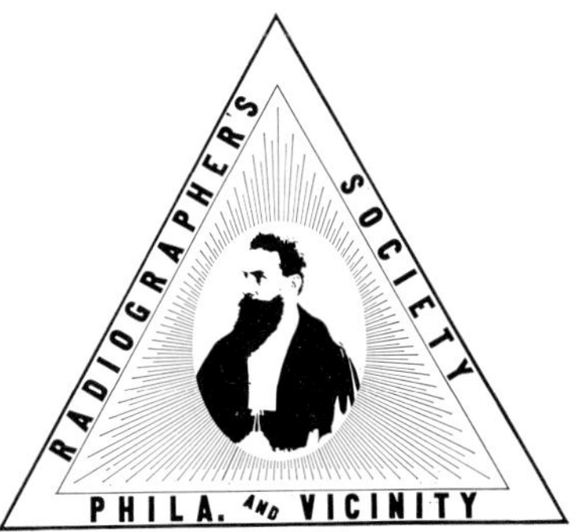

Courtesy: Charles W. Smith

PHILADELPHIA RADIOGRAPHERS. This society was created by Charles Smith and Thomas Gallo, on their return trip from the 1933 ASXT meeting in Rochester (New York). This seal was designed by Gallo, who was one of George Pfahler's technicians. Röntgen's portrait in this seal comes from Pfahler's collection, the triangle is the well known masonic symbol.

apolis in February of 1961, the Board of Trustees of the Registry unanimously agreed to give the ASXT equal representation: henceforth the Registry Board will consist of eight Trustees, four of whom will be licensed physicians, representing the ACR, and four will be registered technicians, representing the ASXT.

In July of 1963 several semantic readjustments took place. The American Society of X-Ray Technicians changed its name to American Society of Radiologic Technologists, its journal became *Radiologic Technology,* and the Registry returned to its original radio-root, and is now called the American Registry of Radiologic Technologists, meaning that the initials RT now stand for Radiologic Technologist. And the Society's Journal, which had been published by the Bruce Company of Minneapolis-St. Paul was relocated in the care of Williams & Wilkins. The reason given was that technicians have currently many nuclear assignment which exceed the x-ray label. This is, of course true, but in many respects the change is simply an expression of the semantic upheaval in radiology which has been so characteristic for its Atomic Phase.

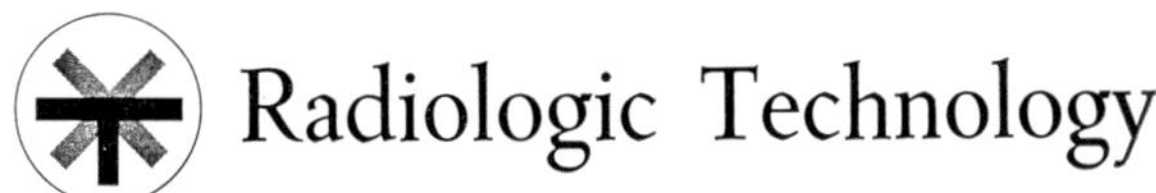

OFFICIAL JOURNAL OF THE AMERICAN SOCIETY OF X-RAY TECHNICIANS

VOLUME 35 July, 1963 NUMBER 1

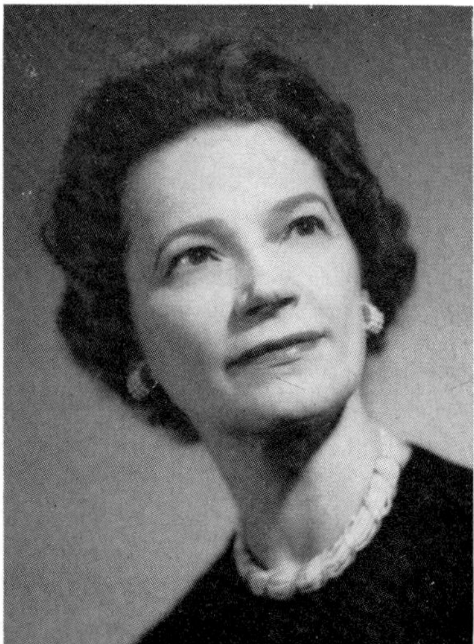

JEAN INGLIS WIDGER, editor of *Radiologic Technology.* Is it just a coincidence that the editors of the Yellow Journal and of the Gray Journal are also in Detroit?

"OTHER" X-RAY TECHNICIANS

Not everybody calls the x-ray technician by this name.

In 1958, appeared a US Air Force "on the job training" book, called *Radiology Specialist* – meaning almost X-ray technician. The book also revealed that the AFSC (Air Force Specialty Code) recognizes five positions on this particular ladder: medical helper, apprentice radiology specialist, radiology specialist, radiology

VOL. 20 JANUARY, 1963 Issue No. 84

Authorized as Second Class Mail Post Office Department, Ottawa, and for payment of Postage in Cash. Postage Paid at Hamilton. Ontario, Canada.

THE FOCAL SPOT

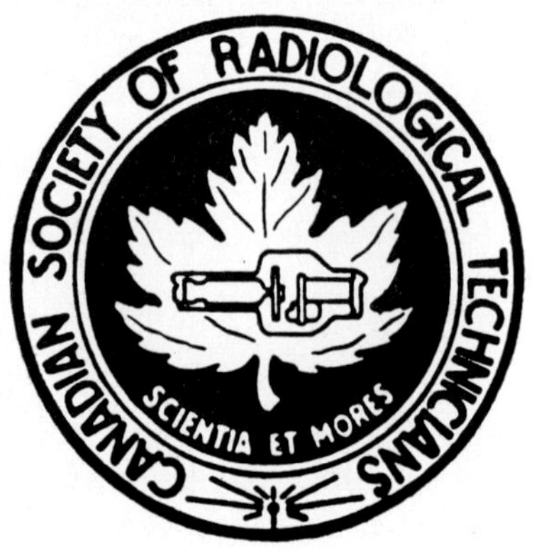

technician, and medical superintendent (the latter is the chief technician, actually a warrant officer, but not a medical graduate).

In South America, the x-ray technician is called *tecnico de radiologia,* in France he is a *manipulateur radiologiste,* while in Russia the term is *rentgentekhnik.*

The Canadian Society of Radiological Technicians was organized in 1943. They hold periodic international conventions with the ASXT, for instance the

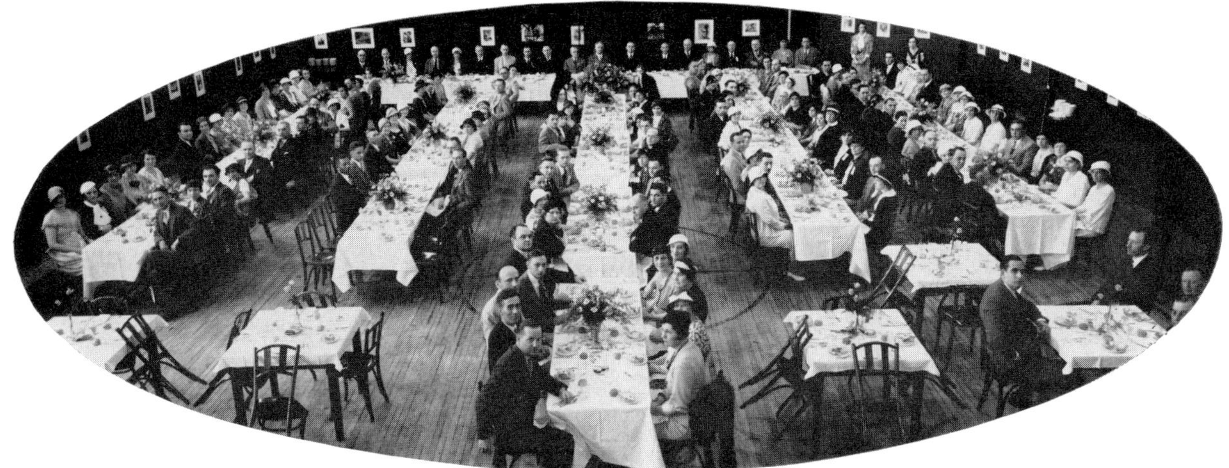

ASXT LUNCHEON June 2, 1933 in Rochester (New York). Its president for that year was Claude J. Bodle of Winnipeg. This explains (1) the continued British usage in the title American Society of Radiographers, imprinted on the Eastman Kodak photograph from which this reproduction was made, (2) the name given by Smith and Gallo to the Philadelphia Radiographers, and (3) the fact that I could obtain this picture from John Coones of Toronto, an old friend of Bodle's.

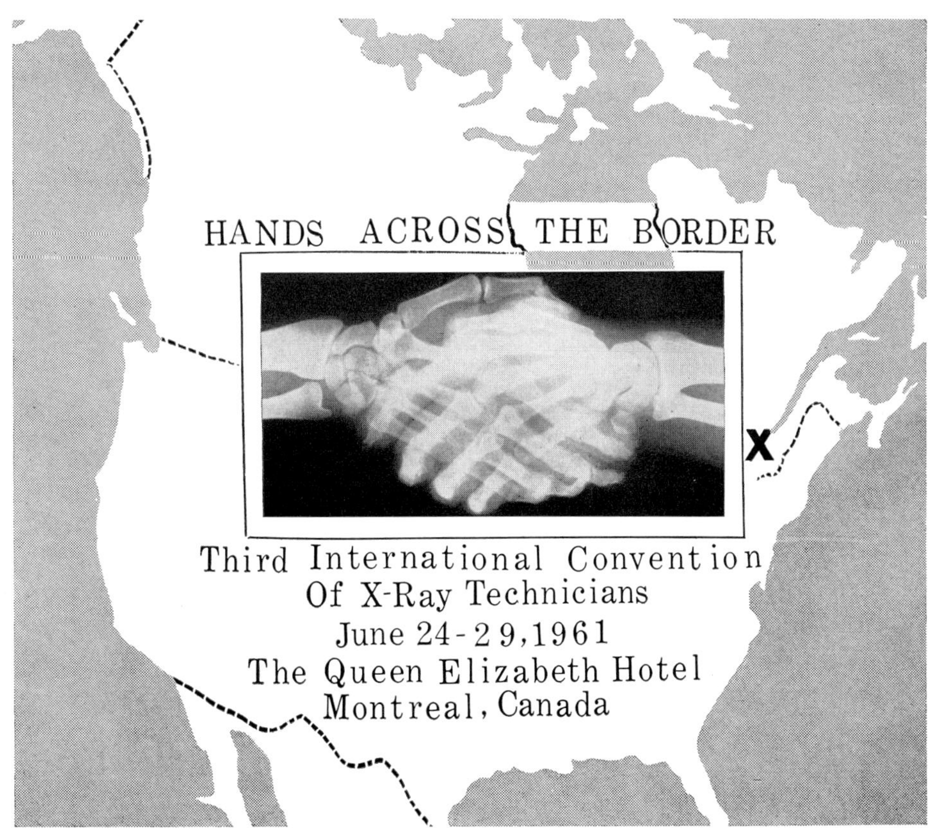

third such assembly was held in June of 1961 in Montreal, when they "clasped radiographic hands across the border."

Regarding the formation of the Canadian Society of X-Ray Technicians, this is the information received from its first president, John Howard Coones of Toronto:

"The first committee which attempted to organize the Canadian x-ray technicians was formed during the meeting of the American Society of Radiographers, held in Rochester (New York) on June 2, 1933. The president was Bodle of Winnipeg, and he was a member of our committee, the others being Sam Cox, Sadie Storm, and myself. We met with very little success. Toward the end of 1934 another committee was formed. It consisted of George Reason, Robert Bradley, J. Gutherie, and myself. At first we organized the Ontario Society of Radiographers, and from it was developed the Canadian Society."

The popular appelation *x-ray man* or *x-ray doctor* is used mostly by the laity. This is not the same with radio doctor, currently a favored designation for television and radio repair men.

For the sake of confusion it may be specified that Victor's radioliers were neither technicians nor radiologists; they were a short-lived club of (broadcast) radio hams, recruited in 1920 among employees of the Victor X-Ray Corporation.

BACK TO RADIOLOGIST

During a banquet address, printed in the *Journal of Radiology* of March, 1922, Frank Smithies (1880-1937) a gastro-enterologist from Augustana Hospital in Chicago, and general secretary of the American College of Physicians, suggested that everybody in the profession be called an *actinologist*.

This is actually the significant part of the title of the Greek Radiologic Society, ΕΛΛΕΝΙΚΗ ΑΚΤΙΝΟΛΟΓΙΚΗ ΕΤΑΙΡΕΙΑ (transliterated as *Elleniki Aktynologiki Etairya*). It was formed on October 31, 1933 – its first president being Dimitros Vassilidis, the secretary Athanase Leonidas Lampadaridis. During the Golden Age of Radiology, among the better known Greek radiologists were Christos Kalantidis (1875-1947); Felix Harth (1885-1953), who was professor of radiology in Athens and died of leukemia; and P. Gregoratos, who is alive. The younger generations of Greek radiologists are mainly pupils of Apostololos Yiannakopoulos, who is the current professor of radiology in the University of Athens, known for his original work in tomography.*

*This information was obligingly provided by Dr. K. B. Kotoulas, secretary of the Greek Radiological Society.

In the USA, the term actinologist never caught on. Radiologist remained the accepted word, even though the ARRS tried hard to promote the German transliteration *roentgenologist.*

In 1924, Josef Wetterer of Mannheim (Germany) made an unsuccessful attempt to organize and publish (with Beclere's help) an international *Index Radiologorum.* Generally, though, Germans were quite definite in their preference for *Roentgenologe.**

Where in use, the term radiologist carries more or less the same connotation as that of radiology in the territory considered. In France, Italy, Spain, Roumania, and South America the radiologist is a diagnostician, while the practitioner who uses ionizing radiations in treating patients is called a *radiotherapist* or *radiotherapeutist.* In Russia, and in most of its satellite countries, the therapist is called

*One of my overseas friends, the sparkling biologic philosopher, excellent diagnostician, and unorthodox expert in summation shadows, Dr. Heinrich Chantraine, resides in Neuss-am-Rhein (Germany) where he engages in the private practice of medicine with the title *Facharzt für Röntgen- und-Lichtheilkunde.*

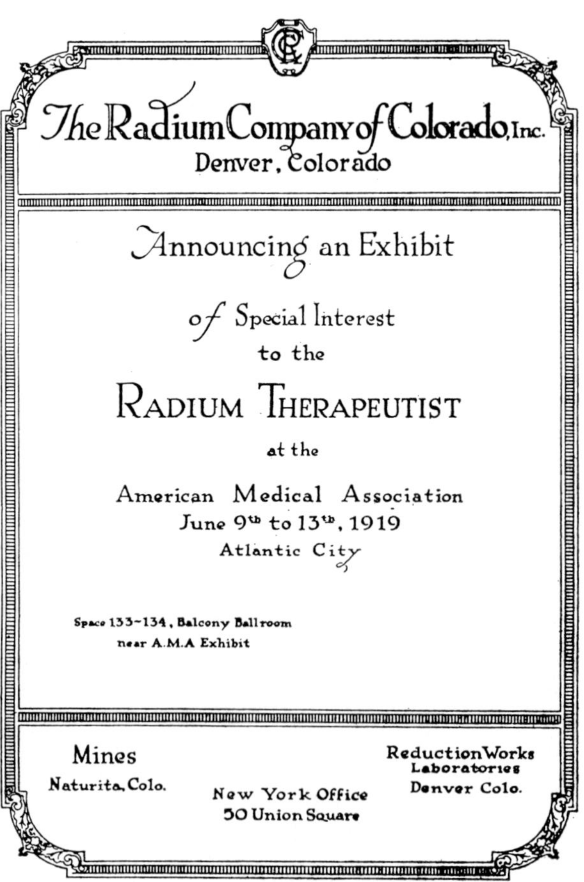

a radiologist while the diagnostician is called a roentgenologist. In Central Europe, the term roentgenologist is more generic (it includes both the diagnostic and the therapeutic use of x rays), and approaches the sense conveyed in English by the term radiologist, except that the European term roentgenologist does not cover the use of radioactive substances.

A semantic concession was made in the inscription on the obelisc of the roentgen martyrs, erected in the garden of St. Georg Hospital in Hamburg: it is dedicated both to roentgenologists and to radiologists who were "victimized" by the rays (even by radium rays).

Today the term radiologist is firmly established in all English-speaking countries, where its coverage is all-encompassing.

In the 1956 souvenir number of the *Indian Journal of Radiology,* G. Stead retraced the history of *Radiological Education in the United Kingdom.* The Cambridge diploma had been created through the efforts of the British Association for the Advancement of Radiology and Physiotherapy (BARP), which later became the BIR. Stead, a physicist, was for many years the secretary of the Committee for Medical Radiology and Electrology, responsible for the course leading to the Diploma in Medical Radiology and Electrology (DMRE), conferred between 1922 and 1942. Another DMRE was granted in Liverpool until 1944 when it was suspended because of war difficulties and re-instituted in 1946 with separate degrees for diagnosis DMR (D), and therapy DMR(T) — this is when they finally removed electrology from the syllabus. Since 1925, there was a DR (Diploma in Radiology) at the University of Edinburgh. In 1946, they, too, came to a separation into DMRD and DMRT. An Academic Diploma in Medical Radiology (ADMR) was instuted by the University of London in 1932. In the same year a Diploma in Medical Radiology (DMR) was created by the conjoint board of the Royal College of Physicians and Surgeons.

There exists in England the Faculty of Radiologists, which has its own periodical, the *Journal of the Faculty of Radiologists,* first issued in July of 1949. Since January, 1960 it is called *Clinical Radiology.*

The BIR had always been a heterogenous association. In 1934 was founded the British Association of Radiologists, with membership limited to licensed physicians who practiced radiology exclusively. They established a higher radiological qualification, and in 1935 a special class of members was created to be known as *fellows.* The medical presidents and past presidents of existing radiological societies were made *founder fellows.* Other members were given permission to apply for fellowship by December, 1937 (something like the "grandfather clause" in early American Board certification.) The same privilege was extended until the end of 1938, although the first fellowship examination (for those who could not qualify as "grandfathers") was held in December, 1937.

The (British) Society of Radiotherapists, with likewise exclusively medical membership, was founded in November, 1935. In 1939 the British Association of Radiologists and the Society of Radiotherapists merged under the title of the Faculty of Radiologists. It had first been located at 32 Welbeck St., together with the BIR. In 1944 the Faculty moved to new quarters (literally and perhaps figuratively) into the building of the Royal College of Surgeons.

The Faculty was incorporated in 1940, and was granted a Royal charter in 1953. Their membership covers also the former overseas British territories, for instance they include members of the Australasian College of Radiology.

In 1961 the Faculty of Radiologists received its

Clinical Radiology

The Journal of
The Faculty of Radiologists

Editor: DAVID SUTTON, M.D., M.R.C.P., F.F.R.

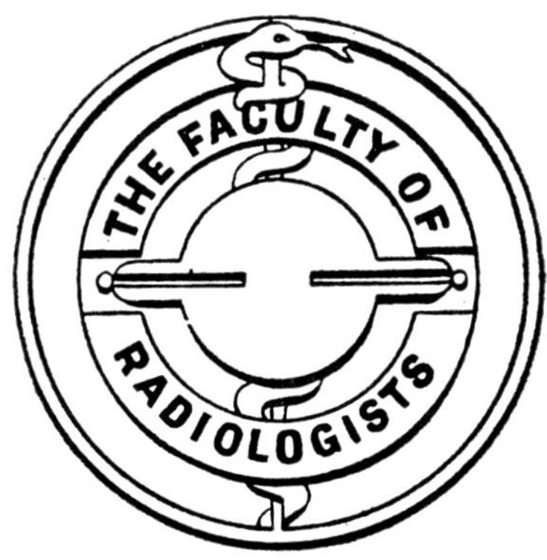

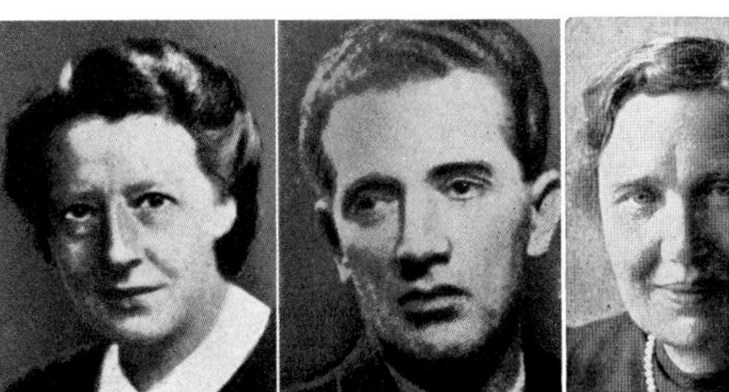

EDITH PATERSON BOB MCWHIRTER CONSTANCE WOOD

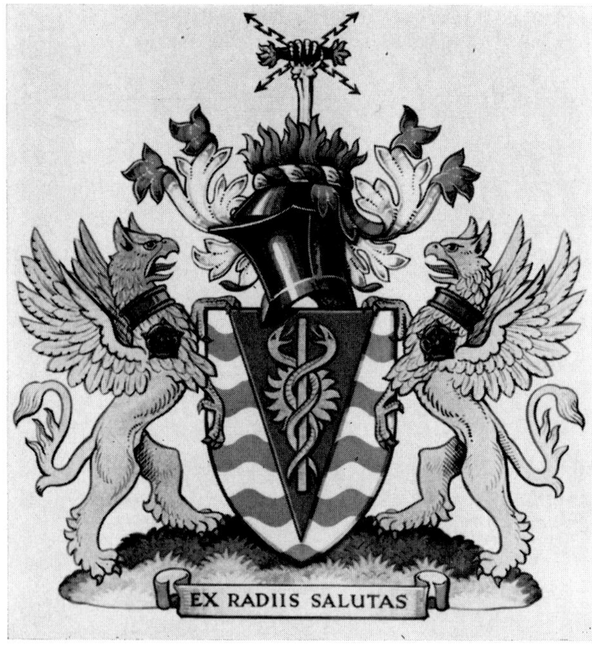

Coat of Arms, with the subscript *"ex radiis Salutas."* It is officially described as follows:

Arms. Barry wavy of ten Argent and Gules on a Pile Azure an X-ray Tube Or irradiated at the centre also Or and entwined of two Serpents Gold.

Crest. On a Wreath of the Colours Issuant from Flames alternately Gules and Or a Skeletal Cubit Arm proper the Hand grasping a Thunderbolt fessewise also proper.

Supporters. On either side a Griffin Or collare Azure and charged on the shoulder with a Rose also Azure.

According to information received from Maurice Weinbren, one of the senior radiologists in Johannesburg, the South African Radiological Association (of which he was the first president) was formed in 1932. The organizational committee consisted of Weinbren, R. W. Charlton (who was appointed secretary), Fram, Findlay, and Gus Friedland. The only other organization in this specialty in South Africa is the Faculty of Radiology of the South African College of Physicians and Surgeons, started in the late 1930s. They have no seal. The South African Radiological Society has several branches, the Transvaal Branch, the Cape Branch, the Natal Branch, and the Free State Branch. There is no periodical devoted to radiology, but since last year the South African Medical Journal devotes a copy to the specialty, and it is known as the Radiological Issue, the first one of which was published in April of 1963.

In the USA several associations of radiologists were created in the last decade.

The Association of University Radiologists was formed at the University of Chicago on May 23, 1953. The organizational meeting was actually brought about through the offices of Hugh Wilson of Washington University (St. Louis), Paul Hodges of the University of Chicago, Fred Hodges of the University of Michigan, and Russell Morgan of Johns Hopkins. At that first meeting, Russell Morgan was elected president; Henry S. Caplan, president-elect; and William B. Seaman, secretary-treasurer.*

SYMPOSIUM NEURORADIOLOGICUM

The following information was prepared by James William Douglas Bull, for inclusion in this text:

"In 1938 Lysholm (Stockholm), Ziedses des Plantes (Amsterdam), and Thienpont (Antwerp) decided to organize a symposium on cranial radiology. It was held in Antwerp, in July, 1939. That two-day informal meet-

*This information was supplied by their current secretary-treasurer, Robert D. Moseley, Jr., who succeeded Paul Hodges as professor of radiology in the University of Chicago.

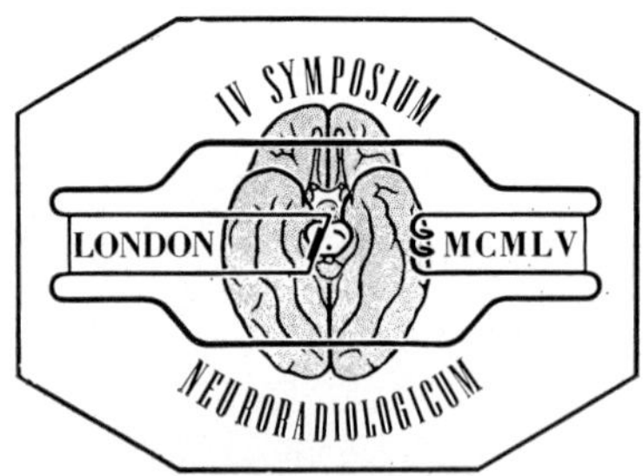

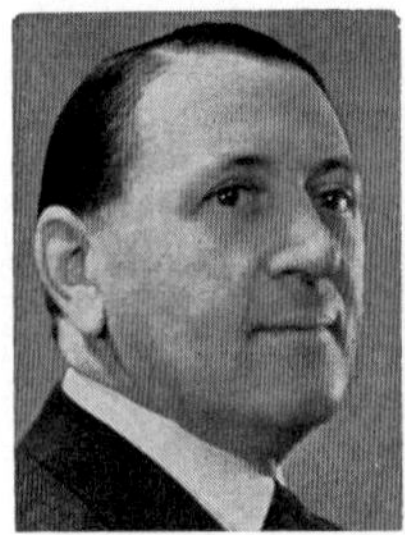
BRIAN WINDEYER

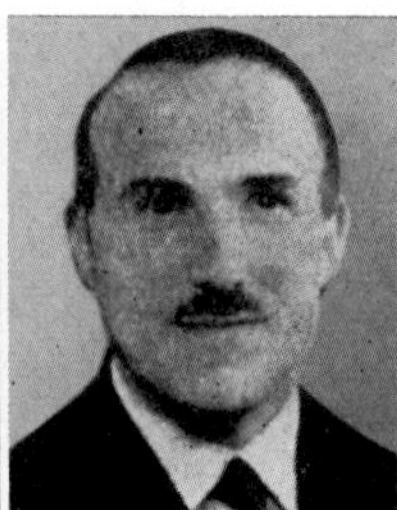
KEMP-HARPER

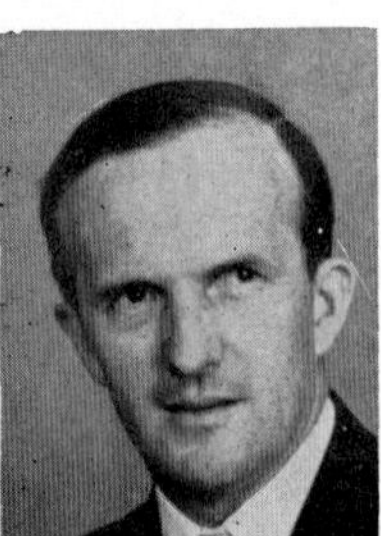
ERIC SAMUEL

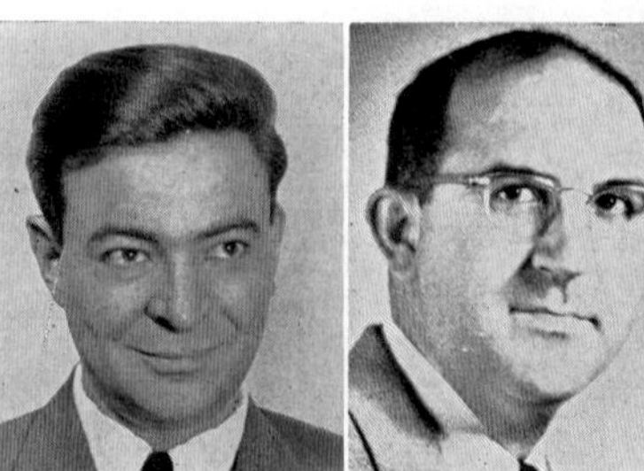
MANNIE SCHECHTER JUAN TAVERAS

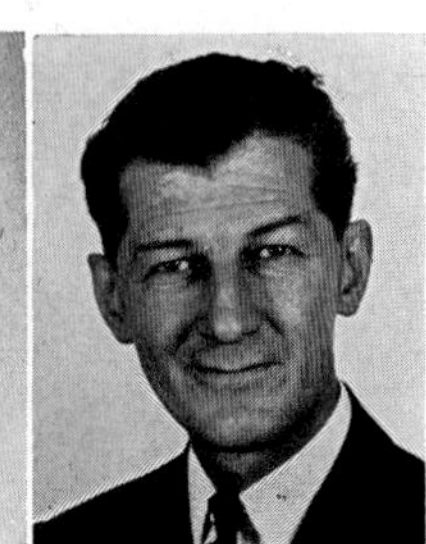
JAMES BULL

ing of about seventy radiologists was very successful (its papers were never published). Most of the people came from Belgium, Holland, France, and Germany. Lysholm was the only Swede. There were two Englishmen, Graham-Hodgson and Bull. An otologist from Paris, Chaussé, showed his apparatus and the ear projections named Chaussé I, II, III, and IV.

"The next meeting was to be held three years later, but it was postponed because of World War II. In 1947 Lysholm and Ziedses des Plantes called another meeting (Thienpont was dead), but in the same year Lysholm died. Ziedses des Plantes, the only survivor of the original triumvirate, now supported by Lindgren and Bull, arranged a second Symposium in Rotterdam in late summer of 1949. The city was still showing the effects of Allied bombings, but the meeting of about 150 people was very successful. The 1939 meeting had been part neuroradiology and part ENT (because Thienpont was an ENT specialist). The 1949 meeting was devoted to neuroradiology only, and it set the pattern.

"The third Symposium Neuroradiologicum (SN) was held in Stockholm in September, 1952 with Lindgren presiding, with over 200 in attendance. At that meeting the Swedish neuroradiologists presented the SN with a beautiful gavel.

"The fourth SN was held in London in September of 1955, under the presidency of Bull. 250 members enrolled and there were many visitors. Seventy papers were read, and the meeting lasted five days. The English neuroradiologists presented the SN with a lectern having engraved on its face a seal with two cerebral hemispheres.

"The fifth SN was held as a section of the International Congress of Neurology in Brussels in July of 1957, with Donald McRae as section president. The formula was not well accepted, and the sixth SN, held in Rome in September, 1961 – under the presidency of Giovanni Ruggiero – returned to the earlier formula, which had proved so successful. The seventh SN is being held in New York City in September, 1964, with Juan Taveras as president, and Mannie Schechter as secretary.

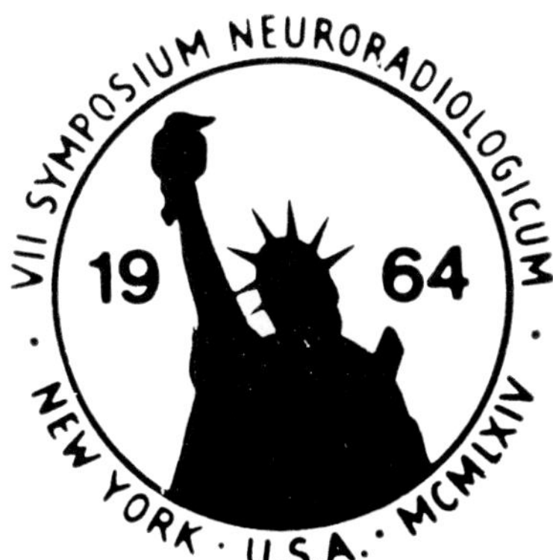

"The proceedings of the second through the sixth SN were published in *Acta Radiologica*."

COUNCIL ON RADIOLOGICAL HERITAGE

The Gas Tube Gang was first organized in 1955, then formally founded in 1956 by William Walter Wasson, a radiologist from Denver. The only qualification for membership was to have used gas tubes at some time in the past. This implied a certain age group because very few gas tubes had been in operation after (say) 1935.*

The first gatherings of the Gas Tube Gang were social occasions, with the obligatory recollections of the "early x-ray man" and his "x-ray machine." In 1960, the Gang broadened its objectives, and opened its membership to include anyone interested in the history and heritage of radiology. At a preliminary meeting held on November 27, 1961 at the Palmer House (Chicago) during the RSNA convention, the name Gas Tube Gang was changed to History Council for Radiology, then to Council for Radiological Heritage. Wasson preferred not to become its leader, and the Council chose Edwin Ernst, Sr., to be the director, with Orndoff as vice-director. The organizational meeting of a National Conference for Radiological Heritage (sponsored by the Council) took place on June 24, 1962 at McCormick House (Chicago) during the AMA convention. The Council's objectives are to encourage the collection and preservation of radiologic memorabilia, records, relics, biographies, writings, even advertisements and descriptions of early equipment.

The preservation and utilization of source material is one of the key problems in the history of science. In the wider perspective of the History of Science Society, a Conference on Science Manuscripts met in the Powell Auditorium of the Cosmos Club in Washington (D.C.) on May 5-6, 1960.

Its proceedings were published as a separate issue of *Isis* (March, 1962). It is today clearly understood that adequate source material must be secured shortly (or at least as soon as practicable) after the actual occurrence. In 1957 the AEC decided to write an official history of its activities. As a pilot study they prepared the first experimental breeder reactor (EBR-1) built in Idaho.

"The story of its operation, even more than its development, lies in the mainstream of reactor history. EBR-1 made possible the refinement and verification of basic data on the fission properties of "fast" or un-

*Gas tubes can still be purchased (for demonstration purposes) from the British manufacturer Cuthbert Andrews. The tubes are not stocked, but made on order.

moderated neutrons. It was the first reactor to use a liquid-metal coolant with a steam generator for the production of useful heat power. It was the first reactor system in the world to produce a significant amount of electrical power for continuing use. Most important of all, it demonstrated for the first time that a reactor could be designed to "breed" or to produce more fissionable material than it consumed." (Hewlett). The EBR-1 had been conceived by Walter H. Zinn while still at the MET Lab in 1945. He became Argonne's first director.

No major difficulties appeared in the pilot study of the history of EBR-1, which was easily completed. Thereupon work proceeded steadily and the first volume of the History of the AEC was published in 1962 as *The New World, 1399-46* by Richard C. Hewlett and Oscar E. Anderson, two physicists who are professional historians of science.

The importance of the preservation of historical source material for the development of science is increasingly recognized. Some of the drug manufacturers, for instance Ely Lilly in Indianapolis, even industrial giants such as DuPont in Wilmington (Delaware) have now organized their own historical archives.

In 1962 the ACR appointed an Ad Hoc Committee (composed of Lewis E. Etter, E. R. N. Grigg, and Linneus Gottfried Idstrom, with Maxwell Poppel as chairman) to study the feasibility of creating a Museum of American Radiology, and to make preliminary arrangements for the preparation of the History of American Radiology. Later on, Edith Quimby was appointed as member of the same committee. But in 1963, the appointments were left "dormant."

On February 8, 1963 — during the annual meeting of the ACR—the National Council for Radiological Heritage held its (last?) dinner reunion at the Drake Hotel in Chicago when it was decided that the Council will become part of the American College of Radiology Foundation, with the three initiators (Ernst, Orndoff, Wasson) acting as a permanent guidance and advisory committee for the historic activities of the ACR Foundation.

American radiology is maturing, both chronologically and intellectually. This is apparent in the growing awareness of, and interest in, the radiologic past. The late Arthur Fuchs (best known as an expert radiographer) made valiant efforts to establish a

History Council for Radiology
FOUNDED AS THE GAS TUBE GANG - 1950
Roentgen
Curie

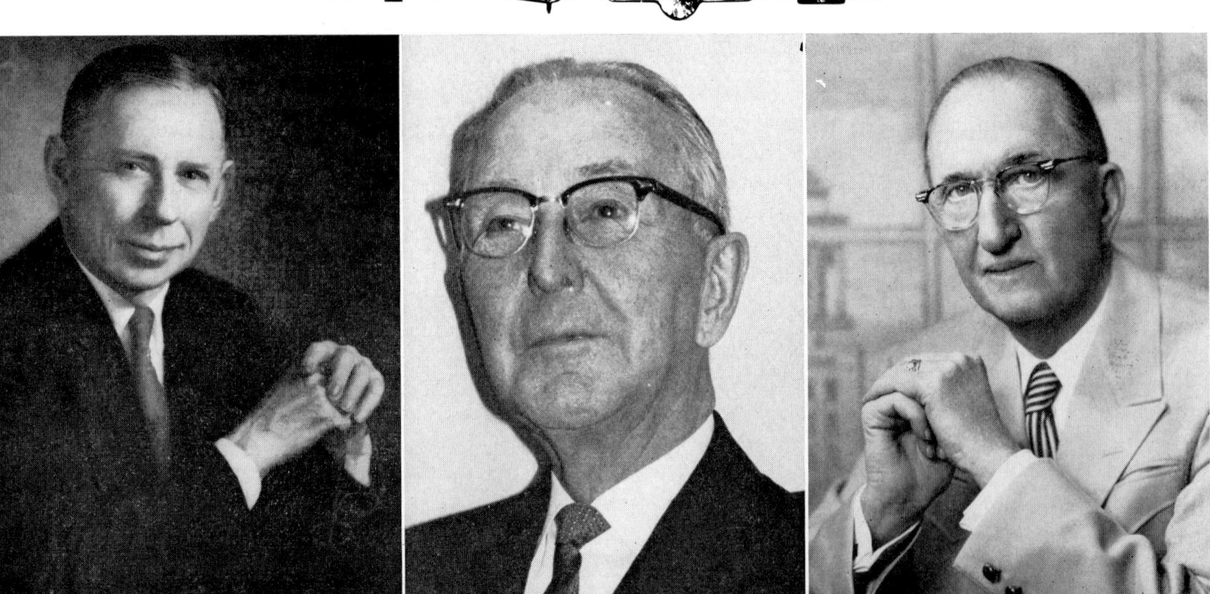

SENIOR (RADIO-HISTORIC) SPONSORS. Ben Orndoff in the middle, Walter Wasson holding his glasses, and Eddy Ernst looking through his spectacles. All three "topped" by the earliest letterhead of their organization.

museum of radiology at the Eastman Kodak House in Rochester (New York).

Late in 1963, the ACR reorganized its historic endeavors, retained the Ernst-Orndoff-Wasson triumvirate in a strictly edvisory capacity, and formed several subcommittees, one of them assigned to supervise the writing of the "history." For the writing itself, the ACR hired two science writers, the husband-and-wife team of Edward and Ruth Brecher from West cornwall (Connecticut). Another subcommittee, headed by Maxwell Poppel, was given the task of helping the "museum." One of the recently appointed members of poppel's subcommittee is Robert Morrison, the radiologic advisor of the George Eastman House (he took the place of the late Arthur Fuchs). Incidentally, Poppel himself has a collection of about 80 gas tubes, in storage in his department Bellevue Hospital.

In an editorial in the *Bulletin of the Atomic Scientists* of November, 1963, Eugene Rabinovitch wrote: "History is a long, long tail that helps to make the social

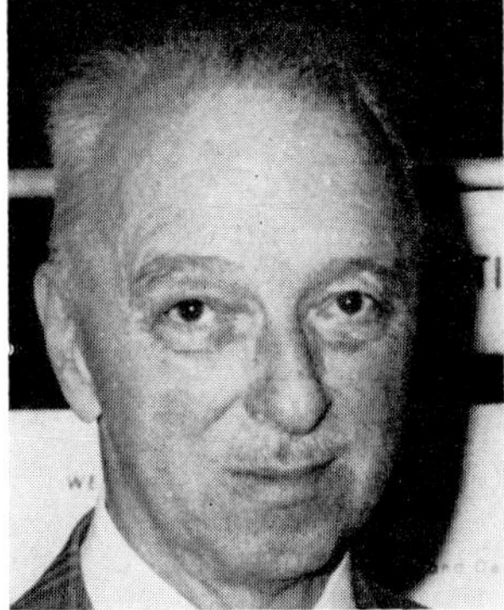

ROBERT MORRISON

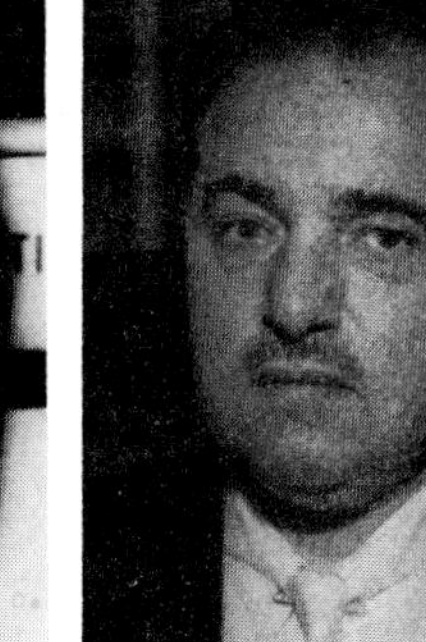

MAXWELL POPPEL

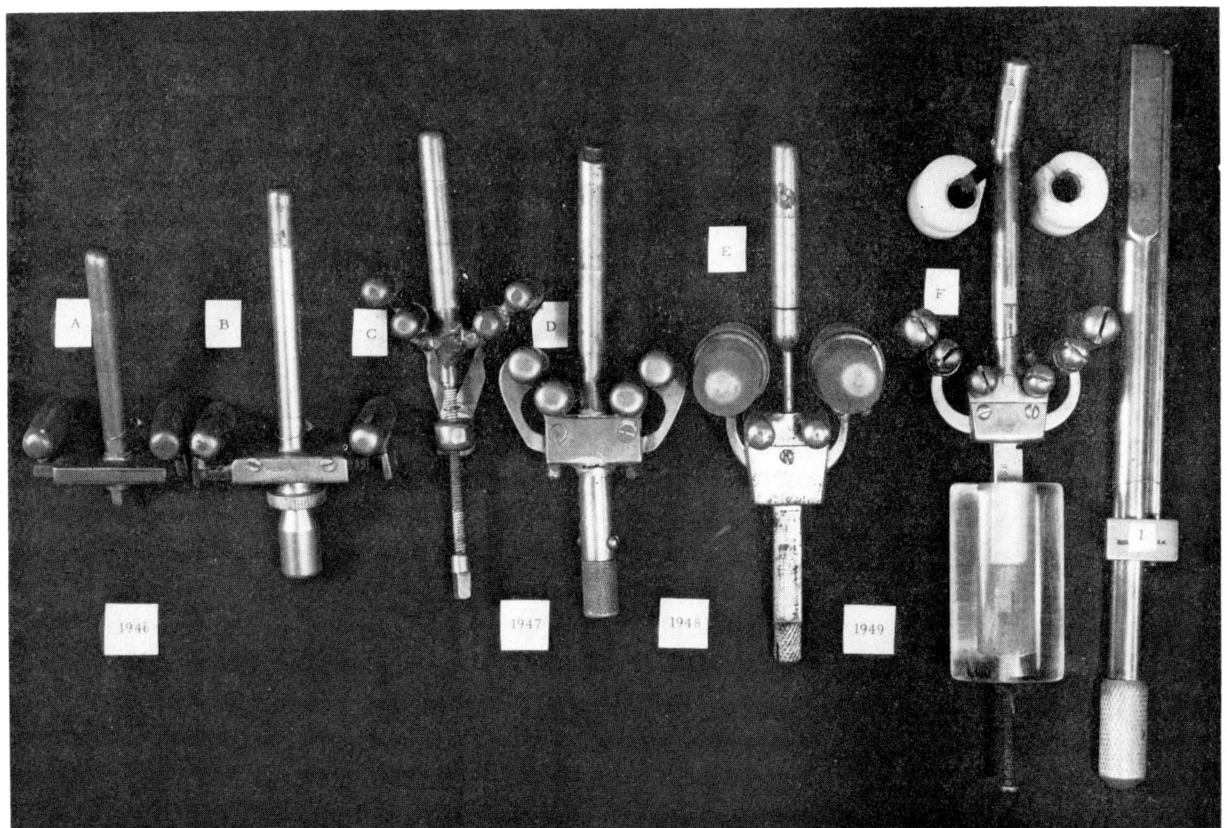

Courtesy: Eddy Ernst, Sr.

GENEALOGIC TREE OF ERNST'S APPLICATOR. The first expanding type of cervico-uterine radium applicator carries the eponym of Edwin Charles Ernst, Sr. who showed his first model in 1946 to the second Mexican Cancer Congress in Guadalajara. That first model had two vaginal sources connected to a stem placed in the uterine canal. At the 2nd IACR (Havana), in 1946, Ernst showed an applicator with four vaginal capsules. At the RSNA meeting in 1948 in Chicago, the stem had been increased to three capsules, and six vaginal capsules, a total of nine capsules for the entire applicator. A full set of dosage measurements appeared in the *American Journal of Roentgenology* of May, 1961, and were also distributed to the profession in a brochure printed by Ansco.

body ponderous, cumbersome, not readily maneuverable. But it is not a tail that can be docked without great danger. The impatient and the cocksure can disregard the past only at the cost of grave error, frustration, and futility."

CHARLIE SMITH

To exemplify what a single person can do in terms of collecting important historic material, I am reproducing a letter received from Charlie Smith, owner of the Pennsylvania X-Ray Corporation of Philadelphia:

"January 24, 1963

"Dear Dr. Grigg:

"The box containing the old manufacturers' catalogues was picked up by Railway Express today. I have sent you the complete collection as follows:

1. American X-Ray Equipment Co., New York City. Manufactured a Coil Dental Machine and Tubestand. 1915
2. The Baker Electric Co., Hartford, Conn. Static Machine & Tesla Coils also called Baker X-Ray Co. 1912 ?
3. Geo W. Brady. X-Ray Accessories. Paragon Plates. 1916 ?
4. Campbell Brothers, Lynn, Mass. 1905. X-Ray Coils, later became Campbell Electric Co., still in business
5. O. Carliczek & Co., Chicago. X-Ray Tubes. Letter in catalog to Dr. Pfahler, dated 1910
6. Otis Clapp & Sons, Boston, Mass. agent for Scheidel Coil, 1900, 1902. Sold Gundelach tubes
7. Clapp-Eastham Co., Boston, Mass. Coils 1908. Quality coil, Standard Coil, Ceco Coil.
8. Jno. V. Doehren Co. The X-Ray House, Chicago. Coils, Green & Bauer Tubes. 1909 ?
9. Electro-Radiation Co., Boston, 1905. Hercules Coil, Ajax Coil.
10. The Friedlander Co., Chicago, 1906 ? Complete line of coils, tubes, accessories.
11. Wm. Gaertner & Co., Chicago, 1912. Static machines, coils, tubes
12. Electric Conversion Co., Brookline, Mass. 1913. Cabot High Potential D.C. Converter.
13. The Engeln Electric Co., Cleveland, 1921. Complete line of x-ray Kelley-Koett representatives.
14. High Tension Transformer and Equipment Corporation, Union Hill, N. J. X-Ray generators, 1920 ?
15. Keystone Electric Co., Philadelphia. Manufacturer's Agent. Electro-Therapy. Scheidel-Coil Distributor. 1904.
16. Kelley-Koett Mfrs. Co., Inc. Covington, Kentucky, 1909 ? Table and nr. 6 Tubestand showing Kelley as model; also letter written by Ed. Geise and Wilbur Werner to C. W. Smith announcing death of J. Robt. Kelley.
17. Kesselring X-Ray Tube Co., Chicago, 1906 ? Tube manufacturer.
18. X-Ray Tube Co., New York City. Manufacturer of "standard" x-ray tubes, 1915.
19. The Kny-Scheerer Co., New York City, 1905. This company had a complete line in the beginning. Later they became Keleket distributors, discontinued x-ray activity about 1920, but were still in business in 1922.
20. Heinz-Wandner X-Ray Tube Co., Chicago, 1910 ? Tube manufacturer; catalog shows glass blowers at work.
21. Paul Luckenbach & Co., New York City, 1925 X-Ray Measuring instruments.
22. Macalaster-Wiggin Co., 1906. X-ray tubes and accessories, later fused & Victor
23. E. Machlett & Co. X-Ray Tube manufacturers 1902 ? 1914 catalog shows glass blowers at work.
24. McIntosh Battery and Optical Co., Chicago, 1912. Manufacturer of the Hogan Silent X-Ray Transformer.
25. The Wm. Meyer Company, Chicago, 1912. Manufacturers of x-ray apparatus.
26. E. B. Meyrowitz, New York City, 1906. X-Ray apparatus
27. V. Mueller & Co., Chicago, 1911. Distributor

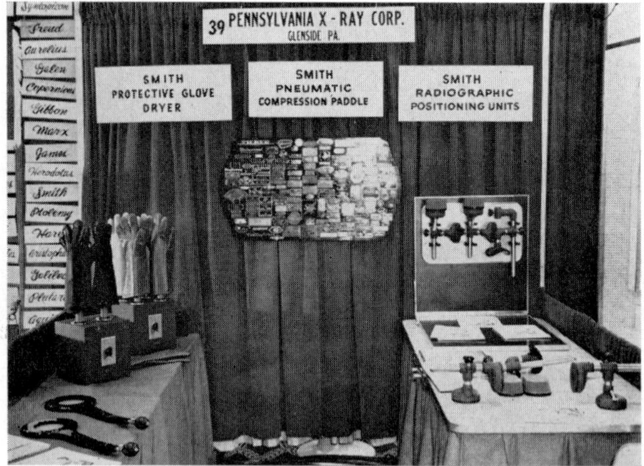

Charlie's own exhibit. This is the way it appeared at the RSNA meeting in Chicago (1962). At that convention I showed Charlie (in the presence of Tom Rogers from Machlett) some of my slides on the history of radiology. Thereupon Charlie decided to let me take a look at his collection of old x-ray catalogs.

for Victor (Wantz), Scheidel and Western.

28. Queen & Co., Philadelphia, 1899; manufacturers of coils, tubes, and accessories.
29. General Electric Co., Edison Decorative and Miniature Lamp Dept., Harrison, N.J. x-ray coils and tubes.
30. W. Scheidel Coil Co., Chicago, 1906. X-Ray apparatus, joined with Western.
31. Snook-Roentgen Manufacturing Co., Philadelphia 1907. Snook first worked for Queen, then Homer Snook founded the Roentgen Manufacturing Co. Made first interrupterless transformer.
32. X-Rays and Snook, 1916. The only copy of this brochure I have ever seen. Complete story of the Snook transformer.
33. Standard X-Ray Company, Chicago 1918. The Story of Standard, x-ray equipment.
34. Swett & Lewis, Boston, Mass., 1902. Manufacturers of the Kinraide Coil.
35. Victor Electric Corporation, Chicago, 1908 ? roentgen apparatus and high frequency outfits. The Wantz Radiographic Coil.
36. R. V. Wagner & Co., Chicago 1899, Electrical Supplies. This is a classic. Full page on how x-ray examinations are made (illustrated). Also why induction coils produce burns and static machines do not.
37. Wandner and Son, X-Ray Tube Co., Chicago, 1911 ? Tube makers
38. Waite & Bartlett Mfg. Co., Long Island City, 1905, x-ray apparatus.
39. Wappler Electric Mfg. Cp., 1914, x-ray apparatus.
40. Williams, Brown & Earle, Dealers in x-ray coils, 1906. Sold Victor and W & B.
41. also (belatedly) James G. Biddle, Philadelphia, complete line of coils, x-ray tables, tubes.

"I also included all of the early European catalogs found in Dr. Pfahler's collection at the time of his death. There are four very early books on x rays, Morton's (1896), Meadowcroft's (1896), Kolle's (1898), and the *Elements of Static Electricity,* which was published in 1895, but has a chapter on electrical currents in vacuum, which makes very interesting reading. Two of these books contain advertisements of x-ray material.

"The original photographic glass plates of Kassabian's hands, which he took himself, as well as the newspaper clippings which appeared in the Philadelphia papers at the time of Kassabian's death, are included.

"I have sent you a photograph of John Carbutt, and a picture of Dr. Newcomet and Sarah Kingston (his technician), taken at the Moore School of Electrical Engineering when he demonstrated my Queen Coil to the Society for Non-Destructive Testing of Metals, a group of men engaged in industrial x-ray work around Philadelphia.

"I will try and find for you a picture of myself but I have had very few taken and it may not be easy.

"I have a picture of the Franklin Head Unit taken the first time we showed it at Cincinnati in 1949, and one of the bi-plane angio (Wampus) unit, designed by Dr. E. Chamberlain of Temple University. The very first Head Unit that I have any knowledge of was designed by Dr. Willis Manges of Jefferson Medical College. It was a wooden frame on which was mounted an x-ray tube which allowed the patient to stand or sit against an angulating cassette holder. The tube could then be angulated to the proper position as well as raised or lowered for height.

"The first head unit produced in this country by a manufacturer was designed by Paul Hodges of the University of Chicago. It was made by Angabright and was known as the Hodges Head Stand.

"With the advent of the rotating anode tube it was found that the vibration of the early rotors caused vibration in the tube arm of the Hodges unit, mess-

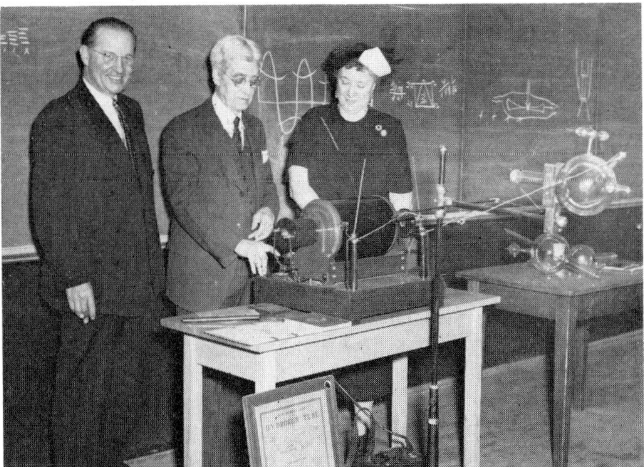

Demonstration of a Queen coil (1954). Charles Smith smiles while William Stell Newcomet, assisted by his longtime x-ray technician, Miss Sarah Kingston, pushes the contact which actuates the coil, and energizes the hydrogen tube, placed on the other table. This coil, which is in perfect operating condition, is still in the possession of Charles Smith. The demonstration took place at the Moore School of Electrical Engineering of the University of Pennsylvania, in Philadelphia.

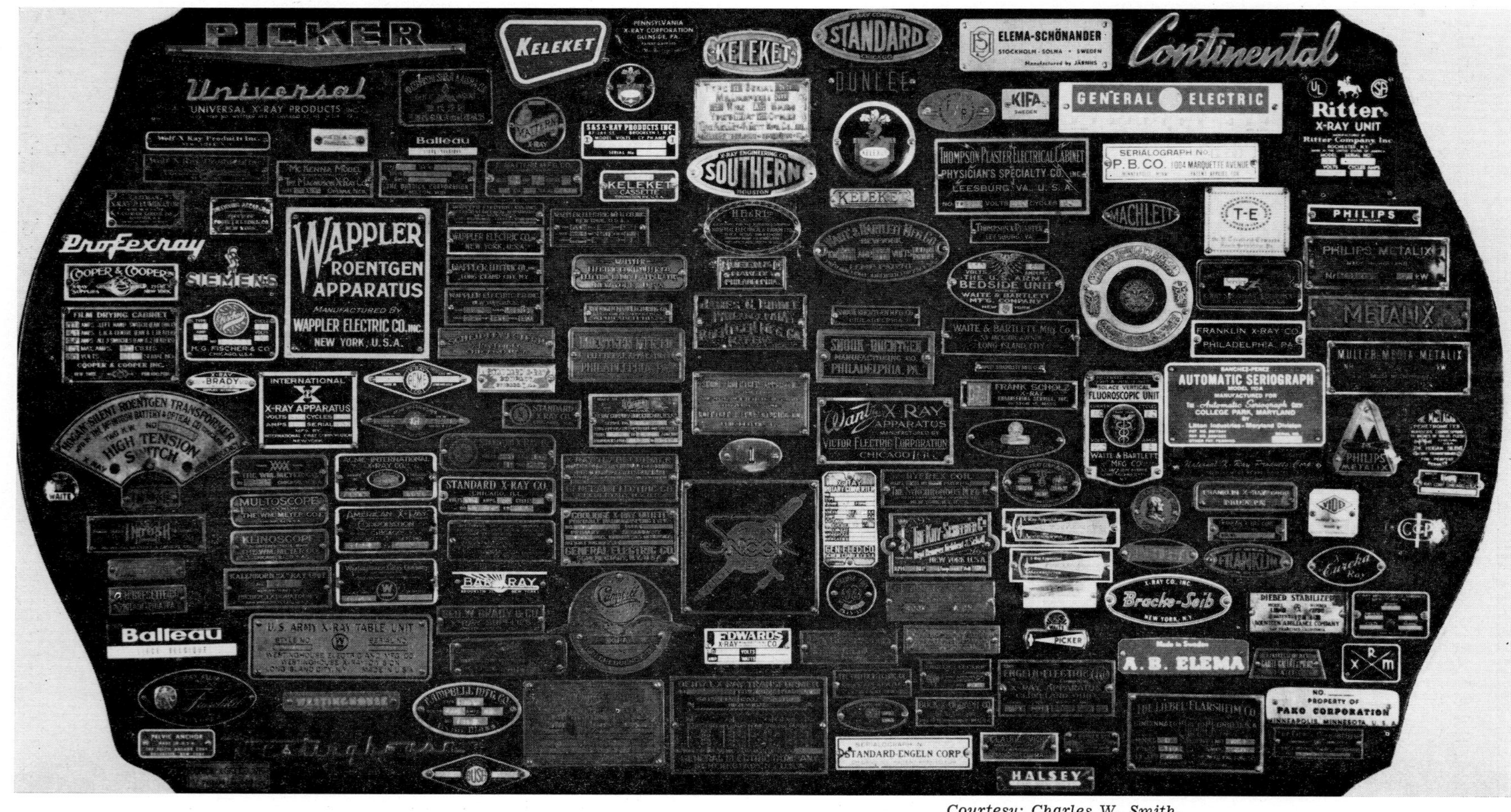

Courtesy: Charles W. Smith.

CHARLIE'S X-RAY MARKS. Interesting collection of plates of various American (and of a few foreign) manufacturers of x-ray equipment, both old and new, which is always part of the technical exhibit of the Pennsylvania X-Ray Corporation. Every year the collection is a bit more crowded, maybe next year the supporting plate will have to be "made bigger."

ing up the focal spot diameter. That was when the Franklin Head Unit came into being.

"It was designed by Wm. J. Hogan of Franklin X-Ray, and I can still see Herman Spranger, Franklin's shop foreman, cutting out the patterns for the component castings with his pocket knife.

"If you have not heard from Franklin by the time you receive this letter, let me know and I will try to have them write the history of Franklin for you.

"Dr. George Wohl, chief of the Department of Radiology at the Philadelphia General Hospital, has asked me to work with him as consultant on the George E. Pfahler memorial room (Pfahler Sanctum) at the hospital. It is to be equipped with early apparatus, contemporaneous with Pfahler's time as chief there, and will be used as a meeting room for 'Old Blockley' residents in radiology, past and present.

"In the box I sent you is Pfahler's caliper (he was one of the first to advocate a technique involving measurement of the part), please treat it as he has inscribed it for his technicians: 'don't be careless, and don't drop it on the floor!' The caliper will be placed in the Pfahler Sanctum.

"I was engaged by Dr. George Pfahler Keefer (Dr. George Edward Pfahler's nephew), heir to the Pfahler offices, to dismantle and appraise the equipment. Hence I fell heir to many things which otherwise would have been destroyed. One of the things most painful to remember was the taking of an acetylene torch to a ten year old GE 250 kvp therapy machine. At the time of its installation, it had to be derricked three floors up from Chestnut Street into the office. There was no other way to get the sizable oil-filled head containing tube and transformer into Pfahler's office. To get it out would have meant to derrick it out the way it had come in, at a cost of $2500, with tying up traffic on Chestnut Street for all of a Sunday afternoon. We had no choice but to put the torch to it, and cut it into small pieces small enough to load on a junk dealer's truck.

"Enclosed find a casting of the first membership pin of the ARRS. The original is owned by the son of Dr. Stewart, an early Philadelphia radiologist.

"Incidentally, I have an original Ruhmkorff Coil made in Paris by the Carpentier Co. in 1886. It was used at the Drexel Institute (Philadelphia) in pre-Roentgen experiments.

"I have a Queen Coil in Al condition. It is with tubestand and tube made in 1898, as an x-ray machine. It produces roentgen plates as satisfactorily as it did back in 1898 when it was purchased by Dr. Stewart, Sr.

"If and when a Museum of American Radiology were to be established, I would be glad to donate all this material to them for safe-keeping and utilization in a proper environment. Yours truly (ss) Charles W. Smith."

OTHER RADIOHISTORIC INDIVIDUALISTS

It has become a modern trend to regard teamwork as the solution to most problems. Five, seven, or eleven heads are certainly better than one, but could a committee have written Hamlet? Even in the peculiar world of today, one head, supported by one income, can still achieve things which to a committee might appear to be a staggering, impossible task.

William Shehadi (known for his cholecystographic endeavors, crystallized in a recent text, entitled *Radiology of the Biliary Tract*) has over 100 gas tubes, many of them of very early vintage, collector's items. Herbert Pollack (specialist not only in the x-ray examination of patients, but also in that of paintings and pottery) organized the roentgen section of the Hall of Fame of the International College of Surgeons in Chicago. Linneus Idstrom (a radiologist from Minneapolis, with a special interest in audio-

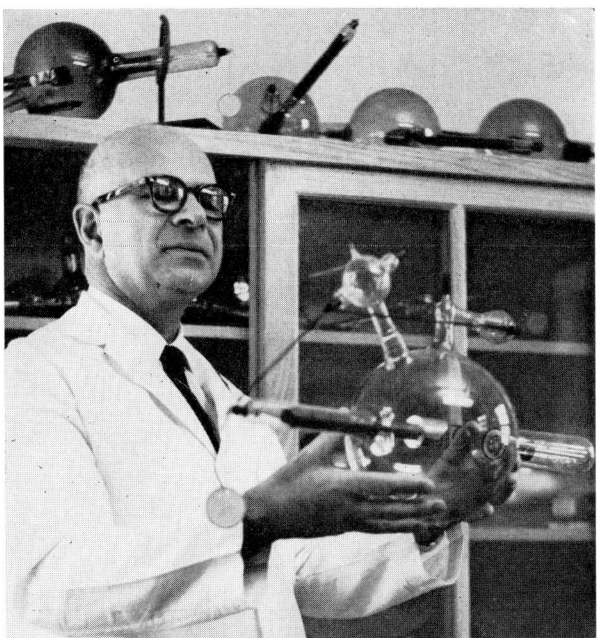

William Henry Shehadi and his tubes. The specimen shown is a gas tube with magnetic ring for "focusing" purposes (by changing the position of the anode). In the background are some of the cold cathode tubes from Shehadi's collection.

visual teaching techniques) has recorded a large number of taped interviews with great men in radiology (and para-radiology). Stanley Paul Bohrer (a former Page Boy in the House of Representatives in Washington, who has recently completed a residency in radiology in Massachusetts General Hospital) has a large collection of stamps, cachets, covers, and other philatelic *objets d' art* on the subject of radiology, including both apparatus and portraits - he had exhibited some of his most significant items at radiologic conventions, and several of them have been reproduced in these pages. And Egon George Wissing (a radiologist from Boston) has a goodly number of old books, manuscripts, and diverse memorabilia from both American and other roentgen pioneers.

I have summarized the *History of American Radiology* on 56 14x17″ panels, each containing five 5x7″ transparencies and one caption. This exhibit was shown in 1963 at the meetings of the ARRS in Montreal, and of the RSNA in Chicago. It will become part of the collection of the projected Museum of American Radiology. The material served as a basis for a brief text, entitled *The New History of* (American) *Radiology.*

Howard Doub is the RSNA's official historian. There is no officer assigned to such a task in either the ACR or the ARRS. Nevertheless, more historic articles have appeared in *The American Journal of Roentgenology* (both absolutely and proportionally) than in *Radiology.*

Among the radio-historic writers in this country, Otto Glasser occupies a pioneering position of preeminence; he has produced less during the Atomic Phase, but his biography of Röntgen is an indelible source of facts, and so remains his volume *Science of Radiology* (soon to be re-issued by Lewis E. Etter). Kenneth Allen (Wasson's office partner) of Denver edited the *History of Radiology in World War II,* soon to be published by the Federal Government. The late Percy Brown's *American Martyrs to Science through the Roentgen Rays* will have a new edition including radio-martyr Percy Brown's own biography (editor: E. R. N. Grigg). Stephen Bronson Dewing, a radiologist from Flemington (New Jersey), has recently authored a text on *Modern Radiology in Historical Perspective,* a lean (*i.e.,* meaty) review of important materials from the earliest days to the present. Andre Bruwer, a radiologist from South Africa who worked for some time at the Mayo Clinic,

RÖNTGENKUNDE IN EINZELDARSTELLUNGEN

HERAUSGEGEBEN VON
H. H. BERG-DORTMUND UND K. FRIK-BERLIN
BAND 3

WILHELM CONRAD RÖNTGEN
UND
DIE GESCHICHTE DER RÖNTGENSTRAHLEN

VON
DR. OTTO GLASSER
CLEVELAND CLINIC FOUNDATION

MIT EINEM BEITRAG
PERSÖNLICHES ÜBER W. C. RÖNTGEN
VON
MARGRET BOVERI
BERLIN

MIT 96 ABBILDUNGEN

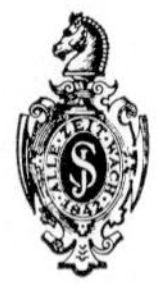

BERLIN
VERLAG VON JULIUS SPRINGER
1931

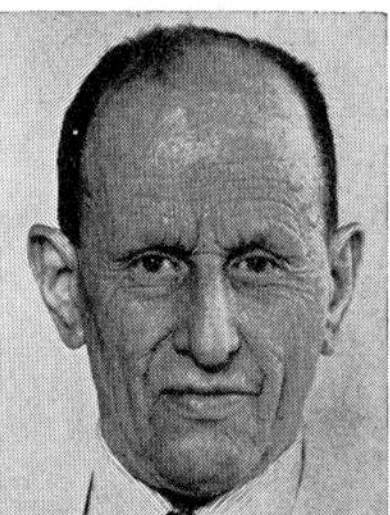

EGON WISSING KENNETH ALLEN

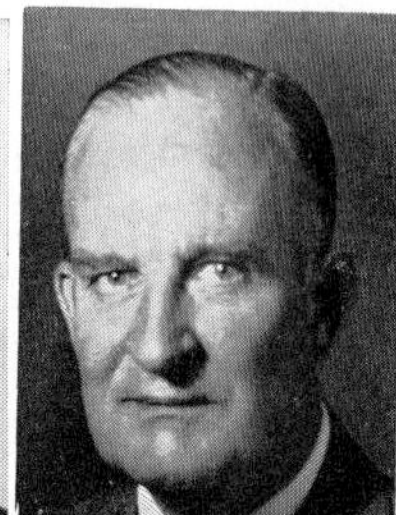

HOWARD DOUB

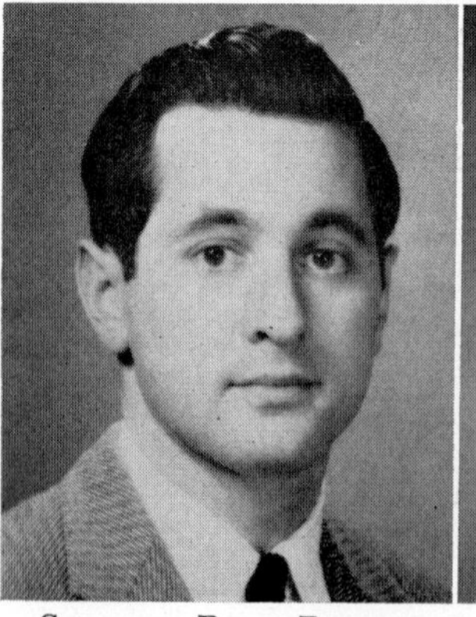

STANLEY PAUL BOHRER

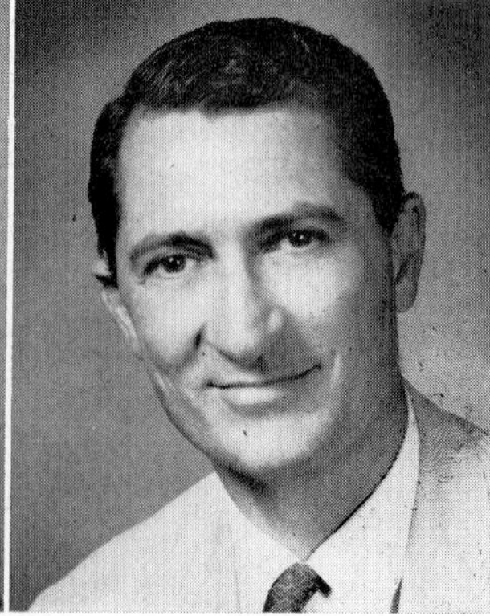

ANDRÉ BRUWER

then established himself in Tucson (Arizona), has edited *Classic Descriptions in Diagnostic Roentgenology,* which contains both original texts and comments on the significance of the respective passages. It is more than a coincidence that all the books mentioned in this paragraph have been or will be issued by the (truly "radio-publishing") house of Charles C Thomas, Publisher.

The house was established in 1928 by Charles Crankshaw Thomas, and was changed into a partnership about 1945; the three partners are Charles, his wife Nanette Payne Thomas, and their son, Payne Edward Lloyd Thomas. The latter is currently the actual head of the firm, which recently moved its headquarters (but not its sales and advertising offices) from the Bannerstone House in Springfield (Illinois) to the Natchez Plantation House in Fort Lauderdale (Florida).

Joseph Burns, Sr., who was born in Relay, an old railroad town in Maryland, once told me of a solid stone curved bridge over the Patapsco river, which is the dividing line between the Baltimore and Howard counties. That stone bridge – the Thomas Viaduct (completed in 1835) – is named after Philip Evan Thomas (1776-1861), the first president of the Baltimore and Ohio Railroad. Relay is the home town of the Thomas family – Philip Thomas and the great-grandfather of Charles Thomas were brothers.

The Bannerstone House, built by the famous architect Frank Lloyd Wright (1869-1959), derives its name from one of those perforated twin-winged stones (found only in America), which could be slipped over a staff to serve as banners in ancient tribal rites. Charles Thomas always cherished this particular bannerstone – he called it the "scarab of Stone Age chieftains of the Mississippi Valley" –even placed its image on his mandala. Payne is quite modern – as a seasoned pilot he flies the firm's twin engine plane (a Riley-modified Cessna 310).

RADIOLOGIC BEST-SELLERS

Regarding the quantity and quality of radiologic books marketed, Charles C Thomas, Publisher is well ahead of all American publishers. But quality in a book is not the most important factor in deciding whether or not it will sell properly. I asked the Thomas company which had been, over the past twenty years, their three radiologic best-sellers? They named (1) *The Head and Neck in Roentgen Diagnosis* by Pendergrass, Schaeffer, and Hodes; (2) *The Fundamentals of X-Ray and Ra-*

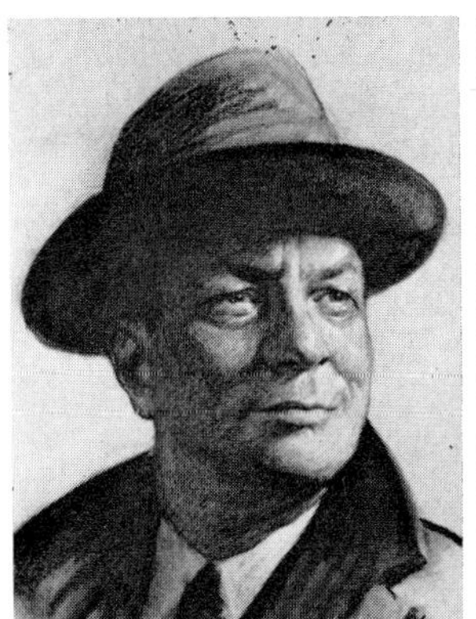

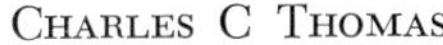

Charles C Thomas

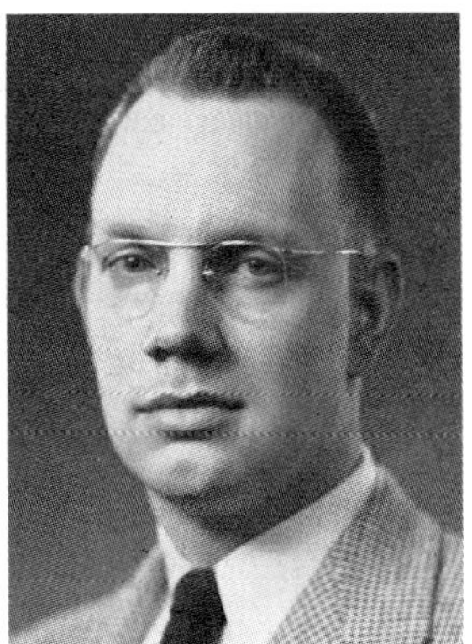

Payne E. L. Thomas

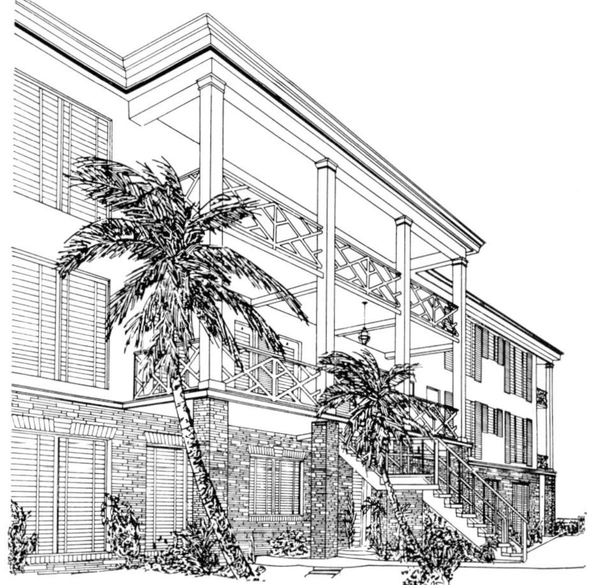

Natchez Plantation House

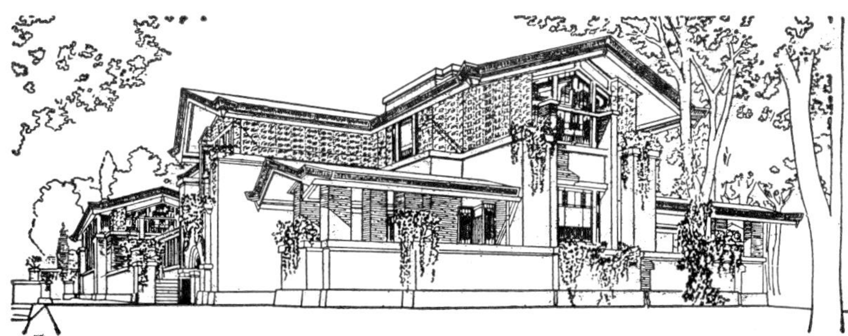

Bannerstone House

dium Physics by Selman; and (3) *The Physics of Radiology,* by Johns. Their all-time radiologic best-seller was Glenn Files' *Medical Radiographic Technic.*

The same question was submitted to other American publishers, to determine whether a definite "trend" could be elicited. J. B. Lippincott Company of Philadelphia – publishers since 1792 – listed (1) Buckstein's *Digestive Tract in Roentgenology;* (2) Rigler's *Outline of Roentgen Diagnosis;* and (3) Stein, Stein and Beller's *Living Bone in Health and Disease.*

Lea & Febiger of Philadelphia – the oldest publisher in the USA (since 1785) – noted their radiologic best-sellers as (1) Jaffe's *Tumors and Tumorous Conditions of Bones and Joints;* (2) Quimby, Feitelberg and Silver's *Radioactive Isotopes in Clinical Practice;* and (3) Ennis' *Dental Roentgenology.*

Williams & Wilkins Company of Baltimore explained that many of their radiologic books which sold well were British imports, such as Brailsford's *Radiology of Bones and Joints* or Cade's *Malignant Disease and Its Treatment by Radium.* In 1951 Williams & Wilkins purchased the Medical Department of Thomas Nelson and Sons of New York City – including Golden's *Diagnostic Roentgenology.* Now Williams & Wilkins best is Traveras & Wood's *Neuroradiology.*

The Year Book Medical Publishers, of Chicago, specified (1) Caffey's *Pediatric X-Ray Diagnosis;* (2) Kjellberg et al.'s *Diagnosis of Congenital Heart Disease* (a Swedish contribution); and (3) the *Year Books of Radiology.*

Grune & Stratton, Inc., of New York City indicated that their radiologic best-sellers had been Case's translations of (1) Schinz *et al.'s Roentgen-Diagnostics;* and of (2) Köhler's *Borderlands of Normal and Pathologic in Skeletal Roentgenology.* Then they had (3) Buschke's *Progress in Radiation Therapy.*

Little, Brown & Company – a relative newcomer in the medical field – mentioned (1) Abrams' *Angiography;* (2) Wilson's *Anatomical Foundation of Neuroradiology of the Brain;* and (3) Walter and Miller's *Short Textbook of Radiotherapy.*

C. V. Mosby Company, of St. Louis, placed (1) Merrill's *Atlas of Roentgenographic Positions* ahead of (2) Jacobi-Hagen's *X-Ray Technology,* and of (3) Ackerman and Del Regato's *Cancer,* but thought that before long Jacobi-Hagen's text would become their best-seller.

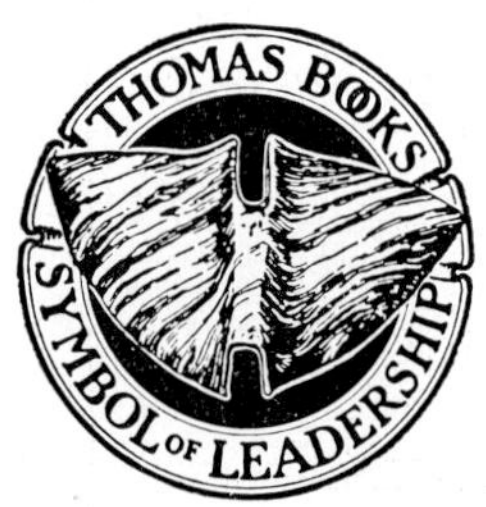

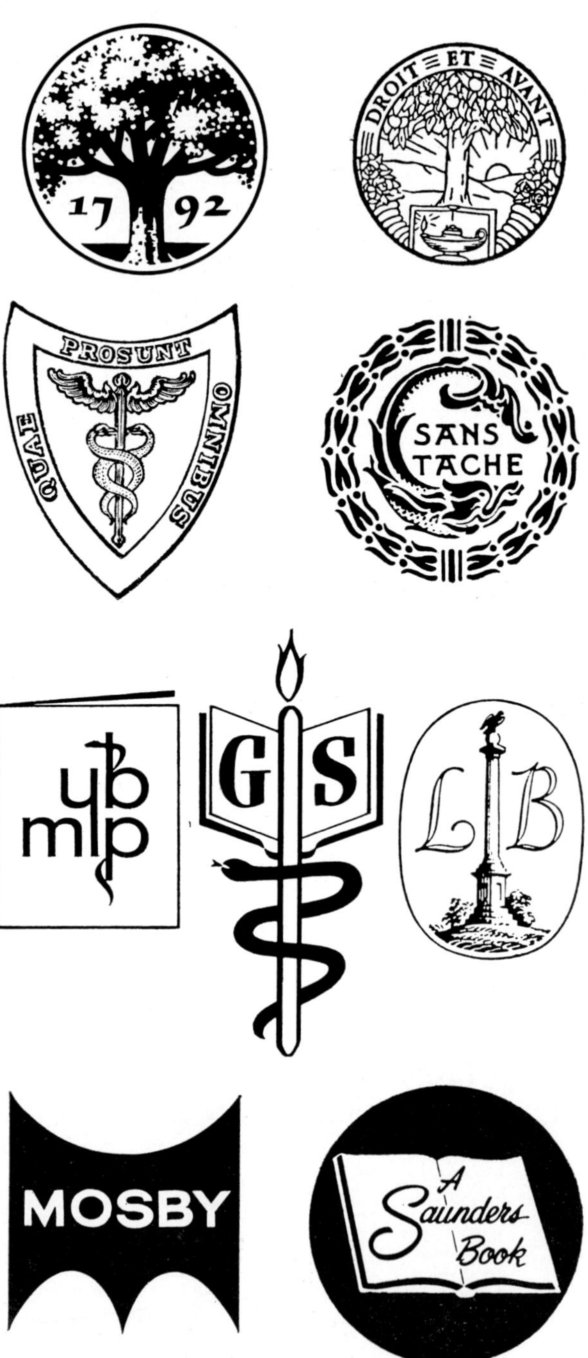

AMERICAN PUBLISHERS' MANDALAS. The two "trees" are Lippincott's. The curvacious triangle belongs to Lea & Febiger. The spotless dolphin is the mark of Williams & Wilkins. Initials are used by the Medical Year Book Publishers, by Grune & Stratton, Inc. and by Little, Brown & Company, while Mosby and Saunders spell their names.

W. B. Saunders of Philadelphia has among its radiologic best-sellers (1) Meschan's *Normal Radiologic Anatomy;* (2) Felson's *Chest Roentgenology;* and (3) Stafne's *Oral Roentgenographic Diagnosis.*

Hoeber-Harper is the way the Hoeber Medical Division of Harper & Brothers of New York City calls itself on the title page of a leaflet on "books in Radiology and Roentgenology." My letter(s) regarding their radiologic best-sellers must have been lost in the mail, because they never answered. I know two of them, (1) Glasser & al.'s *Physical Foundations of Radiology;* and (2) Paul & Juhl's *Essentials of Roentgen Interpretation.*

What makes a radiologic best-seller? It helps if the book is "good," meaning it has both worthwhile and readable text, its illustrations are excellent, and its other typographic assets within acceptable standards. But this is not enough. Even more important is (1) that the author be well known, (2) that the topic be of the "bread-and-butter" type, usable in actual practice, and (3) that there be a large potential "audience" for that book. With fifty thousand x-ray technicians in the USA, it becomes understandable why so many technical texts are among radiologic best-sellers.

The difference between a "good" medical publisher and a "great" one is that the latter – while not forgetting that he is in business to make money (a *sine-qua-non* for survival) – regards it as his moral obligation to accept for publication not only potential best-sellers, but also a number of manuscripts which are just scientifically valid, or otherwise worth to be preserved in print. In this respect, perusal of past performance of the Thomas Company demonstrates that it is a truly great publishing house from a medical viewpoint, and particularly from our restricted radiologic viewpoint. And since the publishing business has its own, ever-present intangibles, once in a while a so-called prestige book will turn out to be, if not a best, at least a "good-seller."

ISR, ICR, FRPCL, CORD, EAR, ACTR

Returning now to the discussion of post-World War II radiologic associations, it is necessary to mention the International Society of Radiology, created at the seventh ICR in Copenhagen (1953); it is actually an office (with Fleming Norgaard as secretary), which bridges the gap between successive meetings of the ICR.

In 1962 the ISR computed a total of 14 thousand radiologist-members in its 44 component societies.

In the Atomic Phase, the ICR resumed its meetings in 1950 in London (6th ICR), with Ralston Paterson as president, and J. W. McLaren as secretary. At the 7th ICR, Flemming-Moller was president, and Flemming Norgaard was secretary. The 8th ICR was held in Mexico City, Manuel Madrazo presided, and José Noriega was secretary.

The ICR with the largest attendance (so far) was the 9th in München (1959), under the presidency of Boris Rajevsky, with Heinrich von Braunbehrens as secretary. The 10th ICR, held in Montreal, had Arthur Singleton as presiding officer, and Carleton Peirce conducting the secretariat. The next (11th) ICR will con-

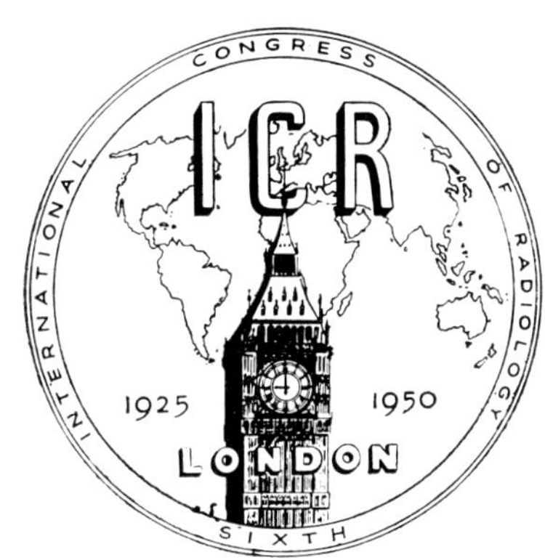

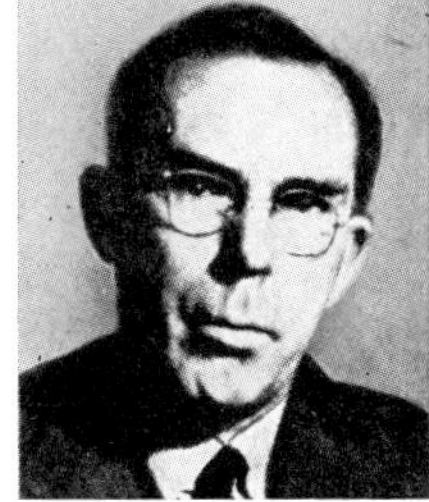

J. R. K. Paterson

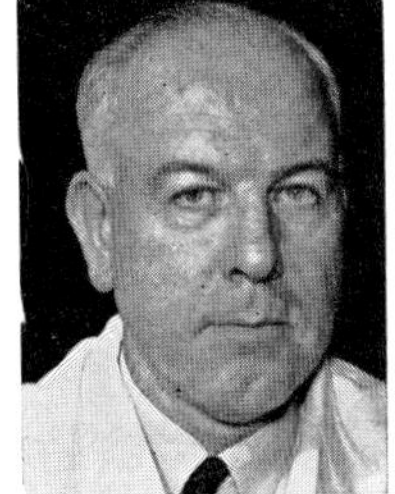

J. W. McLaren

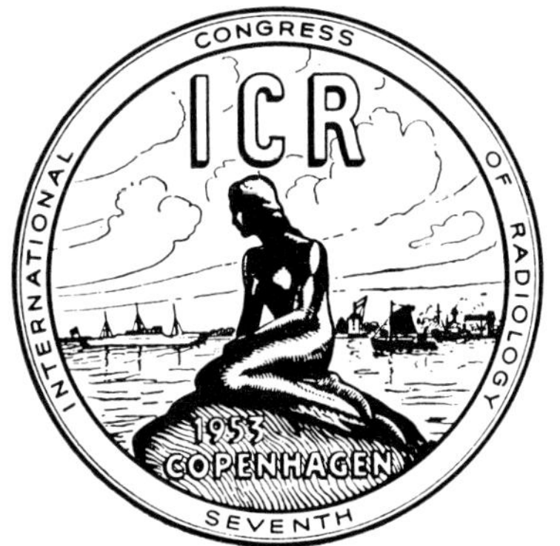

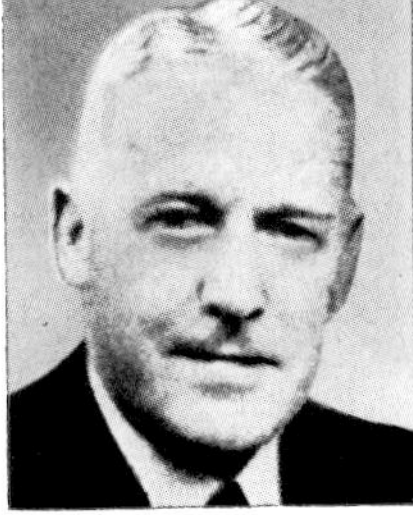

Flemming Møller

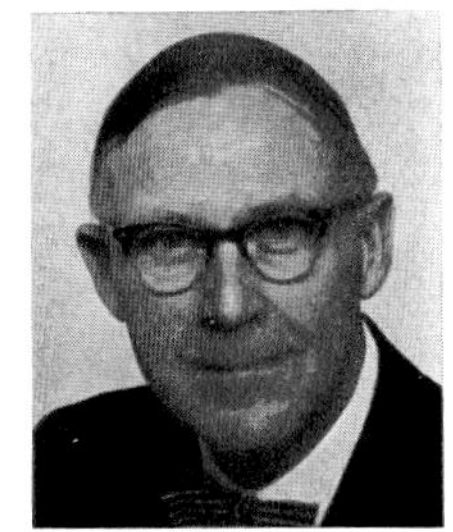

Flemming Nørgaard

vene – in 1965 – in Rome, the organizing officers being Luigi Turano (president) and Arduino Ratti (secretary). The decision was reached to hold thereafter the ICR every four years (instead of every three as was done until now), so as not to interfere with the IACR: there will then be one really international ICR every four years, while at mid-time there will be in America a continental meeting, and at the same time in Europe a meeting of the Radiologists of Latin Culture, an assembly which seems to acquire truly all-European coverage (it may soon change its name to underline this fact).

The next best thing to changing the name of an old organization is to create a new one. The European Association of Radiology was founded in Strassbourg on December 15, 1962. The statutes had been prepared by a committee which had met in Paris, in 1961, during the meeting of the Fédération Latine. The first slate of officers of the Association Européene de Radiologie were B. Rajewski of Frankfurt/Main (president); Cr. Gros of Strassbourg (secretary); A. Zuppinger of Bern (treasurer); S. Masy of Louvain, E. Benassi of Turin, and von Ronnen of Leiden (vice-presidents). The four former presidents of the Fédération des Radiologists des Pays de Culture Latine – R. Coliez, C. Gil y Gil, J. Maisin, and A. Saldanha – were elected as honorary members.

A World Association of Academic Professors of Medical Radiology was created in Switzerland in the year 1961. It held its organizational meeting at the Cantonal Hospital in Zurich, having been called by Hans Schinz (who had presided over the fourth ICR) and by his associate, Umberto Cocchi. It is called (in Latin) Collegium Orbis Radiologiae Docentium.

The ICR is all-inclusive, and yet it lead to the creation of a very exclusive group, the International Club of Radiotherapists.

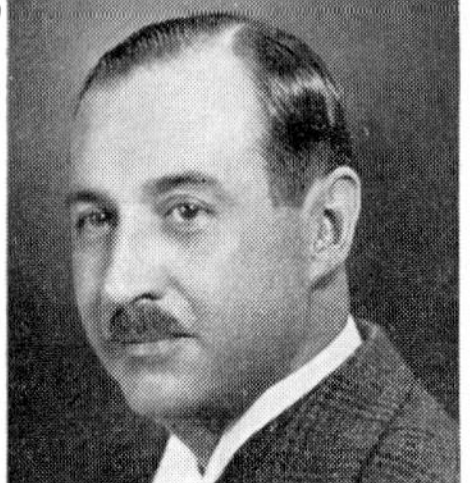

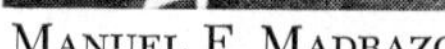

MANUEL F. MADRAZO

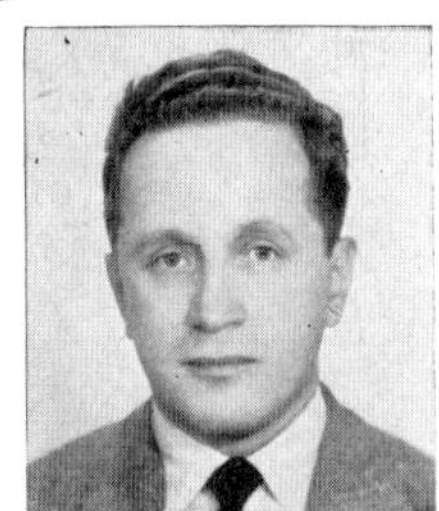

JOSE NORIEGA

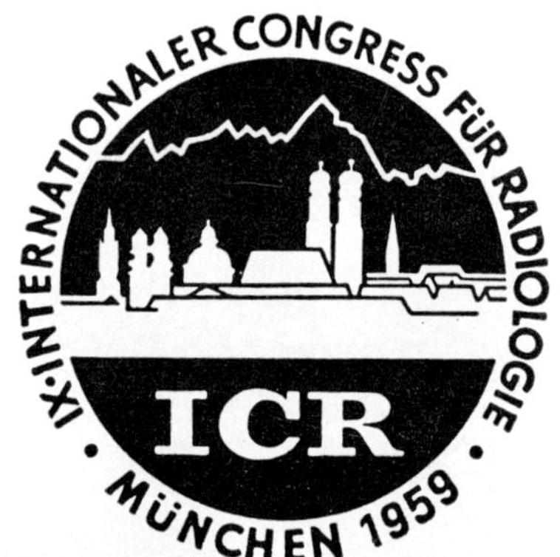

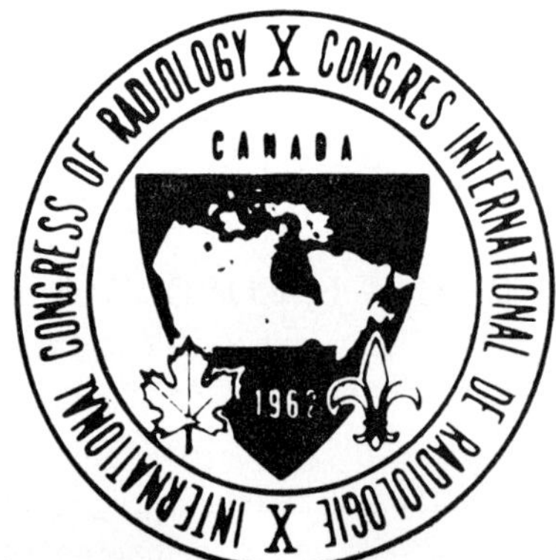

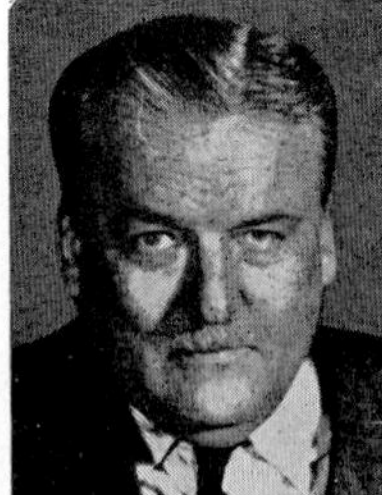

BORIS RAJEVSKY

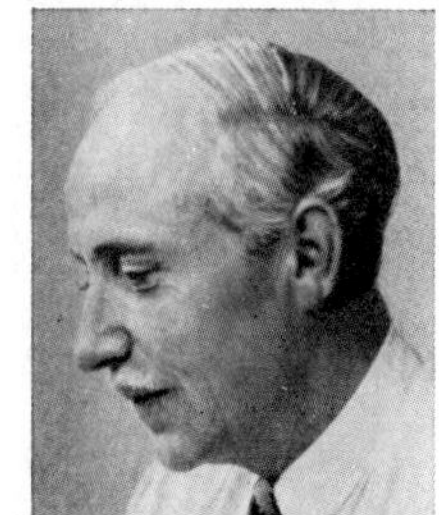

HANS VON BRAUNBEHRENS

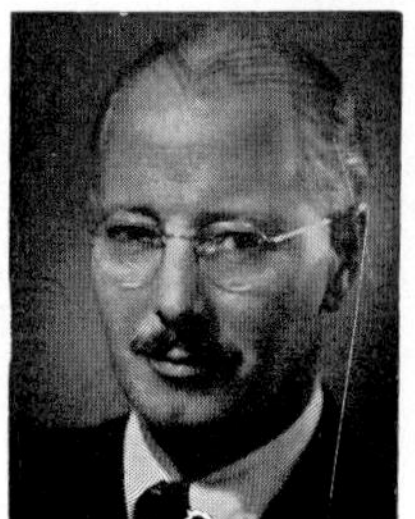

ARTHUR SINGLETON

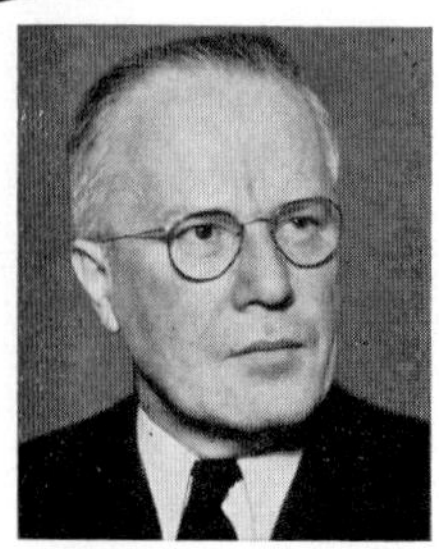

CARLETON PEIRCE

The International Club of Radiotherapists was organized in Copenhagen during the 1953 ICR. The suggestion and the organizing luncheon were offered by Jens Nielsen of Copenhagen. A Founders' Agreement was drawn by an elected steering committee consisting of Ralston Paterson (Manchester), Simeon Cantrill (Seattle), and Jens Nielsen. The agreement stipulated a club with membership limited to one hundred, the maximum number from the United States and England being 14 members for each. Subsequently the figures for other countries were set at maximum membership of one for each six million population. The Club has an elected president, a European secretary, and a secretary for the Americas (including Asia and the South Pacific). Juan del Regato is the secretary for the Americas. The first president was Paterson, the second was Jens Nielsen, and the present one is Jean Bouchard (Montreal). The Club meets once every three years during the ICR. It is usually an informal social exchange followed by a short pre-arranged scientific discussion.*

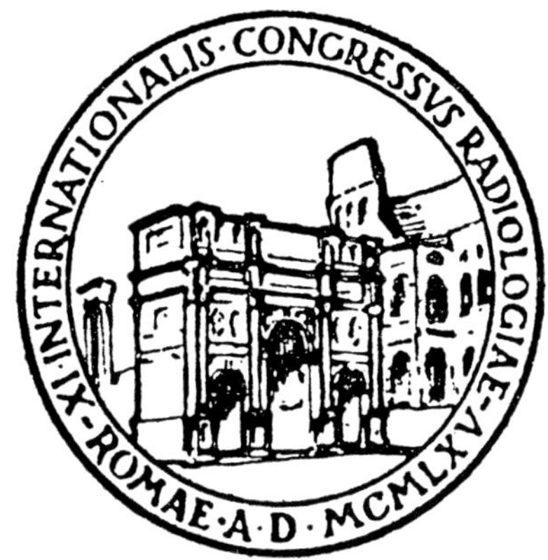

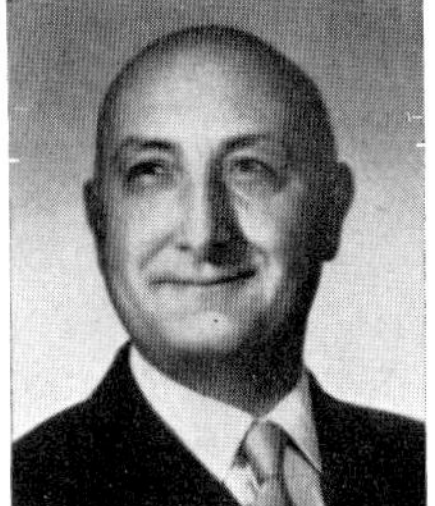
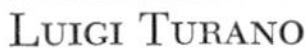
Luigi Turano

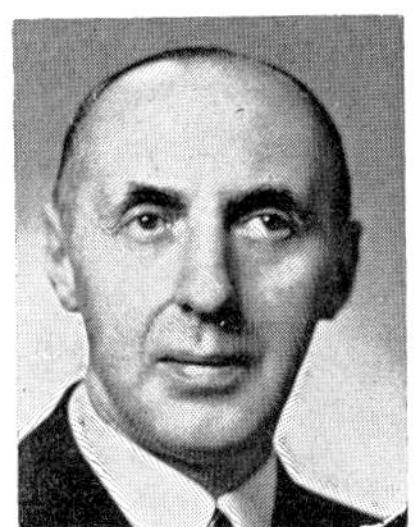
Arduino Ratti

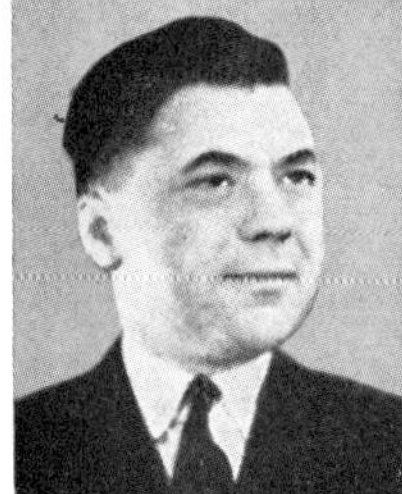
Robert Morrison

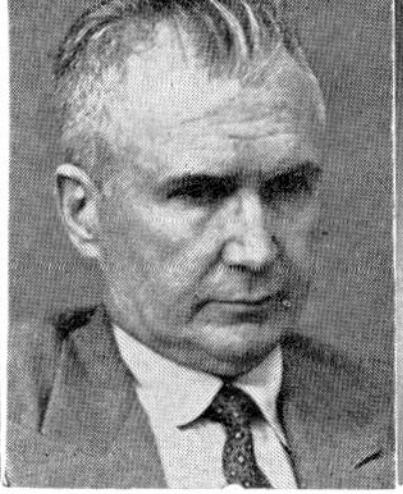
Juan del Regato

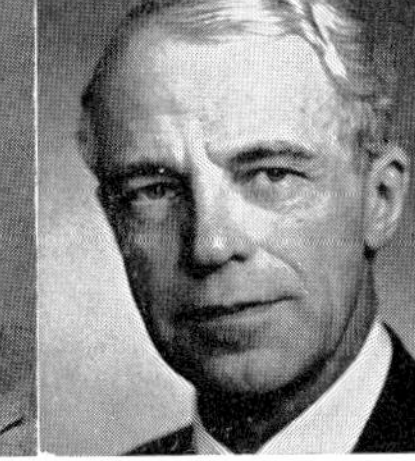
Jens Nielsen

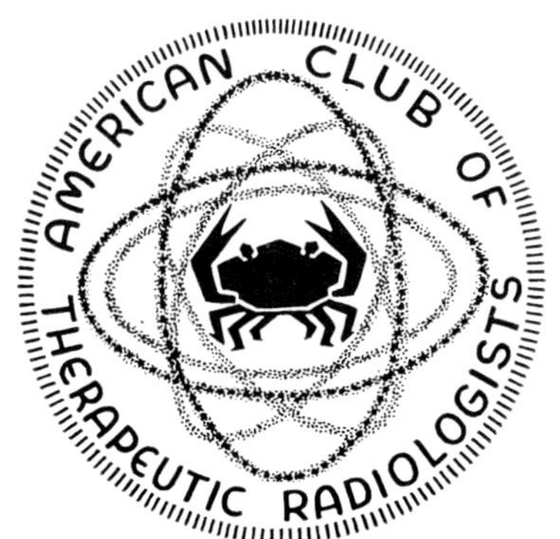

Several American therapeutic radiologists, who were refused admission to the International Club, met for dinner on December 5, 1955 and decided to form an American Club of Therapeutic Radiologists.

A tentative plan was discussed in Hollywood (Florida) on March 29, 1958. On November 18, 1958 in the Palmer House (Chicago) the final text of the Founders' Agreement was approved by a group of fifty-four radiotherapists from the United States, Canada, and Latin America. The first president was Simeon Cantril from Seattle; the first vice-president was James Carpender from the University of Chicago; the (quasi-permanent) secretary was and is Juan Del Regato from Colorado Springs – who recently promoted another of his pet projects, called *Radiologia Inter-Americana.*

The fairly informal club meetings are restricted to members and guests. Recently their discussions centered around the membership's wish to separate completely the residency training in therapy from the training in diagnosis. The club's seal contains a king-size number of atomic orbits, revolving around a cancer crab. What if a chemotherapeutic approach to cancer therapy were to remove this disease from the scope of radiation therapy?

ELECTRO-RADIO-SCISSION

In the early days, the radiologic fraternity was anxious to prevent the entrance of non-medical members. Today the trend is reversed, and efforts are being made to prevent non-medical personnel from leaving the fraternity.

The Roentgen Pioneers were a mixed group. Among their medical members were many neuro-psychiatrists, who had joined the roentgen business because they knew more about electricity than most of their fellow

*This information was courteously given by Juan del Regato (Colorado Springs).

physicians.* Electrotherapy was then a part of neurology, and well into the 1930s a Wimshurst machine was a must in any respectable neuro-psychiatric office. New "electrical" procedures have since been developed, but mostly for diagnostic purposes, such as the electroencephalogram, which requires specialized knowledge. Conversely, therapeutic applications of static electricity and most of diathermy are today all but obsolete. What remained (a "radarized" version of short waves), or was added (ultrasound), came almost entirely into the hands of general practitioners.

During the Golden Age many radiologic organizations discarded their electric prefixes, since the latter had become as outdated as the word electrolier (a contraction from electric chandelier). Electrology had been vernacularized by non-medical people, for instance in Illinois the electrologists are technicians, licensed to use electrolysis in the removal of unwanted hair. In certain radiologic circles the very term electrotherapist is now (almost) a dirty word. In 1962 appeared in Philadelphia (Lea & Febiger) the second edition of the *Manual of Electrotherapy* by Arthur Watkins, but its author is currently specializing in neurology at the Massachusetts General Hospital.

In Europe a quack is a quack. Short of claiming to be a physician, the European quack can easily be spotted with the naked eye. Not so in this country, where quacks have a training (of sorts), are called cultists, possess a framed degree, often a license. In the early days many believed that radiology was a branch of electrotherapeutics. There existed the very ethical *Americal Journal of Electrotherapeutics and Radiology*, edited in 1918 by William Benham Snow and Mary L. H. Arnold Snow, a man-and-wife team of reputable physicians. But the then extant American schools of electrotherapeutics accepted most comers, not only medical graduates. According to Orndoff, this was the main reason for the early separation of radiology and electrology in this country. In South America and In Europe, where only physicians were in the electrotherapeutic business (with the exception of recognizable quacks), the electric "cousins" and the respective prefixes still cling to radiology, here and there. The full title of the French national radiological society is Société Française d'Electro-Radiologie Médicale.

Others changed very early, for instance the Nederlandsche Vereeniging voor Electrotherapie en Röntgenologie, founded on April 14, 1901 by J. K. A. Wertheim-Salomonson (1864-1922), changed its name in 1906 to Nederlandse Vereniging voor Radiologie. This information was given by Bernard Ziedses des Plantes, who mentioned that Wertheim-Salomonson was the first in

*When a Roentgen Pioneer is herein called an internist, a neurologist, or a surgeon, it means simply the medical territory in which he practiced prior to devoting more or less time to radiology.

The Electrical Institute of Correspondence Instruction

Teaches Applied

ELECTRO-THERAPEUTICS AND X-RAYS ENTIRELY BY CORRESPONDENCE.

The courses have been prepared by Prof. W. J. Herdman, Professor of Nervous Diseases, University of Michigan and ex-President of the American Electro-Therapeutic Association, and other leading experts. The Instruction Departments of this Institute are in charge of recognized Electro-Therapeutic and X-Ray authorities. Our courses are endorsed by the leading electro-medical experts of America. This method of instruction is now being followed successfully by thousands. Study can begin at any time. For catalogue containing full information, address

REGISTRAR,

The Electrical Institute of Correspondence Instruction,

1900 Dept. F., 120-122 Liberty St., NEW YORK.

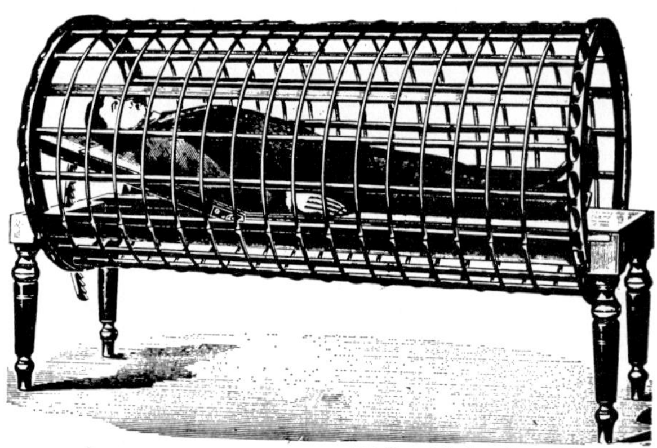

AUTOCONDUCIVE CAGE. Helicoidal solenoid.

ILLINOIS SCHOOL OF ELECTRO-THERAPEUTICS.

INCORPORATED.

OFFICERS: C. S. NEISWANGER, Ph. G., M. D., Pres. EMIL H. GRUBBE, M. D., Vice-Pres. A. B. SLATER, Sec'y and Treasurer.

FACULTY:

FRANKLIN H. MARTIN, M. D., Electricity in Gynecology.
W. FRANKLIN COLEMAN, M. D., M. R. C. S., (Eng.) Electricity in Diseases of the Eye.
ALBERT H. ANDREWS, M. D., Ear, Nose and Throat.
C. S. NEISWANGER, Ph. G., M. D., General Electro-Therapeutics.
EMILE H. GRUBBE, M. D., Electro-Physics, Radiography and X-Ray Diagnosis.
MAY CUSHMAN RICE, M D., Electrolysis.
EDWARD B TAYLOR, M. D., Neurology.
GORDON G. BURDICK, M. D., Radio-Therapy and Photo Chemistry.

This School is for physicians and is equipped with the most modern, up-to-date apparatus. All the rudimentary physics will be profusely illustrated and made plain even to the uninitiated in electro-therapy. No mail courses will be given and no degrees will be conferred, but a handsome engraved certificate of attendance can be obtained, if desired, after the completion of a course. The courses will be of three weeks' duration, and consist of both clinical and didactic instructions. A two weeks' course will make you self-dependent. Write for further information, terms and printed matter.

ILLINOIS SCHOOL OF ELECTRO-THERAPEUTICS, 1301-2-3 Champlain Bldg, Chicago, Ill.

Europe for whom a regular chair (Ordinarius) of radiology was created, in 1899.

In times past, the *American Journal of Physical Therapy* (edited in Chicago by Charles Raymond Wiley from 1924 to 1936) contained many radiologic contributions, quite a few written by Trostler. Now the term physical therapist is used only by para-medical personnel, while a physician in this category is called a physiatrist. The philosophy and technics of physiotherapy (the accredited terminology, as used in the title of their official journal, is *Physical Medicine and Rehabilitation*) are such a departure from the realm of ionizing radiations as to be forbidden ground to most radiologists.*

RADIOBIO(ETYMO)LOGIC SUBSPECIALTIES

Radiobiology - with its puzzling etymologic subspecialties - might soon seem just as forbidding.

In 1959, at the ACR Conference of Teachers of Radiology, Titus Evans explained his concept of the radiobiologist. He prefers the term radio-biophysicist, meaning a cross-pollination between a radiation physicist and a biologist. Few physicians qualify in this category, largely because today a majority among clinicians (dis)regard meticulous animal experimentation as being too fastidious for their taste.

On the vernacular scale of values, physicians have always been classified as men of science. Conversely, since or before Hippocrates, medicine was defined by its practitioners as an art. The latter notion was so well publicized that in "scientific" circles physicians are not included among the scientists. There is a general tendency to grant the qualification of "scientific" only to those areas in medicine in which a PhD degree is sufficient for full coverage of the subject (the so-called basic sciences).

This attitude prevails also in the manner in which medical achievements are selected for the Nobel prize. First of all, the "medical" prize itself is classified as Physiology and Medicine, which fitted in well with the achievements of the neurologic integrationist Sir Charles Scott Sherrington. The relatively few clinicians selected for the Nobel Prize were among those with pharmacologic achievements, *e.g.*, the Austrian malariotherapeutic psychiatrist Julius Wagner von Jauregg, or the American internist who connected pernicious anemia and liver extract, George Hoyt Whipple. Except for Finsen,* the only kin to radiology ever to receive this distinction was the Portuguese creator of neuroradiology, Egas Moniz. Röntgen's Nobel prize was not in medicine; it was in physics.

The practitioners of radiology were regarded from the start with a benevolent eye by the "scientific" community, and there existed the tendency to classify the radiologists with the "genuine" scientists. But medicine is still an art and needs radiologic clinicians (rather than clinical physicists). True clinicians are seldom willing to indulge in theoretical physics, or to perform finicky computations. This is why they had to hire a knowledgeable hand, known generically as a physicist. Until 1950 this hand, however knowledgeable, could advance no further than to the rank of health physicist, or some such sideline of radiophysics. After 1950, his

*There are exceptions to this rule. Irvin Franklin Hummon, Jr., director of the Department of Radiology in Cook County Hospital, teaches Physical Medicine at Stritch Medical School (Loyola University), and is also director of the Department of Physical Medicine in Cook County Hospital.

*The fourth International Photobiology Congress is scheduled to convene in Oxford (England) on July 26-30, 1964. The first three were at Amsterdam (1954), Turin (1957) and Copenhagen (1960). Their subjects of discussion cover first of all the phenomena due to absorption of light by molecules, but they are also trying to come to terms with the quanta theory, and with the principles of photochemistry.

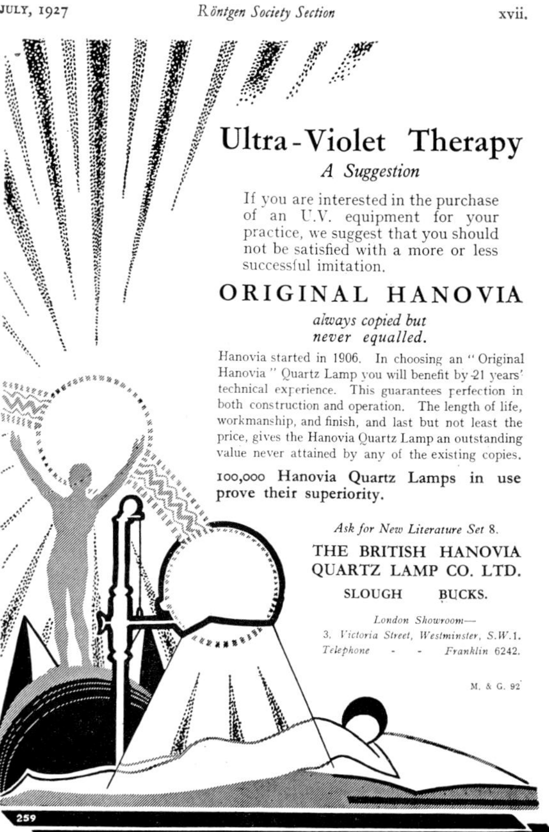

potential territory has expanded with several new trials leading into the growing field of radiobiology.*

*Radiobiology's etymologic "kissing cousin" (electro-biology) is just a fancy synonym for witchcraft.

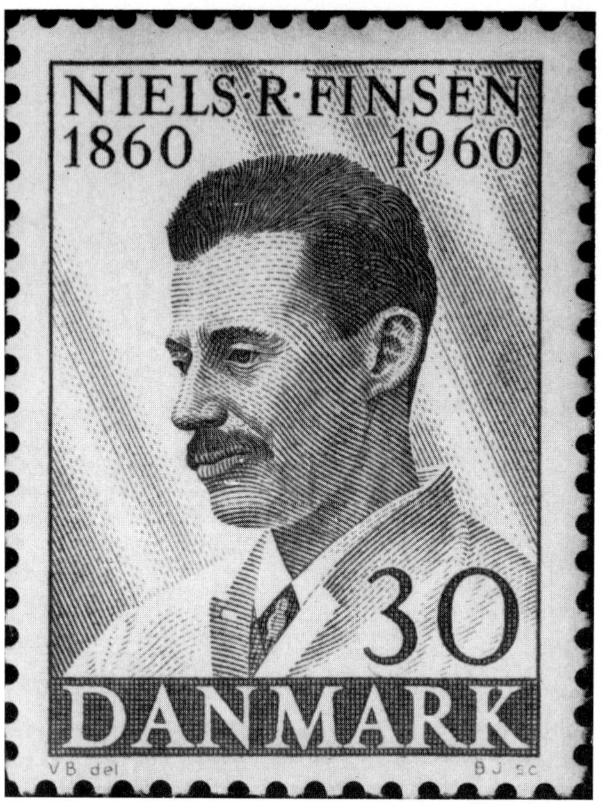

Courtesy: Stan Bohrer.

NIELS RYBERG FINSEN. The "apostle" of actinotherapy was born on the Faeroe Islands, earned his MD in Copenhagen in 1890, discovered the therapeutic benefits of red light for smallpox and ultraviolet for lupus, and in 1896 founded the Light Institute (Medicinske Lysinstitut) in Copenhagen. Finsen's arc light for generation of ultraviolet rays is still in use in some quarters. Finsen received the Nobel Prize for Physiology and Medicine in 1903.

At above mentionel ACR Teachers Conference of 1959 everybody agreed that radio-biologists are egg-heads (which is today a laudable characteristic). Outside of this basic statement they could find no common ground for a more specific definition of the term. Richard Hall Chamberlain explained the difficulty as being due to the inherent tendency of contemporary science toward fragmentalization (specialization) of knowledge. Few problems can be solved with the means available to a limited specialty, and genuine researchers have to reach over the barriers onto "strange" ground. How do you call a surgeon who had to become an experimental pathologist before he could begin to understand his particular research problem? And if you find a name for his specialty, how are you going to define it?

The radiobiologic subspecialties have no serious etymologic difficulties. All those who are active in the field of radiant energy may be called radiologists, thus including non-physicians by definition. Radiobiologists are those radiologists who concern themselves with the effects of radiant energy on the biosphere. This subgroup contains likewise both physicians and other specialists.

Those among the radiobiologists who have received medical training might be called medical or clinical radiobiologists. Their currently accepted designation is radiologists, at times (seldom) with the qualification medical or clinical radiologists. Another semantic subdivision is coming to the fore, that of diagnostic radiologists (formerly called roentgenologists, a classification recently abandoned even by the American Board of Radiology, and therapeutic radiologists or radiotherapists (an abbreviation of radiation therapists). The latter category includes radium therapists (rather than radiumologists as Dorland called them), and roentgen therapists (a term which is today almost obsolete).

The other "comrades-at-arms," of physico-chemical

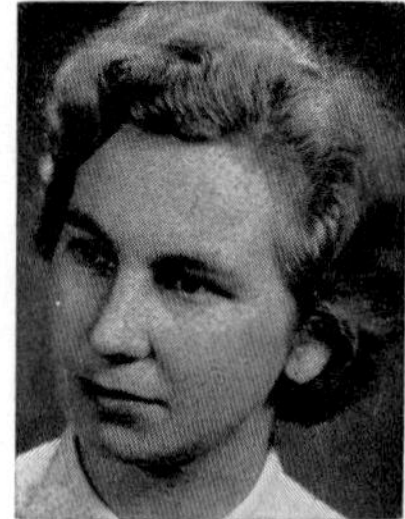
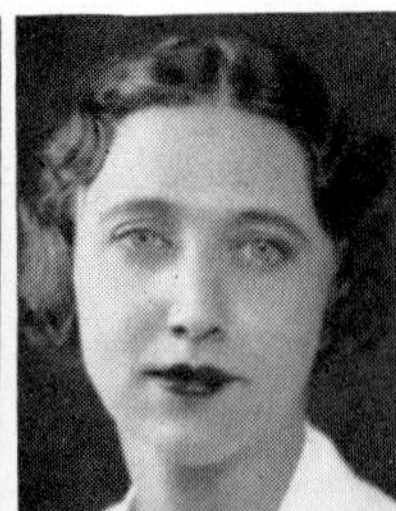
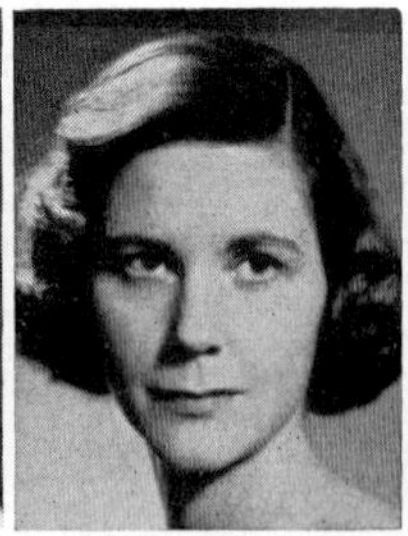
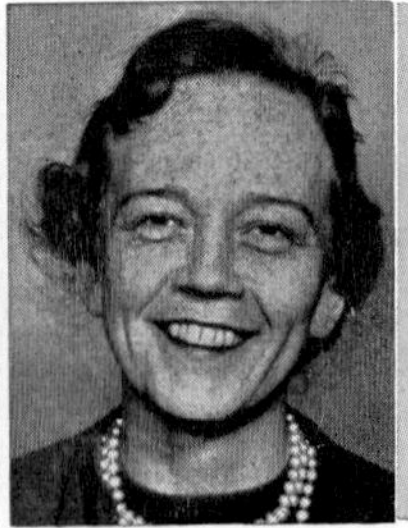
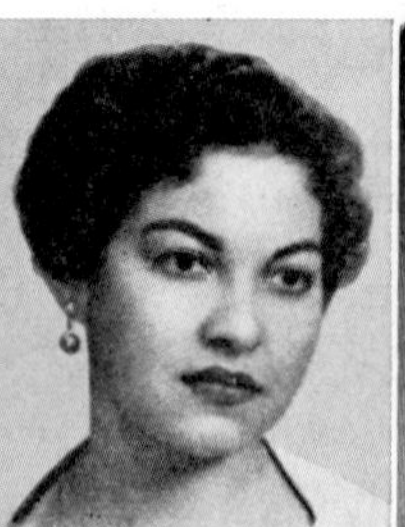
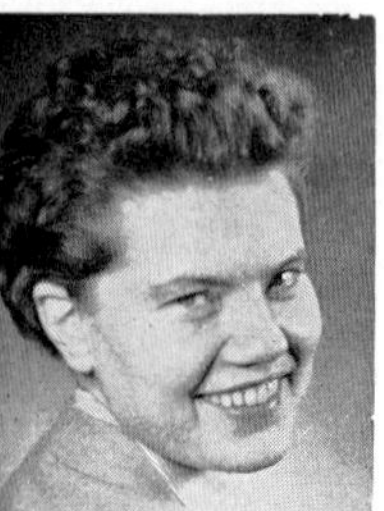

ZDENKA RUNOVIC ISABEL KNOWLTON PATRICIA FAILLA ELLEN ASKEVOLD GRACIELA SERNA ELISABETH PETRI

Good-looking radiologists can be found all over the globe. In this sampling of international "radio-cuties," Zdenka is from Yugoslavia; Isabel is of English ancestry; Patricia is from tbe USA; Ellen is Norwegian; Graciela a Mexican; and Elizabeth a German.

extraction, may be classified by the name of the respective field of endeavor. Not all of them would have to be radiobiologists (albeit they are radiologists): the designations vary from radio(bio)physicist to radio(bio)chemist, and from radiozoologist to radiogeologist.

In recent years, though, the term radiobiologist has been assigned more or less restrictively to non-medical personnel involved in experimentation on sub-human organisms. During the Era of the Pioneers "roentgenbiology" was almost exclusively medical territory. One of the characteristics of the Atomic Phase is the growing number of experimental (non-medical) radiobiologists.

It is undoubtedly wise to retain within the large group of radiologists — and this is an organizational, not an etymologic suggestion — all those who are active in the field of radiation as applied to the biosphere. Even while the specialty was growing, several lay practitioners acquired (in Percy Brown's words) a "right of eminent domain," for which they were "given" medical degrees and official recognition. After all, in the opinion of the religious philosopher and philosophic historian Dagobert D. Runes, we are all laymen, only some more so than others.

At the ninth ICR (Munich, 1959) the president was a physicist, Boris Rajevsky. This illustrates that today an open-door policy among radiologists is not only in order, it is a necessity. Natural selection will weed out those who do not belong. The French *mousequetaires* prospered by following a similar motto: *entre qui veut, reste qui peut!**

RADIO- PENETRATES THE IRON CURTAIN

At the beginning of the Atomic Phase the prefix roentgeno- remained entrenched in most of Central Europe.

In 1948, were printed in Budapest the two volumes (text and atlas) of Nandor Ratkoczy's *Rontgenologia* (reprinted in 1954 with enlarged editorial participation). In 1951, appeared in Praha a text by J. Slanina, called *Roentgenem Technika.*** A more substantial compilation, *Zarys Techniki Rentgenovskiej* (1954) by Ernest Matuszek (1897-1952) was re-edited in Warszawa, at the same time with the third edition of *Rentgenologia Kliniczna* (1954) by Czeslaw Murczynski.

Roumania, having a predominantly Romanic language and being still under a French cultural influence of sorts, remained loyal to the prefix radio-. In 1954, appeared in Bucharest the *Probleme de Radiologie,* edited by M. P. Baran; and in 1956 Amilcar Georgescu authored a *Technica Radiografica.* Semantic creativity became apparent with the approach of the nuclear age. In 1960 appeared in Bucharest the monograph by Octav Costăchel, entitled *Boala de Irradiere,* the disease of irradiation, with two subtitles, the actinic disease and the atomic disease.

Surprisingly, Spain has never been completely sold on the advantages of the radio-root; in 1955 appeared in Madrid the third edition (958 pages) of Ernesto Castillo's *Technica de la Exploración Roentgenoscópica y Roentgenográfica.* But on its frontispiece the author calls his office building *Instituto Radiologico.*

The first "break" in the solid Central European roentgen front occurred in 1948 in Vienna, which was then a divided frontier town: the sophisticated Austrians had never completely subscribed to the German Roentgen Edict.

Prior to World War I, Austrian roentgen specialists were members of the respective German societies. In 1922 was founded the Wiener Röntgengesellschaft, its first president being Guido Holzknecht, with Martin Haudek (the one who "discovered" the ulcer niche)

Radiologia Austriaca

Herausgegeben von der

Österreichischen Röntgen-Gesellschaft

Band I

Mit 82 Abbildungen im Text

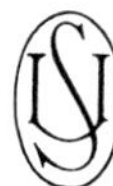

1948

Urban & Schwarzenberg / Wien

*Enter who wishes, remain who can!

**Two years later, also in Prague, appeared another technical text, Marie Ungarova's *Standardisovane polohy pri skiagrafii* — the skigraphic root is still very acceptable in the Czech language. The Australian E. G. Robertson uses skiagram and skiagraphy in *Pneumoencephalography* (Thomas, 1957).

as second in command. Then the need arose to have international representation at the various congresses. This is why the Austrian Roentgen Society was finally organized in 1934, with Robert Kienböck as president. When the Germans overran Austria in 1938 that Austrian society was dissolved, and its members were (re-)incorporated into the Deutsche Röntgengesellschaft. After World War II the Oesterreichische Röntgengesellschaft was reorganized in 1947, its first president being Kienböck's disciple and successor, Konrad Erwin Wilhelm Weiss (professor of radiology in the University of Vienna). In 1948, appeared the society's official organ, and it was called *Radiologia Austriaca.**

After the retirement of Weiss, his position was occupied by one of his pupils, Bruno Thurnher, who published with Hellmut Hubert Ellegast (another Weiss pupil) a paper on the beginnings of Vienese roentgenology. Today in Holzknecht's former department in the Allgemeines Krankenhaus in Vienna, the chief is Ernst Georg Mayer, among whose 200 or so publications the best known are those in which he describes his eponymized view for the temporal bone. And there is the radiologic internist who teaches at the University of Vienna, Anton Leb. In the *Wiener klin. Wcschr.* of November 14, 1958, Mayer remarked that the implementation of proper protection practices is now part of the radiologist's ethical precepts, just like any other rule of medical ethics.

At the University of Innsbruck — located in the beautiful Inn Valley of the Tyrolese Mountains — the professor of radiology is Ernst Ruckensteiner, a good friend of American radiology, who completed a lengthy post-graduate spell in Omaha. Ruckensteiner is today one of the leading European radiologists; his publications range all the way from roentgen signs in bone malignancy and in pulmonary eosynophilic granuloma, to the combined surgical and radiotherapeutic approach in the treatment of carcinoma of the breast. In the radio-historic field, Ruckensteiner has published a biography of the Austrian therapist Leopold Freund.

After Austria, the "radiologic fire" spread to Hungary.

The Hungarian Roentgen Society was founded in 1913 by the previously mentioned "plastic" roentgenologist Bela Alezander, who was at the time professor of radiology in Budapest. The first Magyar specialty periodical in this field was called *Röntgenologia:* it was a commercial venture, under the editorship of Andor Nagy, started in 1922 as a quarterly, went eventually to six yearly numbers, and terminated its existence in 1929. On December 1, 1924 Bela Mayer published *Radio, Röntgen es Egyeb Sugarzasok* (. . . and other radiations); its next and last number appeared in June, 1925. The official organ of the Hungarian Roentgen Society was the *Magyar Röntgen Közlöny,* edited by Béla Kelen (successor of Alexander in the chair of radiology in Budapest), with Jozsef Vegh as publisher; it was started in 1926 and eighteen volumes appeared until 1944 when the Russian occupation supervened. In

*This information was courteously supplied by Prof. Konrad Weiss himself.

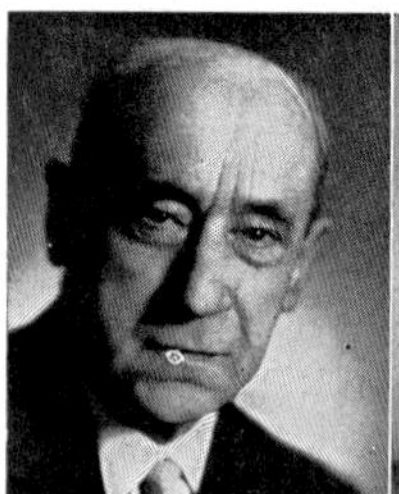

ANTON LEB

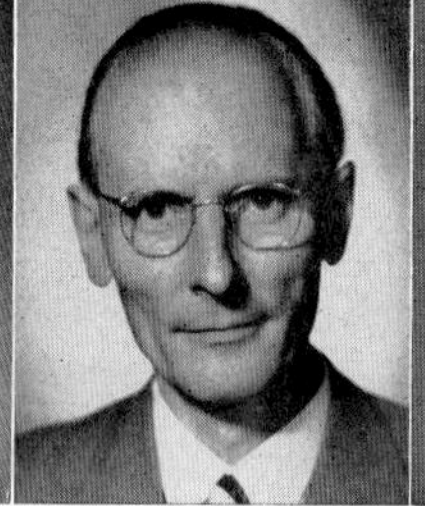

RENE DU MESNIL DE ROCHEMONT

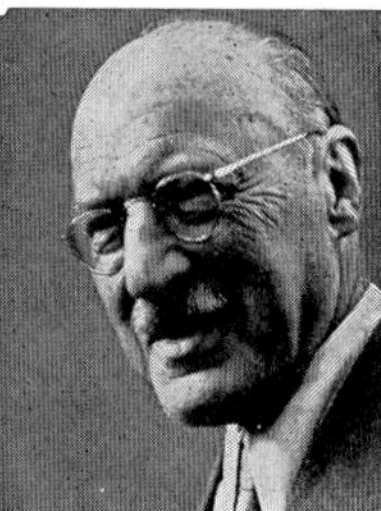

PLEIKART STUMPF

MAGYAR RÖNTGEN-KÖZLÖNY

A RÖNTGEN- ÉS ROKON SUGÁRZÁSOKAT TÁRGYALÓ TUDOMÁNYOS FOLYÓIRAT. A MAGYAR ORVOSOK RÖNTGEN-EGYESÜLETÉNEK HIVATALOS KÖZLÖNYE. SZERKESZTŐSÉG: BUDAPEST VIII. ÜLLŐI-ÚT 26. EGYETEMI RÖNTGEN-INTÉZET.

IV. ÉVFOLYAM. 1930 JÚLIUS—AUGUSZTUS 7—8. SZÁM.

KÖZLEMÉNY A BUDAPESTI KIR. MAGYAR PÁZMÁNY PÉTER TUD. EGY. II. SZ. SEBÉSZETI KLINIKÁJÁRÓL
(IGAZGATÓ: *DR. BAKAY LAJOS* EGYETEMI NY. R. TANÁR).

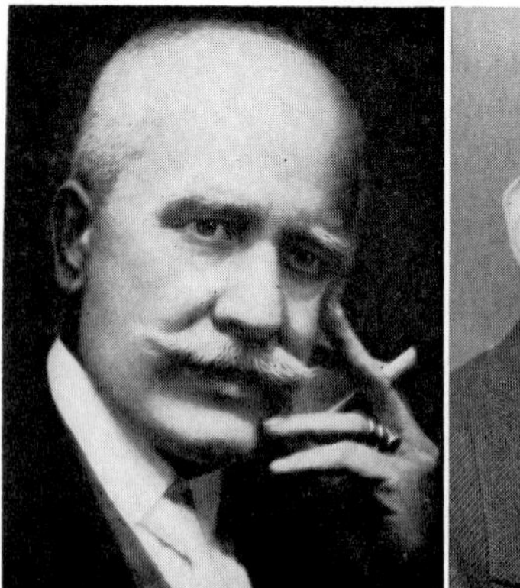

BÉLA ALEXANDER — JOZSEF VÉGH.

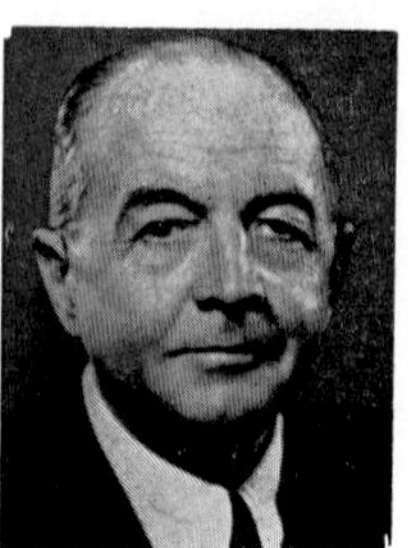

NANDOR RATKOCZY

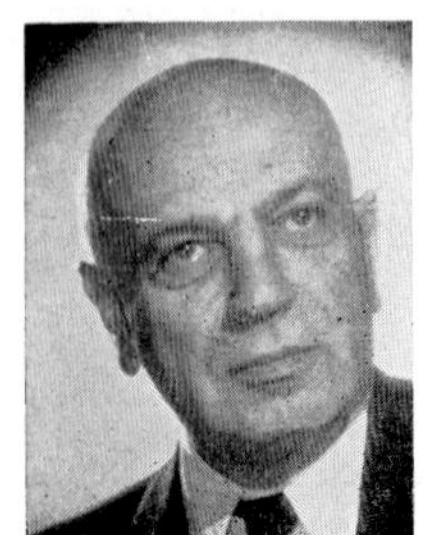

ERWIN ÖTVÖS

1949, the official organ of the Hungarian Roentgen Society re-appeared as the *Radiologia Hungarica,* under the editorship of Nandor Ratkoczy (Kelen's successor as professor of radiology); the publisher was the same Jozsef Vegh. One year later, in 1950, it was reorganized, the name was changed to *Magyar Radiologia,* and an associate editor came in, Zoltan Zsebök. In 1959 appeared in Budapest the 475-page textbook by Nàndor Ratkoczy, entitled simply *Radiologia.* In September of 1961 came out the first issue of *Radiologiai Közlemenyek* (edited by Laszlo Fried and Pal Deak), which contains mainly abstracts.* The current historian of Hungarian radiology is the polyglot Balasz Bugyi, who published recently a lengthy paper on their roentgen pioneers. Bugyi (one of Végh's pupils) has also a variety of scientific publications, including studies on the size of the sella turcica.

In Warszawa there had existed since 1926 the *Polski Przeglad Radiologizny,* edited by the inexhaustible French-oriented Witold Zawadowski, who re-issued the journal under the same title after World War II. In 1954, appeared a second Polish periodical, the *Postepy Radiologii.* And in 1956 was printed in Warsaw a technical text on both roentgen procedures and isotopes, by Jozef Domanus, under the plain title *Radiologia.*

I asked Czeslaw Murczynski, who is professor of radiology in Szczecin, to give me some information on the history of Polish radiology. He referred my request to Witold Zawadowski, professor of pediatric radiology in Warsaw (and uncontested dean of Polish radiologists).

*This information was obligingly provided by Professor Jozsef Vegh.

BUDAPEST 1949. I. ÉVFOLYAM 1. SZÁM

CAT. BY L. C.

RADIOLOGIA HUNGARICA

A MAGYAR ORVOSOK SZABAD SZAKSZERVEZETE RADIOLOGUS SZAKCSOPORTJÁNAK HIVATALOS FOLYÓIRATA

TARTALOM:

FŐSZERKESZTŐ:
RATKÓCZY NÁNDOR

TÁRSSZERKESZTŐK:
HRABOVSZKY ZOLTÁN ÉS WALD BÉLA

FELELŐS SZERKESZTŐ: HAJDU IMRE
FELELŐS KIADÓ: VÉGH JÓZSEF

Kiadóhivatal: Budapest, V., Nádor-utca 26. Telefon: 127-752 és 124-072.

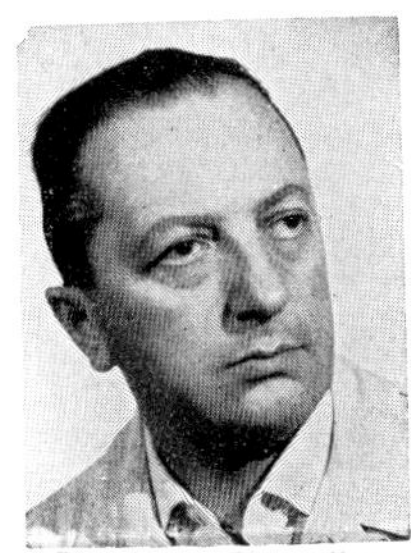

ZOLTAN ZSEBÖK

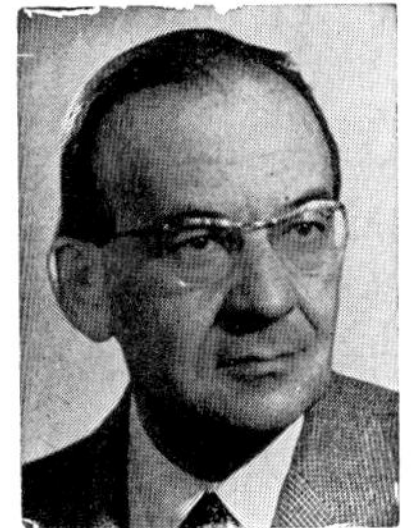

BELA WALD

POLSKI

PRZEGLĄD

RADJOLOGICZNY

ORGAN POLSKIEGO LEKARSKIEGO TOWARZYSTWA RADJOLOGICZNEGO I FIZJOTERAPEUTYCZNEGO

ZAŁOŻONY PRZEZ

DOC. DRA Z. GRUDZIŃSKIEGO

TOM VIII i IX

REDAKTOR
DOC. DR W. ZAWADOWSKI
WARSZAWA

KOMITET REDAKCYJNY: DR E. BRUNER (Warszawa), PROF. DR A. CIESZYŃSKI (Lwów), DOC. DR A. ELEKTOROWICZ (Warszawa), DR S. GĄDEK (Warszawa), DR E. MEISELS (Lwów), DR N. MESZ (Warszawa), PROF. DR K. MAYER (Poznań), PROF. S. PIEŃKOWSKI (Warszawa), DR B. SABAT (Warszawa), DR A. SOŁTAN (Warszawa), DR Z. STANKIEWICZ (Warszawa), DR H. WACHTEL (Kraków), DR M. ZALESKI (Warszawa).

SEKRETARZ REDAKCJI
DR M. WERKENTHINÓWNA
WARSZAWA

ADMINISTRATOR
DR J. KOCHANOWSKI
WARSZAWA

NAKŁ. POLSKIEGO LEKARSKIEGO TOW. RADJOL. I FIZJOTERAP.

WARSZAWA 1934

Following are excerpts from Zawadowski's letter: "The first x ray specialists in Poland appeared around 1910 in the then extant medical schools, for instance in 1910 Bronislaw Sabat (1871-1953) of Lwów pioneered kymography, and in 1916 Karol Mayer (1882-1946) of Kraków published his first paper on the x ray plates of the heart, made with a moving x ray tube. That was the beginning of tomography. After World War I, the until then separate Polish provinces were reunited into independent Poland. Among the extant five medical schools, the first chair of radiology was that of Karol Mayer, at Poznan, in 1923. Since 1913 Warsaw radiologists met more or less periodically, and from that first regional group was formed the national radiological society in 1925 in Warsaw. The founders were the previously mentioned Mayer (who was also the first president, many times re-elected); Zygmund Grudzinski (1870-1929) of Warsaw; Adam Elektorowicz (1887-?) of Warsaw; Bronislaw Sabat of Lwow; and Gregorz Drozdowicz (1871-1934). In 1939, the Germans occupied Poland, and the library of the Polish Radiological Society was destroyed by an incendiary bomb during the first siege of Warsaw. In 1925 there were 50 members in the Society. The number had increased to 170 by 1939. During the war about half of them were killed, others emigrated, and by 1945 there were again only about 50 radiologists in all of Poland. After World War II, new medical schools were organized (or reorganized as in Szczecin, the former Prussian metropolis Stettin), the total number being now eleven, each with a chair of radiology, in addition to eleven clinical radiology departments attached to university hospitals."

POSTĘPY
RADIOLOGII

TOM I

Pod redakcją
PROF. DRA W. ZAWADOWSKIEGO

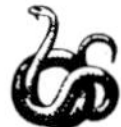

WARSZAWA 1954
PAŃSTWOWY ZAKŁAD WYDAWNICTW LEKARSKICH

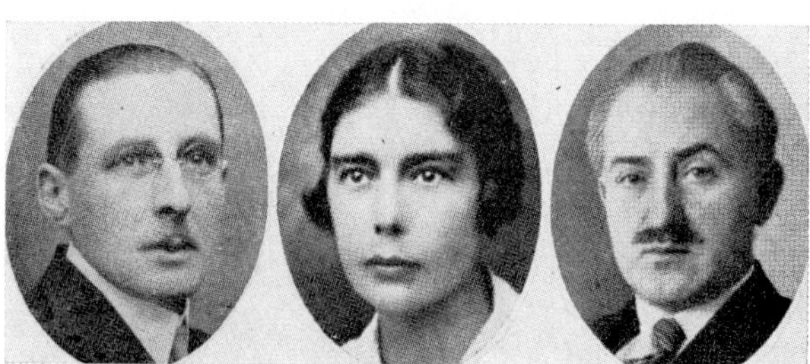

ADAM ELEKTOROWICZ — MARIE WERKENTHIN — WITOLD ZAWADOWSKI

"Specialization in radiology in Poland demands first of all one year of general practice, followed by three years of formal training, after which the candidate is examined, and if he passes he becomes a specialist of the first degree, which entitles him to work as a junior radiologist. If he wishes to advance, he returns for another three years of study, and another, much more demanding examination for the title of second degree specialist in radiology. The Polish Medical Society of Radiology has currently about 650 members, most of them first degree specialists. National meetings are held every two years, the next being slated for 1964 in Kraków, as that medical school is part of the Jagellonian University, which celebrates its 600th anniversary (it was founded in 1364). The *Postepy Radiologii* (= advances) was discontinued in 1956. The other journal, originally founded by Zygmund Grudzinski, has recently added (an atomic tailpiece) to its title, and is now the *Polski Przeglad Radiologii i Medycyny Nuklearnej.* An English edition of the latter (*Polish Review of Radiology*) is in the planning stage.*"

The "father of radiology" in Czechoslovakia, Rudolf Jedlicka (1869-1926), is also regarded as the founder of their specialty society, the Ceskoslovenske Spolecnosti pro Rentgenologii a Radiologii. Their official organ was first issued in 1938 under joint sponsorship with the Anti-Cancer League (Liga protiv Rakovine), and was therefore called *Acta Radiologica et Cancerologica Bohemoslovenica.* The title varied, and sometimes it appeared as *Ceskoslovenske Rentgenologie,* with *Acta Radiologica* as a subtitle.

After having unsuccessfully requested information on Czechoslovakian radiology from their unofficial historian, Frantisek Bilek, and from the secretary of their society, I wrote to Vladimir Teichmann, chief-radiologist of the second Medical Service in the Charles University Hospital in Prague. Following are excerpts from his letters: "The first roentgen plates in Prague were made by physicists. Zedlicka believed that the very first one was made in Puluj's lab by an amateur photographer named Paspa: the subject was a hedgehog. Then Cífka, the owner of the hotel called *The Black Horse* in Prague, purchased an x ray outfit, and used it, part as a publicity gimmick, but also for the needs of certain patients. Toward the end of 1896, Jedlicka, who was then an assistant in the University Surgical Service, used Cífka's installation to demonstrate a nail swallowed by one of his patients. Finally, in 1897, Jedlicka

*Prof. Zawadowski was also trying to find some photographs, but their archives had been destroyed during the war.

was allowed to install the first x ray equipment in a university hospital, in his surgical place of work. It was a Max Kohl installation with induction coil."

It is interesting to note that Albert Alexander (1857-1916), who practiced in Kezmarok, a small town in Middle Slovakia, purchased in 1897 a Reiniger, Gebbert & Schall x ray machine (the machine is preserved in the Municipal Museum of Kezmarok). His work became so well known that the Hungarian Government (who controlled that territory during the reign of the Austrian Habsburgs) sent him to the German Röntgenkongress (1905), then called him to Budapest" (indeed, this is the Béla Alexander, mentioned in the section on Hungary).

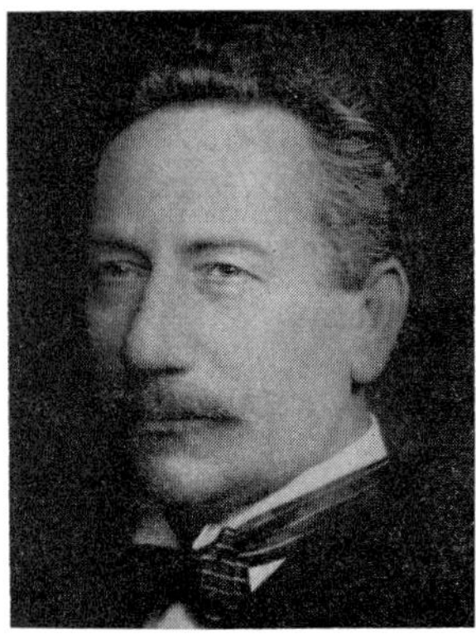

Rudolf Jedlicka.

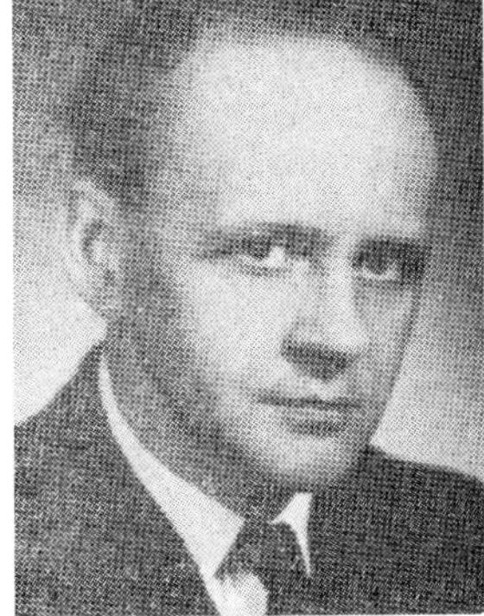

Vladimir Teichmann

ROČENKA

ČSL. SPOLEČNOSTI PRO RÖNTGENOLOGII A RADIOLOGII V PRAZE

SVAZEK I. 1927.

ANNUAIRE

DE LA SOCIÉTÉ TCHÉCOSLOVAQUE POUR LA RÖNTGENOLOGIE ET LA RADIOLOGIE À PRAGUE

TOME I. 1927.

JAHRBUCH

DER TSCHECHOSLOWAKISCHEN GESELLSCHAFT FÜR RÖNTGENOLOGIE UND RADIOLOGIE IN PRAG

BAND I. 1927.

NÁKLADEM ČSL. SPOLEČNOSTI PRO RÖNTGENOLOGII A RADIOLOGII V PRAZE.

"The Czechoslovakian Society for Roentgenology and Radiology was founded on June 28, 1924 (*cf.*, page 1138 in the *Casopis Lekaru Ceskych* of 1924). The first meeting took place in May, 1926 in Prague, with Jedlicka as president. The first specialty publication was *Rocenka Ceskoslovenské Spolecnosti pro Röntgenologii a Radiologii,* which appeared in three volumes (1927, 1929, and 1936). It contained mainly papers presented at the national meetings. The *Acta Radiologica et Cancerologica Bohemoslovenica* appeared first in 1938, and continued until 1940. It was re-issued after World War II, but in 1955 changed its title to *Ceskoslovenska Roentgenologie.* Finally, in 1964, the name was changed to *Ceskoslovenska Radiologie.*"

This is a sign of the nuclear age, but it seems to come from above. The rank-and-file prefer the old roentgen root, for instance in 1961 appeared in Praha the *Rentgenova Diagnostika,* edited by Ferdinand Marx. A Czechoslovakian peculiarity is in fact that even though the terms *radioskopia* and *radiografia* have occasionally been used (as by O. Frankenberger in the very first issue of 1899 of the *Casopis*), Jedlicka popularized the terms *skiaskopia* and *skiagrafia,* and they have remained to this day the accepted terminology.

While the Czechs exhibited a continued (perhaps even renewed) preference for the roentgen-root, the Yugoslavs seemed to orbit the other way (at least temporarily). There had appeared in Zagreb, beginning in 1927, the *Izdanja* of the Centralni Rentgenologiski Institut. After World War II a slim manual called *Radiografska Tehnika* (1956) was published in Zagreb, authored by Vladimir Kolmikov.

USSR

In matters of protocol and nomenclature there is in the Soviet Union a very conservative and traditionalistic approach.

Today's rank and file Sovietic communist is closer to a Western law-abiding citizen than to the subversive type of communist encountered on this side of the Iron Curtain. As the satellite countries were being occupied, Sovietic intellectuals appeared to be closer in mentality to, and capable of communicating easier with, the occupied bourgeoisie than with the local communists (who had just graduated from the terrible life of the underground). Because of lengthy indoctrination, the Sovietic intellectual may at times appear suspicious, at least during his first meeting with a Western counterpart. After a while, though, especially if person-to-person rapport can be achieved, as long as political differences are left out of the picture, a common threading ground can easily be established.

As previously stated, within ten years after the October 1917 revolution, seven major radiologic centers were created in the Soviet Union (Leningrad, Moscow, Kiev, Kharkov, Baku, Erevan, and Rostov-on-the-Don). In the beginning the most important was the one in Leningrad.

Ever since Czarist times, St. Petersburg, later Petersburg, and later yet Leningrad had been a cultural center, more refined, luxurious, and progressive than the rest of the country. This was true also from a radiologic viewpoint until well into the 1930s, when it was overtaken by Moscow. In the 1920s the Roentgenologic and Radiologic Institute in Leningrad, founded and directed by Mikhail Isaevich Nemenov (1880-1950), constituted the most advanced teaching and research place in the Soviet Union. Nemenov published also diagnostic studies (for instance, one on the detection of cardio-esophageal malignancies), but his main interest was in therapy. Already in 1896 the (previously mentioned) physiologist Tarkhan-Muravov had reported certain effects of roentgen rays on the nervous system of experimental animals. Aside from the conventional type of roentgen and radium therapy, Nemenov studied extensively the "indirect" manner of applying radiation to the sympathetic chain, and reported encouraging results in cases of peptic ulcer (the latter was also irradiated directly), hypertension, angina pectoris, frost bite, etc.

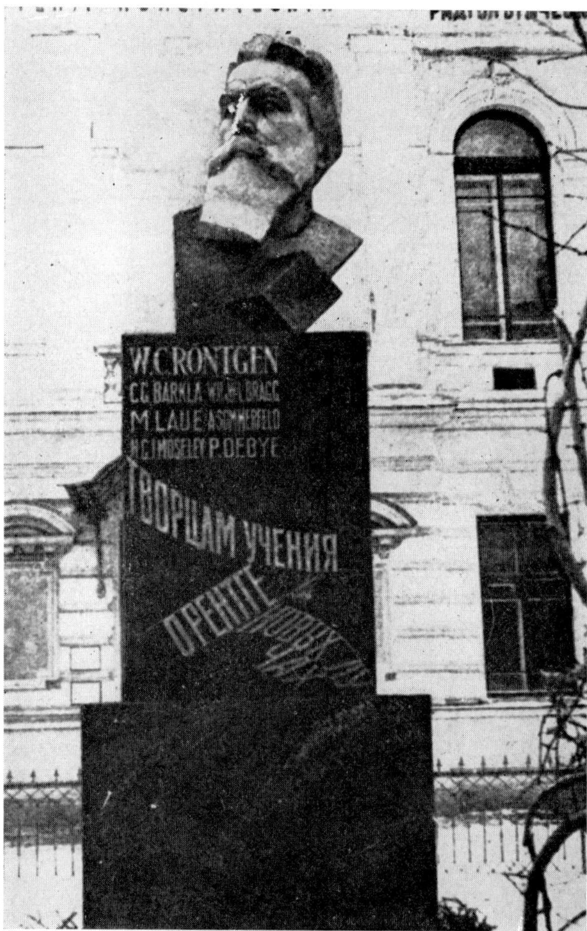

Sovietic Roentgen Monument, erected in front of the Institute of Roentgenology, Radiology, and Oncology in Leningrad, unveiled on January 29, 1920. The sculptor's name is N. S. Altmann. On the base are engraved the following names: C. C. Barkla, W. H. and W. L. Bragg, M. Laue, A. Sommerfeld, H. G. J. Moseley, P. Debye, P. and M. Curie, Becquerel, Rutherford, W. Ramsay, Crookes, J. J. Thomson, Lenard, H. A. Lorentz, C. T. R. Wilson, Millikan, M. Planck, and N. Bohr.

Contributions to therapy were made also outside Leningrad. Jakov Grigorievich Dilon (1873-1952), professor of radiology in the second Moscow Medical School, perfected a method of irradiation with multiple small ports distributed in circular fashion around the thorax. These seemed to prolong survival after treatment of bronchogenic and esophageal carcinoma.

The most important figure to come out of Nemenov's group was undoubtedly Samuel Aronovich Reynberg. Being a voracious reader in addition to his facility for handling foreign tongues, Reynberg never lost contact with the universal radiologic literature. His scientific contributions are many, for instance at the first ICR in London in 1925 Reynberg offered a valuable contribution on bronchial peristalsis.

The earliest attempt to opacify living bronchi was reported on February 1, 1906 by Springer before the Medizinisch-Biologische Sektion of the Lotos in Prague: he had inserted an elastic catheter into the trachea of dogs, and insufflated powder of iodoform and bismuth, which resulted in satisfactory fluoroscopic visualization, as described in the *Prager Medicinische Wochenschrift* of March 22, 1906. It was then not uncommon to opacify the bronchial tree post-mortem, for instance Kennon Dunham reproduced delicate "stereo-chest plates" of this type in the *American Quarterly of Roentgenology* of July, 1911. It is difficult to find who was the first who visualized – inadvertently – the bronchial tree when bismuth mixture spilled from the esophagus, either because of paralysis, or through a fistula. The latter instance occurred in the presence of William Stewart in 1915, but he did not do that on purpose until 1921. In 1918, Chevalier Jackson in Philadelphia became the first to purposely opacify the bronchial tree in the human being, as he insufflated bismuth powder, and reported it in the *American Journal of Roentgenology* of that year. In February, 1921, appeared in the same journal the communication of Henry Lynah and William Stewart, who had injected bronchiectases with a mixture of bismuth in olive oil by using a bronchoscope.

Bronchography became a clinical tool only after the introduction of adequate contrast media. Around the turn of the century Guerbet, a professor in the Paris School of Pharmacy, succeeded to suspend iodine in poppyseed oil, intended for the treatment of syphilis. Because of his faculty appointment, Guerbet could not appear as a commercial producer. He arranged with a colleague to have the product issued under the latter's name, and this is why to this day it is called the Lipiodol Lafay. Lipiodol was put on the market in 1901 but it did not achieve radiologic importance until two decades later, when the Parisian neurologist Jean Athanase Sicard (1872-1929) finally succeeded in finding a student willing to accept as the subject of his doctoral thesis a study of the possibilities of using Lipiodol as an opaque medium; that pioneering paper was presented on (and published as of) March 17, 1922 in the *Bulletin et Mémoires de la Société Médicale des Hôpitaux de Paris.* The paper discusses not only bronchography, myelography, as well as fistulous opacification, but practically all other radio-opacifying possibilities are at least considered. That princeps communication by Sicard together with his pupil Jacques Forestier constitutes the basis of modern radiologic contrast procedures. Bronchography soon became a popular procedure around the globe. Reynberg's communication of 1925 is the first to mention the existence of bronchial peristalsis.

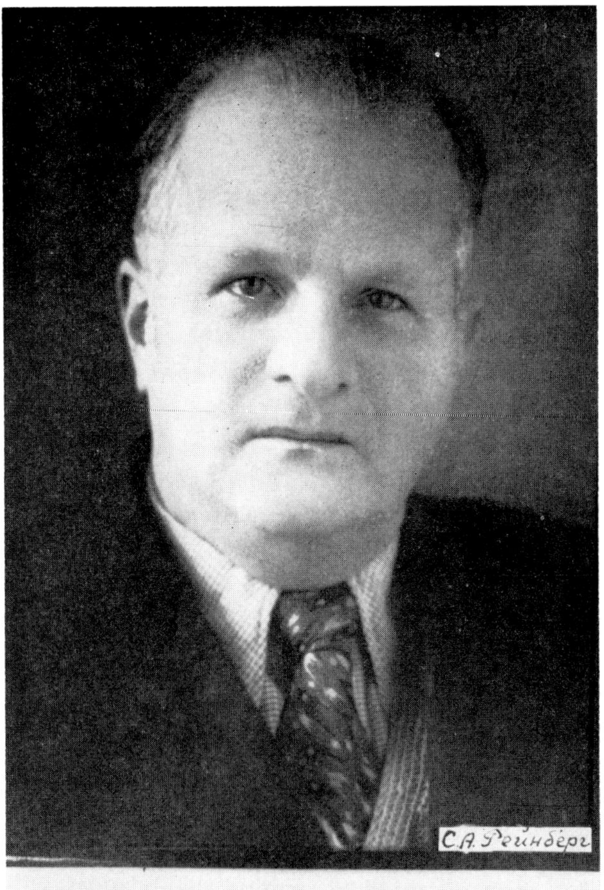

Sam. A. Reinberg

Other occurrences in Reynberg's scientific life were a text on osteo-articular roentgen diagnosis, which appeared in 1928; the demonstration of bronchial obstruction as a significant factor in the evolution of pulmonary tuberculosis, reported to the ICR in Zurich in 1934; and the editorship of a textbook on roentgen diagnosis with multiple authors, published in 1938. He coined many clinical concepts, for instance the "roentgen masks" of bronchogenic carcinoma, known to be capable of simulating most any chest condition. Today, Reynberg teaches at the Central Post-Graduate Institute in Moscow. He is also the (unofficial) historian of Sovietic radiology.

By the mid-1930s, several centers had developed teaching and research facilities.

In Erevan (Soviet Armenia) Vartholomeu F. Fanardjian was the radio-chief; aside from many pupils, his interest included particularly gastrointestinal roentgen diagnosis. G. O. Kharmandaryan, director of the Ukrainian Roentgenologic and Radiologic Institute in Kharkov, studied the influence of hypnosis on the gastric mucosal folds (1939). In Moscow the radiotherapist B. M. Ioffe treated actinomycosis quite often successfully by a combination of actinolysat and radiotherapy. At the time radiation was quite frequently used in the treatment of inflammatory conditions, from pneumonitis and tonsillitis to pulmonary abscess and osteomyelitis.

As far as periodicals were concerned, Nemenov's *Vestnik* continued unabated, and a few others were added such as the *Voprosy Rentgenologii,* started in Kiev in 1936. Then came World War II, to which Sovietic authors often refer as the "traumatic epidemic." Interest was focused on roentgen diagnosis of war injuries and on roentgen therapy of infected

Вестник
РЕНТГЕНОЛОГИИ
и
РАДИОЛОГИИ

(or potentially infected) wounds. An extensive Sovietic bibliography on the radiation treatment of gunshot wounds was published in a 1948 monograph by Lew D. Podlyashuk, who then became the chief of radiotherapy in the Central Radiologic Institute in Moscow.

A monograph on osteo-articular trauma, this one purely diagnostic, was published in 1944 by Gheorg Artemovich Zedguenidze, at the time the professor of radiology in the Medical Academy in Leningrad.

Among Zedguenidze's many publications are two particularly interesting monographs, one on fistulography (1945), the other on sialography (1953). Today Zedguenidze is in Moscow, at the Radiological Institute of the Sovietic Academy of Medical Sciences, of which he is a member. He is also currently president of the all-Sovietic Association of Roentgenologists and Radiologists.

Among Zedguenidze's latest endeavors are acute radiation sickness, and pulmonary radiation reaction. One of his books, *Emergency Roentgen Diagnosis*, was published in 1957, in collaboration with one of his pupils, Leonid Davidovich Lindenbraten.* Another book, *Dental Roentgenology*, appeared in 1962.

Leonid Lindenbraten seems to be a rising star in Sovietic radiology. He is now professor of radiology in the first Lenin Medical Institute in Moscow. He has publications on various phases of radiology, both in therapy and in diagnosis, including intravenous cholangiography and angiocardiography. His current interests involve also the teaching of radiology, and on this he has prepared a substantial report, printed as a monograph in 1961.

One of today's leading Sovietic radiologists and radiologic teachers, Dmytri Gherasimovich Rokhlin, had also been one of Nemenov's, associates. Rokhlin has published extensively, but is best known as an osteoradiologist, and is said to be able to tell the sex and age of a patient from the sole inspection of the film of a long bone. He is chief radiologist of the first Medical Institute in Leningrad, where he has created a teaching center. In keeping up with the trends of the Atomic Phase, Rokhlin recently published (with two associates) a paper on radio-iodine in the treatment of thyroid malignancy.

*According to Russian custom, the middle name is the father's first name, combined with the suffix *itch* (patronymic). The father of Lindenbraten, Jr. is the physician David Lindenbraten. In the case of females, the suffix used for the middle name is *evna*. In either case, it is considered proper (since Czarist times) to address a person of any rank by using the first and second name only, *e.g.*, Leon Davidovich.

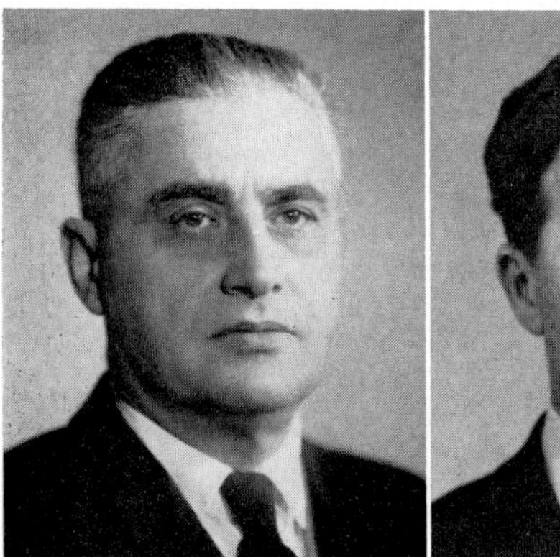

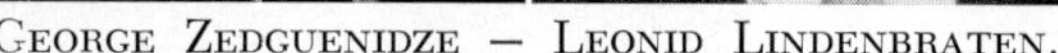

George Zedguenidze — Leonid Lindenbraten.

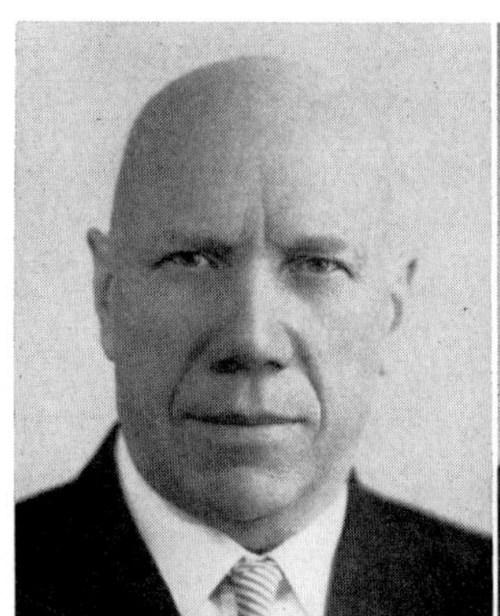

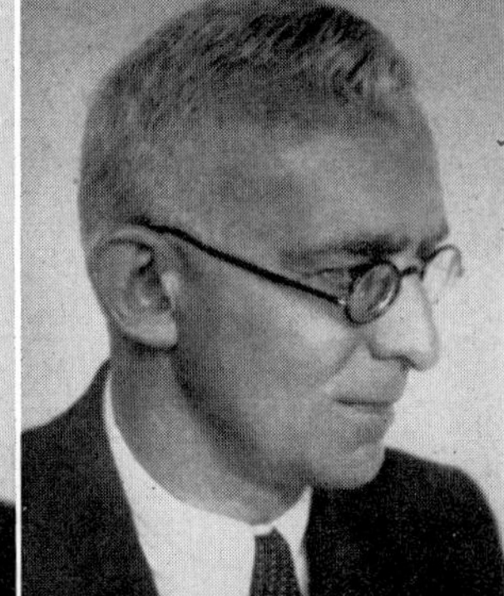

Fedor Krotkov — Dmytri Rokhlin.

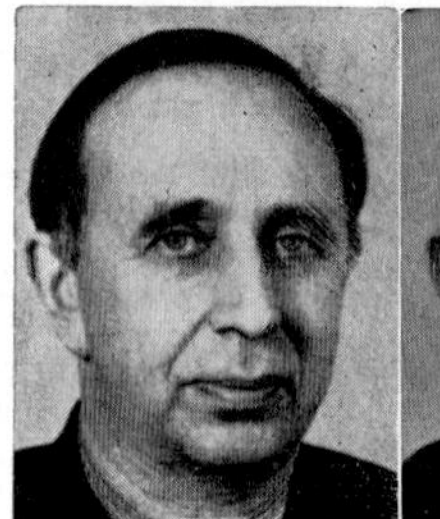

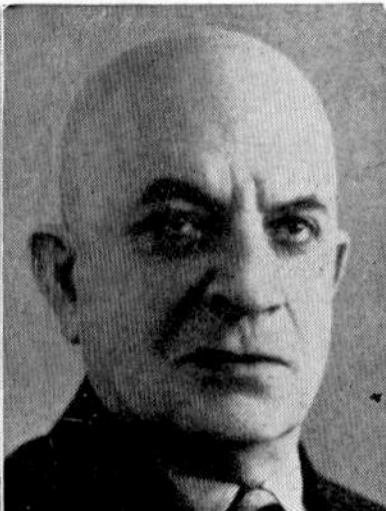

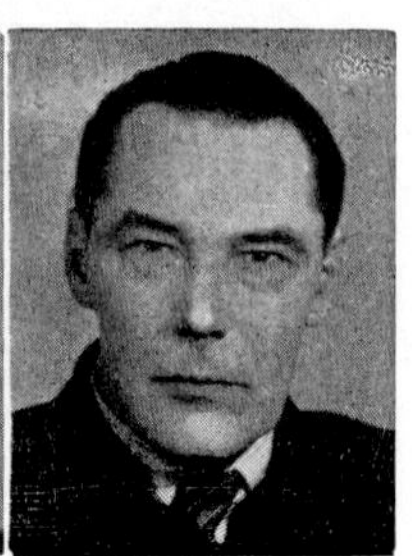

K. Aglintsev   Boris Shtern   M. Pobedinsky

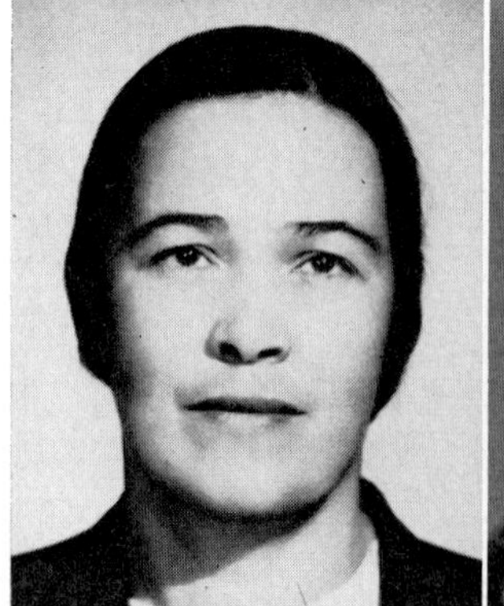

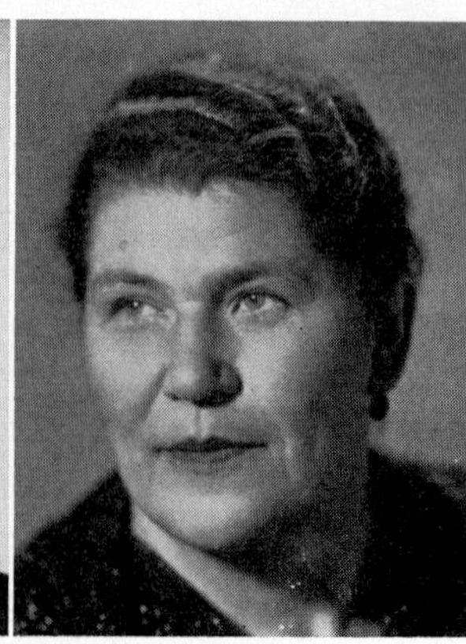

Anna Kozlova — Irina Lagunova.

Another associate of Nemenov's was July Arkussky, who is regarded as a pioneer in cardio-radiology in the Soviet Union. Catheterization became established in Moscow in 1949 with the work of E. N. Meshalkin. Their contrast media include the earlier Arbogen and the more recent Cardiotrast.

In 1948, M. S. Ovoshnikov developed tomofluorography, meaning the replacement in a body section device of the cassette with a photofluorographic pyramid. In 1954, he used the same method for registering on a single photographic plate the fluoroscopic image of a patient's entire body. The desirability or advantages of this procedure are not quite clear, it seems that there had been the intention to use it for the detection of foreign bodies or perhaps for rapid survey of the extent of systemic bone diseases (metastases?).

The proportion of female physicians in the Soviet Union exceeds that encountered in other countries. Irina Gheorghievna Lagunova is the director of the Public Roentgenologico-Radiologic Institute of the Ministry of Health in Moscow; she has written on fibrous dysplasia and other (for instance neurotrophic) bone changes. Anna Vasilevna Kozlova is today one of the leading radiation therapists in the Soviet Union — her *Principles of Radium Therapy* appeared in 1956; Kozlova's publications cover the entire field of therapy, but she devoted particular interest to the problem of avoiding radiation reaction, for which she has developed a method of procaine block of the territory under consideration. In 1960 Kozlova published a monograph on radioisotopes.

Nemenov's immediate successor in Leningrad was Mikhail Nicolaevich Pobedinsky; among his contributions is a study on the combined radium and roentgen therapy of carcinoma of the cervix. Pobedinsky has recently retired.

Nemenov's successor as editor of the *Vestnik* is Yuri Nicolaivich Sokolov, a radiologist who teaches in the Post-Graduate Institute in Moscow; he is

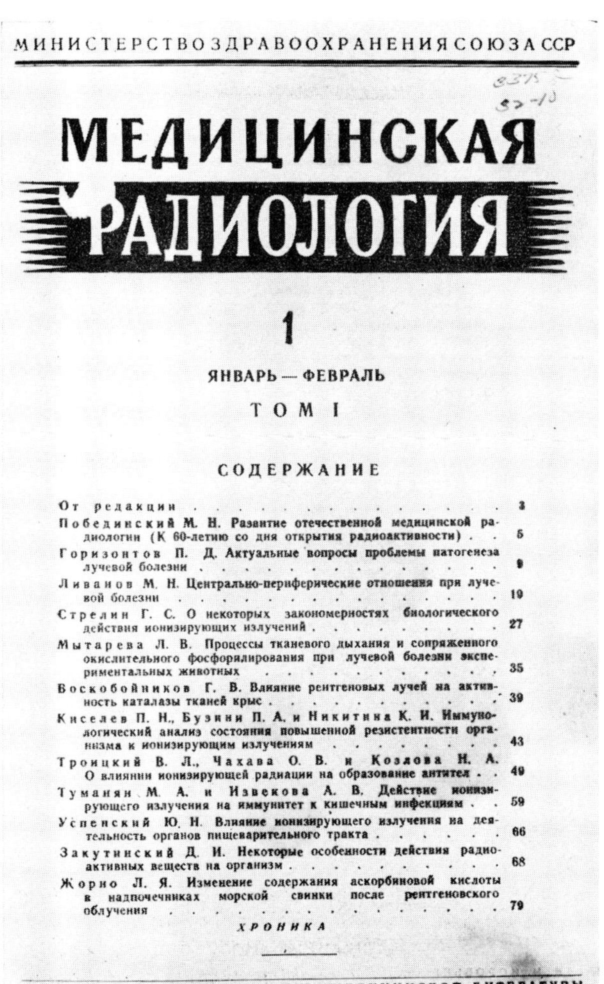
МИНИСТЕРСТВО ЗДРАВООХРАНЕНИЯ СОЮЗА ССР

МЕДИЦИНСКАЯ РАДИОЛОГИЯ

1

ЯНВАРЬ — ФЕВРАЛЬ

ТОМ I

СОДЕРЖАНИЕ

ГОСУДАРСТВЕННОЕ ИЗДАТЕЛЬСТВО МЕДИЦИНСКОЙ ЛИТЕРАТУРЫ
МЕДГИЗ — 1956 — МОСКВА

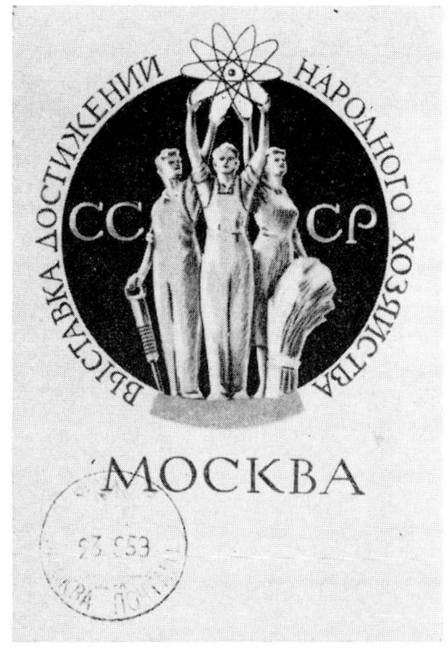

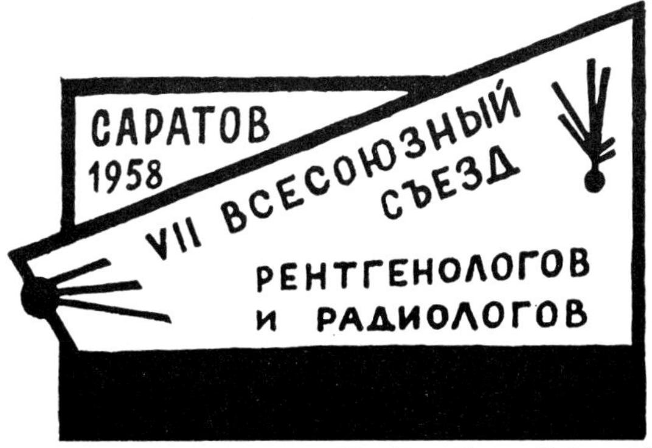

Courtesy: Georg Zedguenidze.

SARATOV 1958. Seal of the 7th All-Union Convention of Roentgenologists and Radiologists.

known for studies of *pneumosclerosis,* also called the "second disease" (the first being tuberculosis); it is a generic name which includes interstitial pulmonary fibrosis, bronchiectasis, scars, etc.

As previously stated, Sovietic terminology changes very slowly. Their meaning of radiology (today as well as twenty-five years ago) is identical with what the ABR defines as therapeutic radiology. The Sovietic term roentgenology corresponds to ABR's former definition of diagnostic roentgenology.*

In 1955, appeared in Moscow, under the editorship of A. V. Lebedinsky, a text for physicians, and students, entitled *Radiatzionnaya Medizyna.* In 1956 Fanardjian started his own periodical in Erevan (Soviet Armenia): it was called *Voprosy Rentgenologii i Onkologii.* In January of 1956 appeared the first issue of *Medizinskaya Radiologya,* edited in Moscow by the hygienist Fedor Grigorievitch Krotkov. Today its editor is Zedguenidze.

Radiology is today on the move in the Soviet Union. British advertisements have begun to appear in Sovietic radiologic periodicals. In some territories of the Soviet Union the Atomic Phase has taken over with such rapidity that they had to skip the Golden Age. Correspondingly, the root radio- is gaining momentum also in the Soviet Union. They have now, for instance, the *Voprosy Radiobiologii,* published in Leningrad since 1956. As previously stated, though, the root roentgeno- is still very much entrenched in the Soviet Union. But as long as there is life, there is hope*: a living language does things to the meaning of any given vocable.

*This was still the situation when the Washington (D. C.) radio(bio)logist Gerald McDonnell visited Russia in the Fall of 1959.

*A cancer quack had worked up a sizable clientele in the Soviet Union, then their Health Ministry heard of it, and promptly put him out of business. But the physicians of Leningrad objected violently, not in support of the quack. They asserted the right of physicians to discipline their own house, and in this respect they were ultimately sustained by the Central Committee of the Communist Party (which in the USSR is the "court of last resort").

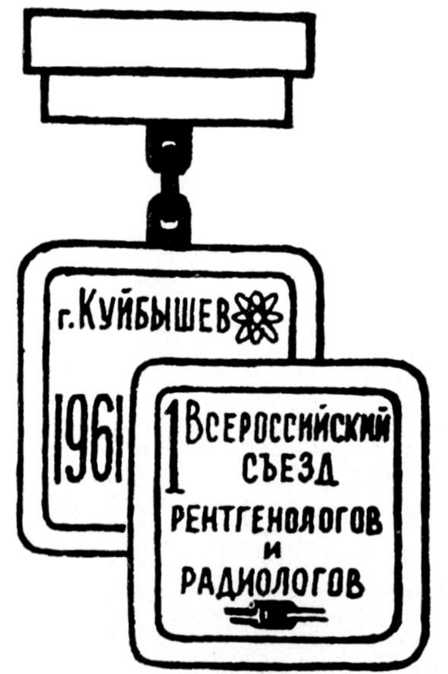

Courtesy: Georg Zedguenidze.

KUIBISHEV 1961. "Atomized" seal of the All-Russian Convention of Roentgenologists and Radiologists.

ПОСЛЕДНИЕ ДОСТИЖЕНИЯ

в изготовлении радиоизотопов—

Имеющиеся новые Изотопы. Постоянные усовершенствованные процессы в Амершам и других местах привели к тому, что на рынке появились новые изотопы для всеобщего употребления, в том числе:

- **Берилий-7**
- **Кальций-47**
- **Кобальт-57**
- **Йод-124/125**
- **Йод-132**
- **Стронций-85**

Более высокая специфическая активность. В настоящее время мы имеем возможность предложить Хлор-36 и Хром-51 следующих качеств:

- **Хлор-36 — удельная активность 0,5 мс/грам.**
- **Хром-51 — удельная активность 100 кюри/грам.**

Некоторые из этих препаратов имеются на складе, другие изготовляются через регулярные и частые промежутки времени, Мы с удовольствием дадим котировку цен нужных Вам препаратов.

По запросу мы готовы выслать подробные каталоги.

Все запросы относительно доставок радиоактивных препаратов и обслуживания просим направлять по адресу:

THE RADIOCHEMICAL CENTRE

AMERSHAM, BUCKINGHAMSHIRE, АНГЛИЯ

Мировой Центр для РАДИОХИМИЧЕСКИХ ПРЕПАРАТОВ

Телефон: Little Chalfont 2701 *Телеграфный адрес: Active, Amersham* 83141

Адрес для кабелей: Activity, Amersham Telex

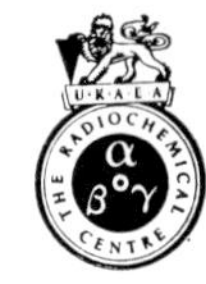

1958

TAS/RC/0

Импорт товаров в СССР осуществляется в соответствии с законоположениями о монополии внешней торговли.

BRITISH AD IN SOVIETIC RADIO-MAGAZINE.

RADIO- IN GERMANY

There had always been dissenters to the Roentgen Edict of 1905.

Lenard was one of them, and not the least articulate. His "establishment" in Heidelberg was called *Deutsches Institut für Radiologische Forschung.* At the ceremony during which Lenard received the Nobel prize he gave a talk on *Kathodenstrahlen,* a term which he used instead of x rays.

In classic German texts, the Roentgen Ordinance was strictly respected.

Such were Rieder's *Lehrbuch der Röntgenkunde;* Grashey's *Atlas typischer Röntgenbilder;* the sixteen odd German (and numerous foreign) editions of Alban Köhler's *Grenzen des Normalen und Anfänge des Pathologischen im Röntgenbilde;* or Werner Teschendorf's twin volumes of the *Lehrbuch der Röntgenologischen Differentialdiagnostik* (its monumental fourth edition is in preparation).

But the years went by, and the old guard of Teutonic Roentgen Pioneers exchanged their earthly abodes for what might well be an exclusive subdivision of Valhalla — hosted (figuratively) by Röntgen himself.* The younger generations have little respect for the old roentgen edict. Indeed, a recent monument dedicated to Röntgen is so modern that all it shows is a bundle of symbolic rays. With the *radioaktive* orientation of the Atomic Phase, the root radio- began to creep up in recent German scientese. The semantic efforts of copy writers are generally an excellent indicator of the vernacular used by the profession to whom the advertiser wishes to speak.

In 1959, in the Swiss *Radiologia Clinica* the Italian firm Barazzetti referred to itself (in a German ad) as *Spezialfabrik für Rontgenapparate*. In 1962 in the Panamenian *Radiología,* Siemens advertised its machines (in Spanish) for use in *radiodiagnostico* and *radioterapia.*

In pre-World War II Germany, the name of the firm Radiologie had been the only significant infringement of the roentgen ordinance by the German x-ray industry. Today Cosmas Röntgenerzeugnisse offers an automatic film processor called Radiomat; Fritz Hoffman GMBH had a spotfilm device named Radiograph; Agfa's very latest developer is called the Radional; and the otherwise quite historically minded C. H. F. Müller Co. stresses the advantages derived from their

*In *Röntgenblätter* of August, 1959 Friedrich Alt (of München) reported that Röntgen's bust received a place of honor in the grandiose *Walhalla Tempel.* That monumental edifice had been built in 1842 at Donaustauf (on the Danube) by Ludwig I (1786-1868) of Bavaria, who is remembered mainly for his active patronage of arts and artists (such as Lola Montez).

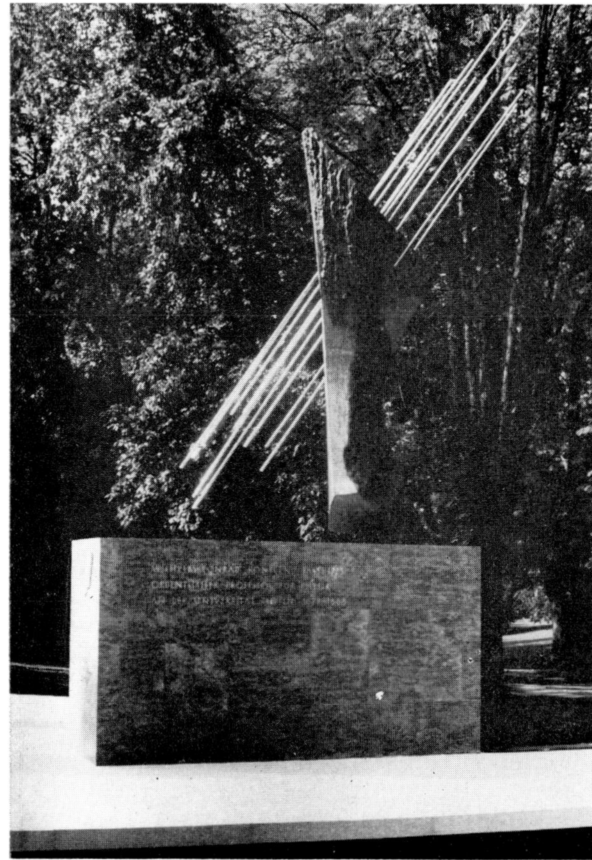

Röntgen monument in Giessen (1962)

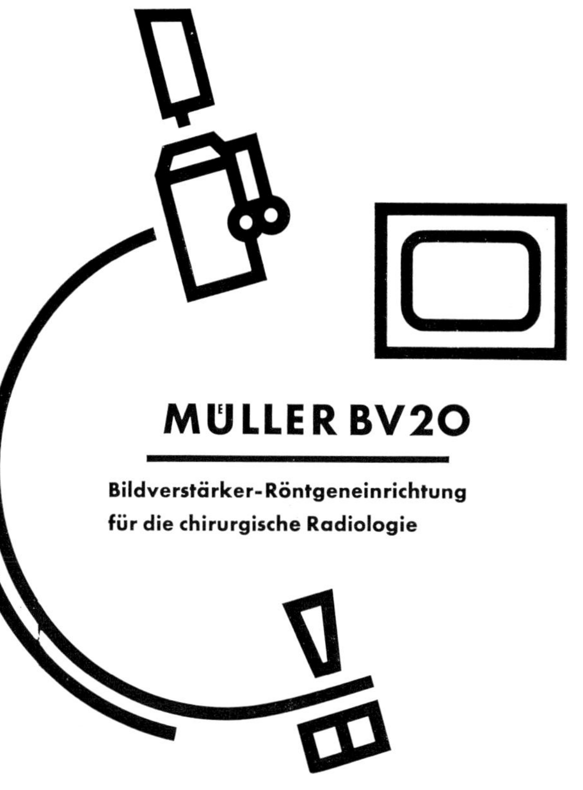

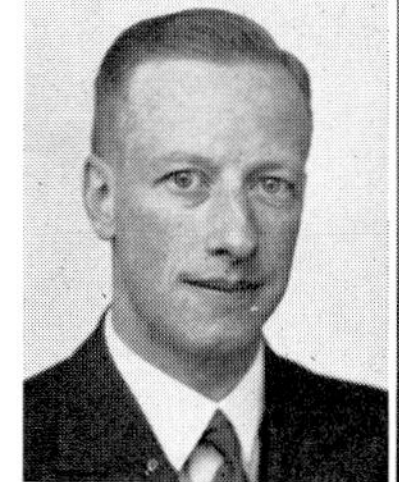

Georg Ziedses des Plantes

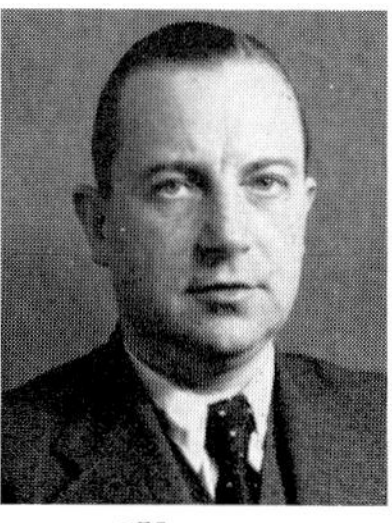

Werner Teschendorf

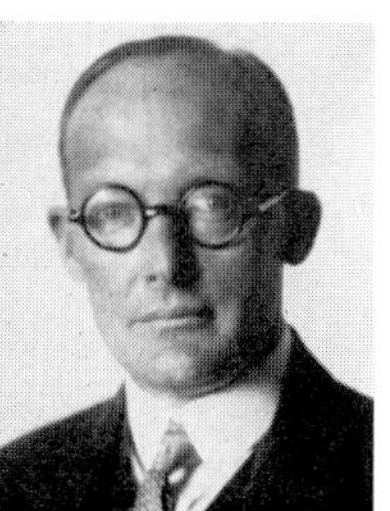

Hermann Holthusen

mobile television unit in the practice of *chirugische* (surgical) *Radiologie* (history does not record whether the remains of C. H. F. started spinning in his grave at the time such roentgen-blasphemous copy was issued with the Müller name on it.

There exists now in Germany a Vereinigung Medizinischer Assistentinnen in der Radiologie. They have – since October, 1961 – a periodical of their own, called *Die Medizinisch-Technische Assistentin in der Radiologie.* With the ninth issue they have added an orbited abbreviation, *MTA Radiologie,* but they have bowed to the roentgen root in the subtitle, Zeitschrift für Röntgen-Assistentinnen. Obviously, times have changed.

The titles of books and periodicals are also excellent gauges for evaluating the popularity of certain terms.

The Georg Thieme Verlag is conservative, and most of their titles are orthodox, such as the *Technik der Röntgendiagnostik* (1959) by the radiologist Hanno Poppe (Göttingen), in collaboration with his x-ray technician Ilse Lohstoeter, and with the physicist Philippe Lauwers (director of Gevaert's X-Ray Department in Anvers): When Daniel Routier's *Radiologie Cardiaque* was translated from French into German it became *Röntgenbild des Herzens* (1960). Conversely, an international gastro-enterologic monograph (in the spirit of the Common European Market) by Pierre Porcher (Paris), H.-U. Stössel (Bern), and P. Mainguet (Bruxelles) came out as *Klinische Radiologie des Magens und des Zwölffingerdarms* (1959). The monograph by Sabino Di Rienzo (Córdoba) and Hellmut Hermann Weber (Bern) is called *Radiologische Exploration des Bronchus* (1960). In the same way, *Klinische Neuroradiologie* (1960), with international contributions edited by Kurt Decker (München), clearly uses the word *Radiologie* in its "forbidden" sense of diagnostic discipline. Incidentally, Thieme issued several of the twenty monographs published between 1924

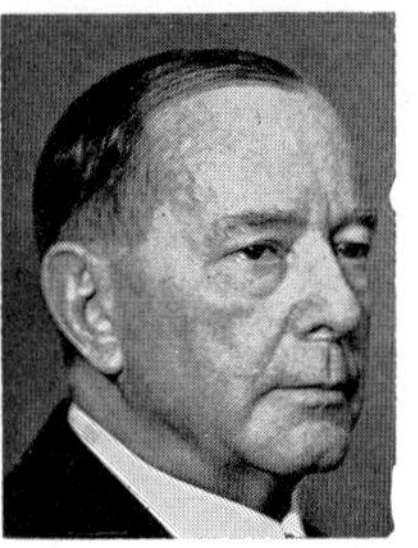

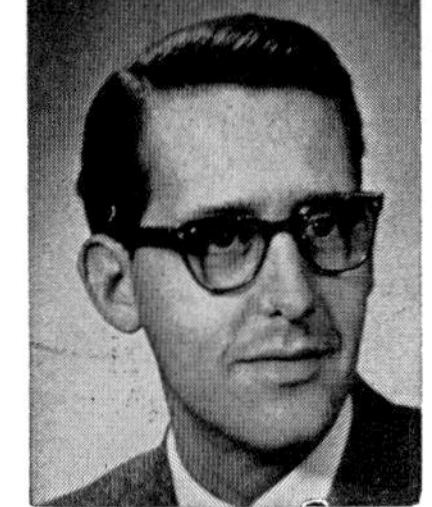

BRUNO HAUFF, SR. GÜNTHER HAUFF, JR.
OFFICIALS OF THE GEORG THIEME VERLAG.

Zeitschrift für Röntgen-Assistentinnen

MTA RADIOLOGIE

Die Medizinisch Technische Assistentin in der Radiologie

MODERN GERMAN X-RAY TECHNICIANS. The "traditional" name, *Röntgen-Assistent(in),* has been preserved but the "progressive" appelation and its orbited background have found their way onto the cover of this most recent German technical x ray journal.

DER RADIOLOGE

HERAUSGEGEBEN VON

R. HAUBRICH, KARLSRUHE · O. OLSSON, LUND · F. STRNAD, FRANKFURT/M. · H. VIETEN, DÜSSELDORF

WISSENSCHAFTLICHER BEIRAT

J. BECKER (HEIDELBERG) · L. DIETHELM (KIEL) · J. FRIMANN-DAHL (OSLO) · CH. M. GROS (STRASBOURG) K. LIDÉN (LUND) · J. NIELSEN (KOPENHAGEN) · L. OLIVA (GENUA) · G. J. VAN DER PLAATS (MAASTRICHT) S. DI RIENZO (CORDOBA) · E. RUCKENSTEINER (INNSBRUCK) · H. J. SCHÄFER (PENSACOLA) V. SVÁB (PRAG) · S. TAKAHASHI (NAGOYA) · E. M. UHLMANN (CHICAGO) · F. WACHSMANN (ERLANGEN) Z. B. ZSEBÖK (BUDAPEST) · A. ZUPPINGER (BERN)

JAHRGANG 1 · HEFT 1 · APRIL 1961

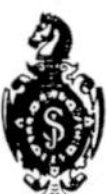

SPRINGER-VERLAG · BERLIN · GÖTTINGEN · HEIDELBERG

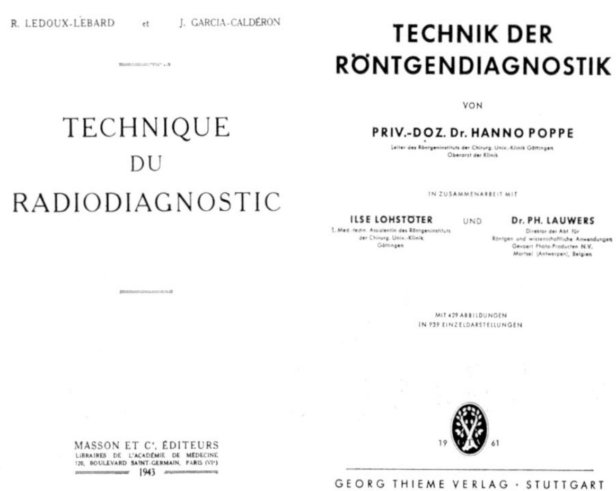

R. LEDOUX-LEBARD et J. GARCIA-CALDÉRON

TECHNIQUE
DU
RADIODIAGNOSTIC

MASSON ET Cie, ÉDITEURS
LIBRAIRES DE L'ACADÉMIE DE MÉDECINE
120, BOULEVARD SAINT-GERMAIN, PARIS (VIe)
1943

TECHNIK DER RÖNTGENDIAGNOSTIK

VON

PRIV.-DOZ. Dr. HANNO POPPE
Leiter des Röntgeninstituts der Chirurg. Univ.-Klinik Göttingen
Oberarzt der Klinik

IN ZUSAMMENARBEIT MIT

ILSE LOHSTÖTER
1. Med.-techn. Assistentin des Röntgeninstituts der Chirurg. Univ.-Klinik Göttingen

UND

Dr. PH. LAUWERS
Direktor der Abt. für Röntgen und wissenschaftliche Anwendungen Gevaert Photo-Producten N.V. Mortsel (Antwerpen), Belgien

MIT 429 ABBILDUNGEN
IN 939 EINZELDARSTELLUNGEN

1961

GEORG THIEME VERLAG · STUTTGART

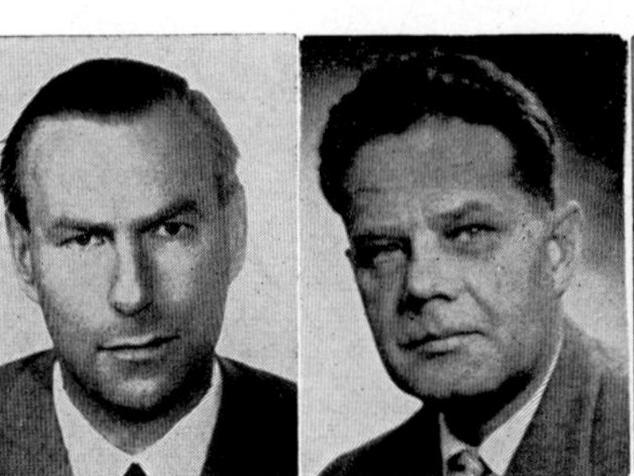

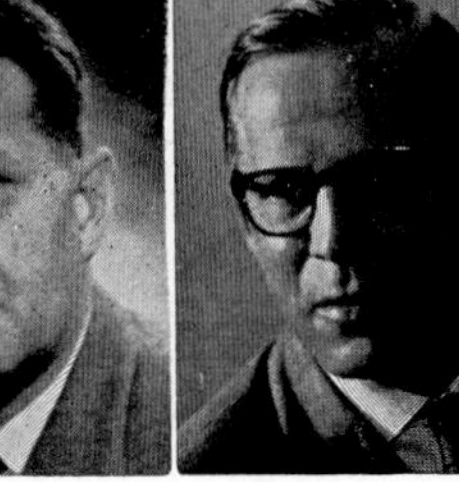

OLE OLSSON F.-J. STRNAD HEINZ VIETEN

and 1933 under the title *Radiologische Praktika* (the collection had been started in Frankfurt-am-Main by another publisher, Keim & Nemnich).

The ninth ICR (München, 1959), called in German *Internationaler Kongress für Radiologie,* published its papers under this name in the Thieme Verlag. And yet Thieme's catalog of specialty books continues to carry the twin title *Roentgenologie und Strahlenheilkunde* (therapeutic radiology).

By contrast, the catalog of the Springer Verlag has the all-encompassing catchword *Medizinische Radiologie.* In 1961, they started a new German periodical, called *Der Radiologe*: as used therein the sense of the term is all encompassing. They have in preparation a monumental, 15-20 volume, bilingual *Handbuch der Medizinischen Radiologie/Encyclopedia of Medical Radiology,* edited by Olle Olsson of Lund (Sweden), Franz-Josef Strnad of Frankfurt-am-Main (Germany), Heinz Vieten of Duesseldorf (Germany), and Adolf Zuppinger of Bern (Switzerland).

In 1963 Springer published Hermann Büchner's *Radiometrie,* which carried the "appeasing" (?) subtitle *Theorie und Praxis Roentgenologischer Messmethoden.* The German *Altmeister* in roentgen measurements, Wilhelm Ernst, would never have used such "apocryphal" terms. Interestingly enough, Theophil Christén's report on the half-value-layer in the *Archives of the Roentgen Ray* was entitled *Radiometry.* To confuse the issue (hopelessly!), the radiometer manufactured in 1963 by the Danish firm Radiometer has nothing to do with radioactivity, it is simply a pH measuring device.

And to top it, in October of 1961 the venerable *Fortschritte* announced that their abstract section will henceforth be called *Berichte aus der Radiologischen Weltliteratur.*

NUCLEAR MEDICINE MEDECINE NUCLÉAIRE

NUCLEAR-MEDIZIN

ISOTOPE IN MEDIZIN UND BIOLOGIE
ISOTOPES IN MEDICINE AND BIOLOGY
ISOTOPES EN MÉDECINE ET BIOLOGIE

EDITORES:
J. Becker, Heidelberg; K. Fellinger, Wien; D. Jahn, Nürnberg

CO-EDITORES:
R. Bauer, Tübingen; H. v. Braunbehrens, München; G. Domagk, W.-Elberfeld; B. N. Halpern, Paris; L. Heilmeyer, Freiburg/Br.; A. Herve, Liège; W. Horst, Hamburg; A. Jakob, Nürnberg; G. Joyet, Zürich; H. W. Knipping, Köln; J. Kühnau, Hamburg; L. F. Lamerton, London; K. Lang, Mainz; J. H. Lawrence, Berkeley; E. Odeblad, Stockholm; H. Oeser, Berlin; M. Perey, Strassburg; H. Pette, Hamburg; H. Schoen, Karlsruhe; A. Vannotti, Lausanne

REDACTORES:
K. E. Scheer, Heidelberg; H. Vetter, Wien

NUCLEAR-MED. VOL. 1, No. 1 15. III. 1959

FRIEDRICH-KARL SCHATTAUER-VERLAG STUTTGART POSTVERLAGSORT STUTTGART

RADIO- IN THE USA

In the country, during the Atomic Phase, usage of the root radio- was promoted by the publicity given to the threat of impending radiologic warfare.

In the *Bulletin of the Atomic Scientists* of November, 1961, W. H. Clark discussed very seriously a Doomsday Machine, which might consist of 1000 tons of heavy water, with a boron blanket. The device could be towed in by an enemy submarine, and sunk to the bottom of the sea near one of our Coast lines. When detonated, the resulting tidal wave, 100 feet high, would wreck the cities from Maine to Florida. As an alternative the 20 tons of neutrons (produced by the 1000 tons of heavy water) could radio-contaminate 200,000 square miles into a landscape of lunar desolation.

In the *Bulletin of the Atomic Scientists* of February, 1962, Gerard Piel calculated that one 1000 megaton Hydrogen bomb, exploded at satellite altitude above the USA, could produce a firestorm that would sear six Midwestern states into a similarly bare desert.

Seymour Melman's concept of the "overkill" (*cf., Saturday Review* of May 4, 1963) is based on the as-

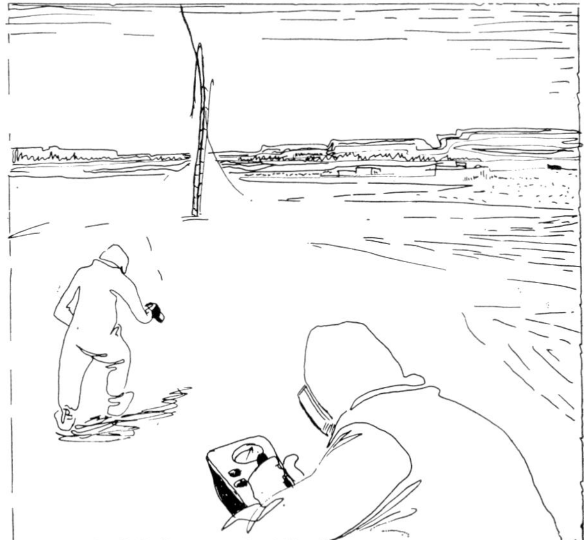

LANDSCAPE OF LUNAR DESOLATION. Compare with N. O. Hines (page 846).

sumption that both the USA and the USSR each have an atomic arsenal large enough to "more than kill" all but a fraction of the adversary's entire population. It is doubtful whether any stockpile is big enough, or any delivery system accurate enough, to complete such a task — but that is beside the point. Melman's conclusions — that we must start to dismantle our atomic weaponry, step by step, whereupon the USSR would be convinced of our intentions, and should follow us on the peace path — such conclusions are puerile. The only thing that deters a full-scale atomic conflict is the adversary's certainty that there could be no true winner of such a conflict. In my opinion there will be other wars, and perhaps tactical atomic devices might come into use, but no city-busters will be dropped, at least not in the foreseeable future. For those who wish to read a more technical reply to Melman's dreamy assumptions, there has appeared Amrom Harry Katz's *The Myth of Overkill* in the *Air Force and Space Digest* of February, 1964.

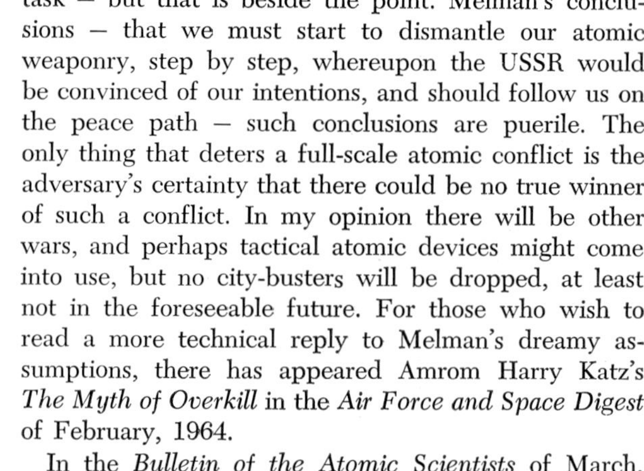

In the *Bulletin of the Atomic Scientists* of March, 1962, Freeman John Dyson defined several new units. The "Beach" (nomenclature originated at the 1960 Summer Study on Arms Control, by courtesy of the late Nevil Shute) is a quantity of fission energy which, if exploded in the atmosphere, would produce enough global fallout to give a lethal dose of radiation to one-half of the earth's inhabitants.

Estimates vary from 10^6 to 10^7 megatons, with the value 3×10^6 megatons presumably correct within the stated uncertainty of a factor of three. The "Kahn" (from the name of the physicist of Rand Corporation, author of a report on potential bomb casualties and desirability of fallout shelters) is the quantity of fission

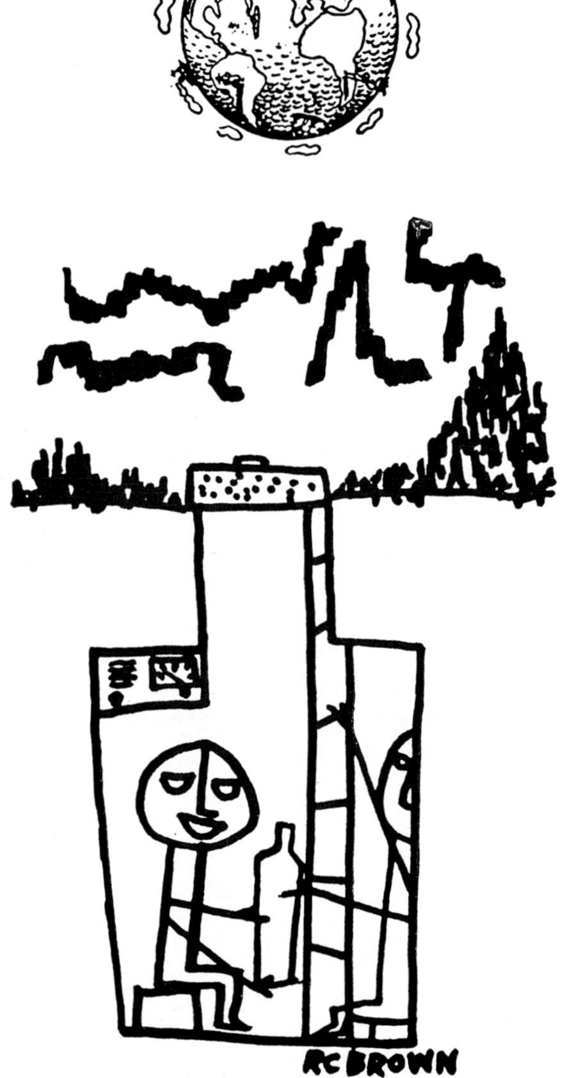

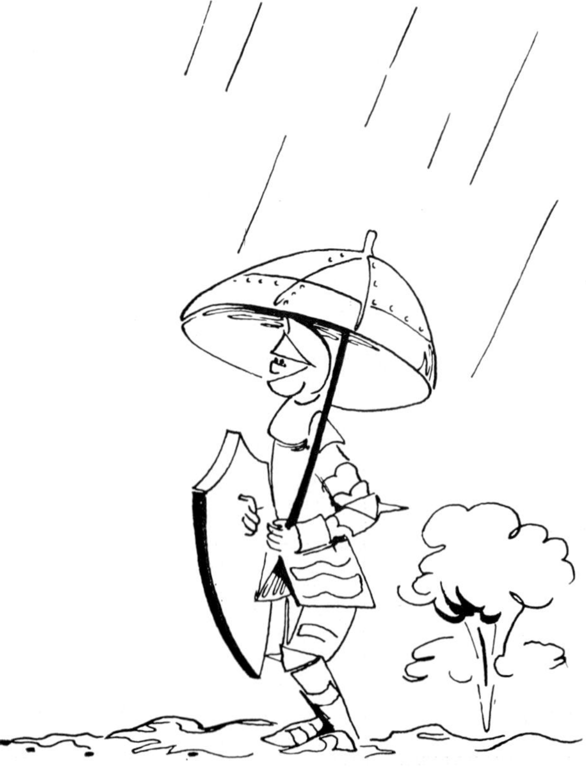

energy delivered to ground targets in a major country which would kill essentially all the inhabitants of that country by local fallout, in the absence of bomb shelters; estimates of the "Kahn" range from 3000 to 30,000 megatons. The third unknown number is called the "Stockpile," meaning the potential of nuclear bombs which a country could muster if it were to transform all its stored uranium into bombs. The USA "Stockpile" is estimated at 1.3 "Beach," with a similar quantity presumably available in the USSR.

Such apocalyptic perspective conjures the image of a tired St. Michael in full armor, strolling wearily through the rain, with a lead parasol for protection against the fallout.

So much potential fallout suggests the need for Radiological Health Specialists but so far these have very little to do with the fallout.

The Radiological Health Specialists are not physicians. They are intended to do a job of "preventive maintenance." They would staff the Radiological Health Divisions of the various agencies planned, or already legislated at federal, state, county, and city levels for the "control" of all sources of ionizing radiation. Of course, first in line are the tools of the medical radiologist.

Several scary radio-vocables became part of the language, for instance the self-explanatory radio-shock.

The older radio-toxaemia has been practically replaced by the newer radio-contamination. The latter evolved into a new discipline: on the grounds of Colorado State University in Boulder, on September 11-15, 1961 a Symposium on Radio-ecology was held . . . an ominous thought about future environments.

Radio-iodotherapeusis sounds and is fancy but there is no doubt about what it means. Radio-cardiography, however, is not an x-ray method of gauging the size of the heart; it is an isotopic procedure for evaluating blood flow to the heart and other parts. Radio-capsules (not to be confused with radiocaps) are miniaturized battery-powered FM broadcast transmitters which, when swallowed by the patient, can (re-) transmit internal physiologic data to an extracorporeal monitoring device.

On May 11, 1961 — during the ARS meeting in Colorado Springs — Joseph L. Morton (Indianapolis) moderated a Symposium on Radiosensitivity and Radiocurability, as judged by microscopical technics.

The panel members used mostly conventional terms, such as radioresistance, radioresponsiveness, radiopathology, radiohistology, even at one time radiocolloid. Nobody mentioned radiesthesia (divination by the so-

THE ACCRA ASSEMBLY — THE WORLD WITHOUT THE BOMB 21st. TO 28th. JUNE 1962
6d
GHANA

HIROSHIMA
PEACE FOREVER
1949
FIRST DAY OF ISSUE
IN COMMEMORATION OF ESTABLISHMENT OF HIROSHIMA CITY OF PEACE.

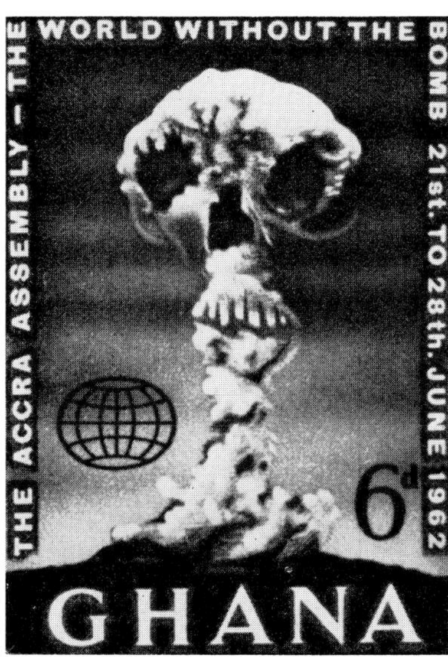

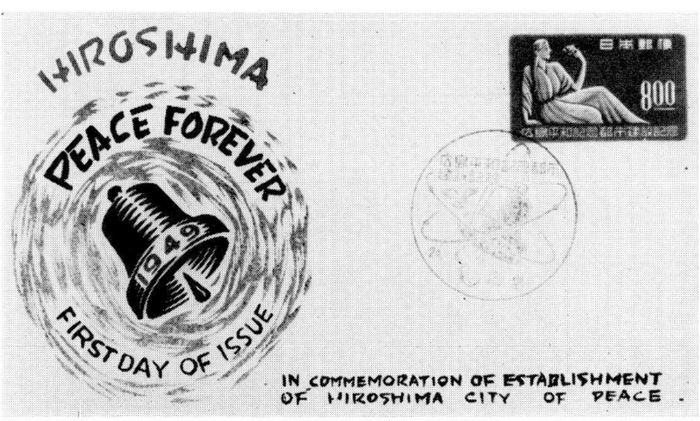

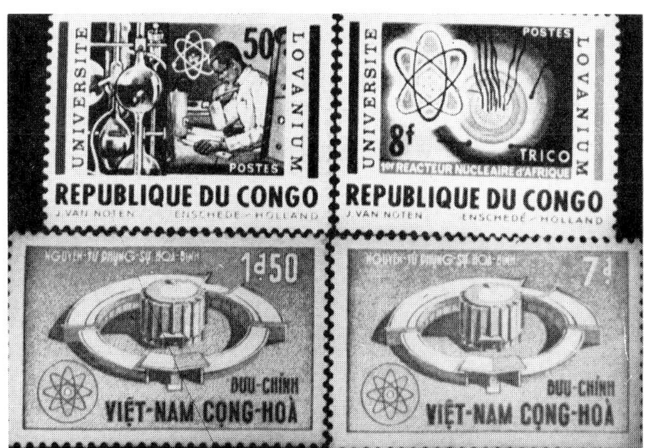

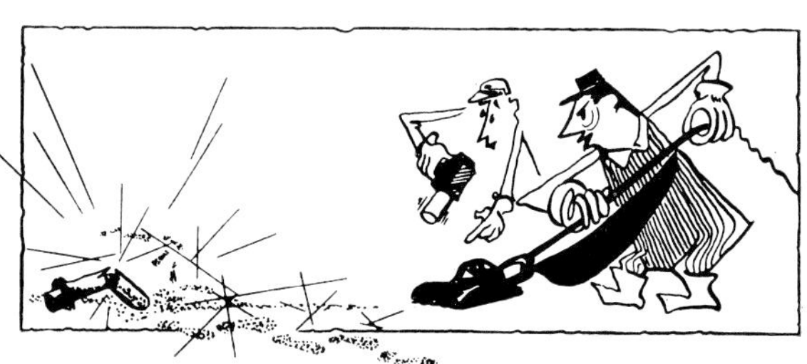

called pendulum) although this might have sounded quite appropriate as an appellation for those who wish to predict the outcome of an irradiated tumor from the morphology of its cells.

In this country the term x ray is today quite common, for instance it appears in the names of many hospital (X-Ray) departments.

It may be recalled that several textbooks use "x-ray" in their title, for instance Max Ritvo's *Chest X-ray Diagnosis* (1951), or John P. Caffey's classical *Pediatric X-ray Diagnosis,* of which the 5th edition is being prepared.

In the underworld slang (Eric Partridge), x ray means a $10 thousand bill (while X is a $10 bill). In the same slang, a large diamond is called a radiator, sometimes spelled ray-diator, because it "emits rays of light." In English slang, x-legs are knock knees (genu valgus).

In the Atomic Phase, as the word radiology and its radioactive particles became well known, their popularity was utilized — in reverse — by the "broadcasting cousins," the most often heard or seen being a play on words over a given radio station getting to be "radioactive."

X-ray, in the aviator's phonetic alphabet stands for the letter x. The VOR airways are called Victor (for instance V 161 or V 38) for the same reason, Victor is the letter v in the phonetic alphabet.

There is in the *AMA Journal* a monthly "X-ray Seminar," sponsored by the Massachusetts General Hospital — the first in this series was published as of July 22, 1961.

An exhibit entitled "X-Ray Detective" is on display in the Hall of Fame of the ICS in Chicago.

The collection consists of thirty-one radiographs exemplifying the non-destructive examination of rare objects, art work, stamps, and so on, for the demonstration of authenticity, or for the detection of forgery. The material was donated by Herbert C. Pollack (a Chicago radiologist) and Charles F. Bridgeman (an Eastman Kodak executive).

It is not generally known that the x-ray examination of paintings was performed in Vienna as early as March, 1896. In the *Scientific American* of January, 1940 Charles Wisner Barrell claimed that x-ray examinations of Shakespeare portraits supported the (also otherwise very sensible) view of the Oxfordian school, *i.e.,* that Shakespeare was the pseudonym used by the mysterious Elizabethan courtier and lyric poet Edward de Vere, later Bulbeck (1550-1604).

No doubt exists in the case of the master art forger Hans van Meegeren (1889-1947). He was very

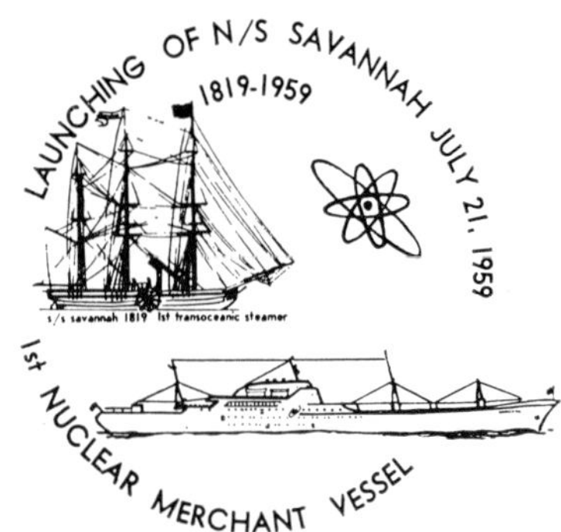

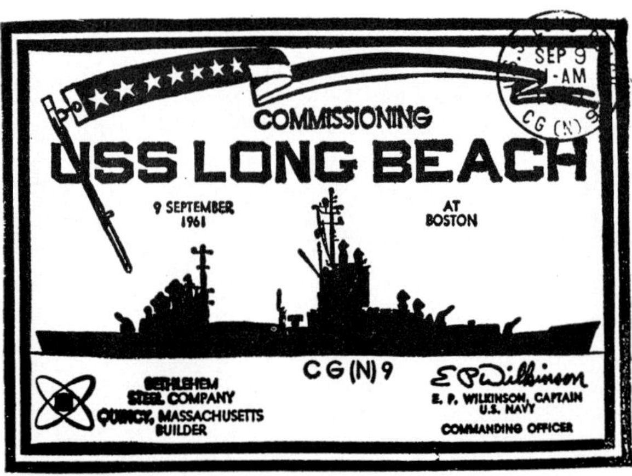

Courtesy: Stan Bohrer.

WORLD'S FIRST NUCLEAR CRUISER. The atomic powered guided missile cruiser USS Long Beach CGN-9 was first underway on October 27, 1961.

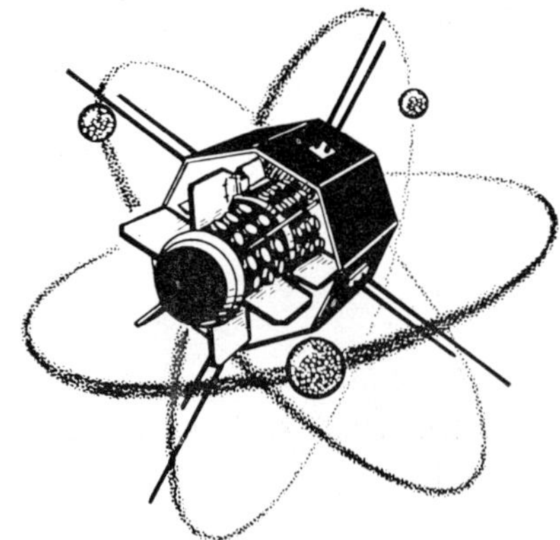

ATOMIES IN ORBIT. Symbol borrowed from *Nucleonics,* wherein it indicates the intended use of nuclear power in space.

CBS
ATTENTION! THIS AREA IS RADIO ACTIVE
turn YOUR DIAL TO 1400
WDWS The News-Gazette STATION
For the FINEST in MUSIC NEWS and SPORTS

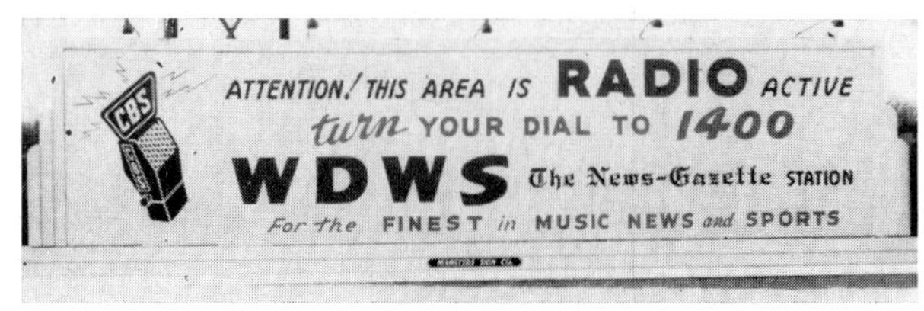

talented, but art works signed with his own name never were more than mildly successful.

Van Meegeren became a specialist in the painting style and technic of the famous *genre* master Jan Vermeer (1632-1675) – and sold alleged Vermeers for a total of $2 million. Most of these paintings changed hands during the Nazi occupation of Holland; therefore, after the end of World War II, Van Meegeren was hauled into court for having sold national art treasures to the enemy. That is when he defended himself by revealing he had duped the Nazis. He proved it by painting another "almost authentic" Vermeer. X-ray examinations of his previous exploits proved the forgery. He was then sentenced to one year in prison, where he died of coronary occlusion.

American physicians, both in and outside the radiologic profession, employ many colloquial forms derived from x ray, including the (proscribed) verbs to x-ray, and to reray. Such unorthodox forms can be found quite often in x-ray (roentgen) reports. More restraint is generally applied in the case of articles, especially when the manuscript is intended for the Yellow Journal. The *American Journal of Roentgenology* is the last bastion of the Roentgen Edict, but their editors have more and more difficulty to enforce such rules.

In the *American Journal of Roentgenology* of May, 1954 GE stressed that its Imperial can be used very easily for tall individuals; the caption reads, "Could you x-ray Mr. Basketball in this position?" In a December, 1960 editorial Arthur Stiennon wondered whether it is justifiable to regard prolapse of the gastric mucosa as a "clinical-radiologic" entity. The words medical radiology can be found in the conclusion of an article on "x-ray image intensification" by Wilfred F. Niklas, published in February of 1961. And in March, 1961 Eugene P. Pendergrass – in the eulogy of William Stell Newcomet (1872-1960) – wrote, ". . . Dr. Newcomet became interested in the employment of x-rays in the study of the chest . . ."

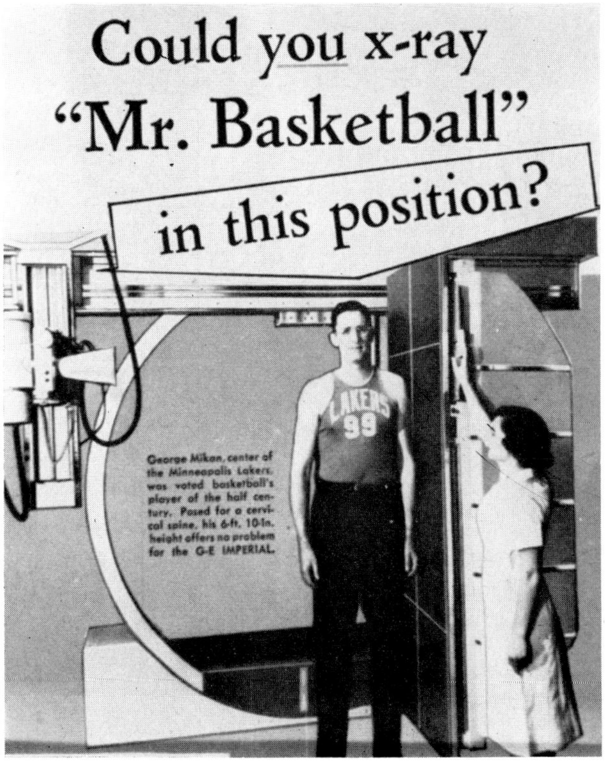

As a matter of fact, in 1919 and 1920, the terms radiology and its derivates (radiographic, radioscopic, etc.) were freely used in the columns of the Yellow Journal. Today's strict policy was not introduced until late in the 1920s.

The editors of the Yellow Journal insist also on using roentgenoscopy and roentgenography (which are practically obsolete in the spoken language), and roentgenogram (instead of radiograph or x-ray). Words are the clothes that thoughts wear — only the clothes (Samuel Butler). There is no urgency to change the policy of the *American Journal of Roentgenology*. It may even be desirable to retain (by force) some of these antiquated vocables, if only for their historic flavor. The next generation of radiologists, or maybe the one after the next, will take care to eliminate the excessively outdated relics.

The etymologies employed in the names of regional radiologic associations are at times interesting, and often confusing.

In September, 1933, Garland, Newell, and Stone founded in the Bay area (a) the *X-ray Study Club of San Francisco* which, by a process of budding and fission, acquired after 1946 three (scientific) sister organizations: (b) the *South Bay Radiological Society* in Menlo Park, (c) the *East Bay Roentgen Society* in Oakland, and (d) a *Northern California Radiological Society* in Sacramento. They also have (e) the *San Francisco Radiological Society* (created for economic purposes), and (f) a city-wide *Section on Radiology* of the San Francisco Medical Society (revived to give radiology a mouthpiece in local organized medicine). In addition, San Francisco furnishes headquarters for the (g) state-wide *Pacific Roentgen Society,* which is the Section on Radiology of the California State Medical Association.* In July, 1962 the Pacific Roentgen Society changed its name to California Radiological . . .!

---

*This information was courteously supplied by Dr. John Harvey Heald, a San Francisco radiologist who is the present secretary of the *X-Ray Study Club*. At least partial fusion seems to be in progress because (a), (e), and (f) are now holding combined quarterly meetings.

The radiologic organization in Milwaukee changed its name at least twice. At the meeting of November 25, 1963, on the occasion of its 40th anniversary, John Edwin Habbe (one of its senior members) recalled the history of the society's beginnings. On December 21, 1923, Harry Bernard Podlasky (1884-1935), radiologist at Mount Sinai Hospital and first professor of roentgenology at Marquette University, called a few colleagues to meet in his office for the purpose of organizing a new society, rather than (as the minutes said) to attempt to reorganize the old one. Habbe tried hard to locate some information on that pristine group, but efforts "led to naught." In 1922, Fouts listed that "old" society as the Milwaukee X-Ray Club. Podlasky's group decided to call themselves the Milwaukee County Radiological Society. Its first president was Frank Mackoy (1880-1954), who succeeded Podlasky in the position of head of the teaching service in roentgenology at Marquette. The secretary was Clarence Geyer, the radiologist of the Marquette University Hospital. Habbe came to Milwaukee in 1927, one year after Geyer's death. At some unspecified date, the organization

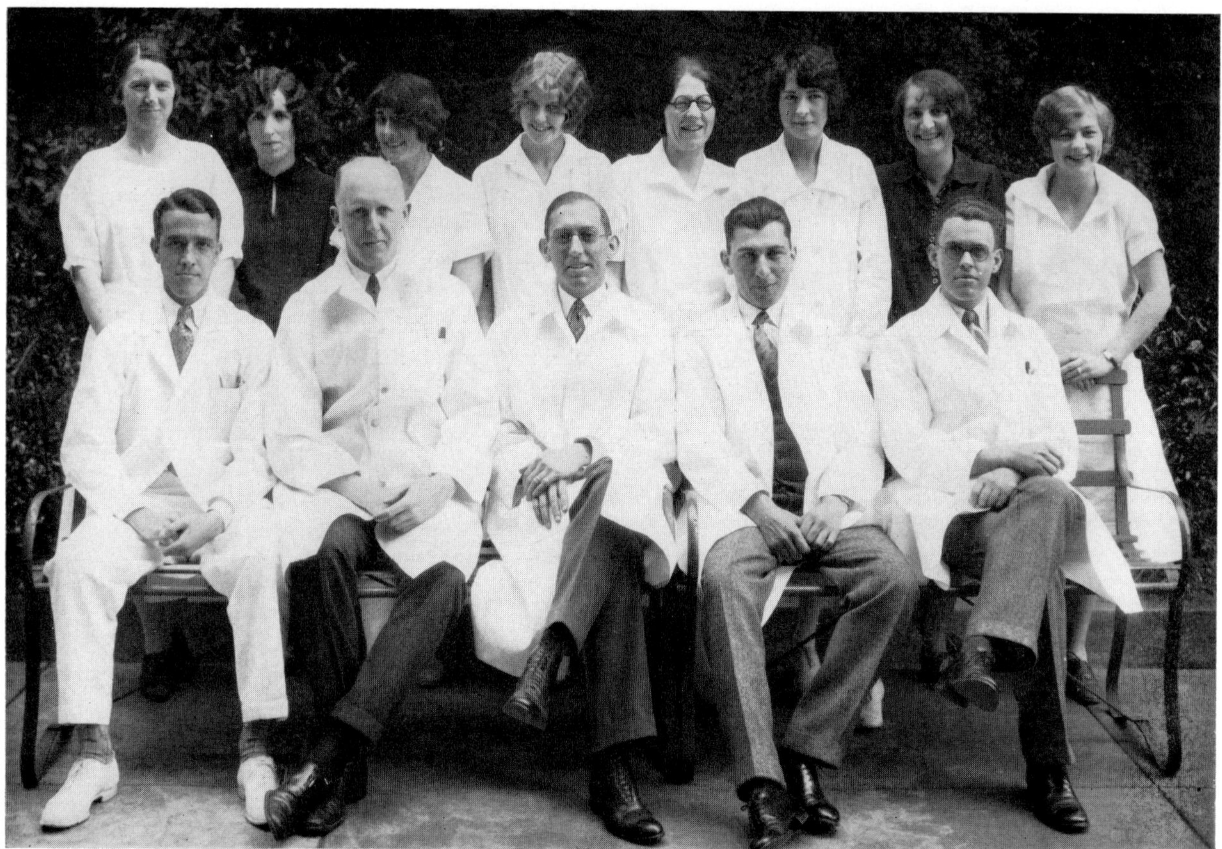

RADIOLOGY AT STANFORD (1927). From the left (sitting): Garland, Bob Newell, Ed Chamberlain, Frank Rice, and Wm. Taylor. Writes Garland: "Chamberlain and Newell were dynamic and not prone to silence at staff meetings, which made for a minimum of torpor at ward rounds and CPC's. The lateral chest film was coming into vogue, and there were mighty arguments on its usefulness, if any. Intravenous cholecystography was a moderately major procedure. Intravenous urography was just on the horizon. Pneumoencephalography required strong backs and considerable endurance on all sides. There was endless debate as to the most reliable measure of radiation dosage (the E unit of Duane; the R unit of Solomon; while the pastille was still in use). Meantime, milligram-hours and milliampere-minutes permitted reasonable documentation of exposure. In retrospect, radiology at Stanford Hospital in those days was in the happy era of clinical practice (the Golden Age), after having overcome the mechanical difficulties inherent in early apparatus. In 1927, Ed Chamberlain made some x ray movies of the heart, using 10x12 films exposed sequentially at 4 to 8 frames per second. The noise, the radiation, and the ensuing 35 mm or 16 mm reproductions entertained all hands. *Eheu fugaces labuntur anni!*"

changed its name to the one currently in use, the Milwaukee Roentgen Ray Society.

The radiologic organization in Denver underwent its own two changes in name, but they were of a different nature. On October 23, 1930 Frederick E. Diemer, a Denver radiologist, held an organizational meeting at his home, and those present decided to form the Denver Radiological Club, which met on November 18, 1930 and adopted a constitution and by-laws. The first president was Samuel Childs, with Diemer as secretary. At the September, 1933 annual meeting of the RSNA, Walter Wasson proposed that the 1935 RSNA meeting be held in Denver, but Rollin Stevens objected to that by claiming it would be too cold and snowy in Denver, and so he succeeded to get that meeting place for his home town, Detroit. Thereupon, at Wasson's suggestion, the Denver Radiological Club decided to organize its own regular Summer Radiologic Conference: the first one was held on August 29/30, 1935. In 1941 they changed that name to Rocky Mountain Radiological Society, which could then include members from adjoining states. And on October 15, 1948 the Denver Radiologic Club voted to change its name to Colorado Radiological Society.

The name was no problem in Missouri. In June, 1957 Gwilym Lodwick, the professor of radiology in the University of Missouri at Columbia, called an organizational meeting, at which both Wendell Scott (of St. Louis) and Ira Lockwood (of Kansas City) spoke in favor. But when the constitution and by-laws were to have been adopted, the Greater St. Louis Society of Radiologists stood firm against the organization of a state society, for reasons that matters of representation would be very difficult if members joined a state society, and that problems of out-state Missouri and Kansas City were quite different from those in St. Louis. Thereupon the project "went to sleep for a few years," and was revived by the same Lodwick in the summer of 1960. At that time the organizational committee met for several times until they solved the "matter of representation," and the Missouri Radiological Society was officially incorporated on January 6, 1961, with Gwilym Lodwick as its first president. He even worked with the artist on the design of the society's seal.

MILWAUKEE ROENTGEN RAY SOCIETY
FOUNDED 1923

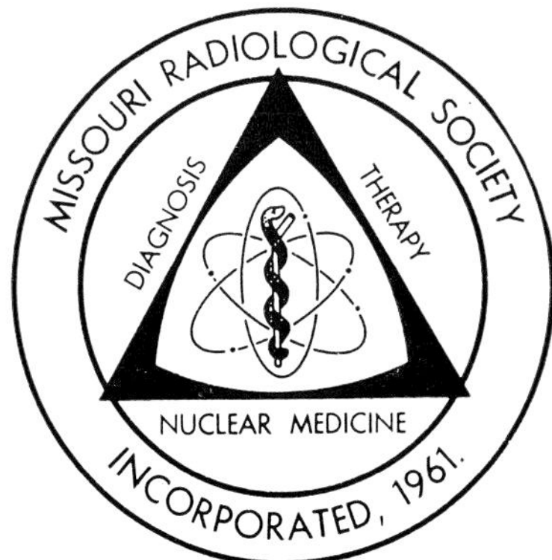

A variety of roots was used in the Bay area as a means of differentiation. Such a mixture may be less desirable in a text.

In Great Britain it is perfectly dignified to use the term x-ray (both colloquially and in writing) either as a verb, noun, or adjective.

An etymologic purist might object to some features found in the "British" translation (1955) of the Dutch text from T.J.J.H. Meuwissen's well illustrated and competently captioned gastro-enterologic atlas. But the translated text is quite clear, so that matter is one of

X-RAY IT ON *Ensign* FILM

BARNET ENSIGN LTD., FULBOURNE ROAD, WALTHAMSTOW, LONDON, E.17

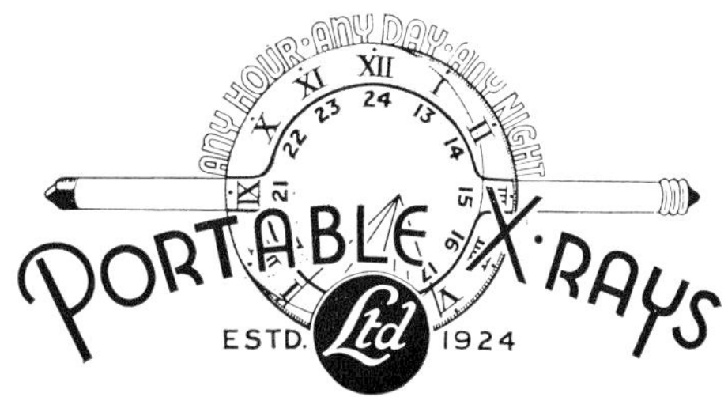

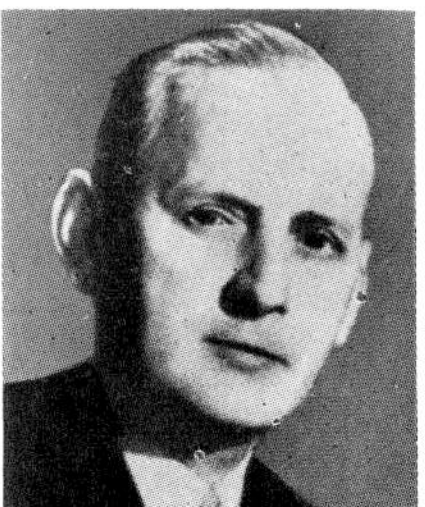

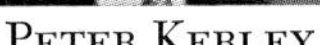
PETER KERLEY

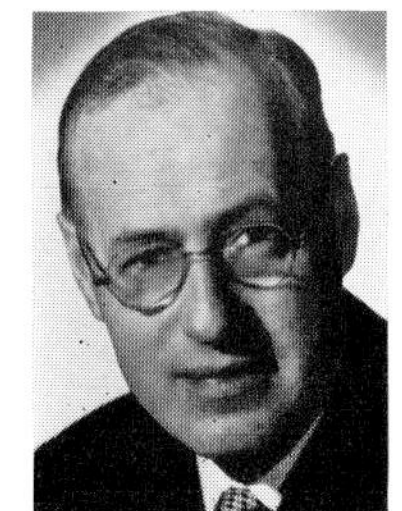
COCHRANE SHANKS

esthetics, *i.e.*, debatable, as people are entitled to differ in matters of taste.

There is the physicistic text *X-ray Microscopy* (Cambridge University Press, 1960) by the two British specialists in "flying spot technics," V. E. Cosslett and W. C. Nixon.

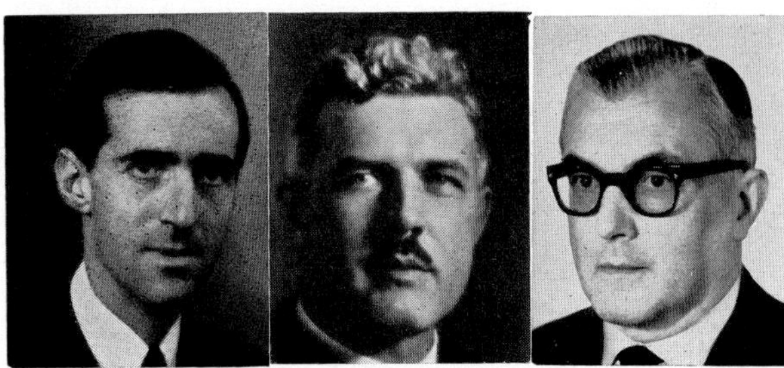

MAURICE TUBIANA URSUS PORTMANN WILHELM ERNST

APRIL 1963

VOLUME I NUMBER 1

THE RADIOLOGIC CLINICS OF NORTH AMERICA

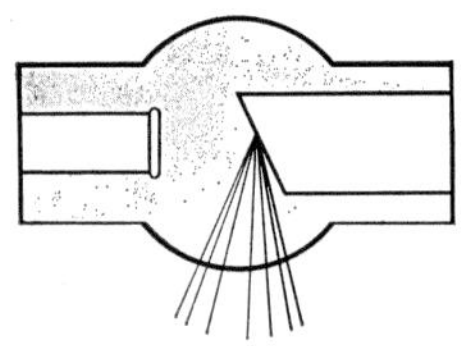

Symposium on

RECENT CLINICAL ADVANCES IN RADIOLOGY

Philip J. Hodes, M.D.
Guest Editor

W. B. SAUNDERS COMPANY
PHILADELPHIA AND LONDON

The title of the standard British textbook by Shanks and Kerley is *X-ray Diagnosis.* A similar American work, originally edited by Ross Golden, and now re-edited by Laurence Robbins, is called *Diagnostic Roentgenology.* When Englishmen write for American consumption they are not beyond using the term roentgenology, as did the well-known physicist George William Clarkson Kay (1880-1941).

But neither are all American book titles uniform in this respect.

Ursus Victor Portmann edited in 1950 the *Clinical Therapeutic Radiology* (a new edition of this classic text is long overdue); its very title implied the existence of diagnostic radiology. In recent years post-graduate courses in "diagnostic radiology" are being offered in several places, *e.g.*, in Indiana, in California, and in Kansas.

In 1952, Bernard S. Epstein, chief radiologist of the Long Island Jewish Hospital, published a book on the *Clinical Radiology of Acute Abdominal Disorders.* The following year, with Leo M. Davidoff, Epstein issued an *Atlas of Skull Roentgenograms.*

Until 1959, the cards in the Catalog of the Army Medical Library, published in book form, were indexed separately under roentgenography, radiography, radiotherapy, and roentgentherapy. Since 1960 — when the National Library of Medicine (NLM) took over — roentgenography was abandoned (after being retained for one more year as a cross reference to radiography). The same thing happened to roentgentherapy in favor of radiotherapy.

More recently there is in this country the tendency to use the term radiology in the (French and British) sense of purely diagnostic endeavor.

The (abortive) Society for Investigative Radiology wa the dream of Thomas R. Marshall of the University of Louisville (Kentucky), but his efforts were "nipped in the bud" during the 1963 ARRS meeting in Montreal.

The (apocryphal) American Society of Clinical Radiology was organized in California in 1961. Its pro-

THE REGISTRY OF RADIOLOGIC PATHOLOGY

Sponsored by

THE AMERICAN COLLEGE OF RADIOLOGY, THE AMERICAN ROENTGEN RAY SOCIETY, and THE RADIOLOGICAL SOCIETY OF NORTH AMERICA,

At the

ARMED FORCES INSTITUTE OF PATHOLOGY

Washington, D. C.

motional leaflets indicate clearly that no reference to any form of radiation therapy was implied by its title.

There is also the (very legitimate) Society for Pediatric Radiology.

It was organized during the ARRS meeting of September, 1958 in Washington (D.C.). The first president of the "pediatric radiologists" was Edward D. Neuhauser of Boston and their first secretary was Richard Lester of Minneapolis. Upon inquiry, the latter stated that they had never given any particular thought to a precise definition of the term radiology in their title, but since they have members interested both in the diagnostic and in the therapeutic aspects of radiology, he believes that the broader sense might apply. Actually, their scientific sessions are (almost) entirely devoted to diagnostic problems.

There is finally a title in which no equivocation is possible. It is the Registry of Radiologic Pathology, at the Armed Forces Institute of Pathology in Washington (D.C.), sponsored jointly by the ACR, ARRS, and RSNA. In this title the term radiologic is obviously used in a purely diagnostic connotation.

CONCLUDING THOUGHTS

Shakespeare's rose would certainly smell as sweet by any other name. Scientific terminology may be no more than an academic exercise in semantic futility, but understanding demands some agreement over the meanings given to what words are utilized. Therefore syllables govern the world (John Selden), especially the modern world, which has put such a price on both the national and the international communication of ideas.

Most of the time it is useless to lay down etymologic rules and regulations. Words are like leaves; some wither every year, and every year a younger race succeed (Roscommon). But it is necessary to review at periodic intervals the semantic content of important (or perhaps of all) disciplines. Successive terminologic baselines are the best available method for grasping the relationship between words, underlying ideas, and past as well as current scientific and popular concepts. Modern medical history (regardless whether it investigates Galen, Paracelsus, or Röntgen) is inconceivable without the careful etymologic analysis of all catchwords encountered at the time and place under consideration.

We have seen the epic battle of the radio-prefix and the roentgen-eponym. We have noticed the past and present geographic variations in the meaning of the terms used in radiology. Many times the reasons for these variations were outright preposterous, yet differences will continue to exist: we cannot remove them by ignoring their existence. In 1867, the aristocratic jurist George Douglas Campbell, 8th Duke of Argyll (1823-1900), remarked caustically that "words, which should be the servants of thought, are too often its masters!"

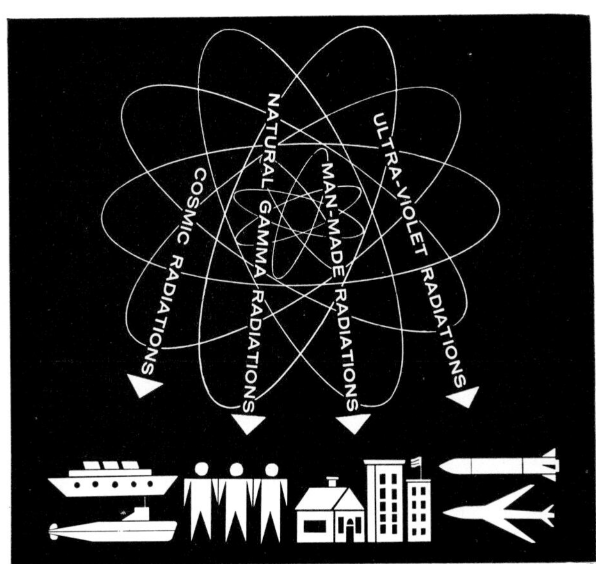

Chapter 4

A PLEA FOR PALLIATION*

Thou shalt not kill, but need'st not strive
Officiously to keep alive!
ARTHUR HUGH CLOUGH

WHILE THE biologic age of the population advances, there occurs an increase in the incidence of malignant neoplasms.** As the perfect oncolytic agent is still wanting, there also occurs a proportional rise in the number of "hopeless" cancer patients. And yet, in medical schools few hours of formal teaching - if any at all - are devoted to the management of "incurable" situations.

Over the past fifty years, medical curricula have suffered more and more from the inroads of specialization. Teachers have waged serious battles over their allotted portion of the student's time. But since for a given timespan there is a limit to what one person can accumulate in the way of information, even general subjects had to be trimmed to make place for the bandwagon of those who want to teach more and more about less and less.

As a result, many physicians experience a feeling of inadequacy and despair when they must approach a patient in whom - as in the metaphor of Metastasio† - "The Canker, which the trunk conceals, is revealed by the leaves, the fruit, or the flower."

Some day, oncologic surgery may be proscribed; today it remains a necessary evil, and is therefore performed in practically all teaching hospitals. Most surgical residents are adequately seasoned, both scientifically and psychologically, to excise neplasms. In terms of increased survival time, the radical surgery of malignancies has proved satisfactory when limited to reasonable, now classic, indications in carefully selected instances.

The obvious logic behind cancer surgery is the desire to extirpate the tumor with one magistral stroke. This concept needs considerable revision. Warren Cole and his associates at the University of Illinois in Chicago, have demonstrated the frequency with which clumps of viable neoplastic cells are encountered in the blood stream of patients during the surgical removal of *clinically localized* malignancies. Actually, five-year survivals are not exceptional among patients in whom cancer cells had been found in the blood. One must presume that most of these circulating cell clumps never amount to much - deposited somewhere in the body they remain dormant for extended periods of time. But any of these metastases may "revive" at any time, even a quarter of a century after "successful" mastectomy or nephrectomy. If we would only find a method by which the indefinite latency of these metastatic cell deposits could be assured, currently available surgical and radiologic procedures should take care of most of the problems encountered at the primary site.

The ominous implications (manipulation = metastasis) of Cole's findings do not appeal to men of action, who prefer to "do something* about it." That"something" may turn out to be an extensive dissection, or some other mutilating procedure. They may thence labor assiduously to keep the patient alive, and will not desist from endoscoping, injecting, draining, transfusing or perfusing until the last rasping breath and flickered pulse.

At the other end of the residential spectrum there are some who verbalize eloquently their honest belief that specialized training periods must not be "wasted"

---

*Excerpts from this chapter have appeared as an editorial in the *American Journal of Roentgenology* of November, 1958, and are herein reprinted with the kind permission of the editor, and of the publisher, Charles C Thomas, Publisher, of Springfield (Illinois).

**The relationships between the biologic (which is not necessarily identical with the chronologic) age of a demographic group, and the frequency of cancer in the latter, have been discussed in the article *Age, Biology, and Carcinoma,* published in the *Journal of the International College of Surgeons* of February, 1962.

†Literary pseudonym of the Italian poet Pietro Antonio Domenico Bonaventura Trapassi (1698-1782).

*The medical lexicographer J. E. Schmidt believes that *ergasiomania* stands for excessive eagerness to perform aurgery; this precious hybrid derives from the Greek *ergasia* (work) and the Latin *mania* (madness).

on the care of "terminal" patients, whether exenterated or not. Officially or otherwise, the least experienced man on that team, a new intern if available, is left in charge of the "incurables." It is tacitly assumed that these patients have passed the point of no return, and cannot be further harmed, in the same way in which infinity cannot grow any bigger, regardless how many finite quantities are added to it.

The average radiologist in medium-sized and smaller hospitals is sufficiently familiar with conservative oncotherapy, but he can seldom devote the time required for its completion. More often than not, after ten or fifteen "morale building" irradiations, he returns the patient to the referring physician. The average general practitioner is emotionally mature, aware of the demands of, and willing to care for, patients with operable or inoperable malignancies. But many "modern" technologic and other medical developments are not everywhere available. Without them, one may have to revert to fundamentals. Thus, in many instances, patients with incurable malignancies receive little more than opiates and reassurance.

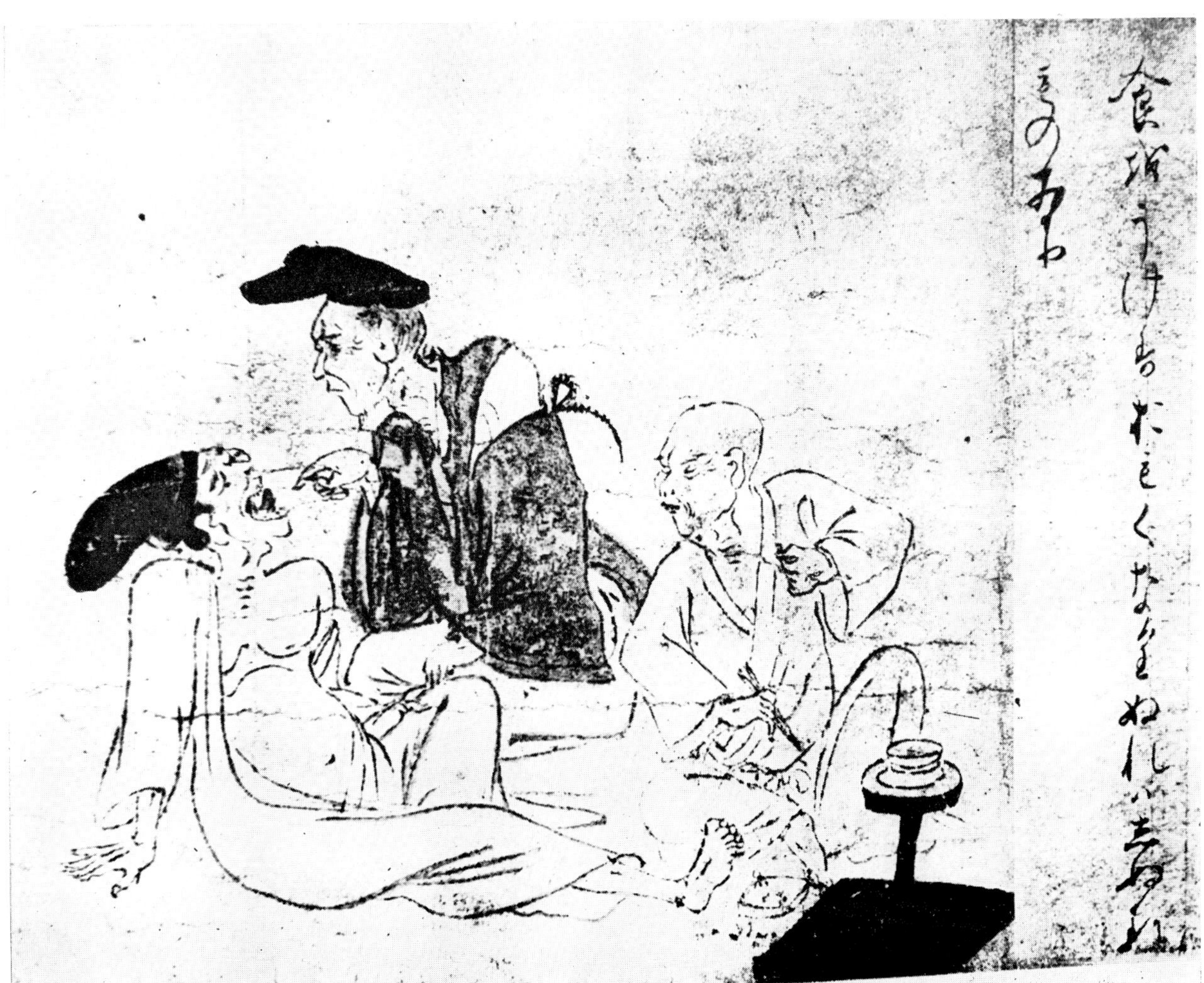

Courtesy: Masaaki Nishida.

THE SECOND TONGUE. This frame is from a 12th century Japanese scroll called *Yamai-no-Sôshi* (unusual diseases). The reclining man complained that he was growing an additional tongue. The physician tried (unsuccessfully) to burn the growth with the instrument which his bald helper had heated up. The second tongue kept on growing, and in the end killed its host by obstructing the passage of either food or drink. The suggestion has been made that it was a ranula (cyst caused by accumulation of saliva following occlusion of a salivary canal), but the protracted course, and fatal outcome indicate a more malignant type of tumor. Neoplasms have been with us since times immemorial.

Palliation is a delicate and complex art, albeit it makes one feel akin to the legendary ferryman of Hades. It cannot offer the "scientific" incentive of the presumed (or rather, desired) completeness of an evisceration. Nor does it promise spectacular results, even though it may achieve them, if unexpectedly.

The basic philosophy of palliation is built upon the knowledge that human misery is never infinite; it can always grow a little worse, and hurt a little stronger than the day before, until the very end. Clinical judgment, technical proficiency, and personal experience must be accumulated before one can perform successfully in this territory which encroaches upon the borderlines of so many specialties. Individualization of approach is nowhere so essential: a single overdosage can spoil, irremediably, the fleeting benefits of a carefully planned and executed program. Not the disease *per se,* but the patient's own problems and sufferings must be met. Wihle continuous warmth and sympathetic understanding are very desirable assets, the patient-physician relationship must never be stained, not even with a trace of the so often and so wrongly displayed commiseration.

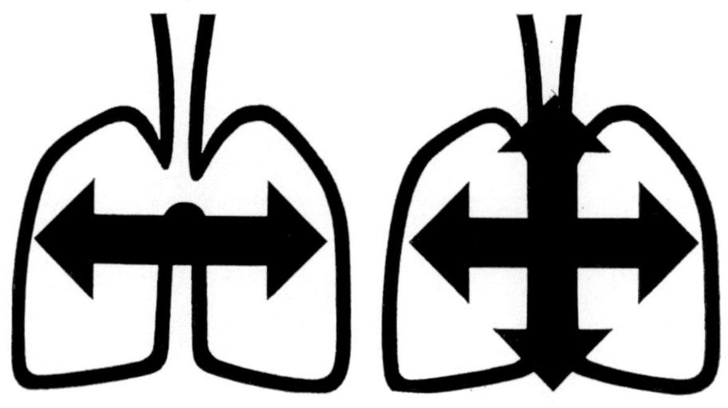

Medical historians have demonstrated that theoretical principles are easier grasped after linguistic identification of the catchwords used in their definition. Etymologic analysis, with its synonyms and analogies,

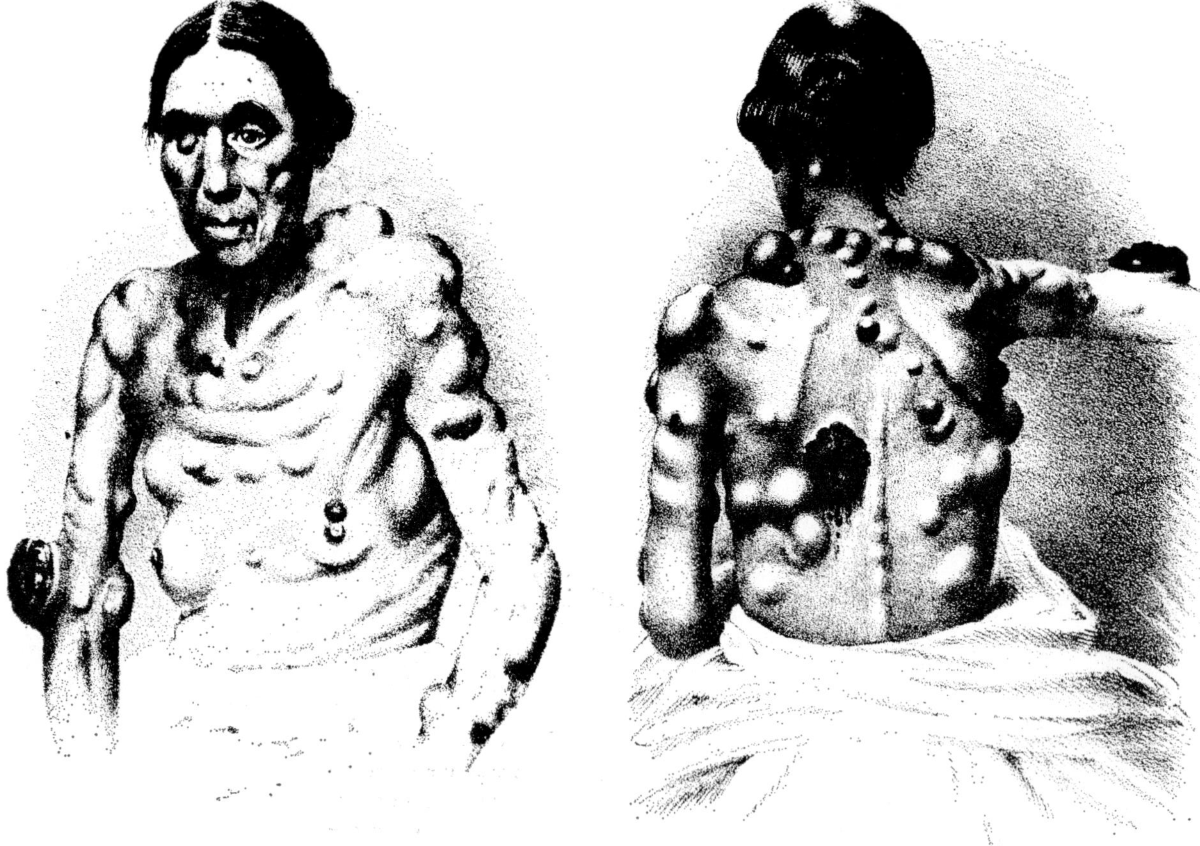

Courtesy: John Crerar Library.

MELANO-SARCOMATOSIS (FROM THE IRIS?). The right eyeball of this fifty-two-year old woman had been removed in October, 1857. The skin nodules appeared first in 1861, whereupon her disease was called "melanosis, non-cancerous (sebaceous)." She died in June of 1863. The sketches are from M. H. Collie's text *On the Diagnosis of Cancer,* published by John Churchill in London in 1864.

provide a fascinating insight in the tedious ways in which cognate meanings can create strange associations of ideas. In the case of *palliation,* the primary word or etymon is the Latin *pallium* (the respective Greek vocable was *himation,* which means a loose mantle or cover, a much simpler and less formal attire than the toga).

Today, according to English dictionaries, a pallium is in anatomy the cerebral cortex, which covers the brain; in zöology it is the mantle of a bird, brachiopod, or mollusk, and as an adjective it defines several species, for instance the American oyster-catcher *(Haematopus palliatus).* In meteorology, a pallium is an extended sheet of clouds. In its ecclesiastical significance it represents a woolen garment worn by the Pope, and conferred by him to archbishops and selected bishops.

The specifically feminine counterpart of the Roman pallium was a wide mantle or ample tunic, the *palla.* The shorter English word *pall* (except for the meanings derived from its other root, appall) evolved mainly toward the signification of cloth, such as that used to cover the coffin, whence *pallbearers* were originally assigned to hold up the corners of the pall draped over the coffin. Other garments with names derived from pall are the *paletot* (overcoat); its Middle English correspondent, the paltock; and the tarpauline (from tar and palling), a waterproof material. The verb pall, meaning to cover, cover up, to clothe, was also used, both in prose and in poetry.

The English verb *palliate* comes from the Latin *palliare,* which originally meant to cover with or as with a cloak.* As time went on, three main groups of synonymies developed, the earliest of which was related to the sense of hiding, *i.e.,* (A) to palliate was to put out of sight, or beyond ready observation or approach, that is to *hide, cloak, cover up, conceal, disguise, veil,* or *screen.* Within the significance of medical palliation, this includes the various prosthetic devices intended to replace functionally (speech, breathing, eating), or at least esthetically, the necrotized and/or excized pieces of skin, muscle, or bone from the face and other parts. Likewise, when "in the sweetest and most forward bud the eating canker dwells" (Shakespeare), and the bud

**Cloak* is a transliteration from the Old French *cloke,* akin to the Medieval Latin *clocca,* the bell (*Glocke,* in German) in the sense of wide, shapeless garment.

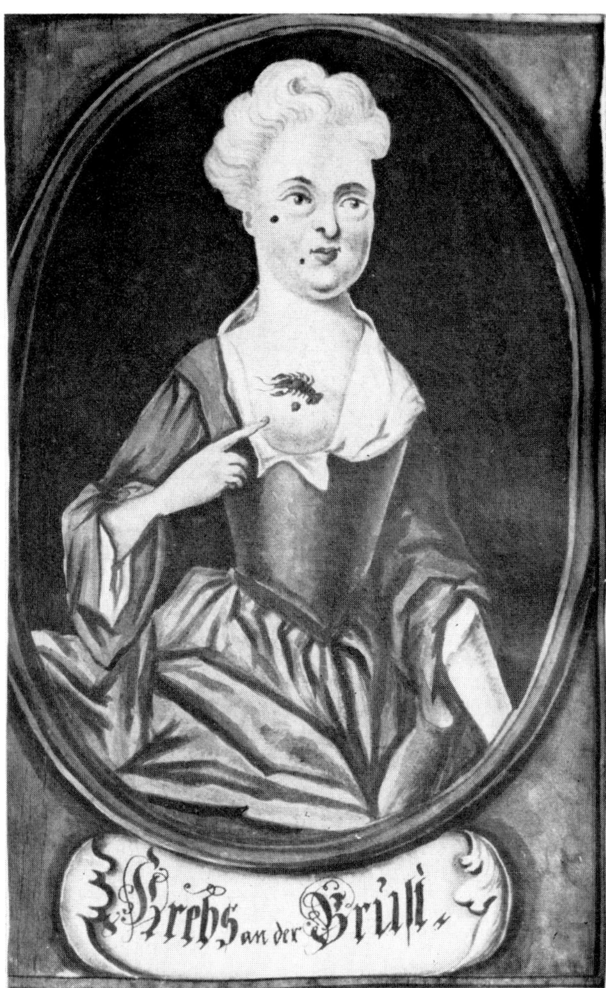

Courtesy: Wellcome Medical Library, London.

CZECH CANCER CRABFISH. This painting comes from a sixteenth century manuscript, preserved in Prague. The inscription is in German, and means cancer on the breast. This rare illustration was made available by Edgar Ashworth Underwood, one of Great Britain's most respected living medical historians.

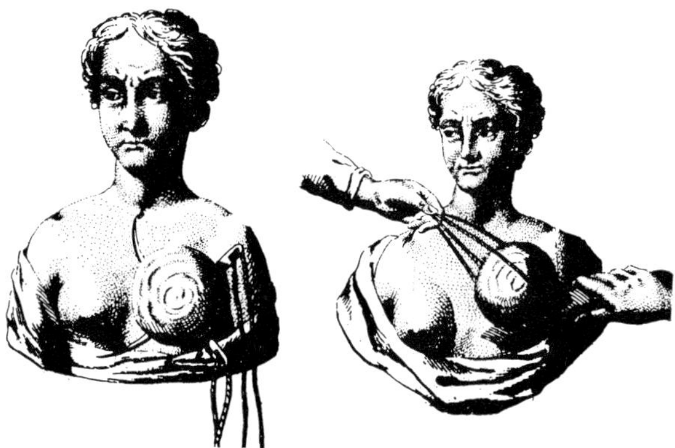

Courtesy: John Crerar Library.

MASTECTOMY 17TH CENTURY STYLE. These woodcuts are from Diderot' grandiose *Dictionnaire Universel de Médecine* (1746), but therein they were redrawn from the *Armamentarium Chirurgicum* (1655) of Johann Schultes (1595-1645). The Diderot version reproduces somewhat better than the originals in the Scultetus.

has to be removed, one can always improve the patient's spirits by reshaping her profile with an appropriate form. (Correspondingly, patients with carcinoma of the prostate, scheduled for orchiectomy, often request the surgeon to refill the emptied bursa with two plastic balls). As a corollary comes the hard and fast rule that all patients must maintain, as long as practicable, a decent outward appearance (clothing, make-up, smile), since this will improve their inward look as well.

Another analogy of the word hide is to *shelter,* which implies giving temporary cover from something that might harm. Patients may sometimes be given actual *refuge* in adequate (not only custodial) facilities, but to shelter means also to protect them from the cruel knowledge of what is considered an irremediable condition. In this respect, one may decide to cloak (which means to hide completely, as behind a pall), or just palliate (*i.e.,* to veil or screen so as to make the outlines indistinct).

The patient who harbors an "incurable" malignancy must be told he is seriously ill, the nature of his illness being then described either as (a) non-neoplastic (naming instead any popular disease with similar symptomatology), or (b) as a benign growth (with details concerning the potential severity of local extensions), or (c) as a malignant tumor (never using the word cancer, always emphasizing how amenable it often is to therapy). The degree of disclosure should be adjusted to the patient's personality. He is entitled to the benefit of the doubt, one may always downgrade at first, and preserve another step of revelation for a later date, when added symptomatology will require further explanations. There are very few individuals who can or ought to be forewarned of their impending death (even then, the cold facts must be palliated by attaching the theoretical chance of eventual stabilization) for, as Keats once wrote, "to bear all naked truths, and to envisage circumstance, all calm, is the top of sovereignty."

The next group of synonyms is based on the sentence (B) to palliate is to cover with a mantle of excuses. When we palliate a wrong, we seek to *extenuate* it in part. Either to palliate or to extenuate is to admit the existence of the evil under consideration, but to extenuate is rather to *apologize* for the offender, while to palliate is to disguise it (circumstances which cannot change the inherent wrong, may be extenuating, can never be palliating). Likewise, to *gloze* or *gloss over* something is to attempt to *excuse* it by concealing its true disagreeableness.

These varied meanings can be applied to the qualified halftruths, proffered in reply to pointed questions, asked by patients who are under treatment for advanced malignancies. Since the final episode may be protracted over several years, it takes much inventiveness, as well as common sense, and beyond that experience, to say just the right words. Busy therapists may find it convenient to formulate standard answers to certain, often heard queries, if only because patients discuss their problems between themselves. It also helps in avoiding contradictions in the course of later interviews.

For the same reason it may be worthwhile to incorporate in the records any unusual euphemisms offered to the patient. This will save time and brainwork needed to reassure the patient who discovers inconsistencies in subsequent comments, for when faith is lost, everything is lost. The accomplished therapeutist knows that the right word at the right time is more effective than one sixth of morphine, while the loss of hope proves to be, in Milton's words, "as killing as the canker to the rose."

In (Cromwell's) England, *canker* was derived from the Latin word for crabfish *(cancer);* it also indicated the fourth zodiacal constellation; a plant, the dog-rose; a plant disease, caused by the canker-worm (caterpillar); and a spreading, corroding, decaying ulcer in man.

As so often, the name given to malignancy comes from the Greek, who called it after the crabfish *kar-*

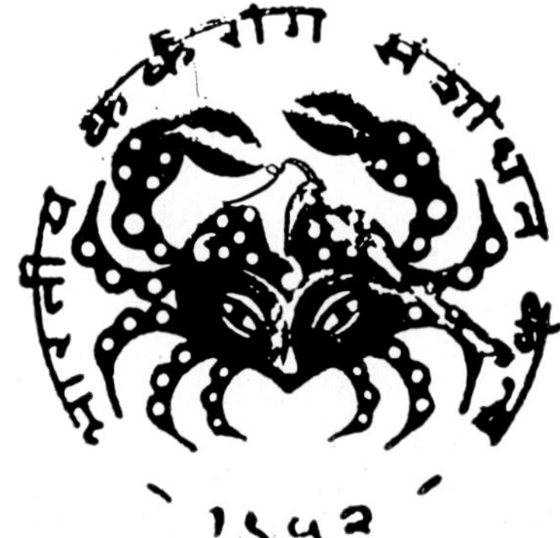

INDIAN CANCER CRAB. Beautifully stylized seal of the Indian Cancer Association.

PENROSE CANCER HOSPITAL
Sisters of Charity

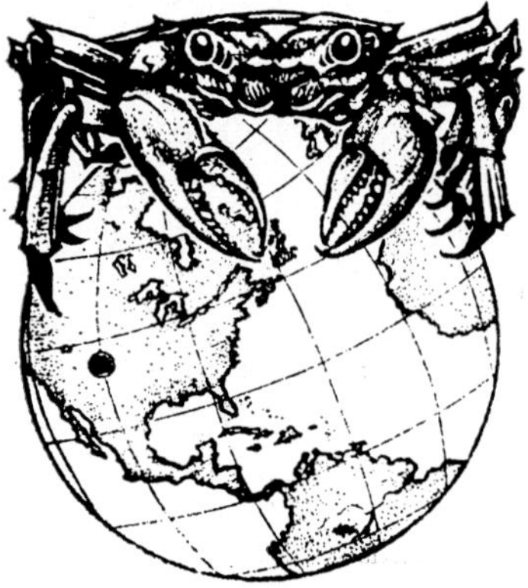

2215 North Cascade
Colorado Springs Colorado

kinos, (καρκίνος). It was subsequently translated and/or transliterated into most languages, *cancer* in Latin, French, English, Spanish, Portuguese, and Roumanian, *cancro* in Italian, *Krebs* in German, *kreeft* in Dutch, *kråfta* in Swedish, *pak* (rhahk) in Russian. All of them are homonyms, each means both lobster (or a cousin of it) and malignant neoplasm. Stylized versions of one or the other of these pincered crustaceans serve as trade-marks in the seals of several "cancer-combatting" organizations. One of these crabs can be seen climbing on top of the world; when another did the same thing in Brazil, it was transfixed by a dagger.

A slightly different style of crab appeared on Gauthier-Villars' elegant *maquette* for the transactions of the Franco-Sovietic radio-bio-conference on leukemia, held in Paris (at Quai d'Orsay) in September of 1961. The chief delegates were: for the French, Lacassagne; for the Soviets, Zedguenidze.

In my editorial, I had derived carcinoma from *karkinos* (crab) and *nemein* (νεμειν) or *nomi* (νωμη), meaning to spread by creeping around. This version had been used in the *Real-Encylopaedie der Gesammten Heilkunde* (ed. 3, Vienna 1894; iv, 273), in Jacob Wolff's monumental *Lehre von der Krebskrankheit* (Jena, 1907; i, 5), and in Pachyrembel's *Klinisches Woerterbuch* (Berlin, 1944), to mention only three sources. After reading my editorial, John Lewis Heller, (chairman of the Department of Classics in the University of Illinois in Urbana) advised me that said version was erroneous, if only because it would have lead to the spelling *karkinonoma.* He cited the best authority in the matter, the *princeps edition* (1572) of the *Thesaurus Linguae Graecae* by Henri Estienne (1528-1598).

COLLOQUE FRANCO-SOVIETIQUE
cancer
leucémie ET
radiobiologie
gv GAUTHIER-VILLARS ET Cie ÉDITEUR PARIS

It is therefore proper to assert that the Latin word *carcinoma* is the transliterated Greek *karkinoma* (καρκίνομα), which comes from the verb *karkinoon* (καρκίνωον), to cause to spread like a crab or, in the passive voice, to spread like a crab.

To differentiate the "gelatinous" mesodermal growths from the "bony" epidermoid tumors, the English surgeon John Abernethy (1764-1831) coined the term *sarcoma* for the "soft" type of malignancy. It comes from the Greek word *sarkoo* (σαρωο), which means to make or to become fleshy.

Morris Leider and Morris Rosenblum (in the *Journal of Investigative Dermatology* of October, 1947), and Harry Keil (in the *Bulletin of the History of Medicine* of August, 1950) have shown that use of the suffix *-oma* to designate tumor came about by a somewhat complicated process, the main reasons being similitude and the desire for linguistic contractions.

The reasons for equating "crabbification" with "cancerization" have been stated (and interpreted) by many authors such as Cl. (for *clarus,* meaning brilliant, not Claudius) Galen (A.D. 130-201), who stressed the "hardness" of the crab's back. The most "comprehensive" explanation may have been given by the 17th Century English surgeon John Brown in his *Compleat Treatise on Praeternatural Tumours* of 1678 (on page 156); ". . . it is called . . . by us a Cancer, from the resemblence it has with a Sea-Crab. For as the one hath expanded claws and feet in several places, being of a livid or cinerish colour; so also is this *Tumour* of a

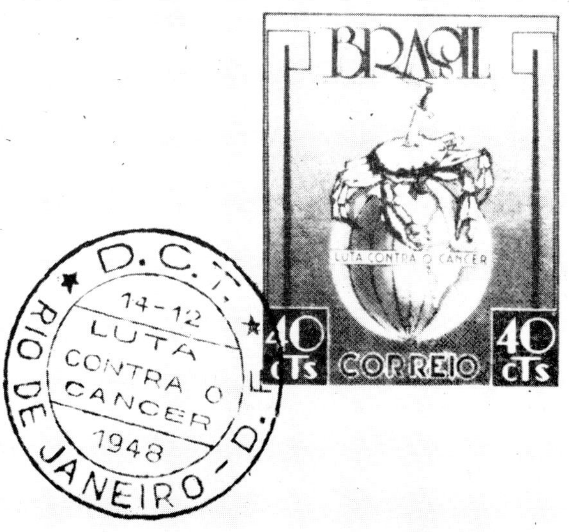

round Figure, of a livid Colour, and sticketh or adhereth so close to the part affected as a Key to a Door, or a claw of a Crab in its gripping, having *in it* by some reported to carry *in it* exalted Veins; but this is more fabulous then (sic) true, for not in four of a hundred as Falloppius observes, can you see them thus apparent." As a modern parallel, Jacob Gershon-Cohen (a radiologist from Philadelphia) emphasizes that on the mammogram the appearance of a spreading carcinoma resembles that of a crab with expanding limbs.

The French translator and editor of the Hippocratic Canon, the positivist philosopher Max Paul Émile Littré (1801-1881) believed that to the ancient Greeks *karkinoma* meant "incurable" ulceration (v, 221). The Arabic authors, for instance Avicenna (the Persian prince of medicine and philosophy), are credited with the concept of the *frigid tumor* (swelling without inflammation). The Greeks knew of the existence of crypto-carcinoma (hidden, or occult tumors without

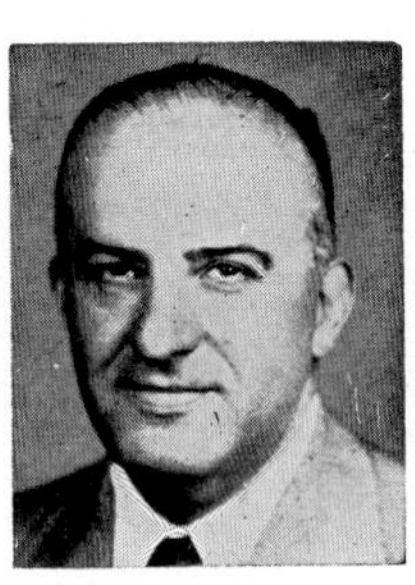

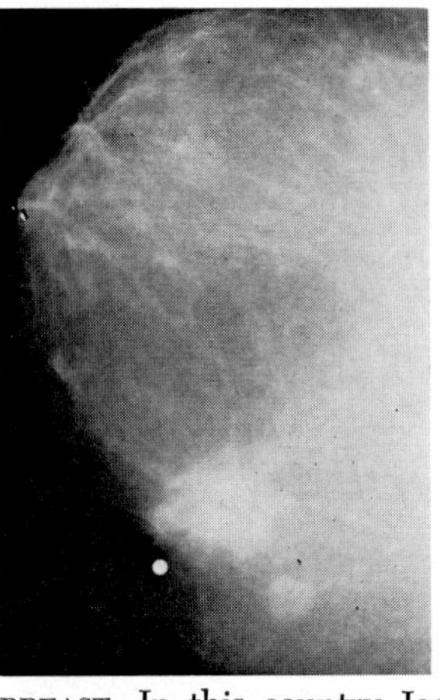

ROENTGEN-CRAB IN THE BREAST. In this country Jacob Gershon-Cohen — who teaches radiology in the Albert Einstein Medical Center (Philadelphia) — has pioneered but did not succeed in making popular the x-ray examination of the breast. In his opinion, the roentgen appearance of a malignancy in the breast often resembles the outline of a crab. This reproduction is from one of his patients. The lead shot on the skin marks the mass which the fifty-two-year old patient had first noticed one week before this x-ray study was performed. It shows a typical malignancy of the scirrhous type, with tentacles and spicules infiltrating into the surrounding tissue. A satellite tumor (also malignant) is seen adjacent to the main mass. The histologic examination of the surgical specimen confirmed entirely the radiologic prediction and — hopefully — there seemed to be no evidence of axillary, or of any other metastases.

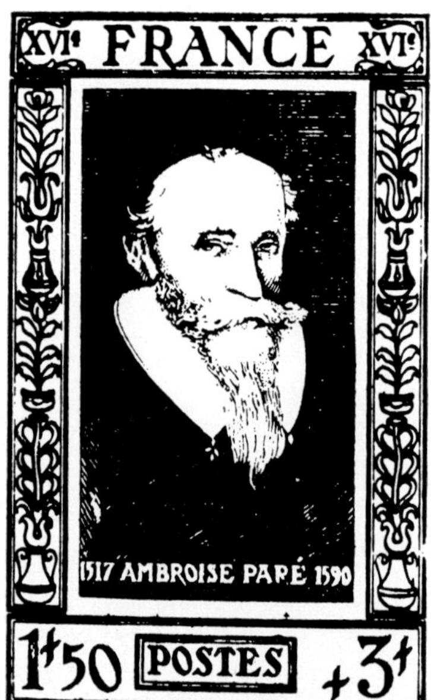

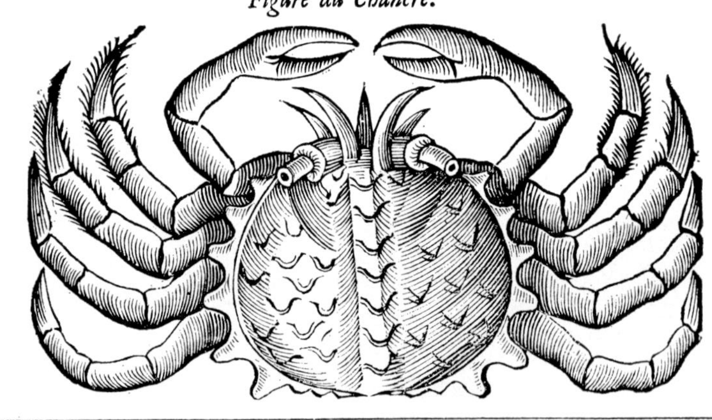

212 Le ſeptieſme Liure,

Figure du Chancre.

Des cauſes, eſpeces, ou differences, & prognoſtics de chancre.

CHAP. XXVIII.

CRAB = CHANCRE = CANCER. Ambroise Paré (1517-1590) was a barber's apprentice who became one of France's great surgeons, for which he was honored with a commemorative stamp. In his *Oevvres* (princeps edition, Paris, 1575), Paré inserted the woodcut of a fancy crustacean, in the midst of chapters which discuss the diagnosis and treatment of malignant growths. Note the vernacular spelling *chancre,* which in French means crab as well as ulceration, and presently designates a benign venereal disease. Thence, *cancer* was a *chancre* which had the consistency of a *crab,* and which proved to be incurable.

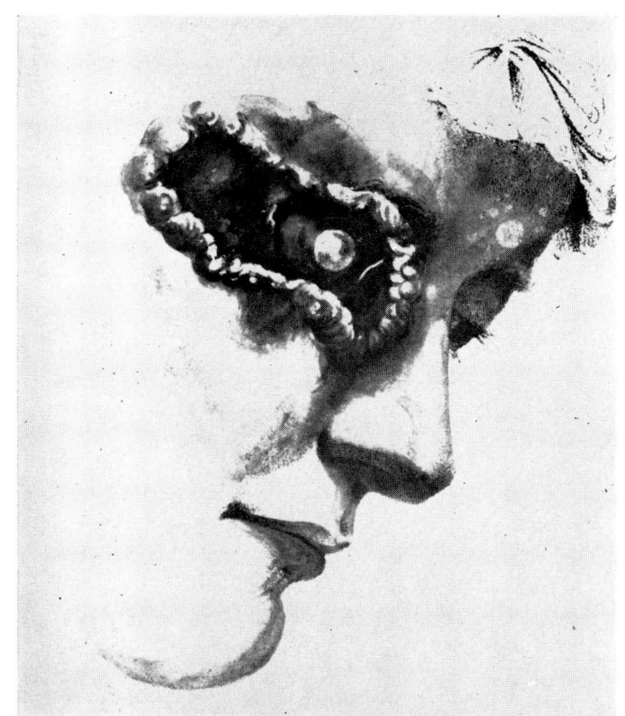

Courtesy: John Crerar Library.

NOLI ME TANGERE! This is the illustration which appeared in the princeps article on rodent ulcer by Arthur Jacob (1790-1874), published in the *Dublin Hospital Reports* (1827). Until World War I, basal-cell carcinoma around the eyelid was called Jacob's ulcer. This specimen is shown after four years duration, but in the same paper, Jacob mentioned one that had lasted for twenty-three years.

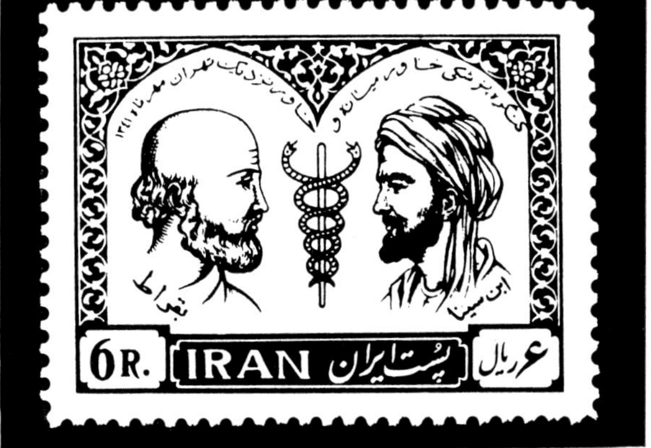

PERSIAN POSTAL STAMP. Bald Hippocrates (460-377? B.C.) and abu-Ali al-Husayn ibn-Sina Avicenna (980-1037) – with an interposed Caduceus (symbol of Mercury, the god of communication and commerce) – are honored on the occasion of the World Medical Congress (1962).

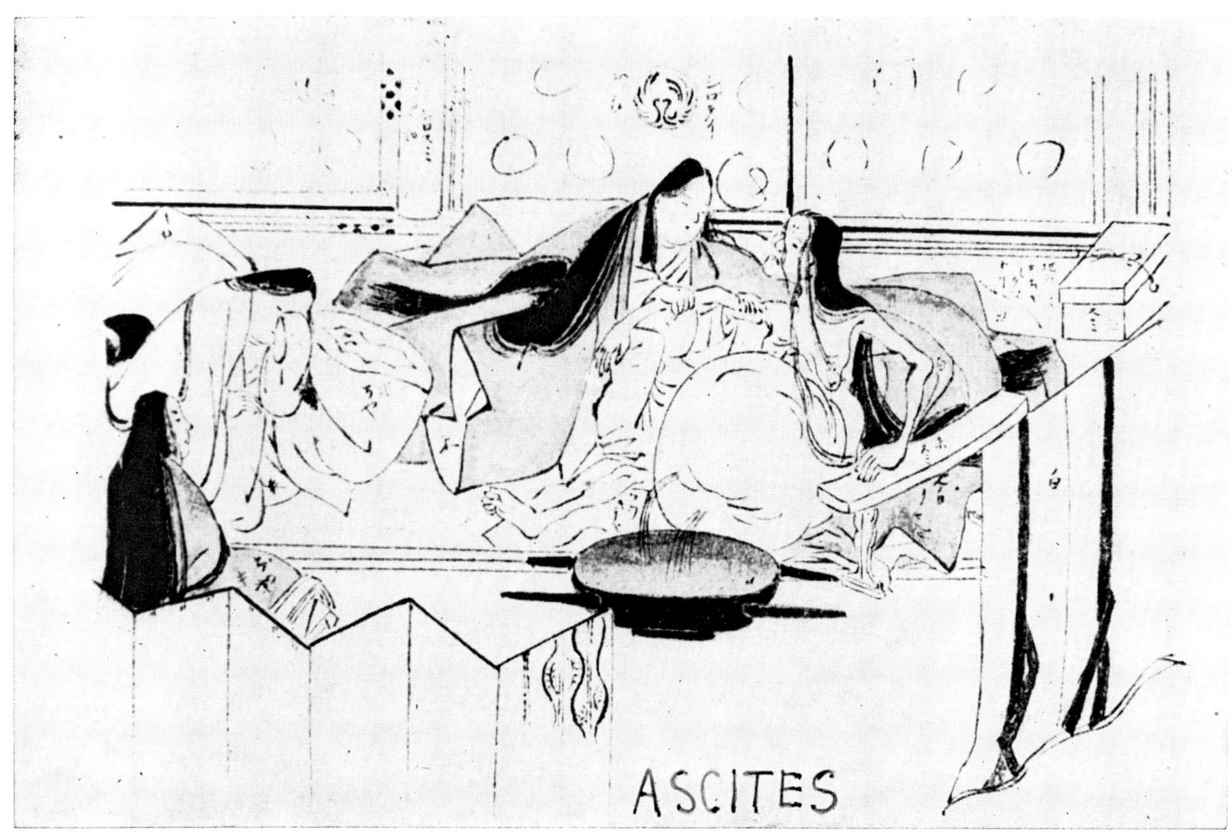

external ulceration), indeed Hippocrates advised in a famous aphorism (vi, 38) that (over-)treatment of crypto-carcinoma may shorten, rather than prolong, the patient's life. This evolved later into the doctrine of *Noli me tangere.* The latter expression was first printed in 1484 in the *Sermones Medicinales,* authored by Niccolló Falcucci (?-1412).

The expression was actually used, centuries earlier, in Medieval medical manuscripts. In the surgical treatise of Guy de Chauliac (1300-1370), *Noli me tangere* (don't touch me!) is the very name given to *ulcus rodens* (basal-cell carcinoma of the skin) as a warning that excision is inadvisable because of the frequency of local recurrence. Ironically, this particular variety of "cancer" practically never metastasizes but can, and often does, kill by local extension (and intercurrent disease).

The last and largest group of synonyms of palliation revolved around the strictly medical connotation (C) to palliate is really to diminish the violence of a disease. The term which includes most of these meanings is (i) to *alleviate,* that is to lift a burden, or at least to lighten it, and thus make it more bearable, which is not quite as much as to *relieve* a sufferer, and certainly less than to *remove* the cause of suffering. (ii) to *allay* is to lay to rest, for instance we allay suffering by using means to *soothe* (to assent to, to humor) that which is excited, or otherwise *appease, pacify, mollify* (soften), *assuage* (sweeten), *calm, quiet, still,* in one word, *tranquilize.* (iii) To *mitigate* is to make milder, or less severe, such as to *moderate, lessen, attenuate, decrease, reduce* anything from fever and swelling to anxiety and pain. (iv) Among the cognates of soothing is to *solace, console, comfort, sympathize,* which in turn contain meanings easily blended into the significations hereunto expounded. (It may be stated parenthetically that the four above listed groups of analogies carry a more or less obvious undertone of provisorial or transient, similar to the effectiveness of today's cytostatics, *e.g.,* Triethylene melamine in Hodgkin's disease.)

Above array of terms could cover every possible facet of palliation in medicine, from analgesic x-ray

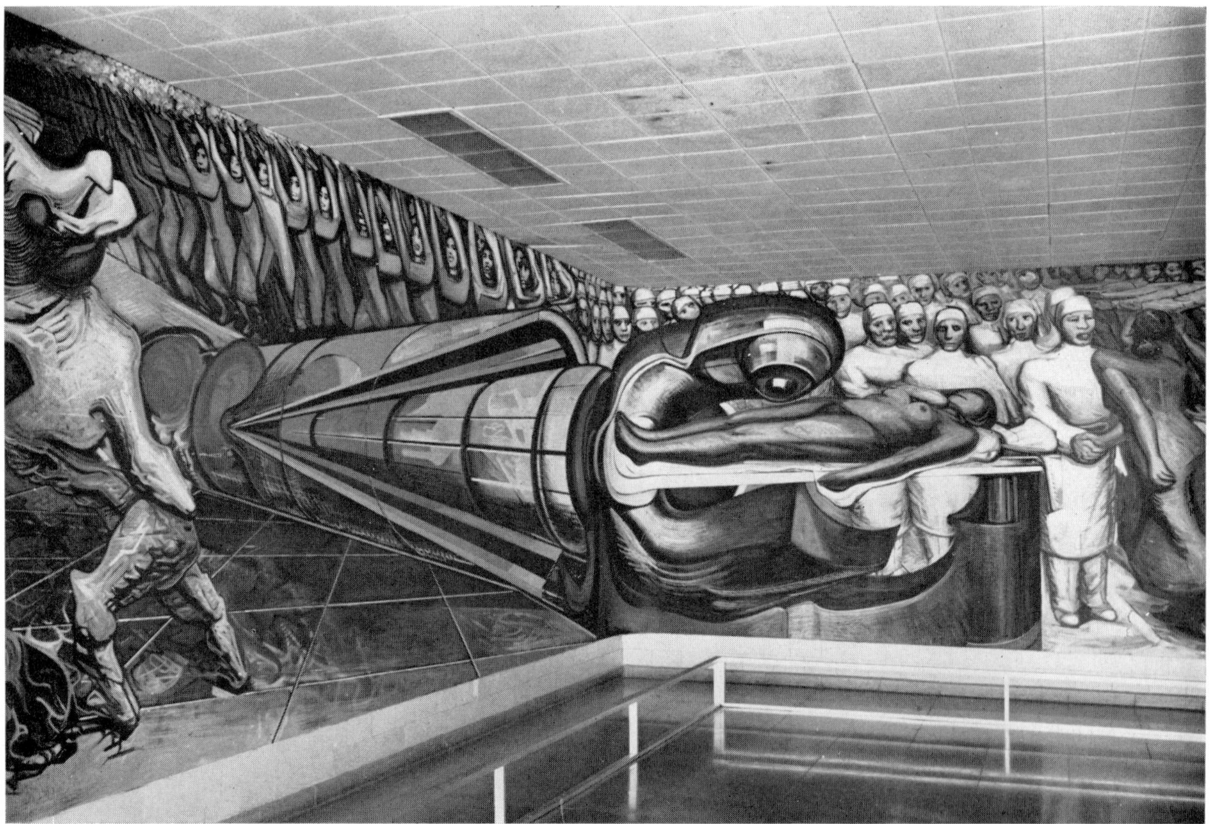

COBALT MURAL, spanning two walls in the Mexico City Medical Center. One patient is shown between the "claws" of the machine. The other patient is a representative of a group of dark-clad patients thanking a representative of the white-clad therapists. The author of this mural is David Alfaro Siqueiros, a patriarchal painter who is currently a fervent Communist rabble rouser (for which he recently served a prison sentence in the Black Palace in Mexico City).

therapy, administered to lessen the discomfort of bone metastases, to posterior rhizotomy, for the suppression or at least attenuation of intractable pain; from the radioactive colloidal Au 198 (or Nitrogen mustard), instilled intraperitoneally to lighten the burden of ascites, to bypass operations for the relief of intrinsic or extrinsic bowel obstruction of malignant origin; and from the blood transfusions (the knowledgeable prefer packed red cells) given to allay the dyspnea of leukemics with anemia, to the supervoltage radiation which alleviates dysphagia as it re-opens an esophagus shriveled with carcinoma (for a while it was fashionable to insert a plastic tube instead). Furthermore, since most of these patients have both "the canker, and the grief" (Byron),

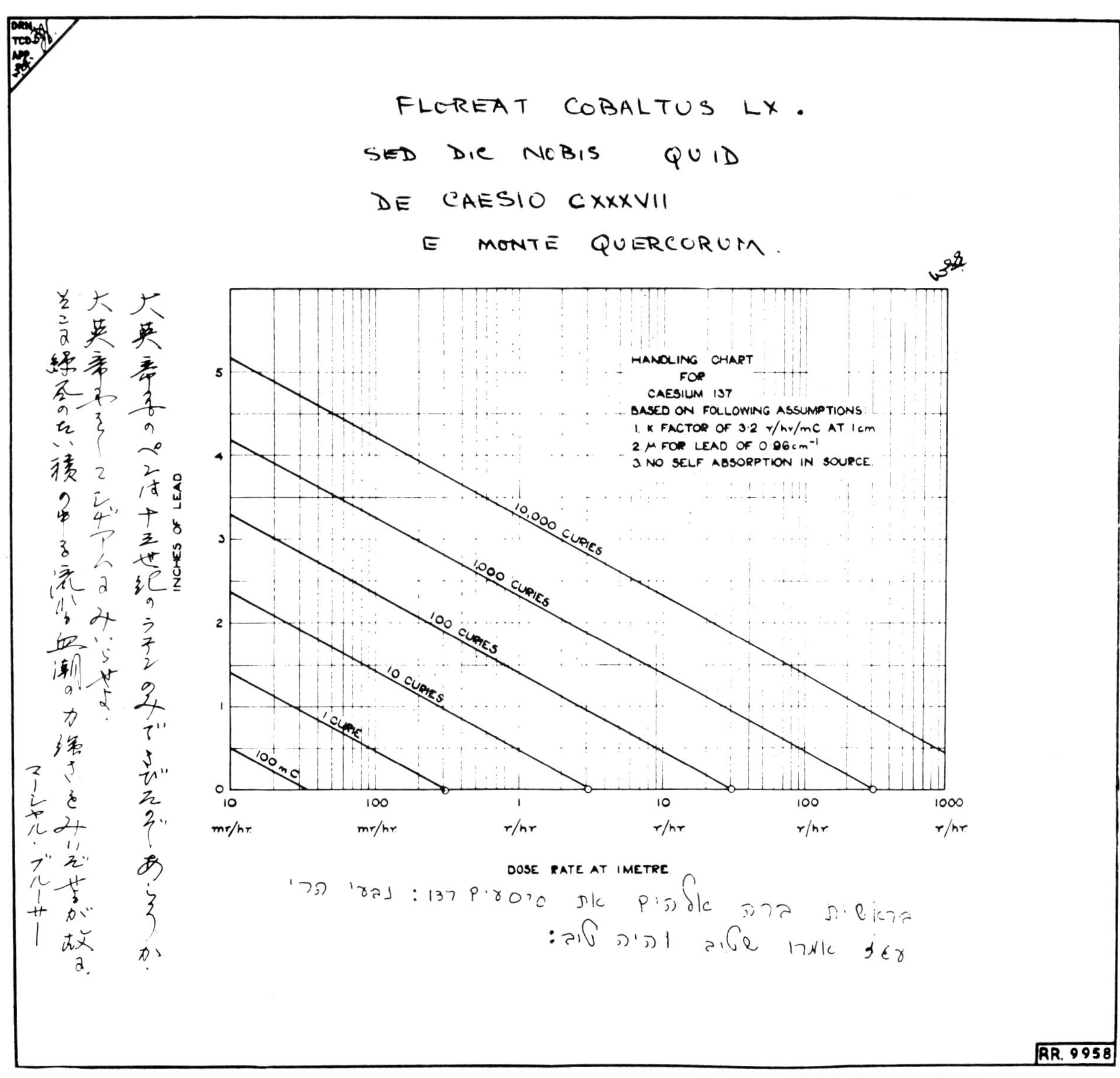

Courtesy: ORINS, Medical Division.

Polyglot radio-cesium graph. The inscription in Latin, by Alexander Thomas Eastwood of London (Ontario), asserts that not only does (the use of) cobalt flourish, but we have also cesium-137 at Oak Ridge *(Mons Quercorum)*. The Japanese sentences are a Marshall Brucer witticism, transposed into a poetic tirade, purporting that 13th century Latin has rusted the pens of the Great British, who ought to learn that cesium has the strength of the blood of young people. The notation in Hebrew is a play on the first words in the Old Testament, stating that in the beginning the Lord created cesium, and decided it was good, because gas (radiation) was coming out of it.

their anxiety must be mitigated, that is tranquilized, a task which the drug companies have certainly facilitated.

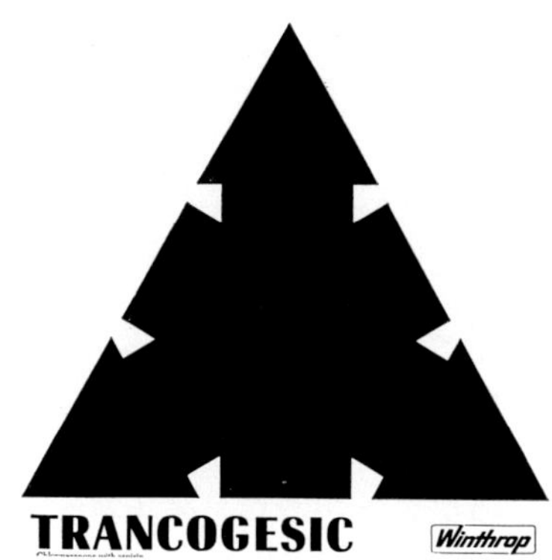

Today, adequate facilities for oncologic palliation require both a surgical and a radiologic orientation. The world-wide utilization of Co^{60} teletherapy sources - and the comparatively slower spread of supervoltage and megavoltage apparatus, with their (initially) inconspicuous skin and other reactions, have provided very desirable instruments for palliation. Increased use of other radioactive (even fission) products, such as Cesium-137 and added refinements might in the future decrease the cost of high energy irradiation.

In general, though, to paraphrase Leo Henry Garland's "law of radiocurability" - re-iterated in the *American Journal of Roentgenology* of October, 1961 - radio-palliation depends 60 percent on the treated tumor's radio-sensitivity, 30 percent on the treating radiologist's skill and radio-ability, and only 10 percent on the available radio-modality.

For the *Science of Radiology* (1933), Ursus Victor Portmann prepared an excellent review of the beginning of roentgen therapy. Regarding onco-radio-therapy, little more than palliation was done until well into the Golden Age of Radiology. Emile Grubbé in Chicago was probably the first who applied x rays to a malignancy of the breast, but did not report it in print until

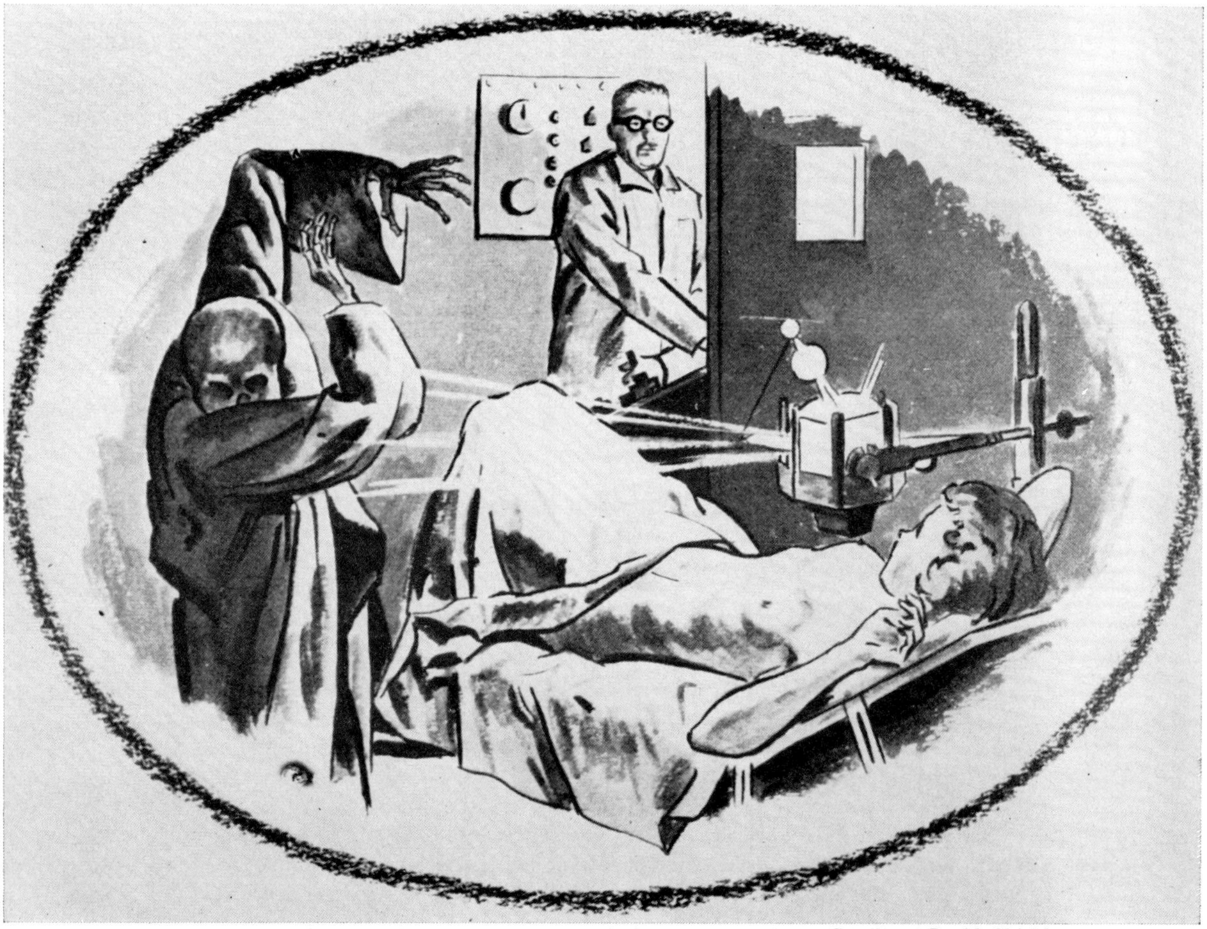

Courtesy: David Shields.

RONTGEN THERAPY (ABOUT 1903). Even death is afraid of such inordinate amount of scattered radiation. This poster appeared in a Keleket advertisement of the 1930's.

very much later. The first paper on the radiation therapy of carcinoma of the breast was published by Hermann Gocht in the very first issue of *Fortschritte auf dem Gebiete der Roentgenstrahlen* (1897), but with the soft radiation available at that time, he could hardly have reached much further than skin-deep. In 1900, William Benham Snow (a former associate of William James Morton) published his *Manual of . . . Radiotherapy,* which contained photographs of patients "before and after" roentgen therapy for disfiguring malignancies of the face. Leopold Freund's *Grundriss der Radiotherapie* (Wien, 1903) carried indications for the treatment of malignancies, but the emphasis was on non-tumoral, mainly on dermatologic, conditions. In 1904 appeared in Philadelphia (Lea Brothers & Co.) the *Radiotherapy and Phototherapy* by Charles Warrenne Allen, which contained significant material on the treatment of carcinoma, as well as on apparatus utilized in "radiology."

Portmann never intended to offer a detailed history of the beginnings of radiotherapy. In the *Archives d'-Electricité Médicale* of January, 1898 M. Schonberg claimed — belatedly — he had employed x-ray treatment in two cases of lupus, during the month of March, 1896. The Chicago surgeon Nicholas Senn is credited with the first x ray therapy of leukemia — he called it "pseudoleucaemia" in his paper on the subject, published in the *New York Medical Journal* of April 25, 1903.

At the turn of the century, treatment of tuberculosis was quite a problem. Any new threapy that appeared on the medical horizon was sooner or later tried also on phthisics, and the invisible rays were no exception. The following question-and-answer, reprinted *verbatim* from the *American X-Ray Journal* of December, 1902, will provide a good idea of just how this was being done:

"Dr. H. P. Pratt:

I have been treating two cases of consumption. Have given twelve treatments. How long treatments can I give and what distance should the tube be kept from the patient? I have been giving seventeen inches distance. How far away do you have the tube when treating cancer? Does the patient feel the heat from the tube? A. F. R.

[The first treatment for tuberculosis should be very short, particularly if the patient is in an advanced stage of the disease; say five minutes at a distance of 15 to 20 inches. This distance may be gradually lessened and the length of time increased, as the patient begins to improve. The limit will depend entirely upon the condition of your tube, and the resisting power of the patient. In treating cancer begin the same way, but if the cancer is small, and particularly if very malignant, begin with seven or eight minutes exposure at ten inches and gradually increase the time. It is seldom necessary to use a tube closer than 10 inches but put it closer if you cannot otherwise obtain sufficient intensity of the x-rays. There is no sensation from the tube, unless it becomes very hot by using a strong current.—Editor]"

Not mentioned by Portmann is the fact that in 1906 Mihran Krikor Kassabian surveyed by letter the leading x-ray therapists in this country, and a few abroad. He published the results of that survey in an Appendix to his classic *Röntgen Rays and Electro-Therapeutics* (Lippincott, 1907). Those appended pages (a delight for the historian) show that there was no uniformity of either dosage, scope, or philosophy of treatment. Opinions were about evenly divided on whether an erythema should be produced or avoided, with a few calling it an incident, others an accident. Estimation of the hardness of the rays was made more often than not by the green light of the gas tube. Caldwell utilized in therapy only tubes that were no longer satisfactory for diagnosis (because of excessive hardness). Quite "modern" sounds the reply of Reginald Morton, "radiologist to the London Hospital," who specified that superficial cutaneous lesions, including rodent ulcer, are treated in the department of dermatology, while cases of malignant and constitutional disease are referred to the Electric Department under his supervision (incidentally, Reginald Morton believed that the more severe the lesion, the more necessary it is to bring about definite erythema, but no severe reaction).

Homogenous irradiation of the entire body is today one of the modalities of palliation for leukemia and other generalized types of malignancy: in the Medical Division of the ORINS this is done with six sources of Cesium-137. Total body irradiation in the hope of

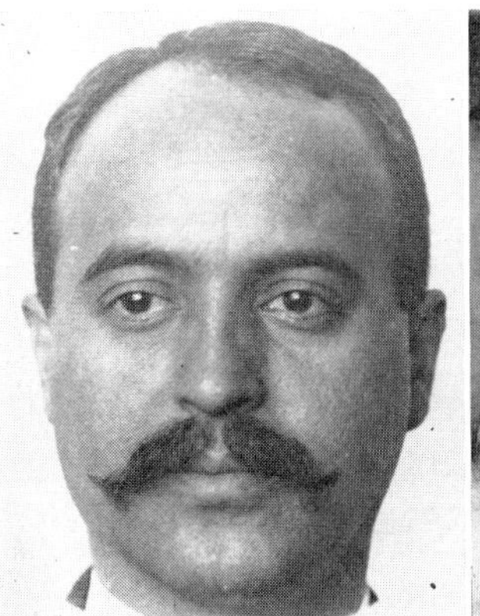

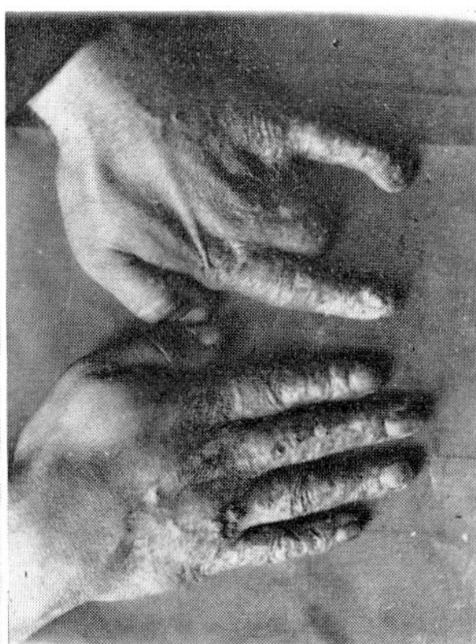

Courtesy: Charles W. Smith.

Kassabian and his hands. This is an inedit photograph which I have printed from the original glass plates, preserved in Philadelphia.

achieving homogeneity was originated sometime in 1905 by the German physicist Friedrich Dessauer: in the *Muenchener Medizinische Wochenschrift* of June 16, 1908, he defended his priority claim against Holzknecht who retorted that the basic idea for homogenous radiation had actually been developed by Georg Perthes (1869-1927).

Significant advances in radiotherapy were soon made in many countries, in Sweden by Thor Stenbeck and Tage Sjögren; in Austria by Robert Kienboeck; in England by Robert Knox and Hall-Edwards; and in France by Antoine Béclère, Jean Alban Bergonié, and later by Claude Regaud.

Before the Congrès International d'Oto-Rhino-Laryngologie (Paris, 1922), Regaud and Coutard reported six cases of advanced laryngeal malignancy, stabilized with the sole help of x-ray therapy. This caused quite a stir, and that is when roentgen therapy "graduated" as a primary method of controlling as yet (clinically) localized malignancies, rather than being accepted only when there was no other choice.

In 1901, at a meeting of German dermatologists in Breslau, Leopold Freund declared that roentgen therapy shall not come of age unless and until the doses administered, and the effects resulting from them, could be reproduced at will. Decades were to pass before this problem was (almost) settled: of great importance to the solution was the concept of half-value layer (HVL), developed by Franz Theophil Christén (1875-1920) of Switzerland.

As a spot check for the height of the Golden Age of Radiology I used the second edition (1936) of *Practical X-Ray Treatment* by Arthur Wright Erskine (1885-1953). It revealed that the majority of radiologists had not yet realized that, with fractionated irradiation, the average malignant neoplasm cannot be controlled with less than 5000 roentgens. Should this mean that at the time few patients received more than palliative dosages? In the matter of actual palliation - the so-called "Treatment of hopeless cases" - Erskine wrote, "the question of how far to go in the treatment of patients whose cases are almost certainly hopeless is one which every physician

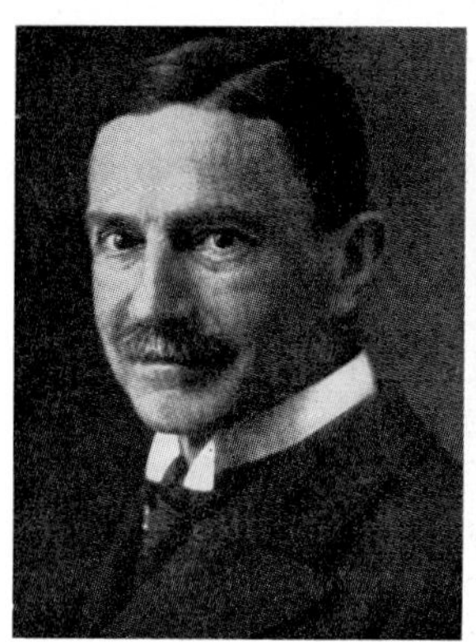

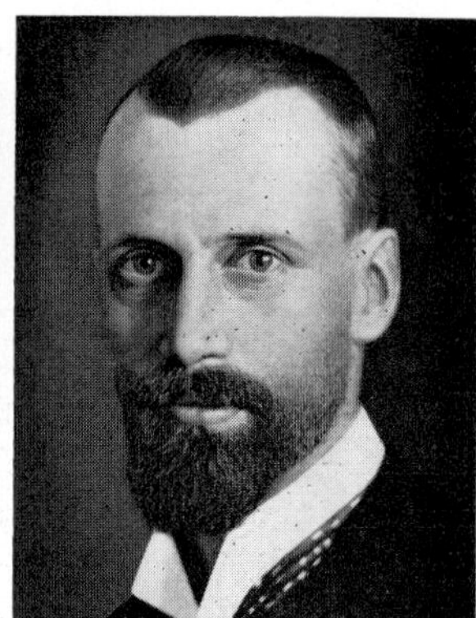

Courtesy: Georg Grössel - Agfa.

GEORG PERTHES, a surgeon who pioneered cross-firing in roentgen therapy through multiple ports, using hard x-ray tubes and filtered beam. On the right is goateed FRANZ THEOPHIL CHRISTÉN. Physician, physicist, mathematician, economist, revolutionary — remembered in radiology as the creator of HVL, the half-value-layer.

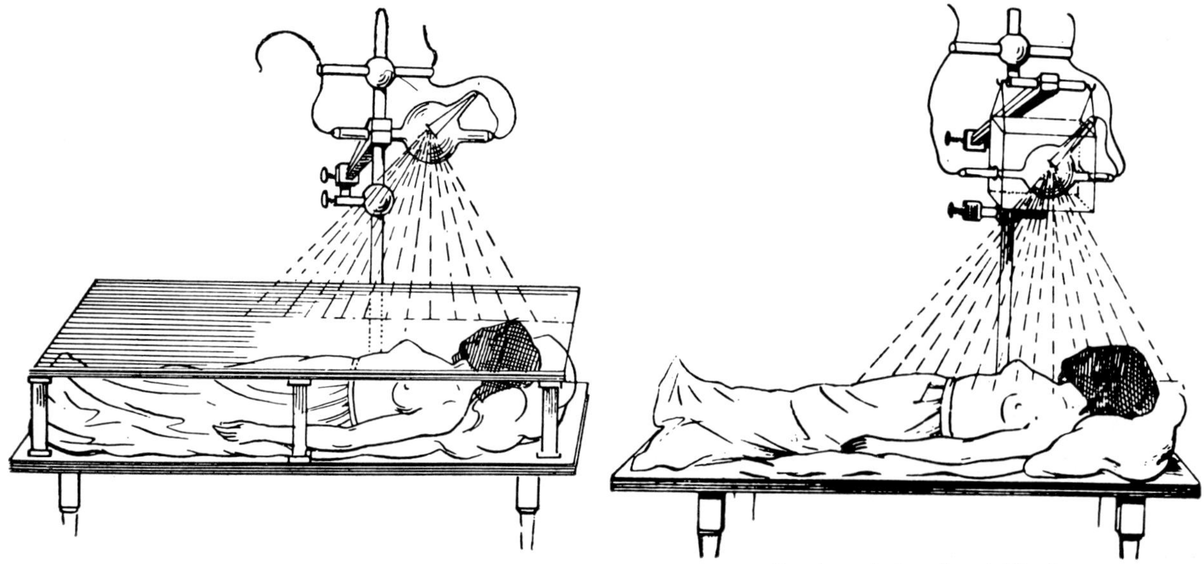

Courtesy: University of Illinois.

FILTRATION 1908 STYLE. Josef Wetterer utilized either a king-size glass plate, or else he encased the tube in a glass box, but patient's face was screened in both instances.

must decide for himself . . . we know that brilliant results are occasionally achieved in the most unpromising cases."

At the 10th ICR in Montreal (1962), Franz Buschke insisted that protraction beyond six weeks is just as effective as when the dose has been given in less than six weeks. He explained that the so-called cancerocidal dose of 6000 r was simply the average limit of tolerance of the vasculo-connective tissue, *i.e.*, the maximal safe dose. He added two witticisms: (1) Radical medium volt therapy for curable cancer is — with some exceptions — mainly of historic interest, and (2) The greatest single (radiation) hazard remains the poorly trained radiation therapist. He finally quoted the British therapist Manuel Lederman, who contended that "generally the patient who does not suffer during treatment rarely encounters complications after treatment."

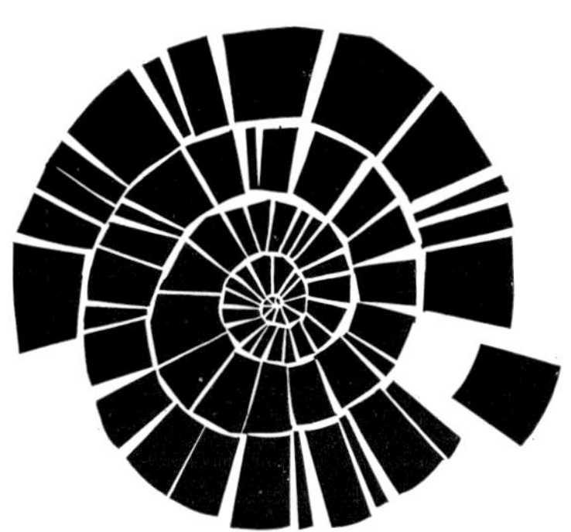

In general, quotations tend to be used out of context. Often cited in articles on palliation is the one by Shakespeare (*King Henry VI*, pt. 2; iii, 3), in which Salisbury stops Warwick from verbally importuning the dying Cardinal Beaufort, "disturb him not, let him pass peaceably." Even the quote used as a motto for this chapter sounds a bit different in its original setting, in the *Latest Decalogue* by Arthur Hugh Clough (1819-1861):

Thou shalt not kill, but need'st not strive,
Officiously to keep alive.
Do not adultery commit;
Advantage rarely comes of it.
Thou shalt not steal;
An empty feat,
When it's so lucrative to cheat.
Bear not false witness;
Let the lie
Have time on its own wings to fly.
Thou shalt not covet;
But tradition
Approves all forms of competition.
The sum of all is, thou shalt love,
If anybody, God above;
At any rate, shalt never labour
More than thyself to love thy neighbour!

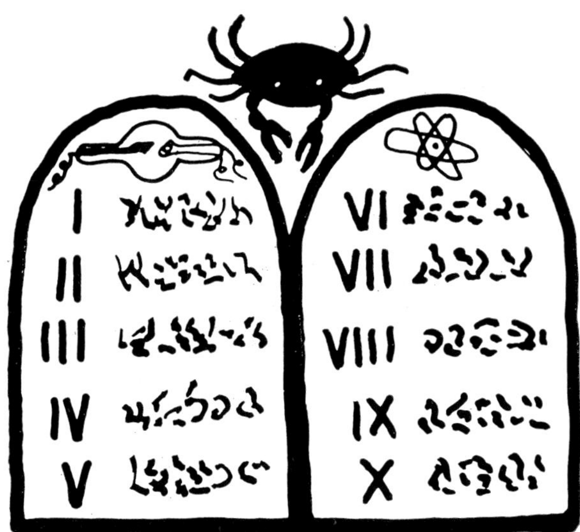

It is difficult to establish a firm set of rules, which would apply in each and every case. Still, a tentative *Decalogue of Palliation* might be of help in providing a basic philosophy for the management of "incurable" malignancies:

I. *Thou shalt be the only physician in charge of the patient.* Other consultants might be called in to help in the evaluation and disposition of the case, a surgeon could be delegated to perform a certain procedure, a dentist may be requested to extract a few teeth, but the overall responsibility for the treatment of the patient's body and mind must be "jealously" preserved in the hands of one physician.

II. *Thou shalt not profane the sense of palliation.* It should not be regarded as a mixture of small talk and analgesic medication. In fact, iatrogenic drug addiction can seldom be justified - except in the last month of life expectancy, when it may become a desirable feature. Life is made enjoyable by the satisfaction of many small, and of a few big, cravings. When the usual desires can no longer be satisfied, the white father may be allowed to create an artificial craving, the satisfaction of which will make the patient's life somewhat more tolerable. For that final stretch, Hayward offered in the *Medical Journal of Australia* of January 3, 1959, his formula for rose-colored spectacles: tincture of opium 15 minims, camphorated tincture of opium 15 minims, and chloroform water to 2 drachms. This, then, becomes (in his words) the elixir of the gods as it produces the cool detachment of the opium smoker: the patient never comes out of it (if properly administered), and when the time arrives he just fades away, peacefully!

III. *Thou shalt give the patient his sabbath.* The forty hour week, which applies today to almost everyone in the hospital - with the exception of patients and physicians - makes it often unavoidable to interrupt the series of irradiations for one or two days out of every week. In fact Franz Buschke - at the ICR in Montreal (1962) - insisted that he detected no difference in the (satisfactory) tumor response of controllable malignancies when "curative" irradiations were fractionated to the rate of thrice weekly. It is also otherwise good medical practice to insert, between periods of active treatment, intervals of "rest," during which injections, pill-pushing, even strict diets, are discontinued. This will make for easier handling of the patient's morale. Walter Alvarez believed that restrictions actually shorten rather than prolong life.

IV. *Thou shalt honor the work of the patient's previous attending physician(s),* otherwise the premiums for professional liability insurance might increase at an even steeper rate than they presently do. Everybody makes mistakes at one time or another: your turn may be next. It is of no help to the patient to be told that the treatment might have been easier, or more successful, had he come earlier, first of all because this is not always true. In point of fact, the only effective cancer prevention method known today is exeresis: if by miracle, we could elicit ahead of time which patient is going to develop a sarcoma of the humerus, in the present state of knowledge, nothing short of amputation could prevent its development.

V. *Thou shalt not kill.* This precept goes deeper than simple ethics, or religious determinants. It has been said that if we were to kill a patient who is incurable today, it is possible that tomorrow a cure might be found for that very illness.

This argument is not likely to hold water for very long. In most incurable situations of non-infectious etiology there is usually considerable destruction of vital tissue: even if the original disease were to become controllable, the patient's survival would hardly be possible or worthwhile. And such unexpected "cure" regimens or medications are more often announced than actually achieved.

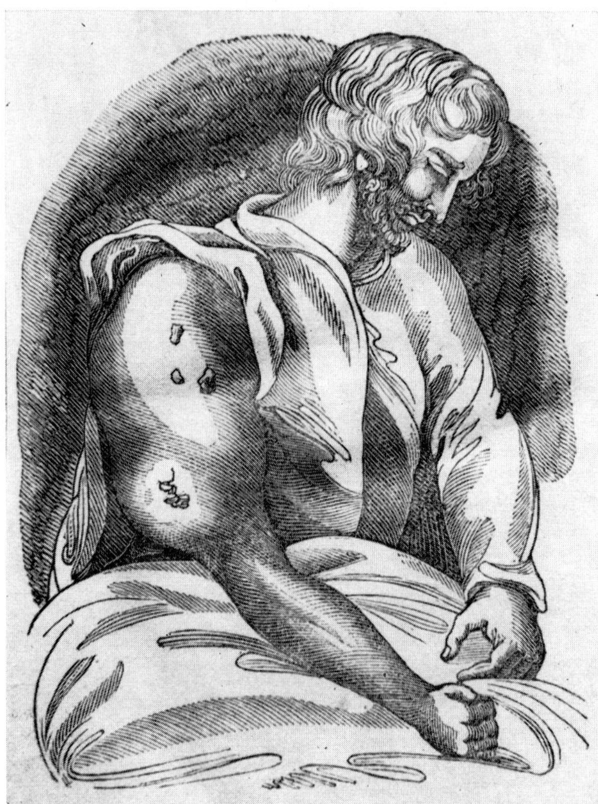

Courtesy: University of Illinois

OSTEO-SARCOMA OF THE HUMERUS. This was the literal diagnosis made pre- as well as post-operatively by Alexander H. Stevens, a surgeon from New York City. The first swelling was noted below the insertion of the deltoid, about six months before this sketch was made. While the tumor was still smaller than a hen's egg, it was repeatedly blistered. Then an "ignorant practitioner" punctured it, but only blood and bloody serum was discharged, and the puncture marks never closed. On June 15, 1821 Stevens performed a disarticulation. Upon "dissection" of the specimen, the "knife encountered spicula of bone," and there was a "separation of the humerus" (pathologic fracture), which had caused atrophy of disuse of the forearm. The wound took long in healing, a small fistula persisted in the axilla, and six months after surgery there occurred a "return of the ulceration (with fungus shooting out)." This woodcut is reproduced from the American edition of Samuel Cooper's *First Lines of the Practice of Surgery* (with notes by Alexander Stevens) published in Philadelphia by John Grigg in 1830.

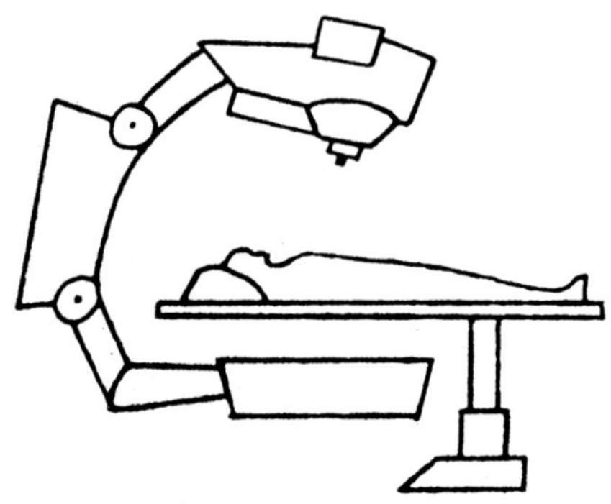

The real reason for maintaining this precept in the most hopeless instances is the difficulty of deciding who has reached the point of no return: who is going to be preserved, and who shall be destroyed? Our diagnostic procedures are still much too coarse to permit an accurate determination in the majority of cases. And there are so many more factors involved — the frailty of human judgment, and other "moral" vagaries, to mention just two — that, as long as proper safeguards against abuses were adopted, such an ultimate "health and death tribunal" would prove to be so time-consuming as to remain ineffectual.

But the world's population is continually increasing. Unless war can be abolished* the time is coming closer when shortages of "vital space" and of food could force the legalized extermination of hopeless "non-productive" segments of the population. Many of us (I for one) may not wish to be around if and when such measures were to become the law of the land.

For the time being, though, "mercy-killing" is a crime, regardless of circumstances. Its commission must not be condoned, no matter how compelling the

*It is generally stated and believed that war reduces the number of a nation's population. Nothing could be further from the truth. It is not merely death, but mainly fertility which determines the de- or re-pletion of a given nation. West Germany has today a larger total population than the pre-war German Reich ever had. Naturally, it might take a long time to replenish the world's population if and when strategically delivered H-bombs were to deplete it. But I firmly believe that future wars will not be fought with *strategic* atomic weapons. And since "conventional" wars increase the number of population in the affected areas, the only way to decrease the speed with which the world's population increases is to abolish war, while at the same time improving the living conditions in "underdeveloped" areas (such "improvement" has always been associated with a dropping fertility). For additional details on this topic—which is perhaps the truism most misunderstood by scientists and politicians alike—see the *Essay on a Fundamental Law of Life* in *Human Biology* of February, 1956.

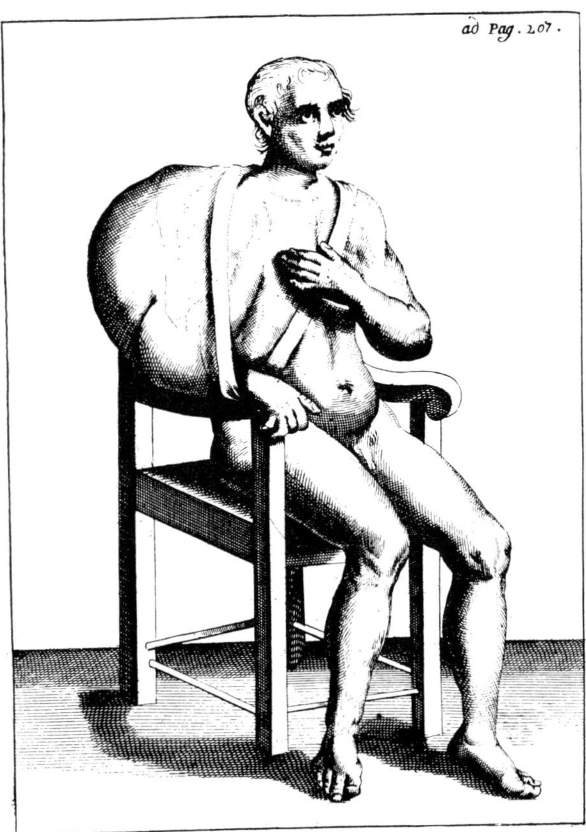

Courtesy: National Library of Medicine.

TUMOR OF THE SCAPULA? Patient was a young Spaniard, his arm became very swollen, and the tumor was regarded as incurable — these are all the details of this case as given by the comparative anatomist Marco Aurelio Severino in what is regarded as the first textbook of surgical pathology, *De Recondita Abscessum Natura,* published in Naples in 1632. This is another sample from my collection of (more or less) artistic representations of neoplasia.

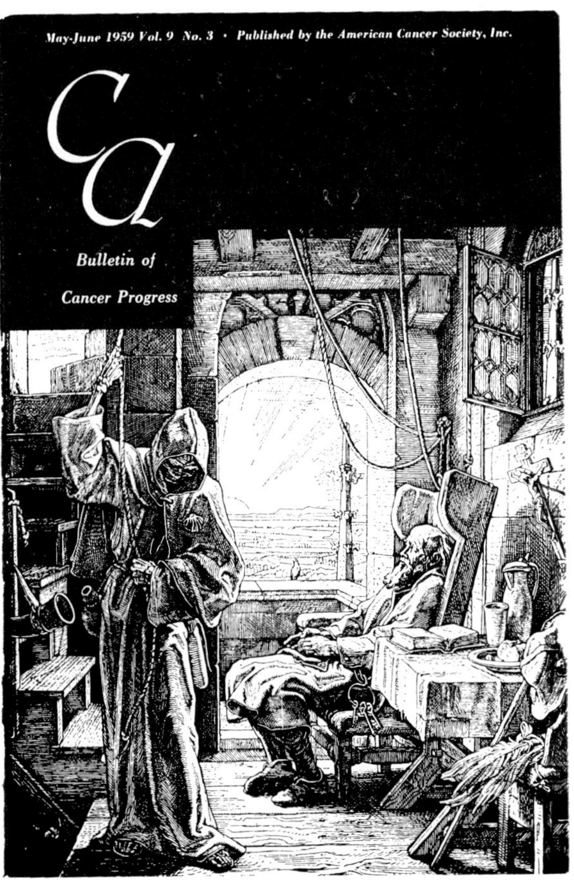

motives would seem to be. Omission, however, has been advocated in some of the most knowledgeable quarters.

In the American Cancer Society's *Bulletin of Cancer Progress* of May-June, 1959, appeared an article by Edward Harper Rynearson (from the Mayo Clinic). He contended that "if these two things are certain: first, that the patient is dying of a malignant process, for which there can be no treatment, and second, that the patient, his relatives, and his spiritual adviser are aware of the situation, then what I am suggesting is the physician should do all he can to alleviate the patient's suffering and make no effort to prolong his life." Rynearson's editorial, and for some obscure reason also the cover illustration of that issue of the *Bulletin of Cancer Progress**, provoked violent protests. So much so that another number of the same publication (January-February, 1960) had to be devoted to the same subject of palliation. That other issue contained a very "conventional" editorial by David Karnofsky (from the Sloan-Kettering Institute in New York City) and a *Symposium*, which consisted of five dissenting and thirty-four concurring opinions (*i.e.*, favoring "omission" of treatment under certain circumstances). These opinions had been given in spontaneous or invited letters to the *Bulletin's* editor, William H. Stoner.*

Death the Friend, by Alfred Rethel (1816-1859), depicts a room in the church tower. The old man, who was supposed to ring the church bell, has just died while quietly sitting in his chair. The implication is that he has lived a full life (the pilgrim's hat indicates a trip to Jerusalem, a "must" for the respectable Christian), and the time had come for him to "go." In the old man's stead, the "friendly skeleton", hooded and palled, is pulling the ropes, which death is doing anyway, though this time perhaps with a glance toward improving public relations.

The main difficulty lies in the definition of inoperable, incurable, terminal, or whatever vocable the respective essayist were to choose.

Perhaps the most realistic is the term uncontrollable, suggested by the Washington (D.C.) onco-surgeon Murray Marcus Copeland in a comprehensive paper (150 references) in the *Journal of Chronic Diseases* of August, 1956.

Lord Horder quotes Samuel Gee as having remarked that over-insistence in hopeless cases does not prolong life so much as it prolongs the act of dying. Most people will agree that a comatous patient,

*In this chapter I have utilized also additional material from a *Bibliography on Palliation in Cancer,* graciously compiled for me by Dr. Sourya Henderson, who is the medical librarian of the American Cancer Society.

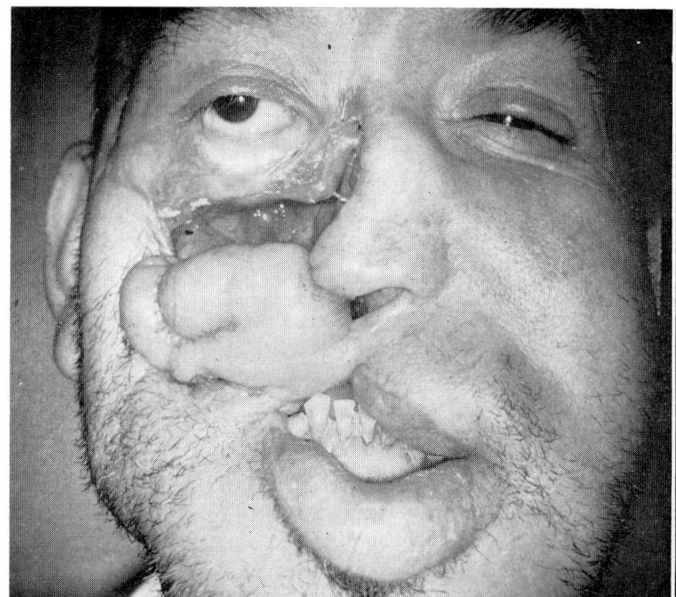

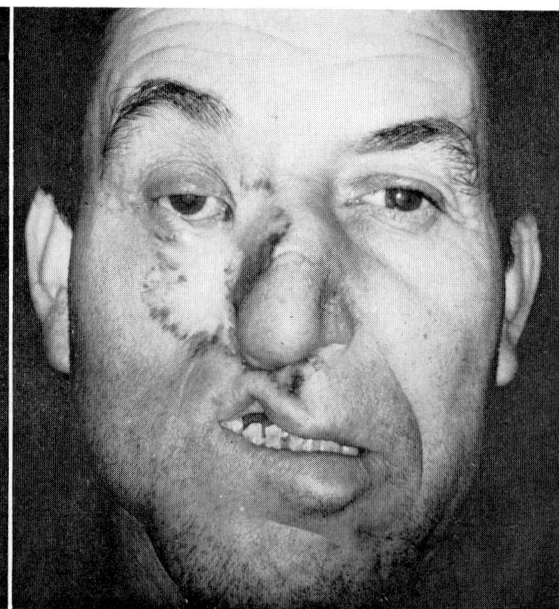

Courtesy: Marion Frank Magalotti.

Antral carcinoma. The right maxillary antrum was first "surgically cleaned out." It recurred, the skin graft broke down, and the tumor mass began flowing freely from the opening. After maximal, but carefully protracted irradiation with both external and interstitial irradiation, excellent result was achieved. Had radiation been given from the beginning, there would have been little if any deformity. The entire radiation treatment was given at the Radiation Center of Cook County Hospital.

known to have generalized carcinomatosis with brain metastases, ought to receive nothing beyond bare supportive therapy. As Edwin Davis (the Omaha urologist) puts it, "passive euthanasia" means to give sedatives and withhold stimulants. In less obvious cases the physician's conscience may be heavily taxed when he must decide where to draw the line. But it is, it should be, and it always will remain, his responsibility. The church has in general agreed with this stand, *e.g.*, the English prelate Thomas Fuller (1608-1661) stated, "when he (the physician) can keep life no longer in, he may fare an easy passage for it to go out."

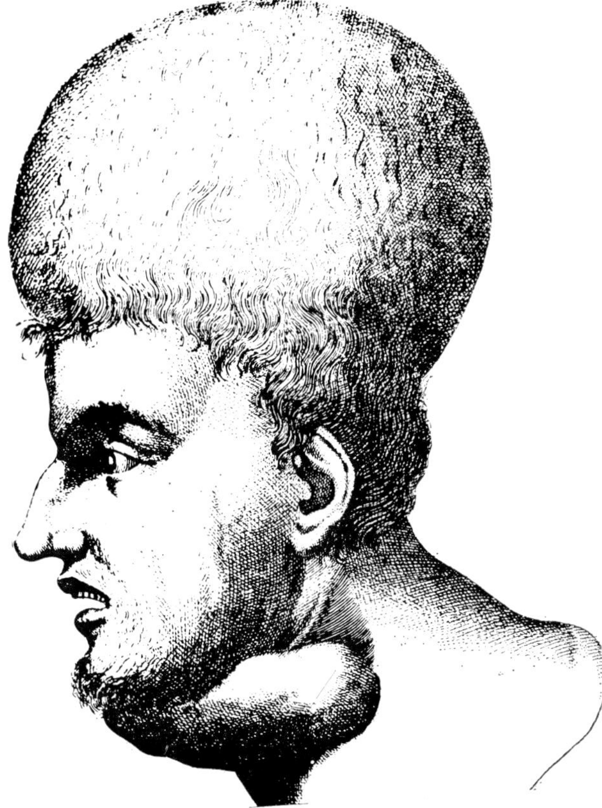

Courtesy: John Crerar Library.

MENINGIOMA. Lorenz Heister inserted this woodcut into his *Chirurgie*, not in its first edition (1712), in the one printed in 1752 in Nürnberg. He had operated in previous years two patients with similar tumors. Both had bone tumors of the calvarium, extending all the way to, but not into the dura, and both had died after the operation. Therefore Heister refused to operate on the 40 year old man shown in the drawing. Among the ancient Incas, such hyperostosis qualified its bearer as a sacred person, perhaps leading to the job of minister. Eugene Pendergrass once told me he had seen a young girl with meningioma who developed just as impressive a forehead. Being "benign" and slow growing, when accessible, meningioma can be extirpated (cured!).

VI. *Thou shalt not adulterate the meaning of palliation.* Life must not be prolonged at the price of added discomfort or excessive disability. When the primary has been in the uterine cervix, the terminal stages of carcinomatous extension (with ureteral compression) are often accompanied by uremia. With a clouded sensorium, the patient passes peacefully from drowsiness to death; ureterostomy, if painfully successful, would reawaken her to the mental anguish of several frightening "last weeks" prior to the unavoidable finish. There undoubtedly are sensible indications for surgical drainage of the ureters, with due regard for the life expectancy in the contemplated case. Operative palliation must never be allowed to become a *routine* procedure of last resort in the preterminal stage of any given malignancy.

VII. *Thou shalt not purloin the patient's right to make his own decisions.* This is especially imperative when the projected extensive removal of organs will result in the artificial drainage of excreta, and in other consequences leading to invalidism. Even in less compulsory situations, the expected degree of disability and inconvenience of the projected palliative procedure must be sincerely explained to the patient. After all, the patient is the one who must give his *informed consent,* without which dire legal consequences may ensue.

Sometimes, if he were to know that he harbors a malignancy, the patient might submit to an operation which he would otherwise refuse. Still, one must avoid, whenever possible, the word cancer, and use substitute terms such as tumor; new, adventitious, unrestrained growth; and so on.

VIII. *Thou shalt protect the patient's peace of mind.* Information regarding his illness must be offered to the patient in a package commensurate with his understanding and receptivity. Beyond that, this eighth commandment provides for the treatment of the psychosomatic aspects of advanced malignancies. It seems that "symptoms originated in the mind" are more numerous and bothersome than is generally suspected. At times these "sensations" outweigh the discomfort caused by the incurable process itself. Habb (in the *Canadian Medical Association Journal* of September, 1951) emphasized that the dying patient is usually more occupied with symptoms than with portents. Fortunately, these side-tracking occurrences can often be successfully treated: in so doing (fitting a new denture, or removing a nevus), the patient's attention is mercifully focused away from his main problem, to the obvious advantage of all concerned.

IX. *Thou shalt protect the patient's family life.* As long as feasible, the patient must be encouraged to live in his familiar environment, to go after his occupation, and to keep enjoying his hobbies, with the least possible disruption. The family must be told the truth about the patient's condition, but experience has shown that divulgation to the spouse of all the sordid and repellent details is not recommendable, at least not in the large majority of cases. A running account of the progress made, and mention of the expected survival time (which is rarely more than a vague approximation, even for an experienced observer) must be offered, not necessarily to the nearest of the patient's relatives, but rather to the most responsible member of the family.

X. *Thou shalt protect the patient's estate.* When the patient expires, the family wants to be told everything within human reach has been done to prevent, to postpone, or at least to alleviate, the final outcome. In charity institutions (where a physician incurs less frequently the hazard of being compared with the money-hungry Charon), the extent of this "everything" is determined by the equipment available, by the oncologist's judgement, and by the patient's consent. In private (or semi-private) practice, when most everything constitutes a "cash" proposition, another very important factor enters into consideration: the expected benefits must be evaluated against the costs, not only with respect to what can be commandeered from the family, but also with due regard for what will be left over when it is all over. Should the savings be spent on senseless repletion, or on a futile hypophysectomy (there exists the still more crippling bilateral adrenalectomy) only to see the surviving spouse go on public relief after the patient's inevitable death? Honest appraisal of the situation, and frank discussion with a responsible relative (or friend of the family) will help in bringing forth the proper decision.

THE FACE OF DEATH. The ulceration on the lip proved to be "incurable," because patient succumbed with metastases from an histologically ill-defined retroperitoneal malignancy, before radiation could have controlled the squamous-cell carcinoma on his lip.

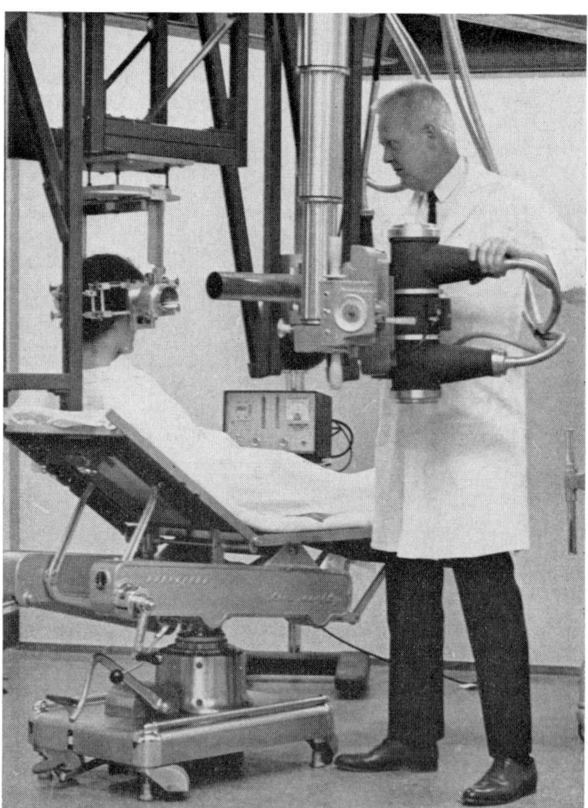

RADIO-ABLATION OF THE PITUITARY. In Harvard's Biomedical Lab, 160 mev protons accelerated by MIT's electron-cyclotron are employed to "remove" the function of the hypophysis, a procedure used in the palliation of metastatic malignancy. This requires considerable accuracy in positioning (a truly "dead aim"), which is achieved by first sending an x-ray beam from the x-ray tube, shown here supported by a telescopic ceiling mount.

What price palliation? This utilitaristic query cannot be adequately answered until after the compilation of a list with price-tags attached to the various degrees of human misery. Such a price schedule might some day be prepared, if only to facilitate the task of the courts, at a time when it has become an all-pervading trend to attempt to translate (even alleged) physical or psychological damage into monetary advantage. In the meantime, as long as euthanasia remains ethically unacceptable, a growing number of people will demand and require the impalpable, immeasurable, but nonetheless very real benefits of palliation.

In general, a more realistic attitude in oncology is quite desirable, if merely to separate the facts from fancy fallacies. Contrary to common slogans (and today's methods are certainly more efficient than Chaucer's astrological "sygne of the cancre"), early detection does not necessarily insure a favorable therapeutic response. When the patient was able to reach a relatively advanced stage before the appearance of symptoms, his chances of prolonged survival are often better than those of another patient in whom the first symptoms appeared during the early phases of tumor growth. This rule, which is consistent with Ian Macdonald's concept of the biologic predetermination of neoplastic development, can be confirmed in everyday practice, time and again. It becomes particularly evident in lymphomata, especially in the so-called follicular variety, which for this reason has been labeled "benign" by some obviously wishful thinker. Cases which enter in that category have been maintained in fairly good health for more than twenty years after obtaining the histologic proof of the disease. Judicious council, and adequate therapeutic efforts, can keep many of these "hopeless" patients afloat for long intervals of time. Otherwise, as Maggy Magalotti puts its, one helps "the tumor to survive the patient."

Since all humans are mortal, there is in essence only a quantitative, not a qualitative difference between the results obtained in "curable," and the results obtained in "incurable" patients, *i.e.,* the survival time. From this vantage point, palliation acquires a deeper meaning, and grows in stature so that – if all nosologic entities could be reduced to a common denominator – one might be inclined to agree with the immortal G. B. Shaw, who claimed that "the only difference between one man and another is the stage of the disease at which he lives."

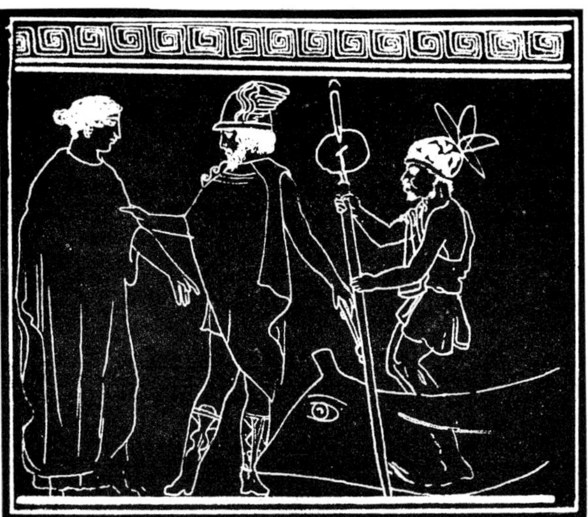

Entering the underworld. The Greeks pictured the soul (Psyche) as a female clad in a shapeless himation (palla), escorted (delivered) by Hermes Psychopompus (conductor of souls) to Charon, who ferried the souls into the underworld across the river Styx – for a fee! This is why at burial the Greeks placed a coin (obolus) in the deceased's mouth. With no obolus for Charon, the soul would wander aimlessly on the wrong side of the Styx, and never find peace. Charon made some exceptions: he is shown wearing Leucippus' fancy headgear, taken in exchange for a one-way passage. The vase from which this interesting frame was copied had been unearthed in Sicily, near the town of *Bugia Sfrontata.*

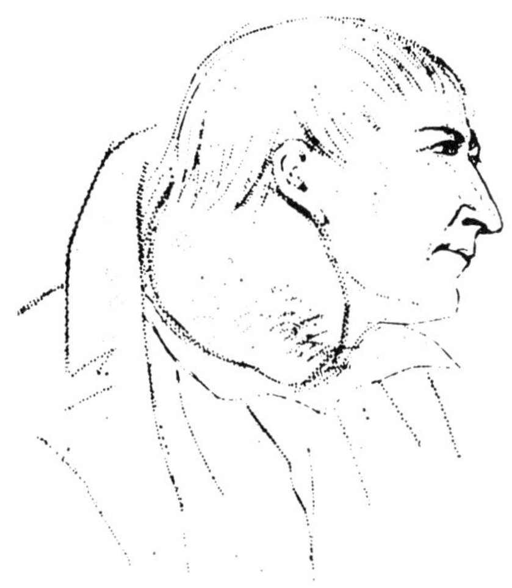

Courtesy: John Crerar Library.

Follicular (benign?) lymphoma. The patient herein shown was a respectable, fifty-two-year old farmer, who had this "lymphatic tumor" for over thirty years. The drawing (the original is in pale colors) comes from the classic *Surgical Observations on Tumors* (Boston, 1837), written by John Collins Warren, a surgeon from Massachusetts General Hospital, who is also famous for having performed the first operation with anesthesia given by W. T. G. Morton.

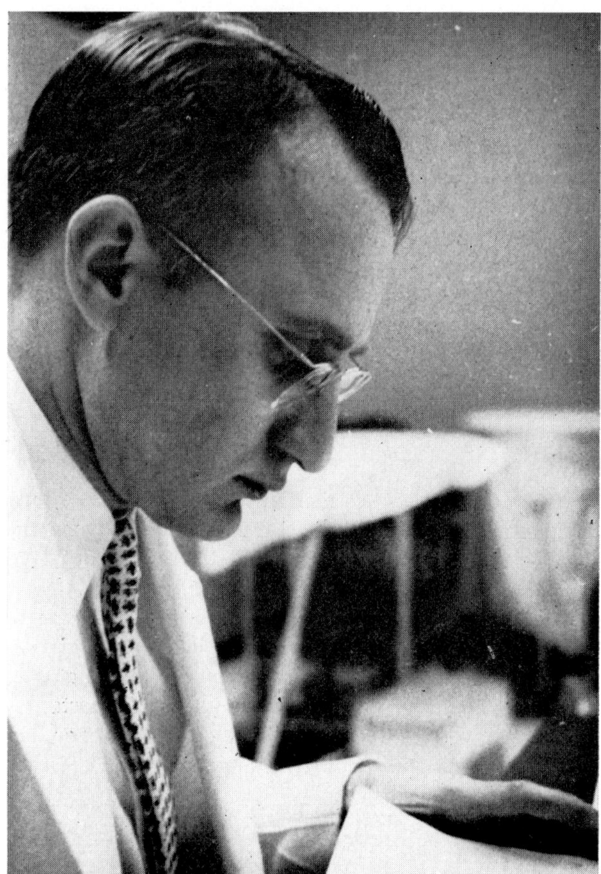

Marion Frank Magalotti. Director of the Radiation Center in Cook County Hospital (Chicago), master radiotherapist (in general) and expert in the therapeutic use of radioiodine (in particular).

It seems that many of the recognized experts in palliation can say with Virgil's Aeneas - *Quaeque ipse miserrima vidit* - that they, too, had at one time or another reached the depths of misery. Maybe the therapist, just like any other artist, must first go through a period of personal suffering before he can achieve his measure of professional maturity.

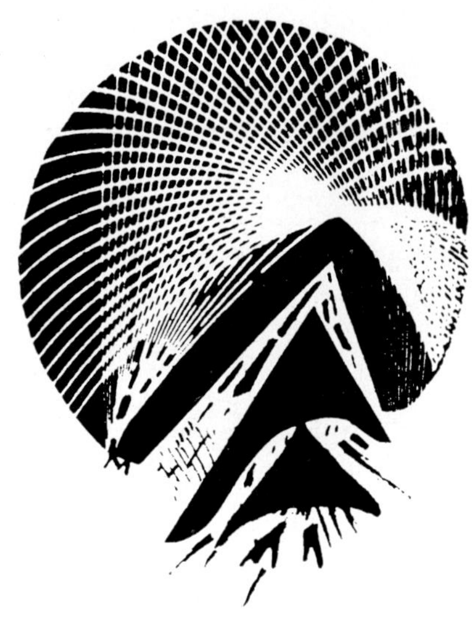

Chapter 5

THE POWER OF WISHFUL THINKING OR, HOW TO (MIS)LABEL POSITIVE, NEGATIVE, AND NORMAL SHADOWS*

Many of the mischiefs that vex
this world arise from words
EDMUND BURKE

RADIOLOGY is a relatively fast moving discipline. Its routines—including the preparation of roentgen reports—must therefore be reappraised at periodic intervals. Such reappraisal ought to start with a retrograde review of the procedure under consideration. Dialectic analysis of the essentials thus uncovered is educational and otherwise rewarding. It should go as far back as bare truisms, since re-emphasis placed on some antique tenet—so self-evident as to be disguised in, and disregarded as, a platitude—may give the old routine a new lease on life.

BEHEST FOR A MORE RIGHTEOUS LABELING OF SHADES

Referring specialists often wish to make their own interpretations, a privilege which must never be challenged. Knowing more about the particular patient, and perhaps more about the roentgen minutiae of the area under considerations, they seem to get more out of (or read more into) the films. A few of these gentlemen, on the other hand, discard the roentgen reports without so much as glancing at them, which again is their privilege. As a result, though, contrary to the graphorrhea of private roentgen practice, in some highly regarded teaching institutions, roentgen reports for certain departments (orthopedics, urology, and the like) are issued in a sloppy, bureaucratic manner—just to have something on paper. While nobody is perfect, by comparison with a radiologist the orthopedist is more likely to miss gallstones, the urologist more prone to overlook osteolytic lesions, the internist more apt to ignore prostatic calcifications. But when these neglected shadows finally come to the fore, the old roentgen report is checked, and it is then better to have *all* its shadows labeled, correctly if possible. Under existing circumstances, it is not as incongrous as it seems to remind the radiologic fraternity that reporting is the most essential of its diagnostic tasks.

At first glance, a fluoroscopic examination is less glamorous than Hamlet's sarcastic tirade, aimed at his queen-mother:

Come, come, and sit you down; you shall not budge;
You go not till I set you up a glass
Where you can see the inmost part of you.

The British physicist Silvanus Phillips Thompson (1851-1918) "discovered" this quotation (Act 3 scene 4) before 1897, and regarded it almost as a Shakespearian premonition of fluoroscopy. Ever since, the triplet has tantalized many others in radiology, *e.g.*, Kells (1926), Kaye (1928), Garland (1945), Le Wald (1952), Jones (1954), Bleich (1960). It is bound to "re-appear" whenever "newcomers" begin to peruse old radiologic texts. One of the established fans of this triplet, the radio-historian Isadore Trostler asked twice

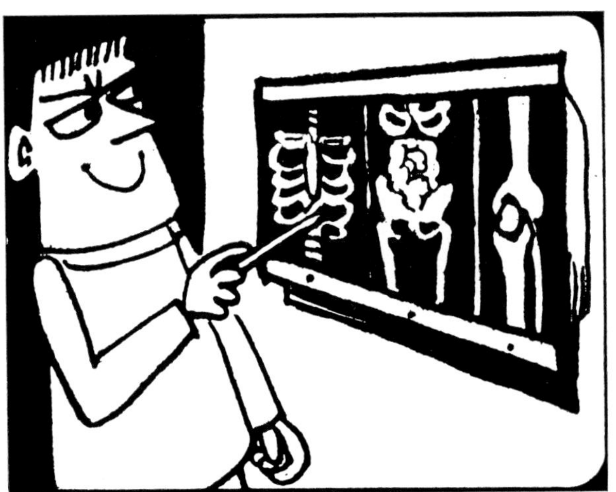

*The beginning of this chapter appeared as an editorial in the April, 1961 issue of *Radiology,* and is herein reprinted with their gracious permission.

(in 1930, and again in 1931) what – else than the proverbial crystal ball – it meant.

On the surface, a roentgen ritual may seem less dramatic than the lonely Dane's vindictive misdemeanors. And yet, on the simple strength of its prognostic implications, a roentgen examination is just as much a matter of life and death. Besides, it leaves two mementoes, the technician's processed film (or set of films), and the radiologist's report.

The films belong to the hospital, or to the physician in whose (private) office they were made. This has been acknowledged by the courts. The first such case *(Hurley Hospital vs. Gage)* was successfully tested on April 21, 1931, in the Circuit Court for the County of Genesee (Michigan).

In their private offices, the radiologists will retain only a few films, selected from unusual cases. Most films are either sent to the referring physicians or are discarded, albeit not immediately. Eugene Lutterbeck (of Chicago) justifies this procedure by referring to clinical laboratories, which do not preserve samples of blood or urine, even if this were practicable. Conversely, in private offices, copies of the roentgen reports are invariably kept for decades —"indefinitely" if sufficient storage space is available.

In large hospitals and clinics, all (except the current and the teaching) films are eventually destroyed (Carman, 1921), at times only after some of them have been "filed" (Sutherland, 1941) in the guise of miniaturized substitutes. In the Department of Radiology of Cook County Hospital (Chicago), since 1957 (shortly after Irvin Franklin Hummon, Jr., became director of the department) all roentgenograms are copied on microfilm (as a last step in processing, after sorting but before the reporting). With the volume on hand, this exceeds one million frames (*one mega-frame*) every two years. It poses in itself a serious storage problem, if single frames are to remain available for reference. The original roentgen reports, attached to the hospital records, are stored for a longer time. Furthermore, hospital records are also microfilmed, page by page, and microfilms of hospital records are preserved much longer than microfilms of roentgenograms.

Roentgen reports prepared before 1920 are scarcer than incunabula, but the *average* roentgen report of today survives just a little longer than all the other vestiges of a given roentgen examination.

Indeed, it takes only a few weeks and the alibis, excuses, and related incidents—from (*a*) the processing solutions which were too hot or too cold, (*b*) the films fogged in transit, and (*c*) the patient's inadequate preparation and/or lack of co-operation, to (*d*) the hasty viewing blamed on lack of time due to lengthy personal consultations, (*e*) the defective dictating device and/or the inattentive secretary, and (*f*) the fleeting wet-film remarks not incorporated in the report—are all forgotten. At that stage of procedural amnesia, retrospective judgment of roentgenologic valor rests on pure, unmitigated documentary evidence, *i.e.*, on the roentgen report.

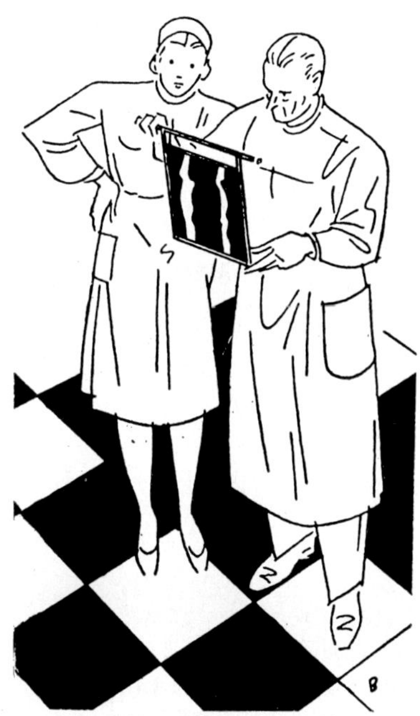

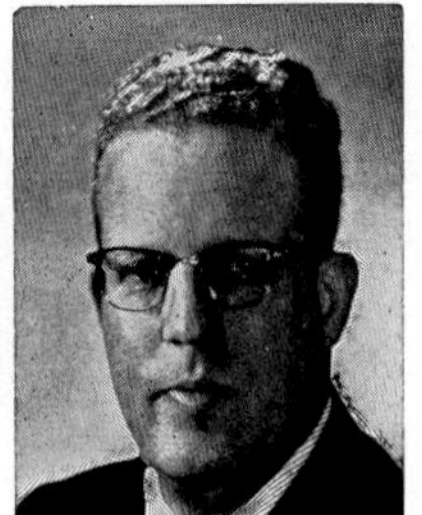

EUGENE LUTTERBECK

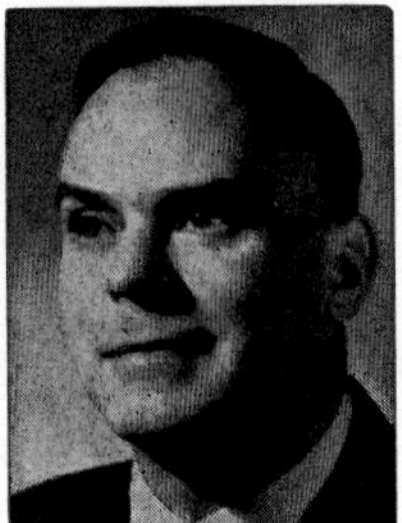

IRVIN HUMMON

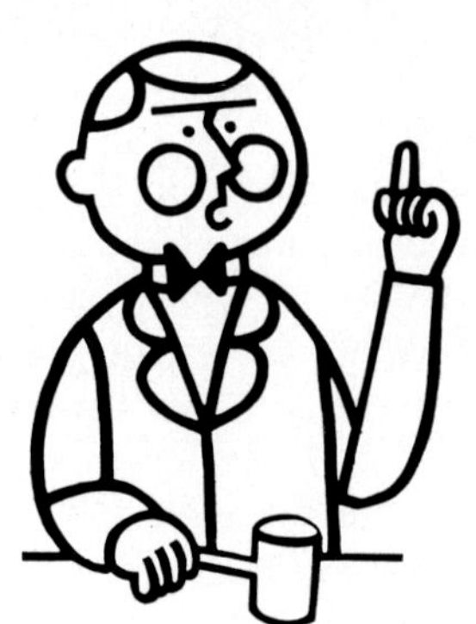

Considering the obvious (and even more so the latent) significance of proper reporting for an adequate practice of radiology, one wonders why is it that so little importance has been attached to this phase in the graduate teaching of radiology? Perhaps one of the February teaching sessions of the American College of Radiology should be devoted to this problem.

In 1918, Albert Soiland (1873-1946) who, at the time, was one of the experts in forensic radiology, contended that if requested by court he must furnish either "a print, a copy, or a written report." In the opinion of one of the all-time authorities on such matters - the Ann Arbor roentgenologist Samuel Wright Donaldson (1891-1961) - microfilms are admissible in court, at least as secondary or best evidence. In actual instances, when films were no longer available, the courts have accepted instead the sole opinion, that is to say *the report,* of the radiologist (Trostler, 1934).

When it is subpoenaed in court (Barrow), or before the discriminating audience of a surgical conference, or summoned by the clinico-pathologic tribunal of last resort, or simply by the attending physician for a quizzical retrospective glance, the (carbon copy of the) roentgen report must be both crisp and stalwart: it faces ever-present wordmongers, always ready, willing, and able to indulge in lingual dissection.

At that decisive moment, be the report concocted in a few, *swept* terms, or *garnished* with many uncouth vocables, if it should fail to come up with an adequate answer, it remains but *empty* prose, that is, what the Kit-Kat (Cushing) physician-poet, Sir Samuel Garth (1661-1719), would have called "a barren superfluity of words!" Whereas, if the words had been offered by weight, not by number nor with haste, and if they had solved *(at least some of)* the points in question, those particular shadows were correctly labeled and would never come back to haunt the radiologist.

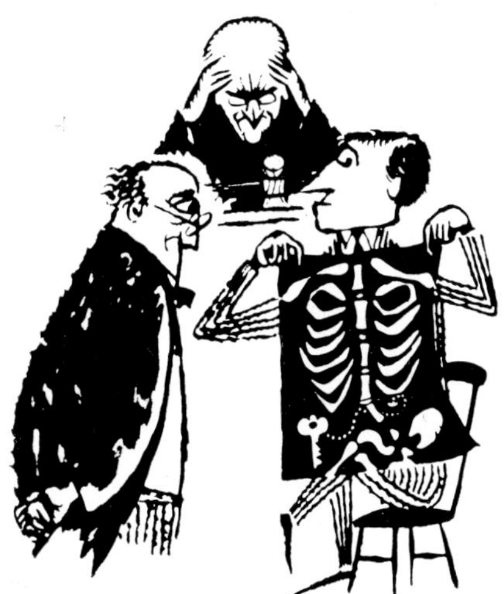

"When your x-rays go on trial." This is the very title under which this copyrighted cartoon appeared in *Medical Economics* (of November, 1957), herein reproduced with their kind permission.

CONSULTANTS

The galley proofs for the sections on reporting have been critically reviewed by three radiologists: (1) Don Bauer, a private practitioner in Klamath Falls (Oregon) who has his own office, makes the rounds of several hospitals, and has recently published a chapter on *Radiologic Report Writing;* (2) George Miller, a partner in a group practice, the Carle Clinic in Urbana (Illinois), whose studies on the high kv technique in examination of the colon set a pattern currently accepted as a standard; and (3) Roscoe Miller, associate professor of radiology in the University of Indiana and full-time teacher and researcher in the Medical Center in Indianapolis, the one who described the "football sign" in perforated viscus (the falciform ligament contrasted by the oval-shaped accumulation of air in the peritoneum).

The consultants were in agreement with most of my presentation. They offered, however, certain comments, and voiced certain exceptions, and these were incorporated in the text.

DEFINITION AND DESIGNATIONS

The *roentgen report* is a text in which the roentgenologist describes and interprets - either impersonally, or for the benefit of the patient's attending physician - the findings elicited during a diagnostic roentgen examination.

Many alternate terms have been (or are still) in use, for instance the extended *roentgenologic* (preferably without the supererogatory suffix *-al* as in the redundant *roentgenological*) report. The Francophile *radiologic*(al) report could conceivably cover even an iodine uptake, while more specialized vocables, such as *fluoroscopic, radiographic, roentgenographic, kymographic, roentgenphotographic, roentgencinematographic, stratigraphic, autoradiographic,* etc., report would be limited to the respective, circumscribed territory.

In the past, several other terms were concurrently employed, such as *notes, findings, diagnostic comments, remarks, memoranda, protocol,* usually preceded by either *roentgen, radiologic,* or *x-ray*. These are all more or less obsolete. The vernacular *x-ray report* has survived, but a number of people consider it objectionable, for traditionalistic reasons explained in the Semantic Treatise.

Similarly, a variety of designations can be found in foreign languages, including *protocole, rapport, compte-rendu* in French, *Befund, Röntgen-Diagnostik-Protokoll* in German, *reperto, relazione, registrazione, rendi-conto* in Italian, *zakhluchenya, protokol* in Russian, *registro, protocolo, relación* in Spanish.

All of these carry at least to some extent the connotation of report, which means an account of something witnessed or investigated, given by one person to another.

Reporting of roentgenograms is a common practice all over the world. It has also attracted the attention of certain (European) legislative organs.

A regulation of the *Sécurité Sociale* in France (which dates there from 1930) provides in art. 45, ch. 13 *(Électro-Radiologie et Physique)* that all "electro-radiologic" examinations must be recorded with a written "commentary" signed by the performing physician.

For some time, Italian regulations offered a peculiar re-definition of the roentgen report. When the radiologist forwarded it to the referring physician, it was regarded as an inter-professional communication, and as such it was tax-exempt (duty-free). But when the radiologist handed the report directly to the patient (for pre-employment, pre-marital, and similar requirements), it became a certificate; as such it had to be written on a special, pre-stamped (pre-paid) blank, or else a stamp of identical monetary value had to be pasted onto the stationery used.

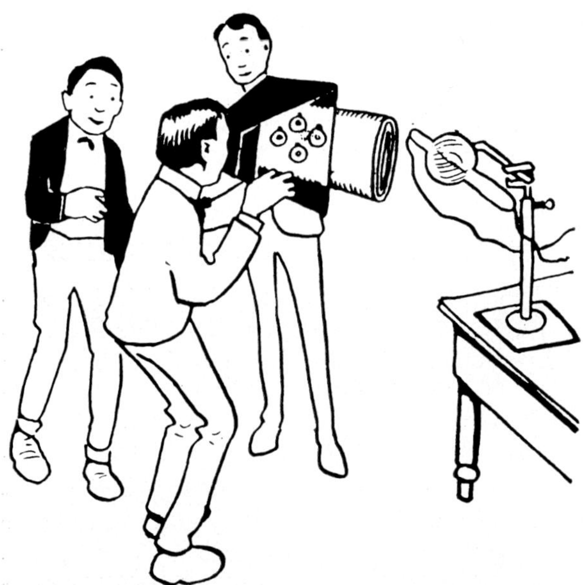

AND FOR COUNTERBAND WATCHES, TOO! In the beginning it used to be said that "x rays are good for bullets, bones, and gallstones." Here, in a sketch from an article by Fred O'Hara in the *American X-Ray Journal* of July, 1902, is shown the dramatic moment of truth when a St. Louis custom agent found Swiss watches on "crypto-scoping" a bolt of cloth.

In the very beginning, the reports were simple letters, on the physician's regular stationery. Special forms were introduced before the turn of the century. Typed reports did not become the rule until after World War I. Elaborate blanks, with spaces provided for pasted-on positive prints, were in use around 1910 by successful private radiologists in the large cities around the world, for instance on Park Avenue in New York City. Prior to World War II, in Central Europe, some reporting forms contained cutouts for the insertion of trimmed spotfilms (of bulb or cecum). After World War II, the pendulum whirled around once more, and it is now *bon ton* for private radiologists to issue roentgen reports typed on their regular (simple, *i.e.,* dignified) stationery.

REVIEW OF THE LITERATURE

A rather extensive search yielded comparatively few bibliographic titles dealing specifically with what should be included in or deleted from the roentgen report, or the manner in which it ought to be formulated. The diminutive text with the alluring title *X-ray Reports* (Buckley) turned out to be a manual for radiographers (current British appellation for x-ray technicians) and clerks: it was built mainly on the nomenclature found in Shanks & Kerley's textbook, and is therefore less elaborate than the excellent *Glossary* of Etter (1960). Both have chapters on how to prepare reports.

From a simply chronologic viewpoint, the first book to contain a full-fledged section on roentgen reporting was published in 1925 by a radiologist from Louisville, (Kentucky), Charles Darwin Enfield. The U. S. Army X-Ray Manual, printed in 1918, contained several paragraphs on how to report foreign bodies. There might have existed other "bookish" precursors.

Five practical hints on the essence of reporting (one of them a multi-headed maxim by Grashey) can be found in the princeps edition (1928) of a Swiss *Lehrbuch* (Schinz, Baensch, and Friedl): these hints appear unchanged through its fifth edition (1950), despite the acquisition of an additional senior author (Uehlinger), and of an American translation (by the collaborators of

Case). More substantial chapters on reporting are found in a German treatise (Glasscheib) of 1936, and in a Russian volume (Reynberg) of 1938. Shorter comments on this topic are contained in a British textbook (Bull) of 1935 (simply reprinted in its 1951 re-issue), in a South-American compendium (Esguerra-Gómez) of 1939, and in a North-American syllabus (Hodges & Peck), first published in 1939, then in 1947 and again in 1959.

An excellent chapter, entitled *Radiologic Report Writing* (pp. 180-197) appeared in Donald de Forest Bauer's *Practice of Country Radiology* (Thomas, 1963) As a motto he uses a few sentences from the ACR's radiologic Code of Ethics: "It shall be considered ethical to give an opinion to a physician in consultation on films regardless of their origin. The radiologist shall interpret films regularly only when the radiology department is under his supervision and where his official status is evident."

More often, though, basic texts in diagnostic radiology – whether originated in Germany (Kaestle), Canada (Harrison), France (Gibert), Belgium (Van Pée), or in this country (Sante) – bring only perfunctory remarks on reporting. In some instances (*cf.*, De Lorimier), succinct enunciation succeeds in covering at least the essentials.

Papers containing remarks on roentgen reporting, or on some of its phases, are not uncommon. A true survey of the field is nevertheless very difficult, if at all possible. In most instances, the subject is merely broached, incidentally as it were, while the main topic is sailing under a completely different title. When specifically devoted to reporting, the papers were usually editorials and as such, at least in the past, considered ephemeral and deleted from the annual table of contents. But even those which are indexed, appear under a baffling variety of bibliographic captions.

(a) No such heading as *report* or *reporting* occurs in any of the first four excellent volumes published to date as a *Cumulative Index* of the journal *Radiology*. In writing, one must actually specify what kind of report is meant, because most people conceive the vocable in terms of committee or meeting report. On the other hand, the article alluringly entitled *Reports of Findings* (Trostler, 1932) turned out to be a discussion on the future of radiology as a specialty, said to depend on the radiologist's ability to *tell more* from the film than other physicians.

(b) The catchword *interpretation* is much too general, even for early titles, *e.g.*, Hickey (1904), M'Kendrick (1912). There is the classic *Roentgen Interpretation*, currently in its ninth edition, first issued in 1919 by George Winslow Holmes (1876-1959) of Boston and Howard Edwin Ruggles (1886-1939) of San Francisco. More recent items so titled – Rigler (1959) – are actually concerned with reporting.

(c) Quite a few papers are classified under the captions *nomenclature* and *terminology*,* one by the professor of radiology at Tufts, in Boston, Arial Wellington George (1882-1948), another by the Evansville (Indiana) radiologist Stephen Nathaniel Tager. These are usually recommendations for the use of "correct" language, as emphasized also by Sidney Thomas or Robert Barden.

(d) *Reading* of films is another equivocal heading, found in both French (Cluzet) and Swiss (Jaeger)

*These vocables are not interchangeable, except loosely. *Nomenclature* is a system of names, especially those derived from a classification, as distinguished from *terminology*, which signifies the technical or special terms used in a given discipline. The difference is about the same as that between strategy and tactics, or between a state's constitution (nomenclature) and its laws (terminology).

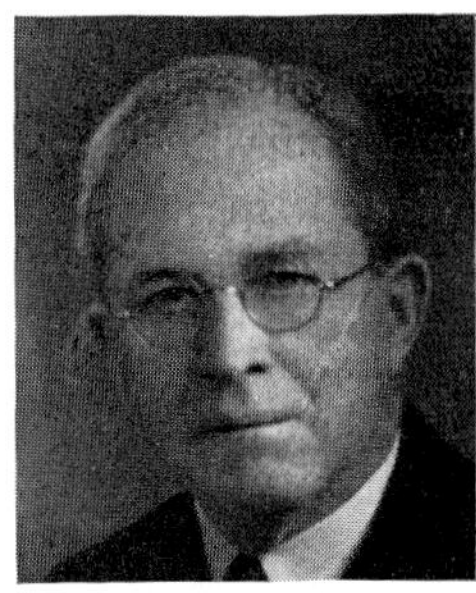

George W. Holmes

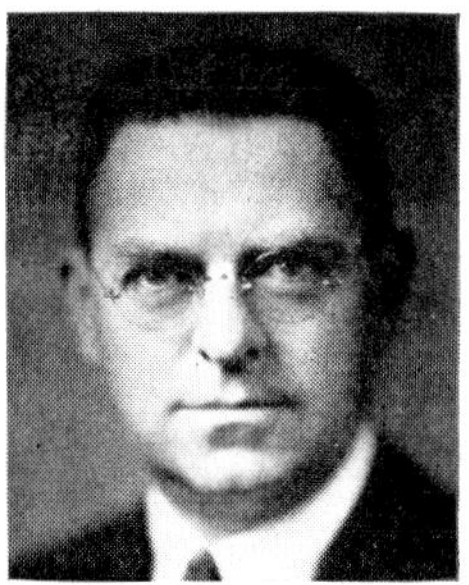

Howard E. Ruggles

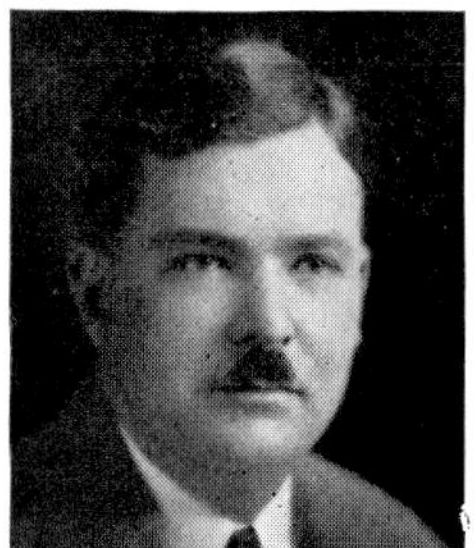

LeRoy Sante

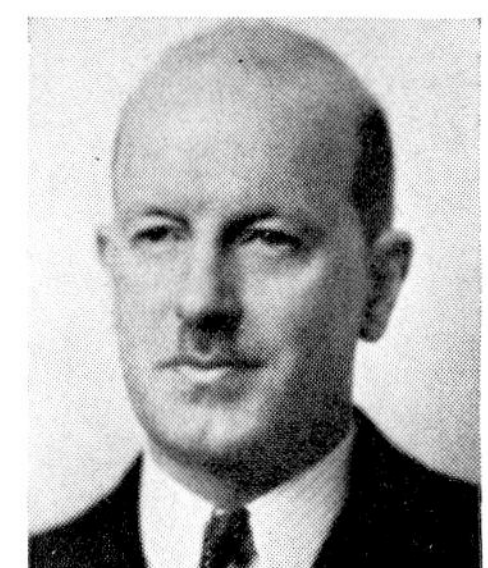

Bede James Harrison

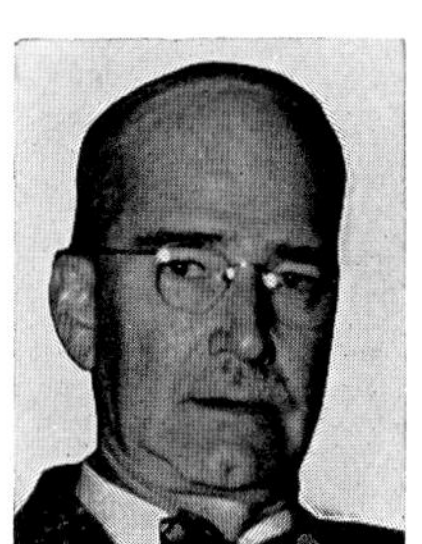

Alfred de Lorimier

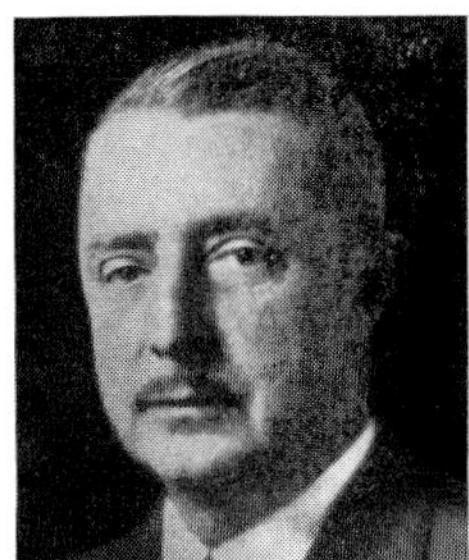

Arial W. George

articles, occasionally also in contributions from Canada (McRae) as well as from this country (Dunham, Pirkle).

(e) *Diagnosis* is (in this context) a very vague notion, but under such a title are indexed several valuable contributions to the problem of reporting, for instance one by Carman (1922) of Mayo's, another by Sosman (1950) of Peter Bent Brigham (Boston) Hospital fame, or the 1958 Caldwell Lecture given by Rigler while still in Minneapolis (he is now in Los Angeles).

(f) Under *records* are listed articles – *cf.*, one by Charles Goldie Sutherland (1877-1951) from the Mayo Clinic – dealing with blanks for easy cross-checking of diagnostic roentgen findings (1929). Under *classification* come the methods of indexing reports and other roentgen records (Sante, 1926).

(g) Incidental (and yet significant) remarks on reporting can also be found in papers which explore the basic tenets of roentgenology in its relationship with other specialties, as in an editorial by Sherman, or in Roscoe Miller's *Attending Physician in the Radiological Team,* published in *Medical Times* of July, 1963.

(h) Some papers, while concerned mainly with reporting, carry titles (*e.g.*, the one by Rees) which defy a listing germane to this topic.

HOLZKNECHT

As far as could be ascertained, the very first paper on roentgen reporting was prepared by Guido Holzknecht* (1872-1931): it appeared in 1919 in friable postwar newsprint in the *Jahreskurse für ärztliche Fortbildung,* a non-radiological "postgraduate" journal published in Münich. Almost all questions which to this date have arisen in connection with roentgen reporting, are at least mentioned in that truly *princeps* article on the subject (Holzknecht, 1919).

Insistent efforts were made to obtain one of the reports holographed by Guido Holzknecht, but to no avail. Ernst Georg Mayer, whose eponym is associated with the thrice angulated temporal view, and who is today the director of the *Zentral-Röntgen-Institut* in the *Allgemeines Krankenhaus* in Vienna (where he has worked in various capacities since 1921) declared categorically that he had never seen Holzknecht writing (or dictating) an actual roentgen report. Holzknecht must have reported films sometimes before 1921, but all those records had been destroyed.

Konrad Weiss, the former secretary of the *Oesterreichische Röntgengesellschaft* (both Weiss and Mayer also teach radiology in the University of Vienna) – who had been associated since 1918 at the Vienna *Poliklinik* with Robert Kienböck (1871-1954) – had never seen the latter preparing a roentgen report.

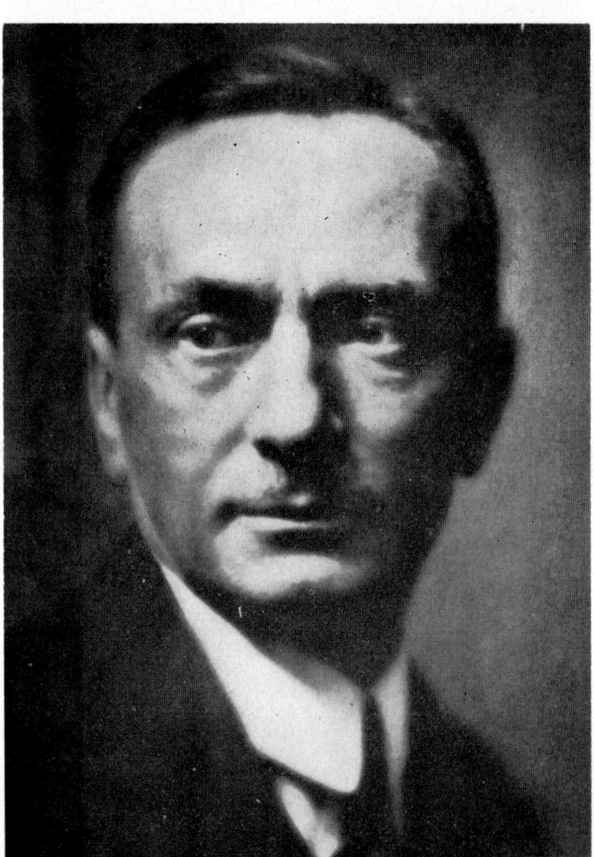

GUIDO HOLZKNECHT.

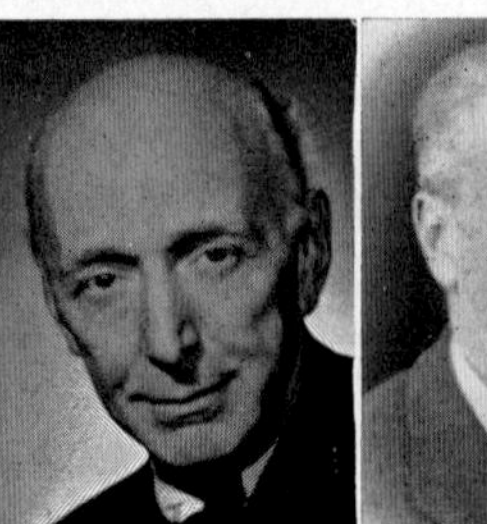

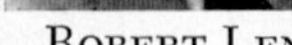

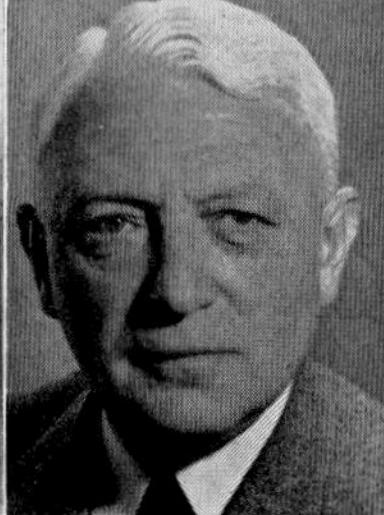

ERNST MAYER ROBERT LENK FELIX FLEISCHNER

*At the September, 1959, meeting of the ARRS in Cincinnati, I interviewed a score of roentgen pundits, on the subject of reports. Felix Georg Fleischner (at the time the radiologist of Beth-Israel in Boston, formerly in Vienna) recalled that the Swedish pioneer Gösta Forssell (1876-1950), while offering the eulogy at Holzknecht's burial, mentioned that the Viennese roentgen philosopher had inaugurated modern roentgen reporting. Following Fleischner's suggestion, a (never acknowledged) inquiry was sent to another Holzknecht pupil, Robert Lenk, who is living in Israel. The search was then shifted to the old, reliable bibliographic treasure chest, the *Index Catalogue*: naturally, that first paper (Holzknecht, 1919) was found in the ninth volume of its third series (1931), pigeon-holed under the non-committal heading *Roentgenography and roentgenoscopy!*

Indeed, it seems that most of the modern "big roentgen chiefs" act only as consultants!

HICKEY

In this country, the first significant contribution to roentgen reporting was made by Hickey.

Hickey's original paper (1922) was found – lo and behold – under the heading *Reports, roentgen ray* in the first (1903-1937) of the five volumes of the *Consolidated Indices* of the *American Journal of Roentgenology.* The second volume (1938-1942) of these *Indices* contains again the heading *Reports,* but these carry only reports of various committees, and the following three volumes no longer include any such bibliographic caption.

In 1922, Hickey surveyed the members of the ARRS, and requested samples of their roentgen reports, in an attempt to reach some sort of standardization.* For reporting of fractures Hickey adopted the wordings of Harold Jesse Pierce** (1882-1960), a radiologist from Terre Haute (Indiana). Such adoption is specifically mentioned in Hickey's magistral paper, published in the *Americal Journal of Roentgenology,* and abstracted in the *Journal of Radiology* (1922).

In 1923, Enfield published in the *AMA Journal* his article on roentgen reporting. It was going to be reprinted, almost verbatim, in his previously mentioned book (1925) - which brings us back to the previous bibliographic starting point.

*At the previously mentioned Cincinnati meeting of the RSNA, I discussed this matter with the then still fiery James Thomas Case (1882-1960) who proclaimed on the spot that Hickey had actually appropriated his (Case's) own scheme of reporting. Case explained that one of his (Case's) secretaries switched bosses in 1915, and went to work for Hickey, and this is allegedly how the "transfer of information" took place. Even though Case gave me specific permission to be quoted, the authenticity of this anecdote is highly doubtful. Old-timers have repeatedly assured me that (for some now no longer identifiable reason) there had always been hard feelings between Hickey and Case—ever since the latter replaced the former in the position of editor of the *American Journal of Roentgenology.*

**In the fall of 1959 I made a special trip to visit the country squire Pierce, at his estate and orchards in Brasil (Indiana). In that pastoral environment the conversation was naturally interspersed with reminiscences, as nostalgic as those of a well-tempered clavichord. On the specific question of reporting, Pierce confirmed Hickey's (but laughed off Case's) statement, and promised to look for a copy of the samples which he (Pierce) had been using in the early 1920's. My second visit to Pierce's orchards never materialized because the country squire had unexpectedly departed for points unreachable (coronary thrombosis). Inquiries with Pierce's estate went unanswered.

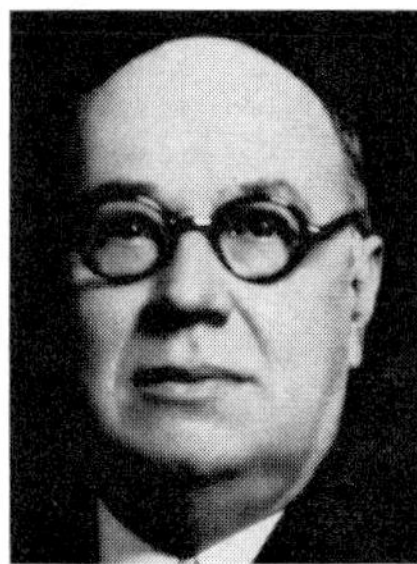

Preston Hickey

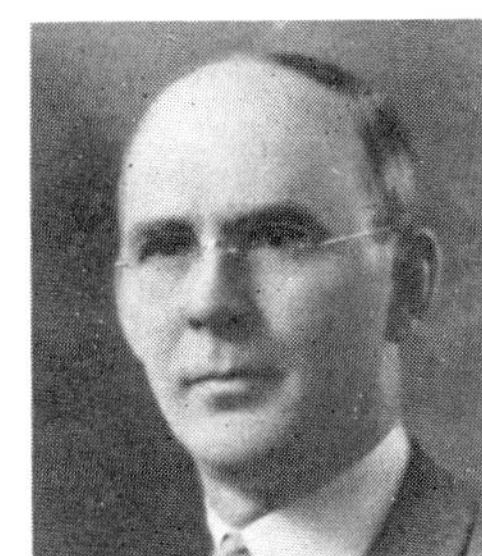

Harold Pierce

WORDS AND SHADOWS

With the exception of time spent in actual consultations, in a small hospital the dictation of roentgen reports is performed in solitude. By contrast, this ritual is often quite spectacular in teaching centers, where audience is provided by residents, students, and "visiting firemen." In a typical stance, several heads are draped in a semi-circle around a viewbox while, in the center of attention, the officiating soothsayer busily perorates into his microphone. As this knight-of-the-shade uses a wide range of anatomic and nosologic terminology to bark his way through a more or less rapid succession of reports, he seems to re-enact Oliver Goldsmith's parson:

While words of learned length and thundering sound
Amaz'd the grazing rustics rang'd around,
And still they gaz'd, and still the wonder grew,
That one small head could carry all he knew.

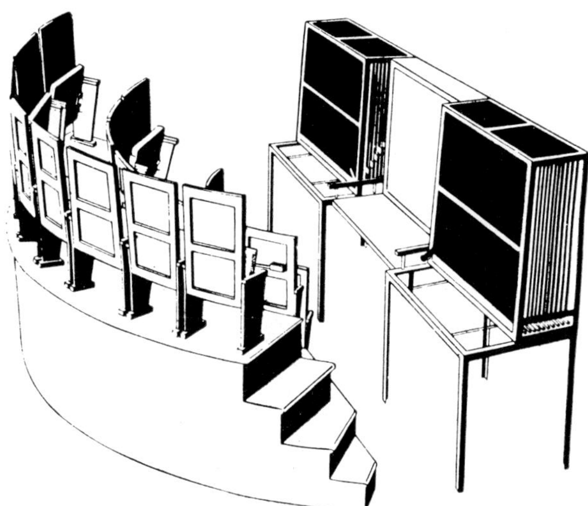

Roentgen reporting room. Diminutive amphitheatre built around the Elema-Schönander Dekaskope viewbox.

An audience may want to believe that an actor's work consists only of facile recitation in the glow of spotlights. By comparison, the radiologist reads most of his lines without the benefit of a rehearsal (although he is sometimes beseeched by uninvited prompters). Nevertheless, few people are acutely aware of the fact that, while a roentgen report is made of words, obviously, words alone do not a roentgen report make. Shadows (some visible, most of them invisible) constitute its other main ingredients.

Fritz Pordes (1890-1936), who suffered severe radiation damage, but ultimately died of tuberculosis, was one of Holzknecht's most articulate pupils. Residing in Freud's Vienna, he acquiesced in 1921 that there had been a tendency to equate the interpretations of roentgenograms with the interpretation of dreams. Noticeable improvements have been made since the advent of *Röntgen's silhouettes* (editorial of 1896), but it is still true what Mihran Krikor Hassabian (1870-1910), the Armenian electro-radiologist from Philadelphia, had written in 1907: "There are numerous shadows on the negative that defy all efforts at interpretation and are as little understood today as they were when skiagraphy was first presented to the notice of the medical profession." Although the number of these "unexplainable" shadows is shrinking as visibly as a space-diminishing process, some radiologists still resort to the psychoanalytical undertones derogatorily summarized by Pordes as *Schattenwissenschaft* (science of the shadows.) A few colleagues even try to emulate Nostradamus — Michel de Notre-Dame (1503-1566) a French astrologer who published rhymed prophesies — and offer roentgen interpretations "thin" enough to fit practically anything that could happen to the patient.

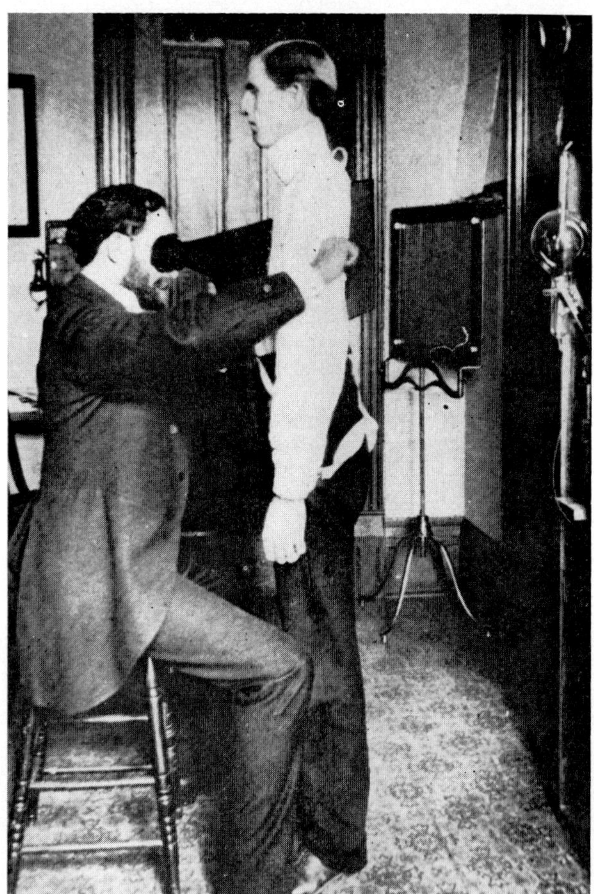

CRANE WITH CRYPTOSCOPE. The "paddle" held against the patient's back is a Crane skiascope. It consisted of stripes of varied x-ray density, and served as a standard of comparison for the radio-opacity of adventitious parenchymal shadows encountered during the examination. The close proximity of patient and operator in the pathway of the x-ray beam, typical for that time, caused many deaths among the roentgen pioneers.

A very significant improvement in the way to describe the shadows was emphasized as early as 1899 by Augustus Warren Crane (1868-1937), a private radiologist from Kalamazoo (Michigan). He had inquired both searchingly and fruitfully into the *density* of the shadows. Crane proposed also an instrument for the measurement of these density differentials - the *skiameter* - and, ever since, this instrument has been repeatedly re-discovered. Excerpts from Crane's original article were reprinted by Hickey in 1916.

John Caffey - the pediatric radiologist *par excellence,* formerly of New York, then of Denver - pictured Röntgen's pallid shades as dark holes carved within radiant streams. These shadows are cold, silent, and empty (twisted rifts beyond the substance), meaningless in themselves. To acquire some meaning, they must first be translated into (roentgen) evidence!

STAGES IN REPORTING

During their Era, the Roentgen Pioneers were blunt in labeling the shades. They would name with-

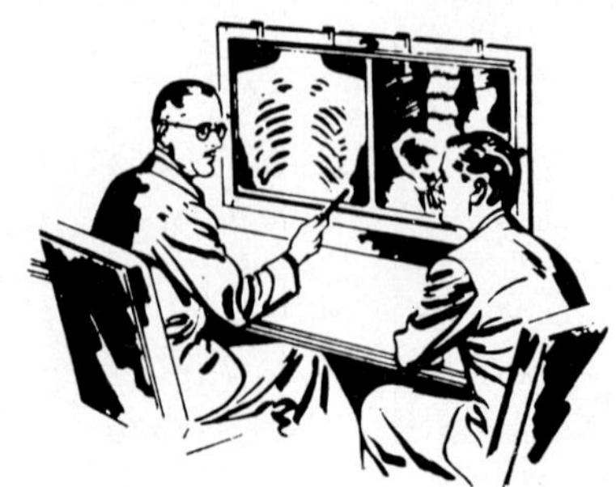

out hesitation the organ, disease, or foreign body supposed to have produced the incriminated shadow(s). They added references to the patient's history, or to non-radiologic examinations to which they had subjected that patient, whenever they thought it was pertinent.

During the Golden Age of Radiology, the reports tended to be puristic, with the accent placed on description of the shadows (and of nothing else). The conclusions offered were those that could be drawn from the roentgen findings proper, leaving out all "extraneous" matter.

The Atomic Phase was well established before the "modern" way of reporting began to take shape: now it appears desirable to provide certain specific answers extending beyond the immediate range of the actual roentgen findings. In practice, this means to reply to hypothetical questions asked by the referring physician. "Modern" requisition slips contain concrete questions such as "what exactly do you suspect?" or "state specifically what you are looking for," or - in a more diplomatic way - "what do you want to rule out?"

SEARCHING FOR REPORTS

I spent several years in trying to collect actual roentgen reports, old or new, of either American or other provenience.

To begin with, letters were sent to many senior confrères. The few replies received contained (if anything at all) relatively recent items. Then, inquiries were mailed to various medical periodicals,* but this was even less rewarding. Later requests were directed to museums, finally to general practitioners in the senior category. *Most of the letters were never so much as acknowledged.* Slowly, though, old reports began to trickle in, and a few of these are reproduced in the following pages. Evidently, there became available a large selection of recent roentgen reports.

*Letters requesting (copies of or information on) old roentgen reports were graciously accepted for publication by the editors of the *British Medical Journal* and *Lancet* (London), *Minerva Medica* (Torino), *South African Medical Journal, Medical Journal of Australia,* etc. In this country, similar letters appeared in the *New England Journal of Medicine,* and in the *New York State Journal of Medicine.* The only rejections came from the *AMA Journal* and from the French *Presse Médicale.* While the reply from the former was unnecessarily blunt, the latter evaded the issue by referring the inquiry to the (always very helpful) Miss Antoinette Béclère.

PFAHLER

Several correspondents had suggested that there might exist reports by George Edward Pfahler (1874-1957), the first formal teacher of radiology in this country (in the University of Pennsylvania).

During his lifetime Pfahler had saved all his records, beginning with those from his first year in private practice (1902). After Pfahler's death, his office was taken over by a nephew (the radiologist George Pfahler Keefer) who discarded all but the current records.*

Additional inquiry revealed that none of the early (presumably handwritten) reports given by Pfahler in the Philadelphia General Hospital had survived.**

GRUBBE

I interviewed Emile Herman Grubbé (1875-1960) on July 22, 1959, in the Swedish-Covenant Hospital (on Chicago's North Side).

Grubbé's left ala nasi was gone (with exposure of the nasal septum), as was his upper lip (with exposure of the dental plate); his left forearm and several fingers from the right hand had been amputated years before, and now he was hospitalized because of a mass in the right axilla (it turned out to be a metastatic lymph node, removed the next day). Grubbé had moderate loss of both vision and hearing, yet he was relatively easy to contact, He tended to wander off into digressions, but seemed lucid as well as cooperative.

When asked about early reports, Grubbé stated that he had written many such reports during his tenure as director of the X-ray Department at the Hahnemann Hospital in Chicago. He reminisced that in the very

*The pioneer's widow—Mrs. George (Muriel) Pfahler—was extremely obliging. She had gone through all his documents, and had saved many of them (used in publishing a book of reminiscences) but there were no reports among them.

**This information was obtained from Pfahler's student, friend, and successor as chief-radiologist (therapist) in Philadelphia General Hospital, Bernard Pierre Widmann.

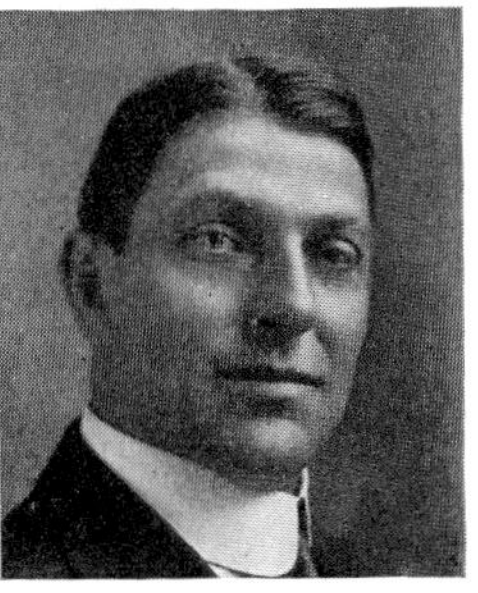

M. J. Hubeny

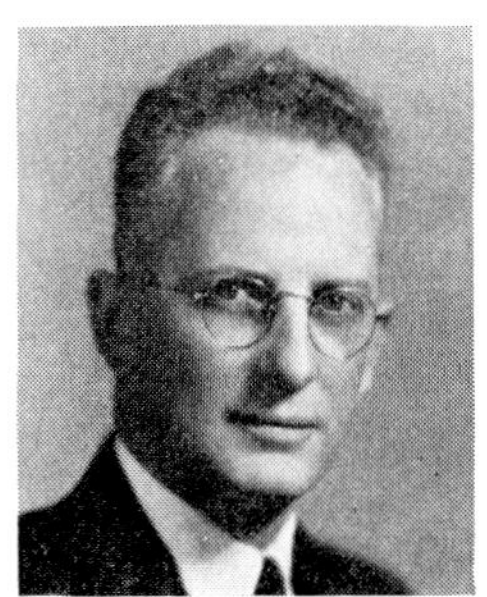

Fred Jenner Hodges

year 1896 he had been promoted to "professor of X-rays" in Union Medical College (which owned Hahnemann Hospital). He seemed to think that some of those records might still be in existence. He also volunteered the information that he had saved old documents in his home, and he invited me to come and visit with him, and perhaps search through those documents.

As it turned out, the (homeopathic) Union Medical College had been absorbed by Loyola University, while the Hahnemann Hospital became Chicago Memorial Hospital, which was later absorbed by Wesley Memorial Hospital. More than thirty years had passed since those old records had been destroyed.

On November 24, 1959 I visited Grubbé in the latter's apartment on Chicago's Far North Side, overlooking Lake Michigan. Things were different, Grubbé could not recollect anything from the previous interview, he now denied having done much diagnostic radiology (which is not true: Orndoff and Hummon had seen Grubbé writing diagnostic roentgen reports in longhand). When asked why he had not written reports, he evaded the issue by retorting that he was afraid of exposing himself to malpractice suits* and this is why he let his "assistant" do it. That assistant turned out to have been Max Hubeny who – according to Grubbé – was scribbling the "diagnosis" on paper slips, subsequently glued to the (then used) glass plates.

CASE AND GRUBBE

Jimmy Case, who lived his last years in Santa Barbara (California), had not answered any of the letters regarding roentgen reports. I buttonholed the ebullient Case during the (now discontinued) Picker cocktail hour at the September, 1959 meeting of the ARRS in Cincinnati.

When asked about reporting, Case specified that he had been writing such reports ever since he could remember, at least since 1902. He had none of his own files because they were preserved as records in the offices in which he had worked. He knew for sure that all the early records of the Battle Creek (Michigan) Sanitorium had been destroyed.

*To this day, in the State of Illinois, no radiologist has ever been hauled into court because of a diagnostic procedure, but this (of course) is no guaranty for the future.

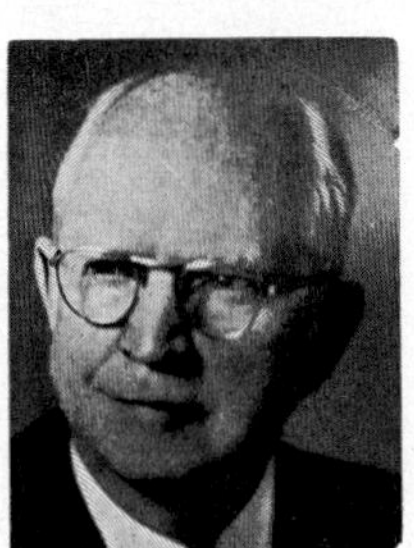

James Thomas Case

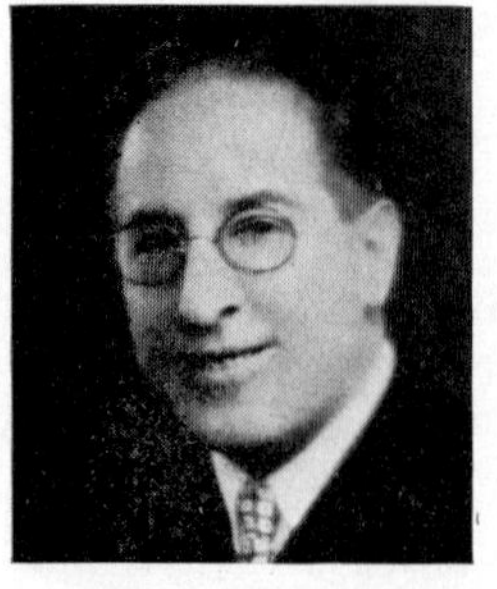

Emil Grubbe

When asked to comment on Grubbé's statements, Case refused to discuss the subject altogether. To him, Grubbé was not a *bona-fide* pioneer, and he declared that he (Case) had just helped to thwart an attempt by some ARRS members who wanted to offer a commemorative gold medal to Grubbé.

It is undoubtedly true that the assay chemist Grubbé (who had been "given in 1898 a so-called medical degree by his homeopathic diploma mill) did not have the inventiveness of the electrical engineer Caldwell (who had been "given" his medical degree in 1905 by the Bellevue Medical College). Nor did Grubbé have the pleasant personality of the practical pharmacist Dodd (who had been "given" his medical degree in 1908 by the University of Vermont, after Harvard had turned him down). And Grubbé most certainly did not study anatomy, physiology, or pathology the thorough way the elevator operator Zingroni would (Zingroni refused to go through a simulated course, and thus never was granted the medical degree offered him by Loyola University).

Grubbé, in his more publicitary than scientific testament (published in 1949 by Bruce in St. Paul) claims at least three priorities: (1) he had experimented with Crookes tubes in the last few months of 1895, and therefore incurred the first roentgen skin reaction on record. That first skin reaction appeared in mid-January 1896. He showed that skin reaction to a physician who wondered whether such a powerful agent might not be effective in cancer, and referred him a patient for treatment. Thus (2) on Wednesday, January 29, 1896 Grubbé administered the first x-ray therapy session to a 55-year old lady with a malignancy of the breast. Moreover (3) he used (introduced ?) lead foil both as protection against, and to circumscribe the area treated with, x rays. As a matter of fact, Orndoff recollected that in the early 1900's, the famous dermatologist and roentgen therapist William Allen Pusey (1863-1940) spoke of Grubbé as having been one of the pioneers in x-ray therapy. Aside from such chronologic priorities, Grubbé made no scientific contributions to either roentgen diagnosis or therapy. And the text of his early advertising handbills was certainly not such as to endear him to the medical roentgen pioneers.

SIDETRACKING

At this point the question was raised whether in the very beginning there were any reports at all.

The problem was submitted (at that same 1959 convention in Cincinnati) to the yachtsman* Hollis Elmer Potter, a former president of the ARRS. He reminisced about the period when, in 1906, while still a medical student, his time off would be spent producing roentgen plates in a room located beneath the surgical amphitheatre in Cook County Hospital.

Potter stated categorically that he did not start writing reports until after 1910, *i.e.,* long after he had replaced (in 1906) the first radiologist of the Presbyterian Hospital in Chicago, the so-called X-ray Smith. The latter's name was Joseph F. Smith, an orthopedist who moved to Milwaukee, thus vacating the spot, which was accepted by Potter before he had actually graduated (in 1908 from Rush Medical School, located at that very Presbyterian Hospital). Inquiries with the record librarian of the now merged Presbyterian-St. Luke's Hospital (in Chicago's Medical Center) revealed that their oldest preserved records are from the 1920's: all previous papers have been destroyed!

Potter is, of course, the eponymic half of the Bucky-Potter diaphragm. Gustav Bucky — a German-born radiologist in New York City, known also for his contributions to *Grenzstrahlen*-therapy — had shown his model of the stationary grid to the German Roentgen Society, during its meeting in Berlin in March, 1913. That contraption never became popular in Europe (or anywhere else) until Potter made it movable, thus creating a practically indispensable tool. But the original idea was Bucky's!

On October 14, 1922, while speaking at a Bull Moose meeting in Milwaukee, Theodore Roosevelt was shot in the breast by a crazed assailant. Teddy (who was then a former president) came on the train to Chicago, to be treated by John Benjamin Murphy (1957-1916), the "stormy petrel of surgery" (Loyal Davis).

Just about that time John Baptist Zingroni had been promoted from elevator electrician to x-ray technician. He exposed and developed that famous roentgen plate of Teddy Roosevelt's thorax, showing the bullet - the plate is now preserved in the collections of the American College of Surgeons. Extensive search failed to locate a copy of the respective x-ray report. Finally, Zingroni's brother Nicholas (who kept on working as an x-ray technician in Zingroni's former office) was interviewed, and cleared up the mystery: no x-ray report had been prepared on that occasion.*

*The *Chicago Tribune* photograph of Commodore Hollis Potter's yacht, winning on August 31, 1926 the third dash of twelve miles of a race on Lake Michigan, was reproduced in the August, 1928 issue of *Radiology* (11:161).

DESPAIR

In 1907, Kassabian noted casually that the "report of the x-ray negative should be written or oral" - and oral reports are inherently ephemeral. Even after World War II, various authors, for instance Hernaman-Johnson (1919), Barclay (1920), Case (1924), urged that written reports be prepared. Orndoff remembers that in the early 1900's everybody was so interested in the procedure, and so few patients were referred for roentgen examination, that it was quite common for the referring physician to accompany his patient to the "x-ray laboratory." After they all gazed at the plate together with the specialist, the preparation of a report might have seemed superfluous.

Similarly negative responses were received from several foreign institutions. Neither the *Röntgen-Museum* in Remscheid-Lennep (Germany) nor the *Centre Antoine Béclère* in Paris, or the *Wellcome Historical Medical Museum* in London had early roentgen reports. Of course, the latter's vaults contain a beautiful selection of incunabula!

Likewise unsuccessful were inquiries with American institutions, such as the *John Crerar Library* (Chicago), the *Howard Dittrick Museum of Historical Medicine* (Cleveland), the *National Library of Medicine,* and the *Medical Museum of the Armed Forces Institute of Pathology* (both in Washington, D.C.).

*John Edwin Habbe, the historian of the Milwaukee Roentgen Ray Society, tells me that Teddy Roosevelt was shot at during the Bull Moose meeting, on October 12, 1912, the pioneer roentgen-photographer from Milwaukee, Jake Janssen (1869-1937) made glass plates of the ex-president's chest, and demonstrated that the bullet had not penetrated very deeply. The story goes that the notes which Theodore Roosevelt had prepared for his speech, and which he carried in his breast pocket, attenuated the speed of the bullet.

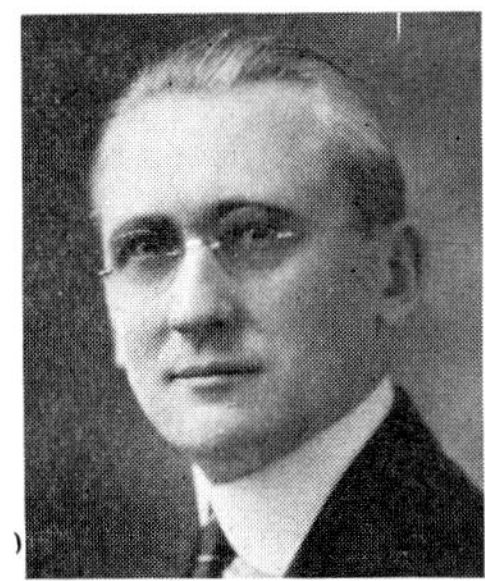
JOSEPH LITSCHGI

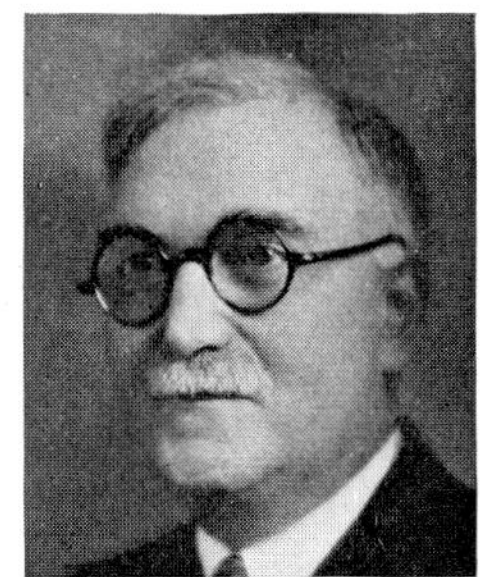
LEON LEWALD

Among the numerous individuals queried, several tried hard to find early reports, for instance Benjamin Felson searched the hospitals in Cincinnati; Henry George Moehring, then of Duluth (Minnesota), inserted a notice in his County Medical Bulletin; Robert Reid Newell combed the San Francisco territory. It all seemed to no avail, the situation was desperate!

At that point I interviewed Joseph John Litschgi (born in 1882) who had been for many years the radiologist of Grant Hospital (Chicago). He must have learned the secret of eternal youth because he is now (after his retirement from Grant's) one of the more active members of the staff of the Department of Radiology in Cook County Hospital. Litschgi had attended postgraduate courses at Cook County Hospital in 1912, and he remembers perfectly that they *were* writing roentgen reports at that time. Inquiry with the Cook County Hospital record librarian disclosed that nothing prior to 1935 had been preserved.

EUREKA

The first hint of a find came from California - a state which happened to have as its motto the alleged Archimedean interjection used as a title for this section.

Several letters had been sent to the New York University professor of roentgenology (emeritus) Leon

OFFICE
DR. WILLIAM JAMES MORTON,
NO. 19 EAST 28TH STREET,
CONSULTATION HOURS, 10-1.

NEW YORK CITY, May 20 1896

Dear Doctor Stieglitz

The X ray shows plainly that there is no stone of an appreciable size in the kidney. The hip bones are shown & the lower ribs and the lumbar vertebrae, but no calculus. The region of the kidneys is uniformly penetrated by the X ray & there is no sign of an interception by any foreign body.

I only got the negative today and could not therefore report earlier. I will have a print made tomorrow. The picture is not so strong as I would like but it is strong enough to differentiate the parts.

Yours very sincerely
W. J. Morton.

Gift Dr. Leopold Stieglitz through friends 1/16/52

TEXT: May 25, 1896. Dear Doctor Stieglitz: The X ray shows plainly that there is no stone of an appreciable size in the kidney. The hip bones are shown and the lower ribs and the lumbar vertebrae, but no calculus. The region of the kidneys is uniformly penetrated by the x ray and there is no sign of an interception by any foreign body.— I only got the negative today and could not therefore report earlier. I will have a print made tomorrow. The picture is not as strong as I would like but it is strong enough to differentiate the parts. Yours very sincerely (signed) W. J. Morton.

Theodore Le Wald (1874-1962). He had exposed roentgen plates in the very year 1896, while serving an internship in the Knickerbocker Hospital in New York. Le Wald was the first to identify colonic diverticula on the roentgenogram (in 1914), and the first to demonstrate in the same way congenital pyloric stenosis. Perhaps the most interesting among his many contributions is a long forgotten roentgen study of the aviator's heart, under conditions simulating high altitude (1920). Because of ill health, Le Wald never answered any of my letters.*

A letter of inquiry had been sent to Robert Reid Newell, the former professor of medical radiology at Stanford who, having reached retirement age, had become a physicist (one of the best!) in the Naval Radiological Laboratory. Newell sent back a file on West Coast pioneers. In the file was also a letter to Newell, in which Le Wald alluded to one of his own historic articles, published in 1952 in the *Academy Bookman,* a house organ of the New York Academy of Medicine.

That article (Le Wald 1952) was consulted as a matter of routine and it carried the text of a roentgen report handwritten in May, 1896, by William James Morton himself. Le Wald had prepared his article as a background to the announcement that said report and an accompanying letter had been presented to the Academy. Both documents are now owned by, and preserved in the manuscript section of, the New York Academy of Medicine which consented graciously** to have them herein reproduced.

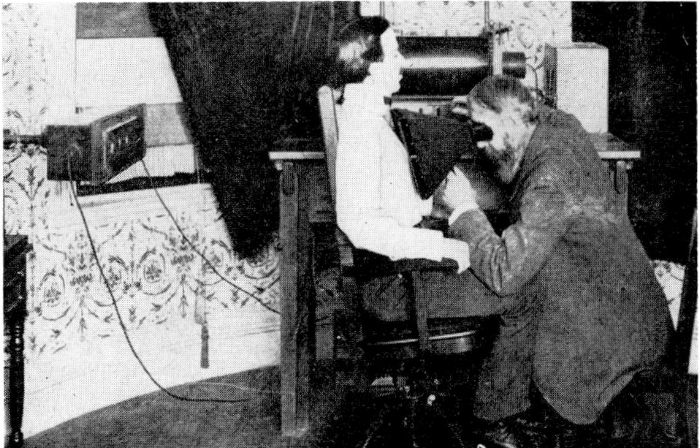

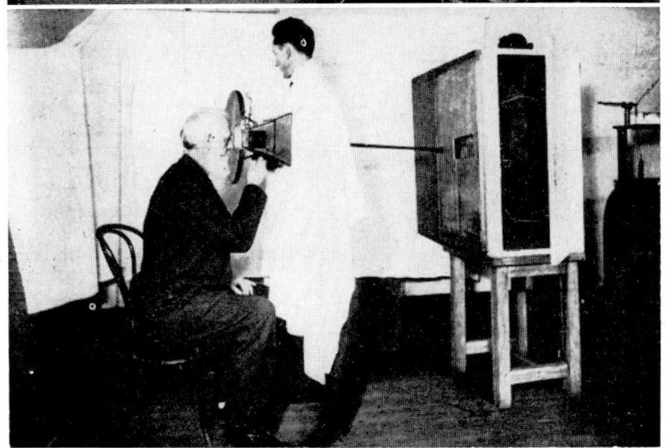

Francis Williams at the cryptoscope. The upper half shows him in 1896, with dark hair. Note the distance between x-ray tube and patient. In the lower photograph — almost four decades after the other — a white-haired Williams is seen using a stereo-fluoroscope. Despite heavy and repeated exposure, he did not become a radiation casualty, which shows that there are individual variations in the susceptibility to ionizing radiation.

EARLY ROENTGEN REPORTS IN HOSPITALS

The procedure used before the turn of the century at Boston City Hospital is adequately described in the classic text of Francis Williams (1901):

"The blank (filled out by the house officer and signed by the visiting physician or surgeon) gives the name of the patient, the ward and bed number; also the volume and page of the medical or sugical record. The negatives are seen by the surgeon, or the physician, as the case may be, and a print of each is inserted in the record book as a part of the record of the patient. When an examination with the fluorescent screen has

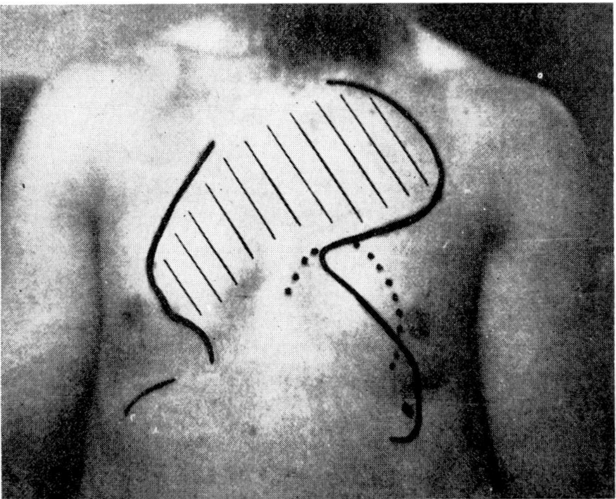

Francis Williams *dixit*: About 1892 patient became suddenly unconscious for one minute. No warning, recovery immediate. About June, 1896 began to get

*The then professor of radiology in the New York Polyclinic Medical School and Hospital, William Henry Shehadi, kindly obtained for me a set of reprints from, and the herein reproduced portrait of, Le Wald.

**Through its chief-librarian, Miss Gertrude Louise Annan.

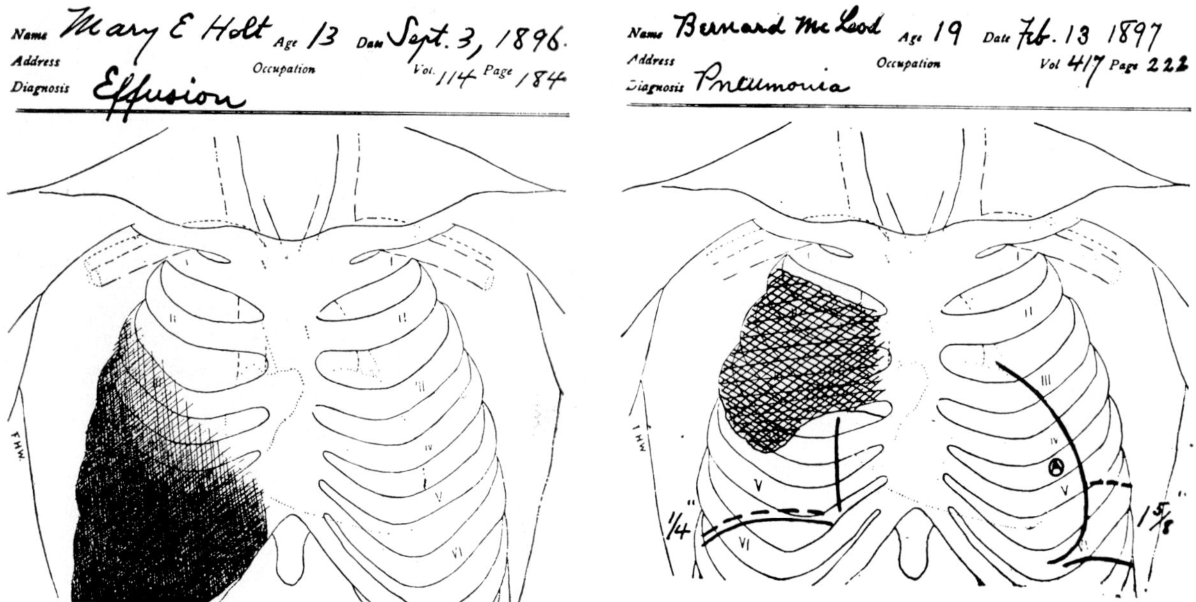

MEDICAL X-RAY REPORTS BY FRANCIS WILLIAMS (1897). Note the terse *Diagnosis.*

been made, a memorandum of it, and a tracing if desired, is inserted in the record book."

In those early days, in hospitals, actual roentgen reports were prepared only when fluoroscopies had to be described. Even so, at times, Williams' only report of the fluoroscopy was the tracing of the contour of the heart and/or diaphragm, inscribed in wax pencil directly on the patient's skin. The roentgen plates were regarded as self-explanatory, at least by (and for) the referring physician or surgeon.

MASSACHUSETTS GENERAL

Through the good graces of Laurence Lamson Robbins, the radiologist of Massachusetts General Hospital, a search of the old archives of that institution was made by Miss Mary E. Converse (their record librarian), and this is what she found:

"The medical volumes of 1896-97 made no reference to x-rays. . . None of the cases of pneumonia or pul-

hoarse, and grew rapidly worse, and had some cough, and dyspnea. On July 15 first raised a little blood. Father had died of consumption at 72 – it was usual for males in their family to develop tuberculosis after 59 years of age, and this is what they (including the family physician) thought the patient had. X-ray examination with screen made October, 1896 showed that the patient had a large thoracic aneurysm as shown in the drawing made on his skin. A few weeks later, after returning from a drive, death occurred suddenly.

". . NOW, LET US CONSIDER THE NEXT WELL-KNOWN CANDIDATE . . '

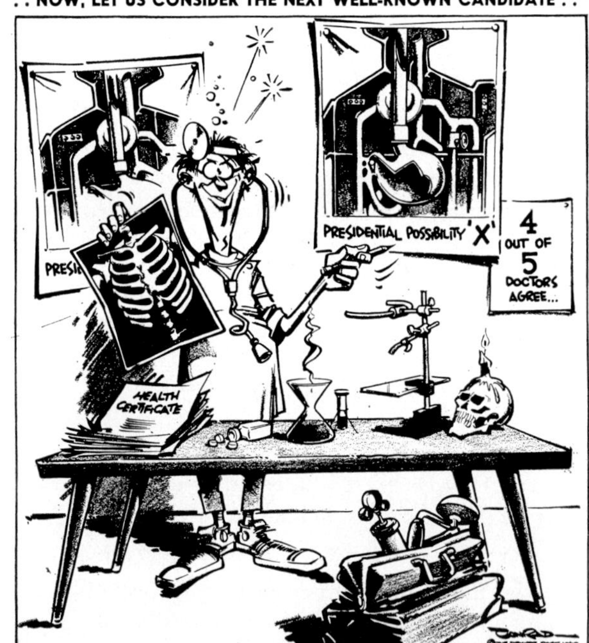

SELF-EVIDENT RADIOGRAPHS. In the Era of the Roentgen Pioneers it was often held that "x-ray pictures" are as obvious in their interpretation as photographs. Another "basic fact" accepted in the popular mind is that no medical examination can be complete without an "x-ray." These two premises are illustrated in this spoof on the flurry of medical certificates offered during the 1960 presidential campaign. This cartoon appeared first in the *Denver Post* (of July 6, 1960), and is herein reproduced through the courtesy of the artist, the editorial cartoonist Paul Conrad.

monary tuberculosis mentioned x-rays although there was an abundance of laboratory data and pathology reports were becoming quite popular. . . In the surgical volumes of 1897 we did find x-ray references (of which) the earliest entry was May, 1897."

Some of these notations were quite to the point, such as *"X-ray shows a piece of needle between 4th & 5th metatarsal"* but more elaborate wordings are also included, for instance one of a Colles fracture dated December 22, 1897:

". . .X-Ray taken showing slight deformity of ulna 1 in. above lower end-displacement of styloid (ulna) inwards & oblique fracture outer half of lower end of radius with styroid process. Displacement ¼ in. upwards."

Another passage, which is striking, and has a drawing to boot, is herein reproduced as a vivid exemplification of the anonymous scribe's descriptive predicament.

JOHNS HOPKINS

A sample of the (roentgen) record book, as used in Johns Hopkins Hospital (Baltimore) at the beginning of the century, was provided by courtesy of Russell Hedley Morgan, who is today their professor of radiology. The technical director of his department,* Richard Alexander Olden, combed their antiques,

*It is gratifying to see that x-ray technicians are receiving greater recognition, not only in monetary ways, but also by adequate job designations. In some places, the more deserving are granted academic faculty status. This is all to the better: in a scientific team, the stature given to each individual should not be determined by his rank but by the degree of responsibility!

[illegible]. negro: chest negative: at middle of thigh is a fracture, demonstrated by abnormal mobility, crepitus & shortening: by Xray, line of fracture is from before backward, transverse: from without inward, slightly oblique upward: displacement of lower fragment is inward & upward.

Ether J. W. York. Ward.

On extension displacement reduced completely & fragments easily controlled: extension straps applied: posterior wire splint: bandage: internal & external splints & long Dessault: coaptations over upper fragments: reduction complete: position good: [illegible] 18 lbs. weight to extension: recovery from ether good.

Surgical x-ray report from Massachusetts General Hospital. The page in the register is 163, the date August 30, 1897, and the diagnosis "thigh fracture (left)." The passage which is of interest for our purposes reads, "by X-ray, line of fracture is from before backward, transverse, from without inward, slightly oblique upward: displacement of lower fragment is inward & upward."

Date	X Ray No.	Surg. No.	Ward	NAME AND ADDRESS	DIAGNOSIS	REMARKS
1898						
Dec 19th	92		D	R. J. Warner	Fracture of humerus	Exp. 20 mins Fair.
July 4	101 (8x10)		"	" "	" three weeks old –	Exp. 14 min. good
20	93	Dispensary		J. Dainaker	Colles' Fracture (?)	Exp 15 min Fair
23	17 x 20 94	7204	D	Sidney Saunders	Dislocation of hip (osteomyelitis - tubercular)	Exp. 50 mins { Very good New tube
27	95		D	James B. Andrews	Pott's fracture	Exp 15 mins New tube Fresh Battery
29	8x10 96		C	John C. Field	Bullet in arm	Exp 15 mins - very good.

X-RAY REGISTER FROM JOHNS HOPKINS (1898).

and offered for reproduction a page from a record book of 1898. For a better grasp of the significance of this particular register one may refer to a citation from Percy Brown (1936):

"Most interesting is the origin of Baetjer's devotion to the . . . roentgen-rays, so closely to be associated with the colorful history that attaches to the old "x-ray room" at the Johns Hopkins, wherein the primitive static-machine was rotated or electrical switches were thrown by men whose later lustre in other fields, among them the renowned Harvey Cushing, sheds a retroflective glow upon its aging walls. When routine had become established, it was customary for the work to be assigned in rotation to one of the house-officers. In due course, this duty fell to Baetjer and thus, in "looking after the x-ray room," was his enthusiastic interest engendered and his career moulded. . ."

RONTGENAUFNAHMENPROTOKOLLBUCH

This lengthy title is the German spelling of roentgen record book, cited from the reminiscences (1937) of Alban Köhler (1874-1947). This particular record book, dated from October 20, 1898, to March 9, 1901, carried its inscriptions as usual in columns, for instance *20 X* (date: 20th of October) - *R. K.* (patient's name) - *Osteomyelitis cruri sin.* (osteomyelitis left femur) - *Röntgographie* (meaning no fluoroscopy was performed) - *18/24* (size of the plate in centimeters) - *3 Min.* (time of exposure in minutes).

FALLACIOUS ROENTGEN REPORTS

The change-over from those scanty notations in the early record books to the substantial roentgen reports, currently *en-vogue* in some institutions (like the one-page essay at Columbia-Presbyterian in New York City) followed the devious trail of the so-called x-ray fallacies.

Cartoons and other references from the very early days show that in many circles, roentgen rays were thought to allow three-dimensional viewing of the innards of the body (object) under scrutiny.

The experts knew better (Dumstrey and Metzner) but it took some time to convince the majority - even today there are a few doubters. In 1897, under

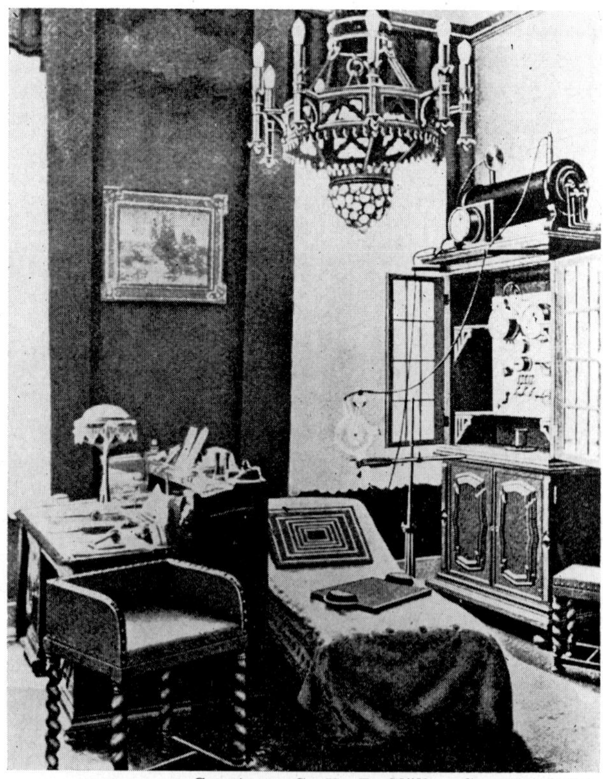

Courtesy: C. H. F. Müller Co., Hamburg.

ALBAN KÖHLER'S OFFICE (ABOUT 1900). This is the diagnostic corner. The register was kept on the desk.

the provocative caption *The Fallacies of X-Ray Pictures,* Edward Aloysius Tracy (1863-1935) of Boston insisted that "the position of the tube may modify the resultant plate so much that diagnosis can be mistaken."

Thence, Tracy exchanged a round of printed rejoinders with Louis Andrew Weigel (1854-1906), an orthopod from Rochester (New York) who was to become a *roentgen saint.*

Carl Beck (1856-1911), a surgeon from New York, specified that "a distinct skiagraphic plate will always tell the truth, but only if accompanied by the details of operation." Others, for instance Henri Lucien (1843-1907), a surgeon from Lille (France), spoke of radiographic illusions.

Samual Howard Monell (1857-1918) of Brooklyn ideated an ingenious procedure which inscribed on the plate itself all the data needed in court. Harry Preston Pratt of Chicago was willing to testify in court in order to establish the legal identity of his roentgen production.

Francis Williams advocated that "the position of the part, of the plate, and of the tube should be accurately determined and stated." In the beginning, this must have been something like virtue — often preached but seldom practiced — because in 1901 Holzknecht remarked that, remonstrances in the literature notwithstanding, such technical details were not routinely included in roentgen reports.

Most of the confusion arose actually - but not exclusively - from the pitfalls of unrecognized principles of photographic perspective, as outlined in 1902 by the British roentgen pioneer Wililam Cotton (?-1936) of Bristol. The request that physical data be included in the report was particularly stressed in France by the forensic radiologist, pioneer in pelvimetry, and roentgen martyr Maxime Ménard (1872-1926) from the Hôpital Cochin in Paris.

FILM IDENTIFICATION

It is self-evident that substitution of the patient's name (by mistake or otherwise) introduces a cardinal error in the actual report. While there is as yet no foolproof method, photographing on the film a card with the patient's essential data seems to be a fairly adequate method.

For historic interest it may be mentioned that Monell (1902) had a very similar procedure. In 1917 C. D. Blachly of Drumright (Oklahoma) used glue in water to write the patient's name on a card; lead powder sprinkled on it would stick to the glue, then the card could be radiographed directly on the film. This procedure was independently re-discovered by the musical professor of radiology in the Medical College of South Carolina, Robert Burbidge Taft (1899-1951) who, at the time — in 1924 — was a roentgen intern at Bellevue Hospital in New York: he added mucilage to ink, then sprinkled his writing with lead powder.

William Johnson Manning (1868-1948), a radiologist from Washington, (D.C.), had a more elaborate procedure whereby the patient's fingerprint was made on the film holder, using a mixture of white lead in oil and barium sulphate. That fingerprint, radiographed on the film, was said to be sufficiently clear for (legal) comparison with the fingerprint on the film holder (envelope).

WILBERT

On December 10, 1902, at the Chicago meeting of the ARRS, Wilbert addressed the membership on the subject of systematic records. He said, among other things:

"At the German Hospital, Philadelphia, written records of the x-ray work have been kept for upward of

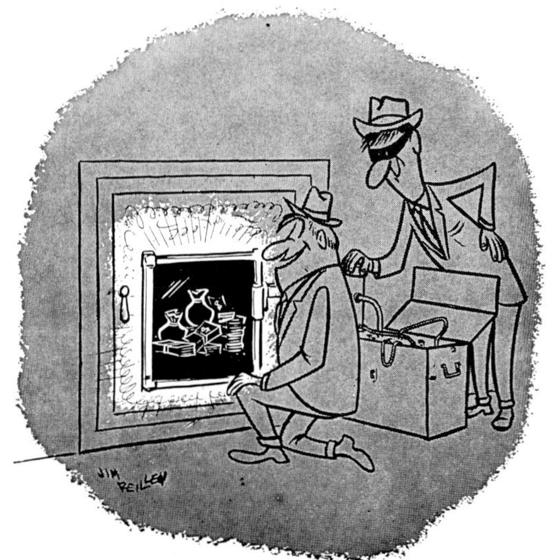

"These Du Pont screens sure give you detail, huh?"

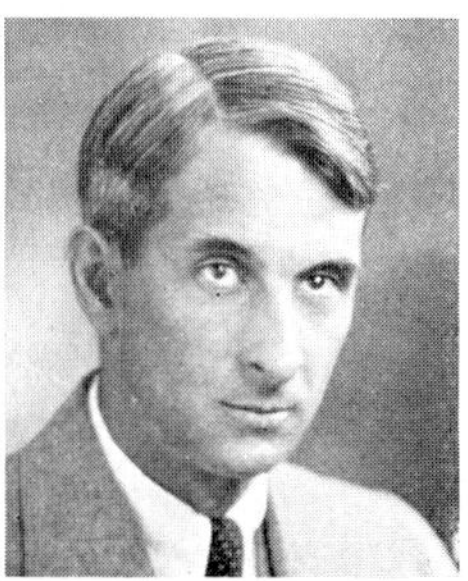

ROBERT B. TAFT

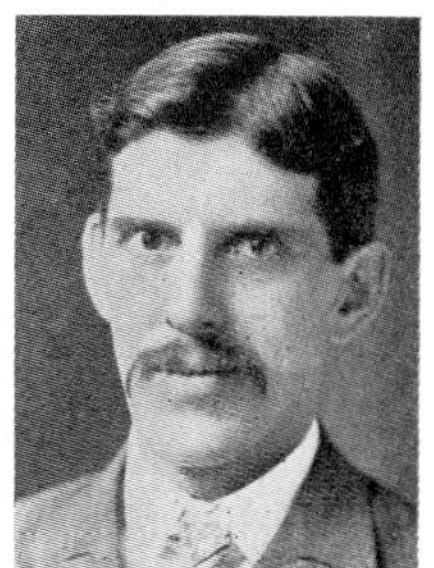

MARTIN I. WILBERT

six years. . . The records have been continued in book form, in preference to using cards. . . The records . . . are in triplicate, and are arranged (1) under the serial number of the radiograph, (2) under the alphabetical index of names of patients, (and) (3) under an analytical reference to the part of the body involved. . . . ."

"Under the main, or serial number entry, we record the number of the exposure, the month and date, the part of the body exposed, the side of the body, the direction of exposure, the size of the plate used, the name of the patient, the age of the patient, the number of the tube, the spark gap on which the tube is working at the time, the distance of the anode from the plate, the time of exposure, a short history of the accident, or an outline of the condition, and an account of the x-ray findings. . ."

"For reporting the findings of the x-ray examination two separate blanks are used. For hospital cases a special blank form is filled out, and this becomes an integral part of the record or history of the case. For reports to the out-patient department, we use the record card of the patient."

There is little doubt that this procedure (or a reasonable facsimile thereof) was in operation at that time. Hence, a search was begun to locate some (any!) of those records.

I wrote to Barton Rogers Young, the chief-radiologist of Germantown Hospital. He replied that Germantown Hospital had nothing to do with the (old) German Hospital. The latter had changed its name to Lankenau Hospital, and moved to a suburban location. Further inquiry revealed the by now familiar fact that, in the process of moving, all the old records had been destroyed.

The venerable *College of Physicians* of Philadelphia had catalogued many hospitals' and physicians' records, and therefore an inquiry was sent to them in the hope they might have seen (perhaps preserved) one of those reports. The answer was no but, as a compensation, they had a file on Wilbert*:

Martin Inventius Wilbert (1865-1931), of German stock, came to the German Hospital in 1891 as apothecary. He was (also) placed in charge of its Radiographic and Photographic Laboratory at the time of its inception (about the middle of 1896), and filled the job very successfully until October, 1908, when he resigned to become assistant in the Division of Pharmacology of the U. S. Public Health Service. In 1905 he was one of the founders and original members of the AMA Council on Pharmacy and Chemistry, and became in 1911 its secretary (it was then called the Section on Pharmacology and Therapeutics).

As a "lay roentgenologist" Wilbert had been excellent, which proves again that a good man will do a good job in most any place he happens to be. The obituary in the *AMA Journal* contains no information on his early roentgen work. Its final sentence reads: "He spent his life in trying to stem the tide of commercialism (in both the medical and the pharmaceutic professions), and the full measure of his influence at Washington in behalf of public health will never be fully known."

ET ALTERA

The oldest roentgen report with physical data included (which I was able to locate) is signed by Charles Edmund Kells, Jr. (1856-1930), a well polished Southern gentleman, scholar, and dentist from New Orleans. Having suffered considerable radiation damage, he developed radio-carcinomatosis, and ultimately took his own life.

Despite Holzknecht's quip, the inclusion of technical details on the roentgen reports became a widespread practice, both in Europe and in this country. As an exemplification could serve the report blank, reproduced in facsimile in the textbook of Franz Maximilian Groedel (1881-1951), a German cardio-roentgenologist who lived the second half of his life in New York City.

Even today, in many institutions, the printed forms on which roentgen reports are typed have spaces

DENTAL SKIAGRAPH.

By DR. C. EDMUND KELLS, Jr.

No. 523 Date May 26-1901

Of Mrs H. W. B.

Age adult ~~Upper~~ Lower

Examined for Molar root fillings and xtent of abscess.

Make of Film Seed's Special

Distance 12" Time 1 Minute

Tube Gen'l Electric

Developer Metol-Hydro.

Notes

*Courteously submitted by Mr. W. B. McDaniel, 2nd, the curator of their historical collections.

allotted for the technical factors used (kvp, ma or mas, time, distance, position). This is commonly verbalized as being done to facilitate duplication (which it would, if the technician could refer the next time to the old report) or punitive action (when the films are poor and the data indicate that the patient was not measured). It is more likely, though, that the reason for including such data is the subconscious ("atavistic") reminiscence from the old times when one needed all the help he could get to forestall the fallacies of the aboriginal x-ray pictures.

SAGITTAL REPORTING

After reading my letter to the editor (in *Lancet*) inquiring about x-ray reports, Paul Coling - a medical practitioner from Odiham (Hampshire) in Great Britain - sent me the following message:

"I found this (envelope) at Guy's Hospital in the early 1940's soon after a heavy air-raid had damaged many of the hospital buildings."

The envelope contained a faded positive paper print showing a subcapital fracture of the femoral neck - and the fracture site is indicated by a coarse arrow, traced in wax pencil. Coling also wondered whether the arrow might not have been the "entire" report. That paper print was much too faded for a meaningful reproduction.

The envelope is dated July 16, 1906. The referring physician was one of Guy's surgical pillars, Louis Albert ("John") Dunn (1858-1918) who had practically lived and died at the Hospital. This particular fracture, judging from its date, must have been one of the cases used

No. in Skiagraph Register 895
Patient's Name Percy Frith
Physician or Surgeon Mr Dunn Ward Bed
Nature of Injury Old Fracture Neck of Femur
Date 16/7/06 1906
L A Dunn Esq

Courtesy: Peter Coling

SKIAGRAPHIC ENVELOPE (1906). This relic from Shenton's times at Guy's Hospital in London brings up the question who started the custom of writing the "diagnosis" on the envelope? I suspect that this habit started in the very first year, 1896, but I cannot prove it.

CASE TO BE SKIAGRAPHED.

Name and age of Patient
Address
Physician or Surgeon Mr Kaye *Ward* OP *Bed No.*
A short statement is to be inserted below of the character of the lesion of which a Skiagraph is required, and of any particular point which it is desired to elucidate. If the presence of a foreign body is suspected, its probable site and nature should be indicated.

STATEMENT.

Date 19/12/00 *Signed* E. F. Reeve

No. 207 See 192 Date July 16th
Physician, Surgeon, or House-Surgeon Mr Lucas Ward Department Bed
Name and Age Occupation
Address
Nature of Case and what is required to be shown Wired patella One wire broken
Exposure Distance Tube
Plate Size How many taken
Current in Ampères No. of Volts
Result Very good negative
Remarks

X-RAY REQUEST AND REPORT FROM GUY'S HOSPITAL (1900). Note the use of the verb to skiagraph. The patella had been wired, and one of these wires broke. After the caption *result* appears the statement, "very good negative."

by Guy's famous first *radiographer* (at the time, the term was used also for physicians) – Edward Warren Hine Shenton (1872-1955) – in the preparation of the article (1907) in which he first described what is now known as Shenton's line.

In one of Shenton's earlier papers (1902), appeared a similar arrow, pointing therein to a renal calculus.

The question of whether at that time (1906), roentgen reporting at Guy's used to be done with "arrows" was submitted to the current director of their X-ray Department; in reply, Thomas Henry Hills sent a selection of eleven reports taken from a "volume of x-ray records" dated 1900. One of these reports is herein reproduced. The accompanying letter stated:

"I was actually at this hospital all through the War, and the X-ray Department itself was not directly bombed. This volume of x-ray records was, in fact, in the basement of one of the oldest parts of the hospital, which was totally destroyed by fire with one incendiary bomb, which lodged itself in the roof. Unfortunately, at that time there were so many fires burning, that no water was available, and we had to watch the fire slowly working its way down through the building. There was plenty of time to rescue the furniture, pictures and records. As far as I can remember, this was the only x-ray volume removed from the building, and I think it probable that the later volumes must have been thrown away at some earlier date."

It is hard to say when people began marking the "diagnosis" on the envelopes. In 1913 Sir Archibald Douglas Reid (1871-1924) mentioned that this was the custom at St. Thomas's Hospital (London), even though "cards were (also) being filled in with the x-ray opinion of the case."

FUCHS

Another bowman if not a sagittarian was the Chicago roentgen pioneer (a former electrician for the Aurora Railroad) Wolfram Conrad Fuchs (1865-1908). Although lacking formal medical training, he became quite a diagnostician — one of his noteworthy achievements was the roentgen demonstration of an aortic aneurysm. But he paid his price, and made a place for himself in Percy Brown's roentgen martyrology (1936).

In one of his papers, Fuchs "arrows" biliary calculi and the spleen. As a rule, lay roentgenologists avoided writing reports, but would indicate the pathology with an arrow right on the plate.

COLE

Quite fortuitous was the "discovery" of an original report by Lewis Gregory Cole (1874-1954), professor of roentgenology at Cornell and president of the ARRS.

To one of my routine inquiries (the secretary of) Roy Demarest Duckworth, a roentgenologist at the *Medical Centre* in White Plains (New York) replied that two original Cole reports "done up in the style of a diploma" were being preserved in the office of a surgeon in the same "centre." The reports were in the possession of Edwin George Ramsdell, who graciously consented to their reproduction.

The reports had been prepared after a bismuth meal (April 25, 1912) and a bismuth enema (April 30, 1912), performed on a patient referred by William Francis Honan, a physician from New York. Of interest is the fact that, aside from the "scrolled" reports, there is a booklet with pasted-in positive prints made from spotfilms of the duodenal bulb. These were exposed with the serialograph, a device perfected by Cole in that same year. Orndoff remembers that Cole was always so convinced of the accuracy of his findings that he spoke of the *positive diagnosis* of ulcers (Cole got into a heated argument with Kennon Dunham and George Johnston over it). Also of interest are Cole's peculiar classification of stomach types (text-book, cow-horn, fish-hook, drain-trap, and deformed), his "adaptations" gastric systole and diastole, and Cole's own "x-ray tube" seal (trademark!).

An excellent way of getting acquainted with the spirit of the cantankerous Cole is by perusing his scientific testament, *Lung Dust Lesions versus Tuberculosis,* of which my own copy is an autographed specimen. That book was (more or less) privately printed. In its preface, Cole gives a lot of credit to his then just deceased son, William Gregory Cole (1902-1948), who had also been a radiologist. The son's name did not appear as a co-author because it was a testament.

The book contains also incidental material, such as old reprints of articles on tuberculosis – in this respect Cole has an authenticated title, dated 1907, on the roentgen detection of pulmonary tuberculosis. Cole was somewhat amateurish in his approach to physics: as a sample may be quoted his chapters on the x-rays of *specific absorption (i.e.,* virtually monochromatic) and x-rays of *selective absorption (i.e.,* polychromatic). He had sired this theory many years ago, but all he achieved was to incur physicistic wrath. The theory boiled down to the fact that Cole, like many pioneers, preferred the films produced with a gas tube energized

LEWIS GREGORY COLE M.D.
103 PARK AVENUE
NEW YORK

April 25, 1912.

Mr. Burchard Dutcher,
39 Pierrepont Street,
Brooklyn, New York.

Dr. William F. Honan,
15 West 73rd Street,
New York City.

X-Ray findings:

A series of plates of the stomach, the first one made immediately after the bismuth had been given, show its size, shape and position distinctly.

Type:- Text-book.
Size:- Slightly dilated.
Position:- Moderately prolapsed.
Peristalsis:- Active; three wave type; equal on the greater and lesser curvatures; unobstructed.
Systole and diastole:- Shown distinctly.
Jejunum:- Shown distinctly.
Second and third portions of the duodenum:- Abnormally distended.
Triangular cap(or first portion of the duodenum):- Slightly contracted and assymmetrical.
Pyloric sphincter:- Wide open in all of the plates, the lumen being at least three times as large as the average lumen, and centrally located.

Diagnosis:

From a study of these plates one is justified in stating that the stomach is of the type, size and position described in the findings. The active peristalsis and the large lumen of the pyloric sphincter probably account for the unusual dilitation of the second and third portions of the duodenum. While the cap is not perfectly normal, I do not feel that there is sufficient variation to justify one in making a diagnosis of a lesion in this region.

Respectfully submitted,

Lewis Gregory Cole

Courtesy: Edwin George Ramsdell.

X-RAY REPORT BY LEWIS GREGORY COLE (1912). Cole coined the term "duodenal cap." In this report he explains its meaning as it was not to come into popular (medical) use until much later.

by coil and interrupter (with consequently wider range of wave lengths) to the films produced with a hot cathode tube, energized by a transformer. The sin was that he tried to explain this preference in a personal way.

Cole had been a pupil (intern) and admirer of the famous pathologist Francis Delafield (1841-1915) and – by the testimony of Robert Earl Pound (*cf.* preface to the "testament") – Cole himself was quite well versed in both macro- and micro-scopic studies. The main body of the "testament" consists of detailed correlations between the crystallographic demonstrations of intrapulmonary silica (using a very personal method developed by Cole) and its roentgen-anatomo-histologic appearance.

But while his physicistic elucubrations provoked at least some controversy, Cole's theories on silicosis met the worst fate that can befall a scientific endeavor: they were completely ignored! In the meantime, silicosis is slowly becoming a (relatively) rare condition, so that the entire problem is gradually receding toward the highly academic level of medical history.

There are today several mail-order houses in New York City, which specialize in salacious literature. The current gimmick is to send out half-and-half listings wherein the erotica are interspersed with "serious," preferably medical items, so as to qualify that mailing for a "professional" audience. There must have remained many unsold copies of Cole's *Lung Dust Lesions* because over the past year it was offered at one dollar a copy, while on the same sheet were advertised cheap reprints of *Fanny Hill* and of the *Contes Drôlatiques* at $3.95, or expensive "art" reproductions of *Amor-Roma* and *Eros Kalos* in the $30 category. In a nostalgic mood (and to see whether it was a bona-fide ad) I sent them one dollar and in due time received a (second) copy of *Lung Dust Lesions* for my library.

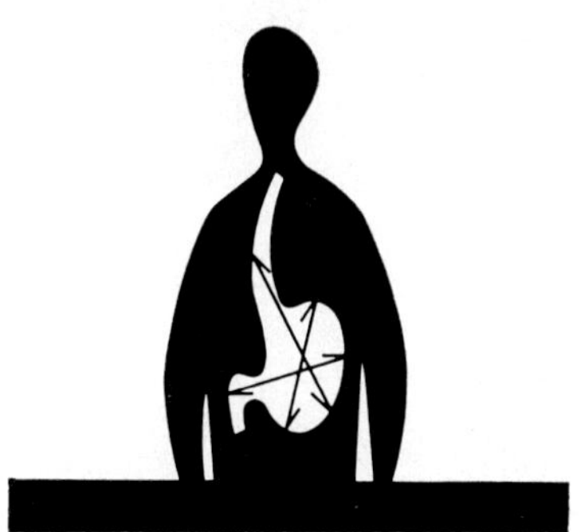

Some day, there will appear a biographer willing to illuminate Cole's varied contributions to medicine in general, to radiology in particular. He had been very successful in practice, and had received external recognitions (gold medals), but his scientific work was never adequately credited. And yet, ideas such as Cole's "multiple type of pulmonary tubercle" concept (adapted from Delafield) might offer a surprisingly fresh approach to the understanding of granulomata.

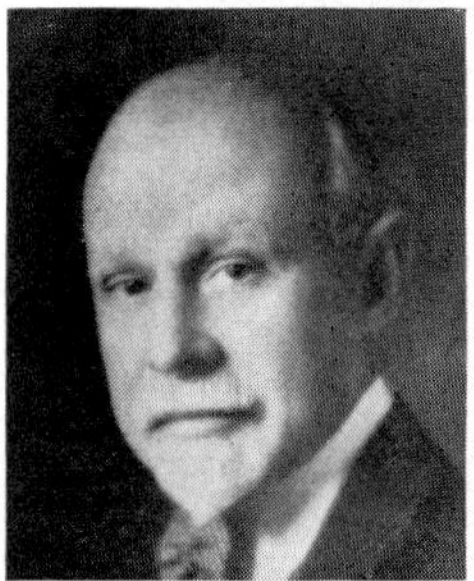

Lewis Gregory Cole

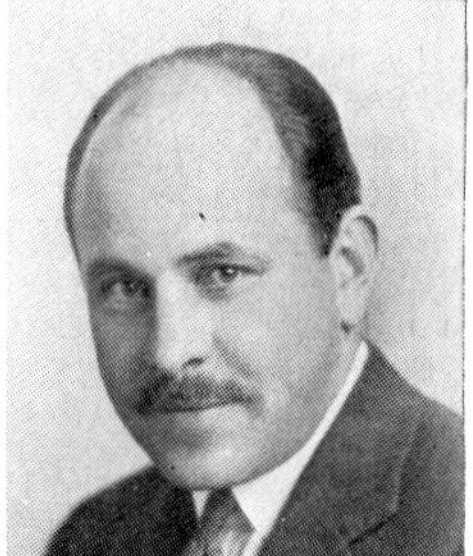

Wm. Gregory Cole

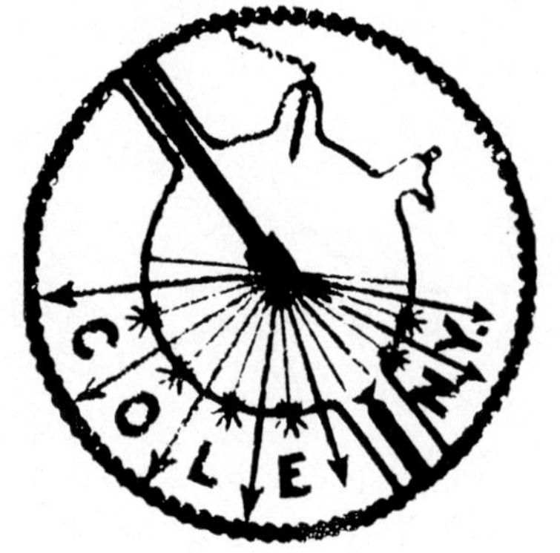

ORNDOFF

A roengten report by Orndoff is also reproduced in facsimile. The subject was a "bleeding pregnancy" investigated with diagnostic pneumoperitoneum. The pelvic mass was larger than a three months pregnancy. Thereupon Orndoff inserted a peritoneoscope - similar to the glorified cystoscope, first used for such a purpose in 1910 by the Danish surgeon Hans Christian Jacobaeus (1879-1937) - and saw a tumor, in addition to the pregnancy. Subsequent surgery confirmed it to have been a dermoid cyst, and Orndoff presented the case on January 14, 1920 to the

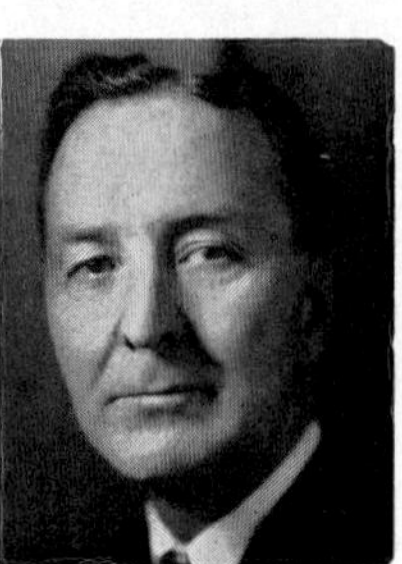

Ben H. Orndoff

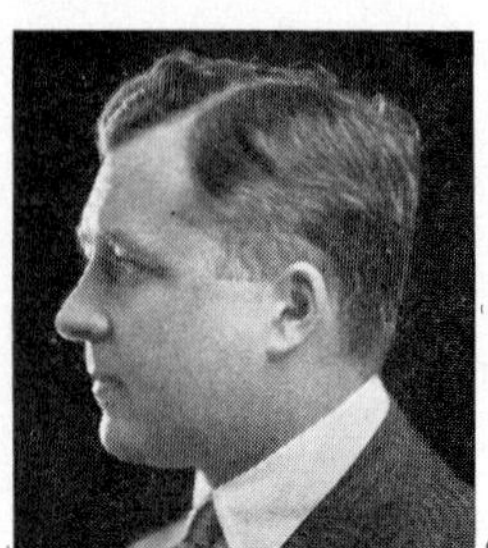

Edward Smith Blaine

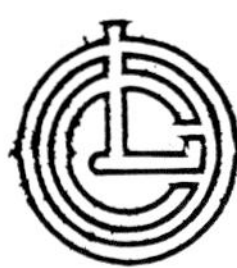

THE ORNDOFF CLINICAL LABORATORY

FRANCES WILLARD HOSPITAL

710 SOUTH LINCOLN STREET

CHICAGO

BENJAMIN H. ORNDOFF, M.D.
25 E. WASHINGTON STREET
PHONE: CENTRAL 5129
HOURS: 1:30 TO 3:00

LOLITA GOODHUE, M. D.
25 E. WASHINGTON STREET
PHONE: CENTRAL 5129
HOURS: 3:00 TO 4:00

TELEPHONE . . WEST 6167

Jan. 9, 1920.

Dr. C. C. Rogers
25 East Washington St.
Chicago, Ill.

Nr. 4109

Dear Dr. Rogers:

I wish to report to you upon the Roentgen examination of your patient, Mrs. Anna Kowaleski, 1/8/20.

Patient indicated absence of menstrual periods for past three months, and menorrhagia for the past two years. She complained of more or less constant nausea and vomiting.

X-ray observations after pneumoperitoneum show mass in the pelvis, larger than the uterus with three months pregnancy.

The peritoneoscope was then introduced and showed the presence behind the uterus of another mass, approximately the size of an orange. The mass was pale gray in color with peritoneum showing the usual shiny appearance, while the uterus was dark red in color. There were only few adhesions.

In my opinion there is in addition to the pregnancy also a tumor attached to (or growing from) the uterus. It could be a dermoid cyst.

Thanking you very much for the opportunity to serve you, I remain,

Very truly yours,

B H Orndoff

B.H.O.-L.B.

B. H. Orndoff, M.D.

Loyola Research Society in Chicago, and published it in the first issue of the *Journal of Roentgenology.*

Diagnostic pneumoperitoneum, including *pelvigrams* (views obtained in Trendelenburg to show the uterus), had been introduced in this country by William Holmes Stewart (1868-1954) of New York. Stewart presented

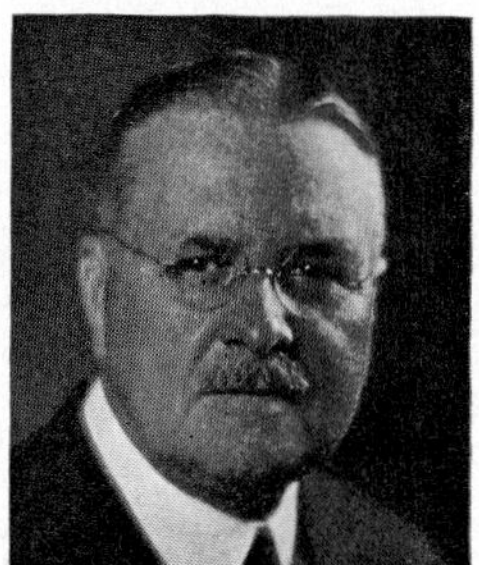

Wm. H. Stewart

his first set of cases on June 9, 1919 to the American Association for Thoracic Surgery, and the next day to the American Gastro-Enterological Society. Orndoff was the first who combined the pelvigram with peritoneoscopy.

Orndoff's report is also of interest because it brings up the often discussed problem whether, and if so how many, non-radiologic procedures can or should be performed by the radiologist, in either diagnosis or therapy?

Orndoff's innate facility for acquiring new skills enhanced his willingness to learn all sorts of procedures, radiologic or others, as long as their use promised to be of help to some patients (he has done numerous hystero-salpingograms). But this was one of the reasons why, even in his time of glory, he had not been in the graces of all the notabilities of the day. A few regarded him simply as a general practitioner with some interest in radiology. Edward Smith Blaine (1882-1958) of Chicago advised him repeatedly and relentlessly not to seek admission to the ARRS. Only in 1926, when Orndoff's good personal friend, Russell Carman, acceded to the presidency of the ARRS (Carman was the only one who had been president both of the RSNA and of the ARRS), was Orndoff asked to submit his application for membership in the ARRS, and Carman shouldered it through the committee. A few months later Carman - who was working on a paper on carcinoma of the stomach - diagnosed his own case as an inoperable gastric malignancy (confirmed by biopsy), and died without completing his term in office.

GENERAL PRACTITIONERS OF RADIOLOGY

Most specialists would like to (be able to) perform as well as to interpret all customary procedures within their circumscribed area of anatomy or pathology. He who can correlate all (clinical, laboratory, and roentgen) findings in a given case, will acquire a better understanding of the situation (than if he had to rely on separate interpretations given by the respective specialists). The roentgen pioneers, not bound by either tradition or agreement, used from the very beginning just that (horizontal!) all-encompassing approach. Nobody ever quite persuaded them to accept a change.

The inevitable accumulation of (vertical!) knowledge in the so-called subspecialties forced a re-distribution of tasks. In the process, the radiologist was asked to limit himself to his shadowy empire, even though the other (and especially the surgical) specialists tended to acaparate their respective portions of shadowland.

Since none of these sub-specialists can or will accept responsibility for seeking out on "his" films all the potential abnormalities belonging to other specialties, it is obvious that the *general practitioner of radiology* - who sees "all" the films - is here to stay (at least for some time). As to the problem of who is doing what, that is best solved in accordance with local circumstances.

The all-around, polyvalent super-roentgen-man — who would give the barium meal, do the fluoroscopy, interpret the films, diagnose a gastric malignancy, resect the stomach, and administer ultimate palliative roentgen therapy to the (already "empty") epigastrium — is today (almost) extinct.

Here and there it seems as if the trend has been reversed, and a number of radiologists shy away from performing certain procedures. This is often verbalized

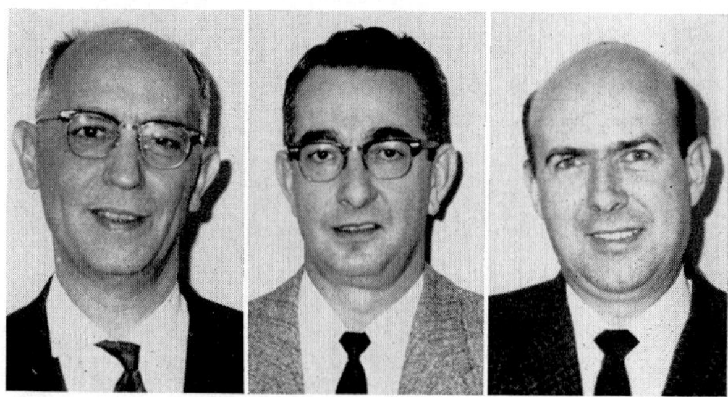

Radiologists at the Carle Clinic. From the viewer's left: Cesare Gianturco, George Miller, and Howard Neucks.

– at times rightly so. Is it proper to do myelograms in a hospital which does not have an active "disc surgeon" on the staff? If a protruded disc is identified (the patient is symptomatic or else he would not have been referred for myelography in the first place), the patient will be sent to a surgeon in another hospital. Quite often, this new surgeon believes only in myelographies performed at his institution, and will ask for a repeat.

When far away from a medical center, patients may want to take in stride even a potential repeat, rather than choose the extensive trip. Once they get to that center, they are usually subjected to a *really* complete work-up. Is such completeness always necessary?

When doing angiographies, whether cerebral, cardiac, or peripheral, the radiologist is often a spectator until "the light is turned off" but there are exceptions to this rule. In the (excellent) Carle Clinic in Urbana (Illinois), Cesare Gianturco and his associates (especially George Andrew Miller) insert all the needles – and today there are few places in the body where opaque material could not be carried through a careful puncture. Moreover, in Gianturco's department the radiologists personally proctoscope all patients referred for barium enema and, while this might not work elsewhere, *their* proctologists *are* satisfied with this arrangement.

Speaking in very general terms, the fact that a radiologist wishes to acquire a new skill cannot and should never be regarded as intrinsically wrong. Whether or not this skill can be routinely utilized in actual work will have to be decided on the strength of local circumstances, especially on interpersonal and intraprofessional relationships. Almost any situation may be justified - from the radiologist not doing any kind of punctures (not even for intravenous urograms) to his needling of the aorta or carotid - as long as the *golden rule* is observed: what is best for the patient!

INCREASED BRONCHOVASCULAR MARKINGS

An original letter-report, handwritten in 1918 by Hollis Potter was located in the private archives of a referring physician.*

Today one may rightfully object to the terminology used in his report, but since bronchiectases were subsequently demonstrated, Potter's concluding statement was actually confirmed. Besides, in 1918 these terms were considered adequate, even if today they are no longer acceptable.

In 1904, Preston Hickey (then in Detroit) made the pioneering remark that on chest films the linear shadows which radiate from the hila are probably ves-

*With the consent of Potter, Sr., search for this report was successfully conducted by his son. Dr. Robert Morse Potter, Jr., who is also a radiologist, practices in the office of his (retired) father. That radiologic office has now been in operation, in the same location, for over fifty years.

8-14-18.

HOLLIS E. POTTER, M.D.
1410 PEOPLES GAS BLDG
CHICAGO

Dear Dr Coleman,

X-Ray, lungs, Mrs. Hathaway Watson show no typical tb deposits in lungs but show a rather diffuse peri-bronchial and hilus increase. The peri-bronchial shadows are wide as if the seat of a temporary ~~pos~~ inflammation. This is compatible with a bronchitis more than tb.

Yrs Potter

ORIGINAL POTTER REPORT (1918). The text reads: "X-ray, lungs, Mrs. H. W. show no typical tbc deposits in lungs but show a rather diffuse peri-bronchial and hilus increase. The peri-bronchial shadows are wide as if the seat of a temporary inflammation. This is compatible with a bronchitis more than tbc."

sels. Almost one quarter of a century later, in 1927, the American Trudeau Society commissioned Pancoast, Baetjer, and Dunham – Henry Kennon Dunham (1872-1944), the tuberculosis specialist from Cincinnati – to investigate the roentgen features of 280 "healthy chests," cleared by both clinicians and bacteriologists. The trio obtained the assistance of two additional experts – the pathologist Eugene Lindsay Opie (from New York), and the internist Frederick Maurice McPhedran (from Philadelphia), both of whom, at the time of this writing, are alive. It so happened that, with the help of the physicist Charles Weyl, McPhedran had made particularly detailed studies of the hila, and knew how to differentiate calcified nodules from vessels seen on end.

Subsequent advances, especially in angiocardiography (more precisely in what the Portuguese, the French, and the Italians call angiopneumography), have proved conclusively that bronchi, unless calcified and/or viewed in cross-section, are *not* visible on plain chest films. Differentiation of the so-called interstitial (peribronchial ?) fibrosis is still a moot problem, but the term *broncho-vascular* must go! These linear shadows are usually vessels, and their prominence is simply related to the degree of pulmonary ventilation, and/or pulmonary congestion. With advancing emphysema, the vessels become more apparent, without acquiring any other significance.

The fact that hilar and perihilar nodularity is due most often to vessels seen on end was quite well known to Baetjer. Recent roentgen reports, originated at Johns Hopkins, prove that this is still common knowledge among the residents in radiology in Baetjer's old bailiwick.

PIRIE

William Alfred Jones of Kingston (Ontario), the respected "grand old man" of English-Canadian radiologists, delivered the Richards Lecture before the Canadian Association of Radiologists on January 11, 1955 in Ottawa. The subject of his masterful address was the eulogy of Gordon Earle Richards (1885-1949), published in the *Journal of the CAR* of March, 1955. Jones mentioned in that speech that Richards developed a method of making miniature

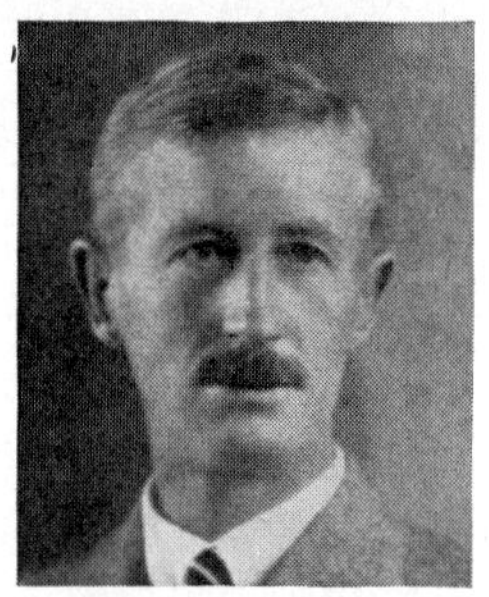

Alexander Pirie

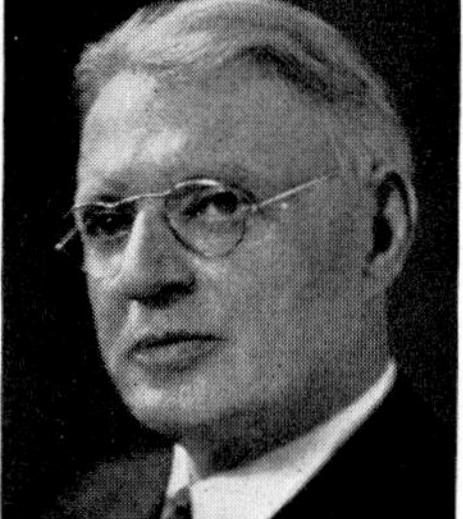

Kennon Dunham

X. Ray Department,
No. XI Canadian General Hospital!
Record No. 10145
3.3.1919.

M.O, wd. 3.
No. XI. CGH.

Kelly. T. J. Pte.,
2130345. C.A.M.C., English. 23.
left ankle.

Negative to fracture. There is an extra navicular bone in ~~the~~ both right and left foot which must not be mistaken for fracture of the navicular bone.

................................MAJOR, C. A. M. C.
OFFICER I/c X RAY [illegible]
No. XI CANADIAN [illegible] HOSPITAL, MOORE BARRACKS,
SHORNCLIFFE.

prints of the x-ray plate, to accompany the x-ray report - indeed, Richards published an article about it in 1917. Jones then said:

"This brings to mind that during World War I it became routine to make prints of x-ray plates. The x-ray report was typed or written upon the backs of these prints, and so passed on to the surgeon. I well remember doing this, and reporting plates in such a way. I still have in my possession the print of an injured foot, with the report typed on the back and signed by Pirie."

Thereupon I wrote to Jones, and asked him whether he would consent to have Pirie's report reproduced. The gracious answer was yes, even though those original prints by Alexander Howard Pirie (1885-1944) were pasted in a copy of Quain's *Osteology*.

Pirie's report is seen in facsimile. What he calls an extra navicular bone is today the talo-navicular.

SHADOW GAZERS

In a dialogue with Glaukon — reported in Plato's *Republic* — Socrates hypothesized a tribe of imaginary cave dwellers, permanently immobilized (chained) so that they could look only straight forward at one of the cave's walls. Behind the dwellers was a source of light (fire), and people passed between the fire and the chained tribe. Throughout their lives, these hypothetical cave dwellers would see only shadows, their own, those of their companions, of the passers-by and of various objects carried by the passers-by.

To the shadow gazers, shadows were the only recognized reality. Had their curse been lifted, and had they been allowed to inspect at the same time both the shadows and the objects which projected these shadows, they would have undoubtedly used the shadows as an orientation point to evaluate the original objects.

This is an inescapable human trait. At a roentgen-pathologic confrontation, the radiologist will time and again think out loud in his shadowy terms, rather than refer to the macroscopic appearance of the actual organ. There is, of course, always the possibility that changes had taken place between the time of exposure and the moment of death or necropsy.

In the case of bone tumors, the radiologist's evaluation is generally more accurate than that of the pathologist, in part because of the non-destructive qualities of the roentgen method, and also because of its comprehensiveness. In fact, many pathologists obtain soft films of the lungs, after removal from the thoracic cage, before the actual sectioning.

In certain quarters, the (often so very fleeting) roentgen shadows have become an accepted reality, which has spilled over into the vernacular. References to "having a shadow on the lungs" are common in the slang of patients from tuberculosis sanatoria.

In his continuing question-and-answer session with Glaukon, Socrates asserted that his hypothetical shadow gazers, being accustomed to their "station" in life, ought to have been relatively satisfied, *i.e.*, adjusted to their sort. Had an outsider tried to tell them that all objects have three, rather than their shadowy two dimensions, he would have been met with scorn and ridicule. "What then," asked Socrates, "were to have been that indiscreet outsider's fate, if the shadow gazers had the power to enforce their decision?" "Death," replied Glaukon.

This may be a bitter but accurate view of the public attitude toward "new" things, as well as toward those who dare to search for hidden explanations. Four centuries after Miguel Serveto (1511-1553), the penalty of death is seldom if ever incurred because of alleged (or even authenticated) scientific "heresies." But even if one were to face professional ostracism, he should have the courage to iterate and re-iterate that *roentgen shadows are only shadows* — not the *real* thing — and as such they may be, and quite often are, very fallacious.

In 1903, Théodore Guilloz (1868-1916) – a pharmacist from Lyon (France) who became a physician; turned to radiology; and terminated as a radiation casualty – affirmed that "in radiography, as in photography, microscopy, and many other observations, the appearance which seems the most obvious does not always correspond with the real condition." To some extent, this can be regarded as one of the earliest statements of what is now being called observer error in roentgen interpretation.

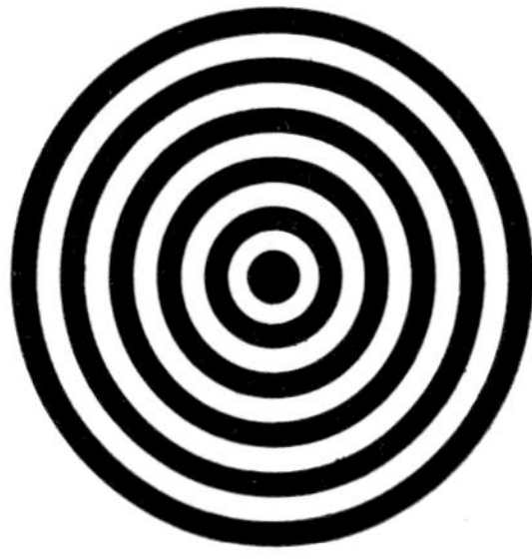

Analysis of the factors which may influence the quality of the roentgen reports can be time- and space-consuming. For the sake of convenience, these factors shall be summarized in the following table.

FACTORS INFLUENCING THE QUALITY OF ROENTGEN INTERPRETATION (X-RAY REPORTS)

(A) *The Patient*

1. Factors related to the patient's physical condition.
2. Factors related to the patient's mental condition.

(B) *The Technique of Examination*

1. Availability of equipment (including adequate viewing facilities) and specialized procedures.
2. Quality of films; number and timing of views, and similar details.

(C) *The Observer*

1. The observer's physical and psychological make-up.
2. The observer's radiological make-up: skill, knowledge, judgment.

THE PATIENT

The patient's *physical condition* may alter significantly the (text of the) roentgen report.

On the day of examination, a gastric ulcer crater may be filled with a blood clot, and thus remain invisible. A full term fetus, in breech position during pelvimetry, may turn spontaneously and make a "heady" appearance in this world. Fleeting pulmonary infiltrations and transient atelectases appear and disappear within the span of a few hours. After seemingly interminable protraction, a ureteral calculus may complete in a few minutes its journey into the bladder or beyond. Whether meteorologic influences are capable of producing reversible roentgen changes is debatable (the affirmative is quite likely). Stretcher patients, who cannot stand up for their examination, start out with a definite handicap as far as the accuracy of the final interpretation is concerned.

In a similar category is the patient's *preparation.*

When polypi must be demonstrated, improper cleaning usually invalidates the findings. This applies also to dehydration before intravenous urography or cholangiography, to removal of chest tapes before evaluation for rib fractures, and to removal of plaster cast before recheck of fractures for callus formation. There is also the forewarning which must be given to the patient, so that s(he) knows what to expect: in most instances it will result in better all-around cooperation.

This brings up the patient's *mental condition.*

Inability to co-operate (infants, patients during acute psychotic episodes) may prevent the performance of anything but a sketchy, that is incomplete (inadequate, inconclusive) examination. At the other end of the spectrum is the intelligent, highly motivated patient who permits anything, even the head-down position needed to see an atelectatic lobe otherwise obscured by pleural exudate.

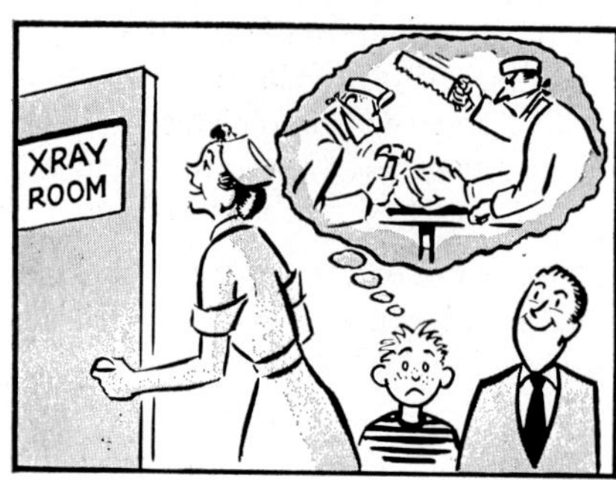

"Has that skull been fixed yet?"

Any of these (or similar) situations must be indicated in the roentgen report. Otherwise, the interpretation would remain hopelessly incomplete. A few examples are offered.

BARIUM ENEMA. In the absence of anal sphincteric action, patient expelled the retention catheter twice, and then refused to have it re-inserted, forcing discontinuation of the procedure. Barium suspension had penetrated only to the transverse colon . . .

CHEST FLUOROSCOPY. Patient was acutely disturbed (both resistive and aggressive), and physical restraint was needed to keep her behind the screen. Only a cursory glance of the lung fields was obtained, barely permitting identification, but not localization of.

In charity and teaching institutions, it occurs occasionally that patients are sent for routine examinations in disregard of their precarious general condition. The radiologist must never forget that he is first and foremost a physician, and does not have to perform the roentgen examination if he feels that the inevitable manipulations might jeopardize the patient's remaining strength. The following report relates just such a situation.

BARIUM MEAL. From the stretcher, patient was rolled into prone recumbency on the fluoroscopy table, and barium suspension was administered through a drinking tube. The first few swallows were seen passing through the cardia, then patient's respiration became stertorous, and at the same time contrast material appeared laterally to, and to both sides of, the distal esophagus. The roentgen beam was widened, and a single glance showed an extensive bilateral (barium) bronchogram. The lights were immediately turned on, the patient had already expired. Prone chest film was exposed, and confirmed the fluoroscopic findings.

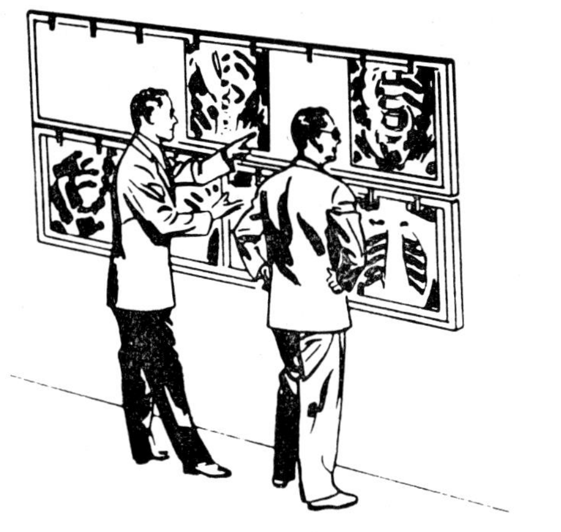

IMPRESSION:Bilateral bronchogram, due to pre-agonal aspiration of barium.

It is just as important to mention any significant difficulties or unusual situations encountered by the technician (in the absence of the radiologist). It is good practice to have the technician scribble this information on a slip attached to the films, and then incorporate this information in the final roentgen report.

Single frontal view of the cervical spine was obtained, because the attending physician had indicated that the patient must not be moved from the (radiolucent) stretcher. It shows . . .

Routine views of the upper G. I. tract are blurred by respiratory motion, because patient was unable to hold his breath, despite repeated coaching. . .

George Miller insists that it is good practice to have a radiologist view the films of most (if not of all) patients before they leave the x-ray department. This is especially valuable in emergency situations in both the chest and abdomen. It is also important in the fact that immediate retakes can be requested to adequately identify a fracture line, or see whether a para-ureteral concretion is a phlebolith or a calculus.

In modern teaching departments there is now a special job, assigned to a senior resident in radiology, who sits at the lighted end of an automatic roller processor, and looks at the films as they come out. If this resident is given the authority to request as many re-examinations or additional views as he sees fit, and if the patient does not leave the x-ray floor until this resident has seen the films, the quality of the x-ray work performed in the department will inevitably improve.

It is imperative to describe the incidental pathologic findings, observed during the examination, as this might help both the patient and his physician. An elderly lady had been referred for a barium meal because of alleged hematemesis. When placed in prone recumbency, she began to cough and had a frank hemoptysis. This information was extremely valid to the referring physician: it established the actual site of bleeding (it finally turned out to be a bronchogenic carcinoma) — and thus belonged into the report of the barium meal!

MEDICO-LEGAL IMPLICATIONS

Obviously, all accidents and incidents related to the roentgen procedure must be reported in as much detail as necessary. This is mandatory, not only for the possibility of future litigation, but simply because nowadays good practice of medicine is inconceivable without adequate records. The following report was prepared by Archie Fine:

BARIUM ENEMA IS PERFORMED: The patient expelled the Bardex catheter and it was re-inserted by me. Barium was seen to enter the rectum. Suddenly, to my consternation, a sort of flood of barium was seen advancing rapidly up the abdomen toward the diaphragm. Immediately the technician was told to stop the enema. The patient's breath became gasping and with the tube still in her, I attempted to perform artificial respiration. At the same time the technician was told to call for one of the medical residents. The patient took two or three breaths and then ceased voluntary respiration. I continued the artificial respiration for three or four minutes by compressing the chest wall and relaxing it until the medical resident arrived. He attempted to start the heart beating by injecting adrenalin but to no avail. The patient had expired within a minute or so after the entrance of barium into the vessels. At this time, I ordered the technician to take AP and lateral views of the chest and abdomen in order to definitely confirm what I thought was the entrance of opaque material into the blood vessels of the rectum.

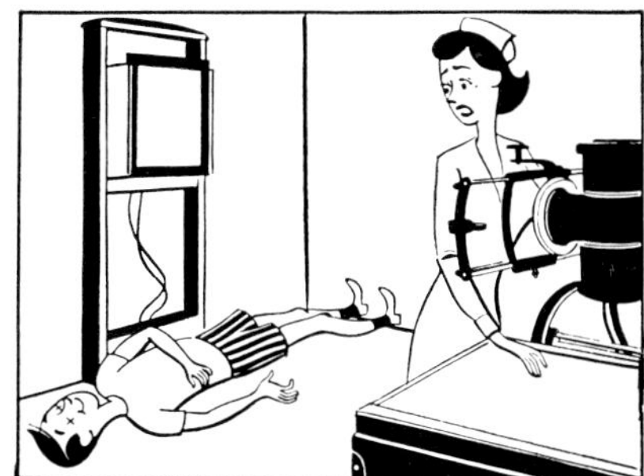

Abusive apnea. This delightful cartoon captioned "Oh . . . you can breathe now, Mr. Snodgrass!" – is one of a series published at irregular intervals in the *Du Pont X-ray News*. Several among these cartoons have been reproduced in this book, through the gracious courtesy of the Du Pont Company.

CHEST REPORT: Examination of the chest disclosed the presence of barium in the inferior vena cava, right atrium, right ventricle, and pulmonary arteries.

ABDOMEN: Examination of the abdomen revealed barium in the portal radicles.

This is the roentgen report, as it was inserted into the patient's record. A more detailed account appeared in *Radiology* (Rosenberg and Fine*). It serves as a reminder that even the most innocuous appearing procedure is potentially lethal. A similar instance was observed quite recently (1960) by Truemner, White, and Vanlandingham in Rockford (Illinois).

FELSON

Under different circumstances, a report may provoke chuckles, as in the following instance:

G. I. SERIES: All the barium ingested in the ward six hours earlier was in the colon, as expected. At this time, inadvertently, plaster of Paris suspension was administered to the patient instead of barium. No gross abnormalities were demonstrated in the esophagus, stomach, or duodenum. At the end of twenty-four hours, essentially all of the plaster of Paris suspension has remained in the stomach. It appears to have solidified or "set" and has formed a cast within the stomach. Close observation is indicated, with abdominal films made at least daily.

The text of this report was obligingly reconstituted by the master diagnostician and chronic jester, Benjamin Felson, professor of radiology at the University of Cincinnati. The actual incident — during which four patients swallowed plaster of Paris suspension (the plaster was in the fluoroscopy room because it had been used to seal light leaks) — took place at a U. S. Army Hospital in England, just before D-Day in World War II.

Felson recounted this episode in a refreshing note, entitled *Radiologist on the Rocks,* but none of those witty remarks can be quoted, because that is a copyrighted item. Moreover, he did not mention therein whether any of the examinees, when told what they had swallowed, recited the not so well known sestet from the *Nonsense Book* of Frank Gellett Burgess (1866-1951):

PARISIAN NECTAR for the Gods
A little thick, but what's the odds?
Many people seem to think
Plaster O' Paris good to drink;
Though conducive unto quiet,
I prefer another diet!

The gastroliths eventually crumbled, and were spontaneously eliminated, though not before giving the plaster-dispensing radiologist a few anxiety-ridden days with intervening sleepless nights. Otherwise the episode had only humorous consequences for all concerned.

In a more recent issue of *Medical Economics,* Felson related the radio-scato-graphic events which took place – in his X-ray Department at the University Hospital – during the non-destructive testing of a reluctant cow.

As a recognized expert in "chest radiology," Felson has described the *paracardiac silhouette* sign (hazy cardio-phrenic angle means posterior pulmonary consolidation if the heart contour is sharp, anterior if the cardiac silhouette is indistinct), the *open bronchus* sign (visibly patent brochus leading into atelectatic segment or lobe indicates that the atelectasis is post-inflammatory, rather than occlusive, the latter being usually equated with neoplastic), and the *air bronchogram* (bronchial ramifications cannot be seen in either pleural or mediastinal lesions, thus allowing differentiation from intrapulmonary processes). Felson has also popularized that excellent educational exercise called "case of the day" (of the week or of

*Permission to print the text of this report was graciously granted by Archie Fine, radiologist at the Jewish Hospital in Cincinnati.

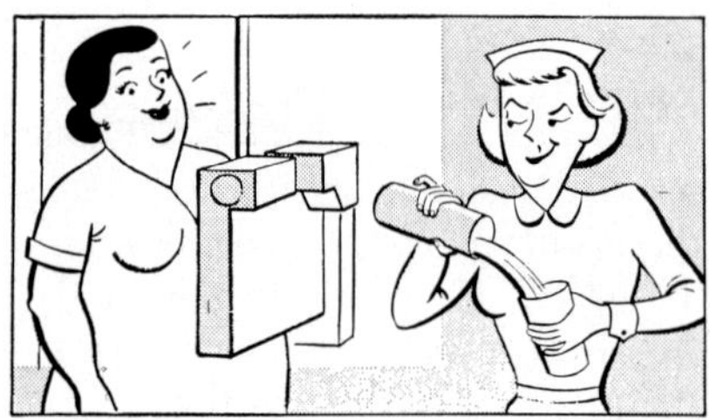

"Ooh, a milkshake . . . and I'm on a diet, too!"

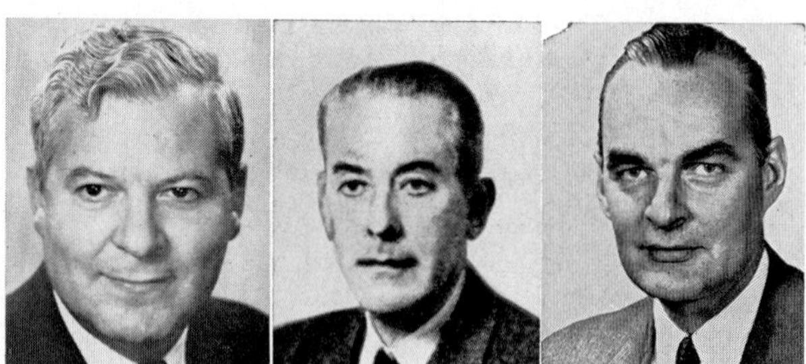

B. FELSON WILLY BAENSCH DONALD MCRAE

A trio of "uncanny" roentgen-diagnosticians, the pneumoradiologist Felson from Cincinnati, the gastroenteroradiologist Baensch from Washington (D.C.), and the neuroradiologist McRae from Montreal.

the month, as that particular case may be). He is an eternal seeker of new methods in radiologic education. He went so far as to become a "programmer" in the hope of introducing this new procedure (B. F. Skinner developed programmed learning at Harvard around 1954.) Felson set up a controlled experiment, reported in *Radiology* of November, 1963: the result was a tie, students did not seem to advance significantly faster with any procedure. This, of course, was nothing new to me. As a father of (many) schoolchildren I found out that the most elaborate teaching aids and the most involved systems are no substitute for the pupil's personal motivation. No matter how well and how much one were to teach, in the final analysis it is the pupil who must do the learning.

Felson is recognized not only for his chestmanship (he was guest editor of the August, 1963 — Chest — issue of the *Radiological Clinics of North America*). He is an expert at bloody (and sanguine) repartees, and is perhaps better known yet for ascribing to his many children a remarkable number of *bon mots.* Actually Felson just tries, and often succeeds, in making his presentations more palatable by the inclusion of a few irreverent remarks.

BRIEF ASIDE

To be able to see the humorous side of one's own inadvertencies (as long as they occur rarely), and to be willing to admit one's own inadequacies (assuming they are few), means to remain candid under all circumstances, which is a mark of intellectual maturity.

In the original manuscript of one of my papers (published in 1952) – which dealt with the transient analgesic effects of intracutaneous injections – I had used the following words: "On one occasion, by mistake, distilled water, and another time saline, was injected instead of procaine – and the analgesic effect was the same." A surgeon of my acquaintance consented to edit the manuscript, and simply deleted the words "by mistake." As I rechecked it, I replaced the crossed-out "by mistake" with "inadvertently."

That surgeon just happened to see the galley proofs, and his face became congested. He took great pains in explaining to me that one must never *(never, ever!)* admit a mistake, nay an inadvertency. I gave in *(mea culpa!)* and settled for replacing "inadvertently" with "incidentally," which is how it finally appeared in the *South Dakota Journal of Medicine.*

The inclusion in roentgen reports of an occasional (but more than homeopathic) retrospective self-castigation is quite likely to improve relations between the radiologist and the referring clinicians. This theme will be dealt with in a subsequent paragraph.

TECHNIQUE OF EXAMINATION

The availability of certain equipment and/or gadgets might have to be alluded to in the report. An example follows:

AORTO-RENAL ANGIOGRAM. A polyethylene catheter was inserted percutaneously (with the help of a "piano" wire) through the right femoral artery into the aorta to a distance of 30 cm. from the inguinal ligament. Anteroposterior view of the abdomen, exposed after the injection of 3 cc. of contrast medium, showed the tip of the catheter overlying the body of L2. Following injection of 30 cc. of Hypaque 50 per cent, two films were exposed at brief interval. An excellent renal arteriogram was obtained showing extrinsic pressure on the lower pole of the right kidney (confirming what was seen on the excretory urogram). Two additional (late) films were exposed but the venous phase had passed, the pyelo-calyceal system was visualized, and there was no residual staining in the lower pole of the right kidney.

IMPRESSION: Under these circumstances . . .

Obviously, this examiner had neither an image intensifier to check the position of the catheter, nor a seriograph (or cineroentgenography) to expose an adequate number of films during both the arterial and the venous phases of the renal angiogram. And since the pathology extant was not definitely identified, the examination went only so far — *in all fairness to the patient,* and to those who would have to re-evaluate (perhaps repeat) this procedure, *when pertinent, one must indicate in the report the limitations of the equipment utilized.* An indirect if verbose mention (as in above report) is perfectly adequate for the connoisseur at the other end (the uninitiated is of less importance). Hardier souls, unhampered by institutional pride, may insert straightforward wording such as "*. . . in the absence of a device for obtaining serial views only four films were exposed at relatively brief intervals . . .*"

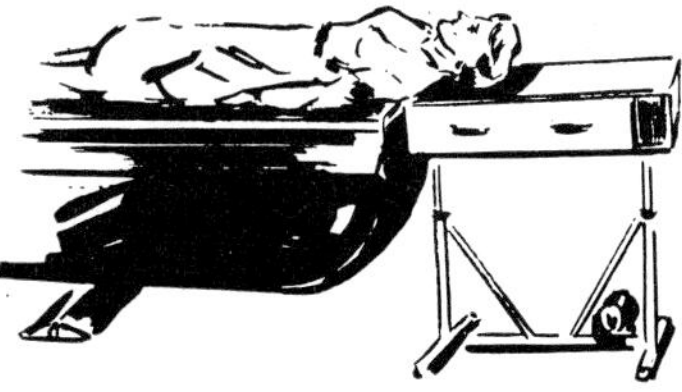

SERIOGRAPH. This is an older Sanchez-Perez model, sitting next to a Picker table.

The importance of adequate technical help for the success of a radiologic department cannot be overemphasized. Often there develops a team spirit, with a dose of personal friendship injected into the initially business-like relationships. Such a relationship cannot be severed without psychologic trauma.

BYRON MONTELLE SMITH (1924-1963)

An old Turkish proverb describes death as a black camel that kneels once at every man's door. The inevitability of death is a commonplace, but it offers no consolation, certainly not for the sudden, irreparable departure of a dear friend.

Byron Smith finished high school in his home town, Tuscola (Illinois). In 1947 he graduated from the Edgewater Hospital School of Radiography in Chicago, got married, passed the ARXT test, and then accepted a job as x-ray technician with the hospital in Paris (Illinois). This is where I met him in 1956.

By then, Byron had become a consummate master at both radiography and photography. He produced the radiographs from which he made the photographic reproductions for the section on reporting in this text. Byron was chief-technician of both the Paris Hospital and the Paris Clinic. He had designed the excellent x-ray department at the clinic, and displayed unusual administrative ability, and a gift for teaching. He gave refresher courses to the technicians from "my" other hospitals. Word got around, and Byron received several offers for teaching positions in big centers, but he preferred the smaller town of his choice. Although aware of his usually asymptomatic aortic stenosis, Byron was always "on the go," always looking for "new" procedures: in his last six months he became familiar with mammography, urine radiography, and cineradiography, and introduced all three at the Paris Hospital.

Byron, having become a fervent Baptist, organized a Men's Choir. The first performance was set for Father's Day, June 16, 1963. On that Sunday in church, in the midst of a resounding hymn, Byron unexpectedly collapsed, and in the sudden silence died of a fulminating ventricular fibrillation. He was laid to rest in Tuscola, the next-of-kin survivors being his wife and son.

Byron and I were working on several scientific projects, yet the task was unequally divided: his part was bigger than mine and thus far I have not found the time to resume that work. But what hurts most is the loss of a good, honest, irreplaceable friend, a typical representative of the American Middle West in which he was born, bred, and buried. Whenever I fly over the Tuscola cemetery (presently about three times a week, on my way from the University to the Coles County Airport), I spot Byron's grave from the air, I recall his eternally cheerful grin, I bank each wing

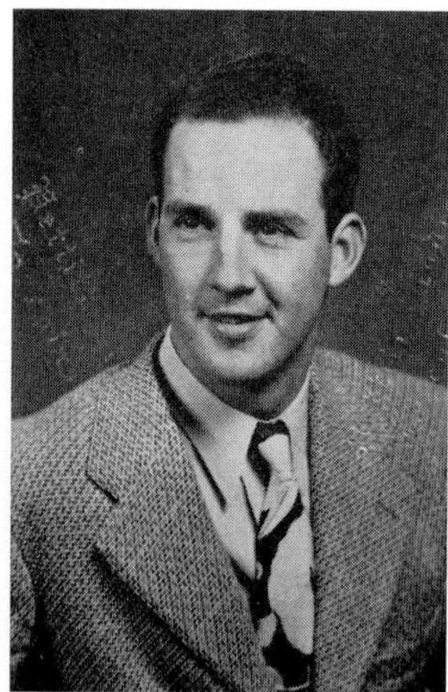

EAST

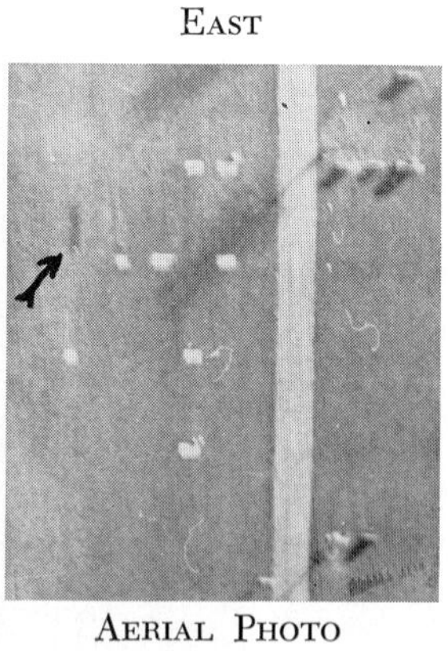

AERIAL PHOTO

BYRON MONTELLE SMITH and his grave (arrow), an East-West oriented slit, as yet bare of grass, seen in the early morning sun, which obliques the shadows from the southeast. The white dots are grave stones.

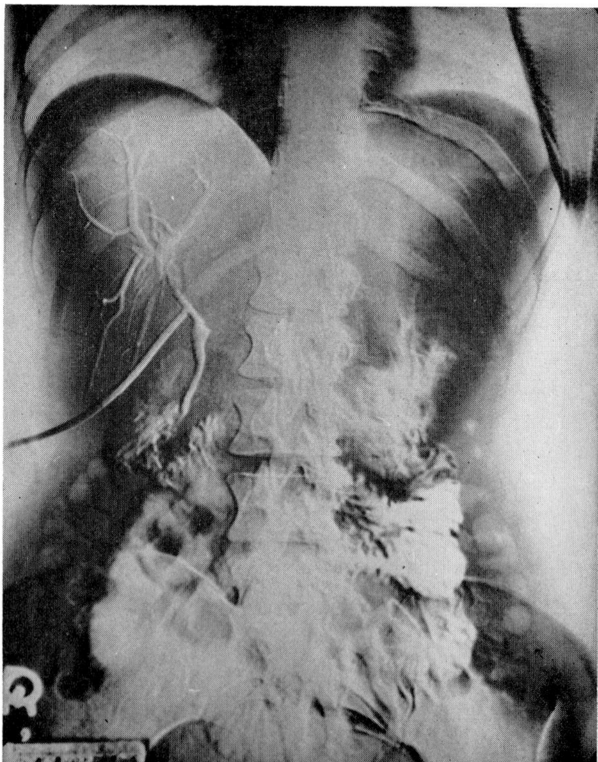

PLASTIC CHOLANGIOGRAM. Excellent filling, also of hepatic radicles, with facile passage into the duodenum — accentuated by "plastic-ization."

RADIOLOGY

67 EAST ROUTE 14
CRYSTAL LAKE, ILLINOIS

HOURS BY APPOINTMENT

E. R. N. GRIGG, M.D.

PHONE 459-4217 - AREA CODE 815

February 27, 1963

Patient: Mrs. Beatrice Huxtable - age 54 years
4532 Lakeview Lane
Crystal Lake, Illinois

Examination #547/63

Referred by Paul C. Wilson, M.D.

Dear Doctor Wilson:

GALLBLADDER SERIES: About sixteen hours after the ingestion of five grams of Telepaque, there is a fair concentration by the gallbladder, sufficient to demonstrate at least two radiolucent gallstones. Even in retrospect no gallstones are visible on the peroral cholecystogram dated 5-17-61.

BARIUM MEAL: In prone recumbency, the gastric fundus herniated (in a sliding fashion) through the esophageal hiatus; spontaneous reduction occurred in the erect position. The duodenal bulb was contracted most of the time; it is seen well filled on several spotfilms and on one of the routine radiographs. Palpation of the bulb produced no discomfort. There was spot tenderness on pressure over the still opacified gallbladder fundus. Evacuation of the stomach proceeded with no hesitation. The small bowel pattern was not unusual. Progress film of the abdomen, about one hour after ingestion of contrast substance, shows the head of the barium column in the terminal ileum. A walnut-sized cluster of calcifications is seen in the pelvic inlet.

IMPRESSION:

1. Cholelithiasis, developed within the past two years; tenderness on pressure over gallbladder indicates inflammation.
2. Sliding type of hiatus hernia with esophageal irritability, perhaps an early stage of peptic esophagitis.
3. Calcified pelvic tumor, probably uterine myofibroma.
4. In the presence of hiatus hernia and gallstones, if clinically desirable, the third in Saint's triad (in this case diverticulosis of the colon) might have to be investigated.

With many thanks for the referral of this patient, I remain

Yours very cordially

E.R.N. Grigg

ERNG: jd

P.S. This report does not mention: (1) a few shadows which were not seen because they were not looked at, nor (2) those shadows which may have been looked at, but were not seen because of their small size, lack of contrast, or similarly obscuring factors, and certainly not (3) the shadows which (although both looked at and seen) were ignored because the signer of this report has not yet learned what significance, if any, they have.

to honor his memory, and then I again bid him a restful peace.*

SPOT FILMS AND OTHER TECHNICALITIES

While the adequacy (or inadequacy) of equipment, if significant, should be mentioned in the report, exaggerations must be avoided, as a matter of course.

A radiologist yearned for a spotfilm device, but the hospital board refused to buy such a devious contraption. He had to convince the staff first, so for the next six months, all negative barium meal examinations terminated with something like

IMPRESSION: in the absence of spotfilms with graded compression, crater in antrum or bulb cannot be definitely excluded. . .

That particular radiologist got (away with it and got) a spotfilmer, but only because he was otherwise well liked. The roentgen report is not a medium for publicity, for rancor, or for the exhibition of anything that is not directly related to that particular patient.

Don Bauer had a similiar experience with a hospital board composed of physicians, who threatened to fire him because they feared potential liability if the records contained the proof that they had been informed of the inadequacy of their x-ray equipment (it was so old, with exposed, overhead conduits, that no spotfilmer could be adapted to it). Roscoe Miller sided likewise with the radiologist, being a firm believer that without adequate spot films the examination is inadequate except for large lesions. They both agreed that the x-ray report is not a medium for rancor, etc., but insisted that whenever no spot films are made during a barium examination, this fact must be incorporated in the respective report. So be it!

Modern developments have come to qualify this statement. The proper way of doing gastrointestinal examinations today is with the image intensifier. I have been doing this since 1956, and I can attest to the fact that "intensified" fluoroscopy, especially with a television monitor, has greatly reduced the need for spotfilming. And in those cases in which spot films are still needed for either clarification, or for the recording of an otherwise fleeting image, cineradiography will easily provide a few hundred spotfilms, which can then be inspected in peace, frame by frame.

When special radiographic positions have been used, such as Hampton's technique, or the trans-

*This is the text of the obituary which I wrote for *Radiologic Technology* of January, 1964, reproduced with their kind permission.

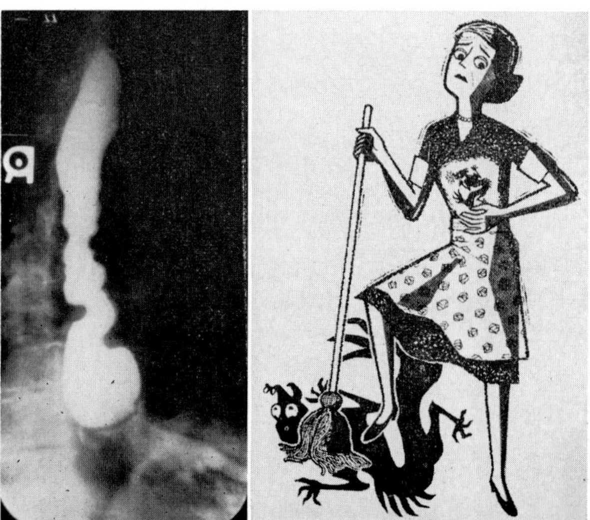

PEPTIC ESOPHAGITIS. Tertiary contractions indicate esophageal irritability. The vignette is from a Smith, Kline, & French advertisement with the caption, "The battle won in the house is lost in the stomach."

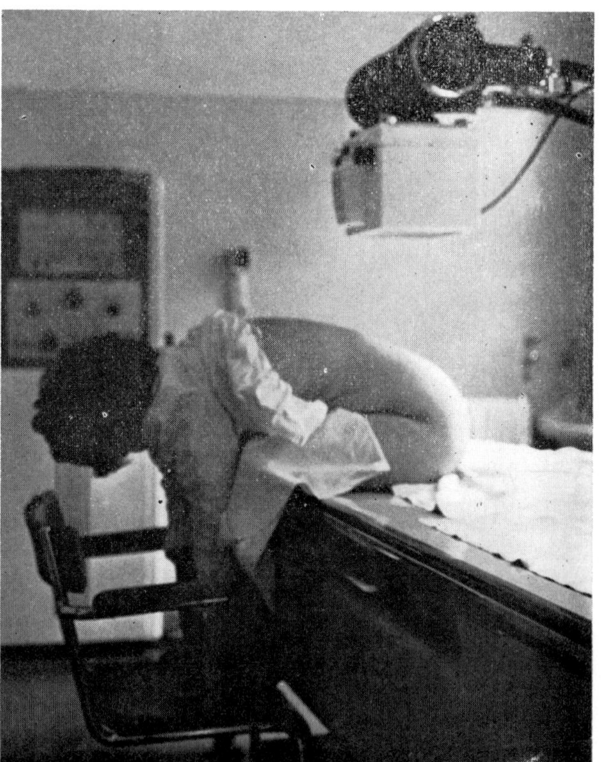

SQUAT SHOT. This peculiar position has been suggested by many authors and was used for several contrast examinations in the pelvis. It is herein reproduced from an article by Garavaglia, Guzzon, and Romanini, published in *Minerva Medica* of March 28, 1961 – they all are given this courtesy line for having sent us their original glossy for the etching.

sacral projection for the bladder, this should be mentioned in the report. The number of views available may some day acquire medico-legal significance. In many institutions the report is typed on forms which contain blank spaces for the number of views and related technical details. In other institutions the forms are white (real blank), and then it is preferable to begin the report with a statement regarding the number of projections available for interpretation, such as

Three views of the left elbow show . . ., or *Four views of the facial bones (including exaggerated Waters' position) reveal . . .*, or *Three views of the right heel (one being an axial projection of the calcaneus) disclose . . .*

Whenever positive or negative contrast media have been used during an examination, it is of advantage to indicate that by intercalating in the report a title in capital letters (*BARIUM MEAL, RETROGRADE PYELOGRAM, PERCUTANEOUS AORTOGRAM,* and so on). When two or more such procedures have been performed on one patient, and all are reported in continuation, the capital captions serve as convenient dividers.

The date on which the interpretation was dictated — when different from the date of examination — must be mentioned in the report. In pertinent instances, such as progress films for suspected bowel obstruction, it is proper to specify the hour when the film(s) had been exposed. Similar importance should be given with certain contrast media to time intervals between films. The proprietary (instead of the often less well known chemical) name of the contrast substance ought to be used. Its concentration and amount are preferably spelled (rather than given in figures). Another general rule is to avoid all but the most obvious and generally accepted, abbreviations (it is not redundant to spell even the latter).

CHOLECYSTOGRAPHIC SAMPLES

GALLBLADDER SERIES. At eight a.m., about fourteen hours after alleged ingestion of three grams of Orabilex, the gallbladder is not seen, and no opaque calculi are identified. There is no visible contrast substance in the bowels. Speckled costal cartilage calcifications are seen.

IMPRESSION: non-visualization of gallbladder after presumed ingestion of single dose of cholecystographic material.

A few lines could be shaved off, but further editing (down to "*non-visualized gallbladder*") would fail to tell the whole story. Ingested contrast material is almost always visible in the bowel. Orabilex used to cause fewer, but still identifiable shadows. From the above report, one could not tell whether the patient had ever ingested the tablets, whether the tablets had been regurgitated, or whether they had failed to reach the proper places at the required time. The wording *single dose* when incorporated in a *non-visualizing* report is usually sufficient to suggest a repeat with double dose, without having to say so explicitly.

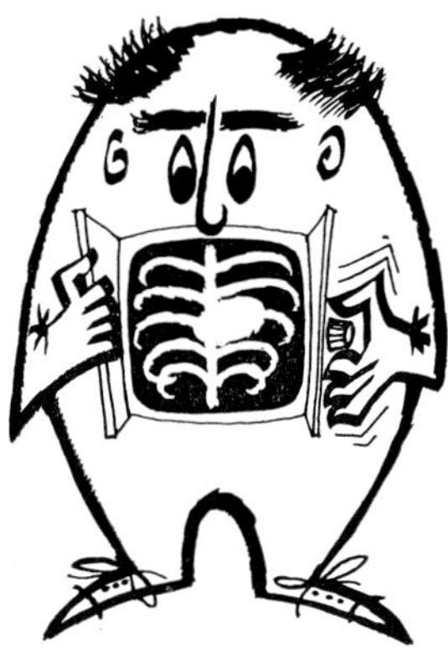

Ectopic gallbladder. British ad for Winthrop's Telepaque.

REPEAT GALLBLADDER SERIES. Fourteen hours after ingestion of six grams of Telepaque, which is also thirty-eight hours after the ingestion of three grams of Telepaque, a large amount of contrast substance fills the bowels. The gallbladder is only faintly visible, sufficient to rule out opaque (but not lucent) calculi. No layering is identified on the upright or on the lateral decubitus views. The film exposed one hour after fatty meal stimulation shows no change in either size or shape of the gallbladder.

IMPRESSION: Because of poorly concentrating gallbladder, radiolucent gallstones are not definitely excluded; functional disturbances suspected.

If the various views, the fatty meal stimulation, and other details had been deleted from the report, and the patient were to consult another physician after a brief lapse of time, it would not be possible — on the strength of the sole roentgen report — to determine whether layering had or had not been searched for. That other physician may then feel justified in requesting a repeat examination (from another radiologist, of course!)

Pointers on terminology, as in all of medicine, relate to the state of the art. In reporting cholecystograms, it might be desirable to avoid the term *contract(ion)* until the pundits have reached some sort of agreement on whether the gallbladder empties actively or by (intestinal) suction.

UROGRAPHIC SAMPLES

The term intravenous pyelogram is very often utilized; it is nevertheless etymologically improper. It simply means study (or visualization) of the kidney pelvis: who would settle for that only?

INTRAVENOUS UROGRAM. Preliminary anteroposterior view of the abdomen shows multiple phleboliths, and one of these, projected above the level of the ischial spine, could be in the distal left ureter. Following intravenous injection of thirty cc of Hypaque fifty per cent, there occurred prompt and excellent concentration by the collecting system of the right kidney, with good visualization of properly cupped calyces. On the left, visualization was delayed, and dilated calyces appear only on the film exposed thirty-five minutes after the injection; pelviectasis is faintly visible on the one hour view. On none of these films is the left ureter identified. The right ureter, and the urinary bladder revealed no abnormalities.

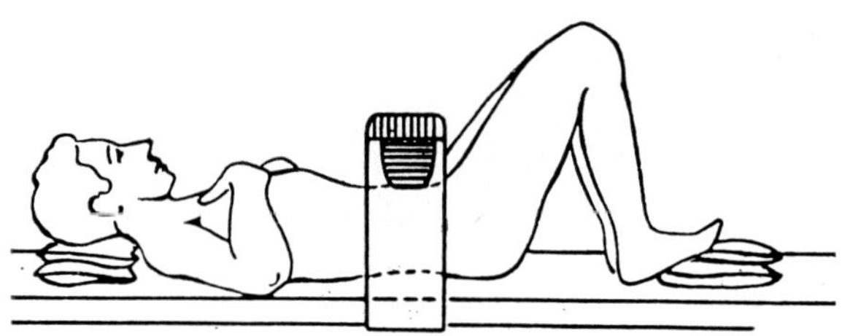

IMPRESSION: Left pelviectasis with calyectases; suspicion of calculus impacted in distal left ureter, perhaps demonstrable on retrograde examination.

At this point, another general rule may be clarified. Physicians usually resent being told what to do, even when they come to the radiologist for advice. They want the advice, but it has to be presented in a palatable container. The recommendations must not be given in a mandatory way: this is why in the wording of the report one should try to avoid outright terms such as *". . . it is suggested,"* or *". . . it appears indicated."*

In this particular example, the same advice could have been conveyed by saying (in the impression), *". . . Impacted ureteral calculus could be present; if clinically in doubt, or otherwise desirable, additional (retrograde) investigation may be considered."* Over and above the legal implications, such a report places the responsibility for the decision in the hands of the referring clinician — and that is where it belongs; a clinical decision ought to be reached on the basis of more than a single examination.

Roscoe Miller added two "palatable containers," in use at the Indiana Medical Center: such and such examination "may be informative," or "may give further information."

While the term urography is certainly more appropriate for the intravenous procedure, the term retrograde pyelography is less improper, since that examination is less comprehensive. Even so, retrograde urography remains the preferred term.

RETROGRADE UROGRAPHY. Preliminary anteroposterior view of the abdomen shows the left ureteral catheter in place. The questionable concretion, described on the previous examination as projected above the level of the left ischial spine, is again seen but it is not in contact with the catheter; besides, its central rarefaction is now well visible which identifies it as a phlebolith. Instillation of three cc. of Hypaque twenty per cent into the catheter results in excellent filling of the pyelo-calyceal system of the left kidney, with no evidence of pathologic alterations. After removal of the catheter, there is good filling of the left ureter, while traces of contrast material coat the left kidney pelvis and calyces.

IMPRESSION: No abnormalities in the retrograde examination of the left reno-ureteral system; as previously stated, a radiolucent calculus may have been impacted in the left ureter; if so, it was probably eliminated prior to the start of this examination.

A bit of humility never hurts. Such advice as is given must be offered in sentences less than categorical — even though (perhaps more so when) the evidence seems quite obvious. Only a few things are certain in medicine, and those few things do not stay that certain for very long.

The baron Jean Nicolas Corvisart des Marets (1755-1821) is remembered as the father of pathologic anatomy; he introduced percussion as a method of examination, and was Napoleon's private physician. Corvisart — a medical giant in his days — knew less about the basic physiology and pathology of the human body than does the lowest-ranking medical student of today. There is no doubt that to the generation of a century hence the great medical pundits of today will appear as "innocent" (ignorant?!) as Corvisart seems to us. This is why one can take with a grain of salt what all the pundits say. But some of Corvisart's aphorisms on generic medical subjects are today just as fresh and valid and eternal as they would have been when Hippocrates first coined his transcendental sentence about life being short and medical art much longer (than anticipated).

FILMS NOT DIAGNOSTIC

Should a detailed report (or any report at all) be prepared on the basis of technically inadequate films? The answer is a qualified yes. Even when the examination is to be repeated without additional cost to the patient (thus acknowledging that the poor quality of the films was not due to the patient's condition, but to a technical error), some information can often be gained for subsequent corroboration. Sometimes, a certain finding may be perfectly visible only on an otherwise unusable film. An underpenetrated lateral view of the skull may show an unsuspected fracture of the nasal bone, and an overpenetrated frontal projection of the chest can demonstrate a calcified gallbladder or a staghorn.

How should one report these "inadequate" films? It is inexcusable to place the blame - in the report - on the x-ray technician. Even a thorough investigation might not be conclusive in proving that it had been his fault (voltage drops, and contaminated developer can always be invoked). Just as improper would be a statement such as *"Two views of the right wrist are not diagnostic. Repeat is advised also because of suspicion of Colles fracture."* It is better to say *"Two views of the right wrist, exposed with light technique* (or *as viewed through a strong light,* if that should be the case), *reveal a deformity of the radius, resembling impacted fracture. Additional views might be of help for adequate evaluation."* A nimble wording is desirable if merely because re-examination may not always be feasible.

In most situations (except *perhaps* in wartime or during physical combat), it is preferable to adopt a neighborly attitude. Few mortals are perfect, the one who reports films for a living is just as fallible as the others. All of us have the government and the technicians we deserve.

INCOMPLETE EXAMINATIONS

Similar recommendations are valid when (some of) the films were lost, double exposed, or never made. Here is an example:

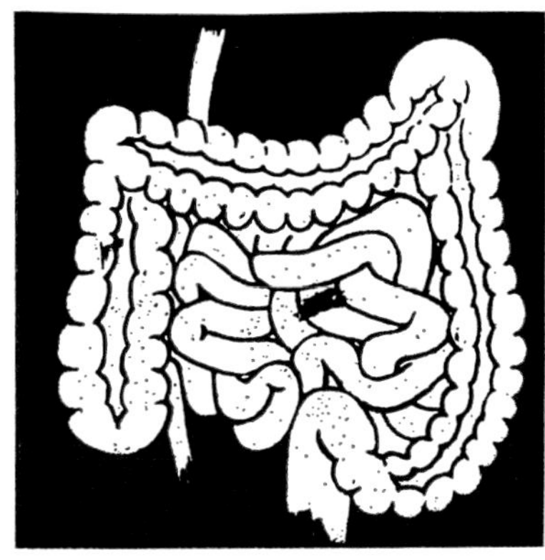

BARIUM ENEMA. Barium suspension, introduced per rectum, penetrated through a collapsed colon, and reached the cecum, but despite insistence and local massage, never entered the terminal ileum. The appendiceal stump was filled. Routine post-evacuation film is not available for interpretation, and spotfilms of sigmoid and cecum are very light. Routine pre-evacuation film is blurred by breathing during the exposure.

IMPRESSION: technically inconclusive examination, suggesting (transient?) obstruction at the ileo-cecal valve; repeat desirable.

It is more time-consuming than to say *"Inadequate examination, advise repeat!"* but if, for one reason or another, the patient is not returned for another try, the initial roentgen report remains the only source of information; even a little bit of information can go a long way, when clinically corroborated. It all depends on the reporting radiologist's degree of intestinal fortitude. Is he mainly concerned with being (always?) right or does he worry more about actually helping the patient? Of course, fluoroscopy must have been carefully (not perfunctorily) performed. How often, and how many of us stand by in a sort of daze — while the barium column rolls counterclockwise around the abdomen — relying for the ultimate report on a sigmoid spot and on the routine views?

There are many possible examples of partial reporting. Take for instance lengthy procedures, such as body section radiography:

CHEST STRATIGRAPHY. Seven body section films were exposed over the left perihilar area at one, three, five, seven, nine, eleven, and thirteen cms. from the posterior wall. Most of the films were light, but a cavity is fairly well delineated at three and at five cm. Calcifications were neither seen, nor excluded.

IMPRESSION: Not entirely conclusive chest tomography, indicative of cavity in apex of left lower lobe; if further information is desired, additional tomograms at two, four, and six cm. may be requested.

In that case the need for further investigation will usually depend on bacteriologic confirmation. With unequivocal proof of virulent tubercle bacilli in the sputum, a pulmonary cavity is tuberculous until and unless proven otherwise. Without bacteriologic confirmation, the demonstration of a cavity raises more problems than it solves. I know of no specific signs by which tuberculosis can be differentiated from histoplasmosis when only chest films are available. Single malignant nodes (whether primary or secondary) have also been known to excavate, and acquire a fluid level.

FACTS RELATED TO THE OBSERVER

The reporting radiologist's *physical* and *psychological* condition influences considerably the quality of his roentgen reports. Refraction errors and large scotomata are so obvious that they cannot be a very long time "overlooked" by the one who carries them. Conversely, marital and ethylic vicissitudes, although often just as significant, are usually taken in stride until the "readers" of the respective roentgen reports begin to complain.

Let us now turn to more transient — *i.e.*, easily reversible — psychologic disturbances, from over-exuberant mornings to moody afternoons (wide affective swings). It has been established beyond any doubt

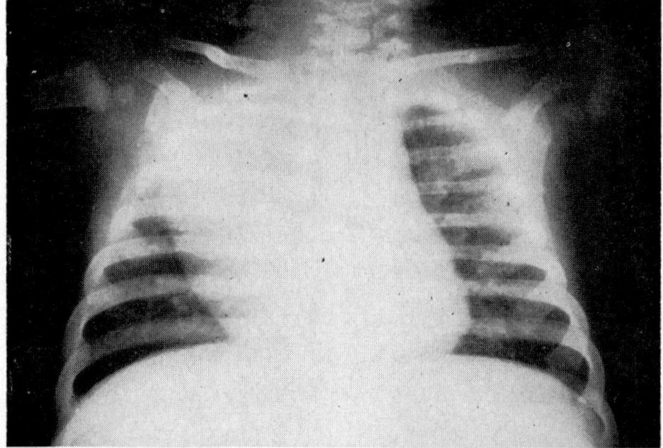

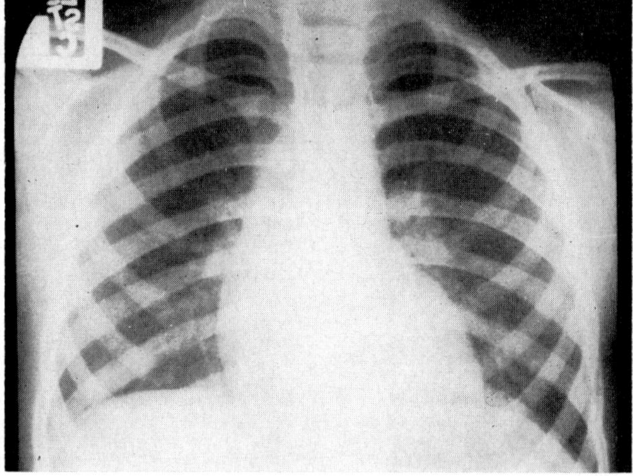

TITANIC THYMUS. This is the film of my three-months old daughter Susan Kathlyn, exposed (in December, 1954) the day after she had developed a sudden, afebrile dyspnea. Several grave consultants shook their heads in horror, and spoke of roentgen therapy to be followed by exploratory thoracotomy. I balked, and showed the film to a pediatric radiologist (Harvey White at Children's Memorial in Chicago), who discounted the large thymus as non-pathologic, but pointed to the basilar blebs as indicative of partial bronchial obstruction. It turned out to be a severe bronchiolitis. A week later Susan was much worse, although the pediatrician-in-charge (Robert Gustafson, Sr., then in Kankakee, now in Houston) had exhausted most of his pharmacologic arsenal; seeing my wife's and my own desperate looks, he tried something that made no sense, a blood transfusion. The cutdown and everything else was very messy, but after the first few cc. of blood entered her veins, Susan began to breathe easier. Whether coincidental or not, that transfusion was the turning point; three days later we brought Susan back home. The thymus took three years to disappear. Today Susan has no discernible residuals from that episode. The bottom film was exposed in 1958.

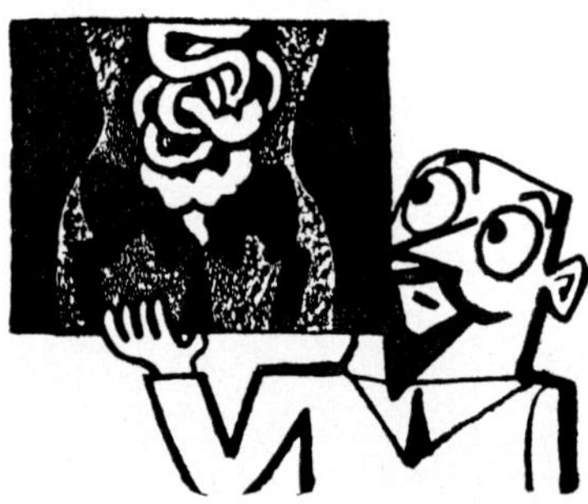

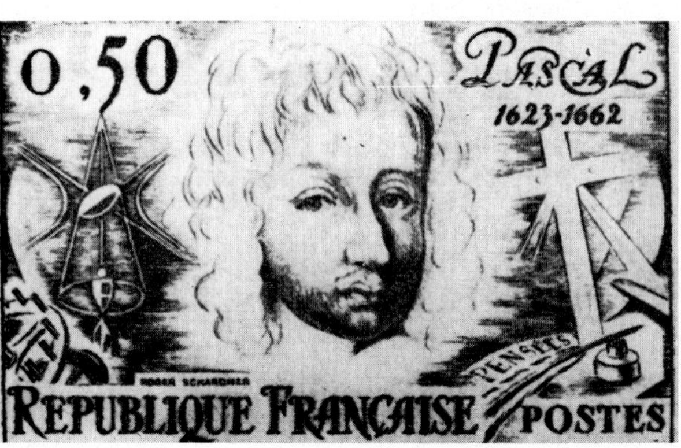

that these swings can widely affect the efficiency of any pursuit. A good rule, similar to advice given automobile drivers, is that danger lurks at both extremes of the affective swing: when either too elated or too depressed, don't drive and don't read films!

Evidently of greatest importance is the reporter's *radiologic make-up,* which consists of *skill* (dexterity acquired through training), *knowledge* (information, more or less comprehensive), and *judgment* (correlation of the previous two with experience).

Blaise Pascal (1623-1662), the French mathematical philosopher, was convinced that atheists – if forced to go regularly through the motions of praying (even without understanding) – would begin to believe.* The human mind being as frail as it is, this happens to be, indeed, a very valid method of teaching. Therefore, in a residency, as long as proper supervision is available, fledgling radiologists should begin to report films at a very early stage, so as to *acquire* the necessary skill, *i.e.,* the mechanics of the procedure, and to learn to manipulate its terminology. The needed knowledge may take time to *accumulate,* and later it will have to be *refilled* at periodic intervals. As to *developing* judgment – of what is good and what is evil in roentgen reporting – one may have to wait longer than the four years, currently required for a blessing by the American Board of Radiology.

In actual practice, the younger members of the profession cover up their deficiencies in judgment by excelling in knowledge and skill. After a few years, they tend to become rusty in certain areas of information, but their judgment has improved, and they function much better than at the time when they were able to recite in one breath the differential diagnosis of (so-called) interstitial pulmonary fibrosis. Judgment can conceal (substitute for) many deficiencies, which is demonstrable also in roentgen reporting.

ANALYSIS OF AN INTERPRETATION

At times, based seemingly on a single glance, the radiologist can reassure a worried pediatrician that the menacing opacification of almost the entire right lung field is merely a garden variety of overgrown (but otherwise non-pathologic) thymus. It may take a little longer to pick out a faintly visible fracture line in the head of the radius, and longer yet to decide whether an intracranial calcification is a tumor or a (unilaterally) calcified glomus.

*The French usually quote Pascal as having said, *"A force de parler d'amour, on devient amoureux,"* talking constantly of love makes one (to become) a lover.

If all previously mentioned factors (those related to patient and technique) are eliminated, the reporting observer must go through three stages, *detection, identification,* and finally actual *interpretation* of the incriminated shadow(s).

DETECTION

The first step is to pick out the "shadow(s) of annoyance" (Shelley). Newell and Garneau have postulated the existence of an absolute physical threshold, below which detection with conventional means is not possible. It might also be important to think of a threshold for a given observer, depending on his eyesight and ability to discriminate between various photographic densities. So far most, if not all, of the statistical studies have been based on the detection of opacities which were well within the reach of the un-

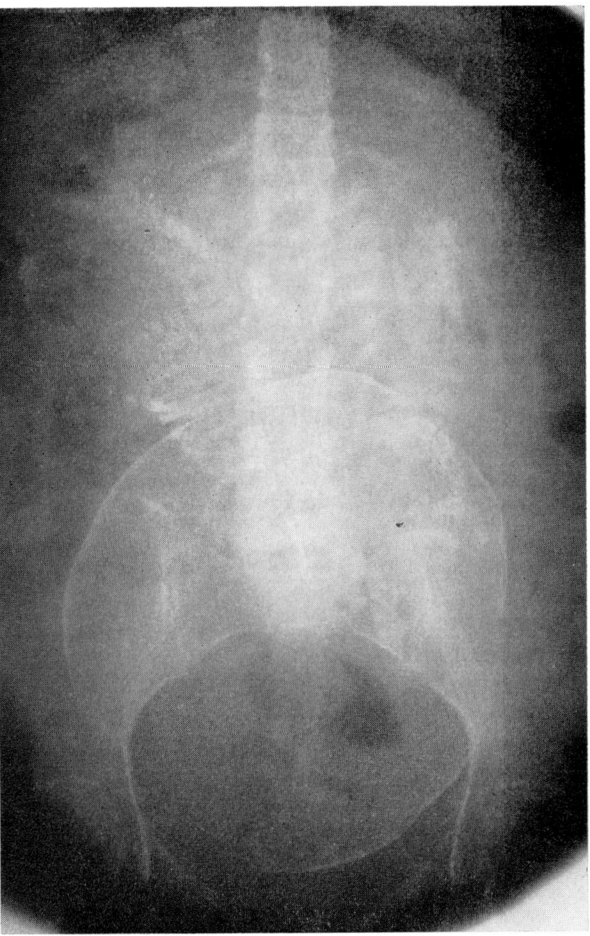

HYDROCEPHALUS IN UTERO. At the time this "obvious diagnosis" was made, the fetus was dead. It was extracted after craniostomy, with no detectable injury to the mother.

trained eye. This is true even in the case of the much more elaborate psychophysiologic studies in roentgen image perception, made by Bill Tuddenham of Philadelphia.

The trained observer has in addition the so-called *insight.* Any professional bird (or girl) watcher can testify to the fact that, for best results, one must know where to look, and have a good idea of what there is to be seen. As the baron and philologist Wilhelm von Humboldt (1767-1835) put it, "to behold is not necessarily to observe" (Garland, 1959). By implication, there is no place left for the unbiased observer. Complete lack of bias can be offered only by one totally ignorant of the topic under consideration (which is obviously undesirable).

In practice, many tangibles and several intangibles play a role, such as overlapping, summation, and/or chance configuration of the shadows. The incidence of "unseen" (undetected, missed) shadows — called *observer error* — has received serious consideration in California, by Garland (1949), and by a mathematican who teaches statistics in the University of California School of Public Health, Jacob Yerushalmy.

On small chest survey films, about one third of suspicion-worthy pulmonary shadows may be overlooked by competent readers. This can be remedied — in part — by double reading (same films read independently by two observers). Since 1958, in this country, large scale chest surveys have become a thing of the past. Should the number of qualified radiologists continue to increase at the rate it does now, double reading may soon be suggested also for large films.

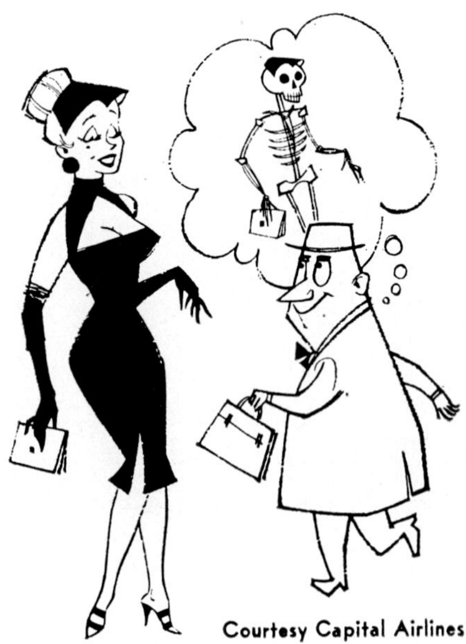

Courtesy Capital Airlines

MISTAKES

If more people were to know of the frequency with which observer errors occur among competent observers, the referring clinicians would become (f)rightfully suspicious of the radiologist who never admits any mistakes. Shrewd roentgen practitioners know that, when an observer (reporting) error is uncovered, the best — indeed, the easiest — way out is to acknowledge it freely, with a statement such as:

Three views of the right foot were re-examined at the request of the referring physician, who pointed out a fracture in the middle phalanx of the fourth toe. This fracture had not been mentioned in the previous report. Its fragments are in good position . . .

Another, somewhat touchier, example might be:

Upright postero-anterior view of the chest was reviewed in the presence of the attending clinician, who requested additional information on the obliterated right costo-phrenic angle, a finding which had not been discussed in the previous report. Moreover, at this time, on close scrutiny, a few ill-defined opaque patches are recognized in the right base.

IMPRESSION: Contrary to the previously issued (esentially negative) report, the appearance is now interpreted as being due to acute, presumably nonspecific inflammatory process, involving both pleura and parenchyma in the right lower hemithorax.

And when the occasion is even more serious than that, it is wise — if only for the sake of good public relations — to use a very hot iron:

Re-examination of the films made after barium meal was prompted by the biopsy report of adenocarcinoma. Surgical exploration had been performed despite the negative report. The operation revealed inoperable gastric malignancy. At this time, in retrospect, a ragged filling defect can be identified . . .

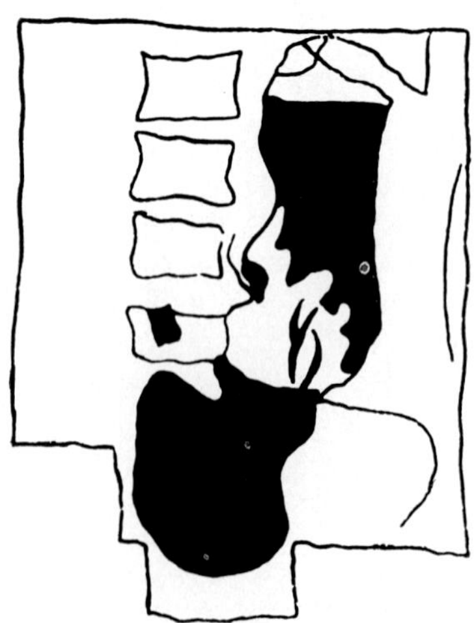

One of Roscoe Miller's favored sentences — used especially under such circumstances — is "don't ride a dead horse!"

As long as such introspective and self-castigating re-adjustments remain relatively infrequent, they are much better received (and a much closer interpersonal relationship with the clinicians can be established) than if futile attempts are made to stick to one's guns and claim that the lesion was below the threshold of visibility.

IDENTIFICATION

Many times, the problem hinges on the accurate recognition of the shadows. A post-bulbar ulcer may be confused with a duodenal diverticulum, and a large diverticulum may resemble a gallbladder (filled with barium through a cholecysto-duodenal fistula).

A linear radiolucency overlying the parietal bone may be a suture, a vessel, or a fracture. Late re-opacification of the right heart chambers during angiocardiography could be due to a left-to-right shunt, or simply to an otherwise insignificant storage of contrast material in the hepatic circulation.

In any of these instances, the wrong choice would seriously affect the quality of the roentgen report.

INTERPRETATION

In 1946, Birkelo *et al.* evaluated the usefulness of photofluorograms versus conventional 14x17 in. films, and found them equally satisfactory for the actual detection of lung "abnormalities." They were appalled, though, by their inability to agree consistently on the presence or absence of a lesion, and even less on its state of activity or inactivity.

Studies published in 1954 by three consummate diagnosticians and teachers of radiology — Newell, Chamberlain, and Rigler — demonstrated a just as obvious lack of reliability (dependability of attaching the same label to a given density) when one set of films had been reviewed by several observers. There was also a tendency toward self-contradiction, when the films were re-interpreted by the same observer after a lapse of time. They could not agree on whether the lesion was active or inactive, sometimes not even on whether it had improved or not!

Apparently, these roentgen shadows are very fallacious, perhaps *abysmally fallacious,* certainly more so than the pioneers had ever suspected them to be.

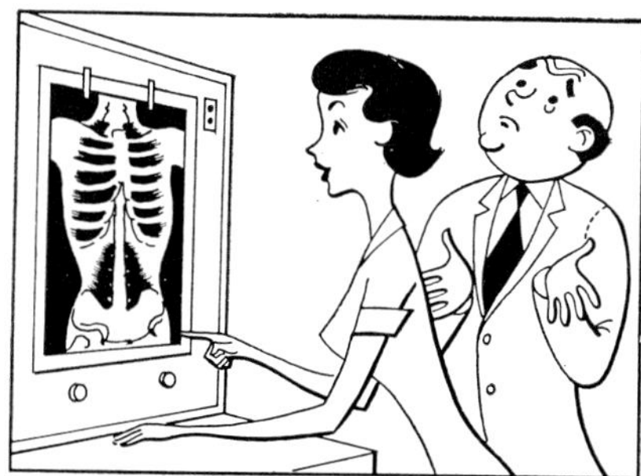

"Oh . . . so it's Mrs. Wintergreen again. She's *really* photogenic, isn't she, doctor?"

RADIO-PATHOLOGIC CONFRONTATION

George Miller wanted it mentioned that when a pathologist (1) sends slides from a patient to another pathologist (2), he always sends along his report. The radiologist (1) seldom if ever sends his interpretation along with requested films. But when the pathologist (2) returns the slides to the first pathologist (1), he attaches his own reading of the slides, if he has made one. The radiologist (2) practically never reports films which were not made under his direct or indirect supervision. Not having performed the respective fluoroscopy is a valid excuse for radiologist (2) in those many instances in which fluoroscopy constitutes an important part of the procedure.

DIAGNOSIS

With shadows so fleeting and deceitful, one wonders how such a thriving "x-ray business" was ever built up? In actual practice these shadows, however fleeting and deceitful, must have had, or may have acquired, a measure of respectability, if not outright dependability.

The term *diagnosis* – διάγνωσιδ – can be found in the Hippocratic Canon. It appears therein in a book on diets, together with the related vocable, *prognosis* – spelled *prodiagnosis,* προδιάγνωσιδ. The Hellenic diagnosis was simply transliterated into Latin, and can be found as such, for instance in the 17th Century (Savona). In Murray's *Dictionary on Historic Principles,* its earliest known usage in English is in a 1681 translation of the *Pharmacopeia* of Willis.

In Eric Partridge's *Origins* of the English Language (1958), the word *diagnosis* is derived from the stem *gnom-* with the root *gno* as in the Greek γνοδιδ (knowledge), a seeking to know, a means of knowing, whence the erudite English *gnosis.* "To diagnose" is regarded (by Partridge) as a back-formation from the Greek *diagnosis* which, in turn, is said to come from διαγιγνώσκειν (in Littré's Hippocrates, it is spelled without the second γ), to distinguish, literally to know through ($\delta\iota\alpha$), something like knowledge in depth.

Consequently, *diagnosis could be defined as the determination of the nature of a condition* (which may but must not necessarily be caused by disease), *as well as the opinion* (more or less formally stated) *which results from the investigation of such a condition.*

PHASES IN ROENTGEN DIAGNOSIS

Over the years, obvious changes became noticeable in the phrasing of roentgen reports, reflecting both the advancement of knowledge, and the changing philosophies of a budding discipline.

Ben Orndoff remembers that a favored saying around 1905 was "x rays are good for bullets, bones, and gallstones."

During the Era of the Roentgen Pioneers, the approach to everything (reporting included) was largely pragmatic. The appearance of a given shadow was equated with a certain condition (whether pathologic or otherwise). Once that given shadow was (thought to have been) detected, the detective felt perfectly justified in inserting at the end of his report the magic caption *diagnosis,* followed by such simple statements as gallstone, pneumonia, or fracture.

Soon, though, the radiologic fraternity began to realize that the shadows could be equated only, if at all, with certain anatomic (macroscopic) modifications. As a result, in the Golden Age of Radiology, they went one step further and, at the bottom of the roentgen report, the final caption (which previously had read diagnosis) was changed to *conclusions.**

During the Atomic Phase further sophistication took place. It became quite clear that similar shadows can be produced by different conditions. It seems more appropriate to interpret these shadows in terms of possible or probable (rather than definite) cause. Thence another change was made in the title of the terminal sentence(s) of the roentgen report. This is why — among knowledgeable reporters — the final paragraph(s) of the roentgen report will now be called (diagnostic) *impressions.*

Two points must be stressed. The correlation between stages in radiologic history and the reporting captions used is inevitably schematic. There are always people ahead and people behind their times. The basic verities of roentgen interpretation had been discovered by the pioneers. Widespread "acceptance" of the "modern" sense of roentgen interpretation came about much later, and gradually.

The other point is that use of the term impression is tantamont to admitting (potential) fallibility. This must not be deplored as an abdication from a position of strength. It is simply an acknowledgment of existing realities. Clinical radiology had been called a scientific discipline. It may eventually reach that stage, but today it is still very definitely a part of medicine, and as such it is not (yet) a science, only an art!*

CONTENT OF A REPORT

It is almost redundant to say that a report consists of: (1) a description of the findings, (2) their interpretation, and (3) recommendations derived therefrom. The most important part is undoubtedly the final sentence of the interpretation, and this is sometimes the only one which survives in the extremely compressed roentgen reports, found here and there.

In times past, many radiologists — for instance, Murray Cass Morrison from London (Ontario) — used to make rather short roentgen reports.

Frederick Henry Baetjer (1874-1933) was the first radiologist and teacher of radiology at Johns Hopkins.

*Don Bauer's main objection centered on the fact that he likes the term *conclusions.* His philosophy is that the radiologist offers a consultation, not a film reading, and is therefore entitled to present his conclusions. That implies utilization of all available methods of examination. In actual practice, the radiologist could not possibly examine all the patients on whom he sees films (I couldn't). Should *conclusions* be used when reporting on patients on whom a physical was done by the radiologist, and *impressions* on the others? And if one starts doing physicals, how detailed must they be? Without a physical examination of the patient, I only dare to offer channels for the diagnostic thoughts of the attending clinicians, and for such a purpose I feel *impressions* suffice.

*When it comes to the prerogatives of radiology, George Miller is as sensitive as a gouty toe. On the margin of my "artistic" quip, he pencilled the sentence, "Radiology is perhaps not perfect, but it certainly is not all art!" Shall we fight about percentages?

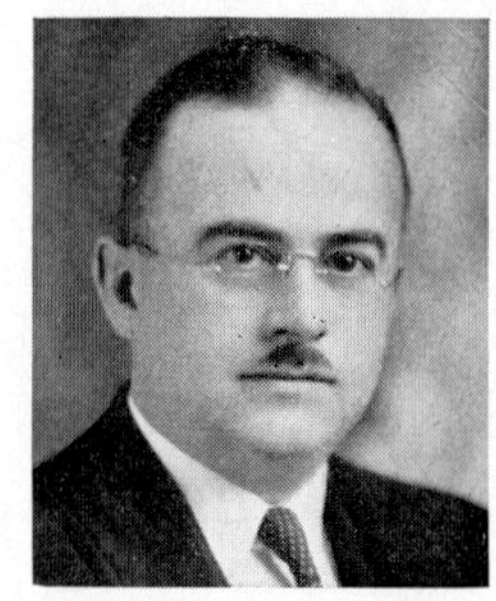

MURRAY CASS MORRISON

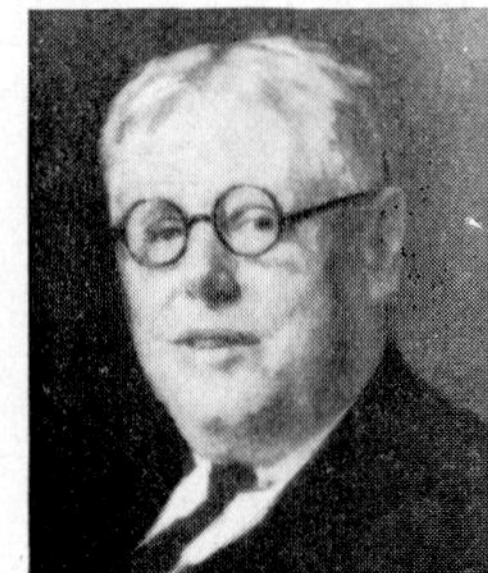

FREDERICK BAETJER

Despite his handicap (only one eye), he was unquestionably what the trade calls an "uncanny" diagnostician. His reports exhibited a telegraphic style, consisting of single (sometimes incomplete) sentences, as in the following example.*

Elliott, Thompson #151775
Head: Posterior clinoid very indistinct.
Sinuses: Clear
L. Tibia: Periostitis of tibia, probably luetic.
Dr. Baetjer.

Use of such a clear-cut etiologic diagnosis (lues!) makes one feel like quoting the first English printer, William Caxton (1422-1491): "He maketh non euidence for in neyther side he telleth what moeueth him so for to saye!"

Even when a negative report contains a *single word,* it still implies that (a) no findings worthy of mention were encountered, which (b) was interpreted as meaning absence of pathology, thus (c) no further recommendations are necessary.

NORMAL

Unfortunately, that famous single word—*normal*—is still very often employed in summarizing the results of a negative examination. Such abuse is a totally unwarranted positive assumption, *i.e.,* the observer has no basis of fact for it.

The word comes from the Latin *norma,* a carpenter's square, hence a rule of conduct, or *norm.* The corresponding Latin adjective, *normalis* (patterned after or made with a carpenter's square) acquired also a figurative meaning, likewise accepted in the English language. In the *Glossographia,* a dictionary of difficult words published in London in 1656 by Thomas Blount (1618-1679), *normal* is given as right by rule, made by the square or rule! Since early 19th Century, normal is also used popularly as constituting, conforming to, not deviating or differing from the usual, the common type or standard, the general, regular, familiar, ordinary, natural, typical, customary, habitual, and so on.

Biologists – including radiologists such as Lusted (and his mathematician, Keats) – are happier when they can obtain numerical guidelines to substantiate their statements. When measurements performed on many individuals are plotted on a system of coordinates, the result is always a *normal* curve, *i.e.,* a bell-shaped frequency distribution. Actually, both legs of the curve are asymptotic to the base line, and thus *theoretically* have no limited range.

This curve of normal probability was discovered by Abraham de Moivre (1667-1754), a Huguenot refugee in England. Being renowned as a mathematician, he was chosen to arbitrate between Newton and Leibniz, after both claimed the invention of infinitesimal calculus. While in London, de Moivre, who needed money, is said to have solved, for an adequate compensation, gambling problems submitted by wealthy clients. He discovered the *normal* curve in the course of just such a mathematical analysis of the probabilities involved in tossing a coin. De Moivre's* normal curve is currently providing the mathematical basis for most of the statistical computations in biology.

In science, the normal range is the computed or estimated deviation from the median (mean, average), determined by one of de Moivre's bell-shaped curves. Whatever falls within the (more or less arbitrarily) accepted range of deviation is normal. Since there is an all-or-none principle in biology, those who fall right on the median line are not any more normal than the others.

NON SEQUITUR

Chest examinations comprise about 30-35 per cent of the workload of the average (normal?) radiologist. Many of these chest films are taken as a matter of routine. This may be why a very tempting, and possibly the more frequent, use of the term normal is in *normal chest.*

What the observer actually wants to say is that he had found nothing unusual. When pressed, he might qualify his initial statement by specifying *radiographically normal chest,* or by the (semantically nonsensical) *chest within normal limits.* The inevitable

*Personal communication from Russell Morgan, currently professor of radiology in Baetjer's place.

*Marshall Brucer told me that the normal curve had been described long before de Moivre, perhaps as early as the 15th Century.

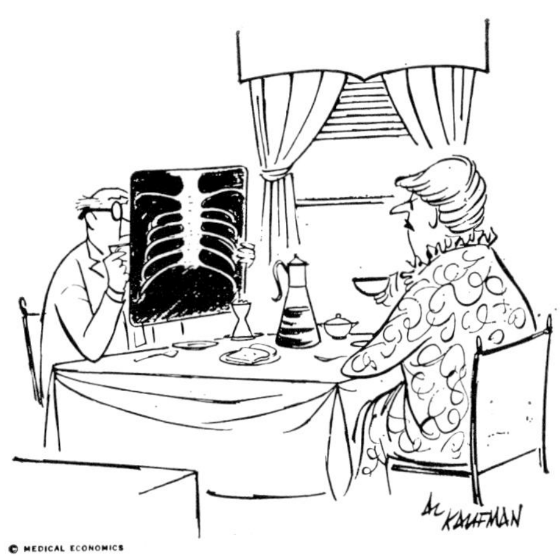

MEDICAL ECONOMICS · APRIL 11, 1960

question arises: what are the limits of the normal chest? In this context four categories of findings may be discussed.

1. There exist minute, easily detected deviations, such as hilar calcifications (when not confused with vessels seen on end), minimal pleuritic scarring, healed rib fractures, one isolated apical or cardiophrenic bleb, or calcified aortic knob (without enlargement of the heart). Can these be called, in all honesty, *normal?* Are asymptomatic senescent features *normal?*

When hilar calcifications are said to be within normal limits, is that based on some established *norm,* such as number and/or size per square (or rather per cubic) inch of hilar tissue – or does that go by feel?

Small, easily disregarded changes may actually be the residual of an extinct (but not necessarily healed) inflammatory process. When partial pneumonectomy (segmental resection) is performed without removing any ribs, its only obvious reminder may be healed rib fractures (due to overactive spreading during surgery). Of course, an experienced observer (who has seldom the time to do that) could follow the vascular pattern and discover that a branch is missing. Can such a lung stump (however uninvolved) ever be called normal?

When a pulmonary "coin lesion" remains unchanged on films taken over a period of several years, it is commonly discounted and labeled as *normal.* But a surgeon can get tired of nostalgically looking at the "coin" especially because – as iterated and reiterated by Larry Rubenstein of Cook County and Michael Reese Hospital – even an eight or ten year old "coin" may turn out to be a (latent?) squamous cell carcinoma, which had failed to act the way a "normal" malignancy is supposed to (overact?!).

2. There are minute changes which cannot be given a definite pathologic significance, as least not on the first film seen. But when examined with Leo Rigler's *retrospectoscope* (1950), after a "lesion" has been discovered, a prominent vascular marking or some such triviality can often be found on the very spot on which the subsequently obvious organic alteration was to develop.

3. In the third category are findings which become evident only with the help of additional investigation (be it a simple lateral view, a tomographic study, or such complicated procedures as bronchography or angiocardiography). The lesions were there all the time (so that chest was obviously not normal).

4. Certain anatomo-pathologic (usually histologic, but sometimes macroscopic) lesions are simply below the threshold of demonstrability by any of the currently available roentgen methods. Indeed, no lesion will become roentgen visible unless and until there appears within it one or more areas with x-ray absorption coefficients different from the immediate vicinity.

Wilhelm Max Wundt (1832-1920), a German psychologist, physiologist, and philosopher, called *negative sensations* those produced by stimuli below the threshold of *positive sensations.* Unfortunately, the existence of such subclinical sensations is today no longer accepted, but in roentgen interpretations the play on words can still be used and is offered for just such a facetious purpose.

Non-sequitur — in Dagobert Runes' *Dictionary of Philosophy* (1942) — is any fallacy in which there is a lack of connection between the premises advanced and the conclusions drawn. How can anyone take as a premise his failure to detect (what he considers significant) abnormalities on a single, frontal view of the chest, and conclude that its owner has a *normal* chest? The fact that this unwarranted assumption

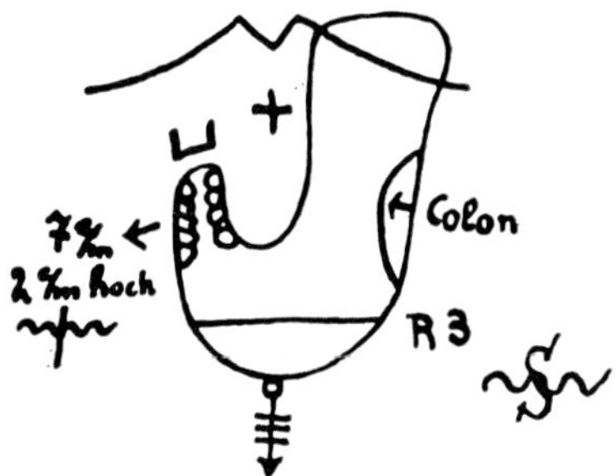

Pictorial reporting. Several schemes had been proposed for the summarization of roentgen findings by means of line drawings interspersed with brief notations. To be successful, such a method must be self-explanatory, as well as easy to memorize. The above example is from a method devised by E. Rosenthal, and used at the time of World War I in the first Department of Internal Medicine in the University of Budapest (the method was explained in a paper by Erwin Kolta, in 1924). The arrow with the three cross hatches means that this (hook shaped) stomach is located three finger breadths above the umbilicus. The indentation by the colon is self-explanatory. The fluid level indicates residual secretion, three finger breadths high. The wave symbol, with the capital S (for *schwach,* puny) signifies sluggish overall peristalsis. The cross is the location of pain on pressure over the epigastrium, but not over a specific location referable to the gastro-intestinal tract. Finally, there is a filling defect in the antrum, seven centimeters long, and two centimeters tall, with no peristalsis going through it. None of these logographic attempts lasted much longer than, or spread beyond the working place of, their authors.

turns out to be usually (because of statistical probability) correct cannot justify the continued usage of such a fallacious statement.

NORMAL = HEALTHY?

Pancoast, Baetjer, and Dunham investigated in 1922 the "chests of normal children." They realized the liabilities of the term *normal,* and this is why, in 1927, they suggested its replacement with the term *healthy.* Their suggestion was accepted, and *healthy* became part of the standard nomenclature of the National Tuberculosis Association. But it had been an unfortunate semantic choice, and had to be discarded.

It was actually a patent boner. Health — just as life (Grigg, 1956) or happiness — cannot be defined, except in retrospect *(a posteriori).* If normalcy* could be divided into a finite number of qualifications, and if every one of these qualifications were measurable (to determine the respective normal ranges), then normalcy might be "defined." Even then, a healthy individual with six fingers could hardly be called normal!

A priori, neither normalcy, nor healthy, can be determined in any other way than by exclusion. This leaves an inherent margin of error, which depends on the comprehensiveness of the examination.

"A very markedly healthy chest" is the definition given for *healthy chest 4* in the system of stenographic roentgen reporting, conceived in the late 1930's by Duncan McRae, at the Tuberculosis Sanatorium in Ninette, Manitoba.**

Healthy chest 2 meant "slight bronchial thickening." *Subminimal chest* signified "suspicion of tuberculosis, but film-shadows are not sufficient in themselves and lack adequate confirmation." There were also many outright cryptic notations, such as *RD up 2, tied* (right hemidiaphragm elevated and fixed) or *Th W cav up 4, fl* (very large thick-walled cavity at the apex with a fluid level).

Actually, it would be correct to use the word *normal* in roentgen reports, but only when applied to numbers *e.g., normal heart measurements.* In such instances, though, the term *average* approximates much more closely the intended sense, because it implies a statistical correlation, which is not so obvious in the word *normal.*

Knowing the limitations of diagnostic radiology, introduction of the term *normal* in roentgen reports (except with reference to actual measurements) is an obvious *non sequitur.*

RADAR NORMALCY

When flying a light plane into an area of restricted visibility, the pilot might want to contact the nearest FSS (Flight Service Station), to find out whether there is any other aerial traffic in the vicinity. The controller (who, at least in this respect, is shrewder than "normal" radiologists) will never answer "there is no traffic!" The typical (negative) reply is "no traffic reported."

Even if the contacted air traffic controller were to sit in front of a radar scope, he would not make a

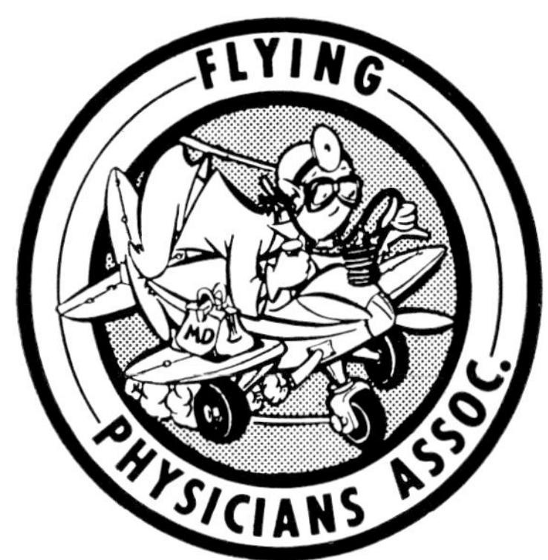

positive statement (absence of other planes in the area), but only something like "no (other) traffic identified." Of course, visualized blips will be properly reported, *e.g.,* target ten o'clock four miles *(from your present position),* northeast bound, altitude unknown."

NEGATIVE

This term, which is of pure Latin origin, has a long tradition in the English language. It can be found in translation of the bible (1380) by John Wicklyffe (1320?-1384). For our purposes, an adequate definition was given by the English philosopher Isaac Watts (1674-1748): ". . . a negation is the absence of that which does not naturally belong to the thing we are

---

*One of the premises, on which Eugene Ionesco based his surrealistic play *Rhinoceros,* is that normalcy cannot be defined.

**Edward Ross, medical director of the Manitoba Sanatorium Board, and Alfred Paine, thoracic surgeon and superintendent at Ninette, graciously explained that the method was used for some time at Ninette, then dropped as too time-consuming. Duncan McRae, although in his seventies and greatly incapacitated by tuberculosis, was still doing part-time medical work at Ninette in 1961.

speaking of." A more modern version is "devoid of, or lacking in, distinctly positive attributes."

The negation may be all encompassing, such as

Four views of the right ankle, including one axial projection for the calcaneus, are negative for evidence of dislocation, of recent fracture, or of any other visible bone abnormalities, which does not rule out soft tissue injury or disease.

The phrase carries a redundancy of negatives, one more than the four of which Shakespeare's clown (*Twelfth Night* v, 1, 24) complained they might yield two affirmatives, and that he felt was ill counsel. In roentgen reports, though, it is advisable to circumscribe one's statement very carefully, otherwise — should the case wind up in court — the always ill-intended opposing counsel will grasp at any straw which might help him stir up a controversy.

The all-encompassing *roentgen negative* statement appeared very early in the history of radiology. A classic example can be found in 1897: "Negatively, we are assured (by comparison of this print with other prints of the normal skull) that no deviations, malformations, or abnormal growth, dental or otherwise, exist" (Morton).

Actually, when reporting a skull examination — in a patient who had been exposed to trauma — one must specify whether the *skull proper* and/or the *facial bones* had been radiographed. In this territory, the term *linear fracture* is preferable to *recent fracture* — for instance, *five views of the skull proper (including a basilar projection) reveal no linear fracture . . .* — because some of these fracture lines persist indefinitely.

NORMAL = NEGATIVE?

Most radiologists are perfectly aware of the fact that the word *normal* is highly objectionable when used in roentgen reports. Some think they can avoid the issue by speaking of a *negative chest,* a *negative gallbladder,* or simply of *negative findings.* Not only do they continue to convey the meaning of *normality,* they also add insult to injury by using a wrong word: *normal* is by its very sense a positive concept and cannot be expressed by a negation!

In the final analysis, when reporting a "normal" case, all the radiologist can say is that he did not find anything of that which (in Watt's opinion) does not belong there. If this is the only thing he can say, this is all he should say — *the examination was negative for . . .* (for whatever they were looking). But *Essentially negative peroral cholecystogram* is a radio-

L. HENRY GARLAND, M.B.
HAROLD A. HILL, M.D.
M. E. MOTTRAM, M.D.
M. A. SISSON, M.D.
J. H. HEALD, M.D.

REPORT ON ROENTGEN EXAMINATION
OF

Mrs. Marian Chan

AT THE REQUEST OF DR. G. W. Douglas

REGION Barium Enema DATE August 5, 1959

The colon outlines readily. No constant defects are seen. On attempted evacuation it empties well.

Conclusion: No x-ray evidence of organic lesion.

g/f

FRED O. COE, M.D.
EDGAR M. MCPEAK, M.D.
JAMES E. WISSLER, M.D.
RALPH M. CAULK, M.D.
C. E. BICKHAM, JR., M.D.
U. VINCENT WILCOX, M.D.
KARL C. CORLEY, M.D.
F. V. SCHUMACHER, M.D.
GREGORY T. HENESY, M.D.
ALBERT J. MIELE, M.D.

TELEPHONE REPUBLIC 7-4600

DRS. GROOVER, CHRISTIE AND MERRITT
1835 EYE STREET, N. W.
WASHINGTON 6, D. C.

RADIOLOGISTS TO
DOCTORS HOSPITAL AND WASHINGTON HOSPITAL CENTER

THOMAS A. GROOVER, M.D. 1916-1940
EDWIN A. MERRITT, M.D. 1919-1946
ARTHUR C. CHRISTIE, M.D. 1916-1956

Report of roentgen findings in the case of Mrs. Mary Brown
1-6-61 for Dr. Arnold McNitt
1835 Eye St., N. W., Washington, D. C.

Examination of the chest shows no evidence of abnormality of the bony framework, heart, great blood vessels, lungs or pleurae. foc/aam

Fred O. Coe

transparent fake for *Essentially normal gallbladder (study).*

One may actually delete the very word negative, as long as its sense is preserved — by substituting absence of evidence:

Five views of dorsal and lumbar segments of the spine reveal no evidence of metastatic bone activity, nor any other visible changes in bone texture.

NAF (no abnormalities found) is the formula used by A. J. Cawley (who is both MD and DVM), professor and chairman of the Department of Radiology in Ontario Veterinary College in Guelph (Canada).

HEDGING

Henry Cecil Herbert Bull of London wrote in 1935: "There are three sorts of reports; positive, negative, and indeterminate." Bull's third category of roentgen reports might be just the thing of which complained, in 1550, the Bishop of Ossory, John Bale (1495-1563): "But I founde therein no answere appoynted to be made, neyther by affirmacion nor yet negacion!"

To hedge (synonym: to fence) meant originally – according to the *Oxford Dictionary* – to surround oneself with a hedge for purposes of defense. Among its figurate meanings, given in the *Webster Dictionary,* is to safeguard oneself from loss (on a bet or speculation) by making compensatory arrangements on the other side. The meaning to which we are going to refer herein is to arrange ways of escape from any position taken, specifically to use reservations and qualifications so as not to commit oneself definitely one way or another.

The use of reservations and qualifications in roentgen reports is a very honorable and time-honored, practice. It is also very necessary because it reminds everybody that the roentgen method itself is fallible. Perhaps every blank (used for typing roentgen reports) should have imprinted on the bottom of the page a few words of warning, as a sort of post-scriptum: *P.S. This report does not mention: (1) a few shadows which were not seen because they were not looked at, nor (2) those shadows which may have been looked at, but were not seen because of their small size, lack of contrast, or similarly obscuring factors, and certainly not (3) the shadows which (although both looked at and seen) were ignored because the signer of this report has not yet learned what significance, if any, they have.*

Anyone unwilling to sign such a statement is unaware of the limitations of roentgen reporting, and may not be ready to report films without adequate supervision.

All those hedging vocables (essential, significant, apparent, visible, gross, probable, assumed, and so on) should only be used to emphasize the fallaciousness of roentgen shadows in general. They are of no help (nor were they intended to serve) as a built-in face-saving device for the eventuality that initially "unseen" shadows were to come to the fore at some later date.

On seeing the very first film of a certain patient, one might have used the phrase *no essential abnormalities in the examination of the chest.* A barium meal, performed the next day, demonstrates a big hiatus hernia. The first chest film is then re-viewed – perhaps in the

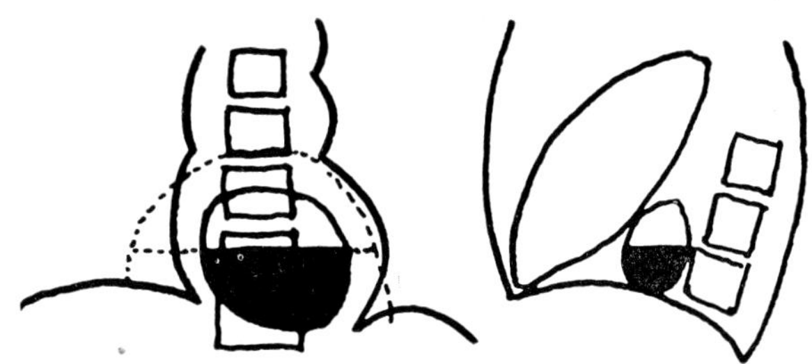

presence of the attending clinician – and now (like Banquo haunting Macbeth) the horrible shadow of the thoracic stomach is *lurking in a double shade* (Wordsworth) behind the heart. It would be both foolish and ridiculous to point to the term *essential* and claim it had covered just such contingencies. *It would have covered* the hiatus hernia (or an aneurysm of the descending aorta) – *if the incriminating shadow(s) could not be identified, in retrospect,* on the original chest film.

Likewise, when reporting the films of a single extremity of a youngster with growing epiphyses, instead of refusing to interpret before viewing films of the opposite side, it is preferable to say *Two views of the . . . show no gross evidence of dislocation or of recent fracture . . . but, if in doubt, comparison with the opposite side may be requested to exclude epiphyseal separation.* If an obvious fracture turns out to have been missed on the initially interpreted views, one must never try to hide behind the *no gross evidence.* It was not intended for this purpose; such an ill-advised attempt would only make things worse.

RETREAT

A special type of negative hedging is the tendency (which may become a habit) to dodge issues by demanding repeat examination(s). It is sometimes done with the subconscious (?!) hope that — in the interim — the clinician might stumble unaided over the answer. In large institutions, the next time around, that case could befall another member of the staff.

Pertinent in this respect is a piece of doggerel, culled from the admonition of an anonymous instructor (working in a well-known Midwestern institution) as offered to incoming residents in radiology:

First you look at all those shades,
Then describe them in charades,
Mixed with negative tirades.
Finally, to make it neat,
Order also a repeat!

When the bulb is very small,
Or defects sprawl in its wall,
Or there is no bulb at all
Show that you are quite discreet,
Sternly ask for a repeat!

Is that stone now on the go?
Is that kidney high or low?
Do you see its pelvis? No?
Never ever grant defeat,
Call instead for a repeat!

Of course, there are very legitimate instances in which the request for a repeat examination is mandatory (rather than permitted). This applies especially to the so-called "surgical" cases.

RARE BIRDS

There is another sort of *negative fencing,* or, rather, a negative fencing of sorts. Its psychologic infra-structure is the fact that it often appears easier to say what it is not — instead of having to commit oneself to saying what it is.

In obscure cases, the more numerous the *negative* possibilities listed in the differential diagnosis, the better the chances are for having included the right one. This exercise in futility is typical for a certain breed of (negative?) radiologists, interested mainly in nosologic rarities. Every teaching center has at least one represensative specimen of this radiologic mutant.

A trivial pneumonitis, a Pott's fracture, a duodenal ulcer cannot commend their undivided attention. They are interested only in "exciting" items such as agenesis of the lung, renal rickets, or perhaps ulcerated ("bull's eye") melanosarcomatous deposits in the intestine. When asked for a consultation, the "rare-bird" radiologist will always throw in, like *pearls before swine,* the mention of some such remote alternative.

To crowd the differential diagnosis with alternates fits in well with what the transcendental idealist Immanuel Kant (1724-1802) called a *noumenon* (anti-phenomenon), that is an object of purely intellectual intuition, devoid of all phenomenal (realistic) attributes. A naughty internist once defined such a *noumenon* as the maladive figment of a negative radiologic imagination.

GLORIFIED GUESSERS

The film reading session is a time-tested function at radiologic meetings. A moderator presents a series of films to a panel of three or four radiologists, who are supposed to make the diagnosis on the basis of sketchy or misleading additional information. There is usually a thick crowd in attendance, especially when the moderator is as popular as the pungent Garland or the hilarity-seeking Felson.

The teaching value of these guessing games remains debatable. The cases shown are usually of the "rare bird" variety, often include instances resembling "unique" case-histories published in the literature during the preceding year or two.

In many ways, film reading sessions are show business. Television's rigged $64 Thousand Question and the phony wrestling matches have shown that the audience likes to see the underdog win, in this case the panelist. They do not enjoy seeing the guesser stumped, and if there is need for collusion to avoid such a stunning, the intelligent moderator will find an avenue of communication with the panel.

It has been said that the brilliant differential diagnosis offered by the panelists are the really important part of those sessions. That reminds me of Peter of Abano (1250-1315), one of the most respected medical teachers in the University of Padua (Italy), who was renowned for his sharp scholastic analysis. In the presence of a very critical audience, one of his adversaries (to make collusion impossible) would read a letter from a patient describing his symptoms, whereupon Peter would analyze those symptoms in terms of humors (water, blood, bile, black bile) and other qualities (warm, cold, dry, humid), make a full differential diagnosis, and indicate the "appropriate" treatment, basely solely on the symptoms described in the letter. Peter's medical advice was quite sought-after and very well paid, so it must have achieved "some" results.

Consider a film reading session in the 1950s, during which a panelist made a diagnosis of malignancy of the bone whereupon — to the enthusiastic applause of the audience — the pathologic report called it chondrosarcoma. But many of those chondrosarcoma cases survived ten and fifteen years after diagnosis, which is why we have created a benign subgroup among these tumors, and labeled them chondroblastoma. The similarity between this panelist and Peter of Abanao is one of degree. One of my favored sayings is that a diagnosis is valid only for a given generation, a given time, and a given place.

Is anybody willing to predict how posterity is going to judge today's "glorified guessers." (who are really "kissing cousins" of the previously mentioned negative radiologists?

NEGATIVE RECOMMENDATIONS

Since the discovery of tubercle bacilli there had existed a widespread tuberculophobia, which is just subsiding. Its only justified remnant is the chest film, required as part of the routine pre-employment examination in most public, and in many private, organizations. Certain industries include also roentgen studies of the lumbo-sacral spine, because of the medico-legal pressure of numerous compensation claims based on allegedly service-connected injury with low back pain. In all such cases, the pre-employment examination is supposed to eliminate those regarded as bad risks, and to establish a baseline for the others.

In any pre-employment examination, the radiologist is expected to make a clear statement on whether the applicant should or should not be employed. But the films have to be correlated with clinical, laboratory, and other findings before they acquire definite validity. Hence, a semantic way must be found to convey the information derived from the films, without making unwarranted assumptions. One of three situations may arise:

1. *Nothing special was found.* A simple negation will suffice. For those employers who still cling to the myth of thus detecting tuberculosis, a good formula is *No evidence of active pulmonary tuberculosis, on the chest examination, nor of any other visible contraindication to employment.*

2. *Obvious findings warrant rejection.* After describing those findings (in detail or sketchily, whichever is demanded by local custom), the impression should contain another type of negative statements, *e.g., employment cannot be recommended.*

3. *The findings are pathological but not decisive.* This is when the eternal demand for clinical correlation comes into legitimate play. Suppose fibrotic appearing inflammatory residuals are found in the upper lobes. Experience has shown that inactive lesions are at times contagious, while active lesions may never spill virulent micro-organisms. It is difficult (if not impossible) to determine from a single film whether visible lesions are or are not active and/or contagious. The statement suggested for the impression would then be: *In view of the presence of pulmonary lesions, suspicious of acid fast origin, applicant cannot be recommended for employment unless and until adequate clinical and bacteriologic work-up rules out activity and/or contagiousness.* The clinician will then decide what is *adequate* in that particular instance.

TELLER

These negative statements of positive facts are culled from wordings used under similar circumstances by Ernest Teller (1900-1959), late chief of the Tuberculosis Control Service of the Department of Public Welfare, with jurisdiction over all public mental institutions in the State of Illinois.

In that office Teller had been preceded by several specialists, each of whom claimed to have initiated (fathered) the anti-tuberculous program in Illinois' mental hospitals. With so many "fathers" the progeny

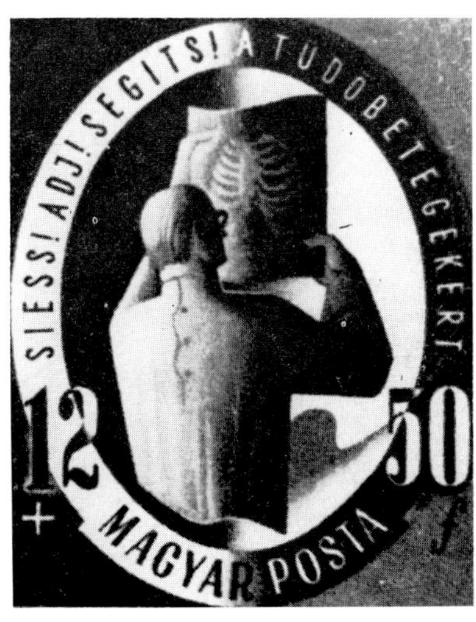

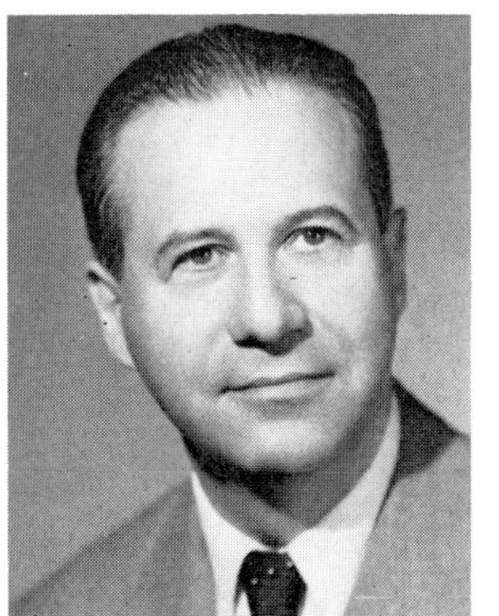

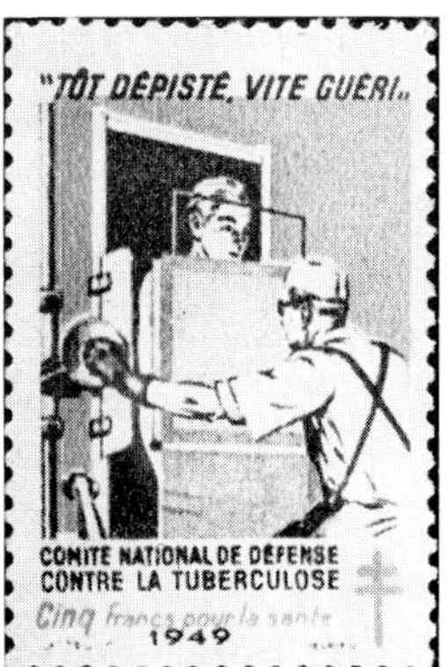

Courtesy: Illinois Tuberculosis Association.

Ernest Teller. After so many "fathers," "mother" had a coronary.

had not fared too well. Teller never claimed paternity: rather, as a good "mother," he only wanted to make a go of it, and in this he succeeded beyond any doubt. As a Vienna-trained pediatrician, he had a thorough background of general medicine. While reading over two hundred thousand chest films in Illinois mental institutions during World War II, he developed a "chest eye" (as keen as Vidar's, the mythical Scandinavian sage who could see through everything): Teller's other eye was usually focused on a bedspread or some such potentially tuberculo-contaminated object.

Teller was not always eager to partake of his knowledge (or of his intuition), and he exhibited frequently a streak of sardonic wit ("Your speed is improving, you may soon be reading films before they are developed!"). Among his other characteristics was a slightly waddling gait and, above all, an indomitable energy, which carried him through his first myocardial infarction. One year later came a second (fulminatingly fatal) episode of coronary occlusion. On the very last day of his earthly sojourn, Teller was so busy and intent on working that – for all we know – he may still be reporting chest films, and waddling after bedspreads, somewhere beyond the visible horizon.

EVIDENCE

When used correctly in roentgen reports, *negative* stands either for *negative result of examination* or *negative for evidence of* as in *Negative for evidence of recent bone trauma.*

George Holmes used to say "The longer the report, the more mistakes one is likely to make." (Shehadi)* Even more so, in the absence of positive findings, when pressed for time, one may want to shorten the report, and delete the negative description. As soon as a significantly larger number of qualified radiologists will be(come) available for interpretation, such a justification will no longer be timely.

In many ways, redundant reporting is akin to a check list. When the radiologist says, either into the microphone or to his secretary, *both breasts are visualized,* he is less likely to merely glimpse into the "straight Hellespont between the Sestos and Abydos of her breasts."** He is then also much less likely to overlook a missing breast.

When a breast has been amputated, that chest is no longer a subject fit for a negative report. The patient may have been referred for a routine check-up* but the surgeon expects a statement regarding possible metastases. The typical report, when the examination was negative, would be:

Upright postero-anterior view of the chest shows absence of the right breast shadow and of part of the outline of the right pectoralis major, while these structures are well identified on the opposite side. Hypertrophic changes are seen in the acromio-clavicular joints, and cervical spine, but the osseous texture is otherwise unremarkable. The aortic knob is calcified. The heart is not enlarged.

IMPRESSION: 1. Right (presumably radical) mastectomy; no evidence of metastatic activity in either lungs or bones. 2. Senescent features.

*Personal communication.

**The quote is from John Donne (1571?-1631): *Elegies* No. 18.

EVIDENCE OF SIGHT

In following modern statisticians the radiologist Steven Ernest Ross (formerly of San Francisco, now in Pittsburgh) gauges the accuracy of biologic investigations by counting separately the *false positives* and the *false negatives.* In the preceding pages, a (fairly) strong case was made for including certain "uncertainties" in all negative reports (negative hedging) as a built-in reminder of the existence of *false negatives,* meaning negative reports offered while existing positive findings remained "unseen." *False positive*

*The need to "educate referring physicians (in the hope of obtaining more information) is as old as radiology. In a discussion which followed a paper by Batten (1930), a British confrère, Miles, told of the patient who came to him with the clinician's notation "Query, chest" to which he returned the answer "*Chest present, but feeble.*"

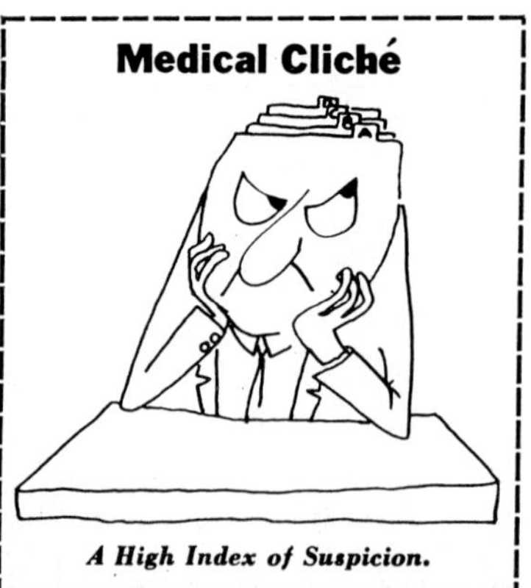

Cartoon by Olden. It was first published in the *Medical Tribune* (New York City) on October 9, 1961 and is herein reproduced with their and the artist's gracious permission.

roentgen reports, *i.e.*, trivial findings given undue significance, come under the caption of over-reading.

There is also another type of *false positive* reports, as when traumatic origin is assumed in the case of a predominantly pathologic fracture. Of special interest are instances classified as roentgen malingering. To detect them one needs not only a very high index of suspicion, but also a thorough knowledge of (all?) existing possibilities.

During the occupation of Belgium in World War II, deportees to forced labor camps had routine chest films prior to departure. One of the underground physicians, using barium suspension, painted cavities (with fluid level, surrounding infiltration, and all) right on the skin of some of the prospective deportees. The "candidates" were also instructed to mention blood-tinged sputa during the anamnesis. Their films were dutifully interpreted as showing cavitary tuberculosis. History does not record how many were thus saved from concentration camps, nor whether the deception was ever perceived.

Some circumstantial evidence is very strong, as when you find a trout in the milk (Thoreau). Under less extreme circumstances, those *who in the shades of sorrow dwell* (Wordsworth) should add a dose of humility to the certainty of their roentgen interpretations.

C. A. Good *(et altera)* reported an instance when easily demonstrable pulmonary cavities, with sputum smears positive for acid-fast organisms, were not due to tuberculosis. This occurrence is no longer unusual. It is currently called *mycobacteriosis*, a condition caused by chromogens and other strains of acid-fast (and yet non-tuberculous) micro-organisms.

Terms such as resembling, have the appearance of, compatible or consistent with, will convey the same information, without assuming a degree of infallibility. Remember that the *evidence of sight* must always be *corrected by the judgment!*

SIGHT OF EVIDENCE

In 1393, John Gower said of theology that it "giveth evidence of thing which is nought bodily." Radiology bases at least some of its evidence on faith (in the reporter's shadow-recognizing abilities).

In 1922, Alfred Rosario Potvin, who was then teaching radiology in Université Laval (Quebec) — he is now the Registrar of Tumors — coined a beautiful sentence to describe the characteristics of roentgen symptoms: "These symptoms are often proteiform, a few times paradoxical, but never contradictory and seldom pathognomonic."

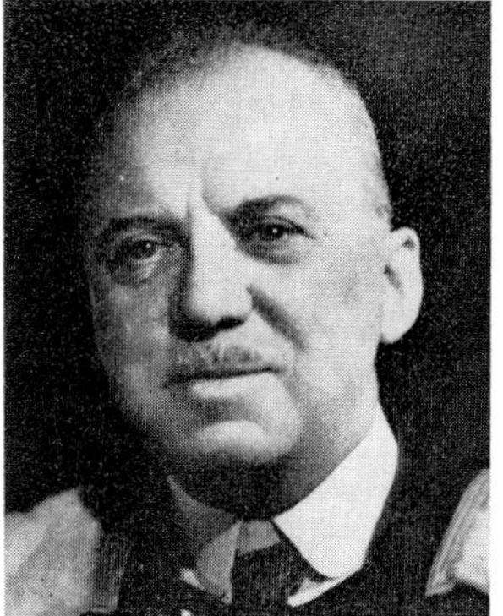
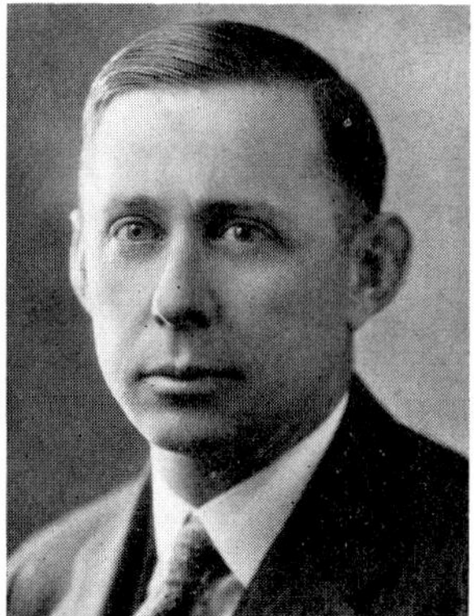

ALFRED ROSARIO POTVIN. A request for a portrait had been modestly refused; thereupon I asked René Bureau, professor of geology in Université Laval, to provide me with this likeness of our common friend. The "youngster" is WILLIAM WALTER WASSON.

In 1936, William Walter Wasson of Denver — who in 1922 had compared the roentgen method with microscopy — developed the idea further, and discussed roentgen syndromes.

It follows that the "fleeting image of a shade" *(the thing nought bodily)* must first be translated into a sign before it can be accepted in evidence. And when it is finally accepted, it is no longer regarded as a shadow, but as the representation of an anatom(o-patholog)ic situation. Such acceptance demands a solid dose of circumspection: in 1866 John Stuart Mill had emphasized that evidence is not that to which the mind does, or must yield to, but that to which it ought to yield.

RADIOLOGIC (ROENTGEN) DIAGNOSIS

By definition, a radiologic (roentgen) diagnosis is the more or less formal statement issued as a result of the radiologic investigation. Actually, a summarizing account can be given after any of the three steps, previously described. In the stage of *detection,* one might offer a *descriptive,* or a (roentgen) *symptomatic* diagnosis. After *identification* of the shadow, one should arrive at a *morphologic* or *anatomic* diagnosis. Finally, during the *interpretation,* which includes causal considerations, one may reach an *etiologic,* if not *histologic,* diagnosis.

Examples are *triangular opacity right base* (descriptive diagnosis) – *consolidation of middle lobe* (anatomic diagnosis) – *non-specific pneumonitis* (etiologic diagnosis), or *ragged narrowing in mid-esophagus* (symptomatic diagnosis) – *incomplete organic obstruction* (morphologic diagnosis) – *probably squamous-cell carcinoma* (histologic diagnosis). Some of the twin appellations, such as *anatomic* and *morphologic*, are almost interchangeable.

Several roentgen symptoms may be united into a roentgen syndrome, for instance *radiolucent areas in ribs, vertebral facets, and pelvis; absence of right breast shadow with deformity of pectoralis major and linear opacities in projection of periphery of second right anterior interspace* (roentgen symptoms) – *amputation of right breast with fibrosis right upper lobe and disseminated osteolytic lesions* (roentgen syndrome) – *bone metastases following* (despite) *irradiation of right axilla and amputation of carcinomatous right breast* (histologic diagnosis).

At times – as with a *staghorn calculus* – no description is needed, and the symptomatic diagnosis coincides with the morphologic identification, which also implies a certain nosologic classification, *i.e.*, nephrolithiasis. Evidently, this could be but the symptom of a systemic disease.

Such a tri-partite view is obviously schematic, and may not fit all situations. In most fracture cases, the etiology is obviously traumatic, and therefore automatically deleted. And yet, just by thinking of bone-softening etiologies, one will miss fewer pathologic fractures than otherwise.

On occasion, the intermediate diagnosis seems superfluous. After a descriptive statement such as *calcifications surrounding large niche carved within extensive gastric filling defect,* it may seem redundant to interpose *ulcerated tumor* instead of going directly to *possible leiomyo(sarco)ma.* But the redundant way may be the safer way (*cf., American Journal of Medicine* of October, 1961).

Despite its shortcomings, the triple gradation of roentgen diagnoses is very useful. It clarifies certain basic issues, and is all-around helpful also for didactic purposes. It can be used as a rule of thumb in evaluating a given case. In this respect it compares favorably with that other recommendation for solving obscure cases which is to try to explain the findings by assuming (by excluding) in succession a developmental, inflammatory, degenerative, and neoplastic process.

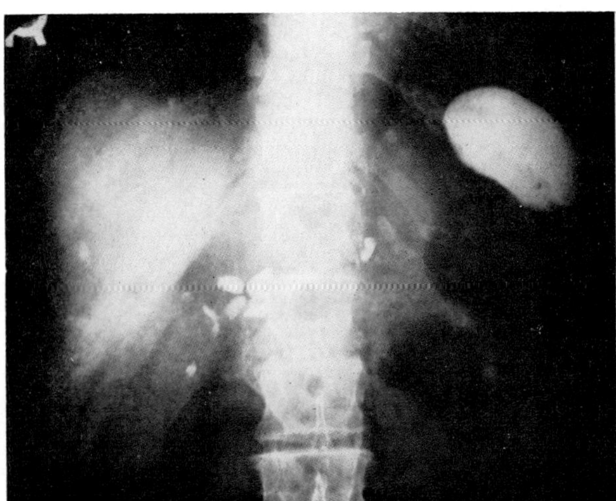

Tarrying Thorotrast. *Antero-posterior view of the abdomen shows no evidence of obstruction. Minor hypertrophic spurring is seen in the spine. Both the liver and the spleen are opacified, having a sort of metallic tinge, exhibited also by mesenteric lymph nodes. IMPRESSION: the appearance is typical of thorotrast deposition.* Patient was a seventy-seven year old female, referred to the X-ray Department of the Charleston (Illinois) Hospital for a barium enema because of rectal bleeding (due to hemorrhoids). Insistent interrogation of the patient failed to disclose when, where, and why she had been given an intravenous injection of Thorium dioxide.

POSITIVE IMPRESSIONS

It would be correct to use *roentgen diagnosis* as a caption for the final, summarizing sentence(s) in the radiologist's report. But it would lead to the inevitable confusion with the unqualified term diagnosis. Just as in biochemistry, there are pathognomonic findings in diagnostic radiology. In problem cases, though, the radiologist can seldom offer more than tentative diagnoses (hypotheses in the opinion of Van Pée), and this is why the summarizing lines in this report are preferably labeled (diagnostic) impressions.

The proper way is to state firmly (positively!) the most advanced stage of diagnosis reachable. From there on, one simply indicates the range of existing alternatives (by definition, the patient has only one alternative). An example of such a partial diagnostic impression would be *gastric ulcer, probably benign (peptic?).*

As long as a crater has been positively identified, one can be sure that at least the first part of his statement is accurate. The same words could have been arranged as *probably benign (peptic?) gastric ulcer.* That, however, would have meant to forego the semantic advantage of being at least halfway correct. One must also consider the vantage point of practical psychologics: the second version does not imply as much as the first one that there exists also a malignant alternative!

Then there is the exclusion method, *e.g., pelvic*

mass — in the absence of distended bladder — may be the enlarged uterus or ovary.

The more likely possibility is mentioned positively, while the other is offered for exclusion. In newborns, especially prematures, one may say, *periosteal elevation in both humeri and femora, presumably without significance, after excluding trauma and lues.*

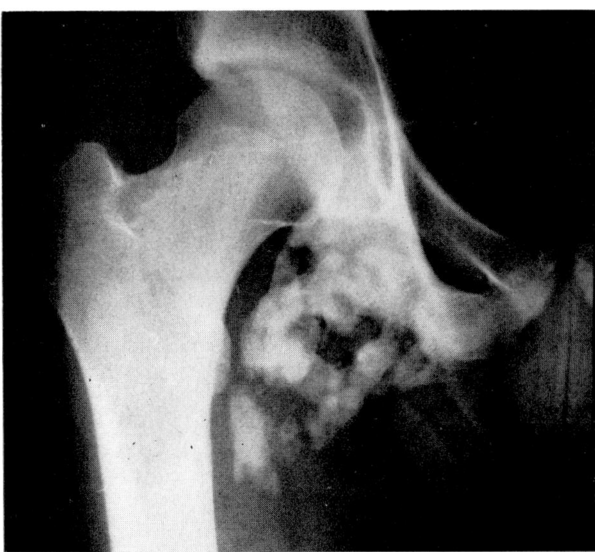

CHONDROBLASTOMA. The film is from a sixteen year old boy referred to the X-ray Department of the Paris (Illinois) Hospital because of a painful swelling in the right buttock, which appeared about three months after an ill-remembered injury. *Three views of the right hip, exposed in various obliquities, reveal a conic mass, consisting of bone substance, interspersed with lucent areas (cartilage?), growing from the ischial tuberosity. The bone at the base of the tumor is less opaque, but the rarefied area — which seems to have "eaten" into the tuberosity — is sharply defined. IMPRESSION: chondroblastoma; no signs of malignancy.* With this report the boy, who had been vacationing in that town, returned to San Francisco where an orthopedist chided the radiologist for having labeled it a tumor, and called it "avulsion of the ischial apophysis." During surgical ablation the cone was found to consist of mature bone, as hard as ivory, with cancellous bone as a core, the whole thing imbedded in a fibrous reaction which had the consistency of tough rope. The pathologist reported microscopic findings suggestive of chondro-sarcoma. The following year (1962) the boy returned to Paris (Illinois) for a vacation, and re-examination showed that the "thing" had regrown to almost exactly the size and shape seen on this film (it would have been utter duplication to reproduce the recheck). The young man went once again to San Francisco, and had it surgically removed. So far (March, 1964) it has not recurred.

Regardless how certain one may feel about the etiologic diagnosis in a given case, it is preferable — in almost all instances — to precede that definite statement by a qualifying (mollifying) term, such as *probable.* As a matter of fact, the shadows being as fleeting as they are, the qualifying term might preferably be selected from a lower certainty level, *likely, possible, suggestive, remote,* and so on.

Remember that the clinician, the bacteriologist, and the pathologist cast their diagnostic vote usually after the radiologist has filed his report. In bone tumors, a qualified radiologist (with his non-destructive testing) has the advantage over the pathologist, who must rely on tissues heavily altered by maceration (demineralization.)

PARTICULARIZATION

How many details must be included in roentgen reports? The simple answer is that a text is best received when it is made to "agree with" the prospective reader(s).

In the tendon of the gastrocnemius exists a fibrocartilage *(fabella)* which, when ossified, is visible on films of the knee. In a roentgen report intended for an orthopedist, it is sufficient to say *fabella is present.* For a general practitioner, the phrase might read *the smooth bone fragment, projected over the popliteal region, is a fabella, a sesamoid without known pathologic significance.* If the fabella is not mentioned in the report, it may be "found" (unwittingly) and (temporarily) interpreted as a fracture. The sole (unexplained) mention of the term fabella in the report usually elicits a telephone call from the referring physician who demands a "translation" — it is a time-saver to explain the whole thing from the beginning. This is also true of accessory tarsal or carpal ossicles, actually of all ununited secondary ossification centers.

For the neuro-surgeon it is enough to list the intracranial calcifications visible on skull films, but for a generalist it is preferable to indicate their importance, for instance *calcium deposits are seen in the pineal gland and falx (neither of which is deviated), as well as in the choroid plexuses and meninges; all other findings are likewise noncontributory.*

Whenever in doubt, one should lean backward, and be redundant. This is better than to force the reader into looking up the "term" and its significance in a dictionary. The latter procedure is unquestionably educational, but it will hardly create good will.

RECOMMENDATIONS

The advice included in roentgen reports must be adjusted to the knowledge and experience of the referring physician. At no time must these recommendations be expressed in terms stronger than a casual suggestion. After all, things may not turn out as they should, and when court proceedings become inevitable, an irate and irresponsible counsel may castigate the referring physician for having disregarded the advice of the roentgen specialist. It would then take time, effort, and considerable persuasion to make it clear to the court and/or jury that clinical decisions, whether diagnostic or therapeutic, must be made on the basis of all available (not only from the single roentgen) data.

For these (and for a few other, more or less obvious) reasons it is always wise to qualify the roentgen suggestions with a conditional clinical corroboration.

When a "coin" lesion is discovered in the lung, a decision must be made on whether to have a go at it or not. The radiologist could say *in the absence of visible calcifications (if such absence is confirmed by planigraphy), it remains a clinical decision whether biopsy of the "coin" should be considered.*

This brings up what may be called *surgical hedging.* In my experience, large filling defects in esophagus, stomach, or colon, have "disappeared" from one week to another. This was more often a matter of food retention, or wrong identification of the films. For the past years, I have therefore "hedged" on the first roentgen report of potentially surgical cases.

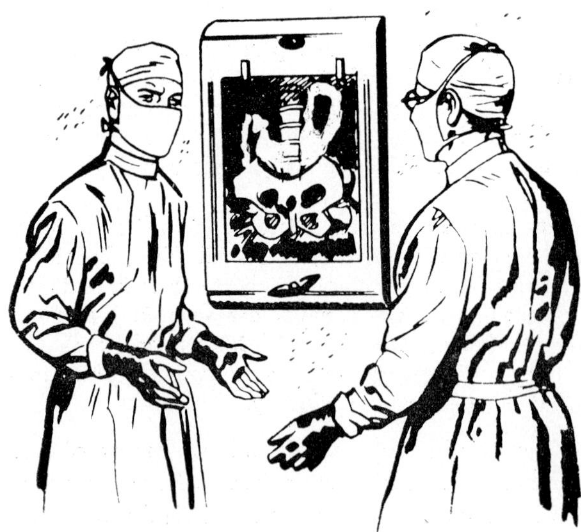

What ever happened to THAT "tumor"?!" Are you the radiologist in this cartoon?

A practical formula, which can be adapted equally well to any segment of the gastro-intestinal tract, is *apparently constant filling defect in the transverse colon, possibly a malignancy: if surgery is contemplated, please return patient for repeat barium enema, after thorough cleansing of the bowel, and prior to final decision regarding operation.*

The second time around, if the roentgen appearance is the same, one is much more justified to state *negative filling defect, visualized on two separate examinations, highly suggestive of malignancy.* At this point, further mention of surgery is unnecessary.

The radiologist's main job is to provide pathways for the clinician to channel his thoughts. In most instances, the referring physician would gladly settle for a simple (but then, of course, unequivocal) statement on whether the problem at hand is "medical" or "surgical."

In his marginalia, Roscoe Miller emphasized that it is the radiologist's prerogative and duty to receive the x-ray request as a consultation, which means to accept responsibility and to show initiative. The radiologist must insist on adequate preliminary patient preparation, but he must also try to answer the clinician's questions, if at all possible, at the first examination. In the above cited colon case, Roscoe Miller would have solved the problem right then and there by giving the patient a cleansing enema in the x-ray department, followed by repeat barium enema with multiple spot-films. Their attending staff is delighted when cases are so handled. Only the new, insecure radiology resident finds any fault with such a procedure, and even he begins to like it, just as soon as he overcomes his insecurity.

I was delighted to learn that things are so well organized at the Indiana Medical Center. The radiology residents at Cook County Hospital are still fighting the "battle of the feces." After lengthy trial and error, it appears that the best method is to give the patient a drastic dose of Dulcolax the night before, followed on the morning of the examination by cleansing enemata — to the point of clear return. But that must be done on the ward. Still, about one in every three patients cannot be called adequately prepared. In the course of a working day, over seventy-five patients undergo barium enema at Cook County Hospital: if one third of them had to receive cleansing enemata in the x-ray department, the latter would be more like a "defecatorium." In a private hospital, I would not give a cleansing enema to a patient unless and until the specific consent of the patient's attending physician had been secured, and that is time-consuming. Roscoe Miller's is undoubtedly the ideal way of handling such a situation, but I doubt whether it is applicable except under special conditions, for instance in a group practice (clinic). Even then, existing facilities and available personnel in the x-ray department usually limit its applicability to the occasional, isolated instance.

That reminds me of the private "scato-salon," which a registered nurse has recently opened in Rochester (Minnesota). All she does there – for a fee – is to thoroughly cleanse the colon of patients scheduled for special examinations at the Mayo Clinic. At last report her business was booming, figuratively, of course.

DON'T BE MEAN!

Shortly after World War I, Frederick Earl Diemer (1885-1938), who was then a captain in the U. S. Army medical corps and later practiced radiology in Denver, stated: "An adverse report is given in all fracture cases until the reduction is anatomically, rather than functionally, correct. These cases have been radiographed repeatedly until the results were satisfactory. Special stress in our reports has been laid on displaced weight bearing, axis, angulation, and thrust."

This may have seemed desirable in the military establishment in which Diemer was then working. In private practice, "adverse" reports must never be issued! Evidently, no information should be withheld from inclusion in the report, but such terms as improper (position), inadequate (apposition), or poor (alignment) are forever banned.

Provided there exists an accurate description of the initial traumatic situation with all its comminutions, impactions, and displacements – when in "semantic need" – one can always report that *no significant change* or *slight improvement in position* (whichever applies) has taken place since the date of that initial description. Such an euphemism (together with a personal phone call to the referring physician) should take care of all contingencies.

George Miller wanted it emphasized that it must be no tongue-in-cheek x-ray reporting, otherwise the radiologist was accused of trying to white-wash "guilty" colleagues. I fully agree that pertinent facts should never be concealed. Whatever valid information can be "squeezed" out of the film(s) has to be incorporated in the report. This means all the facts, not necessarily all possible interpretations. As far as grading of results goes, only laudatory remarks are permitted, for obvious reasons. When a progress eamination shows the fractured fragments in anatomic position, it is self-evident that all the problems have been solved, and the term *excellent position* is in order. But when only partial reduction has been achieved or none at all, it is not proper to call it *abominable alignment*, because any such qualification may injustly reflect on the "manipulator." Adequate evaluation of the result must take into consideration not only the manipulator's ability, but also several other factors, such as the patient's age, occupation, state of health, willingness to submit to painful procedures or to general anesthesia, and so on. Since the radiologist usually bases his statements on the sole (flattened) dimensions of his films, he should abstain from passing judgment without having all the data.

While all derogatory words are irrevocably banned from the reporting radiologist's dictionary, he must accumulate a large supply of "good" words. When pertinent, he should liberally spill such terms as *excellent reduction, anatomic restoration, perfect alignment, complete apposition,* and so on. With the uncertainty inherent in shadow-gazing, one can always use friends!

STYLE

Among those who write for a living (diagnostic radiologists belong in this category), there are some who have an innate talent for fitting words together: this means they have *style!* Most other people work hard before they learn to express their ideas, and a few never quite succeed at it.

There have been many top stylists in the radiologic past, for instance in 1909 the famous Charles Lester Leonard (1861-1913) of Philadelphia used the sentence *"when the swallows homeward fly"* to describe the passage of opaque material through the esophagus.

TERMINOLOGY

In this respect, the (actually age-old) advice given by Alexander Pope (1688-1744) is just as fresh today as when he first wrote it into his *Essay on Criticism:*

In words, as fashions, the same rule will hold:
Alike fantastic, if too new, or old:
Be not the first by whom the new are tried,
Nor yet the last to lay the old aside.

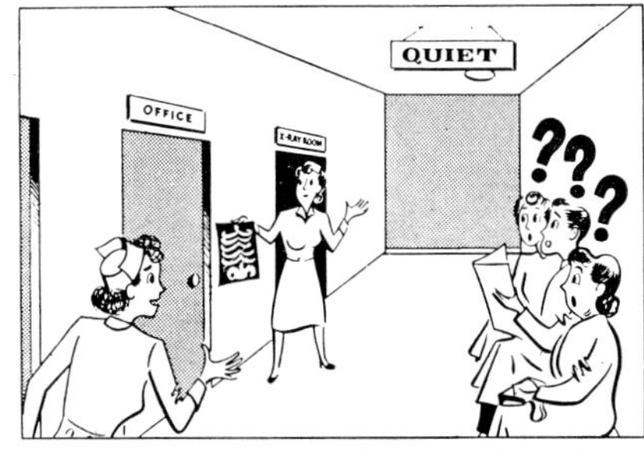

"How many stomachs does Dr. Ditmar have today?"

Indeed, who would be justified to use nowadays the terms *central pneumonia* (Williams, 1898) or *x-ray fracture* (E. C. Koenig). They were originally aimed at preserving the professional pride of touchy clinicians, when faced with the necessity of accepting "unexpected" roentgen findings.

During the Golden Age of Radiology, especially in Europe, there was the reverse tendency to translate roentgen features into clinical concepts, for instance the *increase in vascular lung markings* was called in French *tramite,* as if it were an inflammatory process.

A British confrère coined his own pet phrase *sino-bronchitic catarrhal changes,* which pervades many of his chest reports — on the assumption that every patient whose cough deserves a chest film, should also have his paranasal sinuses investigated. My own doctoral dissertation had been devoted to the *naso-pulmonary syndrome,* and the existence of such a pathologic relationship has been repeatedly demonstrated. But its incidence in the antibiotic era is uncommon. Besides, there are no specific signs which would permit one to identify it from the chest film alone.

As a group, radiologists are prone to adopt words from other specialties — which in itself would be no "crime" — only they give them special, "radiologic" meanings. A typical example is *osteogenic,* which originally meant boneforming, but is used to designate a tumor (believed to be) arising from bone cells (Sutherland, 1938).

The urologists used to inject phenolphthalein intravenously: a few minutes later they would watch it reddening the drops which came from the ureteral catheters, as a rough measure of kidney function. Radiologists adopted the word *dye* for opaque (iodinated) media, especially in urography and cholestography.

It is sometimes possible to gauge the success in the radiologic literature of an original paper or monograph by evaluating the speed with which its terminology appears in daily roentgen reports. Hickey (1922) may have been the first to observe this phenomenon after the publication of the celebrated classic on the mastoids by Frederick Manwaring Law (1875-1947) of New York City.

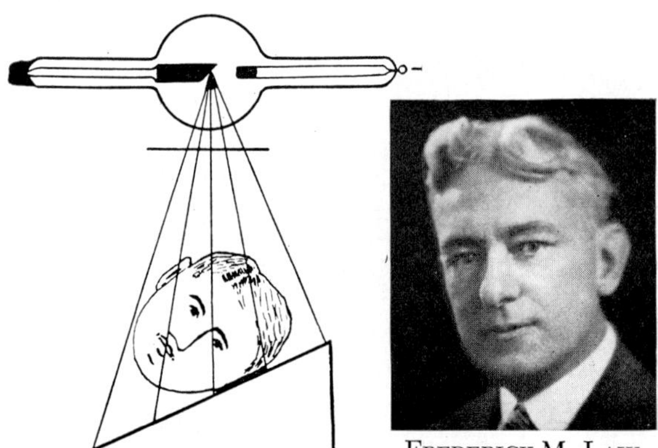

Frederick M. Law

The habit of using the term *dye* in reporting a cholecystography was certainly fostered by the fact that this term appeared in an otherwise excellent and quite early article on the subject (Pendergrass and Hodes).

Obviously inappropriate is *extravasation of dye* when intended to describe the spilling of iodinated substance from the urinary tract: neither is the contrast substance a dye, nor is it spilled from vessels!

Today the suffix *-oma* is correctly employed only with the meaning of tumor (Harry Keil). But there are blatant misuses, such as in *hygroma* (not to speak of the differently derived tsroma, scotoma, and coloboma), the post-cholecystectomy amputation neuroma (called *muñon cistico* by Lidio Mosca), or the highly ambiguous granuloma.

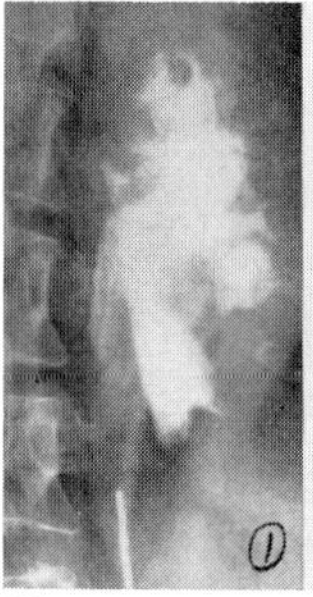

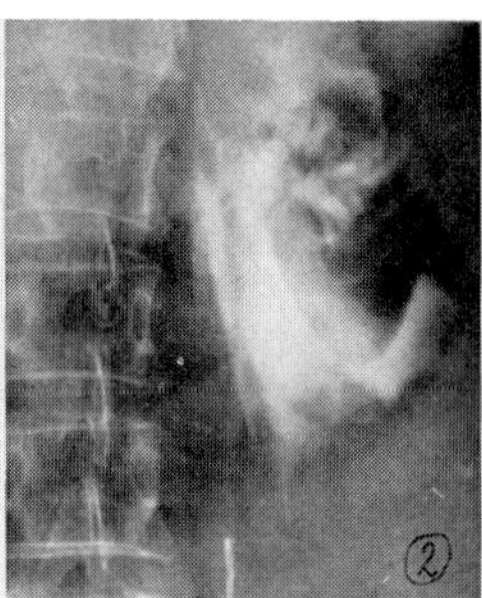

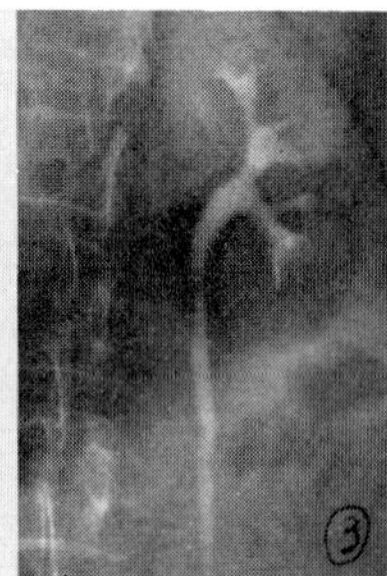

Unfledged urologist. This examination was *not* done at the Paris (Illinois) hospital. The retrograde was requested because an intravenous urogram (not shown) revealed a questionable obstruction in the proximal left ureter. During instillation of contrast material into the left ureteral catheter, a young "plumbing confrère" (*nomina odiosa*) encountered some resistance for which he "bore down on the barrel." The resulting film (1) caused sufficient anxiety to make him request a second view, which showed an outline of the kidney capsule (2). Such "iatrogenic perforation" is often done with impunity: another intravenous urogram (3), one week later, disclosed no visible pathologic alteration, and no trace of the material spilled. My report merely stated that the *instilled material filled the pyelo-calyceal system on the left, with pyelo-renal reflux and outline of kidney capsule,* while the *IMPRESSION* indicated *no evidence of obstruction in left ureter and otherwise inconclusive examination.* Of course, the report of the subsequent intravenous urogram specified *absence of retained urographic media, and apparent integrity of the visualized pyelo-calyceal system.*

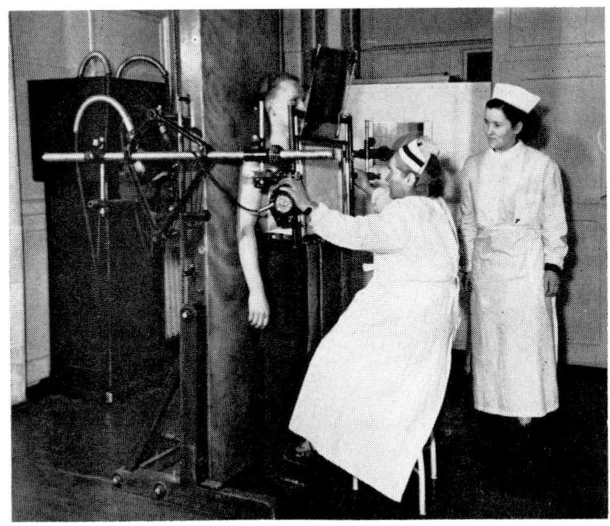

Courtesy: Sovfoto

POLISH ROENTGEN NURSE (1954). This photograph (#PO-36469/6), circulated by the official Polish agency, carried the following caption: "Nurse Alina Zagorska giving the patient an x-ray examination in the department of anti-tubercular clinic of the General Clinic at the State Factory of Railway Cars in Wroclaw – one of the best equipped establishments of this kind."

As a term, tuberculoma is worse than granuloma. The Russians prefer instead, of all things, the suitably transliterated *cazeoma!* This information was contained in a paper written in Roumania (1956) by two phthisiologists (Popper, Kaufman) and one radiologist (Zibalis).

The senior man, Maximilian Popper (1898-1960) – like his Parisian counterpart of a previous generation, Émile Sergent (1867-1940) – was often able to predict on the basis of clinical information the extent of involvement of the patient's lungs which was to be found on roentgen examination. One day, though, in the late 1930's Popper gave a patient a clean bill of health, the patient was not satisfied, went the same afternoon to another physician, who ordered a chest film, and proved the existence of a large (mute!) cavity! Next day Popper had a fluoroscope installed in his office. Popper was quite well versed in reporting chest films, but he is remembered first and foremost as a "healer." This was also the impression left during his visit to this country, in 1946.

It is very interesting to observe how the advent of certain concepts is reflected in the terminology prevalent in the roentgen reports of a given era.

In a nostalgic article (1960) Frederic Silverman, a radiologic pediatrician from Cincinnati, recalled that

Hospital Number: 6509

Date Entered: 12-3-55

Diagnostic File

DEPARTMENT OF RADIOLOGY

Veterinary Hospital — State College of Washington

Radiograph Number: A-226

Date Radiograph Made: 12-5-55

NOTE: This form must be filled out legibly and as fully as possible as it is preserved as a permanent record. Use ink.

Owner FABIAN, FELIX — Address 1907 INDIANA, PULLMAN, WN.

Species Feline — Age 10 yr — Sex F — Color or Breed Domestic

Referred by Dr. [illegible] — Student Maycumber

History Last Sunday drooling saliva, pained expression on face, rough hair coat, Tried a few times to vomit – as if something caught in throat. Scratches at throat region.

Clinical Diagnosis

Examine for

Radiograph - Date	Region	View	Thickness	KvP	Ma	F.T.D.	Exposure	Film Size	Develop. Temp.	Develop. Time	Machine	By	Remarks
1. 12-5-55	Skull	Lateral	6 cm	40	400	36 in	1/30	5x6	63	4¼	Standard	[illegible]	
2.	(Head and neck	V.D.	5.5	40	400	36 in	1/30	5x6	63	4¼	Standard	[illegible]	
3.	region)												
4.													

Diagnosis Foreign body (chicken wishbone) Oesophagus

Reported to — Date — Charge $5.00 Paid — Reported by [illegible]

Albert Friedlander (1871-1939), an internistic pediatrician from Cincinnati, had performed his first thymic irradiation in 1905 (reported in 1907). In the ensuing four decades, a multitude of thymus glands were more or less gently raised to varying radiation levels, until the atomic phase "spoiled" it all.

In 1959, Latourette and Hodges reviewed some of the roentgen reports on thymus films prepared between 1932 and 1951 in the University Hospital at Ann Arbor: "The degree of deviation or angulation of the trachea, particularly posteriorly, was the subject of considerable comment. Occasionally, the trachea was described as being narrowed or notched by the increased pretracheal soft tissues. The summary of the reports frequently included the words 'enlarged' or 'hyperplastic thymus' and in the older children the term 'persistent thymus' was used. There were of course a gamut of clinical symptoms mentioned on the requisitions . . .; after radiation . . . check-ups were often interpreted as showing reduction of the thymic enlargement."

Another facet of this all-important problem — terminology in roentgen reports — was discussed by Arnold and Washko (1958) of Honolulu: they pointed out the emptyness of the hopelessly outdated term *flat plate* (meaning: not stereoscopic!). The correct wording is simply *anteroposterior view of the abdomen* (or posteroanterior view of the chest, as the case may be). In veterinary reporting, however, Newton Tenille (1954) of Oklahoma prefers DV (dorsoventral) and VD (ventrodorsal), which is self explanatory.

QUOTES WITHOUT COMMENT

This title is correct in so far as the actual quotes are concerned. I could not insert the section without offering an introductory comment.

For several millenia, intellectual maturity has been the monopoly of a small elite. Less than two hundred years ago, more than 99 per cent of the world's population could neither read nor write. Today, in civilized countries, the majority of the people have lived through several generations of literacy, and therefore signs of intellectual maturation are beginning to appear on a "popular" level. One of these signs is the formation of large groups, not only in the arts and sciences, but also among professionals and tradesmen, willing to recognize, record, and respect the contributions to their particular endeavor, made by previous generations.

This general trend is just as clearly apparent among radiologists, but it is not yet shared by a significant number of the officers of specialty organizations. That is so partly because of the scarcity of contact (inadequate intra-organizational communications) between rank-and-file and officers, and mainly because most such officers do not have the historian's contemplative state of mind, or else these "pushers" never would have become officers in the first place. The following brief "radio-anthology" has been included with the precise intent to foster the profession's regard for its history. This anthology (cross section) of views on roentgen reporting and related topics covers about six decades in the life of the specialty.

Augustus Warren Crane (1868-1937) of Kalamazoo (Michigan): "In roentgenology . . . the differential diagnosis lies between different physical conditions rather than between different diseases." (1899)

Francis Henry Williams (1852-1936) of Boston: "In making examinations with this new method, as with

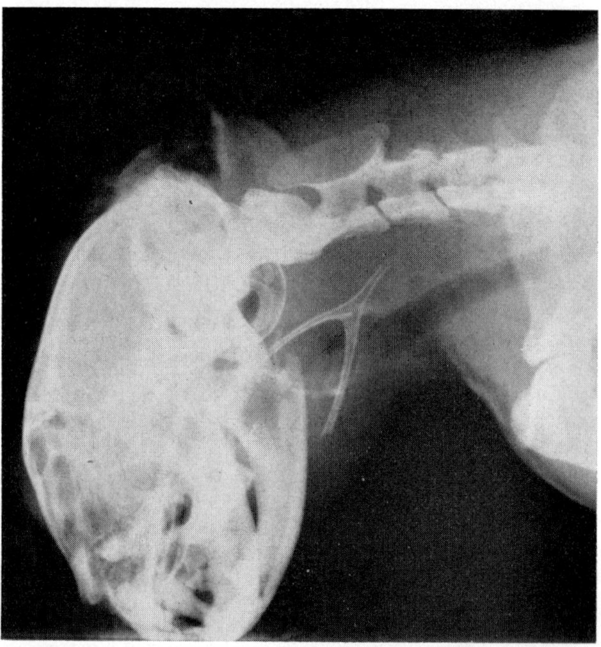

Courtesy: Fred Lester Williams

CHICKEN WISHBONE IN A CAT'S THROAT. This is the film mentioned in the attached veterinary x-ray report. The wishbone is formed by the chicken's united clavicles. The fused portion of the wishbone was in the cat's esophagus, but the chicken's *dorsal* clavicle (dorsal with respect to the cat's body) got stuck in the cat's soft palate, the chicken's *ventral* clavicle (ventral to the cat's body) had perforated the cat's larynx. As described in the *Journal of the Veterinary AMA* of June 1, 1956 by Richard Ott, the wishbone was removed piecemeal, its dorsal clavicle directly with a forceps, the ventral clavicle through an incision into the larynx, finally the fused portion through a gastroscope. The cat did fine, and went home five days after surgery.

the older ones, the three following stages should be kept distinctly and separately in mind: (1) Attention should be given to observing carefully the appearances which present themselves. (2) A careful record should be made of these appearances in some simple and direct way which shall be a record of facts, not of opinions. (3) The observations should be well considered by themselves and in connection with the information furnished from other sources, the evidence from each source being given just, but not exclusive consideration before making the diagnosis" (1901).*

John Nesbit Scott (1871-1922) of Kansas City: "X-rays are like figures in that they are always correct, (but) we may make a mistake in adding up a column of figures" (1902).

Antoine Béclère (1856-1936) of Paris: "Radiologic documents (plates, prints, etc.), all assumptions to the contrary notwithstanding, are neither self-evident, nor easy to read. . . There are no true radiographic errors – the method itself is never at fault – there are only errors of interpretation . . ." (1906).

Mihran Krikor Kassabian (1870-1910) of Philadelphia: "The (roentgen) report should be made as intelligible as possible. . ." (1907)

Rudolf Grashey (1876-1950) of Hamburg: "Have you ascertained that the abnormalities (which you are about to report) are neither artefacts, nor developmental variations?" (1908).

Francis Hernaman-Johnson (1879-1949) of London: "The final reputation of an x-ray diagnostician is determined neither by pretty pictures nor an engaging manner; but by the general correctness or otherwise of the opinions he gives" (1919).

Guido Holzknecht (1872-1931) of Vienna: "There exists no roentgen diagnosis. There are, of course, roentgen signs as well as pathognomonic groupings of such signs, but this is not enough to make it a method of diagnosis. Roentgenology is only a method of examination" (1919).

Arthur David Dunn (1873-1934) of Omaha: "The roentgenologist is in the position of a manufacturer who has one product to sell but who has not as yet determined to whom or through what channels he shall permanently market his product . . .; the 'stuff' he sells to a . . . general practitioner (ready-made diagnosis) differs from what he sells to a specialist (raw material of a finer quality) . . . Furthermore . . . the lure to sell directly to the patient becomes at times pretty strong . . . As a purchaser of roentgenological wares, I desire to discuss what goods I, as an internist, think I want . . . Only by a discussion of our needs will the function of the x-ray man be gradually determined . . ." (1919).

Alfred Ernest Barclay (1876-1949) of London: "The place of the radiologist in medicine . . . (demands that) his department be lifted out of the cellar into a more central position in the hospital" (1920).

Russell Daniel Carman (1875-1926) of Rochester (Minnesota): The roentgenologist can refrain from advice which he is not qualified to give . . . confine his diagnosis to cases presenting diagnostic signs, and if he is uncertain frankly admit it . . . Recently, one of my assistants, after examining the colon, ventured this report 'Appendix visible, segmented, and fixed.' A few

*Richard Schatzki of Brookline (Massachusetts) told me that a very pertinent maxim is on permanent exhibit in the roentgen reading room at Massachusetts General Hospital. It was placed there by George Holmes. Upon request, Laurence Robbins graciously provided the text, and its origin; it was first printed in the classic textbook by Williams, of which the princeps edition appeared in 1901.

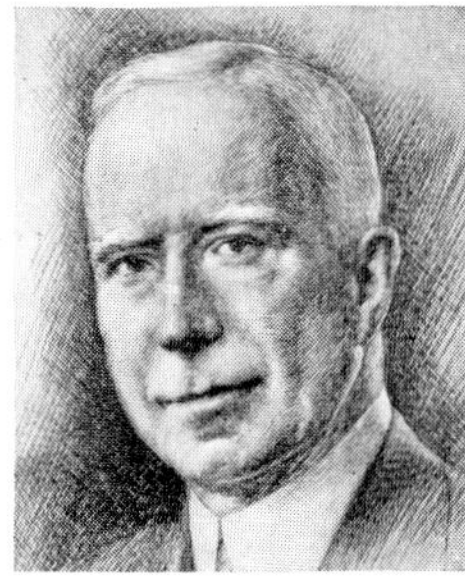

August W. Crane

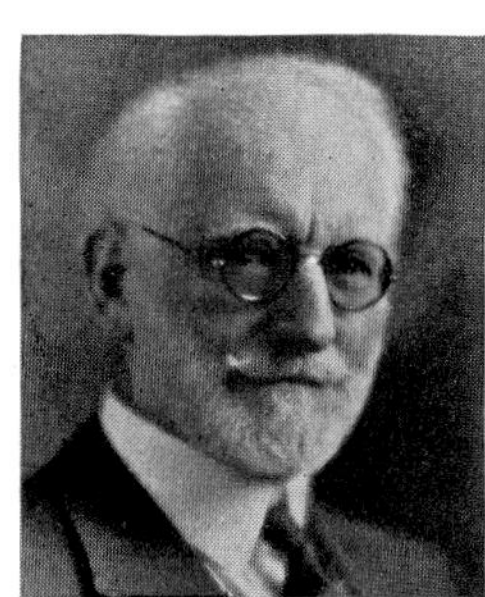

George Pfahler

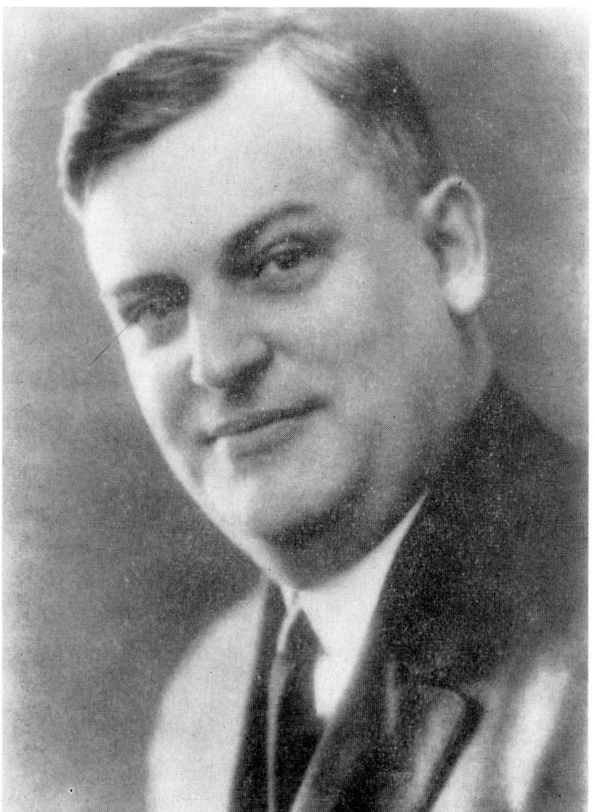

Russell Daniel Carman (1875-1926)

days later, W. J. Mayo — William James Mayo (1861-1939) — operated the patient, and having the x-ray report in mind as he explored the appendiceal region, remarked: 'Yes, the appendix is fixed to the extent that he cannot wipe his nose with it' " (1922).

Charles Darwin Enfield (1887-1946) of Louisville (Kentucky): "There are two recognized extremes (in reporting) . . . The one . . . is typified by the report which describes in detail all that the roentgenologist sees . . . but does not tell what he thinks about it . . . (which is) at its best a perfect word picture without meaning . . . (as) it commits the roentgenologist to nothing. . . At the other extreme is the report which gives merely a diagnosis . . . in a sentence; it is economical of time and effort, it commits the roentgenologist absolutely, but I think it is even worse . . . (because) it utterly fails to give his grounds for that opinion. The ideal report is one that (combines) both the types mentioned. It paints the word picture . . . and it gives conclusions, nay, even perhaps a diagnosis . . . It puts the roentgenologist out in the open where the clinician can shoot at him, and then provides the ammunition. But it does offer a fair chance to correlate the (roentgen and the) clinical aspects . . ." (1923).

Maximilian John Hubeny (1880-1942) of Chicago: ". . . in correlating x-ray and other findings it is very tempting to make definite conclusions on findings other than roentgenological. This method reads a diagnosis into the plate rather than reading it out of the plate" (1926).

John Magnus Redding (1889-1930) of London: "In no branch of medicine is the 'spot-diagnosis' a more fruitful source of error than in radiology" (1927).

George Beckett Batten (1860-1942) of London: "It has been said that they (the radiologists) must 'suffer fools gladly' and treat the clinicians with consideration and kindliness" (1930).

REPORT, X-RAY DIGESTIVE TRACT.

Case No. A 88404 X-Ray No. 23298 Phy. Graham Mussey Date 7-23-13

Name Henry Miller Sex male Age 58

STOMACH
- Tonus: Hypertonic
- Filling defect: None
- Form: Steer horn
- Position: Oblique
- Size (1, 2, 3, 4) (1. Small. 2. Medium. 3. Large. 4. Very Large.): 1 — Peristalsis: Vigorous
- Incisura: None
- Residue in Stomach after 6 hrs. (0, 1, 2, 3, 4): 0
- Pylorus
  - Position: Normal
  - Patency: Free
  - Opening: Immediate

DUODENUM
- Duodenum Visualized: Yes — Dilated — Obstructed — Residue: Yes
- Cap: Irregular — Residue (0, 1, 2, 3, 4): 3

DIAGNOSIS: Probable Duodenal Ulcer. Hypertrophic arthritis of spine. Question of a filling defect in pars cardiaca.

Signed Carman

X-RAY REPORT BY RUSSELL DANIEL CARMAN AT MAYO'S (1913). Carman is remembered as the creator of gastro-intestinal fluoroscopy in the modern sense of the word. His major work with Albert Miller was the classic *Roentgen Diagnosis of Diseases of the Alimentary Canal* (Saunders, 1917). Sutherland, and later Kirklin, became chief of radiology at Mayo's. This original report was graciously provided by the current chief of diagnostic radiology at Mayo's, Clarence Allen Good.

George Edward Pfahler (1874-1957) of Philadelphia: "If I have in mind anything that will be helpful in getting the patient well, I believe it is my duty as a radiologist to make my suggestion. The man in charge can throw away all my advice if he so chooses" (1932).

Byrl Raymond Kirklin (1888-1957) of Rochester (Minnesota): "But the radiologist is an adviser to clinician, surgeon, and specialist, shares in the responsibility to the patient, and to meet that responsibility squarely must give the best and most complete advice of which he is capable. It may not always be accepted, but advice that is respectable will usually be respected" (1937).

Samuel Aronovich Reynberg (1897-) of Moscow: "The physician who accepts the impression on a roentgen report as a definite diagnosis is unfair to his roentgenologist as well as to medical science" (1938).

William Alfred Jones (1892-) of Kingston (Ontario): "Perhaps one of the great mistakes of our time is the tendency to expect the radiologist to hand out a typed diagnosis, reading the type as it were directly from the film and transferring it to paper as something turned out of a machine, mechanically correct, and purporting to be infallible" (1938).

Gonzalo Esguerra Gomez (1902-) of Bogotá (Columbia): "The description (of the position of fractured bone fragments) must be so precise and detailed as to suffice even when prescinded from the films" (1939).

James Frederick Brailsford (1888-1961) of London: "Interpretation of radiographs without knowledge is a major sin" (1945).

Ross Golden (1889-) of New York City (at the time): "Clarity in writing is obviously based on clear thinking and accurate observation" (1946).

Sidney Frissell Thomas (1912-) of Palo Alto (California): "The word 'prespondylolisthesis' implies . . . that . . . there will inevitably be a slip. . . . Other examples of unjustifiable implication are to be found in reports. . . . Pressure is frequently brought to bear upon the radiologist to turn his roentgenographic findings into clinical diagnosis, as 'mucous colitis' or 'chronic appendicitis.' (To yield is to) endanger the scientific approach that is the radiologist's privilege and obligation to medicine" (1946).

Leo Henry Garland (1903-) of San Francisco: "There are times when an expert 'sees' a 'seeable' lesion clearly and times when he doesn't. . . That this should happen to amateurs is accepted, but that it should happen to experts is now . . . thoroughly proved statist-

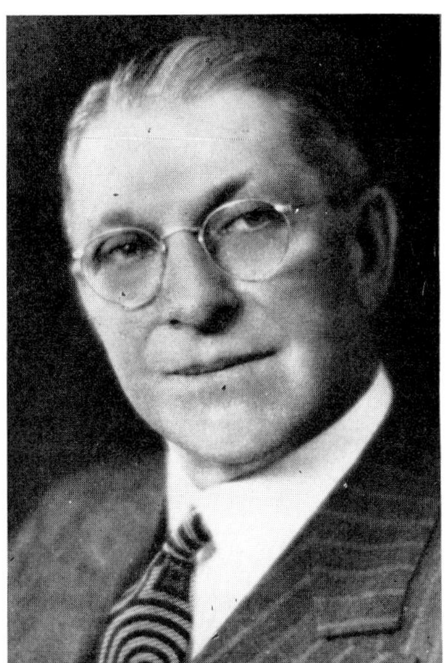

MAXIMILIAN JOHN HUBENY
OCTOBER 12, 1880 – JULY 2, 1942
THIS PLAQUE IS DEDICATED
TO THE MEMORY OF ONE
WHO DURING HIS LIFE
CONTRIBUTED MUCH TO THIS
DEPARTMENT AND TO THE
SCIENCE OF ROENTGENOLOGY.

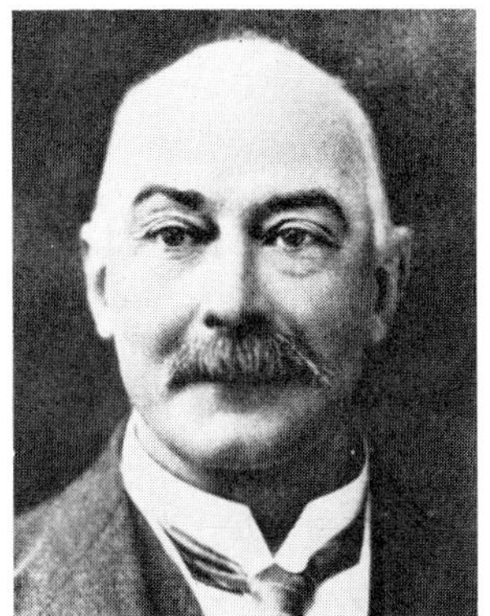

George Becket Batten

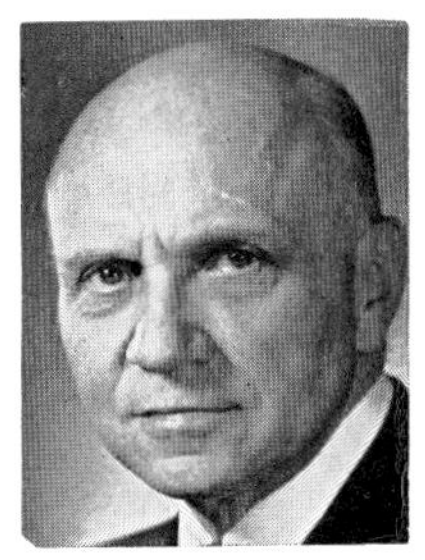

Ross Golden

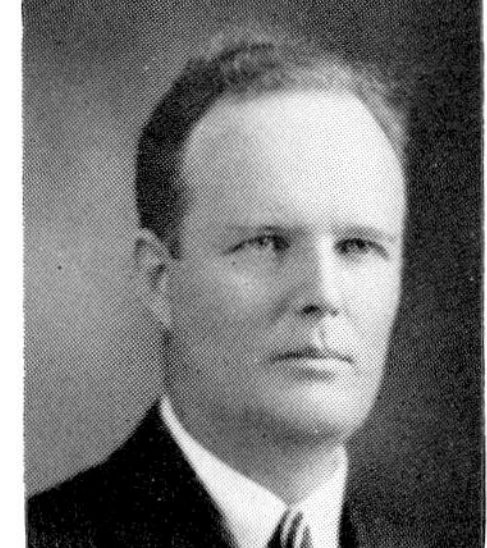

Wm. Alfred Jones

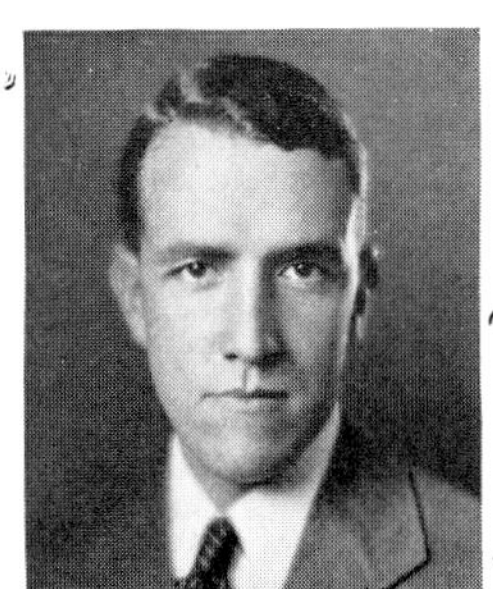

Henry Garland

ically. . . The interpretation of roentgenograms is subject to a certain degree of error . . . or variation (which) is significant, but (which) compares favorably with that found in other clinical methods and diagnostic aids . . . This fact is no reason for deprecating either the experts or the method" (1949).

Leo George Rigler (1896-) of Minneapolis (at the time): "The long-winded report . . . without conclusions . . . too often represents an evasion of clinical responsibility . . . (while) a simple dogmatic statement without explanation carries with it a connotation of infallibility which is unjustified . . . (but) . . .If we are to withhold a conclusion until complete certainty can be established, few diagnoses will be made premortem" (1950).*

Merrill Clary Sosman (1890-1960) of Boston: "Our diagnoses are based on gross pathology in the great majority of cases — certainly well over 90 per cent. As roentgenologists I am sure that much of our accuracy depends on mathematical probabilities in a given case or set of circumstances" (1950).

Harry Zachary Mellins (1921-) of Brooklyn: "*Definition of a Diagnostic Roentgenologist.* The roentgen diagnostician is a clinician who has sacrificed one of the greatest glories of the practice of medicine and its greatest responsibility — the daily contact with the ill and with their families — in order to concentrate the more on the other essence of our profession, the pathology of the living. This he sees through the medium of shadows, which has left him open to the charge of not quite being a real doctor. But shadows, after all, are real. What are we to one another and what is the world to any of us but an inverted image on the retina. Seeing is done with the mind. The camera does not see; it records. The radiologist perceives a shadow, sees a lesion, and imagines the man. The bedside physician sees the man, perceives the signs, and imagines the lesion. They practice from the outside in, and we practice from the inside out. Both are clinicians, for in truth there is no other kind of doctor worthy of the name. The decisive test for all is finally and always at the bedside. This, then, is one concept of the radiologist — with a film on the viewbox, but the bedside on his mind" (1953).*

*In 1916, Carman and Miller wrote: "Extreme limitations of diagnostic latitude are not truly conservative, but are reactionary. They would seem to rest on the assumption that a diagnosis is a statement of fact, not an expression of opinion. Yet, every diagnosis implies the exercise of opinion and the rendition of judgment, and even the pathologist, who has the last word in this respect, is not infallible."

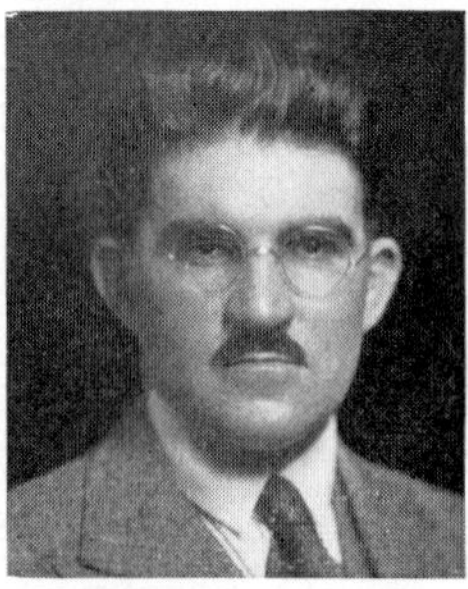
Leo G. Rigler

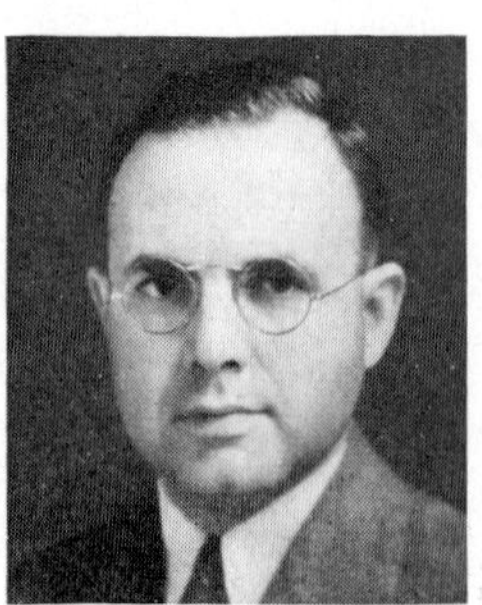
John D. Camp

John Dexter Camp (1898-) of Los Angeles: "People have become accustomed to, and expect specialization. . . William Mayo once defined a specialist as one who knew more and more about less and less, and the general practitioner as one who knew less and less about more and more. Where that leaves the radiologists — who is sometimes referred to as the general practitioner of the specialists — I do not know. . . The patient is now apt to credit a new drug or a device . . . rather than the person who selected it. He credits the electrocardiogram with discovering his heart disease, and the x-ray film with disclosing his ulcer. We can hardly blame him when we tell a traffic cop that we did not know we were speeding because our speedometer was broken . . . let us try to put a little warmth and feeling in the use of both (drugs and machines), and recover a little of the art and practice of medicine which today is too frequently left in the hands of the psychiatrist." (1954).

Christian Virgil Cimmino (1916-) of Fredericksburg (Virginia): "To some clinicians, the radiologist is still the 'puller of switches and blower of fuses,' and not to be regarded seriously when he talks about clinical medicine from his realm of shadows. To others, his ray is endowed with magic properties such as allow the circumvention of the cerebral cortex. To still others (and it is to be hoped the largest group), he is a valued consultant, whose opinion and findings, like those of other consultants, must be woven into the fabric of the whole clinical pattern" (1956).

Lieba Buckley (-) of London: "An x-ray report, like a will, should always be signed at the end" (1957).

Robert Stanton Sherman (1909-) of New York: " 'I don't know' or 'impossible to tell' are neglected statements in x-ray reporting; yet such opinions constitute a form of positive knowledge. . . Playing hunches (or deliberately guessing in order to gain easy glory) can

*I first heard this beautiful definition quoted by Leo Rigler in his *Next 50 Years,* an address delivered on February 7, 1963 before the Chicago Roentgen Society on its 50th anniversary. I wrote to Mellins, who since 1956 is professor and chairman of the Department of Radiology in the Medical College of the State University of New York in Brooklyn. He answered from The Johns Hopkins Hospital, where he is spending a sabbatical year. This definition had been written in 1953, for a gathering of senior medical students, as a brief explanation of the radiologist's point of view. It was then printed in ACR's *Monthly Newsletter* of March, 1954.

eventually undermine the . . . roentgenologist's reputation. . ." (1958).

Roger Allen Harvey (1910-) of Chicago: "I am just wondering how many of us . . . are writing (roentgen reports) for other radiologists rather than for other doctors? I was brought up in an era when there was a pattern and terms that we had to use that only radiologists understood . . . (Do) you have the impression that you are slanting (your roentgen reports) toward people who do not understand them?" (1959).

Frederick Esterbrook Elliott (1881-1963) of Brooklyn (New York): "It has long been my conviction that only a radiologist should undertake interpretation of x-ray imagery, though it should not be within his province to reach a final diagnostic conclusion. The latter, I firmly believe, is the province of the attending doctor" (1959).

Lewis Elmer Etter (1901-) of Pittsburgh: "It seems that some undesirable terms in radiologic etymology are here to stay and will become embedded in the medical language and be accepted through continuous usage. Many other words too often in everyday use, principally ill-considered use by the profession, are amenable to correction. Terms and phases should be carefully chosen to convey the exact meaning of our thoughts in the tradition of best scientific and medical practice" (1959).

Clarence Allen Good (1907-) of Rochester (Minnesota): "Reports made today at the Mayo Clinic are generally brief, often limited to the diagnosis. We say, 'Negative lumbar spine and pelvis,' 'Duodenal ulcer with central crater,' 'Annular ulcerating carcinoma of the transverse colon limb of the splenic flexure,' 'Functioning gallbladder with cholelithiasis,' 'Small cavitating lesion situated posteriorly in the L.U.L. at the level of the 4th and 5th ribs. Exclude T.B.' 'Atelectasis with marked contraction of L.L.L. and compensatory emphysema of the lingula. Thickened pleura in the left base. Suggest bronchogram to confirm impression of bronchiectasis,'. . .and so on. We seldom list or describe negative findings and we try to limit descriptive reports to those cases in which we are at a loss for proper diagnosis" (1959).

Heinrich Chantraine (1891-) of Neuss-am-Rhein (Germany): "It is often fun to watch internists reading roentgen films, as they introduce their clinical preconceptions (prejudices?) into the reports. In an asymptomatic patient, a pulmonary opacity may be discounted as non-contributory, and a very similar opacity in a febrile patient will be labeled with profuse pathologic pseudonyms. I have always held that films from different patients with identical findings must be given at least identical descriptions. – Every physician knows that all humans are subject to errors. The pathologist knows it, and the roentgenologist is acutely aware of it. Nevertheless, you must have the courage to stand up and voice your opinion. You should never forfeit this privilege, because attempted eschewal will not preserve your tranquility. If you want to stay in the game, you must play, or else you will soon be counted out" (1959).

Robert Reid Newell (1892-) of San Francisco: "Having described the roentgen evidence, the report should then evaluate it diagnostically. Probabilities just on roentgen evidence should be distinguished from diagnostic suggestions based on the entire evidence. Clinical data ought to be given their just weight, but *not* have their weight doubled by being first applied by the radiologist and later again by the clinician" (1959).

Steve Ernest Ross (1920-) of San Francisco: "According to William James, a great scientist *and* philosopher, philosophy is nothing but an unusually obstinate effort to think clearly; in this sense most radiologists are practicing philosophers. The approach of "operations research" (analysis of *true positives, true negatives, false positives, and false negatives*) promotes clarity by stressing, among others, the need for meaningful standards of performance and for examining the consequences of alternate courses of action. Since this is what responsible roentgen reporting rests upon, one could assert, alliteratively, that the approach of operations research often results in optimal radiology" (1959).

Lee Browning Lusted (1922-) of Rochester (New York): "The probabilistic concepts in medical diagnosis arise because a diagnosis can rarely be made with absolute certainty. The end result . . . is, rather, a 'most probable' diagnosis. Thus, the purpose of the probabilistic considerations is to determine which of the

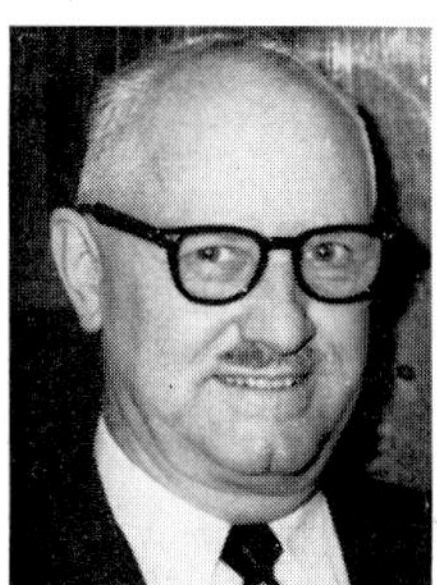
LEWIS E. ETTER

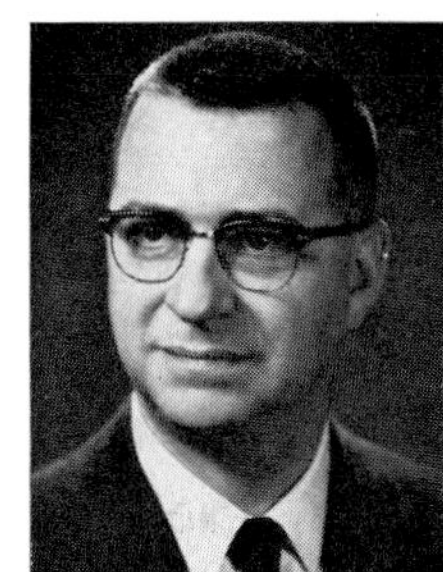
C. ALLEN GOOD

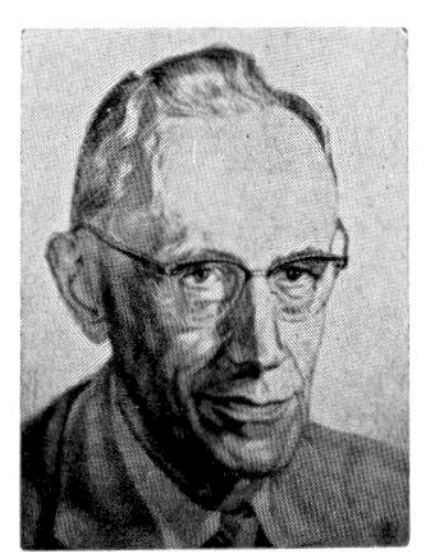
HEINRICH CHANTRAINE

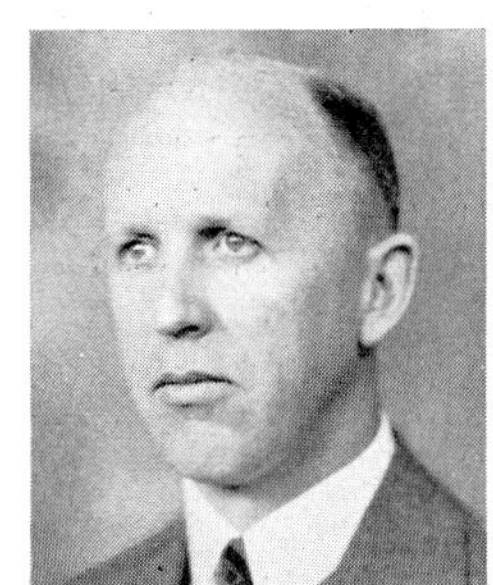
ROBERT NEWELL

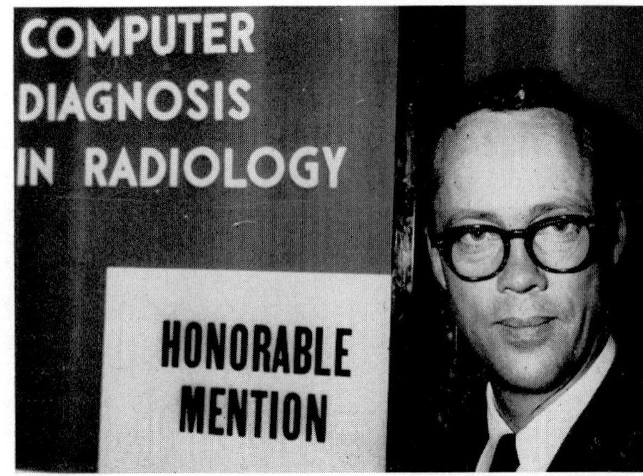

GWILYM LODWICK (a flying physician) is professor and chairman of the Department of Radiology in the University of Missouri in Columbia. He is perhaps best known for his continuing attempts at systematizing the roentgen symptomatology of bone tumors, from his study of juvenile unicameral cysts in the *American Journal of Roentgenology* of September, 1958 to the exhibit on the coding of roentgen images for computer diagnosis, shown at the 1963 RSNA meeting in Chicago.

alternative disease complexes is 'most likely' for a particular patient. . . Symbolic logic and probability contribute to our understanding of (such reasoning processes). . . The device which might be developed as the radiologic counterpart of the Cytoanalyzer. . .would be . . . an electronic 'scanner-computer' to look at chest photoflurograms and to separate . . . the abnormal chest films . . . (which) would be marked for later study by the radiologist" (1962).*

COMMENT WITHOUT QUOTES

Above title is a second thought. The first one had been the ostentatious *Aphorisms on Roentgen Reporting*. Most of the paragraphs in this section are too long to qualify in that category. Besides, antique medical apophthegms have a certain transcendental, everlasting quality, which is hard to match — in a discussion restricted to one specialty. A classic all-encompassing example is herein offered from the "genuine" works of Hippocrates (*Aphorisms,* vii, 87): *Those diseases which* (the internist's) *medicines do not cure, iron cures*: *those which* (the surgeon's) *iron cannot cure, fire cures; and those which* (the radiologist's) *fire cannot cure, are to be reckoned wholly incurable.*

☆

It is relevant — when (w)riting roentgen reports — to recognize, remember, and respect the limitations of diagnostic radiology, as well as your own!

☆

In order to pick up a rare condition, one must constantly think of it and watch for it. In the absence of pathognomonic findings in myelofibrosis, is it permissible to miss that unique case as likely as not ever to cross one's path, or is it preferable to report every bone change as suspicious for myelofibrosis? What most radiologists actually do — for one month from the date of publication of that paper on myelofibrosis — is to call (almost) everything *possible myelofibrosis;* then they get tired, and forget all about it!

☆

Try hard not to overlook the *first* fracture! Having accurately labeled (in one patient) the fractures in the seventh, eighth, and ninth ribs, while missing the fracture in the tenth rib — or in a Colles having described the radial fracture and missed the fragmentation of the ulnar styloid — is seldom of more than academic significance. This, however, does not obtain if you reported the broken ribs while missing the Colles altogether. Let us therefore complete the initial statement: try hard not to overlook the *first* fracture in any single anatomic territory surveyed!

☆

When reporting, refrain from describing first the eye-catching pathologic alteration. Instead, look over carefully the presumably uninvolved territory. This is time-consuming, but it will pay off in lowering the incidence of significant oversights. Except in far advanced disease, significant findings are seldom eye-catching!

☆

Every radiologist possesses books, but most of these serve only for decorative purposes.* While reporting,

*In reading the section "Quotes Without Comment," Roscoe Miller was reminded of his old Chief, Paul C. Hodgez, who often remarked about the interpretation of films of patients whose anatomy had been altered by surgery, "Once the surgeon has been in, all bets are off!"

*In his erudite *Anatomy of Bibliomania* (1931), the witty British bibliophile Holbrook Jackson (1874-1948) included a chapter on *Books as Furniture.*

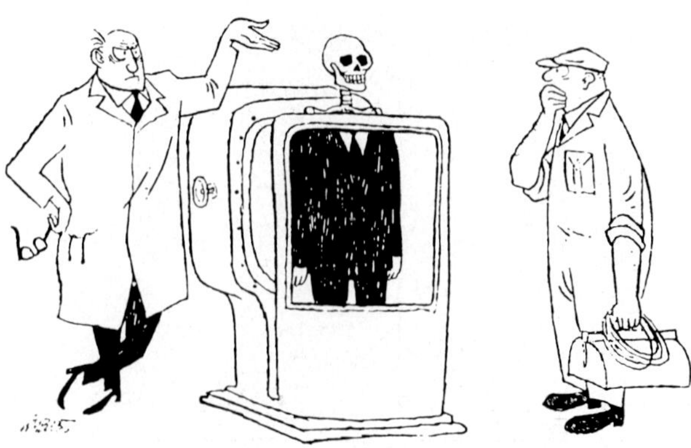

reputable reference works should be within easy grasp (*i.e.*, reachable without having to get up!). Certain radiologists (almost) never feel the need, during their film reading, to "look up" some detail — these gents should be admired (or suspected). In a single day's work, most radiologists *(me too)* will consult several times one or more radiologic "good books."

☆

A hospital administrator told me that when interviewing candidates for the job of roentgen-report-typing-secretary, he seldom asks them how well they spell medical terms. With a modicum of good will, they can always pick that up. He confessed wrily of being more worried over their spelling of common English, which had to be at least as good as that of the radiologist whose dictation they were supposed to transcribe.

☆

Typing errors may be embarassing — *e.g., revolving* (instead of resolving) *pneumonitis* — especially when they reverse the intended meaning, or when they result in grotesque combinations, such as *views of the mandible reveal fracture of the right ankle* (instead of angle). The solution is simple: read carefully your reports before signing (or before applying the signature stamp).

☆

I prefer dictating machines with magnetic tape. How often did you say *numerous pulmonary calcifications* (when *several* would have been perfectly adequate)? How often did you report *considerable gastric dilatation* (when *minimal,* or at best unqualified gastric dilatation would have sufficed)? How often did you describe severe degenerative changes (when there were actually three of four barely lipping fringes holding on to the lumbar vertebrae)? As long as the correction of a flaw remains a complicated procedure, one may be inclined to let it ride — but with the facile erasure permitted by magnetic recording, such *overzealousness* is more likely to be deleted from the final roentgen reports.

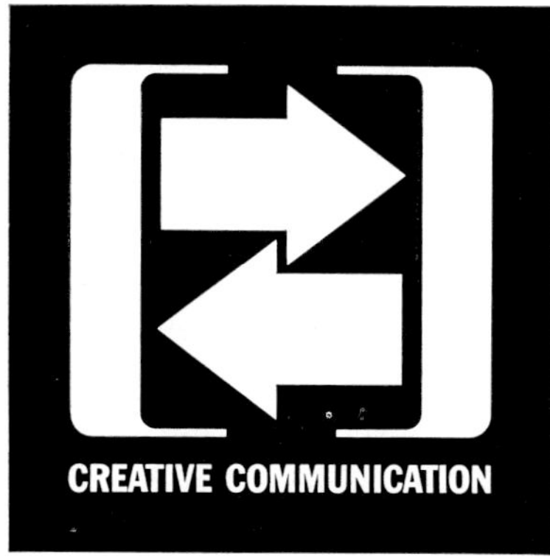

Based on repeated usage and tradition, some terms are more suggestive than others, for instance *clear lungs, calyceal cups, ureteral spindles, intact trabeculation, pulmonary reticulation, patulous sphincter, redundant sigmoid, Phrygian cap,* and so on. Such "standard" wordings may be given preference in roentgen reports, but any others are acceptable, provided they are combined from words accepted in current usage.*

☆

Private agreements with referring physicians can never justify the use in roentgen reports of invented terms, nor of standard terms with meanings different from those found in current dictionaries. Only a few years after having dictated such a "ciphered" report, the respective radiologist, who had lost or forgotten the "key," wasted an uncomfortable hour with the patient's complete chart in trying to understand just what he had wanted to say in that "ciphered" report.

☆

In roentgen reports, the term *except* is fraught with many pitfalls. I once saw (maybe even dictated) a report which contained the sentence *lungs clear, except for infiltration in the right upper lobe.* This is like stating in a psychiatric report that a paranoid patient is "sane," except for a strong desire to kill his wife.

☆

No mammalian body has absolutely symmetrical halves. For practical purposes, though, it is permissible to report *symmetrical apices*, or to use other statements of the sort (*e.g., equidistant vertebral bodies*) — but only if and when the inherent limitation (inaccuracy) of such a wording is of no practical significance.

☆

The sentence *no change from previous films* is obviously incorrect, because living organisms undergo constant changes. *No gross* (or *no essential*) *change* sounds better, but is not good enough. If the proper expression would demand time-consuming explanations, simpler (or above) forms might be acceptable. But it requires no additional effort to use the correct wording, which is *no detectable* — or any of its equivalents *(no visible, no demonstrable)* — change.

☆

Whenever previous films are available for comparison, a statement to the effect that such comparison was made, must be incorporated in the roentgen report. Chest films are preferably numbered chronologically (with a wax pencil, right on the bottom of the film, which facilitates subsequent re-arrangement by date). With gastro-intestinal series, such numbering

*Bergen Evans has in this respect a favored quotation from Shakespeare's *Richard II* (2, ii, 76), "Uncle, for God's sake, speak comfortable words!"

is more time-consuming (and usually unnecessary). References to previous examinations should include specific dates. Changes in the radiologist's opinion of the case must also be mentioned. For that, it may become necessary to re-read one's own previous prose, which can be depressing, but is always educational.

☆

It is not only permissible or desirable, but mandatory to comment in the roentgen report on the reason for the patient's referral, even when this reason had not been indicated on the referral slip (*e.g.*, post-mastectomy recheck for metastases). All the more, when a definite request had been forwarded, *i.e. please evaluate for epigastric mass,* one must indicate in the reply whether there were findings referable to that mass.

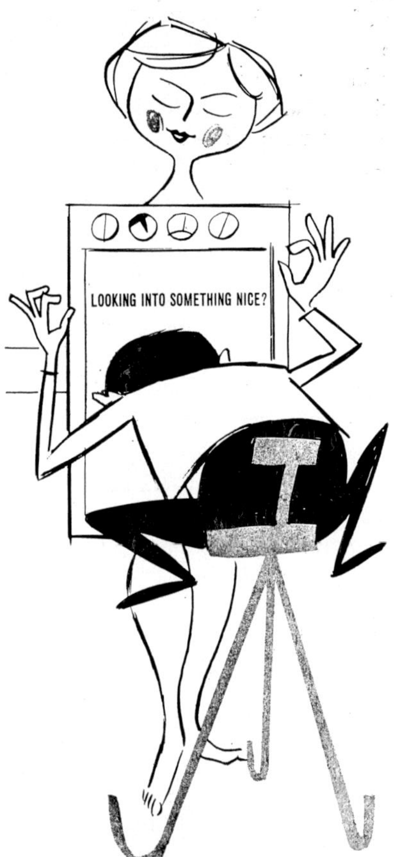

FLUOROSCOPIC DIAGNOSIS. Swedish chest fluoroscopic practices notwithstanding, conventional fluoroscopy must be used only for functional, never for morphologic evaluation. Miliary tuberculosis, thin-walled cavities, many non-calcified "coin" lesions are well below the fluoro-visual threshold. Intensified fluoroscopy has brought within the reach of the fluoroscopist some but not all of these formerly "invisible" items. Even so, I make it a practice *never ever* to declare absence of pathologic alterations in the examination of a chest unless and until I can look (at least) at a conventional 72" posteroanterior radiograph of that chest. This cartoon is from a Brazilian poster for the 7th IACR in São Paulo — which, of course, is what they asked you to look into!

☆

Normal stomach may seem like a well justified abbreviation of a lengthy description of a negative examination, but from a semantic viewpoint it is violently incorrect. When summing up (the result of) a negative examination, the only thing you can honestly say is that *no pathologic alteration was identified.* If you want to be very brief, why make any unwarranted assumptions beyond that — *i.e.,* why say anything else?

☆

In the USA, a person is innocent until proven guilty in court. The fifth amendment to the Constitution grants everybody, especially the accused, the right to refuse to incriminate himself. It seems preferable to let ninety-nine guilty go free rather than unjustly convict a single innocent. The reverse is true in medical diagnosis. It seems preferable to suspect ninety-nine healthy people rather than fail to detect a single sick patient. Hence the physician in general, and the radiologist in particular, should be on the lookout for disease rather than for its absence. This is the type of approach (*there is no evidence of disease* rather than *there is evidence of health,* which must receive its semantic reflection in radiologic reporting.

☆

Hedging in roentgen reports is a sacrosanct privilege. But it is granted only as a built-in reminder that these shadows are inherently fleeting as well as deceitful. *Possible gastric malignancy* will actually commit the radiologist just as strongly as if he had said *carcinoma of the stomach.* The former wording is preferable only because it emphasizes that a roentgen diagnosis is seldom as "final" as the pathologist's "ultimate" evaluation. Equivocation is no sure cure against getting caught on the wrong side of the diagnostic barrier. In fact, when verbal fencing is too freely and too frequently used, it inevitably backfires.

☆

At teaching sessions it is very desirable to discuss as complete a differential diagnosis as can be listed. In practical roentgen reporting, this would serve no useful purpose. It could never be as comprehensive as a reference manual, and even if it were, this would not advance the "cause," which is to pinpoint the most likely eventuality. As a rule, among the more common possibilities, two (at the most three) choices should be offered to the referring clinician.

☆

Hi(gh)-fi(delity) reproduction demands a redundancy of harmonics. Likewise, a roentgen report acquires sophistication only when it is, at least to some extent, redundant. The same argument can be used the other way around: an ordinary telephone offers only a few octaves, but these are enough for the trained listener to recognize the sound. He may then provide (in his imagination) as many additional harmonics as he wishes.

Roentgen reports from private offices are usually longer than those issued in teaching institutions. An instructor in radiology, as he opened his private office, prepared a number of standardized reports, thinking he would merely tell his secretary to type no. 5, 12, or 24, as the case would require. After the office opened, he had at first only a few reports and all the time he wanted. Later, when business increased, he had "grown up" and knew better than to put out pre-fabricated roentgen reports. Even when adequately prepared and properly seasoned, so as to look and taste (almost) like the real thing, pre-cooked meat will never fool the connoisseur.

☆

A right middle lobe may legally harbor a malignancy,

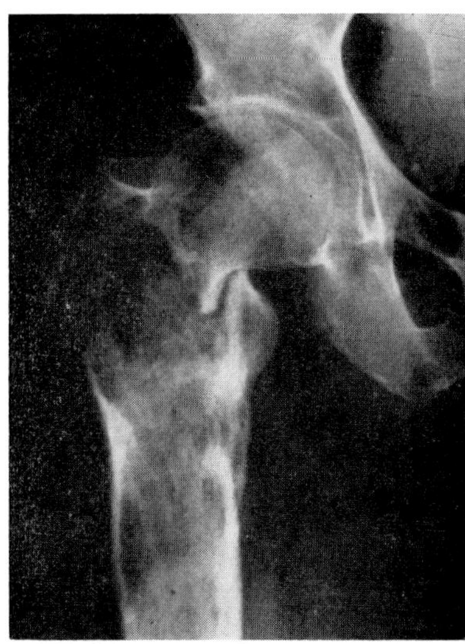

PATHOLOGIC FRACTURE. This seventy-seven-year old male was admitted with arteriosclerotic heart disease in failure. The urologist suspected prostatic malignancy, and the biopsy confirmed his suspicion. The right femoral fracture was discovered during the retrograde urography (patient had been bed-fast for several months). The roentgen report of the retrograde contained also the following sentence: *Osteolytic* process is *visible in the right upper femoral shaft and trochanteric region, with pathologic intertrochanteric fracture; no displacement of the fragments; it has the appearance of a metastatic lesion, possibly though not very likely from the prostatic carcinoma.* Autopsy demonstrated instead – of all things – a primary osteosarcome in the right femur.

but such an occurrence is thought to be exceedingly rare. When you find atelectasis in the middle lobe, chances are it is benign. In such an instance, mentioning in the report the malignancy first, is like betting at the roulette table on a single number.

There was a radiologist who boasted of a secret weapon, which he called the time-bomb. His reports were so long that few readers ventured beyond the impression. Occasionally, he would slip into the report – *but not into the summary* – some item intended only as an alibi, just in case things were to turn that way. The method was "successful" and this radiologist enjoyed several "free bites" – but when he finally found another job he resolved to renounce the use of weapons concealed in roentgen reports.

From an aerodynamic viewpoint, the bumble bee is absolutely unfit to fly, but not having been so told, it keeps on flying. Also in radiology, *empiricists* (in the pure sense of the word) are often successful. It is possible to correlate a given configuration of shadows – without knowing why and wherefore – with a certain disease. Later, when one recognizes (in another patient) that same configuration of shadows, he is perfectly entitled to mention that certain disease in the respective roentgen report, as long as the whole thing is identified as what it is: a hunch.

As a group, the Ph.D.'s have added so much to our knowledge that radiology is forever indebted to them. But their influence has also fostered the (excessive) use of numerical yardsticks. When pelvimetric measurements are significant, one way or another, this is usually so obvious that it can be told in the roentgen report without checking or involving actual figures. In borderline cases, the figures are equivocal, and clinical evaluation is usually needed to determine the degree of *functional* cephalo-pelvic disproportion. Quite a few times, the matter is finally settled in a sensible (natural) way, by labor trial.

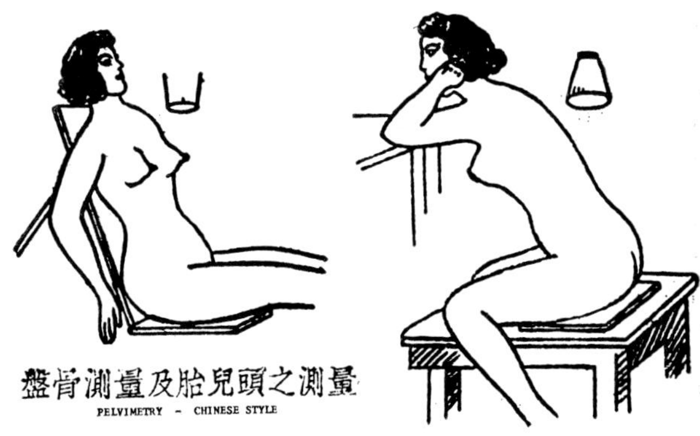

A well known hospital radiologist proudly referred to himself as the cock whose crowing (the consultations and roentgen reports) provided the ingredient needed to impregnate the minds of the (hens forming the) medical staff. Another confrère – the difference has obvious Freudian overtones – complained that he is treated like a courtesan, who must satisfy the requests of anyone on the staff, at any time, the most bothersome demands being made in the midst of roentgen reporting. Even if one feels that way, there is still a choice between being as cultured, refined, and diplomatic as a hetaira of ancient Greece, or behaving like a common harlot.

☆

A small town surgeon, who sees the same people over and over again, is usually more candid, cautious, cheerful, considerate, and conscientious than a big city operator. Similarly, to his constant customers (the referring physicians), the radiologist must offer true professional courtesy, not only polite countenance. Nobody is perfect: if given sufficient time and patients, the best of radiologists will send a few misleading roentgen reports to each of his referring physicians. This is expected to happen, and no serious clinician will become querulous over sporadic oversights or occasional misinterpretations. As long as the radiologist remains cogent, composed, congenial, consistent, and co-operative with his captive clientele, nobody will clamor for another, perhaps more charming captor.

ROUND-UP OF ROENTGEN REPORTS

In this sampler no attempt was made to cover the entire diagnostic field, or even a circumscribed portion of it. The reports have been selected (almost) at random. Some have ancient, respectable dates, others are quite recent. Several carry the names of famous radiologists, while as many or more are the work of residents in training. The list contains a few excellent, and a slight majority of satisfactory, reports; others are not quite so good. A number of gross errors have been "weeded out," but — as in all human endeavor — there is still room for improvement. Besides, there are always several correct ways of reporting a given situation or occurrence.

Plans are being made to re-print the entire chapter as a separate publication. In that case it would have a sizable appendix with roentgen reports selected so as to cover all anticipated contingencies. Those wishing to have their creations considered for inclusion in that king-size sampler, are herewith invited to submit as many typical (and/or outstanding) report specimens as they believe to be suitable for such a purpose. An occasional film might also be reproduced in that sampler, provided it stressed a particular reporting point.

Form I-91 (11-12-58)
Inspection Dept. X-RAY REPORT

PT.NAME I.P. CYL. OUTER LOWER NO.OF PCS. 1 DATE 3-9-58
ORDER NO. 2-0304-20562 GROUP NO. 0600-002 INSP. Ausloos *Ausloos*
DRAWING NO. 03-509-180-002 TEST NO. W52699 PATTERN NO TE 16093-2
CUSTOMER Wis. Electric Power Serial 157 P.O.NO. 298614

AREA	TECHNIQUE		INDICATIONS		DISPOSITION
153	120R	6'	7 x17A		OK
154	110R	6'	14 x 17A		OK
155	40R	6'	14 x 17A		OK
156	40R	6'	14 x 17A		OK
157	40R	6'	14 x 17A		OK
158	40R	6'	14 x 17A	gas, sand	Repr.
159	30R	6'	14 x 17A	gas, shrink	Repr.
160	40R	6'	14 x 17A	sand, gas, shrink	Repr.

Courtesy: Allis-Chalmers.

BETATRON REPORT. Radiographic examinations made at the Allis-Chalmers in Milwaukee are reported with simple technical data, and include – on the same line– the advice offered.

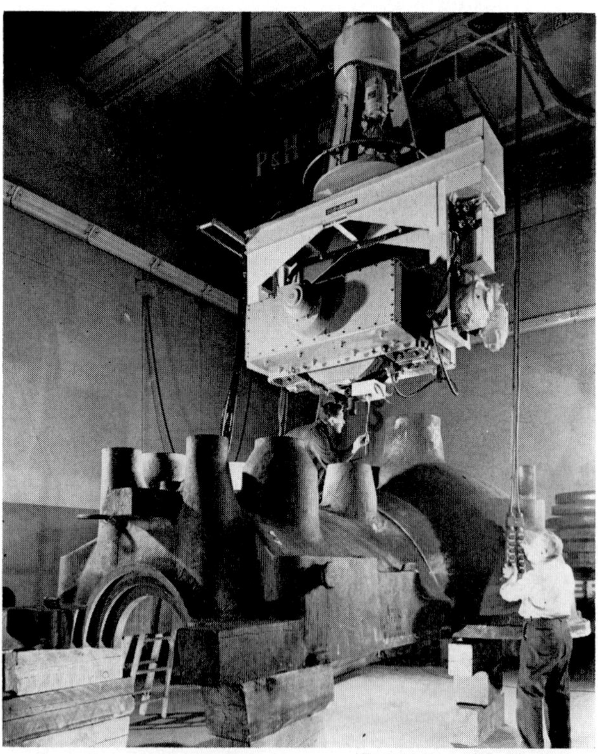

Courtesy: Allis-Chalmers.

BETATRON IN INDUSTRIAL ACTION. This is the IP (intermediate pressure) cylinder, mentioned in the preceding report, being subjected to betatron radiography in the Allis-Chalmers laboratories. The cylinder is from a 125,000 kw cross-compound reheat steam turbine.

Cook County Hospital, Chicago, September 21, 1939.

Four views of the skull proper reveal a non-depressed fissure fracture in the right occipital bone. The fracture measures about three inches in length.— EDWARD WARNICK, M.D.

☆

San Francisco, Calif., May 5, 1959

SINUSES. The nasal and accessory sinuses are well developed. The left maxillary sinus is clear. There is a polyp or cyst in the roof of the right maxillary sinus, and thickening or scarring in the floor of this sinus. This was well seen on the Waters' view.

There is a 4 mm diameter opacity in the roof of the right frontal sinus, in about its mid portion. This could be a small osteoma. There is an extra loculus extending cephalad from the upper portion of the frontal sinuses, actually connected with the left frontal.

Incidentally, there is benign hyperostosis of the inner table of the frontal bones. The ethmoidal and sphenoidal sinuses are clear. — J. H. HEALD, M.D.

☆

University Hospitals, Cincinnati, August 24, 1959

AP AND LATERAL SKULL: No unusual findings are noted with the exception of the enlargement of the sella turcica which is probably on the basis of the previously treated pituitary tumor. — DR. LESSURE

☆

Johns Hopkins Hospital, Baltimore, Md., September 1, 1959

SKULL: The calvaria, sella, petrous pyramids and base show no particular abnormality. There has been no real change in the appearance of the skull since the previous examination of 8-5-57; however, there may be a borderline shift of the pineal to the left. This shift amounts to only two millimeters as far as I can ascertain. It is of questionable significance, but the pineal did not appear shifted on previous films. Accordingly, contrast studies of the brain may be entertained. — DR. LANG

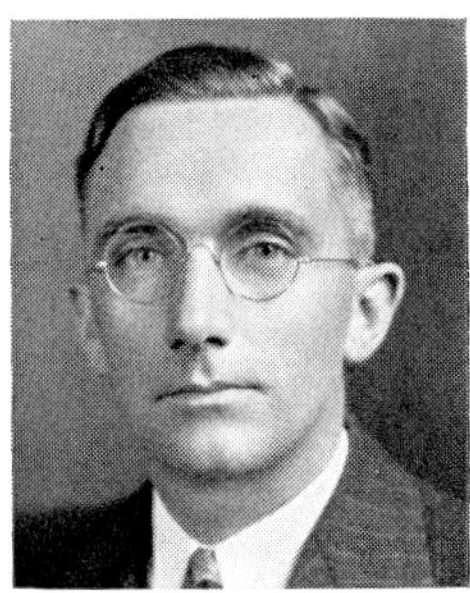

BARTON YOUNG

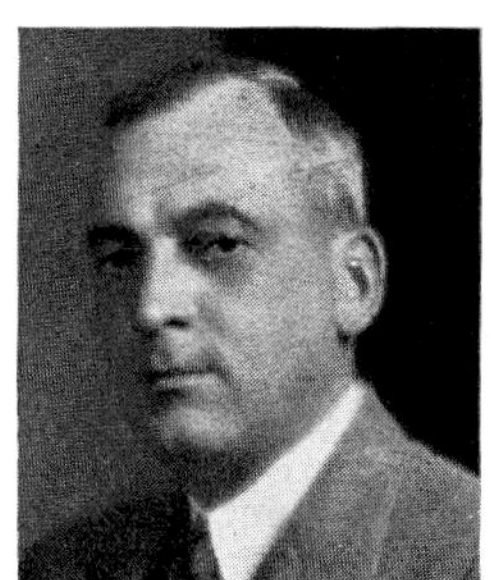

CHARLES A. WATERS

☆

Germantown Hospital, Philadelphia, September 13, 1959

MANDIBLE AND SKULL: The mandible is fractured in three places, namely in the region of the right and left condyles and at the symphysis. The distal or major fragment of the right condyle is displaced posteriorly and the same statement is true on the left although displacement is not as marked as on the right. There is very little displacement of the fragments of the fractured symphysis. A gap several millimeters wide is plainly demonstrated. The extent of damage to the teeth cannot be easily evaluated because intraoral examination is not yet possible.

The cranium is free of evidence of fracture. The cranial bones and sutures are intact.

CONCLUSIONS: We have demonstrated fractures of the mandible in the region of the symphysis and right and left condyles. — BARTON R. YOUNG, M.D.

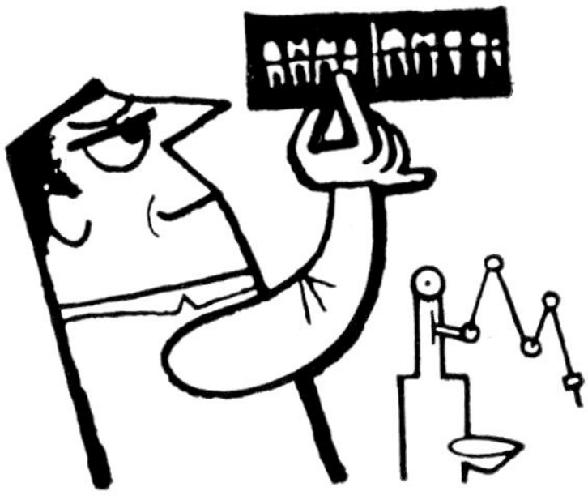

Bellevue Hospital, New York City, April 18, 1960

Examination of the right mandible reveals periseptal widening of the second molar, with noticeable alveolar recession. A lucent area (granuloma?) is seen near the apex of the root. — DR. THORNHILL

☆

Western Psychiatric Institute, Pittsburgh, November 16, 1961

SKULL & ORBITS: Additional examination with special attention to the right orbit, using posteroanterior and lateral plane laminagraphic cuts at one half centimer interval, confirms the previous finding of tumor mass, involving the orbital surface of the greater wing on the right side of the sphenoid bone. On laminagraphic studies made in the coronal plane, the tumor is shown to have destroyed the orbital plate on the right, extending posteriorly to the greater and lesser wings of the sphenoid bone, with destruction of the cerebral surface of the greater wing, and of the anterior wall of the right middle cranial fossa. These findings are also confirmed by four-fold enlargement studies which, in addition, reveal to better advantage the osteoblastic qualities of the process. There are no changes in the pituitary fossa or sella turcica to suggest increased intracranial pressure.

IMPRESSION: Tumor in right orbit, probably metastatic prostatic carcinoma, involving the orbital surface of the right sphenoid bone, the orbital plate above it, and the anterior wall (cerebral surface of the greater wing) of the right middle cranial fossa.— LEWIS E. ETTER, M.D.

☆

Bellevue Hospital, New York City, May 21, 1951

Pneumoencephalography shows a marked deviation of the ventricular system to the right. Even the left ventricle (which is otherwise of average size and shape) has crossed the midline over to the right. The right ventricle is markedly dilated, in a uniform fashion. The third and fourth ventricles are not dilated. There is no air in the subarachnoid space.

CONCLUSION: Hydrocephalus ex-vacuo to the trophic side, which in this case is the right. — S. L. BERANBAUM, M.D.

☆

Leningrad, January 3, 1941

Patient was referred for roentgen examination with the diagnosis, "concrement in Wharton's duct, right." Preliminary views of the skull show a rounded, fair-sized calculus in the soft tissues of the right inframandibular region. The stone is best seen in the vertico-submental projection.

SIALOGRAPHY. The oral orifice of the right-sided Wharton's duct was located at the level of the first incisor, and appeared markedly dilated. Salivary secretion was noticeably diminished. In order to empty the duct, patient was advised to chew a slice of lemon. After two minutes of chewing, salivation from the right Wharton's duct ceased. One milliliter Iodolipol was instilled into the orifice of the duct.

The sialograms reveal good filling of the basal branch of the duct, and of its subdivisions within the body of the submaxillary gland. A round filling defect is clearly noticed at the junction of proximal and middle thirds of the duct. This filling defect is sharply circumscribed, and coincides with the location of the concrement, seen on the preliminary films. The lumen of the duct distal to the calculus is visibly narrowed. Below the calculus there appears a cavity, well filled with opaque medium. The lumina of the small ramifications of the duct within the salivary gland are slightly dilated — presumably because of the occlusion of the duct, but otherwise show no pathologic alterations.

CONCLUSION: Concretion in the right-sided Wharton's duct, with abscess in the right sub-mandibular gland. — G. A. ZEDGUENIDZE, M.D.

☆

University Hospital, Ann Arbor, Mich., November 12, 1959

NASO-LACRIMAL INJECTION: Injection of the naso-lacrimal ducts bilaterally shows that there is an adequate flow of the duct system into the nasal cavity on the right. Pooling of the contrast material is seen in the naso-lacrimal canals on the left without evidence of flow into the nasal cavity. No significant dilatation is seen in the sac system on either side.

IMPRESSION: Apparent obstruction of naso-lacrimal duct system on the left. — J. C. SPENCER, M.D.

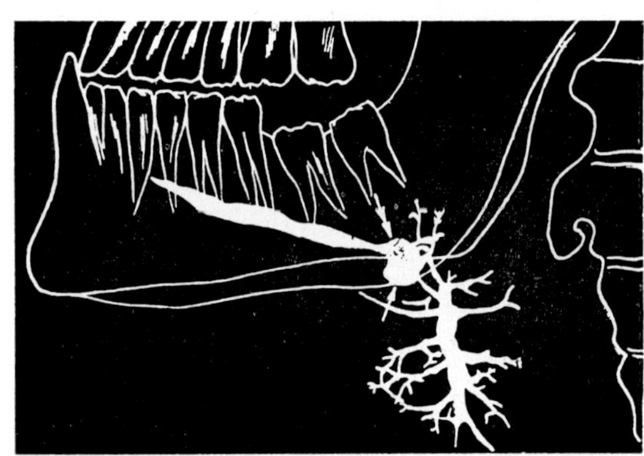

SIALOGRAM. The stone in Wharton's duct is marked with a twin-pointed arrow. Immediately below the calculus is the (larger) abscess cavity, marked with a single-pointed arrow. This case was included by Zedguenidze in his monograph on sialography, published in Moscow in 1953 – this sketch is therein Figure 38 (on page 86), and is herein reproduced through courtesy of its author, and of the publisher, Medgiz.

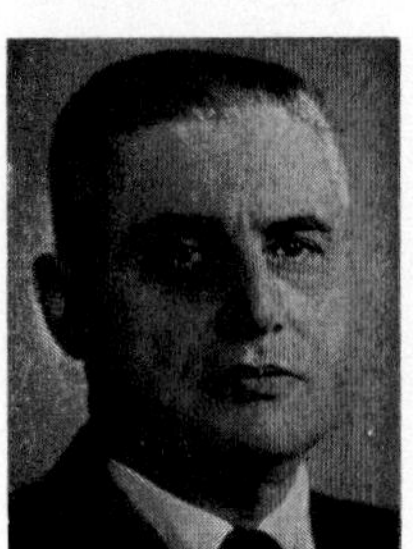

GEORGE ZEDGUENIDZE

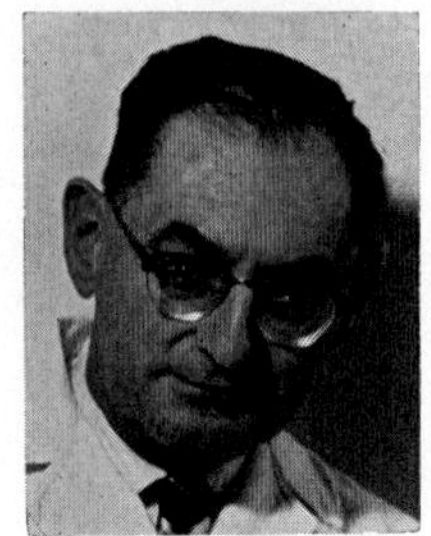

ERNST RUCKENSTEINER

Washington, D.C., February 2, 1920

Small oval rarefied area about one inch above lower articular surface of tibia, one-half inch from inner surface and same distance from posterior surface. Some increased density of entire end of bone, probably due to congestion. Probably localized abscess (Brodie's abscess). Edwin A. Merritt, M.D.

☆

Cook County Hospital, Chicago, March 8, 1955

Two views of the right ankle show a tri-malleolar fracture, with comminution into the articular surface of the tibia. The fibula is widely separated. There is talo-tibial subluxation, with the astragalus displaced laterally, as well as posteriorly.

Two other views of the right ankle, made after manipulation, reveal that the previously described fragments have been reduced to almost anatomical

19 3/1 41г

Протокол рентгенологического исследования

Возраст— М. Ж.

Фамилия, и., о. Б-ов, 21 года

Адрес:

Больной направлен на рентгенологическое исследование с диагнозом "конкременты прав.вартонового протока".

На обзорной рентгенограмме черепа в боковой проекции определяется: овальной формы, довольно крупный конкремент в мягких тканях правой подчелюстной области. Этот конкремент более отчетливо виден на рентгенограмме нижней челюсти в подбородочном положении.

Сиалография

Выходное отверстие правого вартонова протока расположено на уровне первого правого резца, резко расширено.

Слюноотделение значительно уменьшено.

С целью опорожнения вартонова протока больному предложен кусочек лимона для сосания. Через 2 минуты слюноотделение из отверстия прав.вартонова протока прекратилось. Через выводное отверстие в вартонов проток введено около 1 мл иодолипола.

На сиалограммах определяется: контрастное вещество хорошо заполняет основной ствол протока и все его разветвления в толще железы. На границе средней и проксимальной трети протока отчетливо виден овальной формы дефект наполнения, имеющий четкие, хорошо очерченные контуры. Дефект наполнения по местоположению соответствует обнаруженному на рентгенограммах конкременту. Дистально от конкремента определяется значительное сужение просвета протока. Непосредственно под конкрементом видна довольно крупная полость, заполненная контрастным веществом.
Внутрижелезистые разветвления вартонова протока патологических изменений не обнаруживают, за исключением небольшого расширения их просвета в результате затруднения оттока.

Заключение: Конкремент в прав.вартоновом протоке.
Абсцесс прав.подчелюстной железы.

Профессор [signature] (Г.А.Зедгенидзе)

Report by Zedguenidze. The (liberal) translation is incorporated in the sampler.

relationship. The limb is encased in plaster cast, with walking irons.

IMPRESSION: Pott's fracture right ankle, reduced, and casted in excellent position. — George Podlusky, M.D.

☆

Cook County Hospital, Chicago, December 12, 1956

Anteroposterior view of the pelvis, including both hips, and single (oblique) view of the left hip, show again the previously described subcapital fracture of the left femur, with a Smith-Petersen nail in place. Super-imposition of the latest films upon those exposed on September 8, 1956 reveals that noticeable additional impaction has occurred in the femoral neck. The fragment of femoral head is apparently more opaque than before. On the latest film, the tip of the nail "protrudes" in projection beyond the cortex of the acetabular rim.

IMPRESSION: Devitalization of the fragment of femoral head suspected. — Morris Sokoloff, M.D.

University Roentgen Institute, Innsbruck, Austria, July 27, 1957

RIGHT UPPER THIGH: Just above the right femoral mid-shaft, the bone has expanded in the

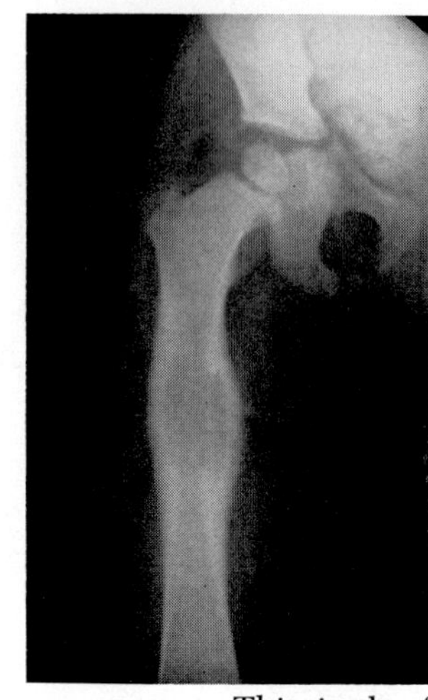

Eosinophilic granuloma. This is the film described in Ruckensteiner's report.

Aus dem **Zentralröntgeninstitut der Universitätskliniken Innsbruck**

Prof. Dr. Ernst Ruckensteiner

Bericht an Herrn Dr. Medizinalrat Dr. Ganner.

über M o n o t t Franziska. Die Untersuchung erfolgte am 27.6.1957.

Rechter Oberschenkel:

Ein ca 4 cm langer, knapp oberhalb der Mitte des Schafts gelegener Bereich des rechten Oberschenkelknochens ist spindelig aufgetrieben. Die Cortikalis dieses Bereichs ist größtenteils erhalten, wohl aber örtlich verdünnt. Der Bereich ist zentral aufgehellt. Diese Aufhellung geht cranial- und caudalwärts in die der Markhöhle über. Sie ist aber intensiver als letzterer, so daß eine scharf gezeichnete Grenzlinie zustande kommt. Dadurch wird offenbar, daß ein umschriebener, gut begrenzter, osteolytischer Herd vorliegt. Die Periostlinie ist ebenmäßig und die den Herd benachbarte Knochenstruktur hat keine Änderung erfahren.

Differentialdiagnostische Erwägungen legen weder die Annahme eines maligen osteogenen Knochentumors nahe, noch die eines umschriebenen Entzündungsherdes; entsprechende Röntgensymptome fehlen. Es kann sich auch nicht um eine blande Knochencyste handeln, da eine solche anders lokalisiert und anders gestaltet aufzutreten pflegt. Besonders mit Rücksicht auf das Alter des Kindes ist an die Wahrscheinlichkeit zu denken, daß ein eosinophiles Granulom vorliegt.

Ruckensteiner

C-Stoff 70 g - 20 m - 1. 62 - Frohnweiler 28557

Report by Ruckensteiner. The (liberal) translation is in the sampler.

shape of a spindle. The cortex is preserved, if thinned out in places. The expanded bone segment contains a central radiolucency, which extends into the medullary canal, both craniad and caudad. In the latter extension the radiolucency is more pronounced, and results in a demarcating line. This is a localized, well circumscribed, osteolytic process. The periosteal line is smooth, and the surrounding bone texture has undergone no alterations.

Neither malignant osteogenic bone tumor, nor localized inflammatory process should be included in the differential diagnosis, because the respective roentgen symptoms are lacking. A benign bone cyst would be expected to appear in a different shape and location. Especially with regard to the child's age, the probability of an eosinophilic granuloma ought to be considered. — Ernst Ruckensteiner, M.D.

Cook County Hospital, Chicago, February 23, 1958

Two views of the right knee, including the proximal thirds of tibial and femoral shafts, after removal of plaster cast, show additional new bone formation about the previously described plateau fracture. The bone fragments are apparently "glued," but the fracture line is still identified.

IMPRESSION: Progress examination of fracture of plateau of right tibia, healing in good position. — Hyo Hyun Byun, M.D.

University Hospitals, Cincinnati, August 25, 1959

AP PELVIS: The right acetabulum is poorly developed and shallow, and the femoral head is located superiorly and laterally to its expected position. There is rotation and coxa vara deformity. Large bony spurs are present on the right ilium. It is not known whether this is a result of old trauma or surgery, such as a bone graft. The left hip joint shows no abnormality.

LEFT FOOT: There is hallux valgus deformity. The relationships of the tarsal bones appear somewhat distorted but this is probably due to the angle

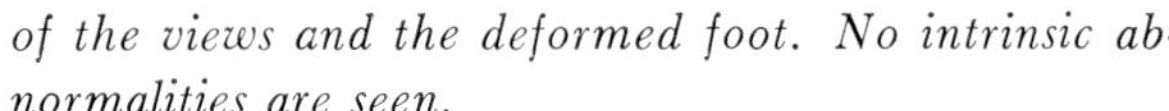

of the views and the deformed foot. No intrinsic abnormalities are seen.

IMPRESSION:
1. *Coxa vara deformity right hip.*
2. *Shallow poorly developed right acetabulum.*
3. *Large bony spurs in the right ilium, the etiology of which is not known.*
4. *Deformity of the left foot, with no intrinsic bony abnormalities seen.* — Dr. Smith

☆

Chicago Osteopathic College and Hospital, September 26, 1959

Postural study made with the patient in the weight bearing position with shoes on, and with one quarter inch lift under the right heel, reveals the left femoral head to be twelve millimeters lower than is the right. There is no significant variation in the base of the

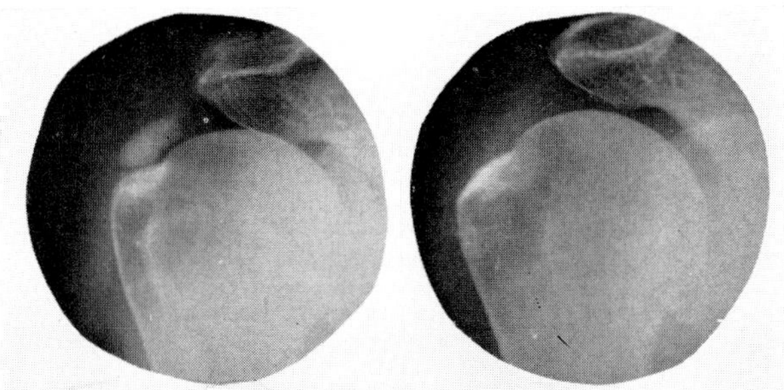

Evanescent calcification. Patient came to the Medical Clinic in Paris (Illinois) because of pain in the shoulder. The visible opacification was interpreted as a calcification in the subdeltoid bursa. After a few applications of ultrasound to the point of maximum pain, a recheck showed that the "calcification" had faded. The opacification must have been due to the calcium content of the intrabursal fluid, because a true-to-goodness calcification is not very likely to disappear on such a short order.

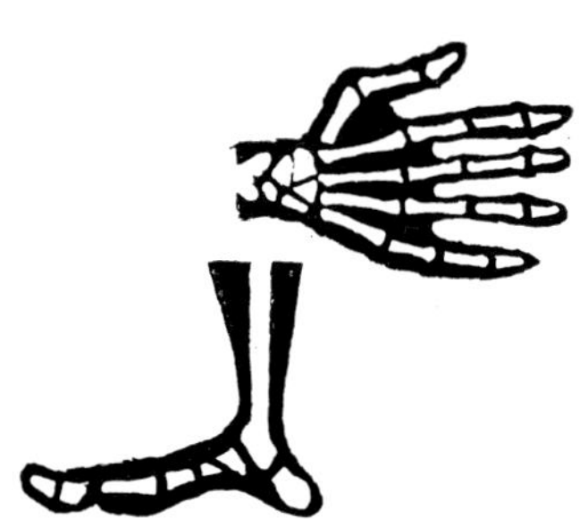

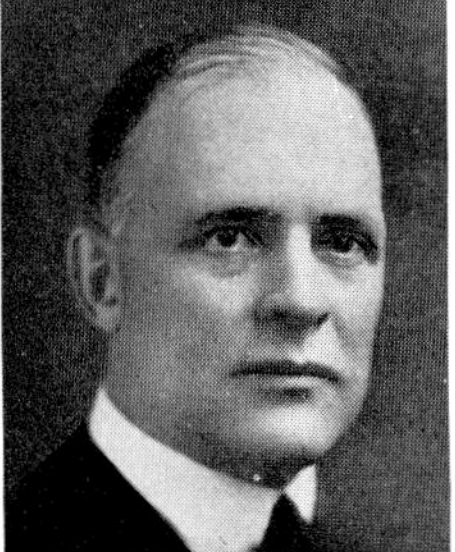

Thomas Burcham

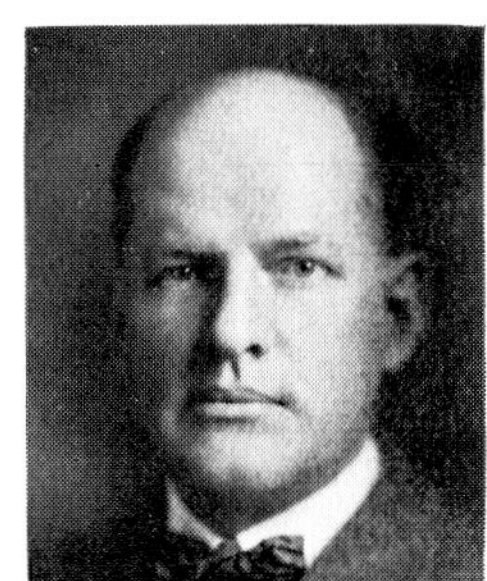

Edwin A. Merritt

sacrum, however a definite rotoscoliosis of the lumbar spine to the right is identified.

IMPRESSION: Pelvic tilt down on the left with definite rotoscoliosis of the lumbar spine to the right. — Ray E. Bishop, D.O.

☆

Presidio Division Hospital, July 27, 1898

Radiograph of the chest, viewed from the back, shows lodged Mauser bullet, which has passed through the spine, lying two inches to the right of the spine over the third intercostal space. — E. F. Ascheim*

☆

Iowa Methodist Hospital, Iowa City, December 4, 1916

Right lung good condition. Glands on right slightly calcified. Lower left lobe — lower portion — firm. Lung partially covered with fibrous tissue; there is also a cavity 1½ inches in diameter. Upper lobe seems to be replaced by fairly dense tissue which resembles tuberculosis. Both the fourth and the fifth ribs posteriorly on the left side are destroyed. This had the appearance of malignancy. — Thomas A. Burcham, M.D.

☆

Montreal General Hospital, December 15, 1924

X-ray examination of the chest shows the presence of coarse mottling with blurring occupying the upper half of the right lung field. The hilar shadows are enlarged. Heart small and vertical. Inner halves of diaphragm flattened. — W. A. Wilkins, M.D.

☆

Montreal General Hospital, April 28, 1925.

Single plate was made of the chest. Both lungs show diminished ventilation practically throughout, although the right lower lobe is not so much involved. Both costo-phrenic angles clear and distinct. Both root shadows show heavy increase and contain fibrotic glands and lymph nodes. Marked generalized bronchial and peri-bronchial thickening seen. Marked infiltration throughout the right upper and middle lobes, the entire left upper lobe and part of the lower lobe. There are some areas of consolidation seen in both upper lobes. DIAGNOSIS: Marked evidence of tuberculosis of a broncho-pneumonic type with consolidation and possible cavitation. W. L. Ritchie, Roentgenologist.

New York University, New York City, January 24, 1935

Diffuse hazy cloud over the lower half of the left pulmonic field and portions of the right pulmonic field, as a result of partial infiltration and consolidation. Progress examination of known case of yeast infection. Improvement noted. — Lewis J. Friedman, M.D.

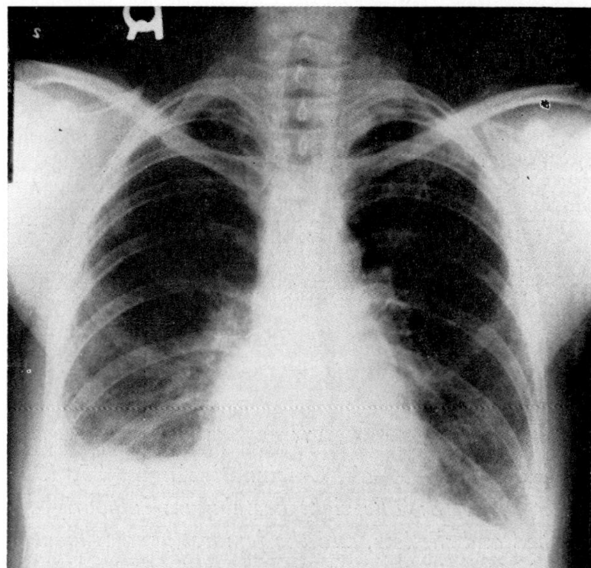

Stage five. This forty-three-year old female had been treated with a full course of intracavitary radium plus external roentgen therapy for a small ulceration of the cervix which, on biopsy, proved to be a carcinoma. One year later she was back with a frozen pelvis. She also coughed, and the description of her chest film was *Posteroanterior view of the chest shows bilateral pleural effusion, presently a large amount on the right. Increased linearity is seen in both bases, compatible with pneumonitis, and yet not at all typical. The outline of the heart is somewhat irregular, as if there were pleuro-pericardial adhesions. IMPRESSION: knowing that patient has recurrent carcinoma of the cervix, with extensive pelvic involvement, one wonders how the findings in the chest could be related to the malignant pelvic tumor.* The answer was not long in coming. Patient died in the Paris (Illinois) Hospital, and at autopsy — performed by James Falker, the gynecologic consultant — patient proved to have metastases from the carcinoma of the cervix to the heart and right lung.

*Elizabeth Fleischmann Ascheim (1859-1905) was not a physician, but she is one of the roentgen martyrs listed by Percy Brown (1936). This report was preserved in an illustrated text printed after the Spanish War in 1900 by the then captain and assistant surgeon William Cline Borden (1858-1934). The suggestion to use some of the reports from Borden's text was made by several radiologists, including Charles Wesley Blackett and Howard Leary of Boston, and James Jay Clark of Atlanta.

shape of a spindle. The cortex is preserved, if thinned out in places. The expanded bone segment contains a central radiolucency, which extends into the medullary canal, both craniad and caudad. In the latter extension the radiolucency is more pronounced, and results in a demarcating line. This is a localized, well circumscribed, osteolytic process. The periosteal line is smooth, and the surrounding bone texture has undergone no alterations.

Neither malignant osteogenic bone tumor, nor localized inflammatory process should be included in the differential diagnosis, because the respective roentgen symptoms are lacking. A benign bone cyst would be expected to appear in a different shape and location. Especially with regard to the child's age, the probability of an eosinophilic granuloma ought to be considered. — Ernst Ruckensteiner, M.D.

☆

Cook County Hospital, Chicago, February 23, 1958

Two views of the right knee, including the proximal thirds of tibial and femoral shafts, after removal of plaster cast, show additional new bone formation about the previously described plateau fracture. The bone fragments are apparently "glued," but the fracture line is still identified.

IMPRESSION: Progress examination of fracture of plateau of right tibia, healing in good position. — Hyo Hyun Byun, M.D.

☆

University Hospitals, Cincinnati, August 25, 1959

AP PELVIS: The right acetabulum is poorly developed and shallow, and the femoral head is located superiorly and laterally to its expected position. There is rotation and coxa vara deformity. Large bony spurs are present on the right ilium. It is not known whether this is a result of old trauma or surgery, such as a bone graft. The left hip joint shows no abnormality.

LEFT FOOT: There is hallux valgus deformity. The relationships of the tarsal bones appear somewhat distorted but this is probably due to the angle of the views and the deformed foot. No intrinsic abnormalities are seen.

IMPRESSION:
1. *Coxa vara deformity right hip.*
2. *Shallow poorly developed right acetabulum.*
3. *Large bony spurs in the right ilium, the etiology of which is not known.*
4. *Deformity of the left foot, with no intrinsic bony abnormalities seen.* — Dr. Smith

☆

Chicago Osteopathic College and Hospital, September 26, 1959

Postural study made with the patient in the weight bearing position with shoes on, and with one quarter inch lift under the right heel, reveals the left femoral head to be twelve millimeters lower than is the right. There is no significant variation in the base of the

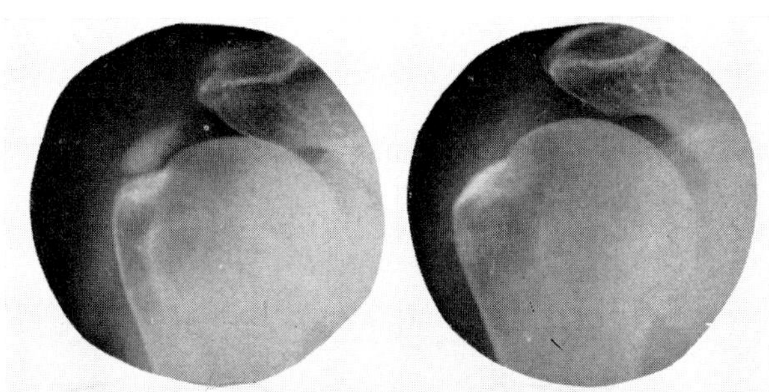

Evanescent calcification. Patient came to the Medical Clinic in Paris (Illinois) because of pain in the shoulder. The visible opacification was interpreted as a calcification in the subdeltoid bursa. After a few applications of ultrasound to the point of maximum pain, a recheck showed that the "calcification" had faded. The opacification must have been due to the calcium content of the intrabursal fluid, because a true-to-goodness calcification is not very likely to disappear on such a short order.

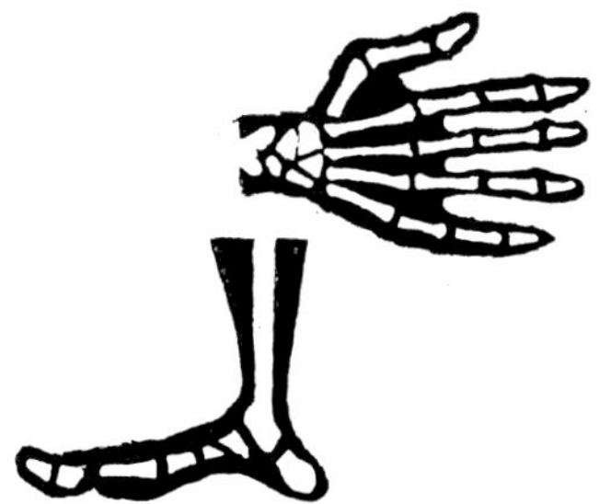

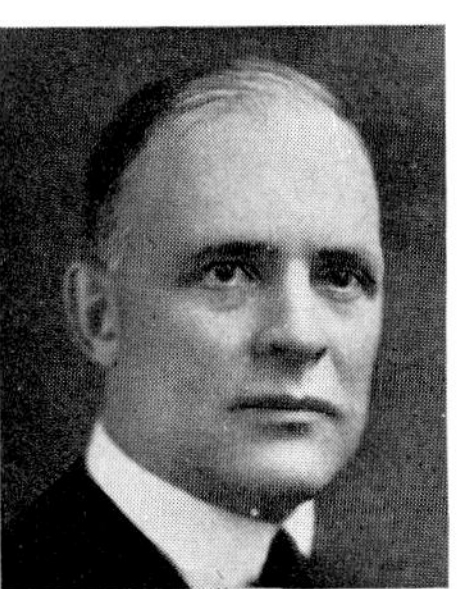

Thomas Burcham

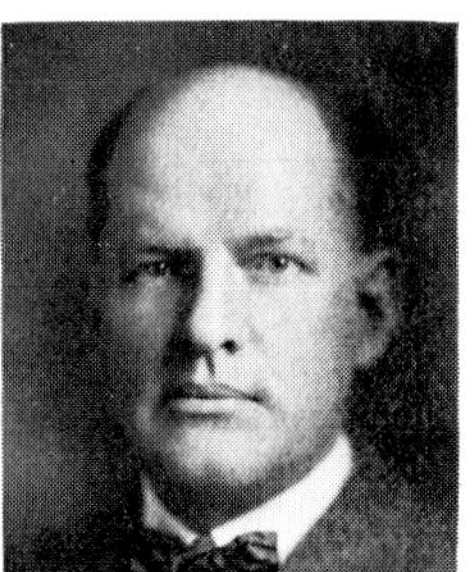

Edwin A. Merritt

sacrum, however a definite rotoscoliosis of the lumbar spine to the right is identified.

IMPRESSION: Pelvic tilt down on the left with definite rotoscoliosis of the lumbar spine to the right. — RAY E. BISHOP, D.O.

☆

Presidio Division Hospital, July 27, 1898

Radiograph of the chest, viewed from the back, shows lodged Mauser bullet, which has passed through the spine, lying two inches to the right of the spine over the third intercostal space. — E. F. ASCHEIM*

☆

Iowa Methodist Hospital, Iowa City, December 4, 1916

Right lung good condition. Glands on right slightly calcified. Lower left lobe — lower portion — firm. Lung partially covered with fibrous tissue; there is also a cavity 1½ inches in diameter. Upper lobe seems to be replaced by fairly dense tissue which resembles tuberculosis. Both the fourth and the fifth ribs posteriorly on the left side are destroyed. This had the appearance of malignancy. — THOMAS A. BURCHAM, M.D.

☆

Montreal General Hospital, December 15, 1924

X-ray examination of the chest shows the presence of coarse mottling with blurring occupying the upper half of the right lung field. The hilar shadows are enlarged. Heart small and vertical. Inner halves of diaphragm flattened. — W. A. WILKINS, M.D.

☆

Montreal General Hospital, April 28, 1925.

Single plate was made of the chest. Both lungs show diminished ventilation practically throughout, although the right lower lobe is not so much involved. Both costo-phrenic angles clear and distinct. Both root shadows show heavy increase and contain fibrotic glands and lymph nodes. Marked generalized bronchial and peri-bronchial thickening seen. Marked infiltration throughout the right upper and middle lobes, the entire left upper lobe and part of the lower lobe. There are some areas of consolidation seen in both upper lobes. DIAGNOSIS: Marked evidence of tuberculosis of a broncho-pneumonic type with consolidation and possible cavitation. W. L. Ritchie, Roentgenologist.

New York University, New York City, January 24, 1935

Diffuse hazy cloud over the lower half of the left pulmonic field and portions of the right pulmonic field, as a result of partial infiltration and consolidation. Progress examination of known case of yeast infection. Improvement noted. — LEWIS J. FRIEDMAN, M.D.

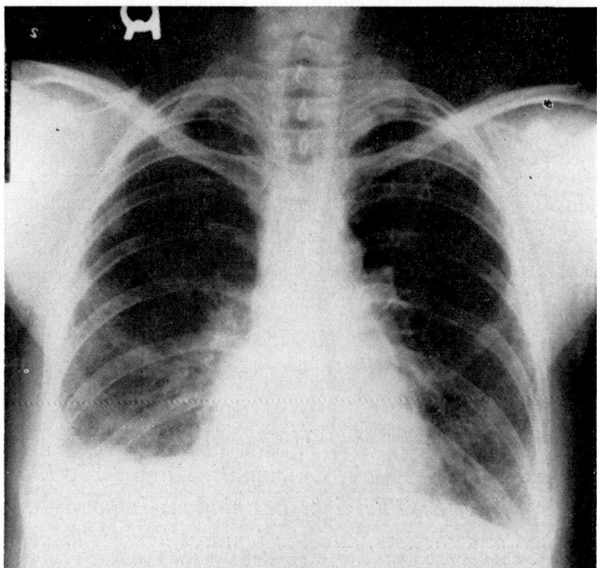

STAGE FIVE. This forty-three-year old female had been treated with a full course of intracavitary radium plus external roentgen therapy for a small ulceration of the cervix which, on biopsy, proved to be a carcinoma. One year later she was back with a frozen pelvis. She also coughed, and the description of her chest film was *Posteroanterior view of the chest shows bilateral pleural effusion, presently a large amount on the right. Increased linearity is seen in both bases, compatible with pneumonitis, and yet not at all typical. The outline of the heart is somewhat irregular, as if there were pleuro-pericardial adhesions. IMPRESSION: knowing that patient has recurrent carcinoma of the cervix, with extensive pelvic involvement, one wonders how the findings in the chest could be related to the malignant pelvic tumor.* The answer was not long in coming. Patient died in the Paris (Illinois) Hospital, and at autopsy — performed by James Falker, the gynecologic consultant — patient proved to have metastases from the carcinoma of the cervix to the heart and right lung.

*Elizabeth Fleischmann Ascheim (1859-1905) was not a physician, but she is one of the roentgen martyrs listed by Percy Brown (1936). This report was preserved in an illustrated text printed after the Spanish War in 1900 by the then captain and assistant surgeon William Cline Borden (1858-1934). The suggestion to use some of the reports from Borden's text was made by several radiologists, including Charles Wesley Blackett and Howard Leary of Boston, and James Jay Clark of Atlanta.

St. Louis City Hospital, St. Louis, Mo., May 27, 1946

Re-examination of the chest within one week after radiation therapy reveals marked regression of the consolidation previously present throughout the upper portion of the lungs. This would indicate that the condition is probably a new growth of the lymphoblastoma type. At this examination the tumor seems to take on the appearance of a more rounded mass in the upper mediastinal region similar to that seen in the examination of 1942. There is no visible pathology elsewhere in the lungs. — LeRoy Sante, M.D.

☆

Kankakee State Hospital, Kankakee (Illinois), March 16, 1959

CHEST RECHECK: Light productive densities in the right upper lobe. Very likely acid fast in nature. No appreciable change since 1947. Hilar calcium deposits bilaterally. Advise periodic bacteriologic work-up, and clinical observation. Recheck in 3 months. — Ernest Teller, M.D.

☆

San Francisco, Calif., March 3, 1959

CHEST: There are several circular opacities scattered throughout the lungs, ranging from 3 to 5 mm. in diameter. The left hemidiaphragm is obscurred by fluid or thickened pleura.

THORACIC SPINE: Moderate hypertrophic changes are present on the margins of most of the thoracic bodies. There is thinning of the 10th and 11th discs.

SKULL: There are multiple areas of increased and decreased density in the calvarium, mostly about 1 cm. in diameter. The sella is of average size and shape. The pineal is not displaced.

CONCLUSION: Metastatic lesions, lungs and skull. — L. H. Garland, M.D.

☆

University Hospital, Ann Arbor (Michigan), April 5, 1959

The previously described pneumonitis in the right base has cleared entirely since 5-14-59. The pulmonary markings are somewhat prominent. This has been a feature of this chest throughout all our examinations and is probably a non-pathologic variant There is no evidence of active pulmonary parenchymal diseases at this time. — J. A. Tobin, M.D.

☆

Houston, May 23, 1959

Anteroposterior view of the chest, exposed with mobile equipment, is not diagnostic for heart size because of short focal distance, but the transverse cardiac diameter seems enlarged. Absence of a segment of the left sixth rib indicates recent thoracotomy. No pneumothorax can be identified, but hazyness over the left lung field may represent pleural effusion in declive location. A few linear opacities in the left base may be resolving areas of atelectasis. For further information please request chest x-ray recheck in upright position when feasible with the patient's general condition. — Dr. Johnson

Germantown Hospital, Philadelphia, September 19, 1959

There is still no evidence of metastatic disease in this patient's lungs and ribs. The lungs remain clear and the rib cage is intact. The heart and great vessels continue to present their usual appearance.

Another finding of interest is deviation of the trachea to the right at the level of the thoracic inlet, probably due to an adenoma of the left lobe of the thyroid.

CONCLUSIONS: The chest remains clear and free of evidence of metastatic disease. Incidentally, the trachea is deviated to the right, presumably due to a mass in the left lobe of the thyroid which is most likely an adenoma. — Robert B. Funch, M.D.

University Hospital, Cincinnati, April 11, 1960

PA TELEO CHEST: Comparison is made with the examination of 4-7-60. Also at this time the heart

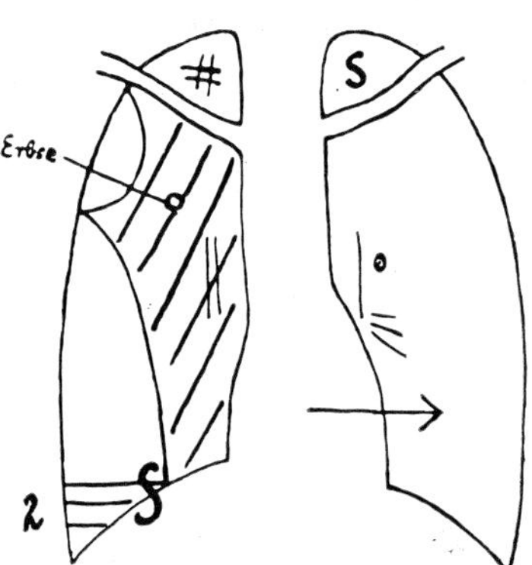

Radio-stenography. This is another of Erwin Kolta's samples from Rosenthal's shorthand image reporting. *Slight clouding left apex; thick left hilar strands, with calcified lymph node. Right apex markedly beclouded, with sero-pneumothorax and adhesions; lung incompletely collapsed. Pea-sized* (Erbse) *subclavicular cavity. Right hemi-diaphragm almost fixed* (S), *two-finger* (2) *width fluid level in the sinus, and heart displaced to the right.*

obscures the left base making examination of this area difficult. Elevation of the right hemidiaphragm is again noted, but the naso-gastric tube is no longer in place. The infiltrate in the left lung has cleared up. Calcification in the aortic knob and descending aorta is irregular with respect to the outline of the vessel. One wonders whether or not this patient has had a dissecting aneurysm at some time in the past.— DR. SPITZ

St. Anne's Hospital, Chicago, July 23, 1961

Two views of the cervical spine show a metallic coin (probably a quarter) lodged in the cervical portion of the esophagus, at the level of C6 and C7. — JOSE SUGRANES, M.D.

Indiana University Medical Center. Indianapolis, January 10, 1964.

ESOPHAGEAL EXAMINATION. Fluoroscopy by R. E. Miller. At fluoroscopy there was an irregular constricting lesion of the esophagus just above the aortic arch. The esophagus expanded to normal diameter at the end of the constriction, which appeared about 5.0 cm long. Cineradiography and six conventional radiographs, including spot films, confirm the fluoroscopic findings. IMPRESSION: irregular constricting lesion in the upper thirs of the esophagus, almost surely a squamous cell carcinoma. — R. E. MILLER, M. D.

☆

Washington, D.C., December 26, 1913

Bismuth passes through esophagus more slowly than usual, and there is slight delay at the cardiac end. Shadow of the entire pyloric end of stomach is replaced by long, thin line of bismuth. Marked deformity of cap. The appearance is that of a large carcinoma involving much of the pyloric end of the stomach and producing obstruction with consequent dilatation of the cardiac end. Presumably inoperable. — ARTHUR C. CHRISTIE, M.D.

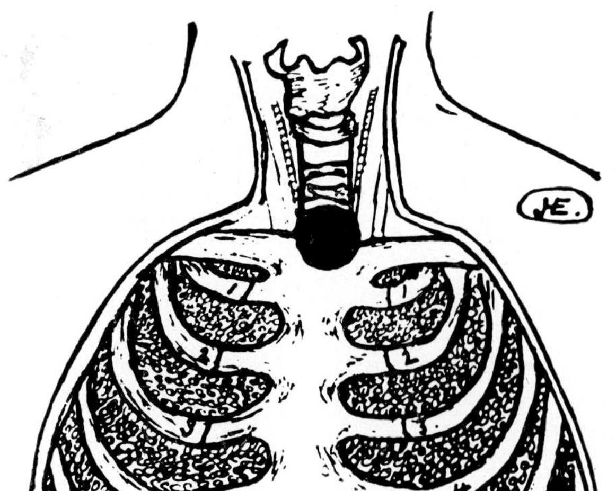

COIN IN THE ESOPHAGUS. This illustration appeared in the *American X-ray Journal* in 1898.

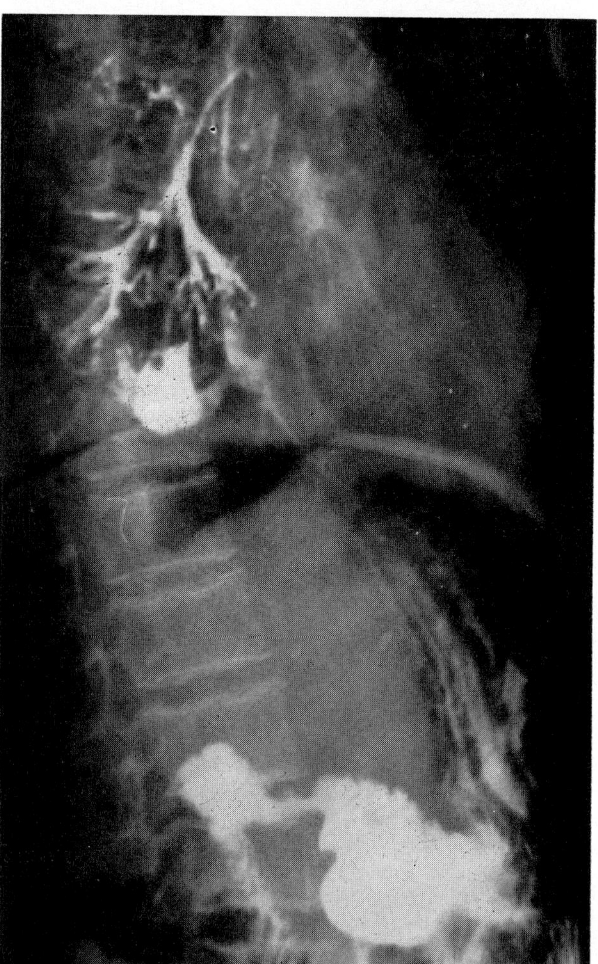

PATHOLOGIC POT-POURRI. This emaciated fifty-year old female was admitted to Paris (Illinois) Hospital for suspected partial gastric obstruction. She was blind, apparently as a result of long-standing syphilis. Ingested barium suspension penetrated through an esophageal fistula into an abscess in the posterior basilar segment of the right lower lobe. A well-functioning gastro-jejunostomy was found, whence a narrowing in the post-pyloric region was interpreted as recurring duodenal ulcer. Exploration revealed what was thought to be cicatricial stenosis in the duodenum. Patient died suddenly of myocardial infarction, and post-mortem examination confirmed the previous findings, except for the "duodenal stenosis" which was due to carcinoid.

Washington, D.C., March 18, 1916

Stomach occupies fixed position below and to the left of unbilicus. Ragged deformity in bismuth shadow along lesser curvature near pylorus. Constant "cut-out" along lower part of the greater curvature appears in all positions and remains same in extent and shape under manipulation before the screen. No cap demonstrable. Large six-hour residue. These findings point to extensive infiltrating growth of walls of stomach, probably carcinoma. — Thomas A. Groover, M.D.

Robert W. Long Hospital, Indianapolis, December 17, 1916

X-RAY GALL BLADDER & STOMACH: No calculi detected. Stomach unusually active. Emptied in 2¼ hours. After stomach was almost empty, deformity of bismuth appeared along this portion. This is indicative of ulcer. — De. L.

☆

Kansas City, Mo., December 4, 1918

A barium meal in mother's milk was given at 1:30 p.m. to the seven week old patient. Fluoroscopic and plate examination at 5 p.m. showed stomach contents retained except small amount visualized in the small bowel surrounded by gas, occupying the right chest cavity, displacing the chest contents entirely to the left half of the chest. The heart was against the left chest wall. The clear gas filled bowel convolutions showed a sharply defined path through the diaphragm to the right of the liver area. At the eighteen hour period, the stomach and small bowels were found empty, the colon being visualized on the pelvic floor.

ROENTGEN CONCLUSIONS: stomach of usual size, shape, and location. Ninety per cent rentention at three hour period due to pylorospasm. Small bowel entering chest cavity through diaphragmatic opening along right chest wall. — Oliver Howard McCandless, M.D.

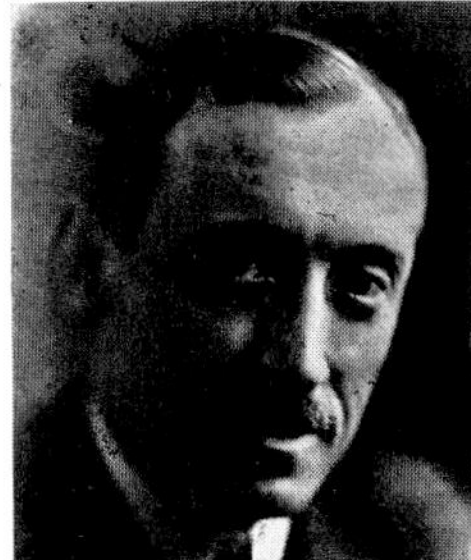

Oliver H. McCandless

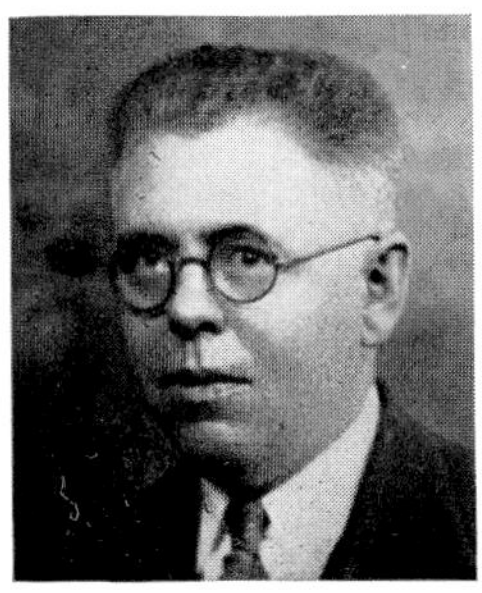

Lewis Friedman

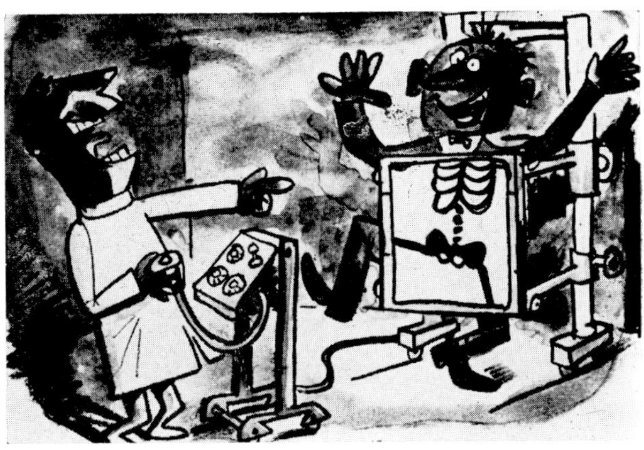

New York City, June 30, 1952

Examination of the gastro-intestinal tract shows no fluoroscopic or radiographic abnormality of the esophagus. The stomach is hypertonic in type, and of

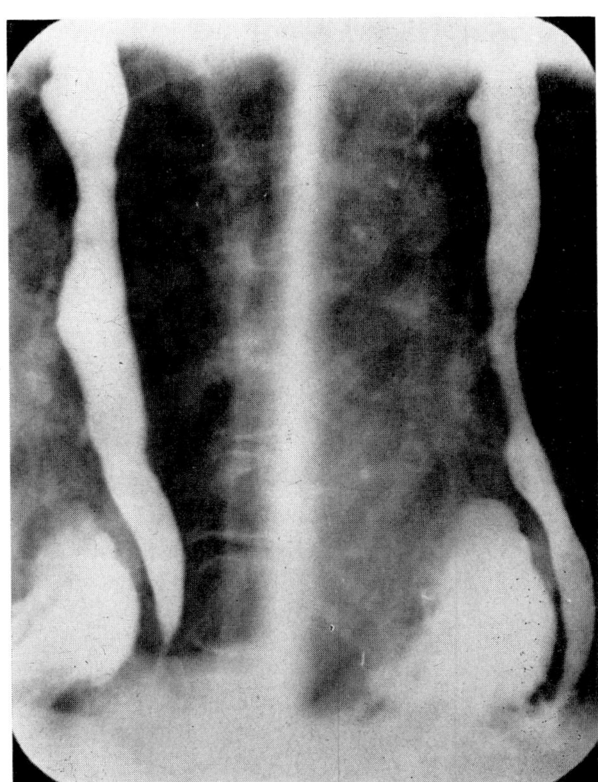

Rolling hernia. Patient was referred with the suspicion of duodenal ulcer, and the barium meal revealed a crater in the cap. But there was also what I once called the "rolling" type of hiatus hernia (*cf., Diseases of the Chest* of September, 1954). There was no evidence of esophageal irritability, therefore this herniation was regarded (for the time being) as an incidental finding, but the referring clinician was alerted to the possibility that a peptic esophagitis might develop at some time in the future.

active tone. There is hypertrophy of the gastric mucosa. The stomach is displaced anteriorly and there is a defect on its lesser curvature, due to pressure from the pancreas. The bulb is large, and slightly irregular. The upper loops of the jejunum are dilated. The extensive calcification in the pancreas has been previously reported.

The stomach is empty before six hours. The head of the barium column has reached the transverse colon.

Additional film is available, which shows a large, round, smooth cavity filled with opaque material, measuring about four inches in diameter, located anteriorly to the second and third lumbar vertebrae. This represents a pancreatic cyst which has been aspirated, and then injected with diodrast. — R. ABRAMS, M.D.

☆

Carle Hospital Clinic, Urbana (Illinois), September 24, 1952

Patient had by-pass surgery for carcinoma of the common duct, one month ago. ESOPHAGUS negative for significant alterations. STOMACH—marked deformity of the antrum, of the pyloric canal, and of the duodenal cap, with destruction of the mucosal pattern of the antrum, probably due to continued growth of the tumor with invasion of the antral wall. — CESARE GIANTURCO, M.D.

☆

Bellevue Hospital, New York City, April 8, 1953

Examination of the small bowel pattern particularly in the three hour film shows evidence of segmentation, dilatation, and an ironing out of the contour of the loops. The pattern is similar to that seen in Sprue, but it may well be of tuberculous etiology. — DR. BUCKSTEIN

☆

Boston, Mass., October 4, 1958

UPPER GASTRO-INTESTINAL TRACT: Studies of the esophagus reveal no evidence of obstruction, displacement, or irregularity of outline. There is herniation of a portion of the cardia of the stomach through the esophageal orifice of the diaphragm. This hernia measures about 3 cm. in diameter and reduces itself as the stomach empties.

The stomach is high, atonic, with sluggish peristalsis; its outline is regular. The duodenal cap is smooth and there is no localized tenderness over it on fluoroscopic palpation. An ulcer crater is not demonstrable. There is slight angulation and narrowing of the duodenum in the region of the junction of the first and second portions. Six hours later, the stomach is entirely empty, small bowel loops are partially filled, and are unremarkable.

At twenty-four hours, the head of the barium meal is at the rectum. The cecum is high, well filled, smooth in outline, and non-tender. The colon is atonic.

REMARKS: There is a small reducible esophageal hiatus hernia. There are adhesions about the duodenum. — MAX RITVO, M.D.

☆

Washington, D.C., August 15, 1959

Examination of the upper gastro-intestinal tract shows no abnormalities in the esophagus. There is mucosal coarsening and irritability of the prepyloric antrum, pylorus, and first portion of the duodenum. No ulceration is demonstrated and the findings are attributed to antral gastritis and duodenitis with scar tissue formation in the first portion of the duodenum. There is no delay in the emptying of the stomach. — FRED O. COE, M.D.

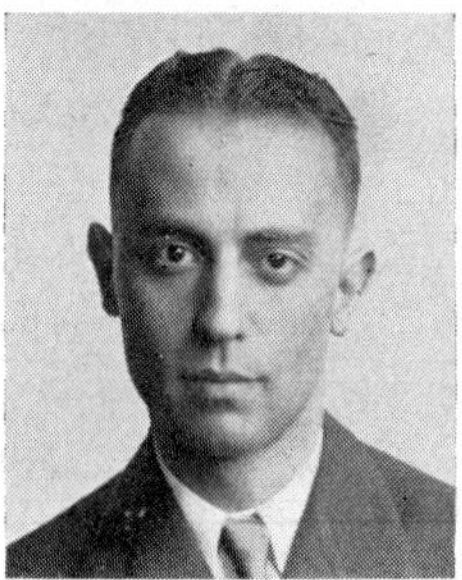

CESARE GIANTURCO

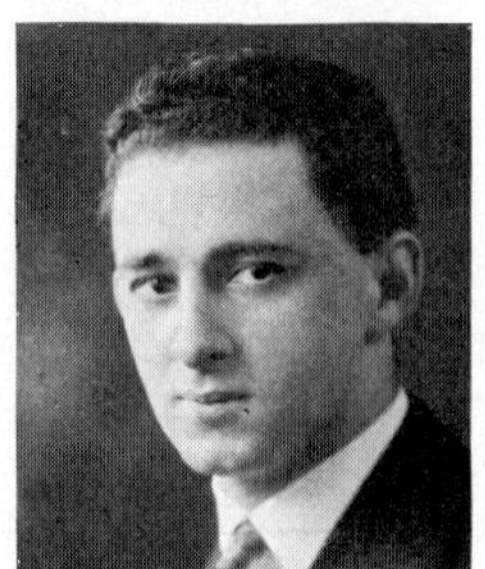

MAX RITVO

Johns Hopkins Hospital, Baltimore, Md., September 2, 1959

G. I. SERIES: We were unable to demonstrate any significant abnormality in the esophagus, stomach, or duodenum. Several of the spot films are rather light, but it is felt that the study is adequate for interpretation. — D. J. Torrance, Jr., M.D.

☆

Germantown Hospital, Philadelphia, Pa., September 12, 1959

G. I. SERIES FOR COMPARISON WITH 7-22-54: Re-examination of the stomach and duodenum again reveals marked deformity of the duodenum because of chronic ulcer disease. In addition, the pyloric canal and antral portions of the stomach are narrow and elongated. This area is quite rigid. Since it has not changed a great deal in the last five years we feel that it represents cicatrix secondary to an inflammatory process rather than neoplasm. The duodenum was found to be irritable at the time of fluoroscopy and in all probability we are dealing with active ulcer disease.

CONCLUSIONS: We have demonstrated roentgen evidence of chronic duodenal ulcer disease with probable activity. The actual morphology of the distal end of the stomach and duodenum has not changed a great deal in the past five years. — Jay W. MacMoran, M.D.

☆

New York Polyclinic Medical School & Hospital, New York City, October 5, 1959

RADIOGRAPHY AND RADIOSCOPY: G. I. SERIES: Barium administered by mouth passes through the esophagus without delay. Gastric peristalsis is active, evacuation proceeds readily. There is a marked mushroom shaped deformity at the base of the duodenal cap. This changes in its extent during varying periods of the examination. There is marked

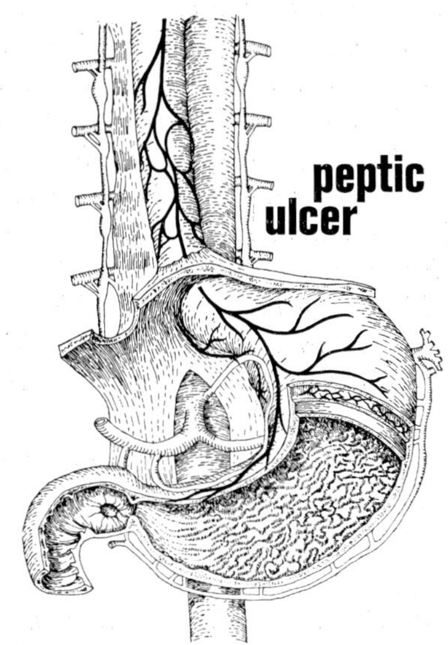

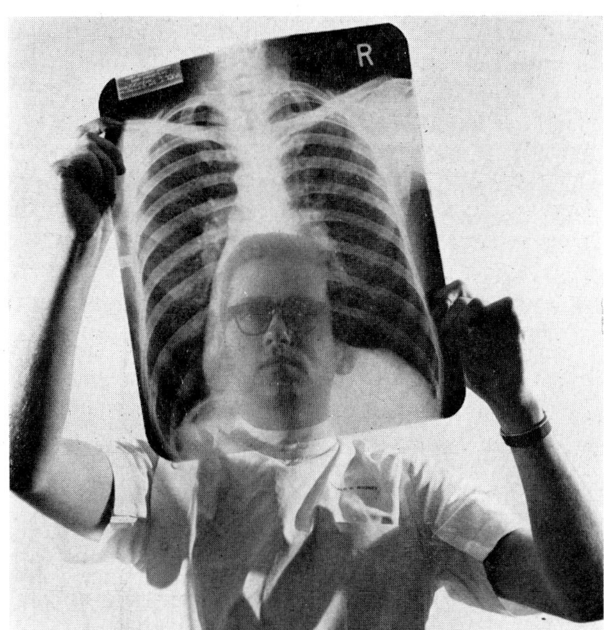

Don Rooney by Leigh. Ted Leigh in Atlanta is not only a specialist in the radiology of meningioma and of the mediastinum. He is also a recognized amateur photographer who has had one-man exhibits. The photograph shows one of his residents – Donald Rooney, currently a radiologist in Marietta (Georgia) – examining the film of a patient with mitral (rheumatic) heart disease. This "snapshot" made the cover of *Newsweek*.

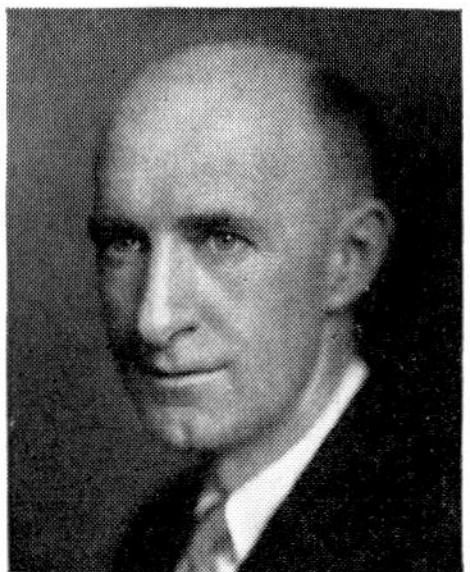

Fred Oscar Coe

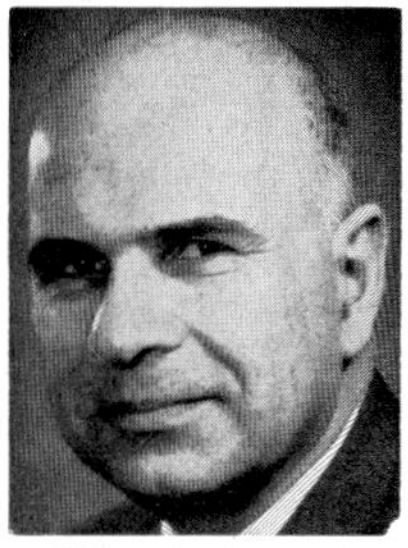

Wm. Shehadi

Fred Coe is an expert in vaginography, as can be seen from the *American Journal of Roentgenology* of October, 1963. Shehadi, who was formerly at the American University in Beirut, has numerous publications on cholecystographic and other opaque media, including a book on the *Clinical Radiology of the Biliary Tract* (Blakiston, 1963).

swelling of the mucosa of the entire duodenum. Some of the films show a 1 cm. barium fleck at the posterior wall of the duodenal cap, consistent with an ulcer crater at that level.

Gastric evacuation is complete before 6 hours and the progress of barium through the small and large intestines is not remarkable. Incidentally, the appendix is visualized and irregularly filled, moveable and not tender.

CONCLUSION: Marked duodenitis. Marked prolapse of the gastric mucosa through the pylorus. Deformity of the duodenal cap with a posterior wall ulcer. — WM. H. SHEHADI, M.D.

☆

Veterans Administration Hospital, Hines, Illinois, October 26, 1961

The esophagus shows no abnormalities fluoroscopically. The stomach reveals a projection in the middle third, measuring 1.5 cm. in diameter and 1.3 in depth. It is not associated with a filling defect, and the mucosal folds in its vicinity are not unusual. The duodenal bulb and duodenal curve are smooth and well filled.

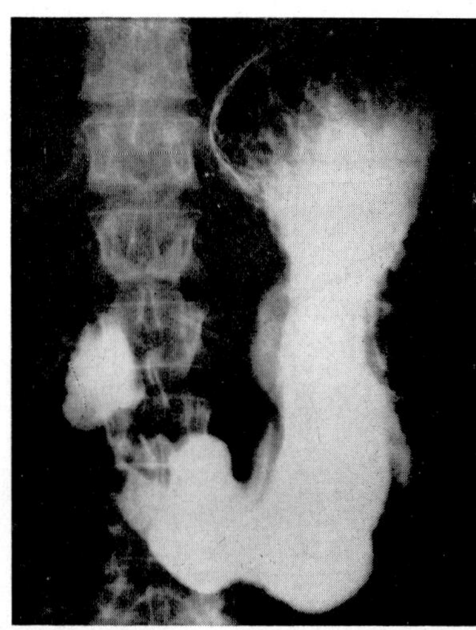

GIANT GASTRIC ULCER. This thirty-five-year old female had been followed for three years at the Charleston (Illinois) Hospital. The crater herein reproduced represented the fourth recurrence in the same location. At this size, one can hardly call it ulcer, the proper term is walled-off perforation. To Israel Kirsh (from the Veterans Administration Hospital in Hines) goes the credit for having re-popularized the notion that these large craters are most of the time (but not necessarily) benign, *cf.*, *Radiology* of March, 1955. This patient had resisted heroically for three years: a few days after above film was taken, she underwent a gastrectomy, and has been doing fine ever since.

IMPRESSION: Gastric ulcer, benign, - I. E. KIRSH, M.D.

☆

New York City, April 30, 1912

X-RAY FINDINGS: Series of plates, the first one made immediately after the bismuth had been given, show the size, shape and position of the colon distinctly. The caecum is extremely prolapsed, even with the patient in the prone posture. The ascending colon is long. The hepatic flexure is slightly prolapsed. The transverse colon traverses the abdomen about on a level with the umbilicus, and then passes down to the left iliac fossa. It then ascends to the splenic flexure, which is held up in position. The sigmoid and caecum are in such close apposition that it is diffifult to identify the one from the other.

DIAGNOSIS: From a study of these plates the extreme prolapse of the caecum is the most important finding. - LEWIS GREGORY COLE, *M.D.*

☆

Chicago, June 8, 1949

BARIUM ENEMA: The sigmoid filled easily. Several diverticula in this area are identified on the spotfilm. Annular narrowing, about two centimeter's long, was seen in the apex of the splenic flexure. It is well identified only on the oblique view, ordered in addition to the conventional anteroposterior projection.

IMPRESSION: diverticulosis of the sigmoid; localized, so far incomplete obstruction at the splenic flexure, very possibly of malignant nature. - MARION F. MAGALOTTI

☆

Cook County Hospital, Chicago, August 14, 1955.

BARIUM ENEMA: Somewhat deliberate retrograde flow of barium through the otherwise distensible bowel. No intrinsic or extrinsic lesions demon-

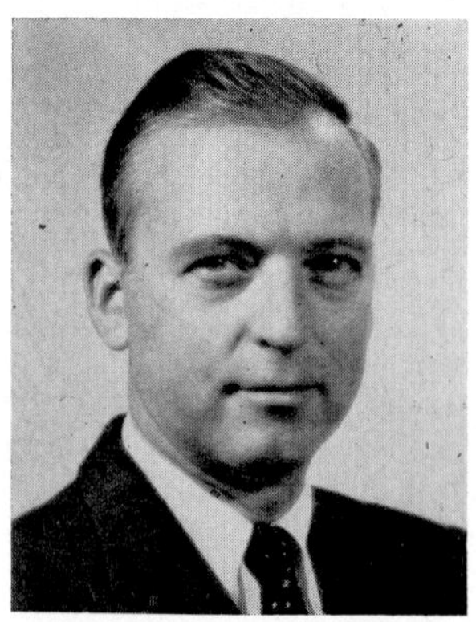

TED FLOURNOY LEIGH.

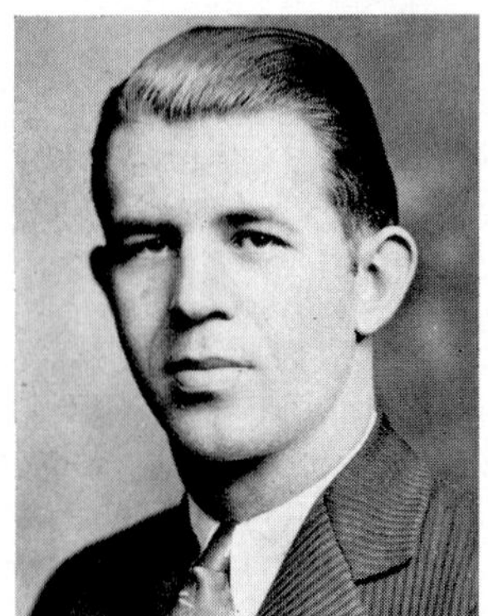

RALPH CAULK

strated. Satisfactory evacuation.—GEORGE I. PAPRIKOFF, M.D.

☆

Bellevue Hospital, New York City, November 7, 1955

Fluoroscopic and film examination of the colon was made by means of a barium enema, with barium introduced both through the rectum, and through a colostomy in the mid transverse colon. A large, irregularly narrowed segment was visualized in the sigmoid portion of the colon, which permitted only slight flow from the rectum. The cecum was poorly visualized by retrograde flow. Numerous diverticula were demonstrated in the descending and sigmoid portions. Leading from the lesion, several fine tracts of barium are demonstrated, suggesting the presence of fistulae. - R. GROSS, M.D.

☆

Washington, D. C., April 25, 1959

Examination of the colon by barium enema and air contrast shows the presence of a questionable filling defect in the region of the ileocecal valve, but apparently slightly cephalad to the actual location of the valve. While this may still represent hypertrophy of one of the valve lips, this cannot be definitely determined in the available films, and the examination should be repeated. No other abnormality is noted from the cecum to the rectosigmoid. The patient will be asked to return for re-examination of the colon with particular reference to the cecal and ileocecal region. - KARL C. CORLEY, M.D.

☆

University Hospital, Cincinnati, August 26, 1959

Repeat air contrast enema fails to demonstrate polyps or other intrinsic or extrinsic lesions of the colon. - DR. GRAHAM

☆

Johns Hopkins, Baltimore, Md., September 18, 1959

BARIUM ENEMA: No evidence of significant intrinsic or extrinsic abnormality of the large bowel is

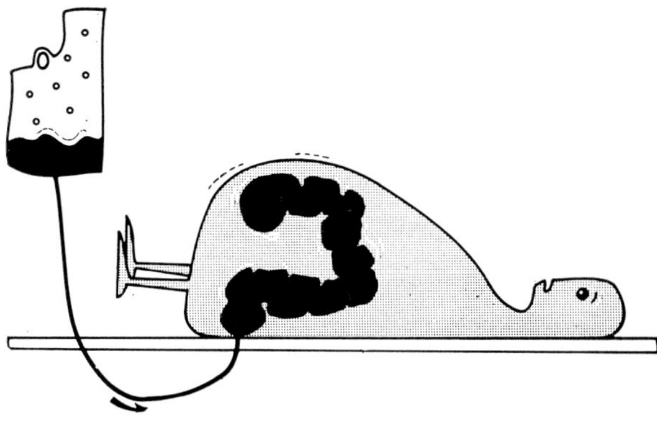

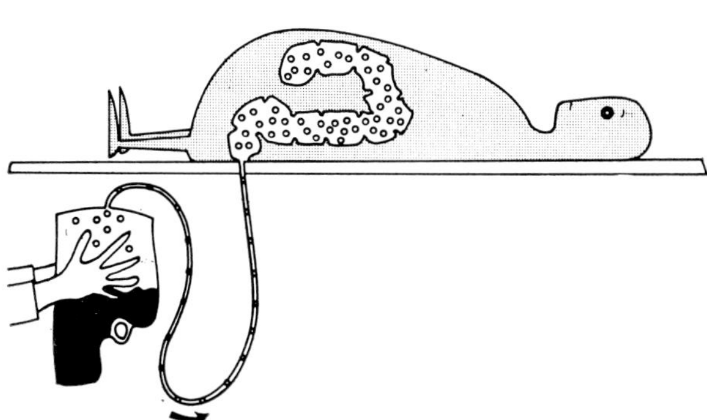

BARIUM IN THE BAG. The "modern" – and very convenient – way to execute double contrast studies is to use a single stage, closed system with a disposable, prepackaged barium enema kit, reproduced here from the original publication by Rubem Pohaczevsky and Robert Stanton Sherman, from the Sloane-Kettering Cancer Center at the Memorial Hospital in New York City.

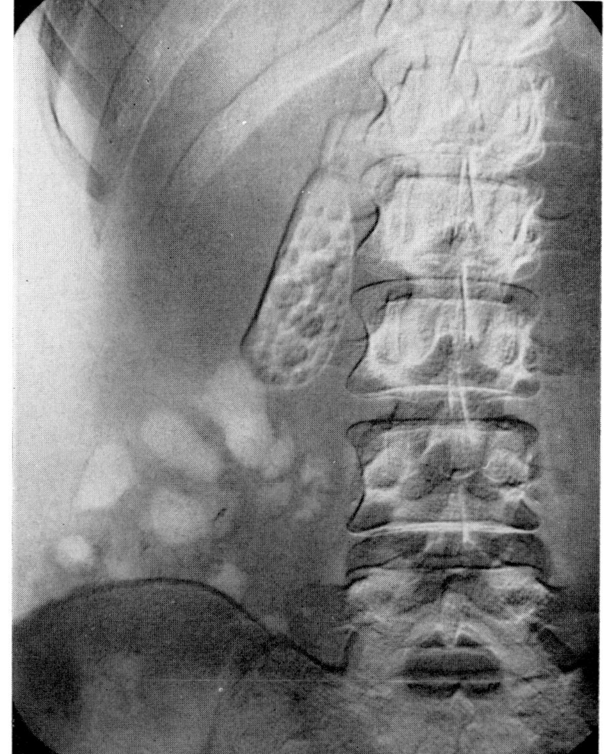

BLADDER-ROCKS IN BAS-RELIEF. "Plastic-ization" adds no information, but sometimes it gives a beautiful picture. This specimen was masterfully executed by my good friend Byron Smith, the chief x-ray technician in Paris (Illinois), who processed the photographic prints of radiographs used in this chapter.

demonstrated. There is some decrease in haustral markings in the descending colon which is sometimes seen in individuals who have been accustomed to taking large doses of laxatives for many years, but which is not definitely abnormal. - Dr. Washburn.

☆

St. Elizabeth's Hospital, Boston, January 20, 1913

The gallbladder presents a faint nebulous mass which could be produced by a single large gallstone of low specific gravity. - Percy Brown, M.D.

☆

Battle Creek Sanitarium, Battle Creek, Mich., February 18, 1915

On several occasions a large ovoid shadow was seen in the gallbladder region, suggestive of gallstones, but not sufficiently clear for a definite diagnosis of cholelithiasis. Annular pyloric stenosis. - James Thomas Case, M.D.

Cook County Hospital, Chicago, July 18, 1954

CHOLECYSTOGRAM: well functioning gallbladder with cholelithiasis. - Dr. Ignacio Iglesias

☆

Bellevue Hospital, New York City, January 27, 1955

Average size gallbladder full of biliary calculi. No organic lesion of the stomach or duodenal bulb. Some delay in the passage of barium beyond the junction of 1st and 2nd portion of duodenum, with dilatation of this area. No evidence of organic pathology. — Dr. Craig

☆

Washington, D.C., August 9, 1959

Cholecystogram shows excellent function of the gallbladder. There is a filling defect about 2 mm. in diameter in the fundus of the gallbladder which probably represents a so-called papilloma and is not sig-

SERVICIO CENTRAL DE RADIOLOGIA

HOSPITAL CORDOBA

Jefe: Dr. LIDIO G. MOSCA

PROF.DR.JORGE ORGAZ.-
Paciente:Sr.Jorge Arduna
11 Nov. de 1961

COLANGIOGRAFIA INTRAVENOSA.-

Se administraron 20 cc. de Biligrafina Forte y 1 cg. de morfina, tomándose radiografías a los 40, 60 y 80 minutos.

Se comprueba un colédoco de 14 mm. de calibre y, a nivel del tronco del hepático, una imagen redondeada, transparente, que corresponde a un cálculo biliar.

Una imagen de aspecto diverticular que aparece junto al borde derecho de la via biliar principal debe ser interpretada como correspondiente a un muñón cístico.

En síntesis: litiasis residual de la vía biliar principal y considerable dilatación de la misma por hipertrofia del esfínter de Oddi; muñón cístico de escasa extensión.

Salúdale cordialmente,

L.G. Mosca

Dr. Lidio G.Mosca

Translation: "20 cc Biligrafin Forte and 1 cgm of morphine were injected, and radiographs were exposed at 40, 60, and 80 minutes. A 14 mm wide common duct was demonstrated, with a rounded, transparent image at the level of the hepatic trunk, interpreted as a biliary calculus. An image of diverticular aspect, connected to the right border of the common duct, must be interpreted as corresponding to the cystic stump. SYNTHESIS: residual lithiasis of the common biliary duct, which is noticeably dilated because of hypertrophy of the sphincter of Oddi; relatively short cystic stump."

nificant. There is no other evidence of abnormality. —RALPH M. CAULK, M.D.

☆

Mary Hitchcock Memorial Hospital, Hanover, N. H., August 17, 1959

EXCRETORY UROGRAM. Both kidneys show good function and the upper urinary tract reveals no pathologic findings. The bladder is slightly trabeculated, but not definitely elevated. There is a 2.5 cm diverticulum on the left side. Several small calcific densities project just above the right transverse process of L2, probably pancreatic calculi. There is moderate hypertrophic spurring in the lumbar spine. —LESLIE K. SYCAMORE, M.D.

☆

University Hospital, Cincinnati, August 25, 1959

PELVIMETRY: Pelvic measurements are as follows: true conjugate 12.5, transverse 10.9, total 23.4. Midpelvis: AP diameter 13.5, interspinous 9.0, total 22.5. Pelvic outlet: post sagittal 6.5, intertuberous 8.5, total 15. The AP view shows full term fetus Breech presentation with breech engaged as far as the midpelvis. The position left sacrum transverse. The pelvic inlet has a rather flat posterior segment. The inlet plane is in the near oblique. Uterine axis is oblique. The promontory of the sacrum is medial. The sacrum is fairly short and curved convexly. Spines are medium size. There is no evidence of acetabular bulge. There is definite conversion of the lateral walls but subpubic notch is large. Unfortunately the fetal head size cannot be determined on this film because the top portion does not show. However, with the narrowed measurements of the inlet total of 15, it is thought that labor with repeated labor trials and the fact that this patient is a 16 year old primipara totally are in agreement with this finding.

IMPRESSION: Cephalopelvic disproportion is most probable. This is a breech presentation. — DR. SCHLUETER

☆

M. D. Anderson Hospital, Houston, September 2, 1960

MAMMOGRAMS. Left breast: in the upper outer quadrant, 4 cm above and 5 cm lateral to the nipple, is a 0.7 x 1 cm. infiltrative lesion containing fine stippled calcification, producing minimal retraction of the overlying skin.

Right breast: In the upper outer quadrant, in the subcutaneous adipose tissue, is a smooth-bordered oval mass 1.2 x 1.0 x 2.0 cm in size. No other nodules are demonstrated, and there are no signs of carcinoma in this breast.

IMPRESSION: 1. 0.7 x 1.0 cm carcinoma upper outer quadrant of left breast. 2. 1.2 x 2.0 benign lesion in right breast, either sebaceous cyst or hematoma. — ROBERT L. EGAN, M.D.

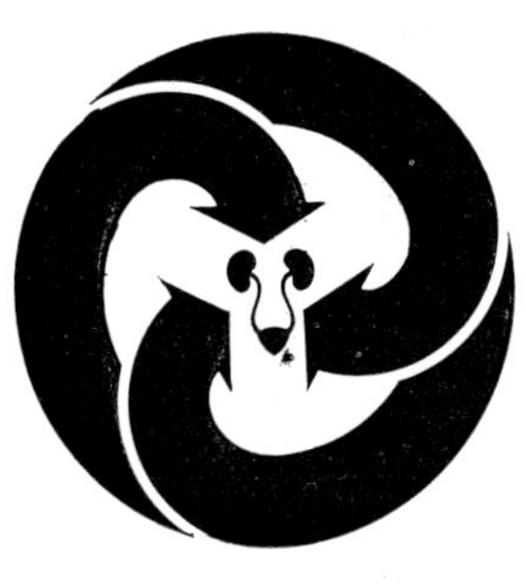

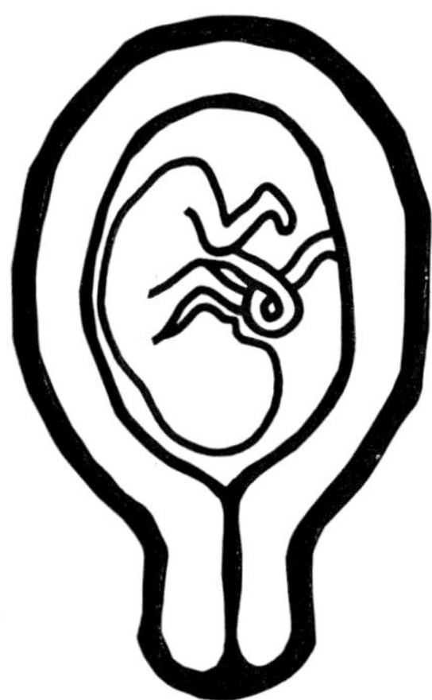

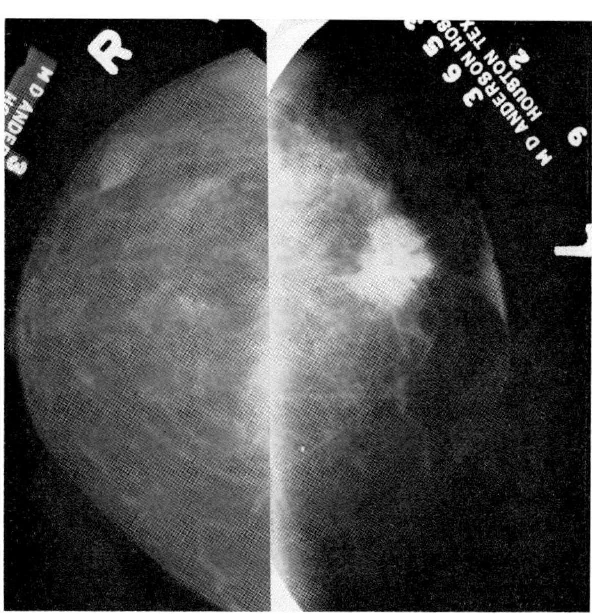

Courtesy: M. D. Anderson Hospital, Houston.

MAMMOGRAMS TO EGAN'S REPORT.

Indiana University Medical Center, Indianapolis, May 14, 1960

SELECTIVE RETROGRADE LEFT VENTRICULOGRAPHY AND AORTOGRAPHY was done utilizing a #8 polyethylene catheter and 80 per cent Ditriokon contrast media, with 6 kg/cm² pressure injection.

With the catheter tip in the left ventricle and the patient in 45° RAO position, an injection of 50 cc of contrast media shows a moderately enlarged left ventricular chamber and a tremendous reflux of media across the mitral valve into the dilated left atrium. The left atrium is estimated to be four or five times the average size. There is a great delay in the emptying of the atrial cavity. The pulmonary veins are dilated.

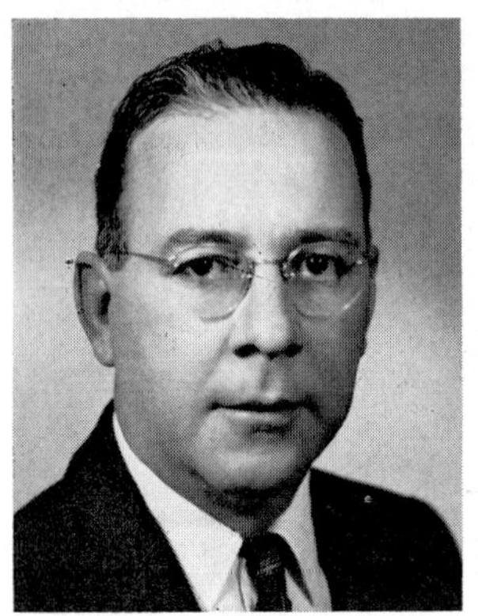

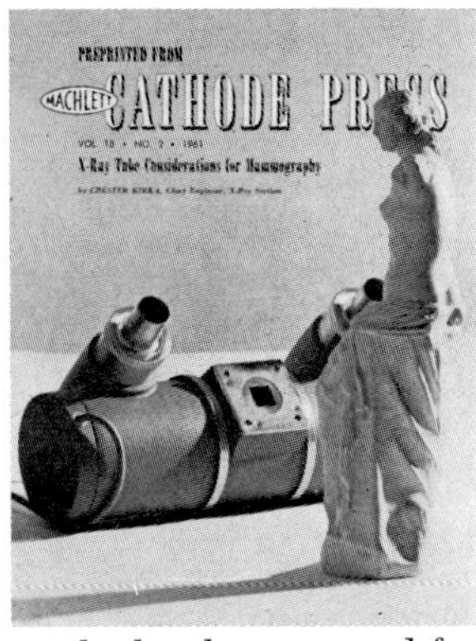

ROBERT LEE EGAN. Mammography has been around for a long time. The pioneer in this field was the German surgeon A. Salomon (see *Arch. klin. Chir.* of 1913). In 1931, in Portugal, Bénard-Guedes and his associates revived the method. Leborgne in Montevideo and Gershon-Cohen in Philadelphia were doing it while Egan was still in high school. When Egan joined the act at the M. D. Anderson Hospital (Houston) at the University of Texas, he insisted on using industrial film, extreme soft-tissue technics, and large statistical series with plenty of histologic correlation. He proved the value of the method, and popularized it. Whatever the pioneering merits of the precursors, until Egan's advent, mammography was a dead issue. It turned out to be a "sleeping beauty," and now Egan has a reputation, a new job (at Methodist Hospital in Indianapolis), and a superb book on the breast (published in 1964 in Charles C Thomas' *American Lectures in Roentgen Diagnosis,* edited by Lewis Etter). And since the breast has become a bandwagon, everybody is trying or at least considering to "use" it. The available x-ray tubes, however, do not take very kindly to 1800 mas, repeated at brief intervals, and this is why the tube companies, for instance Machlett, have issued bulletins on the subject.

With the catheter tip in the proximal aorta and the patient in LAO position, a 25 cc. injection shows a relatively small aortic caliber with slight reflux of opaque media across the aortic valve into the left ventricle. The left ventricle rather quickly rejects the reflux however.

IMPRESSION: Marked mitral insufficiency with some stenosis. Evidence of slight aortic regurgitation, probably of a functional rather than organic type. — EUGENE C. KLATTE, M.D.

☆

Indiana University Medical Center, Indianapolis, April 29, 1960

SELECTIVE CINECARDIOANGIOGRAPHY is performed using a #5 R-A catheter and Ditriokon contrast medium, with 8 kg/cm² pressure injection.

With the catheter tip in the left ventricle and the patient in 70° LAO position, there is demonstrated an average sized chamber with shunting and a high interventricular septal defect into the right ventricle. A repeat injection of 3 cc. into the left ventricle shows to better advantage left to right shunt through the septum.

With the catheter threaded through the septal defect into the aorta and the patient in the PA projection, 2 cc injection shows a relatively small aorta, which descends on the left.

With the catheter in the right ventricle and the patient the 30° RAO position, a 3 cc. injection shows a large patent right ventricular outlet and main pulmonary artery. No valvular stenosis is seen.

With the catheter tip in the right ventricle and the patient in a 30° LAO position, a 3 cc injection also shows the large right ventricular cavity and patent outflow tract.

IMPRESSION: Eisenmenger's complex with large ventricular septal defect. — JOHN A. CAMPBELL, M.D.

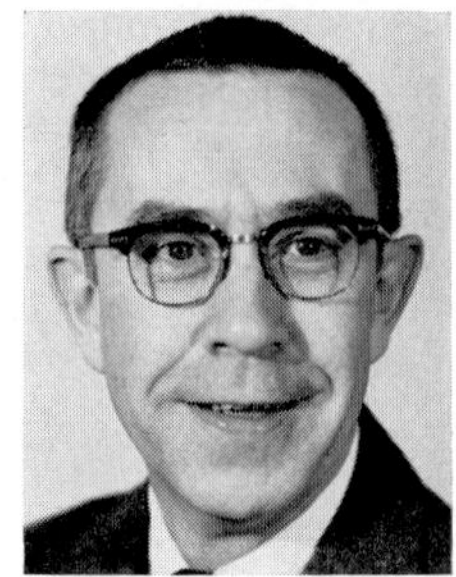

JOHN CAMPBELL

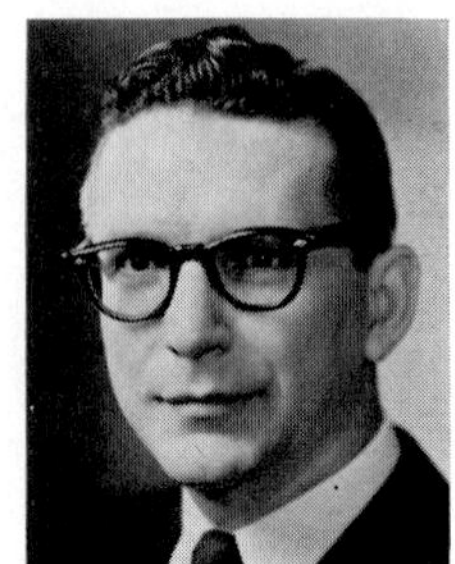

ROSCOE MILLER

PARTING ADVICE

After peripateticating through the labyrinthine detours of this chapter on roentgen reporting, a few choice words of final admonition are in order. For this purpose I asked the help of a wise radiologic master from Quebec. With Gallic wit and wryness, Alfred Rosario Potvin suggested, "Above all, never report what you did not see!"

I was still trying to decipher all the meanings hidden in Potvin's sibylline, though seemingly so simple, sentence when I stumbled over a bitter phrase, written by the sage from Baltimore, Henry Louis Mencken (1880-1956). His utterance actually illustrates one of the main problems in roentgen reporting: "The public demands certainties; it must be told definitely, and a bit raucously, that this is true and that is false. But there *are* no certainties!"

As always, there is place for a note of moderation. There exists a philosophy which will assure success in the preparation of roentgen reports (indeed, it will assure success in most anything on this planet): nothing pleases so much as (and meets with the approval of more people than) does plain dealing and common sense!

4¢
POSTAGE
The UNITED STATES
Fear to do ill, and you need fear Nought else.
B Franklin
OF AMERICA
Credo

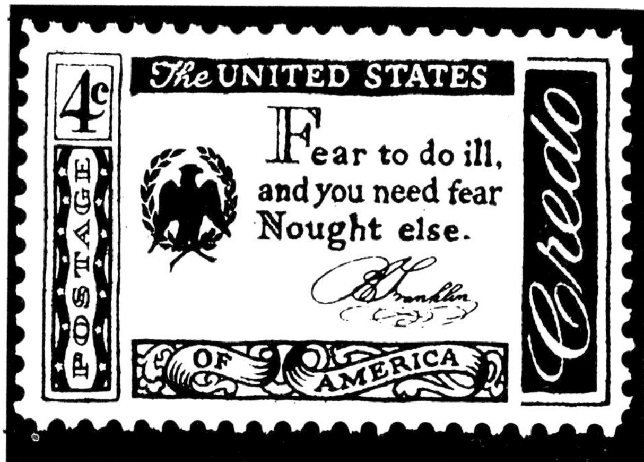

REFERENCES ON ROENTGEN REPORTING

Arnell, S.: An apparatus for making sketches of radiograms. *Acta radiol., 3*:176-179, 1924.

Arnold, H. L., and Washko, P. J.: "Flat film" of the addomen. *J.A.M.A., 167*:773-774 (June 7) 1958.

Baetjer, F. H.: The x-ray diagnosis of thoracic aneurysms. *Bull. Johns Hopkins Hospital, 17*:24-27 (January) 1906.

Barclay, A. E.: The place of the radiologist in medicine. *Brit. M. J., 2*:385-387 (September 11) 1920.

Barden, R. P.: Clear writing. *Radiology, 72*:875-876 (June) 1959.

Batten, G. B.: The requirements of the clinician from the radiologist and vice-versa. *Brit. J. Radiol., 3*:259-268 (June) 1930.

Bauer, D. deF.: *The Practice of Country Radiology.* Springfield, C. C. Thomas, 1963, pp. 180-197.

Beck, C.: Errors caused by the false interpretation of the roentgen rays, and their medico-legal aspect. *Med. Rec. (New York), 58*:281-285 (August 25) 1900.

Béclère, A.: Des prétendues erreurs radiographiqes. *Bull. et Mém. Soc. de méd. d. hôp. de Paris, 23*:948-949 (October 19), 1906.

Béclère, A.: Necessité de ne confier qu'à des médecins la direction des services de radiologie. *J. de radiol & électrol., 2*:564-567 (May-June) 1917.

Bergmann, H.: Vordrucke zum Eintragen von Roentgenbefunden. *Fortschr. a. d. Geb. d. Rstrhlen, 26*:193-195, 1919.

Blachly, C. D.: A comvenient method recording data on roentgen-ray plates. *J.A.M.A., 69*:999 (September 22) 1917.

Blaine, E. S.: The relation of the roentgenologist to the physician and surgeon. *Illinois M. J., 30*:338-342 (November) 1916.

Bowen, D. R.: Roentgen index, bibliography. *Am. Quart. of Roentgenol.,* July 1909 through June, 1910.

Buckley, G. L.: *X-Ray Reports. Their Importance in the Diagnostic Department.* London, H. K. Lewis, 1957, 72 pages.

Bull, H. C. H.: *X-Ray Interpretation.* London, Oxford University Press, 1935, p. xxxiii.

Carman, R. D.: The making and filing of records in the section on roentgenology in the Mayo Clinic. *Am. J. Roentgenol., 8*:372-382 (July) 1921.

Carman, R. D.: Limitations of roentgenologic diagnosis. *New York State J. of Med., 22*:302-305 (July) 1922.

Case, J. T.: Some statistics on the negative and positive roentgen diagnosis of gallstones. *Am. J. Roentgenol., 3*: 246-252 (May) 1916.

Case, J. T.: Los requisitos fundamentales de un buen servicio roentgenológico en los hospitales. *J.A.M.A. (Spanish edition), 12*:58-60 (July 1) 1924.

Cerné, A., and Aubourg: Schemas radiologiques du tronc. *J. de radiol. et d'électrol., 1*:340 (June) 1914.

Christie, A. C.: *Bulletin on Studies in X-Ray Diagnosis.* Washington, Government Printing Office, 1915, 35 pages.

Cimmino, C. V.: The radiologist and his fellow physicians. *Virginia M. Monthly, 83*:270-271 (June) 1956.

Cimmino, C. V.: On the nature of the roentgenologic examination. *Virginia M. Monthly, 85*:220-221 (April) 1958.

Cluzet, M. J.: Sur la lecture des images radiographiques. *Lyon méd., 120*:126-128 (January 19) 1913.

Cole, L. G.: Skiagraphic errors: their causes, dangers, and prevention. *New York M. J., 79*:59-592 (March 26); 635-641 (April 2); 678-680 (April 9) 1904.

Cole, L. G.: Serial radiography in the differential diagnosis of carcinoma of the stomach, gallbladder infection, and gastric or duodenal ulcer. *Archives of the Roentgen Ray, 17*:172-181 (October) 1912.

Cole, L. G.: Roentgenology as a method of studying the natural history of disease. *Am. J. Roentgenol., 6*:72-74 (February) 1919.

Contremoulins, G.: Méthode générale de metroradiographie, pp. 17-20; 32-48 *in Premier Congrès International pour l'Étude de la Radiologie et de l'Ionisation* (Liège). Bruxelles, L. Severeyns (1906).

Cotton, W.: The true and false perspective of x-ray representation. *Archives of Skiagraphy, 7*:25-34 (July) 1902.

Crane, A. W.: Skiascopy of the respiratory organs. *Philadelphia Monthly M. J., 1*:154-170 (March) 1899.

Crane, A. W.: What every roentgenologist knows. *Radiology, 2*:50-51 (January) 1924.

Crane, A. W.: Negative x-ray findings. *Radiology, 12*: 252-254 (March) 1929.

Deutschberger, O.: *Fluoroscopy in Diagnostic Roentgenology.* Philadelphia, W. B. Saunders, 1955, p. 731.

Diemer, F. E.: Report of the department of roentgenology, U. S. Army Base Hospital, Camp Lewis, Wash. *J. Roentgenol., 2*:34-41 (March) 1919.

Donaldson, S. W.: A code system for cross indexing records. *Am. J. Roentgenol., 13*:81-87 (January) 1925.

Donaldson, S. W.: *The Roentgenologist in Court.* Ed. 2, Springfield, Charles C Thomas, 1954, 349 pages.

Dunn, A. D.: Roentgenology from the standpoint of the internist. *J. Roentgenol., 2*:292-298, 1919.

Elliott, F. E.: Radiology and the radiologist of the future. *New York State J. of Med., 37*:1647-1651 (October 1) 1937.

Enfield, C. D.: The scope of the roentgenologist's report. *J.A.M.A., 80*:999-1001 (April 7) 1923.

Enfield, C. D.: *Radiography. A Manual of X-Ray Technique, Interpretation, and Therapy.* Philadelphia, P. Blakiston's Son & Co., 1925, p. 279.

Esguerra Gomez, G.: *Radiodiagnostico.* Tomo II. Sistema Oseo. Bogotá, Editorial Cromos, 1939, p. 46.

Etter, L. E.: *Glossary of Words and Phrases used in Radiology and Nuclear Medicine.* Springfield, Charles C Thomas, 1960, 203 pages.

Etter, L. E.: X Rays and You. *Radiol. Technology, 35*:32-33 (July) 1963.

Etter, L. E.: The Language of Radiology. *Am. J. Roentgenol., 90*:656-658 (September) 1963.

Euphrat, E. J.: Polaroid photography as a practical method of providing illustrations of radiographs for clinical records. *New England J. Med., 252*:628-630 (April 14) 1955.

Folet, H.-F.: Illusions radiographiques. *Echo méd. du Nord, 4*:568-569 (December 9) 1900.

Fossati, F.: *Dizionario Tecnico di Radiologia.* Italiano-Français-Deutsch-English-Español. Milano, Wassetmann, 1952, 489 pages.

Fossati, F., and Gallone, P.: *Radiologia Schermografica.* Milano, Garzanti, 1949, p. 272.

Gaitskell, C. E.: *Radiological Terminology.* London, J. & A. Churchill, 1935, 90 pages.

Gamble, F. O.: *Applied Foot Roentgenology.* Baltimore, Williams & Wilkins, 1957, p. 217.

Garland, L. H.: The roentgen diagnosis of duodenal ulcer. *Radiology, 14*:482-487 (May) 1930.

Garland, L. H.: On the scientific evaluation of diagnostic procedures. *Radiology, 52*:313-328 (March) 1949.

Garland, L. H.: Studies on the accuracy of diagnostic procedures. *Am. J. Roentgenol., 82*:25-38 (July) 1959.

George, A. W.: Is the practice of roentgenology above criticism? *Radiology, 34*:376-377 (March) 1940.

Glasscheib, S.: *Allgemeine Röntgenkunde.* Wien, Julius Springer, 1936, vol. I, p. 272.

Goin, L. S.: Science and solitude vs. clinical consultation. *Radiology, 68*:319-326 (March) 1957.

Golden, R.: Comments on the preparation and presentation of medical papers. *Am. J. Roentgenol., 55*:495-502 (April) 1946.

Good, A. C., Carr, D. T., and Weed, L. A.: Positive roentgenograms plus positive smears do not always equal pulmonary tuberculosis. *Am. J. Roentgenol., 81*:187-195 (February) 1959.

Grashey, R.: Fehlerquellen und diagnostische Schwierigkeiten im Röntgen-Verfahren. *Muenchen. med. Wchschr., 52*:807-810 (April 25) 1905.

Grashey, R.: Röntgenologie pp. 64-97 *in Handbuch der Aerztlichen Erfahrungen im Weltkriege* 1914-18. (Ed.: Otto v. Schjerning) Leipzig, J. A. Barth, 1922.

Grigg, E. R. N.: On the labeling of shadows. *Radiology, 76*:644-646 (April) 1961.

Groedel, F. M.: Röntgentechnik, vol. I, p. 68 *in Lehrbuch und Atlas der Röntgendiagnostik in der inneren Medizin und ihren Grenzgebrieten.* Ed. 4, München, J. F. Lehmann, 1924.

Guilloz, T.: Interpretation d'une illusion radiographique. *C. R. de la Soc. de biol. de Paris, 55*:1689-1691 (December 14), 1903.

Gunning, R.: Clear writing, pp. 34-48 *in Proceedings of the ACR Annual Clinical Conference of Teachers of Radiology,* mimeographed, Chicago, American College of Radiology, 1959.

Habbe, J. E.: The roentgenologist's report: who should receive it. *Radiology, 38*:618-619 (May) 1942.

Harrison, B. J. M.: *A Textbook of Roentgenology.* Baltimore, Wm. Wood & Co., 1936, p. xxiii.

Hernaman-Johnson, F.: The place of the radiologist and his kindred in the world of medicine. *Arch. Radiol. & Electrol., 24*:181-187 (November) 1919.

Herrick, J. F.: The radiologist as a consultant. *Radiology, 18*:1011-1012 (May) 1932.

Hickey, P. M.: The interpretation of radiographs. *J. Michigan M. Soc., 3*:496-499 (November) 1904.

Hickey, P. M.: Standardization of roentgen-ray reports. *Am. J. Roentgenol., 9*:422-425 (July) 1922.

Hodges, F. J., and Lampe, I.: Filing and cross-indexing roentgen-ray records. *Am. J. Roentgenol., 41*:1007-1018 (June) 1939.

Hodges, F. J., Lampe, I., and Holt, J. F.: *Radiology for Medical Students.* Chicago, Year Book Publishers, 1947, p. 52.

Hodges F. J., and Peck, W. S.: *Introduction to Radiology.* Ann Arbor (Michigan), Edwards Bros., 1939, p. 19.

Holman, E.: Concerning more effective medical reporting. A plea for sobriety, accuracy, and brevity in medical writing. *J.A.M.A., 181*:245-247 (July 21) 1962.

Holmes, G. W., and Robbins, L. L.: *Roentgen Interpretation.* Ed. 8., Philadelphia, Lea & Febiger, 1955, p. 16.

Holzknecht, G.: *Die röntgenologische Diagnostik der Erkrankungen der Brusteingeweide.* Hamburg, Lucas Gräfe & Sillem, 1901, p. 26.

Holzknecht, G.: Der Röntgenbefund. *Jahreskurse f. aerztl. Fortbildung (München), 10* (nr. 8):32-49 (August) 1919.

Holzknecht, G.: *Einstellung zur Röntgenologie.* Wien, Julius Springer, 1927, 115 pages.

Holzknecht and Kienböck: Ueber die Einrichtung des Plattenarchivs. *Fortschr. a. d. Geb. d. Röstrahlen, 5*:308-310, 1902.

Hubeny, M. J.: Power of suggestion. *Radiology, 6*:167-168 (February) 1926.

Jaeger, W.: Das Lesen des Röntgenbildes. *Schweiz. med. Wchschr., 72*:1429-1431 (December 26) 1942.

Jones, W. A.: Points of mutual interest to the general practitioner and the radiologist. *Canadian M.A.J., 39*:152-157 (August) 1928.

Kassabian, M. K.: The early diagnosis of pulmonary tuberculosis by roentgen rays. *Am. X-Ray J., 12*:105-110 (April) 1903.

Kassabian, M. K.: *Röentgen Rays and Electro-Therapeutics.* Philadelphia, J. B. Lippincott, 1907, p. 242.

Kästle, C.: Roentgendiagnostik und Roentgentechnik, vol. I, p. 122 *in Lehrbuch der Röntgendiagnostik.* (Ed.: A. Schittenhelm). Berlin, Julius Springer, 1924.

Kienboeck: Ueber Methoden der Deutung und Reproduktion von Radiogrammen. *Wien. Klin. Rundschau, 16*: 825-831 (October 26) 1902.

Kienboeck, R.: Ueber die technischen Bezeichnungen von Rumpfaufnahmen. *Fortschritte a. d. Geb. d. Röstrahlen, 25*:446-449, 1918.

Kirklin, B. R.: Responsibilities of the radiologist. *Am. J. Roentgenol., 38*:677-680 (November) 1937.

Koenig, C. E.: Some misinterpretations of x-ray plates and fluoroscopic screens. *Northwest Med., 24*:136-139 (March) 1925.

Koenig, E. C.: Fractured skull without clinical symptoms. *Am. Atlas of Stereoroentgenol., 9*:246-247, 1920.

Kolle, F. S.: Roentgenogram ethics. *Am. X-Ray J. 2*:210-211 (March) 1898.

Kolta, E.: Ueber eine einfache Zeichenschrift bei der internen Röntgen-Diagnostik. *Fortschritte a d. Geb. d. Röstrahlen, 32*:365-368, 1924.

Lacaille, E.: La radiographie, en tant qu'élement diagnostic est oeuvre médicale et, comme telle, doit rester entre les mains des seuls médecins. *Rev. de méd. légale,* (Paris) *9*:121-127, (March) 1902.

Landau, G. M.: 68 roentgenologists tell to whom x-ray films may be shown. *Hosp. Management, 30* (nr. 5):80-86 (November) 1930.

Lanphear, E.: X-Ray negation leads to positive diagnosis. *Am. X-Ray J., 5*:678-679 (December) 1899.

Lapirot: Calques radioscopiques rapides et precis. *J. de radiol. et d'électrol., 3*:80, 1918.

Latourette, H. B., and Hodges, F. J.: Incidence of neoplasia after irradiation of thymic region. *Am. J. Roentgenol., 82*:667-677 (October) 1959.

Ledoux-Lebard, A., and Garcia-Calderon, J.: *Technique du Radio-Diagnostic.* Paris, Masson & Cie, 1943, p. 90.

Legros, G.: Les erreurs d' interpretation en radiographie. *Progrès méd., (Paris) 24*:470-472 (June) 1908.

Leonard, C. L.: The technique of the positive and negative diagnosis of ureteral and renal calculi by the aid of the roentgen rays. *Ann. of Surgery, 31*:163-169 (February) 1900.

Long, F. A., and Lloyd, P. T.: *The Use of the Roentgen Ray in the Study of Vertebral Mechanics with Special Reference to its Adaptability in Osteopathic Procedures.* Philadelphia College of Osteopathy, 1938, 94 pages.

Lorimier, A. A. de, Moehring, H. G., and Hannan, J. R.: *Clinical Roentgenology.* Springfield, Charles C Thomas, 1954, vol. I, p. 9.

Lusted, L. J.: Logical analysis in roentgen diagnosis. *Radiology, 74*:178-193 (February) 1960.

McCandless, O. H.: Diaphragmatic hernia. *J. Roentgenol., 2*:82-89 (March) 1919.

M'Kendrick, A.: Insufficient data as a cause of faulty interpretation of radiographs. *Edinburgh M. J., 8*:521-524 (June) 1912.

McRae, D.: A system for reading x-ray films for use in sanatoria. *Am. Rev. Tuberc., 21*:811-818 (June) 1930.

Manning, W. J.: Roentgenograms as evidence. *J. Radiol., 6*:376-377 (September) 1925.

Ménard, M.: Lecture et interprétation des radiographies au point de vue médico-legal. *Ann. d'hyg. publ. et de méd. légale, 16*:253-268 (April) 1911.

Meschan, I., and Farrier-Meschan, R. M. F.: *Roentgen Signs in Clinical Diagnosis.* Philadelphia, Saunders, 1956, p. 45.

Miller, R. E.: Radiograph filing facilties and loan service at the Indiana University Medical Center. *Med. Radiography & Photogr., 38*:55-79, 1962.

Miller, R. E.: The attending physician in the radiological team. *Med. Times,* July 1963.

Monell, S. H.: Letter on "Standards." *Am. Electrotherap. & X-Ray Era, 1* (nr. 3):9-10 (August 15) 1901.

Morton, W. J.: The x-ray picture of the living human head. *Am. X-Ray J., 1*:89-91 (October) 1897.

Newell, R. R., and Garneau, R.: The threshold visibility of pulmonary shadows. *Radiology, 56*:409-415 (March) 1951.

Newell, R. R., Chamberlain, W. E. and Rigler, L.: Descriptive classification of pulmonary shadows. A revelation of unreliability in the roentgenographic diagnosis of tuberculosis. *Am. Rev. Tuberc., 69*:566-584 (April) 1954.

Nogier, T.: Precautions pratiques pour éviter les interprétations erronées basées sur le seul examen des radiographies positives. *Arch. d'electr. méd., 22*:263-264 (March 10) 1913.

Ottolengui, R.: Interpretation of dental roentgenograms. *Am. J. Roentgenpl., 3*:169-170 (March) 1916.

Pancoast, H. K., Baetjer, F. H., and Dunham, K.: Clinical and x-ray findings in chests of normal children. Report of the x-ray group. *Am. Rev. Tuberc., 6*:338-340 (July) 1922.

Pancoast, H. K., Baetjer, F. H., and Dunham, K.: The healthy adult chest. A clinical and roentgenological report. *Am. Rev. Tuberc., 15*:429-471 (April) 1927.

Pendergrass, E. F., and Hodes, P. J.: Oral cholecystography: evaluation of the method and suggestions for a new nomenclature. *Radiology, 25*:261-266 (September) 1935.

Pfahler, G. E.: Discussion. *Radiology 18*:1012-1013 (May) 1932.

Pirkle, H. B.: A method of recording roentgen-ray readings. *Am. Rev. Tuberc., 27*:311-314 (March) 1933.

Popper, M., Kaufman, S., and Zibalis, S.: Diagnosticul radiologic al tuberculomului pulmonar. *Radiologia (Bucharest), 1*:121-128 (September-October) 1956.

Pordes, F.: Methodenwahl in der Röntgendiagnostik. Die

unzweckmässigen und die zweckdienlichen Wege. *Med. Klinik (Wien), 17*:1520-1522 (December 15); 1552-1555 (December 22); 1577-1579 (December 29) 1921.

Pothérat, E.: Illusions radiographiques. *Bull. et mém. de la Soc. de chir. de Paris, 31*:370-371 (April) 1905.

Potvin, A. R.: Le symptôme radiologique. *Bull. méd. de Quebec, 23*:120-122 (November) 1922.

Proseus, F. W.: The responsibility of the radiographer regarding interpretation of radiograms. *Internat. J. Orthodontia (St. Louis), 10*:433-437 (July) 1924.

Ramsey, G. S.: The negative x-ray report in cancer of the colon. *Brit. J. Surg., 43*:576-579 (May) 1956.

Redding, J. M.: *X-Ray Diagnosis.* New York, Wm. Wood & Co., 1927, p. 2.

Rees, T.: Platon und die Röntgenärzte. *München. med. Wchschr., 83*:671-673 (April 24) 1936.

Reynberg, S. A.: Obshaya methodika rentgenologicheskoye isledovannye, pp. 90-95 in *Kurs Medicinskoye Rentgenologii.* Moskva, Narkomzdrav, 1938.

Richards, G. E.: X-Ray Reports. *J. Royal Army Med. Corps,* (August) 1917.

Rigler, L. G.: Roentgen diagnosis and clinical responsibility. *Radiology, 54*:884-885 (June) 1950.

Rigler, L.: A critique of roentgen interpretation. *Radiology, 72*:431-433 (March) 1959.

Rigler, L.: Functional roentgen diagnosis: anatomical image — physiological interpretation. *Am. J. Roentgenol., 82*:1-24 (July) 1959.

Robertson, H. E.: Teamwork between the roentgenologist and the pathologist. *J. Radiol., 3*:308-310 (August) 1922.

Rose, H. M.: *Medical Radiographic Terminology.* Ann Arbor (Michigan), Edwards Brothers, 1955, 108 pages.

Ross, S. E.: Operations research and optimal radiology. *Radiology, 73*:618-620 (October) 1959.

Ross, W. L.: The value of negative roentgen findings of the stomach. *J. Roentgenol., 2*:217-226 (May) 1919.

Sandberg, L. B.: *Atlas und Axis.* Statische und funktionelle Röntgenbildanalyse der Halswirbelsäule als Grundlage für die chiropraktische Behandlung (HTO-Therapie). Stuttgart, Hippokrates-Verlag, 1955, 124 pages.

Sante, L. R.: An indexing system for the cataloguing of pathological films. *Radiology, 7*:149-163 (August) 1926.

Sante, L. R.: *Principles of Roentgen Interpretation.* Ed. 10, Ann Arbor (Michigan), Edwards Brothers, p. 1.

Sante, L. R.: Index classification for a pathological file, pp. 480-495 *in Manual of Roentgenological Technique.* Ed. 16, Ann Arbor (Michigan), Edwards Brothers, 1956.

Saupe, E.: *Die Roentgenbildanalyse* (ed.: W. Teschendorf), ed 3, Stuttgart, G. Thieme, 1956, p. 283.

Schinz, H. R., Baensch, W. E., Friedl, E., and Uehlinger, E.: *Lehrbuch der Röntgendiagnostik.* Ed. 5, Stuttgart, Georg Thieme, 1950, vol. I, p. 96.

Schreiber, M. H.: The clinical history as a factor in roentgenogram interpretation. *J.A.M.A., 185*:399-401 (August 3) 1963.

Scott, J. N.: How some of the mistakes are made in radiography. *Am. X-Ray J., 10*:1046-1049 (May) 1902.

Shenton, E. W. H.: Roentgen-ray diagnosis of renal calculus. *Guy's Hosp. Rep., 56*:91-97, 1899 (1902).

Sherman, R. S.: On making a roentgen diagnosis. *Radiology, 70*:98-99 (January) 1958.

Sherman, R. S.: The roentgenologist as a consultant. *Radiology, 75*:293-295 (August) 1960.

Soiland, A.: The medico-legal status of the roentgenologist. *An J. Roentgenol., 5*:173-175 (March) 1918.

Sosman, M. C.: The specificity and reliability of roentgenographic diagnosis. *New Egland J. Med., 242*:849-855 (June 1) 1950.

Spirko, C.: *Radiologic Records.* Springfield, Charles C Thomas, 1960, 304 pages.

Stein, A. E.: Die Einordnung und Buchung der exponierten Röntgenplatten. *Fortschritte a. d. Geb. d. Röstrahlen, 5*:183-185,1901.

Stover, G. H.: The radiographer's property right in the radiogram. *Am. Quarterly of Roentgenol., 3*:131-136 (July) 1911.

Stevens, R. H.: X-ray work in hospitals. *Am. Quarterly of Roentgenol., 2*:107-112 (March) 1910.

Sutherland, C. G.: The value of the x-ray in general practice. *Minnesota Med., 21*:839-846 (December) 1938.

Sutherland, C. G.: A proposed new method: the filing of roentgenograms. *Hospitals, 15*:93-98 (October) 1941.

Taft, R. B.: Film marking by a new method. *Am. J. Roentgenol., 12*:390-391 (October) 1924.

Tager, S. N.: The terminology of the roentgenologist. *Radiology, 35*:369-371 (September) 1940.

Takiuchi, S.: *Hoshasen Sho Jiten* (Radiological Dictionary). Tokyo, Kimpodo, 474 & 78 & 44 pages.

Tennille, N. B.: Survey of veterinary radiography. *North Amer. Veterinarian, 35*:195-198 (March) 1954.

Thomas, S. F.: The radiologist's report. *Radiology, 47*:404-405 (October) 1946.

Thompson, E. A.: *Text on Chiropractic Spinography.* Ed. 4, Chicago, W. B. Conkey Co., 1923, p. 34.

Tracy, E. A.: The fallacies of x-ray pictures. *J.A.M.A., 29*: 949-951 (November 6) 1897.

Trostler, I.: Reports of findings. *Radiology, 19*:110-112 (August) 1932.

Trostler, I. S.: The legal aspect of identification and interpretation of roentgenograms. *Am. J. Roentgenol., 32*:680-693 (November) 1934.

Trostler, I. S.: Legal liability for error in diagnosis. Roentgenologist and his employer held liable for a mistaken diagnosis. *Radiology, 48*:282-283 (March) 1947.

Tuddenham, W. J.: Visual search, image organization, and reader error in roentgen diagnosis. Studies of the psychophysiology of roentgen image perception. *Radiology, 78*: 694-704 (May) 1962.

Tuddenham, W. J.: Problems of perception in chest roentgenology: facts and fallacies. *Rad. Clinics of North America, 1*:277-289 (August) 1963.

Van Pée, P.: *Précis de Radio-Diagnostic.* Liège, Editions Desoer, 1944, p. 46.

Walker, S. F.: Classification and filing in the department of roentgenology. *Radiology, 40*:603-604 (June) 1943.

Wasson, W. W.: The x-ray as a microscope. *J. Radiol., 3*: 268-271 (July) 1922.

Wasson, W. W.: Roentgenologic syndromes. *Radiology, 27*: 500 (October) 1936.

Wheaton, C. L.: Radiographic studies in shadow density, from the standpoint of the clinician. *Illinois M. J., 38*: 138-140 (August) 1920.

Wilbert, M. I.: Systematic records and the routine use of the x-rays. *Amer. X-Ray J., 12*:38-39 (February) 1903.

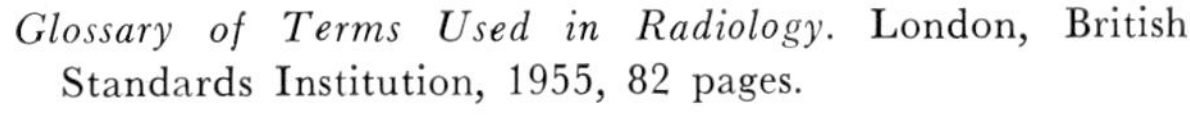

Wilbert, M. I.: A comparative study of fractures of the extremities. *Transactions of the ARRS, 4*:195-204 (December 9) 1903 (1904).

Williams, F. H.: A method for more fully determining the outline of the heart by means of the fluorescope *(sic)* together with other uses of this instrument. *Boston M. & S. J., 135*:335-337 (October 1), 1896.

Williams, F. H.: The roentgen rays in thoracic diseases. *Am. J. M. Sciences, 114*:665-687 (December) 1897.

Williams, F. H.: *The Roentgen Rays in Medicine and Surgery.* New York, Macmillan, 1901, p. 99.

English-French Glossary of X-ray Terms. A Compendium of Words and Phrases for the Use of Radiologists of the Allied Forces in France. Tours, E. Arrault & Cie, 1918, p. 43.

Glossary of Terms Used in Radiology. London, British Standards Institution, 1955, 82 pages.

Lay radiographers and medical reports. *Radiology, 6*:344 (April) 1926.

Legal status of hospital records. *Radiology, 14*:520-521 (May) 1930.

Ownership of roentgenograms. *Radiology, 18*:332 (January) 1932.

Termini Radiologici (Deutsch, English, Français, Español). *Deutscher Medizinischer Sprachendienst.* München, Urban & Schwarzenberg, 1959, 78 pages.

United States Army X-Ray Manual, prepared under the direction of the Division of Roentgenology. New York, Paul B. Hoeber, 1919, p. 212.

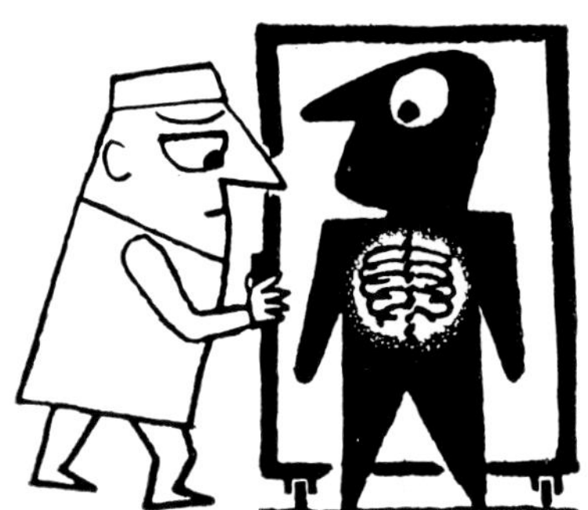

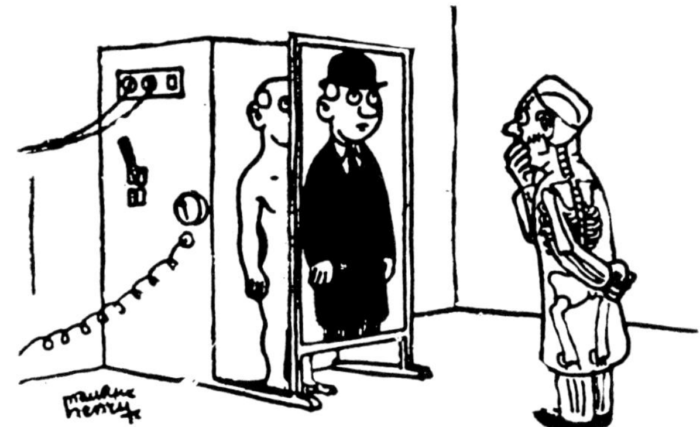

Chapter 6

WILLIAM JAMES MORTON (1845-1920), FIRST MEDICAL ELECTRO-RADIOLOGIST IN AMERICA

There is properly no history;
only biography!
RALPH WALDO EMERSON

FEW PAGES FROM the radiologic past are more interesting, instructive and inciting, or more involved, than the fascinating life of the "neurologist and electro-therapeut" William James Morton. The qualifications given in the preceding sentence are actually incomplete because Morton was — above everything else — the *earliest* (American) *x-ray specialist.*[1]

SOURCES

Fairly accurate information (on the first fifty years of Morton's life) was offered by Morton himself for inclusion in a source-book, compiled by the now forgotten American medical biographer, Irving Allison Watson (1849-1918).[2]

Watson's sketch[2] served as an unnamed source for the *Cyclopaedia*[3] and for a well known medico-biographic dictionary.[4] A belated, and at that half-hearted, eulogist – the historian of neurology Charles Loomis Dana (1852-1935) – misled by the death notice[5] in the *AMA Journal,* and by a misprint in Watson,[2] came

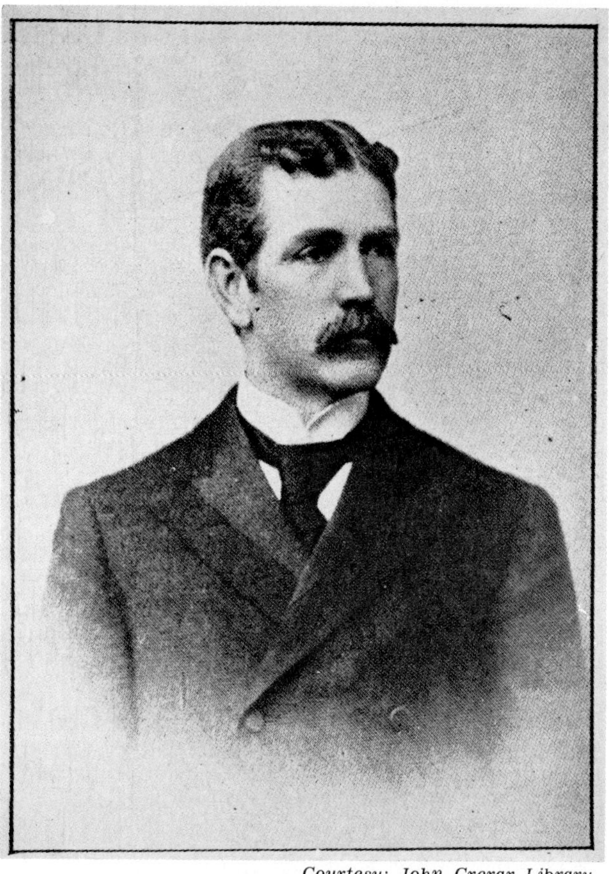

Courtesy: John Crerar Library.

WILLIAM JAMES MORTON. This photograph, made in the 1880's, was offered by Morton himself for reproduction in Watson's biographic sketch.[2] A sketch made from the same photograph appeared in the *Cyclopaedia.*[3] The walrus *(deuxième république)* type mustache, and the *fin-de-siècle* lapels add a measure of masculinity to his initially delicate facial features.

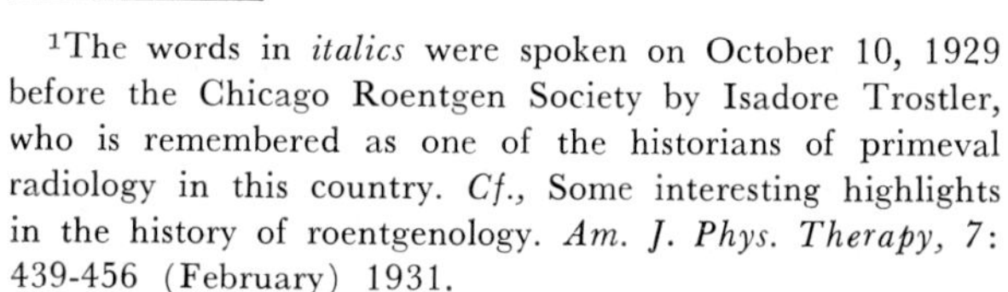

[1]The words in *italics* were spoken on October 10, 1929 before the Chicago Roentgen Society by Isadore Trostler, who is remembered as one of the historians of primeval radiology in this country. *Cf.,* Some interesting highlights in the history of roentgenology. *Am. J. Phys. Therapy, 7:* 439-456 (February) 1931.

[2]*Physicians and Surgeons of America. A Collection of Biographical Sketches.* Concord, N. H., Republican Press Association, 1896, pp. 806-809.

[3]*The National Cyclopaedia of American Biography.* New York, James T. White & Co., 1900, vol. 8, p. 333.

[4]Kelly, H. A., and Burrage, W. L.: *Dictionary of American Medical Biography.* New York, Appleton & Co., 1928, p. 878.

[5]Deaths. *J.A.M.A., 74:*1113 (April 17) 1920.

up with a wrong birthplace and wrong birthyear,[6] which creeped also into a subsequent panegyric.[7]

Information on Morton's pioneering roentgen work was deleted from several obituaries, [6, 8], or mentioned in an obsolete fashion, obscure to anyone but the historian,[9] while in the Webster,[10] Morton is given credit only for his therapeutic achievements.

Morton's latest biography was again written by a neurologist, Smith Ely Jelliffe (1866-1945).[11] It is more serene (objective?), and more complete than any of those previously published. Nevertheless, it contains only perfunctory references to Morton's radiologic endeavors.

BACKGROUND AND EDUCATION

William James Morton was born in Boston on July 3, 1845[12] of pure colonial New England stock.

His father – the practical dentist[13] William Thomas Green Morton (1819-1868) of ether *(letheon)* fame – was the great-grandson of Robert Morton, who had come from Scotland to Mendon (Massachusetts) and who later founded Elizabeth(town) in New Jersey.

W. J. Morton's mother – the former Elizabeth Whitman of Farmington, Connecticut – descended in direct line from the famous John Whitman of Weymouth.[14]

Young Morton graduated from the excellent and aristocratic Boston Latin School, entered Harvard in 1863, and got his M.A. in 1867. He grew up at a time when his family suffered many psychologic, as well as financial, frustrations.

The last decade in old W. T. G. Morton's life had been a continuous battle to establish his claim as the discoverer (or at least as the revealer) of anesthesia, and to fight alleged infringements against his (never recognized) ether patent. He lost his health, the dental practice, the "model farm," and whatever fortune he had possessed.[15] Creditors bedevilled him to the very last, and when he died, the widow – left with five children – had a hard time to make ends meet.[16]

W. J. Morton must have resolved then and there (a) to vindicate his father's memory, *i.e.*, to uphold his scientific claims. So as to avoid making the old man's mistakes, young Morton determined (b) to strive for palpable (monetary!) rewards, and (c) to attach chronologically indisputable claims to all his own (future) scientific contributions. Such resolves cannot justify or excuse his subsequent behavior, but at least they explain much of what haunted him for the balance of his life. He was endowed with considerable innate intelligence—indeed, he had a touch of genius — and was capable of sustained work. His handsome face, trim frame, and charming, eternally optimistic, personality contributed to his tremendous success, and helped him considerably during, and after, his downfall.

In 1867, Morton, Jr., interrupted his studies and taught for one year in the Gardiner (Mass.) High School. After his father's death (July 15, 1868) he matriculated in Harvard Medical School, and supported himself by residing (as a medical officer) in the Discharged Soldiers' Home (1869), then as house pupil (and after 1871 as house surgeon) in Massachusetts General Hospital, where memories and friends of Morton, Sr., lingered on for many decades.

At the time of his graduation (M.D., 1872) from Harvard, Morton was physician of Boston Dispensary. He remained there for another year, practicing at 1 Park Square, an address which he gave on his first paper,[17] a brief article on typhoid fever (2).[18] Shortly thereafter, Morton went to Europe.

---

[6]Dana, C. L.: The career and accomplishments of the late Dr. W. J. Morton, *J. Nerv. & Ment. Dis., 53*:255-256 (March) 1921.

[7]*Semi-Centennial Volume of the American Neurological Association* (Eds.: F. Tilney & S. E. Jelliffe). Albany, N. Y., Boyd Printing Co., 1924, pp. 208-209.

[8]Obituary notes. *Med. Record, 97*:617 (April 10) 1920. —Recent deaths, *Boston M. & S. J., 182*:416 (April 15) 1920.

[9]Obituary. *New York M. J., 111*:718 (May 11) 1920.

[10]*Webster's Biographical Dictionary*. Springfield, Mass., G. & O. Merriam Co., 1943, p. 1061.

[11]*Dictionary of American Biography*. New York, Scribner's Sons, 1934, vol. 13, pp. 267-268.

[12]Morton's birthyear in Watson is misprinted 1846, but given correctly nine lines above, on the same page.[2] Morton's parents were married in May, 1844, and their second child (Marion Aletha Morton) was born on February 2, 1847: W. J. Morton's birthday could not have been on July 3, 1846.

[13]Rice, N. P.: A grain of wheat from a bushel of chaff. *New York Monthly Magazine, 53*:133-138 (February) 1859.

[14]Farnam, C. H.: *History of the Descendants of John Whitman of Weymouth, Mass.* New Haven, Tuttle, Morehouse, & Taylor, 1889, pp. 526-527.

[15]Beecher, H. K., and Ford, C.: Nathan P. Rice's *Trials of a Public Benefactor*. A commentary. *J. Hist. Med., 15*: 170-183 (April) 1960.

[16]She succeeded, as they had many friends. The youngest child, Bowditch Morton, graduated from Harvard Medical School in 1881.

[17]Watson[2] mentions a Boylston Prize essay, allegedly written by Morton in 1872 under the title 'Anaesthetics.' This is strange, because in that year — *cf.*, Boylston prize. *Boston M. & S. J., 86*:380 (June 6) 1872 — the Com-

TRAVELS

Before the turn of the century, Wm. J. Morton crossed the Atlantic at least ten times.

He stayed in Vienna through May of 1874, and then went all the way to Kimberley (South Africa), where diamonds had been found in 1871. Morton became the medical officer of a mining concern, and in addition established a profitable private practice, to the point where he had to import an assistant from England (another American physician, who subsequently took over the entire practice). Morton made journeys into the "interior," hunted big game, and staked his own diamond claims (worked with the help of local labor gangs).

The South African adventure must have been fairly rewarding, because in 1876, Morton toured England, France, and Germany before returning, at the end of the year, to America. He joined the American Geographical Society, published a travelog (3), and was marking time in New York City when a fortuitous occurrence placed him on a neuro-psychiatric pathway.

A German immigrant, who made a financial success in America, learned that his bride-to-be, left behind, had been committed to a mental institution. In the summer of 1877 he asked Morton to go to Germany as a "sanity expert." The self-styled expert returned triumphantly to America after a few months, bringing the "patient" with him. This episode induced Morton to settle in New York City in 1878, and open an office at 33 East 33rd Street.

In 1879, Morton became clinical assistant to the Chair of Diseases of the Mind and Nervous System in the University of the City of New York (today's Cornell). That particular chair was then occupied by William Alexander Hammond (1828-1900), the former Surgeon General (1862), who had been court-martialed and dismissed (1864), then reviewed (1878), re-instated and retired. Together they issued in April, 1879, the short-lived *Neurological Contributions* (1879-1881), which appeared to be little more than a personal outlet for case-reports (5, 10), or fancies.[19]

In 1877, the "Southern" gynecologist James Marion Sims (1813-1883)[20] supported the chronologically valid, but otherwise insignificant, claim of the Georgia surgeon Crawford Williamson Long (1815-1878). The latter had actually operated under ether enesthesia in 1842 (six years before Morton, Sr.), but only on a few occasions, and without publishing anything about it at the time. In 1879, Morton Jr., attacked Sims for his "unjust, sophistical, and Quixotic" efforts (9, 11) in behalf of Long. But Southern senators must have had more "pull" with the Postmaster, because Long's portrait was reproduced on a topical stamp, while no such honor was granted to Morton, Sr.

At periodical intervals, throughout his life, W. J. Morton (40, 47, 48, 49, 91, 96) would crusade for his father's recognition as the discoverer of anesthesia.

On November 6, 1879 Morton, Jr., was elected a Fellow of the New York Academy of Medicine.[21] In June, 1880 he married Elizabeth Campbell — the daughter of Col. Washington Lee Campbell of Wilkesbarre (as it was then spelled) in Pennsylvania — and went for an extended honeymoon to Paris.

mittee met on June 3, and awarded $200 to John Collins Warren (1842-1927) of Boston for an essay on 'Malignant and semi-malignant pathology' and $150 to Horatio Charles Wood, Jr. (1841-1920) of Philadelphia, for an essay on 'Sunstroke.' In search for a clarification, an inquiry was mailed to the Boylston Prize Committee, and Prof. Harry Trimble (special consultant to the Dean of Harvard Medical School) obligingly searched the minutes of the Boylston Medical Society for that period: on February 9, 1872 was the entry "The Committee on prize dissertations have decided unanimously that none of the essays submitted to them this year is worthy of a prize, signed F. Minot, Chairman," and "Dr. Fitz (President) stated that there were three dissertations handed in." They must have changed their minds subsequently, since they awarded at least two prizes. Unfortunately, the Archives of Harvard have not preserved a list of the Boylston Prize Awards.

[18]The figures in parentheses refer to Morton's bibliography, found at the end of this chapter.

[19]Hammond, W. A.: The therapeutical use of the magnet. *Neurol. Contrib., 2*:44-58, 1880.

[20]The discovery of anesthesia. *Virginia Med. Monthly, 4*:81-100 (January) 1877.

[21]This and several other details have been graciously contributed by Miss Gertrude Louise Annan, chief-librarian of the New York Academy of Medicine.

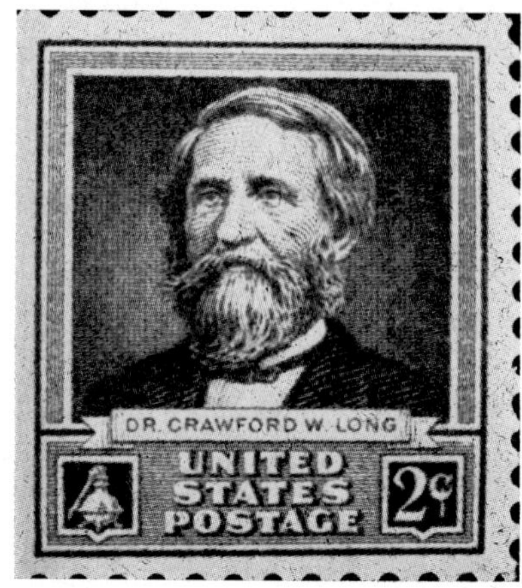

Being firmly committed to neuro-psychiatry, he used the journey to "study" with Jean Martin Charcot (1825-1893), whose "hysterical" patients were at that time very much *en-vogue*. Incidentally, Morton sent (for the folks back home) several carefully composed 'Letters to the Editor' (12, 13, 14), aimed to keep his name within the reach of public attention.

After a few side trips (15), the newly-weds returned to New York. The urge to travel was still there, but occasions (21) were fewer. In 1888 they went to Mexico City (36), and in 1894 to Rome (Italy), where Morton was an official U. S. delegate to the International Medical Congress. By that time, he was already famous, had written a chapter for a popular textbook (43), and was twice called to Germany (1894) for *bona-fide* medical consultations.

ACHIEVEMENTS IN NEUROLOGY

After the honeymoon, Morton stayed on until 1882 as assistant to Hammond, while from 1880 through 1885 he spent most of his summer time at Burlington, teaching neuro-psychiatry in the University of Vermont.

The turning point in his career came at the end of 1881, when Morton purchased (perhaps with part of the dowry?!) the *Journal of Nervous and Mental Diseases* from James Stewart Jewell (1837-1887), the neurologist of Chicago Medical College. With the January, 1882 issue Morton became the editor of that journal, and by the same token a figurehead in American neuro-psychiatry.

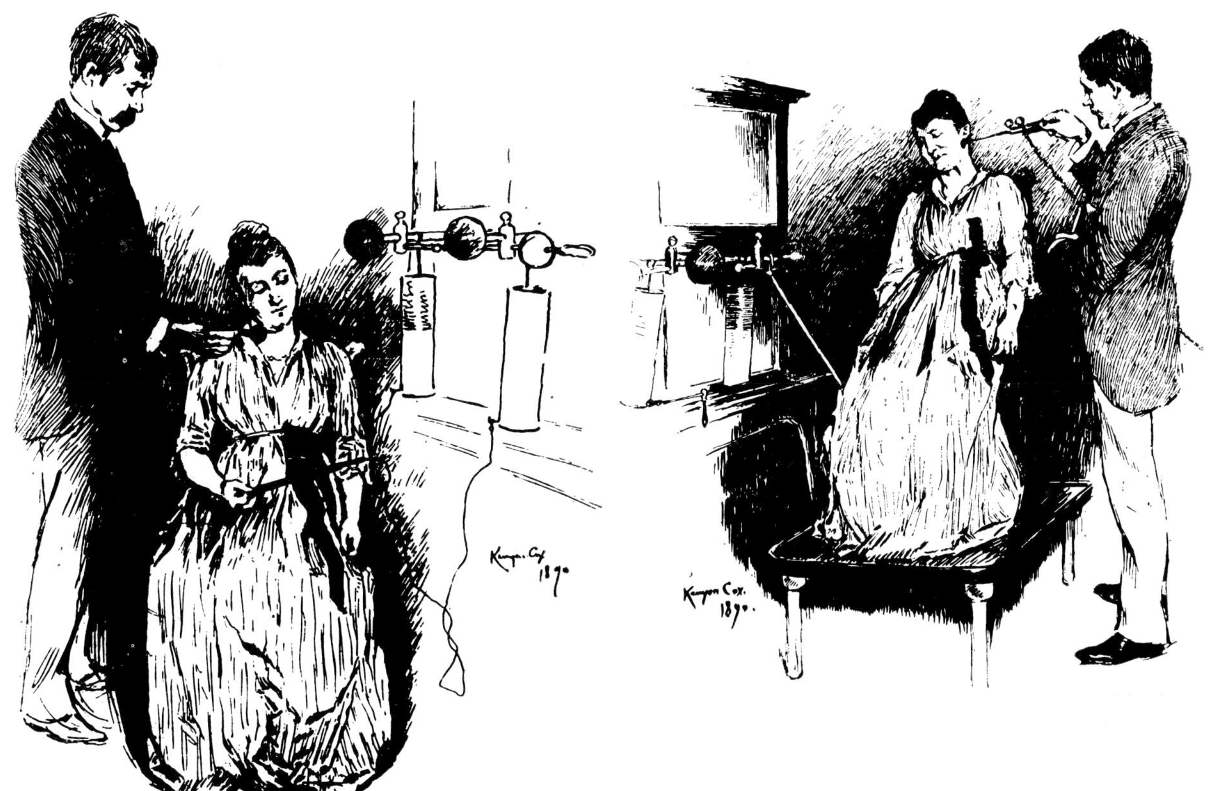

Courtesy: Midwest Inter-Library Center, Chicago.

MORTON AND "HIS" CURRENT. Both sketches were made by the aristocratic painter Kenyon Cox (1856-1919), another heir to a famous name. The static machine with its Leyden jars is well recognized. Morton is applying his eponymic[22] static induced (a sort of high frequency) current. He is shown using a wet sponge electrode over the facial nerve (with resultant rictus), and a gun-shaped electrode (of his own design) over the sterno-cleido-mastoid (leading to transient torticollis). Each of these drawings appeared as full-page illustrations in the reputable *Medical Record* (38). Reprints of that article were actively circulated among referring physicians, as well as among potential patients.

Together with twenty (or so) other physicians, he watched Daniel Smith Lamb (1843-1929) perform the autopsy of Charles Guiteau (1840-1882), the executed assassin of President Garfield: then, Morton assigned himself to report on the examination of Guiteau's brain. For this job, he acquired an associate (22, 23), a young physician named Charles Dana (a nephew of Morton, Sr.'s lawyer), the same one who, decades later, was slated to become Morton, Jr.'s somewhat reluctant eulogist.[6]

In 1882, Morton was named adjunct professor of Diseases of the Mind and of the Nervous System in the New York Post-Graduate Medical School and Hospital. He attained full professorship (which included the teaching of electro-therapeutics) in 1890, and this remained his main academic title for almost thirty years.

His clinical contributions to neurology, while initially promising,[11] carry little significance. The papers on 'Tea-drinker's disorder' (5, 8), and on 'Nerve-stretching' (7, 19, 20, 35, 41) are of some interest, but they are as grossly overplayed as most of his prose. Reprints of his articles were skillfully circulated, and properly displayed in the waiting room of his office, moved about that time to 15 East 45th Street.

Morton's style, often pompous but never obscure, tended toward the pontifical, especially in editorials (29, 30, 31, 32), or in the presidential address (28) delivered to the New York Neurological Society.

In December, 1885 Morton sold the *Journal of Nervous and Mental Diseases,* which meant abdication from the editorship (34). His original investment had paid off handsomely, and there was no need to continue to subsidize a losing venture. He had then a booming practice, and a luxurious home at 36 West 56th Street.[6]

ACHIEVEMENTS IN ELECTROTHERAPY

Morton had undoubtedly an inventive and mechanical (albeit a bit preposterous) turn of mind, *e.g.,* in the 1880's he was working on a water motor, intended to revolutionize dynamics.

In 1881 Morton devised an arrangement by which a Holtz or other influence machine, coupled with Leyden jars, would turn out series of condenser discharges. He called these discharges "static induced currents," and referred to the procedure as "Franklinism" (16).

He ascribed to these condenser discharges curative effects in so many situations, he promoted the method so effectively, and defended his priority in the mat-

Again, I quote from the Transactions of the American Institute of Electrical Engineers, November, 1893, p. 604, the following, which also accurately describes the same "arrangement":

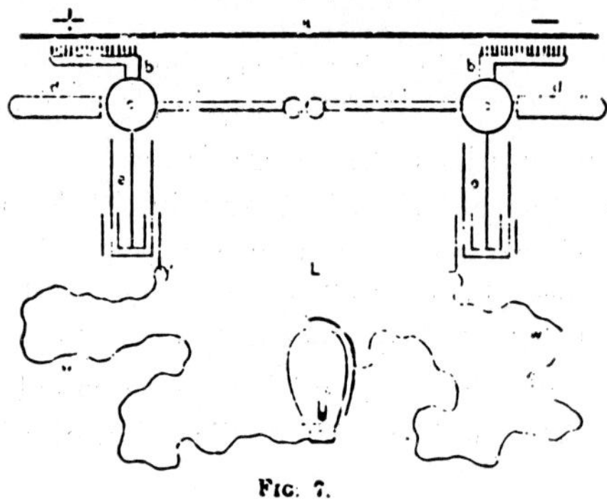

" Fig. 7. Parts of influence machine and condensers, as before described; L an Edison 16 candle-power lamp with broken filament; a piece of tinfoil laid against a portion of the bulb, w, w'; w, wire leading to filament; w', leading to the tinfoil.

" Now that the lights in the hall are turned down, you see that the glow is most brilliant for a glow lamp effect. As we increase the size of the Leyden jars and cut down the length of the spark crossing the air gap, the purple color changes to whitish, and the effect is intensified."

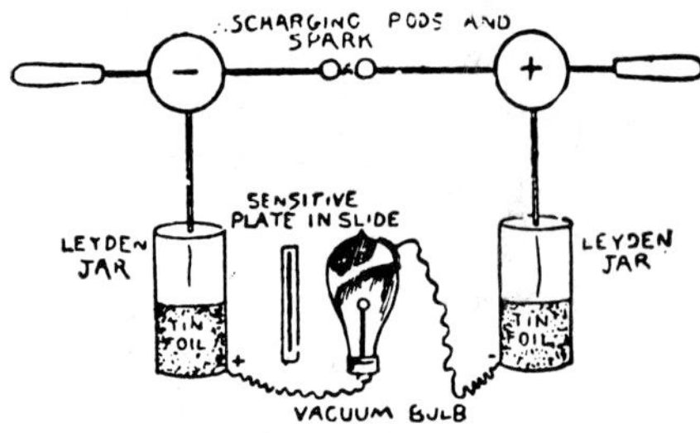

DR. MORTON'S NEW ARRANGEMENT FOR PRODUCING ROENTGEN RAYS.

"One of Dr. William J. Morton's experiments is for demonstrating that the cathodic rays may be produced in vacuum tubes by a static machine. The use of the vacuum tubes of any construction excited by a static machine is a novel proposition in Roentgen photography, and its adoption may extend the facilities for work in this new field.

Courtesy: John Crerar Library.

MORTON AND HIS PRIORITIES. The drawing called Figure 7 was first published by Morton in 1893 (42), and then reproduced by Morton in 1896 (55) to prove that said arrangement was his own, even though — because of its simplicity — it might have been used by others.[23] From the caption to Figure 7 it becomes clear that Morton was one of the many who had produced x rays — unknowingly — prior to Röntgen's announcement. With that same arrangement, Morton probably produced x-rays in the very first week of February, 1896.

ter so strenuously that the procedure is eponymized in the universal literature under the title *Morton's current(s)*.[22]

He employed oversized influence machines (17), which produced more impressive sparks, further magnified by a clever publicity.

Cataphoresis (as he called it) was Morton's other major electric preoccupation. He used it, for instance, to stain tissues for microscopic examination (46), to anesthetize peridental tissues (52), and – obviously – to treat a variety of diseases (50).

As a matter of fact, Morton is also regarded as one of the pioneers of what today is called ionization, and his tract on this subject (68) has remained a classic.

THE ADVENT OF ROENTGENOLOGY

On January 8, 1896 appeared the first mention in New York newspapers of Roentgen's discovery.

For several weeks, public response barely exceeded the level of passing interest. Medical circles never paid real attention to the "invisible" rays until after favorable editorial comment was printed as of February 1, 1896 in both the *New York Medical Journal* and in the *Medical Record.*

On February 6, 1896 Morton came up with what seemed to be a hoax: roentgen effects produced without a vacuum tube (53).

He had merely stumbled upon *brush discharge effects,*[23] a phenomenon already described in popularization papers.[24] Actually, the British physicist Sylvanus Phillips Thompson (1951-1916) believed in "spark x-rays" (162), while the American inventor Amos Emerson Dolbear (1937-1910) recalled in 1896 that – twenty years earlier – the "telephonist" Alexander Graham Bell (1947-1922) thought that "some" spark effect could be demonstrated even though a plaque of ebonite, provided exposure was sufficiently protracted.[25]

A few days later, Morton obtained (real) roentgen rays by connecting a vacuum tube to his giant influence machine (54). He used for this purpose a burned-out electric bulb, to which he had attached an external armature — and called it promptly *Morton's tube.* The manner in which the bulb was connected to the static machine was christened Morton's arrangement (55). And when the paternity of "his" arrangement was questioned,[23] Morton proved that he had published just such a diagram in 1893, at which time he had used it to produce his (Morton's) static induced currents (42).

This fact (56) explains the otherwise mysterious reference of an anonymous necrologist: "By the aid of his (Morton's) current, x-ray pictures are produced".[9] It also qualifies Morton for that very select club of scientists who — however unwittingly — had produced roentgen rays long before Roentgen's more

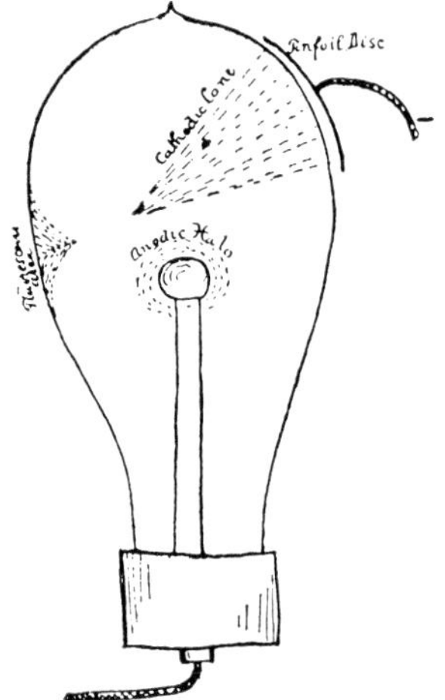

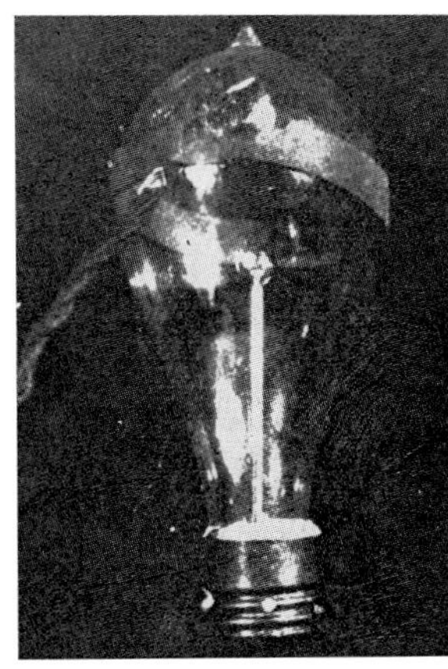

Courtesy: John Crerar Library.

MORTON'S TUBE. Morton had witnessed the demotion of his father (W. T. G. Morton) from "discoverer" to "revealer" of anesthesia. Young Morton therefore had, throughout his life, the obsessive urge to brand (eponymize) whatever he regarded as original in his publications. This tube was made on order from Morton by J. L. Somoff in October, 1894 (one year before Röntgen's experiments): its fore-runner was an "Edison 16 candle-power lamp with broken filament (and) a piece of tin-foil" as external armature (55). On Sunday, February 9, 1896 Pupin[23] visited Morton in the evening, and found him "fussing with . . . a mass of (cast-off) incandescent lamps with broken filaments." After Morton had reversed to conventional x-ray tubes, Edison began to use modified Crookes tubes as light bulbs, calling them "fluorescent lamps." The results were disastrous: ". . . I (Edison) started in to make a number of these lamps, but I soon found that the x-ray had affected poisonously my assistant, Mr. Dally, so that his hair came out and his flesh commenced to ulcerate. I then concluded it would not do, and that it would not be a very popular kind of light, so I dropped it. . ."

---

[22]Fischer, I.: *Biographisches Lexikon.* Wien, Urban & Schwarzenberg, 1933.

[23]Pupin, M. I.: Communication to the editor. *Electricity 10*:90 (February 19) 1896.

[24]Dolbear, A. E.: Electricity and photography. *Cosmopolitan 16*:765-766 (April) 1894.

[25]Dolbear, A. E.: Roentgen's photographs. *Electr. World, 27*:147 (February 8) 1896.

deliberate endeavors of 1895. After all, even Molière's gentlemanly *bourgeois,* Mr. Jourdain, had been speaking prose for forty years, and did not become aware of it until told by his master of philosophy.

ANIMADVERSIONS

Morton had been subjected to printed criticism on several occasions, but never before or after was the attack so vituperative as in the case of the Serbian immigrant, Michael Idvorsky Pupin (1858-1935), who was teaching physics at Columbia.

Pupin[23] accused Morton not only of ineptitude, but also of crass ignorance, as well as of plagiarism. He blasted the "famous doctor" and "pompous Electro-Therapist" as being accustomed to stalk "clumsily along on borrowed stilts from which he threatens to tumble down at every moment."

A few years prior to that episode, Morton had defended his arrangement of condenser jars, connected to an influence machine (45) against a similar device,

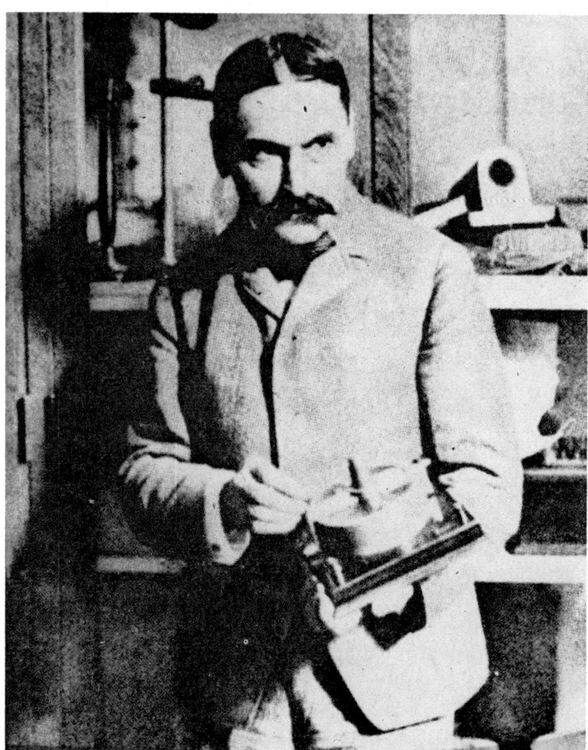

Courtesy: David Shields.

MORTON'S VILLAIN. Michael Idvorsky Pupin (1858-1935) may have acted "evil" toward Morton, but otherwise Pupin was a true research physicist, who inspired many famous pupils, including Robert Millikan. Besides, Pupin himself is remembered as the first user of intensifying screens.

(re-) discovered by Ambrose Loomis Ranney (1848-1905).[26]

The use of giant influence machines for the production of roentgen rays was quite common in the beginning[27] and soon the matter reached competitive commercial levels, permitted by the absence of patents. Thus the Van Houten & Ten Broeck Company (300 Fourth Avenue, New York City) marketed the Morton-Wimshurst-Holtz influence machine (with a Monell static tube), while the Waite & Bartlett Mfg. Co. (108 East 23rd St., New York City) brought out the Ranney-Wimshurst-Holtz generator, as can be seen from advertisements in the 1899 issues of the *American X-Ray Journal.*

Morton was also tackled by his electro-therapeutic predecessor (at Post-Graduate), Alphonso David Rockwell (1840-1925), of whom he disposed fairly easy (72, 73). Indeed, to prevent any further arguments, Morton requested the appointment of a special committee of the American Electro-therapeutic Association. Such a committee was actually appointed — on September 27, 1900 — and it recognized (178) "officially" Morton's paternity over his static currents.

THE EARLIEST AMERICAN "X-RAY SPECIALIST"

In the first months of 1896, the mature Morton was at the height of his career; he had both the "electrical know-how" and the desire to become an expert at "picturing the invisible" (53).

Morton demonstrated the presence of a needle in a foot: the foreign body was then removed by (a former heavy-weight boxer, and subsequent urologist) the surgeon Ramon Benjamin Guitéras (1859-1917), and duly reported (58). Morton published the plate of his own hand, including the shadowgraph of a ring (60). For the pediatrician Henry Dwight Chapin (1857-1942), Morton produced the "roentgen picture" of the whole body of a nine-week old infant, after it had succumbed to dehydration (61).

By the end of April, 1896 Morton had become so well know in this new field, that Thomas Commerford Martin (1856-1924) selected him as the only physician (162) in a Symposium on X-Rays: the panel included, among others, the "electrician" Elihu

[26] A new form of a statical converter for medical use. *J. of Electrotherapeutics, 12*:146-150 (July) 1894.

[27] *Cf.,* illustration of such an arrangement *in* Walther, K.: Der erste Roentgenpionier in Schottland, John Macintyre (1857-1928). *Roentgen u. Laboratoriumpraxis, 11*: 1958.

Thomson (1853-1937), the Canadian physicist John Cunningham McLennan (1867-1935), and the inventor-foreman Thomas Alva Edison (1847-1931).

Morton's elegant offices – located since 1891 at 19 East 28th Street – still contained the huge influence machine, but he now preferred to use the induction coil for the production of roentgen rays.

From that period dates the herein reproduced letter sent by Morton to a New York general practitioner, Leopold Stieglitz (1867-1956).[28] Its text, previously printed,[29] conveys an outdated philosophy which, however obsolete, is still encountered, here and there. It denotes insecurity, and is thus "dangerous."

[28]His twin, Julius Oscar Stieglitz (1867-1937) was professor of chemistry in the University of Chicago, while another brother was the famous photographer Alfred Stieglitz (1864-1946).

[29]LeWald, L. T.: X-ray discovery excites New York. *The Academy Bookman 5* (nr. 3):1-13 (Fall) 1952.

CONTRIBUTIONS TO ROENTGEN DIAGNOSIS

During 1896, Morton published a dozen articles about roentgen rays. He was the first to suggest a workable method for making roentgen plates of the teeth (63). At the beginning of July, 1896 he summarized the existing status of medical applications of roentgen rays: that particular paper (64) contained the footnote:

"Photographic prints of my negatives, now a fairly large collection, may be obtained of Mr. E. B. Meyrowitz, 104 East 23rd St. A descriptive catalog will be furnished upon application to him."

While the publicity angle, included in this statement, is not even concealed, one must also admit that there was—at that time—a real need for making such a collection available to medical practitioners. In the early days, diagnostic problems were often solved by comparing the roentgen plate under consideration with plates from the interpreter's collection. Under

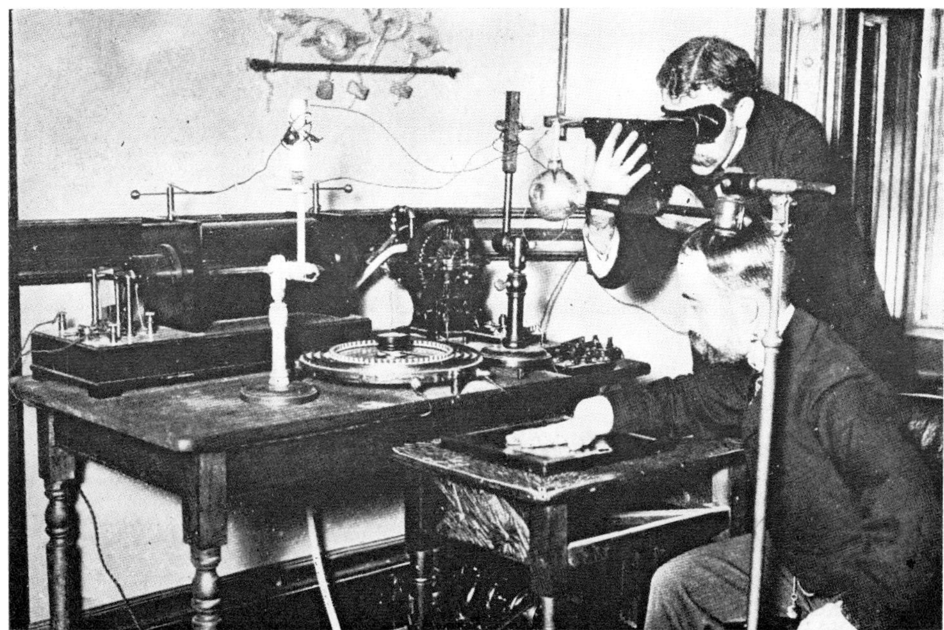

Courtesy: National Library of Medicine.

Morton the radiologist. Morton soon abandoned the static machine, and began using the induction coil, shown with its "break wheel", and the four spare gas tubes on the rack. With the exposure in progress, Morton is checking the operating tube for hardness by looking at his hand through an Edison cryptoscope. Many serious injuries were caused in this way, yet Morton never suffered any ill effects, perhaps because he did not stay very long in the exclusively diagnostic field. He complained, though, of unusual ocular symptoms, said to have appeared after prolonged gazing at "roentgen-fluorescent substances" (radium), but this was – in Percy Brown's opinion – simple retinal irritation.

such circumstances, the larger the collection, the wiser the diagnostician.

Before the end of 1896, Morton published—together with the electrical engineer, Edwin Wesley Hammer (1867-1951 — a tract on *The X Ray* (65).

Hammer had an even more interesting Stepbrother, William Joseph Hammer (1858-1934), who served a few commercial tours of duty abroad, with the English Edison Company (1881) and the German Edison Company (1883). In 1890, he resigned from the Edison Company, and became a free-lance consulting engineer in New York City. Among his many inventions are a luminous preparation of radium for watch dials, and various types of motor-driven flashing electric signs. He was allegedly the first to suggest and apply radium therapy in malignancies (perhaps with Robert Abbe). Incidentally, Hammer assembled a fine collection of photographs of pioneer airplanes and aviators.

Among other innovations, their book contains the first combined photograph-roentgenogram. It also carried two advertising pages, which reveal that the distribution of Morton's *prints* had been passed along to another company.

The following year, Morton established another first, the roentgenogram of the entire body of a healthy, thirty-year old woman, with the shoes on,

OFFICE
DR. WILLIAM JAMES MORTON,
NO. 19 EAST 28TH STREET,
CONSULTATION HOURS, 10-1.

NEW YORK CITY, June 10th 1896

Dear Doctor Stieglitz.
In regard to a proper charge to make to your patient. I find it difficult to decide and I am most willing to be guided to a great extent by you.
My usual charge to radiograph through the entire body is $100. But like all physicians services a negative result is harder to charge for than an affirmative one. If we had found the stone in the kidney it would have been worth that money. but we didn't. I think therefore it will be fair to say $75.

Courtesy: New York Academy of Medicine.

MORTON'S AUTOGRAPH. This letter, dated June 10, 1896, reads: "Dear Doctor Stieglitz: In regard to the proper charges to make to your patient, I find it difficult to decide and I am most willing to be guided to a great extent by you. My usual charge to radiograph through the entire body is $100. But like all physicians' services a negative result is harder to charge for than an affirmative one. If we had found the stone in the kidney it would have been worth that money, but we didn't. I think therefore it will be fair to say $75." Such a reasoning, if applied today in orthopedics and other surgical specialties, is tantamount to inviting malpractice suits.

but without corset. The technique used is given herein in Morton's own words:

"The apparatus employed was that with which I have worked from the first (except when using a static machine), namely a 12-inch induction coil whose primary was supplied from the 117-volt Edison current of the street mains and "made" and "broken" by means of a break wheel causing about 5,000 breaks per minute. Both condenser and blower were employed to keep down the spark on the break wheel. At 5,000 RPM of the break wheel, the coil discharged sparks across a five-inch air gap. A focus x-ray tube was used; its vacuum at the start corresponded to a spark of two inches, and gradually rose until at the end it was eight inches. The platinum anode was run at continuous red-heat. The distance of the tube from the sensitive film was 4 feet and 6 inches. The tube was run the first ten minutes steadily; then the current was turned off several times during a minute to allow it to cool. The total time consumed, including stoppages to take the picture, was thirty minutes.

THE X RAY

OR

PHOTOGRAPHY OF THE INVISIBLE

AND

ITS VALUE IN SURGERY

BY

WILLIAM J. MORTON, M.D.

Professor of Diseases of the Mind and Nervous System and Electro-Therapeutics in the New York Post Graduate Medical School and Hospital; Member of the Medical Society of the County of New York: Permanent member of the Medical Society of the State of New York; of the New York Academy of Medicine; American Electro-Therapeutic Association; American Neurological Association, Harvard Medical Society of New York City; American Medical Association; Societe Francaise d'Electro-Therapie; New York Electrical Society, Etc., Etc.

WRITTEN IN COLLABORATION WITH

EDWIN W. HAMMER

Electrical Engineer

NEW YORK

AMERICAN TECHNICAL BOOK CO.

45 VESEY STREET,

1896

A sensitive film 6 feet long by 3 feet wide, furnished by the Eastman Film Company of Rochester, New York, was employed. Its development by the Eastman Company was procured by the firm of E. B. Meyrowitz, of this city, who also rendered other aid in regard to the preliminary mounting of the film" (66).

These details were included not only for their obvious historic interest, but also because someone might possibly want to compute the total body dose to which the subject was raised in the process. History did not record, however, whether she experienced any ill effects from this radiation exposure.

In his original paper, Morton expressed the hope that "Roentgen pictures of the entire adult skeleton at one exposure (might soon) become a part of the ordinary curriculum of x-ray work in our hospitals" a suggestion which—for obvious reasons—has never been widely followed. Even so, this remarkable stunt won him a substantial measure of international fame —as the "picture" was exhibited at the inaugural meeting of the British Roentgen Society.[30]

CONTRIBUTIONS TO RADIATION THERAPY

About 1898, Morton's acute interest in roentgen diagnosis was waning, and he returned to his old passion, the electrostatic current, for which he found as "incendiary" utilizations as in sexual impotence and uterine fibroids (70). His pronouncements might not have appeared acceptable to the chairman of a puritanic ethical practice committee; for instance, in one of his papers, Morton concluded that "the pain of neuritis is temporarily relieved from the first (electrostatic) treatment, and the case it totally cured in a minimum of time (69)."

Soon Morton "discovered" that the unseen radiance offered an even vaster therapeutic territory, easier to explore (and exploit) because of the general lack of knowledge in the matter. This allowed him to go in print with sweeping statements such as:

"What is accomplished by the x-ray? 1. Relief from excruciating pain and constant suffering, often immediately. 2. Reduction in the size of the growth . . ."(77).

He published also papers with photographs, taken "before" and "after" treatment (79, 82, 89)—and yet, when Morton wanted, he could be very scientific. Some of the words he spoke before the Harvard

---

[30]Thompson, S. P.: Presidential address. *Arch Roentgen Ray, 2*:23-30 (November 5) 1897.

Medical Society, on January 7, 1905, have remained valid to this day:

"1. Radiation treatment exerts a retarding effect upon the growth of some cancers. 2. It cures some cases — the ratio to operative measures is not here discussed. 3. Preoperative radiation will increase the ratio of cures by operation. 4. Preoperative radiation transforms some cases into operable ones (89)."

After the turn of the century, Morton pursued several interesting projects, such as that related to *artificial fluorescence.*

In his preliminary announcement (81) of 1903, subsequently amplified (83), translated in foreign tongues (85), as well as published in British journals (94), Morton theorized that (a) the natural (spontaneous) fluorescence of the tissues and fluids of the body is modified (decreased?) under pathologic circumstances (*i.e.*, disease!): since (b) radium and/or roentgen rays were known to cause artificial fluorescence, he assumed that in favorable therapeutic situations, radium (or roentgen) therapy merely restores the level of natural fluorescence. As a corollary, Morton wanted (c) to use it not only as a diagnostic method, but also as a treatment procedure: he would "flood the entire living organism with a fluorescible solution (quinine, aesculin, fluorescein, eosin, orcin)" (86) and then irradiate, hoping thus to potentiate the overall effect.

Despite valiant promotion, the "fluorescible" method never really caught on. In the interim, though, Morton had begun to generate another "miraculous" therapeutic tool, the radioactive water (92).

Radon suspended in water was said to be "good for both cancer and tuberculosis" which, inevitably, drew

LIST OF RADIOGRAPHS.

ALL LIFE SIZE, HANDSOMELY MOUNTED.

Negatives by Prof. William J. Morton, M. D., New York.

Dr. Morton's collection of X-Ray pictures is without doubt the largest and finest in this country. It covers a great variety of subjects, especially those relating to surgical diseases, injuries, and malformation of the bones. His work is characterized by its great accuracy in definition, and many of his pictures taken months ago have not yet been equalled. He has particularly excelled in large work like the pictures of the trunk, etc. His pictures, many of which are here enumerated, are constantly being added to by unique cases brought to him by physicians for X-Ray diagnosis. The value of the X-Ray to the surgeons is scarcely yet appreciated.

Infant Nine Weeks Old, Life Size.—Showing with beautiful detail the bones of the skeleton, the stage of ossification, the location of the liver, stomach, heart, etc. $2.00

Adult Trunk, Life Size, From Chin to Pelvis.—Showing vertebrae, the shoulder joints, the ribs, the bones of the arm and elbow joint, the lung cavities, the heart 2.00

Adult Trunk, Life Size, Tubercular Disease of Head of Humerus.—Showing a normal and diseased shoulder joint in contrast with each other Otherwise same as above. The finest picture of the trunk thus far produced 2.00

Adult Trunk and One Shoulder Joint 1.00

Adult Head, Side View, Showing Skull and Cervical Vertebrae with Spineus Processes .... .60

Adult Head, Side View .... .60

Portion of Skull, Showing Roots of Teeth .... .60

Adult Neck, Shoulder and Chest, Showing Location of a Bullet in the Chest and Behind the Sternum 1.00

Abdominal Cavity in Region of Kidneys.—Showing negatively the absence of calculus in the kidney. Patient lying face downward, so that vertebrae and hip bones showed but obscurely .... .60

Abdominal Cavity and Lumbar Spine.—A case of suspected Potts disease in an adult .... .60

Adult Female Pelvis.—Showing Lumbar vertebrae, hip and thigh bones. Exposure 5 minutes .... .50

Pair of Large Adult Knees.—Medico-legal case. Trolley car accident: undetected fracture and osseous growth on head of tibia. Showing value of the X-Ray and of comparing in the same picture the injured and the normal bones .... .75

Knee Joint, Child Aged 12.—Showing skin, muscles, tendon of patella and bones. Case of partial anchylosis revealing that it was fibrous rather than osseous. A beautiful radiograph .... .60

Adult Ankle Joint.—Showing old un-united fracture of the internal malleolus separation of tibia and fibula. Distortion of astragalus, bone and adhesions. Upon seeing this picture, the surgeon exclaimed, "This is a wonderful revelation; my entire plan of operation must be changed. I could not have known that the bone had failed to unite." .... .75

Adult Elbow Joint.—Old fracture, one year standing; fracture of lower end of humerus and union in malposition. Anchylosis and osseous adhesion between radius and ulna. Three minutes exposure .... .60

Normal Adult Foot in Shoe.—Showing leather of shoe, nails and metal shank, flesh, tendons, and the bones of the leg and ankle, the tarsal bones and the phalanges; in short the entire osseous structure. Exposure 5 minutes. .75

Child's Ankle.—Anchylosis and active disease of the bone .... .50

Adult Foot.—With needle in it; foreshortened, top view .... .60

Adult Foot, Same Patient.—Side view showing the needle in length, operated upon with immediate success by aid of picture .... .60

Adult Foot.—Female, normal, view from sole of foot .... .60

Adult Forearm.—Blacksmith, showing location of two pieces of steel .... .60

LIST OF RADIOGRAPHS.—Continued.

Adult Forearm and Hand.—Showing an un-united fracture of the radius. Taken while within half-inch board splints and bandages, the pins shown fastened the dressings of the splint .... .75

Elbow Joint of Child.—Anchylosis, the result of fracture and dislocation showing bands of osseous tissue. A very clear and instructive picture .... .60

Elbow Joint of Child.—Right and left, restricted motion. Picture shows it was probably due to fracture .... .50

Normal Adult Wrist and Hand.—A perfect radiograph, showing wrist joint, carpus, metacarpus and phalanges in perfect detail while still preserving throughout a ghost-like and *even* representation of the flesh .... .60

Positive of the Same. Bones show White .... .60

Two Wrists and Hands on One Plate, Adult, Female.—Comparative method. Colles's fracture, one year's standing. Thought to be dislocation. Impaction of both radius and ulna. This picture is a revelation to surgeons. The injured may be inspected in contrast with the normal bones ... .75

Two Wrists and Hands on One Plate.—Tubercular disease of phalanges of left hand. Dr. White's case taken before the Medico Society .... .75

Two Wrists and Hands on One Plate.—Chronic Rheumatism of one year's standing of left wrist, distortion of carpal bones .... .60

Hand, Adult, Female.—With needle in it. Taken at a meeting of the County Medical Society, April, 1896. Needle shows with great clearness. Operation unsuccessful before picture; by its aid immediately successful .... .60

Wrist and Hand, Adult, Female.—With diamond ring. Showing the easy penetrability of the diamond by the X-Ray .... .60

Wrist and Hand, Adult, Female.—With bracelet and ring. Two seconds exposure .... .60

Hand, Adult.—Showing location of bullet unsuccessfully probed for .... .60

Child's Hand.—Webbed fingers, prior to operation, juncture of bones. Congenital deformity .... .60

Child's Hand.—Y-shaped metacarpal bone, webbed fingers. Operation. Congenital deformity .... .60

Wrist and Hand, Adult, Normal.—A piece of Fluorescent screen has been laid upon a portion only of the plate, shows comparatively the effect of the Tungstate of Calcium screen in taking X-Ray pictures 50

Metallic Objects in a Box.—An early picture, taken with Static Machine .. 50

Handwriting of a Will Within a Sealed Envelope.—Showing the possibility of reading the contents of sealed documents 50

Large Flounder.—Showing the bones of the fish and smaller shell fish in the stomach. Makes a beautiful lantern slide in which by varying the focussing distance of the stereopticon lens, different planes of osseous structure are revealed 75

Trout, Showing Bones 50

Normal Kidney and Kidney containing Calculus on Same Plate, Showing Density of Calculi 50

Two Kidneys Containing Uric Acid Calculi upon Same Plate Showing Calculi 50

Calculi of Kidneys and Bullets, Etc., on Same Plate, Showing Calculi to be Relatively about Equally Obstructive to the X-Ray 50

Living Kidney, Partially Exposed in an Operation for Calculus of this Organ by Dr. Willy Meyer, and X-Rayed by Dr. Morton.—X-Ray showed absence of a Calculus which was verified by incision by the operator. Patient fully recovered 50

Foreign Body in Scrotum 60

Human Teeth in Situ.—Showing the roots and fillings. Also the pulp chambers and location of disease at the roots and in the bone, exostoses, etc. 50

An Unsuspected Canine Tooth in an Adult which had never Erupted.—Demonstrating the value of the X-Ray in dentistry 50

Any of the above will be sent on receipt of price and 5c. each for postage by

AMERICAN TECHNICAL BOOK CO.,
45 VESEY STREET, NEW YORK.

Courtesy: John Crerar Library.

MORTON'S ADVERTISEMENTS. These appeared in his first x-ray tract (65). At that time the teaching value of his plates was beyond any question. And such selling of plates was in common use, for instance Walther Petersen's orthopedic x-ray prints were for sale by the publishing house of Renger in Leipzig (*cf.*, the article by Helferich in *Fortschritte der Medicin* of April 1, 1896).

objections, as from the Philadelphia psycho-electrologist and onco-roentgenologist George Betton Massey (1856-1927); to the criticism, Morton replied very caustically: "In regard to Dr. Massey's remarks, they are not exactly justified – that these emanations are intangible, implying by that, that they might not be of value, I may say that, of course, they are not as tangible as a case of hobnails, but quite as tangible as burns from the sun, or arc light or any kind of heat, tangibility meaning sensibility of touch. But any such sensibility is not a necessity for the cure of disease as I take it (92)."[31]

The Edinburgh embryologist John Beard (1858-1924) preconized enzymatic oncotherapy,[32] and this seemed so promising that Morton went all out, and in 1906 reported that he had obtained satisfactory results by treating cancer with trypsin (97, 98). This important "literary" contribution was immediately translated into German by Emil Ekstein, a gynecologist from Teplitz i. B. (which is today part of Czechoslovakia). As published in the *Prager medizinische Wochenschrift,* the translation had acquired a significant postscript:

"Through Prof. Morton's courtesy, Dr. Ekstein has received a large amount of Trypsin, with which he (Ekstein) has started to treat some patients (97)." Was that the pre-arranged translator's fee?

The validity of Morton's observations (in general) is open to question when discovering how blatantly he had misrepresented one of the breast cancer cases, treated with trypsin.[33] And yet, while the enzyme story was slowly fading away, on October 13, 1907, Morton delivered a memorable, and very well received, therapy lecture before the 2nd International Congress on Physiotherapy, meeting in Rome (Italy).

In his later years, the treatment of cancer was more and more often on his mind. In 1912, he issued a rehash of the "artificial fluorescence" idea:

"May it not be possible to administer to the patient by the mouth separate drugs at separate times, counting upon their curative reaction within the cancer cell itself by chemical combination made within the body instead of outside of it?" (105) In practice he meant by this the ingestion of one of several dyes, followed by radium and/or roentgen therapy. Can it be regarded as a premonition of modern activation of boron?

This paper (105) caused a sensationalistic outburst in the daily press, to the point where Morton had to "disclaim having a ready cure for cancer (106)." At that time Morton, his proud demeanor notwithstanding, was already in deep personal trouble, inexorably involved in a "down-draft."

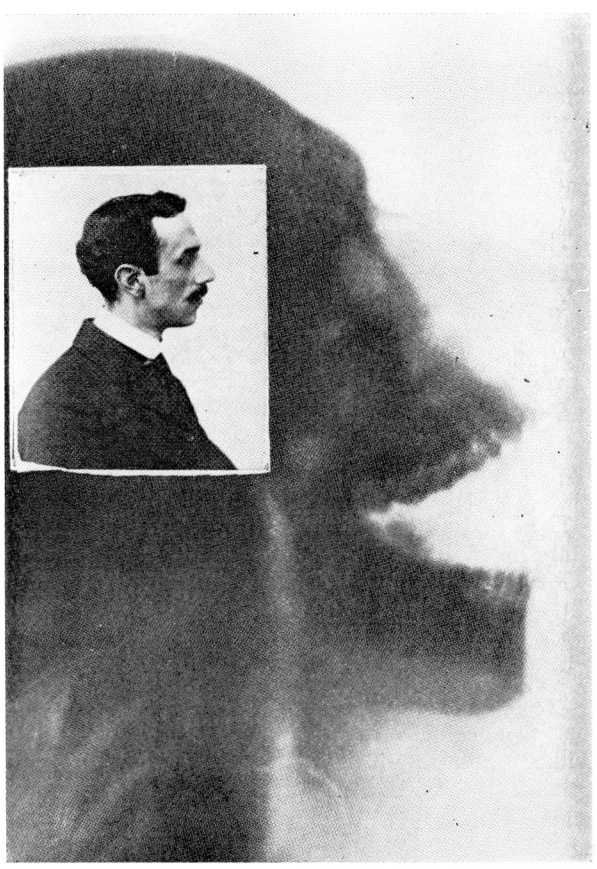

Courtesy: John Crerar Library.

MORTON'S FIRST PHOTO-ROENTGEN-MONTAGE. Very many "firsts" appeared in 1896: this was an illustration in Morton's x-ray primer (65).

---

[31]The ingestion of radon is always senseless and may be dangerous (depending on dosage). Surprisingly enough, *Trink-Kur* with emanation is still mentioned by two Austrian authors in a recent German textbook, as if the procedure were in current usage, *cf.*, Tappeiner, J., and Wodniansky, P.: Radium, pp. 149-165 in *Dermatologie und Venerologie* (Eds.: H. A. Gottron & W. Schoenfeld), Vol. 2, part 1. Stuttgart, Georg Thieme, 1958, p. 156.

[32]Later, Beard assembled all his papers under one cover: *The Enzyme Treatment of Cancer and its Scientific Basis.* London, Chatto & Windus, 1911, pp. 290.

[33]Edward Wright Peet (1862-1943), of New York, wrote a strongly worded Letter to the Editor: Trypsin for the cure of cancer. *Med. Record, 71*:69 (January 12) 1907, contending that one of the patients, reported as improved, had actually worsened. Morton's answer (98) carried the patient's own letter, stating she feels better, and declaring to be no longer under Peet's care, as if that had anything to do with (objective) improvement or worsening. Evidently, patients — especially those called "hopeless" — *want* to believe!

THE DEBACLE

Surprisingly, it all started with a strong, spirited, and seemingly successful scheme of soliciting subscriptions for a seething stock, supported somewhat strenuously by secret subterraneous spadings. Soon, slates of simpletons (usually stingy, but seeking speedy silver) were serenely separated from their savings. Suddenly, the stock-exchange stepped in to stop the sale of such spurious securities. So many had been slighted, so much specie had switched sides, and this stupendous scandal had spread so scathingly, that society sought to soothe its stirred subjects, not simply by sconcing somebody, but by slapping a stiff sentence, shackling one or, better still, several scapegoat(s).

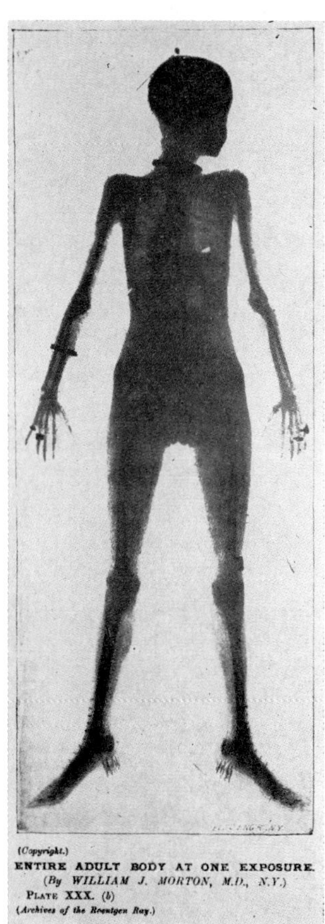

(Copyright.)
ENTIRE ADULT BODY AT ONE EXPOSURE.
(By WILLIAM J. MORTON, M.D., N.Y.)
PLATE XXX. (b)
(Archives of the Roentgen Ray.)

Courtesy: University of Illinois, Chicago.

MORTON'S FULL-BODY FEAT. "The subject was a woman, thirty years of age, five feet four inches in height and weighing 120 pounds. She was in perfect health, well developed and muscular, particularly about the hips. . . In making the attempt I (Morton) had hoped to be able to use two or more tubes at the same time, but . . . each tube occasioned independent pictures, whose outlines did not coincide, and (it was impossible) keeping two tubes . . . whether in series, or in parallel . . . up to an equal degree of work. . . The resulting negative would have been better if longer exposure had ben given, particularly about the region of the hips, but . . . this region . . . is extremely difficult to portray under the best of circumstances" (66). Eastman Kodak could have used this full body exposure for publicity purposes: this is why in the 1930's and 1940's Arthur Wolfram Fuchs searched for a better copy, but none could be located.

Among Morton's personal friends was Julian Hawthorne (1846-1934), son of the famous novelist. Hawthorne, Jr. matriculated in Lawrence College (Harvard), and later at Dresda (Germany), but never graduated. He was for some time a civil (hydrographic) engineer, and then became a successful writer.

An enterprising New York promoter, Albert Freeman, induced Hawthorne to participate in the organization of four companies, created to operate (worthless) mining properties in the Canadian Cobalt region. These four companies merged into the *Hawthorne Iron & Silver Mines Company,* which floated considerable stock.

Hawthorne himself prepared the advertising copy, and his friend Morton was placed on the Board of Directors. Another scion of Hub aristocracy (the great-grandson of a famous revolutionary leader) and former Harvard graduate, the lawyer Josiah Quincy (1859-1919) former mayor of Boston, member of the Massachusetts House of Representatives, and one time Assistant (U. S.) Secretary of State – acted as counsel for Hawthorne's and Freeman's organization.

The advertising claims, leaflets circulated by mail, were grossly exaggerated, but investors subscribed over $3½ million.

When the affair came into the open, the Federal Government indicted Freeman, Hawthorne, Morton, and Quincy, charged them with use of the mails in aid of a scheme to defraud, and brought them to trial before a federal jury in U. S. Court in Manhattan.

The proceedings opened on November 28, 1912. A total of 106 witnesses gave testimony during six weeks, at a cost to the Government of over $50,000.[34] Then Judge Charles Merrill Hough (1858-1927) took ill, and the case was assigned to Judge Julius Marschuetz Mayer (1865-1925). The Assistant District Attorney Henry Alexander Wise (born 1874) provoked the court's objections through vehemence and use of epithets such as "bunko steerers," and "green goods men." He also said that Freeman's "trained seals" (Morton and Quincy) had been sent to Maine to incorporate the "company." Wise emphasized that most of the

---

[34]Hawthorne defense opens. *New York Times,* January 8, 1913, 3:5.

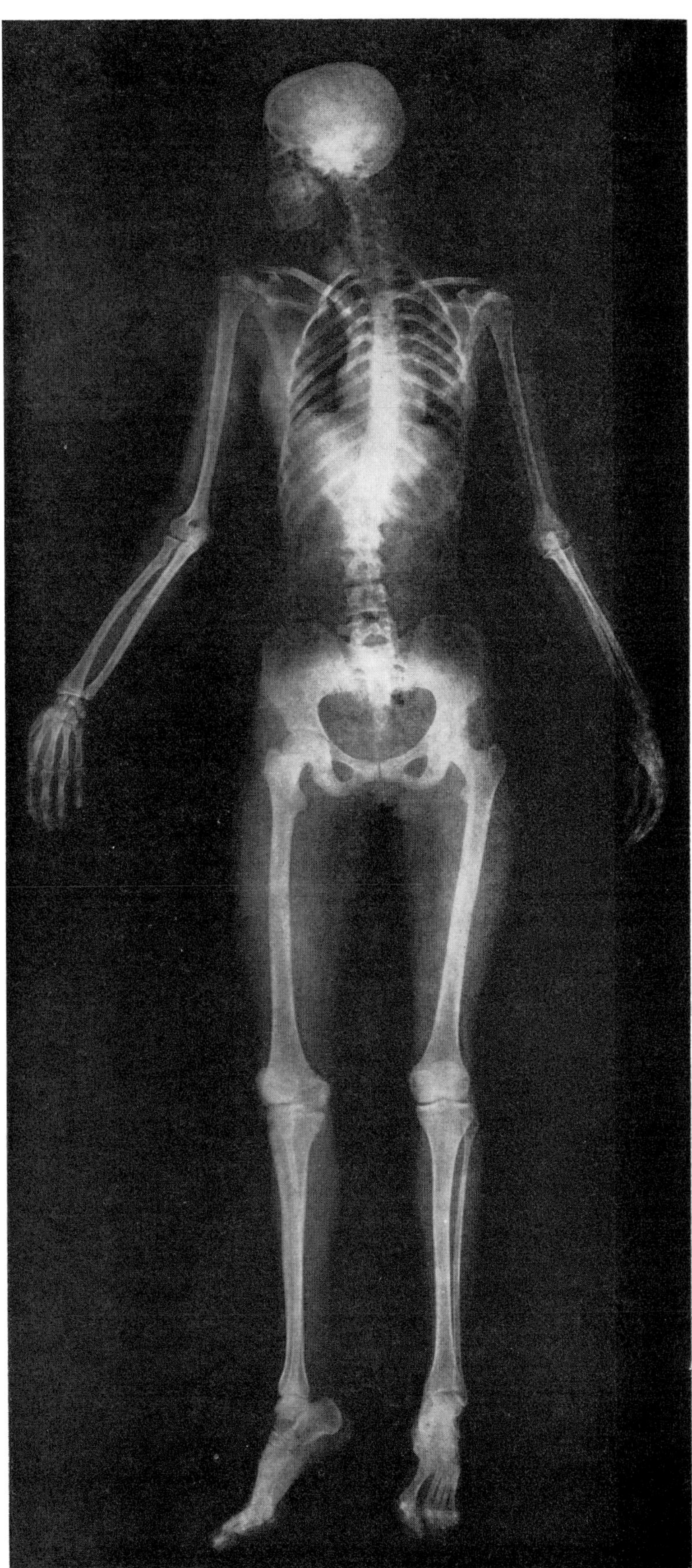

Courtesy: *Robert Janker*

MODERN FULL-BODY ROENTGENOGRAM. This is from the collection of Robert Janker of Bonn (Germany), the radiologist known as one of the creators of photofluorography and indirect roentgen-cinematography. At one time it was thought that full-body radiographs might be of use in the rapid evaluation of the extent of systemic bone involvement, but the technique for that had never been satisfactorily worked out.

embezzled were white collar people from relatively low income groups, and demanded severe punishment.[35]

The jury deliberated twenty eight hours, then acquitted Quincy,[36] but found both Hawthorne and Morton guilty on seventeen counts each: they were sentenced to one year and one day in prison. Freeman, found guilty on twenty three counts, was sentenced to five years in prison.[37] Hawthorne and Morton agreed to waive their right to appeal, in exchange for the promise they will stay only one day in prison, long enough to be given a parole. Indeed, they were smiling as they boarded the train for the Atlanta penitentiary.[38]

With the twosome safely bagged behind prison bars, the U. S. Attorney General, James Clark McReynolds (1862-1946), dug out an old regulation, whereby granting of parole was prohibited before at least one-third of the sentence had been served. In prison, Hawthorne became the editor of the prison's newspaper, and Morton was assigned to the office. They served six months and a few days, and came out sputtering: they would accept no pardon, only apologies, and they also demanded prison reforms.[39]

That was no more than idle talk. Hawthorne's rights were not restored. He moved to California, married (his secretary), and returned to his career as a very successful writer.

RESURRECTION

Conversely, medical and other responsible organizations intervened in Morton's behalf, and on December 16, 1913 he was granted pardon by President Wilson. It restored his civil rights, but more was needed before he could return to medical practice.

Morton's main, if not only, guilt was that of having been a dupe. Valiant efforts were made by his brilliant attorneys, the famous lawyer and diplomat Joseph Hodges Choate (1832-1917), and his son, J. H. Choate, Jr. The latter pointed out on December, 1913 in a pamphlet addressed to the members of the New York Legislature, that Morton had been convicted on the theory (not well understood before his time) that every man who has an important connection with any enterprise is responsible for its conduct, whether the offenses committed are or are not morally due to his own personal action or neglect.

Additional details are herein given from a personal letter written by Choate, Jr.:

"I (Choate, Jr.) have always been convinced of his (Morton's) innocence and that his conviction was as gross a miscarriage of justice as ever happened. How a jury could believe that a man of his professional reputation (and income) could knowingly have taken part in the fraud I never could understand. Probably, after four months of trial, in all of which the D. A. incessantly insisted that "they" (meaning all four defendants) did everything that was done by any of them, the jurors found themselves unable to distinguish one from the other.

"The trial judge (Mayer) shared my belief. Before sentencing the convicted men he called up the attorneys for Morton and Hawthorne, and stated plainly that he thought no punishment was called for. He suggested that if we would not appeal, he would sentence them to a year and a day, dating from the beginning of the trial, which would make them eligible for parole at once. He added that both he and the D.A. would recommend the parole and that he had never known such a recommendation to fail. In view of the colossal effort and cost of even a successful appeal, and new trial, this proposition was agreed to by Dr. Morton.

"Unluckily McReynolds, then U. S. Attorney-General, had been under heavy newspaper attack for approving parole of convicts in a most conspicuous case, and he frankly told me he had had all he could take and would approve no application for parole at that time.

"To complete the miscarriage of justice, Quincy (clearly as guilty as his client Freeman) was acquitted after the jury (standing 10 to 2 against him) became convinced that the two (jurors) would never yield. This turnabout occurred because they (the 2 jurors) mistakenly supposed that to acquit one of the alleged conspirators would spoil the verdict against the rest and nullify the whole long trial."[40]

Yielding to public pressure, the New York Legislature passed a special act, signed into law by Governor Martin Henry Glynn (1871-1924), which permitted the New York Board of Regents to reinstate Morton as a practicing physician.[41] On that occasion St. Clair

---

[35]Wise flays Hawthorne. *New York Times,* March 13, 1913, 3:5.

[36]He was in 1917 the Democratic candidate for Attorney General of Massachusetts.

[37]Convict three men in Hawthorne case. *New York Times,* March 15, 1913, 1:7.

[38]Hawthorne goes to prison. *New York Times,* March 24, 1913, 1:6.

[39]Hawthorne seeks apology. *New York Times,* October 17, 1913, 20:2.

[40]Quoted from a very gracious, personal communication, dated June 24, 1960, written by Mr. Choate, Jr. (born 1876), who is now the senior partner of the New York law firm Choate, Ronald, Reynolds, & Hollister.

[41]Dr. Morton reinstated. *New York Times,* June 26, 1914, 13:6.

McKelway (1845-1915), Chancellor of the University of the State of New York, published an editorial in the *Brooklyn Daily Eagle,*[42] in which he hailed it as a "case which redresses the balance which was (formerly) against justice." It may be of interest to quote a few passages from this editorial:

"One of the defendants, Josiah Quincy . . . a man of distinguished ancestry . . . was acquitted on the same trial in the same court on the ground that he had only been counsel . . . and as counsel was not required to disclose his confidence to any tribunal.

"Dr. Morton has not, so far as has ever been known or charged, been addicted in science to the sensational recourses of Julian Hawthorne in, let us say, 'journalism.'

"The presiding judge, and the officiating D.A. both thought that Dr. Morton could have been acquitted, or could as well have had no sentence imposed upon him, his formal acquittal being difficult in conditions which did not permit his case to be technically differentiated (from the others) . . .; these letters (from Mayer and from the D.A., were) in the hands of the Governor . . . and (when) the Regents did become possessed of them, the Board acquiesced in their conclusions and freely restored Dr. Morton to the avenue of honor and activity which should not, in the opinion of the trial court, ever have been closed to him."

THE FINANCIER

Freeman's fate is reminiscent of the fable in which two mice were trapped in a milk container: one of them gave up, sank, and drowned, while the other kept on kicking until the milk eventually turned to butter, thus providing both firm support, and ample nourishment.

Freeman's counsel consisted of several legal giants – including the very learned Wade Hampton Ellis (1866-1948). Even though at the time of the trial they had given their fully stipulated consent, subsequently they appealed on the ground that Judge Mayer had been substituted for Judge Hough in the middle of the trial. They used deleting tactics; when Freeman was finally granted a new trial, and was again arraigned, they invoked double jeopardy (*i.e.,* being tried twice for the same offense), but this was thrown out.[43]

The case came to trial at a time when public opinion was occupied with World War I. The jury could not agree on a verdict (7 to 5 for conviction), and was dismissed on December 3, 1916. The trial had cost the Government and Freeman upward of $100,000 each. The "weary assailants" made a "deal" whereby the Special Prosecutor Frank Swacker (born 1879) accepted Freeman's plea of guilty, with the proviso that punishment should not be imprisonment.

When sentencing time finally rolled around, Judge Augustus Noble Hand (1869-1948) told Freeman that the latter's case was very aggravated, that it is difficult to understand why the jury had not agreed upon a verdict, but that under these circumstances all he (Hand) could do was to impose a fine of $3,000. Whereupon, notes the court reporter, "Freeman drew a big roll from his pocket, stripped from the roll three $1,000 notes, handed them to the clerk, and walked out"[44] as a free financier.

Indeed, when Freeman died in 1929—in Paris (France), where he had gone from Bad Nauheim (a German spa "for cardiacs")—the *New York Times* made no mention of the mining affair, but when Morton had died, in Miami, on March 26, 1920, of heart disease, the *New York Times* made it a point to dwell upon his prison sentence,[45] and was going to do the same in 1934, at Hawthorne's passing.

AFTERMATH

When Morton returned (after the term in prison) to his practice in the old office at 19 East 28th Street, he was a different man. Advancing age, and a weakened myocardium contributed to slow him down. He published two other articles (107,108), both dealing with radiation therapy, and both very well written, but he had lost his old stamina. Even his style was changed, as if he had made peace with the world.

In the closing years of his life, Morton did not forget his perennial efforts to insure Morton, Sr.'s immortality (*i.e.,* a decent place in medical history). In 1918, he donated to the New York Academy of Medicine a portrait and an autographed letter of W. T. G. Morton.[46] He hoped Morton, Sr. would be elected to the Hall of Fame, but Morton, Jr. did not live long enough to see it happen.

A very few months after W. J. Morton's death, Sigard Adolphus Knopf (1857-1940) requested that W. T. G.

---

[42]Copies of this editorial and of the Choate pamphlet are preserved in the collection of the New York Academy of Medicine; *cf.,* footnote.[21]

[43]Freeman must go on Trial. *New York Times,* October 12, 1916, 11:6.

[44]Freeman pays $3,000 fine. *New York Times,* December 21, 1916, 13:3.

[45]Dr. William J. Morton dead. *New York Times,* April 4, 1920, 22:2. His address was then given at 65 Central Park West, in New York City.

[46]Philip van Ingen: *The New York Academy of Medicine. Its First Hundred Years.* New York, Columbia University Press, 1949, p. 361. Also, *cf.,* footnote.[21]

Morton be given a place in the Hall of Fame on University Heights in New York City.[47] This was decided on November 6, 1920 – and a replica of W. T. G. Morton's bust is therein on permanent display.

That replica is from a sculpture by Helen Farnsworth Mears (1876-1916), of which the original is in the Smithsonian Institution in Washington (D.C.). The sculpture was commissioned by Morton, Jr., and was shown by him to the staff of the Massachusetts General Hospital during a special festivity, on October 16, 1909.[48]

[47]Knopf, S. A.: William T. G. Morton, the discoverer and revealer of anesthesia, and his place in the Hall of Fame. *Med. Record 97*:1086-1087 (June 26) 1920.

[48]Morton commemoration exercises. *Med. Record, 76*:695 (October 23) 1909.

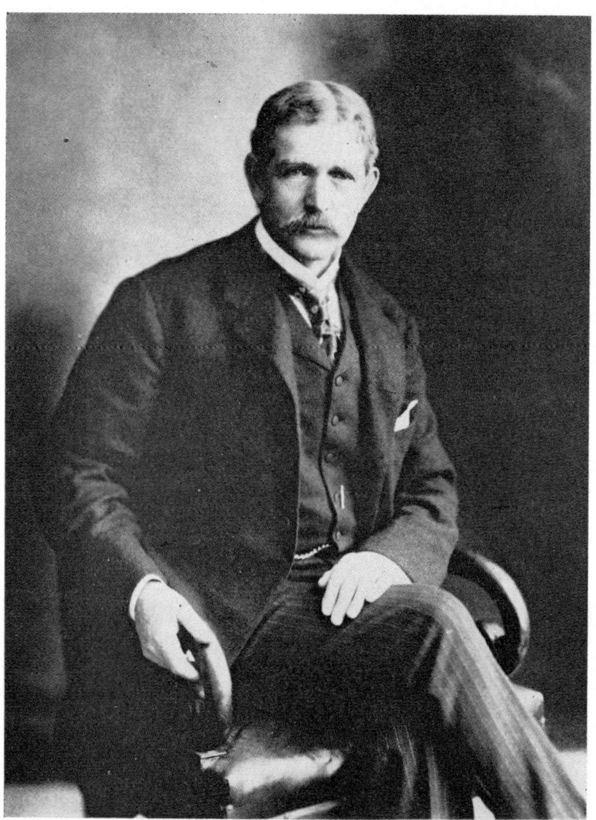

Courtesy: New York Academy of Medicine.

MORTON MATURE. Good physicians (like good wines) keep improving as they approach maturity. Moreover, maturity merely added a few wrinkles to Bill Morton's aristocratic physiognomy. This excellent portrait – executed by Davis & Sanford (246 Fifth Avenue, in New York City) – brings out a pleasant trait about the subject's mouth. Gertrude Annan dates this portrait as being after 1900, perhaps closer to 1910, but certainly prior to the debacle.

The family of Morton, Jr. inherited the latter's concern for Morton, Sr.'s spiritual immortality. In March of 1942, Elizabeth Campbell Morton wrote to the New York Academy of Medicine, requesting help in raising the sum of $942 needed to prevent the leveling of Morton, Sr.'s grave in the Mount Auburn Cemetery in Cambridge, Massachusetts. In 1948, she sold to the same Academy the portrait of Morton, Jr., a huge oil painting made by the same Kenyon Cox (in 1899). That portrait is now on permanent display in one of the Academy's meeting rooms.

Further information on Morton's "widow" was obtained through the gracious investigations made by Gertrude Annan. From 1948 through 1953, Elizabeth Morton lived in the home of a family, and was their son's baby sitter. Ellen Morton died in May, 1953 in Roosevelt Hospital in New York City.

Thereupon I wrote to the record librarian of the Roosevelt Hospital, and my inquiry was referred to her personal physician (Loton H. Rasmussen), who advised that Elizabeth (Ellen) Morton had succumbed with carcinoma of the stomach, which had metastasized to regional lymph nodes, to the liver, and to the peritoneum. His files gave her birth date as 1888, which indicates that she was not Morton's widow (Morton was married in 1880), she was his daughter. From a letter written by the family for whom she had worked, I take the following sentences:

"Ellen Morton had worked for us for five years, coming to us at the birth of our son, in 1948. . . At death, Mrs. Morton left an estate of some $60 thousand in investments, which she wanted to leave to us, but was persuaded to bequest it to her own (Elizabeth Morton's) relatives living in Germany. . . The last five years of her life (the period she was with us) revolved entirely around her love and adoration of my son . . . when she had to leave to go to the hospital, it nearly broke her heart. . . In many ways Mrs. Morton was a fine and unusual person."

FINAL JUDGMENT

What, then, should be William Morton's place in the history of radiology?

He did not expose the first roentgen plate in America, but he made some plates in the first or second week of February, 1896. In the following three months (until April, or May of 1896), the collection of plates accumulated by Arthur Willis Goodspeed (1860-1943) might have been larger than Morton's, but Goodspeed was a physicist.

In this country—from a chronologic viewpoint—the first truly scientific roentgenologist was the physician Francis Henry Williams (1852-1936), but he did not get started in the new field until several weeks after Morton. Besides, at least in the beginning, Williams restricted his roentgenologic endeavors to the Massachusetts Institute of Technology, and then to the Boston City Hospital. On the other hand, Morton was not only the first medical man who accumulated a sizable collection of roentgen plates, but also the first one who devoted a large portion of his private office practice to roentgenology.

A few years later, as the "rays" were adapted for treatment purposes, Morton achieved a similarly pioneering position in roentgen and radium therapy, even though by that time he had lost what initially was a practical monopoly in the diagnostic domain. Quite often, pathfinders are unwilling or unable to explore thoroughly the territory they had entered (there are many exceptions to this rule), which is probably due to their personality make-up.

Turning now to Morton's private life, one must realize that—preachers, poets, and prejudices notwithstanding—actual people are seldom, if ever, either "good" or "bad," but rather a mixture of both these (as well as of several other) ingredients. It is fair to say that Morton, in his skirmish with the Law, was neither a crook, nor a martyr who suffered only because of his friendship for Hawthorne. Basically, Morton had been imprudent, and perhaps gullible. His position is also hard to defend because of the at-

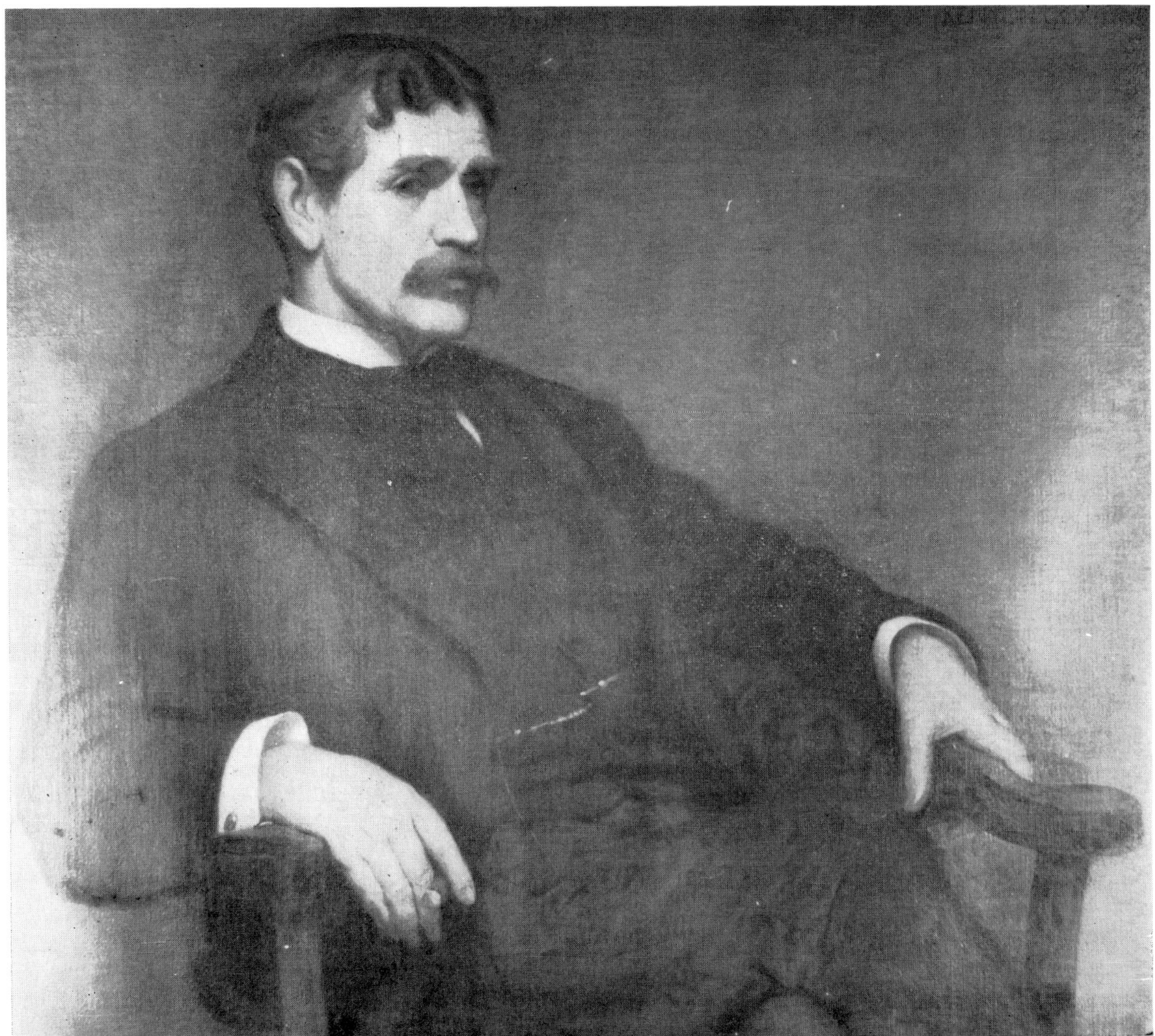

Morton Academicus. This oil painting (by the same Kenyon Cox) graces the walls of the New York Academy of Medicine. It is the way in which I think Morton should be remembered, serene, detached, intelligent, and shrewd, a dignified fellow of the New York Academy of Medicine.

tendant pecuniary motivation. Whatever guilt may be attributed to Morton, derives not so much from having started, as for having continued, the unfortunate association with Freeman's group.

By the testimony of several contemporaries, Morton was an excellent diagnostician. He inspired great confidence because he was above all an accomplished *healer.*[49] In his marginal behavior regarding professional ethics, Morton was neither a rascal, nor a saint, simply because medical mores in his time were more relaxed. Still, his eternal publicity antics, his thinly veiled strive for monetary rewards, and his (shall we say) wishful thinking applied to therapeutic case-reports, cannot be condoned, and will not come out in the (white-)wash, regardless how many euphemisms were to be employed.

One may want to accept or disregard Morton's sketchy scientific achievements. One may choose to be attracted or repulsed by Morton's flamboyant personality, and by his successes as a *healer.* One may wish to excuse or condemn Morton's minor medical, and more serious, extracurricular misdemeanors. But nobody can deny that—having been the first to build up, in succession, a private practice in diagnostic roentgenology, and then in roentgen and radium therapy—he was, beyond any doubt, the first medical radiologist in this country. Of course, as a token of respect for the terminology in use long after the turn of the century, William James Morton should go down in history as the *first American medical electroradiologist.*

But this is not all. Underneath his roguish features, there was more than the contemporaries could grasp. In 1896 Pupin snorted with reference to Morton: "Genius is a wonderful thing; it works unconsciously where we poor mortals have to guide our steps by clear and exact knowledge."[23] This, of course, is not entirely correct, because no matter how much intuition one were to display, it could never function properly, unless there is available a sufficient amount of basic, underlying information. Obviously, Morton had both the information, and a spark of genius, or else he could not have written—in 1915!—the following words which, being the last paragraphs in his last article (108), are tantamount to being his scientific testament. These paragraphs are reproduced in facsimile:

MEDICAL RECORD. [March 6, 1915

11. Comparing the present success of external radiotherapy to the reasonable expectations of internal radiotherapy, the writer is of the opinion that the latter will in time far outstrip the former in successful medical service to the human race.

12. Radiotherapy in its fulfillment and radiochemicotherapy in its embryo are illustrations of the thought that the scoffs of yesterday are the medical practice of to-day, while those of to-day will be the practice of to-morrow.

13. In particular, in this line of work designated by the writer as radiochemicotherapy, it has been his aim to treat cases of cancer by causing a metallic or other radioelement to become "fixed" in the cancer tissue as iodine, for instance, becomes fixed in thyroid tissue and there exert a prolonged and intimate radiation effect, the more effective by reason of being able to utilize the highly ionizing alpha rays.

[49]There have been *healers* since times immemorial. The healing faculty being innate, *healers* are found at all levels of the "health" professions, from the primitive medicine man to the quack, and from midwife to the well trained physician. The only prerequisite for the qualification of *healer* is performance of (real or imaginary) "cures." Oribasius (325-400), Avicenna (980-1037), Boerhaave (1668-1738) are now famous for their intellectual (theoretical) exploits, but in their lifetime, they were renowned only because of the high incidence of "satisfied customers." Even today, very few treatments, are specific (whatever that is), but the lack of an effective therapy seldom interferes with the *healer's* success. While practising radiology, one often finds that the referring physician who controls the largest number of patients is seldom the best-trained, or the most up-to-date. And yet, when the radiologist himself happens to have a personal medical problem, he is prone to discover that (much to his surprise) the concise, unexplained, but eminently practical advice of the *healer* (usually) makes better sense than the elaborate, elusive, and disconcerting suggestions of a "scientific" colleague. There is no ready explanation for these facts. Maybe the *healer's* art consists in finding the most realistic (practical?) approach, with knowledge currently (commonly?) available. A more tantalizing alternative is to admit that the psychologists are correct in assuming a median mental age of the population (scientists and the professions included) equal to that of a fourteen-year-old. William Osler said that "this is yet the childhood of the world, and a supine credulity is still the most charming characteristic of man."

BIBLIOGRAPHY OF WILLIAM JAMES MORTON

1. Anesthetics (in manuscript). Boylston Prize Essay (?), 1872 (*cf.,* footnote[17]).

2. Mount desert and typhoid fever during the summer of 1873. *Boston M. & S. J., 89*:421-426 (October 30) 1873.

3. South African diamond fields, and a journey to the mines. Paper read at the meeting of the American Geographical Society, March 13, 1877. *Bull. Amer. Geogr. Soc., 9*:66-83, 1877. Also in *Bull. Nr., 4*:3-30, 1877. Also issued

as a booklet, New York, Printed for the Society, 1877, pp. 28.

4. "To South Africa for diamonds." *Scribner's Monthly, 16*:551-663 (August); 662-675 (September) 1878.

5. Toxic effects of tea, and other case-reports. *Neurol. Contributions, 1*:79-89, 1879.

6. Anaesthetic inhalation; rival claimants to the discovery. Dr. Long's claim criticised; the priority of Dr. Morton's announcement maintained. *New York Times*, September 8, 1879, *2*:4. Also reprint.

7. Traumatic dislocation of the fifth cervical vertebra; one week's duration; immobility and distortion of head and neck; paralysis of arms and legs; inability to swallow food; reduction by suspension by the head and rotation of the body. *Med. Record, 16*:320-321 (September 27) 1879.

8. Tea drinker's disorder, or toxic effects of tea. *J. Nerv. & Ment. Dis., 6*:586-602 (October) 1879.

9. "The discoverer of anesthesia." The claims made of Dr. Long criticised. *Med. Record, 16*:428-431 (November 1) 1879.

10. Clinical cases reported from the Clinic for Diseases of the Mind and Nervous System of the University Medical College. *Neurol. Contributions, 1* (nr. 2):61-96, 1880.

11. The invention of anaesthetic inhalation or, "Discovery of anaesthesia." *Virginia Med. Monthly, 6*:949-985 (March) 1880. Also reprint (with additions and alterations), New York, D. Appleton & Co., 1880, pp. 48.

12. Hystero-epilepsy: its history, etc. (Letter to the editor). *Med. Record, 18*:246-248 (August 28) 1880.

13. Hystero-epilepsy, or hysteria major (Letter to the editor). *Med. Record, 18*:388-390 (October 2) 1880.

14. Induced hysterical somnambulism and catalepsy. Muscular hyperexcitability — indeed delusions and aphasia — phenomenon of suggestion — universal muscular contracture — method of inducing these conditions (Letter to the editor). *Med. Record, 18*:467-470 (October 23) 1880.

15. The town of Gheel, in Belgium, and its insane; or, occupation and reasonable liberty of lunatics. *J. Nerv. & Ment. Dis., 8*:102-123 (January) 1881. Also — in French translation |La cité de Gheel, en Belgique, etc.) — in *Rev. internat. d. sciences biol.,* (Paris) 7:431-449 (October) 1881.

16. On statical electrotherapeutics, or treatment of disease by Franklinism. Abridgement of paper read before the New York Academy of Medicine on March 3, 1881. *Med. Record, 19*:367-371 (April 2):395-398 (April 9) 1881. Also reprint.

17. Size and kind of Holtz machine adapted to medical uses. *Med. Record, 19*:472 (April 23) 1881.

18. A new current of induction electricity; or, a new method of producing electrical nerve and muscle reaction. *Med. Record, 20*:62-63 (July 9) 1881.

19. A contribution to the subject of nerve-stretching; in 1. lateral sclerosis; 2. paralysis agitans; 3. athetosis; 4. chronic transverse myelitis; 5. sciatica; 6. reflex epilepsy. *J. Nerv. & Ment. Dis., 9*:133-163 (January) 1882. Also reprint.

20. A contribution to nerve-stretching in lateral sclerosis, paralysis agitans, athetosis, chronic transverse myelitis, sciatica, reflex epilepsy. *Med. Record, 21*:240-243 (February 25) 1882.

21. Colony treatment of the insane: a visit to Fitz-James, at Clermont, in France. *J. Nevr. & Ment. Dis., 9*: 343-348 (April) 1882.

22. Preliminary notes of autopsy held upon the body of Charles J. Guiteau. *Med. Record, 22*:53-55 (July 8) 1882 (with C. L. Dana).

23. Microscopical appearance of Guiteau's brain. *Med. Record, 22*:134-135 (July 29) 1882 (with C. L. Dana).

24. Remarks on the treatment of migraine. *Med. News, 42*:744-745 (June 30) 1883.

25. The treatment of migraine. *Med. Gaz., N. Y., 10*: 342-344 (July 7) 1883. Also in *J. Nerv. & Ment. Dis., 10*: 513-516 (July) 1883.

26. A contribution to traumatic neuritis illustrated by a case following dislocation of the humerus. *Med. Gaz., N. Y., 10*:327-329 (July 14) 1883.

27. Neuritis following dislocation. *J. Nerv. & Ment. Dis., 10*:455-461 (July) 1883.

28. Neurological specialism. Presidential address delivered at the annual meeting of the New York Neurological Society on May 1, 1883. *J. Nerv. & Ment. Dis., 10*:618-629 (October) 1883.

29. Jury trial for the insane (editorial). *J. Nerv. & Ment. Dis., 11*:103-104 (January) 1884.

30. Americano-philism in English alienists (editorial). *J. Nerv. & Ment. Dis., 11*:104-105 (January) 1884.

31. Philanthropy vs. science (editorial). *J. Nerv. & Ment. Dis., 11*:288-290 (April) 1884.

32. Half truth on the witness stand (editorial). *J. Nerv. & Ment. Dis., 11*:290-291 (April) 1884.

33. Case of morbid somnolence. *J. Nerv. & Ment. Dis., 11*:615-618 (October) 1884.

34. Card from Dr. Morton. *J. Nerv. & Ment. Dis., 13*: 53 (January) 1886.

35. Suspension treatment of locomotor ataxia and other diseases of the nervous system with remarks and an illustrative case. *Med. Record, 35*:403-406 (April 13) 1889.

36. A flying visit to Mexico (1888), 1889. Quoted in Watson.[2]

37. The place of static or frictional electricity in medicine. *Med. Record, 37*:609-610 (May 31) 1890. With (subsequent) Letter to the editor: Actual work represented by a spark of static electricity. *Ibid., 37*:668 (June 7) 1890.

38. The Franklinic interrupted current or, my new system of therapeutic administration of static electricity. *Med. Record, 39*:97-104 (January 24) 1891.

39. Upon a possible electric polarity of metabolism, and its relations to electro-therapeutics and electro-physiology. A suggested basis and guide for medical treatment by electric energy. *Med. Record, 42*:265-273 (September 3) 1892. Also reprint.

40. The introduction of anaesthesia. *Med. Record, 42*: 719-720 (December 17) 1892.

41. Writer's cramp. *J. Nerv. &Ment. Dis., 10*:503-504 (July) 1893.

42. A brief glance at electricity in medicine. Lecture given before Columbia College on May 17, 1893. *Tr. Am. Inst. Electr. Engineers, 10*:555-602 (November) 1893.

43. Diseases of the Spinal Cord, pp. K-71-132 *in International System of Electro-Therapeutics.* (Ed.: H. R. Bigelow). Philadelphia, F. A. Davis & Co., 1894, pp. 1147. Elso Ed. 2, 1901.

44. Ozone and its uses in medicine. *New York M. J., 59*:779-783 (June 23): 807-819 (June 30) 1894. Also reprint (pp. 58).

45. Note on a "new?" form of static converter for medical use. *Tr. Amer. Electrotherap. Assn., 4*:347-349 (September 27) 1894.

46. Electro-chemical method of staining tissues preparatory to microscopical examination. *Tr. Amer. Electrotherap. Assn., 4*:349-354 (September 27) 1894.

47. Memoranda relating to the "Discovery of anaesthesia." New York, 1895. Four galley sheets (National Library of Medicine, Washington, D. C.).

48. Origin of the term anaesthetic. *Med. Record, 46*: 799-800 (December 22) 1894.

49. Discovery of anaesthesia. *Hartford Times,* April 12, 1895, *8*:1.

50. Electrical medicamental diffusion. Metallic electrolysis, cataphoresis, soluble metallic electrodes, with illustrative cases of tinnitus aurium, trachoma, nasal and post-nasal catarrh, urethritis, tonsillitis, vascular tumor, dermoid cyst, naevi, sycosis, etc. Read before the American Electrotherapeutic Association, meeting at the New York Academy of Medicine on September 26, 1894. *J.A.M.A., 24*:676-682 (May 4) 1895. Also reprint.

51. Electricity in medicine from a modern standpoint. Read before the New York State Medical Society at its 89th Annual Meeting. *New York M. J., 61*:488-492 (April 20): 595-563 (May 4) 1895. Also *Tr. Med. Soc. N. Y.,* Philadelphia, 1895, 245-267. Also reprint.

52. Guaiacol-cocain cataphoresis and local anesthesia. *Dental Cosmos, 38*:48-53 (January) 1896.

53. Photography of the invisible without the aid of a Brookes *(sic)* tube. *Electr. Engineer, 21*:140-141 (February 5) 1896.

54. Roentgen's discovery. *New York World,* February 10, 1896 and February 12, 1896 - quoted in (55).

55. Communication to the editor. *Electricity, 10*:89-90 (February 19) 1896.

56. Cathodographs by the discharge of Leyden jars and other disruptive discharges of static electricity—a new method of producing Roentgen rays. *Electr. Engineer, 21*: 186-187 (February 19) 1896.

57. A Roentgen picture from a medical point of view. *New York M. J., 63*:333 (March 14) 1896.

58. A needle in the foot demonstrated by Roentgen rays. *Med. Record, 49*:371-372 (March 14) 1896 (with R. Guitéras).

58b. May not the x-rays proceed from fluorescence? *Electr. Engineer, 21*:311 (March 25) 1896.

59. The x-ray detection of deformities of bones. *New York M. J., 63*:479-480 (April 11) 1896.

60. A Roentgen picture of the bones of the wrist and hand. *New York M. J., 63*:516 (April 18) 1896.

61. A Roentgen picture of a marasmic infant. *New York M. J., 63*:540-541 (April 25) 1896 (with H. D. Chapin).

62. Photographing the unseen. A symposium on the Roentgen rays. *The Century Magazine, 52*:120-131 (May) 1896 (with T. C. Martin, R. W. Wood, Elihu Thompson, S. P. Thompson, J. C. McLennan, and T. A. Edison).

63. The x-ray and its applications in dentistry. *Dental Cosmos, 38*:476-486 (June) 1896.

64. The x-ray and some of its applications in medicine: demonstrations of apparatus at work and exhibition of stereopticon views. *Med. Record, 50*:9-11 (July 4) 1896.

65. *The X-Ray or Photography of the Invisible and Its Value in Surgery.* New York, American Technical Book Co., 1896, pp. 196 (with E. W. Hammer).

66. X-ray picture of an adult by one exposure. *Electr. Engineer, 23*:522 (May 19) 1897. Also *in Arch. of the Roentgen Ray, 2* (nr. 1):17 (July) 1897.

67. The x-ray picture of the living human head. *Items of Interest, N. Y., 19*:313-315 (July) 1897. Also *in Amer. X-Ray J., 1*:89-91 (October) 1897.

68. *"Cataphoresis" or Electrical Medicamental Diffusion as Applied in Medicine, Surgery, and Dentistry,* New York, American Technical Book Co., 1898, pp. 267.

69. Cases of sciatic and brachial neuritis and neuralgia; treatment and cure by electro-static currents. Cases compiled from records by W. B. Snow. *Med. Record, 55*:521-527 (April 15) 1899. Also reprint (pp. 24). Also—in French translation (Cas de névrites brachiale et sciatique, etc).—*in Rev. internat. d'Électrothér. et de Radiothérapie,* (Paris) *10*:102-114 (February) 1900.

70. Electrostatic currents and the cure of locomotor ataxia, rheumatoid arthritis, neuritis, migraine, incontinence of urine, sexual impotence, and uterine fibroids. *Med. Record, 56*:845-849 (December 9) 1899. Also reprint.

71. "Is static electricity a specific for organic and structural nervous disorders?" (Letter to the editor). *Med. Record, 57*:43-44 (January 6) 1900.

72. The static induced current and Dr. Rockwell (Letter to the editor). *Med. Record, 57*:294-295 (February 17) 1900.

73. The static induced current (Letters to the editor). *Med. Record, 57*:520 (March 24): 746-747 (April 28) 1900.

74. The use of electricity in chronic rheumatism. *Med. Record, 57*:674-676 (April 21) 1900.

75. A case of multiple neuritis with atrophy, fibrillar twitchings, cramps, and exaggerated reflexes: two years duration and recovery. *J. Nerv. & Ment. Dis., 27*:605-608 (November) 1900.

76. The treatment of malignant growths by the x-ray, with a provisional report on cases under treatment. *Med. Record, 61*:361-365 (March 8) 1902. Also reprint.

77. Radiotherapy for cancer and other diseases. *Med. Record, 61*:801-805 (May 24) 1902. Also reprint.

78. Static induced currents. *Arch of the Roentgen Ray, 7*:67 (January) 1903.

79. Primary and recurrent mammary carcinoma treated by the x-ray. *Med. Record, 63*:845-851 (May 30) 1903.

80. The x and violet radiations in the treatment of cancer and other diseases. *Med. Brief, St. Louis, 31*:842-844 (June) 1903.

81. Not on artificial fluorescence of living human tissue. *Electr. World & Engineer, 41*:1058 (June 20) 1903.

82. Some cases treated by the x-ray. Facial cancer, carbuncle, cheloid, acne, alopecia areata, sychosis *(sic.),* fibroid tumor, psoriasis, lupus. *Med. Record, 64*:121-127 (July 25) 1903. Also reprint.

83. Artificial fluorescence of living human tissue. *Med. Record, 64*:215-216 (August 8) 1903.

84. Treatment of cancer by the x-ray, with remarks on

the use of radium. *Internat. J. Surgery, 16*:289-294 (October) 1903.

85. Fluorescence artificielle des tissus vivants. *J. de Physiothérapie,* (Paris) *2*:3-5 (January) 1904.

86. Artificial fluorescence of living tissue in relation to disease. *New York M. J., 79*:300-303 (February 13); 353-356 (February 20) 1904. Also reprint. Also abstracted in *J.A.M.A., 42*:612 (February 27); 677 (March 5) 1904. Also *in Arch. Roentgen Ray, 8*:194-197 (April) 1904.

87. Galvanization. Properties of the galvanic current. *Post-Graduate, N. Y., 20*:35-41 (January) 1905.

88. Local anesthesia by cataphoresis and by mechanical pressure. *Med. News, 86*:495-498 (March 18) 1905.

89. Radiotherapy and surgery, with a plea for preoperative radiations. Read before the Harvard Medical Society, on January 7, 1905. *Med. Record, 67*:443-447 (March 25) 1905. Also reprint.

90. Recent advances in electrotherapeutics. *New York M. J., 81*:634-637 (April 1) 1905.

91. Memoranda relating to the discovery of surgical anesthesia and William T. G. Morton's relation to this event. *Post-Graduate, N. Y., 20*:333-353 (April) 1905.

92. Radioactive water and other fluids and their preparation. *J. of Advanced Therapeutics 23*:582-593 (October) 1905. Also reprint.

93. New high potential high frequency "cataphoric" electrode or phoric medicamental electrode. *Med. Record 68*:843 (November 18) 1905.

94. Fluorescence artificially produced in the human organism by the x-ray, by radium, and by electric discharges, as a therapeutic method. *Med. Press & Circ.,* (London) *80*:670-672 (December 27) 1905.

95. Improved cataphoric electrode for high potential currents. *Med. Record, 69*:995 (June 16) 1906.

96. Geschichtliche Beitraege zur Entdeckung der Anaesthesie in der Chirurgie und ueber die Beziehungen Dr. William T. G. Mortons zu derselben. *Wiener med. Presse, 47*:1888-1897 (September 16) 1906.

97. Trypsin for the cure of cancer; with report of the microscopic examination of a cancerous tumor of the breast thus treated. *Med Record, 70*:893-900 (December 8) 1906. Also—in German translation (Trypsin zur Karzinombehandlung, etc.)— *in Prager med. Wchschr., 32*:211-213 (April 25); 224-225 (May 2); 239-240 (May 9) 1907.

98. Trypsin for the cure of cancer. *Med. Record, 71*:110-111 (January 19) 1907.

99. A case of cancer treated by trypsin. *New York M. J., 85*:443-444 March 9) 1907. Also—in German translation (Ueber einen mit Trypsin behandelten Fall von Krebs) —*in Prager med. Wchschr., 32*:240-241 (May 9) 1907.

100. Preoperative radiation and surgical treatment of cancer. *Med. Record, 71*:815-817 (May 18) 1907.

101. Radium for the treatment of cancer and lupus. Read at the 2nd International Congress of Physiotherapy in Rome, October 13, 1907. *Med. Record, 72*:760-766 (November 9) 1907. Also—in Italian translation (Il radium nel trattamenta del cancro e del lupus) — *in Riv. internaz. di terapia fisica, 9*:160-182, 1908. Also abstracted in *Arch of the Roentgen Ray, 12*:278-281 (March) 1908.

102. The wave current and high frequency currents. *J. Advanced Therapeutics, 26*:227-239 (May) 1908. Also abstracted in *Arch. of the Roentgen Ray, 13*:67-70, 1908. Also—in French translation (Le wave current et les courants de haute fréquence)—*in Arch d'Électr. méd.,* (Bordeaux) *16*:331-343, April 1908.

103. Static electricity: its methods of application and therapeutic value. *Post-Graduate, N. Y., 23*:331-343 (April) 1908.

104. Note on fluorescence excited within human tissues as a method of treatment. Read at the 12th Annual Meeting of the American Therapeutic Society, Boston, May 13, 1911. *Monthly Cycl. & Med. Bull.,* (Philadelphia) *4*:705-710, 1911.

105. Some problems in the chemotherapy of cancer. *New York M. J., 95*:625-627 (March 30) 1912.

106. Baseless and cruel newspaper sensationalism (Letter to the editor). *New York M. J., 95*:777-778 (April 13) 1912.

107. Imbedded radium tubes in the treatment of cancer. With report of a case of sarcoma remaining cured nine years after radiation. *Med. Record, 86*:913-915 (November 28) 1914.

108. Radiochemicotherapy; the internal therapeutics of the radio-elements. *Med. Record, 87*:381-390 (March 6) 1915.

Chapter 7

RADIOLOGIC PERIODICALS

Providence . . . permitted the invention of printing as a scourge for the sins of the learned.
ALEXANDER POPE, *The Dunciad* (1728)

The graphomania, which seems to be so prevalent in this day and age, is all but a recent development. Martin Luther (and others before him) complained that "the multitude of books is a great evil. There is no limit to this fever for writing (as if) everyone had to be an author."

This list of radiologic periodicals was compiled for the etymologic purposes explicated in the Radio-Semantic Treatise. An obviously malevolent tendency can be recognized in the very existence of such a multitude of radiologic titles—but then even the most modest of these periodicals carries occasionally certain bits of information of interest at least to the historian.

The attempt to compile as complete a list as possible is also otherwise justified. Hard pressed bibliographers often select for inclusion in annual listings only those items which they regard as being worthy of remembrance. But history has shown the frequency with which contemporaries were unable to discriminate between what has and what has no lasting value: how many famous authors received their first significant recognition as a posthumous gesture?

METHOD OF COMPILATION

As a starter I went to the John Crerar Library in Chicago, and obtained copies of all the cards listed in their files under the heading Radiology (diagnosis and therapy).*

To this basic list were added titles from various sources. No such catalogue card copies could be obtained from the NLM because its subject catalogue is restricted to the last 25 years with the exception of a few items, such as bibliographies. Many titles were found in the *Index Catalogue* of the old Army Medical Library. The recently published card catalogues of the NLM were consulted. The (American) list of *Union Serials* and the (British) *World List of Periodicals* contained some items which were neither at Crerar, nor at NLM. A few esoteric titles were found at the New York Academy of Medicine, or at the College of Physicians in Philadelphia. Finally, my listing contains a few periodicals—such as the TÜRK RADYOLOJI MECMUASI, ROENTGEN-EUROP, and RADIAZIONI DI ALTA ENERGIA — which in 1963 were not included in any of the above catalogues.

*Of much help in this, as in so many other instances, was Mr. Walter Shelton, who heads the card catalogue and also chairs Crerar's Acquisitions. The cards were photographed on a 16 mm. negative, printed thereafter on a continuous roll of heavy paper (card stock), which was then cut to the original size. Valuable assistance in this matter (as well as on several other occasions) was offered by Mrs. Carole Swain, chief of the Photoduplication Department at Crerar.

PERIODICITY

By definition, a periodical is a publication which appears at more or less regular (periodic) intervals. For our purposes, the avowed or implied intention of periodic re-issue was considered sufficient for including the respective titles. There is, for instance, James Case's translation of ROENTGEN DIAGNOSTICS: PROGRESS VOLUME. One might have questioned also Franz Buschke's PROGRESS IN RADIATION THERAPY, but then a second volume of the latter has just been published.

In recent years, in this country the papers presented at the annual radiologic conventions are published during the following year in the respective society's journal. In Italy and in other European countries, convention reports are often published as a separate volume. The respective Italian title is ATTI, CONGRESSO NAZIONALE DI RADIOLOGIA MEDICA. At times these reports are published as a supplement to an existing journal, as in Poland—ZJAZD RADIOLOGOW POLSKICH.

ELECTRIC AND ATOMIC ADULTERATION

In the Era of the Roentgen Pioneers, specialty journals were geared to electrology as much as (or more than) to radiology. From 1916 to 1925 PHYSICAL THERAPEUTICS called itself THE AMERICAN JOURNAL OF ELECTROTHERAPEUTICS & RADIOLOGY. Some of these actually started out in the 1880's and 1890's as journals devoted entirely to "electric" topics.

A number of physicistic titles were deleted, for instance the famous JAHRBUCH DER RADIOAKTIVITAET UND ELEKTRONIK, of which the first seventeen volumes were edited by the renowned Johannes Stark, the other three by H. Seeliger; the publisher was S. Hirzel in Leipzig (1905-1924). Likewise beyond the scope of this listing were considered the BOLETIN DE RADIACTIVIDAD, issued since 1909 by the Instituto Nacional de Geofisica in Madrid, and the TRAVAUX, edited shortly after the revolution in what was then still called Petersburg (today's Leningrad) at the Physical & Technical Roentgen Institute by Abraham Joffé, who became famous for his contributions to solid state physics. THE JOURNAL DE PHYSIQUE ET LE RADIUM had to be included, if only because it had absorbed a reputable publication with definite radiologic connotation.

In the Golden Age of Radiology the schism between radiologists and electrologists deepened. Today electrology has become a minor branch of what is called Physical Medicine or Physical Therapy, and is usually connected with the idea of Rehabilitation. This is reflected in the respective journal titles, but the line is not always easy to draw. If true to its name, the ARCHIV FUER PHYSIKALISCHE THERAPIE was not supposed to contain radiologic material, except incidentally. Yet, as a supplement to that ARCHIV, there appeared in 1956 a Symposium on Biophysics and Radiology, edited by Walther Friedrich and Hans Schreiber (Leipzig, Thieme).

Physicistic contamination recurred in the Atomic Phase when "nuclear" attachments blossomed in ever-increasing numbers. Again valuable titles had to be deleted, such as the excellent but clearly nonmedical NUCLEAR SCIENCE AND ENGINEERING, the official publication of the American Nuclear Society, or their less formal NUCLEAR NEWS, both appearing in Chicago since 1957. NUCLEONICS was retained because of its many contributions to medical isotopology.

Neither were included the (Sovietic) ATOMNAYA ENERGIYA, nor the (German) ATOMKERNENERGIE. The (likewise German) KERNTECHNIK indicates in its subtitle that it is intended for engineers. And the (American) ISOTOPES AND RADIATION TECHNOLOGY, published for the AEC at Oak Ridge, since 1963, is a quarterly technical progress review.

RADIO-DELETIONS

During the compilation, journal titles in various listings were scanned for "radio-content." The title RADIATOR was used in 1848-1849 in Clinton (New York) by a "weekly miscellany," in 1891-1899 in Kansas City by an "insurance advertiser," in 1918-1919 in France by the official newspaper of the U. S. Army Ambulance Service, and more recently in Detroit by a firm engaged in central heating.

Nor were included in this listing such titles as RADIOMANIA (a 1936 publication of Cuban broadcasters), the RADIOIST (a radio ham paper from Omaha), the RADIOGRAM (a similar sheet from Elmira, New York), not even the RADIOGRAPH (a 1920-1921 organ of the Radio Officers Union of London, who soon changed its name to SIGNAL). A number of radio-titles, such as the RADIONIC QUARTERLY, are issued by the various societies of Radiesthesia. However willing to oblige, those items could not possibly be included.

As a bonus feature will be mentioned the Partenopean journal RADIOCHIRURGIA, which was first issued in Naples in 1909 with the significant subtitle LA CHIRURGIA DELL'ERNIA E DELL' ADDOME (surgery of hernia and of the abdomen), devoted to the promotion of electric operations. Also deleted were the ARCHIVES DE RHUMATOLOGIE, alias AIX-LES-BAINS MÉDICAL, despite the alluring SUBTITLE ARCHIVES CLINIQUES RADIOLOGIQUES ET THÉRAPEUTIQUES, and the existence, at Aix-les-Bains, of the Hôtel du Radium. Strangely enough, there was even an item entitled X-RAY which had to go: its subtitle was A BEACON FOR TAXPAYERS AND HONEST LABORERS, printed prior to World War II in Muncie (Indiana).

BORDERLINE DELETIONS

A few items almost made the grade, but not quite, such as the BOLLETINO SCHERMOGRAFICO, which contains reports on mass chest surveys performed by

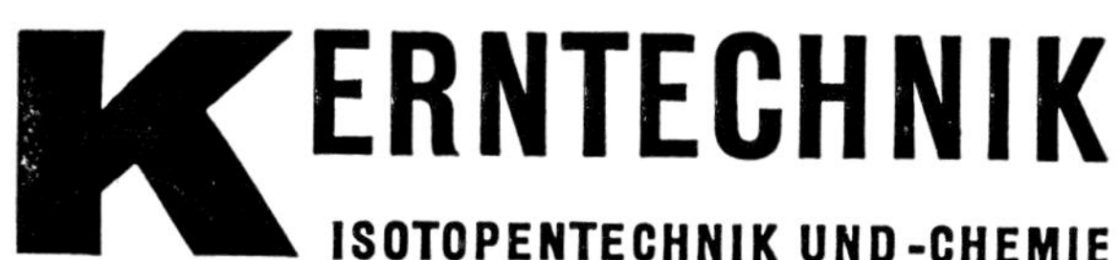

the Italian Health Ministry. The PEORIA FLUOROSCOPE is the house organ of the Municipal Tuberculosis Sanitarium in Peoria (Illinois). The LIBRARY INFORMATION BULLETIN, mimeographed since 1954 (?) by the Commonwealth X-Ray and Radium Laboratory of Melbourne (Australia) had to be deleted just as STRAHLUNGSWERTE (Atmospheric Radiation Levels Resulting from Fallout), published as a supplement to the MEDIZIN-METEOROLOGISCHER BERICHT, printed in Hamburg (since 1954?) by the Meterological Service.

COMMERCIAL HOUSE ORGANS

Several "prepaid" publications are outstanding because of the seriousness of their editorial policy, meaning they carry chiefly non-commercial contents. There is for instance in this country Eastman-Kodak's MEDICAL RADIOGRAPHY & PHOTOGRAPHY, in Germany C. H. F. Mueller's ROENTGENSTRAHLEN. Others are included to avoid confusion with similar titles, such as the RIVISTA DE RADIOLOGIA, which sounds just like the name of several non-commercial Italian periodicals.

Many more house organs (for instance WATSON'S X-RAY NEWS) have appeared than are herein listed. Some of the companies have printed a large number of these rather short-lived titles. Only the X-ray Division of General Electric has issed at one time or another BUSHEL BASKET, MARKET BASKET, X-RAY SALES GENERATOR, IDEAS, GEXRAY NEWS, GEXTRA, in addition to the better known RADSIDIAN or GEXCO NEWS.

METHOD OF LISTING

First comes a listing of periodicals by country of origin. A peculiar position retains the RADIOLOGISCHE RUNDSCHAU, published in Berlin until Hitler's coming to power; it was then transplanted to Switzerland where it is currently published in Basel as the RADIOLOGIA CLINICA. In that first listing there is also an entry called *International,* which includes journals published in more than one language, or with avowed international background.

In the second part, journals are indexed under their names in alphabetical order (introductory prefixes such as the English the, the French *le* or *la,* the German *der, die,* or *das,* the Spanish *el,* or the Italian *il* were deleted). All names under wich the respective journal had been circulated are given as cross-references. In the full listing the main title of the periodical appears in CAPS AND SMALL CAPS, followed by the other titles under which it is known (those other titles are introduced by the words 'title varies'). When a journal continued numbering its volumes while changing the title on the frontispiece, it was considered as being the same journal. But when the title changed as well as volume numbering, even though there was the same editor and/or publisher, the journal was regarded as a new venture, reference to its predecessor being made with the words superseded or replaced. In this respect, difficulties arose with the ZEITSCHRIFT FÜR MEDIZINICHE ELEKTROLOGIE, which changed its name every two years until 1910 when it split into two distinct sets, with different names, each of them continuing the volume numbering of the original journal. By contrast, in the case of the (German) ROENTGEN-BLAET-

Röntgenstrahlen

Geschichte und Gegenwart

1

1 9 5 1

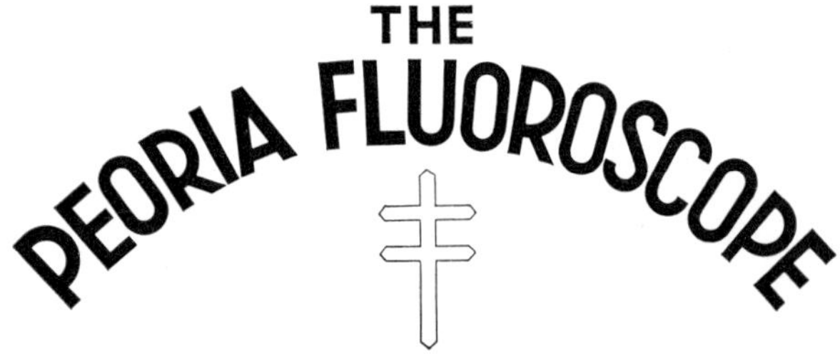

The PEORIA
FLUOROSCOPE

TER, and the Italian QUADERNI DI RADIOLOGIA, they reappeared after World War II with the same name but with different volume numbering and different publishers.

In the main listing, a star preceding the name of the publication, as in *RADIOLOGY, signifies current publication. Whenever the title is sponsored by a society, the latter's name appears in *italics*. After the place of publication is given the name of the publisher (if available). Whenever the imprint varies, this is also noted. For defunct publications, the total number of volumes (if known) is mentioned after the imprint. Otherwise, and in the case of current titles, only the date of the first volume is given with a small hyphen, indicating that the "terminal" figure is (as yet) unknown.

The multitude of radiologic periodicals may be a "great evil," but it should be easier to bear if currently available indices would simplify the identification of any single title. Indeed, as the Roman historian Titus Livius (59 B.C.—17 A.D.) noticed, "the evil best known is also the most tolerable."

ARGENTINA

Acta radiologica interamericana
Anales. Instituto Municipal de Radiología, Buenos Aires
Jornadas Radiologicas Argentínas
Memoria. Instituto Municipal de Radiología, Buenos Aires
Radiodoncia
Radiología, Buenos Aires
Revista de la Sociedad argentina de radio y electrología
Revista practica de radiumterapía

AUSTRALIA

Journal of the College of Radiologists of Australasia
Radiographer
Report of the Queensland Radium Institute

AUSTRIA

Mitteilungren aus dem Institut für Radiumforschung, Wien
Mitteilungen aus dem Laboratorium für radiologische Diagnostik, etc.
Mitteilungen aus der k. u. k. Kuranstalt für Radiumtherapie, St. Joachismthal
Radiologia austriaca
Röntgenologie
Safety Series, International Atomic Energy

BELGIUM

Annales internationales de médecine physique et de physiobiologie
Journal belge de radiologie
Radiologie et chirurgie

BRASIL

Revista brasileira de radiologia
Revista de radiologia clinica

CANADA

Canadian X-Ray News Letter
Focal Spot
Journal of the Canadian Association of Radiologists
Ontario Radiographer
Rayons X, Montréal
X-Rays, Kentville

CHINA

Chinese Journal of Radiology

COLOMBIA

Archivos, Instituto Nacional de radium, Bogotá
Boletin, Instituto Nacional de radium, Bogota

CUBA

Anales de radiología
Radiología oral

CZECHOSLOVAKIA

Československá radiologie
Referatovy vyber z rentgenologie
Ročenka československé společnosti pro rentgenologii a radiologii

DENMARK

Beretning og Regnskab
Dansk radiologisk selskab

ECUADOR

Revista de radiología y fisioterapía

FRANCE

Annales de radiologie
Année électrique, électrothérapique et radiographique
Archives d'électricité médicale
Atomes et radiations
Bulletin d'information, Centre Antoine Béclère
Bulletin officiel de la Société française d'électrothérapie et de radiologie médicale
Bulletin et mémoires de la Société de radiologie médicale de France
Cahiers de radiologie et d'électrologie
Cliniques radiologiques
Journal de physique et le radium
Journal de radiologie et d'électrologie
Métalix
Radiodiagnostic et radioanatomie de précision
Radiographie
Radiologie, Paris
Radiologie pratique
Radiophysiologie et radiothérapie
Radium, Paris
Radium, La radioactivité, etc.
Radiumculture
Rayonixar

Rayons X, Paris
Revue d'actinologie et de physiothérapie
Revue de physiothérapie chirurgicale et de radiologie
Revue générale internationale d'électroradiologie et d'actinologie
Revue internationale d'électrothérapie et de radiothérapie
Revue pratique de radiumthérapie
Roentgen-Europ

GERMANY

Agfa Röntgen Hausmitteilungen
Archiv für physikalische Medizin und medizinische Therapie
Archiv für physikalische Therapie
Archiv und Atlas der normalen und pathologischen Anatomie in typischen Röntgenbildern
Atompraxis
Biophysik
Ergebnisse der medizinischen Strahlenforschung
Fortbildungskurse auf dem Gebiete der Röntgenstrahlen
Fortschritte der angewandten Radioisotopie
Fundamenta radiologica
Internationale Radiotherapie
Jahrbuch für Röntgenologen
Jahresbericht Radiologie
Kongressbericht über die Tagung der medizinisch-wissenschaftlichen Gesellschaft für Röntgenologie
Medizinisch Technische Assistentin in der Radiologie
Medizin Technik
Nuclear Medizin
Radiobiologia, radiotherapia
Radiologe
Radiologische Rundschau
Radiologia diagnostica
Radiologische Mitteilungen
Radiologische Praktika
Radium in Biologie und Heilkunde
Radium Therapie
Revista de radiología - X
Röntgenblätter
Röntgendiagnostik, Ergebnisse
Röntgenkunde in Einzeldarstellungen
Röntgenliteratur
Röntgenpraxis
Röntgenstrahlen
Röntgen-Taschenbuch
Röntgentechnische Berichte
Röntgen- und Laboratoriumpraxis
Röntgographie in der inneren Medicin
SRW-Nachrichten
Strahlenbiologie, Strahlentherapie, Nuklearmedizin und Krebsforschung
Strahlentherapie
Verhandlungen der deutschen Röntgengesellschaft
Zeitschrift für medizinishc Elektrologie und Röntgenkunde
Zeitschrift für Röntgenologie
Zentralblatt für die gesamte Radiologie
Zentralblatt für Röngenstrahlen, Radium, etc.
Zwanglose Abhandlungen aus dem Gebiete der medizinischen Elektrologie und Röntgenkunde

GREAT BRITAIN

British Journal of Radiology
Clinical Radiology
International Journal of Radiation Biology
Journal of the Röntgen Society
Medical Electrology and Radiology
Proceedings of the Royal Society of Medicine; Section on Radiology
Progress
Radiography
Report, Medical Research Council
Report, Mt. Vernon Hospital and Radium Institute
Report, National Radium Commission
Report, London Radium Institute
Report, Radiobiological Laboratory
Statistical Report, Christie Hospital
Watson X-Ray News
X-Ray Supplement (The Practitioner)
Year Book, British Institute of Radiology

HUNGARY

Magyar radiologia
Magyar röntgen közlöny
Medicor News
Radiologiai közlemények
Radio, röntgen és egyéb sugarzások
Röntgenologia

INDIA

Indian Journal of Radiology

INTERNATIONAL PERIODICALS

Acta isotopica
Acta radiologica interamericana
Actas, Congresso interamericano de radiología
Annales internationales de médecine physique et de physiobiologie
Archivio internazionale di radiobiologia generale
Atti del Congresso degli elettro-radiologi di cultura latina
Comptes-rendus des séances du Congrès international d'électrologie et de radiologie
Comptes-rendus des séances du Congrès international pour l'étude de la radiologie et de l'ionisation
Comptes-rendus des séances du Congrès international de radiologie et d'électricité
Comptes-rendus du Congrès annuel des médecins électro-radiologistes de langue française
Congrès international de radiophotographie
Fundamenta radiologica

International Journal of Applied Radiation and Isotopes
International Journal of Radiation Biology
Medical Electrology and Radiology
Proceedings, Interamerican Congress of Radiology
Proceedings, International Conference on Radiobiology
Proceedings, International Congress of Radiology
Proceedings, Symposium on X-Ray Microscopy
Radiazioni di alta energia
Radiobiologia, radiotherapia
Radiobiologica latina
Radiografía y fotografía clínicas
Radiología, Pánama
Radiologia, Roma
Radiologia clinica
Radiologia diagnostica
Radiologia Interamericana
Radiquéno
Revista de radiología - X
Revista de radiología y fisioterapía
Revue générale internationale d'électroradiologie et d'actinologie
Revue internationale d'électrothérapie et de radiothérapie
Safety Series, International Atomic Energy Agency
Symposium neuro-radiologicum

ITALY
Acta isotopica
Actinoterapia
Annali di radiologia diagnostica
Archivio di radiologia
Archivio internazionale di radiobiologia generale
Atti del Congresso degli elettro-radiologi di cultura latina
Atti del Congresso nazionale di radiologia medica
Diario radiologico
Letteratura radiologica italiana
Minerva fisioterapica e radiobiologica
Minerva nucleare
Nuntius radiologicus
Quaderni di radiologia
Radiazioni di alta energia
Radiobiologica latina
Radiologia, Roma
Radiologia medica
Radiologia pratica
Radiologia sperimentale
Radioterapia, radiobiologia e fisica medica
Rivista di radiologia
Rivista italiana di radiologia clinica
Roentgen-Europ
Scritti italiani di radiobiologia
Stratigrafia

JAPAN
Hoiken Nyusu
Hoshasen Igaku Saikin No Shinpo
Irigaku Ryoho Zasshi
Irigaku Shinpo
Journal of Radiation Research
Kanazawa Ika Daigaku Gyosekishu
Kanazawa Irigaku Sosho
Keiko
Nippon Acta Radiologica
Nippon Hoshasen Gijutsu Gakkai Zasshi
Nippon Rentogen Gakkai Zasshi
Nippon X-sen Gishikai Kaiho
Osaka Furitsu Hoshasen Chuo Kenkyusho, Sakai
Rentogengaku Nippon Bunken
Rinsho Hoshasen
Saishin Chiryo
Shimadzu Rentogen Jiho
X-rays, Nakanoshima

MEXICO
Revista mexicana de radiología

NETHERLANDS
Camera radiologica
Excerpta Medica, Section 14, Radiology
Journal Belge de Radiologie
Medica Mundi
Old Delft (Odelca) Bulletin

PANAMA
Radiologia, Panamá

PERU
Revista peruana de radiología

POLAND
Polski przeglad radiologiczny
Postepy radiologii

PORTUGAL
Acta iberica radiológica-cancerológica
Boletim da sociedade portuguesa de radiologia

ROUMANIA
Radiologia, Bucuresti
Supplement, Revista stiintelor medicale

SPAIN
Acta iberica radiológica-cancerológica
Anales, Instituto radioquirúrgico de Guipúzcoa
Boletin, Sociedad española de radiología y electrologia
Revista de diagnostica y tratamiento físicos
Revista de medicina física
Revista española de electrología y radiología medicas
Revista general de roentgenologia (supplement)

SWEDEN
Acta radiologica
Berättelse fran styrelsen

SWITZERLAND
Archives, Centre anticancéreux et radium institut de Genève

Bibliotheca radiologica
Radiologia clinica

TURKEY
Türk radyoloji mecmuasi

U. S. S. R.
Annales de roentgenologie et de radiologie
Izvestya Kievskoye rentgenovskaya kommissya
Materialy po toxicologiy radioaktivnich veshest
Medizinskaya radiologia
Pitannya onkologiy
Radiobiologiya
Radiokhimiya
Rentgenovsky viestnik
Uchenye zapiski
Vestnik rentgenologiy i radiologiy
Voprosy nevrorentgenologiy
Voprosy obshei
Voprosy radiobiologiy
Voprosy rentgenologiy i onkologiy
Voprosy rentgenologiy i smezhnyk oblastei

U. S. A.
Abstracts and Proceedings, Conference on Radiation Cataracts
Acme Bulletin
American Atlas of Stereoroentgenology
American Journal of Physical Therapy
American Journal of Physiologic Therapeutics
American Journal of Progressive Therapeutics
American Journal of Roentgenology
American Lectures in Radiation Therapy
American Lectures in Roentgen Diagnosis
American Radiography Technologists Journal
Annals of Roentgenology
Archives of Electrology and Radiology
Archives of Physical Medicine and Rehabilitation
Archives of Physiological Therapy
Biological Defense Briefs
Bulletin, American College of Radiology
Bulletin of the Atomic Scientists
Bulletin of the Electro-Therapeutic Laboratory, University of Michigan
Bulletin, Intersociety Committee for Radiology
Bulletin, Radium Emanation Corporation
Cathode Press
Dental Radiography and Photography
Dunlee Digest
DuPont X-Ray News
Engeln X-Ray Special and Physiotherapy
Gexco News
Health Physics
International Journal of Applied Radiation and Isotopes
Isotopics
Journal of Nuclear Medicine
Journal of Physical Therapy
Journal of Roentgenology
Journal of the American Radiotherapy Society
Medical Radiography and Photography
Memorial Hospital, New York
Nucleonics
Physical Therapeutics
Picker News
Proceedings, American College of Radiology
Proceedings, Medical Radioisotope Conference
Proceedings, Symposium on X-Ray Microscopy and Microradiography
Progress in Radiation Therapy
Radiance Medical Journal
Radiation Research
Radiation Therapy
Radiografía y fotografía clínicas
Radiographic Aids for the Veterinary Practitioner
Radiologia Interamericana
Radiological Clinics of North America
Radiological Health Data
Radiological Health News
Radiological Review
Radiologic Technology
Radiology Reporter
Radiquéno
Radium Abstracts
Radium. Devoted to the chemistry, physics and therapeutics of radium, etc.
Radium Digest
Radium Quarterly
Radium Light
Radium Therapist
Radsidian
Report, US Atomic Energy Commission
Revista de radiología y fisiotherapía
Roentgendiagnostics, Progress Volume
Roentgen Economist
Scintillator
Supplement on Roentgenology (Interstate Medical Journal)
Transactions, American Electrotherapeutic Association
Transactions, American Medical Association, Section on Radiology
Transactions, American Roentgen Ray Society
Victor News
World Radiology Current Abstracts
X-ray Studies
X-ray Technician
Year Book of Radiology
Your Radiologist

YUGOSLAVIA
Izdanja. Centralni rentgenologski institut.
Primena radioaktivnih izotopa
Radioloski glasnik

Acme Bulletin, Chicago, commercial house organ.
Acta Isotopica, Subtitle: Rivista di medicina e bio-

logia nucleare, also translated in French, English and German; Padova, vol. 1- (March 1961-).

Acta radiologica interamericana, official organ of the *Colegio Interamericano de Radiología* (Interamerican College of Radiology); Buenos Aires, vol. 1-(1951-); summaries in English, French, Spanish, and Portuguese.

*Actas, Congresso interamericano di radiología; 1-Buenos Aires (1943), 2-Habana (1946), 3-Santiago de Chile (1949), 4-Mexico City (1952), 5-Washington, D. C. (1955), 6-Lima (1958), 7-Sao Paulo (1961).

Actinoterapia, Revista internazionale di terapia dei raggi, Parco Margherita, Napoli, vol. 1-10 (1915-1931).

Advances in Radiobiology, see Proceedings, International Conference on Radiobiology.

*Agfa Röntgen Hausmitteilunger, commercial house organ.

American Atlas of Stereoroentgenology; a quarterly, edited and published under the sole auspices of the *New York Roentgen Society;* Troy, N. Y., the Southworth Co., Vol. 1-3 (January 1916-July 1920); paged continuously; in slide cases.

American Electro-Therapeutic and X-Ray Era, see Archives of Electrology and Radiology.

American Journal of Electro-Therapeutics and Radiology, see Physical Therapeutics.

American Journal of Physical Therapy (title varies: . . . and Ambulant Therapy, Including Scientific Food Advances), official journal of the *American Assn. of Medical Hydrology and Physical Therapy;* Chicago, Professional Press, Inc., vol. 1-13 - through nr. 5 - (April 1924-May 1936); absorbed in January 1933 the Journal of American Medical Hydrology; merged in 1936 into Clinical Medicine and Surgery.

American Journal of Physiologic Therapeutics, A Journal of Progress in Non-Medicinal Therapy; Chicago, vol. 1-2 - through nr. 4 - (May 1910-November/December 1911).

American Journal of Progressive Therapeutics (title varies: American X-ray Journal (col. 1-15) with subtitle A Monthly Devoted to the Practical Application of the New Science and to the Physical Improvement of Man (vol. 1-12); published in St. Louis (vol. 1-11), then in Chicago; vol. 1-18 (May 1897-January 1906); in January 1905, the American X-ray Journal united with the Archives of Electrology and Radiology into the above title.

*American Journal of Roentgenology, Radium Therapy, and Nuclear Medicine (title varies: 1913-1922 American Journal of Roentgenology, 1923-1951 . . . and Radium Therapy), organ of the *American Roentgen Ray Society* and (since 1921) *American Radium Society;* published in New York City, Paul B. Hoeber (1913-1929), then in Springfield, Illinois, Charles C Thomas; superseded American Quarterly of Roentgenology; Consolidated Indices: I (1903-1947), II (1938-1942), III (1943-1947), IV (1948-1952), V (1953-1957), VI (1958-1962).

*American Lectures in Radiation Therapy; Springfield, Illinois, Charles C Thomas, Publisher ((1949-); monographs, not numbered.

*American Lectures in Roentgen Diagnosis; Springfield, Illinois, Charles C Thomas, Publisher (1949-); monographs in book form, not numbered.

American Quarterly of Roentgenology, organ of the *American Roentgen Ray Society;* Detroit, vol. 1-5 (October 1906-September 1913); superseded Transactions of the American Roentgen Ray Society; was replaced by American Journal of Roentgenology.

American Radiography Technologists Journal; Enid Oklahoma, vol. 1-(March 1956-).

American X-Ray Journal, see American Journal of Progressive Therapeutics.

Abstracts and Proceedings, Conference on Radiation Cataracts and Neutron Effects, Held under the auspices of the National Research Council's Division of Medical Sciences for the U. S. Atomic Energy Commission (title varies slightly); Washington, D. C., 1st- (1950-).

*Acta ibérica radiologica-cancerologica, Organ of the *Sociedad Espanola de Radiología y Electrología Médicas* (founded 1945); Madrid, vol. 1- (January/March 1952-); contributions in Spanish or Portuguese; superseded Radiológica-Cancerológica.

*Acta radiologica, Published conjointly by the *Associations of Medical Radiology in Denmark, Finland, Holland, Norway, and Sweden;* Stockholm, P. A. Norstedt & Söner (first volume by Marcus' Boktryckeri-Aktiebolag), vol. 1- (1922). Separated in 1963 into Diagnosis (red-lettered title) and Therapy - Physics - Biology (blue-lettered title).

*Acta radiolorica, Supplementum; Stockholm, P. A. Norstedt, vol. 1- (1927-); monographs in book form.

*Acta radiologica et cancerologica bohemoslovenica, see Československá roentgenologie.

Anales de radiología, official organ of the *Sociedad Cubana de Radiología y Fisioterapia;* Habana, vol.

1-2 - through nr. 3 - (1929-July 1930).

ANALES, Instituto Municipal de Radiología y Fisioterapía Buenos Aires vol. 1- (1934); have seen 1935 and 1938.

ANALES DEL INSITUTO RADIOQUIRGICO DE GUIPUZCOA, San Sebastian, Spain.

ANNALES DE LA SOCÍETÉ BELGE DE RADIOLOGIE, see JOURNAL BELGE DE RADIOLOGIE.

ANNALES DE MÉDECINE PHYSIQUE, see Annales Internationales de Médecine Physique et de Physiobiologie.

*ANNALES DE RADIOLOGIE, radiologie clinique-radiobiologie; Paris, La Semanine des Hôpitaux (Expansion Scientifique Francaise), Vol 1- (1958-).

ANNALES DE ROENTGENOLOGIE ET RADIOLOGIE, organ of the *Association de Radiologie de l'URSS* et de l'Institut d'État de Roentgenologie et de Radiologie a Pétersbourg (subtitle varies); published in Petersbourg (vol. 1), then in Paris, Presses Universitaires de France; vol. 1-3 - of the latter only part 1 - (1922-1928); English, French, or German text; international edition of Vestnik Rentgenologiy i Radiologiy.

ANNALES INTERNATIONALES DE MÉDECINE PHYSIQUE ET DE PHYSIOBIOLOGIE (title varies, vol. 1-4: Annales de la Société de médecine physique d'Anvers; vol. 5-19; Annales de médecine physique), organ of the *Société de médecine Physique d'Anvers* (vol. 9-30, also of *Société Belge de Physiothérapie*, vol. 29-30, also of *Association Internationale de Médecine Physique et Physiobiologie*); Anvers, Vol. 1-30 (1903-1937).

*ANNALI DI RADIOLOGIA DIAGNOSTICA, (title varies; vol. 1-7, 1929-33: Rivista di radiologia e fisica medica; vol. 8-12, 1934-38: Annali di radiologia e fisica medica); Bologna, Licinio Capelli, vol. 1- (1929-).

ANNALI DI RADIOLOGIA E FISICA MEDICA, see Annali di radiologia diagnostica.

ANNALS OF ROENTGENOLOGY; numbered monographs published irregularly in book form; New York, Paul B. Hoeber, vol. 1-21 (1920-1953).

ANNÉE ÉLECTRIQUE, ÉLECTROTHÉRAPIQUE ET RADIOGRAPHIQUE, Revue annuelle des progres électriques en 1900 (-1913); Paris, C. Béranger, vol. 1-14 (1901-1914).

*ANNUAL CONFERENCE OF TEACHERS OF RADIOLOGY, see Proceedings, Annual Conference of Teachers of Radiology.

ANNUAL REPORT(S), see Report(s).

ARCHIV FÜR PHYSIKALISCHE MEDIZIN UND MEDIZINISCHE TECHNIK, nebst Beiblatt "Fortschritte und Neuheiten der physikalisch-chemischen und photographischen Industrie in ihrer Anwendung auf das Gesamtgebiet der praktischen Medizin," Publikationsorgan of the Medizinische Abteilung des radiologischen Institutes an der Universität Heidelberg; Leipzig, Otto Nemnich, vol. 1-8 (1906-August 1914).

*ARCHIV UND ATLAS DER NORMALEN UND PATHOLOGISCHEN ANATOMIE IN TYPISCHEN RÖNTGENBILDERN (title varies, vol. 1-4: Atlas der normalen und pathologischen, etc.), considered a supplement (Ergänzungsband) to Fortschritte auf dem Gebiete der Röntgenstrahlen; monographs, (numbered consecutively) published in book form, with individual title-pages; vol. 1-35 published in Hamburg, Lucas Gräfe & E. Sillem, then in Leipzig, Georg Thieme, vol. 1- (1900-).

ARCHIVES D'ÉLECTRICITE MÉDICALE, Électrologie, radiologie, curielogie et physiothérapie du cancer (title varies, until 1915 Archives d'électricité médicale experimentales et cliniques; 1916-1923 Archives d'électricité médicale et de physiothérapie; 1924-1931 Archives d'électricité médicale et de physiothérapie du cancer); published in Bordeaux, then in Paris, J. B. Baillière, vol. 1-42 (1893-1932); merged into Journal de radiologie et d'électrologie.

ARCHIVES DE L'INSTITUT DU RADIUM DE L'UNIVERSITÉ DE PARIS, see Radiophysiologie et radiotherapie.

ARCHIVES OF CLINICAL SKIAGRAPHY, see British Journal of Radiology.

ARCHIVES OF ELECTROLOGY AND RADIOLOGY (title varies; vol. 1, nr. 1: Electro-Therapeutic and X-Ray Era; vol. 1, nr. 2: American Electro-Therapeutic and X-Ray Era); Chicago, R. Friedländer, vol. 1-4 (June 1901-December 1904); in 1905 united with American X-Ray Journal to form American Journal of Progressive Therapeutics.

ARCHIVES DU CENTRE ANTICANCÉREUX ET DU RADIUM INSTITUTE DE GENÈVE, sponsored by *Société Médicale de Genève, Association des Médecins de Genève,* and *Section Genévoise de la Croix Rouge;* Genève, Switzerland (1941-).

*ARCHIVES OF PHYSICAL MEDICINE AND REHABILITATION (title varies: 1920-1925 Journal of Radiology; 1926-1937 Archives of Physical Therapy, X-Ray, Radium; 1938-1944 Archives of Physical Therapy; 1945-1952 Archives of Physical Medicine), official organ of the *Radiological Society of North America* (1920-April 1924), of the *Ameri-*

can College of Radiology and Physiotherapy (May 1924-1925), of the *American Congress of Physical Medicine and Rehabilitation* (1926-) - the latter having had several names, American College of Physical Therapy (1926-1929), American Congress of Physical Therapy (1929-1944), American Congress of Physical Medicine (1946-1952) - jointly with the *American Society of Physical Medicine* (1953-); Chicago, Vol. 1-(1920-); absorbed in March 1933 Physical Therapeutics.

ARCHIVES OF PHYSICAL THERAPY, X-RAY, RADIUM, see Archives of Physical Medicine and Rehabilitation.

ARCHIVES OF PHYSIOLOGICAL THERAPY, with subtitle in vol. 3-4 only (devoted to the diagnostic and therapeutic uses of electricity, radiant energy, heat, water, mechanical vibration, dietary regulation, exercise, psychic suggestion, etc.); Boston, B. G. Badger, vol. 1-4 (February 1905-December 1906); in 1907 merged into the Journal of Inebriety.

ARCHIVES OF RADIOLOGY AND ELECTROTHERAPY, see British Journal of Radiology.

ARCHIVES OF SKIAGRAPHY, see British Journal of Radiology.

ARCHIVES OF THE RÖNTGEN RAY, see British Journal of Radiology.

*ARCHIVIO DI RADIOLOGIA; Napoli, Tipografia Francesco Giannini & Figli, vol. 1- (1925-).

ARCHIVIO INTERNAZIONALE DI RADIOBIOLOGIA GENERALE (title varies: vol. 1 Atti, Congresso internazionale di elettro-radio-biologia), organ of the *Società internazionale di Radiobiologia;* Bologna, Licinio Capelli, vol. 1- (1934-); superseded Radiobiologia generalis.

*ARCHIVOS, Instituto Nacional de Radium, Universidad Nacional; Bogotà, Colombia, vol. 1- (1941-); summaries in Spanish, French and English.

ATLAS DER NORMALEN UND PATHOLOGISCHEN ANATOMIE IN TYPISCHEN RÖNTGENBILDERN, see Archiv und Atlas der normalen und pathologischen Anatomie, etc.

ATOMES ET RADIATIONS, physique, biologie, médecine; Paris, Expansion Scientifique Française, vol. 1 - nr. 1-10-(October 1946-December 1947).

*ATOMPRAXIS, Monatszeitschrift für angewandte Atomenergie in Technik, Industrie, Naturwissenschaften, Medizin, Landwirtschaft und Grenzgebieten; Karlsruhe, Germany, G. Braun, vol. 1- (October 1955).

*ATTI, CONGRESSO DEGLI ELETTRO-RADIOLOGI DI CULTURA LATINA, 3rd (Rome, 1954), published with 18° Congresso della Società italiana di radiologia medica.

*ATTI, CONGRESSO NAZIONALE DI RADIOLOGIA MEDICA (title varies, Congresso italiano di radiologia medica), *Societa Italiana di Radiologia Medica,* 1st- (October 1913-).

BERETNING OG REGNSKAB, Afgivet af Forretningsutvalget, Radiumfondet; København, vol. 1- (?); have seen 1914-1915.

*BERÄTTELSE FRAN STYRELSEN FÖR CANCERFÖRENINGEN I STOCKHOLM ÖVER VERKSAMHETSARET Radiumhemmet; Stockholm, K. L. Beckman, (1930-); includes Index of papers published at Radiumhemmet (1909-), and Report on cases treated and controlled at Radiumhemmet (1921-).

*BIBLIOTHECA RADIOLOGICA, supplement to Radiologia clinica; Basel, S. Karger, Fasc. 1- (1959-); monographs in German.

BIOLOGICAL DEFENSE BRIEFS, Preventive Medicine Division, Office of the Surgeon General, US Air Force; Washington, D.C., vol. 1-4 (July 18, 1951-December 17, 1954).

*BIOPHYSIK; Berlin, Springer Verlag, vol. 1- nr. 1- (February 1963-).

BOLETIM DA (official organ of the) *Sociedade Portuguesa de Radiologia Medica;* Lisbon (1932-1950); superseded by Acta ibérica radiológica-cancerológica.

BOLETIN, Instituto Nacional de Radium, Universidad Nacional, Bogotà, Colombia, vol. 1-2 - nr. 1-13 - (August 1948 - June 1950); superseded by Revista Colombiana de Cancerología.

*BOLETIN, Sociedad Espanola de Radiología y Electrología Medicas; Madrid; quarterly.

BOLLETINO DI MARCONITERAPIA, see Radioterapia, radiobiologia e fisica medica.

BRITISH JOURNAL OF RADIOGRAPHY, see Radiography.

*BRITISH JOURNAL OF RADIOLOGY (title varies: Archives of Clinical Skiagraphy since May 1896, Archives of the Röntgen Ray since 1897, Archives of Radiology and Electrology since 1915, British Journal of Radiology (British Institute of Radiology Section) since January 1924, then merged with British Journal of Radiology (Röntgen Society Section), which was the successor of the Journal of the Röntgen Society, and since January 1928 appears in a new series in present form), official organ of the *British Institute of Radiology* incorporated with the *Röntgen Society* (founded 1897); London, vol. 1-32 (May 1896 - December 1927), new series, vol. 1- (January 1928-).

*British Journal of Radiology, Supplement, London, nr. 1- (1947).

Bulletin de radiologie du service de santé militaire, supplement to Journal de radiologie et d'électrologie, nr. 1- (January-February 1918-).

Bulletin of the Electro-Therapeutical Laboratory of the University of Michigan; Ann Arbor, Inland Press, vol. 1-4 (1894-1897); quarterly, caption title, no index.

*Bulletin d'information pour les sociétés nationales de radiologie, Centre Antoine Beclere; Paris, no. 1/3- (January-March 1952-).

Bulletin officiel de la Société francaise d'électrotherapie et de radiologie médicale: Paris, vol. 1-28 (January 1893-December 1920); now published in the Journal de radiologie, d'électrologie, et de médicine nucléaire.

Bulletin of the American College of Radiology; Chicago, 1932-1936. Published in American Journal of Roentgenology, 1937-1940 (?).

*Bulletin of the Atomic Scientists, The Magazine of Science and Public Affairs; University of Chicago Press, vol. 1-, January 1945-.

Bulletin of the Intersociety Committee for Radiology; Chicago (August 1937-).

Bulletin of the Memorial Hospital, see Memorial Hospital, New York.

Bulletin of the New York Society of AMA approved roentgenologists, see Roentgen Economist.

Bulletin of the Radium Emanation Corporation; New York City, vol. 1-2 (1928-1929); commercial house organ.

Bulletins et mémoires de la Sociéte de radiologie médicale de France; (title varies: before 1913, Société de radiologie médicale de Paris) Paris, G. Steinheil, then Masson & Cie, vols. 1-5 - nr. 1-50 - (1909-1913).

Cahiers de radiologie et d'électrologie (Supplement to Gazette médicale de France); Paris, nr. 1- (January 1930-).

Camera radiologica, Dagra, Ltd., Dept. of Clinical Pharmacology; Amsterdam, vol. 1- (195-); text in English; summaries in English, French, German, Italian, Spanish and Portuguese; commercial house organ.

Canadian X-Ray News Letter, Canadian Industries Limited; Montreal (1945-); commercial house organ.

*Cathode Press, Machlett Laboratories; Springdale (Connecticut), vol. 1- (1943-); commercial house organ.

Centralblatt für Röntgenstrahlen, see Zentralblatt für Röntgenstrahlen.

*Československá Radiologie (title varies, 1938-1940 Acta radiologica et cancerologica bohemoslovenica; latter became subtitle when title was changed in 1948 (publication suspended 1940-1948) to Ceskoslovenská rentgenologie; current title since 1964). Official organ of *Československé Společnosti, pro rentgenologii a radiologii* (until 1940 also organ of the *Liga proti Rakovině*). Praha, published by Státní Zdravotnické Nakladatelství. Articles in Czech and Slovakian, with summaries in Russian and English. Started anew with vol. 1- in 1948-.

Chicago Medical Recorder, see Radiological Review.

*Cinese Journal of Radiology, (Chung hua fang she hsueh tsa chih), published by the Fang-she-hsueh-hui of the Chung-hua-ihsueh-hui; Peiping, vol. 1-(1953-).

Chiryo Igaku, see Saishin Chiryo.

*Clinical Radiology, (title varies: until October 1959, Journal of the Faculty of Radiologists), organ of the *Faculty of Radiologists* (London); Edinburgh, E. & S. Livingstone, vol. 1- (July 1949-).

Clinical Studies, Memorial Hospital, see Memorial Hospital, New York City.

Cliniques Radiologiques; Paris, ser. 1- (1959).

Comptes-rendus du Congrès international d'électrologie et de radiologie médicales; 1st (Paris) 1900; 2nd (Berne), 1902.

Comptes-rendus du Congrès international pour l'étude de la radiologie et de l'ionisation, (title varies: 2nd was Congrès international de radiologie et d'électricité); Bruxelles, L. Severeyns, 1st, 1905 (1906?); 2nd, 1911.

*Comptes-rendus du Congres annuel des médecins electro-radiologistes de langue francaise; vol. 2- (1935-); supersedes Réunion des médecins électro-radiologistes de langue française; published in Journal de Radiologie (vol. 18, 1934).

Congrès international de radiophotographie, *International Society of Photofluorography;* 1st Paris 1951; 2nd Milano; 3rd Stockholm 1958 (published as a special issue of Excerpta Medica).

Congresso interamericano de radiologia, see Actas, Congresso interamericano de radiología.

Congresso internazionale di electro-radio-biologia, see Archivio internazionale di radiobiologia generale.

CONGRESSO NAZIONALE (ITALIANO) DI RADIOLOGIA MEDICA, see Atti, Congresso nazionale di radiologia medica.

*DANSK RADIOLOGISK SELSKAB, Forhandlingar (supplement to Hospitalstidende); København (1920-).

*DENTAL RADIOGRAPHY AND PHOTOGRAPHY, Eastman Kodak Company; Rochester, N.Y., vol. 1- (1927-); also edition in Spanish; commercial house organ.

DIARIO RADIOLOGICO; Torino, Ospedale Maggiore (later published by Minerva Medica), vol. 1-12 (1921-1933).

*DUNLEE DIGEST, Dunlee Corporation; Bellwood (Illinois), vol. 1- nr. 1 (1957-); commercial house organ.

*DU PONT X-RAY NEWS, E. I. Du Pont de Nemours Co., Photo Products Department; Wilmington, Delaware, Nr. 1- (1956?-); commercial house organ.

ELECTRO-THERAPEUTIC AND X-RAY ERA, see Archives of Electrology and Radiology.

ENGELN X-RAY SPECIAL AND PHYSIOTHERAPY, Engeln Electric Company; Cleveland, vol. M 1-8? (1922-1929); commercial house organ.

ERGEBNISSE DER MEDIZINISCHEN STRAHLENFORSCHUNG (Röntgendiagnostik, Röntgen-, Radium- und Lichttherapie); Leipzig, Georg Thieme, vol. 1-5 (1925-1931).

*EXCERPTA MEDICA, SECT. 14, RADIOLOGY; Amsterdam, vol. 1- (June 1947-); contains abstracts.

*FOCAL SPOT, Organ of the *Canadian Society of Radiological Technicians;* Toronto, vol. 1- (1944?-).

*FORTSCHRITTE AUF DEM GEBIETE DER RÖNTGENSTRAHLEN UND DER NUKLEARMEDIZIN, Diagnostik, Physik, Biologie, Therapie (title varies: 1897-1948 Fortschritte auf dem Gebiete der Röntgenstrahlen; 1949-1954 Fortschritte auf dem Gebiete der Röntgenstrahlen vereinigt mit Röntgenpraxis), organ of the *Deutsche Röntgengesellschaft;* published first in Hamburg, by Gräfe & Sillem, then in Stuttgart, by Georg Thieme, vol. 1- 1897-; publication suspended with vol. 70 (1944), resumed with vol. 71 (1949), after absorbing Röntgenpraxis; index for vol. 1-11 (1897-1907) in vol. 11 (1907).

FORTSCHRITTE AUF DEM GEBIETE DER RÖNTGENSTRAHLEN, SUPPLEMENT (Ergänzungsbände), see Archiv und Atlas der normalen und pathologischen Anatomie, etc.

*FORTSCHRITTE DER ANGEWANDTEN RADIOISOTOPIE UND GRENZGEBIETE; Heidelberg, A. Hütnig, vol. 1- (1957-).

FORTSCHRITTE UND NEUHEITEN DER PHYSIKALISCH-CHEMISCHEN UND PHOTOGRAPHISCHEN INDUSTRIE IN IHRER ANWENDUNG AUF DAS GESAMTGEBIET DER PRAKTISCHEN MEDIZIN, Supplement, see Archiv für physikalische Medizin und medizinische Technik.

FUNDAMENTA RADIOLOGICA (title varies: vol. 1-3 as Radiologica, then quadrilingual, with title translated in four languages, such as Internationale Zeitschrift für Biophysik, Photochemie, Photobiologie und Strahlenmedizin, International Journal of Biophysics, Photochemistry, Photobiology and Medical Radiobiology, etc.); Berlin, de Gruyter, vol. 1-5 - only through nr. 5-6 - (1937-1940).

GENERAL ELECTRIC X-RAY NEWS, Gexco News (title varies: 1929 Victor News); imprint varies Chicago, then Milwaukee, vol. 1-19 (1929-June 1947); commercial house organ.

*HEALTH PHYSICS, organ of the *Health Physics Society;* New York, Pergamon Press, vol. 1- (June 1958-); vol. 1 (1958) includes abstracts of papers presented at meetings of the society and of the International Conference on the Peaceful Uses of Atomic Energy.

HEALTH RAYS (title varies: X-rays); Kentville, Nova Scotia, vol. 1- (1928-).

*HOIKEN NYUSU (Hoiken News Bulletin); Chiba Japan), Hoshasen Igaku Sogo Kenkyusho, vol. 1- (1958-).

*HOSHASEN IGAKU SAIKIN NO SHINPO (Recent advances in radiology): Tokyo, vol. 1- (1959-).

*INDIAN JOURNAL OF RADIOLOGY, official organ of the *Indian Radiological Association;* Madras, vol. 1- (February 1947-).

INTERNATIONAL ARCHIVES OF RADIOBIOLOGY AND NUCLEAR MEDICINE, see Radiobiologica latina.

INTERNATIONAL CONGRESS OF RADIOLOGY, see Proceedings, International Congress of Radiology.

*INTERNATIONAL JOURNAL OF APPLIED RADIATION AND ISOTOPES; New York, vol. 1- (July 1958-); articles in English, French, German, or Russian, with summaries in four languages.

INTERNATIONAL JOURNAL OF BIOPHYSICS, PHOTOCHEMISTRY, PHOTOBIOLOGY AND MEDICAL RADIOBIOLOGY, see Fundamenta radiologica.

*INTERNATIONAL JOURNAL OF RADIATION BIOLOGY AND RELATED STUDIES IN PHYSICS, CHEMISTRY AND MEDICINE; London, Taylor & Francis, vol. 1- (1959-).

INTERNATIONALE RADIOTHERAPIE, Besprechungswerk auf dem Gebiete der Röntgen-, Curie, Licht und Elektrotherapie; Darmstadt, L. C. Wittich, vol. 1-3 (1925-1928).

INTERNATIONALE ZEITSCHRIFT FÜR BIOPHYSIK, PHOTOCHEMIE, PHOTOBIOLOGIE, UND STRAHLENMEDIZIN, see Fundamenta radiologica.

INTERNATIONALE ZEITSCHRIFT FUER DAS GEBIET DER ROENTGENDIAGNOSTIK, see Radiologia diagnostica.

IRIGAKU RYOHO ZASSHI (Journal of medico-physical therapy); Tokyo, vol. 1- (1914-).

IRIGAKU SHINPO (Journal of physical medicine & radiotherapy); Osaka, vol. 1-11 (shigatsu 1932 - rokugatsu 1942).

*IRIGAKU SOSHO (Radiography series) - title varies: vol. (maki) 1-9, 1922-1930 Keio Rentogengaku Sosho; vol. 10-32, (rokugatsu) 1931-1940 Jissen Irigaku Sosho (Practical radiography series) - Tokyo, vol. 1- (1922-).

ISOTOPE IN MEDIZIN UND BIOLOGIE, see Nuclear Medizin.

ISOTOPE TECHNIQUES CONFERENCE, see Proceedings, Radioisotopes Conference.

ISOTOPICS, Announcements of the Isotopes Extension Division, Atomic Energy Commission, which are of civilian application; Oak Ridge, Tennessee, vol. 1-6 - of the latest only nr. 1-2 - (1951-1956).

IZDANJA, Centralni Rentgenoloski Institut, Zagreb Universitet; Zagreb, vol. 1- (February 1927-).

IZVESTYA KIEVSKOYE RENTGENOVSKAYA KOMMISSYA, Kiev, 15 issues, 1916-1918.

JAHRBUCH FÜR RÖNTGENOLOGEN; Berlin, W. de Gruyter & Co., vol. 1-2, 1930-1931.

*JAHRESBERICHT RADIOLOGIE, bibliographisches Jahresregister des (yearly index of the) Zentralblattes für die gesamte Radiologie; Berlin, J. Springer, vol. 1- (1926-).

JISSEN IRIGAKU SOSHO, see Irigaku Sosho.

JORNADAS RADIOLOGICAS ARENTÍNAS; 1st- (?); have seen the 4th (Rio Cuarto, 1947), Buenos Aires, El Ateneo, 1948.

*JOURNAL BELGE DE RADIOLOGIE, Annales de la *Société Belge de Radiologie* (title varies: April 1908-1923 Journal de radiologie); Bruxelles, vol. 1- (1907-). Since 1958 also official organ of the Dutch Society of Radiology.

JOURNAL DE L'ASSOCIATION CANADIENNE DES RADIOLOGISTES, see Journal of the Canadian Association of Radiologists.

*JOURNAL DE PHYSIQUE . . . ET LE RADIUM (title varies: Journal de physique théorique et appliquée through series 5, vol. 9 when it absorbed Radium (Paris)[2] and changed to latest title); Paris, series 1, vol. 1- (1872-); latest (fifth) series, vol 1- (January 1920-).

JOURNAL DE RADIOLOGIE, see Journal belge de radiologie.

*JOURNAL DE RADIOLOGIE, D'ÉLECTROLOGIE ET DE MÉDICINE NUCLÉAIRE, Revue médicale mensuelle; Paris, Masson & Cie, vol. 1- (1914-); absorbed Archives d'électricité médicale; contains also Bulletin de la *Société Française d'Électroradiologie Médicale* (and affiliated societies); publication suspended September 1914-April 1915.

JOURNAL OF ADVANCED THERAPEUTICS, see American Journal of Electrotherapeutics and Radiology.

JOURNAL OF ELECTROTHERAPEUTICS, see American Journal of Electrotherapeutics and Radiology.

*JOURNAL OF NUCLEAR MEDICINE, official publication of the *Society of Nuclear Medicine;* Chicago, Samuel N. Turiel & Associates, vol. 1- (1960-).

JOURNAL OF PHYSICAL THERAPEUTICS, see Medical Electrology and Radiology.

JOURNAL OF PHYSICAL THERAPY; Hammond, Indiana, F. S. Betz, vol. 1-2 - through nr. 7 - (September 1905 - March 1907); commercial house organ.

JOURNAL OF RADIATION RESEARCH, organ of the *Radiation Research Society;* Japan vol. 1- (1960-).

JOURNAL OF RADIOLOGY, see Archives of Physical Medicine and Rehabilitation.

JOURNAL OF RADIOLOGY AND PHYSICAL THERAPY, see Kanazawa Irigaku Sosho.

JOURNAL OF ROENTGENOLOGY, organ of the Western Roentgen Society; quarterly; Iowa City, vol. 1-2 (May 1918 - December 1919); superseded by Journal of Radiology.

*JOURNAL OF THE AMERICAN RADIOTHERAPY SOCIETY, Drown Laboratory of Radiotherapy; Hollywood, California, vol. 1- (June 1949-); superseded Journal of the Drown Radiotherapy.

*JOURNAL OF THE CANADIAN ASSOCIATION OF RADIOLOGISTS, also called Journal de l'*Association Canadienne de Radiologistes,* organ of the *Canadian Association of Radiologists;* quarterly; Montreal, vol. 1- (March 1950-).

*JOURNAL OF THE COLLEGE OF RADIOLOGISTS OF AUSTRALASIA, supersedes the Proceedings of . . .; official organ of the College of Radiologists of Australasia; Sydney; vol. 1-, 1957-.

JOURNAL OF THE DROWN RADIOTHERAPY, Drown Laboratory of Radiotherapy; Hollywood, vol. 1-3 (1940-1942), irregular; superseded by Journal of the American Radiotherapy Society.

JOURNAL OF THE FACULTY OF RADIOLOGISTS, see Clinical Radiology.

JOURNAL OF THE RÖNTGEN SOCIETY, for the Study and Discussion of X-Rays and Allied Phenomena in their Relation to Medicine, the Arts and Sciences, organ of the (British) Röntgen Society; London, vol. 1-24 (1904-1928); in 1927 the Röntgen Society and the British Institute of Radiology were amalgamated and the Journal of the Röntgen Society merged into the British Journal of Radiology.

KANAZAWA IKA DAIGAKU GYOSEKISHU (collected papers . . . on radiology); Kanazawa (Japan), Rigakuteki Shinryoka Kyoshitsu (1934-).

*KANAZAWA IRIGAKU SOSHO, Journal of Radiology and Physical Therapy, Kanazawa Medical University; (Kanazawa Japan), Rigakuteki Shinryoka Kyoshitsu, vol. 1- (gogatsu 1946-); table of contents and abstracts of articles in English.

KEIKO (Fluorescence); Japanese technical x-ray journal; 1927-1942.

KEIO RENTOGENGAKU SOSHO, See Irigaku Sosho.

KONGRESSBERICHT über die Tagung der *Medizinisch-Wissenschaftlichen Gesellschaft für Röntgenologie der Deutschen Demokratischen Republik;* Berlin (1955-).

LABORATORY AND CLINICAL STUDIES, see Memorial Hospital, New York.

LETTERATURA RADIOLOGICA ITALIANA, Indice bibliografico dei lavori italiani di radiologia; Milano, vol. 1 (1895-1935); vol. 2 (1936-1940) published as special number of Radiologia medica; 1946-1950 published as supplement to Radiologia medica.

*MAGYAR RADIOLOGIA, (title varies: vol. 1, Radiologia hungarica), organ of the *Orvos-Egeszségügyi Szakszerveset,* Radiologus Szakesoport; Budapest, vol. 1- (1949-).

MAGYAR RÖNTGEN KÖZLÖNY, organ of the *Röntgenverein Ungarischer Aerzte;* Budapest, Barta & Szekely, vol. 1-19 (1926-1944).

*MATERIALY PO TOXYKOLOGIY RADIOAKTIVNICH VESHEST, Trudy, Institut Gigieniy, Akademia Medizinskiy Nauk; Moskva vol. 1- (1957-); English translation (Materials on the Toxicology of Radioactive Substances), published at Oak Ridge, Tenn. 1- (1959-).

MEDICAL ELECTROLOGY AND RADIOLOGY, an International Quarterly Review (title varies: vol. 1-3, Journal of Physical Therapeutics); London, vol. 1-8 (1899-1907); absorbed by Proceedings of the Royal Society of Medicine, Section on Radiology.

*MEDICAL RADIOGRAPHY AND PHOTOGRAPHY (title varies: until July 1930 X-Ray Bulletin and Clinical Photography, published in Detroit; 1930-46 Radiography and Clinical Photography), Eastman Kodak Company; Rochester, New York, vol. 1- (May 1925-); index for vol. 1-10 (1925-1934) with vol. 10; commercial house organ; also edition in Spanish.

*MEDICA MUNDI, Philips Gloeilampenfabrieken; Eindhoven, Netherlands, vol. 1- (1955); commercial house organ.

*MEDICOR NEWS, Budapest; commercial house organ.

*MEDIZINISH TECHNISCHE ASSISTENTIN IN DER RADIOLOGIE, Zeitschrift für Röntgen-Assistentinnen. Organ of the *Vereinigung Deutscher Medizinisch Technischer Assistentinnen in der Radiologie;* Aachen; vol. 1-, 1961-.

*MEDIZIN TECHNIK, published by Vereinigung Volkseigener Betriebe Mechanik, Leipzig; (East German) commercial house organ; vol. 1-, 1961-.

*MEDIZINSKAYA RADIOLOGYA, Ministerstvo Zdravookhranienya S. S. R.; Moscva, Medgiz, vol. 1- (January-February 1956-).

MEMORIA, Instituto Municipal de Radiología y Fysioterapía; Buenos Aires (1934-).

MEMORIAL HOSPITAL FOR THE TREATMENT OF CANCER AND ALLIED DISEASES, NEW YORK CITY (title varies: Laboratory and Clinical Studies, Laboratory studies, Clinical Studies, sometimes sponsored by Collis P. Huntington Fund for Cancer Research, Bulletin, Radium Therapy, Radium Reports); New York (1905-); Laboratory and Clinical Studies 1-3 (1905-1912), 5-6 (1919-1925), 7-17 (1926-1936); Bulletin 1-2 (March 1929-May 1930); Clinical Studies 1 (1919-1923) and 2 (1924-1925); Radium Report(s) of the Memorial Hospital; New York, Paul B. Hoeber (1917-).

MÉTALIX, Philips, S. A., Department Métalix; Paris, vol. 1- (1951-); commercial house organ.

*MINERVA FISIOTERAPICA E RADIOBIOLOGICA Torino, vol. 1-; luglio 1956-.

*MINERVA NUCLEARE, supplement to Minerva medica, organ of the *Società Italiana di Biologia e Medicina Nucleare;* Torino, Edizioni Minerva Medica, vol. 1- (1957-).

MISSISSIPPI VALLEY MEDICAL JOURNAL, see Radiological Review.

MITTEILUNGEN AUS DEM INSTITUT FÜR RADIUMFOR-

---

*Its first report is of historic significance. The complete title was Radium Therapy in Cancer at the Memorial Hospital, by Henry H. Janeway . . . with the Discussion of Treatment of Cancer of the Bladder, by Benjamin S. Barringer . . . and an Introduction upon the Physics of Radium, by Gioacchino Failla.

SCHUNG; Wien, nrs. 1-228 (1911-1928); monographs, separately bound.

MITTEILUNGEN AUS DEM LABORATORIUM FÜR RADIOLOGISCHE DIAGNOSTIK UND THERAPIE, K. K. Allgemeines Krankenhaus, Wien; Jena, G. Fischer, nr. 1-2 (1907).

MITTEILUNGEN AUS DER KÖNIGLICH-KAISERLICHEN KURANSTALT FÜR RADIUMTHERAPIE IN ST. JOACHIMSTHAL; Wien, W. Braumüller (1915).

NEW YORK, MEMORIAL HOSPITAL, see Memorial Hospital, New York City.

*NIPPON ACTA RADIOLOGICA, Nippon Igaku Hoshasen Gakkai Zasshi, organ of the *Nippon Societas Radiologica* (Japan Radiological Society); Tokyo, vol. 1 (1940-); title in Japanese and Latin, text in Japanese with English or German abstracts; formed from merger of Nippon Hoshasen Igakkai Zasshi and Nippon Rentogen Gakkai.

*NIPPON HOSHASEN GIJUTSU GAKKAI ZASSHI (Japanese Journal of Radiologic Technology), supersedes Nippon Rentogen Gijutsu Gakkai. Kyoto, maki 2-, ichigatsu 1947- (Index for maki 1-8, 1944-1953 with maki 8).

NIPPON RENTOGEN GAKKAI; Tokyo, vol. 1-17 (1923-1940); had also a supplement, Rentogengaku Nippon Bunken (q.v.); merged with Nippon Hoshasen Igakkai Zasshi to form Nippon acta radiologica.

*NIPPON X-SEN GISHIKAI KAIHO (official organ of the *Japanese Association of X-Ray Technicians*). Tokyo, vol. 1- (1950-).

*NUCLEAR MEDIZIN, Isotope in Medizin und Biologie; Stuttgart, Friedrich-Karl Schattauer Verlag, vol. 1-, März 1959- (subtitle translated in French and English).

*NUCLEONICS, New York, vol. 1-, 1943-.

*NUNTIUS RADIOLOGICUS; published in various places, Firenze, Siena, latest is Belluno, Istituto di Radiologia dell'Università di Roma, vol. 1- (1933-).

ODELCA BULLETIN; Old Delft Bulletin issued separately; commercial house organ.

ONTARIO RADIOGRAPHER; vol. 1- (1940-).

OSAKA FURITSU HOSHASEN CHUO KENKYUSHO, SAKAI; annual report; Osaka, vol. 1-, 1960-.

PHYSICAL THERAPEUTICS (title varies: 1883-1889 Medical Library; 1890-1901 Journal of Electrotherapeutics; 1902-1915 (after absorbing Transactions, American Electrotherapeutic Association, and New York Lancet) Journal of Advanced Therapeutics; 1916-1925 American Journal of Electrotherapeutics and Radiology), organ of the *American Physical Therapy Association;* Elmira New York, vol. 1-50 (1883-1932); merged into Archives of Physical Medicine and Rehabilitation.

PICKER NEWS; Picker X-ray Corporation; Cleveland, vol. 1- (1937-); commercial house organ.

PICKER INTERNATIONAL COURIER; Picker X-ray Corporation; White Plains, New York; vol. 1- (1947?-); vol. 1, nr. 11 is dated April, 1949; commercial house organ.

POLISH REVIEW OF RADIOLOGY, see Polski Przeglad Radiologiczny

*POLSKI PRZEGLAD RADIOLOGICZNY, organ of *Polskiego Lekarskiego Towarzystwa Radiologicznego i Fizjoterapeutycznego;* pre-1938 issues have also subtitle Revue polonaise de radiologie; Wárszawa, Pánstwowy Zaklad Wydawnictw Lakarskich, vol. 1- (1926-); publication suspended with vol. 13 (1938), resumed after World War II; articles in Polish with summaries in French (before 1938), and after World War II with summaries in English and Russian. With tom 25 (1961), title changed to Polski Przeglad Radiologii i Medycyny Nuklearnej. It is now the official organ of *Polskie Lekarskie Towarzystwo Radiologiczne.* The journal was scheduled in 1963 to start a parallel English edition, the Polish Review of Radiology.

*POLSKI PRZEGLAD RADIOLOGICZNY, SUPPLEMENT - have seen nr. 2 (1953), which was XVI Zjazd Radiologow Polskich w Warszawie (May 21-23, 1953).

POSTEPY RADIOLOGII (Advances in radiology), Warszawa; vols. 1-3 (1954-1956); table of contents in English, Polish, and Russian. No more published.

PRIMENA RADIJAKTIVNIH IZOTOPA I JONIZUJUCIH ZRACENJA U MEDICINI; BILTEN, Beograd; Savezna Komisya za Nuklearnu Energiju i sekretarijat za Narodno Zdravijo; vol. 1-, 1960-.

PROBLÈMES DE ROENTGENOLOGIE ET DOMAINES ATTENANTS, see Voprosy Rentgenologiy i Smezinshnykh Oblastei.

*PROCEEDINGS, ANNUAL CONFERENCE OF TEACHERS OF (CLINICAL) RADIOLOGY; Chicago, *American College of Radiology,* sporadically numbered)21st, (1954-).

*PROCEEDINGS, COLLEGE OF RADIOLOGISTS OF AUSTRALASIA, see Journal of the College of Radiologists of Australasia.

PROCEEDINGS, INTERAMERICAN CONGRESS OF RADIOLOGY, see Actas, Congresso interamericano di radiología.

PROCEEDINGS, MEDICAL RADIOISOTOPES CONFERENCE

(OXFORD); New York City, Academic Press (1954-).

*PROCEEDINGS, INTERNATIONAL CONFERENCE ON RADIOBIOLOGY, with French subtitle Comptes-rendus de la Conférence internationale de radiobiologie (title varies: 1st meeting (1952) was informal; 2nd (1953) appeared in the Invited papers of the 7th International Congress of Radiology (Copenhagen); 3rd (1954) was called Proceedings of the Radiobiology Symposium; 4th (1955) was published as Progress in Radiobiology, and 5th (1956) as Advances in Radiobiology); New York, Academic Press (1953-); articles in English or French.

*PROCEEDINGS, INTERNATIONAL CONGRESS OF RADIOLOGY, 1st- (1925-).

PROCEEDINGS OF THE RADIOBIOLOGY SYMPOSIUM, see Proceedings of the International Conference on Radiobiology.

*PROCEEDINGS, RADIOISOTOPE CONFERENCE (1951 issued as Isotope Techniques Conference), sponsored by the Atomic Energy Research Establishment, Harwell (England); London, Butterworth Scientific Publications, 1st- (1951-).

*PROCEEDINGS, ROYAL SOCIETY OF MEDICINE, RADIOLOGY SECTION; superseded Medical Electrology and Radiology.

*PROCEEDINGS, SYMPOSIUM ON X-RAY MICROSCOPY AND MICRORADIOGRAPHY, sponsored by the International Union of Pure and Applied Physics; New York Academic Press, 1st- (1956-).

*PROGRESS, organ of the *Society of X-ray Technology;* Loughton (England), vol. 1- (February 1957-).

PROGRESS IN RADIATION THERAPIE; New York, Grune & Stratton (1958); 2nd volume (1963).

PROGRESS IN RADIOBIOLOGY, see Proceedings, International Conference on Radiobiology.

QUADERNI DI RADIOLOGIA, Collana di monografie, Instituto di Radiologia dell'Università di Pavia; Padova, vol. 1- (1955-).

QUADERNI RADIOLOGICI, Instituto Radiologico dell' Ospedale Civile di Belluno; Belluno, Cartolibreria, vol. 1-7 (1930-1936); a new series vol. 1- (1937-) was issued as Quaderni di radiologia, then re-issued after World War II.

RADIANCE MEDICAL JOURNAL; probably of osteopathic origin; mentioned in American X-Ray Journal of 1900.

*RADIATION RESEARCH, organ of the *Radiation Research Society;* New York, Academic Press, vol. 1- (February 1954-).

RADIATION THERAPY, Tumor Institute, annual supplement to the Staff Journal of the Swedish Hospital; Seattle, vol. 1- (February 1940-).

RADIAZIONI DI ALTA ENERGIA (pentalingual); Roma, vol. 1- (1962-).

RADIOBIOLOGIA GENERALIS; Venezzia vol. 1-? (?-1933); superseded by Archivio internazionale di radiobiologia.

*RADIOBIOLOGIA, RADIOTHERAPIA; Berlin, vol. 1- (March-April 1960-); articles in German, French, or English with summaries in the three languages.

*RADIOBIOLOGIYA, bimonthly; Moskva, Akademia Nauk., vol. 1-, 1961-.

*RADIOBIOLOGICA LATINA, Archivio internazionale di radiobiologia e di medicina nucleare, International Archives of Radiobiology and Nuclear Medicine; Milano, Istituto per la Diffusione di Opere Scientifiche, vol. 1- (January-March 1958-); articles in French, Italian, German, Spanish, Portuguese, and English, with summaries in several languages.

RADIOBIOLOGY SYMPOSIUM, see Proceedings, International Conference on Radiobiology.

*RADIO-DIAGNOSTIC ET RADIO-ANATOMIE DE PRÉCISION; Paris, Masson & Cie (1955?-); series of monographs.

RADIODONCIA, revista semestral, organ of the *Sociedad Odontológica Argentina de Radiología;* Buenos Aires, vol. 1- (1940-).

*RADIOGRAFÍA Y FOTOGRAFÍA CLINICAS (title varies: until vol. 4, nr. 2 (April-June 1938) it was called Radiografía), Eastman Kodak Company; Rochester, New York, vol. 1- (July-September 1935); Spanish edition of Radiography and Clinical Photography; commercial house organ.

RADIOGRAPHER, Journal of the Australasian Institute of Radiography; Sydney, vol. 1- (1948?-).

RADIOGRAPHIC AIDS FOR THE VETERINARY PRACTITIONER; quarterly; Chicago, Quaker Oats Co., vol. 1-, 1960-.

RADIOGRAPHIE, Revue mensuelle des applications médicales et industrielles des rayons de Roentgen; Paris, Payen, vol. 1- (1897-).

*RADIOGRAPHY, organ of the *Society of Radiographers;* London, vol. 1- (1935-); issued with the British Journal of Radiography.

RADIOGRAPHY AND CLINICAL PHOTOGRAPHY, see Medical Radiography and Photography.

RADIOISOTOPE CONFERENCE (TECHNIQUES), see Proceedings, Radioisotope Conference.

RADIOKHIMIYA, MOSKVA, Akademia Nauk SSSR; appears in English translations in Washington, D.C., and in Israel; vol. 1-, 1959-.

RADIOLOGE; Berlin (Göttingen-Heidelberg), vol. 1- (April 1961-).

*RADIOLOGIA (BUCURESTI), organ of the *Sectiunea de Radiologie, Societatea Stiintelor Medicale din România;* Bucuresti, Editura Medicală, vol. 1- (July-August 1956-); summaries in English, French, German, and Russian.

RADIOLOGÍA (Buenos Aires), organ of the *Sociedad Argentina de Radiología y de Difusion de la Radiología Sudamericana,* Revista medica bimestral; Buenos Aires, vol. 1- (1937?-); have seen vol. 5 (1942).

*RADIOLOGÍA (Panamá), started as organ of the *Sociedad Radiologica Panaména,* since 1960 it is the organ of the *Associación de Radiólogos de Centro-América y Panamá,* vol. 1- (1950-).

*RADIOLOGIA (ROMA), Rassegna internazionale trimestriale di radiobiologia, radioterapia, radiodiagnostica, terapia fisica e fisica applicata alla medicina; Roma, Istituto Bibliografico Italiano, vol. 1- (1941-); quarterly.

*RADIOLOGIA AUSTRIACA, organ of the *Oesterreichische Röntgengesellschaft;* Wien, Urban & Schwarzenberg, vol. 1- (1948-).

*RADIOLOGIA CLINICA (title, imprint, and sponsor vary; the only thing in common is the publisher; until February 1937, it was published in Berlin as Radiologische Rundschau, organ of the *Bayerische Gesellschaft für Röntgenologie und Radiologie*), Internationale radiologische Rundschau, International radiological review (also translated in French and Italian), organ of the *Schweizerische Gesellschaft für Radiologie und Nuklearmedizin* (until 1958 the *Schweizerische Röntgengesellschaft*); Basel, S. Karger, vol. 1- (June 1932-).

*RADIOLOGIA DIAGNOSTICA; Berlin, vol. 1- (January-February 1960-); text in German, with summaries in German, English, or French. Subtitle, Internationale Zeitschrift fuer das Gebiet der Roentgendiagnostik.

RADIOLOGIA E FISICA MEDICA, see Radioterapia, radiobiologia e fisica medica.

RADIOLOGIA HUNGARICA, see Magyar Radiologia.

RADIOLOGIA INTERAMERICANA, Colorado Springs, vol. 1, nr. 1, 1962; organ of the *Interamerican College of Radiology.* No more published.

*RADIOLOGIAI KÖZLEMENYEK, organ of the Landesröntgen- und Strahlenphysikalischen Institut; Budapest, vol. 1- (1959?-); mimeographed; mostly abstracts.

*RADIOLOGIA MEDICA, organ of the *Società Italiana di Radiologia Medica;* previously published in Milano, now in Torino, Minerva Medica, vol. 1- (1914-).

RADIOLOGÍA ORAL, organ of the Catedra de Radiología, Escuela de Odontología; Habana, vol. 1- (March 1948-).

RADIOLOGIA PRATICA; Genova, vol. 1- (May 1951-).

RADIOLOGIA SPERIMENTALE; Parma Maccari Editore, vol. 1-3 (1937-1939).

RADIOLOGICA, see Fundamenta radiologica.

*RADIOLOGICA-CANCEROLOGICA, Revista ibérica de ciencias médicas, organ of the *Sociedad Española de Radiología y Electrología Médicas;* Madrid, vol. 1-6 (1946-1951); superseded by Acta ibérica radiologica-cancerologica, also organ of *Sociedade Portuguesa de Radiologia Medica.*

*RADIOLOGICAL CLINICS OF NORTH AMERICA, Philadelphia, W. B. Saunders, vol. 1- (1963-).

*RADIOLOGICAL HEALTH DATA, Quarterly (now monthly) report, U. S. Public Health Service, Division of Radiological Health, Washington, D.C., vol. 1- (1960-); superseded (mimeographed ?) Monthly Radiological Health Data Reports.

RADIOLOGICAL HEALTH NEWS, Berkeley (California) Bureau of Radiologic Health; vol. 1-, October 1961-.

*RADIOLOGICAL REVIEW AND MISSISSIPPI VALLEY MEDICAL JOURNAL, (title varies: appeared as Radiological Review until 1927 when it united with Chicago Medical Recorder, and continued as Radiological Review and Chicago Medical Recorder, with volume numbering of the latter; with vol. 58 it changed to Radiological Review and Mississippi Valley Medical Journal); Quincy, Illinois, Radiological Review Publishing Company, vol. 1-5 (1924-1927), then vol. 49- (1927-).

*RADIOLOGIC TECHNOLOGY, Detroit; organ of the *American Society of Radiologic Technologists* (name of sponsor changed from American Association of Radiological Technicians in 1930 to American Society of Radiographers, then American Society of X-Ray Technicians). Name of publication was X-Ray Technician from vol. 1- (1929-) until July 1963 when current name was adopted.

RADIOLOGIE, Supplement to Bulletin Medical; Paris, nr. 1-8 (June 29 - December 14, 1910) and new series nr. 1-6 (January 15 - June 24, 1911).

Radiologie et chirurgie; Bruxelles, Chambier, vol. 1 - through nr. 5 - (January - May 1925).

Radiologie pratique, Documentation analytique et pratique radiologique; Lyon, Editions Médicales Cartier, Vol. 1 - nr. 1-4 - (1946-1948).

Radiologische Mitteilungen; Kreuznach, Germany, vol. 1- (?).

Radiologische Praktika, monographs in book form, first published at Frankfurt am Main, by Keim & Nemnich (the first being S. Hirsch's *Die peripheren Blutgefässe im Röntgenbilde,* 1924), then published in Leipzig, by Georg Thieme (for instance Karl Goldhamer's *Normal Anatomy of the Head as Seen by X-ray,* in a German translation, 1930-31), vol. 1-20 (1924-1933).

Radiologische Rundschau, see Radiologia clinica.

*Radiology, a monthly journal devoted to clinical radiology and allied sciences, organ of the *Radiological Society of North America;* published first in Chicago, then in St. Paul, now in Syracuse (New York), vol. 1- (September 1923-); Cumulative Indices: vol. 1-39 (1923-1942), vol. 40-49 (1943-1947), vol. 50-59 (1948-1952), vol. 60-69 (1953-1957), vol. 70-79 (1958-1962).

Radiology Reporter, Published monthly by Winthrop Laboratories to report some of the significant data given at medical meetings of interest to radiologists; New York, vol. 1 - only nr. 1-10 - (January - October 1959); commercial house organ.

*Radioloski Glasnik, Review of Yugoslav radiology (translated on face page, also in German and French); Zagreb, vol. 1- (1937-).

Radiophysiologie et radiothérapie; Recueil de travaux biologiques, techniques et thérapeutiques, also called Archives de l'Institut du Radium de l'-Université de Paris et de la Foundation Curie: Paris, Les Presses Universitaires de France, vol. 1-3 - through nr. 4 - (1927-1939); irregular.

Radio, Roentgen es Egyeb Sugarzasok, organ of the *Radioklub der Budapester Polytechnischen Hochschule* and of the *Röntgengesellschaft der Ungarischen Aerzte;* Budapest, vol. 1 (December 1924-June 1925).

Radioterapia, radiobiologia e fisica medica (title varies: formed by merger of Radioterapie e fisica medica, Scritti italiani di radiobiologia, and Bollettino di marconiterapia; 1934-1938 Radiologica e fisica medica; 1939-1943? Radioterapia e fisica media), organ of the *Associazione Italiana di Radioterapia;* Bologna, Licinio Cappelli, third series, vol. 1 - (1946-).

Radiqueno, General Electric Company; Chicago (1946-); Spanish edition of the Radsidian; commercial house organ.

Radium (New York), Abstracts of selected articles on radium and radium therapy, compiled by American Institute of Medicine for United States Radium Corporation; New York City, printed by Adams & Grace (1922-).

Radium (Paris)[1], Publication mensuelle; Paris, vol. 1 - through nr. 6 - (January - June 1904).

Radium (Paris)[2], La radioactivité et les radiations, les sciences qui s'y rattachent et leurs applications, Publication mensuelle; Paris, vol. 1-11 (July 1904-December 1919); suspended publication from July 1914 through April 1919; merged into Journal de physique et Le radium.

Radium (Pittsburgh), devoted to the chemistry, physics and therapeutics of radium and other radio-active substances; Pittsburgh, 1st series, vol. 1-18 (1913-1922); new series vol. 1-3 (1922-January 1925); third series 2 numbers only (April and October 1925).

Radium Commission (Great Britain), see Reports, National Radium Commission.

Radiumculture; Paris (?)

Radium Digest, Radium Service Corporation of America; Chicago vol. 1-2 - through nr. 7 - 1929-1931.

Radium in Biologie und Heilkunde, Monatsschift für biologisch-therapeutische Forschung; Lepizig, J. A. Barth, vol. 1-2 (May 1911-December 1913); united with Strahlentherapie.

Radium Light; St. Louis (?).

Radium Quarterly; Chicago, vol. 1 - only nr. 1-2 - (January-April 1917).

Radium Report(s), see Report(s); see also Memorial Hospital, New York, City.

Radium Therapie; Dresden, vol. 1-2 (1913).

Radium Therapist, a publication devoted to his interest, Radium Company of Colorado; Denver, vol. 1-2 (1922-1933).

Radium Therapy, see Memorial Hospital, New York City.

Radsidian, General Electric Company; Chicago (1946-); commercial house organ; had also a Spanish edition (Radiqueno).

*Rayonixar, Compagnie Générale de Radiologie; Paris (1952-); publication suspended 1936-1951; previous title: Revue de la CGR; commercial house organ.

Rayons X (Montréal), l'Electricité médicale et la

physicothérapie, Revue mensuelle illustree; Montréal, vol. 1 - through nr. 7 - (1910).

RAYONS X (PARIS), Annales de radiologie théorique et appliquée; Paris, vol. 1 (February 5, 1898 - April 22, 1899); weekly!

*REFERATOVY VYBER Z ROENTGENOLOGIE; Praha, Ustav pro Zdravotnickou Dokumentaci, vol. 1- (1957-).

RENTGENOVSKIY VIESTNIK; Odessa, vol. 1 - only three issues - (1907).

*RENTOGENGAKU NIPPON BUNKEN, Supplement to Nippon Rentogen Gakkai; Tokyo, vol. 1- (1924-).

REPORT(S), MEDICAL USES OF RADIUM, Summary of reports from research centers, prepared by Medical Research Council; London, H. M. Stationery Office (1924-); special report series nr. 90, 102, 112, 116.

REFORT(S), MOUNT VERNON HOSPITAL AND THE RADIUM INSTITUTE; Northwood, Middlesex, vol. 1- (192-); combination narrative and statistical report of the English national center for the treatment of cancer.

REPORT(S), NATIONAL RADIUM COMMISSION; London, H. M. Stationery Office (1930-).

REPORT(S), QUEENSLAND RADIUM INSTITUTE; Brisbane (1945?-).

REPORT(S), RADIOBIOLOGICAL LABORATORY, Agricultural Research Council; Wantage (England), nr. 1- (1959-).

REPORT(S), RADIUM INSTITUTE; London vol. 1-12 (1913-1924); the first, reprinted from the British Medical Journal (January 25, 1913), covers period August 14, 1911 - December 31, 1912; reports for 1925-1927 issued as monographs; later reports not published.

*REPORT(S), UNITED STATES ATOMIC ENERGY COMMISSION, prepared by the Radiological Laboratory, University of California (San Francisco); Oak Ridge, AEC Technical Information Service Extension, nr. 1- (1946-); several classified.

REVIEW OF YUGOSLAV RADIOLOGY, see Radiološki Glasnik.

*REVISTA BRASILEIRA DE RADIOLOGIA, organ of the *Colegio Brasileiro de Radiologia;* Sao Paulo, vol 1- (1958-); papers in Portuguese, with summaries in English; includes abstracts.

REVISTA DE LA SOCIEDAD ARGENTINA DE RADIO Y ELECTROLOGÍA, Crónica de sesiones, Publicatión de la Asociación médica argentina; Buenos Aires, vol. 1- nr. 1-2 - (May-December 1925); minutes of sessions, previously published in Revista de la Asociación médica argentina; continued in Revista de especialidades.

REVISTA DE MEDICINA FÍSICA, Instituto Nacional de Radium, Universidad Nacional; Buenos Aires, vol. 1- (March 1932-).

REVISTA DE RADIOLOGIA E CLINICA (title varies slightly; first eight numbers called Revista de radiologia clinica); Porto Alegre (Brasil), vol. 1-3 (1932-1934).

REVISTA DE RADIOLOGÍA - X, Revista de roentgenología, Periodico cientifico mensual en lengua castellana; Berlin, vol. 1-4 (1923-1926).

REVISTA DE RADIOLOGÍA Y FISIOTERAPÍA, General Electric Corporation; Chicago, vol. 1- (1934-); commercial house organ.

REVISTA DE RADIOLOGÍA Y FISIOTERAPÍA, official organ of the Sociedad Educatoriana Ecuatoriana de Radiología y Fisioterapia; Guayaquil, vol. 1- (1954-).

REVISTA ESPAÑOLA DE ELECTROLOGÌA Y RADIOLOGÍA MEDICAS, Valencia; vol. 1-, 1910 ?-

REVISTA GENERAL DE ROENTGENOLOGÍA, Supplement to Revista de ciencias médicas de Barcelona; Barcelona (June-July 1911 - May-December 1913).

*REVISTA MEXICANA DE RADIOLOGÍA, organ of the *Sociedad Mexicana de Radiología y Fisioterapía* (current appelation is without "y Fisioterapia"); Mexico, D. F., vol. 1- (1947).

*REVISTA PERUANA DE RADIOLOGÍA, organ of the *Sociedad Peruana de Radiología;* Lima, vol. 1- (1946-).

REVISTA PRACTICA DE RADIUMTERAPÍA, organ of the *Associacion Argentina de Radium;* Buenos Aires, vol. 1- (1926-).

REVUE D'ACTINOLOGIE ET DE PHYSIOTHÉRAPIE (title varies: 1925-1927 Revue de physiothérapie, 1928 Revue d'actinologie, 1929- combined title); Paris, Expansion Scientifique Française, vol. 1-15 (1925-1939).

REVUE DE LA CGR, Compagnie Générale de Radiologie; Paris, vol. 1-6 (1930-1935); continued in 1952 as Rayonixar; commercial house organ.

REVUE DE PHYSIOTHÉRAPIE CHIRURGICALE ET DE RADIOLOGIE; Paris, vol. 1- (1910?-); have seen issues from May 1911 through January 1913 (New York Academy of Medicine).

REVUE DES ÉTABLISSEMENTS GAIFFE-GALLOT ET PILON Gaiffe-Galot & Pilon; Paris (1922?-); commercial house organ.

REVUE GÉNÉRALE INTERNATIONALE D'ÉLECTRORADIOLOGIE ET D'ACTINOLOGIE: Bordeaux vol. 1- (1928-); abstracts.

REVUE INTERNATIONALE D'ÉLECTROTHÉRAPIE ET DE RADIOTHÉRAPIE; title varies, Revue internationale d'Electrotherapie (vol. 1-6); A. Maloine, Paris, vols. 1-14 (August 1890-June 1905). Vols. 2-3, official organ of the *Société Française d'Electrotherapie.*

REVUE POLONAISE DE RADIOLOGIE, see Polski przeglad radiologiczny.

REVUE PRATIQUE DE RADIUMTHÉRAPIE, Rayonnements, émanations, substances radioactives diverses, et Archives générales de thérapeutique physique réunies; Paris, vol. 1- (May 1914-).

*RINSHO HOSHASEN (Clinical Radiology); Tokyo, Kanehara Medical Book Co., vol. 1-, shigatsu 1956-.

RIVISTA DI RADIOLOGIA, Officine Elettrotechnice Italiane Arcioni; Milano, vol. 1-2 (May-June 1947 - January-April 1949); publication suspended during 1948; commercial house organ.

RIVISTA DI RADIOLOGIA; Official organ of the *Associazione Romana di Radiologia e di Electrologia,* Roma, Editura Universo, vol. 1- (1961-).

RIVISTA DI RADIOLOGIA CLINICA, see Rivista italiana di radiologia clinica.

RIVISTA DI RADIOLOGIA E FISICA MEDICA, see Annali di radiologia diagnostica.

RIVISTA ITALIANA DI RADIOLOGIA CLINICA (title varies: first volume issued as Rivista di radiologia clinica); Pescia, vol. 1- (1951-).

ROCENKA ČESKOLOVENSKÉ SPOLECNOSTI PRO RENTGENOLOGII A RADIOLOGII, annual meeting publications of the Ceskoslovenské Spolecnosti pro rentgenologii a radiologii; Praha, vols. 1-3, 1927, 1929, 1936.

*RÖNTGEN BLÄTTER, Zeitschrift für Röntgen-Technik und medizinisch-wissenschaftliche Photographie; published in Berlin, vol. 1-10 (1931-1940); after World War II, issued again as vol. 1- (May 1948-) in Baden-Baden, by Verlag für Kunst und Wissenschaft; published since August 1949 in Wuppertal-Elberfeld by Verlag W. Girardet; now bimonthly.

ROENTGENDIAGNOSTIK, ERGEBNISSE; Stuttgart, Georg Thieme (1952-1956-); published also in English translation as Roentgendiagnostics, Progress Volume (Grune & Stratton, 1958).

ROENTGEN ECONOMIST (title varies: started as a mimeographed Bulletin), organ of the *New York Society of A.M.A. approved Roentgenologists;* New York, vol. 1-6 - through nr. 4 - (January 1933-April 1938).

ROENTGEN-EUROP (trilingual); Paris, vol. 1- (1962-).

RÖNTGENHILFE, see Zeitschrift für Röntgenologie.

RÖNTGENKALENDER, see Röntgentaschenbuch.

RÖNTGENKUNDE IN EINZELDARSTELLUNGEN; Berlin, J. Springer, vol. 1-4 (1928-1931); monographs.

RÖNTGENLITERATUR, im Auftrage der Deutschen Röntgengesellschaft und unter Mitarbeit des Literatursonderausschusses; Stuttgart, Ferdinand Enke Verlag, vol. 1-15 (1911-1936).

RÖNTGENOLOGIA; Budapest, vol. 1-9 (1922-1929).

RÖNTGENOLOGIE, eine Revision ihrer technischen Einrichtungen und praktischen Methoden; Wien, vol. 1 (1918) and 2 - only 2 issues - (1924).

RÖNTGENPHOTOGRAPHIE, MEDIZINISCHE PHOTOGRAPHIE UND MEDIZINISCHE LABORATORIUMPRAXIS, see Röngten- und Laboratoriumpraxis.

RÖNTGENPRAXIS, Diagnostik, Röntgen-, Radium-, Lichttherapie, organ of the *Deutsche Röntgengesellschaft;* Berlin, Georg Thieme, vol. 1-17 - through nr. 6-7 - (March 1929-1948); suspended 1945-1947; appeared originally as a supplement to, but later merged with, Fortschritte auf dem Gebiete der Röntgenstrahlen.

RÖNTGENSTRAHLEN, Geschichte und Gegenwart, C. H. F. Müller, G. M. B. H.; Hamburg, vol. 1- (1951-); commercial house organ.

RÖNTGENTASCHENBUCH, (title varies: first volume called Röntgenkalender), zugleich ein kleines "Jahrbuch für die Fortschritte auf dem Gebiete der physikalischen Therapie" (subtitle varies); Frankfurt-am-Main, Keim & Nemnich, vol. 1-9 (1908-1924).

RÖNTGENTECHNISCHE BERICHTE, Gevaert (?); Braunschweig (1930-1932), commercial house organ.

*RÖNTGEN- UND LABORATORIUMPRAXIS (title varies: until vol. 3, nr. 6 (September 1950) called Röntgenphotographie, medizinische Photographie und medizinische Laboratoriumpraxis); Stuttgart, S. Hirzel, vol. 1- (October 1947-).

RÖNTGOGRAPHIE IN DER INNEREN MEDICIN; Wiesbaden, J. F. Bergmann, vol. 1-5 (1901-1902).

SAFETY SERIES, International Atomic Energy Agency; Vienna, nr. 1- (1958-).

SAISHIN CHIRYO, Therapie der Gegenwart (Radium); Tokyo, vol. 1-17 (junigatsu 1924-1941); united with Ijin, Chiryo Iakuho, and Yamanouchi Tokuho into Chiryo Igaku (1941-1943-).

SCRITTI ITALIANI DI RADIOBIOLOGIA, organ of the *Associazione Italiana di Radiobiologia;* Bologna, vol. 1-10 (1934-1946); merged into Radioterapia, radiobiologia e fisica medica.

*SCINTILLATOR; Picker X-Ray Corporation; White

Plains, New York, vol. 1- (1952?-); commercial house organ.

SHIMADZU RENTOGEN JIHO (Shimadzu roentgen news), 64 issues 1912-1942; then merged into Shimadzu Hyoron; commercial house organ.

*SRW-NACHRICHTEN, Siemens-Reiniger Werke; Erlangen, Germany, vol. 1- (?-); commercial house organ (also issues SRW-Mitteilungen).

STATISTICAL REPORT(S), CHRISTIE HOSPITAL AND HOLT INSTITUTE, Manchester (title varies slightly); imprint varies, published 1932-1933 in Stockport by Rowland Berry & Co., later in Edinburgh, by E. & S. Livingston, vol. 1- (1932/1933); have seen also 1946 volume, with 5 and 10 year assessments (prepared by Ralston Patterson, Margaret Tod, and Marion Russel).

STAHLENBIOLOGIE, STRAHLENTHERAPIE, NUKLEARMEDIZIN UND KREBSFORSCHUNG; Stuttgart, Georg Thieme, vol. 1- - covering 1952-1958 - (1959-).

*STRAHLENTHERAPIE (ORIGINALE), Mitteilungen aus dem Gebiete der Behandlung mit Röntgenstrahlen, Licht und radioaktiven Substanzen; zugleich Zentralorgan für Krebs- und Lupusbehandlung, organ of the *Deutsche Röntgengesellschaft,* of the *Gesellschaft füe Lichtforschung,* and of the *Deutscher Zentralausschuss für Krebsbekämpfung und Krebsforschung;* Berlin, Urban & Schwarzenberg, vol. 1- (June 1912-); indexes: vol. 1-6 (1912-1915) in vol. 6; vol. 1-25 (1912-1927), vol. 1-50 (1912-1934), and vol. 51-100 (1935-1956) as separate volumes.

STRAHLENTHERAPIE (REFERATE); Berlin, Urban & Schwarzenberg, vol. 1 - covering 1914 - (1916); abstracts; no more published.

STRAHLENTHERAPIE (SONDERBÄNDE); Berlin, Urban & Schwarzenberg, vol. 1- (1912-); monographs, in book form, with separate title-pages.

STRATIGRAFIA; Roma, vol. 1- (1956?-).

SUPPLEMENT ON ROENTGENOLOGY, published quarterly in the Interstate Medical Journal; St. Louis (1910?-); have seen 1915 and 1916 issues.

SYMPOSIUM NEURO-RADIOLOGICUM; 3rd - Stockholm (1952), 4th - London (1955), 5th - Bruxelles (1957).

SYMPOSIUM ON X-RAY MICROSCOPY AND MICRORADIOGRAPHY, see Proceedings, Symposium on X-Ray Microscopy and Microradiography.

THERAPIE DER GEGENWART, see Saishin chiryo.

TRANSACTIONS, AMERICAN ELECTROTHERAPEUTIC ASSOCIATION; Annual meeting; imprint varies; vol. 1-10 published in Philadelphia, the others in New York, vol. 1-19 (1891-1910); continued as Journal of Advanced Therapeutics.

TRANSACTIONS, AMERICAN ROENTGEN RAY SOCIETY; first two meetings never published, nr. 3 published in Louisville, nr. 5 in Philadelphia, the others in Pittsburgh, vol. 3-9 (1902-1905); indexed in Consolidated Indices, American Journal of Roentgenology I (1903-1937); superseded by American Quarterly of Roentgenology.

TRANSACTIONS, SECTION ON RADIOLOGY, AMERICAN MEDICAL ASSOCIATION, actual title: Transactions of the Section on Miscellaneous Topics, Radiology, of the A.M.A., at the 76th annual session, Atlantic City, May 25-29, 1925; Chicago, 1925; *Section on Radiology of the A.M.A.* was created in 1925; no more published in this form.

TRUDY, KIEVSKOGO GOSUDARSTVENNOGO RENTGENO-RADIOLOGICHESKOGO INSTITUTA, see Voprosy Rentgenologiy i Smezhnykh Oblastei.

*TÜRK RADYOLOJI MECMUASI, organ of the *Türk Radyoloji Cemiyeti* (founded 1924); Istanbul, vol. 1- (1955-).

*UCHENYE ZAPISKI, Rentgeno-Radiologicheskii i Onkologicheskii Institut; Kiev, vol. 1- (1949-).

*VERHANDLUNGEN, DEUTSCHE RÖNTGENGESELLSCHAFT; Stuttgart, Georg Thieme, vol. 1- (1905); since 1922 issued as supplement to Fortschritte auf dem Gebiete der Röntgenstrahlen; transactions of the meetings of the *Deutsche Röntgengesellschaft.*

*VESTNIK RENGENOLOGIY I RADIOLOGIY, Jurnal Gosudarstvennogo Rentgenologicheskogo i Radiologicheskogo Instituta; imprint varies, Petersburg, Gosudarstvennoe Izdatelstvo, then Leningrad, vol. 1- (1919-); had a French edition, Annales de roentgenologie et radiologie.

VICTOR (SEMI-) MONTHLY X-OGRAM, Victor X-Ray Corporation; Chicago, vol. 1- (August 1, 1916-); superseded by Victor News; commercial house organ.

VOPROSY NEVRORENTGENOLOGIY; Kiev, Gosudarstvennoye Medizinskoye Izdatelstvo, 1939; no more published.

VOPROSY OBSHCHEY I CHASTNOE RENTGENOLOGIY, Gosudarstvennoe Institut dlya Usovershenstvovanniya Vrachey; Moscva, Izdatelstvo Akadsemiy Nauk S.S.R., vol. 1- (1935-).

*VOPROSY RADIOBIOLOGIY, Centralniy Nauchno-Issledovateskiy Rentgeno-Radiologicheskiy Institut; Leningrad, vol. 1- (1956-).

*VOPROSY RENTGENOLOGIY I ONKOLOGIY, Nauchno-Isseldovatelskiy Institut Rentgenologiy i Onkologiy;

Erevan, vol. 1- (1950-).

VOPROSY RENTGENOLOGIY I SMEZHNYKH OBLASTEI, (on added title-page: Problèmes de roentgenologie et domaines attenants), Trudy Kievskogo Gosudarstvennogo Rentgeno-Radiologicheskogo Instituta; Kiev, Gosudarstvennoe Meditsinskoe Izdatelstvo, vol. 1- (1936-); French summaries.

WATSON X-RAY NEWS; North Wembley, Middlesex (England); commercial house organ.

WORLD RADIOLOGY CURRENT ABSTRACTS, Mallinckrodt Chemical Works; St. Louis, vol. 1- (1958-); commercial house organ.

X-RAY BULLETIN AND CLINICAL PHOTOGRAPHY, see Medical Radiography and Photography.

X-RAYS (KENTVILLE), see Health Rays.

X-RAYS (NAKANOSHIMA); Osaka, vol. 1- (1940-1956).

X-RAY STUDIES, Research Laboratory, General Electric Company; imprint varies: first volume in Schenectady, New York (1919), later volumes in Chicago, vol. 1- (1919-); reprints of papers by staff members, previously published in scientific periodicals.

X-RAY SUPPLEMENT, in Practitioner; London, vol. 1- (7-).

X-RAY TECHNICIAN, see Radiologic Technology.

*YEAR BOOK, BRITISH INSTITUTE OF RADIOLOGY, incorporated with the *Röntgen Society;* London, vol. 1- (1930-); list of members and other information.

*YEAR BOOK OF RADIOLOGY; Chicago, Year Book Publishers, vol. 1- (1932-); abstracts.

*YOUR RADIOLOGIST, American College of Radiology; Chicago (Spring 1956-); for the laity.

ZEITSCHRIFT FÜR DIE GESAMTE PHYSIKALISCHE THERAPIE, see Zentralblatt für die gesamte Radiologie.

ZEITSCHRIFT FÜR MEDIZINISCHE ELEKTROLOGIE UND RÖNTGENKUNDE (title varies: vol. 1-3 Zeitschrift für Electrotherapie und ärztliche Electrotechnik; vol. 4-6 Zeitschrift für Elektrotherapie und physikalische Heilmethoden; vol. 7-8 Zeitschrift für Elektrotherapie und Elektrodiagnostik einschliesslich der Röntgendiagnostik und Röntgentherapie, vol. 9-11 Zeitschrift für medizinische Elektrologie und Röntgenkunde); Leipzig, J. A. Barth, vol. 1-11 (1899-1910); in 1910 it was divided into two distinct sets: Zeitschrift für medizinische Elektrologie und Zeitschrift für Röntgenkunde und Radiumfoschung, each periodical continuing the volume numbering of the original journal; also imprint varies: vol. 1-3 Coblenz, W. Groos, vol. 4-5 Berlin, Vogel & Kreienbrink.

ZEITSCHRIFT FÜR RÖNTGEN-ASSISTENTINNEN, see Medizinisch Technische Assistentin in der Radiologie.

ZEITSCHRIFT FÜR RÖNTGENKUNDE UND RADIUMFORSCHUNG, continues volume numbering of Zeitschrift für Elektrologie und Röntgenkunde; Leipzig, J. A. Barth, vol. 12-15 (1910-1913), ceased publication.

ZEITSCHRIFT FÜR RÖNTGENOLOGIE (title varies: vol. 1-3 Röntgenhilfe); Berlin, C. F. Pilger & Co., vol. 1-13 (1921-1933).

ZEITSCHRIFT FÜR RÖNTGENTECHNIK, see Röntgen Blätter.

*ZENTRALBLATT FÜR DIE GESAMTE RADIOLOGIE; until 1930 appeared as Zeitschrift für die gesamte physikalische Therapie, Abteilung B, Referatenorgan of the *Deutsche Röntgengesellschaft;* Berlin, Julius Springer Verlag, vol. 1- (1926-); has supplement Jahresbericht Radiologie (1926-1944), resumed after World War II (1952-).

ZENTRALBLATT FÜR RÖNTGENSTRAHLEN, RADIUM UND VERWANDTE GEBIETE; Wiesbaden, J. F. Bergmann, vol. 1-10 (1910-1919); ceased publication.

ZISSEN IRIGAKU SOSHO, see Irigaku Sosho.

ZJAZD RADIOLOCOW POLSKICH, see Supplement to Polski Przeglad Radiologizny.

ZWANGLOSE ABHANDLUNGEN AUS DEM GEBIETE DER MEDIZINISCHEN ELEKTROLOGIE UND RÖNTGENKUNDE (title varies: nr. 1-7 Zwanglose Abhandlungen aus dem Gebiete der Elektrotherapie und Radiologie und verwandter Disziplinen der medizinischen Elektrotechnik); Leipzig, J. A. Barth, nr. 1-11 (1904-1912); no more published.

Chapter 8

ANNOTATED "RADIO-HISTORIC" BIBLIOGRAPHY

The images of men's wits and knowledge
remain in Books, exempted from the wrong of time,
and capable of perpetual renovation.
FRANCIS BACON, *The Advancement of Learning* (1605)

"THE ENORMOUS multiplication of books in every branch of knowledge is one of the greatest evils of this age; since it presents one of the most serious obstacles to the acquisition of current information by throwing in the reader's way piles of lumber in which he must painfully grope for the scraps of useful matter, peradventure interspersed." This quotation—dated 1845—comes from the pen of the "unhappy" Edgar Allan Poe (1809-1849). The same thought had occurred, in a more constructive way, to Miguel de Cervantes Saavedra (1547-1616) who—back in 1615—knew of no book so bad that something good could not be found in it.

A staggering amount of lumber went into such printed matter as is considered pertinent *to t*he history of radiology: much less has been written *about* it. The following bibliography is restricted to "radio-historic" titles proper. An earlier version contained several adulterating "radio-philosophic" items, but those have since been transferred to the roentgen reporting references, posted at the end of the chapter on Wishful Thinking in the labeling of shadows.

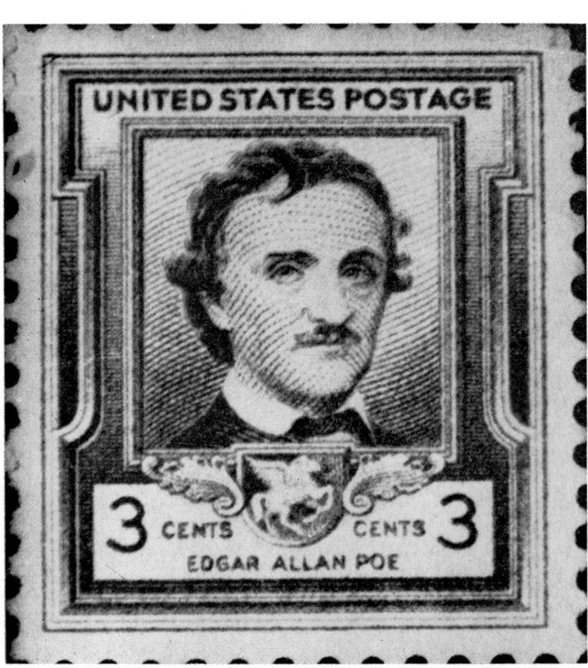

Perusal of the names in this bibliography proves that a representative sample of the choicest brains in the specialty can be compiled simply by listing those who have written on the history of radiology. To achieve nominal representation, a few titles—which are neither historically valid, nor instructive, perhaps not even amusing—had to be included for their signature only. Their lack of significance has been disguised by non-committal annotations (sufficiently clever, I hope, to defy immediate recognition). In this respect I follow—most of the time—the policy of the *National Geographic Magazine* which is never to print any thing definitely derogatory.

A number of bibliographic titles are self-explanatory: no notation was added, *i.e.,* no "gilding of the lily." No biographies were included, except those of Röntgen. This rule has been broken for a few eulogies which contained special material.

Historic compositions, much like "comprehensive" examinations, bring out a certain amount of factual material, eagerly displayed by any self-respecting examinee or would-be historian. They also reveal the depth to which the subject under consideration has been explored. Most of all, they provide clues to the author-candidate's general (especially cultural) background, or to the lack of it, as the case may be.

"Excerpted bibliography" might have seemed more correct for some of the titles in this chapter, but "annotated" was preserved, just because it "sounded better to the naked eye."

The AMA, in order to facilitate the location of a journal requested on loan from its library, insisted on getting the following indications: name(s) of author(s), full title of paper, name of periodical (abbreviated as in the *Index Medicus*), volume number, first and last pages of paper, finally the paper's date of publication with month (and day, if possible). This then became the "American way" of giving a bibliography. It is not altogether inadvertent, as it often obliges one to really "look up" the original. Such information is seldom needed when trying to locate the item in a library: as soon as it is bound, the (German) *Fortschritte auf dem Gebiete der Röntgen-Strahlen* displays no dates other than for the volume and the year. The (Italian) *Annali di Radiologia Diagnostica* uses only volume numbers, but not the year of publication, except in the printer's mark.

In the ensuing (but not in the roentgen reporting) references, the month has been omitted. First and last page numbers have been included, as they permit a rough estimate of size. Size alone may actually be misleading: a lot of material can be crowded into a few pages, or less than that diluted into a redundant monograph.

The first draft of this "radio-historic" bibliography was heavily annotated. It burst at the seams with cross-references and footnotes, in the manner of that scholarly exercise in academic futility, which is so endeared to "real" historians.*

In 1642, the English clergyman Thomas Fuller (1608-1661) remarked sadly that "learning hath gained most of those books by which the printers have lost." Today things are different, at least in this country. If properly advertised, any professional book (meaning one of which the cost is deductible for income tax purposes) can be printed and sold in the USA with a reasonable profit - unless said book is hopelessly abstruse, its binding defective, or its cover unattractive.

After a bit of hesitation I decided to shave off the excess of hopelessly abstruse marginalia. Their limited "contribution to learning" failed to compensate for the annoyance which such excess might have produced in the majority of readers. Most of all, the shaving helped in its own, however diminutive, way to reduce a fraction from this inevitable addition to radiologic lumber.

**Et in Arcadia ego!* I, too, have committed such "futilities." My note in *Isis* (of December, 1957) contained more substance in the footnotes than in the supernatant text. In the last decades of his life, George Sarton (1884-1956), the "father of the history of science," was literally unable to write without footnotes: he used them in his personal letters, even in the notes he wrote for himself. *Quod licet Jovis . . .* Sarton's digressions were so rich that appending a footnote seemed the simplest way of bracketing that bit of information away from the main stream of thought.

Abreu, M. de: The bearers of shadows. *Dis. of Chest, 11*:639-647, 1945. History of the development of fluorography.

Aebersold, P. C.: The development of nuclear medicine. *Am. J. Roentgenol., 75*:1027-1039, 1956. Excellent survey, from Rutherford and Cockroft-Walton, over Lawrence, Fermi, and Hertz (first radioiodine treatment) to J. H. Müller (first intracavitary use of radiogold in 1945 in Switzerland), Grimmett, and Marshall Brucer.

Aebersold, P. C.: Radioisotopos (1947-1957); una decada de rapido progreso. *Radiología, (Panama), 8*: 103-108, 1958. Chronologic review, translated from *Nucleonics.*

Albers- Schönberg, H.: *Die Röntgentechnik* (ed.: R. Grashey), ed. 6, vol. I, Leipzig, Georg Thieme, 1941, 701 pages. Individual chapters (by various authors) contain a wealth of historical material on technical developments, with many references to contributions by authors from outside the German sphere.

Albert-Weil: Les débuts de la radiologie *Paris médical, 14* (suppl.):193-201, 1914. Abbé Nollet, Crookes, and Röntgen with excerpts from the latter's first communication on x rays; Oudin exposed his first roentgen plate by "promenading" the tube (held with a forceps) for twenty-five minutes at a distance of about three centimeters from the dorsum of the patient's hand.

Alexander, B.: Historische Momente; Lenard und Röntgen. *Pest. med.-chir. Presse, (Budapest), 49*:409-413; 418-421, 1913. Factual account of the development of gas tubes. Faraday was the first who studied electrical discharges in rarefied gases, then Plücker described in 1858 the *Glimmlichtstrahlen,* which Goldstein was to re-discover and name cathode rays.

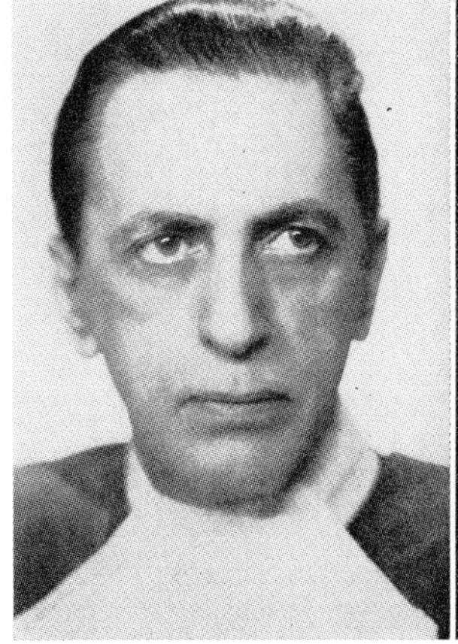

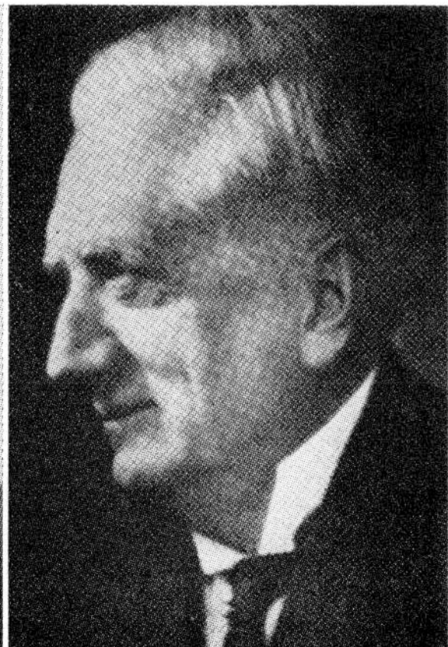

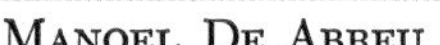

MANOEL DE ABREU GÖSTA FORSSELL

Allardice, C., & Trapnell, E. R.: *The First Pile*. Argonne (Illinois), Argonne National Laboratory, 1961, 21 pages. Reprint of AEC Report TID-292, March, 1955—the writing was actually completed on November 17, 1949. It contains a list of those present, and photographs of scale models of Fermi's first reactor, CP-1 (Chicago Pile one). It went critical on December 2, 1942 at 3.25 p.m. (Chicago time), operated for twenty-eight minutes, and was then shut down. Thereupon Arthur Compton called James B. Conant at Harvard, by long-distance telephone. Their code was not pre-arranged. "The Italian navigator has landed in the New World," said Compton. "How were the natives?" asked Conant. "Very friendly!"

Anderson, C. C.: Radiology in New-Zealand. *Bull. d'Inf. Centre A. Béclère, 5* (nr. 57):3-6; (nr. 58) 9-12, 1956. Lists important names, from pioneers to martyrs. The Radiological Section of their Medical Society met in Dunedin during the 3rd Intercolonial Meeting of the British Medical Association: at that meeting, the radiological highlight was Ed Jerman, representing the Victor X-Ray Corporation of Chicago.

Anderson, E. B.: *Ten Years With the Peaceful Atom*. Oak Ridge, ORINS, 1956, 16 (pages mimeographed). A warm, personal account of people and events in the atomic town, by a sensitive witness.

Andrews, J. R.: Planigraphy. *Am. J. Roentgenol., 36*:575-587, 1936. Very documented account, including Bocage, Vallebona's *stratigraphy,* Ziedses des Plantes' *planigraphy,* Bartelink, Grossmann's *tomography* - and the *laminagraphy* of the (Frenchman) Jean Kieffer from Norwich (Connecticut).

Arrieta Sanches, L.: Revue historique de la radiologie au Panama. *Bull. d'Inf. Centre A. Béclère, 4* (nr. 40):4-5, 1955. Homage to Joaquin José Vallarino.

Ashworth, W. J.: Links in the chain. *Radiography, 22*:225-231, 1956. The chain: Guericke, Nollet, Hauksbee, Crookes, Hittorf, Faraday, Roentgen, and J. J. Thomson. Quotation: ". . . the television craze, by holding huge numbers of the population in a state of total inactivity for many hours every week, may produce much more serious mutations than ionizing radiations ever could!"

Astier, C.: Evolution de la radiothérapie. *Marseilles méd., 62*:1636-1656, 1925. At the Moscow Congress of 1897, Oudin, Barthélemy, and Darier reported on sixty cases of radiodermatitis, attributed first to the heat given off by the x-ray tube. In 1900 Kienböck showed the real cause of this to be the roentgen rays. In 1902 Williams reported the first case of carcinoma of the lip successfully treated with x rays, and in 1903 Nicholas Senn published two cases of lymphoma (Hodgkin and myeloid leukemia) controlled by x ray.

Barclay, A. E.: History and future of British radiology, *Brit. J. Radiol.* (Roentgen Society Section), *21*:3-20, 1925. Classic source of information on British radiology, including the genealogy of their specialty journals.

Barros, R. de: Os primordios da radiologia em São Paulo. *Rev. brasil. de radiol., 5*:113-120, 1962. At the Escola Politécnica, in 1896, Silva Ramos produced the first x-ray plate in São Paulo. The first x-ray equipment in the city was installed in 1906 in the office of Walter Seng, a surgeon of Austrian descent. The first hospital x-ray installation was that of Arnaldo Vieira de Carvalho in 1909—his x-ray technician was Henrique Gruska. Rafael Penteado de Barros studied with Antoine Béclère in Paris, then returned in 1912 as the first formally trained radiologist to work in São Paulo. Among his associates were Cabello Campos (who excelled in Jiu Jitsu, and wrote in 1928 a thesis on cholecystography, which reported his experiences with Graham-Cole's procedure); Eduardo Cotrim (who wrote a thesis on the alterations of the sella turcica); Paulo de Toledo (who later wrote a *Tratado de Radiologia Clinica do Aparelho Digestivo; Jose* Moretzsohn de Castro (the expert in cineradiography); and Walter Bonfim Pontes (who is professor of radiology in the Faculty of Medicine of Sorocaba, and editor of the *Revista Brasileira de Radiologia*). In 1941, Barros created the first organization of radiologists in São Paulo. In 1948, through the efforts of Cabello Campos, and Walter Pontes, was organized the first Jornada de Radiologia in São Paulo, as a result of which was created the Colegio Brasileiro de Radiologia on September 18, 1948.

Becker, J.: Entwicklung der Therapie mit energiereichen Strahlen. *Med. Klin., 54*:1337-1339, 1959. The betatron was developed in the USA, but its

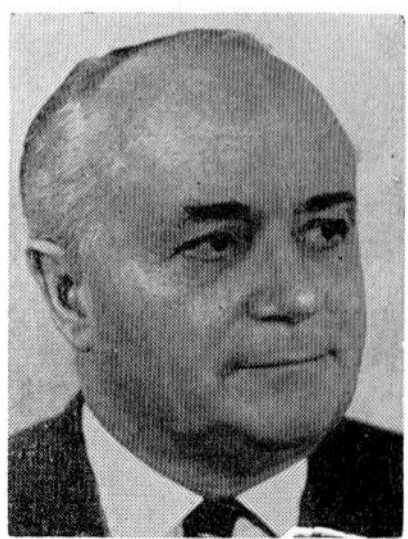
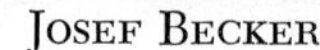
JOSEF BECKER

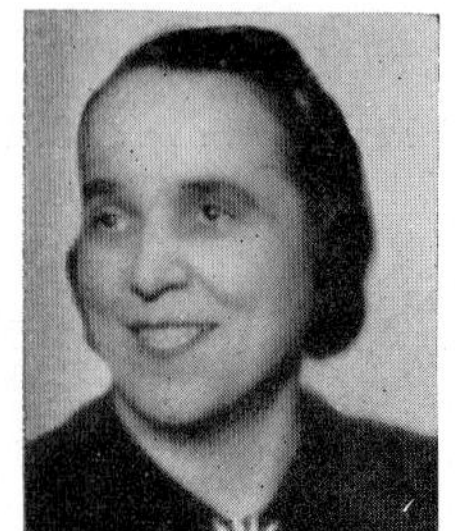
ANTOINETTE BÉCLÈRE

fundamental theory was based on Wideröe's theoretical considerations of circular acceleration. Wideröe built Brown-Boveri's Asklepitron. In Europe the first betatron was a 6 mev model, placed in operation in Göttingen (Germany) in 1946; it was first used for medical therapy in 1949. Also at SRW, Gund developed a 15 mev betatron.

Béclère, A.: Premières notions de radiologie medicale; la découverte de Röntgen. *Sem. d. hôp., 1*:513-526, 1925. Röntgen's merit was great, but could not compare with that of Maxwell who, by reasoning and calculus, predicted the existence of electric oscillations twenty years before Hertz's actual proof; from Nollet to Crookes, and from Röntgen to early changes in gas tubes.

Béclère, A.: 10 années d'activité du Centre Antoine Béclère. *J. de radiol. & d'électrol., 43*:X-XXX, 1962. The author is Antoinette Béclère (daughter of Antoine, author of the previous article), who created the *Centre* in Paris, named after her father. This is the report of the *Centre's* first ten years of activity.

Bélisle, L.-P.: Histoire de la radiologie au Canada français. *Union méd., 88*:40-52, 1959. A sentimental, but accurate account of French-Canadian pioneers, from LaFlamme to Perron, Potvin, Pariseau, and Origène Dufresne.

Belot, J.: La röntgenologie en France. *Fortschritte a. d. Geb. d. Rstrlen, 10*:87-94, 1906. Villard's osmoregulator, Sabouraud and Noiré's radiometer, Béclère's equivalent spark, Benoist's radiochromometer, and early fights against *empirisme* (x-ray examinations performed by lay, *i.e.*, unqualified observers).

Bender, G. A.: Röntgen: invisible rays that save lives. *Therapeutic Notes* insert with no pagination, 1962. Text and production by Bender, with painting by R. A. Thom, as part of the remarkable *A History of Medicine in Pictures,* sponsored by Parke, Davis & Co. This particular painting (and the story) present Röntgen's first public address on his rays.

Berg, H. M.: Swedish contributions to radiology, *Radiology, 78*:471-473, 1962. Gösta Forssell ("father of scientific radiology" in Sweden), Åke Åkerlund ("the" pediatric radiologist), Ellis Berven (the radiotherapist), James Heyman (the radiumtherapist), and Erik Lysholm (the skull and sinuses specialist).

Berg, S.: History of the first survey of the medical effects of radioactive fallout. *Military Medicine, 124*: 782-785, 1959. With Shields Warren as co-chairman, a joint (civil and military) commission was set up on September 29, 1945, to investigate the situation in the Nishiyama District of Nagasaki. The same desire to minimize (if possible) the effects of fallout prompted reactivation of the commission, after the mishap (radioactive exposure) of the Marshall Islanders following the detonation of the second experimental fusion device on the Bikini Atoll on March 1, 1954.

Bernardi, E. de: Étude sur la radiologie en Italie. *Bull. d'Inf. Centre A. Béclère, 2* (nr. 19-20):1-6, 1953. Concise, precise, authoritative.

Berven, E.: The development and organization of therapeutic radiology in Sweden. *Radiology 79*:829-841, 1962. A masterly, well illustrated account by the senior Swedish therapist, a shorter version, with text only, appeared in *Röntgen-Blätter* of September, 1962.

Besio, G. L.: *Index Stratigraficus.* Raccolta di Voci Bibliografiche sulla Stratigrafia dal 1930 al 1959. Genova, Edizioni Universitarie, 1962, 275 pages.

Bilek, F.: The beginning of Czech medical x-ray science, 1897-1900. *Cas. Lek. ces., 97*:409-412, 1958. The Czech title is Počátky Česke lékarské rentgenologie. The text was used for the respective section in the *Semantic Treatise.* Aside from Jedlicka, prominent place is given to the internist Vesely, and to the ophthalmologist Chalupecký.

Bischopp, K.: 40 Jahre Drehstromapparat. *Röntgen-Blätter, 9*:401-412, 1956. From Siemens & Halske's first triphasic therapy generator, shown to the Berlin Medical Society by K. Lasser in 1916, over Koch & Sterzel's 2000 ma Titanos (1927) and Siemens' 2000 ma Gigantos (1929), to the 1956 SRW Tridoros with up to 1000 ma or 150 kvp.

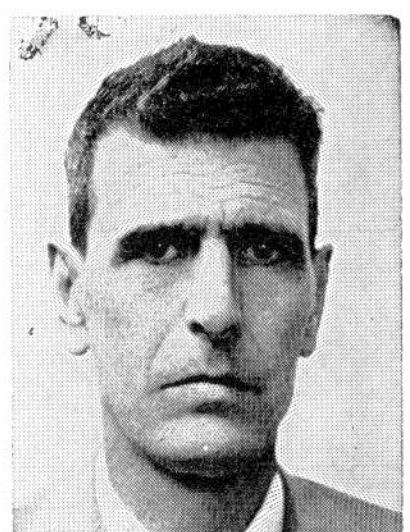
E. de Bernardi

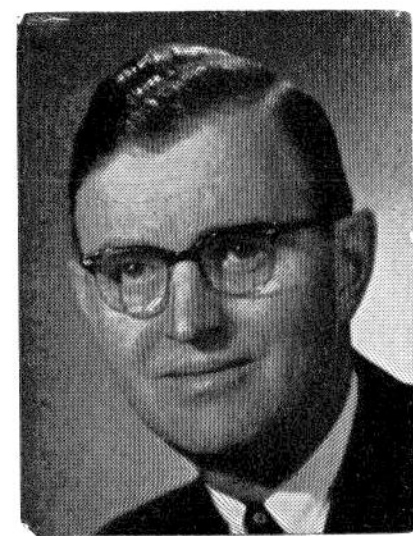
L. P. Belisle

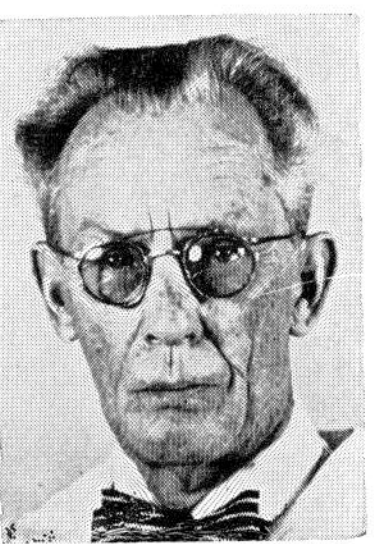
Elis Berven

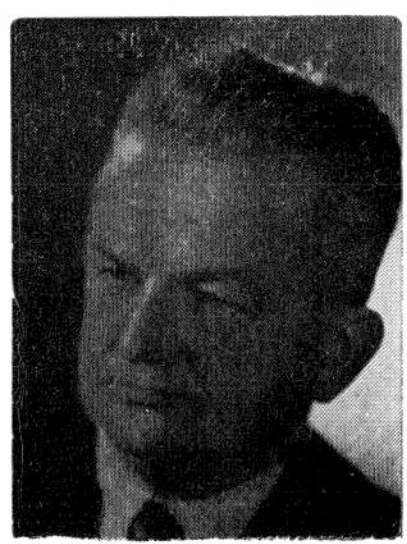
Kurt Bischoff

Bischopp, K.: Die Entwicklung der medizinischen Röntgentechnik in den letzten 12 Jahren. *Elektrotechnische Zeitschrift, 10*:526-536, 1958. SRW's chief-engineer analyzes "atomic phase" improvements in high kvp technics, phototimers, photofluorography, image intensification, television monitoring, and electronic contrast modifiers.

Blackman, S.: Dental radiology, past, present, and future. *Brit. Dent. J., 107*:83-86, 1959. "Röntgen was an expert engineer who designed and made his own apparatus and instruments. . . The greater part of the practical improvements in the production of the x-rays were made here in England by Herbert Jackson of King's College, who designed the first focus tube. . . In January, 1896, Dr. Frank Harrison informed a meeting of the BMA that he had constructed a special vacuum tube for dental use with the x-rays. . . on June 26, 1896, (Harrison submitted) x-ray photographs of teeth taken from dry specimens and from life—all with a reduced exposure of ten minutes. Then Harrison quoted Wm. J. Morton's . . . the covered now has become uncovered, the concealed has been revealed, and the invisible is now visible." This paper is a corrected transcript of the first presidential address given on March 19, 1959, before the then newly formed British Society of Dental Radiologists, assembled at the Royal Dental Hospital in London.

Bleich, A. R.: *The Story of X-Rays from Röntgen to isotopes.* New York City, Dover, 1960, pp. 186. Popularization paperback.

Bloomfield, J. A.: Half a century of progress in radio-diagnostic protection. *Med. J. Australia, 1*:289-292, 1959. The author is a radiologist from Tasmania who, after discussing somatic x-ray martirdom, remarked that in diagnostic radiology, epilation and x-ray dermatitis have been eliminated, while the leukemogenic effect is negligible.

Bohrer, S. P.: Radiology on stamps. *Topical Time, 13* (nr. 3): 12-15; *13* (nr. 5): 11-19, 1962. Listing which served as source material for Radiología y Filatelia by Miguel Dao D., printed in 1964 in the Venezuelan (?) journal *Radiología y Medicina Nuclear.*

Brailsford, J.: Röntgen's discovery of x-rays. *Brit. J. Radiol., 19*:453-461, 1946. "Deservedly they should be called roentgen rays and not x rays—since they were an unknown quantity only until he had taught us their characteristics."

Bromer, R. S.: History of radiology in Philadelphia; history of Philadelphia Roentgen Ray Society. Part II: 1920-1954. *Amer. J. Roentgenol., 75*:23-32, 1956. The first part of that article, appearing in the same issue, was from the pen of George Pfahler.

Brown, P.: A short history of roentgen rays. *New York M. J., 102*:1269-1271, 1915. From Röntgen to Bleyer, and from Williams to Leonard, with final quotation by Abraham Lincoln: "I am not bound to win, but I am bound to be true; I am not bound to succeed, but I am bound to live up to the Light. I have!"

Brown, P.: *American Martyrs to Science Through the Roentgen Rays.* Springfield (Illinois), Charles C Thomas, 1936, 276 pages. Biographies of radiation fatalities, beginning with Dally (Edison's glassblower), and ending with G. F. Parker, a radiologist from Iowa. This book is a classic in the history of radiology.

Brown, P.: Debt of radiology to the Thomsons and the Thompsons. *Am. J. Roentgenol., 44*:409-422, 1940. Contributions of physicists to the growth of radiology, as viewed by the historian of the ARRS, who starts this superb article by analyzing Shotwell's interpretation of the term and concept of history as an instrument of investigation.

Brown, P.: The inception and development of fluoroscopy. *Radiology, 38*:414-425, 1942. Holzknecht was one of the originators of the method. In this country both Williams and Crane accumulated fluoroscopic experience in the early days, but by 1905 Pfahler had discarded screening "because of its inaccuracy, and of the dangers attending its use." In 1910 Fedor Haenisch reported on the meager use of fluoroscopy in the USA. Then came Carman who may be regarded as the true popularizer and developer of the fluoroscopic method in the USA.

Brucer, M.: The therapeutic limitations of radioisotopes in urology. *Lederle Bulletin, 1* (nr. 2):1-14, 1957. Delightful (though a bit naughty) history of the r, the rep, and the rad.

Brucer, M.: Brachytherapy. *Am. J. Roentgenol., 79*:1080-1090, 1958. In 1901 Pierre Curie gave a small tube with radium to Danlos (a physician), suggesting that it be inserted into a tumor—and this is

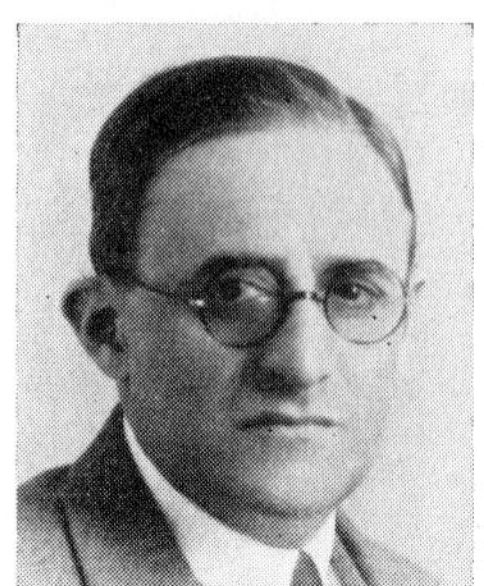

GUSTAV BUCKY

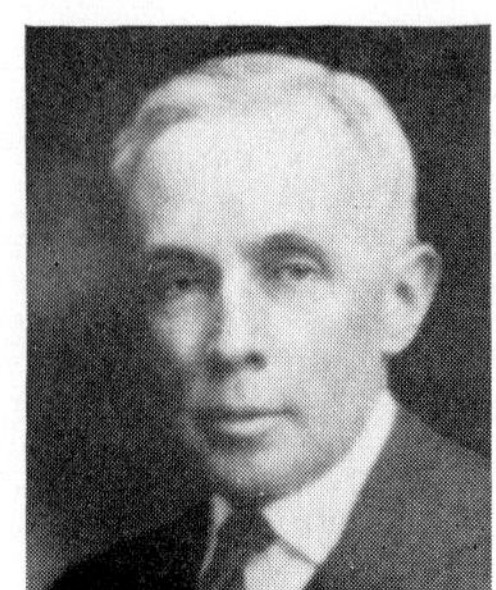

PERCY BROWN

how brachytherapy was born. Includes also a review of modern (isotopic) sources available in different countries.

Brucer, M.: A history of the Society of Nuclear Medicine. *In preparation.* Quotation: "The first man to study the x rays was probably Professor Miller at King's College in Cambridge (England). He was mapping out the far ultraviolet region beyond visible light. He probably produced and maybe even measured some soft x rays, but this was in 1854, and he did not know he was approaching a new subject in physics."

Bruner, E.: Radioterapia dermatologiczna w Polsce w latach 1899-1939. *Przegl. Derm. Wener. 8*(45): 461-481, 1958. From epilation to carcinoma, and then back to epilation—but in a very documented way.

Bryant, F.: Radiotherapy. *Boston M. & S. J., 181*: 270-276, 1919. Excessively enthusiastic address read before the Thurber Medical Society in Milford (Massachusetts), discussing the history of radium therapy, and concluding with the quotation from Gauss: "At Freiburg (Germany) we no longer operate, we radiate!"

Buckstein, J.: Historical development of the roentgen diagnosis of the pathological appendix. *Am. J. Roentgenol., 27*:236-239, 1932. Factual, but dated as far as conclusions are concerned. Buckstein had a similar paper, on the history of the peptic ulcer niche, in the same journal in October, 1928.

Bucky, G.: *Grenz Ray Therapy;* Bibliography. No date, no publisher (New York City, about 1938), 46 pages. Authoritative, because Bucky originated the method. This item appeared later in book form, issued by Bucky with an associate. Incidentally, Bucky's first paper on the Bucky diaphragm was published in the (British) *Archives of the Röntgen Ray* of June, 1913.

Bugyi, B.: Zur Geschichte der Röntgenologie in Ungarn (1896-1916). *Zschr. f. Gesch. d. Naturwissensch., Technik u. Med., 1* (3):87-114, 1962. Very documented paper, beginning with the first notice of Röntgen's discovery, which appeared in the *Pester Lloyd* on January 16, 1896; continued with Klupathy, Eötvös, Högyes, Kiss, Holzwarth, Pekar, Karolyi, and especially Béla Alexander. Blasius Bugyi is Hungary's unofficial historian of radiology, with a dozen or so papers on the subject, including one on the Hungarian roentgen martyrs in the *Orvosi Hetilap* (1960), and one on the first fifty years in Hungarian radiology in the *Horus Medicorum* (1957).

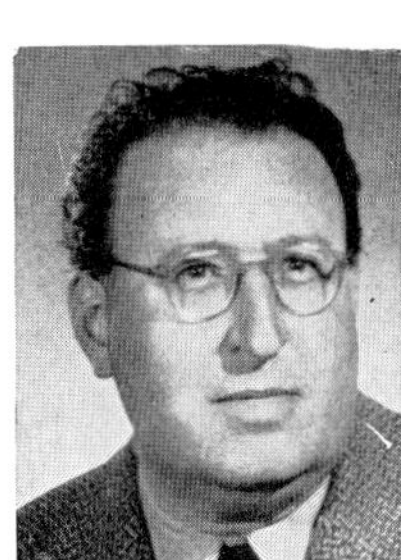

Blasius Bugyi

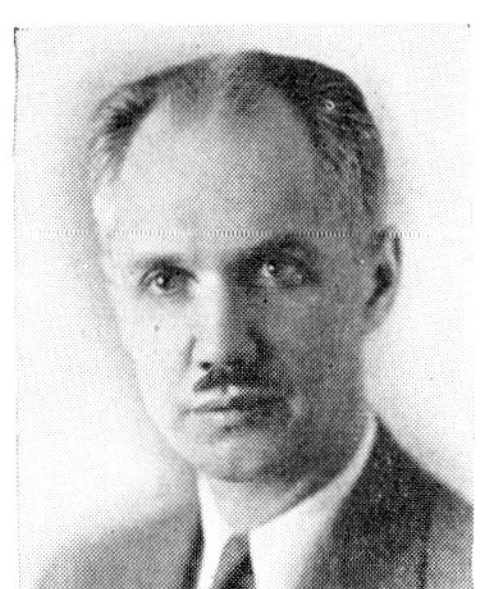

H. Milton Berg

Burnam, C. F.: Early experiments with radium. *Am. J. Roentgenol., 36*:437-452, 1936. Janeway Lecture, excellent source material on early radium-biologic endeavors of Howard Kelly (Burnam had been Kelly's associate): many other interesting details, such as the mention that the first case of skin cancer as a result of roentgen irradiation was reported in 1906 by De Beurmann, Dominici, and Gougerot—by 1911, Krause collected fifty-four similar cases from the literature.

Burns, E. E.: The story of Professor Roentgen's discovery. *Pop. Scient. Monthly, 73*:554-556, 1908. This is the princeps source for the tale with the key, the book, and the (energized but neglected) Hittorf tube.

Cade, S.: Radiological achievement 1937-1950. *Brit. J. Radiol., 24*:119-122, 1951. This paper, read at the 6th ICR (London, 1950), is a special tribute to Barclay. In the same paper the radium therapist Cade declared that the separation of radiodiagnosis and radiotherapy had been accepted in most countries since 1937 (one wonders what he meant by most countries).

Caffey, J.: The first sixty years of pediatric roentgenology in the United States—1896 to 1956. *Am. J. Roentgenol., 76*:437-454, 1956. The first roentgen department in America organized for the exclusive use of infants and children was set up at Boston's Children Hospital in 1899. The first such department in Canada was set up in 1902 in the Hospital for Sick Children (Toronto) in 1900, with A. H. Rolfe as radiologist. In Detroit, similar facilities were installed at the Children's Hospital in 1904, with Hickey in charge. In Philadelphia this was done in 1921, in New York City at Babies' Hospital in 1922. In 1906, P. E. Brown was replaced by Arial Wellington George, who may be regarded as their first bona-fide American pediatric radiologist: he collaborated with Thomas Morgan Rotch and furnished the illustrations for (but his name was not included on the title page of) the pediatrician Rotch's *Roentgen Method in*

Pediatrics (1910). In 1914 Percy Brown replaced Arial George.

Case, J. T.: A brief history of the development of foreign body localization by means of the x-ray. *Am. J. Roentgenol., 5*:113-124, 1918. Excellent, and very documented, just like other diagnostic reviews by Case, *e.g.,* the one on twenty-five years of progress, published in the same journal in October, 1931 (this is when he mentioned that no less than 125 roentgen books and atlases were dated 1905 and earlier). Also in the Yellow Journal (of December, 1945) Case reviewed fifty years of gastro-entero-roentgenology, and offered 230 references.

Case, J. T.: Evolution of radiology in Latin America. *Radiology, 48*:517-526, 1947. This is a smoothed-out version of his address before the 2nd IARC in Havana in 1946. On April 24, 1955—in his inaugural address to the 5th IARC in Washington (DC)—Case summarized the history of the IARC, which was then published in *Radiology* of April, 1956.

Case, J. T.: Early history of radium therapy and the ARS. *Am. J. Roentgenol., 82*:574-585, 1959. At the 1953 meeting of the ARS, Case had summarized the history of the ARS, printed in the same journal as of September, 1953: that was an editorial, and did not make the indices. The 1959 version is broader in scope, and remains an indispensable source material on this topic.

Castellanos, A.: La angiocardiografia; revision general. *Radiología, (Panama), 9*:47-66, 1959. Polished version of author's presentation before the International Congress of Cardiology in Bruxelles (1959)—with adequate bibliography.

Castellanos, A.; Garcia, O., and Pereiras, R.: La angiografía en Cuba. *Radiología, (Panama), 6*:127-159, 1956. History of the development of angiocardiography for congenital heart disease in pediatric patients. Paper includes annotated bibliography.

Chadwick, J. (ed): *The Collected Papers of Lord Rutherford of Nelson.* New York, Interscience (Wiley), 1962, 931 pages. The first volume covers only the New Zealand period (1894-1906). The second volume will be his Manchester period (1907-1919), the third will be Cavendish (1919-1937), while the fourth volume will contain miscellaneous items. The editor is Sir James Chadwick (discoverer of the neutron) one of Rutherford's most distinguished pupils. It was indeed high time to publish Rutherford's papers after the collected papers of so many atomic scientists had been published.

Chamberlain, W. E.: Fifty years of progress. *Am. J. Roentgenol., 76*:177-178, 1956. Since the *American Quarterly of Roentgenology* became the *American Journal of Roentgenology* there occurred many changes and advances, for instance it was somewhat painfully realized that visceroptosis is a physiologic position of the bowels, not the dreadful drop of yore.

Chase, C.: American literature on radium and radium therapy. *Am. J. Roentgenol., 8*:766-778, 1921. Accurately annotated list of books and articles published before January 1, 1906.

Christensen, H.: Die Röntgenologie in Dänemark. *Röntgen-Blätter, 12*:201-207, 1959. With portraits; excellent.

Christie, A. C.: Roentgenology in North America. *Acta radiol., 6*:281-295, 1926. The pioneers: Williams, Cannon, Kassabian, Leonard, Caldwell, Dodd, etc. Another version of this paper appeared in the *American Journal of Roentgenology* of October, 1931.

Christie, A. C.: The American Roentgen Ray Society. An historical sketch—"Lest we forget." *Am. J. Roentgenol., 76*:1-6, 1956. Introducing the golden anniversary volume of the Yellow Journal.

Chwolson, O.: Die Bedeutung der Entdeckung Roentgens für die Physik. *Ann. de roentgenol. et radiol., (Petersbourg), 1*:247-234, 1922. As seen through the eyes of one of the Russian roentgen pioneers.

Cipollaro, A. C.: The earliest roentgen demonstration of a pathological lesion in America. *Radiology, 45*:555-558, 1945. Edwin Frost exposed the plate

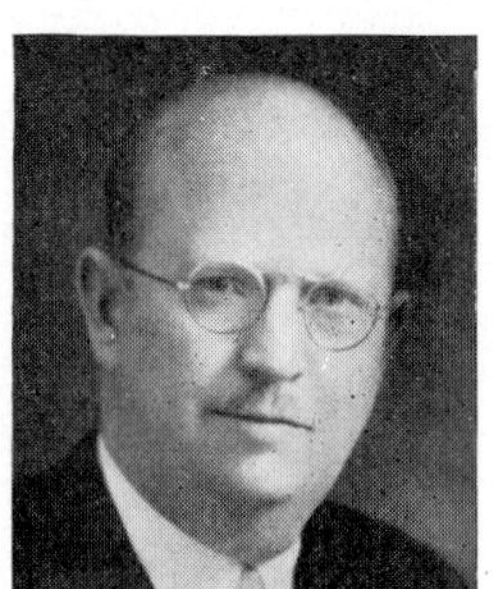
JAMES CASE

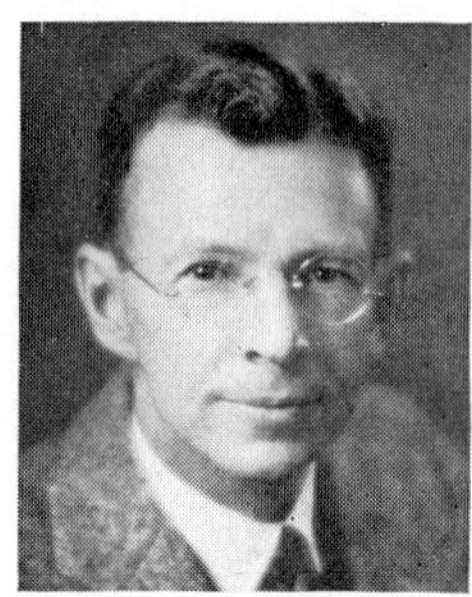
WM. D. COOLIDGE

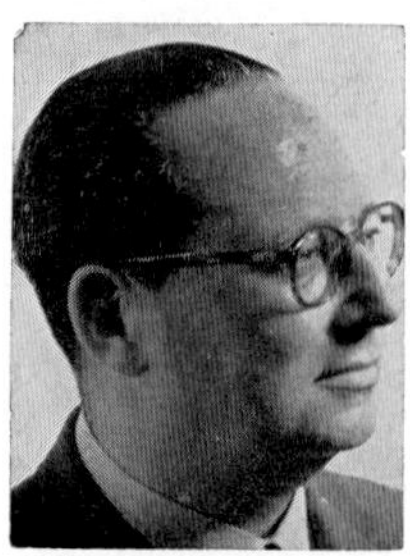
UMBERTO COCCHI

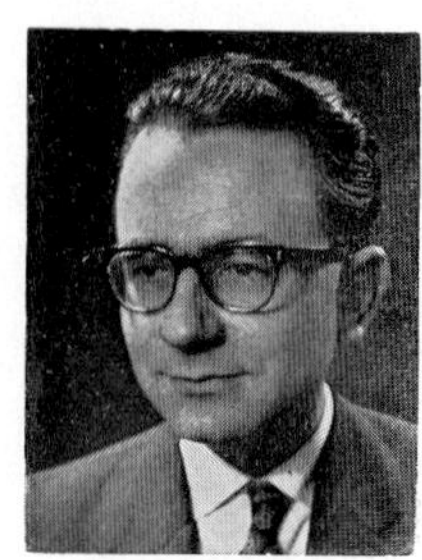
JAN COBBEN

of a Colles fracture at Dartmouth College on February 3, 1896.

Clark, G. L.: Half century of roentgen rays in industry. *Radiology, 45*:539-548, 1945. Condensed account (for more details see introduction to *Applied X-Rays* by same author); just as authoritative is the chronologic timetable of development of x-ray tubes and electron physics in the *American Journal of Roentgenology* of October, 1931.

Clemmesen, C. A.: *Radiumfondet, Oprettet til Minde om Kong Frederik VIII, 1912-1929.* København, 1931, 110 pages. History of the Danish Royal Radium Institute.

Cobben, J.: Nederlandse pioniers in de radiologie. *J. belge de radiol., 42*:738-745, 1949. Three biographies, that of Wertheim Salomonson; of P. H. Eykman (1862-1914); and of Nicolaas Voorhoeve (1879-1927).

Cocchi, U.: Geschichte der Röntgendiagnostik. *Praxis, 48*:617-622, 1959. Inaugural lesson as professor of radiology, held in June of 1958, covering a large "diagnostico-historic" territory.

Cole, L. G.: *Lung Dust Lesions Versus Tuberculosis.* White Plains (New York), American Medical Films, 1948, 474 pages. This was Cole's scientific testament, containing much of his own history, including elucubrations on the rays of selective absorption.

Cole, W. H.: Historical features of cholecystography. *Radiology, 76*:354-375, 1961. The "last" Carman Lecture of the RSNA by surgeon Cole of the Graham-Cole test came after the historico-biographical preamble by radiologist Wachowski.

Compton, A. H.: Modern physics and the discovery of x-rays. *Radiology, 45*:534-538, 1945. Thoughtful pages by the then director of the Metallurgical Laboratory where Fermi had achieved the first chain reaction. Compton recalled that in 1894, at the building of a Physics Laboratory in the University of Chicago, A. A. Michelson contended that the physics of the future lays in the 4th decimal place, meaning that all fundamental principles of physics had been established, so that further research meant only more precise measurements. But one year later, in 1895, came Röntgen, in 1905 Einstein, and today (in 1945) we have all sorts of radio and the atom bomb to boot.

Coolidge, W. D.: Development of modern roentgen-ray generating apparatus. *Am. J. Roentgenol., 24*:605-620, 1930. Caldwell Lecture, crisp, cursive, competent.

Coolidge, W. D. and Charlton, E. E.: Roentgen-ray tubes. *Radiology, 45*:449-466, 1945. Ample, accurate, and authoritative; another article (signed by Coolidge alone in the *American Journal of Roentgenology* of December, 1945) contains the story of the first demonstration of the hot cathode tube on December 27, 1913 in a New York City hotel, before a select audience of radiologists.

Cornacchia, V.: Storia della radiologia medica. *Riv. d. storia d. medicina, 5*:261-274, 1961. The following installments appeared in the same periodical, *6*:114-132, 223-236, 1962; *7*:73-93, 1963, and so on. The author, Vio Cornacchia, is a retired x-ray technician who resides in the (independent) Repubblica di San Marino (on the Italian peninsula). He acquired not only radiation damage, but also an intense love for the history of radiology, and has written several papers on the subject, for instance a history of pediatric roentgenology in the USA, published in the *Rev. med. Rio Grande do Sul,* in two installments, between July and December of 1961.

Curie, M.: *Pierre Curie, With the Autobiographical Notes of Marie Curie.* Translated by Charlotte and Vernon Kellogg, with an introduction by Mrs. Wm. Brown Meloney. New York, Macmillan, 1923, 118 pages.

Cuthbert, A.: Half a century of shadows. *Radiography 22*:250-254, 1956. Remembrances: "It was in 1903 that I had my first contact with the subject—and that is 53 years ago—whereas it was in 1909 that I came definitely in the business . . . Amongst the shadows of the earliest days of our Society (of Radiographers) I have grateful memories of C. E. S. Phillips. He was the tall distinguished Englishman of the French stage, and a veritable amateur Admirable Crichton. A physicist of no small attainments, he formulated radium standards and experimented with selenium cells. He exhibited at the Royal Academy, made, remade, and played violins and spinets, and did a marvelous "nigger minstrel" turn with the bones . . . Then there was Campbell Swinton, a

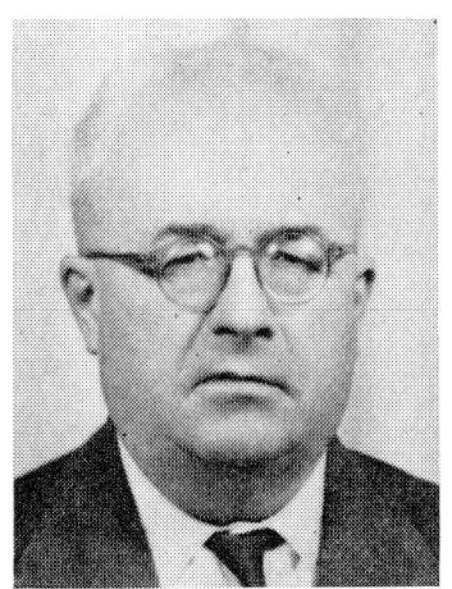

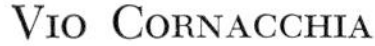

Vio Cornacchia

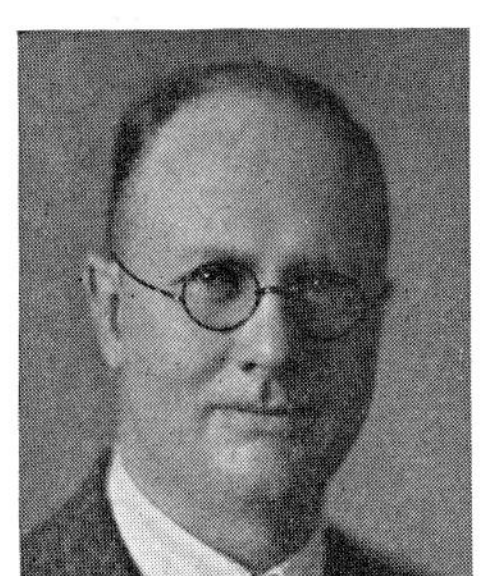

Kenneth Davis

rather dour personality with an unfortunate nose . . . Sir Clifford Patterson, although one of the Society's sponsors, drifted to the purely electrical industry, becoming head of the General Electric Company's great research department at Wembley."

Davis, K. S.: History of radium. *Radiology, 2*: 334-342, 1924. Important source material, including full text of letter by Alexander Graham Bell (first printed in the *American Magazine* of August, 1903), suggesting interstitial use of radium for therapeutic applications. Same suggestion had been made previously by Rollins.

Davis, L.: Neurological surgery, so to speak, out of roentgenology. *Am. J. Roentgenol., 76*:217-225, 1956. Hickey lecture—with portrait; pantopaque and Dandy; Edward Blaine at Wesley Memorial Hospital; James Case at Battle Creek, and then at Northwestern University; quotation: ". . . the graduate nurse who roentgenized the patients . . ."

De . . ., see under last name (*e.g.,* instead of De Abreu, M., see Abreu, M. de).

Dessauer, F.: *Wilhelm C. Roentgen, die Offenbarung einer Nacht.* Frankfurt/Main, Knecht, 1945, pp. 167. Biography written while author was in exile.

Dewing, S. B.: *Modern Radiology in Historical Perspective.* Springfield (Illinois), Charles C Thomas, 1962, 189 pages. Excellent condensation with particular emphasis on scientific advances, quoting mainly American authors. Radiologic organizations, and similar items are schematically considered.

Dmokhovsky, V. V.: Ways and trends of development of roentgen engineering in the Soviet Union. *Indian J. Radiol.,* (souvenir number) 615-622, 1956. Factual account of problems encountered, and solutions adduced.

Donaldson, S. W.: *Roentgenologist in Court,* ed. 2. Springfield (Illinois), Charles C Thomas, 1954, 215 pages. Classic text with numerous historic recalls, and adequate bibliographic support, by the former historian of the ACR, and all-time expert in forensic radiology.

Dormer, B. A.: Miniature radiology, its early history. *Med. Proc., (Johannesburg), 4*:605-607, 1958. In 1929 Dormer (a physician) and Capt. K. G. F. Collender produced miniature chest survey films, using machinery developed by Collender in 1927, when he applied for South African provisional patent nr. 698 (granted in April, 1928). Although that first attempt was successful, they did not try it again until 1935 (when they used 60 mm. film) after which they published the first article on miniature radiography to appear in the English language—in *Lancet* of June 10, 1939. On March 14, 1942 Collender filed the South African provision patent nr. 166/42, which was based on the use of a concave mirror. I wrote to Dormer, who is the head of the Health Department in Durham (South Africa), and he promised to send me more detailed information. That was in 1963, and I still have no answer.

Doub, H. P.: Radiology; its twenty-fifth anniversary. *Radiology, 51*:455-458, 1948. Subdued comment for a milestone of pride, by the longtime editor of the Gray Journal. He has published several other historic papers, for instance the biography of Augustus Crane in *Radiology* of July, 1955 or Radiology in this Century in the *Illinois Medical Journal* of November, 1963. In *Radiology* of November, 1964 appeared Doub's excellent *RSNA, 50 Years of Progress.*

Eggert, J.: Die Anschauungen über das latente Bild im Wandel der Zeiten. Pp. 13-31 *in 100 Jahre Schleussner.* Frankfurt/Main, Schleussner, 1960. In the 100th anniversary of the photographic house of Schleussner, the master roentgen photographer John Eggert calls in physicistic spirits (from Herschel and Daguerre to Einstein and Mott), and asks them to discuss the development of the concept of the latent photographic image.

Ellegast, H. H., and Thurnher, B.: Die Anfänge der Röntgenologie in Wien. *Fortschritte a. d. Geb. d. Rstrlen, 96*:145-158, 1962. Viennese roentgen pioneers, discussed by Atomic Phase disciples of Konrad Weiss.

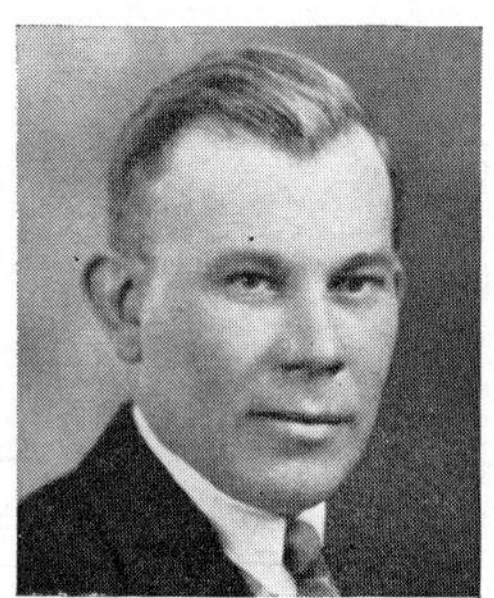

Sam Donaldson

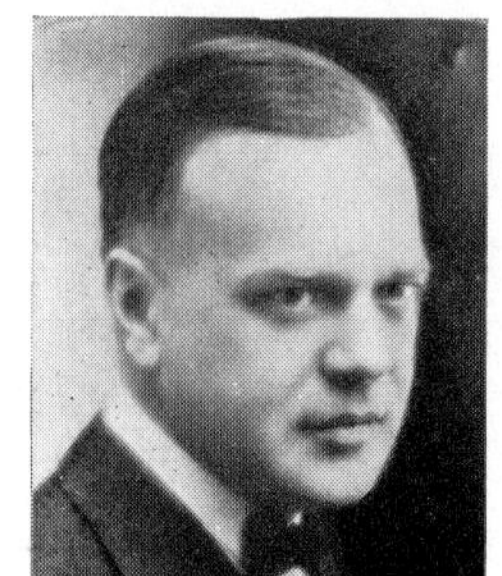

Arthur Wright Erskine

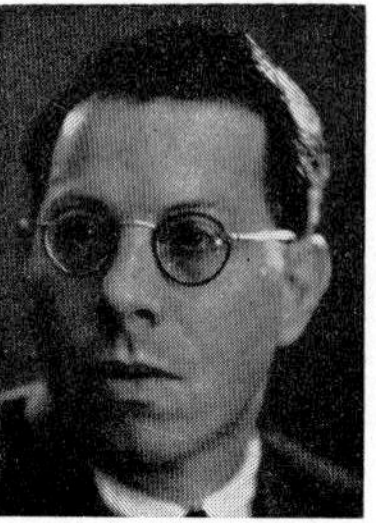

Bruno Thurnher

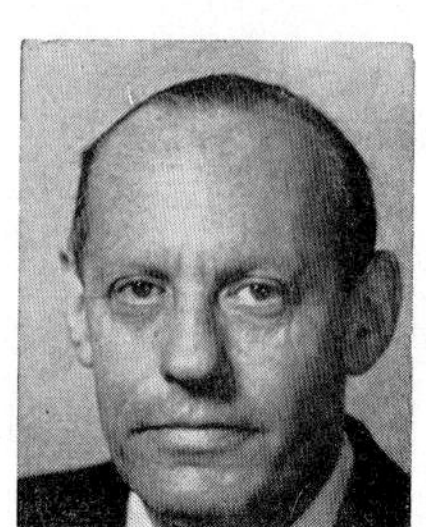

Friedrich Ellinger

Ellinger, F.: *Medical Radiation Biology.* Springfield (Illinois), Charles C Thomas, 1957, 945 pages. Treasure mine of bibliographic information.

Ellis, L. E.: Some modern developments in roentgenology, *M. J. South Africa, 13*:15-20, 1917. Read before the Witwatersrand branch of the BMA, This address (by a pupil of Reginald Morton) ended with a prediction: "When the present destructive and devastating war culminates, as we all feel sure it will, in the vindication of the high ideals of justice and liberty aimed at by the Allied Powers, then under an uninterrupted Peace, Science will be enabled calmly to work her sure and certain course. Roentgenology will, at that time, receive a due share of consideration, and a resulting advance will take place which will justify such a paper as I have laid before you this evening being regarded as very elementary, if not absolutely antiquated."

Elward, J. F.: The midwinter conference of Eastern radiologists (historical). *Am. J. Roentgenol., 42*:903-907, 1939. Factual account with group picture of 1911 meeting.

Ernst, E. C.: Reminiscences of roentgenology during the last war, 1917-1919. *Radiology, 36*:421-438, 1941. Includes samples of reports, pictures of equipment, and pages from registries.

Erskine, A. W.: Organized roentgenology in America. *Radiology, 45*:549-554, 1945. Diplomatic account, based on Skinner's writings, but omitting a few delicate details.

Esguerra Gomez, G.: Tribute to Wilhelm Conrad Röntgen. *Am. J. Roentgenol., 60*:96-103, 1948. Address delivered on November 20, 1946 during a commemorative session at the 2nd IACR in Havana. Esguerra spoke on the same topic to the Academia Nacional de Medicina in Bogotá (Colombia) on September 10, 1940.

Eston, V. R. de, and Eston de Eston, T.: A medicina nuclear no Brasil. *Rev. brasil. de radiol., 4*: 140-143, 1961. This man and wife team (Tede and Veronica) organized in 1949 a radioisotope lab at the University of São Paulo. It was the first such organization in South America, indeed they gave the first South American course in radioisotope methodology (under UNESCO sponsorship) in 1953. In 1959 the lab's name was changed to Centro de Medicina Nuclear. So far about 100 physicians have received postgraduate instructions at the Center—Veronica (livre-docente de Química Fisiologica) is in charge of the educational program. In Brasil there are nuclear reactors at São Paulo and at Belo Horizonte, but production of biological products is far below demands.

Etter, L. E.: Postwar visit to Röntgen's laboratory. *Am. J. Roentgenol., 54*:547-552, 1945. Sentimental pilgrimage to the old master's former locales of activity; with appropriate references to relics and recorded recollections.

Etter, L. E.: Some historical data relating to the discovery of the roentgen rays. *Am. J. Roentgenol., 56*:220-231, 1946. Lenard's frustrations and his attempts to grab at least some glory for himself; with several historic letters in facsimile and translation.

Evans, W. A. (Sr.): Michigan's contribution to early roentgenology. *J. Michigan State Med. Soc., 33*:243-249, 1934. Reminiscences of local pioneers, including Crane.

Ewing, J.: Early experiences in radiation therapy. *Am. J. Roentgenol., 31*:153-163, 1934. This was a Janeway Memorial Lecture given during the American Congress of Radiology in Chicago (1933). Kelly

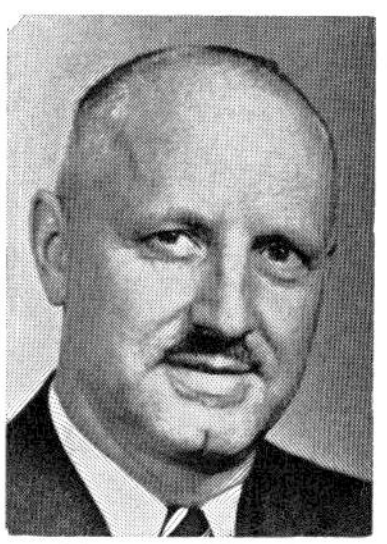

Lewis Etter

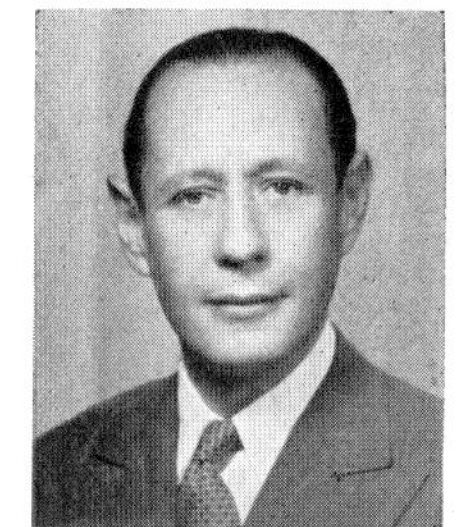

Gonzalo Esguerra-Gomez

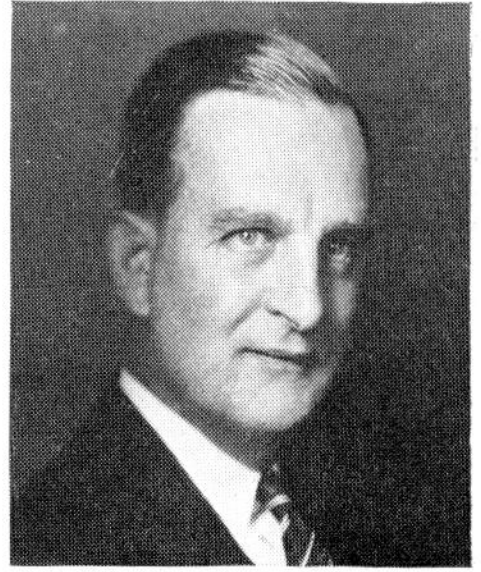

Howard Doub

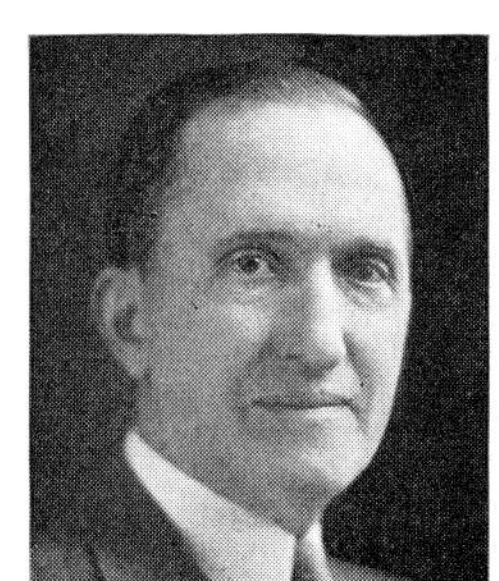

Ed. C. Ernst

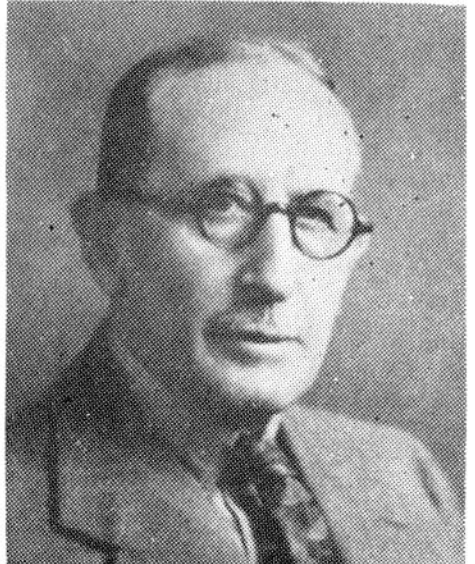

James Ewing

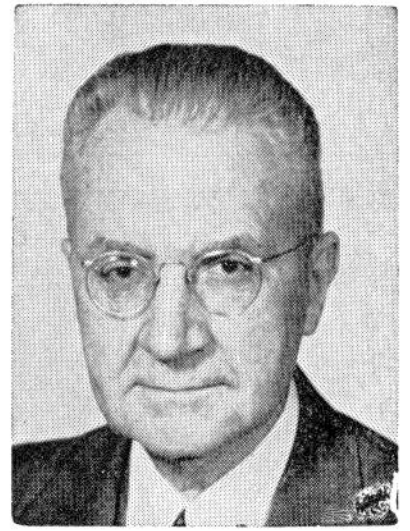

Gioacchino Failla

and Burnam began the systematic treatment of uterine ca (meaning cervix) in 1912, and reported their results in the *J.A.M.A.* of November 27, 1915. "I (Ewing) believe that the first cure of any considerable number of carcinomata of mucous membranes was accomplished by Janeway with his glass seeds of radon, but these glass seeds gave terrific local reactions, and this is why they were replaced by gold radon seeds." Janeway entered the radiation field in 1910. Another Ewing quotation: "Much confusion arose from the multiplication of terms, the conflict of theories, and the striking differences in the effects of different doses. There was the stimulating dose, the erythema dose, the epilation dose, the vesicating dose, and all too often the necrotizing dose."

Failla, G.: 25th anniversary of the discovery of radium. *Radium, (Pittsburgh), 3*:124-128, 1925. The beginnings of Janeway's "buried emanation" can also be found in Failla's paper on the filtered radon implants in the *American Journal of Roentgenology* of December, 1926. Janeway's own article on "buried emanation" appeared in the Yellow Journal of July, 1920.

Farr, L. E.: Role of a nuclear reactor in medical research and therapy; short-lived isotopes, activation analysis, neutron therapy, and neutron capture therapy. Pp. 442-463 *in Application of Radioisotopes and Radiation in the Life Sciences* (Hearings before the Congressional Committee on Atomic Energy, May 27-30, 1961). Washington (DC), Government Printing Office, 1961. History of neutron therapy from Robert Stone (1938) to the neutron capture modality (first performed at Brookhaven National Laboratory on February 15, 1951).

Fermi, L.: *Atoms in the Family,* Chicago University Press, 1954, 267 pages. This is the biography of Enrico Fermi, written by his wife Laura. While sentimental, it is a significant contribution, and brings many interesting details from the life of the "Italian navigator" who first reached the "new" (atomic) world. Enrico Fermi was also a semantic genius (the neutrino was conceived by Wolfgang Pauli, but "christened" by Fermi), even a mechanical genius (Fermi built a trolley for transporting the target in a cyclotron). Incidentally, the book contains the facsimile of Einstein's letter to Roosevelt.

Finzi, N. S.: The early days of radiology. *Clinical Radiology, 12*:143-146, 1961. Wonderfully simple and poignant summary of personal recollections.

Forssell, G., Berven, E., Reuterwall, O., and Sievert, R.: King Gustaf V's Stockholm Jubilee Clinic for Radiotherapy and Research in Cancer. (Suppl. 38 to *Acta radiol.*) Stockholm, P. A. Norstedt and Söner, 1939, pp. 80. Description of the Radiumhemmet, the Radiopathology Institute, and the Radiophysics Institute, which together constitute the Jubilee Clinic—all transferred by King Gustaf to the Karolinska Hospital on June 11, 1938.

Freundlich, M. M.: Origin of the electron microscope. *Science, 142*:185-188, 1963.

Friend, F.: 25 Jahre Röntgen-Frühdiagnose der Lungentuberkulose. *Wien. klin. Wchschr., 71*:519-520, 1959. Before 1928 it was a dogma that pulmonary tuberculosis starts in the apices, and advances toward the bases. This theory has been obsolete for 35 years, but how many still believe in it subconsciously?

Fuchs, A. W.: Evolution of roentgen film. *Am. J. Roentgenol., 75*:30-48, 1956. One of the fundamental papers on the subject, well documented, well written, and well illustrated. It complements Fuchs' chapter on Radiographic recording media and screens in *Science of Radiology* of 1933.

Fuchs, A. W.: Radiography of 1896. *Image, 9* (1): 4-17, 1960. This is not Roche's *Image,* it has the subtitle Journal of the George Eastman House of Photography. A genteel article, interspersed with perfect reproductions of old plates, portraits, and posters, comparable both in style and in shape with this all-time master radiographer's paper on Edison and roentgenology, published in the *Am. J. Roentgenol.* of February, 1947.

Fujinami, K.: *Literaturregister der Strahlenkunde und allgemeinen physikalischen Therapie in der japanischen Medizin.* Bericht über 1912-1929. Tokyo, Keio University, 1931. Classified bibliography, with author index, text in Japanese (part I), German or English (part 2). Fujinami, who trained with Kienböck in Vienna, published in 1911 in the *Fortschritte,* a paper on ossification times of carpal bones, based on observation of 200 subjects.

Fulton, H.: 60 years of cardiovascular roentgenology. *Am. J. Roentgenol., 76*:657-663, 1956.

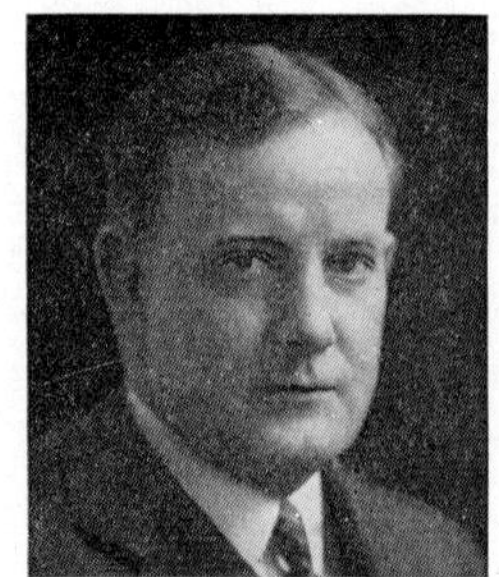
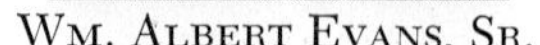

Wm. Albert Evans, Sr.

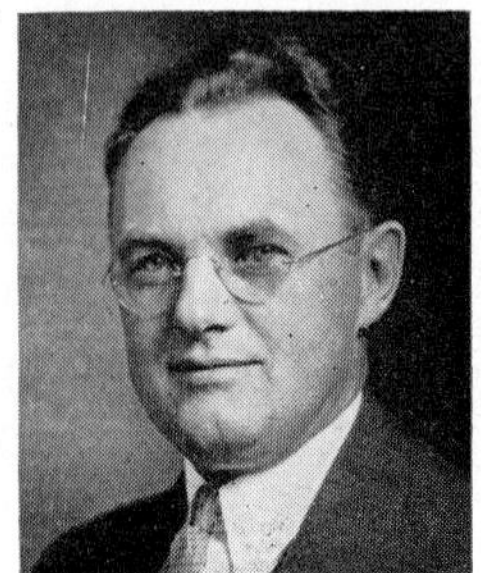

Arthur Fuchs

Garcia, P. J.: History of radiology in the Philippines. *J. Philipp. Federation Priv. Med. Practit., 11*: 686-688, 1962. The author, a radiologist by trade, is the former "boss" of the Philippine Atomic Energy Board. The first physician to use x rays in Manila was Jose Maria Salinas, shortly after 1900. Their "father of radiology" was Ramon Fernandez, who for a long time was professor of radiology in both the University of the Philippines and the University of Santo Tomas. A surviving old-timer, Daniel Ledesma, was for a long time the only radiologist for the southern islands. The Philippine Radiological Society was founded on August 14, 1948, with Paterno S. Chikiamko as its first president. He was succeeded in that position by Paulino Garcia (the author of this article). The Society has currently about forty radiologist-members.

Gardiner, J. H.: The origin, history, and development of the x-ray tube. *J. Röntgen Soc., 5*:66-80, 1909. Pioneers, from Crookes and Röntgen to Jackson and Thomson. Basic paper on history of gas tubes.

Garland, L. H.: History of radiology in California. *Bull. d'Inf. Centre A. Béclère, 4* (nr. 45):1-6, 1955. On February 19, 1897 T. M. McCoy examined a patient's eye for a retained metallic foreign body; the oval bald spot, which appeared on the scalp where it had touched the x-ray tube, was explained as idiosyncrasy to x rays. In February, 1902 Soiland reported improvement in a case of carcinoma of the breast treated with x rays; whereupon George Lasher remarked that this speaks in favor of the microbian origin of cancer. George Painter, a pioneer radiologist who practiced in the Butler Building (San Francisco), was killed in 1917 by the bomb thrown during the Preparedness Days Parade. In 1928 Charles Lauritsen built a high-voltage tube (a so-called "cold tube") at the California Institute of Technology in Los Angeles; when it was found that it produced fluoroscopic images of the hand through concrete walls several rooms away, no therapeutic use was (then) made of this machine (it was used in 1929). California firsts: development of the first light flexible fluoroscope (Rieber, 1916); radon plant (Laurence Taussig, 1919); 200 kvp therapy in San Francisco (Rehfisch and Kilgore, 1920); cardiac x-ray movies (Chamberlain and Dock, 1926); 1000 kvp therapy unit in Los Angeles (Mudd, Costolow, 1929); P-32 radioisotope therapy (Lawrence, 1936); and neutron therapy (Stone, 1938). In a personal communication, Garland added one paragraph to the above summary: "The 200 kvp machine installed by Rehfisch was a GE Snook cross-arm rectified unit. He brought in a Dauvillier dosimeter from Paris to calibrate it, and I (Garland) spent many an hour moving the Xenon chamber around the large water phantom. That was between 1929 and 1931, before the international roentgen unit was fully agreed upon. Our roentgen was strictly national, if not local. Needless to say, the racket made by the sparks on the large cross-arm rectifier was of immense therapeutic benefit to patients with non-neoplastic disease."

Garland, L. H.: Forensic skiagraphy. *California Medicine, 87*:295-297, 1957. An individualistic, indomitable, and informed Irishman inquires into the etymologic motivation for radiologic injustices. Quotation: "The late Judge George H. Buck of San Mateo County would not allow the introduction of roentgenograms into his court. He believed that they were not intelligible to the average juror, and that jurors could better be informed by hearing or reading the expert interpretations of the films made by persons qualified to do so. The good judge was far ahead of his time."

Gauducheau, R.: La radiologie en France. *Bull. d'Inf. Centre A. Béclère,* 12 (nr. 137, 138, 139 & 140): 11 pages, 1963. Inedit details on the *Fondateur de la Radiologie Française,* Antoine Béclère; on the scientific achievements in France; and on the growth of the Société Française d'Électro-Radiologie Médicale, which was founded by Béclère in 1908.

Gebauer, A.: Historical development of radiological tomography. *Indian J. Radiol.,* (souvenir number) 213-227, 1956. Well documented and illustrated (by SRW).

Ghent, P.: *Roentgen, a Brief Biography.* Toronto, Hunter-Rose, 1929, 28 pages. Contains long excerpts from 1896 interview of Dam (London correspondent of *McClure's Magazine*) with Röntgen. Quotes at length from Middleton's book and key affair. This biography was printed on the occasion of RSNA's 15th annual meeting in Toronto (1929). It carried

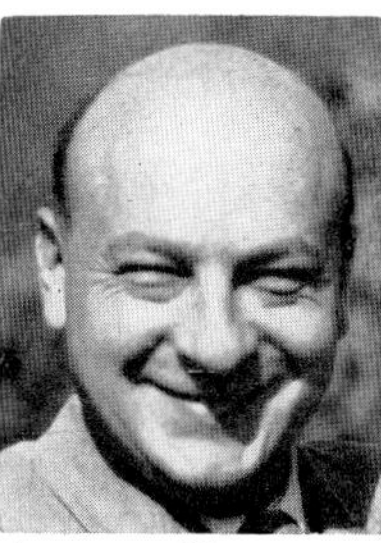
Alfred Gebauer

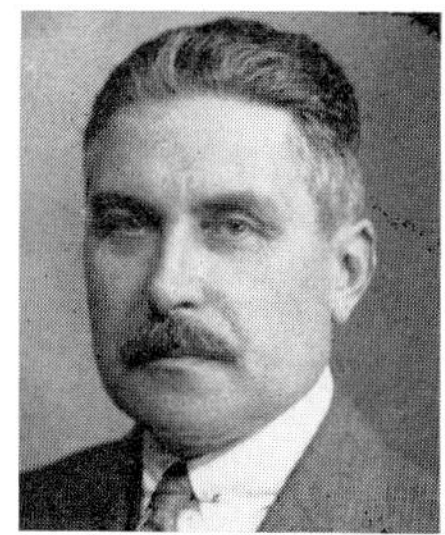
Rene Gauducheau

a foreword by Gordon Richards (Percy Ghent was Richards' x-ray technician).

Ghent, P.: A journalist talked to Röntgen. *Ontario Radiographer, 1* (nr. 3):8-12, 1940. Anecdotic.

Gilbert, R.: *A propos du cinquantenaire de la découverte des rayons X.* Lausanne, Royge, 1946, pp. 23. Part of this material appeared in the January, 1946 issue of *Alma Mater* (Lausanne). Gilbert signed the obituary for his friend Mario Ponzio in the *Acta Radiologica Interamericana* of July-September, 1956.

Glasser, O.: *Wilhelm Conrad Röntgen und die Geschichte der Röntgenstrahlen.* Berlin, Springer Verlag, 1931, 337 pages. This is an excellent, deeply documented biography, of which there are several versions (including two translations in English). It contains also a list of over one thousand titles of publications on roentgen rays printed during the year 1896.

Glasser, O. (ed.): *Science of Radiology.* Springfield, Charles C Thomas Publisher, 1933, 450 pages. Twenty six authors issued the most comprehensive survey of the history of the specialty, brought up to (that) date. Collector's item.

Glasser, O.: Early American roentgenograms. *Am. J. Roentgenol., 54*:590-594, 1945. Result of a letter survey on who got the first clinical film in this country: contest undecided! Otto Glasser published several other papers in both the Gray and in the Yellow Journal (see the respective cumulative indices).

Gocht, H.: Röntgographie oder Diagraphie. *Fortschritte a. d. Geb. d. Röstrlen, 2*:138-139, 1899. Early etymologic endeavors: reizend!

Gocht, H.: *Röntgenliteratur,* vols. 1-15. Stuttgart, Ferdinand Enke Verlag, 1911-1936. Tremendous collection, best on Central-European sources; contains bibliographic information of all sorts (meetings, journals, books).

Gökmen, M.: Baslarken. *Türk Radyoloji Mecmuasi, 1*:3-4, 1955. The Turkish Radiological Society was founded in 1924 as the Türk Elektro-Radyoloji Cemiyeti.

Goldstein, A. E., and Abeshouse, B. S.: A historical and practical consideration of pyelographic media. *Am. J. Roentgenol., 33*:165-175, 1935. It should have been specifically called . . . *for retrograde urography.* Earliest attempts were made by Tuffier in 1897. Schmidt and Kolischer in 1901, and Fenwick in 1905. The very first visualization of the ureter through a retrograde catheter was achieved in 1904 by B. Klose who reported it in the same year in the *Deutsche Ztschr. f. Chirurgie.* The term pyelography was introduced by Voelcker in the *München. med. Wchschr.* in 1906.

Gonzales, A.: *La posicion de la radiología en sus cincuenta anos de vida.* Guatemala, Universidad de San Carlos, 1946, 53 pages. Thesis.

González, G.: *Historia de la Radiología Española,* University of Madrid, 1961, 158 pages & 9 pages of references. This thesis was sponsored by Carlos Gil y Gil, who mentioned it in one of his letters. He had no copy in his possession, so I wrote to the Faculty of Medicine, but they said their only exemplar is mimeographed, and must be retained in their files. I was told that the author, Gabino González González, had returned to his native Colombia. Thereupon I wrote to Jorge Henao Echavarria in Baranquilla, and he made extensive inquiries in the town of Cali (Colombia) and with the medical librarian of the University of Antioquia (Colombia), but to no avail.

Goto, G.: Honpo nikkan shimbun ni hozerareta rentogen-sen no hakken. *Rinsho hoshasen, 8*:308-312, 1963. Account of 1896 Japanese newspaper reports of Röntgen's discovery. Goro Goto, who possesses unusually vast documentary material, is currently preparing a formal history of Japanese radiology.

Gray, A. L.: A brief review of the progress of roentgenology in the past decade. *Amer. J. Roentgenol., 2*:869-871, 1915.

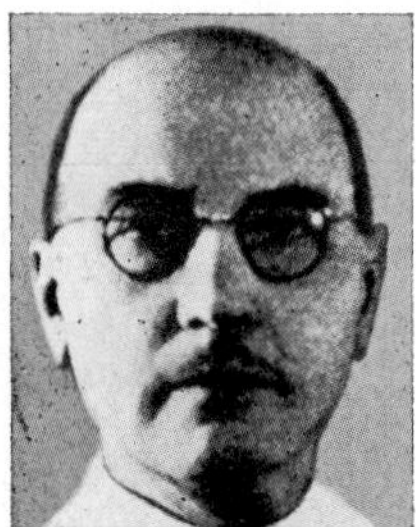
René Gilbert

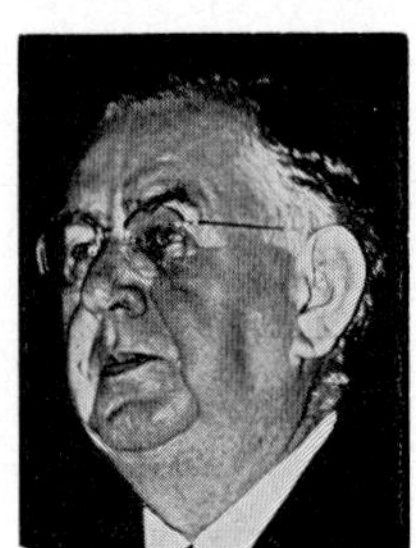
Otto Glasser

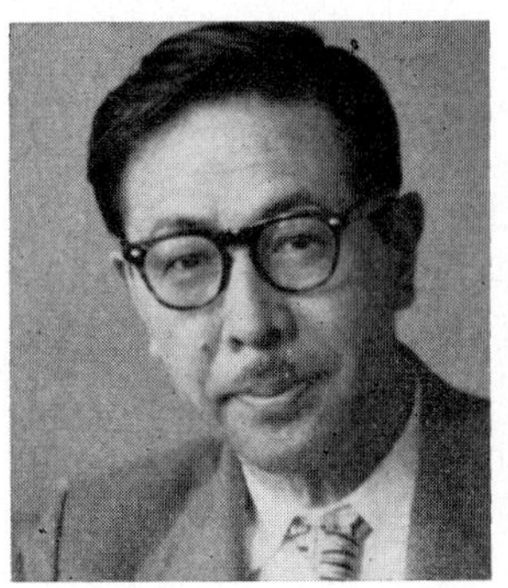
Goro Goto

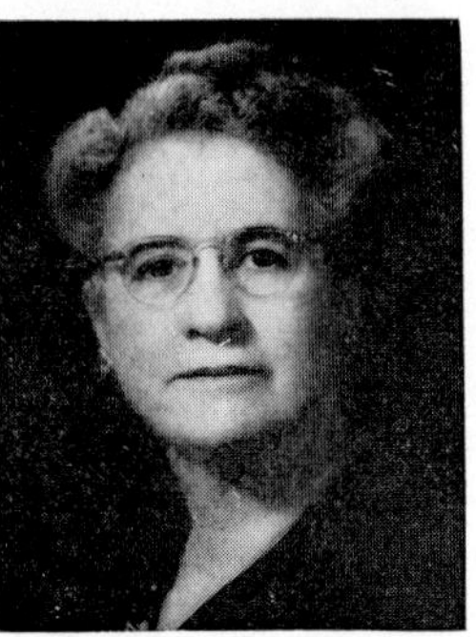
Margaret Hoing

Green, A. B.: Quo fata vocant. *X-Ray Technician, 26*:76-88, 1954. History of the American Registry of X-Ray Technicians, factual and accurate.

Grigg, E. R. N.: Prelude to the classics *in Classic Descriptions in Diagnostic Roentgenology* (ed.: A. J. Bruwer). Springfield (Illinois), Charles C Thomas, 1964.

Grigg, E. R. N.: The "New History" in American radiology. This paper, based on my historic exhibit *(American Radiology in Historical Perspective)*, was printed in *Radiologic Technology* of January, 1965. In 200 B.C., Polybius demanded that historic knowledge be made a prerequisite for those wishing to engage in public affairs. Similar requirements ought to prevail in the selection of officers of radiologic societies. Without an adequate knowledge of the radiologic past, one cannot understand the radiologic present, and is probably unfit to plan for the radiologic future.

American radiology has progressed as a result of the tripartite collaboration of radiologic clinicians, radiologic technicians, and radiologic artisans. No meaningful history can be written without recognizing that present high standards of radiologic care would not have been achieved without the increasing availability of graduate x-ray technicians (*i.e.*, radiologic technologists), without the acceptance of the physicist as a significant member of the radiologic team, and without the active co-operation of the x-ray industry.

Karl Lamprecht's *What is History?* (1905) started the arguments which led in the 1920s to the formulation of the dynamic discipline called "The New History." It has remained to this day the most sensible and widely accepted historiographic concept, in opposition to Sir John Robert Seeley's outdated view of "history as past politics" (1890), anecdotically selected and episodically expounded. The application of the New History to radiology requires a division into historic stages.

Three stages, separated by the first two world wars, are recognized in the history of radiology: (1) *The Era of the Roentgen Pioneers,* (2) *The Golden Age of Radiology,* and (3) *The Atomic Phase.* The martial interludes swelled both the medical and the technical ranks of the specialty. War exerted a significant influence on the x-ray industry as well. And had there not been the military desire for an A-bomb, we might yet be dreamily sailing through a protracted Golden Age of Radiology.

It is worth mentioning that most roentgen "novelties" were described, or at least ideated, within the first year after Röntgen's discovery. Only in the first half of 1896 was Europe ahead of America (by about one month) in terms of medical roentgen applications. The situation was later reversed, especially in terms of technical roentgen advances. Both the Golden Age of Radiology, and the Atomic Phase were "made in the USA."

The first established American radiologist was Wm. James Morton, a neuropsychiatric electrologist in New York City. This illustrates the close connection between the roentgen pioneers and electrology, a pseudo-science which at the time was quite legitimate, even if that could not be said of all its practitioners. The electrotherapists had the technical knowledge and the machinery needed to produce roentgen rays, and there was an industry catering to their needs. This is how the static machine and its manufacturers —for instance, the colorful Rome Vernon Wagner and mica plate creation—came into the x-ray business, albeit the static machine never really displaced the induction coil.

The electrologists provided the first formal (and often less than formal) roentgen teaching. They supported the first *American X-Ray Journal* (1897), and participated in the creation by Heber Robarts of the first Roentgen Society of the United States (1900), today's ARRS. Thence an epic battle was fought to divorce roentgenology from its electrologic partners. This professional separation was completed in the USA before the end of the Era of the Roentgen Pioneers: like many divorces, it caused bitter words and hard feelings, which often did not fade until the death of the participants.

In the attached chronologic table—entitled *Historical Synopsis of Radiology in the USA and Canada*—the transitional events are those which seemed most responsible for shaping the "next" stage. Due to erratic time-schedules in actual history and to the fact that for some events only approximate dates were available, the transitional occurrences did not always take place just before or after the end of the "previous" stage. A recording functionary would violently object to the chronologic incongruity of grouping such disparate events into the same transitional stage. But then, this is what separates historians from recording clerks.

HISTORICAL SYNOPSIS OF RADIOLOGY IN THE USA AND CANADA

	TECHNICAL ADVANCES IN DIAGNOSIS	DIAGNOSTIC ADVANCES
THE ERA OF THE ROENTGEN PIONEERS	—Reproduction of W. C. Röntgen's experiments (1896) —Intensifying screen of M. I. Pupin (1896) —Fluoroscope improved by T. A. Edison (1896) —Photographic x-ray plate of J. Carbutt (1896) —Photofluoroscope of J. M. Bleyer (1896) —Stereo-roentgenography of E. Thomson (1896) —Oil-immersed x-ray tube of J. Trowbridge (1896) —Idea of x-ray tube with rotating anode by R. W. Wood (1896) —High-tension rectifying switch of H. Lemp (1897) —Skiameter of A. W. Crane (1897) —Orbital foreign body localizer of W. M. Sweet (1898)	—First dental x-ray plate by C. E. Kells (1896) —First x-ray diagnosis of osteosarcoma by S. H. Monell (1896) —First full-body radiograph on single film by W. J. Morton (1897) —Gastric opaques investigated by J. C. Hemmeter (1896), W. B. Cannon (1898), and F. H. Williams (1901) —Description of roentgen findings in gastric carcinoma by G. E. Pfahler (1911) —Serial gastric radiography by L. G. Cole (1912) —Paranasal sinuses view of C. A. Waters (1914) —Insufflation of bismuth as an attempt at bronchography by Chevalier Jackson, reported in 1918
TRANSITION I	—Motor-driven cross-arm rectifier of H. C. Snook (1907) —Motor-tilted fluoroscopic table of E. W. Caldwell (1912) —Antiscatter diaphragm of G. Bucky (1912) and H. E. Potter (1916) —Hot cathode x-ray tube of W. D. Coolidge (1913) —Oil-immersed transformer and tube of H. F. Waite (1919) —Dental angle meter of H. R. Raper (1919)	—R. D. Carman re-introduces gastrointestinal fluoroscopy (1912) —Retrograde pyelography with thorium dioxide by J. E. Burns (1914) —Collargol salpyngography by W. H. Cary (1914) —X-ray detection of pulmonary tuberculosis in recruits by L. G. Cole (1917) —Air ventriculography (1918) and air myelography (1919) by W. E. Dandy
THE GOLDEN AGE OF RADIOLOGY	—Microradiography improved by G. L. Clark (1928) —First chest survey using paper radiography, made by F. T. Powers (1931) —Kymography improved by I. S. Hirsch (1934) —Laminography improved by J. A. Andrews (1936) and by J. Kieffer (1938)	—Pelvigraphy (pelvic pneumoperitoneum) by W. H. Stewart and A. Stein (1921) —Urography of L. G. Rowntree (1922) —Cholecystography of E. A. Graham and W. H. Cole (1923) —Fatty meal of E. A. Boyden (1925) —Nomenclature and classification of bone tumors by E. A. Codman (1925) —Lymphangiography of L. J. Menville (1931) —Stereographic pelvimetry of W. E. Caldwell and H. C. Moloy (1932) —Regional enteritis of B. B. Crohn described in 1932 —Study of pulmonary infarction by A. O. Hampton and B. Castleman (1940)
TRANSITION II	—Phototimer of R. H. Morgan (1942) —Automatic hanger x-ray film processor of G. Dye (1943) —X-ray image intensifier tube of J. W. Coltman (1948)	—Angiocardiography in adults by G. P. Robb and I. Steinberg (1936) —Introduction into USA of photofluorography by H. E. Potter (1938) —Venography improved by E. C. Baker and F. A. Miller (1940) —Pelvimetry by H. Thoms (1943)
THE ATOMIC PHASE	—Electro-kymography of G. C. Henny and W. E. Chamberlain (1947) —X-ray image intensification with television (1949) —Cine-fluorography with image intensification (1954)	—Diagnostic classification of bone tumors by G. S. Lodwick (1958) —Use of computer in facilitating x-ray diagnosis by L. B. Lusted (1959) —Continuing refinements in diagnosis with opaque media (including cine-fluorography)

HISTORICAL SYNOPSIS OF RADIOLOGY IN THE USA AND CANADA

FIRMS AND DIAGNOSTIC MACHINERY

—The Sayen self-regulating x-ray tube made by Queen & Co. (1896)
—The Thomson Inductorium and Standard x-ray tube made by GE's Edison Co. (1896)
—The Morton-Wimshurst-Holtz machine made by Van Houten & Ten Broeck (1896)
—The glass plate static machine made by the Wagner Co. (1897)
—The positive x-ray film made by the M. A. Seed Dry Plate Co. (1899)
—The upright fluoroscope made by Waite & Bartlett (1906)
—The Grosse Flamme coil made by Kelley & Koett (1906)
—The Premier American intensifying screen made by H. Threlkeld-Edwards (1912)
—The improved fluoroscopic screen made by the Patterson Screen Co. (1913)
—The cloverleaf tungsten transformer tube made by Green & Bauer (1913)

—The first commercial tilting table (Clinix) made by the Campbell Co. (1915)
—Coolidge tube in Shearer's (Army) bedside unit, made by Waite & Bartlett (1916)
—The Victor merger (1916); the Acme defection (1918); GE purchases Victor (1920)
—The double-coated x-ray film made by the Eastman-Kodak Co. (1918)
—The X-ograph dental packets made by the A. W. Buck Co. (1919)
—The first commercial Bucky-Potter, made by the Geo. Brady Co. (1920)
—The Carman revolving radiographic table made by the Keleket Co. (1924)
—First American hot valve-rectified transformer made by the Wappler Co. (1924)

—The all-metal SimpleX, DupleX, and TripleX made by the Engeln Co. (1925)
—The Dushman hot-cathode kenotron (1915) made by GE (1926)
—The Picker Co. purchases Waite & Bartlett (1929) and opens Cleveland plant
—Line of shockproof x-ray equipment introduced by GE (1929)
—American X-Ray Co. and Wappler Co. purchased by Westinghouse (1930)
—Only American triphasic x-ray transformer made by the Picker Co. (1933)
—Liebel-Flarsheim begins large-scale manufacture of Bucky-Potter (1934)
—The Micronex tube for microsecond radiography made by Westinghouse (1937)
—The first American rotating anode x-ray tube made by the Machlett Co. (1938)
—The Patterson Screen Co. purchased by the Du Pont Co. (1943)

—The Army Field X-ray Unit made by the Picker Co. (1942)
—The Supertilt table made by Keleket for the US Army (1943)
—First commercial phototimer made by the Westinghouse Co. (1945)
—High-kv ratings in American-made x-ray transformers (after 1950)
—The 360° Imperial x-ray table made by the GE Co. (1952)
—The Fluorex with image intensifier tube made by the Westinghouse Co. (1953)
—The automatic roller film processor made by Eastman Kodak (1956)
—Thoriated tungsten valves made by the Dunlee Co. (1957)

—Spotfilm devices made by the Scholz Co. (1950?) and the Leishman Co. (1953)
—The ceiling tube support made by the Blair X-Ray Co. (1954)
—The radiographic collimator with lighted field, made by Howdon-Videx (1954)
—The portable Fexitron made by the Field Emission Co. (1959)
—The remote-controlled Teletrol made by GE, and Satellite by Picker (1959)
—The tiltable tube-Bucky Verta-Vue made by the Continental Co. (1960)
—The Superfine 133 line/in. stationary grid made by Liebel-Flarsheim (1961)
—The pulsating, grid-controlled rotating anode made by the Machlett Co. (1962)
—The rotating anode, 125 kvp, selenium-rectified, mobile EP-300 made by GE (1962)
—The Mammograph made by the XRM Co. (1963)

THERAPEUTIC ADVANCES AND MACHINERY

—First therapeutic use of roentgen rays by E. H. Grubbé (January, 1896)
—Roentgentherapy of series of breast carcinoma reported by G. W. Hopkins (1901)
—First x-ray therapy of leukemia reported by N. Senn and W. A. Pusey (1903)
—First x-ray therapy of enlarged thymus reported by A. Friedländer (1907)
—First constant potential x-ray transformer made by the Keleket Co. (1918)

—Saturation method of roentgentherapy of L. B. Kingery (1920)
—First American deep therapy x-ray unit made (for J. T. Case) by GE (1921)
—Landauer's roentgenometer (ionto-quanitmeter) made by Standard (1924)
—Condenser dosimeter, built by O. Glasser, U. V. Portmann, & V. B. Seitz (1929), made by the Victoreen Co. as the Condenser R-meter

—Dee's deep therapy tilting tube container made by the Standard Co. (1925)
—Constant potential Quadrocondex made by Wappler (1926), then by Westinghouse
—First 1200 kvp unit, built in Pasadena by C. C. Lauritsen (1928)
—600 kvp GE unit, with Coolidge cascade tube, at Memorial Hospital (1931)
—Cyclotron at Berkeley, ideated and built by E. O. Lawrence (1931)
—800 kvp GE units at Mercy (Chicago) and Swedish Hospital (Seattle) in 1933
—First electrostatic generator, built by R. J. Van de Graaff (1933), first used in therapy in 1937
—Oil-immersed Maximar 200 kvp (1936) and 1000 kvp Maxitron (1939), made by GE

—Supervoltage therapy results reported by S. G. Mudd & C. K. Emery, and by H. Schmitz (1935)
—E. H. Quimby & G. C. Laurence: Technical Bulletin No. 1 (1940) of the Committee on Standardization of the RSNA
—Betatron built at the University of Illinois (Urbana) by D. W. Kerst (1940)
—Beryllium window x-ray tube for contact therapy, made by Machlett (1944)

—First experience with megavoltage therapy (betatron) reported by R. A. Harvey (1951)
—First experience with fast electron therapy (from betatron) reported by L. Haas (1954)
—High voltage sources (electrostatic generators made by HVEC, and linacs made by Varian) available for both electron and x-irradiation

HISTORICAL SYNOPSIS OF RADIOLOGY IN THE USA AND CANADA

	RADIUM AND ARTIFICIAL RADIOISOTOPES	EDUCATION
THE ERA OF THE ROENTGEN PIONEERS	—Correspondence between S. T. Lockwood and P. Curie (1902) —J. R. Lofftus finds and begins to mine radium-containing carnotite in Utah (1903) —First radium treatment of carcinoma of cervix uteri by M. A. Cleaves (1903) —R. Abbe first implanted radium in a tumor, exophthalmic goiter) in 1905 —W. J. Morton advocates radiochemicotherapy, meaning ingestion of radium followed by external roentgentherapy (1906) —W. Duane first suggested use of emanation (radon) in tumors (1908) —J. M. Flannery organized Radium Chemical Co. (1911) —H. A. Kelly & J. Douglas start the National Radium Institute (1914)	—W. J. Morton's educational positive x-ray prints, sold by E. B. Meyrowitz (1896) —Brooklyn Post-Graduate School of Clinical Electro-Therapeutics and Roentgen Photography — S. H. Monell, M.D. (1896) —Chicago College of X-Rays and Electro-Therapeutics—H. P. Pratt, M.D. (1898) —Instruction in X-Ray Work, St. Louis X-Ray Lab—Mr. M. E. Parberry (1899) —New York Electrical Institute of Correspondence Instruction in X-Rays and Electro-Therapeutics—W. J. Herdman, M. D. (1900) —Scientific and technical exhibits at first meeting of ARRS (1900) —First use of roentgen aids in teaching anatomy in Milwaukee—C. R. Bardeen (1910)
TRANSITION I	—H. H. Janeway "buries emanation" permanently (implantation of radon glass seeds) into tumors (1915) —First commercial manufacture of platinum-iridium needles for interstitial implantation, made by the US Radium Co. (1918) —Cheaper uranium for Belgian Congo forces discontinuation of refining of American radium ores (1923) —Radium dosage tables prepared by E. H. Quimby (1928)	—G. E. Pfahler, first legitimate professor of radiology (1911) in Philadelphia —First examination by American Registry of Radiologic Technicians (1922).
THE GOLDEN AGE OF RADIOLOGY	—Radon gold seeds first made by G. Failla (1926) —Four-gram radium pack ("bomb") constructed by G. Failla (1928) —H. S. Martland first reported on radioactivity in radium dial painters (1931) —R. S. Stone unsuccessfully treated leukemia with cyclotron-produced radiosodium while J. H. Lawrence succeeded in 1938 with radiophosphorus. —S. Hertz begins animal studies on thyroid with cyclotron-produced radio-iodine (1938) does uptakes in 1939, and treats hyperthyroidism (1942) —R. S. Stone first used cyclotron neutrons on human tumors (1939)	—Prevalence of preceptorship training in medical radiology by recognized authorities (J. T. Case, P. M. Hickey, W. H. Stewart, L. G. Cole), advertising in radiologic journals —First three schools of x-ray technicians, approved by the ARRT (1933)
TRANSITION II	—First sustained nuclear chain reaction produced in the E. Fermi & L. Szilard CP1 (Chicago Pile One) in 1942 —Reactor-produced isotopes more plentiful than if cyclotron-produced: first shipment from Oak Ridge to Barnard Free Cancer Hospital (1946) —The cervico-vaginal radium applicator of E. C. Ernst, Sr. (1946) —Co-60 as substitute for radium in teletherapy: irradiator conceived by L. G. Grimmett (1949): first completed model in Regina (Sask.) 1951	—Creation of American Board of Radiology (1934) —First course in the Oak Ridge School of Radioisotope Technique (1948) —Inclusion of radiation physicist as a member of the radiologic team, after radiophysics is made part of the required ABR examination
THE ATOMIC PHASE	—Co-60 depth dose teletherapy curves by H. E. Johns (1952) —Co-60 as a radium substitute in brachytherapy: in flexible nylon tubing by J. L. Morton & al (1950); in steel needles by I. Meschan et al. (1951) —W. G. Myers & U. K. Henschke investigate radiogold in flexible tubing (1951) —B. Cassen; L. Curtis & C. W. Reed: Scintillation scanner (1951) —P. R. Bell's Medical Scintillation Spectrometer (1955) —M. A. Bender: autofluoroscope (1960). —H. O. Anger: scintillation camera (1961). —Since 1961, intracavitary applications of radiogold obsolete (or almost)	—Growth of training programs in ABR approved radiology residencies —Radiologic teaching and research modified by growing dependency on federal and other grant-supported programs

HISTORICAL SYNOPSIS OF RADIOLOGY IN THE USA AND CANADA

RADIATION PROTECTION

—First report on x-ray epilation by J. Daniel (April, 1896)
—First protective use of lead foil by E. H. Grubbe (May, 1896)
—Self-inflicted experimental radiation injury by E. Thomson (June, 1896)
—W. A. Price produces lead rubber gloves (1898?)
—R. Friedländer Co. x-ray catalog lists protective devices, including lead rubber hoods, aprons, and gloves (1899)
—First determination of "safe" x-ray intensity: less than needed to fog a photographic plate in seven minutes—W. H. Rollins (1902)
—S. H. Monell proposes Committee on Standards of the ARRS (1903)
—First radiation fatality in the USA: C. M. Dally (1865-1904)

—First report on roentgen-induced mutations in toads by C. R. Bardeen (1907)
—First standing Roentgen Ray Protection Committee, ARRS (September, 1920)
—First whole body "tolerance" dose—72 r/year—by A. Mutscheller (1925)

—Formation of CXRP—Advisory Committee on X-Ray and Radium Protection (1928)
—Demonstration of genetic effects of radiation by H. J. Muller (1930)
—CXRP's first NBS Handbook 15 on X-Ray Protection (1931)
—"Safe" whole body exposure to radium (and hard x rays)—36 r/year—established by G. Failla (1932)
—"Safe" radium dose to fingers—5 r/day = 1500 r/year—by G. Failla (1932)
—Failla's "safe" dosage included in CXRP's NBS Handbook 18, Radium Protection (1934)
—P. Brown: American Martyrs to Science through the Roentgen Rays (1936)

—First A-bomb (1945); with resultant studies on late leukemogenic effects; on mutagenic effects; on fallout, etc.
—1946: CXRP becomes NCRP (National Committee for Radiation Protection)
—1948: NCRP creates concept of "permissible" whole body exposure, established for occupational circumstances to 15 r/year
—1950: NCRP's "permissible" dosage endorsed by AEC

—1958: decrease of "permissible" occupational whole body exposure to 12 r/year
—1962: decrease of "permissible" exposure to 5 r/year
—1962: radiation statutes adopted by various state legislatures

MEMORABLE BOOKS

—W. J. Morton: X-Ray or the Photography of the Invisible (1896)
—F. H. Williams: Roentgen Rays in Medicine and Surgery (1901)
—S. H. Monell: System of Instruction in X-Ray Methods (1902)
—W. A. Pusey & E. W. Caldwell: Roentgen Rays in Therapeutics and Diagnosis (1903)
—W. H. Rollins: Notes on X-Light (1904)
—C. W. Allen: Radiotherapy and Phototherapy (1904)
—C. Beck: Roentgen Ray Diagnosis and Therapy (1904)
—M. K. Kassabian: Roentgen Rays and Electro-Therapeutics (1907)
—T. M. Rotch: Diagnosis of Diseases in Early Life by the Roentgen Method (1910)
—H. R. Raper: Elementary and Dental Radiography (1913)
—W. S. Newcomet: Radium and Radiotherapy (1914)

—R. D. Carman & A. Miller: Roentgen Diagnosis of the . . . Alimentary Canal (1917)
—Army X-Ray Manual (1917)
—G. W. Holmes & H. E. Ruggles: Roentgen Interpretation (1919)
—F. M. Law: Mastoids Roentgenologically Considered (1920)
—F. H. Baetjer & C. A. Waters: Injuries and Diseases of Bones and Joints (1921)
—F. E. Simpson: Radium Therapy (1922)
—H. Wessler & L. Jaches: Clinical Roentgenology of Diseases of the Chest (1923)
—G. L. Clark: Applied X-Rays (1927)

—L. R. Sante: Manual of Radiological Technique (1928)
—G. Bucky: Grenz Ray Therapy (1929)
—C. F. Geschickter & M. M. Copeland: Tumors of Bone (1931)
—B. J. M. Harrison: Textbook of Roentgenology. Diagnosis and Therapy (1936)
—R. Golden (Ed.): Loose-leaf Diagnostic Roentgenology (1936)
—S. W. Donaldson: The Roentgenologist in Court (1937)
—E. A. Pohle: (Ed.): Clinical Roentgen Therapy (1938)
—H. K. Pancoast, E. P. Pendergrass & J. P. Schaeffer: Head and Neck in Roentgen Diagnosis (1940)
—W. Snow: Clinical Roentgenology of Pregnancy (1942)

—J. Buckstein: Clinical Roentgenology of the Alimentary Tract (1940)
—O. Glasser & al.: Physical Foundations of Radiology (1944)
—J. Caffey: Pediatric X-Ray Diagnosis (1945)
—G. Files: Medical Radiographic Technic (1947)
—L. V. Ackerman & J. A. del Regato: Cancer (1947)
—F. Buschke, S. T. Cantril & H. M. Parker: Supervoltage Roentgentherapy (1950)
—U. V. Portmann (Ed.): Clinical Therapeutic Radiology (1950)
—G. A. Andrews, M. Brucer & E. B. Anderson (Eds.): Radioisotopes in Medicine (1953)

—V. Merrill: Atlas of Roentgenographic Positions (1949)
—I. Meschan: Normal Radiographic Anatomy (1949)
—W. F. Braasch & J. L. Emmett: Clinical Urography (1951)
—H. E. Johns: The Physics of Radiology (1953)
—A. A. de Lorimier, H. G. Moehring & J. B. Hannan: Clinical Roentgenology (1954)
—H. L. Abrams & H. S. Kaplan: Angiocardiographic Interpretation (1956)
—E. H. Quimby & al.: Radioactive Isotopes in Medicine and Biology (1958)
—W. D. Claus (Ed.): Radiation Biology and Medicine (1958)
—G. H. S. Ramsey & al.: Cinefluorography (1960
—McC. Wilson: Anatomical Foundation of Neuroradiology of the Brain (1963)
—J. M. Taveras & E. H. Wood: Diagnostic Neuroradiology (1964)

HISTORICAL SYNOPSIS OF RADIOLOGY IN THE USA AND CANADA

	SOCIETIES	IMPORTANT PERIODICALS
THE ERA OF THE ROENTGEN PIONEERS	—American Roentgen Ray Society (1900) —Philadelphia Roentgen Ray Society (1906) —New York Roentgen Society (1912) —Chicago Roentgen Society (1913) —American Radium Society (1916) —Detroit Roentgen Ray and Radium Society (1921)	—American X-Ray Journal (1897) —Archives of Electrology and Radiology (1901) —Transactions of the American Roentgen Ray Society (1902) —American Quarterly of Roentgenology (1906) —Rayons X, Montreal (1910) —American Journal of Roentgenology (1913) —Radium, Pittsburgh (1913) —American Atlas of Stereoroentgenology (1916) —Journal of Roentgenology (1918)
TRANSITION I	—Radiological Society of North America (1915) —Canadian Radiological Society (1920) —American Society of Radiological Technologists (1920) —American Registry of Radiological Technologists (1922)	—Journal of Radiology (1920)
THE GOLDEN AGE OF RADIOLOGY	—Milwaukee Roentgen Ray Society (1923) —American College of Radiology (1923) —Section on Radiology of the AMA (1924) —Société Canadienne-Française d'Electro-Radiologie Médicale (1928 —American Congress of Radiology (1933) —Canadian Association of Radiologists (1937)	—Annals of Roentgenology (1920) —Radiology (1923) —X-Ray Technician (1929) —Medical Radiography and Photography (1930) —Year Book of Radiology (1932) —Roentgen Economist (1933) —Focal Spot (1944)
TRANSITION II	—American Board of Radiology (1934) —Inter-American College of Radiology (1943) —Canadian Society of Radiologic Technicians (1943) —Radiation Research Society (1952)	—Nucleonics (1943) —Isotopics (1951)
THE ATOMIC PHASE	—Association of University Radiologists (1953) —Society of Nuclear Medicine (1954) —Health Physics Society (1956) —Society for Pediatric Radiology (1958) —American Club of Therapeutic Radiologists (1958) —Missouri Radiological Society (1961)	—Bulletin of the Atomic Scientists (1945) —Journal of the Canadian Association of Radiologists (1950) —Radiation Research (1954) —Health Physics (1958) —Radiological Health Data (1960) —Journal of Nuclear Medicine (1960) —Radiologia Interamericana (1962) —Radiological Clinics of North America (1963) —Radiologic Technology (1963)

HISTORICAL SYNOPSIS OF RADIOLOGY IN THE USA AND CANADA

HISTORIANS AND HISTORICAL TEXTS	CATCHWORDS
—H. C. Snook: A Brief History of Roentgenology (1916) —F. H. Williams: Reminiscences of a pioneer in roentgenology (1925) —P. M. Hickey: The first decade of American roentgenology (1928) —I. S. Trostler: Highlights in the history of roentgenology (1931) —E. Thomson: Work in the first decade of roentgenology (1932) —W. W. Wasson: Radiologic Pioneers in Colorado (1934) —A. W. Fuchs: Edison and roentgenology (1947) —C. W. Smith: X-ray technician of 1900 (1952)	—roentgeno- —roentgenology —skiagraphy —x ray —invisible ray(s) —cathography —x-ray photography —radium —emanation
—W. F. Manges: Camp Greenleaf School of Roentgenology (1919) —C. H. Viol: History and development of radiumtherapy (1921) —P. Brown: The inception and development of fluoroscopy (1942)	—radiography —radiotherapy —electron
—O. Glasser: Wilhelm Conrad Röntgen (1931) —American Journal of Roentgenology, October 1931 —O. Glasser (Ed.): The Science of Radiology (1933) —A. W. Erskine: Organized roentgenology in America (1945) —Radiology, November 1945 —D. G. Shields: Fashion parade of x-ray apparatus —X-Ray Technician, November 1945	—radiology —radiodiagnosis —radon —supervoltage
—L. Reynolds: History of the use of the roentgen ray in warfare (1945) —E. H. Skinner: The organization of the Roentgen Society of the US (1950 —A. B. Greene: Quo fata vocant (1954) —M. Brucer: History of the Society of Nuclear Medicine (1965?)	—A-bomb —atomic (pile) —image amplification —neutron
—M. Hoing: History of the ASXT. 1920-1950 (1952); 1951-1960 (1961) —L. H. Garland: History of radiology in California (1955) —I. M. Woolley: Roentgenology in Oregon; the First Fifty Years (1955) —American Journal of Roentgenology, Golden Vol. 75, 1956 —A. R. Bleich: The Story of X-Rays from Röntgen to Isotopes (1960) —S. B. Dewing: Modern Radiology in Historical Perspective (1962) —A. Bruwer (Ed.): Classic Descriptions in Diagnostic Roentgenology (1964) —E. R. N. Grigg: Trail of the Invisible Light (1964) —L. E. Etter (Ed.): *The Science of Ionizing Radiation* (1965)	—H-bomb —nuclear (reactor) —image intensification —radiobiology —radiopathology —radioisotopology —megavoltage —autofluoroscope

After the bitter experience with the electrologists, the American Roentgen Ray Society (ARRS) became very selective with applicants for membership. In 1915, Fred O'Hara and Miles Titterington formed the Western Roentgen Society (WRS), to give status to roentgen workers who had not been accepted by the ARRS. Benjamin Orndoff, the WRS president for 1918, changed its name to Radiological Society of North America (RSNA), thus granting rank to the term radiology. In 1920 the Victor Co.—through Ed Jerman—sponsored the creation of the American Society of Radiological Technicians, later called ASXT, now again ASRT. In 1922, the RSNA sponsored the creation of the Technicians' Registry Board. Coolidge's hot cathode tube and Snook's rectifying switch (later the valve-rectified transformer) and Eastman's double-coated films permitted the duplication of an x-ray exposure simply by following numerical guidelines. All these radio-social and radiotechnical changes "democratized" the specialty. Thereupon radiology became (just like Plato's democracy) charming, full of variety, vigor and disorder, imparting a sort of equality to equals and unequals alike.

North of the USA border, most anything is bilingual, including radiology. The first English-Canadian radiologist was Gilbert Girdwood, the first French-Canadian radiologist was Henri Lasnier, who edited the first Canadian roentgen periodical, *Les Rayons X* (1910). The first all-Canadian Radiological Society was formed in 1920, Leo Pariseau founded the Société Canadienne Française d'Électro-Radiologie in 1928. Gordon Richards organized the second, *i.e.,* the current (all-)Canadian Association of Radiologists in 1937.

In 1923, Albert Soiland founded the American College of Radiology (ACR) as an exclusive club of one hundred among America's foremost radiologists. Within a few years it became the "State Department" of American radiology. The ACR organized the American Congress of Radiology (1933) with Henry Pancoast as president, and the Fifth International Congress of Radiology (1937), with Arthur Christie as president. Both these congresses were held in Chicago, with Ben Orndoff as secretary. Soiland willed that his remains be cremated and scattered in the fjord next to his Norwegian birthplace; as that was being done (1946), extrinsic pressure and a different climate had already forced the old ACR into giving up its original substance for the perpetuation of the radiologic life cycle.

The transitional events which led to the Atomic Phase show once more how fate can twist things around. The left-leaning German-born pacifist Albert Einstein made the A-bomb possible by conceiving in 1905 that $E=mc^2$, and by signing in 1939 the famous letter to the president, in which he alerted Franklin Roosevelt to the danger that Germany might develop atomic explosives. Thereupon the Manhattan Project was organized with the intent of "getting there first." In 1942, in Chicago, Italian-born Enrico Fermi brought to criticality the first nuclear reactor. And in 1945 the atomic "Little Boy" was exploded over Hiroshima, proving loudly that, indeed, $E=mc^2$. The nuclear detonation upset Japan, and then the rest of the world. From that moment on, also in radiology, things could never again be the same. The Atomic Energy Act of 1946 changed the military Manhattan Project into the civil, but still federal, Atomic Energy Commission (AEC's regulatory powers had a tremendous impact on radiology, through the simple expedient of gradually lowering the level of permissible exposure to radiation.

During World War II, governmental support of specialized production lines was instrumental in furthering the growth of Machlett Laboratories, the x-ray tube maker. During that war, so many of Picker's Army Field Units went to such far away places that the attendant publicity—and the move of GE's x-ray plant from Chicago to Milwaukee in 1946—permitted peacetime Picker to challenge GE's supremacy in the production of x-ray equipment, a supremacy undisputed since Victor times.

Of considerable importance to the profession was the change of the ACR from the old cap-and-gown fraternity (1923), through the Inter-Society Committee for Radiology (1937)—chairman of the chancellors being Ed Chamberlain—into the new ACR (1939), with lay executives, and other attributes of a strong business association.

George Pfahler, in 1911, was the first formal professor of radiology in the USA. Teaching at the graduate level became common only toward the end of the Golden Age, with the advent of teachers such as George Holmes in Boston, Ross Golden in New York City, Paul Hodges in Chicago, LeRoy Sante in St. Louis, or Howard Ruggles in San Francisco. The American Board of Radiology (1934), ably directed by its long-time secretary Byrl Kirklin (the American radiologic educator *par excellence*), fostered the growth of residency programs which provided ever-growing cohorts of young radiologists, without whom neither American radiology in general, nor the ACR in particular, could have ever reached or maintained the current level of achievement.

In 1948 the "atomic physician" Marshall Brucer organized at the Oak Ridge Institute for Nuclear Studies a medical research and teaching center, and gave it some of his brilliance and controversy. Nuclear knowledge is also being imparted at other centers, such as the Argonne National Laboratory, where Leonidas Marinelli perfected whole body counters; and at Brookhaven National Laboratory, where Lee Farr tried hard to prove that the nuclear reactor can be a medical tool.

Artificial radioisotopes are still most often used as biologic and other type of tracers. As for their therapeutic applications, Co-60 has replaced radium in many brachytherapy devices. Intracavitary Au-198 is almost obsolete, peroral P-32 has yet a few supporters, only I-131 is solidly extrenched, both in diagnosis and in therapy.

The scintillation counter has all but replaced the Geiger-Müller tube in medical applications. The scanner, introduced in 1949, is just now in the process of being superseded by the so-called autofluoroscope (the scintillation camera). The medico-nuclear needs are served by an active, though financially still unsettled, industry which makes apparatus (the largest in this field is Nuclear-Chicago), and bottles radiochemicals (the oldest in this category is Abbott Laboratories).

Angiocardiography was introduced in 1936 in pediatric patients by Agostin Castellanos and Raul Pereiras (Havana) and—at the same time, independently—in adults by George Robb and Israel Steinberg in New York City. The recent improvements in cardiovascular surgical technics have led to demands for improvements in opaque medis, methods and machinery for use in both central and peripheral angiography.

King-sized mobile units, with rotating anodes, have been developed for use in the operating room. GE's mobile has silicon rectifiers instead of valves (when economically feasible, solid state rectification will replace the kenotrons in most applications). These mobiles are much too heavy to be misnamed "portables"—it takes an athletic constitution just to caster them around. But true portables can be useful under combat and other emergency conditions, which is why James Kereiakes and Adolph Krebs built for the US Army—at Fort Knox (Ky.)—an isotopic Th-170 radiographic unit with a shutter made of gold (a metal which is becoming scarcer even there).

With the coming of the Atomic Phase, certain rearrangements occurred in the x-ray tube business. Westinghouse discontinued its line of x-ray tubes; Machlett gave more attention to power tubes than ever before; GE continued and increased its x-ray tube production; and a new firm joined the industry, the Dunlee Corporation.

Currently in the USA, with the exception of dental and other special applications, all diagnostic x-ray tubes are of the rotating anode type. They come in various, ever-higher ratings, with optional grid control for use in pulsed cineradiography. Among non-rotating x-ray tubes is the beryllium-window model which permits high-intensity emission, suitable for contact therapy or for George Clark's microradiography.

In 1952 GE introduced its startling ring-mounted 360° Imperial table. The idea was very successful, even its name was imitated. There has recently been somewhat more restraint in offering 90/90 or 180° tilt in tables. Very desirable is the ceiling-mounted, uncluttered radiographic tube, a feature which has become the accepted standard in this country. Spot-filmers have been used in the USA more often since the advent of the Atomic Phase—particularly since the introduction of phototimers. Photoroentgenographic equipment is no longer actively advertised in this country (although it can be purchased), partly because of the radiation scare, and mainly because of the procedure's low yield (Henry Garland). It is still being used in large hospital admissions, and in certain health department surveys.

A fluoroscopic screen is viewed by looking straight toward the patient. Mirror-type image intensifiers brought an oblique viewing angle. With television, the observer watches a monitor and that or any additional monitors can be placed anywhere, to the delight of radiologic instructors and referring clinicians. The next step is to move the radiologist out of the room by providing remote control and servo-motors for table motions, as in GE's Teletrol (1959) or Picker's Satellite. What the radiologist's "looking away," and now the "moving away," from the patient will do (if anything) to the philosophy of radiology is as yet uncertain.

X-ray equipment—any x-ray equipment—is only as good as the service available. Only the "Big Four" American x-ray manufacturers maintain (almost) nation-wide service organizations. GE, after losing ground in 1946, has made a strong comeback since the mid 1950s. The Picker family has sold their firm to a financial concern, but Harvey Picker (son of the founder) remained the firm's chief-executive: over the past years, the Picker Co. has steadily expanded, and has created Picker-Nuclear and a German subsidiary. Westinghouse somehow did not take the expected advantage from its priority in image intensification, then discontinued the manufacture of x-ray tubes; now they are once again making a powerful bid for their share in the market. Keleket suffered a substantial setback because of changes in ownership and location (they moved from Covington to Boston); some of the equipment they now advertise is made for them in Europe.

Until now, for several reasons, there is in the USA no significant volume of imported x-ray equipment. A few special items are being brought in, such as Philips-Massiot's remarkable Polytome; the Planigraph of Siemens-Reiniger; or Elema-Schönander's set of twin rollfilm changers.

In 1907, Charles Bardeen was the first to show that roentgen rays may cause undesirable effects in the offspring (of toads). Since 1929 there exists in the USA a National Committee for Radiation Protection (Lauriston Taylor has been its chairman since the very beginning). The general public, even some of the radiologists, did not become aware of the protection problem until the mid 1950s, when certain political pressure groups demanded that testing of atomic weapons be discontinued to avoid potential genetic hazards from fallout. That the radiation background in the Northern Hemisphere has been raised in recent years is indubitable—paper is now so often radioactive that Du Pont advertised this as the main reason for introducing non-interleaved x-ray film.

To the leftist attacks based on test-generated fallout, "conservative" physicists retorted that medical radiation sources (mainly radiologic examinations) contribute a larger (estimated) dose than existing fallout. This did not solve the dilemma "to test or not to test," but it has effectively involved in the controversy the entire radiologic fraternity. That radiation may cause damage has been demonstrated in fast-reproducing insects and small mammals. This led often to daring, and sometimes to hysterical extrapolations. No genetic mutations have as yet been demonstrated in humans, despite the (often indiscriminate) use of diagnostic radiology for more than six decades. In the children and children of the children of women whose ovaries had been irradiated by Ira Kaplan (for sterility) in the 1920s, none had as yet developed any demonstrable malformation. Maybe most of the radiation-induced mutations are incompatible with survival, or else weeded out by natural selection. After the radiogenetic problem came the controversy over fallout shelters, which again brought the Atomic Phase radiologist closer to his times and to politics, much closer than the pioneers, or the Golden Age people had ever been.

Each radio-historic stage had its predominant professional organization, the ARRS in pioneer days, the RSNA during the Golden Age, while the ACR is radiology's mouthpiece during the rigors of the Atomic Phase. Meanwhile other organizations are being formed, most of them admittedly exclusivistic, such as the Association of University Radiologists (1953), the Society for Pediatric Radiology (1956), or the American Club of Therapeutic Radiologists (1958). Among established congregations, the ARS, in the quest for survival, expanded its scope into that of a therapeutic society: it worked, the ARS is now once more in full bloom.

Radiology is today in a state of flux, which is the way it has been for most of its existence. The proportion of radiologists in private offices has decreased, while the proportion of radiologists who practice in hospitals has risen. Also higher is the percentage of radiologists on straight salary—whether in government, in teaching, or in some "unethical" relationship with a busy hospital.

The three radio-historic stages are of help to the radiologic official also in sizing up his "constituents." There are practically no living roentgen pioneers in the USA, but belated ones may still be found in foreign lands. They are usually recognizable by the semantic attachment to their former electrologic partners. Golden Radiology men are, of course, quite abundant, here and abroad. They can be identified by their reaction (or absence of reaction) to such things as concern over unnecessary exposure to radiation, and insistence on personnel and patient protection; the use in radiography of filters, of collimators, of high-kv technics, and of high-speed screens; the utilizations of therapeutic radiation for malignancies only (a dwindling few acceptable exceptions to this rule are still on the books); and the adjustment of thinking to such terms as rads, rems, reps, or whatever new units are being proposed. Age in itself is not a deciding factor (although it helps) in recognizing that "Golden" man: it is his unwillingness to change with the times!

Groves, L. R.: *Now it Can be Told. The Story of the Manhattan Project.* New York, Harper & Brothers, 1962, 465 pages. A lucid, vivid, candid, and yet sensitive account of the dramatic years from 1942 until 1947 when the civilian AEC took over the Manhattan Engineering District (MED), and Groves changed from head of the MED to chief of the Army's Special Weapons Project (he retired in 1948). Before Groves became the boss at MED, he was made a brigadier general; a wise move, because "strangely enough, it often seemed to me (Groves) that the prerogatives of rank were more important in the academic world than they are among soldiers." —The famous letter from Einstein to Roosevelt was not written by Einstein, but only signed by Einstein: it had been written by Alexander Sachs, a Wall Street economist—"(In the selection of a chief for Los Alamos) Oppenheimer had two major disadvantages —he had almost no administrative experience of any kind, and he was not a Nobel Prize winner . . . The security organization, which was not yet under my complete control, was unwilling to clear him (Oppenheimer) because of certain of his associations, particularly in the past . . ." Thereupon Groves personally read all the documentation on the case, and requested that clearance be issued on his responsibility. "I, (Groves) have never felt that it was a mistake to have selected and cleared Oppenheimer for his wartime post." "The most disastrous break in security was that resulting from the treasonable actions of the English scientist, Klaus Fuchs . . . Our acceptance of Fuchs into the project was a mistake. But I am at a loss when I try to determine just how we could have avoided that mistake without insulting our principal war ally, Great Britain, by insisting on controlling their security measures."—As D-Day (landing in Normandy in 1944) approached, the possibility was considered that the Germans might use "radioactive poisons" against Allied troops, therefore a supply of portable Geiger counters was ordered, and a directive was issued requesting immediate reporting of all cases in which x-ray film used anywhere would have been fogged or blackened with no apparent cause. The Germans had never planned such attacks, indeed subsequent investigation showed that their scientists considered it unlikely that a workable weapon could be developed from an uranium pile.—The Japanese city of Kyoto was spared serious destruction by conventional bombers because it had been (tentatively) selected as a potential atomic target.—The senseless destruction of five Japanese cyclotrons (after capitulation) is described in a whole chapter, and called just what it had been, a blunder caused by a break-down in communications, coupled with misinterpretation of orders; to this Groves adds: ". . . the basic truth was demonstrated again, that honest errors, openly admitted, are sooner forgiven."—During the interim period, before takeover of the MED by the AEC, Groves offered to help with any advice that he might be able to give, but the AEC almost never sought his advice. In his final chapter in the book, Groves hypothesizes that if the USA had not developed the A-bomb in 1945, it would have been "discovered" somewhere in the world within the following two or three years. If a power-hungry nation were the developer, it would have dominated the world completely and immediately.—"When I (Groves) was a boy, I lived with my father at a number of the Army posts that had sprung up during the Indian wars throughout the western United States. There I came to know many of the old soldiers and scouts who had devoted their active lives to winning the West. And as I listened to the stories of their deeds, I grew somewhat dismayed, wondering what was left for me to do now that the West was won . . . Those of us who saw the dawn of the Atomic Age that early moring at Alamogordo will never hold such doubts again . . . when man is willing to make the effort, he is capable of accomplishing virtually anything."

Grubbé, E. H.: Priority in the therapeutic use of x-rays. *Radiology, 21*:156-162, 1933. Referral of first patient for x-ray treatment of extensive, ulcerated carcinoma of breast. Story repeated in his book (see next reference).

Grubbé, E. H.: *X-Ray Treatment. Its Origin, Birth, and Early History.* St. Paul, Bruce Publishing Company, 1949, 154 pages. Personal recollections, including the "first x-ray burn."

Habbe, J. E.: Milwaukee's radiologic heritage. *Wisconsin M. J.* in publication. This is the revised text of the talk given before the Milwaukee Roentgen Ray Society on November 25, 1963, on its 40th anniversary. It contains the mention that Wisconsin's first radiologist was Jacob Janssen (1869-1937), a registered pharmacist who produced the roentgen plate

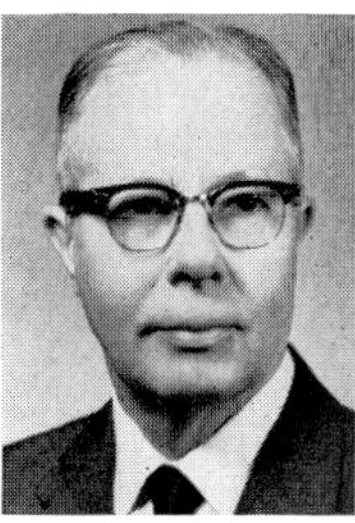

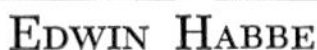

EDWIN HABBE

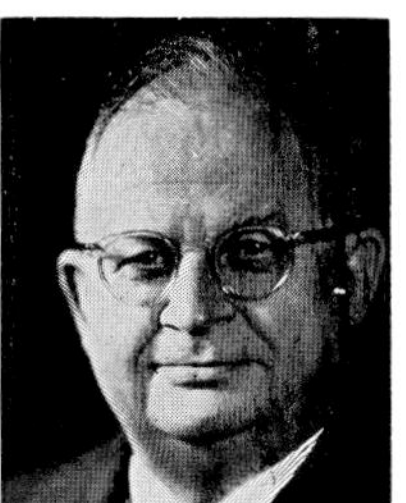

PAUL CHESLEY HODGES

of a hand (allegedly) during February of 1896. A print of that plate is in the possession of the Milwaukee Hospital. Janssen served as radiologist to that hospital until the time of his death.

de Hevesy, G.: Marie Curie and her contemporaries. *J. of Nuclear Med., 2*:169-182, 1961. The Becquerel-Curie Memorial Lecture by one of the pioneers of radioactive tracer technics: Marja Sklodowska, Becquerel, Rutherford, and Bohr.

Hewlett, R. G., and Anderson, Jr., O. E.: *The New World,* 1939/1946. University Park, Pennsylvania State University Press, 1962. pp. 766. First volume of the history of the AEC, written by two professional historians, apparently unhampered by classified documents; epic account of the Manhattan Project, ending with the creation of the AEC by the US Congress; excellent!

Hickey, P. M.: The first decade of American roentgenology. *Am. J. Rentgenol., 20*:150-157; 249-356, 1928. A delightful combination of personal recollections, bibliographic correlations, and direct informations from other contemporary witnesses. Example: a physician, Harry Tetrell, published with Goodspeed a paper in which they suggested using the word skiagram instead of x-ray picture.

Hickey, P. M.: Caldwell Lecture, 1928. *Am. J. Roentgenol., 25*:177-195, 1931. Published posthumously: pleasant, polished presentation in which the dying eulogized the dead.

Hille, H.: From the memoirs of a student in Röntgen's laboratory in Würzburg half a century ago. *Am. J. Roentgenol., 55*:643-647, 1956. For a number of (planned) speaking engagements in the USA, a business representative offered five-figure sums in dollars first to Röntgen, then to the latter's assistant, Otto Stern, but was turned down by both of them.

Hines, N. O.: *Proving Ground. An Account of the Radiobiological Studies in the Pacific, 1946-1961;* Seattle, University of Washington Press, 1962, 366 pages. Applied Fisheries Laboratory was the code name for the Laboratory of Radiation Biology, created in 1943 in the University of Washington. It began investigations of the biological effects of nuclear radiation even before the first A-bomb was exploded at Alamogordo. It has been in continuous operation since 1943, and this is the factual story of its activities. Neal Hines, the author, was a member of the Bikini-Eniwetok survey group of 1949, and of the ocean survey team aboard the U.S.S. Walton in 1951. Quotation (page 308): "The Laboratory had developed a confidence in the healing powers of the natural environment. Members of the field team had examined the effects of nuclear blasts. They had seen islands swept clean, water churned, and the damage created by heat, pressure and radioactivity. Yet they failed to find in the natural environment evidence of gross population or morphological change definitely ascribable to the effects of residual radioactivity alone. They realized that changes probably did occur, but neither in the ocean nor on land were examples discovered, and nowhere that they had studied the long term effects of radioactivity as a separate phenomenon was there evidence that normal regrowth was not occurring. . . The probabilities of remote radiation effects could not be denied, but positive evidence of such effects was not found at the test atolls or anywhere else in the Pacific."

Hirsch, I. S.: Wilhelm Corad Röntgen; his life and work. *Radiology, 4*:63-66; 139-142; 249-253, 1925. "Röntgen's last years were sad and lonely. He died of carcinoma of the rectum. It was asymptomatic until the very last . . . From the distance of centuries Röntgen will be seen as one of the towering figures of our time."

Hirsch, I. S.: William *(sic)* Konrad Roentgen; a biographical sketch. *New York M. J., 102*:1266-1269, 1915. The book, key, and lunch story accepted without reservation, and the date of Röntgen's discovery retro-set to 1893 *(sic)*.

Hodges, P. C.: Development of diagnostic x-ray apparatus during the first fifty years. *Radiology, 45*: 438-448, 1945. Changes are discussed by considering each of successive five decades. Hodges returned with the "seventh decade" of radiology in the *American Journal of Roentgenology* of December, 1955, and in 1964 with a Grubbé biography (Univ. of Chicago Press).

Hoing, M.: *A History of the ASXT,* 1920-1950. St. Paul, Bruce Publishing Company, 1952, 87 pages. Detailed, dependable, diligent, decorous. Volume 2 (1951-1960), by the same author, appeared in 1961, 82 pages.

Holinger, J.: The early history of x-ray in Chicago.

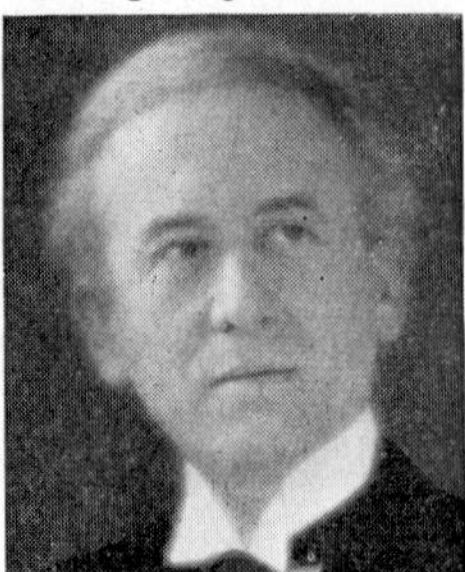

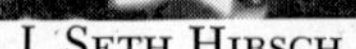

I. SETH HIRSCH

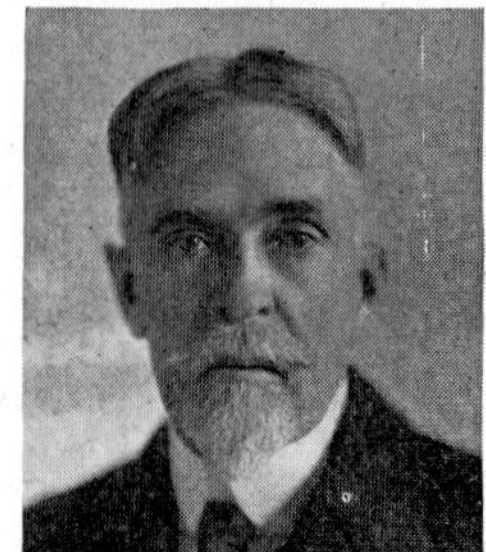

ED JERMAN

J. of Roentgenol., 1:426-431, 1918. Trostler asked Jack Holinger (who was an oto-rhino-laryngologist, and one of the founders of the German Medical Society of Chicago) to record the story of the first x-ray office in Chicago, owned successively by Harnisch, O. L. Schmidt, P. Latz, and Fuchs. A lumber dealer from Blue Island was brought to the office intoxicated, and with a leg injury. Patient moved during exposure, so three attempts (each of 35-40 minutes exposure from tube placed 5-6 inches from the skin) were made to obtain a roentgen plate. Ulceration supervened, the leg had to be amputated, patient sued, and the jury awarded him $10,000 (*cf., American X-Ray Journal* of May, 1899).

Holmes, G. W.: American radiology: its contributions to the diagnosis and treatment of disease. *J.A.M.A., 125*:327-330, 1947.

Holmes, G. W.: Development of the science of roentgen technique. *Am. J. Roentgenol., 45*:163-170, 1941. A brilliant Caldwell Lecture.

Holthusen, H.: Zur Geschichte der Einheit "Röntgen" und der Möglichkeiten ihrer Weiterentwicklung. *Fortschritte a. d. Geb. d. Röstrahlen, 89*:746-752, 1958. The idea of measuring dosage by measuring ionization is not (yet) outdated, but the r is nevertheless obsolete. It will be remembered as an historic step, associated with the name of Manne Siegbahn, the Swedish physicist who chaired the committee which brought the r into life.

Holthusen, H., Meyer, H., and Molineus, W. (eds.): *Ehrenbuch der Röntgenologen und Radiologen aller Nationen*, ed. 2, (*Sonderband* 42 to *Strahlentherapie*). München-Berlin, Urban and Schwarzenberg, 1959, 267 pages. Biographies of 359 professional radiation fatalities from all over the world. The first edition appeared in 1937 (also as a supplement to *Strahlentherapie*), with only 169 names, but *with* portraits.

Holzknecht, G.: Innere Entwicklung der Röntgenologie in Oesterreich. *Strahlentherapie, 36*:403-409, 1930. Welcoming address to the meeting of the Deutsche Röntgengesellschaft in Vienna (April of 1929). The pioneers had technical difficulties, but easy diagnoses (fractures, foreign bodies); with improved technics came (internistic) diagnostic problems.

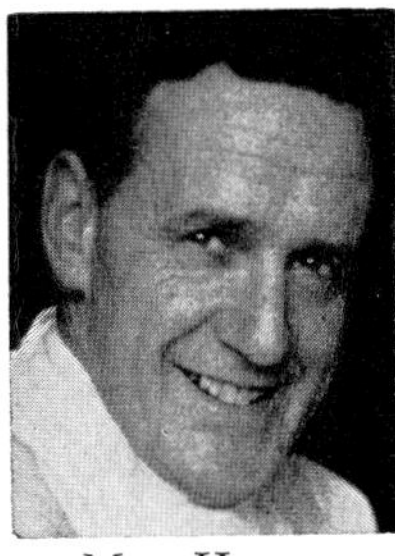

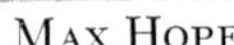

Max Hopf

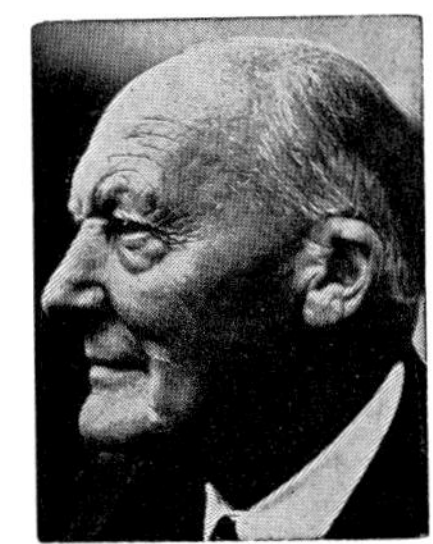

Hermann Holthusen

Hopf, M.: Études sur la Société suisse de radiologie. *Bull. d'Inf. Centre A. Béclère, 11* (nr. 123-124): 1-6, 1962. Excellent; includes a "reference" to Switzerland's scenic beauties, which attracted both Röntgen and Béclère.

Imboden, H. M.: Progress in the development of roentgen ray apparatus. *Am. J. Roentgenol., 26*:517-523, 1931. The Yellow Journal's one-time editor (who had been Caldwell's associate) reminisces about gas tubes (Sayen's modification which became Queen's self-regulating tube), about Snook and Coolidge, and about the first deep therapy apparatus built in the USA by GE (for use by Case at the Battle Creek Sanitarium in Michigan) in 1921.

Isenburger, H. R.: *Bibliography on Filmbadge Monitoring.* Washington, Government Printing Office, 1961, 15 pages. 235 references, issued as NP-10738 by the AEC.

Janker, R.: Die Röntgen-Photographie. Pp. 33-81 *in 100 Jahre Schleussner,* Frankfurt/Main, Schleussner, 1960. Röntgen discovered the x rays on November 8, 1895—but exposed the plate with his wife's hand on November 22, 1895; excellent review from Röntgen's endeavors to roentgen-cinematography.

Jerman, E. C.: X-ray technic; from the old to the new. *Radiology, 5*:245-247, 1925. Magistral summary by the consummate, all-time master x-ray technologist.

Jones, W. A.: Gordon Earle Richards—a little about his life and times. *J. Canadian Assn. of Radiol., 6*:1-7, 1955. The right blend of sadness, sensitivity, and scholarship needed to secure the proper setting for recalling the spirit of Richards.

Jupe, M.: Early days of radiology in Britain. *Clinical Radiology, 12*:147-154, 1961. Third-generation radiologist collected precise documentation on the pioneers, and presented it in a most palatable form.

Jurado Lopez, E.: Los primeros 60 anos de radiología. *Radiología, (Panamá), 6*:111-113, 1956.

Kaye, G. W. C.: Radiology, medieval and modern. *Brit. J. Radiol., 2*:3-28, 1929. All known "electric" precursors, from Toricelli and Guericke to Hauksbee and Morgan.

Kaye, G. W. C.: Röntgen and his forerunners. The 300 years that led to radiology. *Radiography, 27*:406-412, 1961. Reprint of a paper which first appeared in the same periodical in January, 1936 under the title "Some pre-x-ray pioneers." The forerunners:

Guericke, Nollet, Hittorf, Hauksbee, Faraday, Crookes, and J. J. Thomson.

Kirklin, B. R.: American Board of Radiology. *Am. J. Roentgenol., 31*:258-259, 1934. How it was founded, and when it first convened. Same author published in same periodical (December, 1945) the history of cholecystography.

Klason, T.: Svensk förening för medicinsk radiologi 1919-1939. *Svenska Läkaresällskapets Handlingar, 78*:7-18, 1959. Only extant history of the Swedish Association of Radiologists.

Koehler, A.: Aerztlicher Röntgenbetrieb um die Jahrhundertwende. *Strahlentherapie, 60*:283-289, 1937. Personal recollections and relics, for instance an old register. Most of the pioneers were first fluoroscopists and then radiographers. This is why so many of them wound up in Holthusen's *Ehrenbuch.*

Krabbenhoft, K. L.: A history of roentgen therapy. *Am. J. Roentgenol., 76*:859-865, 1956. A review of technical improvements (megavoltage, dosimetry), and of changes in clinical methodology, written for the golden anniversary year of the Yellow Journal by its assistant (now associate) editor who quoted appropriately from Sir Thomas Browne: "Who knows whether the best of men be known, or whether there be not more remarkable persons forgot than any that stand remembered in the known account of time."

Krebs,* A. T.: Hans Geiger. 50th anniversary of the publication of his doctoral thesis, 23 July 1906. *Science, 124*:166, 1956. "Divine curiosity and a childlike impetus to play are, Einstein told us, the driving forces of the true investigator. If any scientist fills the definition it was Hans Wilhelm Geiger." The problem of Geiger's thesis originated in an observation of A. Wehnelt (known for his eponymic interrupter), a professor at the same Friedrich-Alexander University in Erlangen, who had measured electric discharges in vacuum tubes. After graduation, Geiger went to London as assistant to Rutherford, and in 1928 Geiger published in the *Physikalische Zeitschrift* his first paper on a new counting device which was to become the Geiger tube (counter).

Lafferty, R. H.: Some Southern pioneers in x-ray. *Radiology, 7*:257-258, 1926. Story of the three students of Davidson College (North Carolina) who exposed the first glass plate on a Sunday night, allegedly on January 12, 1896.

Lawrence, J. H.: Early experience in nuclear medicine. *Northwest Med., (Seattle), 55*:527-533, 1956. This is the gist of a talk given at the first annual banquet of the Society of Nuclear Medicine, on June 18, 1955 in Portland (Oregon). One of Lawrence's first contacts with radiation was the inadvertent damage done to an early cyclotron when he walked into a powerful magnetic field while carrying a pair of pliers in his pocket: the pliers flew into the Dees, hit, and smashed the vacuum chamber. In 1935 Lawrence visited in Newark (New Jersey) with Harrison Martland, who had accumulated observations on aplastic anemia, osteonecrosis, and osteosarcoma in radium dial painters. In 1935 Lawrence, with Paul Aebersold, put a rat in a small box, and exposed it to neutrons; the rat died in a few minutes; next day autopsy showed the cause of death to be suffocation (not radiation): but the initial scare may have stayed with those who saw the rat die, and it saved some early cyclotron workers, especially their eyes from cataracts (that cyclotrons could cause opacification of the lens was obviously not known in the first years). In 1936 Lawrence introduced P-32 into therapeutics by treating a female patient who had chronic lymphatic leukemia: in 1956 that first patient was alive and well at the age of 74 years.

Leonard, C. L.: The past, present and future of the Roentgen-ray. *Transactions ARRS,* 20-39, 1905/6. Colorful but clear, cool and collected; careful and yet comprehensive!

Leucutia, T.: Integrated radiology. *Am. J. Roentgenol., 86*:803-806, 1961. Presidential address with historic references to name of ARRS journal.

Leucutia, T.: Ionizing radiations in our era. *J.A.M.A., 182*:44-45, 1962. "Sabin A. von Sohocky in 1915 originated the luminous radium-paint formula for watch dials; the paint was used during World

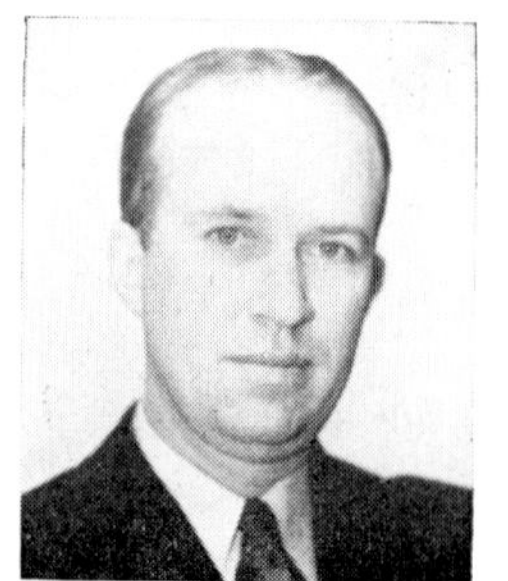

John Hundale Lawrence

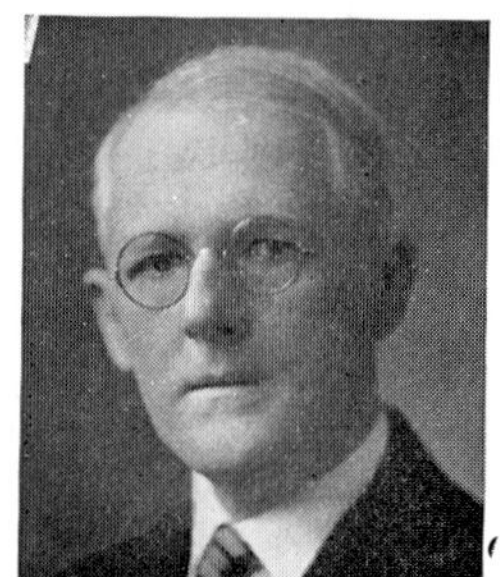

Robert H. Lafferty

*This is the same Krebs who developed in 1941 a *photontube counter* in which a scintillation phosphor was combined with a photo-electric detector. According to Otto Glasser, in 1944 S. C. Curran combined the scintillating crystal with a photomultiplier tube, and in 1950 C. E. Mandeville improved this by placing the phosphor in direct contact with the photo-tube. The result became known under the name of *scintillation counter*.

War I in painting instrument faces for submarines and aircraft. Sohocky died in 1928 at the age of 45 from external and internal radiation injuries. In the early 1920's several of the dial-painter girls died from "mysterious diseases" now known to have been due to the damaging effect of internal irradiation with radioactive substances." Also discussed is the history of radiation protection from the ARRS committee of 1920 to the CAR, including the radium project (Argonne, Massachusetts Institute of Technology, and New Jersey State Department of Health) and the Radiation Registry of Physicians (ACR, College of American Pathologists, National Academy of Sciences and National Research Council).

LeWald, L. T.: X-ray discovery excites New York. *Academy Bookman, 5* (nr. 3):11-13, 1952. W. J. Morton autographs donated to the New York Academy of Medicine bring up old memories.

Lockwood, S. T.: *Radium Research in America, 1902-1914-1939.* Buffalo, 1920, no pagination. This is a complete copy of the *Souvenir* given to Madame Curie by the Buffalo Society of Natural Sciences at the time she visited the city in 1920. Lockwood, who prepared it, was at the time a member of the Board of Managers of that society. He added an Appendix to the souvenir, to bring it up to the period ending March 28, 1939. The whole thing was then bound in silk and limp leather, and deposited in the Society's archives, with another copy going to the Buffalo Public Library. The Souvenir contains the story and photographs of the early carnotite mining in Colorado and Utah (James H. Lofftus, James N. McBride); Lockwood's animadversions with Flannery's vanadium steel (vanadium could be extracted from carnotite (the "radium" ore); Lockwood's testimonies before Congressional committees, The Appendix is a letter from Lockwood to James E. Lounsbury of the Radium Dial Company (New York City), in which Lockwood recalls that he was the one who sent the famous "letter from America" to the Curies, and he (Lockwood) was the one to whom they replied, giving details of the refining process of radium. Quotation: "At present I (Lockwood) would not lift a finger to accelerate the atomic disintegration of Uranium because I would be afraid of being successful; and if I were successful, I would not disclose or publish the results."

Loichinger, C.: Zur Geschichte der roentgenologischen Magendarmuntersuchung. *Fortschr. a.d. Geb. d. Röstrahlen, 38*:1067-1072, 1928. Priority of Hermann Rieder's opaque (bismuth) meal.

Loose, G.: Fortschritte der Röntgentherapie seit meiner Assistenzzeit bei Levy-Dorn. *Fortschritte a. d. Geb. d. Röstrahlen, 31*:441-450, 1924. He remembers the beaming face of Heinz Bauer demonstrating his self-regulating gas tube.

Lossen, H.: *Aerztliche Röntgenkunde und Frankfurt-am-Main.* Frankfurt/Main, Schleussner, 1953, pp. 53. Illustrated story of "local" radiologists, *e.g.,* Walter König, Alban Köhler, Franz Groedel, Karl Ludloff, Ludwig Seitz, and Hans Holfelder. Lossen supplied the information on Röntgen-Kongresse, printed in the *Bull. d'inf. Centre A. Béclère* of December, 1953.

Mabileau, J. F.: Contributions à l'histoire de la reglémentation des substances radioactives. *Rev. Hist. Pharm., (Paris), 47*:1-7, 1959. Following the USA decision, made in 1947, to export "peaceful" radionuclides to friendly nations, in 1948 in France radioactive substances were included among the potentially poisonous substances, so as to come under the regulations governing all dangerous drugs. Further reglementation was done in 1952.

MacDonald, C.: Some reminiscences of Thomas Barlow and Frederick Still. *J. Coll. Radiol., Australasia, 5*:88-91, 1961.

Macintyre, J.: Early x-ray photographs. *J. Röntgen Soc., 3*:137-138, 1907. This Scottish pioneer made his first x-ray exposures in the "Spring of 1896."

Maino, M.: San Michele Arcangelo e le radiazioni. *Pag. Stor. Med., 6* (2):3-16, 1962. Very documented study of St. Michael, the radiologic patron saint: in the Old Testament he was the patron of the Hebrews; he is currently the patron of the Italian parachute jumpers, of the bankers, and of the Brasilian military police. But the radiologists have a special consideration, because they had asked ahead of the others, as confirmed by Pius XII in his *Discorsi e Radiomessaggi.* Finally, on page 128 in the *Acta Apostolicae Sedis* of 1941 appeared the official announcement: *"Sanctus Michaël, Archangelus pro radiologis et radiumtherapeuticis patronus et protector declaratus!"*

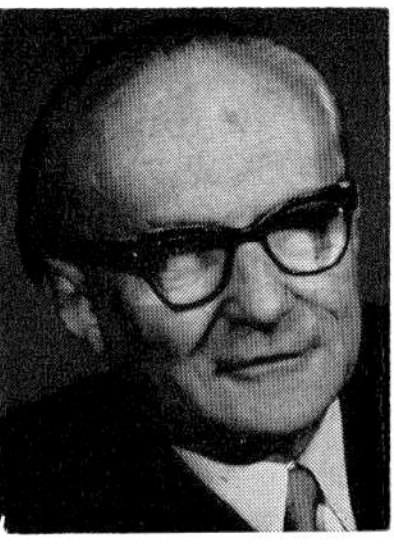

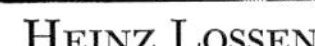

HEINZ LOSSEN

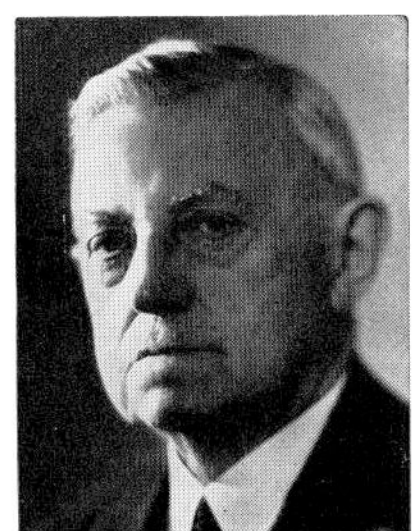

HANS MEYER

Malmio, K.: Bref aperçu retrospectif de l'histoire de la Société finlandaise de radiologie de 1925 à 1954. *Bull. d'inf. Centre A. Béclère, 4* (nr. 37):2-4, 1955. The full name of the Finnish Radiological Society is Suomen Radiologiyhdistys-Radiologforeningen i Finland. First demonstration of privately produced radiographs in Finland was presented to the 1902 meeting of Suomen Laakariseura (their medical society) by the medical roentgen pioneer A. Clopatt.

Manes, G. I.: The discovery of x-ray. *Isis, 47*:236-238, 1956. George Manes (1875-1953) had lived in Germany until the coming of Hitler, after which he emigrated to the USA, and continued to practice psychiatry. This is a posthumous note, published from a manuscript found among the papers left after Manes' death. It reports a conversation with Wolfgang Brendler (one of Röntgen's associates). The discovery took place on the evening of November 8, 1895. Röntgen worked in a very small room, assisted by a *Diener* (servant). The *Diener* was the one who first noticed the light on the screen. After a while the *Diener* went home, but Röntgen spent the whole night in that room, experimenting. When Brendler came to work next morning, Röntgen told him the story, giving the news of the discovery with his usual, amazing calm.

Manges, W. F.: Camp Greenleaf School of Roentgenology. *Am. J. Roentgenol., 6*:305-357, 1919. With many illustrations of men and machines; the highest ranked officer at Camp Greenleaf (located in Chickamauga Park, Georgia) was William Holmes Stewart of New York City.

Maragliano, V.: *Scuola Elettroradiologica Genovese,* 1897-1938, (ed.: P. Amisano and L. Reale). Genova, Ospedale San Martino, 1938, 299 pages. Historic essays, meeting reports, bibliography of works published by teachers and pupils.

Martin, F. C., and Fuchs, A. W.: The historical evolution of roentgen-ray plates and films. *Am. J. Roentgenol., 26*:540-548, 1931. Excellent review of early names in dry plates used in radiography (from Carbutt, Seed, and Schleussner, to Imperial, Cramer, and Eastman Kodak). First dental roentgenogram was produced during January, 1896 in Braunschweig (Germany) by Otto Walkhoff, who exposed his own teeth for 25 minutes, using an ordinary glass plate. First dental plate in America is ascribed to Wm. Morton (Kells was really ahead of Morton).

Martius, H.: Ueber die Entwicklung der Strahlentherapie am Beispiel des Gebärmutterhalskarzinom. *Strahlentherapie, 100*:329-334, 1956. Radiation therapy of carcinoma of cervix from 1938 through 1950 corroborates the fact that overdosage is just as harmful as underdosage.

McCoy, C. C.: Development of roentgenologic examination of the biliary tract. *Radiology, 11*:13-26, 1928. Basic source material, especially for era before introduction of cholecystographic media. The author recognizes the (1) pre-stone period, 1895-1899, (2) the occasional stone period, 1899-1913, (3) the period of stone statistics, 1913-1924, (4) the period of indirect signs, 1911-1925, (5) the gallbladder shadow era, 1915-1925, and (6) the age of cholecystography.

Medelman, J. P.: History of the Section on Radiology. *J.A.M.A., 178*:785-788, 1961. Chairman's address at the 110th annual meeting of the AMA in New York City of June 29, 1961. Manges, Soiland, and Hubeny were the first officers of the meeting of radiologists within the AMA as part of the Section on Miscellaneous Topics, in 1924. That year Trostler moved to give a vote of thanks to Soiland for his efforts toward establishing a "Section on Roentgenology." The Section on Radiology was officially created in 1925 with Hickey, Carman, and Hubeny as officers.

Merrill, A. S.: Brief history of the Department of Roentgenology of the Massachusetts General Hospital. *Am. J. Roentgenol., 36*:727-736, 1936. Based on G. W. Holmes' pages in the memorial volume issued by Massachusetts General in 1921.

Meyer, H.: Geleitwort zum 100 ten Bande. *Strah-*

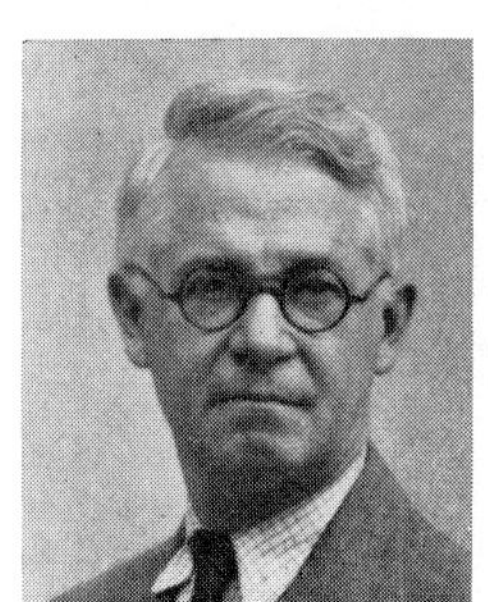
Arthur Mutscheller

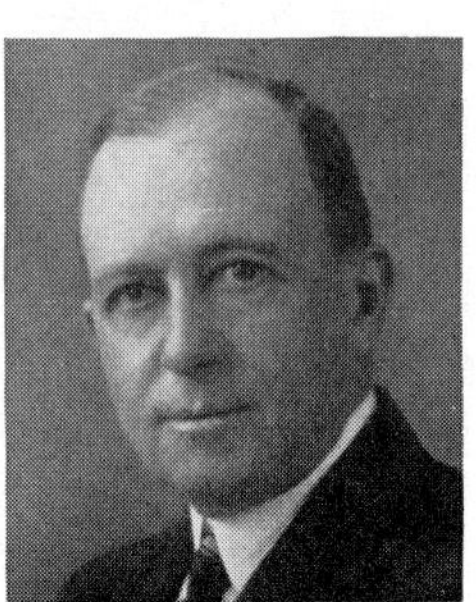
Willis F. Manges

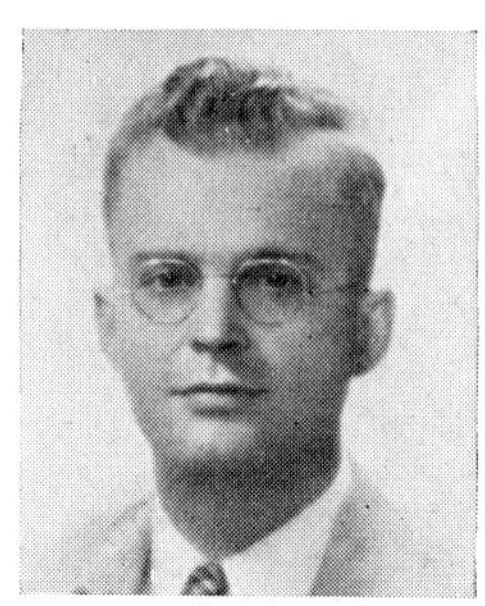
John Paul Medelman

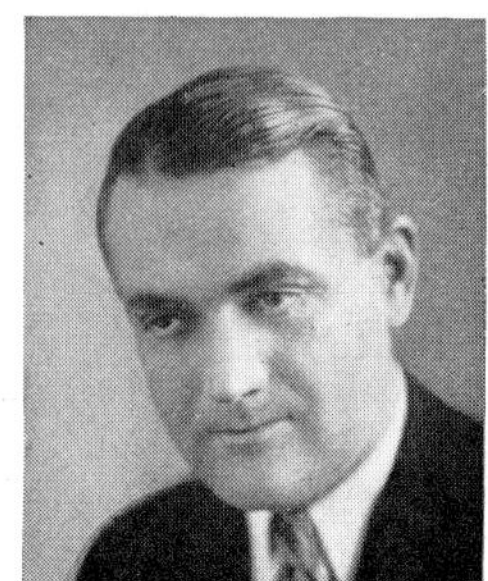
Traian Leucutia

lentherapie, 100:2-4, 1956. That 100th volume is dedicated to the memory of Eduard Urban (1873-1953) of Urban & Schwarzenberg, known medical publishers in the German language. Those 100 volumes stretched over 44 years, and seven thousand papers. It took an entire forest to make that much paper.

Michaescu, G. T.: Serviciul de radioscopie si radiografie din Spitalul Militar Central. *Rev. San. Milit., 3*:614-69; 684-691, 1900. History of the first "military" x-ray department in Roumania, by one of Roumania's first electro-radiologists.

Milani, E.: Der Beitrag Italiens zur Strahlenbiologie. *Strahlentherapie, 65*:517-544, 1939. History of Italy's radiobiologists: Bertolotti, Busi, Balli, Ghilarducci, V. Maragliano, and Perussia; authoritative.

Miller, J. A.: *Yankee Scientist;* Schenectady, Mohawk Development Service, 1963, 216 pages. Biography of William David Coolidge, whose 90th anniversary was recently celebrated, *cf., Med. Techn. Assist. in der Radiol.* of December, 1963.

Mody, K. P.: Development of radiation and its contribution to medical science: the cancer problem. *Indian J. Radiol., 13* (1):1-19, 1959.

Mody, K. P.: The discovery of x-rays and after. *Indian J. Radiol.,* (souvenir number) 197-301, 1956. Quotation: "It will be for the future generation to commemorate the centenary of Röntgen's discovery. We may, however, venture to hope that 15 years hence we shall celebrate the 75th anniversary . . ." Mody died in London, on June 6, 1961.

Møller, P. F.: Radiologiens historie i Denmark. *Bibl. Laeger, 152*:311-340, 1960. Contains portraits of the pioneers, and sizes up both the scientific advances, and the development of professional organizations.

Molotkov, A. E.: *Bibliografia Russkoi Radiologii i Rentgenologii* (ed. M. I. Nemenov). Nr. 6-7 of Monographs of the Leningrad Roentgenologic, Radiologic, and Onkologic Institute. 2 volumes Leningrad, Narkomzdrav, 1938-1941, 684 pages. The first volume contains titles on radium and therapy 1896-1938, the second is on roentgenology and diagnosis, 1896-1940. Excellent compilation, indispensable for any study of Russian or Sovietic radiology.

Morgan, R. H.: The performance of screen intensification and cinefluorographic systems. *Am. J. Roentgenol., 86*:1027-1039, 1961. This was the H. Clyde Snook Annual Oration before the Philadelphia Roentgen Ray Society (November 10, 1960): it started therefore with a well-documented history of Snook and his crossarm rectifier.

Morgan, R. H., and Lewis, I.: The roentgen ray: its past and future. *Dis. Chest, 11*:502-510, 1945. Discussion on need for intensification of fluoroscopic image. Illustrations from the collection of Paul Chesley Hodges.

Morilllo-Atencio, M. A.: In memoriam José Otilio Marmol (1874-1959).*Radiología (Panama), 9*:91-94, 1959. Marmol was the *Padre de la radiología venezolana,* who imported his x-ray machine into Venezuela in 1899.

Mosebach, R.: Wilhelm Conrad Röntgen in Giessen. *Giessener Hochschulblätter,* 10 (2-4: 1-2, 1963. Röntgen had been professor of physics in the Justus Liebig Universität, and he is buried in Giessen. This note appeared on the unveiling of a modernistic monument to the father of radiology. In the same issue is another brief note, by Wilhelm Henle, on Röntgen's scientific achievements.

Murczynski, C., and Sypniewska, M.: *Wilhelm Konrad Roentgen; Dzieje Wielkiego Odkrycia.* Warszawa, Panstwowy Zaklad Wydawn Lekarskich, 1957, 238 pages. Biography.

Mutscheller, A.: Early history of electron emission. *Amer. J. Roentgenol., 31*:244-250, 1934. Scientific filiation of the hot cathode tube, beginning with 1852 when Becquerel found that discharges from hot electrodes do not obey Ohm's law. The most significant among Coolidge's "forefathers" was Wehnelt who in 1903 developed, and on January 15, 1904 filed a patent for, the first practical device embodying a

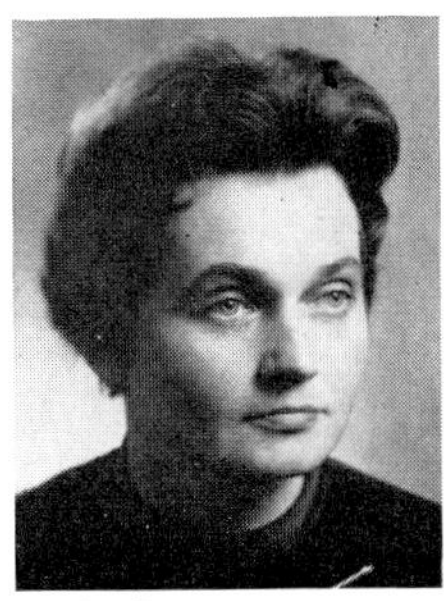
M. Sypniewska

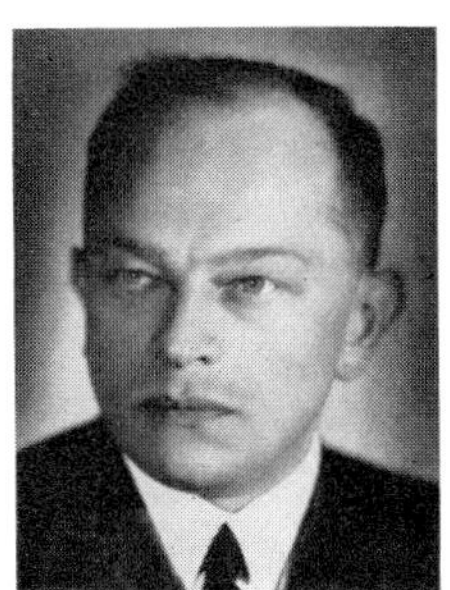
C. Murczynski

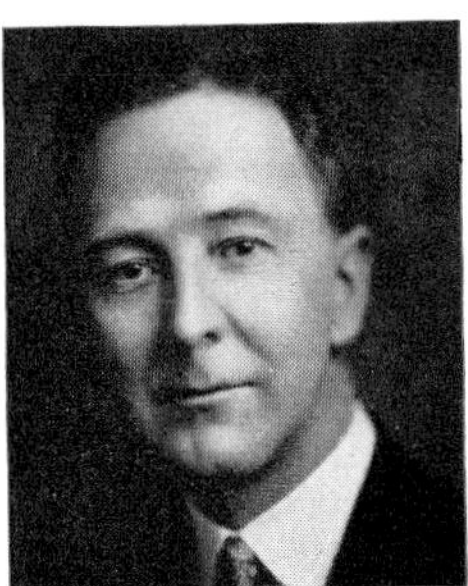
B. H. Orndoff

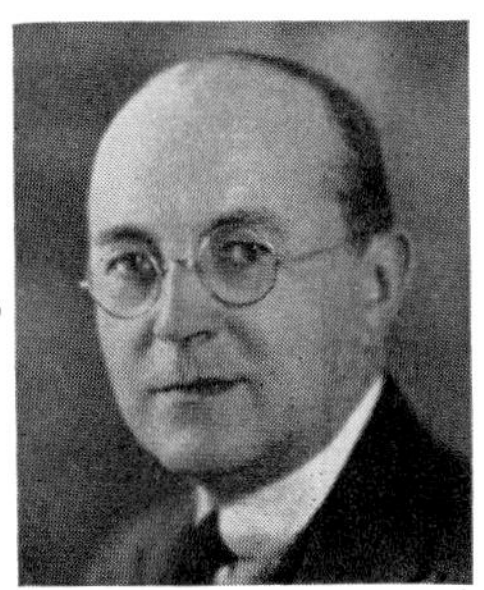
F. W. O'Brien

high degree of vacuum with an electron-emitting heated cathode and a cold anode (that device was made and sold by Emil Gundelach, and can be found in his 1909 catalog), *cf., Wehnelt, A.*: Ein elektrisches Ventrilrohr, *Phys.-Med. Soz., Erlangen, 37*:364, 1905. Then there was the famous tube made by Lilienfeld, J. E., and Rosenthal, W. J.: Eine Roentgenroehre von beliebig und momentan einstellbarem, vom Vakuum unabhaengigem Haertegrad. *Fortschr. a. d. Geb d. Röstrahlen, 18*:256-263. Incidentally, Mutscheller had been brought to this country by the Wapplers; at the time he wrote the article, he was director of research at Westinghouse. Mutscheller is remembered for having initiated the concept of safe dose, *i.e.*, the amount of daily exposure which could be indefinitely tolerated (with no demonstrable effects). Mutscheller's tolerance dose, proposed in 1925 while he was Wappler's physicist, amounted to .01 erythema dose per month, or about 200 mr/day.

Mygge, L. J.: Erindringer fra røntgenstralernes berndom herhyemme. *Ugeskrift for Laeger, 2*:429-431, 1921. Personal recollections culled by Denmark's first radiologist.

Negro, C. C.: L'evoluzione dell'apparecchio radiologico dentario. *Minerva stomat., 10* (1):59-61, 1961.

Nemenov, M. I.: Fortschritte der Röntgenologie in den 25 Jahren. *Ann. roentgenol. et radiol., 1*:255-261, 1922. Summary of international progress in the first quarter century after Röntgen's discovery.

O'Brien, Sr., F. W.: Radium treatment of cancer of the cervix; historical review. *Am. J. Roentgenol., 57*:281-292, 1947. This was a Janeway Lecture at the ARS.

O'Hara, F. S.: Looking backward. *Radiography & Clin. Photogr., 8* (nr. 3):3-9, 1932. Witty but sentimental personal recollections by the founder of the RSNA.

Orndoff, B. H.: An interview with Madame Curie. *Radiology, 71*:750-752, 1958. During 3rd ICR in Paris (1931), Orndoff convinced Mme Curie to accept an invitation of the ACR to a roof-garden ceremony in which she got a gold medal. Usually seclusive, Mme Curie came and cooperated in recording her voice for a sound movie. Einstein once said that, of all celebrated beings, Marie Curie was the one whom fame had not corrupted.

Packard, C.: Roentgen radiations in biological research. *Radiology, 45*:522-533, 1945. Excellent review of early radiobiologic endeavors by a former associate of Francis Carter Wood.

Pakkenberg, H.: *Historisk Oversigt over Danske Hospitalers og Privatklinikkers Først Anskaffere Røntgen-Apparatur, samt over Røntgenafdelingernes Ledere.* Copenhagen, Dansk Røntgen Teknik, 1960, 55 pages. Early apparatus and early radiologists in Denmark.

Palmieri, G. G.: La recognizione radiologica a feretro chiuso dei resti di San Domenico. *Pontificia Academia Scientiarium Commentationes, 7*:733-773, 1943. Radiologic examination of the unopened sarcophagus of Saint Dominic (1170-1221). A total of 137 bony parts were identified, including the hioid and nine teeth (aside from the ten teeth still implanted in the mandible), but not including the calcified cricoid and thyroid cartilages. Missing were the skull, and assorted small bones (phalanges and the like), which had been removed for setting into precious metals as sacred relics.

Pancoast, H. K.: Reminiscences of a radiologist. *Am. J. Roentgenol., 39*:169-186, 1938. Pancoast was one man who could refer to himself as a radiologist, to his place of work as the x-ray department, and not have these etymologies censured in the Yellow Journal.

Pao-Sen, L.: Let science serve the welfare of mankind. In memory of the 60th anniversary of the discovery of x-ray by W. C. Röntgen (in Chinese). *Chinese J. Radiol., 3*:241-242, 1955.

Passalacqua, F.: *Biolography of the Publications of Biological and Medical Applications of Autoradiography,* 1924-1954. Supplement to (*Radio*) *Biologica Latina.* Milano, IDOS, 1954, 30 pages. Relative apparent prevalence of European sources.

Pendergrass, E. P.: Looking backward. *Radiology, 66*:218-224, 1956. Presidential address at 1955 meeting, with data from the history of the RSNA. Pendergrass published also a history of the roentgen examination in occupational lung diseases (*American Journal of Roentgenology* of December, 1945).

Pendergrass, H. P., and St. Aubin, F. M.: Changing patterns in the training and practice of radiology.

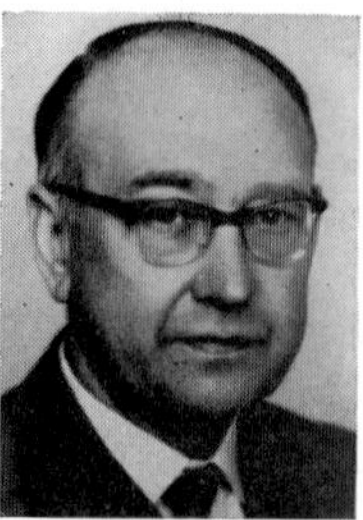

H. Pakkenberg

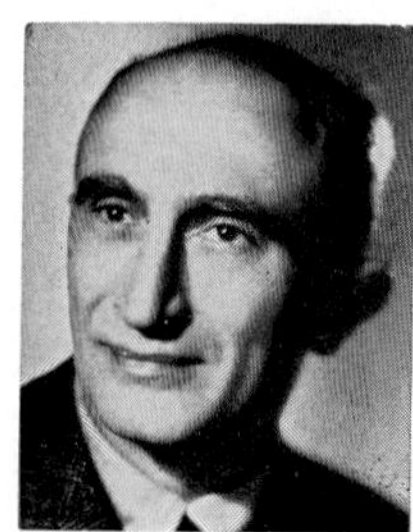

G. G. Palmieri

Radiology, 82:595-601, 1964. "If one extrapolates the results of the recent Health, Education, and Welfare survey of diagnostic radiological examinations . . . it would appear that at least 75 to 80 million diagnostic radiological examinations are performed yearly in the USA. At a low approximate charge of $15.00 per examination . . . radiology may account for over a billion dollars in our health budget. (The technological revolution) is even now making it progressively more expensive to practice radiology. The cost of equipping a modern fluoroscopy room, which was approximately $5,000 in 1935 and $15,000 in 1945, may now amount to over $60,000. In *Radiologic Subjectivity, "Fads," and Objectivity* in that same (April, 1964) issue of *Radiology,* Laurence Robbins editorialized: "Subjectively, we recognize at least three certainties in our lives — death, taxes, and change. Of the former two we are most aware, our appreciation of the last is less keen."

Peter, G.: De la historia de la radiología en Mexico. *Röntgenstrahlen,* 5-24, 1956. Personal recollections: author migrated from Switzerland and started out in Mexico City as a therapist.

Petrovčic, F.: History of the Radiological Section of the Medical Association of Croatia. *Bull. d'inf. Centre A. Béclère, 4* (nr. 43-44):1-4, 1955. Oldest and largest radiological group in Yugoslavia.

Pfahler, G. E.: Development of roentgen therapy during fifty years. *Radiology, 45*:503-521, 1945. Pfahler (just like Jimmy Case) knew how to corroborate reminiscences with printed data from sources contemporary to the events under consideration. Such a point is well demonstrated by this excellent paper from the pen of one of the best known American pioneers in radiotherapy.

Pfahler, M. B.: *The Love of a Physician.* Philadelphia, Dorrance, 1958, 274 pages. Sentimental biography by his widow. Pfahler was the first radiologist of Philadelphia General Hospital, which is by tradition the "first" hospital in the USA (so said their Blockley Radiological Society in 1956). There is a Pfahler Sanctum at Blockley.

Pizon, P.: Soixantième anniversaire du premier travail associant la radiologie à la clinique. *Presse méd., 67* (1):33-34, 1959. It was the doctoral thesis, sustained on December 8, 1898 in the University of Paris by Albert Mouchet. The topic was fractures of the distal humeral extremity.

Phillips, C. E. S.: *Bibliography of X-Ray Literature and Research.* London, Electrician Printing & Publishing Co., 1897, 68 pages. Earliest radio-bibliography extant; author was an "auto-didact," but the listings are accurate, and constitute indispensable source-material (in 1896 there appeared over one thousand radio-titles). Incidentally, Phillips' wife designed the presidential badge, offered by the BIR to the ICR (*cf., Brit. J. Radiol.* of January, 1932): the badge is a variation on the BIR crest, with a topaze, pure gold, and an alloy to provide strength, the whole thing suspended on a silk cord.

Podlyashuk, L. D.: Main trends of the development of radiobiology and radiotherapy in the USSR. *Indian J. of Radiol.,* (souvenir number) 690-702, 1956. Substantive survey, including the story of roentgen therapy of war wounds.

Ponzio, M.: *Società Italiana di Radiologia Medica,* 1913-1940. Torino, Tip. P. Giani, 1930, 18 pages. Only available paper on the founding of the Italian Radiological Society, by its long-time, famous secretary, and dignified radiation casualty.

Popović, L., and Smokvina, M.: *Pregled Naše Rentgenoloske Literature.* Zagreb, Izdanja Centralni Rentgenoloski Institute, no date, 20 pages. Bibliography of Yugoslav titles on radiology.

Porter, D. C.: The new photography. *Ulster M. J., 31*:117-127, 1962. Early radiologists at Royal Victoria Hospital in Belfast, including among others, Robert Maitland Beath, Sir Frank Montgomery, and the radiographer R. M. Leman.

Potter, H.: History of diaphragming roentgen rays

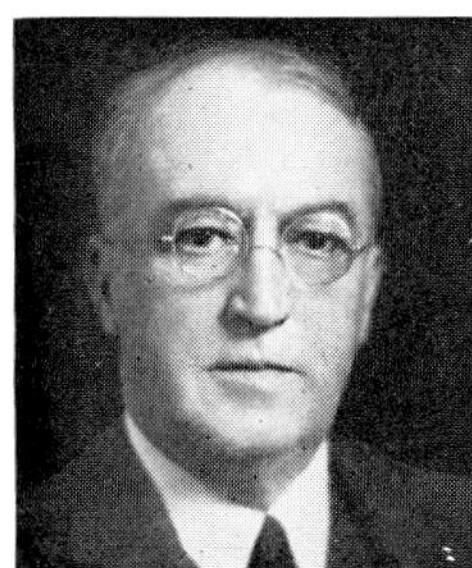
WM. ALLEN PUSEY

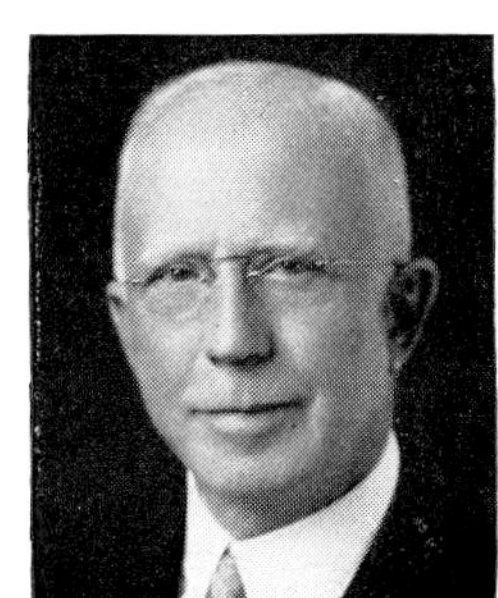
GEORGE PFAHLER

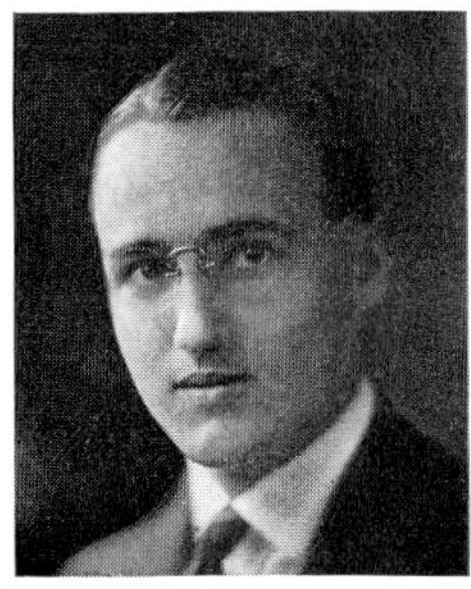
EUGENE PENDERGRASS

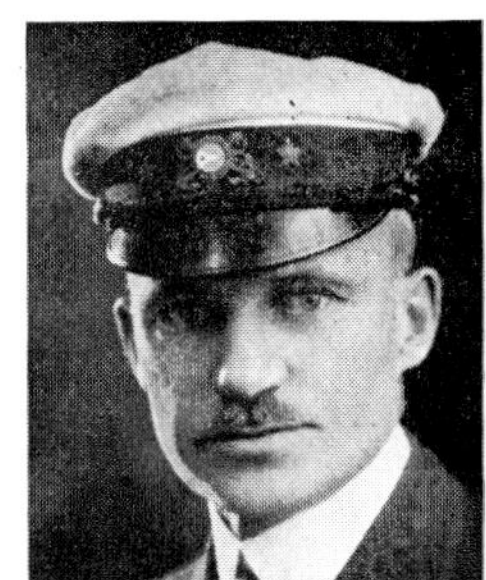
HOLLIS POTTER

by using the Bucky principle. *Am. J. Roentgenol., 25*: 396-402, 1931. Precise, professional, ponderous: Bucky, Caldwell, Potter, and Wilsey.

Prévot, R.: Die Entwicklung der Strahlentherapie seit Rieder's Zeiten. *München. med. Wchschr., 101*: 471-474, 1959. Since 1928 therapy has developed mostly by providing more precise dosages. This article is part of that periodical's 100th anniversary of Rieder's birth, with commemorative papers on the various contributions of Rieder to hematology (Blut-Rieder), to hydrotherapy (Wasser-Rieder), and to radiation (Strahlen-Rieder). There is, of course, also a reminder of the fact that Rieder introduced the opaque meal.

Pullin, V. E., and Wiltshire, W. J.: *X-Rays, Past and Present.* London, Ernest Benn Ltd., 1927, 229 pages. Mostly physicistic, relatively few medical items.

Pusey, W. A.: Roentgen-ray therapy 20 years ago. *J.A.M.A., 81*:1257-1260, 1923. Personal recollections by one of the pioneers in therapy; he treated his first case (hypertrichosis) on February 1, 1900; his first lupus in May, 1900; his first skin epithelioma in January, 1901; and his first carcinoma of the breast by the middle of 1901.

Quimby, E. H.: The background of radium therapy in the United States, 1904-1946. *Am. J. Roentgenol., 75*:443-450, 1956. Personal recollections, including development of the radium industry, by one of the pioneers in radium dosage (and 1940 Janeway Lecturer).

Rajevsky, B., and Hobitz, H.: Radiologie und Biophysik. *München. med Wchschr., 100*:401-405, 1958. A physicist and a physician evoke the events from Leopold Freund (who inaugurated superficial radiotherapy) to radioisotopes.

Ramos, A.: Notes historiques sur la radiologie au Portugal. *Bull. d'inf. Centre A. Béclère, 5* (nr. 55-56):1-8, 1956. Comprehensive. One detail: Egas Moniz always gave credit to his radiologists, for instance to Pereira Caldas (inventor of the "radio-carrossell") for assistance in the development and improvement of angiography.

Ramos, A.: No 25° anniversario da Sociedade Portuguesa de Radiologia Medica. *Médico (Porto), 9*:642-646, 1958.

Raper, H. R.: Notes on the early history of radiodontia; with special attention to its relation to the Indiana School of Dentistry. *Oral Surgery, Oral Medicine, and Oral Pathology, 6*:70-81, 1952. Basic text for history of dental radiology in the USA; scholarly, sensible, and witty. Quotation: "At the 1913 annual meeting of the National Institute of Dental Pedagogics, an Indianapolis competitor of the Indiana Dental College said: 'I question very much whether there is any need for us to teach dental radiography in our schools . . . It seems to me it would be the height of folly to consider the proposition to have every dentist a radiographer . . . The curriculum is crowded with so many more important things!' For the sake of clarity I (Raper) should add that we were not teaching (in 1913) all our students to do the (dental radiographic) work; but we were teaching all who wanted to do the work, and had been since the beginning in 1909. Come to think of it, maybe we never do better than to teach only those who want to learn in any department at any time." Amen!

Reckow, J. B. von: Die Bedeutung Wiener Zahnaerzte fuer die Entwicklung der zahnaerztlichen Roentgenologie. *Oester. Ztschr. Stomatolog., 58*:21-33, 1961. Very well documented, containing the basic data on the development of dental radiology in Central Europe.

Reid, A. D.: History of the x-ray department at St. Thomas Hospital. *Proc. Royal Soc. of Med., 7* (Electro-Therap. Sect.):23-25, 1914. Interesting details from personal recollections.

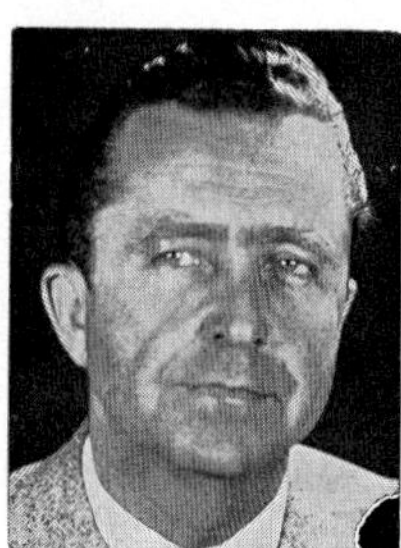
FERDO PETROVCIC

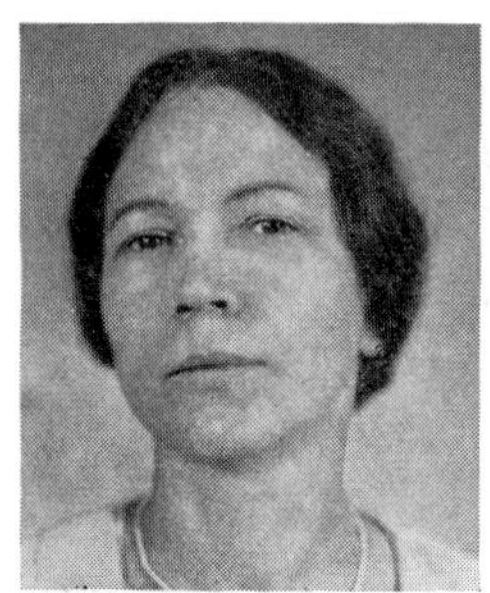
EDITH QUIMBY

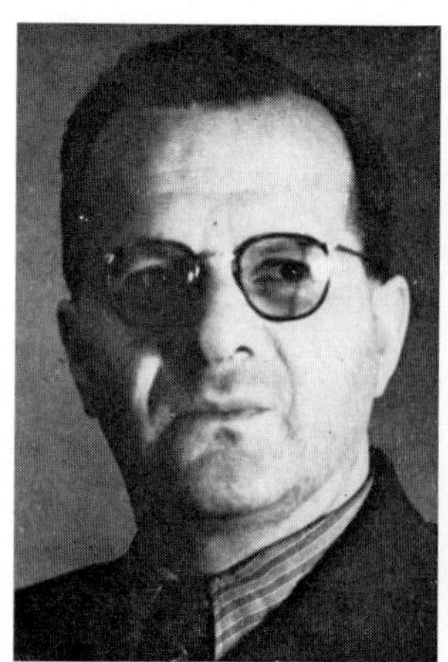
SAMUEL REYNBERG

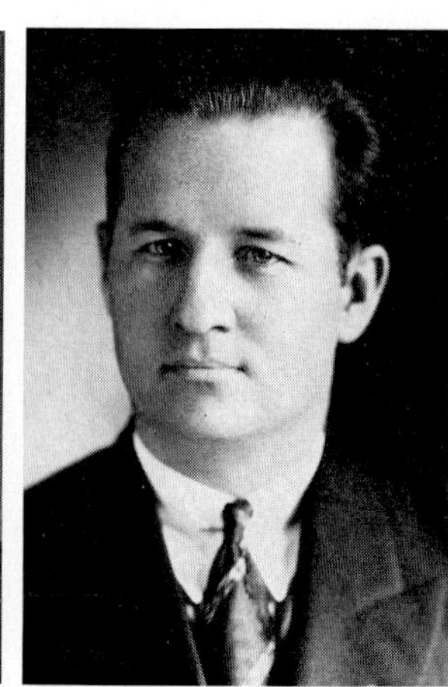
CHARLES W. SMITH

Reynberg, S. A.: Puti razvytya Russkoye i Sovyetskoye rentgenologii. *Sovyetskaya Medyzyna, 10* (nr. 3): 1-7, 1946. On the 50th anniversary (January 23, 1946) of Röntgen's first public presentation of his discovery, Reynberg—the (unofficial) historian of Sovietic radiology—addressed the Academy of Medical Sciences in Moscow. Reynberg summarized the times of the Russian roentgen pioneers, as well as the development of radiology after the advent of the Soviets. Documented and authoritative, a basic text in the history of Sovietic radiology.

Reynberg, S. A. (ed.): *Ocherky Razvytya Medzynskoye Rentgenologii.* Moskva, Medgiz, 1948, 275 pages. Twenty-four essays by various authors covering the development of diagnostic radiology in the Soviet Union; issued on the occasion of the fiftieth anniversary of the introduction of roentgen rays in medicine.

Reynolds, L.: History of the use of the roentgen ray in warfare. *Am. J. Roentgenol., 54*:649-672, 1945. Erudite review by a gentlemanly scholar; it begins with Giuseppe Alvaro (Naples) and the Abyssinian conflict (1896); continues with the Greco-Turkish War (1897); the Tyrah Campaign and Khyber Pass (1897); the River War in the Soudan (1898); the Spanish-American War (1898); the Boer War (1899); then World War I and World War II. A classic text on the topic. Incidentally, this was the unique Caldwell-Carman Lecture, delivered in Chicago in 1944 before the only combined ARRS-RSNA meeting, a transient union prompted by wartime exigencies.

Reynolds, R. J.: Early history of radiology in Britain. *Clinical Radiology, 12*:136-142, 1961. Expanded version of a relatively brief note in the *Bull. d'inf. Centre A. Béclère* of January, 1956. As an adolescent, Reynolds exposed on September 6, 1896 a plate with small specimens of various metals (coil and tube provided by his father, who was a physician); that plate is now on exhibit in the Science Museum in South Kensington (London).

Rieder, H.: Ueberblick ueber die Leistungen der Röntgenstrahlen seit ihrer Entdeckung. *Münch. med. Wchschr., 68*:109-114, 1921. Summary of German achievements at 25th anniversary of Röntgen's discovery.

Rigler, L. G.: Development of roentgen diagnosis. *Radiology, 45*:467-502, 1945. Valiant effort to summarize the tremendous amount of bibliography into readable review pages.

Roberts, J. E.: Radiation measurement and the adoption of the rad as the unit of absorbed dose in radiotherapy. *Indian J. Radiol.,* (souvenir number) 650-662, 1956. Author was one of those who "brought in" the rad; the paper is equally knowledgeable.

Robinson, D.: Early radiology in Savannah, Georgia. *J. Med. Ass. Georgia, 51*:535-537, 1962. John Wesley, the father of Methodism, was also an electrotherapist (he published in 1755 a collection of 829 receipts for the treatment of 288 conditions, utilizing the electrostatic machine. Three Savannah radiologists are mentioned, Eugene Corson (1856-1946), W. A. Cole (1884-1958), and Robert Drane.

Roland, C. G.: Priority of clinical x-ray reports: a classic dethroned? *Canadian J. of Surg., 5*:247-251, 1962. The extraction of a bullet after its demonstration on a roentgen plate, reported by Cox and Kirkpatrick in the *Montreal M. J.* of March, 1896 was not the first clinical roentgen report in the English literature. It was preceded at least by Robert Jones and Oliver Lodge's paper on the discovery of a bullet lost in the wrist, published in the *Lancet* of February 22, 1896.

Rossi, S.: *Capitulo de Radiología en Síntesis Médica.* Barcelona, Wassermann, 1945-56, 35 pages. Bibliography of (internistic) clinico-radiobibliographies.

Rowe, E. W.: A review of American radiology. *J. of Radiol., 3*:386-388, 1922. After the pioneers (Caldwell, Dodd, Robarts, J. N. Scott, Williams, Stover, Cannon, Bardeen, Zwaluwenburg, Hickey, L. G. Cole) and the physicists (J. S. Shearer and Duane), the article mentions creation of the ARRT

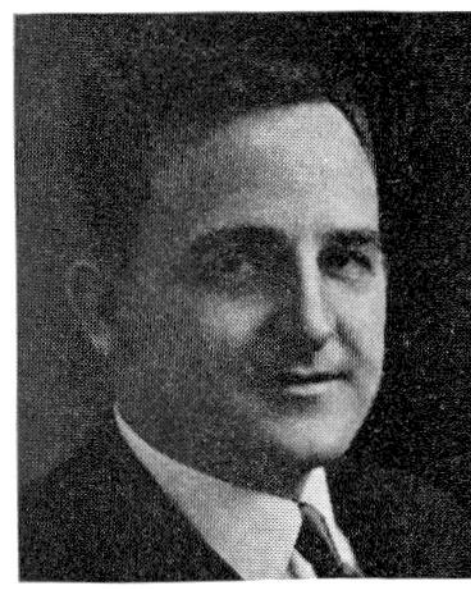
LAWRENCE REYNOLDS

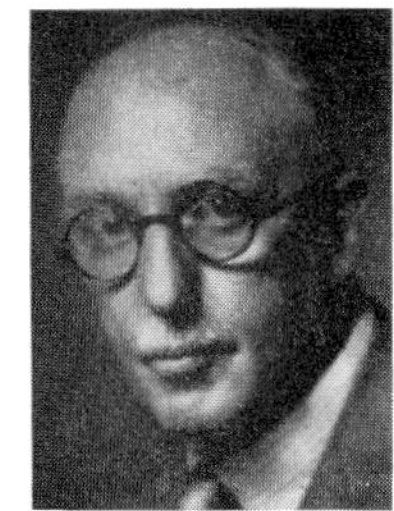
RUSSELL REYNOLDS

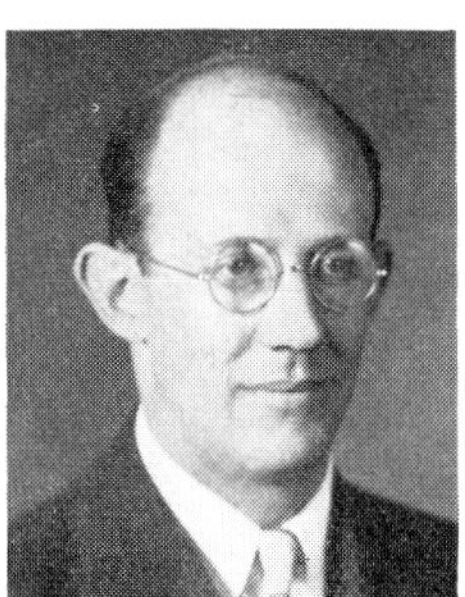
WENDELL SCOTT

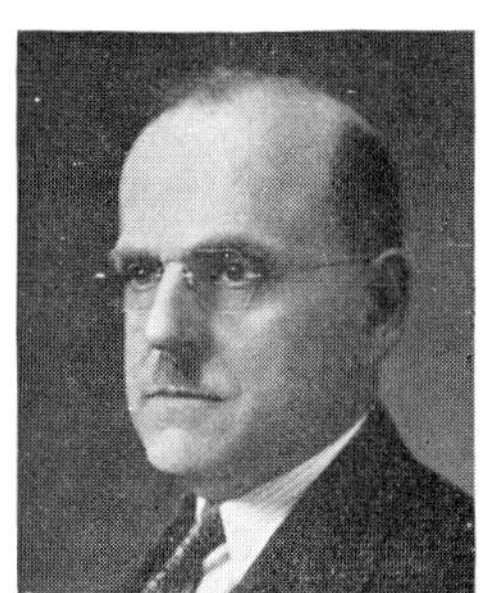
EDWARD ROWE

(American Registry of Radiological Technicians) sponsored by the RSNA. Quotation: "Indicative . . . is . . . the recent action of the Mayo Clinic where a most complete and fully equipped electro-therapeutic laboratory (including the ultra-violet) has lately been installed. . . . The fact is significant when it is remembered that the Mayo Clinic has always been primarily a surgical institution." "Practically half his (Carman's) time is spent in the surgical operating room studying the pathology which he has previously visualized under his fluoroscope."

Ruckensteiner, E.: Anfänge der Röntgentherapie in memoriam Leopold Freund. *Radiol. Austriaca, 12*: 219-234, 1961. Freund's first patient—a child with hairy nevus—on whom he had proved the depilatory effect of roentgen rays, returned in 1961 as a woman (age 65) to be seen by Freund's pupils, Fuchs and Gebauer: she had developed an ulceration at the site of therapy, but it healed and never bothered again. Paper contains also bibliography of Freund until World War I. Incidentally, at the time of first Oesterreichischer Röntgenkongress in 1936 appeared a compilation, entitled *40 Jahre Oesterreichische Forschungsarbeit auf dem Gebiete der medizinischen Röntgenologie* (publishers: Urban & Schwarzenberg).

Rutherford, E.: Development of radiology. *Proc. Roy. Soc. Med., 13* (Sect. Electrotherapy):145-157, 1919-1920. Physicistic view, by Lord Rutherford of Nelson.

Sabat, B.: Zur Geschichte der Röntgenkymographie und Ausarbeitung der Modifikationen der Methode. *Fortschritte a. d. Geb. d. Röstrahlen, 50*:309-312, 1934. Bronislaw Sabat made his first communication on this procedure on July 7, 1911 to the Lemberg Medical Society, and the text appeared in the *Lwowski Tygodnik Lekarski* of July 13, 1911. All subsequent communications (Theodor Gött and Joseph Rosenthal's in the *Münchener medizinische Wochenschrift* of September 17, 1912), however independent, have no chronologic priority. Sabat gives credit for improvements also to Pleikart Stumpf (of München), Pietro Cignolini (of Genova), and Erich Zdansky (of Vienna). What is the scientific significance of a discovery which has gone unnoticed? And if someone (re-)discovers the same thing, on his own, and makes the world understand its value, how much credit should he get for that? What amount of eponymic credit ought to get the one who has the chronologic priority, and how much the other?

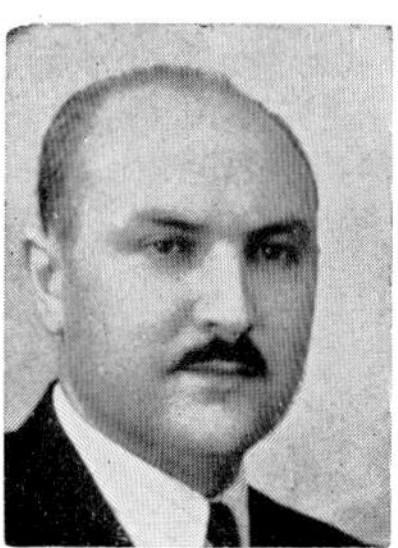

Albano Ramos

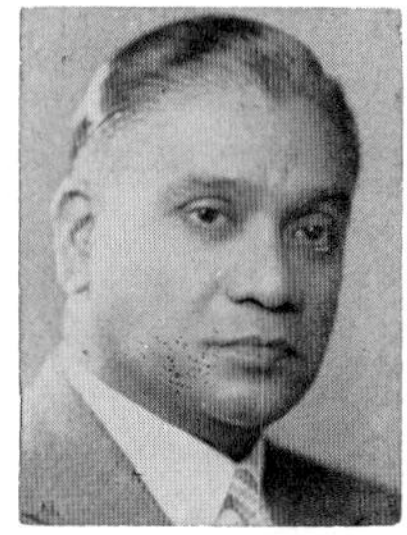

Ayres de Sousa

St. John, A., and Isenburger, H. R.: *Industrial Radiology; X-Rays and Gamma Rays,* ed. 2. New York, Wiley, 1948, 298 pages. Contains the excellent bibliography (pp. 231-289) by Isenburger.

Schinz, H. R.: *60 Jahre medizinische Radiologie, Probleme und Empirie.* Stuttgart, Georg Thieme, 1959, 275 pages. Issued on the occasion of the 9th ICR in München; name re-calling, no bibliography, many portraits.

Schmitz, H.: Development of the forms of treatment in carcinoma of the uterine cervix during the last one hundred years. *Am. J. Roentgenol., 40*:805-816, 1938. Janeway Lecture at the ARS meeting.

Schuster, N. H.: Early days of Roentgen photography in Britain. *Brit. M. J., 2*:1164-1166, 1962. Surgeon Norah Schuster is the daughter of Arthur Schuster, one of the two British scientists who received from Röntgen a letter with a copy of that very first paper on the new rays. The other was Lord Kelvin, who happened to be sick, so he gave his letter to Bottomly who, in turn, wrote a letter to *Nature,* talking mainly of Lord Kelvin's ten year old experiments. Arthur Schuster was more enthusiastic in his letter, published in the *Brit. M. J.* of January 18, 1896. Norah indicates that John Macintyre was responsible for opening the first properly organized radiological department in a British hospital, in the Glasgow Royal Infirmary, *cf., Brit. M. J.* of June 6, 1896.

Scott, J.: Radiography, ancient and modern. *Radiography, 26*:97-107, 1960. This is a Stanley Melville Memorial Lecture. It contains two quotations, one by Churchill (the farther backward you can look, the farther forward you are likely to see), the other by Kelvin (when you are up against an impossibility, you are on the threshold of a great discovery).

Scott, W. G.: Development of angiocardiography. *Radiology, 56*:485-49, 1951. Carman Lecture at the RSNA meeting. For additional historic data, see Dotter & Steinberg's book on Angiocardiography (1951).

Shields, D. G.: Fashion parade of x-ray apparatus 1895-1945. *X-Ray Technician, 17*:348-360, 1945. Excellent review of American makes with beautiful reproductions by a master-photographer. Same illustrations made also into set of slides used (and guarded jealously) by the American representative of the (British) Ilford.

Sievert, R. M.: Medical radiophysics in Sweden 1920-1950. *Acta Radiol., 33*:191-252, 1950. The Institute of Radiophysics started out as the Physics Lab of the Radiumhemmet (with funds from the Stockholm Cancer Society). When Karolinska took over the Radiumhemmet in 1937, the Institute of Radiophysics was moved into a new building, constructed with money from the King Gustav V Jubilee Fund. Operating expenses were tranferred to the state in 1941 when it became the Karolinska Institute of Radiophysics. The paper contains also the history of radiation safety of radiologic installations, strictly controlled in Sweden since 1941, when such legislation was first enacted.

Silverman, F. N.: Thymic irradiation; a historical note. *Am. J. Roentgenol., 84*:562-564, 1960. First thymic x-radiation was applied by Albert Friedländer (1871-1939), a Cincinnati pediatrician, who published the case in the *Archives of Pediatrics* (July, 1907). Patient was alive and well in 1959.

Simon, M.: Stray remarks on the history of medical radiology in Sweden. *Acta radiol., 7*:476-490, 1926. In Stockholm the first roentgen plate was produced on February 9, 1896 by Thor Stenbeck at the Serafimerhospitalet, and reported in *Hygiaea.* Stenbeck also treated and "cured" the first carcinoma of the skin (in 1899). Gösta Forssell became Stenbeck's assistant. In addition, the paper mentions the therapist Tage Sjögren, and other Swedish pioneers.

Singleton, E. B.: Society for Pediatric Radiology. *Amer. J. Roentgenol., 91*:706-707, 1964. Thirty-five radiologists attended the first meeting of the society in Washington (D.C.), but the first membership list included 52 members. About 100 radiologists hold currently active membership. In 1962 the Executive Committee was approached by two French radiologists, regarding the possibility of an international meeting. Thereupon, the First International Reunion of Pediatric Radiologists was held in Paris (France) in May 1963.

Skinner, E. H.: Early American roentgeniana. *Am. J. Roentgenol., 26*:549-555, 1931. Reproductions of covers, and other details by a dedicated student of American radio-history. He praised E. P. Thompson and Williams, but deprecated Monell and the *American X-Ray Journal.* This particular paper contains also the transcript of a letter from Pusey to Skinner (September 17, 1930). Excerpt: "Caldwell was the best trained pioneer in the field, the soundest and the most interested that I met, and I have never felt that he got all the credit he deserved."

Skinner, E. H.: The organization of the Roentgen Society of the United States *in ARRS 1900-1950.* Springfield (Illinois), Charles C Thomas, 1950. Issued at the 50th anniversary of the creation of the ARRS, for its meeting in St. Louis; was printed in 1100 copies, is now a collector's item. Includes text of first presidential address by Heber Robarts.

Smith, C. W.: X-ray technician of 1900; his problems and apparatus. *X-Ray Technician, 23*:278-280; 322; 1952. Anecdote of Goodspeed's pre-Röntgen plate. Snook worked for Queen & Co. before going into business for himself. Paper reproduces letter (dated January 1, 1900) from A. W. Crane to Newcomet: "I have never seen an x-ray burn. In fact I have never seen any effect whatever upon the skin or tissues from exposure to a Crookes tube. When patients have spoken of the possibility of a burn, I tell them the x-ray tube is like a candle—if you come too close you get burned! My times of exposure (for dry plates) vary from three to fifteen minutes (the longest forty-five minutes). I have at least six inches between the tube and the flesh, although of late I have ceased to think of x-ray burns as a real danger."

Snook, H. C.: *A Brief History of Roentgenology.* Philadelphia, privately printed, 1916, 20 pages. History of the Snook Manufacturing Company, and of the Snook rectifier, used as a basis for the biographical remarks made by Morgan during the 1960 H. Clyde Snook Annual Oration.

Snook, H. C.: Development of roentgenology. *Am. J. Roentgenol., 4*:337-342, 1917. Abbreviated text of an address given during a complimentary dinner offered to Snook (and wife) by the Philadelphia Roentgen Ray Society on December 15, 1916. After going through Röntgen's "electric forefathers," Snook mentions that the first State Institute for roentgen work was established in Berlin under Grunmach at nr. 18

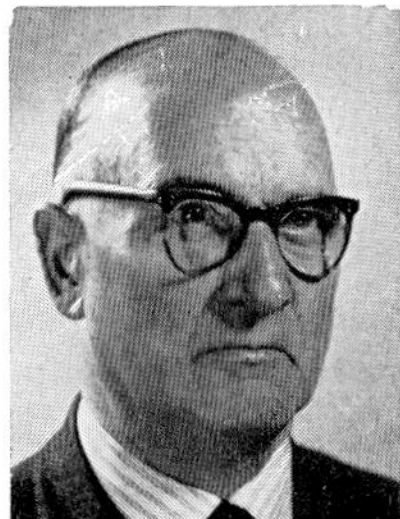

John Scott

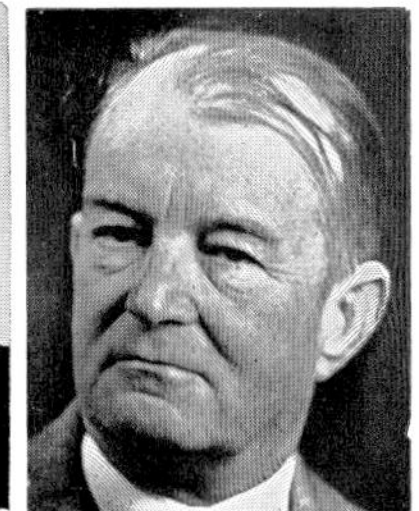

Rolf Sievert

Hans Schinz

on Luisenstrasse, near the Charité Hospital.

Sokolov, Y. N.: Trends of development of roentgenodiagnostics in the USSR. *Indian J. Radiol.,* (souvenir number) 263-277, 1956. Ably summarized by the current editor of the *Vestnik Rentgenologii i Radiologii,* the oldest extant radiologic periodical in the Soviet Union.

Sosman, M. C.: Medicine as a science: roentgenology. *New England J. Med., 244*:552-563, 1951. This is part of a group of papers on fifty years of medical progress, a re-evaluation at half-century. Sosman accepts the fact that the Yellow Journal is a continuation of the *American X-Ray Journal* as the official organ of the ARRS.

Sousa, A. de: Os rayos x na imprensa portuguesa. *Imprensa médica, 11* (nr. 14) :3-20, 1945. Pioneering professional (as well as lay) printed sources on the acceptance of the x-ray discovery in Portugal; reproduction of the roentgen plate of Queen Amelia de França e de Bragança, exposed on February 20, 1905, and facsimile of a remembrancer, handwritten by the Queen on February 28, 1945. Ayres de Sousa—the (unofficial) historian of Portuguese radiology—composed several other historic papers. One of the sources for the review by Alban Ramos (q.v.) was Sousa's article in *Coimbra médica* of January-February, 1946 about the beginnings of radiology in that teaching center. In the *Boletim Clinico* (of January-February, 1948) of the Civilian Hospitals of Lisbon, de Sousa specifies that the first "gabinete de radiologia" in that institution began to operate on October 2, 1898.

Sousa, A. de: Angiopneumografia (resenha historica do metodo). *Gaz. Méd. Portuguesa, 8*:237-245, 1960. Portuguese researchers (Egas Moniz, Lopo de Carvalho, Almeida Lima), while performing angiopneumography (visualization of pulmonary circulation), inevitably obtained dextro(cardio)grams before 1931, ahead of either Castellanos and Pereiras (Havana) or Robb and Steinberg (New York City).

Spear, F. G.: Radiation martyrs (a list). *Brit. J. Radiol., 29*:273, 1956. These are the names later added to the 2nd edition of Holthusen's book.

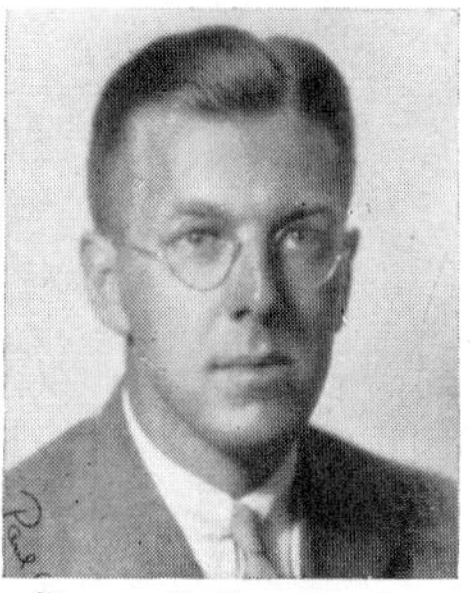

Paul C. Swenson

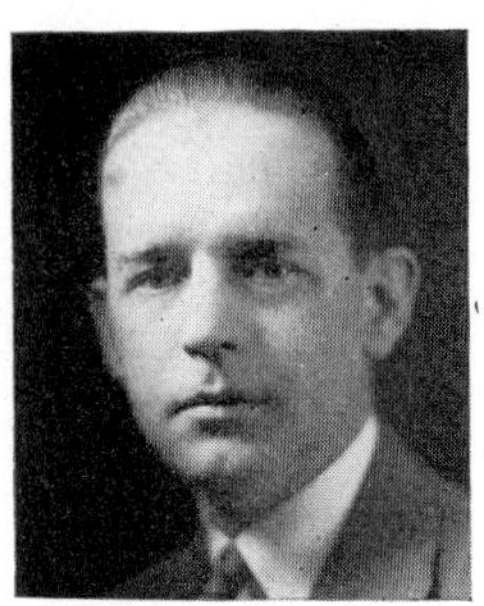

Merrill Sosman

Spear, F. G.: Questioning the answers. *Brit. J. Radiol., 35*:77-89, 1962. Radio-philosophico-historic presidential address, delivered to the BIR on October 19, 1961, as a "second swan song" (after the 35th Mackenzie Davidson Memorial Lecture). The lease of 32 Welbeck Street (residence of the BIR) was bought in 1922 on a bank overdraft guaranteed personally by Melville, Barclay, G. H. Orton, and Archibald Reid. Spear also quotes Hamlet's "looking glass." "Questioning the answers" is the title of two articles written independently of each other for the *British Medical Journal;* one of these articles contained the passage: ". . . in the last 10 or so years various investigators have shown a substantial lack of agreement btween observers independently examining the same patient, or the same radiograph . . .!" With Mayneord, Spear had inspected in the Cairo Museum the symbol of Aten (solar disc), which has stylized hands at the tips of the sun rays (while the BIR device has pointed rays with no hands). Frederick Gordon Spear finally quotes Shelley's Adonais (1821) in which life is likened to a dome of many colored glass where each seeker, attracted by this or that tint, or by this or that degree of brightness, works according to his light and achieves according to his opportunity, but where all make their contribution to that white radiance which belongs to eternity.

Spear, F. G., Russ, S., Andrews, C., and Carling, E. R.: British X-Ray and Radium Protection Committee. *Brit. J. Radiol., 26*:553-557, 1953. As the Committee went out of existence, living participants recorded their reminiscences.

Spillman, R.: Early history of roentgenology of the sinuses. *Am. J. Roentgenol., 54*:643-646, 1945. Caldwell and his associate (Imboden) are properly recognized as pioneers by Ramsay Spillman, former historian of the ARRS, then historian of the New York Roentgen Ray Society.

Stead, G.: Radiological education in the United Kingdom. *Indian J. Radiol.,* (souvenir number) 316-334, 1956. Very good summary of events connected with the Cambridge Diploma, by its long-time secretary.

Stead, G.: Early days of radiology. *Brit. J. Radiol., 32*:468-471, 1959. Abstracts of papers read on December 5, 1958 at the annual meeting of the BIR; authors: Russell Reynolds, Finzi, Russ, and Cuthbert Andrews, with motion to give them a vote of thanks proposed by W. E. Schall.

Stead, G., Reynolds, R. J., Finzi, N. S., Andrews, C., Lacassagne, A., and Case, J. T.: Sixty years of radiology. *Brit. J. Radiol., 29*:233-255, 1956. Combination of personal reminiscences in various fields, supported by data from recorded British radiologic history (with a French inflexion on radiobiology, and an American contribution).

Stephens, S. V., and Tsien, K. C.: *Application of High Energy Radiation in Therapy. Vienna.* Vienna, IAEA, 1960, 86 pages. Global approach to the problem, with adequate bibliography. At the 1961 meeting of the ARS in Colorado Springs, Kia-Chi Tsien presented a world survey of Cesium and Cobalt teletherapy sources, printed in the *American Journal of Roentgenology* of March, 1962.

Stiles, G. L.: From dawn to noon. *Radiography, 22*:137-141, 1956. 18th Stanley Melville Lecture, recounting the founding of the (British) Society of Radiographers in 1920, and its continuing progress.

Streller, E.: Das erweiterte deutsche Röntgen-Museum. *Röntgen & Lab.-Praxis, 13* (8):132-136, 1960. The director of the German Roentgen Museum published in the January, 1960 issue of the same periodical a few less well known portraits of Röntgen.

Stuermer, W.: Zur Geschichte der Röntgen-Leuchtstoffe. *Fortschr. a. d. Geb. d. Röstrahlen, 97*:514-519 1962. Titus Livius mentions that in 186 B.C., in Rome, the bacchantes twirled luminescent batons (presumably painted with phosphorescent CaS). In 1895 Röntgen used a screen made with barium-platinocyanide; in 1896 Pupin reinforced radiographic images with zinc sulfide, Edison came up with calcium wolframate. G. Rupprecht introduced zinc silicate in 1911, and cadmium wolframate in 1914. Guntz developed zinc cadmium sulfide in 1921. In Britain, in 1933, L. Levy and D. W. West used a new process, "silver-activation." In 1939, R. P. Johnson and F. B. Quinlan obtained a U. S. Patent for a screen with potassium iodide. In 1940, F. F. Renwick and H. S. Tasker, in Great Britain, produced a reinforcing screen with lead barium sulfate. Apparently the most successful is calcium tungstate, used for blue-sensitive photographic emulsions, while zinc cadium sulfate gives the greenish light best suitable for fluoroscopy.

Sutherland, C. G.: Röntgen and his discovery. *X-Ray Technician, 8*:143-149, 1937. American pioneers, including Goodspeed's "metallogram" of 1890, and the exploits of the student trio at Davidson College in North Carolina.

Suzuki, M.: A Japanese historical review of radiation protection. *Industr. Med. Surg., 28*:280-287, 1959. In Japan a dermatologist, named Dohi, was the first to use radium—at the beginning of the Taisho Period (before World War I). The Japan Roentgen Society was formed in 1924. In 1934 the ICR in Zürich established what was then called the "tolerance dose" of one r per day total body radiation. The first radiation protection ordinance in Japan was issued in 1937 by the Ministry of Internal Affairs. The Japan Radiology Congress established in 1941 a Japanese Committee for Radiation Protection, which had considerable importance in formulating proper standards of precaution.

Swenson, P. C.: American radiology—1905 to 1955. *Internat. Abstr. Surgery, 101*:313-325, 1955. Relationship and reciprocal influence between radiology and surgery, with substantial survey of aspects and phases (for instance Swenson likens the early 1930's in radiology to the medieval Renaissance). Quotation from Swenson: "Radiology . . . must live as an intact specialty . . . to keep the standards high in (its) various cooperative endeavors. It is so easy to decentralize the diagnostic phases, but the one thing that has kept standards high is the purely ra-radiologic approach in the midst of integrated and cooperative endeavors."

Swinton, A. A. C.: Some early radiograms. *J. Röntgen Soc., 2*:11-12, 1905. Listing of his first plates, beginning with one (the first after Röntgen) dated January 7, 1896.

Taylor, L. S.: Brief history of the National Com-

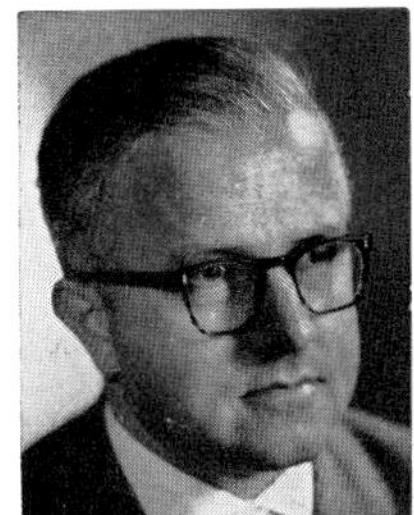
WILHELM STUERMER

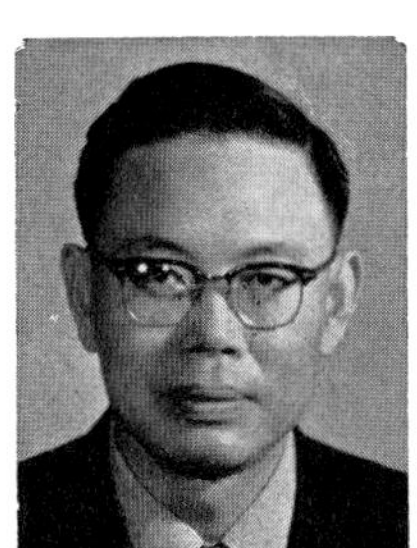
KIA-CHI TSIEN

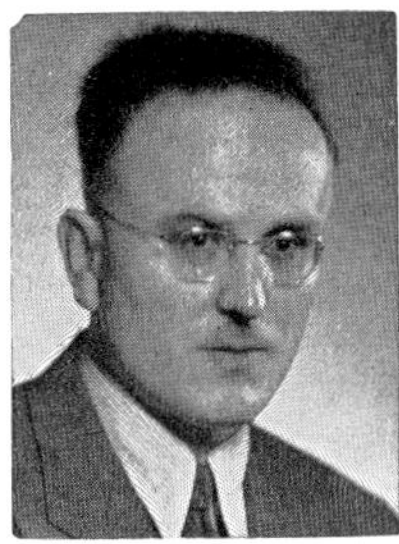
ERNST STRELLER

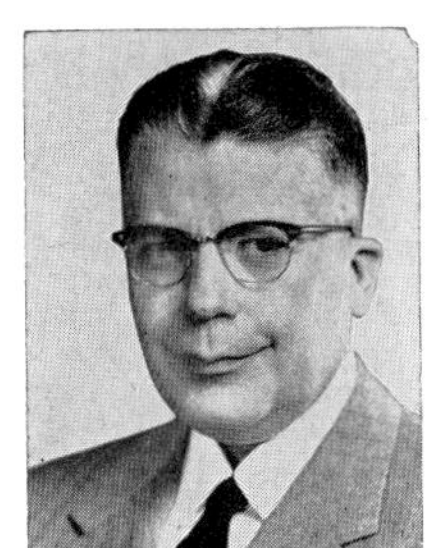
DALE TROUT

mittee on Radiation Protection and Measurements (NCRP) covering the period 1929-1946. *Health Physics, 1*:3-10, 1958. Taylor has been NCRP's secretary since its inception, and knows its history quite well.

Taylor, L. S.: History of the International Commission on Radiological Protection (ICRP). *Health Physics, 1*:97-104, 1958. Development of the basic concept of permissible (rather than tolerance) dose, and progressive lowering of that permissible dose.

Thompson, E. P.: *Roentgen Rays and Phenomena of the Anode and Cathode.* New York, Van Nostrand, 1896, 190 pages. Precise bibliographic indications for contemporary papers (with a concluding chapter by Wm. A. Anthony). Source material of high quality, prepared by a patent attorney.

Thompson, S. P.: Presidential address. *Arch. Roentgen Ray, 2*:23-30, 1897. Concise story, in literary terms, of what happened in "x-ray" until time of delivery of this inaugural speech at formal opening of British Röntgen Society.

Thomson, E.: Work in the first decade of roentgenology. *Am. J. Roentgenol., 28*:385-388, 1932. History of the activities of GE's research lab at Lynn (Massachusetts), including Thomson's standard double focus tube (for alternating current), and Lemp's high tension rectifying switch (forerunner of Snook's interrupterless), for which patents applied in 1896 were granted in 1904 under nrs. 774,090 and 774,138.

Tousey, S.: Origin and development of x-ray therapy. *Am. J. Electrotherap. & Radiol., 41*:52-59, 1923. "In 1885 when I (Tousey) took a degree of Master of Arts, one of my subjects was electrical engineering, and Crookes tubes were familiar subjects of experiment. They were for the passage of a high tension current through a vacuum of about one millionth of an atmosphere, and we did not know that we were generating x-rays every day." Tousey's address had been delivered on October 4, 1922 before the New York Electrotherapeutic Society. He quoted Charles Lester Leonard from the *Am. X-Ray J.* of October, 1898: "Static electricity causes the (so-called x-ray) burns. It is impossible to produce a burn while roentgen efficiency is undiminished. Effect on tissues could be prevented by interposing a grounded grid." Leonard died as a roentgen martyr. Incidentally, Tousey used in this paper the (transliterated German) term roentgencater.

Trainor, J. P.: *Salute to the X-Ray Pioneers of Australia.* Sydney, published by W. Watson & Sons, Ltd., 1946, 81 pages. A genuine history book, put together by the director of a commercial firm (the company's name is mentioned nowhere else but on the frontispiece); unique source of information.

Trostler, I. S.: Original communication of the discovery of the roentgen rays. *Am. J. Phys. Ther., 7*:95-99, 1930. Brief comments on impact of Roentgen's first announcement.

Trostler, I. S.: Some interesting highlights in the history of roentgenology. *Am. J. Phys. Ther., 7*:439-456, 1931. Transcript of a talk given before the Chicago Roentgen Society on October 10, 1929, containing valuable data on the beginnings of radiology in the USA.

Trout, E. D., and Kelley, J. P.: The evolution of equipment for dental radiography. *J. Ont. Dent. Assn., 35*:10-18, 1958.

Trump, J. G.: Radiation for therapy — in retrospect and prospect. *Amer. J. Roentgenol., 91*:22-30, 1964. Van de Graaff's generator, and other supervoltage sources in the Hub area: in Boston, million-volt x-ray therapy was first given to a patient on March 1, 1937 at Huntington Hospital.

Tuddenhsm, W. J.: Fifty years of progress in roentgenology of the chest. *Am. J. Roentgenol., 75*:659-672, 1956.

Underwood, E. A.: Wilhelm Conrad Roentgen (1845-1923) and the early development of radiology. *Canadian M. A. J., 54*:61-67, 1946. Roentgen, his scientific forefathers, and the discovery; summarized

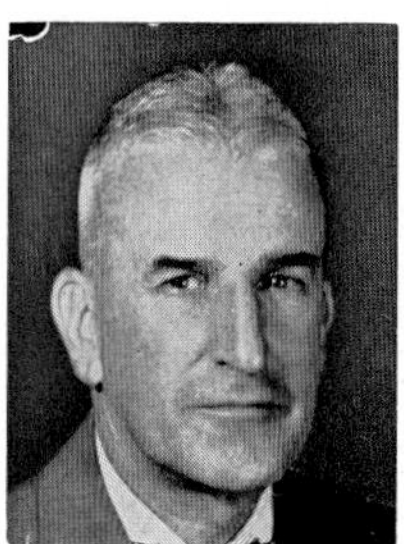
L. S. TAYLOR

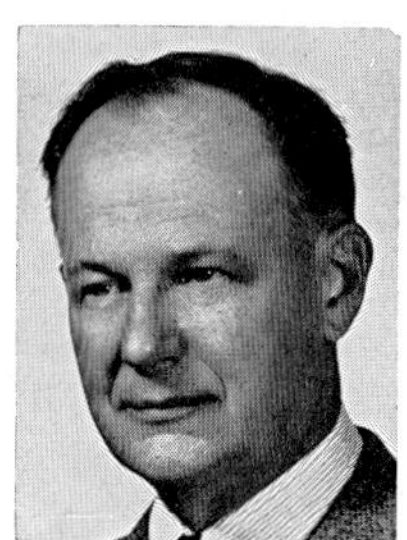
J. G. TRUMP

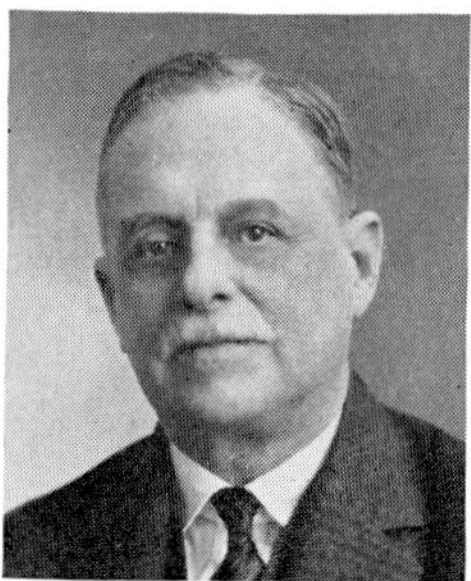
ELIHU THOMSON

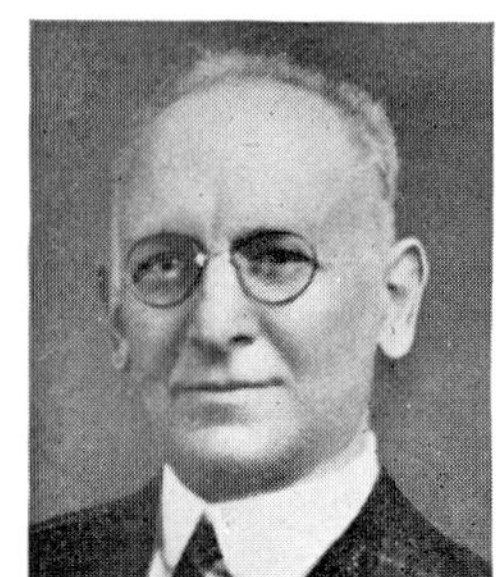
ISADORE TROSTLER

in brilliant style by a professional medical historian (director of the Wellcome Medical Museum, and son-in-law of the famous Charles Singer).

Unger, H.: *Wilhelm Conrad Röntgen.* Hamburg, Hoffman und Campe, 1949, 270 pages. Biography.

Vernar, H.: Historical notes on roentgenology in Slovakia. *Bratisl. lek. Listy, 9*:559-564, 1958.

Vezey, J. J.: The Röntgen Society. *J. Röntgen Soc., 1*:2-8, 1904. Recalls the details surrounding the first meeting of the organizers of the (British) Röntgen Society—Fenton, Harrison Low, and Walsh—at 20 King Street (Strand).

Viol, C. H.: The radium situation in America. *Radium,* (Pittsburgh) *4*:105-120, 1915. Viol of the Standard Chemical Co. summarized the history of Howard Kelly's National Radium Institute of Sellersville, Pennsylvania, and discussed the Radium Company of America, Colorado carnotite, the Federal Bureau of Mines, and the "radium bills." In *Radium* of June, 1921 Viol told the story of the gram of radium, given by the American women to Marie Currie in 1921.

Viol. C. H.: *Compendium of Abstracts of Papers on the Therapeutic Use of Radium.* Pittsburgh, published by Radium Chemical Company, 1920. The first volume is a looseleaf item, with a glossary of terms. Valuable collection.

Viol, C. H.: History and developments of radiumtherapy. *J. of Radiol., 2* (nr. 8):29-34, 1921. Paper read before the Iowa Roentgen Club (in Iowa City) on April 15, 1921; Walkhoff (the same one who took the first dental roentgen plate) recorded for the first time the effect of radium on the skin (in *Photographische Rundschau* of October, 1900); early radium "standards" after the Congress of Radiology and Electricity in Bruxelles (1910), the three tubes (10.11 mgm, 31.70 mgm, and 40.43 mgm) of Hönigschmid in Vienna, and single tube (21.99 mgm) of Marie Curie in Paris (1912).

Voltz, F., and Zacher, F.: Entwicklungsgeschichte der modernen Röntgenröhren. *Fortschritte a. d. Geb. d. Röstrlen, 27*:83-98, 1919. Contains many sketches of early tubes, useful for identifying certain models.

Wachowski, T. J.: Some logistics of the RSNA with thoughts about the future. *Radiology, 76*:480-483, 1961. Presidential address, continuing the presentation of Pendergrass (q.v.), with some figures on RSNA membership.

Walther, K.: Gründer der Deutschen Röntgengesellschaft. *Röntgen-Blätter, 8*:289-352, 1955. Detailed and accurate biographies of the pioneers who founded the German Roentgen Society in 1905, with historic sidelights and bibliographic baselines. Kurt Walther (an internist) is a recognized authority on the history of world radiology. In the *Fortschritte* of August, 1963, Walther published a delightful "diplomatic history" of German-American radiologic relations.

Walther, K.: Ueber die ersten Schritte in Berlin. *Röntgen-Blätter, 9*:297-304, 1956. The German roentgen historiographer often publishes eulogies, and other commemorative pieces, for instance on Béclère, Paul Lazarus, C. H. F. Müller, John Macintyre. He is now working on Evarts Graham. Walther is also the author of a continuing series, called *Röntgenhistorische Daten des Monats,* published monthly in *Der Radiologe;* it recalls briefly individuals as related to events which took place in that particular month at least ten years before the date of publication.

Wasson, W. W.: *Radiologic Pioneers in Colorado.* Compiled in 1934 with the help of Mindell Winter Stein (Wasson's secretary). Exists only in 30 pages of manuscript, from which several photostats have been produced (minus its 66 references). Covers the period 1896-1918, from the "electrician" Colonel C. F. Lacombe (who operated the first—"free"—x-ray laboratory in Denver, at his Mountain Electrical Company) and Chauncey E. Tennant, Jr. (the physician who produced the roentgen plate used in that famous Arapahoe court case in which a radiograph was admitted in evidence), to George Henry Stover (the first medical radiologist in Colorado, who started in

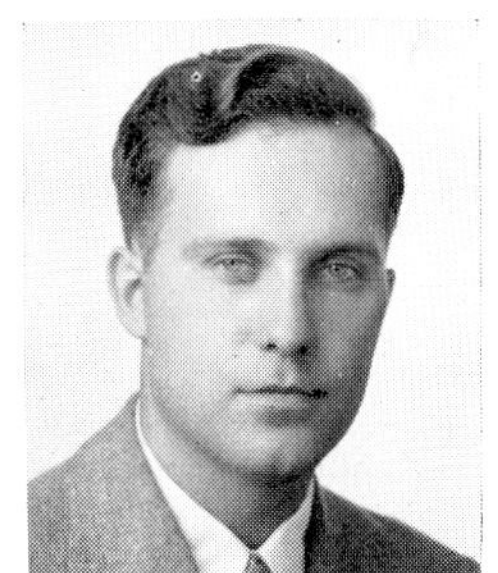
THEODORE J. WACHOWSKI

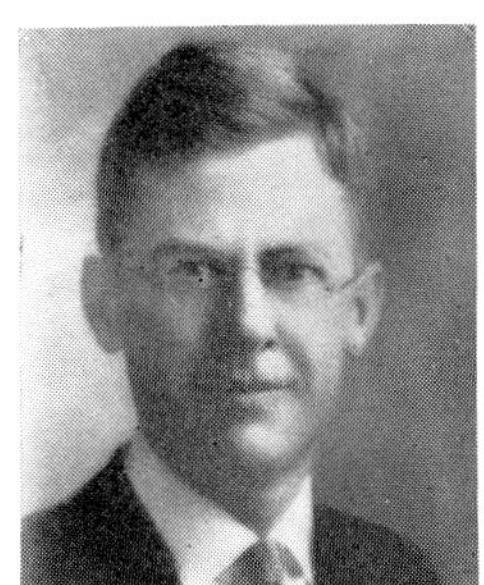
SANFORD M. WITHERS

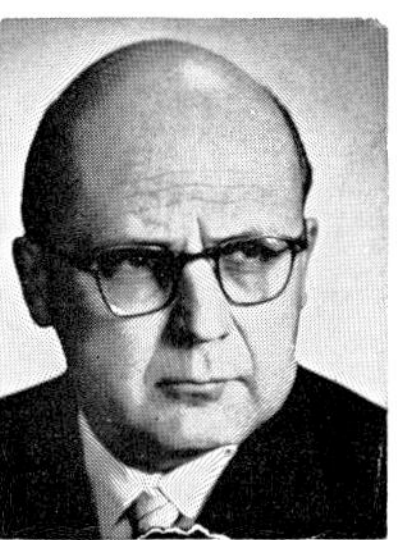
KURT WALTHER

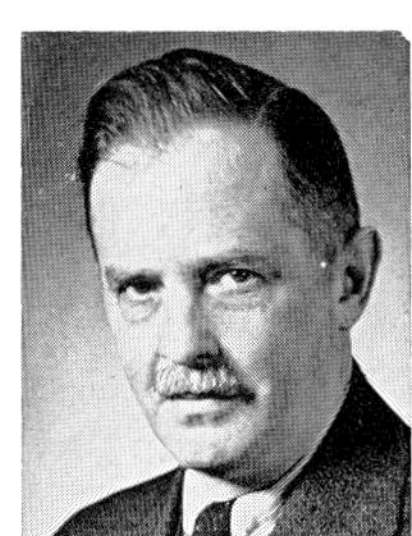
KONRAD WEISS

this field in 1897 and limited his practice since 1903 to the use of x ray, electricity and light), and Samuel Beresford Childs (the best known among Colorado roentgen pioneers, who then became a president of the ACR). The first diagnosis of pneumoperitoneum in the USA was made by W. N. Beggs and W. W. Wasson in March of 1918 from radiographs produced at the Jewish Consumptive Relief Society (air had penetrated into the peritoneum during a "low" attempt at inducing therapeutic pneumothorax). Incidentally William Walter Wasson has several extrahistoric contributions, such as his life-long interest in the "auxiliary heart" (the lungs), crystallized in a text by this name (published in the *J.A.M.A.* of May 14, 1949). Wasson is the founder of the Gas Tube Gang (1955), which became in 1961 the Council for Radiologic Heritage.

Watson, W.: 1895 and all that. *Radiography, 27*: 305-315, 1961. Personal recollections beginning with 1916 wen author was wounded at Ypres and received a roentgen examination. Subsequently author became an x-ray technician, and reminisces all the way to automatic film processors.

Weiser, M., and Eras, Ch. J.: Der Werdegang der Odelka. *Röntgen-Blätter, 12*(6):1-16, 1959. History of Albert Bouwers' De Oude Delft, and of the mirror camera Odelca.

Weiss, K.: Röntgen's Entdeckung im Echo des medizinischen Wien. *Radiol. Austriaca, 9*:67-71, 1956. Address delivered at the 60th anniversary of the discovery, with inedit details on Viennese pioneers. Konrad Erwin Wilhelm Weiss (himself a pupil of Kienböck) reorganized the Austrian Roentgen Society after World War II, and is today the recognized Nestor of Austrian radiology. See also Weiss: Zur Geschichte der Radiologie in Oesterreich in *Bull. d'-inf. Centre A. Béclère* of September-October, 1963.

Whitaker, P. H.: The birth and growth of radiology, pp. 21-33 in *Liverpool Med. Inst. Trans. & Rep.*, 1961. From Röntgen to image intensifiers, with references to early roentgen endeavors in Liverpool, including portraits of Thurstan Holland and Prosper Marsden.

Whyte, L. L.: Essay on Atomism. From: *Democritus to 1960.* Middletown (Connecticut), Wesleyan University Press, 1961, 108 pages. A brilliant introduction to the subject. The view that the ultimate constituents of matter are themselves minute, hard, permanent, indivisible bits of matter of definite sizes and shapes *(atomism)* was conceived in Greece (450-420 B.C.), welcomed in Rome (420-280 B.C.), "slept" throughout the Middle Ages (280 B.C.-1400 A.D.), despite occasional "play" (spontaneous qualitative speculation) as in India (200 A.D.) or among Arab and Jewish thinkers (600-900 A.D.). The Renaissance brought the revival of atomism in Italy (1400-1600), then the first quantitative applications were made in 1600 in Italy, Britain, France, and Holland. The chemical atom was established (1800-1900), but proved misnamed (1900-1930), whereupon its unstable progeny thoroughly confused the issue (1930-1960). The first records of atomistic concepts go back to Democritus (because the *Works* of his teacher Leucippus are no longer extant*). Outstanding contributions to atomism were the concept of *attractive and repulsive forces* of Newton (1686),

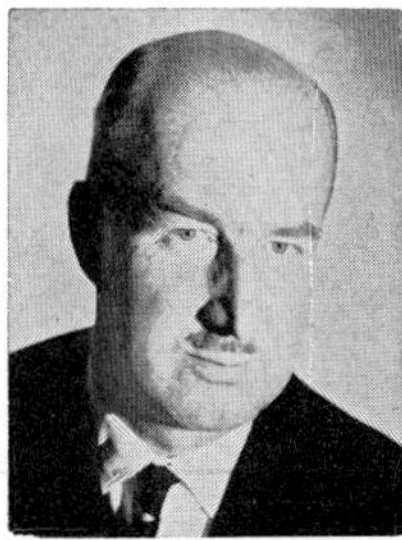

PERCY WHITAKER

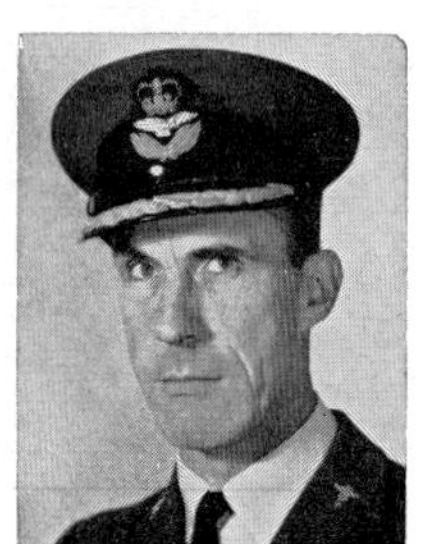

RALPH WYNROE

*Whyte's annotated bibliography contains selected references from German, English, and French authors, published in the past hundred years. I have seen the Italian *Gli Atomisti, Frammenti e Testimonianze* by Vittorio Enzo Alfieri; Bari, Gius, Laterza & Figli, 1936, 410 pages. Alfieri's anthology is a veritable *Corpus Democriteum,* listing all the recognized Hellenic atomists from Leucippus and Democritus down to Metrodorus of Chios, Hecataeus of Abdera, even Diogenes of Smirna. In Collier's *Encyclopedia,* John Wm. Dowling contended that the only authentic sentence by Leucippus is a rigidly deterministic maxim (nothing happens perchance, etc.). That is the maxim which I have placed at the head of the pages of mottoes, preceding *The Author to the Reader.* That sentence is from Περί νοῦ *(On Mind),* and had been quoted by Aetius I, 25, 4. John Lewis Heller, the scholarly classicist from the University of Illinois in Urbana, is also an authority on *Modern Technical Terminology* and on Linnéan texts (which is how we originally met). Heller pointed out to me that another Leucippian relic is mentioned in *Die Fragmente der Vorsokratiker* by Hermann Diels, ed. 6, Berlin, 1952 (ii, 80). That relic consists of the Table of Contents and of several terms—such as ἄtoμοι (atoms) and μέγα κενόν (great vacuum) — from the Méας διάκοσμος *(Great Cosmology),* the lost *magnus opus* which contained Leucippus' *Weltanschaung.* The relics had been found in a papyrus unearthed in the library of the *Casa dei Papiri* of the Epicurean Philosopher of Herculanum. Now this is the kind of footnotes which I have deleted from the radio historic bibliography: I took the liberty to insert this one as a representative sample.

the mathematical scheme for a unified theory of *point-centers* of Boscovich (1758), the identification of the *chemical atom* by Dalton (1803), the suggestion that *all atoms are composed of hydrogen atoms* made by Prout (1815), and the concept of *wave-particles* of De Broglie (1923) and Schrödinger (1926). If Indian speculations are neglected, until 1900 A.D. atomism developed on a tiny strip of land, a mere fiftieth of the earth's surface, extending from Abdera (in Thrace) to Edinburgh. After 1900 an unprecedented empirical harvest was produced in atomistic knowledge in the USA, but no fundamental theoretical advance of the first magnitude, worthy to rank with those of Planck, Einstein, Bohr, or Heisenberg, has yet been made by any one born outside Europe, apart from the New Zealander Rutherford. Today, a generally acceptable statement —in the opinion of Lancelot Law Whyte—is the following: "At a certain level of analysis, physical systems display a discrete or atomic constitution. This level is that of chemical molecules and atoms at normal energies." Such atomic character may not be present at deeper levels, in smaller regions, or at higher energies. Unified field theories are still being proposed in the hope to agree on a basic structure of matter. But since 1850 no claim to finality made on behalf of any theory of fundamental structure has survived more than twenty or thirty years. It is not necessarily true, as has been suggested, that no theory can ever be final and therefore no basic structure can ever be reached. One of my favored atomistic quotations — which I did not find in Whyte's breviar — is from a commentary to Aristotle's *De Caelo*. That commentary is by Simplicius, a neo-Platonic philosopher who lived in the 6th Century A. D.: "They (the atoms) move in the void, and catching each other jostle up together, and some recoil in any direction that may chance, and others become entangled with one another in various degrees, according to the symmetry of their shapes and size and positions and order, and they remain together and thus the coming into being of composite things is effected."

Widger, J. I.: The changing world. *Radiol. Technol., 35*:32, 1963. This is when the *X-Ray Technician* changed both its name and the publisher.

Williams, F. H.: Reminiscences of a pioneer in roentgenology and radium therapy, with reports of some recent observations. *Am. J. Roentgenol., 13*:253-259, 1925. Beginnings at Boston City Hospital, and relations with William Rollins. The "recent observations" concern "good" preliminary results in the treatment of cataract with radium irradiation in homeopathic doses.

Withers, S.: Story of the first roentgen evidence. *Radiology, 17*:99-103, 1931. First case involving radiology tried in a USA court, by Judge Owen Lefevre in Apapahoe County (today District Court of Denver), started in April 1896: sentence (on December 2, 1896) recognized roentgen plates as admissible evidence.

Wöhlisch, E: Fünfundzwanzig Jahre Röntgenstrahlenforschung. *Ergebnisse der inneren Med. u. Kinderheilforschung, 21*:1-46, 1922. I have tried unsuccessfully to figure out why this purely physicistic and theoretic paper, summarizing the advances in roentgen and related radiations, was ever accepted for publication in a periodical devoted to monographs on clinical subjects in internal medicine and pediatrics.

Wolcott, R. E.: X-Ray Horizons. *X-Ray Technician, 17*:337-347; 377, 1945. Kerst's development of the Betatron, Glenn Files' grids, the first automatic film processor, and other important firsts, as viewed by a life-long teacher of x-ray technicians.

Wölfflin, E.: Persönliche Erinnerungen an Wilhelm Conrad Röntgen. *Ciba Symposia, 5*(4):111-119, 1957. Reminiscences.

Woolley, I. M.: *Roentgenology in Oregon; the First Fifty Years.* Portland, privately published, 1955, 95 pages. Many people talk of the need to write such "local" roentgen histories; Woolley decided instead to do something (very good) about it.

Wynroe, R. F.: Oxford, poetry, and radiography. *Radiography, 22*:208-213, 1956. Quotes—with reference to x-ray reports—a line from Samuel Butler: "Life is the art of drawing sufficient conclusions from insufficient premises." Article includes a photograph of an x-ray control stand, rolled in front of a bust of Shakespeare, captioned "A radiographer of originality and distinction."

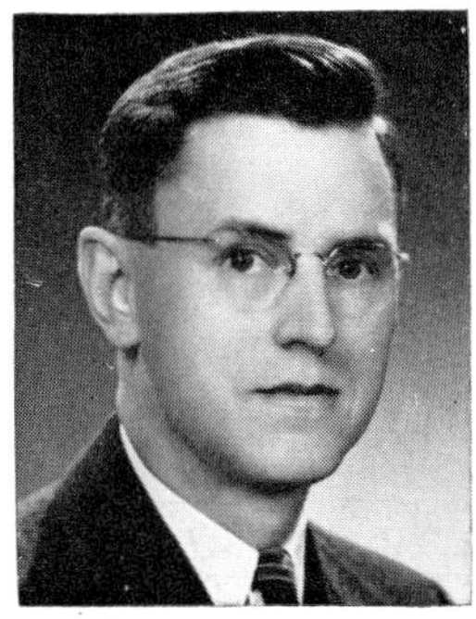

Roy Wolcott

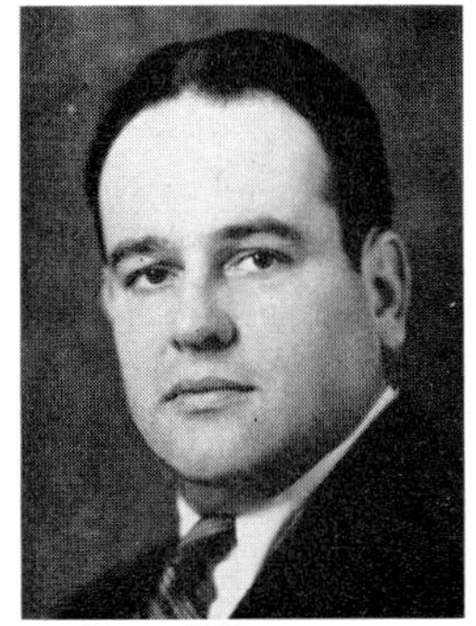

Ivan Woolley

Yakowitz, H., and Cuthill, J. R.: *Annotated Bibliography on Soft X-Ray Spectroscopy.* Washington, Government Printing Office, 1962, 108 pages. 550 references (covering 1950-1960) on application of the method to the study of valence band electronic states in metals and alloys.

Zacher, F.: Zur Entwicklungsgeschichte der Vorrichtungen zur Erzeugung hochgespannter elektrischer Ströme für den Betrieb von Röntgenröhren. *Fortschritte a. d. Geb. d. Röstrahlen., 29*:279-293, 1922. The chief-engineer of Reiniger, Gebbert & Schall (Erlangen) recalls developments of transformers from inductors to the rotary switch.

Zehnder, I.: Persönliche Erinnerungen an Röntgen. *Acta radiol., 15*:557-561, 1934. The first encounter of Zehnder and Röntgen (1886), subsequent joint mountain trips, and other personal recollections. Zehnder published late letters from Röntgen together with a review of physicistic advances in the field.

Zylka, N.: Die Röntgenröhre des Gymnasialprofessors Adolph. Zur Historie der Röntgendiagnostik. *Med. Klin., 54*:1376, 1959. The Elberfeld (Germany) high school physics teacher Adolph used a seven inch coil to reproduce Röntgen's experiment on January 15, 1896 and gave a public demonstration of the method on January 31, 1896. He continued to be interested in the procedure, indeed in 1898 he produced the glass roentgen plate of the knee of a female patient with tuberculosis, and advised amputation (which proved curative).

Die Büste Röntgens in der Walhalla. *Bayerisches Aerzteblatt, 14*:241-242, 1959. Röntgen's bust was placed in the doric temple erected near Regensburg. There were at the time 115 statues in that German Hall of Fame, and the names of 66 historic personalities were inscribed on the walls, but had no statues.

American Roentgen Ray Society, 1900-1950. Springfield, Charles C Thomas Publisher, 1950, pp. 56. Commemorative volume of the ARRS semi-centennial meeting, September 24-29, 1950 in St. Louis.

Bibliography of Titles on Roentgen Rays Contained in the Supplementary Card Catalogue of the Library of the Surgeon General's Office. 1909-1917. Washington, American Research Institute, 1917, 51 leaves. Mineographed.

Bibliography on Radium, compiled by American Institute of Medicine for US Radium Corporation; New York, printed by Adams & Grace, 1922, 132 pages. Listing of articles and books on radium, from the very beginning to January 1, 1922; contained in supplements.

Handbook of the British Institute of Radiology Incorporated with the Röntgen Society. London, 1953, pp. 48. Valuable data about the Institute and all its prizes, collections, and related items.

Katalog over Røntgensammlingen. Kobenhavn, Medicinski-historisk Museum (Copenhagen Universitet), 1953, pp. 87. Interesting collection of about 600 items (tubes, compressors, tubestands, several complete installations, the oldest from 1898, and Helge Christensen's first chest survey apparatus with mirror optic). Text in Danish, English, and German.

"Radiology" wins in court. *Radiology, 2*:352-355, 1924. Story of court battle with Albert Franklin Tyler.

X-Ray department of the London Hospital. *Radiography, 24*:1-11, 1958. History of the department, from its very beginning, with old photographs. Several British hospitals have had their departments so portrayed in *Radiography.*

La Evolucion de la Radiología en sus Primeros Cincuenta Amos. Montevideo, Instituto de Radiología (Universidad), 1949, 131 pages.

Weltliteratur der Radiologie (title translated in English, French, and Spanish). Berlin, Springer, 1959, pp. 71. World list of radiologic books and periodicals available at the time of (and published as an homage to) the 9th ICR in München.

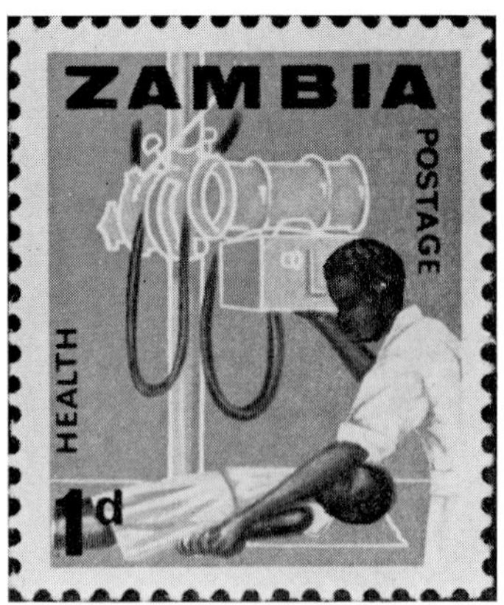

INDEX OF MANUFACTURERS*

So essential did I consider an index to be to every book that I proposed to bring a bill in Parliament to deprive an author who published a book without an index of the privilege of copyright, and moreover, to subject him to a pecuniary penalty

JOHN CAMPBELL (1846)

* This index has been prepared by Mrs. Linda Ayers Whitney, B.A. Where known, addresses are given for manufacturers currently in business.

A

D

E

H

I

J

N

T

U

INDEX OF NAMES*

There are the men who pretend to understand a book by scouring through the index: as if a traveler should go about describing a palace when he had seen nothing but the privy.
JONATHAN SWIFT (1790)

* To reach the level of an abbreviated biographic dictionary of radiology, I first asked Linda Whitney to put on cards all the personal names listed in *The Trail of the Invisible Light,* even the names which appear on reproduced title pages. I then checked her cards against printed sources (Cattell, Marquis, Poggendorff, as well as AMA, specialty, and other directories, various denominations of *Who's Who,* card catalogs of the Library of Congress and of the NLM, and so on). At that point I called for help from old and new friends, such as Abad Valenzuela (Guayaquil), Antoinette Béclère (Paris), Bélisle (Montreal), Bugyi (Budapest), Garland (San Francisco), Holan (the Rumanian expert in *schenerizatie,* which is scanning, phonetically transliterated), Lenzi (Modena), Linton (ACR's public relations officer), McDaniel (Philadelphia), Mosca (Córdoba), Pontes (São Paulo), Sousa (Lisbon) Teichmann (Prague), Uehlinger (Zürich), Zawadowski (Warsaw), and Zedguenidze (Moscow). Data for physicians in the USA were provided by Patricia Witt from the AMA files: their near completeness cannot be matched by past biographic records of any other large medical body, anywhere on this planet. On behalf of manufacturers, data came from several individuals and from Bennett and Goldfield (for Picker), Cornwell (for Eastman Kodak), DePriest (for Westinghouse), Graf (for SRW), Hess (for Standard), Jean Massiot (for Massiot-Philips), Nelson and Newell (for GE), Tasker (for Ilford), Uppenberg (for Elema-Schönander), and Woodall (for the British Watson). Some answers never arrived before press time while a number of replies apologized for "empty" biographic files.

Listings in this index are to include full names, year of birth, year of death for those gone, geographic location or national origin, and occupation. In absence of either year of birth or death, a fl. *(floruit)* has been inserted, to indicate the year in which that person was known to be alive (*i.e.,* flourished). The term American, when applied to this country, was used only for certain immigrants, (*e.g.,* British-American, or Cuban-American); in most instances only the city or state of longest or known residence, or simply USA, is shown. The geographic and nationality listings imply nothing more than an attempt to best identify →

---

those indexed. Occupation is presented mostly in generic terms (radiologist, physicist, technical executive), sometimes with added details (cardioradiologist, radiobiophysicist), seldom including special features of "radiologic" interest, not necessarily characteristic for the individual so listed. Either the adjective medical, or the noun therapist (and certainly any specialty denomination, radiologist, physiatrist—but not electrologist) identify the person as a physician, unless the term lay or non-medical has been attached. Educator, editor, and historian are self-explanatory, while organizer means one active in professional associations. An asterisk after a page number (for instance 459*) indicates a portrait.

When in doubt about family names (Portuguese and Brazilians are unpredictable in this regard), cross-indexing seemed the only solution. The old nobility particles (de, di, von, etc.) caused some problems. Di Rienzo, Sabino is so listed in his native Argentina and in Italy, but in Cuba or in Germany he becomes Rienzo, Sabino di. In the USA, where all aristocratic titles are officially void (on historic revolutionary grounds), people seem fond of nobility particles, and will classify certain Italian immigrants at the letter D, even if the de or di or da in front of their names points only to the town where they or their ancestors were born. Position in this index was assigned on the basis of known (or assumed) usage. I apologize for any errors incurred in that (or any other) manner.

The final version of this index was submitted—for spot checking, revisions, and additions—to Kurt Walther (the German historian and biographer of radiology) and to Charles Roos (who heads the Reference Section of the NLM). Yet, even after receiving the help of these two experts, the index is still incomplete, as are most things on this side of the Styx. Blank spaces have therefore been provided for those knowledgeable readers who might fill in certain data, here and there. I would like very much to receive their communications on this subject, especially because I plan to print in 1967 a few pages of revisions and corrections to this index. Those added pages will be available on request from Charles C Thomas, Publishers, 301-327 East Lawrence Avenue, Springfield, Illinois 62703.

B

C

D

E

F

G

H

I

J

K

M

O

P

Q

R

S

T

U

V

W

X

Y

INDEX OF SUBJECTS*

An index is a necessary implement, and no impediment, of a book except in the same sense wherein the carriages of an army are termed impediments. Without this, a large author is but a labyrinth, without a clue to direct the reader therein.
THOMAS FULLER (1662)

*The asterisk after a page number indicates an illustration.

B

D

E

F

G

H

J

K

L

M

P

Q

R

S

U

V

Y

Z

The chief interest in history lies in the fact that it is not yet finished.

WILLIAM J. ASHLEY (1860-1927)

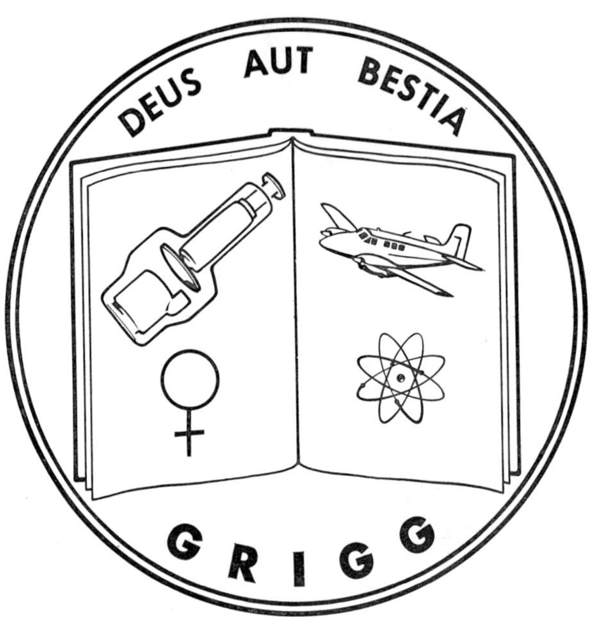